Contemporary Medical-Surgical Nursing

Volume 2

Contemporary Medical-Surgical Nursing

Volume 2

Rick Daniels, RN, PhD
Oregon Health and Science University
Ashland, Oregon

Laura John Nosek, RN, PhD
Frances Payne Bolton School of Nursing
Case Western Reserve University
Cleveland, Ohio

Leslie H. Nicoll, PhD, MBA, RN, BC
Principal and Owner
Maine Desk, LLC
Portland, Maine

THOMSON
DELMAR LEARNING

Australia Canada Mexico Singapore Spain United Kingdom United States

THOMSON
DELMAR LEARNING

Contemporary Medical-Surgical Nursing Volume 2
Rick Daniels, Laura John Nosek, and Leslie H. Nicoll

Vice President, Health Care Business Unit:
William Brottmiller

Director of Learning Solutions:
Matthew Kane

Acquisitions Editor:
Tamara Caruso

Product Manager:
Patricia Gaworecki

Editorial Assistant:
Jennifer Waters

Marketing Director:
Jennifer McAvey

Marketing Channel Manager:
Michele McTighe

Marketing Coordinator:
Danielle Pacella

Technology Director:
Laurie Davis

Technology Product Manager:
Mary Colleen Liburdi

Production Director:
Carolyn Miller

Production Manager:
Barbara Bullock

Art Director:
Robert Plante
Jack Pendleton

Content Project Manager:
Stacey Lamodi
Jessica McNavich

Printed in the United States of America
1 2 3 4 5 6 7 8 XXX 09 08 07 06

For more information, contact Thomson Delmar Learning, 5 Maxwell Drive, Clifton Park, NY 12065
Or find us on the World Wide Web at http://www.delmarlearning.com

Library of Congress Cataloging-in-Publication Data
ISBN 1-4018-3720-4

Notice to the Reader

To Nancy, Luke/Ailie, and Jennie who are the best wife, son/daughter-in-law, and daughter a man could love. I also want to thank my parents and my brother for their love and family support. I am most appreciative to the Lord for His direction in my life.

—Rick

To Frank with deepest appreciation and love for his steadfast support.

—Laura

To EJC, EDM, and JCT . . . good friends forever. Thanks.

—LHN

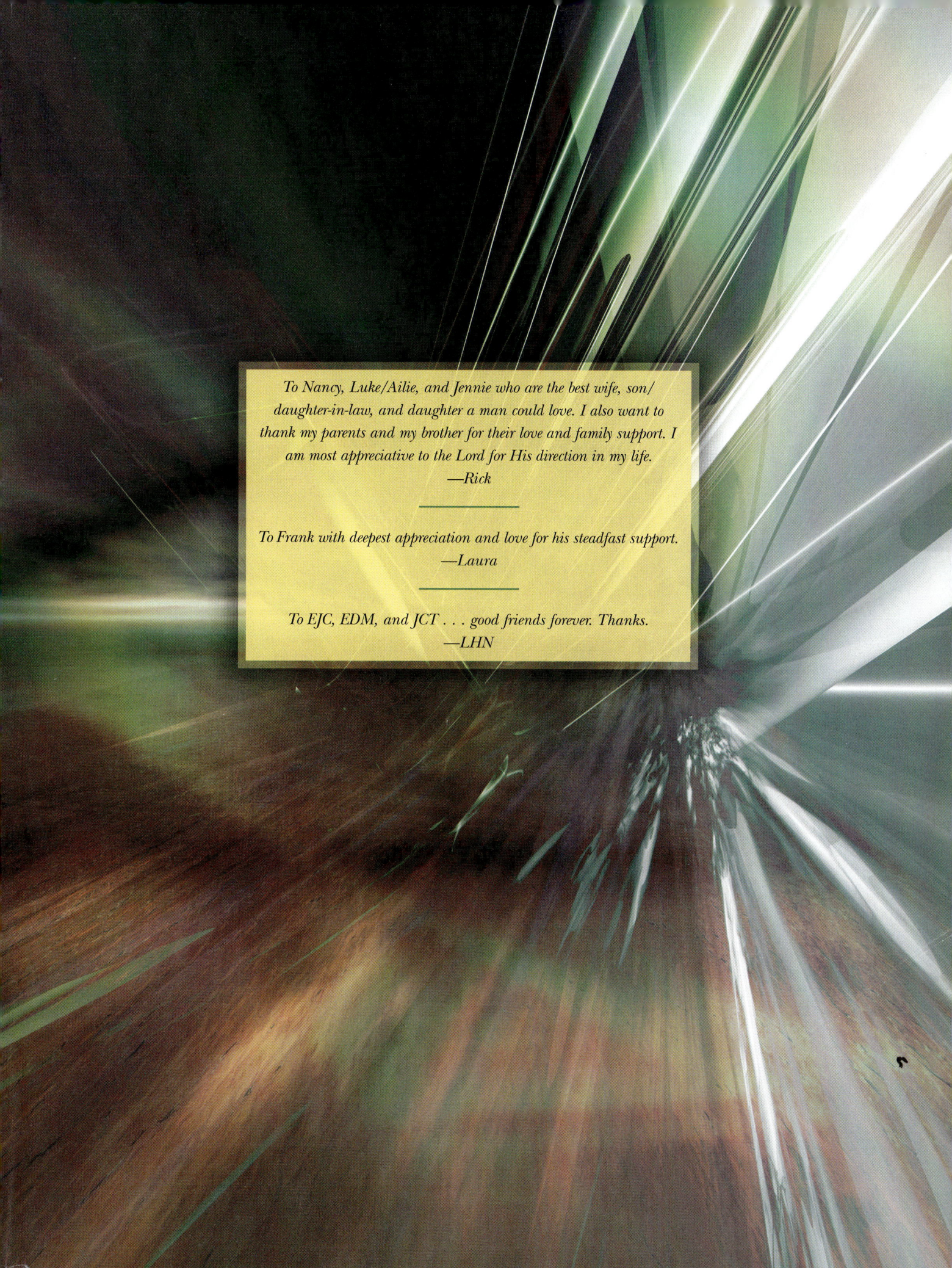

Contents

Preface lxxv
Contributors and Reviewers lxxxii
Acknowledgments lxxxix
About the Authors xc
How to Use This Text xcii
How to Use the CD-ROM xciv

UNIT I: Nursing and the Health Care System 1

CHAPTER 1: The Health Care System and Contemporary Nursing 2

Emergence of the Contemporary Health Care System in the United States 3
Transition from Illness Care to Health Care 3
Emergence of Contemporary Nursing in the United States 9
Contemporary Nursing Practice in the United States 11
Leadership 11
Nursing Education 11
Globalization 12
Changes in Family Structure 14
Risk-Taking Behaviors 14
Transition from Formality to Informality 14
Transition from Nursing as Altruism to Nursing as Business 15
Environment for Contemporary Nursing Practice 17
Culture for Caring 17
Culture for Safety 19

CHAPTER 2: Clinical Decision Making and Evidence-Based Practice 23

Overview of Evidence-Based Practice 24
Knowledge Bases for Clinical Decisions 24
Definition of Evidence-Based Practice 24
Socio-Political Forces in Quality of Care 25
The Process of EBP 25
Applying Evidence-Based Concept 26
EBP in Nursing 27
Examples of Transformation of Knowledge 29
The ACE Star Model of Knowledge Transformation 29
Stages of the Star Model 31
Star Point 1: Discovery 31
Star Point 2: Evidence Summary 31

Star Point 3: Translation 32
Star Point 4: Integration 32
Star Point 5: Evaluation 32
Major Features of EBP 33
Evidence Summary 33
Method for Producing Systematic Reviews 34
Evidence Summaries 34
Sources of Evidence for Clinical Practice 35
Sources of Evidence Summaries 35
Clinical Practice Guidelines 36
Priorities in Evidence-Based Changes in Health Care 39
Use of EBP for Clinical Nursing Practice 40

CHAPTER 3: Health Education and Promotion 43

The Teaching-Learning Process 44
Purposes of Patient Education 44
Facilitators of Learning 45
Barriers to Learning 45
Domains of Learning 46
Teaching Strategies 47
Professional Responsibilities Related to Teaching 48
Legal Aspects 48
Documentation 49
Teaching-Learning and the Nursing Process 50
Assessment 50
Nursing Diagnoses 52
Planning and Implementation 52
Implementation 54
Evaluation of Outcomes 55
Health Maintenance 55
Characteristics of Health Maintenance 56
Health Promotion and Disease Prevention 56
Health Promotion 57
Health Promotion on a Global Level 57
Health Promotion in the United States 58
Assessment 58
Risk Factor Identification in Health Maintenance 59
Diagnostic Tests 59
Nursing Diagnoses 59
Planning and Implementation 60
Needs and Health 60
Evaluation of Outcomes 64

CHAPTER 4: Culturally Sensitive Care 69

Concepts of Culture 70
- Culture 70
- Characteristics of Culture 70
- Ethnicity and Race 70
- Labeling and Stereotyping 71
- Dominant Values in the United States 71

Multiculturalism in the United States 72
- Value of Diversity 73
- Organizing Phenomena of Culture 73

Cultural Disparities in Health and Health Care Delivery 78
- Vulnerable Populations 80
- Environmental Control 82
- Folk Medicine 82
- Biological Variables 82
- Immigrant Population 82

Transcultural Nursing 84

Cultural Competence 85

Cultural Competence and Nursing Process 86
- Assessment 86
- Nursing Diagnoses 88
- Planning and Implementation 88
- Evaluation 89

CHAPTER 5: Legal and Ethical Aspects of Health Care 95

Ethics in Nursing Practice Overview 96

Ethics and Morals 96
- Clinical Ethics 96
- Ethical Issues and Ethical Dilemmas 96

Principles of Clinical Ethics 97

Ethical Theories 98
- Deontology 98
- Teleology and Utilitarian 98
- Rights-Based 98
- Ethics of Care 98

Professional Ethics 99
- Patient's Bill of Rights 100
- Organizational Ethics 100

A Nurse's Role 100
- Moral Distress 101
- Nurse as Patient Advocate 101

Confidentiality 102
Informed Consent 103
Advance Directives 104
Living Will 105
Durable Power of Attorney for Health Care 105
Verbal Advance Directive 106
Surrogate Decision Maker 106
Ethical Decision Making Models 107
Medical Indications 107
Patient Preferences 108
Quality of Life 108
Contextual Features 108
Integrated Model 109
Ethical Issues of Pain Management 109
End-of-Life Care 110
Hospice and Palliative Care 110
Concept of Double Effect 111
Limitation of Treatment 112
Do-Not-Resuscitate Orders 112
Artificial Nutrition and Hydration 113
Right to Die 113
Brain Death and Organ Donation 113
Euthanasia and Assisted Suicide 114
Medical Futility 115
Research Ethics 116

CHAPTER 6: Nursing of Adults Across the Life Span 121

Adult Developmental Stages 122
Theories of Adult Development 122
Contemporary Trends Related to Adult Behavior 123
Dietary Habits 124
Obesity Rates 124
Smoking Trends 125
Suicide Incidence Rates 125
Morbidity and Mortality Trends 125
Evolving Trends in Population Composition 125
The Aging Population 125
Aging Nurse Workforce 126
Minority and Ethnic Population Trends 126
Common Adult Diseases Linked to Contemporary Trends 126
Asthma 126
Metabolic Syndrome 127

Hypercholesterolemia . . . 128
Hypertension . . . 128
Diabetes Mellitus . . . 128
Coronary Artery Disease . . . 129
Cancer . . . 129
Use of Contemporary Treatment Modalities . . . 129
Complementary Alternative Medicine . . . 129
Cosmetic Treatments and Surgery . . . 130
Bariatric Surgery . . . 130
Health and Illness Trends for Young and Middle-Aged Adults . . . 131
Health and Illness Trends for Older Adults . . . 132
Effects of the Aging Process . . . 133
Alzheimer's Disease . . . 134
Subpopulations of Older Adults . . . 134
Homeless Older Adults . . . 135
Older Adult Women . . . 135
Older Adults Living in Rural Areas . . . 135
The Frail Elderly . . . 135
Chronically Ill Older Adults . . . 135
Ethnic Older Adults . . . 136
Trends in Use of Health Care Services by Older Adults . . . 136
Health Promotion . . . 137
Nursing Responsibilities in the Care of the Adult Across the Life Span . . . 138

CHAPTER 7: Palliative Care 143

Overview of Death and Dying . . . 144
Overview of Palliative Care . . . 144
History and Overview of Hospice Care . . . 145
Role of the Hospice and Palliative Care Nurse . . . 146
Role of the Interdisciplinary Team in Hospice and Palliative Care . . . 150
Assessment of the Patient Receiving Hospice and Palliative Care . . . 152
Pain . . . 152
Dyspnea . . . 153
Loss of Appetite, Constipation, Nausea, and Vomiting . . . 154
Urinary Urgency and Incontinence . . . 154
Insomnia, Confusion, and Delirium . . . 154
Anxiety and Depression . . . 155
Nursing Diagnoses . . . 155
Planning and Implementing Care for Patients Receiving Hospice and Palliative Care . . . 156
Managing Pain . . . 156

Managing Dyspnea 162
Managing Loss of Appetite, Constipation, Nausea, and Vomiting. 162
Managing Urinary Urgency and Incontinence 163
Managing Insomnia, Confusion, and Delirium 163
Managing Anxiety and Depression 164
Providing Spiritual Support. 164
Special Considerations in the Home Care of the Dying Patient . . 165
Providing Care in the Active Phase of Dying. 166
Supporting the Bereaved 168

UNIT II: Supportive Patient Care 173

CHAPTER 8: Health Assessment 174

Purpose of Health Assessment 175
Types of Assessment 175
Types of Data 176
Sources of Data 176
The Interview 177
Creating the Climate for the Interview 177
Phases of the Interview Process 178
Methods of Data Organization and Assessment Models 178
Health History 179
Physical Examination 182
Inspection 183
Palpation. 183
Percussion. 184
Auscultation 184
Head-to-Toe Assessment 185
Review of Systems Assessment 185
Laboratory and Diagnostic Data 185
Variations Related to Health Assessment Practices 186
Age 186
Culture 188
Ethnicity 189
Race 189
Gender 190
Physical Variations Related to Gender 190
Genetics. 191
Ethical Considerations Related to Data Collection 191
Patient Rights 192
Informed Consent 192

Confidentiality . . . 192
Advanced Directives . . . 193
Genetic Screening and Counseling . . . 193
Care of the Patient after the Examination . . . 194
Documentation . . . 194

CHAPTER 9: Genetics and the Multiple Determinants of Health 197

Fundamentals of Genetics . . . 198
Structure and Function of Chromosomes and Genes . . . 198
Chromosomal Abnormalities . . . 199
Patterns of Inheritance . . . 203
Mendelian (Single Gene) Inheritance . . . 203
Non-Mendelian (Multifactorial, Polygenic) Inheritance . . . 206
Screening for Genetic Disease . . . 206
Gene Testing . . . 207
Family Screening . . . 209
Population Screening . . . 209
Screening in the Workplace . . . 210
History and Physical Examination . . . 211
Laboratory Studies . . . 211
Genetics Across the Life Span . . . 215
Genetic Contribution to Neonatal and Pediatric Conditions . 215
Genetic Contribution to Adult Conditions . . . 216
Legal, Ethical, and Social Issues . . . 227
Ethical Issues Surrounding Genetics . . . 228
Legal Issues Associated with Genetics . . . 229
The Human Genome Project . . . 232
Gene Therapy . . . 233
Genetic Engineering . . . 233
Pharmacogenomics . . . 234
Expanded Roles for Nurses . . . 235

CHAPTER 10: Stress, Coping, and Adaptation 239

Historical and Theoretical Perspectives . . . 240
Early Civilization Theories and Practices . . . 240
The Germ Theory . . . 240
The Biological Theory . . . 241
Multicausal Theories . . . 241
Stress Stimulus-Response Theory . . . 241
Appraisal-Transaction Theory . . . 244
Life Changes and Illness Theory . . . 244

Stress, Organ Maladaptation, and Disease Theory 245
Psychoneuroimmunoendocrinology 245
Coping 247
Resilience 247
Hope 248
Adaptation 249
Stress and Illness 249
Posttraumatic Stress Disorder 249
Acute Stress Disorder 250
Stress of Chronic Illness 250
Chronic Disease Across the Life Span 252
Additional Risk Factors for Stress-Related Illness 253
Cultural Factors 253
Environmental Stress 253
Caregiver Stress 254
Occupational Stress 254
Nursing Theories and Stress Management 255
Adaptation Model 255
Systems Model 256
Self-Care Theory 257
Significance to Nursing 258
Current Practice Issues 258
Future Nursing Practice Issues 260

CHAPTER 11: Inflammation and Infection Management **265**

Inflammatory Process 266
Leukocytes 266
Chemical Response to Tissue Injury 267
Signs of Inflammation 269
Phagocytosis 269
Resolution and Repair of Tissue 269
Chronic Inflammation 270
Inflammatory Disease 270
Diseases That Result in an Inflammatory Process 270
Diseases Caused by an Inflammatory Effect 272
Nursing Response: Inflammation 273
Risk for Infection 273
Thermoregulation: Ineffective 274
Pain: Acute 274
Nutrition: Imbalanced, Less Than Body Requirements ... 275
Fluid Volume: Risk for Deficit 275

Infectious Disease Control 275
  Transmission Routes 275
Guidelines for Infection Control 279
  Standard Precautions 279
  Transmission-Based Precautions 280
Wound Healing 281
  Types of Wound Healing 282
  Risk Factors for Delayed Wound Healing 282
  Phases of Wound Healing 283
  Dysfunctional Wound Healing 284
  Common Wounds 285
Nursing Response: Wound Healing 286
  Assessment with Clinical Manifestations 286
  Interventions: Wound Management 287

CHAPTER 12: Fluid, Electrolyte, and Acid-Base Imbalances **295**

Fluid Balance 296
  Fluid Gains and Losses 296
  Principles of Concentration Regulation 296
  Electrolytes 298
Control of Fluid and Electrolyte Balance 300
  Kidneys 300
  Cardiovascular System 300
  Respiratory System 301
  Renin-Angiotensin-Aldosterone System 301
  Posterior Pituitary Gland 301
Fluid Imbalances 302
  Fluid Volume Deficit (Hypovolemia) 302
  Fluid Volume Excess (Hypervolemia) 304
Electrolyte Imbalances 307
  Deficient Sodium Ion (Hyponatremia) 307
  Excess Sodium Ion (Hypernatremia) 316
  Deficient Potassium Ion (Hypokalemia) 317
  Excess Potassium Ion (Hyperkalemia) 319
  Deficient Calcium Ion (Hypocalcemia) 320
  Excess Calcium Ion (Hypercalcemia) 322
  Deficient Phosphorus Ion (Hypophosphatemia) 323
  Excess Phosphorus Ion (Hyperphosphatemia) 324
  Deficient Magnesium Ion (Hypomagnesemia) 326
  Excess Magnesium Ion (Hypermagnesemia) 327

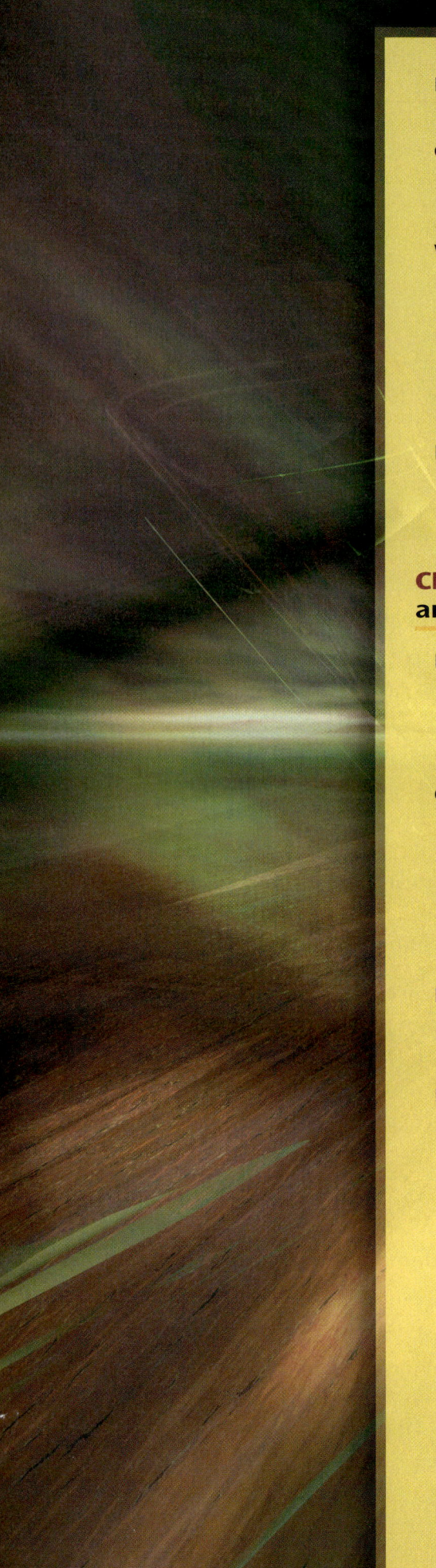

Pharmacology . . . 470
Alternative Therapy . . . 477
Evaluation of Outcomes . . . 478

CHAPTER 17: Pharmacology: Nursing Management **483**

Pharmacological Principles of Drug Action . . . 484
Pharmaceutic Phase . . . 484
Pharmacokinetic Phase . . . 484
Pharmacodynamic Phase . . . 487
Safe Medication Administration . . . 487
Five Rights and Three Checks . . . 487
Geriatric Considerations . . . 490
Pharmacological Resources Available to the Practicing Nurse . . . 491
Ethical Considerations . . . 491
Anti-Infective Agents . . . 492
Penicillins and Cephalosporins . . . 492
Macrolides, Tetracyclines, Aminoglycosides, and Fluoroquinolones . . . 495
Sulfonamides . . . 498
Cardiovascular Agents . . . 499
Cardiac Glycosides . . . 500
Antianginal Agents . . . 502
Antidysrhythmics . . . 504
Diuretics . . . 506
Antihypertensive Agents . . . 508
Medications to Treat Circulatory Disorders . . . 511
Anticoagulants . . . 511
Antilipemics . . . 513
Respiratory Agents . . . 516
Bronchodilators . . . 517
Inhaled Corticosteroids . . . 519
Antiseizure Medications . . . 520
Indications . . . 521
Pharmacokinetics . . . 522
Laboratory Monitoring . . . 522
Side Effects and Adverse Effects . . . 522
Nursing Management . . . 523
Antiulcer Agents . . . 523
Histamine$_2$ Antagonists and Proton Pump Inhibitors . . . 524
Antidiabetic Agents . . . 526
Insulin . . . 526
Oral Hypoglycemic Agents . . . 527

UNIT III: Settings for Nursing Care 531

CHAPTER 18: Health Care Agencies 532

Health Care Cost and Financing 533
Access to Health Care 535
Health Care Quality. 535
Classification of Health Care Agencies 536
Preventive Care Agencies 537
Primary Care Agencies 539
Secondary Care Agencies 540
Tertiary Care Agencies. 541
Restorative Care Agencies. 543
Continuing Care Agencies 544
Indian Health Services 546
The Veterans Affairs Health System 548
The Future of Health Care Agencies 549
Practice Model 550
Synergy Model 551
Outcomes 552
Nurse's Role in Health Care Agencies 553
Assessment 554
Safe Passage 555
Cost, Access, and Quality 555

CHAPTER 19: Critical Care 559

Critical Care Unit. 560
The Critical Care Nurse 560
Delivery of Nursing Care 561
The Critical Care Patient 561
Common Problems of the Critically Ill Patient 564
Infection 564
Nutrition 564
Immobility 564
Pain 565
Anxiety 565
Sleep 566
Communication 567
Family Member Needs 567
Hemodynamic Monitoring 568
Cardiac Output 568
Preload 568
Afterload 569
Contractility. 569

Equipment for Hemodynamic Monitoring 569
Measurement of Hemodynamic Parameters 570
Cardiac Assist Devices 577
Procedure 577
Complications 578
Ventricular Assist Devices 578
Intracranial Pressure Monitoring 579
Types of Intracranial Pressure Monitoring 580
Intracranial Pressure Waveforms 581
Management of Patients with Increased Intracranial Pressure 582
Airway Assistance 583
Oral Airways 583
Nasal Airways 584
Endotracheal Intubation 584
Tracheostomy 585
Mechanical Ventilation 586
Positive Pressure Ventilation 586
Continuous Mandatory Ventilation 586
Synchronized Intermittent Mandatory Ventilation 586
Pressure Control Ventilation versus Volume Control Ventilation 587
Continuous Positive Airway Pressure 588
Pressure Support Ventilation 588
Inverse Ratio Ventilation 588
Airway Pressure Release Ventilation 589
Mandatory Minute Ventilation 589
Proportional Assist Ventilation 589
Nursing Management of Patients Requiring Mechanical Ventilation 590
Complications of Intubation and Mechanical Ventilation . . 593
Ventilator Weaning 599
Withdrawal of Life Support 601

UNIT IV: Perioperative Patient Care 607

CHAPTER 20: Preoperative Nursing Management 608

History of Nursing Contributions in Operative Care 609
Trends 610
Pathways and Diagnosis-Related Groups 612
Short Stay Surgery 612
Remote Assessment 613

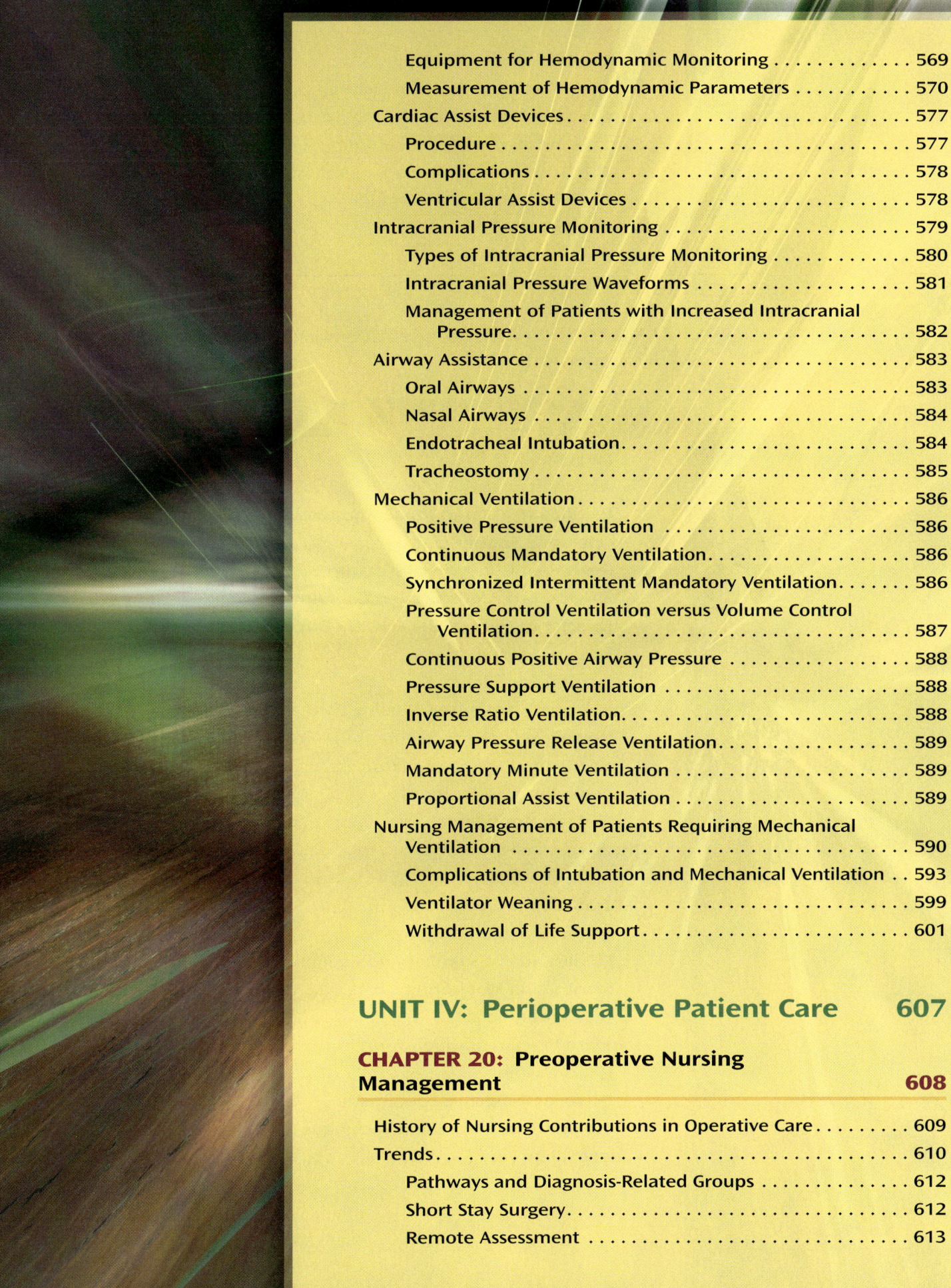

Complementary Therapy 613
The Influence of Religious Faith on Operative Outcomes . . . 614
Electronic Trends 615
Elective and Nonemergency Surgery 616
The Decision to Undergo Surgical Intervention 616
Planning and Implementation 630
Nonelective Surgery 644
Preceding Events 644
Urgent and Emergent Care 644

CHAPTER 21: Intraoperative Nursing Management 653

The Role of the Perioperative Nurse 654
The Surgical Team 656
Surgeon 656
Anesthesiologist 656
Certified Registered Nurse Anesthetist 656
Operating Room Nurse 656
Registered Nurse First Assistant 658
Surgical Services Education Coordinator or OR Educator . . 658
Director of Surgical Services/OR Director 658
Surgical Technologist 658
Surgical Specialties 658
Anticipated Outcomes of Nursing Care 659
Nursing Sensitive Outcomes or Indicators 659
NANDA and the Nursing Process 660
Pediatric Considerations 660
Geriatric Considerations 661
The Surgical Environment 663
Asepsis and Sterility 664
Traffic Control 664
Methods of Sterilization 666
Sterilization of Supplies and Equipment 667
Sterilization Monitoring 668
OR Environment 670
Standard Precautions in the Surgical Environment 671
Hand Washing 671
Personal Protective Equipment 671
Surgical Team Attire and Technique 672
Patient Safety 674
Laser 674
Surgical Fire 675

Latex . . . 676
Cardiac Arrest . . . 677
Anesthesia and Sedation . . . 677
Types of Anesthesia . . . 677
Risks of Anesthesia . . . 678
Intraoperative Complications . . . 680
Retained Objects . . . 680
Hypothermia . . . 681
Intraoperative Fluid Management . . . 682
Safety in Positioning . . . 683
Malignant Hyperthermia . . . 683
Ethics in Perioperative Practice . . . 684
Organ Donation . . . 685
Patient Safety Goals . . . 686
Transportation . . . 686

CHAPTER 22: Postoperative Nursing Management 691

Review of Trends in Postoperative Nursing Management . . . 692
The Post Anesthesia Care Unit . . . 692
Recovery Factors . . . 692
PACU Discharge . . . 702
Nursing Care during the First 24 Hours Post-Surgery . . . 705
The Short-Stay Patient . . . 705
The Patient Receiving Inpatient Care . . . 707
Nursing Care Beyond Transfer . . . 709
Anticipating Complications . . . 713
Recovery Milestones Beyond the Day of Surgery . . . 714
Family and Cultural Aspects of Care . . . 717
The Older Adult . . . 717
Home Planning . . . 718
Discharge Planning . . . 719
Teaching/Learning Principles for the Postoperative Patient . . . 719
Patient and Family Teaching . . . 722
Electronic Resources for the Postoperative Patient . . . 725
Delayed Recovery . . . 726
Predicting and Preventing Outlier Situations . . . 727
The Future of Postoperative Nursing . . . 729

UNIT V: Alterations in Cardiovascular and Hematological Function 733

CHAPTER 23: Assessment of Cardiovascular and Hematological Function 734

Anatomy and Physiology (Hematological System) 735
- Plasma 735
- Erythrocytes 736
- Hemoglobin 737
- Aging of Erythrocytes 739
- White Blood Cells 740
- The Process of Hemostasis 741
- Platelets 741

Assessment 744

Diagnostic Tests 745

Anatomy and Physiology (Cardiovascular System) 747
- Pericardial Layers 748
- Fibrous Skeleton of the Heart. 749
- Chambers of the Heart 749
- Heart Valves 749
- Systemic Circulation 750
- Coronary Artery Circulation 750
- Factors Affecting Blood Flow 751
- Cardiac Cycle. 751

Assessment 753

Diagnostic Tests 762
- Nursing Management 764

CHAPTER 24: Coronary Artery Dysfunction: Nursing Management 769

Coronary Artery Disease 770
- Epidemiology 770
- Etiology 770
- Pathophysiology 774
- Assessment with Clinical Manifestations. 775
- Diagnostic Tests. 777
- Nursing Diagnoses 780
- Planning and Implementation 780
- Evaluation of Outcomes 790

Acute Coronary Syndrome 790
- Pathophysiology 791
- Assessment with Clinical Manifestations. 792
- Diagnostic Tests. 792

Nursing Diagnoses 793
Planning and Implementation 794
Evaluation of Outcomes 797

CHAPTER 25: Heart Failure and Inflammatory Dysfunction: Nursing Management **803**

Heart Failure 804
Epidemiology 804
Etiology 804
Pathophysiology 804
Assessment with Clinical Manifestations 806
Diagnostic Tests 807
Nursing Diagnoses 808
Planning and Implementation 808
Evaluation of Outcomes 811
Heart Muscle Disease and Inflammation Dysfunction 812
Dilated Cardiomyopathy 812
Hypertrophic Cardiomyopathy 813
Arrhythmogenic Right Ventricular Cardiomyopathy 816
Restrictive Cardiomyopathy 817
Carditis 818
Bacterial Endocarditis 818
Myocarditis 820
Pericarditis 821
Valvular Dysfunction and Disease 822
Pathophysiology 822
Mitral Valve Prolapse 823
Mitral Regurgitation 824
Mitral Stenosis 825
Aortic Regurgitation 827
Aortic Stenosis 828
Valvular Surgery 830

CHAPTER 26: Arrhythmias: Nursing Management **835**

Anatomy and Physiology 836
Sinoatrial Node 836
AV Node 836
Purkinje Fibers 836
Electrophysiology 837
ECG Monitoring 838
Monitoring Leads 839
Troubleshooting Cardiac Monitoring Problems 841

The Normal ECG Complex 841
Calculating Heart Rate 841
Determining Rhythm 843
P Waves 844
PR Interval 844
QRS Complex 844
QRS Interval 844
T Wave 845
QT Interval 845
Systematic Approach to Arrhythmia Interpretation 845
Causes of Arrhythmias 845
Reentry 846
Enhanced Automaticity 846
Triggered Activity 846
Sinus Rhythms 846
Normal Sinus Rhythm 847
Sinus Bradycardia 847
Sinus Tachycardia 848
Sinus Arrhythmia 848
Sinus Arrest and Sinus Exit Block 849
Atrial Arrhythmias 849
Premature Atrial Complexes (Contractions) 849
Atrial Tachycardia 850
Atrial Flutter 850
Atrial Fibrillation 851
Supraventricular Tachycardia 852
Junctional Rhythms 852
Premature Junctional Complexes 852
Junctional Escape Rhythm 853
Junctional Tachycardia 853
Heart Blocks 854
First-Degree Heart Block 854
Second-Degree AV Block Type I 854
Second-Degree AV Block Type II 855
Complete Heart Block (Third-Degree Heart Block) 855
Ventricular Arrhythmias 856
Premature Ventricular Complexes 856
Ventricular Tachycardia 857
Torsades de Pointes 858
Ventricular Fibrillation 858
Idioventricular Rhythm 859
Asystole 860
Pulseless Electrical Activity 860

Management Strategies 860
Pharmacology 861
Defibrillation 862
Pacemakers 864
Ablation Therapy 867
Basic Life Support 867
Steps in Basic Adult CPR 868
Airway Obstruction 869
Automatic External Defibrillators 869
Advanced Cardiac Life Support 870
Primary Survey 870
Secondary Survey 870
Ventricular Fibrillation/Pulseless Ventricular Tachycardia 871
Bradycardia Algorithm 871
Unstable and Stable Tachycardia 872

CHAPTER 27: Vascular Dysfunction: Nursing Management 877

Arteriosclerosis and Atherosclerosis 878
Epidemiology 878
Etiology 878
Pathophysiology 878
Genetics 879
Assessment with Clinical Manifestations 879
Diagnostic Tests 879
Nursing Diagnoses 881
Planning and Implementation 881
Evaluation of Outcomes 884
Peripheral Arterial Occlusive Disease 885
Epidemiology 885
Etiology 885
Pathophysiology 885
Assessment with Clinical Manifestations 885
Diagnostic Tests 885
Nursing Diagnoses 886
Planning and Implementation 886
Evaluation of Outcomes 888
Aneurysms and Aortic Dissections 888
Epidemiology 888
Etiology 888
Pathophysiology 889
Assessment with Clinical Manifestations 890

- Diagnostic Tests 890
- Nursing Diagnoses 890
- Planning and Implementation 890
- Evaluation of Outcomes 892

Thrombophlebitis 893
- Epidemiology 893
- Etiology 893
- Pathophysiology 893
- Assessment with Clinical Manifestations 893
- Diagnostic Tests 893
- Nursing Diagnoses 894
- Planning and Implementation 894
- Evaluation of Outcomes 896

Buerger's Disease 896
- Epidemiology 896
- Etiology 896
- Pathophysiology 896
- Genetics 896
- Assessment with Clinical Manifestations 897
- Diagnostic Tests 897
- Nursing Diagnoses 897
- Planning and Implementation 897
- Evaluation of Outcomes 898

Subclavian Steal Syndrome 898
- Etiology 898
- Assessment with Clinical Manifestations 898
- Diagnostic Tests 898
- Nursing Diagnoses 898
- Planning and Implementation 899
- Evaluation of Outcomes 899

Raynaud's Phenomenon 899
- Epidemiology 899
- Etiology 899
- Assessment with Clinical Manifestations 899
- Diagnostic Tests 900
- Nursing Diagnoses 900
- Planning and Implementation 900
- Evaluation of Outcomes 900

Varicose Veins 900
- Epidemiology 901
- Etiology 901
- Pathophysiology 901
- Assessment with Clinical Manifestations 901

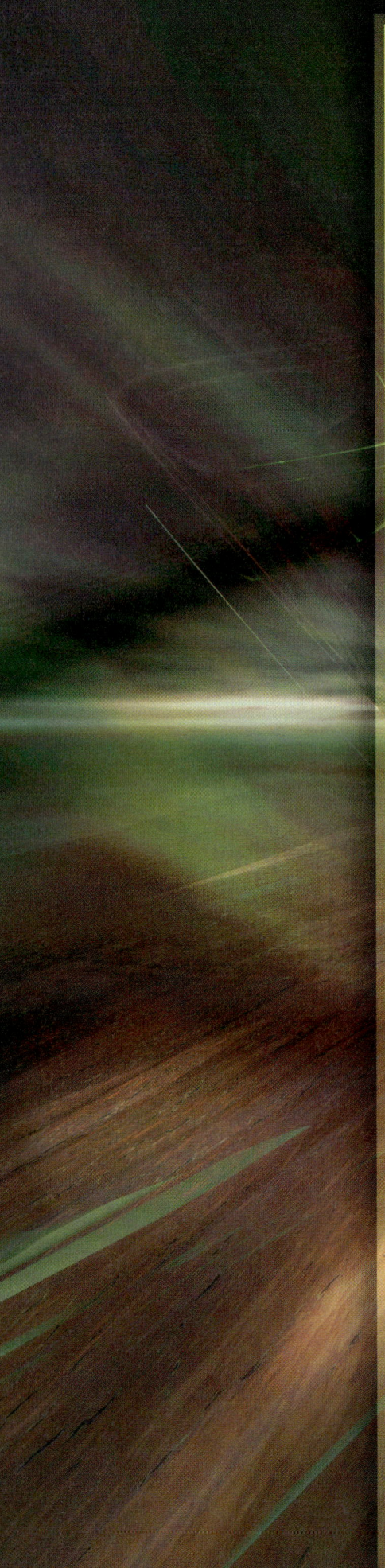

Diagnostic Tests. 901
Nursing Diagnoses 901
Planning and Implementation 901
Evaluation of Outcomes 902
Venous Stasis Ulcer 902
Epidemiology 902
Etiology 902
Pathophysiology 902
Assessment with Clinical Manifestations. 903
Diagnostic Tests. 903
Nursing Diagnoses 903
Planning and Implementation 903
Evaluation of Outcomes 903

CHAPTER 28: Hypertension: Nursing Management **907**

Hypertension 908
Epidemiology 908
Etiology 908
Pathophysiology 911
Assessment with Clinical Manifestations. 912
Diagnostic Tests. 914
Nursing Diagnoses 915
Planning and Implementation 916
Evaluation of Outcomes 926

CHAPTER 29: Hematological Dysfunction: Nursing Management **929**

Anemias 930
Epidemiology 930
Etiology 930
Pathophysiology 930
Assessment with Clinical Manifestations. 931
Diagnostic Tests. 931
Nursing Diagnoses 931
Planning and Implementation 931
Evaluation of Outcomes 932
Hemolytic Anemias. 932
Acquired Hemolytic Anemia. 932
Thalassemia 933
Glucose-6-Phosphate Dehydrogenase Anemia 933
Hereditary Spherocytosis 934
Sickle Cell Anemia. 934

Nutritional Anemias 936
- Iron Deficiency Anemia 936
- Folic Acid Deficiency Anemia 937
- Vitamin B_{12} Deficiency Anemia 938

Platelet and Coagulation Disorders 940
- Thrombocytopenia 940
- Disseminated Intravascular Coagulation 942
- Hemophilia 944

Polycythemias 947
- Primary Polycythemia (Polycythemia Vera) 947
- Secondary Polycythemia 948
- Assessment with Clinical Manifestations 948
- Planning and Implementation 948

Neutropenia 948
- Assessment with Clinical Manifestations 948
- Planning and Implementation 948

Mononucleosis 949
- Pathophysiology 949
- Assessment with Clinical Manifestations 949
- Diagnostic Tests 949
- Planning and Implementation 949

Leukemia 949
- Epidemiology 950
- Etiology 950
- Pathophysiology 950
- Assessment with Clinical Manifestations 950
- Diagnostic Tests 950
- Nursing Diagnoses 951
- Planning and Implementation 951
- Evaluation of Outcomes 953
- Acute Leukemias 954
- Chronic Leukemia 957

Multiple Myeloma 961
- Epidemiology 961
- Etiology 961
- Pathophysiology 962
- Assessment with Clinical Manifestations 962
- Diagnostic Tests 962
- Nursing Diagnoses 963
- Planning and Implementation 963
- Evaluation of Outcomes 964

Malignant Lymphomas 964
- Hodgkin's Disease 964
- Non-Hodgkin's Lymphoma 969

UNIT VI: Alterations in Respiratory Function 973

CHAPTER 30: Assessment of Respiratory Function 974

Anatomy of the Respiratory System 975
- Thorax 975
- Lungs 976
- Upper Respiratory Tract 979
- Lower Respiratory Tract 980
- Pulmonary Mechanics and Musculature 981
- Respiratory Defense Mechanisms 981

Physiology of Respiration 982
- Ventilation and Perfusion 982
- Ventilation-Perfusion Dysfunction 983
- Hypoxemia versus Hypoxia 984
- Hypercapnia versus Hypocapnia 984
- Oxygen Transport 984
- Oxygen-Hemoglobin Dissociation Curve 984
- Acid-Base Balance 986
- Arterial Blood Gas Analysis 987
- Respiratory Adjustments during Exercise, Hypoxia, and in High Altitude 989

Assessment 990
- History Taking 990
- Inspection 993
- Palpation 997
- Percussion 998
- Auscultation 999
- Age-Related Changes in the Respiratory System 1002

Diagnostic Tests 1004
- Laboratory Diagnostic Tests 1004
- Radiographic Diagnostic Tests 1005
- Bedside Monitoring Diagnostic Tests 1009
- Other Diagnostic Tests 1010

CHAPTER 31: Upper Airway Dysfunction: Nursing Management 1017

Allergic Rhinitis 1018
- Pathophysiology 1018
- Assessment with Clinical Manifestations 1018
- Diagnostic Tests 1020
- Nursing Diagnoses 1020
- Evaluation of Outcomes 1023

Viral Rhinitis 1024
Epidemiology 1024
Assessment with Clinical Manifestations. 1024
Nursing Diagnoses 1024
Planning and Implementation 1024
Evaluation of Outcomes 1025
Acute Sinusitis. 1025
Etiology 1025
Pathophysiology 1025
Assessment with Clinical Manifestations. 1026
Diagnostic Tests. 1026
Nursing Diagnoses 1027
Planning and Implementation 1027
Evaluation of Outcomes 1029
Chronic Sinusitis 1029
Pathophysiology 1029
Assessment with Clinical Manifestations. 1029
Diagnostic Tests. 1030
Nursing Diagnoses 1030
Planning and Implementation 1030
Evaluation of Outcomes 1031
Acute Pharyngitis 1031
Epidemiology 1032
Etiology 1032
Pathophysiology 1032
Assessment with Clinical Manifestations. 1032
Diagnostic Tests. 1033
Nursing Diagnoses 1033
Planning and Implementation 1033
Evaluation of Outcomes 1034
Tonsillitis and Adenoiditis. 1034
Etiology 1034
Assessment with Clinical Manifestations. 1034
Diagnostic Tests. 1035
Nursing Diagnoses 1035
Planning and Implementation 1035
Evaluation of Outcomes 1036
Peritonsillar Abscess 1036
Assessment with Clinical Manifestations. 1036
Diagnostic Tests. 1036
Nursing Diagnoses 1037
Planning and Implementation 1037
Evaluation of Outcomes 1037

Acute and Chronic Laryngitis 1037
Pathophysiology 1037
Assessment with Clinical Manifestations. 1038
Planning and Implementation 1038
Obstruction during Sleep 1038
Etiology 1038
Pathophysiology 1038
Assessment with Clinical Manifestations. 1039
Diagnostic Tests. 1039
Nursing Diagnoses 1039
Planning and Implementation 1039
Evaluation of Outcomes 1040
Epistaxis 1040
Etiology 1040
Planning and Implementation 1040
Fractures of the Nose 1041
Assessment with Clinical Manifestations. 1041
Planning and Implementation 1041
Nasal Obstruction 1041
Planning and Implementation 1042
Laryngeal Obstruction 1042
Planning and Implementation 1042
Cancer of the Larynx. 1043
Epidemiology 1043
Etiology 1044
Assessment with Clinical Manifestations. 1044
Diagnostic Tests. 1044
Nursing Diagnoses 1045
Planning and Implementation 1045
Evaluation of Outcomes 1049

CHAPTER 32: Lower Airway Dysfunction: Nursing Management **1055**

Pneumonia 1056
Epidemiology 1056
Pathophysiology 1057
Assessment with Clinical Manifestations. 1058
Diagnostic Tests. 1059
Nursing Diagnoses 1059
Planning and Implementation 1059
Evaluation of Outcomes 1063

Extrapulmonary and Intrapulmonary Restrictive Lung Disorder 1063
Pathophysiology 1063
Assessment with Clinical Manifestations 1063
Tuberculosis 1064
Epidemiology 1064
Pathophysiology 1065
Assessment with Clinical Manifestations 1066
Diagnostic Tests 1066
Nursing Diagnoses 1066
Planning and Implementation 1066
Evaluation of Outcomes 1069
Pulmonary Fungal Infection 1069
Pathophysiology 1070
Assessment with Clinical Manifestations 1070
Diagnostic Tests 1071
Nursing Diagnoses 1071
Planning and Implementation 1071
Evaluation of Outcomes 1072
Bronchiolectasis 1072
Epidemiology 1073
Etiology 1073
Pathophysiology 1073
Assessment with Clinical Manifestations 1073
Diagnostic Tests 1073
Nursing Diagnoses 1073
Planning and Implementation 1074
Evaluation of Outcomes 1075
Lung Abscess 1075
Epidemiology 1075
Etiology 1076
Pathophysiology 1076
Assessment with Clinical Manifestations 1076
Diagnostic Tests 1076
Nursing Diagnoses 1076
Planning and Implementation 1076
Evaluation of Outcomes 1078
Lung Cancer 1078
Epidemiology 1078
Etiology 1078
Pathophysiology 1079
Assessment with Clinical Manifestations 1079
Diagnostic Tests 1079

Nursing Diagnoses . . . 1079
Planning and Implementation . . . 1080
Evaluation of Outcomes . . . 1082
Pneumothorax . . . 1082
Etiology . . . 1082
Pathophysiology . . . 1083
Assessment with Clinical Manifestations . . . 1083
Diagnostic Tests . . . 1083
Nursing Diagnoses . . . 1084
Planning and Implementation . . . 1084
Evaluation of Outcomes . . . 1085
Fractured Rib . . . 1085
Etiology . . . 1085
Pathophysiology . . . 1085
Assessment with Clinical Manifestations . . . 1085
Nursing Diagnoses . . . 1086
Planning and Implementation . . . 1086
Evaluation of Outcomes . . . 1086
Flail Chest . . . 1087
Assessment with Clinical Manifestations . . . 1087
Diagnostic Tests . . . 1087
Nursing Diagnoses . . . 1087
Planning and Implementation . . . 1087
Evaluation of Outcomes . . . 1088
Pulmonary Arterial Hypertension . . . 1088
Epidemiology . . . 1089
Etiology . . . 1089
Assessment with Clinical Manifestations . . . 1089
Diagnostic Tests . . . 1090
Nursing Diagnoses . . . 1090
Planning and Implementation . . . 1090
Evaluation of Outcomes . . . 1091
Cor Pulmonale . . . 1092
Etiology . . . 1092
Assessment with Clinical Manifestations . . . 1092
Diagnostic Tests . . . 1092
Nursing Diagnoses . . . 1093
Planning and Implementation . . . 1093
Evaluation of Outcomes . . . 1094

CHAPTER 33: Obstructive Pulmonary Disease: Nursing Management 1099

Chronic Obstructive Pulmonary Disease 1100
Epidemiology 1100
Etiology 1100
Pathophysiology 1101
Assessment with Clinical Manifestations 1103
Diagnostic Tests 1105
Nursing Diagnoses 1107
Planning and Implementation 1107
Evaluation of Outcomes 1116
Asthma 1116
Epidemiology 1116
Etiology 1117
Pathophysiology 1117
Assessment with Clinical Manifestations 1120
Diagnostic Tests 1120
Nursing Diagnoses 1122
Planning and Implementation 1123
Evaluation of Outcomes 1126
Cystic Fibrosis 1127
Epidemiology 1127
Pathophysiology 1128
Assessment with Clinical Manifestations 1128
Diagnostic Tests 1128
Nursing Diagnoses 1129
Planning and Implementation 1129
Evaluation of Outcomes 1131

UNIT VII: Alterations in Neurological Function 1135

CHAPTER 34: Assessment of Neurological Function 1136

Anatomy and Physiology 1137
Nervous System Cells 1137
Central Nervous System 1139
Peripheral Nervous System 1144
Autonomic Nervous System 1145
Spinal Reflexes 1145
Age-Related Changes 1146

Assessment 1147
History. 1147
Interview. 1148
Physical Examination 1148
Diagnostic Tests 1159
Lumbar Puncture 1160
Radiographic Studies 1160
Electrographic Studies 1164
Ultrasound 1166

CHAPTER 35: Dysfunction of the Brain: Nursing Management **1171**

Cerebrovascular Accidents or Strokes. 1172
Epidemiology 1172
Etiology 1173
Pathophysiology 1174
Assessment with Clinical Manifestations. 1174
Diagnostic Tests. 1174
Nursing Diagnoses 1175
Planning and Implementation 1175
Evaluation of Outcomes 1181
Brain Injuries 1182
Epidemiology 1182
Etiology 1182
Types of Brain Injuries 1183
Pathophysiology 1184
Assessment with Clinical Manifestations. 1186
Diagnostic Tests. 1189
Nursing Diagnoses 1190
Planning and Implementation 1190
Evaluation of Outcomes 1194
Brain Tumors 1195
Epidemiology 1195
Etiology 1195
Pathophysiology 1195
Assessment with Clinical Manifestations. 1196
Diagnostic Tests. 1197
Nursing Diagnoses 1198
Planning and Implementation 1198
Evaluation of Outcomes 1207

CHAPTER 36: Dysfunction of the Spinal Cord and Peripheral Nervous System: Nursing Management 1213

Spinal Cord Injury 1214
- Epidemiology 1214
- Etiology 1214
- Pathophysiology 1215
- Assessment with Clinical Manifestations 1217
- Categorizing Incomplete SCIs 1220
- Nontraumatic SCIs 1221
- Diagnostic Tests 1221
- Nursing Diagnoses 1222
- Planning and Implementation 1222
- Evaluation of Outcomes 1238

Spinal Cord Tumors 1238
- Epidemiology 1238
- Etiology 1239
- Pathophysiology 1239
- Assessment with Clinical Manifestations 1240
- Diagnostic Tests 1240
- Nursing Diagnoses 1241
- Planning and Implementation 1241
- Evaluation of Outcomes 1243

Peripheral Nervous System Dysfunction 1243
- Etiology 1243
- Pathophysiology 1243
- Guillain-Barré Syndrome 1244
- Trigeminal Neuralgia 1247
- Bell's Palsy 1250
- Ménière's Disease 1252
- Peripheral Nerve Injuries 1254
- Carpal Tunnel Syndrome 1256

CHAPTER 37: Degenerative Neurological Dysfunction: Nursing Management 1261

Headache 1262
- Tension-Type Headache 1262
- Migraine Headache 1266
- Cluster Headache 1267

Seizures 1269
- Epidemiology 1269
- Etiology 1269
- Pathophysiology 1269

Assessment with Clinical Manifestations. 1269
Diagnostic Tests. 1272
Nursing Diagnoses 1272
Planning and Implementation 1272
Evaluation of Outcomes 1273
Multiple Sclerosis 1274
Epidemiology 1274
Etiology 1274
Pathophysiology 1274
Assessment with Clinical Manifestations. 1275
Diagnostic Studies. 1276
Nursing Diagnoses 1277
Planning and Implementation 1277
Evaluation of Outcomes 1279
Parkinson's Disease 1279
Epidemiology 1280
Etiology 1280
Pathophysiology 1280
Assessment with Clinical Manifestations. 1280
Diagnostic Tests. 1281
Nursing Diagnoses 1281
Planning and Implementation 1281
Evaluation of Outcomes 1284
Alzheimer's Disease 1285
Epidemiology 1285
Etiology 1285
Pathophysiology 1286
Assessment with Clinical Manifestations. 1286
Diagnostic Tests. 1286
Nursing Diagnoses 1287
Planning and Implementation 1288
Evaluation of Outcomes 1288
Myasthenia Gravis. 1289
Epidemiology 1289
Etiology 1289
Pathophysiology 1289
Assessment with Clinical Manifestations. 1289
Diagnostic Tests. 1290
Nursing Diagnoses 1290
Planning and Implementation 1290
Evaluation of Outcomes 1292
Amyotrophic Lateral Sclerosis 1292
Epidemiology 1292

Etiology 1292
Pathophysiology 1292
Assessment with Clinical Manifestations. 1293
Diagnostic Tests. 1293
Nursing Diagnoses 1293
Planning and Implementation 1293
Evaluation of Outcomes 1294
Huntington's Disease (Huntington's Chorea) 1294
Epidemiology 1294
Etiology 1294
Pathophysiology 1295
Genetics. 1295
Assessment with Clinical Manifestations. 1295
Diagnostic Tests. 1295
Nursing Diagnoses 1295
Planning and Implementation 1296
Evaluation of Outcomes 1296

UNIT VIII: Alterations in Sensory Function 1299

CHAPTER 38: Assessment of Sensory Function 1300

Anatomy and Physiology of the Eye. 1301
External Eye 1301
Internal Eye. 1302
Assessment of the Eye 1303
Present Eye Problem. 1303
Past Medical History 1303
Family History. 1303
Personal and Social History 1303
Examination and Findings 1303
Ophthalmoscopic Examination. 1306
Posterior Segment Structures 1306
Anatomy and Physiology of the Ear. 1311
Ear 1311
Assessment of the Ear. 1312
Present History of Ear Problem 1313
Past Medical History 1313
Family History. 1313
Personal and Social History 1314
Examination and Findings 1314

CHAPTER 39: Visual Dysfunction: Nursing Management 1323

Ocular Movement Disorders 1324
Strabismus 1324
Nystagmus 1324
Ocular Muscle Paralysis 1324
Assessment with Clinical Manifestations and Diagnostic Tests. 1326
Nursing Diagnoses 1326
Planning and Implementation 1326
Evaluation of Outcomes 1326
Visual Acuity 1326
Cataracts 1327
Glaucoma 1329
Retinal Detachment 1330
Macular Degeneration 1332
Traumatic Injuries 1333
Ocular Cancer 1334
Corneal Disorders 1336
Refraction 1337
Pathophysiology 1337
Nursing Diagnoses 1337
Planning and Implementation 1337
Evaluation of Outcomes 1338
Presbyopia 1338
Color Perception 1339
Colorblindness 1339
Inflammatory and Infectious Eye Conditions 1339
Hordeolum 1339
Chalazion 1340
Blepharitis. 1340
Conjunctivitis 1340
Keratitis. 1341
Keratoconjunctivitis Sicca 1341
Iritis and Uveitis 1341
Ocular Disorders Resulting from Other Physiological Processes. 1342
Papilledema 1342
Diabetic Retinopathy 1342
Retinitis Pigmentosa 1343

Low Vision and Blindness 1344
Epidemiology 1344
Planning and Implementation 1344
Assistive Devices 1344
Health Promotion 1345
Safety 1345

CHAPTER 40: Auditory Dysfunction: Nursing Management **1349**

Auditory Dysfunction 1350
Epidemiology 1350
Etiology 1350
Pathophysiology 1351
Genetics. 1352
Assessment with Clinical Manifestations. 1353
Three Classifications of Auditory Dysfunction 1354
Complications of Auditory Dysfunction 1358
Diagnostic Tests. 1360
Nursing Diagnoses 1362
Planning and Implementation 1362
Evaluation of Outcomes 1375

UNIT IX: Alterations in Immunological Function **1379**

CHAPTER 41: Assessment of Immunological Function **1380**

Overview of Immunity 1381
Antigen 1382
Self versus Nonself 1382
Anatomy of the Immune System 1383
Physical Barriers 1383
Leukocytes 1383
Dendritic Cells. 1385
Primary Lymphoid Organs 1391
Secondary Lymphoid Tissue 1391
Chemical Components 1392
Physiology of the Immune System 1394
Innate Immune Response 1394
Adaptive Immunity 1395
Assessment 1401
Age and Developmental Considerations. 1401
Immunizations and Infections 1403

Allergies . . . 1404
Autoimmune Disorders . . . 1405
Cancer . . . 1405
Chronic Illnesses . . . 1405
Surgery . . . 1406
Stress and Social Support . . . 1406
Pharmacology . . . 1407
Lifestyle and Environmental Factors . . . 1407
Physical Examination . . . 1408
Diagnostic Tests . . . 1410
Complete Blood Count with Differential . . . 1410
Radiological Tests . . . 1412
Erythrocyte Sedimentation Rate . . . 1412
C-Reactive Protein . . . 1412
Total Complement (CH50) . . . 1412
Complement C3 . . . 1412
Complement C4 . . . 1412
Phagocytic Cell Function Tests . . . 1413
Protein Electrophoresis . . . 1413
Immunoglobulin Electrophoresis . . . 1413
Radioallergosorbent Test . . . 1413
Antibody Screening Tests . . . 1413
Autoantibody Tests . . . 1413
Antigen Tests . . . 1415
Biopsy . . . 1415
Skin Tests . . . 1416
Anergy Tests . . . 1417
Nursing Management . . . 1417

CHAPTER 42: Immunodeficiency and HIV Infection/AIDS: Nursing Management 1421

Immunodeficiency . . . 1422
Human Immunodeficiency Virus Infection . . . 1422
Epidemiology . . . 1422
Etiology . . . 1423
Pathophysiology . . . 1425
Assessment with Clinical Manifestations . . . 1426
Diagnostic Tests . . . 1426
Nursing Diagnoses . . . 1428
Planning and Implementation . . . 1428
Evaluation of Outcomes . . . 1430
Immunodeficiency Disorders . . . 1431
Graft-versus-Host Disease . . . 1431

Immunosuppressive Therapy 1432
Hypersensitivity Disorders 1433
Autoimmune Disorders 1433
Rheumatoid Arthritis 1434
Sjögren's Syndrome 1441
Systemic Lupus Erythematosus 1441
Progressive Systemic Sclerosis (Scleroderma) 1444

CHAPTER 43: Allergic Dysfunction: Nursing Management 1449

Allergic Dysfunction 1450
Genetics 1450
Pathophysiology 1450
Diagnostic Tests 1452
Nursing Diagnoses 1452
Types of Hypersensitivity 1452
Type 1 Hypersensitivity 1452
Type 2 Hypersensitivity 1453
Type 3 Hypersensitivity 1453
Type 4 Hypersensitivity 1453
Assessment with Clinical Manifestations 1454
Planning and Implementation 1454
Atopic Asthma 1455
Epidemiology 1456
Etiology 1456
Pathophysiology 1456
Assessment with Clinical Manifestations 1456
Diagnostic Tests 1457
Nursing Diagnoses 1457
Planning and Implementation 1457
Evaluation of Outcomes 1460
Anaphylaxis 1460
Epidemiology 1460
Etiology 1461
Pathophysiology 1462
Assessment with Clinical Manifestations 1462
Planning and Implementation 1462
Allergic Conditions 1464
Allergic Rhinitis (Hay Fever) 1464
Allergic Contact Dermatitis 1465
Atopic Dermatitis 1466
Urticaria 1466
Angioneurotic Edema 1467

Food Allergy . . . 1468
Latex Allergy . . . 1469
Serum Sickness . . . 1470
Contact Dermatitis (Dermatitis Medicamentosa) . . . 1471
Hereditary Angioedema . . . 1471

UNIT X: Alterations in Integumentary Function 1475

CHAPTER 44: Assessment of Integumentary Function 1476

Anatomy and Physiology . . . 1477
Epidermis . . . 1477
Dermis. . . . 1480
Subcutaneous Tissue. . . . 1481
Protection . . . 1481
Homeostasis . . . 1481
Excretion . . . 1481
Thermoregulation. . . . 1481
Synthesis . . . 1481
Sensory Perception . . . 1482
Psychosocial Function. . . . 1482
Healing . . . 1482
Skin Changes Throughout the Life Span . . . 1482
Cellular Effects of Aging on the Skin . . . 1483
Factors Regulating Skin and Wound Repair . . . 1483
Assessment . . . 1484
Review of Systems . . . 1485
Assessment of the Skin . . . 1485
Diagnostic Tests . . . 1490
Nursing Diagnoses . . . 1491
The Health Care Team . . . 1491

CHAPTER 45: Dermatological Dysfunction: Nursing Management 1495

General Guidelines for Management of Patients with Dermatological Dysfunction . . . 1496
Debridement . . . 1496
Methods of Treatment . . . 1498
Topical Corticosteroids . . . 1501
Topical Soaks and Wraps. . . . 1501
Moisture Retentive Dressings . . . 1503

Moisturizers and Lubricants 1503
Phototherapy and Photochemotherapy 1504
Common Skin Disorders 1506
Acne 1506
Atopic Dermatitis 1507
Cellulitis 1508
Contact Dermatitis 1508
Folliculitis 1509
Fungal Infections 1510
Furuncles and Carbuncles 1512
Herpes Infections 1512
Impetigo 1514
Pediculosis 1514
Pemphigus 1515
Pruritus 1515
Psoriasis 1516
Rosacea 1517
Scabies 1517
Stasis Dermatitis 1518
Warts 1519
Xerosis 1519
Precancerous and Cancerous Conditions 1519
Sunburn 1519
Malignant Skin Lesions 1520
Nonmelanoma Skin Cancers 1521
Melanoma 1522
Nursing Management 1524

CHAPTER 46: Burns: Nursing Management 1529

Burns 1530
Epidemiology 1530
Etiology 1530
Pathophysiology 1531
Planning and Implementation 1533
Emergent Phase 1534
Prehospital Care and First Aid 1534
Emergency Department Management 1536
Assessment with Clinical Manifestations 1537
Nursing Diagnoses 1540
Planning and Implementation 1540
Evaluation of Outcomes 1545

Acute Phase 1546
Diagnostic Tests. . . . 1546
Assessment with Clinical Manifestations. . . . 1546
Nursing Diagnoses 1547
Planning and Implementation 1547
Evaluation of Outcomes 1556
Rehabilitation Phase. . . . 1556
Diagnostic Tests. . . . 1556
Assessment with Clinical Manifestations. . . . 1556
Nursing Diagnoses 1557
Planning and Implementation 1557
Collaborative Care Management. . . . 1560
Evaluation of Outcomes 1561

UNIT XI: Alterations in Gastrointestinal Function 1567

CHAPTER 47: Assessment of Gastrointestinal Function 1568

Anatomy and Physiology 1569
Mouth, Lips, Cheeks, Tongue, and Pharynx 1569
Esophagus. . . . 1570
Stomach 1570
Duodenum 1570
Pancreas 1570
Liver and Biliary Systems 1571
Jejunum and Ileum. . . . 1571
Cecum and Appendix 1571
Colon. . . . 1571
Rectum and Anus 1571
Assessment 1571
GI Symptom Assessment. . . . 1573
Diarrhea 1576
Constipation 1577
Abdominal Pain 1577
Referred Pain 1578
Assessment 1578
Referred Pain from Abdominal Structures 1584
Diagnostic Tests 1584
Colonoscopy 1585
Laparoscopy 1586
Proctosigmoidoscopy 1586

Paracentesis 1586
Nasogastric Tubes 1587
Esophageal Manometry 1587
Secretin Testing 1587
Equipment for Gastric and Intestinal Intubation 1587
Patient Preparation for Nasogastric and Nasointestinal Intubation 1588
Esophageal Dilation 1589
Feeding Tubes: Gastrostomy and Jejunostomy 1590
Percutaneous Endoscopic Gastrostomy and Percutaneous Endoscopic Jejunostomy Tubes 1591
Barium Studies 1591

CHAPTER 48: Nutrition, Malnutrition, and Obesity: Nursing Management **1595**

The Gastrointestinal Tract and Nutritional Processes 1596
Processes of Digestion, Absorption, and Metabolism 1596
Components of a Nutritionally Adequate Diet 1598
Metabolic Rate 1599
Nutrition and Drug Interactions 1601
Cytochrome P450 1601
Warfarin 1602
Natural Products 1602
Nutrition Support: Alternative Methods of Feeding Patients . 1602
Enteral Feedings 1602
Gastrostomy Feedings 1605
Parenteral Nutrition 1606
Malnutrition 1606
Epidemiology 1606
Etiology 1606
Assessment with Clinical Manifestations 1607
Diagnostic Tests 1607
Nursing Diagnoses 1608
Planning and Implementation 1608
Evaluation of Outcomes 1608
Obesity 1612
Epidemiology 1612
Etiology 1612
Assessment with Clinical Manifestations 1612
Nursing Diagnoses 1613
Planning and Implementation 1613
Evaluation of Outcomes 1614
Nutrition and Aging 1615

CHAPTER 49: Upper Gastrointestinal Tract Dysfunction: Nursing Management 1619

Disorders of the Oral Cavity 1620
Etiology 1620
Planning and Implementation 1620
Nonulcerative Causes of Mouth Pain 1621
Burning Mouth Syndrome 1622
Dysphagia 1623
Esophageal Disorders 1626
Esophageal Pain and Achalasia 1627
Gastroesophageal Reflux Disease 1629
Hiatal Hernia 1631
Esophageal Cancer 1632
GI Tract Pain of Noncardiac and Nonphysiological Origins . . 1634
Noncardiac Chest Pain 1634
Panic Disorder 1635
Functional Gastrointestinal Disorders 1635
Nonulcer Dyspepsia 1635
Epidemiology 1636
Pathophysiology 1636
Assessment with Clinical Manifestations 1636
Diagnostic Tests 1636
Nursing Diagnoses 1637
Planning and Implementation 1637
Evaluation of Outcomes 1637
Peptic-Ulcer Dyspepsia 1638
Etiology 1638
Epidemiology 1638
Pathophysiology 1638
Assessment with Clinical Manifestations 1638
Diagnostic Tests 1639
Nursing Diagnoses 1639
Planning and Implementation 1639
Evaluation of Outcomes 1641
Gastritis, Duodenitis, and Associated Ulcerative Lesions 1641
Stomach Cancer 1641
Epidemiology 1642
Etiology 1642
Pathophysiology 1642
Assessment with Clinical Manifestations 1643
Diagnostic Tests 1643
Nursing Diagnoses 1643

Planning and Implementation 1643
Evaluations of Outcomes 1644

CHAPTER 50: Lower Gastrointestinal Tract Dysfunction: Nursing Management **1647**

Small Intestine 1648
Absorption of Nutrients 1648
Mal-Assimilation Syndromes. 1651
Epidemiology 1651
Pathophysiology 1651
Assessment with Clinical Manifestations. 1652
Diagnostic Tests. 1652
Nursing Diagnoses 1652
Planning and Implementation 1652
Evaluation of Outcomes 1654
Acute Abdomen 1654
Epidemiology 1654
Etiology 1655
Pathophysiology 1655
Assessment with Clinical Manifestations. 1656
Diagnostic Tests. 1659
Nursing Diagnoses 1661
Planning and Implementation 1661
Evaluation of Outcomes 1663
Acute Inflammatory Disorders 1664
Appendicitis 1664
Diverticulitis 1666
Obstruction. 1668
Epidemiology 1669
Etiology 1670
Pathophysiology 1671
Assessment with Clinical Manifestations. 1671
Diagnostic Tests. 1672
Nursing Diagnoses 1673
Planning and Implementation 1673
Evaluation of Outcomes 1675
Colorectal Cancer 1676
Epidemiology 1676
Etiology 1676
Pathophysiology 1678
Assessment with Clinical Manifestations. 1679
Diagnostic Tests. 1679
Nursing Diagnoses 1681

Planning and Implementation 1681
Evaluation of Outcomes 1686
Irritable Bowel Syndrome 1686
Epidemiology 1686
Pathophysiology 1686
Assessment with Clinical Manifestations 1686
Diagnostic Tests 1687
Nursing Diagnoses 1687
Planning and Implementation 1687
Evaluation of Outcomes 1687
Inflammatory Bowel Disorders 1688
Epidemiology 1688
Diagnostic Tests 1688
Nursing Diagnoses 1688
Planning and Implementation 1688
Evaluation of Outcomes 1689
Crohn's Disease 1690
Ulcerative Colitis 1691

CHAPTER 51: Hepatic, Biliary Tract, and Pancreatic Dysfunction: Nursing Management 1695

Hepatic System 1696
Biliary Tract 1698
Pancreas 1699
Diagnostic Tests 1699
Hepatitis 1701
Pathophysiology 1701
Assessment with Clinical Manifestations 1701
Nursing Diagnoses 1708
Planning and Implementation 1708
Evaluation of Outcomes 1708
Alcoholic Hepatitis 1709
Toxic and Drug-Induced Hepatitis 1710
Autoimmune Hepatitis 1710
Hereditary Diseases of the Liver 1710
Cirrhosis 1711
Alcoholic Cirrhosis 1712
Postnecrotic Cirrhosis 1712
Biliary Cirrhosis 1712
Cardiac Cirrhosis 1712
Pathophysiology 1713
Assessment with Clinical Manifestations 1714

Planning and Implementation 1714
Portal Hypertension 1715
Hepatic Encephalopathy. 1717
Hepatorenal Syndrome. 1717
Lecithin-Cholesterol Acyltransferase Deficiencies. 1718
Fatty Liver (Hepatic Steatosis). 1718
Etiology 1718
Pathophysiology 1718
Assessment with Clinical Manifestations. 1719
Diagnostic Tests. 1719
Planning and Implementation 1719
Hepatic Abscesses. 1719
Epidemiology 1719
Etiology 1719
Pathophysiology 1720
Assessment with Clinical Manifestations. 1720
Diagnostic Tests. 1720
Nursing Diagnoses 1720
Planning and Implementation 1720
Evaluation of Outcomes 1721
Liver Trauma. 1721
Etiology 1721
Pathophysiology 1721
Assessment with Clinical Manifestations. 1722
Diagnostic Tests. 1722
Nursing Diagnoses 1722
Planning and Implementation 1722
Evaluation of Outcomes 1722
Cancer of the Liver 1723
Pathophysiology 1723
Assessment with Clinical Manifestations. 1723
Nursing Diagnoses 1724
Planning and Implementation 1724
Evaluation of Outcomes 1724
Liver Transplantation 1725
Etiology 1725
Types of Liver Transplants. 1725
Diagnostic Tests. 1727
Nursing Diagnoses 1727
Planning and Implementation 1727
Evaluation of Outcomes 1729
Diseases of the Biliary Tract 1729
Cholelithiasis. 1729
Cholecystitis 1732

Primary Sclerosing Cholangitis 1733
Primary Biliary Cirrhosis 1733
Cancer of the Gallbladder and Bile Ducts 1735
Pancreatitis 1736
Acute Pancreatitis 1736
Chronic Pancreatitis 1738

UNIT XII: Alterations in Renal Function 1745

CHAPTER 52: Assessment of Renal Function 1746

Anatomy and Physiology 1747
Kidneys 1747
Ureters 1749
Urinary Bladder 1749
Bladder Neck (Posterior Urethra) 1750
Nephron 1751
Renal Tubule 1751
Renin-Angiotensin System 1753
Assessment 1754
Health History 1754
Physical Examination 1755
Diagnostic Tests 1757
Urine Studies 1757
Blood Studies 1757
Urinary Retention Studies 1757
Radiographic Studies 1757
Renal Ultrasound (Kidney Scan) 1757
Renal Biopsy 1760
Cystoscopy 1761

CHAPTER 53: Urinary Dysfunction: Nursing Management 1765

Urinary Tract Infection 1766
Epidemiology 1766
Etiology 1767
Pathophysiology 1767
Assessment with Clinical Manifestations 1767
Diagnostic Tests 1769
Nursing Diagnoses 1771
Planning and Implementation 1771
Evaluation of Outcomes 1771

Interstitial Cystitis 1771
- Epidemiology 1771
- Etiology 1772
- Pathophysiology 1772
- Genetics 1774
- Assessment with Clinical Manifestations 1774
- Diagnostic Tests 1774
- Nursing Diagnoses 1775
- Planning and Implementation 1776
- Evaluation of Outcomes 1777

Pyelonephritis 1777
- Etiology 1777
- Pathophysiology 1778
- Assessment with Clinical Manifestations 1778
- Diagnostic Tests 1778
- Nursing Diagnoses 1778
- Planning and Implementation 1778
- Evaluation of Outcomes 1779

Glomerulonephritis 1780
- Epidemiology 1780
- Etiology 1780
- Pathophysiology 1781
- Assessment with Clinical Manifestations 1782
- Diagnostic Tests 1782
- Nursing Diagnoses 1782
- Planning and Implementation 1782
- Evaluation of Outcomes 1784

Nephrotic Syndrome 1784
- Epidemiology 1784
- Etiology 1785
- Pathophysiology 1785
- Assessment with Clinical Manifestations 1785
- Diagnostic Tests 1785
- Nursing Diagnoses 1786
- Planning and Implementation 1786
- Evaluation of Outcomes 1787

Renal Tuberculosis 1787
- Etiology 1787
- Pathophysiology 1787
- Assessment with Clinical Manifestations 1788
- Diagnostic Tests 1788
- Nursing Diagnoses 1788

Planning and Implementation 1788
Evaluation of Outcomes 1788
Urinary Tract Calculi (Urolithiasis). 1788
Epidemiology 1789
Etiology 1789
Pathophysiology 1789
Assessment with Clinical Manifestations. 1789
Diagnostic Tests. 1790
Nursing Diagnoses 1790
Planning and Implementation 1790
Evaluation of Outcomes 1792
Renal System Trauma 1792
Etiology 1792
Pathophysiology 1793
Assessment with Clinical Manifestations. 1793
Diagnostic Tests. 1793
Nursing Diagnoses 1794
Planning and Implementation 1794
Evaluation of Outcomes 1794
Renal Vascular Disorders 1795
Renal Cancer. 1795
Epidemiology 1795
Etiology 1796
Pathophysiology 1796
Genetics. 1796
Assessment with Clinical Manifestations. 1796
Diagnostic Tests. 1796
Nursing Diagnoses 1797
Planning and Implementation 1797
Evaluation of Outcomes 1798
Bladder Cancer 1798
Epidemiology 1798
Etiology 1799
Pathophysiology 1799
Assessment with Clinical Manifestations. 1799
Diagnostic Tests. 1799
Nursing Diagnoses 1800
Planning and Implementation 1800
Evaluation of Outcomes 1801
Urinary Diversion 1801
Etiology 1801
Assessment with Clinical Manifestations. 1801
Diagnostic Tests. 1802
Planning and Implementation 1802

Urinary Retention 1804
Epidemiology 1804
Etiology 1804
Pathophysiology 1804
Assessment with Clinical Manifestations 1804
Diagnostic Tests 1805
Nursing Diagnoses 1805
Planning and Implementation 1805
Evaluation of Outcomes 1805
Urinary Incontinence 1805
Epidemiology 1806
Etiology 1806
Pathophysiology 1806
Assessment with Clinical Manifestations 1806
Diagnostic Tests 1807
Nursing Diagnoses 1807
Planning and Implementation 1807
Evaluation of Outcomes 1808

CHAPTER 54: Renal Dysfunction: Nursing Management 1813

Pyelonephritis 1814
Etiology 1814
Pathophysiology 1814
Assessment with Clinical Manifestations 1814
Diagnostic Tests 1814
Nursing Diagnoses 1814
Planning and Implementation 1815
Evaluation of Outcomes 1816
Polycystic Kidney Disease 1816
Epidemiology 1816
Genetics 1816
Pathophysiology 1817
Assessment with Clinical Manifestations 1817
Diagnostic Tests 1817
Nursing Diagnoses 1818
Planning and Implementation 1818
Evaluation of Outcomes 1819
Immunological and Vascular Diseases of the Kidney 1820
Alport Syndrome 1820
Small Vessel Vasculitis: Wegener Granulomatosis 1821

Goodpasture's Syndrome 1822
Epidemiology 1822
Etiology 1822
Pathophysiology 1822
Genetics. 1823
Assessment with Clinical Manifestations. 1823
Diagnostic Tests. 1823
Planning and Implementation 1823
Rhabdomyolysis 1823
Etiology 1823
Pathophysiology 1823
Genetics. 1824
Assessment with Clinical Manifestations. 1824
Diagnostic Tests. 1824
Planning and Implementation 1824
Acute Renal Failure 1824
Epidemiology 1814
Etiology 1824
Pathophysiology 1826
Assessment with Clinical Manifestations. 1826
Diagnostic Tests. 1826
Nursing Diagnoses 1826
Planning and Implementation 1827
Evaluation of Outcomes 1832
Chronic Renal Failure 1832
Epidemiology 1832
Etiology 1833
Pathophysiology 1833
Assessment with Clinical Manifestations. 1833
Diagnostic Tests. 1833
Nursing Diagnoses 1833
Planning and Implementation 1834
Evaluation of Outcomes 1842

UNIT XIII: Alterations in Endocrine Function 1847

CHAPTER 55: Assessment of Endocrine Function 1848

Anatomy and Physiology 1849
Glands 1849
Hormones 1849

Regulation of Hormones. 1850
Hypothalamus Gland 1852
Pituitary Gland 1852
Thyroid Gland 1853
Adrenal Glands 1855
Pancreas Gland 1856
Effects of Aging on the Endocrine System 1856
Assessment 1856
Subjective Data 1856
Objective Data. 1858
Diagnostic Tests 1858
Thyroid Scan 1859
Thyroid Ultrasound 1860
Thyroid Biopsy 1860

CHAPTER 56: Endocrine Dysfunction: Nursing Management 1863

Hypersecretion of the Anterior Pituitary Gland 1864
Etiology 1864
Pathophysiology 1864
Hyperprolactinemia 1864
Acromegaly (Gigantism) 1866
Cushing's Disease (Hypercortisolism) 1869
Hyposecretion of the Anterior Pituitary Gland. 1873
Etiology 1873
Pathophysiology 1873
Assessment with Clinical Manifestations. 1874
Planning and Implementation 1874
Posterior Pituitary Disorders 1874
Diabetes Insipidus. 1874
Syndrome of Inappropriate Antidiuretic Hormone 1875
Hyposecretion of the Adrenal Gland 1876
Epidemiology 1877
Etiology 1877
Pathophysiology 1877
Assessment with Clinical Manifestations. 1877
Diagnostic Tests. 1877
Nursing Diagnoses 1878
Planning and Implementation 1878
Evaluation of Outcomes 1879
Hypersecretion of the Adrenal Gland (Hyperaldosteronism) . . 1879
Epidemiology 1880
Etiology 1880

Pathophysiology 1880
Assessment with Clinical Manifestations. 1880
Diagnostic Tests. 1880
Nursing Diagnoses 1881
Planning and Implementation 1881
Evaluation of Outcomes 1881
Pheochromocytoma 1881
Thyroid Disorders 1883
Hypersecretion of the Thyroid Gland 1883
Nontoxic Goiter. 1890
Thyroiditis 1890
Thyroid Nodules and Neoplasms 1890
Hypothyroidism 1891
Myxedema Coma 1895
Hyperparathyroidism 1895
Epidemiology 1895
Etiology 1896
Pathophysiology 1896
Assessment with Clinical Manifestations. 1896
Diagnostic Tests. 1896
Nursing Diagnoses 1896
Planning and Implementation 1897
Evaluation of Outcomes 1897
Hypoparathyroidism. 1897
Epidemiology 1898
Etiology 1898
Pathophysiology 1898
Assessment with Clinical Manifestations. 1898
Diagnostic Tests. 1898
Nursing Diagnoses 1898
Planning and Implementation 1898
Evaluation of Outcomes 1899

CHAPTER 57: Diabetes Mellitus: Nursing Management 1903

Diabetes Mellitus 1904
Pathophysiology 1904
Assessment with Clinical Manifestations. 1906
Diagnostic Tests. 1908
Nursing Diagnoses 1908
Planning and Implementation 1908
Evaluation of Outcomes 1917

Acute Complications of Diabetes 1918
Diabetic Ketoacidosis 1918
Hyperosmolar Hyperglycemic Nonketotic Syndrome 1919
Hypoglycemia 1920
Chronic Complications of Diabetes 1922
Angiopathy or Vessel Disease 1922
Microvascular Complications 1923

UNIT XIV: Alterations in Musculoskeletal Function 1933

CHAPTER 58: Assessment of Musculoskeletal Function 1934

Anatomy and Physiology of the Bony Skeleton 1935
Macroscopic Structure of Bone 1935
Microscopic Structure of Bone 1936
Physiological Processes 1937
Bone Repair/Fracture Healing 1937
Functions of Bone 1938
Aging and the Skeletal System 1938
Anatomy and Physiology of Skeletal Muscles 1938
Nerve and Blood Supply 1939
Tendons, Ligaments, and Bursae 1939
Aging and the Muscular System 1939
Joints 1940
Classifications 1940
Structural Aspects of the Diarthrosis Joint 1940
Motions 1940
Musculoskeletal Assessment 1940
Guidelines for Assessment 1941
Focused Health History 1941
Physical Examination of the Musculoskeletal System 1942
Assessment of Injuries to the Musculoskeletal System . . . 1945
Diagnostic Studies Related to the Musculoskeletal System . . 1948
Laboratory Studies 1948
Radiographic Studies 1948
Special Tests 1951

CHAPTER 59: Musculoskeletal Dysfunction: Nursing Management 1955

Osteoarthritis 1956
Epidemiology 1956
Etiology 1956

- Pathophysiology 1956
- Assessment with Clinical Manifestations. 1957
- Diagnostic Testing 1957
- Nursing Diagnoses 1957
- Planning and Implementation 1958
- Evaluation of Outcomes 1960

Gout 1964
- Epidemiology 1964
- Etiology 1964
- Pathophysiology 1964
- Assessment with Clinical Manifestations. 1964
- Diagnostic Tests. 1965
- Nursing Diagnoses 1965
- Planning and Implementation 1965
- Evaluation of Outcomes 1966

Lyme Disease 1966
- Epidemiology 1967
- Etiology 1967
- Assessment with Clinical Manifestations. 1967
- Diagnostic Tests. 1968
- Nursing Diagnoses 1968
- Planning and Implementation 1968
- Evaluation of Outcomes 1969

Spondyloarthropathies. 1969
- Etiology 1970
- Pathophysiology 1970
- Assessment with Clinical Manifestations. 1970
- Diagnostic Tests. 1971
- Nursing Diagnoses 1971
- Planning and Implementation 1971
- Evaluation of Outcomes 1972
- Ankylosing Spondylitis 1972
- Reactive Arthritis. 1973
- Psoriatic Arthritis 1973
- Etiology 1974

Polymyositis and Dermatomyositis 1974
- Epidemiology 1974
- Pathophysiology 1974
- Assessment with Clinical Manifestations. 1974
- Diagnostic Tests. 1975
- Nursing Diagnoses 1975
- Planning and Implementation 1975
- Evaluation of Outcomes 1976

Fibromyalgia . . . 1976
- Epidemiology . . . 1976
- Etiology . . . 1976
- Pathophysiology . . . 1977
- Assessment with Clinical Manifestations . . . 1977
- Diagnostic Tests . . . 1978
- Nursing Diagnoses . . . 1979
- Planning and Implementation . . . 1979
- Evaluation of Outcomes . . . 1980

Osteoporosis . . . 1981
- Epidemiology . . . 1981
- Etiology . . . 1981
- Pathophysiology . . . 1981
- Assessment with Clinical Manifestations . . . 1982
- Diagnostic Tests . . . 1983
- Nursing Diagnoses . . . 1983
- Planning and Implementation . . . 1984
- Evaluation of Outcomes . . . 1985

Osteomalacia . . . 1985
- Epidemiology . . . 1986
- Etiology . . . 1986
- Pathophysiology . . . 1986
- Assessment with Clinical Manifestations . . . 1986
- Diagnostic Tests . . . 1986
- Nursing Diagnoses . . . 1986
- Planning and Implementation . . . 1986
- Evaluation of Outcomes . . . 1987

Paget's Disease . . . 1987
- Epidemiology . . . 1988
- Etiology . . . 1988
- Pathophysiology . . . 1988
- Assessment with Clinical Manifestations . . . 1988
- Diagnostic Tests . . . 1988
- Nursing Diagnoses . . . 1989
- Planning and Implementation . . . 1989
- Evaluation of Outcomes . . . 1991

Osteomyelitis . . . 1992
- Epidemiology . . . 1992
- Etiology . . . 1992
- Pathophysiology . . . 1992
- Assessment with Clinical Manifestations . . . 1992
- Diagnostic Tests . . . 1993
- Nursing Diagnoses . . . 1993

Planning and Implementation 1993
Evaluation of Outcomes 1994
Tumors of the Musculoskeletal System 1994
Primary Bony and Soft Tissue Tumors 1994
Metastatic Tumors. 1998
Epidemiology 1998
Pathophysiology 1998
Assessment with Clinical Manifestations. 1998
Diagnostic Tests. 1998
Nursing Diagnoses 1999
Spinal Disorders 1999
Scoliosis. 2000
Assessment with Clinical Manifestations. 2000
Kyphosis 2002
Spinal Stenosis 2002
Assessment with Clinical Manifestations. 2002

CHAPTER 60: Musculoskeletal Trauma: Nursing Management **2009**

Sports Injuries. 2010
Overuse Syndrome/Repetitive Motion Injuries. 2010
Dislocation of the Shoulder 2010
Epidemiology 2010
Etiology 2011
Pathophysiology 2011
Assessment with Clinical Manifestations. 2011
Diagnostic Tests. 2011
Nursing Diagnoses 2011
Planning and Implementation 2012
Rotator Cuff Tears. 2012
Epidemiology 2012
Etiology 2012
Assessment with Clinical Manifestations. 2013
Diagnostic Tests. 2013
Nursing Diagnoses 2013
Planning and Implementation 2013
Evaluation of Outcomes 2014
Lateral Epicondylitis 2014
Epidemiology 2014
Etiology 2014
Pathophysiology 2014
Assessment with Clinical Manifestations. 2014

Diagnostic Tests. 2015
Nursing Diagnoses 2015
Planning and Implementation 2015
Evaluation of Outcomes 2015
Carpal Tunnel Syndrome 2015
Epidemiology 2016
Etiology 2016
Pathophysiology 2016
Assessment with Clinical Manifestations. 2017
Diagnostic Tests. 2017
Planning and Implementation 2017
Patellar Tendinopathy 2018
Epidemiology 2018
Etiology 2018
Pathophysiology 2018
Assessment with Clinical Manifestations. 2018
Diagnostic Tests. 2019
Nursing Diagnoses 2019
Planning and Implementation 2019
Ligament Injuries 2019
Etiology and Pathophysiology 2020
Epidemiology 2020
Assessment 2021
Diagnostic Tests. 2021
Nursing Diagnoses 2021
Planning and Implementation 2021
Meniscal Injuries. 2022
Epidemiology 2022
Etiology 2022
Assessment with Clinical Manifestations. 2023
Diagnostic Tests. 2023
Nursing Diagnoses 2023
Planning and Implementation 2023
Evaluation of Outcomes 2024
Ankle Sprain 2024
Etiology 2024
Assessment with Clinical Manifestations. 2025
Diagnostic Tests. 2025
Nursing Diagnoses 2025
Planning and Implementation 2025
Achilles Tendon Injuries 2026
Epidemiology 2026
Etiology 2026

Pathophysiology 2026
Assessment with Clinical Manifestations. . . . 2026
Diagnostic Tests. . . . 2026
Nursing Diagnoses 2027
Planning and Implementation 2027
Evaluation of Outcomes 2027
Plantar Fasciitis. . . . 2027
Etiology 2028
Pathophysiology 2028
Assessment with Clinical Manifestations. . . . 2028
Diagnostic Tests. . . . 2028
Nursing Diagnoses 2028
Planning and Implementation 2028
Evaluation of Outcomes 2029
Stress Fractures. . . . 2029
Epidemiology 2029
Etiology 2030
Pathophysiology 2030
Assessment with Clinical Manifestations. . . . 2030
Diagnostic Tests. . . . 2030
Nursing Diagnoses 2030
Planning and Implementation 2030
Evaluation of Outcomes 2031
Fractures. . . . 2031
Epidemiology 2031
Pathophysiology 2031
Assessment with Clinical Manifestations. . . . 2033
Diagnostic Tests. . . . 2033
Nursing Diagnoses 2033
Planning and Implementation 2034
Evaluation of Outcomes 2036
Hip Fractures 2036
Epidemiology 2037
Pathophysiology 2037
Assessment with Clinical Manifestations. . . . 2038
Diagnostic Tests. . . . 2038
Nursing Diagnoses 2038
Planning and Implementation 2038
Evaluation of Outcomes 2039
Compartment Syndrome 2039
Pathophysiology 2039
Assessment with Clinical Manifestations. . . . 2040
Diagnostic Tests. . . . 2040
Goals 2040

Fat Embolism Syndrome . . . 2040
- Pathophysiology . . . 2041
- Assessment with Clinical Manifestations . . . 2041
- Diagnostic Tests . . . 2041
- Planning and Implementation . . . 2041

Venous Thromboembolism . . . 2042
- Pathophysiology . . . 2042
- Assessment with Clinical Manifestations . . . 2042
- Diagnostic Tests . . . 2042
- Planning and Implementation . . . 2043

Amputation . . . 2043
- Epidemiology . . . 2043
- Etiology . . . 2044
- Pathophysiology . . . 2044
- Assessment with Clinical Manifestations . . . 2044
- Diagnostic Tests . . . 2045
- Nursing Diagnoses . . . 2045
- Planning and Implementation . . . 2045
- Evaluation of Outcomes . . . 2049

UNIT XV: Alterations in Reproductive Function 2053

CHAPTER 61: Assessment of Reproductive Function 2054

Anatomy and Physiology . . . 2055
- Male Reproductive System . . . 2055
- Female Reproductive System . . . 2059

Sexual Response Cycle . . . 2065
- Male Sexual Response Cycle . . . 2066
- Female Sexual Response Cycle . . . 2068
- Interactive Sexual Intimacy . . . 2069
- Sexual Dysfunction . . . 2069

Assessment . . . 2070
- General Health and Medical History . . . 2071
- Sexual Health History . . . 2071
- Intimate Partner Violence . . . 2071
- Sexual Abuse and Assault . . . 2073
- Physical Examination of Male Genitalia . . . 2074
- Gynecological Examination of the Female . . . 2075

Diagnostic Tests . . . 2077
- Male Diagnostic Tests . . . 2077
- Female Diagnostic Tests . . . 2080

CHAPTER 62: Female Reproductive Dysfunction: Nursing Management 2087

Menstrual Disorders 2088
Dysmenorrhea 2088
Amenorrhea 2089
Menopause 2090
Premenstrual Syndrome and Premenstrual Dysphoric Disorder 2091
Polycystic Ovary Syndrome 2092
Dysfunctional Uterine Bleeding 2093
Endometriosis 2094
Assessment with Clinical Manifestations 2095
Diagnostic Tests 2095
Nursing Diagnoses 2096
Planning and Implementation 2096
Evaluation of Outcomes 2100
Infections 2101
Vaginitis 2101
Bartholin's or Skene's Gland Infection 2102
Sexually Transmitted Disease 2102
Herpes Simplex Virus 2103
Human Papillomavirus 2104
Pelvic Inflammatory Disease 2105
Toxic Shock Syndrome 2105
Complications 2105
Assessment with Clinical Manifestations 2106
Diagnostic Tests 2106
Nursing Diagnoses 2107
Planning and Implementation 2107
Evaluation of Outcomes 2110
Structural Abnormalities and Benign Conditions 2110
Polyps 2110
Pelvic Relaxation 2110
Leiomyomata 2111
Ovarian Cysts 2112
Genetics 2112
Assessment with Clinical Manifestations 2113
Diagnostic Tests 2114
Nursing Diagnoses 2114
Planning and Implementation 2115
Evaluation of Outcomes 2116

Female Genital Mutilation 2116
Assessment with Clinical Manifestations. 2117
Diagnostic Tests. 2117
Nursing Diagnoses 2117
Planning and Implementation 2118
Evaluation of Outcomes 2118
Malignancies. 2118
Vulvar Cancer 2119
Vaginal Cancer 2119
Cervical Cancer 2119
Endometrial Cancer 2120
Ovarian Cancer 2120
Assessment with Clinical Manifestations. 2121
Diagnostic Tests. 2121
Nursing Diagnoses 2121
Planning and Implementation 2122
Evaluation of Outcomes 2123
Infertility 2123
Assessment with Clinical Manifestations. 2124
Diagnostic Tests. 2124
Nursing Diagnoses 2124
Planning and Implementation 2125
Evaluation of Outcome 2127
Sexual Dysfunction 2127
Assessment with Clinical Manifestations. 2128
Diagnostic Tests. 2128
Nursing Diagnoses 2129
Planning and Implementation 2129
Evaluation of Outcomes 2131

CHAPTER 63: Breast Alterations: Nursing Management **2135**

Anatomy and Physiology of the Breast 2136
Breast Alterations during Maturational Phases 2137
Assessment and Diagnosis of Breast Problems 2138
Examination of the Breast 2138
Breast Disorders 2139
Mastodynia and Mastalgia 2140
Nipple Disorders 2140
Fibrocystic Changes. 2141
Fibroadenoma 2142
Galactorrhea 2142
Cyst 2142

Abscess 2142
Intraductal Papilloma 2142
Mastitis 2143
Periductal Mastitis 2143
Mammary Duct Ectasia 2143
Breast Tumor 2143
Paget's Mammary Disease 2143
Mammoplasty 2144
Breast Augmentation 2144
Breast Reduction 2146
Breast Cancer 2147
Epidemiology 2147
Etiology 2147
Pathophysiology 2148
Diagnostic Tests 2149
Nursing Diagnoses 2151
Planning and Implementation 2151
Evaluation of Outcomes 2159

CHAPTER 64: Male Reproductive Dysfunction: Nursing Management **2163**

Prostatitis 2164
Epidemiology 2164
Etiology 2164
Pathophysiology 2164
Assessment with Clinical Manifestations 2164
Diagnostic Tests 2164
Nursing Diagnoses 2165
Planning and Implementation 2165
Evaluation of Outcomes 2165
Benign Prostatic Hyperplasia 2166
Epidemiology 2166
Pathophysiology 2166
Assessment with Clinical Manifestations 2166
Diagnostic Tests 2166
Nursing Diagnoses 2167
Planning and Implementation 2167
Evaluation of Outcomes 2168
Prostate Cancer 2169
Epidemiology 2169
Pathophysiology 2169
Diagnostic Tests 2169

- Nursing Diagnoses 2171
- Planning and Implementation 2171
- Evaluation of Outcomes 2173

Testicular Cancer. 2173
- Epidemiology 2173
- Pathophysiology 2173
- Assessment with Clinical Manifestations. 2173
- Diagnostic Tests. 2174
- Nursing Diagnoses 2174
- Planning and Implementation 2174
- Evaluation of Outcomes 2175

Testicular Torsion 2175
- Epidemiology 2175
- Pathophysiology 2175
- Assessment with Clinical Manifestations. 2176
- Diagnostic Tests. 2176
- Nursing Diagnoses 2176
- Planning and Implementation 2176
- Evaluation of Outcomes 2176

Orchitis 2177
- Pathophysiology 2177
- Assessment with Clinical Manifestations. 2177
- Diagnostic Tests. 2177
- Nursing Diagnoses 2177
- Planning and Implementation 2178
- Evaluation of Outcomes 2178

Epididymitis 2178

Hydrocele, Hematocele, and Spermatocele 2178
- Pathophysiology 2179
- Assessment with Clinical Manifestations. 2179
- Diagnostic Tests. 2179
- Nursing Diagnoses 2179
- Planning and Implementation 2179
- Evaluation of Outcomes 2180

Varicocele 2180
- Pathophysiology 2180
- Assessment with Clinical Manifestations. 2180
- Diagnostic Tests. 2180
- Nursing Diagnoses 2180
- Planning and Implementation 2181
- Evaluation of Outcomes 2181

Vasectomy 2181
- Assessment with Clinical Manifestations. 2181
- Nursing Diagnoses 2182

Planning and Implementation 2182
Evaluation of Outcomes 2182
Cryptorchidism 2183
Pathophysiology 2183
Assessment with Clinical Manifestations. 2183
Diagnostic Tests. 2183
Nursing Diagnoses 2183
Planning and Implementation 2183
Evaluation of Outcomes 2184
Phimosis and Paraphimosis 2184
Pathophysiology 2184
Assessment with Clinical Manifestations. 2185
Diagnostic Tests. 2185
Nursing Diagnoses 2185
Planning and Implementation 2185
Evaluation of Outcomes 2185
Balanitis and Posthitis 2186
Etiology 2186
Pathophysiology 2186
Assessment with Clinical Manifestations. 2186
Diagnostic Tests. 2186
Nursing Diagnoses 2186
Planning and Implementation 2186
Evaluation of Outcomes 2187
Urethritis. 2187
Pathophysiology 2187
Assessment with Clinical Manifestations. 2187
Diagnostic Tests. 2187
Nursing Diagnoses 2187
Planning and Implementation 2188
Evaluation of Outcomes 2188
Urethral Stricture 2188
Pathophysiology 2188
Assessment with Clinical Manifestations. 2188
Diagnostic Tests. 2188
Nursing Diagnoses 2189
Planning and Implementation 2189
Evaluation of Outcomes 2189
Epispadias and Hypospadias 2189
Pathophysiology 2189
Assessment with Clinical Manifestations. 2190
Diagnostic Tests. 2190
Nursing Diagnoses 2190

Planning and Implementation 2190
Evaluation of Outcomes 2190
Peyronie's Disease 2190
Pathophysiology 2190
Assessment with Clinical Manifestations. 2191
Diagnostic Tests. 2191
Nursing Diagnoses 2191
Planning and Implementation 2191
Evaluation of Outcomes 2191
Cancer of the Penis (Bowen's Disease) 2192
Pathophysiology 2192
Assessment with Clinical Manifestations. 2192
Diagnostic Tests. 2192
Nursing Diagnoses 2192
Planning and Implementation 2193
Evaluation of Outcomes 2193
Erectile Dysfunction 2193
Etiology 2193
Pathophysiology 2193
Assessment with Clinical Manifestations. 2194
Diagnostic Tests. 2194
Nursing Diagnoses 2194
Planning and Implementation 2194
Evaluation of Outcomes 2195
Priapism 2195
Etiology 2195
Pathophysiology 2196
Assessment with Clinical Manifestations. 2196
Diagnostic Tests. 2196
Nursing Diagnoses 2196
Planning and Implementation 2196
Evaluation of Outcomes 2197

UNIT XVI: Special Considerations in Medical and Surgical Nursing 2201

CHAPTER 65: Multisystem Failure 2202

Inflammatory Immune Response. 2203
Neuroendocrine System Response. 2205
The Renal Response 2206

Shock Syndrome 2208
The Four Stages of the Shock Syndrome 2209
Planning and Implementation 2209
Hypovolemic Shock 2210
Etiology 2211
Pathophysiology 2212
Assessment with Clinical Manifestations 2213
Planning and Implementation 2214
Cardiogenic Shock 2215
Pathophysiology 2216
Assessment with Clinical Manifestations 2217
Planning and Implementation 2217
Anaphylactic Shock 2218
Pathophysiology 2218
Assessment with Clinical Manifestations 2219
Planning and Implementation 2219
Neurogenic Shock 2220
Pathophysiology 2220
Assessment with Clinical Manifestations 2221
Planning and Implementation 2221
Septic Shock 2222
Pathophysiology 2222
Assessment with Clinical Manifestations 2222
Planning and Implementation 2223
Systemic Inflammatory Response Syndrome 2224
Disseminated Intravascular Coagulation 2225
Acute Respiratory Distress Syndrome 2225
Etiology 2226
Diagnostic Tests 2226
Nursing Diagnoses 2226
Planning and Implementation 2226
Evaluation of Outcomes 2226
Multiple Organ Dysfunction Syndrome 2227
Assessment with Clinical Manifestations 2227
Primary Multiple Organ Dysfunction 2227
Assessment with Clinical Manifestations 2227
Secondary Multiple Organ Dysfunction 2228
Assessment with Clinical Manifestations 2229
Planning and Implementation 2229
Populations at Risk 2230

CHAPTER 66: Mass Casualty Care 2235

Emergency Nursing 2236
Triage 2237
START Method of Triage 2239
Military Triage 2240
Mass Casualty Incident 2240
Incident Command 2241
Hospital Emergency Incident Command System 2242
HEICS Activator 2242
Incident Command Education 2243
Hospital Operations Plan 2243
Personal Protective Equipment 2244
Hazardous Materials 2244
Decontamination 2245
Biological Warfare and Biological Agents 2246
Smallpox 2249
Plague 2251
Ebola 2252
Anthrax 2254
Severe Acute Respiratory Syndrome 2255
West Nile Virus 2257
Blast Injuries 2259
Stress Reactions 2260
Posttraumatic Stress Disorder 2261
Critical Incident Stress Management 2264

Boxed Elements Contents

CHAPTER 1 The Health Care System and Contemporary Nursing

Box 1-1: JCAHO Dimensions of Quality Performance 9
Box 1-2: JCAHO Priority Focus Areas 10
Box 1-3: Essential Criteria for a Profession 10
Box 1-4: Do You Know Where Your Plastic Ducky's Been? 12
Box 1-5: Eight Bargaining Units for Hospitals 18
Box 1-6: Clues to the Possibility of Chemical Dependence 20

CHAPTER 2 Clinical Decision Making and Evidence-Based Practice

Box 2-1: Core Competencies for Health Professions 26
Box 2-2: Underlying Premises of Knowledge Transformation . . 30
Box 2-3: Examples of Evidence Summaries from the Cochrane Library and AHRQ 36
Box 2-4: Examples of CPGS 37
Box 2-5: Examples of Knowledge from Various Sources 38
Box 2-6: Strength of Recommendations from the U.S. Preventive Services Task Force 39
Box 2-7: IOM-Priority Areas for National Action 40

CHAPTER 3 Health Education and Promotion

Box 3-1: Beliefs about Learning 45
Box 3-2: Barriers to Learning 46
Box 3-3: Priorities for Health Promotion in the 21st Century . . 57
Box 3-4: Defining Characteristics for Ineffective Health Maintenance 60
Box 3-5: Patient Outcomes for Ineffective Health Maintenance . . 61

CHAPTER 4 Culturally Sensitive Care

Box 4-1: Characteristics of Culture 70
Box 4-2: Ways in Which People Differ . . . . 7[illegible]
Box 4-3: Changes in Racial and Ethnic Demographics . . . . [illegible]
Box 4-4: Organizing Phenomena of Culture . . . . [illegible]
Box 4-5: Wellness and Prayer in Other Cultures . . . . [illegible]3
Box 4-6: Health Disparity Examples . . . . [illegible]9
Box 4-7: Cultural Assessment Factors . . . . [illegible]36
Box 4-8: Cultural Assessment Interview Guide 87

CHAPTER 5 Legal and Ethical Aspects of Health Care

Box 5-1: The ANA Code of Ethics for Nurses 99

CHAPTER 6 Nursing of Adults Across the Life Span

Box 6-1: Profile of Older Americans 133
Box 6-2: Medication Use by Older Adults 134
Box 6-3: Steps of Evidence-Based Nursing Practice 138

CHAPTER 7 Palliative Care

Box 7-1: Dying Patient's Bill of Rights 149
Box 7-2: ABCDE Guide to Pain Assessment 153
Box 7-3: Components of a Comprehensive Pain Assessment . . 153
Box 7-4: Barriers to Pain Management 160
Box 7-5: Spiritual Considerations Related to Dying 165

CHAPTER 8 Health Assessment

Box 8-1: Elements of Health History 180

CHAPTER 10 Stress, Coping, and Adaptation

Box 10-1: Common Complementary Alternative Medicine and Therapies 246
Box 10-2: Posttraumatic Stress Disorder (PTSD) 251
Box 10-3: Orem and Stress Management 258
Box 10-4: Roles of the Nurse Case Manager 259

CHAPTER 11 Inflammation and Infection Management

Box 11-1: Nightingale and Transmission of Disease 281

CHAPTER 12 Fluid, Electrolyte, and Acid-Base Imbalances

Box 12-1: Fluid Volume Deficit 303
Box 12-2: Interpretation of Arterial Blood Gases (ABGs) 334
Box 12-3: An Example of Interpreting Arterial Blood Gases (ABGs) 334

CHAPTER 13 Infusion Therapy

Box 13-1: Add-On Devices for Infusion Therapy 345
Box 13-2: Example of the Three-Step Method 354
Box 13-3: Considerations for Selection of Using a Central Line . . 358
Box 13-4: Nursing Considerations for Parenteral Nutrition . . . 360
Box 13-5: Transfusion Process 366

CHAPTER 14 Complementary and Alternative Therapies

Box 14-1: Basic Massage Techniques 388

CHAPTER 15 Cancer Management

Box 15-1: Warning Signs of Cancer 409
Box 15-2: Common Side Effects of Chemotherapy 421
Box 15-3: Absolute Neutrophil Count Infection Risk Grading System 431
Box 15-4: Nursing Plan for Altered Body Image 437

CHAPTER 16 Pain Management

Box 16-1: Pain Descriptions 458
Box 16-2: Groups of NSAID Drugs 471

CHAPTER 17 Pharmacology: Nursing Management

Box 17-1: Five Rights of Medication Administration 487
Box 17-2: Components of a Complete Drug Order 491
Box 17-3: Nursing Strategies for Administering Penicillins and Cephalosporins 495
Box 17-4: Administration of ACE Inhibitors 511

CHAPTER 18 Health Care Agencies

Box 18-1: National Nursing Home Performance Measures . . . 546

CHAPTER 19 Critical Care

Box 19-1: Intensive Care Unit Admission Criteria 562
Box 19-2: Intensive Care Unit Discharge Criteria 563
Box 19-3: Indications for Mechanical Ventilation 586

CHAPTER 20 Preoperative Nursing Management

Box 20-1: Choosing a Surgeon 617
Box 20-2: Choosing a Hospital or Surgical Center 618
Box 20-3: Observations for Hospital Selection 619
Box 20-4: Touring a Health Care Facility 620
Box 20-5: Couples at Risk: The Frail Elderly 641

CHAPTER 21 Intraoperative Nursing Management

Box 21-1: Perioperative Knowledge and Skills of the Nurse. . . . 654
Box 21-2: Tips for the Student When Observing in Operating Room 655
Box 21-3: Duties of the Scrub Nurse. 657
Box 21-4: PNDS: Examples of Intraoperative Interventions . . . 660
Box 21-5: Sterilization Methods 666
Box 21-6: Electrosurgical Safety Strategies. 676
Box 21-7: Types of Anesthesia 678
Box 21-8: Count Documentation 681
Box 21-9: Management Strategies of MH 684

CHAPTER 22 Postoperative Nursing Management

Box 22-1: Transfer Principles: Body Mechanics and Immediate Patient Comfort 708
Box 22-2: Factors Associated with Delays or Impairment in Wound Healing 711
Box 22-3: Terminology to Describe Ambulation 716
Box 22-4: Discharge Teaching Tips 720

CHAPTER 23 Assessment of Cardiovascular and Hematological Function

Box 23-1: Pain Evaluation. 754
Box 23-2: History of the Cardiovascular System. 756
Box 23-3: Rating Pulses in the Extremities. 757
Box 23-4: Steps of the Precordium Assessment 757
Box 23-5: Assessment of Heart Murmur. 761
Box 23-6: Indications for Exercise Testing 763

CHAPTER 24 Coronary Artery Dysfunction: Nursing Management

Box 24-1: Highlights of the Cardiac Surgery Rapid Recovery Program 788

CHAPTER 25 Heart Failure and Inflammatory Dysfunction: Nursing Management

Box 25-1: Symptoms of Right-Sided Heart Failure 807
Box 25-2: Heart Failure Clinical Manifestations 808
Box 25-3: NIC/NOC for Heart Muscle Dysfunction 813

CHAPTER 26 Arrhythmias: Nursing Management

Box 26-1: Preparing for Placement of Leads 840
Box 26-2: Steps to Set Up Telemetry ECG Monitoring. 840
Box 26-3: Systematic Approach to Arrhythmia Interpretation. 845
Box 26-4: Interventions for Patient with Pacemaker Insertion. . 865
Box 26-5: Maintaining Currency on BLS Certification. 870

CHAPTER 27 Vascular Dysfunction: Nursing Management

Box 27-1: Nursing Diagnoses 881
Box 27-2: Postintervention Care for Patients with Peripheral Arterial Occlusive Disease 888
Box 27-3: Assessments during the Postoperative Period 893
Box 27-4: Assessing Thrombophlebitis 896
Box 27-5: Caring for Patients with Raynaud's Disease 900

CHAPTER 28 Hypertension: Nursing Management

Box 28-1: Potential Causes of Secondary Hypertension. 908
Box 28-2: Hypertension Assessment. 914
Box 28-3: Sources of Sodium 919

CHAPTER 29 Hematological Dysfunction: Nursing Management

Box 29-1: Medications that Heighten the Hemolytic Affects of G6PD 934
Box 29-2: Stages of Coagulation 940
Box 29-3: Three Categories of Hemophilia A 944
Box 29-4: Nursing Measures for Hemophilia 945
Box 29-5: General Nursing Care for Patients with Leukemia . . 953
Box 29-6: Common Problems in Chronic Leukemia with Corresponding Interventions 958
Box 29-7: Clinical Phases of CML 960
Box 29-8: Staging Hodgkin's and NHL 965

CHAPTER 30 Assessment of Respiratory Function

Box 30-1: POLK Method of Interpreting ABGs 987
Box 30-2: Indications for Intubation 998
Box 30-3: Auscultating Lung Sounds 999

CHAPTER 31 Upper Airway Dysfunction: Nursing Management

Box 31-1: Allergy Avoidance Measures. 1021
Box 31-2: Staging System for Cancer of the Larynx-Tumor-Node-Metastasis (TNM) 1046
Box 31-3: Home Care Checklist for the Patient with a Laryngectomy 1050

CHAPTER 32 Lower Airway Dysfunction: Nursing Management

Box 32-1: High Risk Indicators for Acquiring Pneumonia . . . 1058
Box 32-2: Diagnostic Tests for Lung Cancer 1080
Box 32-3: Risk Factors for Pulmonary Arterial Hypertension . . 1089

CHAPTER 33 Obstructive Pulmonary Disease: Nursing Management

Box 33-1: Criteria for Referral for Lung Transplant 1116
Box 33-2: Sample Routine Clinical Assessment Questions . . . 1121
Box 33-3: Nutrition in CF 1130

CHAPTER 34 Assessment of Neurological Function

Box 34-1: Neurological Assessment Questions 1150

CHAPTER 35 Dysfunction of the Brain: Nursing Management

Box 35-1: Modifiable Risk Factors for Stroke Development . . 1173
Box 35-2: Nonmodifiable Risk Factors for Stroke Development 1174
Box 35-3: Clinical Manifestations of Brain Injury 1187

CHAPTER 36 Dysfunction of the Spinal Cord and Peripheral Nervous System: Nursing Management

Box 36-1: Stimuli that Trigger Autonomic Responses. 1231

CHAPTER 37 Degenerative Neurological Dysfunction: Nursing Management

Box 37-1: Headache Diagnostic Studies 1263
Box 37-2: Nursing Diagnoses for Headaches 1264
Box 37-3: Seizure Diagnostic Studies 1270
Box 37-4: Questions Specific for Seizure Assessment 1271
Box 37-5: Medications Administered to Manage Huntington's Disease 1296

CHAPTER 38 Assessment of Sensory Function

Box 38-1: History of the Eye 1304
Box 38-2: Eye Disorders 1304
Box 38-3: History of the Ear 1314

CHAPTER 39 Visual Dysfunction: Nursing Management

Box 39-1: Nursing Diagnoses for Eye Disorders 1326
Box 39-2: Evaluation of Outcomes for Patients with Eye Disorders 1327
Box 39-3: Causes of Blindness 1344

CHAPTER 40 Auditory Dysfunction: Nursing Management

Box 40-1: Assessing a Patient with a Hearing Deficit 1362
Box 40-2: Common Sounds and Associated Decibels Levels. . . 1369
Box 40-3: Types of Hearing Aids 1373

CHAPTER 41 Assessment of Immunological Function

Box 41-1: Common Physical Signs Associated with Impaired Immune Function 1408
Box 41-2: CBC with Differential 1411
Box 41-3: Etiology for Various Infections that Cause Neutropenia 1412
Box 41-4: Diseases Associated with Antinuclear Antibodies (ANA) 1416

CHAPTER 42 Immunodeficiency and HIV Infection/AIDS: Nursing Management

Box 42-1: Classification of Immunological Disorders 1423
Box 42-2: Diagnostic Studies Related to Immunological Response 1427
Box 42-3: Antiretroviral Drug Classifications 1430
Box 42-4: The American College of Rheumatology Criteria for Diagnosis of RA 1437

CHAPTER 43 Allergic Dysfunction: Nursing Management

Box 43-1: Examples of Type 1 Allergic Reactions 1453
Box 43-2: Diseases Manifesting Type 2 Hypersensitivity 1453
Box 43-3: Examples of Human Immune Complex Diseases... 1454
Box 43-4: Assessment of Allergic Disorders 1455
Box 43-5: Pharmacological Management for Symptom Relief... 1460
Box 43-6: Modifiable Risk Factors for Anaphylaxis......... 1461
Box 43-7: Deaths from Anaphylactic Shock 1462

CHAPTER 44 Assessment of Integumentary Function

Box 44-1: Primary Lesions 1487
Box 44-2: Description and Configuration of Selected Group of Lesions 1491

CHAPTER 46 Burns: Nursing Management

Box 46-1: Prehospital Care of Major Burns 1534
Box 46-2: Burn Center Referral Criteria 1536
Box 46-3: Indications for Fluid Resuscitation............. 1543
Box 46-4: Healthy People 2010 1545

CHAPTER 48 Nutrition, Malnutrition, and Obesity: Nursing Management

Box 48-1: Foods High in Vitamin K.................... 1602
Box 48-2: Calculation of BMI 1612
Box 48-3: BMI Categories 1612
Box 48-4: Postbariatric Surgery Diet Progression.......... 1614

CHAPTER 49 Upper Gastrointestinal Tract Dysfunction: Nursing Management

Box 49-1: Dysphagia................................ 1623
Box 49-2: Normal Swallowing......................... 1623
Box 49-3: Assessment of a Patient Who Is Experiencing Difficulty Swallowing............................ 1624
Box 49-4: Techniques of Swallowing Therapy 1626
Box 49-5: Types of Gastric Ulcers 1638
Box 49-6: Nursing Diagnoses for Gastritis, Duodenitis, and Associated Ulcerative Lesions 1641
Box 49-7: Examples of Combination Chemotherapy Used in Treating Stomach Cancer 1644

CHAPTER 50 Lower Gastrointestinal Tract Dysfunction: Nursing Management

Box 50-1: Epidemiology of Lactase Deficiency 1650
Box 50-2: Routine Lab Tests for Mal-Assimilation Disorders . . 1653
Box 50-3: Rovsing's Sign for Appendicitis 1665
Box 50-4: Colorectal Cancer (CRC) 1676

CHAPTER 51 Hepatic, Biliary Tract, and Pancreatic Dysfunction: Nursing Management

Box 51-1: Bilirubin Labels 1698
Box 51-2: Disorders Identified with a Liver Biopsy 1700
Box 51-3: Phases of Hepatitis 1701
Box 51-4: Pathology of Alcoholic Hepatitis 1709
Box 51-5: Dietary Recommendations for People with Wilson's Disease 1711
Box 51-6: Quantity of Alcohol Consumption 1713
Box 51-7: Clinical Manifestations of Liver Disease 1714
Box 51-8: Cadaveric and Live Donor Methods of Procurement 1726
Box 51-9: Conditions to Prioritize Organ Recipients 1726
Box 51-10: Disqualification of a Transplant Recipient 1727

CHAPTER 52 Assessment of Renal Function

Box 52-1: Functions of the Kidney 1749
Box 52-2: Assessment of Urination Patterns: Questions To Ask . 1754
Box 52-3: Potentially Nephrotoxic Drugs and Other Agents . . 1755
Box 52-4: Differentiating Kidney Palpation 1756
Box 52-5: Bladder Abnormalities 1756
Box 52-6: Patient Education For a Renal Ultrasound 1760
Box 52-7: Nursing Care of Patients Having a Renal Biopsy . . 1762

CHAPTER 53 Urinary Dysfunction: Nursing Management

Box 53-1: Summary of Diagnostic Tests for UTI 1770
Box 53-2: Common Medications Used with Patients with UTI . 1772
Box 53-3: Differential Diagnosis of Urinary Frequency, Urgency, or Pain 1775
Box 53-4: Common Medications Used with Patients with IC . . 1776
Box 53-5: Primary Causes of Nephrosis 1785
Box 53-6: Possible Complications of Renal Trauma 1793
Box 53-7: Causes for Renal Cancer 1796
Box 53-8: Diagnostic Tests for Urinary Retention 1805
Box 53-9: Types of Incontinence 1807

CHAPTER 54 Renal Dysfunction: Nursing Management

Box 54-1: Antibiotic Therapy for Infected Cysts in Patients with Polycystic Kidney Disease . . . 1819
Box 54-2: Continuous Renal Replacement Therapy (CRRT) . . 1827
Box 54-3: Management of Hyperkalemia. . . . 1830
Box 54-4: Three Categories of Factors Affecting Progression of CRF . . . 1833
Box 54-5: NIC Care and CRF . . . 1836
Box 54-6: Pharmacological Therapy in CRF . . . 1836
Box 54-7: Management of Vascular Access Devices in Dialysis . . . 1838
Box 54-8: Antibiotic Therapy for PD. . . . 1839
Box 54-9: Live Donor Exclusion Criteria . . . 1841
Box 54-10: Nursing Management for a Renal Transplant . . . 1842

CHAPTER 56 Endocrine Dysfunction: Nursing Management

Box 56-1: Prolactin Levels. . . . 1865
Box 56-2: Advances in Diagnosing Pituitary Secreting Tumor . . 1870
Box 56-3: Caring for the Patient Receiving High-Dose Radioactive Iodine Therapy . . . 1892

CHAPTER 57 Diabetes Mellitus: Nursing Management

Box 57-1: Four Types of Diabetes Mellitus . . . 1904
Box 57-2: Assessment of Patients with Diabetes . . . 1907
Box 57-3: Diagnostic Criteria for Diabetes . . . 1908
Box 57-4: Nutritional Therapy for Patients with Diabetes . . . 1910

CHAPTER 58 Assessment of Musculoskeletal Function

Box 58-1: Orthopaedic Assessment Guidelines . . . 1941
Box 58-2: Health History: Chronic Conditions . . . 1942

CHAPTER 59 Musculoskeletal Dysfunction: Nursing Management

Box 59-1: Care of the Patient with a Total Joint Arthroplasty (Preoperative). . . . 1961
Box 59-2: In Hospital Postoperative Recovery . . . 1962
Box 59-3: After Discharge from the Hospital . . . 1963
Box 59-4: Diagnostic Testing for Osteomyelitis. . . . 1993

CHAPTER 60 Musculoskeletal Trauma: Nursing Management

Box 60-1: Factors Associated with Overuse Syndrome 2010
Box 60-2: Occupations and Sports with High Incidence of Overuse Syndrome 2010
Box 60-3: Risk Factors for Stress Fractures 2030
Box 60-4: Prevention of Stress Fractures 2031
Box 60-5: Causes of Pathological Fractures 2031
Box 60-6: Advantages of External Fixation 2035
Box 60-7: Causes of Acute Compartment Syndrome 2039
Box 60-8: Gurd's Criteria for Diagnosis of FES 2041
Box 60-9: Risk Factors for Developing a DVT 2042
Box 60-10: Guidelines for Positioning a Stump 2048

CHAPTER 61 Assessment of Reproductive Function

Box 61-1: Short Form of Sexual History 2072
Box 61-2: A Short Abuse Assessment Screen 2073

CHAPTER 62 Female Reproductive Dysfunction: Nursing Management

Box 62-1: Criteria for Inpatient Treatment of PID 2105
Box 62-2: Indications for Surgical Management of Fibroids 2115
Box 62-3: Empathy for Others 2118

CHAPTER 65 Multisystem Failure

Box 65-1: Cardinal Signs of the Inflammatory Response 2203
Box 65-2: Characterizations of Chronic Inflammation 2204
Box 65-3: Sequence of Events Involving Anaerobic Metabolism and Metabolic Acidosis 2205
Box 65-4: Cascade of Physiological Events Following an Insult to the Body 2207
Box 65-5: Assessment and Diagnosis of Shock 2211
Box 65-6: Management of Septic Shock 2212
Box 65-7: Assessment and Care of Shock Syndrome 2213
Box 65-8: Selected Manifestations of Hypovolemic Shock . . . 2215
Box 65-9: Management of Hypovolemic Shock 2215
Box 65-10: Selected Manifestations of Cardiogenic Shock . . . 2217
Box 65-11: Nursing Interventions for a Patient in Cardiogenic Shock 2218
Box 65-12: Clinical Manifestations of Anaphylactic Shock . . . 2219

Box 65-13: Pharmacological Shock 2221
Box 65-14: Clinical Manifestations of SIRS 2225
Box 65-15: Clinical Manifestations in Secondary Multiple Organ Dysfunction 2229

CHAPTER 66 Mass Casualty Care

Box 66-1: Katrina Disaster 2241
Box 66-2: Hospital Operation Plan Criteria 2244
Box 66-3: Components of Hospital Hazmat Emergency Response Plan. 2245
Box 66-4: OSHA PPE Levels. 2246
Box 66-5: Potential Biological Warfare Clinical Presentations 2247
Box 66-6: Important Facts Regarding Smallpox Vaccination 2251
Box 66-7: Infection Control Precautions for Potential SARS Patients. 2257
Box 66-8: Signs and Symptoms of PTSD 2261
Box 66-9: The Eight Phases of a Debriefing 2264
Box 66-10: Managing Your Stress during a Disaster 2265

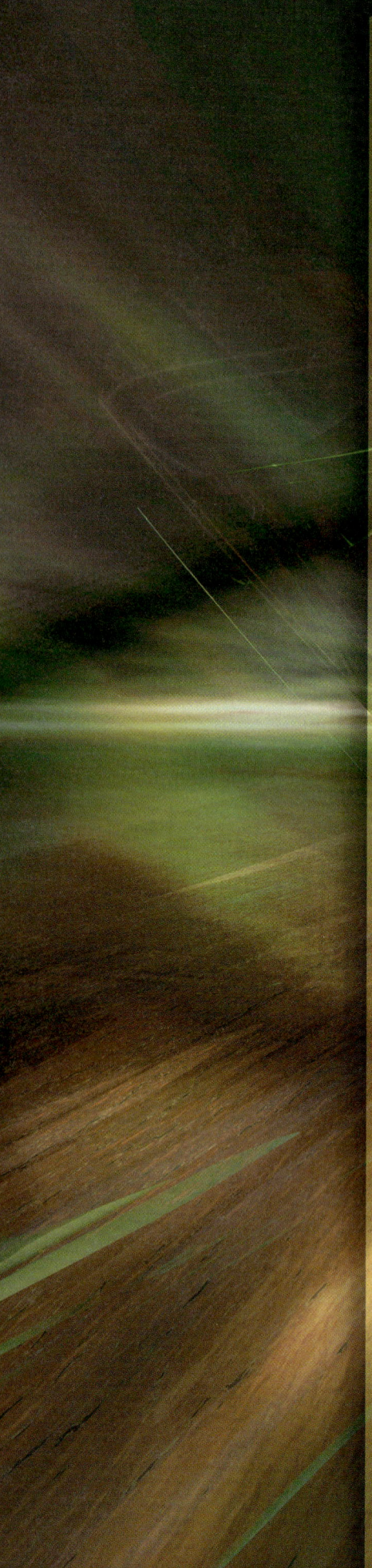

Preface

Contemporary Medical-Surgical Nursing is an exciting new comprehensive text created for nursing students to address the adult health and illness topics that support the most current nursing practice. It provides a reader-oriented, logically organized source of information focused on the knowledge and skill required to become a caring and responsible practitioner.

As the century continues to unfold, the health care delivery system will increase in complexity. Staying abreast of both technological and biotechnological advancements will be challenging, but just as challenging will be ongoing changes in patient situations and in the health care system to which nurses as leaders in care management and system management must adapt. New family structures, increasing prevalence of the diseases of aging and chronic illness, and globalization will refocus the major care requirements of society. Acute care will continue to move from hospitals to community settings, including the home and alternative sites unrelated to health care. Nurses will continue to pioneer new vital roles, and critical shortages of nurse providers across all arenas will challenge the profession toward innovative practice. Nurses must embrace such challenges and prepare students to excel in providing the quality care that is required by a changing society. Our goal in creating this book was to continue Thomson Delmar Learning's commitment to help bridge the gap from nursing student to practitioner. To assist students in making this transition, we provide real-world applications, such as case studies and unique features like Dollars and Sense and Ethics or Law in Practice. In addition, we are proud to feature innovative teaching methods, such as our IV therapy animations and StudyWARE™ games, as well as PDA downloads available on our online companion. And all of this is delivered through a caring approach to the content—a central theme to fostering quality nursing care for generations to come.

CONCEPTUAL APPROACH

The concept for *Contemporary Medical-Surgical Nursing* arose from a need that the authors identified after years of instruction to nursing students, a need for a thorough, organized, and practical approach to its delivery. There is a balance created that presents pedagogical information specifically designed for the nursing student. And there are learning approaches within the text and its additional resources for the various learning styles that are unique to each student. The most current information obtained from a wide variety of sources is the underpinning for this medical-surgical textbook. In addition, there are wide varieties of important features, such as evidence from current research studies, information regarding the ethicolegal practice of nursing, and nursing education approaches that enhance the critical thinking skills of the reader.

The patient is the focus of the textbook, with an in-depth presentation of the many acute care topics that are central to the practice of nursing. There are concept maps and case study presentations throughout the book. In addition, there are review activities and review questions at the end of each chapter styled like NCLEX® questions, which provide the reader with excellent methods of mastering the content. There is a full-color visually appealing design, tables and boxes that emphasize essential points, and additional tutorial references that engage the reader in a user-friendly approach. The information and learning processes in conjunction with the active reader's critical thinking skills foster the development of a caring, ethical, and responsible practicing professional nurse.

ORGANIZATION OF THE TEXT

Contemporary Medical-Surgical Nursing consists of 66 chapters organized into 16 units. A composite of topics provides a comprehensive approach to acute care nursing within these units of study. A unique nursing perspective is threaded through each chapter of study, and the outcome of evidence-based knowledge and evidence-based practice is encouraged. As noticed in most units, the first chapter is an assessment chapter that presents the information necessary for the nurse to begin care for patients in acute care nursing. The chapters that follow in each unit have the phrase nursing management in their titles, which depicts the focus on the relationship of nursing interventions or strategies for most of the topics presented in the 16 units of study.

Unit I: Nursing and the Health Care System, Chapters 1 through 7

These seven chapters introduce the student to the foundational topics of acute care nursing. Chapter 1 is an overview of the health care delivery system. Chapter 2 emphasizes clinical decision making and the value of evidence-based nursing practice. Chapter 3 presents information on health education and promotion. Chapter 4 describes the implications of both the cultural and ethnic backgrounds of patients. Chapter 5 presents the invaluable legal and ethical issues relevant to nursing practice. Chapters 6 and 7 focus on caring for adults across the life span as well as palliative care.

Unit II: Supportive Patient Care, Chapters 8 through 17

The first chapters begin with a review of health assessment (chapter 8), genetics (chapter 9), and stress/coping (chapter 10). In addition, the next seven chapters provide information that is primarily foundational for acute patient care, with such topics as inflammation/infection (chapter 11), fluid/electrolytes (chapter 12), infusion therapy (chapter 13), complementary and alternative care (chapter 14), cancer and pain management (chapters 15 and 16), and pharmacology (chapter 17).

Unit III: Settings for Nursing Care, Chapters 18 and 19

These two chapters present information on two primary settings for acute care nursing. Chapter 18 focuses on health care agencies, and chapter 19 covers critical care nursing.

Unit IV: Perioperative Patient Care, Chapters 20 through 22

The perioperative arena of nursing is essential to acute care nursing. These three chapters present information relative to the three phases of perioperative nursing: preoperative (chapter 20), intraoperative (chapter 21), and postoperative (chapter 22).

Unit V: Alterations in Cardiovascular and Hematological Function, Chapters 23 through 29

These seven chapters present information that involves the cardiovascular and hematological systems. It begins with assessment of the systems (chapter 23) and then presents information on coronary artery dysfunction (chapter 24), heart failure (chapter 25), arrhythmias (chapter 26), vascular dysfunction (chapter 27), and hypertension (chapter 28). Chapter 29 presents information on the hematological system and its acute care topics.

Unit VI: Alterations in Respiratory Function, Chapters 30 through 33

These four chapters explain various topics pertinent to the respiratory system beginning with an assessment of respiratory function in chapter 30. Chapter 31 examines upper airway disturbances, chapter 32 covers lower airway disorders, and chapter 33 describes obstructive pulmonary diseases.

Unit VII: Alterations in Neurological Function, Chapters 34 through 37

These four chapters discuss the neurological system as related to acute care nursing. Chapter 34 describes the assessment of the neurological system. Chapter 35 presents the brain, chapter 36 discusses the spinal cord and peripheral nervous system disorders, and chapter 37 identifies the various neurological degenerative disorders.

Unit VIII: Alterations in Sensory Function, Chapters 38 through 40

These three chapters discuss the important elements organs of sensory function beginning with an assessment of these systems in chapter 38. Chapters 39 and 40 provide information on visual and auditory dysfunctions.

Unit IX: Alterations in Immunological Function, Chapters 41 through 43

These three chapters describe the acute care disorders of the immune system. The unit begins with an assessment of the immune system (chapter 41). Chapter 42 discusses immunodeficient disorders and human immunodeficiency virus (HIV), and chapter 43 presents information on allergic dysfunctions.

Unit X: Alterations in Integumentary Function, Chapters 44 through 46

These three chapters explain disorders of the integumentary system. Chapter 44 presents important information regarding the assessment of the integumentary system. Chapter 45 adds the important nursing implications of dermatological issues, and chapter 46 details an in-depth discussion of patients with burns.

Unit XI: Alterations in Gastrointestinal Function, Chapters 47 through 51

This unit presents a thorough examination of the GI system and begins with assessment strategies in chapter 47. Chapter 48 describes the essentials of nutrition and the disorders of malnutrition and obesity. Chapters 49 and 50 present the variety of upper and lower GI disorders. Chapter 51 concludes the unit with a discussion of the hepatic system, biliary tract, and pancreatic disorders.

Unit XII: Alterations in Renal Function, Chapters 52 through 54

These three chapters discuss the critical diseases of the renal system. Chapter 52 presents the assessment of the renal system. Chapter 53 explores the urinary system disorders, and chapter 54 discusses those affecting dysfunctions of the renal system.

Unit XIII: Alterations in Endocrine Function, Chapters 55 through 57

This unit describes the dysfunctions of the endocrine system; chapter 55 includes in-depth assessment information. Chapter 56 presents the variety of diseases of the endocrine system, along with the nursing strategies. Chapter 57 identifies the specific disorders under the category of diabetes mellitus and the varied implications for patients with this disorder.

Unit XIV: Alterations in Musculoskeletal Function, Chapters 58 through 60

These three chapters address the disorders of the musculoskeletal system. Chapter 58 identifies the assessment of the MS system. Chapter 59 examines MS dysfunctions, and chapter 60 presents MS trauma as it relates to patients and their conditions.

Unit XV: Alterations in Reproductive Function, Chapters 61 through 64

This unit discusses the disorders of the reproductive system, beginning with detailed assessment of the reproductive system in chapter 61. Chapter 62 presents disorders of the female. Chapter 63 presents information on breast alterations, and chapter 64 discusses disorders of the male.

Unit XVI: Special Considerations in Medical and Surgical Nursing, Chapters 65 and 66

These chapters explore complex arenas of multisystem failure (chapter 65) and mass casualty care (chapter 66).

PEDAGOGICAL FEATURES

Enlightening features in *Contemporary Medical-Surgical Nursing* stimulate critical thinking and self-reflection and assist the reader in synthesizing and applying the information provided in the text. These complements to the text information create a supportive learning environment as the student transitions to a practicing professional.

Learning Objectives

Learning objectives are located on the online companion by chapter and provide the primary specific learning goals for the reader. They offer a means of measuring the outcomes of learning the cognitive information contained in each chapter.

Chapter Topics

Chapter topics are placed at the beginning of the chapter to highlight the main points of the text. They help provide direction for study and logically organize the content.

Key Terms

Key terms are bold in the chapters to denote those terms that are of particular importance to the reader. In addition, these terms are defined in the glossary for further reference.

Key Concepts

Key concepts highlight the primary points within the chapter and direct the reader in reviewing pertinent information.

Appendices

Several appendices augment medical-surgical topics. They include the most current NANDA nursing diagnoses, abbreviations and symbols, reference laboratory values, English/Spanish words and phrases, standard precautions, concept mapping, and the detailed glossary.

References

References document a current and varied theoretical basis for the content of the text on a chapter-by-chapter basis and are organized at the back of the text.

Review Questions and Activities

Review questions and answers are located at the end of each chapter and offer readers an opportunity to evaluate their understanding of specific chapter content. There are stimulating questions that are thought provoking and challenging to help develop critical thinking skills.

The Index

The index facilitates access to material and includes special entries for tables and illustrations.

SPECIAL FEATURES

Fast Forward

These provide detailed and informative predictions of new things to come in nursing and health care.

Dollars and Sense

These explore the cost and benefits of a particular nursing intervention. They include relevant statistics, possible solutions, and recommendations.

Real World, Real Choice

These allow for a management strategy scenario discussion that involves a real-life nursing dilemma. The solution and rationale can be found on the accompanying online companion.

Uncovering the Evidence

These present a synopsis of research studies for each chapter, which emphasize evidence-based practice for the concepts fundamental to basic nursing practice. These referred journal sources support the reader in developing a knowledgeable foundation of learning.

Ethics or Law in Practice

These present real-life cases involving legal implications or ethical issues related to chapter content.

Respecting Our Differences

These highlight nursing implications of given cultural backgrounds (e.g., ethnicity, age, race, or gender) in the format of a brief narrative that informs the reader of life span issues and outcome of care.

Red Flag

These provide a concise indication of cautionary information for the nurse, including emergency management of life-threatening and serious situations.

Patient Playbook

These allow concise, relevant teaching interventions for patient, family, or support persons necessary to enhance the individual's health.

Skills 360°

These discuss professionalism, communication, and relevant nursing strategies that are pertinent to the variety of acute care disorders.

Safety First

These identify categories of potential error and outline the problem along with the strategies for nursing management.

Case Studies

These are highlighted in at least one chapter per unit at the end of the chapter and appear in one of two formats: *nursing care plans* and *concept maps*. Both formats include patient examples where pertinent history, physical assessment data, and laboratory findings emphasize the nursing role in the clinical setting. Both engage the reader by humanizing the material and helping readers continue to develop critical thinking skills. In addition, the *case study concept map* challenges the learner to create a concept map at the end of the presented case.

EXTENSIVE TEACHING AND LEARNING PACKAGE

The complete ancillary package was created to achieve two goals:

1. To assist students in learning the skills and information essential to bridging the gap to professional practice.
2. To assist instructors in planning and implementing their programs for the most efficient use of time and other resources.

Clinical Companion (ISBN 1-4018-3721-2)

The *Clinical Companion to Accompany Contemporary Medical-Surgical Nursing* is a practical and convenient manual presented in a concise and alphabetical format for quick clinical reference. Designed for portability, this resource provides nurses fast answers to the questions:

- What is the condition?
- What should I look for?
- What should I do?

Approximately 200 common diseases, disorders, acute care procedures, and treatments are covered in an easy-to-follow format.

Study Guide (ISBN 1-4018-3723-9)

Containing over 1,100 questions, the study guide is an essential tool that reinforces the content presented in *Contemporary Medical-Surgical Nursing*. The variety of questions (multiple response, multiple choice, and fill in the blank) are similar to those found on the NCLEX-RN® and will help the learner build on key concepts presented in the text on a chapter-by-chapter basis.

Electronic Classroom Manager (ISBN 1-4018-3724-7)

Instructor's Guide

Based on each chapter's learning objectives, each chapter in the *Instructor's Guide* contains a variety of instructional strategies, Internet research, discussion questions, homework assignments, and classroom activities.

Computerized Test Bank

This computerized test bank holds over 1,000 questions geared to the text content and follows the NCLEX format. Each answer is accompanied by a rationale explaining right and wrong choices.

PowerPoint Presentations

Almost 1,000 slides are available and designed to support and facilitate lecture and classroom instructions.

Image Library

The image library includes more than 500 files containing images and tables from the text.

Link to Online Companion

An online version of the *Instructor's Guide* is included, as is a wealth of additional information for instructors and students designed to complement core concepts presented in the text. Instructors will also find conversion guides available.

Online Companion

A&P Animations

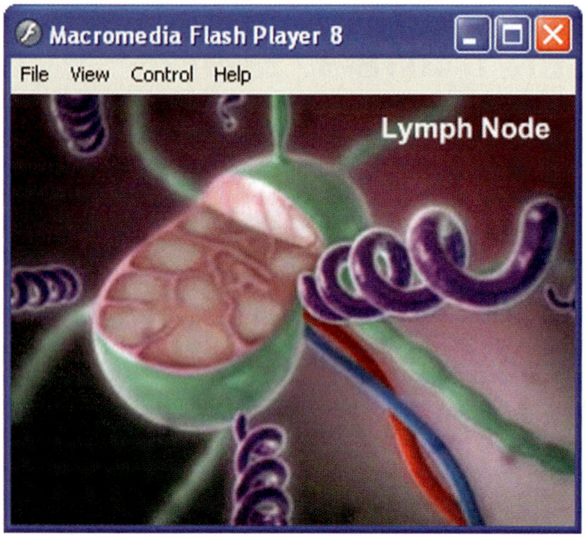

These visually demonstrate detailed anatomy and physiology concepts in an animated environment.

StudyWARE™

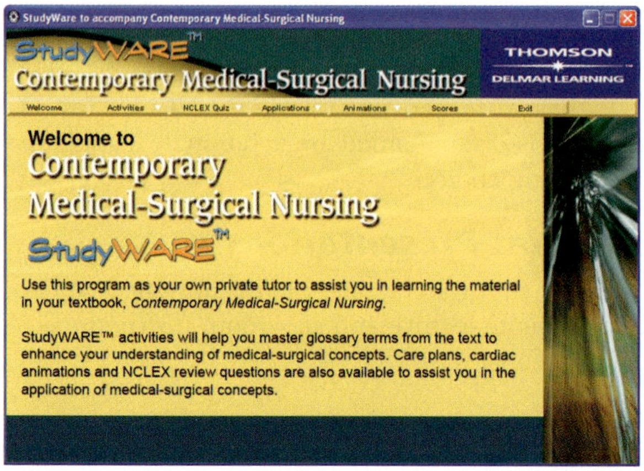

This provides activities and games to enhance the learner's understanding of medical-surgical concepts.

PDA downloads

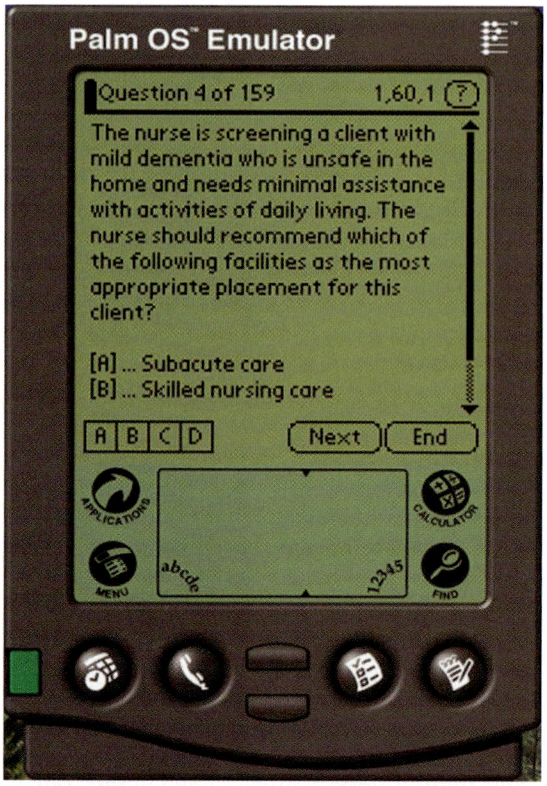

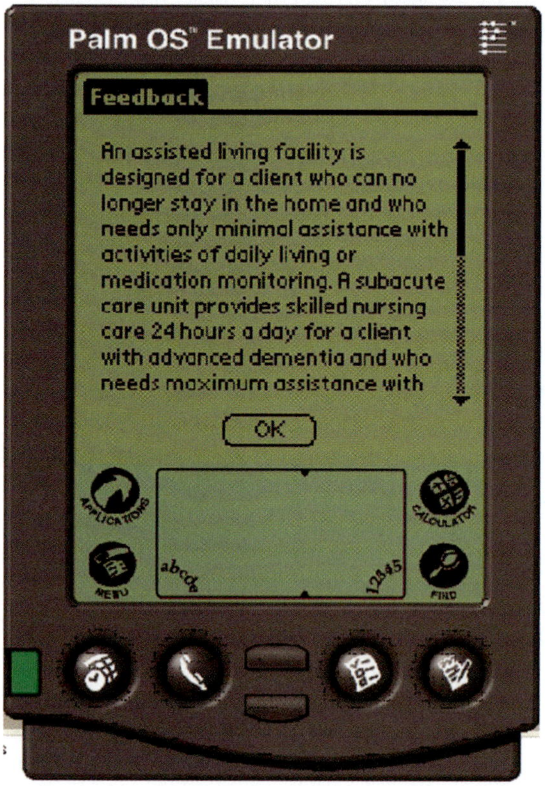

Free PDA downloads of up to 225 review questions in NCLEX style that include rationales as well as test and learning modes.

Additional Reading and Related Web Sites with Hotlinks

These provide a source of additional research on related topics organized in a chapter-by-chapter format.

Instructor's Guide

This is an online version of the *Instructor's Guide* and provides the same variety of instructional strategies, Internet research, discussion questions, homework assignments, and classroom activities.

WebTutor Advantage

Video Clips

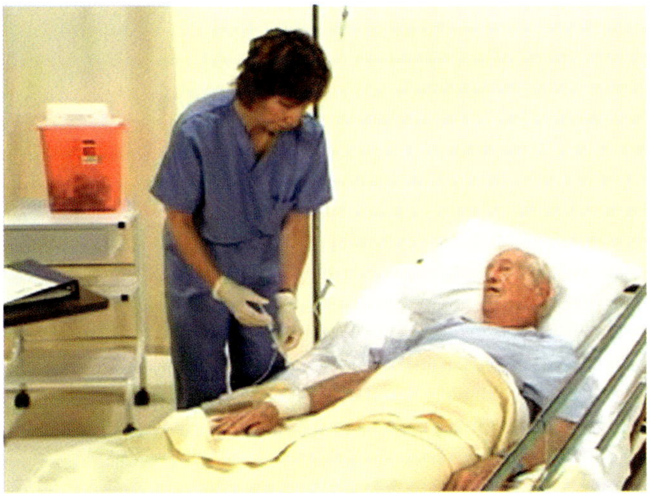

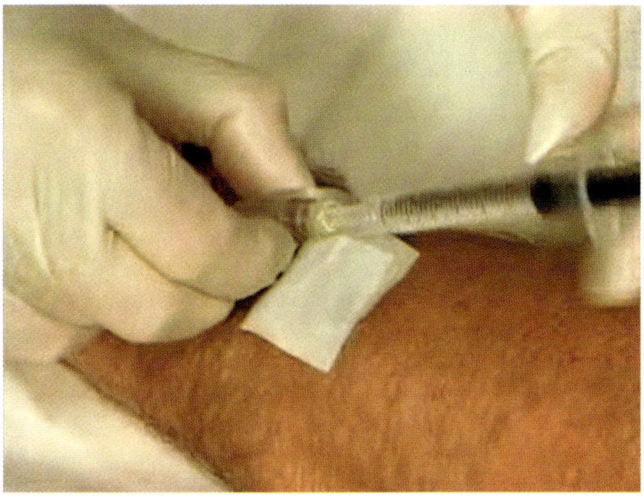

Skills-based video clips that include care of medical-surgical patients, medications administration, and IV therapy skills.

Medical-Surgical Case Studies

Using a body systems approach, this content allows additional opportunities to enhance critical thinking skills while working with medical-surgical patients and conditions.

IV Therapy Animations

Use these two- and three-dimensional animations to watch or participate in a series of specific IV therapy skills. A "Read it," "See it," and "Do it" organization offers a hands-on approach to these important skills and concepts.

Contributors and Reviewers

CONTRIBUTORS

Lisa Anderson-Shaw, DrPH, MA, MSN
Director, Clinical Ethics Consult Service
Assistant Clinical Professor
University of Illinois Medical Center
University of Illinois College of Nursing
Chicago, Illinois
Chapter 5: Legal and Ethical Aspects of Health Care

Crisamar J. Anunciado, MSN, FNP, RN
Senior Specialist
Intermediate Care Unit
Sharp HealthCare
San Diego, California
Chapter 38: Assessment of Sensory Function

Elizabeth D. Archer, MS, DSN, PhD, APRN, BC, CS, ANP, CRRN, CNRN
Clinical Nurse Specialist
Neuro/Ortho Nursing
Northwestern Memorial Hospital
Chicago, Illinois
Chapter 30: Assessment of Respiratory Function

Constance J. Ayers, PhD, RN
Associate Professor
College of Nursing
Texas Woman's University
Houston, Texas
Chapter 36: Dysfunction of the Spinal Cord and Peripheral Nervous System: Nursing Management

Kristi Bennett, RN, ANP, MS
Cardiac Specialist NP
Sharp Memorial Hospital
Escondido, California
Chapter 24: Coronary Artery Dysfunction: Nursing Management

Joyce Campbell, RN, MSN, CCRN, FNP-C
Division of Nursing
Chattanooga State
Chattanooga, Tennessee
Chapter 56: Endocrine Dysfunction: Nursing Management

Martha K. Carlson, MSN
Family Nurse Practitioner
Professor of Nursing
Parkland College
Champaign, Illinois
Chapter 55: Assessment of Endocrine Function
Chapter 57: Diabetes Mellitus: Nursing Management

Sandra K. Cesario, RNC, MS, PhD
Doctoral Program Coordinator
College of Nursing
Texas Woman's University
Houston, Texas
Chapter 9: Genetics and the Multiple Determinants of Health

Paul Chamberland, MSN, APRN, BC, CMSRN
Nurse Consultant
Scarborough, Maine
Chapter 53: Urinary Dysfunction: Nursing Management

Therese M. Clinch, RN, MSN
Academic Coordinator
St. David's Medical Center
Austin, Texas
Chapter 13: Infusion Therapy

Tammy Coffee, MSN, RN, ACNP
MetroHealth Medical Center
Comprehensive Burn Care Center
Cleveland, Ohio
Chapter 46: Burns: Nursing Management

Cecily Cosby PhD, FNP/PA-C
Associate Professor
FNP Program Director
Samuel Merritt College
Oakland, California

Marianne Curia, MSN, RN
Assistant Professor
Staff Nurse
University of St. Francis
University of Chicago
Chicago, Illinois

Connie Frisch, RNMA
Instructor
Department of Nursing
Central Lakes College
Brainerd, Minnesota

Karen K. Gerbasich, RN, MSN
Assistant Professor
Ivy Tech Community College
South Bend, Indiana

Stephanie Johnson, MSN, RN, BC
Assistant Professor
School of Nursing
Morehead State University
Morehead, Kentucky

Mary F. King, RN, MS
Phillips Community College
University of Arkansas
Helena, Arkansas

Anita G. Kinser, EdD, RN, BC
Associate Professor
Nursing Education Resource Specialist
Riverside Community College
Riverside, California

Pam Kohlbry, RN, PhDc
Course Coordinator
College of Nursing
San Diego State University
San Diego, California

Darlene Lacy, PhD, RN, BC
Assistant Professor
School of Nursing
Texas Tech Health Sciences Center
Lubbock, Texas

Miki Magnino-Rabig, PhD, RN
Assistant Professor
University of St. Francis
Joliet, Illinois

Patsy L. Maloney, RN, BC, EdD, MSN, MA, CNAA
Associate Professor
Director
Professional Development and Continuing Studies
Pacific Lutheran University
Tacoma, Washington

Amy Moore, RN, MSN, FNP-C
Instructor
School of Nursing
Texas Tech University
Lubbock, Texas

Jill R. Reed, MSN, APRN
Instructor
College of Nursing
Kearney Division
University of Nebraska Medical Center
Kearney, Nebraska

Amanda Reynolds, MSN, RN
Associate Professor
School of Nursing
Grambling State University
Grambling, Louisiana

Diane Reynolds, RN, MS, OCN, CNE
Assistant Professor of Nursing
Long Island University
Brooklyn, New York

Nancy Jo Ross, RN, BSN, MSN
Instructor
School of Nursing
Central Maine Medical Center
Lewiston, Maine

Bonnie Ruiz, RN, MSN, FNP-C
Instructor
School of Nursing
Health Sciences Center
Texas Tech University
Lubbock, Texas

Jacalyn M. Schaefer, MSN, RN, CNOR
Clinical Associate
College of Nursing
James Cancer Hospital and Solove Research Institute
The Ohio State University
Columbus, Ohio

Linda Schaffer, RN, MN
Chief Nursing Officer
Corporate Director
Health Science Education Programs
U.S. Education Corporation
Mission Viejo, California

Barbara Scheirer, RN, MSN
Assistant Professor
School of Nursing
Grambling State University
Grambling, Louisiana

Krista Susan Sifford, MSN, RN
Assistant Professor
College of Nursing
Arkansas State University
State University, Arkansas

Annette Smith Stacy, MSN, RN, AOCN
Associate Professor of Nursing
BSN Program Director
Arkansas State University
Jonesboro, Arkansas

Kristy Tabor, RN, MSN, AOCN
Clinical Faculty
The Ohio State University
Columbus, Ohio

Annie Thomas, RN, MSN, PhD
Assistant Professor
School of Nursing
Texas Tech University Health Sciences Center
Lubbock, Texas

Elayne Trepel, RN, MSN
Instructor
College of Nursing
University of Illinois at Chicago
Chicago, Illinois

Mary Wcisel, RN, MSN
Assistant Professor
Saint Mary's College
Notre Dame, Indiana

Paige Wimberley, MSN, RN, CS, CNE
Assistant Professor of Nursing
Arkansas State University
State University, Arkansas

Faye G. Zeigler, RN, BSN, MSN
Associate Professor
School of Nursing
Austin Peay State University
Clarksville, Tennessee

Acknowledgments

I would first like to express my appreciation to my two coauthors, Leslie Nicoll and Laura Nosek, for their tenacity and expertise in supervising contributors for this project. Each of these authors has maintained a high level of professionalism as they has pursued the completion of this first edition of this medical-surgical nursing text.

We would also like to thank all of the contributors of this comprehensive book for their time and effort in sharing their knowledge gained through the years. We also thank the reviewers for their time spent in critically reviewing the manuscripts and providing valuable comments that have been added to this text.

We would like to acknowledge and thank the members of the team at Thomson Delmar Learning who have worked with us in making this text a reality. Tamera Caruso, acquisitions editor, and Patty Gaworecki, product manager, are incredible people who have brought their knowledge and professional guidance to assist us with this project.

We particularly want to acknowledge our families for their supportive attitudes and actions as we have undertaken this project. They have encouraged us at each step of the way and enveloped us with their positive thoughts and words. For this we are thankful.

About the Authors

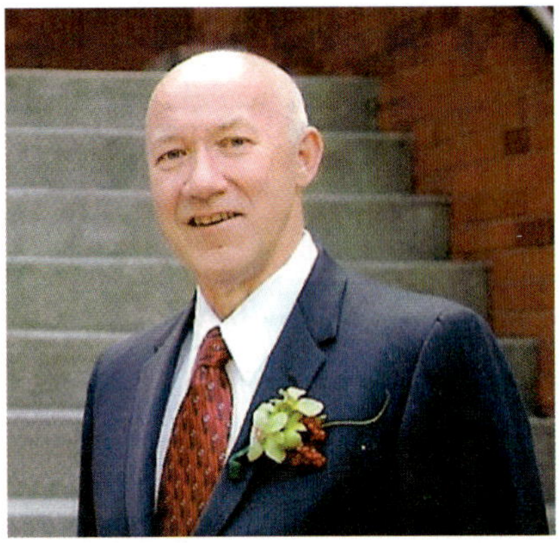

DR. RICK DANIELS

Dr. Rick Daniels obtained a Bachelor of Science in Nursing from the University of Oregon Nursing School, Portland, Oregon; a master of science in nursing from the University of San Diego, California; and a Ph.D. in nursing from the University of Texas in Austin.

He has taught nursing in associate, baccalaureate, and graduate schools of nursing, as well as RN degree completion programs. Dr. Daniels has taught fundamentals of nursing, medical-surgical nursing, pathophysiology, pharmacology, and research in a variety of programs. In addition, he has taught in several venues, including distance learning, correspondence, and traditional classroom settings. He has also taught many adult health and illness topics at seminars and has presented posters for national organizations (e.g., AORN, NLN Educators Conference). Dr. Daniels administers clinical practicum courses in critical care, emergency department, and perioperative nursing arenas.

Dr. Daniels' clinical practice is kept current by practicing nursing as a colonel in the Oregon Army National Guard. He is also serving as the deputy state commander of Oregon under the supervision of the Oregon State Surgeon.

Dr. Daniels' research is primarily associated with the concept of health promotion, and he has received three successive fundings with the Department of the Army to implement health promotion programs with national guardsmen. In addition, Dr. Daniels publishes in nursing journals and authors nursing textbooks. He has membership in a number of professional nursing organizations; such as Sigma Theta Tau and the American Nurses Association.

Dr. Daniels is currently an associate professor with tenure at Oregon Health and Science University, School of Nursing.

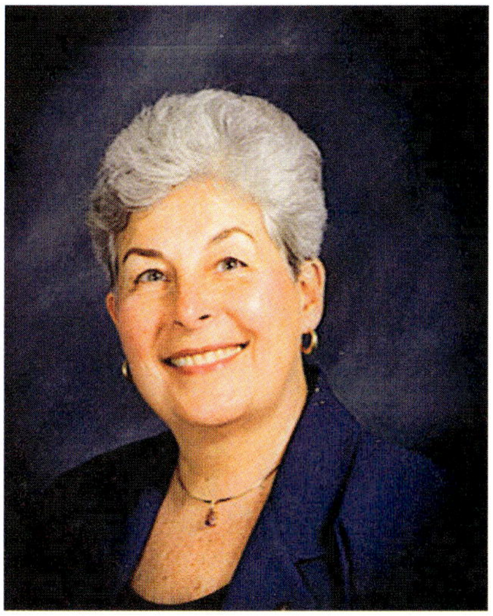

LAURA JOHN NOSEK

Laura John Nosek is a graduate of the Grace New Haven School of Nursing at Yale New Haven Medical Center, New Haven, Connecticut. She earned the bachelor of science in nursing from Frances Payne Bolton School of Nursing, Western Reserve University in Cleveland, Ohio, and the master of science in nursing and the Ph.D. in executive practice from Case Western Reserve University, Cleveland, Ohio.

Dr. Nosek's primary career has been as the chief nursing officer in academic health science centers in the private sector and as the chief nursing officer and chief operating officer in a public sector academic health science center. She currently holds academic appointments at universities in Ohio, Illinois, and New York, where she teaches various aspects of nursing administration and organizational science. She has taught in diploma, baccalaureate, masters, and doctoral nursing programs in four states, focusing on women's health, executive practice, and organizational systems, her areas of research. Dr. Nosek has made numerous presentations nationally and internationally and is published in nursing textbooks and juried nursing journals.

Dr. Nosek has served on national committees of Sigma Theta Tau and the National League for Nursing and has held multiple state and local offices in AONE, NLN, Sigma Theta Tau, and ANA. She currently sits on the national finance committee of NLN and serves as an NLN Ambassador.

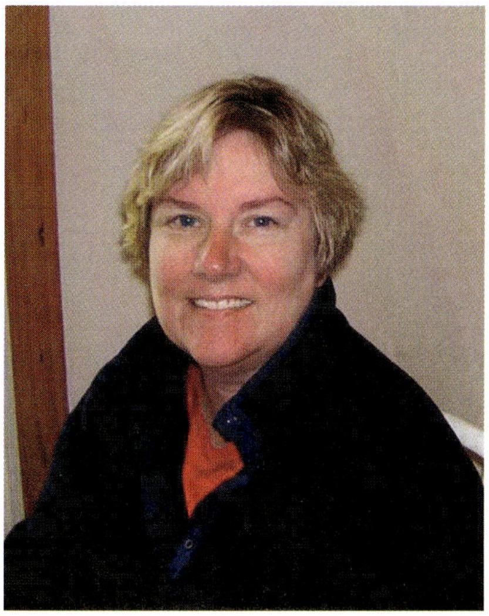

LESLIE H. NICOLL

Leslie H. Nicoll is the President and Owner of Maine Desk, LLC, a consulting and editorial services firm specializing in nursing, health, informatics, and research. Since 1995, Dr. Nicoll has been the editor-in-chief of *CIN* (formerly *Computers in Nursing*). On July 1, 2001, Dr. Nicoll was appointed editor-in-chief of the *Journal of Hospice and Palliative Nursing,* the official publication of the Hospice and Palliative Nurses Association. Prior to founding Maine Desk, Dr. Nicoll held a joint appointment as an Associate Research Professor in the College of Nursing and Health Professions and a Senior Research Associate in the Edmund S. Muskie School of Public Service, both at the University of Southern Maine, Portland, Maine. She is the author of *Nurses' Guide to the Internet* and editor of *Perspectives on Nursing Theory.* In addition, Dr. Nicoll is the author of more than 110 articles, books, editorials, and reviews. On September 8, 2003, she had a crossword puzzle published in *The New York Times,* which many consider a greater accomplishment than all her other articles combined. She is a graduate of Russell Sage College (BS, Nursing), the University of Illinois (MS, Nursing), and Case Western Reserve University (Ph.D., Nursing). As a Commonwealth Fund Executive Nurse Fellow, she pursued MBA study at the Whittemore School of Business and Economics, University of New Hampshire, graduating in 1991.

How to Use This Text

Patient Playbook

PATIENT PLAYBOOK

Coping with Chronic Pain

The patient is not always able to communicate the total impact of chronic pain on functional activities or the quality of life. The family often provides an inappropriate pain assessment due to their inadequate knowledge about the management of chronic pain. Therefore you should teach the patient and family to:

- Learn all they can about the physical condition and understand that there may be no current cure.
- Become actively involved in the customized health care plan.
- Learn to set priorities regarding the activities can help the patient to have a more active life and to set realistic goals appropriate for pain management.
- Understand medication protocol and how to use nonpharmacological interventions, including stress management.
- Recognize when to seek assistance from members of the health care team.
- Recognize that emotions directly affect physical health. Learn how to deal with feelings and ultimately lessen the level of pain.
- Identify a modest and safe exercise program to build strength and tone ...

Patients benefit greatly from knowledge of self-care, and nurses presenting information in a collaborative manner promote health. These boxes present relevant teaching interventions for patient, family, or support people necessary to enhance the individual's health. Instructions on how to equip patients with knowledge of well-being or preparing for procedures or outcomes is vital.

Red Flag

As a professional nurse, you will need to be able to react immediately in selected situations to ensure the health and safety of your patients. Pay careful attention to this feature, as it will assist you to begin to identify and respond to critical situations on your own, both efficiently and effectively.

Red Flag

Ensuring Accuracy of Phlebostatic Measurements

To ensure accuracy of measurements, it is important to eliminate any effect that surrounding atmospheric pressure may have on the monitoring system. This effect is eliminated through zeroing the system. The nurse turns the stopcock off to the patient's pressures, removes the cap on the stopcock connection, and pushes the zero button on the monitor. When the value on the screen reflects zero pressure, zeroing the transducer is completed. The cap and stopcock are returned to their normal monitoring position. Zeroing of the transducer is routinely performed prior to insertion of the catheter, once or twice per shift, or whenever the system is disconnected, changed, or extremes in values are obtained.

ETHICS IN PRACTICE

Ethical Considerations in Using Pain-Relieving Medications

It was not that long ago that health care students were actually taught that the first dose of morphine should also be the last and that no one ever died from pain, they just wished that they could. At least three generations of physicians, nurses, and pharmacists were taught to fear pain-relieving medications derived from opium (opioids).

Undertreatment of pain continues to be a major concern. Access to pain management services are lacking for many, including: people of color, the poor, and those living in rural areas. Protocols have been developed to permit people with terminal illnesses to die with comfort and dignity. However, the field of pain management is still young and evolving. It is essential for health care personnel to have the skills needed for appropriate pain care management. Nurses must also be committed to educating consumers to the facts that pain is treatable and nearly always manageable.

... The Last Word. U.S. Food and Drug ... 10, 2005, from: www.fda.gov.

LAW IN PRACTICE

Medical Marijuana

Marijuana for medical purposes has been approved in 10 states. The FDA has classified it as a schedule I drug, which means that it has a high potential for abuse. It has not been approved by the FDA owing to the lack of evidence from controlled clinical trials regarding its effectiveness as a pain reliever; however, there is great interest in its use by individuals who have not had pain relief from other therapies. It has been used to treat glaucoma, AIDS wasting, neuropathic pain, spasticity of multiple sclerosis, and chemotherapy-induced nausea. Dronabinol (Marinol) is a drug with characteristics similar to those of marijuana; it has FDA approval for controlling nausea and vomiting due to AIDS and chemotherapy-induced nausea.

The U.S. Supreme Court (June 7, 2005) ruled that the federal government can overrule state laws and prosecute seriously ill individuals who continue to use marijuana even when they are doing so under doctor's orders.

Source: McDonald, J. (2005, June 7). Supreme Court decision trumps California law. San Diego Union Tribune. pp. A-1, 8.

Ethics or Law in Practice

Our health care delivery system has many legal and ethical issues for the nurse to consider in the practice setting. These boxes describe patient situations that make it easier for you to see the ethicolegal implications as you provide your patient care. Incorporate these insights into your professional growth and development as an ethical practitioner.

Respecting Our Differences

Respecting Our Differences

Hospitalization and Death Rates of Patients with Asthma

Hospitalization rates for asthma have been highest among African Americans and children. Death rates for asthma are consistently highest among African Americans ages 15 to 24 years old (Tierney, et al., 2004). As a professional, the nurse obviously needs to not discriminate, stereotype, or make judgments regarding the ethnicity of patients who have a higher incidence of a disorder such as asthma.

It is important to recognize the specific implications for your care of patients with different cultural backgrounds. You need to review such things as the physiological and psychological implications of your different patients. This will assist you in delivering individualized nursing care.

Safety First

Safety First 1

Contraindications for Imagery

Imagery is not recommended for patients who are emotionally unstable or have active delusions or hallucinations. Patients with these conditions may become agitated or emotionally upset with imagery. The outcome would not be therapeutic.

Error prevention is a vital consideration in contemporary practice. As you read these boxes, think about how each strategy will improve safe practice and patient care.

Uncovering the Evidence

Evidence-based practice is essential to your development of knowledge and growth as a professional nurse. As you read these boxes, focus your attention on the elements of the research that are presented and incorporate the application as appropriate to your nursing practice.

> **Uncovering the Evidence**
>
> **Survey of Americans Living with Pain**
>
> **Discussion:** To determine the current awareness and understanding of pain and pain management issues among the general population of the United States, a random digit dialing system including all household telephone numbers (listed and unlisted) in the United States was used in 2002 to collect data. Data were collected through 800 telephone interviews with adults experiencing chronic pain.
>
> The findings revealed the following:
> - Seventy-two percent of respondents experiencing chronic pain had lived with it for more than 3 years; 34 percent had lived with pain for more than a decade.
> - Seventy-eight percent of respondents believed that treatment with narcotic medications would cause addiction.
> - Most respondents thought the typical person living with chronic pain was an adult at or above 65 years of age.
> - A majority agreed that some people tend to exaggerate their pain to gain attention, avoid work, or to obtain painkillers. (More of the youngest respondents answered "strongly agree" to this statement.)
> - One-third of respondents reported living with ongoing pain.
> - Workplace Issues:
>   1. Forty-one percent of employed persons who had chronic pain stated that it affected their ability to work a full day.
>   2. Twenty-seven percent stated that the pain affected their ability to get to work.
>   3. Sixteen percent stated that chronic pain affected their opportunities for career advancement.
> - Pain Management:
>   1. Eighty-one percent reported satisfaction with their prescribed plan of medical treatment.
>   2. Eight-six percent of those taking prescription medications also reported using alternative treatments, including physical therapy (58 percent) massage (39 percent), and meditation (23 percent).
>   3. Sixty-four percent of those who used over-the-counter (OTC) medications were satisfied with their relief of pain.
> - Economic Fears: Three of ten persons were unable to have a prescription filled because of its cost or the lack of health insurance; they also felt it would become more difficult to obtain the needed medication in the future.
>
> **Implications for Practice:** Patient education in the many pain-relieving modalities available and encouraging patients and their families to become a principal part of the treatment team are very important aspects of good pain management.
>
> *Source: American Chronic Pain Association (ACPA). (2004). Nurses' pain awareness kit. Retrieved from: http://www.theacpa.org.*

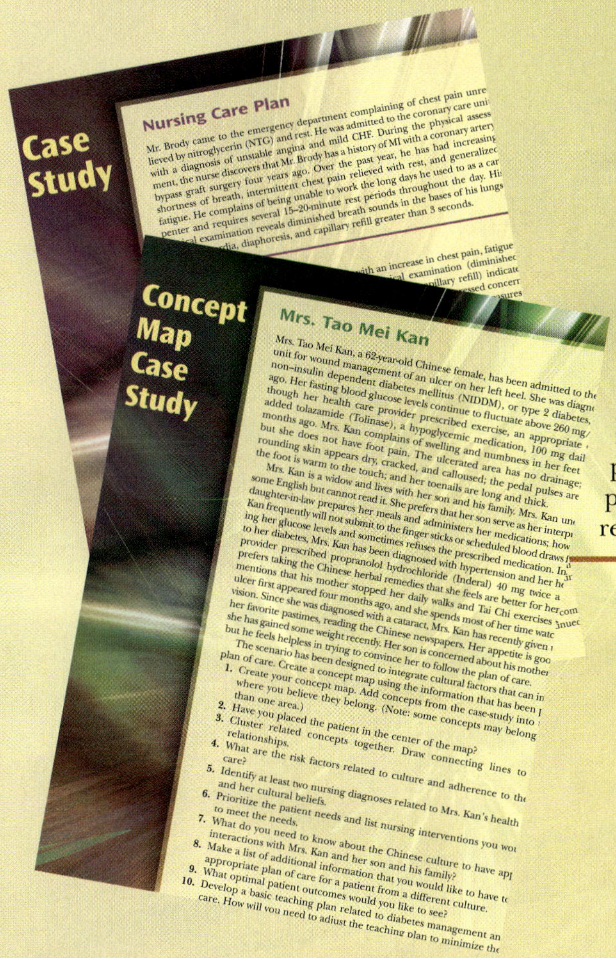

Case Studies

These real-life scenarios present a patient situation followed by nursing responsibilities framed in a nursing process format. Use case studies to provide a focused opportunity to refine critical thinking skills.

Skills 360°

These help to develop and enhance professionalism, communication, and skills in the workplace. Use Skills 360° to expand discussion on patient care.

> **Skills 360°**
>
> **Professional and Caring Communication**
>
> Patients with endocrine disorders may have disfigurement related to their physical appearance (e.g., acromegaly, dwarfism, Grave's disease, or goiter). The nurse must remember to focus on maintaining an objective assessment and still provide a caring and supportive style of communication with the patient.

Review Questions and Activities

As a method of reviewing a chapter, answer the open-ended questions in this box. These activities will stimulate your learning and allow you to synthesize and evaluate the knowledge gained when you study each section.

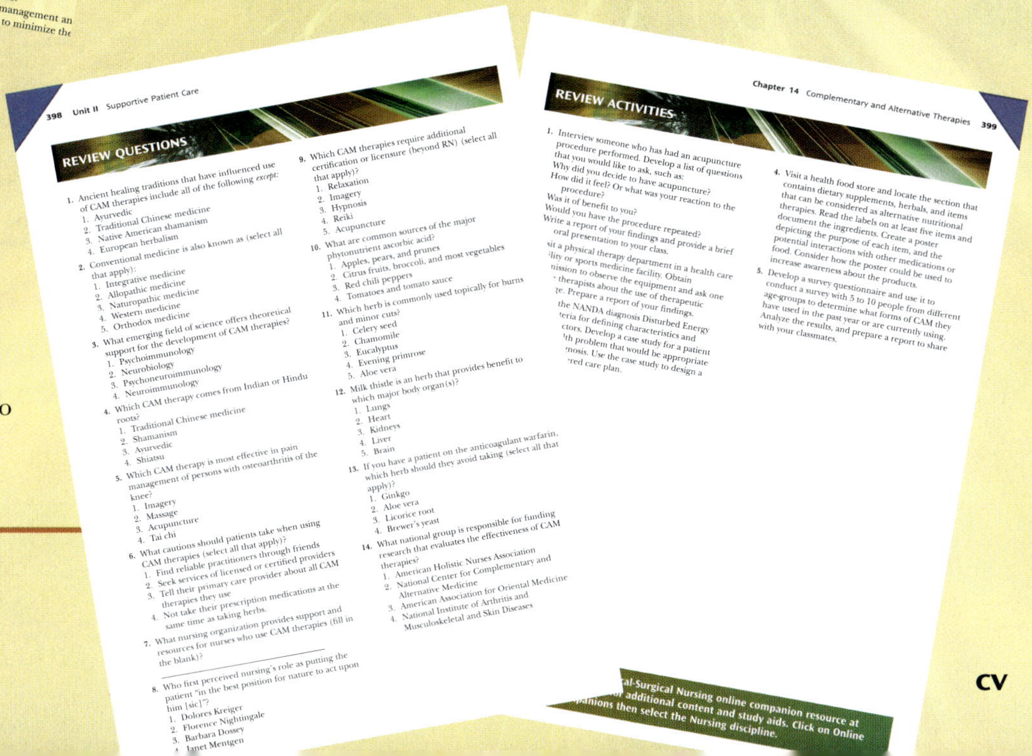

How to Use the CD-ROM

Access a wealth of information designed to enhance the text content

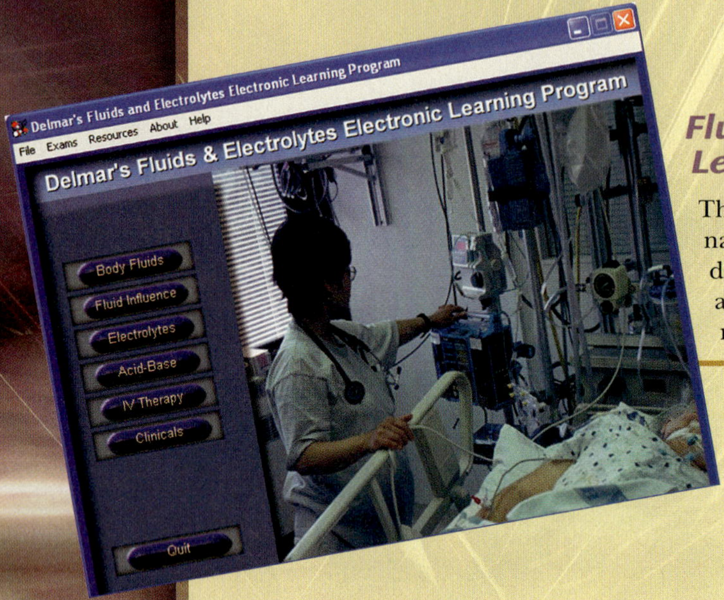

Fluids & Electrolytes Learning Program

This provides an interactive, easy-to-navigate program that simplifies difficult concepts and their application to medical-surgical nursing.

Critical Care Nursing Care Plans

These offer a unique experience to create and customize care plans in an electronic environment for the medical-surgical patient.

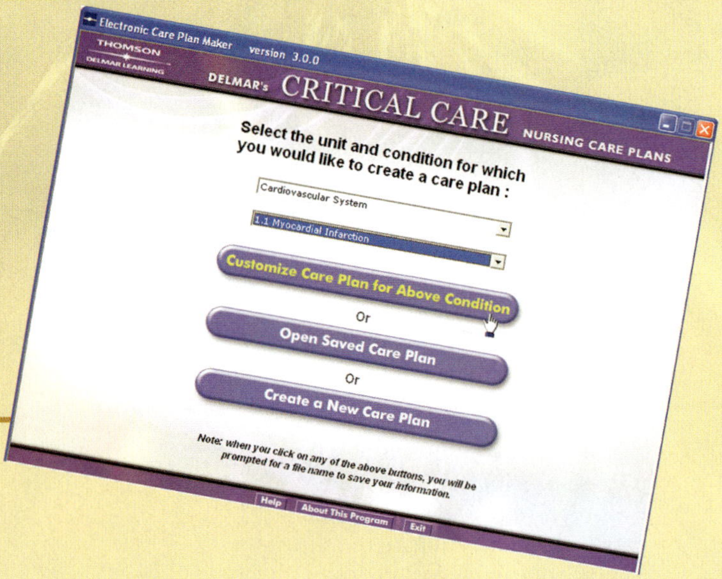

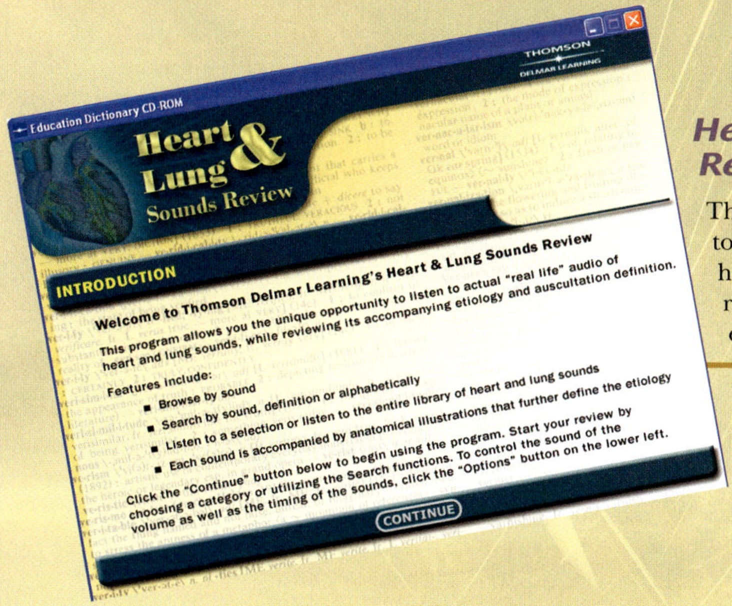

Heart & Lung Sounds Review

This program offers the opportunity to listen to actual real-life audio of heart and lung sounds while reviewing the accompanying etiology and auscultation definition.

NCLEX Review Tests

Two 100-question NCLEX exams are available in a test environment and focus on the areas of delegation and pharmacology. These tests have a rationale for right and wrong choices and are based on the current test plan with an emphasis on the medical-surgical patient.

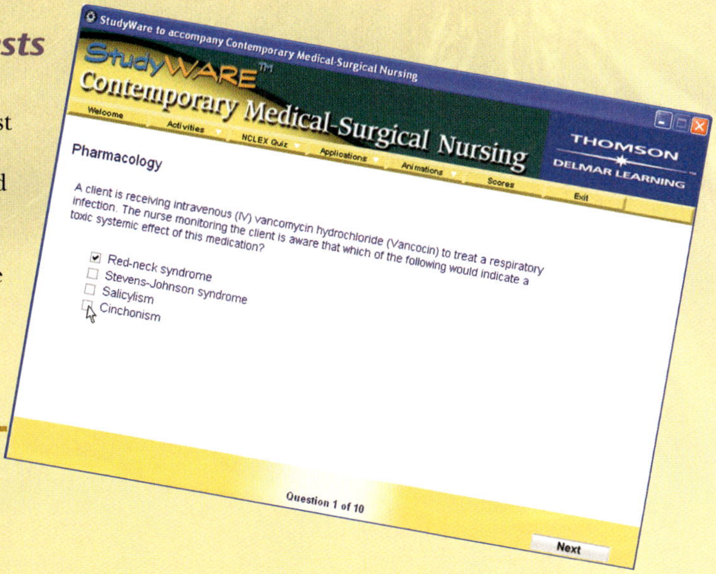

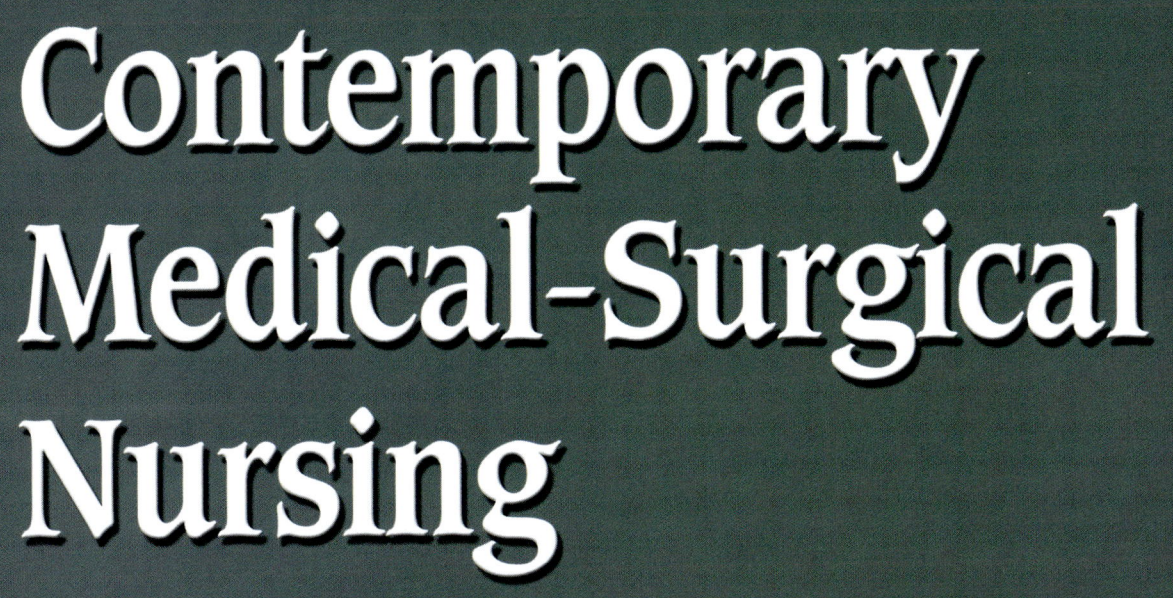

Contemporary Medical-Surgical Nursing

Volume 2

UNIT

VII

Alterations in Neurological Function

Chapter 34 Assessment of Neurological Function

Chapter 35 Dysfunction of the Brain: Nursing Management

Chapter 36 Dysfunction of the Spinal Cord and Peripheral Nervous System: Nursing Management

Chapter 37 Degenerative Neurological Dysfunction: Nursing Management

CHAPTER 34

Assessment of Neurological Function

Doris Denison, MSN, APRN, BC, CCRN

KEY TERMS

Ageusia
Analgesia
Anesthesia
Anosmia
Astereognosis
Ataxia
Diplopia
Dysdiadochokinesia
Dysesthesia
Dysgeusia
Dysmetria
Dysphagia
Dyssynergy
Graphesthesia
Hypalgesia
Hypergesia
Hypesthesia
Hypogeusia
Nystagmus
Paresthesia
Ptosis
Stereognosis

CHAPTER TOPICS

- Nervous System Cells
- Central Nervous System
- Peripheral Nervous System
- Autonomic Nervous System
- Neurological Assessment
- Neurodiagnostic Studies

The nervous system is a complex network of cells, tissues, and specialized organs. It is the center of thinking, judgment, memory, cognition, communication, behavior, emotion, sensation, and movement. There is both direct and indirect control of the body systems. For example, a stroke in the frontal lobe affecting the motor strip may result in seizures and loss of limb movement. The assessment of the nervous system is extremely important for the nurse to apply in the care of the patient in a wide variety of settings.

ANATOMY AND PHYSIOLOGY

The nervous system has two major divisions: the central nervous system (CNS), which consists of the brain and spinal cord, and the peripheral nervous system (PNS), which consists of the cranial nerves, the spinal nerves, and the autonomic nervous system (ANS). The entire nervous system is made up of two types of cells: neurons, which transmit or conduct nerve impulses, and neuroglial cells, which support the neurons.

Nervous System Cells

Neurons are the basic functional unit of the nervous system. They are specialized to gather, integrate, and respond to information from both the internal and external environment. Specialized cells called neuroglia support the neurons. The neuroglia have many functions: axonal insulation, removal of debris and dead cells, assisting with the circulation of cerebrospinal fluid (CSF), and they are a component of the blood-brain barrier.

Neurons

Each neuron consists of dendrites, a cell body, and an axon. The function of the neurons is to transmit impulses. Dendrites are short projections from the cell body that conduct impulses toward the cell body via afferent processes. Dendrites have varying numbers of branches, and each branch synapses with another cell body, axon, or dendrite. The cell body contains the nucleus and cytoplasm. It is the metabolic focal point of the neuron. Most of the cell bodies are found within the CNS. They are clustered together in ganglia or nuclei.

The axon is a long projection that conducts impulses away from the cell body via efferent processes. Axonal length varies from several micrometers to more than a meter, often branching near the end of the projection. The enlarged, distal end of each axon is called the synaptic, or terminal, knob. The synaptic knobs contain the mechanisms for manufacturing, storing, and releasing neurotransmitter substances. Each neuron produces one specific transmitter, capable of either enhancing or inhibiting the impulse.

Many axons, although not all, are covered with a myelin sheath, which is a white lipid substance. Myelinated axons are called white matter. Nonmyelinated axons are called gray matter. The myelin sheath is interrupted at intervals by the nodes of Ranvier. The nodes of Ranvier allow movement of ions between the axon and the extracellular fluid.

Characteristics of neurons include: excitability, conductivity, and the ability to influence other cells. Excitability is the ability to generate a nerve impulse. Conductivity is the ability to transmit impulses to other portions of the cell. Transmission of nerve impulses to other neurons, muscle cells, and glandular cells stimulate changes (Jenner & Olanow, 2006).

Nerve Impulses

The initiation of a nerve impulse involves the generation of an action potential. After the impulse is started, it travels along the axon as a series of action potentials. At the end of the nerve fiber, the impulse is transmitted across the synapse junction between the nerve cells by chemical mechanisms involving neurotransmitters. The nerve impulse moves from axon to axon until it reaches its destination.

Synapses

A synapse is the point where a nerve impulse is transmitted from neuron to neuron, neuron to muscle, or neuron to glandular tissue. The three components needed for transmission are a presynaptic terminal, a synaptic cleft, and a receptor site on the postsynaptic cell. When the nerve impulse reaches the presynaptic terminal, a neurotransmitter is released from tiny storage vesicles.

The neurotransmitter then crosses the synaptic cleft and attaches to receptor sites of the postsynaptic neuron. This alters the membrane permeability and causes a change in the electrical potential of the membrane.

Neurotransmitters

In the CNS, neurotransmitters are chemical substances that inhibit, excite, or modify the responses of another cell. In general, each neuron releases the same transmitter at all of its terminals. Over 30 neurotransmitters have been identified. The general chemical classes are amines (e.g., acetylcholine and serotonin), catecholamines (i.e., dopamine, epinephrine, and norepinephrine), amino acids (e.g., gamma aminobutyric acid [GABA], glutamic acid, glycine, and substance P), and polypeptides (e.g., endorphins and enkephalins). Table 34-1 summarizes the source and actions of the major neurotransmitters.

Neuroglia Cells

The second type of cells in the nervous system are neuroglia. They support the neurons by providing protection, structural support, and nutrition. In the CNS, there are four types of neuroglia: astrocytes, oligodendroglia, ependymal cells, and microglia. Clinically, astrocyte functions include: provision of nutrients, regulating synaptic connectivity, removal of cellular waste products, and control of molecular movement from blood to brain. Oligodendrocytes produce the myelin sheath that protects the neuron. Ependymal cells are found

TABLE 34-1 Neurotransmitters: Site and Action

TRANSMITTER	SITE	ACTION
Amines		
Acetylcholine	Brain, brainstem, basal ganglia, and autonomic nervous system	Usually excitatory Some inhibitory effects of parasympathetic nervous system (e.g., heart by vagus)
Serotonin	Medical brainstem, hypothalamus, and dorsal horn of spinal cord	Inhibits pain pathway of spinal cord Helps control mood and sleep
Catecholamines		
Dopamine	Substantia nigra to basal ganglia	Usually inhibitory
Norepinephrine	Brainstem, hypothalamus, and sympathetic nervous system	Usually excitatory, sometimes inhibitory Some excitatory, some inhibitory
Amino Acids		
Aspartate	Brain and spinal cord	Excitatory
Gamma aminobutyric acid (GABA)	Brain, basal ganglia, cerebellum, and spinal cord	Some excitatory; some inhibitory
Glutamic acid	Sensory pathways	Excitatory
Glycine	Spinal cord	Inhibitory
Substance P	Pain fibers of dorsal horns of spinal cord and hypothalamus	Excitatory
Polypeptides		
Endorphins	Pituitary gland, thalamus, spinal cord, and hypothalamus	Excitatory to systems that inhibit pain
Enkephalins	Spinal cord, brainstem, thalamus, and hypothalamus	Excitatory to systems that inhibit pain

Adapted from Scott, A., & Fong, E. (2004). Body structures and functions *(10th ed.). Clifton Park, NY: Thomson Delmar Learning.*

in the lining of the ventricular system, aid in the production of CSF, and act as a barrier to foreign substances. Microglia play a scavenger role by responding to infection or trauma to the CNS

Central Nervous System

The CNS has two major divisions: the brain and spinal cord. The brain is composed of the cerebrum, the brainstem, and the cerebellum. The spinal cord is the conduit for the ascending sensory and descending motor neurons. This is the pathway for two-way communication between the brain and the periphery. In addition, the spinal cord is the center for reflex action.

Bones

The bones of the skull and the vertebral column prevent injury to the brain and the spinal cord. The scalp moves freely and cushions the head from traumatic injury. The skull is the bony, rigid framework of the head. It is composed of the 14 bones of the face and the 8 bones of the cranium (Figure 34-1). Where the bones of the skull join, suture lines form. The four major suture lines are: sagittal, coronal, lambdoidal, and basilar.

The vertebral column is a flexible, stacked series of bones that support the head and trunk. There are 33 vertebrae: 7 cervical, 12 thoracic, 5 lumbar, 5 sacral fused into one, and 4 coccygeal fused into one (Figure 34-2).

Meninges

The brain and spinal cord are covered with a series of membranes called the meninges. These include: the dura mater, the arachnoid, and the pia mater. The dura mater is the tough, fibrous, outer layer, which lines the skull and vertebrae. The arachnoid is a thin, delicate middle membrane, where CSF is cir-

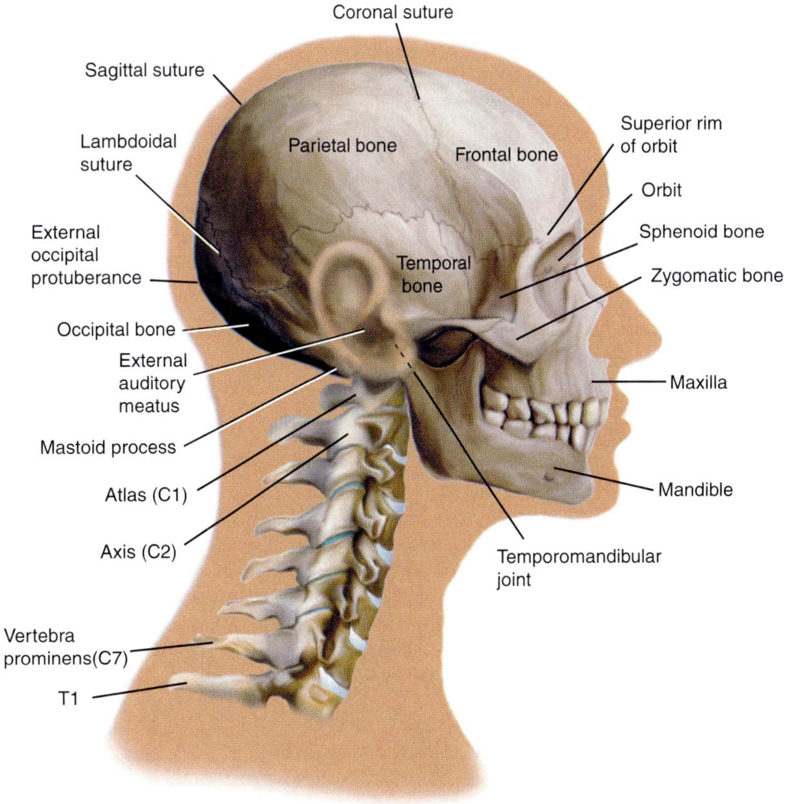

Figure 34-1 Bones of the face and skull (lateral view).

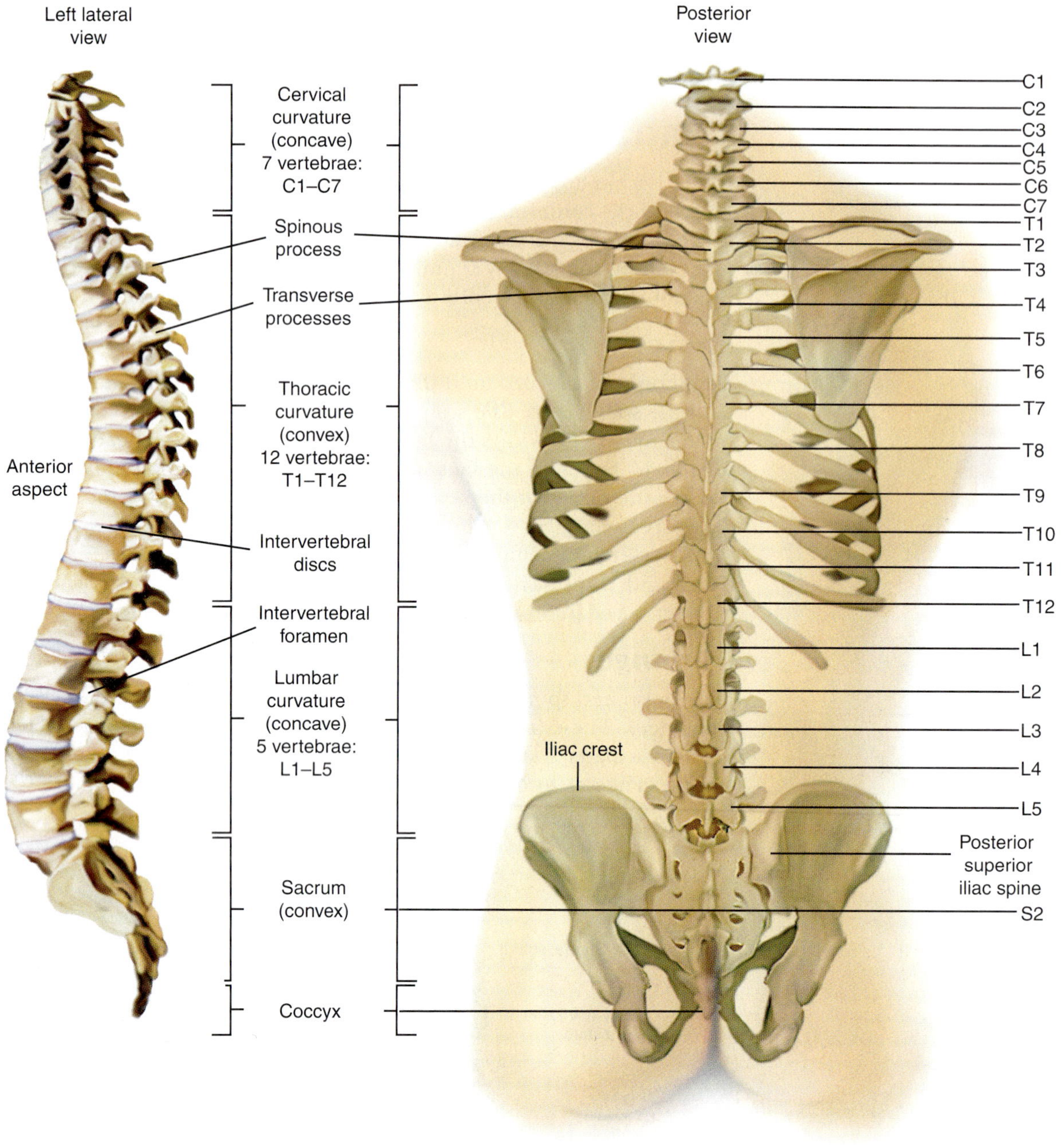

Figure 34-2 Bones of the spine.

culated and absorbed. The pia mater is the thin, vascular inner layer that covers the surface of the brain and spinal cord (Figure 34-3).

Brain

The cerebrum is the largest part of the brain. The surface of the cerebrum is covered by multiple folds or wrinkles, called gyri, which greatly increases the surface area. It is divided into two hemispheres, right and left, by a deep groove. Each hemisphere has an outer layer of neurons called the white matter and an inner layer called the gray matter. These two hemispheres of the cerebrum are connected by a thick band of white fibers called the corpus callosum. The corpus callosum allows the two hemispheres to communicate. Each hemisphere receives sensory and motor impulses from the opposite side of the body. The majority of people are left brain dominant. The left side controls language, while the right side controls perception (Figure 34-4).

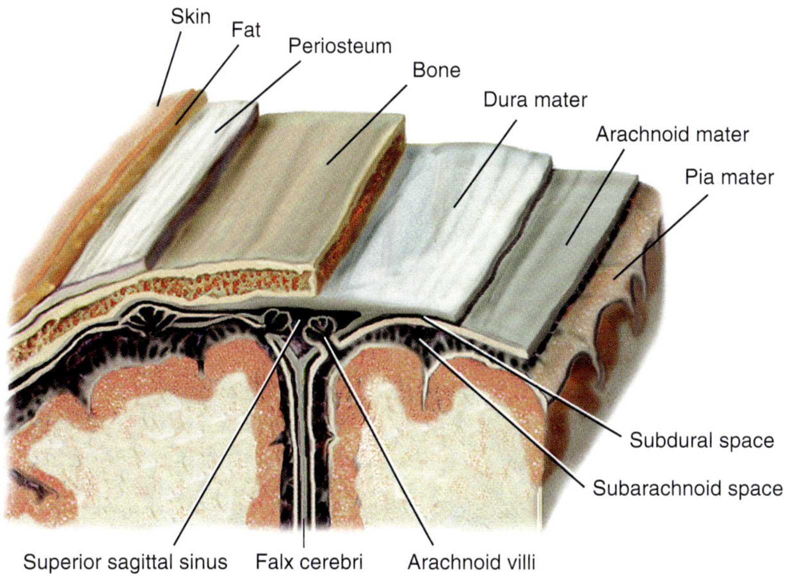

Figure 34-3 The meninges.

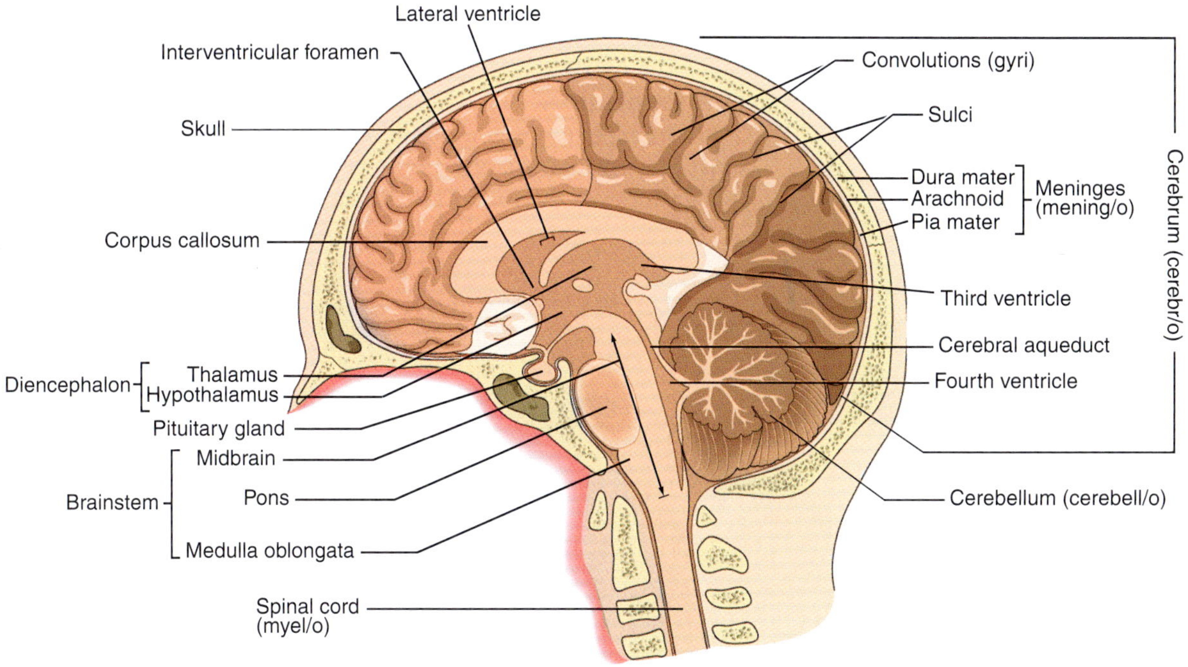

Figure 34-4 Cross-section of the brain.

Ventricles

There are four ventricles (or chambers) within the brain. These include: two lateral ventricles located within each hemisphere, the third ventricle and the fourth ventricle. The chambers are filled with CSF and are linked by ducts (also called foramen), which permit circulation. CSF is a clear, colorless fluid produced by the choroid plexus, located in the ventricles. It circulates through a closed system, which includes the four ventricles and area around the spinal cord. Reabsorption occurs via the arachnoid villi.

Basal Ganglia

The basal ganglia are found deep within the cerebral hemispheres. They consist of several collections of nuclei: the lenticular nucleus, the caudate nucleus, the amygdaloid body, and the claustrum. The lenticular nucleus is composed of the

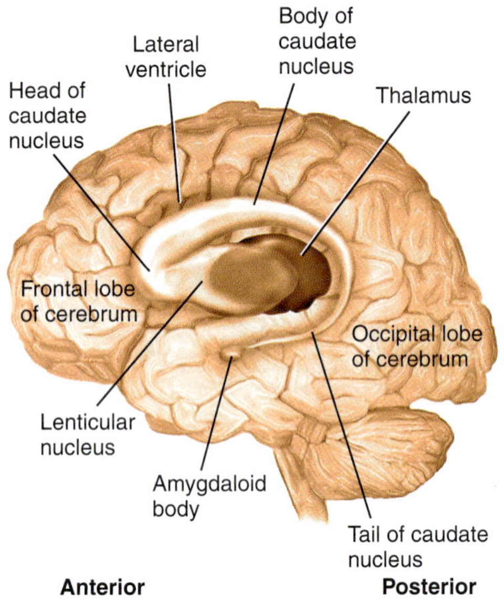

Figure 34-5 Basal ganglia.

globus pallidus and the putamen. The globus pallidus has extensive connections with the striatum, thalamus, and mesencephalon. The putamen is the most common site for intracerebral hemorrhage. Loss of cellular function in the globus pallidus and putamen is a component of Parkinson's disease. The amygdaloid body is an almond-shaped area near the temporal lobe. The claustrum is the barrier between the gray and white matter of the brain. The caudate nucleus is involved the origination of repetitive movements. The basal ganglia coordinate communication between the cerebral cortex and the cerebellum that controls motor activity (Figure 34-5). Lesions of the basal ganglia produce abnormal movements, including chorea, athetosis, hemiballismus, and dystonic posturing.

Lobes

The lobes of the cerebral hemispheres are: frontal, parietal, temporal, and occipital. Major functions of the frontal lobe include: high-level cognitive activities, information storage or memory, voluntary eye movement, basal motor control of breathing, gastrointestinal (GI) function, blood pressure, and motor control of speech in the dominant hemisphere. The parietal lobe is the primary sensory interpretation area. The temporal lobe is the primary auditory reception and interpretation area. Limbic area is part of the temporal lobe and is involved in emotional behavior and self-preservation. The major function of the occipital lobe is visual perception, some visual reflexes, and involuntary smooth eye movements (Figure 34-6).

Diencephalon

The diencephalon is composed of the thalamus, epithalamus, and hypothalamus. The thalamus is the initial processing area for sensory input. The epithalamus forms the roof of the third ventricle and the pineal gland. The hypo-

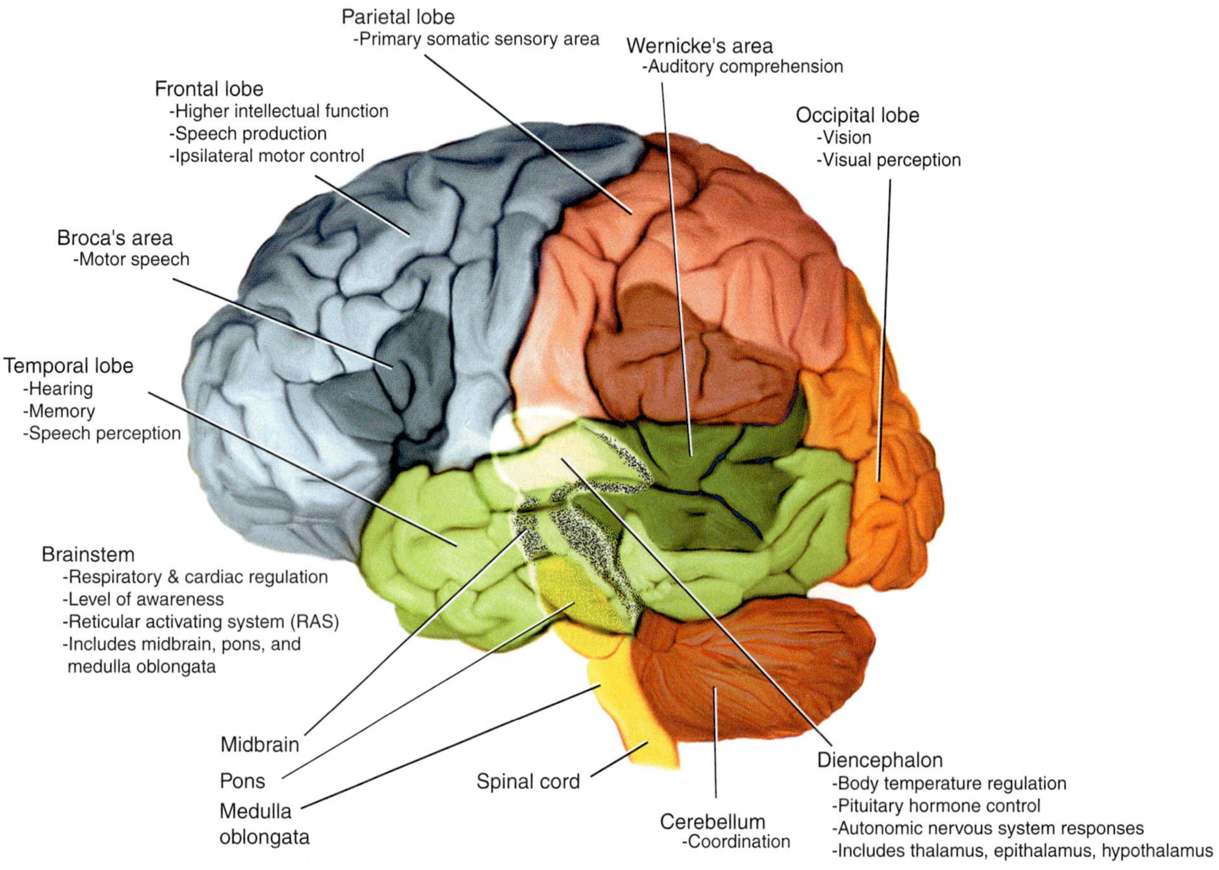

Figure 34-6 The lobes of the brain.

thalamus regulates temperature, appetite, water metabolism, emotional expression, thirst, and a portion of the sleep-wake cycle.

Hypophysis

The hypophysis (pituitary gland) is connected to the hypothalamus by the hypophyseal stalk. There are two lobes, each releasing specific hormones into the systemic circulation. It is controlled by information processed by the hypothalamus. The function of the pituitary gland is discussed in depth in chapter 55.

Brainstem

The brainstem includes the midbrain, pons, and medulla. The midbrain is the center for auditory and visual reflexes. The pons controls respiration. The medulla plays a role in the control of heart rate, blood pressure, respirations, and swallowing.

Cerebellum

The cerebellum is located behind the brainstem and under the occipital lobe of the cerebrum. Functions of the cerebellum include: coordinate voluntary muscle movement, equilibrium, and maintenance of trunk stability. The cerebellum influences motor activity via its axonal connections to the motor cortex, brainstem nuclei, and descending pathways. Sensory information from the cerebral cortex, muscles, joints, and inner ear are used to refine the motor responses.

Cerebral Circulation

The source of blood to the brain occurs via the internal carotid arteries (anterior circulation) and the vertebral and basilar arteries (posterior circulation). These arteries join at the base of the brain to form the circle of Willis (cerebral arterial circle). The two anterior cerebral arteries (ACA) supply the medial portion on the frontal lobes. Two middle cerebral arteries (MCA) supply the outer portions of the frontal, parietal, and superior temporal lobes. The two posterior inferior cerebral arteries (PICA) supply the medial portions of the occipital and inferior temporal lobes. Venous blood drains from the brain via the dural sinuses that drain into the two jugular veins. Knowledge of the major arteries of the brain and the areas supplied is necessary for understanding and evaluating the signs and symptoms of brain tumors, cerebral vascular disease, and trauma. Cerebral aneurysms often occur at bifurcation points along the circle of Willis (Figure 34-7).

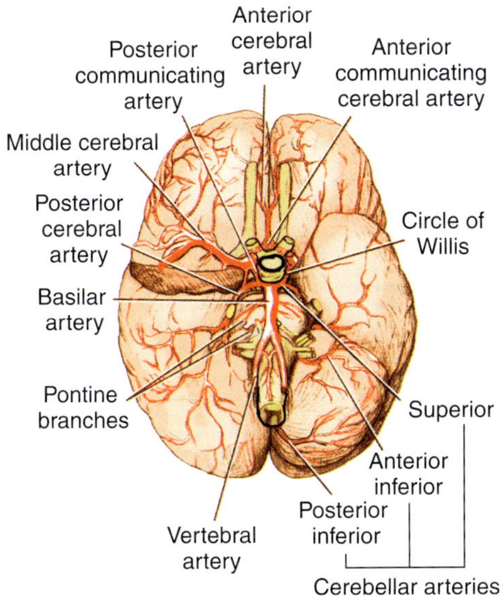

Figure 34-7 Circle of Willis.

Blood-Brain Barrier

The blood-brain barrier maintains a functionally stable environment for the CNS. The barrier is composed of a network of endothelial cells surrounding specialized brain capillaries. This prevents the free movement of material from the bloodstream into the brain and protects the brain from toxic substances that may be circulating in the blood. While protecting the brain, it impairs the effectiveness of many drugs used to treat nervous system problems. For instance, dopamine must be administered in an inactive form (levodopa) and then converted to its active form before it can treat the tremor and rigidity of Parkinson's.

Spine

The spine is a flexible column formed by series of bones called vertebrae. The vertebrae serve multiple functions: protection the spinal cord, support the head, and provide spinal flexibility. Each vertebra consists of a body, arch, and foramen. The body is the anterior portion and contains a central foramen. The stacked vertebral foramina form the canal through which the spinal cord passes. The arch is the posterior segment and consists of two pedicles and two laminae, which support seven processes. The pedicles form intervertebral notches through which the spinal nerves emerge. Processes provide spinal stability and points for attachment of muscles and ligaments.

The intervertebral discs are fibrocartilaginous structures located between the vertebral bodies. They vary is shape, thickness, and size at different levels of the spine. The function of these discs is to cushion movement. Aging, trauma, and poor posture are the most frequent causes of injury to the intervertebral discs.

Spinal Cord

The spinal cord extends from the medulla to the level of the first lumbar vertebrae. It exits the cranial cavity through the foramen magnum. A cross-section of the spinal cord reveals gray matter in an H pattern in the central portion (Figure 34-8). It is surrounded by white matter. The gray matter contains the cell bodies of the voluntary motor neurons, the preganglionic autonomic motor neurons, and interneurons. The white matter contains the axons ascending sensory and descending motor fibers. The myelin surrounding these fibers gives them their white appearance.

The ascending sensory tracts carry specific sensory information to the higher levels of the CNS. The information comes from specialized sensory receptors in the skin, muscles, joints, viscera, and blood vessels. Descending motor tracts carry impulses from the higher levels to the lower motor neurons. The lower motor neurons are the final step of the nerve impulse before stimulation of skeletal muscle. Upper motor neurons are located in the brainstem and cerebral cores and also influence skeletal muscle movement. Damage to the upper motor neurons, sometimes seen in multiple sclerosis (MS), may cause weakness, atrophy, hyperreflexia, or spasticity.

Spinal Cord Circulation

Circulation to the spinal cord comes from three sources: anterior spinal, two posterior spinal, and branches of the descending aorta. The anterior spinal artery comes from the vertebral arteries. The posterior inferior cerebellar or the vertebral arteries are the source of the two posterior spinal arteries. Venous return occurs via both intradural and extradural routes.

Peripheral Nervous System

The preceding part of the chapter discussed the CNS. The nervous system though has two parts. The second part is the PNS. The PNS is composed of the spinal nerves, cranial nerves, and the ANS.

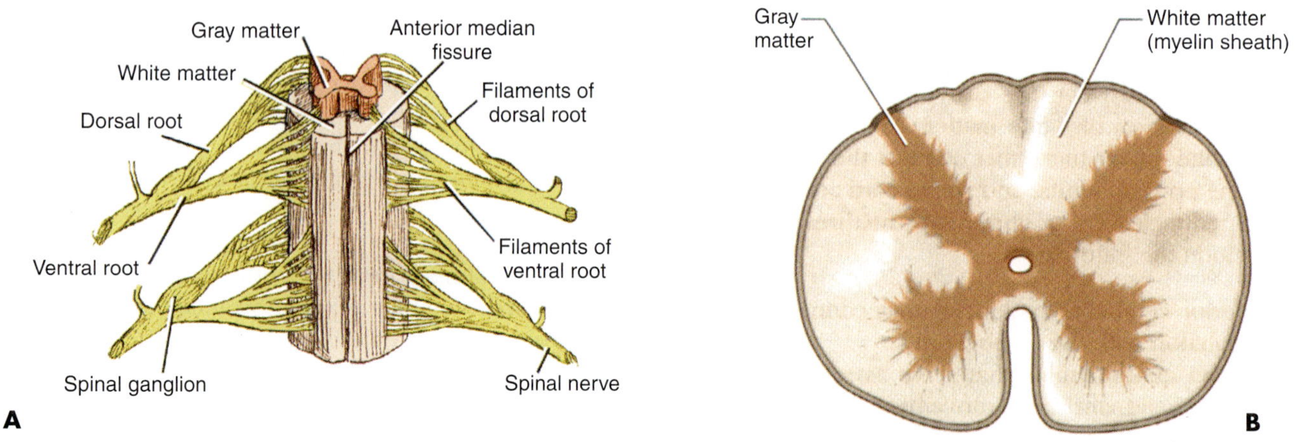

Figure 34-8 Spinal cord: A. Anterior view, B. Cross-section view—white and gray matter.

Spinal Nerves

The spinal nerves consist of 31 pairs exiting from the spinal cord. They include: 8 cervical, 12 thoracic, 5 lumbar, 5 sacral, and 1 coccygeal. Each spinal nerve has both a sensory and a motor component for a specific area of the body. The cervical and thoracic spinal nerves are near the areas they cover. The lumbar and sacral areas are farther away. The specific area for each spinal nerve is represented by a dermatome. For example, the patient with a lesion at L4 and L5 may complain of pain, numbness, or tingling of one or both lower legs, below the knee, including the great toes. When the discomfort is worse on the medial aspects of the legs, the lesion is at L4.

Sensory Receptors

Sensory input is collected throughout the body by receptors of pain, temperature, touch, vibration, pressure, visceral sensation, and proprioception. This information is transmitted to the cortex, along with input from the special senses: vision, taste, smell, and hearing.

Cranial Nerves

The cranial nerves provide both motor and sensory innervation for the head, neck, and viscera. Anatomically they begin in and emerge from the cranium (Figure 34-9). They are called cranial nerves as opposed to spinal nerves, which emerge from the spinal column. Individual nerves may be pure motor, pure sensory, or mixed. Two nerves, oculomotor (CN III) and vagus (CN X), include parasympathetic components. See Table 34-2 for specifics.

Autonomic Nervous System

The ANS has two, semi-independent components: sympathetic and parasympathetic. The two components function together to maintain homeostasis of the body's internal environment. The ANS is responsible for maintaining and regulating glandular function and the smooth muscles. The ANS also coordinates the functioning of the visceral organs. The sympathetic nervous system is responsible for initialing the protective mechanism, called the fight-or-flight response, whenever the body is exposed to stress. The parasympathetic system transmits impulses to the visceral organs and is responsible for those functions that are not under conscious control, called rest and repair or "general housekeeping." Table 34-3 lists the specific systemic responses of the sympathetic and parasympathetic systems to autonomic stimulation for each of the body systems.

Spinal Reflexes

A reflex is a response to a stimulus that occurs without conscious control. One way to classify reflexes is: stretch, cutaneous, and pathological. Muscle stretch reflexes are also called deep tendon reflexes (DTRs). Common DTRs are biceps, triceps, patellar, Achilles, and brachioradialis. Cutaneous reflexes are termed superficial reflexes. Superficial reflexes occur when noxious stimulation is applied to the skin. The response is withdrawal from the irritant. An example is contraction of the abdominal muscles when the skin is stroked. Pathological reflexes should not be present in healthy adults. Presence of a pathological reflex indicates interference with the normal CNS function. The upward movement of the great toe with flaring of the pedal digits is an example of a pathological reflex (Crimlisk & Grande, 2004).

The sensory input may come from muscles, tendons, skin, organs, and the special senses. Sensory information from the specific peripheral location is responsible for the motor impulses that return to the same peripheral location. This is called a reflex arc.

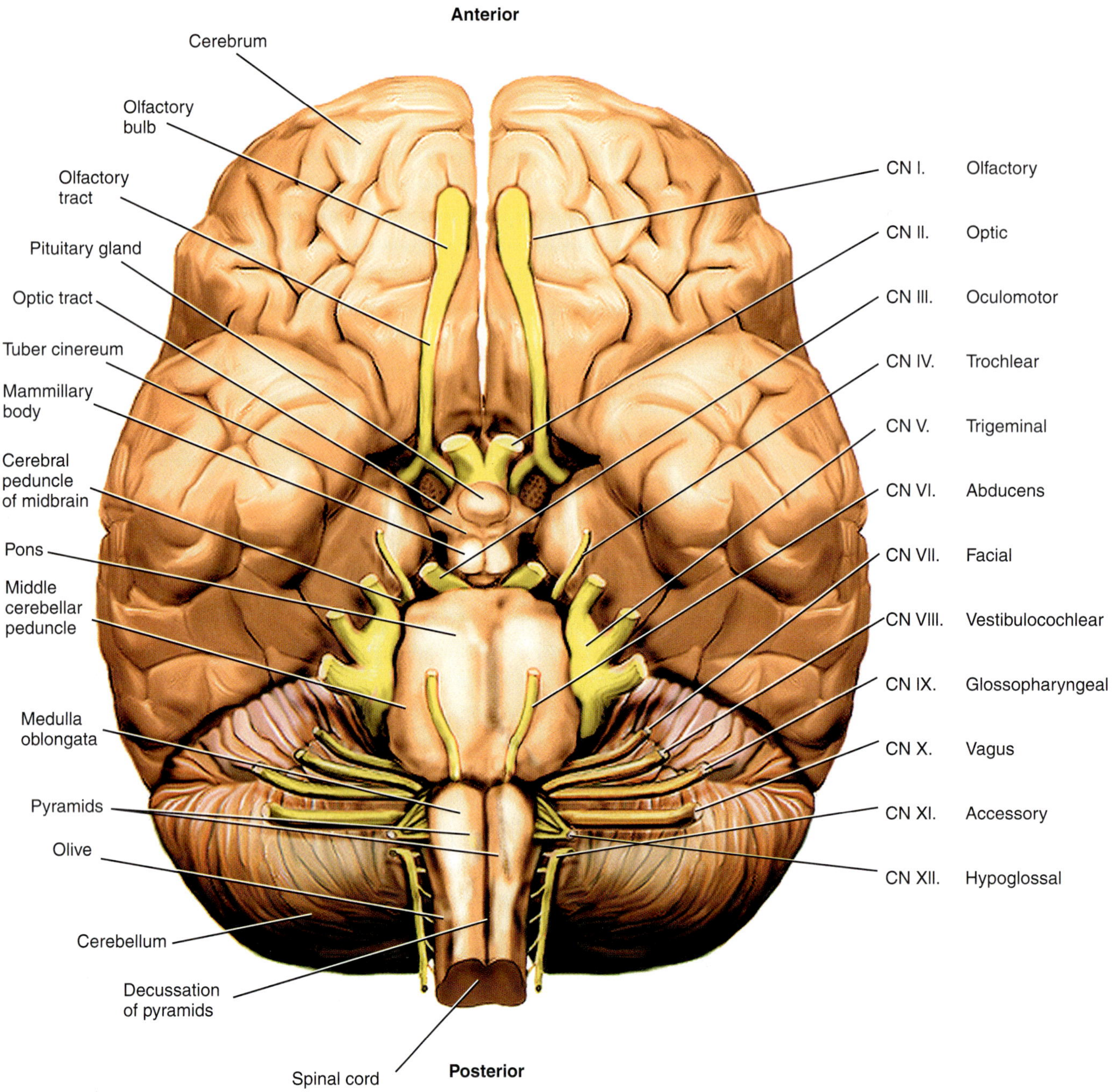

Figure 34-9 Cranial nerves and related structures.

Age-Related Changes

As the human body ages, patients begin to experience both motor and sensory changes. Chronic diseases of the bones, muscles, or joints can have a detrimental effect on the nerves motor function. With aging there is a decrease in both muscle bulk and nerve electrical activity. This causes diminished muscle strength and a decrease in reactions and movement time. Sensory function is diminished due to a decrease in total sensory receptors, decrease in electrical activity, and atrophy or degeneration of the taste buds, olfactory bulb, and vestibular system of the inner ear. Reflexes may diminish because of degeneration of the myelin sheath. Cognitive function continues at the same level as in younger years, unless disease impairs the brain. For example, arteriosclerosis and hypertension may lead to a cerebrovascular accident (CVA) that causes brain damage.

TABLE 34-2 Cranial Nerves

NERVE	FUNCTION
I. Olfactory	Sensory: Smell
II. Optic	Sensory: Sight
III. Oculomotor	Motor: Eye movements; contraction of iris
	Parasympathetic: Smooth muscles of eye socket
IV. Trochlear	Motor: Eye movement
V. Trigeminal	
Ophthalmic branch	Sensory: Forehead, eye, and superior nasal cavity
Maxillary	Sensory: Inferior nasal cavity, face, upper teeth, and superior mucosa of mouth
Mandibular	Sensory: Jaw surface, lower teeth, anterior tongue, and inferior mucosa of mouth
	Motor: Muscles for chewing
VI. Abducens	Sensory: Eye movement
VII. Facial	Motor: Muscles of expression, cheek muscle
	Sensory: Taste of anterior two thirds of tongue
VIII. Vestibulocochlear	
Vestibular	Sensory: Balance
Cochlear	Sensory: Hearing
IX. Glossopharyngeal	Sensory: Pharynx and posterior tongue (including taste)
	Motor: Superior pharyngeal muscles, swallowing
X. Vagus	Sensory: Viscera of chest and abdomen
	Motor: Larynx, middle and inferior pharyngeal muscles
	Parasympathetic: Heart, lungs, most of GI tract
XI. Accessory	Motor: Movement of neck muscles
XII. Hypoglossal	Motor: Movement of tongue

Adapted from Scott, A., & Fong, E. (2004). Body structures and functions *(10th ed.). Clifton Park, NY: Thomson Delmar Learning.*

ASSESSMENT

Knowledge of the anatomy and physiology discussed in the previous section helps the nurse with interpretation of his or her assessment findings. Assessment of the neurological system begins with the history. This interview collects subjective data. The second portion is the physical examination of the neurological system, which collects objective data.

History

A complete neurological health history assists the nurse to identify strengths and weaknesses and determine the extent of any problems involving the nervous system. The focus and extent of the examination is dependent on the patient's symptoms and the probable or actual diagnosis. Assessment begins with observation of the patient's level of consciousness (LOC). The nurse takes note of the patient's speech pattern, mental status, intellectual functioning, reasoning ability, and movement or lack of movement of all extremities while obtaining a health history. When the patient is alert, able to state his or her name, where he or she is, and what day it is, proceed with the health history.

Respecting Our Differences

Patients with English as a Second Language

Assessment of patients for whom English is a second language is often difficult. The lack of the ability to communicate can lead to inaccurate assessments. The nurse may need to involve family or friends to assist with translating. The interpreter or family can assist with the orientation assessment. Orientation is a reflection of the patient's ability to correctly interpret and respond to stimuli. Many institutions keep a record of employees who can act as translators. There are also communication picture boards, which may be helpful.

TABLE 34-3 Sympathetic versus Parasympathetic Response

SYSTEM	SYMPATHETIC RESPONSE	PARASYMPATHETIC RESPONSE
Neurological	Pupils dilated	Pupils normal size
	Heightened awareness	
Cardiovascular	Increased heart rate	Decreased heart rate
	Increased myocardial contractility	Decreased myocardial contractility
	Increased blood pressure	
Respiratory	Increased respiratory rate	Bronchial constriction
	Increased respiratory depth	
	Bronchial dilation	
GI	Decreased gastric motility	Increased gastric motility
	Decreased gastric secretions	Increased gastric secretion
	Increased glycogenolysis	Sphincter dilation
	Decreased insulin production	
	Sphincter contraction	
Genitourinary	Decreased urine output	Normal urine output
	Decreased renal blood flow	

Adapted from Estes, M. (2006). Health assessment and physical examination *(3rd ed.). New York: Thomson Delmar Learning.*

If the patient is comatose or too lethargic to cooperate, the nurse must access secondary sources, such as family or significant others.

When assessing a patient with an altered LOC, use the Glasgow Coma Scale (Table 34-4). The Glasgow Coma Scale is the most widely recognized, standardized LOC assessment tool. The score is based on three categories: eye opening, verbal response, and best motor response. The best possible score is 15 and the lowest score is 3. A score of 8 or less generally indicates a significant alteration in LOC (Crimlisk & Grande, 2004).

Interview

The interview starts with the history of the present problem. The nurse needs to elicit the patient's description of the current problem as shown in the Skills 360°feature.

This information helps the nurse to focus the physical examination. A history of any past illnesses, surgeries, injuries, and medications that the patient is taking may identify related pathology. The social history may reveal exposure to toxic agents, such as viruses, alcohol, tobacco, drugs, or radiation. Family health history may help to identify genetic patterns of disease. For instance, parents or grandparents with chronic diseases or early demise may indicate the patient is also at risk. Prevention of diseases such as myocardial infarction (MI), diabetes mellitus (DM), or CVA may require early intervention by the health care team. Health history questions based on functional health patterns and specific to the neurological system are found in Box 34-1.

Skills 360°

Gathering a Patient History

The nurse asks the following:

Reason for seeking health care?

Symptoms?

When did problem start?

When is it worst?

What makes it worse?

What makes it better?

Associated symptoms?

Physical Examination

The physical assessment examines in detail the function of the CNS. The examination evaluates six areas of neurological function: mental status, cranial nerves, motor, cerebellum, senses, and reflexes. Based on the health history,

TABLE 34-4 Glasgow Coma Scale

CATEGORY	RESPONSE	SCORE
Eyes open	Spontaneous—eyes open without verbal or noxious stimuli	4
	To speech—eyes open with verbal stimuli	3
	To pain—eyes open to noxious stimuli	2
	None—no eye opening with any form of stimuli	1
Verbal response	Oriented—aware of person, place, time, and personal data	5
	Confused—answers inappropriate, but language use correct	4
	Inappropriate words—disorganized, random speech	3
	Incomprehensible sounds—moans, groans, and mumbles	2
	None—no verbal response, even to noxious stimuli	1
Best motor response	Obeys commands—performs simple tasks and repeat on command	6
	Localizes pain—organized attempt to remove noxious stimuli	5
	Withdraws from pain—withdraws from source of noxious stimuli	4
	Abnormal flexion—occurs spontaneously or to noxious stimuli	3
	Abnormal extension—occurs spontaneously or to noxious stimuli	2
	None—no response to noxious stimuli; flaccid	1

Adapted from Estes, M. (2006). Health assessment and physical examination *(3rd ed.). New York: Thomson Delmar Learning.*

the nurse may decide to do a focused or a complete, baseline assessment. The baseline assessment data is useful for future comparison throughout the hospital course.

Mental Status

Subtle changes in mental status are one of the earliest indicators of a potential neurological event. The nurse needs a thorough baseline assessment for comparison, should changes occur. The components of the mental status examination include general appearance, behavior, speech, LOC, mentation, and cognitive function. Much of this information is gathered when doing the health history. When first introduced to the patient, the nurse should observe the patient's gait, posture, and general appearance. The patient's speech patterns, mood, and are evaluated throughout the interviewing and examining process. When assessing the LOC, use questions concerning the time, date or day of the week, location, and situation. To test memory, the nurse should ask questions that require specific answers. For example, "What is the name of the president?" or "What is the name of the last president?" Ask problem solving questions such as, "Subtract 7 from 100, and keep subtracting 7." The nurse should ask the patient to demonstrate simple requests. A simple request might be "Show me two fingers." Then ask the patient to do a more complicated task, such as, "Pick up your pen and write down a list of three words." Instruct the

BOX 34-1

NEUROLOGICAL ASSESSMENT QUESTIONS

Health Perception—Health Management Pattern

Have you ever been diagnosed with a neurologic illness? Seizures? Stroke? Brain or spinal cord injury? Infections of the brain or spinal cord? Brain or spinal cord tumors?
Have you ever been unable to move any body part? If yes, explain.
Any problem thinking clearly? If yes, explain.
Are you having any problems with your ability to see, hear, taste, or smell? If yes, explain.
Have you ever had any diagnostic tests for a neurological problem? If yes, explain.
Do you take any medications for a neurological problem? If yes, explain.
Do you use tobacco products or recreational drugs or drink alcohol? If yes, explain.
What safety practices do you use in a car? On a motorcycle? On a bicycle? Describe.

Nutrition—Metabolic Pattern

Describe your usual dietary intake for a 24-hour period.
Do you have difficulty chewing or swallowing your food?
Are you able to feed yourself? If no, explain.

Elimination Pattern

Has there been any change in your usual pattern of urinary or bowel elimination? If yes, explain.
Do you use laxatives, suppositories, or enemas to assist with bowel elimination? If yes, explain.
Are you able to go to the bathroom independently? If not, explain.
Do you postpone defecation? If yes, explain.
Has your doctor prescribed any medications to manage these problems? If yes, what?

Activity—Exercise Pattern

Describe your typical physical activities in a 24-hour period.
Do you have difficulty with balance, walking, or coordination? If yes, explain.
Do you use any assistive devices for ambulation? If yes, explain.
Do you have any weakness in your arms or legs? If yes, explain.
Do you trip or fall easily? If yes, explain.
Are you able to move all parts of your body? If no, explain.
If you have seizures, describe any precipitating factors, where it begins on your body, and how you feel afterward.
Have you ever experienced shakiness or tremors? If yes, explain.
Does this neurological problem prevent you from performing your activities of daily living? If yes, explain.

Sleep—Rest Pattern

Does your health problem interfere with your ability to sleep and rest? If yes, explain.
Do you take any medications to assist with falling asleep? If yes, what?
Do you ever have pain that awakens you at night? If yes, explain.
Describe your energy level.
Does sleep or rest restore your energy level? If no, explain.

Cognitive—Perceptual Pattern

Do you experience headaches? If yes, describe including frequency, type, location, and precipitating or relieving factors.
Do you ever feel dizzy or faint? If yes, explain.
Do you ever feel like the room is spinning? If yes, explain.
Do you ever experience burning, numbness, or tingling sensations? If yes, describe.
Do you ever experience blurring, double vision, or blind spots? If yes, describe.
Do you ever have problems with your hearing? If yes, explain.
Have you noticed a change in your ability to taste or smell? If yes, explain.
Do you ever have difficulty remembering things? If yes, explain.

Self-Perception—Self-Concept Pattern

How has this problem you are experiencing affected the way you feel about yourself? Describe.
Has the problem changed the way you feel about your life? If yes, explain.
How do you feel about any changes in your life because of this problem? Describe.

Role—Relationship Pattern

Is there a family history of neurological problems? If yes, explain.
Do you ever have difficulty expressing yourself and making others understand? If yes, explain.
How has having neurological problems affected your role in your family? Describe.
How has having neurological problems affected your interactions with family? With friends? At work? In social activities?
Has this problem affected your ability to work? If yes, explain.

Sexuality—Reproductive Pattern

Have your usual sexual activities been altered by this problem? If yes, explain.

BOX 34-1

NEUROLOGICAL ASSESSMENT QUESTIONS—cont'd

Sexuality—Reproductive Pattern—cont'd

Have you ever received information on alternative methods for sexual expression, if this problem impairs your usual sexual activity? If yes, explain.

Describe how having neurological problems makes you feel about yourself as a man or woman.

Coping—Stress Pattern

Describe what you do to cope with stress.

Has this neurological problem affected the way you normally cope with stress? If yes, explain.

Does increased stress make your neurological problems worse? If yes, explain.

What do you believe is the most stressful time you have had with this problem? Describe.

How will you be able to cope with stress from this problem? Describe.

Value—Belief Pattern

Are there activities, practices, or significant others that help you cope with this problem? If yes, describe.

What do you see as your greatest source of inner strength? Describe.

What do you perceive for the future with this problem? Describe.

Adapted from Daniels, R. (2004). Nursing fundamentals: Caring and clinical decision making. *New York: Thomson Delmar Learning; Estes, M. (2006).* Health assessment and physical examination *(3rd ed.). New York: Thomson Delmar Learning.*

Uncovering the Evidence

Evaluating Cognition in Patients

Discussion: The Mini-Mental State Examination (MMSE) is a useful tool for screening mental functioning. The tool measures orientation, immediate memory, short-term memory, and language functioning. There are some limitations to its use, because it is a verbal tool. People from different cultural groups or those with lower levels of education may score poorly.

Implications for Practice: The MMSE is a reliable clinical assessment tool that can be used for a rapid, screening evaluation of mental state or cognitive function. It takes approximately 10–15 minutes to administer. Scoring of points is 0–30. The lower the score, the more severe the alteration of mental state. This tool can be used to track changes over time.

Source: Folstein, M., Folstein, S., & McHugh, P. (1975). Mini-mental state: A practical method for grading the cognitive state of patients for the clinician. Journal of Psychiatric Research, 12*(3), 189–198.*

patient to remember the words, because you will ask him or her what they were in a few minutes. This is a simple way to test memory. Problems with the patient's ability to remember directions have implications for patient education (Crimlisk & Grande, 2004).

Cranial Nerves

Assessment of cranial nerve function is an essential component of the complete neurological examination. Because the cranial nerves are in pairs, each side must be evaluated separately. Findings from each side are then compared for symmetry.

CN I: Olfactory Nerve

This nerve should only be tested if the patient has indicated there is a problem. The sense of smell is tested by having the patient occlude one nostril and close his or her eyes. The examiner then takes a cotton ball soaked with a common, nonir-

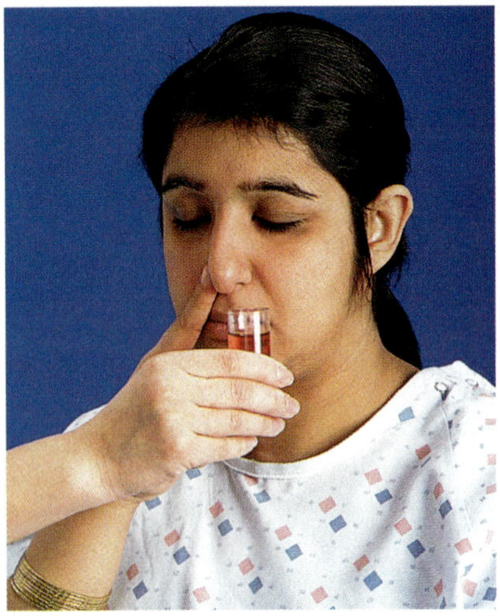

Figure 34-10 Testing of CN I (smell).

ritating substance and places it near the nonoccluded nostril (Figure 34-10). Repeat the process for the opposite side using a different scent.

Some common odors that patients should be able to identify if CN I is intact are: cloves, cinnamon, mint, citrus, or coffee. **Anosmia,** the loss or impairment of smell, can be seen with lesions of the frontal lobe or impaired blood flow to the MCA.

CN II: Optic Nerve

The optic nerve is the only cranial nerve that can be examined directly. Testing includes assessment of both visual acuity and visual fields. Each eye is examined separately while the patient covers the other one.

Visual acuity is tested by having the patient read a Snellen chart from 20 feet away (Figure 34-11). Have the patient start with one eye covered and read the lines from top to bottom (largest to smallest letters). Record the lowest line that the patient can read with 50 percent accuracy. Then have the patient cover the other eye and repeat the test. Lastly, have the patient read the chart using both eyes. You may test the patient who wears glasses with or without his or her glasses. The Rosenbaum pocket vision screener is a portable version of the Snellen chart. It is designed for bedside assessment of visual acuity. If these options are not available, have the patient randomly read from a newspaper or magazine. This will give you a gross evaluation of the patient's visual acuity.

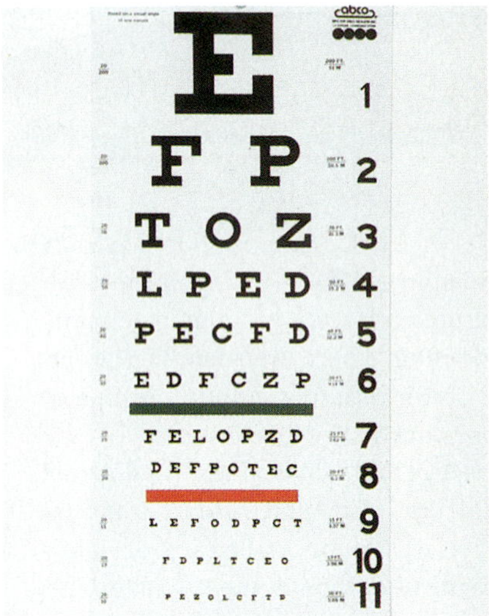

Figure 34-11 Snellen chart.

Testing of the visual fields assesses the peripheral vision and functioning of the macula. One method of testing is called the confrontation test (Figure 34-12). In this test, the examiner stands or sits directly in front of the patient to be tested, at a distance of 18 to 24 inches. Eyes should be at the same level. Ask the patient to cover one eye. The examiner acts as a control and covers his or her opposite eye. Using a penlight, start at the periphery and move toward the center from right to left, above, below, and from the middle of each direction. Both the examiner and the patient should see the penlight move into his or her peripheral vision, at the same time (Estes, 2006). Abnormal findings of blindness or impaired vision in one or both eyes may be found in patients with transient ischemic attacks (TIA) or CVA.

Another assessment technique is called cardinal fields of vision or extraocular movements. For this test, the examiner stands facing the patient. Ask the patient to hold his or her head still and follow the penlight with his or her eyes only. Move the penlight through the six cardinal fields one at a time, returning to the central starting point before proceeding to the next field. Abnormal findings are failure of one or both eyes to follow the penlight in any direction may indicate weakness of the extraocular muscles. **Nystagmus** is an involuntary rhythmic movement of the eyes. It can be associated with neurological disorders or some medications.

CN III: Oculomotor Nerve, CN IV: Trochlear Nerve, and CN VI: Abducens Nerve

These cranial nerves are usually tested together, because they control the function of the extraocular eye muscles. The functions include: eyelid elevation, constriction of the pupils, and movement of the eye through the six cardinal directions. First observe how much of the iris is covered by the eyelid. Normally, about one third is covered. If more is covered, the patient has **ptosis** or drooping of the eyelid, usually from paralysis of CN III, myasthenia gravis (MG), or sympathetic innervation. Second, dim the room lights then assess the size, shape, and constriction of the pupils using a penlight. Have the patient focus on a distant object, hold the light about 8 inches from one eye in the patient's peripheral field of vision, and shine it directly into one of the pupils. Observe for constriction of the pupil in this eye, which is a direct reaction, and observe for constriction in the other eye, which is a consensual reaction. Both pupils should constrict at the same time. Note if the reaction is brisk (4+), less than brisk (3+), slow (2+), very sluggish (1+), or absent (0).

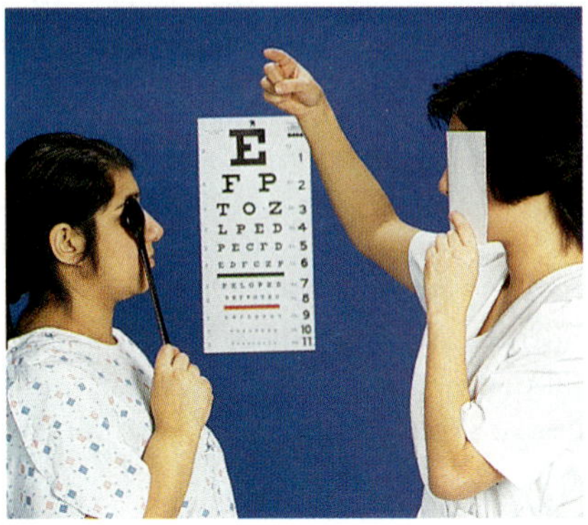

Figure 34-12 Testing visual fields by confrontation.

Repeat the assessment in the other eye. Third, test for convergence (eyes turning inward) and accommodation (pupils constricting with near vision). Hold a finger 8 to 12 inches from the bridge of the patient's nose. Instruct the patient to hold his or her head still, focus on a distant spot, and just move his or her eyes to the commands. Have the patient look at a finger, then the distant spot, and back again. Normally the pupils should constrict and converge equally. Normal findings for CN III, IV, and VI are documented as PERRLA which stands for pupils equal, round, and reactive to light and accommodation. Abnormal findings in patients reveal a dysfunction of these nerves causing them to complain of having difficulty climbing steps, because they are unable to look down or symptoms of **diplopia,** which is blurry or double vision (Almefty, Webber, & Arnautovic, 2006).

CN V: Trigeminal Nerve

The trigeminal nerve is the largest of the cranial nerves and has both motor and sensory components. Testing of the sensory component involves light touch and pinprick in each of the three divisions, ophthalmic, maxillary, and mandibular, of the nerve on both sides of the face. The patient should have his or her eyes closed during the testing procedure. Next, the motor component is evaluated. The strength of the mastication, masseter, and temporal muscles are evaluated by palpating them when the jaw is opened and then closed. The nurse should note differences in the tone or atrophy of the muscles bilaterally. Corneal reflexes, on the conscious patient, can be observed by having the examiner move his or her hand or a small object rapidly toward the patient's face. Observe for blinking. In the patient with a decreased LOC, testing of the corneal reflex involves the light touching of the cornea with a cotton wisp.

Abnormal findings reveal a loss of corneal reflexes indicates lesions of both CN V (sensory) and CN VIII (motor). Patients with lesions of CN V (motor), or after a CVA, may lose sensation or the ability to chew effectively. Severe facial pain is seen with trigeminal neuralgia (tic douloureux).

CN VII: Facial Nerve

The facial nerve is also a mixed cranial nerve with both sensory and motor components. The sensory component includes the sense of taste on the anterior two thirds of the tongue. The testing of the sensory component is often deferred, unless changes are noted in the health history interview. When tested, have the patient stick out his or her tongue and test each side separately. There are four classic modalities of taste: sweet (tip of tongue), sour (sides of tongue), salty (over most of tongue, but concentrated on the sides), and bitter (back of tongue, controlled by CN IX). A fifth taste modality (umami) has been known for approximately 100 years, but was recently added to the list once specific receptors were identified (Ganong, 2003). It is triggered by glutamate, specifically monosodium glutamate (MSG), which is used extensively in Asian cooking. The taste is sweet and pleasant, but different from the standard sweet taste. To test the patient, ask him or her to identify the different tastes as they are applied one at a time to the appropriate location on the tongue. Have the patient rinse his or her mouth with water between tests. Remember that a bitter taste is innervated by CN IX. Taste abnormalities include: **ageusia** (absence of the sense of taste), **hypogeusia** (diminished taste sensitivity), and **dysgeusia** (disturbed sense of taste). Many diseases and certain drugs can produce hypogeusia or dysgeusia (Zavarella, Leblebicioglu, Claman, & Tatakis, 2006).

When testing the motor component of the facial nerve, first observe the face for any asymmetry of the patient's features or facial movements. Observe for facial tics. Then, ask the patient to perform the following movements: raise his or her eyebrows, close his or her eyelids tightly, puff out his or her cheeks, smile, and frown. Observe for weakness or asymmetry of muscle movement. Abnormal findings of upper motor neuron lesions, lower motor neuron lesions, or a stroke can cause weakness or paralysis of the facial muscles (Crimlisk & Grande, 2004).

CN VIII: Acoustic Nerve

The acoustic nerve has two divisions: the cochlear and the vestibular. The cochlear division is involved in hearing. The vestibular division is involved in the sense of balance, which includes equilibrium, coordination, and orientation in space. First, examine the patient's ear canals for obvious blockages or malformations. Also check for excess cerumen (earwax), which may interfere with balance or hearing. Testing of the cochlear division is done by having the patient close his or her eyes and indicate when he or she hears the ticking of a watch or the rubbing of the examiner's fingers. Normal findings are when the patient can hear the watch or rustling 4 to 6 inches away. This test identifies only gross deficits, and deviations are indications for referral for a more comprehensive evaluation.

Next, check for lateralization and air and bone conduction. The Weber's test is used to evaluate lateralization, and the Rinne's test evaluates air-bone conduction. For the Weber's test, vibrate the tuning fork, place it at the center of the patient's forehead, and ask if the sound is heard equally in both ears. If not, ask the patient to describe the differences.

Normally, the sound is heard equally in both ears. In the Rinne test, both air conduction and bone conduction are tested. For the Rinne test, place the base of the lightly vibrating tuning fork firmly on the mastoid process. Ask the patient to note when the vibration is no longer felt. Quickly place the still vibrating tuning fork near the ear with the tines toward the ear. Ask the patient to note when the sound can no longer be heard. Normally, the sound should be heard longer through air than bone. Abnormal findings from either test are indications for further investigation. Testing of the vestibular portion of CN VIII is usually done during testing of the motor or cerebellar systems.

CN IX: Glossopharyngeal Nerve and CN X: Vagus Nerve

The glossopharyngeal and vagus nerves are usually tested together, because they innervate many of the same structures. In the pharynx, CN IX is primarily sensory, and CN X is mostly motor. First, take note of the patient's voice quality. If the patient is hoarse or has a nasal quality, he or she may have vocal cord lesions or paralysis. Second, observe the patient as he or she swallows a small amount of water. Ask if he or she frequently chokes on food or has trouble swallowing. **Dysphagia** (difficulty swallowing) can often be seen after neurosurgical procedures or CVA (stroke). Next, ask the patient to say "ah" and observe his or her uvula. It should move up and not deviate to the side. The palate should also move up when the patient opens his or her mouth. Observe for any asymmetrical movements. Lastly, tell the patient that the gag reflex will be checked next. Use a tongue blade to touch the back of the patient's throat lightly on each side. Loss of the gag reflex occurs with lesions of CN IX and CN X.

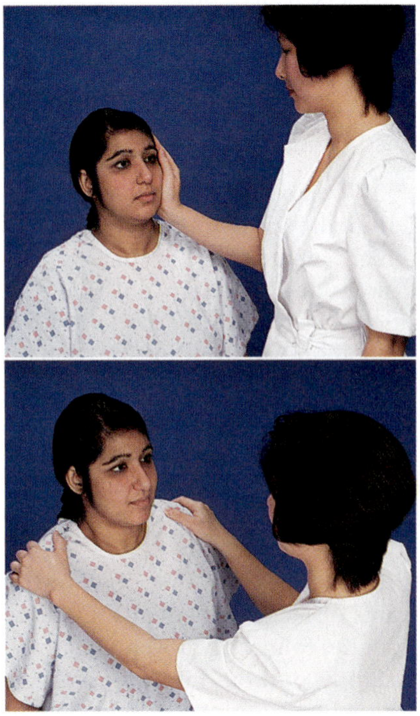

Figure 34-13 Testing CN XI.

CN XI: Spinal Accessory Nerve

The spinal accessory nerve is tested in two segments: trapezius muscles and sternocleidomastoid muscles. Assessment of the trapezius is done by the examiner placing his or her hands on the patient's shoulders. Then, ask the patient to shrug his or her shoulders. Observe for strength and symmetry. The sternocleidomastoid muscles are assessed by the examiner placing his or her hand on one cheek and asking the patient to turn his or her head against a hand as the movement is resisted. (Figure 34-13). Again, observe for strength and symmetry. Repeat the test on the opposite side of the head. Abnormal findings are muscle weakness which can be seen with lower motor neuron disease or in some CVAs.

CN XII: Hypoglossal Nerve

The hypoglossal nerve is tested by asking the patient to open his or her mouth, stick out his or her tongue, and wiggle it side to side. The tongue should be midline. Observe for asymmetry, atrophy, or fasciculations. Carotid endarterectomy is a common cause of dysfunction of CN XII. During the surgical procedure, the nerve can be stretched causing temporary weakness or severed causing permanent dysfunction.

Motor Function

The nerves of the motor system originate from the spinal cord and control muscle movement. The motor examination begins with the neck and proceeds from proximal to distal extremities. Major muscle groups are assessed for specific functions. Each muscle is evaluated for symmetry, size, tone, and strength. First, note the size and contour of each muscle or muscle group. Subtle differences may require measurement of the muscle pair and comparing for differences. Observe for any muscle wasting, atrophy, or hypertrophy. Muscle atrophy is seen with lower motor neuron lesions. Next, assess for tremors and fasciculations. Observe patient movements both at rest and with activity. With the patient relaxed, the examiner puts the joints through normal range of motion. Start with the shoulders and move systematically: elbow, wrist, fingers, hip, knee, and ankle. Compare assessment findings from both sides.

Abnormalities of muscle tone include spasticity, rigidity, and flaccidity. Spasticity, or hypertonia, refers to increased motor tone. The tone is greater with rapid movement than with slow movement. Spasticity is the result of injury to upper motor neurons. Rigidity is increased resistance that persists throughout movement and is related to lesions of the basal ganglia. Flaccidity, or hypotonia, refers to the decrease or loss of muscle tone. The muscle is weak, soft, and floppy. Flaccidity is due to lower motor lesions.

Muscle strength is assessed by having the patient move a specific muscle or group of muscles first against gravity then with resistance provided by the examiner. After each muscle group is assessed, it is graded according to the scale in Table 34-5. Findings are documented as a fraction with the numerator being the patient's score and the denominator as 5 for the maximum score possible.

Possible abnormal findings include weakness, hemiplegia, or paralysis. Weakness is seen with transient ischemic attacks (TIA) and some CVAs. Hemiplegia is found with CVAs. Paralysis is found in patients with MS, MG, and spinal cord injuries (SCI).

TABLE 34-5 Grading Scale for Muscle Strength

GRADE	STRENGTH
5	Active movement against gravity; full resistance; normal muscle movement
4	Active movement against gravity; some resistance; examiner can overcome the patient's muscle resistance
3	Active movement against gravity
2	Active movement of body part when gravity eliminated
1	Weak palpated muscle contraction; no active movement noted
0	No muscle contraction noted

Adapted from Estes, M. (2006). Health assessment and physical examination *(3rd ed.). New York: Thomson Delmar Learning.*

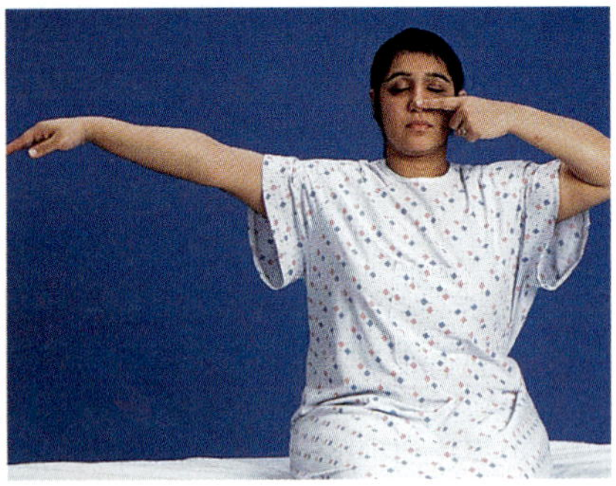

Figure 34-14 Testing coordination.

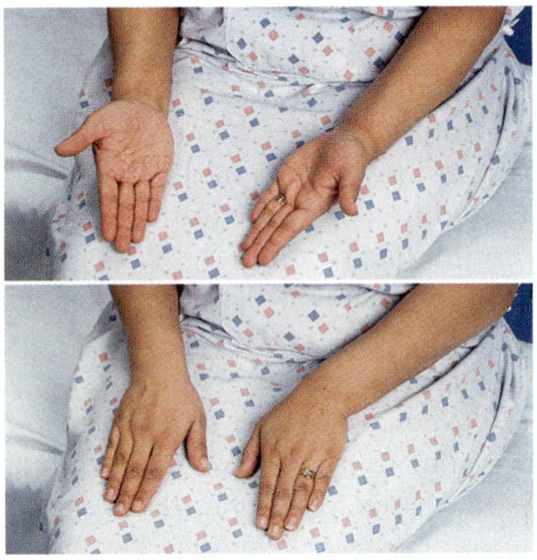

Figure 34-15 Rapid alternating movements.

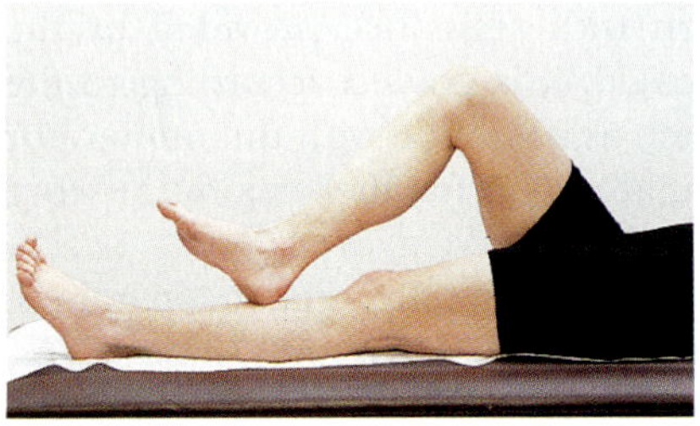

Figure 34-16 Heel slide.

Cerebellar Function

Evaluation of cerebellar function requires the assessment of coordination, balance, posture, and gait. Coordination involves the smooth, precise movement of multiple muscle groups. Testing can be done, using multiple techniques, with the patient sitting up. First, instruct the patient to sit with arms outstretched, eyes open, and facing the examiner. Ask the patient to touch his or her nose with one index finger, then the opposite finger. Have him or her rapidly alternate sides, and then close his or her eyes and continue to rapidly alternate sides (Figure 34-14). Observe for intention tremor or inability to accurately complete the task. Second, ask the patient to rapidly alternate patting his or her knees, first with the palms and then alternating palms with the backs of his or her hands (Figure 34-15). Third, finger coordination is tested by having the patient repeatedly touch his or her thumb to each finger sequentially. Repeat test with opposite fingers. Observe coordination and ability to perform tasks in rapid sequence. Fourth, with the patient either seated or supine, have him or her place one heel on the opposite shin, just below the knee, and slide the heel from the knee to the foot. Repeat on opposite heel (Figure 34-16). Observe leg coordination. Fifth, ask the patient to draw a circle or figure eight with his or her foot either on the floor or in the air. Repeat with the other foot (Figure 34-17). Observe for coordination and regularity of the drawing. Lastly, ask the patient to rapidly flex and extend the toes of one foot. Repeat on the opposite foot. Observe for rate rhythm, smoothness, and accuracy of the requested movements.

Abnormal Findings

Cerebellar disease is the cause of **dyssynergy,** which is a lack of coordinated muscle movement; **dysmetria,** which is impaired judgment of distance, range, speed, and force of movement; and **dysdiadochokinesia,** which is the inability to perform rapidly alternating movements.

The examiner tests balance by having the patient walk heel to toe along a line. Then have the patient walk on his or her toes, only. Follow with walking on his or her heels only. An alternative procedure is to have the patient hop on one foot and then the other. Protect the patient from falls.

Lesions of the cerebellar hemisphere (stroke or tumors) cause the patient to fall toward the affected side, and **ataxia,** a lack of muscle coordination, is observed. Midline cerebellar lesions cause a wide-based gait, and the patient is unable to perform tandem walking.

Posture and gait should be evaluated in ambulatory patients. Posture is the position or awareness of the body in space. Gait is the manner in which the patient walks. The examiner observes the patient walking and whether the patient uses assistive devices. This examination is made without shoes or socks, if possible. The nurse must be prepared to protect the patient from falls or injury. The nurse must ask the patient to walk back and forth in the examination area. Observe and note: gait, smooth or staggering, position of feet, normal or broad-based, symmetry of arm and leg movements, presence of uncoordinated movements or tremors, step height, normal, high, shuffling, and step length (normal, short, or long). Also, make note of the ease of turning and number of steps needed to turn.

Patients with Parkinson's disease stoop over while walking, shuffle their feet, and hold their arms close to their body. Patients with polyneuropathy walk on their heels and then their toes with the feet held wide apart. Often these patients stagger and watch the floor while walking, and their gait becomes worse when asked to close their eyes.

Romberg's Test

Ask the patient to stand erect, feet together, arms at his or her side, and eyes open. Stand close to the patient during the test to protect him or her, should he or she begin to fall. Repeat test with eyes closed. Observe for ability to main-

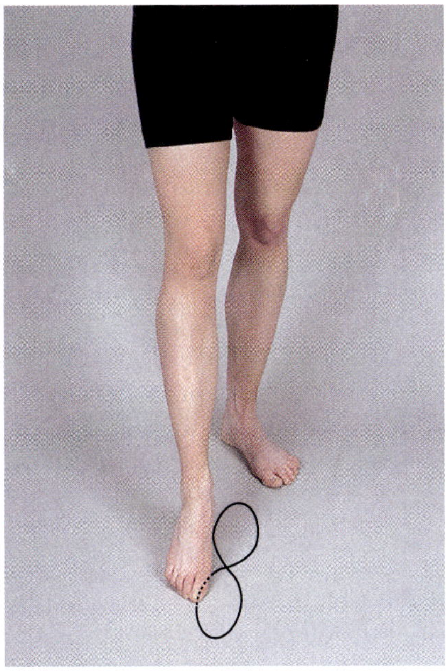

Figure 34-17 Testing coordination (Figure eight).

TABLE 34-6 Sensory Rating Scale

RATING	FINDINGS
Normal	
Present, but diminished (abnormal)	
Absent	

Adapted from Estes, M. (2006). Health assessment and physical examination *(3rd ed.). New York: Thomson Delmar Learning.*

tain balance for 20 seconds with minimal swaying. Abnormal findings of cerebellar lesions (CVA or tumors) cause the unsteadiness.

Sensory Function

Evaluation of the sensory system tests the patient's ability to perceive various types of sensations. The body areas usually assessed are face, neck, deltoid regions, forearms, top part of the hands, chest, abdomen, thighs, lower legs, and top of the feet. See Table 34-6 for rating scale for sensory assessment.

Superficial sensation is tested using various modalities: light touch, pain, and temperature. First, ask the patient to close his or her eyes. The examiner uses a wisp of cotton to touch each of the assessment areas. Instruct the patient to indicate verbally when the stimulus is felt. Vary the stimulation sites to prevent the patient from anticipating subsequent areas. Compare both sides. Second, for assessment of pain use a disposable object (broken wooden applicator or open paperclip) to demonstrate sharp and dull sensations. Be sure to not use an item that will break or puncture the patient's skin. Dispose of your testing object when exam is completed. Ask the patient to close his or her eyes. Instruct the patient to indicate verbally when the stimulus is felt. Vary the stimulation sites to prevent the patient from anticipating subsequent areas. Compare both sides. Third, temperature is tested be using test tubes, one with warm water and one with cold water. Instruct the patient to indicate verbally when the stimulus is felt. Vary the stimulation sites to prevent the patient from anticipating the next area. Compare both sides. This portion of the sensory exam is normal when the patient is able to correctly identify light touch, superficial pain, and temperature accurately.

Abnormal findings of lesions of the peripheral nerves, brainstem, or spinal cord may cause **anesthesia** (absence of touch sensation), **hypesthesia** (diminished sense of touch), **paresthesia** (numbness, tingling, or prickling sensation), or **dysesthesia** (burning or tingling).

Lesions of the thalamus and peripheral nerves may cause: **analgesia** (insensitivity to pain), **hypalgesia** (diminished sensitivity to pain), or **hypergesia** (increased sensitivity to pain).

Deep sensation evaluates vibration, deep pressure pain, position, and discriminates fine touch. To test vibration a vibrating tuning fork is placed on the bony prominences (thumb and great toe). Instruct the patient to indicate verbally when the stimulus is first felt and again when it is no longer felt (Figure 34-18). Compare both sides. Normally, the patient should be able to sense vibration over the bony prominences.

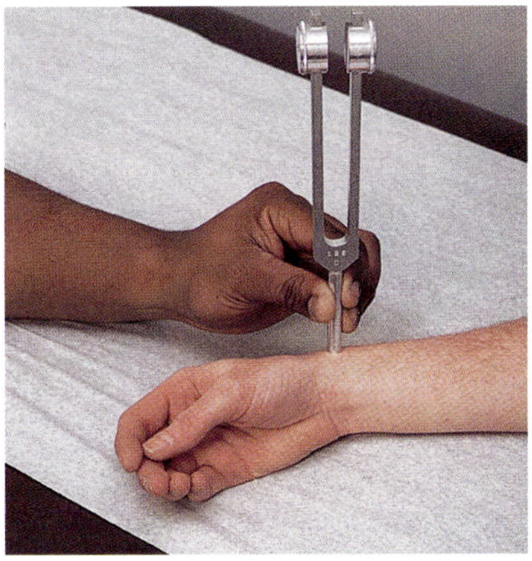

Figure 34-18 Sensory: vibration.

Abnormal findings of some spinal cord lesions and polyneuropathies can cause loss of the vibratory sense. It is normally diminished in the elderly. When testing deep pressure pain the examiner squeezes the Achilles tendon, calf, and forearm muscle. Compare both sides. Note the patient's response. Next, the examiner tests position sense. Instruct the patient to close his or her eyes. Lightly grasp the patient's finger or great toe and gently move it up or down. Instruct the patient to indicate verbally which direction the digit is in. Vary the direction to prevent the patient from anticipating the digit location. Compare both sides. Abnormal findings of lesions of the posterior column of the spinal cord can affect the position sense.

Lastly, assessment of discriminate fine touch involves **stereognosis** (identify objects by touch) and **graphesthesia** (identify letters, numbers, or shapes drawn on hand). To test for stereognosis, ask the patient to close his or her eyes and place an object, such as a coin, paper clip, or key, into the patient's hand. Instruct the patient to feel the object. Ask the patient to name the object. Abnormal findings of dysfunction of the parietal lobe can cause **astereognosis** (lack of ability to identify objects by touch).

To test graphesthesia, first ask the patient to close his or her eyes. Then the examiner draws a letter, number, or shape in the patient's open hand. Repeat on the opposite side. Abnormal findings of lesions of the sensory cortex can cause a loss of the ability to identify letters or shapes when drawn on the palm.

Reflex Testing

Assessment of reflexes provides important information on the status of the CNS in both conscious and unconscious patients. Altered reflexes may be the earliest signs of a pathological condition. There are three categories of reflexes: deep tendon, cutaneous, and pathological. DTRs (muscle-stretch reflexes) occur in response to a sudden stimulus (e.g., tapping with a reflex hammer). It is important to use the correct technique to elicit the specific reflex. With the muscle relaxed and the joint in neutral position and supported by the examiner, the tendon is tapped directly with the reflex hammer. Normally the muscle contracts with a quick movement of the limb or structure. Both sides of the body are tested and assigned a score based on the scale in Table 34-7.

First, test the biceps reflex, by having the patient flex his or her arm slightly, with the palm up. Support the patient's arm at the elbow, with your thumb over the biceps tendon in the antecubital space. Strike your thumb with the reflex hammer. The biceps muscle should contract, and the arm should flex slightly. Repeat on the opposite side. To test the triceps tendon, support the patient's arm flexed at a 90-degree angle and strike the triceps tendon between the epicondyles just above the elbow. The muscle should contract and the elbow extends slightly. Repeat on the opposite side. Next, to test the brachioradialis reflex, support the patient's arm, flexed slightly with the palm down. Strike the radius, about two inches above the wrist. The forearm should rotate laterally and the palm turns upward. Repeat on the opposite side. For testing of the patellar reflex, the legs should be dangling. The examiner places his or

TABLE 34-7 Deep Tendon Reflex Rating Scale

RATING	FINDINGS
4+	Very brisk; hyperactive
3+	More brisk than normal
2+	Normal; average
1+	Diminished; sluggish; minimal
0	No response

Note: All reflexes are documented by a plus sign. There are no minuses used when rating DTRs.

Adapted from Estes, M. (2006). Health assessment and physical examination *(3rd ed.). New York: Thomson Delmar Learning.*

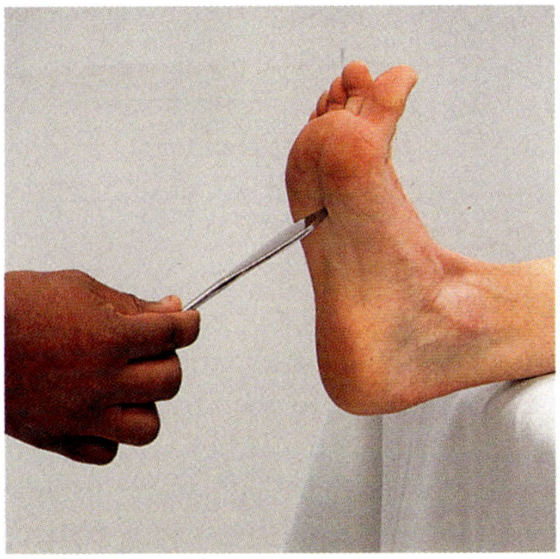

Figure 34-19 Testing of plantar reflex.

TABLE 34-8 Pathological Reflexes

REFLEX	TECHNIQUE
Grasp	Stimulation of palm results in a grasp.
Snout	Stimulation of circumoral region results in puckering of lips.
Sucking	Stimulation of lips, tongue, or palate results in sucking movement.
Rooting	Stimulation of lips results in head moving toward stimulus.
Palmomental	Stimulation of palm results in contraction of the chin muscles.
Glabellar	Eyes blink each time the glabellar area (between eyes) is tapped. Normal: blinking stops after first few taps.

Adapted from Estes, M. (2006). Health assessment and physical examination *(3rd ed.). New York: Thomson Delmar Learning.*

her hand on the patient's thigh and strikes the distal patellar tendon just below the kneecap. The quadricep muscle contracts and the knee extends slightly. Repeat on the opposite side. When testing the Achilles tendon, the examiner supports the patient's foot, slightly dorsiflexed. Lightly strike the Achilles tendon behind the ankle. The foot should plantar flex. Repeat on the opposite side. The plantar reflex (also called Babinski's sign) is tested with the foot in the neutral position. With a moderately sharp object (key or the handle of a reflex hammer), stroke the lateral aspect of the sole from the heel to the ball of the foot, curving medially across the ball (Figure 34-19). Use the lightest stroke required for a response. Normal response is flexion of the toes. Abnormal findings of forsiflexion of the great toe with fanning of the other toes can indicate upper motor neuron pathology.

Cutaneous reflexes are elicited by light, rapid stroking, or scratching of the tissue. The major reflexes tested are: corneal, gag, swallow, upper abdominal, lower abdominal, cremasteric, bulbocavernous, and perianal. Corneal reflexes (CN V or CN VII), gag, and swallow reflexes (CN IX or CN X), were discussed in assessment of the cranial nerves. The cremasteric, bulbocavernous, and perianal are not routinely checked. To test the abdominal reflexes, have the patient supine with clothing moved out of the testing area. Lightly but briskly stroke each assessment area using a tongue blade or warmed handle of reflex hammer. The grading of cutaneous reflexes differs from that used with DTRs. They are graded as either present (+) or absent (0). If present but weak, they are documented as weak. Abnormal findings of absent reflexes can indicate both upper and lower motor neuron pathology.

Pathological reflexes are also called primitive reflexes, because they are seen in infants and then disappear. If these reflexes reappear, they are found in patient's suffering from dementia syndromes or Parkinson's disease. Table 34-8 describes the assessment techniques. Grading of pathological reflexes is documented as presence (+) is abnormal and absence (−) is normal.

DIAGNOSTIC TESTS

Neurodiagnostic tests are performed as adjuncts to a complete history and physical examination. Health care providers can then correlate results from the neurodiagnostic tests with clinical effectiveness of various treatment modalities. Knowledge of the tests, pretest preparation, testing procedure, and necessary follow-up care will facilitate patient teaching by the nurse.

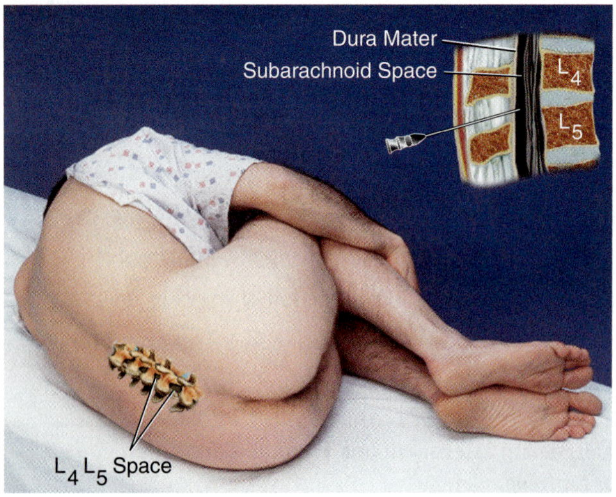

Figure 34-20 Lumbar puncture.

Lumbar Puncture

A lumbar puncture (LP) is the most common method for obtaining CSF for analysis. This test is performed to examine the CSF for pathologies associated with specific diseases (Daniels, 2003).

Nursing Management

Explain the procedure to patient. Inform patient that the test is performed with he or she lying in the lateral recumbent position with knees flexed. Encourage oral fluid intake. Patient is to empty his or her bladder before the test starts. Baseline assessment includes vital signs and neurological status. Blood coagulation values should be checked before the test in all patients taking anticoagulation medications. Administer premedication if ordered.

The patient is placed in the lateral recumbent position with knees flexed (Figure 34-20). Using sterile technique, the practitioner inserts a hollow-core needle into the subarachnoid space, usually at L3–L4 or L4–L5. Once proper placement in the subarachnoid space is confirmed, instruct the patient to relax. Opening and closing pressure readings are documented. Three to five test tubes of CSF are usually collected and numbered sequentially. After the needle is withdrawn, pressure is held for one to two minutes, and a bandage strip applied to the insertion site. The tubes are sent to the laboratory for analysis. See Table 34-9 for a discussion of CSF analysis.

Maintain strict bed rest for a few hours as ordered. Encourage oral fluids. Monitor and compare vital sign and neurological assessment to baseline findings. Administer analgesia as needed.

Radiographic Studies

There are a variety of radiographic studies that are performed as diagnostic procedures. Radiological exams send radiation through the body to form a picture of the internal structures. X-rays turn film black, so areas that allow

TABLE 34-9 Cerebrospinal Fluid Analysis

PARAMETER	NORMAL VALUE	ANALYSIS OF ABNORMAL FINDINGS
Opening pressure	60–200 mm H_2O	Less than 60—dehydration; blocked CSF.
		Greater than 200—brain tumor, abscess, or cyst; subdural hematoma; hydrocephalus; cerebral edema.
Appearance	clear, colorless	Xanthochromia is often due to the breakdown of blood products. Turbidity or cloudiness is often due to increased white blood cells (WBCs), elevated protein levels, or infection.
Red blood cells (RBCs)	none	Cell count of RBCs indicates bleeding; serial reduction of RBCs in tubes sent from lumbar puncture (LP), may indicate a traumatic LP.
WBCs	0–8 μ/L	Elevations may indicate meningitis, tumors, and multiple sclerosis.
Protein	15–45 mg/dL	Elevations with infection, tumor, or hemorrhage.
Glucose	45–75 mg/dL	Elevations are not significant; a decrease indicates infection.
Microorganisms	none	
pH	7.35	
Specific gravity	1.007	

Adapted from Daniels, R. (2003). Delmar's manual of laboratory and diagnostic tests. *New York: Thomson Delmar Learning.*

> **Safety First 1**
>
> **Safety Precautions When Assisting with a Lumbar Puncture (LP)**
>
> When assisting the health care provider with a LP, the nurse needs to ensure the safety of the patient during the procedure. If the patient is unable to maintain a fetal position (knees held close to the chest by his or her arms), the nurse should assist the patient. The patient is positioned on the side, with his or her back close to the edge of the table. Standing on the opposite side of the table, facing the patient, the nurse should hold behind the patients bent knees and neck to gently maintain the examination position. It may be necessary to place a pillow under the patient's head or between his or her knees to maintain body alignment. If the patient is restless or unable to cooperate, two people may be needed to assist.

radiation to pass easily appear dark, while areas that block radiation appear white. Therefore, air-filled lungs appear blackish on X-ray, while bones appear white. X-rays are used in several basic ways; the most common are standard (plain) films, fluoroscopy, and tomography. In addition, when these studies include contrast mediums, they are more invasive. In general, these tests are invaluable to determining the presence of pathology and are often specific in terms of their ability to accurately diagnose a given disorder.

Radiological Examination of the Skull and Spine

Plain X-ray studies of the skull and spine are easy to obtain and noninvasive Damage to the nervous system may include bony fractures, bone erosion, curvature, dislocations, and calcification of soft tissue. Multiple views may be taken. These could include: anteroposterior (AP), lateral, oblique, special views of facial bones, and flexion-extension.

Nursing Management

There is usually no patient preparation needed. The nurse should explain that the X-ray procedure is similar to having a chest X-ray (CXR) done and that the exposure to radiation is minimal. Patients who are immobilized may require the nurse to accompany them to the radiology department. Impaired ambulation may require a stretcher for transport.

Once in the radiology department, the patient is directed to either lie on the examination table or stand, depending on the ordered studies. The patient is positioned for each of the desired views and instructed to not move during each X-ray. There is no required follow-up nursing care.

Computed Tomography

Computed axial tomography (CT scan) is considered one of the most accurate, quickest, easiest, and least expensive method of diagnosing neurologic problems. It combines X-rays with computer technology to produce a three-dimensional picture of thin cross-sections of the body. The X-ray beam rotates around the patient, and then the computer analyzes the data and creates a composite picture. The images may be enhanced by the use of contrast media. CT is sensitive to differences in tissue densities. This allows the neuroradiologist to identify any disease processes in the bones, soft tissue, or fluids. A limitation of the CT scanner is its inability to gather information about functional status.

Nursing Management

Teaching by the nurse should begin with a description of the CT scanner. When contrast media is planned, identification of any allergies to the media, shellfish, or iodine may require premedication. Instruct the patient regarding the need to lie still during the procedure. Identify any need for sedation because of anxiety. The patient is not usually kept to a nothing by mouth (NPO) order. A peripheral intravenous (IV) site may need to be implemented for contrast media injection.

The patient is placed flat on a movable table. His or her head is secured in a holding device. The table moves in and out of the cylindrical scanner. A noncontrast series of pictures is taken first. If contrast medium is ordered, it is administered intravenously, and the series is repeated. The entire procedure usually takes approximately 10–40 minutes.

If contrast agent is given, the nurse should monitor for any delayed reaction. When contrast agent is used, the diuresis that results may require replacement fluids.

Magnetic Resonance Imaging

Magnetic resonance imaging (MRI) is a computer-based imagining method that uses the body's own magnetic energy to visualize disease processes, such as strokes, tumors, trauma, seizures, edema, and brainstem herniation. The magnet causes changes in the radiofrequency signals produced by the body. These changes are detected and interpreted by the computer and then displayed as cross-sectional images. The procedure is noninvasive, unless contrast is required. When visualization needs to be enhanced, gadolinium, a non–iodine-based media, may be used (Daniels, 2003).

Nursing Management

The patient needs to be interviewed regarding any iron-based implanted objects (e.g., artificial joints, pacemakers, bullets or metal fragments, or clips or wires). The powerful magnetic field can cause such devices to move out of position, placing the patient at risk for hemorrhage or bleeding. The magnet can alter the internal settings for pacemakers. Make the patient aware that the procedure is noisy and earplugs are available. Patients who are claustrophobic may need to be sedated. Patients are not usually kept NPO.

The patient needs to remain motionless while enclosed in a tunnel containing the powerful magnet. A two-way intercom is available for the patient to communicate needs. First, a noncontrast series of pictures are taken. If contrast is ordered, it is administered intravenously, and the series is repeated. The procedure may take from 15–90 minutes to complete. If sedation is required, monitor the patient for return to baseline functioning. No further postprocedure nursing care is required.

> **Red Flag**
>
> **Risks to Prevent during a CT Scan**
>
> Prior to sending the patient for radiological scans (CT or magnetic resonance imaging [MRI]), the nurse should assess the patient for potential complications. These complications may include past allergic response to the contrast medium or acute renal dysfunction. Allergy to shellfish, contrast media, or iodine must be examined in detail. Skin testing should be done to test for an allergic reaction.
>
> The health care provider may order premedication prior to sending the patient to radiology. Adequate kidney function testing (blood urea nitrogen [BUN] and creatinine [Cr]) is done before the procedure, and hydration therapy may need to be started. Patients at increased risk of kidney dysfunction are those with multiple myeloma, severe diabetes, or hepatorenal syndrome. Diabetic patients taking metformin must be taken off the medication when radiological studies are anticipated.
>
> During and after the procedure the nurse monitors the patient for the signs and symptoms of an allergic reaction. These include respiratory distress, hives, itching, nausea, vomiting, decreased urine output, and low blood pressure. There is available a noniodianted contrast media, but it is prohibitively costly and not routinely used.

Magnetic Resonance Angiography

Magnetic resonance angiography (MRA) uses the differential signal characteristics of blood flow to visualize the extracranial and intracranial blood vessels. The study provides both anatomic and hemodynamic information. It can be used in conjunction with contrast media (contrast-enhanced MRA [cMRA]). MRA is often used as a less invasive method of screening for and diagnosing cerebrovascular disease.

Nursing Management

The patient preparation for an MRA is essentially the same as the MRI. The time necessary to complete the procedure is about one to three hours to complete. In addition, the follow-up nursing care is also similar to the MRI. The patient should be assessed for boney prominences for pressure areas, and the patient must lie in the same position for most or all of the procedure.

Magnetic Resonance Spectroscopy

Magnetic resonance spectroscopy (MRS) provides information about the chemical composition of tissue. Chemical markers of neuronal integrity are evaluated using MRI techniques. This is often used to differentiate tumor versus abscess or infection versus autoimmune destruction. The patient preparation for MRS is essentially the same as the MRI.

Functional Magnetic Resonance Imaging

Functional magnetic resonance imaging (fMRI) is used to identify changes in cerebral metabolism or blood flow. It looks at chemical changes in response to specific tasks. These tasks consist of periods of activity and periods of rest. The result can functionally map the brain. The patient preparation for fMRI is essentially the same as the MRI.

Cerebral Angiography

Cerebral angiography (angiogram) is an invasive series of radiographic studies involving the injection of contrast medium. This allows the visualization of the intracranial and extracranial blood vessels. It is performed to detect vascular lesions such as, aneurysms, malformations, occlusion, and tumors of the brain.

Nursing Management

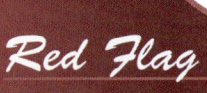

The nurse needs to describe what is involved and identify any allergies to shellfish or iodine. Explain that an IV catheter will be inserted using local anesthetic, usually in the femoral artery. A burning sensation, lasting 20 to 30 seconds, may occur when the contrast media is injected. This is to be expected. The patient needs to be NPO for approximately four to six hours prior to the procedure. IV hydration should be instituted when the patient is NPO. The initial assessment includes baseline vital signs, LOC, and evaluation of all peripheral pulses. Administer premedication when ordered.

The patient is taken to the angiography suite, placed on the examination table, and secured with straps. A headrest is used to immobilize the head. The radiologist locates and cleans the chosen puncture site and then threads the catheter into the artery. Once the catheter is placed, contrast media is injected and a series of radiographic images are obtained that outline the arterial and venous systems. After the catheter is removed, pressure is maintained for at least 5 to 10 minutes to prevent arterial bleeding.

After the procedure, bedrest needs to be maintained for 6 to 12 hours as ordered. Monitor the access site for signs of bleeding or formation of hematoma. A pressure dressing, sandbag, ice bag, or combination need to be maintained as ordered. Vital signs and neurovascular assessment of the area distal to the puncture site are compared to the baseline findings on a 15 minute to hourly routine as ordered. Instruct the patient to minimize movement of the involved limb and avoid flexion at the puncture site. LOC is also assessed for changes, which may indicate circulatory compromise, such as vasospasm, embolism, and thrombosis. Maintain hydration as the contrast media may result in increased osmotic diuresis and places the patient at risk for dehydration and renal tubular occlusion.

Digital Subtraction Angiography

Digital subtraction angiography (DSA) is the combination of X-ray films with computer enhancement to produce images of the cerebral circulation. The procedure is performed using the IV rather than the arterial route. It can be performed as an outpatient test and has few potential complications.

Nursing Management

The nurse needs to describe what is involved and identify any allergies to shellfish or iodine. Food is restricted for two hours before the test, but fluids are not. Instruct the patient to empty his or her bladder. Initial assessment includes baseline vital signs, LOC, and evaluation of peripheral pulses. Administer premedication when ordered.

The patient is taken to the neuroradiology suite, placed on an examination table, and secured with straps. The radiologist selects the puncture site, cleans it, and threads a large angiocatheter into the vein, usually, brachial. IV fluid is administered via a second IV catheter. A baseline X-ray is done to be used as a reference for the remainder of the films. The contrast media is injected, and serial films are compared to the baseline. The computer subtracts the baseline image and generates an angiographic image. DSA is less invasive, less costly, and more convenient for the patient than many other radiographic tests.

The nurse should monitor vital signs and neurovascular status every 15 minutes to hourly as ordered. Regularly evaluate the access site for bleeding. Encourage the patient to increase his or her oral intake for the next 24 hours. There are no activity restrictions.

Positron Emission Tomography

Positron emission tomography (PET) provides a three-dimensional structural and functional view of the brain. It combines CT with radioisotope scanning to measure the metabolic activity of the brain and assess for cell death or damage. The biggest limitation to PET scanning is the need for an on-site cyclotron to prepare the radioisotopes because of their short half-life.

Nursing Management

Explain the procedure to the patient. Instruct the patient to withhold caffeine, alcohol, and tobacco for 24 hours prior to the test. The patient is NPO for 6 to 12 hours before the test is scheduled. If the patient is diabetic, no

Dollars and Sense

Expenses of MRI Scans

With steadily rising health care costs, it is necessary to be aware of the cost of diagnostic tests. An MRI scan, when first available, cost between $2,000 and $5,000 per use. Now with increased use and availability, the cost of an MRI is between $300 to $1,000, depending on how many scans are done each year by the institution. The higher the volume of MRI scans, the lower the cost.

Fast Forward ▶▶▶

The Future of Functional Magnetic Resonance Imaging (fMRI)

Currently the standard test for language lateralization before surgeries planned for seizure disorders or neoplasm resection is the Wada test. This test involves a large medical team, iodinated contrast media, and radiation. It usually involves one to two hours of testing and four to six hours of patient recovery time. In the future, fMRI may replace the Wada test as the preoperative assessment tool for language lateralization. The fMRI usually requires 30–60 minutes of testing time and no postprocedure recovery time. The cost of the Wada test and fMRI were compared and substantial savings with the use of fMRI to evaluate language lateralization were found. Multiple studies have found the results of the fMRI to be equivalent to the Wada test.

antidiabetic medications, such as insulin or oral antiglycemics, are given before the test. Withhold glucose solutions or medications that alter glucose metabolism. Direct the patient to empty his or her bladder prior to the procedure. Instruct patient to not take sedatives or tranquilizers before the test.

The patient is placed on a stretcher and either inhales or is injected with a biologically active radioactive tagged compound made partially of water or glucose, and the mixture is then able to cross the blood-brain barrier. A computerized detector measures the radioactive uptake of these substances and produces a composite image. The areas where the radioactive material is located correspond to areas of cellular metabolism. The patient may be blindfolded if he or she desires and can have earplugs inserted for all or part of the test. The patient is asked to perform specific mental functions to activate different areas of the brain. The total procedure takes two to three hours.

The radioisotope is eliminated by the kidney and requires no special precautions. Encourage the patient to increase oral fluids.

Single-Photon Emission Computed Tomography

Single-photon emission computed tomography (SPECT) overcomes the limitations of PET scanning by using radionuclides that emit gamma rays. These compounds have longer half-lives; therefore they eliminate the need for an on-site cyclotron. The nursing management is essentially the same as for the PET scan.

Myelography

Myelography is an invasive procedure involving the injection of air or contrast media into the lumbar subarachnoid space via a lumbar puncture. After the medium is injected fluoroscopy, conventional radiographs or CT scans are used to visualize selected areas. The spinal subarachnoid space is assessed for obstructions, compression, or herniated intervertebral discs.

Nursing Management

Explain the procedure to patient. Inform patient that the test is performed with him or her lying on an examination table that tilts. Encourage oral fluid intake. Patient is to empty his or her bladder before the test starts. Baseline assessment includes vital signs and neurological status. Administer premedication as ordered.

The patient is placed in the lateral recumbent position with knees flexed. Using sterile technique, the practitioner inserts a hollow-core needle into the subarachnoid space usually at L3–L4 or L4–L5. The selected contrast medium (e.g., air, oil-based, or water-based) is injected. Images are generated by the selected scanner.

Maintain strict bedrest for a few hours as ordered. Encourage oral fluids. Monitor and compare vital sign and neurological assessment to baseline findings. Administer analgesia as needed (Daniels, 2004).

Electrographic Studies

There are several electrographic diagnostic studies that are valuable tests to explore the specific pathologies of diseases. These tests involve either magnetic fields or bioelectric waves produced in the body. The electromagnetic tests measure and record bioelectrical impulses in the body. The brain, heart, nerves, and muscles all produce electrical impulses that can be diagnostic for many different conditions. They prove to be important in the different choices that practitioners have in diagnosing disorders.

Electroencephalography

Electroencephalography (EEG) is a noninvasive method of evaluating the electrical activity of the cerebral hemispheres. This activity is measured be electrodes attached to the scalp. The EEG is used to identify areas of abnormal electrical discharge in the cerebral cortex. There are a wide variety of conditions that an abnormal EEG can identify, for example, seizure activity, tumors, cerebrovascular disease, degenerative brain disease, drug intoxication, or brain death (Ives, 2005).

Nursing Management

Inform the patient that the test is painless and there is no danger of electrical shock. Discuss the purpose and procedure of the test with the patient. Withhold caffeine, tobacco, and alcohol-containing products for 24 hours before the scheduled test. The patient is not to be NPO. Hair should be freshly shampooed, clean, and free of hairpins, sprays, or oils.

CNS depressants and stimulants should be withheld for 24 hours before the test. If a sleep deprived EEG is ordered, the patient should be kept awake from approximately 2 a.m. When anticonvulsants are to be held before the test, the nurse should monitor for any seizure activity.

Either a recliner-type chair or a bed is used to maximize patient comfort. This helps to reduce the need for position changes during testing. Patient movement can interfere with the EEG recording. Electrodes are applied to the patients scalp using a colloidal gel or paste. The patient must lie still during the baseline recording. The remainder of the test involves following directions for various activities: hyperventilation, photo stimulation, or sleep. Hyperventilation by the patient involves breathing deeply 20 to 30 times per minute, for three minutes. This causes cerebral vasoconstriction and alkalosis, which increases the possibility of seizure activity. Photo stimulation uses a strobe light. The patient looks directly at the light, which flashes with varying frequency (1 to 20 flashes per second). This is then repeated with the eyes closed. If the patient's seizures are triggered by changing light frequencies, the EEG will record the location of the activity. Sleep can be natural or induced by the administration of IV sedation. Temporal lobe epilepsy can be demonstrated best during sleep.

The standard test usually takes 40 to 60 minutes to complete. It is preferred that the test be done in the department where external stimuli can be controlled. During administration of the test, all patient movement is recorded, because this can affect the test results. The EEG can be done with portable machinery, but it is more difficult to control the external stimuli. Sleep study EEGs are usually in a video monitored, controlled environment. Instruct patient to wash hair to remove the electrode glue. Administer any medications that were held for the test. Sleep deprivation patients may require a nap.

Magnetoencephalography

Magnetoencephalography (MEG) is similar to an EEG but with the addition of a biomagnetometer. This highly sensitive machine has a passive sensor, which detects small magnetic fields generated by neural activity. It measures both extracranial and scalp electrical fields. It can accurately detect the location of a seizure, stroke, or injury. The nursing management for magnetoencephalography is essentially the same as for an EEG.

Electromyography

Electromyography (EMG) measures the electrical activity of the peripheral nerves by testing muscle activity. An EMG can be performed on specific areas of the muscles throughout the body. For example, an upper EMG would be implemented on the arms and could identify areas of decreased electrical activity associated with various neurological degenerative disorders.

Nursing Management

Explain the procedure to the patient. Inform him or her that there is slight discomfort associated with the insertion of needles into the skin where the test is performed. The patient does not need to be NPO. After making the patient comfortable, the technician cleans the body areas to be tested. Then he or she inserts sterile needles that measure the electrical activity of specific nerve pathways. No follow-up care is required.

Evoked Potentials

Evoked potential (EP) testing measures the electrical activity of nerve conduction along the sensory nerve pathways. Sensors are placed on the skin and scalp and then connected to a computer, which analyzes the incoming data and generates waveforms to depict the electrical activity (Table 34-10 for a description of each type of EPs). The nursing management EP testing is essentially the same as EEG.

Ultrasound

Ultrasound studies use sound waves to produce an image of internal organs, tissue, or fetuses. The sound waves are high frequency and inaudible to the human ear, with a frequency of higher than 20,000 cycles/second (normal human hearing is between 16,000 and 20,000 cycles/second). The ultrasound waves bounce back from the body tissues, producing echoes that the transducer records and displays on a monitor as a picture or into audible sound, which is known as the Doppler method. There are a wide variety of these types of tests and they are relatively noninvasive but are somewhat expensive in practice.

Carotid Duplex Studies

Carotid duplex scanning is a noninvasive method of evaluating for carotid occlusive disease. It is the combination of ultrasound with pulsed Doppler technology. The ultrasound signal is reflected off the moving blood cells and is registered as blood velocity. Stenosis of a blood vessel is indicated when there is increased velocity.

TABLE 34-10 Evoked Potential Types

TYPE	STIMULUS	PURPOSE
Visual		
Visual evoked potential (VEP)	Rapidly changing geometric designs or flashing lights	Locate lesion in visual pathway or visual cortex
Pattern reversal electrical potential (PREP)		
Visual electrical response (VER)		
Auditory		
Auditory evoked potential (AEP)	Multiple clicks to each ear via earphones	Locate lesion; evaluate the central auditory pathways of the brainstem; follow the course of recovery
Auditory brainstem evoked potential (ABEP)		
Somatosensory		
Somatosensory brainstem evoked potential (SBEP)	Electrical stimulation of selected peripheral nerves	Differentiate lesions of the peripheral nerve from those of subcor tical or cortical central sensory pathways
Somatosensory evoked potential (SEP)		

Adapted from Daniels, R. (2003). Delmar's manual of laboratory and diagnostic tests. *New York: Thomson Delmar Learning.*

Nursing Management

Explain the procedure to patient. Patient does not need to be NPO. After the patient is taken to the testing area, he or she is made comfortable on a bed. The technician uses the ultrasound probe, placed on the carotid artery of either side of the neck, to evaluate the blood flow velocity of the blood vessels. A gel is used to enhance the sound. No specific follow-up care is required. The patient may want to wash his or her neck.

Transcranial Doppler Sonography

Transcranial Doppler (TCD) uses the same technology as carotid duplex studies. It records the velocities of the intracranial blood vessels. TCD is a noninvasive method of assessing: vasospasm associated with subarachnoid hemorrhage and altered intracranial blood flow dynamics related to occlusive vascular disease, cerebral autoregulation, the presence of emboli, and brain death.

Nursing Management

Explain the procedure to patient. Restriction of food or fluids is not required. The equipment is similar to the carotid Doppler. In this procedure, the probe is placed on the skin at various windows of the skull. These areas have a thin bony covering. The temporal, orbital, and suboccipital sites are used. The ultrasound signal is recorded as a wave velocities indicate narrowing or occlusion. A gel is used to enhance the signal. No specific follow-up care is required. The patient may want to wash off the gel residue.

KEY CONCEPTS

- The CNS consists of the brain and spinal cord.
- The PNS consists of the cranial nerves, the spinal nerves, and the ANS.
- Neurons transmit or conduct nerve impulses.
- The initiation of a nerve impulse involves the generation of an action potential.
- Neurotransmitters are chemical substances that inhibit, excite, or modify the responses.
- The brain is composed of the cerebrum, the brainstem, and the cerebellum.
- The spinal cord is the conduit for the ascending sensory and descending motor neurons.
- There are four ventricles (or chambers) within the brain and are filled with CSF and are linked by ducts that permit circulation.
- Functions of the cerebellum include coordinating voluntary muscle movement, equilibrium, and maintenance of trunk stability.
- The blood-brain barrier maintains a functionally stable environment for the CNS.
- The spinal cord extends from the medulla to the level of the first lumbar vertebrae.
- The PNS is composed of the spinal nerves, cranial nerves, and the ANS.
- The cranial nerves provide both motor and sensory innervation for the head, neck, and viscera.
- The ANS has two, semi-independent components: sympathetic and parasympathetic.
- Subtle changes in mental status are one of the earliest indicators of a potential neurological event.
- Evaluation of cerebellar function requires the assessment of coordination, balance, posture, and gait.
- Neurodiagnostic tests are performed as adjuncts to a complete history and physical examination.
- LP is the most common method for obtaining CSF.
- fMRI is used to identify changes in cerebral metabolism or blood flow.
- Cerebral angiography is an invasive series of radiographic studies involving the injection of contrast media.
- PET provides a three-dimensional structural and functional view of the brain.
- Myelogram is an invasive procedure involving the injection of air or contrast media into the lumbar subarachnoid space via a lumbar puncture.
- EMG measures the electrical activity of the peripheral nerves by testing muscle activity.

REVIEW QUESTIONS

1. When grading muscle strength, a score of 1 indicates:
1. No muscle contraction
2. Trace of contraction
3. Active movement with gravity eliminated
4. Normal strength

2. What instructions should the nurse give to the patient when performing the Romberg test?
1. Close your eyes and remain still
2. Place your index finger on your nose
3. Jump in place
4. Walk heel to toe

3. The patient who has difficulty choosing the right words and responds hesitantly is displaying symptoms of:
1. Agnosia
2. Homonymous hemianopsia
3. Expressive aphasia
4. Ataxia

4. When the nurse stimulates Babinski's sign in an adult, the big toe moves upward and the other toes fan out. This finding indicates:
1. Normal neurological functioning
2. Upper motor neuron disease
3. Lower motor neuron disease
4. Spinothalamic tract lesion

5. The ability to recognize an object's shape is known as:
1. Graphesthesia
2. Discrimination
3. Stereognosis
4. Visceroptosis

6. Paralysis of lateral gaze indicates a lesion of cranial nerve:
1. II
2. III
3. IV
4. VI

7. Stimulation of the parasympathetic nervous system results in:
1. Dilation of skin blood vessels
2. Decreased secretion of insulin
3. Increased blood glucose levels
4. Relaxation of the urinary sphincters

8. When preparing a patient for an EEG, the nurse should include which of the following statements?
1. Do not take any food or fluids for six hours prior to the test.
2. You must remain absolutely still during the test.
3. Inform the technician if you are allergic to shellfish or iodine.
4. Bright lights will be used during the procedure.

9. The consensual pupillary response is tested by:
1. Asking the patient if he or she has trouble closing his or her eyes
2. Directing a light toward one eye and observing the pupil on the opposite side
3. Instructing the patient to cover one while you observe the opposite eye for extraocular movements
4. Evaluating the ability of the patient's eyes to converge

10. One way to test the vestibular function of the acoustic nerve (CN VIII) is to:
1. Check the auditory studies
2. Ask if the patient experiences dizziness
3. Have the patient shrug his or her shoulders
4. Rub your fingers together near the patient's ears.

11. Which technique is recommended for eliciting a response to peripheral pain?
1. Sternal rub
2 Trapezius muscle squeeze
3. Nail bed pressure
4. Mandibular pressure

12. Cerebrospinal fluid (CSF) is reabsorbed into the venous system via the:
1. Arachnoid villi
2. Aqueduct of Sylvius
3. Foramen of Monro
4. Choroid plexuses

13. What is the significance of the blood-brain barrier?
1. It is thought to result from increased capillary permeability.
2. It allows drugs to diffuse freely from the interstitial space to the intravascular space.
3. It limits the transmission of substances from the blood to the brain.
4. Its disruption is rare in head-injured patients.

REVIEW ACTIVITIES

1. Identify the three neurotransmitters found in the basal ganglia and describe their impact on motor function.

2. Compare and contrast the sympathetic and parasympathetic divisions of the autonomic nervous system.

3. List the six major portions of the physical assessment of the neurological system.

4. Identify your priority nursing interventions when preparing your patient to have a CT scan.

5. Observe several neurological diagnostic studies in the practicum setting.

Visit the Contemporary Medical-Surgical Nursing online companion resource at www.delmarhealthcare.com for additional content and study aids. Click on Online Companions then select the Nursing discipline.

CHAPTER 35

Dysfunction of the Brain: Nursing Management

Beth Hickey, RN, MSN, CRRN, CNA

Carrie A. McCoy, PhD, MSPH, RN, CEN

CHAPTER TOPICS

- Cerebrovascular Accidents
- Brain Injuries
- Brain Tumors

The brain is the central processing unit of the body, similar to what is found in a computer. However, the brain works faster and better than any computer. It houses vast amounts of information throughout the life process. However, when there is a disruption in brain function, there are serious consequences. In this chapter, the nursing management of patients suffering from cerebrovascular accidents ([CVA] strokes), brain injuries, and brain tumors will be discussed.

KEY TERMS

Aneurysm
Aphasia
Cerebrovascular accident ([CVA] stroke)
Concussion
Contracture
Cushing response
Dysarthria
Dysphagia
Emboli
Expressive aphasia (Broca's aphasia)
Global aphasia
Hemiparesis
Hemiplegia
Hemorrhagic stroke
Homonymous hemianopsia
Intracranial pressure (ICP)
Ischemic stroke
Primary brain tumor
Receptive aphasia (Wernicke's aphasia)
Stereotactic radiotherapy (SRS)
Subarachnoid hemorrhage
Thrombus
Transient ischemic attack (TIA)

CEREBROVASCULAR ACCIDENTS OR STROKES

In the United States, every 45 seconds someone has a stroke, every three minutes someone dies from a stroke, and 700,000 new or recurrent strokes occur each year (American Heart Association [AHA], 2003). Strokes are the third leading cause of death in the United States, behind heart disease and cancer, and are the leading cause of long-term disability. Epidemiological studies have determined that 11 states in the Southeast (Alabama, Arkansas, Georgia, Indiana, Kentucky, Louisiana, Mississippi, North Carolina, South Carolina, Tennessee, and Virginia) have a 10 percent higher rate of stroke deaths than anywhere else in the United States (Steefel, 2004).

DOLLARS AND SENSE

The Cost of Stroke Care in the United States

In terms of health care costs, many stroke patients require intensive health care. The United States estimates that in 2004, direct and indirect costs for stroke and cardiovascular disease will be $53.6 billion. These costs include hospital care, nursing home, health care provider(s), medications, durable medical equipment, home health care, and lost productivity (AHA, 2003).

Epidemiology

Strokes also are a health concern worldwide. According to the World Health Organization ([WHO], 2004b), 5.5 million people died from a stroke, making strokes the second leading cause of death worldwide; the first is ischemic heart disease. In terms of disability, strokes rank seventh as a leading cause of disability worldwide and are estimated to move up to fourth by the year 2020 (WHO, 2004b). The countries with the highest mortality rate per 100,000 people are Russia, Romania, and Bulgaria (AHA, 2003).

A **cerebrovascular accident (CVA),** or **stroke,** occurs when a part of the brain is damaged due to a lack of blood flow. The term brain attack has recently been developed by the AHA in an effort to reinforce the importance of knowing the early warning signs (Box 35-1) and seeking medical attention quickly.

There are two main types of stroke, **ischemic stroke** (damage to the brain due to a clogged artery) and **hemorrhagic stroke** (when a blood vessel burst leaking blood into brain tissue or surrounding spaces). An ischemic stroke occurs when a blood vessel to the brain becomes clogged, and brain tissue supplied by that blood vessel begins to die. Approximately 88 percent of all strokes are ischemic in nature, and 8 to 12 percent of all patients die within 30 days of an ischemic stroke (AHA, 2003). Ischemic strokes are caused by either a **thrombus** (a blood clot that blocks a blood vessel) or an **emboli** (a blood clot or other particle plaque that breaks loose and blocks blood vessels). A blood clot may develop because of atherosclerosis, which is a buildup of plaque within a vessel wall. This affects blood flow and causes platelet aggregation, thus forming a clot. An embolic stroke occurs when a blood clot or other particle (e.g., atherosclerotic plaque) breaks loose from a vessel wall and occludes a smaller blood vessel in the brain.

A hemorrhagic stroke occurs when a blood vessel in the brain ruptures, leaking blood directly into the brain tissue or surrounding spaces. While only 12 percent of all strokes are hemorrhagic in nature, 38 percent of patients with hemorrhagic strokes die within 30 days (AHA, 2003). One type of hemorrhagic stroke is called a **subarachnoid hemorrhage** (blood that leaks into the subarachnoid space). This type of hemorrhage is caused by bleeding between the arachnoid meninges covering the brain and the skull, but blood does not invade the brain tissue. An intracerebral hemorrhage occurs when blood enters the brain tissue after a blood vessel ruptures. This can be caused by an **aneurysm** (a weakness in a blood vessel wall) or arteriovenous malformation (Soderman, Andersson, Karlsson, Wallace, & Edner, 2003). The different types of cerebral hemorrhage and management of cerebral hemorrhage will be discussed in greater detail in the section on head injuries.

BOX 35-1

MODIFIABLE RISK FACTORS FOR STROKE DEVELOPMENT

- Hypertension—this is determined by any consistent blood pressure reading above 140/90. Diet changes, medication, and stress management can affect hypertension.
- Hypercholesterolemia—high cholesterol is determined by a blood cholesterol level greater than 240 mg/dL. Dietary changes and medication can influence these levels. High cholesterol also can lead to atherosclerosis.
- Atherosclerosis—is a buildup of plaque in the walls of blood vessels. This plaque can break off, causing an embolic stroke or narrow a blood vessel leading to a thrombotic stroke.
- Atrial fibrillation—is when the upper chambers of the heart do not beat effectively. This causes blood to pool in the chambers and can lead to clot formation. These clots then are released into the blood system and can lead to a stroke. A person with atrial fibrillation is five times more likely to develop a stroke (AHA, 2003). A physician should evaluate atrial fibrillation for the appropriate treatment options. Medications, such as anticoagulants, can be used to decrease this risk factor.
- Obesity—being overweight places additional stress on the body and is usually associated with an inactive lifestyle. Getting into a regular exercise routine and eating properly can address this risk factor.
- Smoking—causes a decrease in oxygenation of the body. This can lead to damage to the blood vessel walls making a stroke more likely to occur.
- Drugs and alcohol—certain illegal drugs (e.g., cocaine and amphetamines), alcohol abuse, and prescribed medications (e.g., birth control pills) can increase the risk of a stroke. Birth control pills are especially risky if the person continues to smoke. Patients should be aware of any medication that may increase their risk of a stroke.
- Other health problems—diabetes and sickle cell anemia are also risk factors for stroke development. Diabetes is a consistent fasting blood sugar above 120 mg/dL. Diabetes affects the vascular system and can have devastating effects. It is important to assist patients with diabetes to properly manage their disease process. With sickle cell anemia, the red blood cells are shaped in the form of a sickle and are less able to carry oxygen to the tissues. These sickle cells can adhere to the lining of the blood vessel walls and form clots (AHA, 2003). Riddington & Wang (2002) reviewed studies evaluating the effectiveness of blood transfusions in the management of sickle cell anemia; they concluded that the risks associated with the blood transfusions caused concerns about the side effects outweighing the benefits of the treatment and noted further research was indicated.
- **Transient ischemic attacks (TIAs)**—are caused by a temporary loss of blood supply to a part of the brain that results in a temporary loss of function. These deficits resolve within 24 hours. They may also be called ministrokes and are a strong predictor of an impending stroke.

Etiology

There are many risk factors associated with a stroke. There are both modifiable and nonmodifiable risk factors (see chapter 24) (Box 35-2). In addition, the combination of these risk factors contributes greatly to the cause of CVAs.

Many people have multiple risk factors. This is why it is so important to educate patients about the risk factors that can be changed. The more risk factors

BOX 35-2

NONMODIFIABLE RISK FACTORS FOR STROKE DEVELOPMENT

- Age and sex—As a person ages, his or her risk for a stroke increases. Patients over 65 years of age are at greatest risk for stroke. While men are at greater risk of a stroke, there are more stroke deaths among women (AHA, 2003).
- Family history and past medical history—having had a stroke within the past year or having a family history of strokes places a patient at greater risk for stroke. This is why it is important to work with patients to address the modifiable risk factors to decrease their risk of another stroke.

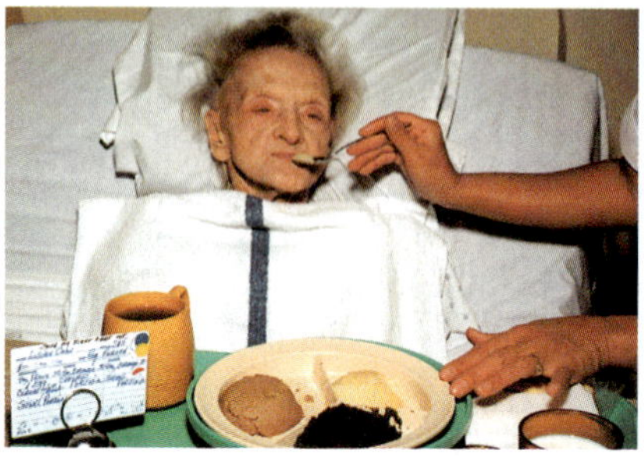

Figure 35-1 This patient with a stroke has multiple risk factors, which adds to her poor prognosis.

a patient has, the higher the likelihood that they will have a stroke in their lifetime (Figure 35-1).

Pathophysiology

To understand the effects of a stroke, it is important to understand what happens to the brain tissue when a stroke occurs. Normally the brain receives blood flow at 60 to 70 mL/100 g of brain tissue/minute, but when that rate is slowed to 25 mL, loss of function begins to occur due to lack of aerobic metabolism. If blood flow is not restored soon, cell death begins to occur. Within a few minutes of blood supply loss, a necrotic core develops. The necrotic core is tissue deprived of oxygen that is permanently damaged. The tissue surrounding the necrotic core, the ischemic penumbra, may continue to survive for a short time even though blood flow has been reduced. The focus of medical management is maintaining blood flow to the ischemic penumbra (Felberg & Naidech, 2003). The location of the tissue damage and the availability of collateral circulation help determine the patient's prognosis. For a more detailed description of the cellular changes that take place as brain tissue becomes anoxic, see the section on head injuries.

Assessment with Clinical Manifestations

The nurse must have keen assessment skills to appropriately assess and manage a stroke patient. The nurse should determine:

- Past medical history—this is important to determine if the patient might have any risk factors or other medical conditions that would affect treatment.
- Current medications—this is important if the patient is taking a medication that would interfere with treatment (e.g., anticoagulants).
- Symptom onset and progression—this is the most important factor, because it affects treatment options and is a factor in differentiating between an ischemic stroke and a hemorrhagic stroke. Patients with ischemic strokes may report a variety of symptoms depending on the location of the stroke; however, if a patient complains of a severe headache with rapid onset, this may be an indication of a hemorrhagic stroke. Some of the most common symptoms of ischemic stroke include weakness or paralysis on one side of the body, inability to maintain balance, blurred vision, dizziness, slurred speech, inability to concentrate, memory deficits, incontinence, fatigue, double vision, and headache. The nurse must remember that each patient may present with slightly different symptoms, because of the part of the brain that has been affected, but quick and effective management of a stroke can mean the difference between a patient returning to functional independence or lifelong disability or death.

Diagnostic Tests

Many diagnostic tools are available for patients suffering from a stroke. But many of these tools take time, which is critical when managing an acute stroke. The most common tool used to diagnose a stroke is a computed tomography (CT) scan. It is widely available in most hospitals and is an important tool to differentiate between ischemic strokes and hemorrhagic strokes. The CT scan can be read immediately, and treatment can begin quickly. The CT scan is done without contrast dye and does not require any preparation on the part of the patient (e.g., nothing by mouth [NPO] or intravenous [IV] access). A magnetic resonance imaging (MRI) may also be ordered, but MRI scans take longer, between 45 minutes and two hours. While an MRI allows the radiologist better imaging of blood vessels and brain tissue, it is contraindicated in patients with metal implants or pacemakers and patients who are claustrophobic.

Laboratory tests will be ordered to assist in diagnosis and to determine treatment options. The most common laboratory tests ordered will include: complete blood count (CBC), electrolytes, blood urea nitrogen (BUN), creatinine (Cr), prothrombin time (PT), and partial prothrombin time (PTT). Other tests may be ordered depending on other presenting symptoms. See Table 35-1 for a list of other tests that may be utilized in the diagnosis and treatment of a stroke.

Nursing Diagnoses

Based on the information gathered, examples of nursing diagnoses in the patient with a CVA may include the following:

- Impaired verbal communication related to different types of aphasia from the CVA.
- Disturbed sensory perception related to the neurological damage from the CVA.
- Impaired physical mobility related to the hemiparesis caused by the CVA.
- Risk for caregiver role strain related to the chronic nature of the resulting CVA.
- Risk for situational low self-esteem related to the variety of changes from the CVA.

Planning and Implementation

The goal of stroke management is to restore function and independence. This is done in with four different management areas: pharmacology, prevention, emergency management, and surgical intervention. The best outcome for

TABLE 35-1 Stroke Diagnostic Tests

NAME OF TEST	REASON
Computerized tomography (CT) scan	Usually the first test done, because it can be done quickly and is readily accessible in most facilities.
	Used to differentiate between hemorrhagic and ischemic stroke
Magnetic resonance imaging (MRI)	Is more sensitive than a CT scan and is detailed in identifying small vessel strokes.
Magnetic resonance angiography (MRA)	Noninvasive test that allows imaging of the blood vessels.
	Especially helpful in determining collateral circulation.
Carotid ultrasound	Determines blood flow to the brain.
	Can detect atherosclerotic buildup.
Nuclear brain scan (cerebral angiography)	Areas of decreased blood flow will have less uptake of the radioactive dye and show damaged tissues.
Transcranial Doppler (TCD)	Noninvasive ultrasound, portable
	Assesses blood flow in cerebral vessels
Electroencephalogram (EEG)	If significant brain tissue involvement, may have little to no brain activity.
Evoked responses	In the area of the brain that is injured, the patient will have a decreased response to the stimuli.
Positive emission tomography (PET) scanning	Determines brain tissue functioning

Adapted from Stanford Stroke Awareness. (2002). Stroke awareness Part II: Diagnosis and treatment options. *Retrieved June 13, 2006, from www.stanford.edu.*

stroke management is not to have one. Prevention and early access to health care are vital to decreasing the number of strokes. In the Healthy People 2010 report (U.S. Department of Health and Human Services, 2002), one of the objectives is to decrease the number of stroke deaths and increase the public's awareness of the signs of a stroke. One of the biggest components to prevention is education. The AHA is playing an important role by having the warning signs of a stroke incorporated into all of their cardiopulmonary resuscitation (CPR) educational training. They have also associated the name stroke with brain attack; making it similar to a heart attack. This was done to encourage people to recognize the importance of seeking medical attention immediately. Many people still do not recognize the warning signs of a stroke and try to lie down, thinking that they will feel better when they get up. This is a serious problem, because delay in seeking health care can lead to devastating results.

Pharmacology

In addition to education, several medications are effective in preventing a stroke. These medications are anticoagulants, antiplatelets, and neuroprotective agents. Anticoagulants, usually heparin and warfarin (Coumadin), are given to prevent blood from clotting. Anticoagulation is especially important for patients with atrial fibrillation (King & LeMaire, 2002). According to the Agency for Health Care Policy and Research (Cohen & De LaMare, 2002), atrial fibrillation causes an estimated 80,000 strokes per year. The increased use of anticoagulant therapy, from 58 to 71 percent, has prevented 1,285 stokes. Antiplatelet medications are used to prevent platelets from clumping together, also known as platelet aggregation, and blocking blood vessels. When a blood vessel is injured, it is normal for the body to send platelets to an area to begin the healing process, but when too many platelets arrive, they can decrease blood flow to the tissues distal to the clot. Antiplatelet agents decrease the number of platelets in the blood stream. Antiplatelet medications include aspirin (acetsalicylic acid) and ticlopidine (Ticlid). Neuroprotective agents have been the focus of many clinical trials over the past few years. According to the National Stroke Association ([NSA], 2006), the objective of these drugs is to decrease the damage to the brain at the necrotic core caused by the ischemic cascade. However, there have been more than 49 different agents studied in over 114 trails without promising results (Murphy, 2003). Some drugs currently being investigated are glutamate antagonists, calcium antagonists, opiate antagonists, gamma-aminobutyric acid–A (GABA-A) agonists, calpain inhibitors, kinase inhibitors, and antioxidants (Beresford, Parsons, & Hunter 2003; Wahlgren & Ahmed, 2004). Investigation of neuroprotective agents will continue to be a focus of research in the future.

> ***Red Flag***
>
> **The Priority Care for the Patient with an Acute Stroke Condition**
>
> Most stroke patients will be admitted through the emergency department (ED). In the acute phase, the nurse is responsible for management of the ABCs, (airway, breathing, and cardiopulmonary support). The patient may need to be assisted with airway management if his or her ability to swallow has been impaired, because he or she is at risk for aspiration of his or her saliva. Also, he or she will have a lot of anxiety and fear over his or her lack of ability to control his or her body. He or she may be confused or lethargic. Safety will be a major concern. The nurse should seek family support and involvement to stay with the patient to keep him or her calm. This also helps to decrease the family anxiety level if they can assist in care.

Emergency Management

In the emergent phase of a stroke it is important for the patient to seek health care attention immediately. Some hospitals have set up stroke teams or a stroke code, which alerts health care providers of a patient who is being admitted for a possible ischemic stroke. Having health care providers who are experts in the diagnosis and management of a stroke can help to expedite treatment and save valuable time, potentially improving patient outcome. It is also important to note that other neurological disorders, such as migraine headaches, epilepsy, syncope, peripheral nerve disorders, intracranial tumors or abscess, subdural hematoma, and metabolic disorders, such as hypoglycemia, may present with symptoms that are similar to those of a stroke. It is vital that the health care team be able to differentiate between these disorders and those of a stroke to accurately administer treatment (Adams, et al., 2003; Institute for Clinical Systems Improvement [ICSI], 2003).

According to the ICSI (2003), tissue plasminogen activator (tPA), which is a drug that helps to break up blood clots, should be administered to appropriate candidates within 60 minutes of the patient presenting to the ED. To achieve this goal, the health care team must work quickly and efficiently to appropriately diagnose the patient. The ED nurse should start the rapid triage protocol. Many hospitals may have a clinical pathway or care map (Figure 35-2) that can

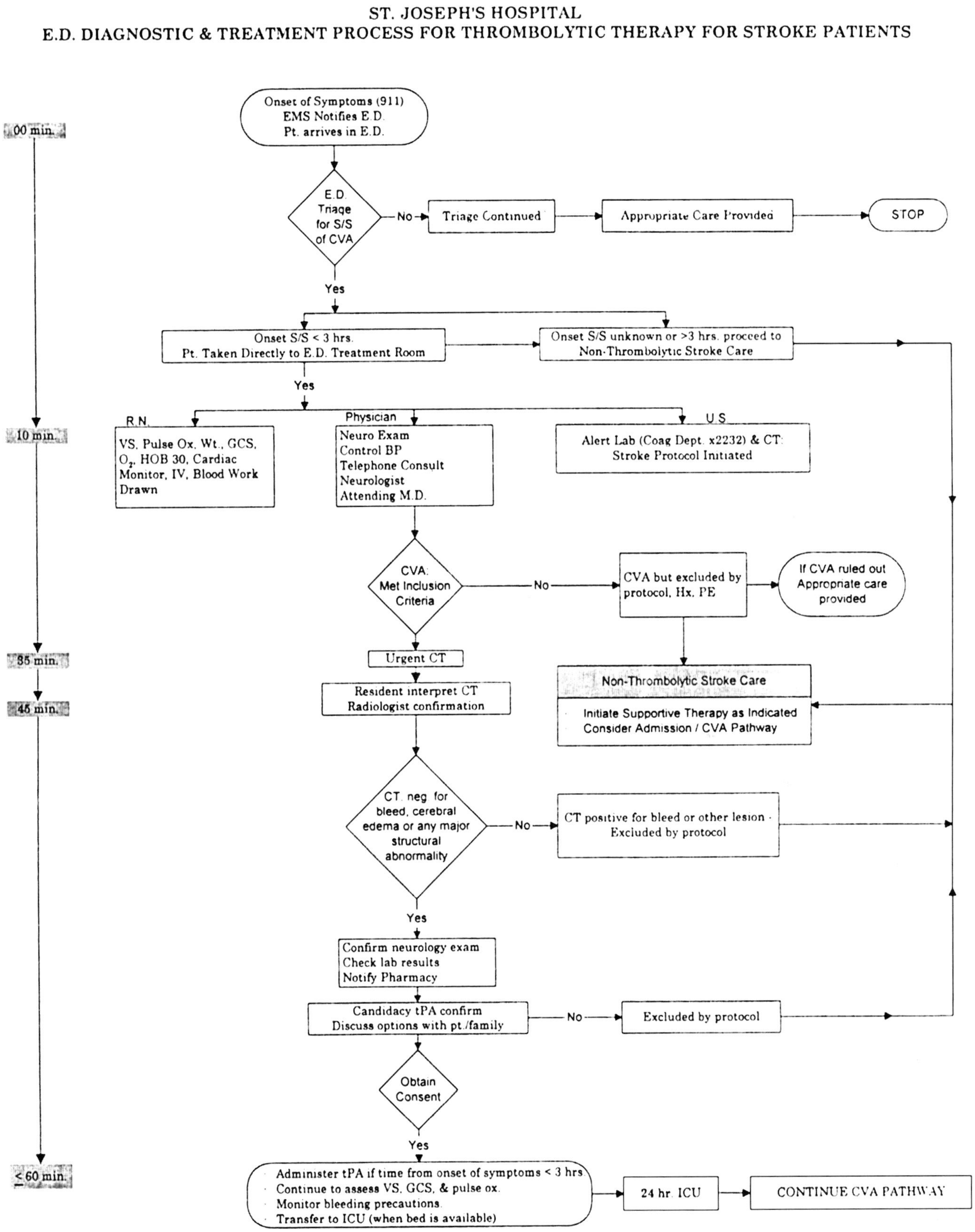

Figure 35-2 St. Joseph's Hospital emergency department diagnostic and treatment process for thrombolytic therapy for stroke patients care map. Courtesy of St. Joseph's Regional Medical Center.

be used to guide patient care in the ED. Patients that present to the ED within three hours of the onset of symptoms should be considered emergent, taken to a treatment room immediately, and the physician notified.

A history of when the symptoms began will be critical. The nurse should determine when was the last time that the patient was observed as normal or at his or her functional baseline. This is when the time begins. For example, if a patient was seen at the grocery store at 9 a.m. and he or she presents to the ED at 11 a.m. with weakness on the right side of his or her body, then the stroke has occurred sometime between 9 and 11 a.m. This is important when looking at the possibility of using certain clot busting drugs. The nurse will also need to determine the location, severity, and length of time the symptoms have been present. After these data have been obtained, the nurse or health care provider will conduct a neurological exam. Using the National Institute for Healthcare Stroke Scale (NIHSS), the patient will be asked to answer a series of questions and to perform simple tasks. The NIHSS is used to evaluate a patient's level of consciousness (LOC), orientation, eye movements, facial movements, motor strength, coordination, sensation, language, comprehension, articulation, and neglect. The exam takes approximately 5 to 8 minutes to administer. The NIH recommends a health care provider first see the patient within 10 minutes of arrival at the ED (ICSI, 2003).

Once the health care provider has determined the possibility of a stroke for a patient, the appropriate diagnostic tests should be completed. The NIH recommends that the CT scan be completed within 25 minutes of arrival to the ED (ICSI, 2003). The nurse should start two IVs in anticipation of administration of thromboembolytic therapy in case the patient is a candidate for tPA. This will allow one IV line to be dedicated to tPA. See Table 35-2 for indications and contraindication for tPA therapy. While the drug of choice for an ischemic stroke is tPA, this drug must be given within the first three hours from the onset of symptoms. This is why it is important for EDs to have a plan for managing stroke patients. All patients presenting with stroke symptoms should be evaluated as a possible candidate for tPA. This clot busting drug can greatly improve a patient's outcome if given within the "golden" three hour window. However, according to the AHA (2003), the average time for a patient to arrive in the ED is three to six hours from the onset of stroke symptoms. The goal of tPA is to restore blood flow to the ischemic penumbra. The dosing for tPA is 0.9 mg/kg intravenously, with a maximum dose of 90 mg. Ten percent of the dose is given in a bolus over 1 to 2 minutes, and the remainder is infused over 60 minutes after the CT results confirm that the patient does not have a hemorrhagic stroke (ICSI, 2003). The nurse must get an estimated or accurate weight to properly dose the patient.

After the patient has received tPA, they are admitted to an intensive care unit (ICU) for close monitoring. The patient will require vital signs and neurological checks every 15 minutes for 2 hours, then every 30 minutes for 6 hours, and then every hour for 24 hours. The nurse should also monitor the patient's blood pressure. The goal, according to the NIH, is to maintain the systolic blood pressure at less than 185 mm Hg and diastolic blood pressure at less than 110 mm Hg (ICSI, 2003). The patient should be closely monitored for central nervous system (CNS) changes, such as decreased LOC, headache, papillary changes, increased blood pressure, nausea, and vomiting. If these symptoms occur, tPA should be stopped and the health care provider contacted immediately. An emergent CT scan may be ordered to evaluate for an intracranial hemorrhage. Lab values (e.g., hemoglobin, hematocrit, PTT, PT, and platelets) should be ordered stat to determine blood volume and clotting factors.

For patients, with an ischemic stroke who are not candidates for tPA, aspirin should be given immediately, except when contraindicated (Klijn & Hankey, 2003). Heparin should be started at 800 to 1,200 units per hour to maintain a PTT between one-and-a-half to two times the patient's baseline.

All acute stroke patients should have close monitoring of blood pressure, hyperthermia, and glucose levels. The goal is to manage the blood pressure.

Red Flag

Nursing Care of a Patient Receiving tPA

A patient who has received tPA must be monitored closely and should be in an ICU or acute stroke unit. These patients are at high risk for intracerebral hemorrhage. Other important interventions are:

- No aspirin, antiplatelets, or anticoagulants should be given for 24 hours after tPA has infused.
- Avoid any invasive procedures (IC or intra-arterial devices or nasogastric tubes)
- Neurological checks should be done every 15 min for 2 hours
- If the patient's neurological status deteriorates, assume an intracranial bleed and notify a physician immediately

TABLE 35-2 Clinical Indications and Contraindications for tPA in Stroke Patients

Indications	Acute onset of neurological symptoms
	Onset less than three hours
	18 years or older
	No evidence of cerebral hemorrhage, sulcal edema, or swelling on CT scan
Clinical contraindications	Onset of stroke greater than three hours
	Rapid improvement of symptoms
	Mild stroke symptoms
	Obtunded or comatose state (involving middle cerebral artery stroke)
	Seizure activity at stroke onset or within three hour window prior to tPA
	Symptoms suggesting subarachnoid hemorrhage
	Uncontrolled hypertension (systolic blood pressure greater than 185 mm Hg or diastolic blood pressure greater than 110 mm Hg)
	Less than 18 years old
History contraindications	Minor ischemic stroke within 30 days
	Major ischemic stroke or head trauma within last three months
	History of intracerebral bleed
	Untreated cerebral aneurysm, arteriovenous malformation (AVM), or brain tumor
	GI or GU hemorrhage within last three weeks
	Lumbar puncture within last 3 days or arterial puncture (at noncompressible site) within last 7 days.
	Patients with international normalized ratio (INR) greater than 1.7 and taking oral anticoagulants
	Patients receiving heparin within last 48 hours and with elevated activated partial thromboplastin time (aPTT)
	Patients receiving low molecular weight heparin within last 24 hours
	Pregnant or anticipated pregnant female
	Known coagulation disorder
	Received tPA within last 7 days
Laboratory contraindications	Glucose less than 50 or greater than 400 mg/dL
	Platelet count less than 100,000 mm^3
	Prothrombin time greater than 15 or INR greater than 1.7
	Elevated APT
	Positive pregnancy test
Radiological contraindications	Intracranial hemorrhage
	Findings suggesting a new or evolving stroke
	Intracranial tumor, aneurysm, or AVM

Adapted from Institute for Clinical Systems Improvement. (2003). Diagnosis and initial treatment of ischemic stroke. *Retrieved June 13, 2006, from www.guideline.gov.*

The drugs of choice are labetalol (Normodyne) or enalapril (Vasotec). Based on current evidence-based practice, hyperthermia has been associated with poor outcomes in patients; therefore, the nurse should treat temperatures above 37.5° C (99.5° F) with Tylenol. For temperatures greater than 39.4° C (103° F), initiation of cooling blankets and ice packs should be warranted.

Managing hyperglycemia is also important. Avoid use of glucose in IV fluids and the use of corticosteroids, and monitor blood glucose levels frequently. Hyperglycemia should be treated with small dose subcutaneous insulin to prevent hypoglycemia (ICSI, 2003).

In the acute phase of stroke care, the nurse also initiates measures to prevent deep vein thrombosis (DVT) and other complications of immobility. Nursing care of the patient who has suffered a stroke will be discussed later in this chapter.

Surgery

For patients who have suffered an intracranial hemorrhage, the prognosis is generally poorer than that for patients who have sustained an ischemic stroke. Treatment for hemorrhagic stroke will depend on the location of the stroke and the blood vessels involved. Recent evidence suggests that in the case of hemorrhage into the ventricle of the brain, fibrinolytic agents injected into the ventricular system may dissolve the clot and improve outcomes (Lapointe & Haines, 2004). However this therapy still needs further investigation. Intraventricular bleeding can cause hydrocephalus, because the clot formed can block drainage of cerebrospinal fluid (CSF). When this complication occurs, a ventricular shunt is required to drain fluid. If the bleeding was caused by an aneurysm, a metal clip can be surgically inserted and placed over the aneurysm to prevent further bleeding. If the bleeding has formed a large clot (hematoma) that cannot be absorbed by the body,

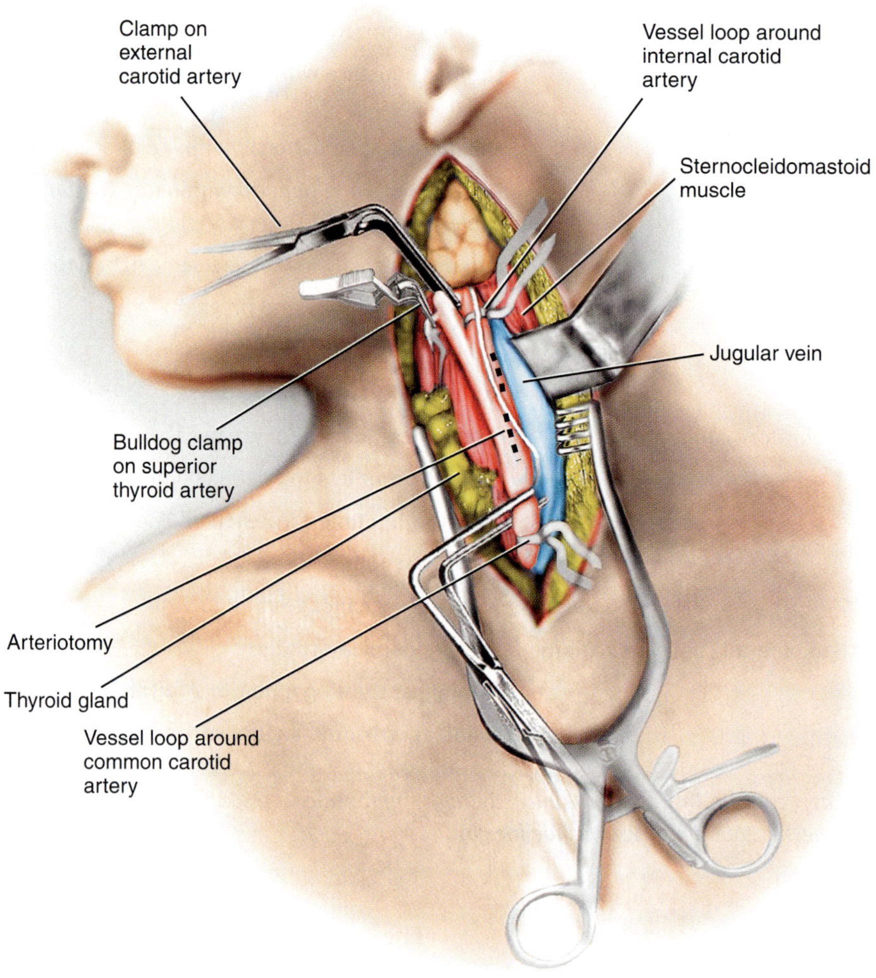

Figure 35-3 A carotid endarterectomy.

the patient may need to have the hematoma surgically removed. Some patients that develop hemorrhagic strokes have a condition called arteriovenous malformation (AVM). These are caused by errors in the development of the blood vessels in the brain that result in a localized arteriovenous shunt. About half of the patients with this condition are unaware that they have the condition until they have a hemorrhagic stroke. The risk of hemorrhage increases with the patient's age. AVMs are a significant risk factor for hemorrhagic strokes in young adults. Depending on the location and the size of the AVM, the patient may be a candidate for surgery, embolization, or radiosurgery (Soderman, et al., 2003).

Other surgical options include carotid endarterectomy to prevent stroke (Figure 35-3). Carotid endarterectomy is a surgical procedure that involves removing plaque from the carotid arteries. The surgeon creates an incision in the carotid artery and removes atherosclerotic plaque that has built up along the artery wall and impaired blood flow. In some cases, a stent is placed in the artery. Stenting is becoming a more popular option for patients with atherosclerotic buildup in the carotid arteries. While this procedure, also known as angioplasty with stent placement, has been done for many years in patients with coronary artery disease, it has only recently been approved for use in carotid arteries. Carotid stenting (Figure 35-4) involves placing a tiny balloon-tipped catheter into the carotid artery, inflating the balloon to improve blood flow, and then leaving a tiny mesh tube in place to keep the artery open (American Stroke Association, 2004; Coward, Featherstone, & Brown, 2004). With risks and complication rates similar to carotid endarterectomy, this procedure will most likely continue to gain popularity with health care providers and patients.

In patients who are ineligible for IV thrombolysis (tPA), catheter-based treatment may be an effective option. Catheter-based treatment involves local thrombolysis and or use of a balloon angioplasty or stenting (Ramee, Subramanian, Felberg, McKinley, Jenkins, Collins, et al., 2004). Ramee, et al. (2004) reported that 56 percent of patients in their study showed marked improvement in their NIHSS score, and 38 percent had independent survival at follow-up. This was a small study and needs further follow-up with larger clinical trials.

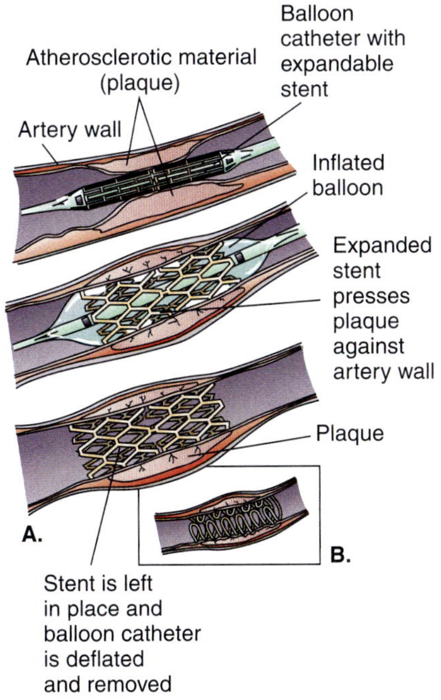

Figure 35-4 Stenting and angioplasty.

Evaluation of Outcomes

Potential patient outcomes for each of the example nursing diagnoses for the patient with the CVA are:

- Impaired verbal communication related to different types of aphasia from the CVA. The patient is able to use a form of communication to get needs met and to relate well with persons and environment.
- Disturbed sensory perception related to the neurological damage from the CVA. The patient achieves optimal functioning within the limits of physical impairments as evidenced by the ability to communicate effectively and to engage in meaningful activities.
- Impaired physical mobility related to the hemiparesis caused by the CVA. The patient performs physical activity independently or with whatever assistive devices are needed.
- Risk for caregiver role strain related to the chronic nature of the resulting CVA. The caregiver demonstrates competence and confidence in performing the caregiver role by meeting care that the patient requires.
- Risk for situational low self-esteem related to the variety of changes from the CVA. The patient recognizes, accepts, and verbalizes positive aspects of the self and his or her performance.

Following a stroke, patients may experience a vast array of complications. Following the initial ischemic episode cerebral hypoxia can result from poor

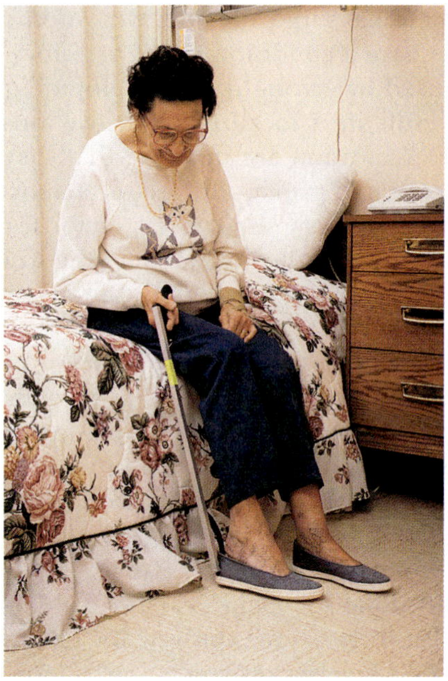

Figure 35-5 A patient in rehabilitation after having a stroke.

oxygenation, decreased cerebral perfusion, and vasospasm of cerebral vessels. The nurse plays a vital role in managing **intracranial pressure** (**[ICP]** the amount of pressure placed on the structures within the brain and promoting cerebral perfusion). In addition, the rehabilitation phase of care for the patient recovering from a stroke is complex (Figure 35-5). These issues will be discussed further in the brain-injured patient.

BRAIN INJURIES

According to the Centers for Disease Control and Prevention, 1.5 million individuals sustain brain injuries annually and another 5.3 million currently live with permanent disabilities associated with brain injuries. While it is estimated that only 74 percent of those with brain injuries are seen in a health care setting (e.g., hospital or clinic); the cost associated with mild brain injuries is estimated at $17 billion.

Epidemiology

The high-risk groups for brain injury are infants, young adolescents, adult males, and the elderly (Brain Injury Association of America [BIAA], 2006). See Table 35-3 for more information on specific behaviors that place these groups at increased risk for brain injury.

Etiology

The major causes of traumatic brain injury are motor vehicle crashes, followed by falls, assaults or firearms, and sports or recreation. Motor vehicle crashes account for 44 percent of traumatic brain injuries. Major contributing factors are not wearing seatbelts and driving while intoxicated. Alcohol intoxication

TABLE 35-3 Causes of Brain Injury by Age-Groups

AGE-GROUP	CAUSES
Infants and young children	Shaken baby syndrome
	Falls (especially under 5 years of age)
	Motor vehicle crashes
	Abuse
	Firearms
Adolescents	Motor vehicle crashes
	Alcohol and drugs
	Inexperienced driving
	Poor use of seatbelts
	Speeding
	Underage drinking
	Illicit drugs (marijuana, cocaine, crack, or inhalants)
	Sports and recreation
Elderly	Falls
	Motor vehicle crashes

Adapted from Brain Injury Association of America. (2006). Retrieved June 13, 2006, from www.biausa.org.

alters perception and reaction time increasing the risk for a motor vehicle crash. Another factor is driver inexperience and high-risk behaviors, e.g., speeding. Several states have implemented a graduated driver licensing system for teen drivers to address the issue of inexperience.

Falls account for 26 percent of traumatic brain injuries. Falls are particularly problematic for the elderly. People over the age of 75 years often have sensory deficits (decreased vision or decreased hearing), generalized weakness, and slower reflexes. These factors contribute to a higher risk for falling. Also, some elderly take medications that can cause lightheadedness or dizziness and affect their balance.

Assaults and firearms accounted for 17 percent of all traumatic brain injuries (CDC, 2006c). Domestic abuse is a significant problem in our society. According to the BIAA, every nine seconds in the United States a woman is assaulted, and researchers have found the primary target for attack in women is the head, thus leading to head or brain injuries. Abuse is not limited to women, it also affects the elderly. In 2001, an estimated 33,000 people age 60 or older were treated in EDs for assault-related injuries (Mitchell, Hasbrouck, Ingram, Dunaway, & Annest, 2003). It is estimated that over half of all the homes in America have a firearm, and greater than 50 percent of firearm owners keep guns loaded and in an unlocked area.

Sports and recreation account for 13 percent of all traumatic brain injuries. Sports, such as boxing, football, soccer, baseball, horseback riding, all types of skating, and skiing, can place a person at risk for a head injury. Colliding with another player, getting hit in the head with a ball, and falling most often lead to mild brain injuries, or concussions; but some injuries lead to more serious brain injury requiring hospitalization.

Types of Brain Injuries

Trauma to the head may result in both primary and secondary injuries to the brain. A primary brain injury is one that is a result of a direct trauma to the brain (Celik, Aksoy, & Akyolcu, 2004). A secondary injury occurs as a result of an injury to the brain (hypoxia, cerebral edema, hypertension, increased ICP, or hypercapnia). A primary injury is called a traumatic brain injury (brain damage as a direct result of an external force). According to the BIAA, a traumatic brain injury is an insult to the brain, not of a degenerative or cognitive nature, caused by an external physical force, which may produce a diminished or altered state of consciousness, and results in an impairment of cognitive abilities or physical functioning. It can also result in the disturbance of behavioral or emotional functioning. These impairments may be either temporary or permanent and cause partial or total functional disability or psychological maladjustment (BIAA, 2004). In 1997, they came out with a definition for an acquired brain injury, stating it commonly results in a change in neural activity, which affects the physical integrity, the metabolic activity, or the functional ability of the cell. Secondary injuries can occur as a result of a primary injury.

Primary injuries to the brain may be classified as either open or closed injuries. An open injury occurs when there is a break in the skull (skull fracture). Skull fractures are caused by direct blows either from an object striking the skull (blunt instrument or projectile) or from the skull striking a surface. A depressed skull fracture results from a blow to the head that causes a part of the skull to be pushed inward, pressing on brain tissue. Patients with open injuries have an increased risk of infection because of the opening created by the fracture. One type of fracture, a basilar skull fracture, is often associated with CSF leakage from the ear or nose.

Closed injuries occur when there is no fracture to the skull but uncontrolled energy is transmitted to the underlying brain tissue causing damage. This damage can occur either at the site of the blow to the skull or to an area in the brain that is remote from the site of the injury. The brain is normally surrounded by CSF, which acts like a shock absorber during normal movement. The fluid protects the brain in the event of minor blows to the head. However, injury forces that cause rapid acceleration and deceleration (fall or motor vehicle crash) force the brain to move rapidly within the skull, causing it to strike rough surfaces that are opposite the site of direct injury. Injuries to sites remote from the impact are called contra-coup injuries.

The brain damage that occurs as a result of primary and secondary injury can be local or involve large portions of the brain. A contusion is a common local brain injury in which the brain tissue is bruised. Contusions can occur in any area of the brain but are most commonly seen in the frontal or temporal lobes of the brain. Diffuse axonal injury is a brain injury that results from rapid acceleration and deceleration forces. These forces produce shearing or tensile stresses that damage the axons of nerves (Smith, Meaney, & Shull, 2003). The damage can involve the brain stem and reticular activating system and result in prolonged coma. Patients with closed head injuries are at particular risk for secondary brain injury, which is brain damage caused by an internal force (e.g., swelling), because the bony skull in the adult is inelastic.

Secondary injuries occur hours to days after the initial injury as a result of the body's response to the initial brain injury. Factors that contribute to secondary brain injury include lack of oxygen, hypotension, or inflammatory processes that result in swelling of brain tissue and release of chemicals that damage healthy brain tissue (Celik, et al., 2004; Jeremitsky, Omert, Dunham, Protetch, & Rodriguez, 2003).

Pathophysiology

When the brain is injured, a number of pathological responses are set in motion. First the primary injury may injure blood vessels and disrupt the neuron axons and cell bodies. Damaged blood vessels, depending on the location of the injury, may bleed into the epidural area located between the skull and the outer covering of the brain, the subdural space, the subarachnoid space, or within the injured brain. Bleeding damages brain tissue by increasing ICP. Symptom onset is usually rapid if the bleeding is from an artery. However, symptoms resulting from venous bleeding can be delayed from hours to weeks.

Next a secondary process of auto destructive factors contributes to additional injury. Factors that have been identified as contributing to this process include: cellular anoxia and depletion of energy stores, cell membrane lipid metabolites, glutamatergic neurotransmission, intracellular calcium overload, release of free radicals, and inflammatory processes (Celik, et al., 2004). Energy is needed to maintain normal intracellular calcium levels. When energy supplies are low because of reduced blood flow and poor oxygenation, mechanisms that maintain normal intracellular calcium levels fail. Release of the neurotransmitter glutamate also leads to an influx of calcium into neurons and results in calcium-mediated cell death. Oxygen free radicals are thought to damage cells during reperfusion after a period of low flow causes ischemia. Oxygen free radicals can result in injury to cellular lipid membranes and damage of deoxyribonucleic acid (DNA), leading to cellular injury.

The normal relationship between brain glucose utilization and blood flow is also altered following head trauma. Directly injured tissue shows reduced glucose utilization, while adjacent uninjured tissue shows increased glucose utilization. The inflammatory processes and cellular edema lead to increased ICP from cerebral edema. The increased pressure results in compensatory mechanisms that raise blood pressure in an attempt to maintain blood flow to the brain. These compensatory mechanisms lead to further increases in cerebral pressure. The increased pressure leads to further injury through compression of brain structures in a closed head injury. As the pressure increases, downward pressure is placed on the brainstem, causing injury to brainstem structures. Pressure on the brainstem leads to damage of the third cranial nerve and results in pupil changes, which may be unilateral or bilateral, and in later stages may dilate pupils. Pressure on the respiratory center leads to changes in respiratory rate and rhythm and eventually leads to respiratory arrest. As pressure increases, other intracranial structures are affected, leading to inability to maintain temperature regulation and fluid balance.

Brain injuries are divided into three levels of severity, mild, moderate, and severe. A **concussion** is a mild form of brain trauma and accounts for 75 percent of all brain injuries (CDC, 2006c). Concussions are characterized by a brief loss of consciousness, period of a loss of memory for before and after the injury event (retrograde and antegrade amnesia), change in mental state (confusion), or change in neurological status (BIAA, 2004). The recovery from a mild brain injury is rapid with no permanent or lasting disability.

A moderate brain injury is characterized by loss of consciousness ranging from a few minutes to hours and days or weeks of confusion. The symptoms may last for months and may be permanent. Individuals with moderate injury usually have a complete recovery or are able to adapt to their disability (BIAA, 2004).

Severe brain injuries are characterized by prolonged loss of consciousness (days, weeks, or months) and severe neurological deficits. Recovery is limited and permanent disabilities are common (Table 35-4 discusses types of severe brain injury).

Complications

A number of complications may occur following brain injury. Hydrocephalus occurs when there is too much CSF in the ventricles. This leads to pressure on the brain tissue and deterioration in neurological status. The treatment is the removal of excess CSF fluid, and in some instances a shunt may need to be inserted (see brain tumors for more information on shunts).

TABLE 35-4 Types of Severe Brain Injury

TERM	DEFINITION
Coma	"State of unconsciousness from which the individual cannot be awakened"
	Little or no response to stimuli
	Does not initiate voluntary activities
	Can last for weeks, months, or years
Vegetative state	Can be awakened but is not aware of surroundings
	Eyes can open
	Responses to pain
Persistent vegetative state	A vegetative state that lasts longer than one month
Minimally responsive state	No longer in a coma or vegetative state
	Some basic reflexes
	Inconsistent in following directions
	Aware of surroundings
Locked-in syndrome	Rare neurological condition in which a person is conscious and able to think, but unable to move any part of their body except their eyes.
Brain death	The brain shows no sign of function

Adapted from Brain Injury Association of America. (2004). Support adequate finding of the traumatic brain injury act in FY 2005. *McLean, VA: Author.*

An infection related to a tear in the dura mater may occur. When a patient suffers an open brain injury or where there is a break in the continuity of the skull, the lining of the dura mater may tear, allowing bacteria to enter the brain. This is a serious complication and may lead to death unless the infection can be managed with antibiotics.

A stroke can occur secondary to intracranial hemorrhage associated with brain trauma or from a clot that develops because of the trauma and lodges in a small blood vessel. Depending on the nature and extent of the injury, a patient may be placed on anticoagulant therapy to prevent a thrombotic or embolic stroke.

Chronic headaches may be lasting sequelae of the brain trauma. A patient may complain of a headache for weeks or months after a brain injury. Treatment with analgesics and narcotics may be used cautiously as narcotics may mask neurological deficits. Also, some patients may experience long-term impairments in memory surrounding the events of the brain trauma.

According to the BIAA (2004), the development of Alzheimer's disease, Parkinson's disease, posttraumatic dementia, and chronic traumatic encephalopathy (dementia pugilistica) have been linked to traumatic brain injuries.

Assessment with Clinical Manifestations

The location and extent of a brain injury will determine the clinical presentation. Nurses must remember that there is no predictability with head injury patients. Patients that initially appear to have minor injuries may later become unconscious and rapidly deteriorate. Two patients presenting with the same mechanism of injury may present with different symptoms and have different outcomes. A patient presenting with a head injury may have all or some of the symptoms described below. It is important that any person with a suspected head injury seek medical attention immediately. Symptoms may occur immediately after injury or be initially absent or subtle with gradual onset occurring days after the initial injury. According to the BIAA (2004) and CDC (2006c), most head injury patients that sustain a brain injury will present with symptoms within three broad categories: physical, cognitive, and behavioral (Box 35-3).

The nursing assessment of the patient with a history of head injury begins with determining the mechanism of injury and whether the patient has a history of loss of consciousness or confusion. If the patient is unconscious on arrival at the hospital, determine if any of the following occurred: the patient was initially unconscious or became alert for a short period of time and then became unconscious again, which is a clue to an epidural hemorrhage (Table 35-5). There are several different locations that result in different clinical manifestations as there are neurological bleeds (Figure 35-6). Many patients with head injury have associated injuries of the neck. If the patient is conscious, ask about neck pain. If the patient is unconscious assume the patient has a neck injury until ruled out with diagnostic X-rays. Also, consider whether the patient might have sustained a neurological or cardiac event that contributed to the injury.

It is important to assess the airway and ventilation while maintaining cervical-spine (c-spine) immobility in the unconscious patient. Patients with brain injury and hypoxia have poorer outcomes. Patients with severe brain injuries will have changes in respirations. In addition, it is also important to assess circulation. Research evidence suggests that brain trauma patients with a history of hypotension have a poorer outcome than brain-injured patients without a history of hypotension (McDermott, Rosenfeld, Laidlaw, Cordner, & Tremayne, 2004; Vavilala, et al., 2003).

The nurse must next assess neurological function. The Glasgow Coma Scale score is used to assess LOC (see Table 34-4). The Glasgow Coma Scale must be obtained through interaction with the patient. A second measure of neurological function is pupil reaction. Assess pupils for pupillary light response,

BOX 35-3

CLINICAL MANIFESTATIONS OF BRAIN INJURY

Physical signs and symptoms include:

- Physical evidence of trauma: wounds, contusions, ecchymosis around the eyes (raccoon sign), or bruising behind the ear (battles sign). Raccoon eyes and battles sign are signs of basilar skull fracture.
- Impaired consciousness: may be brief with rapid recovery or a lengthy loss of consciousness, lethargy, or coma.
- Visual disturbances: blurring, photosensitivity (bright lights are painful), and loss of vision, or inability to move eyes. In addition, the pupillary changes can include: sluggish reaction to light, pupils do not react to light, or one pupil is larger than the other (Note: this is a sign of increasing intracranial pressure).
- Headache and neck pain.
- Leaking CSF from nose or ears: the fluid may appear clear but will have a positive reaction to glucose reagent strip due to high amount of glucose in CSF. If the drainage if bloody, place a drop on a white sheet, if a halo appears around the blood once it is dried, it is cerebrospinal fluid.
- Nausea and vomiting, which may be an early sign of increasing ICP.
- Respiratory distress: may have difficulty breathing and require ventilatory support. Slowing respirations are a sign of increased ICP.
- Dizziness, poor motor control, fatigue, inability to maintain balance, and ringing in the ears.
- **Hemiparesis** (weakness on one side of the body) or **hemiplegia** (inability to move of one side of the body).
- Seizures.
- Impaired speech: expressive or receptive **aphasia** (impairment in the ability to speak or comprehend) or **dysarthria** (difficulty in oral movement to form words).
- **Dysphagia** (inability to swallow).
- Sexual dysfunction.

Cognitive symptoms may include:

- Confusion, inability to concentrate, and shortened attention span
- Impairment in short-term and long-term memory; commonly seen with concussion.
- Difficulty reading and writing, and difficulty with problem solving and reasoning.
- Difficulty with planning, sequencing, impaired judgment, and slowed thought processes.

Behavioral symptoms may include:

- Agitation, irritability, and mood swings.
- Anxiety and restlessness.
- Delusions, paranoia, mania, and explosive behavior.
- Depression and decreased motivation.

size, and symmetry. A pupillary size greater than 4 mm is considered dilated. A measurement difference of more than 1 mm is defined as asymmetry.

The patient must also have an assessment of his or her temperature. Hypothermia has been associated with increased mortality in some studies (Jermitsky, et al, 2003). Hyperthermia may suggest injury to the hypothalamus or infection. Also, the patient must be assessed for other injuries. Patients that have sustained a severe head injury may have sustained other injuries that are overlooked because of the head injury.

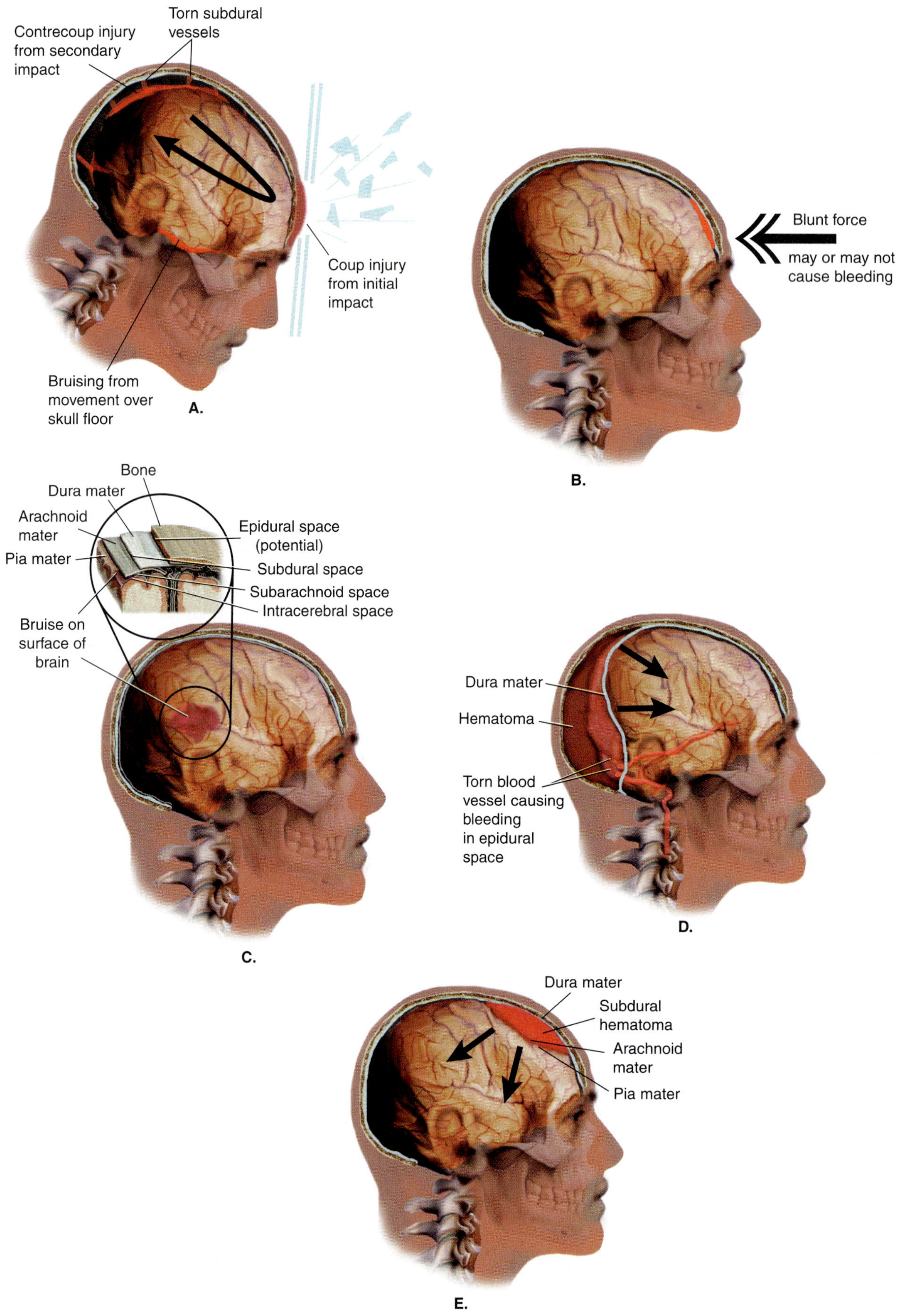

Figure 35-6 Brain injuries: A. Coup/Contracoup, B. Concussion, C. Contusion, D. Epidural hematoma, E. Subdural hematoma.

TABLE 35-5 Neurological Bleeds

TYPE	INCIDENCE OR CAUSE	SYMPTOMS	TREATMENT
Acute subdural hematoma	5–25% of all severe TBI with contusion of laceration Venous blood between dura and brain	Coma Increased ICP	Surgical evacuation of blood Monitor ICP, neuro status, or cerebral perfusion
Subacute subdural hematoma	Higher incidence in elderly related to falls Venous bleed Develops into chronic subdural hematoma	Headache, confusion, aphasia, hemiplegia, seizures, or coma Can appear as late as 2 weeks May be mistaken for stroke	Decrease ICP Surgical evacuation of hematoma Seizure precautions
Epidural hematoma	Young adult males Arterial bleed usually caused by trauma	Brief loss of consciousness but resolves quickly, then a rapid decline in neuro status—nausea, vomiting, headache, seizures, hemiparesis, decreased level of consciousness, respiratory distress, or hypertension	Medical emergency Airway and respiratory management Decrease ICP and monitor cerebral perfusion Requires surgical intervention to remove clot and stop bleeding
Subarachnoid hemorrhage	Happens in males more than females 10–15% die before reaching hospital AVM aneurysm, trauma, drug abuse, or hypertension	Severe headache, decrease in level of consciousness, or neck stiffness	Surgery to repair aneurysm Control ICP Prevent seizures Monitor cerebral perfusion Prevent cerebral vasospasm

Adapted from Reddy, L. S. (2004). Heads upon cerebral bleeds. Nursing Made Incredibly Easy, *2(3), 8–16.*

For the continued rehabilitation of the brain-injured patient, the Rancho Los Amigos Scale is often utilized to evaluate the patient's progress. However, overall nursing care will remain the same whether the patient has a head injury, stroke, or brain tumor.

Diagnostic Tests

Procedures used to diagnose brain injuries include neurological exams, neurological scales, radiological exams, and laboratory studies. During the neurological exam the health care provider will ask the patient some simple questions, ask him or her to follow simple directions, and assess functional ability. This allows the health care provider to determine the extent of the injury and the effect on the patient's ability to interact with the environment.

In the ED a CT will be ordered for all patients that have sustained a head injury. The CT scan will identify skull fractures, bleeding, and contusions of the brain. The CT scan is a screening tool, it cannot rule out some types of brain damage. For example, the CT scan does not provide information on diffusion axonal damage, which occurs at the cellular level, and the CT scan may also not initially detect small amounts of bleeding in the subarachnoid space. A second CT scan may be done later if no injury appears on the first CT scan. If a cerebral hemorrhage is noted on CT scan, an angiogram may be ordered to determine the exact location of the leakage within the vessel. Additional studies that may be ordered after initial treatment include an MRI. CT scans are more effective at detecting bleeding while MRI scans are more sensitive at detecting nonhemorrhagic injuries, such as diffuse axonal damage, cortical contusions, and brainstem injury (McElligott, Greewald, & Watanabe, 2003). A positive emission tomography (PET) scan or a single photon emitting computerized tomography (SPECT) scan may be performed to evaluate brain metabolism. The SPECT scan has the ability to provide a three-dimensional image of the brain.

Several additional imaging techniques are currently under investigation. Several of these techniques make use of the MRI. Diffuse-weighted imaging (DWI) uses MRI to detect subtle changes in the diffusion of water molecules in tissues. Perfusion MRI (pMRI) is used to examine blood flow. Perfusion MRI may be used in the future to determine whether altered consciousness is caused by vascular rather than metabolic, toxic, or infectious causes. Functional MRI (fMRI) measures changes in tissue perfusion based on tissue oxygenation. fMRI can be used to examine regional brain activity in response to sensory, motor, and cognitive stimulation. Proton magnetic resonance spectroscopy (MRS) uses MRI and available software to noninvasively assess brain biochemistry and may be useful in assessing severity of ischemia in traumatic brain injury (McElligott, et al., 2003).

Pulse oximetry is used to assess the patient's oxygen level, and if the patient requires mechanical ventilation, ABGs are ordered to monitor both oxygen and carbon dioxide levels. Depending on the severity of the head injury, and whether the patient also has associated injuries or other medical conditions, additional laboratory studies will be ordered. A CBC will be obtained to assess for infection and hemorrhage, and electrolytes will be obtained to monitor metabolic and renal status. If drug or alcohol intoxication is suspected, toxicology studies will be done, because ingestion of drugs and alcohol can mimic signs of brain trauma. Coagulation studies may be ordered for patients with a history of bleeding disorders or known to be on anticoagulants. Type and cross-matching of blood products may be ordered if the patient has evidence of additional trauma. In severe head injuries an electroencephalogram (EEG) may be ordered to evaluate the electrical activity of the brain. An EEG is one of the diagnostic tools used to evaluate brain death.

Nursing Diagnoses

Based on the information gathered, examples of nursing diagnoses in the patient with brain injuries may include the following:

- Acute confusion related to altered cerebral blood flow or cerebral edema.
- Disturbed sensory perception related to cerebral edema or injury.
- Fatigue related to cerebral edema or injury.
- Impaired memory, short-term or long-term, related to cerebral edema or injury.
- Impaired social interaction related to inappropriate behavior.
- Ineffective tissue perfusion, cerebral edema related to increased ICP.

Planning and Implementation

Head injuries can include patients that are mild to extremely severe in their consequences. On the one hand a patient can have a mild injury without consequences of any substance. On the other extreme a patient can have a head injury that results in increased ICP problems and have a high mortality rate with many complications. Nurses develop excellent methods of planning their care and setting goals, which optimizes the recovery of the patient regardless of the severity of his or her injuries.

Prevention

Most brain injuries can be prevented. Prevention activities include legislation, development of safer products, and education on proper use of safety devices by individuals. The implementation of airbags in vehicles can prevent a person from hitting the steering wheel; but without a seatbelt, the person can be tossed around the car and thrown from the vehicle, leading to a head injury. Legislation has been used to implement helmet and primary seatbelt laws and stricter driving under the influence (DUI) laws in many states. Federal laws have lead to safer automobiles. Education can be used to increase awareness of how alcohol and drug use affect the ability to drive vehicles and operate machinery. Teaching people the importance of wearing seatbelts and helmets is vital. The National Transportation Department and local law enforcement have various programs that educate people, especially teens, on these issues.

Completing a safety assessment of the home can prevent many falls. Removing throw rugs, providing adequate lighting (especially at night), and installing handrails in bathrooms and stairways and tub and shower rails can make for a safer home. Because the elderly are at higher risk for falls, they need to be encouraged to develop a regular exercise routine, such as walking and wearing nonslip, supportive shoes. Exercise keeps muscles and joints flexible and improves balance. Side effects of various medications (antihypertensives, sedatives, or narcotics) will place a patient at greater risk for falls. It is the nurse's responsibility to educate the patient about these side effects.

There are many programs available for people facing domestic violence issues. The nurse should assess all patients for domestic abuse and educate them about available community resources and make appropriate referrals. Many head injuries related to recreation and sports can be prevented though appropriate use of safety equipment. Adults who play sports should be taught the importance of wearing appropriate safety equipment. Properly worn helmets are one of the best ways to protect the head. There are three major programs that receive federal funding from this act. The CDC is responsible for research activities that monitor traumatic brain injuries in each state. They are also involved in community awareness, education, and outreach programs. The Health Resources and Services Administration (HRSA) state grant program works with individuals and their families who have suffered a brain injury, to provide them with services and community resources. The Protection and Advocacy Services State Grants for Individuals with Traumatic Brain Injury is involved in the legal representation and self-advocacy of people who have a traumatic brain injury. To increase community awareness, there are a number of events offered throughout the year related to brain injury safety. The month of October is National Brain Injury Awareness month, and December is National Drunk and Drugged Driving month. Keeping the public informed about the causes of brain injury and ways to prevent them is an important role for the nurse.

LAW IN PRACTICE

Traumatic Brain Injury Act

Because of the impact of traumatic brain injuries on society and the health care system, the federal government passed the Traumatic Brain Injury Act (P.L. 104-166) as part of the Children's Health Act of 2000 (BIA, 2004). This is the only federal legislation specifically designed for people with traumatic brain injury and is a foundation for coordinated and balanced public policy in prevention, education, research, and community living for people living with a traumatic brain injury and their families.

Goals

In general, the following are a variety of goals that nurses can have regarding the management and care of patients with head injuries. The nurse can prevent progression of secondary brain injury (e.g., hypoxia, hypotension, or changes in temperature). The patient can be monitored to ensure a safe environment and receive appropriate patient education in this regard. The patient can be returned to optimal functional status.

Collaborative Management

Patients with moderate to severe injuries will have their care managed either by a neurologist or a neurosurgeon. These are health care providers who specialize in caring for patients with neurological impairments. Other members of the health care team in addition to the physician and patient's nurse may include respiratory therapist, a dietitian, clinical pharmacist, and occupational and physical therapist. Until the patient's condition has stabilized, the patient will be cared for in an ICU. The patient may remain on a ventilator for respiratory support and on a cardiac monitor to evaluate his or her heart rate and watch for any cardiac arrhythmias. An endotracheal (ET) tube is used for short-term ventilation, but if the patient requires mechanical ventilation for an extended period of time, a tracheotomy tube will be inserted. If the patient has any swallowing difficulties, a nasogastric tube may be placed to provide nutritional support.

Management of Head Injury

Most brain injuries are considered mild. The patient will usually return home within 24 hours. Families are instructed to awaken the patient every 2 to 3 hours while sleeping to determine LOC. If the patient develops a headache that increases in severity, nausea or vomiting, visual changes, paralysis of a part of his or her body, or he or she becomes difficult to arouse, the family is instructed to return the patient to the ED or call 911. These symptoms may indicate delayed neurological injury, such as bleeding or developing cerebral edema. Patients who are discharged from the hospital should see their family health care provider for follow-up within a few days.

Care of the patient with a moderate to severe brain injury begins in the prehospital setting (Figure 35-7). Emergency medical personal provide initial airway, breathing, and circulatory management before the patient arrives at the hospital. In the ED airway and breathing management continue to have the highest priority, because some severely injured patients may not be able to breathe adequately on their own. Prepare to assist with intubation of the airway and mechanical ventilation if indicated. Place the patient on continuous pulse oximetry and monitor the patient frequently. The goal is to maintain oxygen saturation at 100 percent (Bader, Littlejohns, & March, 2003). Hypoxia below 90 percent, arterial hemoglobin saturation, is associated with poor outcomes.

The patient is placed on a cardiac monitor and any slowing of the heart rate or cardiac dysrhythmias is reported. IV access is needed to provide fluids and for administration of medications. An IV with an isotonic solution, such as normal saline, so as not to increase ICP is begun. In the instance of multiple trauma, the patient should have two IVs. The blood pressure is monitored closely. The mean arterial blood pressure should be maintained above 90 mm Hg. Episodes of hypotension are associated with poorer outcomes (Jeremitsky, et al., 2003). If the blood pressure falls below this level, notify the health care provider immediately and prepare to intervene with measures to prevent hypotension.

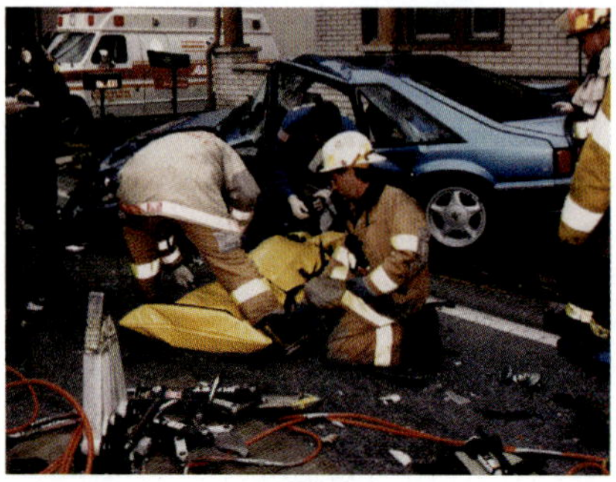

Figure 35-7 Motor vehicle collisions are the most common cause of traumatic brain injury. (Courtesy of David J. Reimer, Sr.)

The patient's neurological status is monitored, and changes in the Glasgow Coma Scale score, changes in pupil response (e.g., asymmetry, sluggish response, or dilation), or a sudden increase in urinary output are also noted. These are all significant signs of increased ICP. Other signs are slowing respirations, slowing heart rate, and increasing blood pressure **(Cushing response)**. Cushing response is a late sign of increasing ICP.

The patient's body temperature is monitored, as damage to the hypothalamus may result in hyperthermia. Some patients may be placed on cooling blankets to lower overall body temperature. For every one degree centigrade that the body temperature rises, the metabolic rate in brain tissue and oxygen needs increases by 7 percent (Celik, et al., 2004). So by lowering the temperature of the body, the metabolic rate in the brain decreases; thus reducing metabolic demands, allowing the brain to begin to recover. Sedative or neuromuscular medications may be needed to prevent shivering and anxiety, which will increase body temperature. A recent study suggests that hypothermia may also be associated with poorer outcomes (Jeremitsky, et al., 2003).

Patients admitted to the critical unit may have a device inserted to monitor ICP. Monitoring ICP is important in the prevention of secondary brain injury. ICP is measured by placing a small tube in the ventricles of the brain. If the pressure gets too high, a ventricular drain (ventriculostomy) may be utilized to remove CSF. The fluid is then collected in a small bag at the bedside. In the past, one way to decrease ICP was through hyperventilation; however, current research now indicates aggressive hyperventilation may actually cause further brain damage by constricting blood vessels and further reducing blood flow to the brain tissue. Another treatment for increased ICP was barbiturate therapy. The use of barbiturates (pentobarbital and phenobarbital) was thought to decrease ICP by producing a sedative and hypnotic effect, but recent research has found that osmotic diuretics, increasing the head of the bed 30 degrees, and draining CSF to be just as effective (Celik, et al., 2004). The osmotic diuretic mannitol may be administered to help manage ICP.

In addition to ICP, the cerebral perfusion pressure (CPP) should be monitored. The CPP is the difference between the ICP and the mean arterial pressure (MAP). CPP is calculated by subtracting the ICP from the MAP. Normal CPP is 70 to 95 mm Hg. (Bretler, 2004). Cerebral blood flow (CBF) is also used to guide treatment in severe brain injury. Normal CBF is about 15 percent of the patient's cardiac output.

Methods are now available in the critical care setting to measure oxygen level in the brain. The goal is for the critical care team to balance the patient's ICP level with the brain oxygen level during the critical phase when the patient is at risk for secondary brain injury. The goal is to keep the oxygen saturation at 100 percent, the $PaCo_2$ between 35 and 40 mm Hg, the brain tissue oxygenation level at least 20 mm Hg, the ICP less than 20 mm Hg, and the CPP greater than 70 mm Hg. During the critical phase, the critical care nurse initiates changes to balance oxygen delivery to the brain and the ICP. This is the primary focus for the critical care nurse during the critical phase until brain swelling is reduced (Bader, et al., 2003).

The nurse plays a vital role in helping to prevent environmental stimuli that might cause an increase in ICP. Keeping lights on a low setting, keeping noise level at a minimum, and providing a calm and restful environment for the patient is important in the recovery process. Visitors may be limited to one or two people at a time for short visits. The family and friends need to be aware of the need to be quiet and not upset the patient. As with all patients who are immobile, the nurse must institute measures to promote healing and prevent complications. Patients with a brain injury should be turned every two hours to prevent skin breakdown. Special attention should be taken, because many patients will need to have the head of the bed at 30 degrees to decrease ICP. This places the coccyx and sacral areas at highest risk for skin breakdown. Also when positioning the patient, make sure to use pillows and support all extremities. Do not stress or hyperextend the neck, as this may increase ICP. Compression stockings or compression boots should be utilized to prevent DVT. The patient may also be placed on anticoagulant therapy to help prevent blood clots from forming.

> ***Red Flag***
>
> **Sympathetic Storming**
>
> When a brain-injured patient becomes stressed, there is an over activation of the sympathetic response and lack of compensatory reaction by the parasympathetic system leading to sympathic storming. The symptoms associated with sympathic storming are hypertension, hyperthermia, papillary dilatation, increased heart rate, cardiac arrhythmias, diaphoresis, increased blood glucose, decreased LOC, and agitation. The episodes usually develop within the first 24 hours after injury and are unpredictable and vary in intensity and duration. Sometimes the symptoms are masked by the use of sedatives and hypnotics being used to manage ICP, but when these drugs are removed, storming symptoms appear. Nurses play a vital role in the diagnosis of sympathetic storming by identifying the triggering agents (e.g., painful procedures, suctioning, and turning the patient). Medications, such as sedatives, opiate receptor agonists, beta-blockers, and CNS depressants, can also help to manage storming. Severe unmanaged storming can lead to a variety of complications.
>
> *Adapted from Lemke, D. M. (2004). Riding out the storm: Sympathetic storming after traumatic brain injury.* Journal of Neuroscience Nursing, 36*(1), 4–9.*

Pharmacology

There are a variety of pharmacological therapy strategies for patients with head injuries. For example, patients with severe brain injuries are also at risk for seizures. Nursing measures should be implemented to reduce the potential for injury in the event of a posttraumatic seizure. Phenytoin, beginning with an IV loading dose may be ordered immediately after the injury and continued for the first seven days to reduce the incidence of posttraumatic seizures (Chang & Lowenstein, 2003).

Heightened alertness and anxiety will increase ICP, thus leading to secondary brain injuries. Antianxiety medication is given to manage nervousness; while antipyschotics are used to manage behavioral issues, such as combativeness, hostility, and hallucinations. However, some recent research investigating pharmacotherapy in behavior management suggests some evidence that beta blockers, such as propranolol (Inderal), pindolol (Visken), and metoprolol (Lopressor), anticonvulsants, such as carbamazepine (Tegretol), divalproex sodium (Depakote), and lamotrigine (Lamictal), and antidepressants, such as sertraline (Zoloft), fluoxetine (Prozac), and paroxetine (Paxil), in high doses may be effective in managing agitation and aggression (Deb & Crownshaw, 2004). However Deb and Crownshaw (2004) suggest further research should be done in this area. They also found some evidence to suggest that psychostimulants may be effective in managing apathy, inattention, and slowness in the brain-injured patient. Again, they suggest further research be conducted. In a study by Whyte, et al. (2004), methylphenidate (Ritalin) was found to be effective in patients with difficulty maintaining attention. They also suggest further research be done.

Surgery

In some cases, surgical intervention is required. A craniotomy may need to be performed to remove a large clot that is applying pressure to brain tissue. Craniotomy will be discussed in further detail with brain tumors. Burr holes may need to be drilled to relieve pressure within the skull cavity when pressure is rising rapidly. When the brain begins to swell after an injury, it only has a small area in which to expand. Burr holes allow the brain some additional room to swell but should be done with caution as this opens the brain up to the risk for infection. If the swelling continues, the brain may herniate (push down) into the brainstem. This is usually indicative of a poor prognosis, and many times the patient is never able to recover.

Patient and Family Teaching

Education of the family is an important role of the nurse in caring for a patient with a brain injury. The family may be experiencing a wide range of emotions. The intensive care unit can be an overwhelming and scary place for most families. Depending on the cause of the injury, they may feel guilt, anger, and frustration; but almost everyone will be anxious and fearful about the outcome of the injury. The nurse must be cognizant of what the family is experiencing and provide emotional support and encouragement. Keeping the family informed of the patient's condition and explaining procedures that are being done will help alleviate some anxiety. Because of patient confidentiality issues, the nurse should limit communication to one or two family members who have been identified as primary caregivers for the patient.

Evaluation of Outcomes

Potential patient outcomes for each of the example nursing diagnoses for the patient with a brain injury are:

- Acute confusion related to altered cerebral blood flow or cerebral edema. The patient will be conscious, oriented, and perform own self-care.
- Disturbed sensory perception related to cerebral edema or injury. The patient will have functional sensory status.

PATIENT PLAYBOOK

Education Topics for a Patient with a Brain Injury

- Inform the patient to return to routine activities slowly and not to return to work too quickly.
- Tell the patient who has employment that requires the operation of heavy equipment that he or she must be given clearance before returning to work.
- Instruct the patient to prevent further injury to the head with the use of safety equipment (e.g., helmets).
- Discuss the importance of avoiding alcoholic beverages and illicit drug use.
- Educate the patient that he or she should inform the nurse of his or her use of any over-the-counter medications and any herbal remedies.
- Encourage the patient to eat a well-balanced diet for healing purposes.

- Fatigue related to cerebral edema or injury. The patient will rest as needed and evidence endurance in their activities of daily living.
- Impaired Memory, short-term or long-term, related to cerebral edema or injury. The patient will recall events (both short- and long-term) accurately.
- Impaired social interaction related to inappropriate behavior. The patient will have control of their aggressive tendencies and participate in normal leisure activities.
- Ineffective tissue perfusion, cerebral edema related to increased ICP. The patient will display intracranial pressure within normal range.

BRAIN TUMORS

The National Institute for Neurological Disorders and Stroke (2006) estimates that in the United States, 40,000 people annually will develop a new brain tumor, and 25 percent of all patients with cancer will develop brain metastasis (where the cancer originates in one part of the body and spreads to another part of the body, as in this case the brain). The cancer usually originates in the lung and breast but can also start in the kidney, prostate, or as lymphoma or melanoma. While malignant brain tumors are only 1 percent of all cancers, they account for 2 percent of all cancer-related deaths (American Cancer Society [ACS] 2004g). While these statistics can appear rather grave, Jemal (2003) noted that patients are living longer with brain tumors than in the 1970s and 1980s.

Epidemiology

The incidence of brain tumors has increased during the past three decades. This is thought to be because of earlier diagnoses rather than an acute rise in actual incidence. There are approximately 17,000 new cases of brain tumors per year, of those, 9,600 are male and 7,400 are female (ACS, 2004g). Secondary brain tumors are more common and occur most frequently in the fifth, sixth, and seventh decades, with a slightly higher incidence in men.

Etiology

Brain tumors are an abnormal growth of cells within the brain tissue. The cause is unknown in many cases, but research is being done to investigate the correlation between exposures to radiation or cancer-causing chemicals. In some cases, genetics may be the cause, especially if the tumor develops in the brain or CNS first, such as neurofibromatosis or tuberous sclerosis.

Pathophysiology

There are several different classifications for brain tumors. Benign tumors are noncancerous and confined to one location or area. Benign tumors are usually slow-growing and usually do not cause much concern in other parts of the body. However because the brain is enclosed within the bony skull, expansion of any kind (tumors or edema) can place pressure on healthy brain tissue, thus leading to neurological compromise. A malignant tumor is cancerous, usually grows quickly, and can spread from one part of the body to another. A grading system has been developed to better understand the different types of malignancy with a grade I being the least malignant and grade IV being the most malignant (Brain Tumor Society, 2004). Use of this type of grading system is also important in determining the type of treatment and how quickly treatment should be initiated. A **primary brain tumor** means that the cancer originated in the brain tissue, however this is rare. A secondary brain tumor is one that started in another location in the body and spread to the brain or CNS.

Another term for secondary brain tumors is metastasis. Brain tumors are also termed for when they develop. Brain tumors present at birth are labeled congenital tumors, and tumors that develop after birth are called a neoplasm.

The most common type of brain tumor is a glioma. These tumors grow from glial cells and usually occur in the cerebral hemispheres of the brain. The most common type of gliomas is an astrocytoma. These tumors are usually seen in children, but if found in an adult, they are usually always malignant. While the choice of treatment is surgery for most astrocytomas, the location, size, and grade of a malignancy often determines the type of therapy. A study by Behin, Hoang-Xuan, Carpentier, & Delattre (2003) suggests that treatment for astrocytomas should only occur once the patient becomes symptomatic and then treatment should include surgery, radiotherapy, and chemotherapy (drugs used to kill cancer cells). While the median survival was only five to eight years, the study did not note any benefit to early treatment with chemotherapy.

Another type of brain tumor is a CNS lymphoma. This tumor develops from lymphocyte cells and is usually located in the cerebral hemisphere. This tumor disseminates tiny seeds throughout the brain and can infect the CSF, therefore diagnosis may involve a spinal tap (lumbar puncture) (Brain Tumor Society, 2004).

Meningiomas are tumors that arise form the covering of the brain and account for 25 percent of all brain tumors and are most common in people over the age of 40 years old. These tumors are slow-growing and nonmalignant, but they can reoccur. Adenomas, also known as pituitary tumors, originate in the pituitary gland and account for 10 percent of all brain tumors. These tumors are usually nonmalignant, curable, and found in younger adults. There are two types of pituitary tumors: nonsecreting and secreting. The secreting tumors cause the most problem by releasing high levels of pituitary hormones, which may lead to impotence, amenorrhea, abnormal body growth, hypertension, and hyperthyroidism. A tumor of the pineal gland accounts for 1 percent of all brain tumors. Primitive neuroectodermal tumors are most often found in children and young adults and are often malignant. Schwannomas are tumors found around nerve fibers and are usually benign. Schwannomas usually involve the eighth cranial nerve, affecting balance and hearing, and may also be called vestibular schwannomas or acoustic neuromas. Vascular tumors are rare and noncancerous, involving the blood vessels of the brain, with the most common being a hemangioblastoma (Brain Tumor Society, 2004).

One of the most common complications of cancer is metastasis to the brain. These cancers are called secondary brain tumors, and they occur in 20 to 40 percent of all oncology patients. The most common originating sites are the lung, breast, colon, kidney, and the skin from melanoma.

Assessment with Clinical Manifestations

The early symptoms of a brain tumor usually are rather subtle and are dependent on the location, size, and type of tumor. Symptoms will usually develop slowly and worsen over time, which is what causes patients to seek a health care provider. If a patient has an occipital tumor, the first symptoms may involve visual disturbances; whereas a patient with a tumor in the frontal lobe may experience personality and memory deficits. However, if the patient is experiencing an increase in ICP, the symptoms may be more generalized and less specific to a region of the brain, because of the fact that the entire brain is now compromised. This is why it is important to complete a thorough neurological assessment to determine the area of the brain being affected.

Headache is usually experienced by 50 percent of people with brain tumors. The pain may last for several minutes to several hours, but is usually more severe in the morning versus the afternoon; with coughing, sneezing, and posture changes are also problematic (Brain Tumor Society, 2004). Seizures may occur because of an interruption in the electrical activity in the brain. In a person without a previous head injury or illness, seizures are an important warning sign. Nausea and vomiting may or may not be associated with the headache, but nausea and vomiting can also be a symptom of increasing ICP. Visual deficits that may include blurred vision, double vision, or partial loss of vision may be related to increasing ICP that is causing reduced blood flow to the eye. Ringing or buzzing sounds in the ear may also be noted as well as balance problems, such as dizziness. Hemiplegia, hemiparesis, or general lack of coordinated movement may be associated with motor or sensory impairment. Behavioral and cognitive changes involving personality changes, inability to concentrate, poor memory, and communication deficits can all be associated with brain tumors.

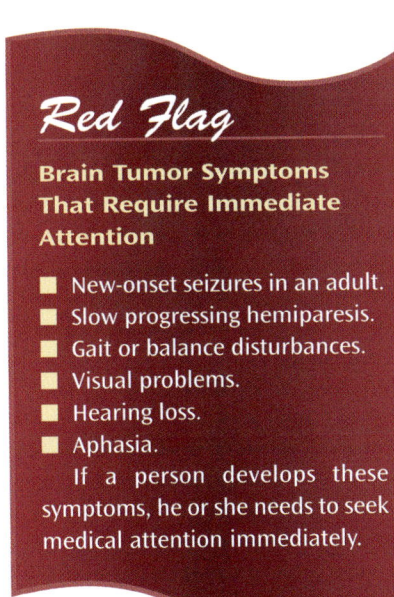

> *Red Flag*
>
> **Brain Tumor Symptoms That Require Immediate Attention**
>
> - New-onset seizures in an adult.
> - Slow progressing hemiparesis.
> - Gait or balance disturbances.
> - Visual problems.
> - Hearing loss.
> - Aphasia.
>
> If a person develops these symptoms, he or she needs to seek medical attention immediately.

Diagnostic Tests

While radiological exams are important in the diagnosis of brain tumors, an extensive physical exam also helps determine the area of the brain being affected and the extent to which the tumor is affecting healthy brain tissue. The physical exam focuses in on a neurological evaluation of the cranial nerves including: eye movement and reflexes, pupillary reaction, hearing, taste, smell, motor reflexes, strength and sensation, and balance and coordination (see chapter 34).

The most common radiological exams used in the diagnosis of a brain tumor are the CT scan and MRI. The CT scan can be used with or without contrast and is readily available in most hospitals. A CT scan can determine the location of the tumor and possibly the tumor type and can detect any associated cerebral edema and bleeding. A CT scan is often used to evaluate the effectiveness of treatment (decrease in tumor size) and whether a tumor is reoccurring. However, an MRI offers better imaging by distinguishing between healthy tissue and diseased tissue and is especially helpful when the tumor is near bone. MRS uses some of the same techniques as an MRI, but does not expose the patient to radiation. Instead, this exam detects the biochemical metabolism of the body and differentiates between healthy tissue and abnormal tissue (Brain Tumor Society, 2004). If the tumor is close to or invading blood vessels, an angiography may be needed. This study involves injecting a patient with dye and then obtaining images of the tumor, to identify the network of blood vessels supplying the tumor, and the blood vessels surrounding the tumor, especially if surgical removal is being considered. An angiography may also assist in determination of the tumor type. An EEG may be obtained to note an abnormal electrical activity in the brain, especially if the patient is having seizures (Daniels, 2003).

While these radiological tests are vital to determine the location and size of the tumor, treatment will depend on the tumor cell type. Determination of cell type is most often done through a biopsy. There are three different techniques used to obtain a biopsy: needle, stereotactic, and open biopsy (American Brain Tumor Association [ABTA, 2004a). A needle biopsy involves aspiration of tissue through a needle. A stereotactic biopsy is similar to a needle biopsy, but it uses the assistance of a computer to locate the tumor and guide the needle into a section of the tumor. Open biopsy involves making a surgical incision into the brain and removing a small piece of tumor tissue; this procedure is usually done during surgical removal of the tumor. The tissue sample is then sent to the pathology lab and evaluated by a pathologist, a health care provider who specializes in the identification of tissue types. Most pathology reports take approximately 24 hours to be completed, but in some cases a frozen section will be taken directly from the operating room and evaluated within 15 to 20 minutes. The pathology report is then given to the surgeon and a decision is made as to how to proceed with the surgical removal. Two of the most important components to the diagnosis of a brain tumor are determination of the origin of the cancer cell (primary site or secondary site) and the potential growth rate. The biopsy results will provide information on whether the tumor is benign or malignant and, if malignant, the malignancy grade. All this information is necessary for the health care provider to appropriately evaluate and develop a treatment plan for the patient.

Nursing Diagnoses

Based on the information gathered, examples of nursing diagnoses in the patient with a brain tumor may include the following:

- Impaired physical mobility related to weakness associated with the brain injuries.
- Risk for injury related to the physical difficulties of the brain injuries.
- Self-care deficit related to weakness or confusion from the brain injuries.

Planning and Implementation

There are three main types of treatment for patients with a brain tumor: surgery, radiation, and chemotherapy. Additional therapies are photodynamic and adjunctive medication therapy. The type of tumor and the grade of the tumor will help determine the course of treatment. In many cases, a patient will require more than one type of treatment (e.g., a patient will have partial surgical removal of the tumor, but need follow-up radiation to destroy the rest of the tumor). A patient's overall general health and past medical history also play a part in determining how the treatment plan will be pursued.

Selection of a health care provider may be one of the first things that a patient is confronted with after learning that they have a brain tumor. The nurse can encourage the patient to look for oncologists who have experience with his or her type of cancer and are willing to discuss all treatment options (including experimental treatments) clearly and fully and able to answer questions and concerns the patient may have. Hospitals affiliated with colleges or universities are more likely to have clinical research trials, if the patient is interested in experimental treatments. The nurse should also provide information on local support groups and community agencies that can provide additional information and services for the patient. Most patients will need a referral to a neurooncologist and possibly a neurosurgeon. A neurooncologist specializes in the management of patients with neurological disorders. Some treatments for cancer located elsewhere in the body are not appropriate for brain tumors. A neurooncologist is knowledgeable about what types of treatments can be used with specific types of brain tumors. A neurosurgeon specializes in surgical procedures involving the CNS.

Management of a patient in the acute phase of a brain tumor is similar to caring for a patient with a brain injury. Patients with brain tumors are at risk for increased ICP, seizures, and other postoperative complications (e.g., infection, pneumonia, or neurological compromise). However, the nurse must also assist in managing the side effects of radiation and chemotherapy (see chapter 15). One of the most frustrating side effects of both chemotherapy and radiation is fatigue. Patients complain that the fatigue is severe, persistent, and unpredictable. It is emotionally draining to be tired all the time. Sometimes the fatigue may have a clinical cause, such as anemia, which may be treated with medications such as epoetin (Procrit). Antiemetic drugs, such as, ondansetron (Zofran), trimethobenzamide (Tigan), or promethazine (Phenergan), may be needed to help control the nausea. These medications can be given before, during, and after the chemotherapy for prevention and management of nausea and vomiting. Patients should be instructed to avoid contact with people who are sick as their immune system has been suppressed by the chemotherapy agents. If a patient wants to become pregnant or becomes pregnant, she should consult her health care provider immediately, as some chemotherapeutic agents may affect her ability to conceive. Mouth and throat sores can be managed with antifungal

Real World, Real Choices

A Patient with Acute Neurological Clinical Manifestations

A 45-year-old office worker with a one-hour history of facial weakness, blurred vision, and left-sided hemiplegia is brought to the ED by life squad. The patient has a past medical history of atrial fibrillation, diabetes, and hypertension. He is a nonsmoker but works in a smoking environment. On assessment, his blood pressure is 210/95 mm Hg, pulse is 110 and irregular, and respirations are 20 per minute. He is anxious, because this is the first time he has been in a hospital. He also shares his concern about missing too much work and losing his job. How should the nurse best handle this situation?

agents, such as clotrimazole (Mycelex), and diet. Appetite changes may lead to significant weight loss; therefore foods should be visually appealing and focus on high caloric and high nutritional value but not large quantities. As with any treatment plan, the patient should be made aware of all the risks and benefits of each therapy and nursing interventions should be focused meeting patient needs.

For a patient who suffers from impaired memory, the nurse should provide orientation cues. Providing a clock and calendar will assist in orientation and provide security in being able to note the date and time. Compensatory strategies may be needed, such as making lists and having a scheduled routine to follow. Teaching should be kept simple and short and may need to involve the caregiver to reinforce learning when the nurse or therapist is not available.

A patient who has suffered brain damage may have deficits in problem solving and decision making. This may lead to problems with his or her ability to maintain a safe environment, manage finances, or keep a job. Strategies to facilitate problem solving need to be practical and applicable to everyday situations. Patients who have a brain tumor need to consider the use of advance directives and identifying a durable power of attorney for health care decisions. In the event that they are unable to make health care decisions for themselves, this person would know their wishes and be able to speak for them. For patients with a brain injury or stroke, the cognitive impairments usually occur quickly and there is no time for setting up a surrogate for health care decisions, but this may not be the case for patients with a brain tumor.

Impulsiveness involves the patient's desire to perform a task without planning the steps to accomplish the task. For example, a patient who has suffered a brain injury may decide that he or she wants to go to the bathroom but not realize that he or she is not strong enough to walk by himself or herself and not remember that he or she needs to put on his or her call light to request assistance. The patient will just act without thinking and place himself or herself at significant risk for injury. Impulsivity is often combined with a lack of judgment, which can lead to disastrous results. The nurse needs to be aware of these patient behaviors and provide a safe environment. The use of rewards or incentives may help to deter some of these behaviors.

Some patients with a brain dysfunction may exhibit explosive outbursts of anger and aggression. Dealing with these patients requires excellent communication skills and a caring attitude. In an effort to calm the patient, the nurse needs to speak in a soft, yet firm manner and attempt to redirect the behavior. The nurse also needs to conduct an environmental assessment to determine what triggered the behavior and, if possible, eliminate the contributing factor. Providing a calm, quiet place, such as the patient's room, may help to relax the patient and allow them to control his or her behavior. Patients may also benefit from a structured environment. Being assigned to the same group of nurses that understand the patient's routine will provide a sense of security and safety for the patient. Limiting the number of visitors, phone calls, and television may be necessary to prevent the patient from becoming overwhelmed. Also, providing frequent rest periods are necessary. While the patient may not have any visual physical impairments, the brain is still recovering. If needed, a medication regimen, including mood stabilizers, antipsychotics, and antidepressants may be helpful (Broyles, Reiss, & Evans, 2007). If the behavior cannot be managed, a patient may need to be enrolled in a structured day program or inpatient psychiatric care.

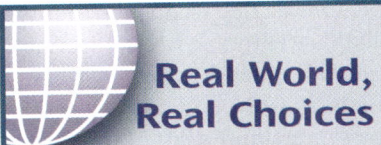

Most stroke patients will have some impairment in communication. Aphasia is when a person is unable to communicate verbally or understand what is being spoken or written. There are three types of aphasia: expressive, receptive, and global. **Expressive aphasia (Broca's aphasia)** is when a patient cannot express what he or she wants to say. The patient knows what he or she wants to say but cannot get the words to form. This type of aphasia may be associated with dysarthria, which is a slurring of speech due to weakness in the facial and oral muscles. **Receptive aphasia (Wernicke's aphasia)** is when a patient is unable to understand what is being said or what is written. It is a comprehension problem. The third type of aphasia is **global aphasia,** which is when a patient has both expressive and receptive aphasia. This type of aphasia is difficult to address because these patients cannot understand what is being said and cannot tell anyone what they need or want. A strategy in working with patients with global aphasia is to use of hand gestures and demonstration. Speech and language therapy will be an important part of a patient's recovery. When caring for patients with a communication deficit, the nurse will need to speak clearly and distinctly. The use of communication boards and gestures may be helpful for patients with severe expressive aphasia. For patients with receptive aphasia, the nurse may need to gesture or direct the patient to perform the task requested (e.g., brushing teeth or combing hair). The patient may be able to perform the task but unable to understand what the nurse is saying. Aphasia can be one of the most frustrating impairments in communication. The nurse must exhibit patience and allow time for the patient to express his or her needs, without jumping in to finish a sentence or help him or her find a word. Some patients may be able to write their needs, so having a pen and paper or chalkboard available will be helpful.

Mobility is one of the biggest concerns for a patient with brain dysfunction. Patients may experience mild weakness of an extremity to total immobility of all extremities. Hemiparesis is weakness on half of the body, while hemiplegia is paralysis (inability to move) on half of the body. Both hemiparesis and hemiplegia place a patient at high risk for falls and the complications associated with immobility. When a patient has hemiplegia or hemiparesis of an upper extremity, he or she is also at risk for subluxation of the shoulder. Subluxation is a partial dislocation of the joint; in most patients it is usually the shoulder. Because of the weight of the arm and his or her inability to move it, the arm tends to hang down pulling on the shoulder joint. This strains the shoulder muscles and over time will pull the shoulder partially out of socket. Some nursing strategies to address subluxation are to support the arm and shoulder with pillows while the patient is in bed and when up in a chair. When the patient ambulates, the use of a sling to support the arm and keep it in alignment with the body will be important. With weakness of the lower extremity, a patient may be in need of an ankle foot orthosis (AFO) or brace to support the ankle and prevent internal or external rotation. The nurse should encourage the patient to wear the AFO during all ambulation or transfers. Spasticity is when a muscle is has an increase in tone that causes an abnormal position or posture.

Spasticity occurs in 65 percent of stroke survivors and can affect activities of daily living, ambulation, and transfers (Ibrahim, Wurpel, & Gladson, 2003). Treatment usually involves stretching, strengthening, splinting, and cold therapy for vasoconstriction. Antispasticity drugs and physical therapy is vital in the management of spasticity. Some medications utilized for spasticity are botulinum toxin, dantrolene sodium, baclofen, diazepam (Valium), tizanidine, and clonidine. Current evidence-based research indicates that the use of intrathecal baclofen (ITB) is effective in the treatment of spasticity related to stroke. The pump is surgically implanted and delivers baclofen directly into the intrathecal space, thus allowing for smaller doses with increased effectiveness. The ITB also allows for frequent titration of the baclofen depending on the level of spasticity. Patients will also need assistive devices for ambulation and transfers. Walkers, canes, wheelchairs, and scooters are all used to assist the patient in mobility. A hemi-wheelchair has a hard seat, which promotes proper sitting posture. A hemi-cane and quad-can are used to help with stability. A walker is used for stability, but the patient must have the upper body strength to lift and maneuver the walker. A wheeled walker may be used, but the patient must be able to maintain some balance.

The nurse must also watch for spasticity, which may lead to the development of a **contracture** (muscle shortening). Contractures occur when a muscle has not been adequately stretched and becomes resistant to stretching. If not treated, contractures can become permanent and disabling to the patient. Nursing care should always include both active and passive range of motion for any patient with hemiparesis or hemiplegia. Edema may occur as a result of an extremity being dependent (hanging below the level of the heart). The nurse should take steps to support and position extremities to promote venous return. Some patients may also experience ataxia. Ataxia is when a person has an abnormal movement pattern. This pattern may appear uncoordinated or jerky. This again places the patient at risk for injury related to falls.

The patient with a brain tumor often has many difficulties with self-care and accomplishing the normal tasks of the activities of daily living. Simple forms of care, such as dressing and grooming, are not easily performed. Therefore, nursing care is needed to assist the patient with his or her daily care.

Sensory-perceptual deficits are in the patient's ability to sense (seeing and feeling) and interpret the data. There are several different types of sensory-perceptual impairments. **Homonymous hemianopsia** is when a patient has lost vision in half of one eye and the nasal half of the other eye. With this visual impairment, the patient is limited in his or her visual field and at risk for falls. Depth perception and a visual field cut may also be impaired, so that the patient does not see anything within that visual field. The patient may walk into a wall or only see the food on half of the plate. Unilateral neglect is when a person is not aware of one side of his or her body. This impairment may lead him or her to only dress one side of his or her body or forget about his or her arm, which is hanging off the chair. Nursing management involves reminding the patient to visually scan his or her environment constantly to watch for environmental hazards and to prevent injury.

Many stroke patients are diagnosed with dysphagia. Dysphagia is impairment in swallowing. It involves the oral and neck muscles and the gag reflex. A patient who cannot swallow properly is at significant risk for aspiration, dehydration, and malnutrition (Rodrigue, Cote, Kirsh, Germain, Couturier, & Fraser, 2002). When a patient with a brain dysfunction is admitted, nurses need to know how to perform a swallowing evaluation at the bedside to determine if further follow-up is needed by a speech therapist. The physician may order a barium swallow study to determine the severity of the dysphagia. Some patients may require a thickened diet, which involves the use of a cornstarch type mixture, to be placed in all their drinks, including water and coffee. The consistency may be like that of nectar or honey, depending on the amount of thickener used. It is important for the nurse to make mealtime as comfortable as possible. The dysphagic patient often has problems with self-concept because of spilling, drooling, and length of time it takes to eat. The nurse should provide a supportive environment by allowing the patient plenty of time to eat (this may entail reheating of foods) and trying to make the foods appealing. Some techniques to assist the patient with swallowing and prevent aspiration include having the patient tuck the chin with each swallow, turn the head toward the weak side to swallow, and hold the breath during a swallow and making sure the patient is in a proper sitting position (Mayer, 2004). For patients with severe dysphagia, enteral tube feeding may be required. The patient may have a nasogastric tube to temporarily provide nutrition with the hopes that the patient will regain some swallowing ability. However, if the patient shows little to no improvement, a gastrostomy tube may need to be placed for nutritional support. When a patient is NPO, it is extremely important to encourage good oral care but be careful of aspiration.

Incontinence is one of the major predictors of discharge disposition for most patients. This not only involves their ability to recognize the need to void or defecate, but also their ability to perform these functions independently. Some stroke patients are aware of the need to toilet but are not able to ambulate or transfer onto the commode without assistance. Also, the ability to manage clothing may be a problem for stroke patients. Making sure the bowel is empty is crucial. Administration of a stool softener and allowing for a regular routine to be established is important. Find out what the patient's routine was at home and then try to accommodate that schedule in the hospital. For bladder management, setting up a voiding schedule and avoiding fluids before bedtime may decrease incontinence. The nurse should also assess the patient for a urinary tract infection (UTI). If the patient had an indwelling catheter at all during his or her hospitalization, he or she is at higher risk for development of a UTI. For patients with a spastic bladder, antispasmodic medications may be helpful. While addressing incontinence, the nurse needs to pay particular attention to skin care issues. Patients who are incontinent are at greater risk for skin breakdown and infection.

Patients who have experienced a brain dysfunction may go through a myriad of emotions from anxiety about what is happening or going to happen to depression and hopelessness that life will never be the same again. In a study by Mukand, Guilmette, and Tran (2003), patients expressed anxiety about dying, changing relationships, loss of independence, change in roles and responsibilities, and financial issues. It is important for the nurse to be aware of all these issues to help the patient work through the emotions and understand how grieving these losses are an important part of the process. Allow the patient to talk about what has happened and how it has affected his or her life; then help the patient to talk about what he or she can do.

Motivation is an important factor in the recovery of any patient. Instead of focusing on what the patient is unable to do, the nurse needs to help him or her focus on what he or she can do. Coaching and encouragement should be a part of every aspect of care. Having the patient do as much as possible, independently, will help increase his or her self-esteem and decrease a sense of powerlessness. In a study by Robinson-Smith (2002), stroke patients who had a higher self-care self-efficacy had less depression. The nurse can help build confidence by helping the patient break the task down into smaller more manageable pieces and then giving them positive reinforcement during each step of the task.

While the stroke patient is struggling with what has happened in their life, the family or caregiver is struggling with change also. For many family members, a change in family roles and structure, financial concerns, time management issues, and dealing with behavior management issues will be a constant struggle. Clark and King (2003) noted that the family or caregiver will go through a sense of loss with a stroke, because their loved one has changed. Instead of the change being a slow and gradual process, such as with dementia, the family has suddenly been thrust into different roles with little to no time to adapt. Clark and King also found a higher level of depression among caregivers of stroke survivors than caregivers of patients with Alzheimer's disease.

They may not even want to assume this new role but are forced into it. It is important for the nurse watch for the signs of elder abuse. These signs may include: physical abuse, sexual assault, neglect, oversedation, or financial abuse (Allen, 2004). A great deal literature has been devoted to exploration of how caregivers are coping with caring for stroke survivors. In a study by O'Connell, Baker, and Prosser (2003), caregivers found the patient relying on them for all activities, including social interactions. The caregivers reported that they would have liked to have more information about the recovery process, emotional changes with the patient, and how to manage these changes. The nurse needs to help the family or caregiver recognizing the stress that a role change can bring and help to build on the strengths within the family unit (Bluvol, 2003). Caregivers are expected to learn a vast amount of information in a short period of time. It is easy for the nurse to overwhelm caregivers. Take time to talk with the family or caregiver to find out what he or she has the most concerns about and address those areas first.

While most patients will be discharged from an acute care or rehabilitation setting, caring for a patient with a brain dysfunction is far from over. With the shortening length of stay for many patients, nurses need to be aware of how to

Uncovering the Evidence

Family Caregivers of Patients with Strokes

Discussion: A study by Bakas, Austin, Jessup, Williams, & Oberst (2004) investigated what caregivers of patients, who had suffered a stroke, identified as the most time-consuming and difficult tasks. They found that while nurses might assume that the actual hands-on care would be the most difficult to master, caregivers felt that administering treatments and medications, providing personal care, running errands, and planning activities were their least difficult task. The most difficult tasks were managing behavioral issues, providing emotional support, carrying out household tasks, and managing finances. The most time-consuming tasks involved providing emotional support, providing transportation, managing finances, bills, health care forms, and doing household tasks. The least time-consuming tasks were finding eldercare, providing personal care, assisting with mobility and administration of treatments and medications, and communicating with the stroke survivor.
Implications for Practice: The implications for nursing care suggest that nurses should provide resources for caregivers to get assistance after discharge. Contacting a social worker or organization for referrals can do this. The nurse should also provide consistent follow-up to see how the caregiver is managing and, if symptoms of depression are noted, to seek psychological counseling. Having an understanding of what tasks are the most difficult and time-consuming for a caregiver will help the family prepare for the adjustments that will be needed once the patient goes home.

Source: Bakas, T., Austin, J. K., Jessup, S. L., Williams, L. S., & Obsert, M. T. (2004). Time and difficulty of tasks provided by family caregivers of stroke survivors. Journal of Neuroscience Nursing, *36(2), 95–106.*

assist these patients within the community. In 1988, the average patient suffering a stroke was in the hospital 11.1 days; in 2002 it has dropped to 5.3 days according to the 2002 National Hospital Discharge Survey (DeFrances, & Hall, 2004). That is a decrease of 5.8 days in the past 14 years. Based on this information, nurses will be caring for stroke patients in multiple health care settings. Some patients may be eligible for home rehabilitation or a type of day rehabilitation program, but insurance companies may not offer coverage for many of these services.

When preparing a patient for discharge to home, it is important to evaluate his or her home environment for safety concerns that were not present before the stroke. Looking at the entrance to the home, staircases, width of doors, and bathroom configurations are essential in helping to make a smooth transition. In some cases, a group of therapists may go into the home to evaluate and recommend modifications before discharge. Socialization is an important part of returning to the community. The patient should be encouraged to return to as many normal and routine activities as possible. The American with Disabilities Act has been instrumental in helping make most public buildings accessible to wheelchairs and other assistive devices. Involvement in support groups may help the patient and family continue to cope with ongoing issues of role change and stress. Support groups are an important part of any rehabilitation program. While these groups provide information on brain injuries and community services, they also give emotional support to family and friend to help them cope with life changes. Nurses should be aware of the resources available to families and of local support groups and encourage family involvement.

Fast Forward ▶▶▶

Gene Therapy in the Treatment of Brain Tumors

There are many therapies currently under investigation for patients with brain tumors. Gene therapy is investigating altering the genes in tissue cells and reprogramming them to self-destruct (suicide gene), slow the growth of the tumor, or to increase sensitivity to certain medications. These genes are injected into tumor cells with the hope that they will replicate and affect the tumor tissue (Castro, et al., 2003). There are studies that examine enhancing the body's own immune system to fight and destroy cancer cells. For example, an immune enhancer gene could be injected into a tumor to activate the patient's own immune response and cause the body to destroy the tumor. While research is promising in many areas of brain tumor management, it is important to note that all potential treatments must undergo extensive well-designed and carefully controlled clinical trials to evaluate the long-term effects on patients before any conclusions can be drawn.

Pharmacology

There are a number of medications used in the management of brain tumors. Corticosteroids are used to decrease cerebral edema and can be used in conjunction with other modalities, but these drugs may interfere with some chemotherapeutic agents. Anticonvulsants may be needed in the management or prevention of seizures, however because it may interfere with some chemotherapy agents, these drugs should not be used routinely (Behin, et al., 2003). Anticoagulants may be utilized to decrease the risk of thrombosis, and antidepressants may be effective in increasing neurological cognition in some patients with brain tumors.

Chemotherapy

Chemotherapy is the use of medications to kill tumor-causing cells, especially those tumors that are malignant. Chemotherapeutic agents may be used alone or in conjunction with radiation and surgery. The type of drug or drugs utilized will depend on the type of tumor, its location, and overall health of the patient. Some patients will receive chemotherapy everyday for weeks or months, and others will receive one dose every week for several weeks; the length and type of treatment will be determined by the oncology health care provider in conjunction with the patient and family. There is significant ongoing research in the development of new medications to treat brain tumors and various delivery methods that will target tumor cells without damaging healthy tissue. The specific drugs used in chemotherapy are divided into two main categories: cell-cycle specific drugs and non–cell-cycle specific drugs. Cell-cycle specific drugs are most effective during a certain part of the cell cycle. Non–cell-cycle specific drugs are effective at any point in the cell cycle (ABTA, 2004b). This is why it is important on biopsy to determine the specific cell type associated with the brain tumor so specific medications can be targeted to kill that cell type. Chemotherapeutic agents are also listed as being either cytotoxic or cytostatic. Cytotoxic drugs (e.g., cisplatin, methotrexate, or rapamycin) actually cause cell death, while cytostatic drugs (e.g., interferon or tyrosine kinase inhibitors) focus on stopping cell reproduction or alter the cell behavior (ABTA, 2004b).

One of the biggest obstacles for chemotherapeutic agents to overcome is attempting to cross the blood-brain barrier, because, while it was designed to prevent harmful agents from entering the CNS, it also prevents helpful medications from reaching the brain. Research is currently being conducted to find medications that can penetrate this barrier, but currently health care providers must use drugs, such as mannitol to help chemotherapeutic agents across the border. Some drugs that can cross the blood brain border include: BCNU (carmustine), CCNU (lomustine), procarbazine, and temozolomide (temdur) (ABTA, 2004b).

Specific information regarding the contraindications and complications in the administration of chemotherapy are described in chapter 15.

Photodynamic Therapy

Another therapy for brain tumor patients involves the use of light and light-sensitive drugs. Photodynamic therapy (PDT) differs from traditional chemotherapy in that it is not histologically cell specific; the treatment is localized (not systemic), and has little effect on healthy tissue. An intravenous photosensitive drug is used and within 48 hours the patient is taken into a surgical suite. In the operating room a laser may be inserted into the tumor tissue or into the cavity after the tumor has been removed. When the laser is turned on, the tumor cells appear to glow green, and the neurosurgeon is able to target the tumor cells with the laser to activate the drug and kill the tumor cells (ABTA, 2004a). Photodynamic therapy is limited to tumors that are visible, accessible, and sensitive to this type of therapy. As with any treatment modality, not all patients will respond to this therapy. Some important risk factors associated with photodynamic therapy include increased risk of cerebral edema, seizures, and extreme photosensitivity to light. The patient must be educated to wear protective clothing at all times, wear sunglasses, and avoid dental and visual exams for four weeks because of the intense exam lights utilized.

Surgery

Surgical removal is often the first line of treatment for brain tumors. The goal of surgery is to remove as much of the tumor as is possible without causing further damage to healthy brain tissue. This is often difficult when the tumor is malignant and surrounds or invades vital brain centers; however, some significant advances have been made in surgical intervention. If the tumor is because of cancer elsewhere in the body, the focus of treatment is on the primary site. Surgery may be utilized to assist with symptom management, but the original site of the cancer must be the focus to prevent further malignancy. Various surgical procedures may also be used to relieve pressure on brain tissue, to relieve seizures, to obtain a biopsy, or to allow direct access to the brain for treatment (ABTA, 2004c). While surgery may be the first line of treatment, some patients may not be good surgical candidates. The most common surgery is a craniotomy. A craniotomy involves removing a part of the skull bone to allow access to the brain tissue, and then the skull bone is replaced. A craniectomy is similar to a craniotomy, but the skull bone is not replaced, leaving a soft spot that will need to be protected (ABTA, 2004c). This type of surgery may be done to allow room for the brain to expand if edema is anticipated. Microsurgery involves the use of a microscope to visualize the surgical area, making it easier for the surgeon to remove the tumor tissue while limiting disruption to healthy tissue. Another type of surgery gaining in popularity is stereotactic surgery. This procedure uses computers to create a three-dimensional image of the brain and allows for precise location of the tumor. In some cases a frame is attached to the patient's skull at four points, and then an angiography is performed to create a picture of the tumor within the context of the frame. With a frameless surgery, tiny markers are taped or glued to the patient's head and then a scan is performed to produce a three-dimensional image. The surgeon uses a wand to touch the markers and then the computer can identify exactly where the surgical instrument is in relation to the brain tumor. While robotic surgery is currently in clinical trials, it is anticipated that this will soon be used to assist in neurosurgery. While embolization may not require a surgical incision, this technique has been useful in preventing blood flow from reaching a brain tumor, thus robbing it of nutrients (ABTA, 2004c). The tumor is then removed a few days later.

Shunts may be inserted in patients experiencing increased ICP due to an increase in CSF. A shunt is a flexible tube that is placed in a ventricle to drain excess CSF. The tube is then rerouted to the abdomen where the CSF empties into the peritoneal cavity. Ultrasonic aspirators use sound waves to vibrate the tumor, causing it to break into small pieces, which are removed with the use of a vacuum.

An important technique that is being used in conjunction with surgery is brain mapping. Brain mapping involves using various methods to draw a map or diagram of the brain. These procedures also may be referred to as stereotaxic procedures. Stereotaxic procedures are especially helpful when dealing with hard to reach tumors located deep in the cortex of the brain.

While surgical intervention is the treatment of choice in the management of brain tumors, it does involve significant risks and needs to be evaluated carefully. As with any brain surgery, patients are at risk for development of infection, hemorrhage, thrombosis, pneumonia, hydrocephalus, stroke, seizures, meningitis, and increased ICP. Goldhaber, Dunn, Gerhard-Herman, Park, and Black (2002) noted the venous thromboembolism (VTE) was the most frequent complication after a craniotomy, leading to DVT and pulmonary embolism. According to their study, enoxaparin or unfractionated heparin, compression stockings, and intermittent pneumatic compression use were found to prevent VTE. Surgical recovery will depend on the patient's general overall health status, age, and location of the tumor, and complexity of the surgical procedure performed.

Radiation Therapy

Radiation therapy uses a concentrated beam of energy to kill tumor cells. The goal of radiation therapy is to decrease the size of the tumor by slowing its growth and preventing tumors from reoccurring. The type and size of the tumor will determine the dose and type of radiation therapy used. Conventional radiation uses high energy X-rays or gamma rays to radiate an area. The dosage is usually the same for each treatment, and treatment lasts for six weeks. However, in the effort to kill tumor cells, healthy cells are also damaged by radiation. Interstitial brachytherapy has been largely replaced by stereotactic surgery, but it may be used in some cases. Interstitial brachytherapy involves surgical implantation of radioactive seeds directly into the brain tumor. It has been effective for recurrent tumors and when other therapy is not effective (Brain Tumor Society, 2004).

Stereotactic radiotherapy (SRS) uses radiation with or without invasive surgery to deliver a precise dose of radiation to a specific location within the brain. It is also called gamma knife, cyclotron, or Cyberknife and can be used for small benign tumors, highly vascular tumors, managing residual tumor that could not be removed surgically, and for recurrent tumors (Witt, Haas, Marrinan, & Brown, 2004). SRS limits damage to the surrounding brain tissue, thus decreasing the risk of posttreatment complications. Stereotactic radiotherapy should be considered for any tumor less than 30 to 35 mm in diameter, patients who are poor surgical candidates, and those who refuse surgery. SRS is most effective on AVM, acoustic neuromas, meningiomas, pituitary adenomas, and grade I and II malignant tumors. Before SRS can be initiated, significant brain mapping needs to occur to determine the exact location of the tumor within the brain and the dosage needed for treatment. After this information is obtained, the actual procedure can take up to four hours to complete. There are some side effects that nurses need to be aware of and are important in the education of the patient and family (e.g., headache, nausea and vomiting, diminished hearing). Two months after treatment an MRI is usually done to evaluate the efficacy of the treatment and determine the need for further management. Radiation therapy is an important tool in the treatment arsenal for brain tumors. Current evidence-based research suggests that patients with single brain metastasis, who have had complete surgical removal of the metastasis, should have follow up with whole brain radiotherapy to decrease the risk of tumor reoccurrence (Supportive Care Guidelines, 2004). Patients scheduled for stereotactic radiotherapy should be assessed for claustrophobia, especially if a frame is to be utilized, any allergy to IV dye, and their knowledge level and comfort with the procedure.

Rehabilitation

The rehabilitation phase begins when the patient arrives at the hospital. Rehabilitation is not a place within an institution; it is a philosophy. It can be done anywhere and anytime—on an acute care unit, in the ICU, clinic, school, and in home care. Nurses should always strive to promote the highest functional independence for a patient. Rehabilitation starts on admission and continues well beyond discharge. The goal of rehabilitation is to return the patient to the highest level of functional independence possible for that person. This will involve training the brain to work differently and adapting to new ways to perform routine activities. Each patient will be assigned specific team members for their unique needs. This team should include multidisciplinary specialists, such as health care providers, physical therapist, occupational therapist, speech-language pathologist, recreational therapist, vocational therapists, psychologists, dietitians, and nurses (Table 35-6). There are several different types of venues for rehabilitation. Acute rehabilitation is usually performed in a general hospital or free-standing rehabilitation hospital. The patient must require

TABLE 35-6 Rehabilitation Team Members and Their Roles

Physiatrist	Physician who specializes in rehabilitation medicine
Physical therapist	Focuses on mobility, balance, gait, strength, and coordination
Occupational therapist	Focuses on activities of daily living (bathing, dressing, etc.), home management
Speech-language pathologist	Focuses on communication (verbal and written), comprehension, memory, and dysphagia
Social worker	Focuses on discharge planning (support systems, financial resources, or community resources)
Psychologist	Focuses on cognitive and emotional status
Therapeutic recreational therapist	Focuses on leisure activities and resocialization
Vocational rehab counselor	Focuses on job retraining and adaptation
Biomedical/Rehab engineer	Focuses on designed adaptive equipment to assist with independence
Family physician	Manages other medical problems outside the realm of the physiatrist
Rehabilitation nurse	Focuses on promoting independence and coordinates follow-through for patient when not with other therapists (PT, OT, etc.)

3 hours of intensive therapy each day and be medically stable. A day treatment program is structured so patients are brought to the rehabilitation facility every day for a full day of therapeutic activities, but the patient returns home at night. Outpatient therapy is when the patient comes to the hospital, daily, for selected therapy times, but then returns home after the therapy sessions are finished. For patients who are homebound, various rehabilitation team members come to the patient's home and provide therapy. Community reentry focuses on helping the patient return to independent living and the possibility of returning to work. They also work with the patient on safety within the community and on financial and household management. Independent living programs help patients to regain as much independence as possible and then provide different levels of assistance as needed. These programs provide housing and a sense of community for patients with a brain injury.

Nurses are a vital component in the recovery process, because they are with the patient 24 hours a day, seven days a week. Patients sometimes feel that therapy stops when they leave the therapy department, however, it is important that therapy continues. It is the nurse's responsibility to make sure the patient continues to progress by following through on the activities he or she was doing in all other aspects of rehabilitation. Nursing care is focused on many different aspects for the patient. Depending on the area of the brain affected, the patient may have more impairment in one area and less in another. It is important for the nurse to understand where the injury occurred in the brain to be able to anticipate the care the patient might need, but remember that each patient is unique. The plan of care will need to be individualized for each patient based on his or her needs.

Evaluation of Outcomes

Potential patient outcomes for each of the example nursing diagnoses for the patient with brain injuries are:

- Impaired physical mobility related to weakness associated with the brain injuries. The patient should begin ambulating and increasing mobility status with success, as well as self-initiating correct body positioning.
- Risk for injury related to the physical difficulties of the brain injuries. The patient will practice fall prevention behaviors and not sustain any injuries.
- Self-care deficit related to weakness or confusion from the brain injuries. The patient will perform activity with coordinated movements and initiate self-care in performing activities of daily living.

Case Study

Nursing Care Plan

Mrs. Lenier, age 77, was admitted yesterday after an ambulance transported her to the emergency department with left-sided hemiparesis. She was treated for a diagnosis of CVA after confirmation with a computed tomography (CT) scan. She was then admitted to the medical unit for follow-up care. Mrs. Lenier's assessment shows that she is normally left-handed and now has difficulty holding eating utensils. In addition, her left leg movements are weak, and her verbalizations are somewhat slow. Her history reveals that she resides in her home with her husband.

Assessment

- "I can't handle a milk carton with one hand."
- "I don't like to use a cane."
- Gait is unsteady and awkward
- Asymmetrical strength in arms and legs
- Unable to hold eating utensils in left hand

Nursing Diagnosis 1: Feeding self-care deficit related to weakness in left hand and inability to hold eating utensils.

NOC: Nutritional status: food and fluid intake

NIC: Nutrition management; Nutritional counseling

Expected Outcomes

The patient will:

1. Attend a teaching session on feeding herself with her left hand at 0930 on 6/15
2. Practice using adaptive spoon at 1330 on 6/15
3. Use adaptive spoon for meals beginning with breakfast on 6/16

Planning, Interventions, Rationales

1. Present a teaching session "feeding with nondominant hand at 0930 on 6/15." *For patients recovering from illness and injury, information about adapting to limitations fosters independence.*
2. Provide the patient with four foods of differing textures, adaptive utensils, and apron for a practice session at 1330 on 6/15. *Providing practice reinforces skills learned and fosters an improved confidence level in the learner.*
3. Notify the dietary department to include a right-hand adaptive spoon with breakfast tray on 6/16. *Using adaptive devices provides safety and promotes independence.*
4. Encourage patient to feed self independently at each meal, beginning on 6/16. *Recognizing and commending success promotes positive self-esteem.*

Evaluation

1. Mrs. Lenier attended the teaching session on 6/15, asked questions, and participated in the practice session.
2. Goal partially met. Mrs. Lenier practiced using eating utensils in left hand to feed self oatmeal, soup, peaches, and pudding on 6/15. Successful self-feeding with all foods except the soup. Continue practice and reevaluate on 6/22.
3. Goal partially met. On 6/16, fed self 80 percent of each meal, used adaptive utensils. Reevaluate on 6/19.

Nursing Diagnosis 1: Risk for injury: Falls related to unsteady, weak gait.

NOC: Risk control; Safety behavior: Home environment; Safety behavior: personal; Safety status: Falls occurrence; Safety status: Physical injury

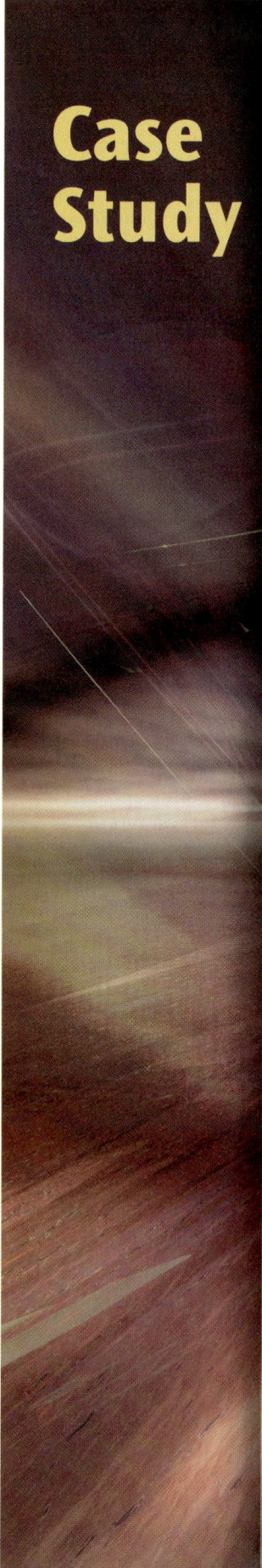

Case Study

NIC: Health education; Behavior modification

Expected Outcomes

The patient will:

1. Participate in physical therapy evaluation of mobility strengths and weaknesses on 6/15 at 1100.
2. Attend a muscle strengthening class on 6/15 at 1500.
3. Perform all strengthening exercises prescribed twice a day at 1000 and 1600, beginning on 6/16.

Planning, Interventions, Rationales

1. Request physical therapy consultation for appropriate assistive devices, strengthening exercises, and gait training on 6/15. Collaboration with other health care providers provides the best care for the patient.
2. Escort patient to muscle-strengthening class on 6/15 at 1600. Provides safety and support as the patient begins to learn new skills.
3. Assigned caregivers will record each exercise, number of repetitions, and patient response twice daily Documenting patient progress toward the achievement of goals aids in outcome attainment and evaluation of care.

Evaluation

1. Goal met. Patient met with physical therapist on 6/15 and "listened well to the therapist."
2. Goal met. Patient attended muscle strengthening class on 6/15 at 1600 and participated fully.
3. Goal met. Patient attended muscle strengthening class and performed exercises as prescribed twice daily.

KEY CONCEPTS

- There are two main types of strokes (i.e., ischemic or hemorrhagic).
- The modifiable risk factors for a stroke include hypertension, hypercholesterolemia, atherosclerosis, atrial fibrillation, obesity, smoking, drugs, alcohol, and other health problems. Nonmodifiable risk factors include age, sex, family history, and past medical history.
- A CT scan is usually the first diagnostic test ordered for a patient suspected of having a stroke. Other tests include: laboratory tests, MRI, PET scan, EEG, and angiography.
- Medical treatment focuses on the ability to administer tPA.
- Complications of a stroke may include cerebral hypoxia related to poor oxygenation, decreased cerebral perfusion, and vasospasm.
- Brain injuries can occur as a direct blow to the brain (primary injury) or as a result of brain swelling, increased ICP, or cerebral hypoxia (secondary injury).
- There are three levels of brain injury, mild (concussion), moderate, and severe (coma).
- The most important signs and symptoms associated with brain injuries are impaired consciousness, visual disturbances and pupillary changes, headache, nausea or vomiting, and impaired cognition.
- Classifications of brain tumors include benign, malignant, primary, and secondary.
- The most common type of brain tumor is the glioma.
- Early symptoms of brain tumors are subtle and depend on the location, size, and type of tumor. The most common symptoms are headaches that get progressively worse as the day progresses, visual disturbances, seizures, weakness, and gait disturbances.
- Surgical intervention is the first treatment choice for most brain tumors. Radiation and chemotherapy may also be needed to prevent reoccurrence or to kill remaining tumor cells.

Continued

KEY CONCEPTS—cont'd

- Stereotactic radiotherapy is a new noninvasive procedure that targets tumor cells using a precise, focused beam.
- Nursing management involves assisting in relieving the symptoms of the tumor and the treatments: surgery (craniotomy), radiation, and chemotherapy.
- Caregiver role strain is a big concern. Nurses must understand the importance of providing caregivers with resources to prevent burnout while caring for their loved one.

REVIEW QUESTIONS

1. The type of CVA (stroke) that occurs when a blood vessel in the brain becomes clogged, usually by plaque buildup is a(n):
1. Ischemic stroke
2. Hemorrhagic stroke
3. Aneurysm
4. Subdural hematoma

2. Select a modifiable risk factor in the prevention of a stroke:
1. Family history
2. Sex
3. Obesity
4. Age

3. An important nursing intervention when caring for a patient receiving tPA is to:
1. Complete neurological checks every 2 hours for the first 24 hours
2. Change the IV site every shift
3. Keep the diastolic blood pressure greater than 110 mm Hg
4. Watch for decreased level of consciousness and increase in blood pressure

4. Usually this radiological test is the first one administered to a patient suspected of having a stroke:
1. MRI
2. CT scan
3. PET scan
4. EEG

5. A primary brain injury is caused by:
1. ICP
2. An external force
3. An abnormal growth of brain tissue
4. An internal force

6. A 16-year-old football player is confused after being struck in the head by another player. He states he does not remember much of what happened, just waking up in the hospital about two hours after being hit. This patient most likely is suffering from a:
1. Concussion
2. Moderate brain injury
3. Severe brain injury
4. Locked-in syndrome

7. The nurse is educating a group of 7-year-old children on preventing brain injury. One of the most important things to tell them is to:
1. Always wear a helmet when riding your bike or skateboard or rollerblading
2. Always wear knee and arm pads when riding your bike or skateboard or rollerblading
3. Look both ways before crossing the street
4. Always wear well-supported shoes when playing outdoors

8. A 67-year-old male is admitted to the intensive care unit following a fall down a flight of stairs. Upon assessment, the patient responds only to pain by withdrawing his hand and curses frequently. Using the Glasgow Coma Scale, the nurse rates this patient as a:
1. 15
2. 4
3. 12
4. 9

9. Your next door neighbor calls you (an RN) at 12 a.m. concerned about her 14-year-old son. She tells you that he fell while horseback riding around 4 p.m., and he struck his head on the ground, but did not lose consciousness. Now he is complaining of a severe headache and blurry vision. You should instruct your neighbor to:
1. Let him rest until morning and then call the physician
2. Give him ibuprofen for pain and some Benadryl for sleep
3. Call 911 or take him to the emergency department
4. Call your family physician and wait for a return call

REVIEW QUESTIONS—cont'd

10. A common medication given to help decrease ICP is:
1. Aspirin
2. Ibuprofen
3. Lasix
4. Mannitol

11. The most important nursing diagnosis when caring for a patient with an open skull fracture is:
1. Risk for infection
2. Risk for impaired skin integrity
3. Risk for impaired swallowing: aspiration
4. Risk for impaired physical mobility

12. A benign brain tumor is:
1. Cancerous
2. Noncancerous
3. Fast-growing

13. A secondary brain tumor:
1. Is only found in the brain or central nervous system
2. Is benign and slow-growing
3. Started somewhere else in the body and spread to the brain
4. Started as a secondary brain injury

14. The most common form of brain tumor is a:
1. Meningioma
2. Glioma
3. CNS lymphoma
4. Adenoma

15. A patient is scheduled for stereotactic radiotherapy in the morning. The patient asks you about the procedure and what to expect. You tell him:
1. It uses special drugs that are sensitive to light.
2. It is effective on large brain tumors.
3. It is a procedure that uses a precise beam of radiation therapy.
4. It is best when used with malignant tumors.

REVIEW ACTIVITIES

1. A 57-year-old bus driver was recently diagnosed with a brain tumor. She has an appointment to talk with her physician tomorrow but is frightened and wants to know what questions she should ask her physician. Identify five important questions you should encourage your patient to ask her physician.

2. You are asked to speak to a group of teenagers about the prevention of brain injuries. What topics would you include in your presentation?

3. A caregiver is concerned about being able to care for her mother, who recently suffered a severe stroke in her home. What are some important nursing interventions to include in your education to this caregiver about caregiver role strain?

4. A 21-year-old patient with a brain injury is admitted to your rehabilitation unit. Identify some appropriate nursing interventions for this patient.

Continued

REVIEW ACTIVITIES—cont'd

5. Identify steps a patient could take to modify various risk factors for a stroke.

CHAPTER 36

Dysfunction of the Spinal Cord and Peripheral Nervous System: Nursing Management

Constance J. Ayers, PhD, RN

CHAPTER TOPICS

- Spinal Cord Injury
- Spinal Cord Tumors
- Peripheral Nervous Disorders

KEY TERMS

Autonomic dysreflexia
Dermatome
Dysesthesias
Lancinating
Lower motor neurons
Neuralgia
Neuropathies
Paraplegia
Paresthesia
Quadriplegia (tetraplegia)
Spinal shock
Tic douloureux
Upper motor neurons

There are a number of central nervous system (CNS) disorders, which exhibit themselves in a variety of ways, often creating long-standing dysfunction. The primary dysfunctions of the CNS described in this chapter are spinal cord injuries (SCIs), spinal cord tumors, and peripheral nerve disturbances. Each disorder creates unique challenges, which affect motor and sensory functioning, and which usually result in long-term adaptation to changes in lifestyle and self-care abilities. A solid understanding of anatomy, physiology, and pathophysiology will contribute to a better understanding of each disorder and an ability to predict the occurrence of alterations, which will result in self-care challenges and painful syndromes. Unique challenges for patients and for their family members are characteristic of these disorders.

SPINAL CORD INJURY

Since 1995 when the actor Christopher Reeve was injured in a horse riding accident, the world has been able to put a "face" on SCIs. After his death in 2004, people became even more acquainted with his heroic activism to support research to find a cure for SCI, especially through stem cell research that has become promising. According to the Christopher Reeve Paralysis Foundation (CRPF), a person injures his or her spinal cord in the United States every 49 minutes. The typical person with SCI is male and between 16 and 30 years of age.

Epidemiology

The face of the person with an SCI has changed in recent years. With the aging of the population, the average age of the person with an SCI has risen from 28.6 in the decade of the 1970s to 38 years of age in 2000 (The University of Alabama National SCI Statistical Center, 2006). The number of people over age 60 who have an SCI has also increased, from 4.7 to 10.9 percent, attributable in part to improved accident response and thus survival rates. The overall incidence rate for SCI is 40 cases per one million people in the United States. This translates to more than 11,000 Americans injured each year. Currently, approximately 250,000 Americans are living with SCI and disability.

Etiology

The life expectancy of a person who has an SCI is somewhat lower than the general population and is increasingly less with higher levels of injury. Higher cervical injuries lead to shortened life expectancy, with ventilator-dependent patients experiencing significant losses to life expectancy. Prior to the 1970s renal failure was the primary cause of death for people with an SCI. Because of improved renal care, however, this is no longer the case. Primary causes of death for people with SCI that have the greatest affect on life expectancy are pneumonia, pulmonary emboli, and septicemia.

Most SCIs are caused by motor vehicle accidents, falls, violence, and sports accidents. Motor vehicle accidents account for 50.4 percent of injuries; falls are the second most common cause for SCI, followed by violence (primarily from gunshot wounds), and sports injuries as primary causes of SCI. Since 2000, SCIs resulting from violence and sports injuries have declined, while injuries from falls have increased.

Primary prevention of drug and alcohol related accidents is also a priority in prevention of SCI. Additionally, sports injuries, especially football injuries can cause SCI; therefore, continuing the education effort about prevention of SCI with the use of protective equipment in sports is warranted. The Think First National Prevention Foundation promotes education for the prevention of SCIs and provides an invaluable resource for nurses, health care providers, and the general public. Their efforts to promote airbags in automobiles have had a tremendous effect on the lowering of spinal injury and mortality rates from motor vehicle crashes.

Accidents are not the only culprits causing SCI. Osteoporosis is strongly linked to SCI in the elderly. In the elderly population, osteoporosis results in compression fractures of the vertebrae, leading to the risk and occurrence of SCI. Spinal tumors may also cause compression and injury of the spinal cord leading to loss of motor and sensory function below the level of the tumor. Other causes of spinal cord dysfunction include cervical spondylosis, myelitis, syringomyelia, and vascular diseases, which result in infarction or hemorrhage leading to spinal cord damage. It is important that nurses understand the leading causes of SCI, so that they can participate in prevention efforts to improve the health care outcomes attributable to SCI.

Safety First 1

Prevention of SCIs

SCIs require the nurse to give serious consideration to primary prevention of accidents in the population, including continued teaching to the public about the use of seatbelts, and regarding the prevention of falls, especially in the elderly. Because falls from bicycles and horses are common causes of spinal injury, public education regarding the necessity of wearing helmets during these activities has helped the safety and prevention effort; however, the likelihood of SCI is not entirely preventable with helmets; the helmet effect is more attributable to the prevention of head injuries.

Pathophysiology

It is important to understand the structure and function of the spinal cord before considering the pathophysiology. Pathophysiological concepts are best understood in the context of the normal anatomy and physiology. Injury to the spinal cord leads to pathology that results because of interruption in the normal structure and functioning of the spinal cord.

One can envision the spinal cord as a power line delivering electricity along its route after leaving the power plant. If damage occurs to the power line, the circuit is broken, and power outages occur in the areas beyond the damaged line. Similarly, the spinal cord carries signals from the brain and CNS to the entire body. Damage or transection of the spinal cord causes loss of transmission of nerve signals beyond the injury resulting in loss of motor and sensory function.

The spinal cord is made up of white matter and gray matter (Figure 36-1). Gray matter is found in the inner areas of the spinal cord and comprises the anterior, lateral, and posterior horns. Sensory functioning arises from the dorsal half of the gray matter, and the ventral half of the gray matter is dedicated to motor functioning. Innervation of visceral and somatic regions of the body arises from the gray matter. Activation of the sympathetic and parasympathetic divisions of the autonomic nervous system occurs in the white and gray matter of the spinal cord.

The sympathetic nervous system is responsible for stimulating the adrenal glands to release epinephrine for the flight-or-fight response. This response will cause vasoconstriction, increased heart rate, and tachycardia. Ventilation and perfusion are also supported by the sympathetic nervous system, and sympathetic responses inhibit digestion and elimination. Sympathetic nervous system responses originate in the gray matter of the spinal cord and are transmitted from the first thoracic through second lumbar sections of the spinal cord. Damage to these areas of the spinal cord will affect the sympathetic nervous system response, causing acute and dangerous physiological issues for the patient.

The white matter of the spinal cord makes up the outer areas of the spinal cord (see Figure 36-1). The pathways for the ascending and descending spinal tracts are located in the white matter of the spinal cord and include the corticospinal tract, the spinothalamic tracts, and the posterior column. The corticospinal tract relays transmissions for motor activity. It originates in the brain, crosses over in the brainstem, and innervates the opposite side of the body. The spinothalamic tract originates in the spinal cord, crosses over within two spinal cord segments, and ascends to the thalamus. This tract transmits pain and tem-

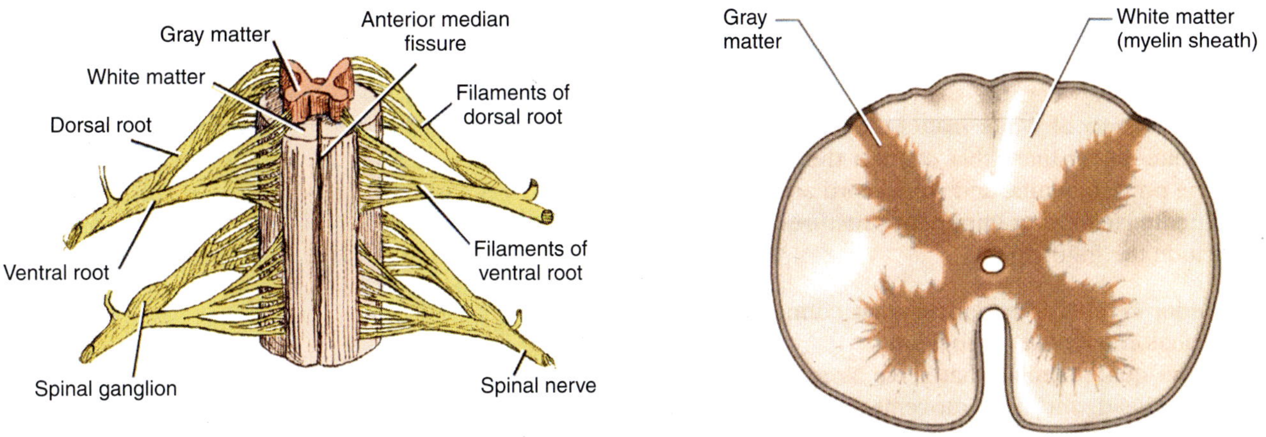

Figure 36-1 Spinal cord: A. Anterior view, B. Cross-sectional view—white and gray matter.

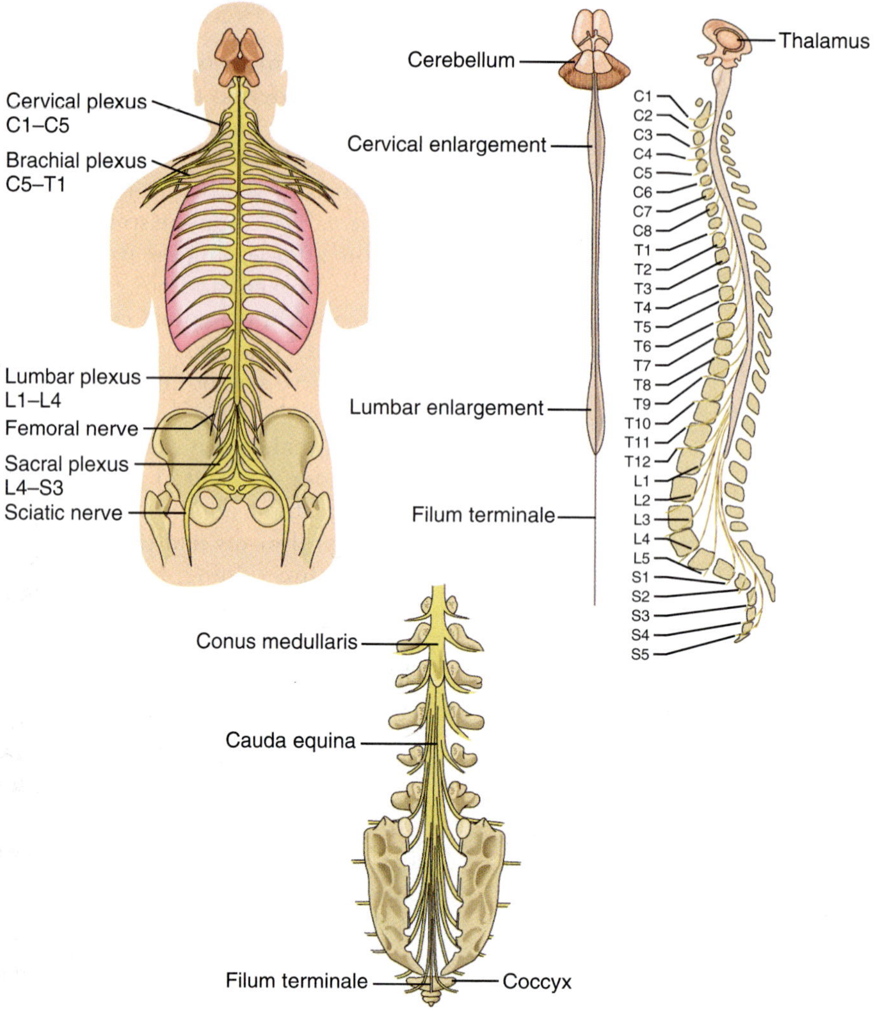

Figure 36-2 Spinal cord and spinal nerves.

perature sensation to the brain and thalamus. The posterior column relays position, vibration, and touch sensation from peripheral sensory neurons.

Activation of the parasympathetic nervous system occurs in the white matter, and originates in the brainstem and sacral areas of the spinal cord. Therefore, parasympathetic responses arise from the cranial nerves and from the sacral segments of the spinal cord. These responses contribute to digestion and elimination through innervation of the viscera, bowel, and bladder. Furthermore, these responses will decrease heart rate.

Spinal nerves corresponding to spinal and vertebral segments also exit the spinal cord. Dorsal roots transmit sensory input to the CNS while the ventral roots transmit motor impulses from the spinal cord to the body. The major plexuses or branches of nerves also innervate specific regions of the body. The cervical plexus innervates the neck and shoulders and houses the phrenic nerve (arising from C3 to C5), which innervates the diaphragm. Therefore, injury to this region of the spinal cord will lead to respiratory crisis if motor impulses from the phrenic nerve to the diaphragm are interrupted.

The vertebral column is made up of 7 cervical, 12 thoracic, 5 lumbar vertebrae, the sacrum, composed of 5 fused vertebrae, and the coccyx, composed of 4 fused vertebrae (Figure 36-2). Correspondingly, there are 8 cervical spinal segments, 12 thoracic spinal segments, 5 lumbar segments, and 5 sacral segments of the spinal cord running through the vertebral canal in the vertebral column beginning at the foramen magnum and ending at the first or second lumbar vertebrae.

Several anatomical mechanisms are present to protect against injury to the spinal cord, which is an extremely vulnerable area. The vertebrae are supported by anterior and posterior ligaments, providing stability to the vertebral column. Acting as cushions against injury are the intervertebral discs, which separate the vertebrae and shield the spinal cord from injury during movement. Even with this protection, because the vertebral column and the spinal cord are in close proximity to each other, injury to the vertebrae and the supportive soft tissue can result in disaster to the spinal cord.

Because the cervical vertebrae must allow for movement of the head and neck, they are innately unstable, thus making this the most vulnerable area of the spinal cord to injury. Logically, the cervical vertebrae are not fixed to the thoracic vertebrae to allow for this movement of the head and neck, but this leads to the danger of injury. Additionally, the mechanism for rotation of the head and neck are provide through the atlas and axis (C1 and C), which increase even more the risk of injury to this area of the spinal cord.

Damage to upper and lower motor neurons contribute to the degree and type of impairment in SCI. **Upper motor neurons,** the descending motor pathways, originate in the brain and synapse with lower motor neurons in the spinal cord. Upper motor neurons suppress firing of lower motor neurons. Without this suppression, lower motor neurons will fire spontaneously. This results in spasticity. Therefore, damage to upper motor neuron pathways will result in loss of control of reflex activity below the level of injury. The inhibition of reflex activity by the CNS by the upper motor neurons is essential in controlling primitive responses that can occur to local stimuli. Consequently, when upper motor neuron is lost through an SCI, spastic paralyses will result because of hyperactive responses to local stimuli.

Lower motor neurons (motor pathways that originate in the spinal cord and continue on as spinal nerves sending impulses to the peripheral areas of the body) originate in the spinal cord and continue on as spinal nerves sending impulses to the peripheral areas of the body. Impulses from stimuli from sites outside the spinal cord travel to the spinal cord and synapse with neurons to form responses back resulting in the classic reflex arc. Flaccid paralysis results from damage to lower motor neurons if interruption of this reflex arc occurs.

Clearly, with an understanding of the anatomy and the physiological functioning of the spinal cord and the CNS, the nurse will be able to anticipate that damage to certain areas of the spinal cord will contribute to or lead to dysfunction of the parasympathetic or sympathetic nervous system, alterations in pain, temperature, vibration, touch, position sense, and to loss of motor activity and sensation. It is possible for life-threatening alterations in ventilation and circulation to occur from an event that will cause interruption of nervous system responses. Furthermore, all systems of the body will be affected, so that nutrition and elimination are also affected, which will be discussed later in the chapter. Hallmarks of nursing care for SCI patients depend on a sound understanding of spinal cord anatomy and physiology.

Assessment with Clinical Manifestations

Assessment of SCI is dependent on an understanding of the manner in which SCIs are classified. Loss of motor and sensory functioning is consistent with the level of SCI, assessment of motor and sensory function will lead to an understanding of the level of SCI and the losses to functioning that may occur as a result. Classification of an SCI, along with the mechanisms of injury, is essential in the assessment of clinical manifestations of the injury. Also important to understanding the patient's situation and extent of injury will be the level of injury, which indicates the expectations for recovery, and the type of fracture that may or may not be present, which will indicate further damage associated with the injury.

Classification of SCI

SCI may be classified as complete or incomplete, depending on the degree of transection or injury to the spinal cord. Complete SCI occurs with complete transection of the spinal cord. This results in total loss of motor and sensory function below the level of injury. The neurological level of SCI is always designated as the lowest segment that has normal functioning. Therefore an injury at C3 indicates that C3 is the lowest segment with normal functioning. Functioning is lost below that level.

Because of the extent of loss of functioning and independence associated with an SCI, this is one of the most devastating types of injuries that a person can experience. Incomplete SCI occurs with partial transection of the spinal cord and results in loss of varying degrees of motor and sensory function below the level of injury. Sensory loss with an incomplete lesion generally follows the spinal tracts with corresponding loss of sensation according to the affected tract. SCI can also occur from an upper or lower motor neuron lesion. Each type of damage creates predictable responses, which require specific nursing care related to the type and level of damage.

Less permanent injury may occur as a contusion, which can cause edema of the affected area of the spinal cord, and results in significant dysfunction of the spinal cord. This usually resolves in days to weeks. Hemorrhage into the gray matter is often a more serious situation, and may create dysfunction consistent with a lower motor neuron lesion. Hemisection of the spinal cord will lead to Brown-Séquard syndrome (discussed later in the chapter).

Mechanism of SCI

Severe SCI occurs as a result of fracture-dislocation during injury. This causes compression, transection, or deformity of the spinal cord. Complete transection of the spinal cord results in immediate flaccid paralysis and loss of sensation below the level of the lesion. Loss of motor and sensory function below the level of injury is an indicator of an SCI that must be identified immediately by health care providers. In the period immediately after injury, reflex activity may be lost and urinary and fecal retention occur. As reflex activity returns, patients experience varying degrees of spasticity and flaccidity, depending on the involvement of upper or lower motor neurons. Spinal cord transection at the cervical cord level results in **quadriplegia (tetraplegia),** paralysis involving upper and lower extremities, whereas, injury of the spinal cord at the thoracic and lumbar areas results in **paraplegia,** paralysis involving the lower extremities (Tierney, McPhee, & Papadakis, 2004).

Lesser degrees of injury to the spinal cord are manifested by varying levels of weakness, urinary dysfunction, and loss of pain, temperature, and position sensation below the level of lesion. Spinal cord disturbances of these types include Brown-Séquard's syndrome, central cord syndrome, and anterior cord syndrome discussed later in this chapter.

Level of Injury

Injuries to the spinal cord can occur at the cervical, thoracic, lumbar, and to a lesser degree, coccygeal areas of the spine. Cervical injuries often result from motor vehicle accidents, football injuries, diving accidents, and falls, while thoracic and lumbar spine injuries may be more related to gunshot wounds as well as falls. In all cases, level of injury can be determined by the loss of motor or sensory functioning below the level of injury. Injury to the cervical spinal cord will result in quadriplegia; however, varying levels of motor and sensory functioning may be present in lower cervical injuries. High cervical injuries above C3 will result in loss of respiratory function and death unless ventilator support is immediately provided.

Cervical injuries result in quadriplegia and loss of movement and sensation below the level of injury, so that movement of the arms and hands are lost along with the potential for loss of head and neck control. C6 injuries are the most common cervical spine (c-spine) injuries because of the greatest mobil-

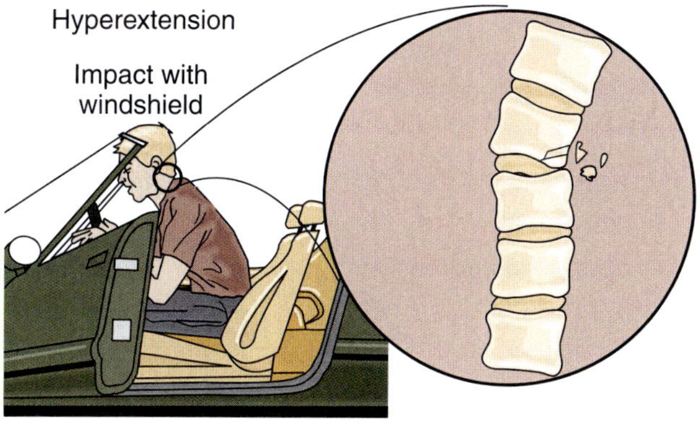

Figure 36-3 Some spinal injuries cause damage to the spinal cord that is immediately evident.

ity of the neck at this area. Injuries at the thoracic level and below allow for movement of the arms and hands. Thoracic injuries allow for increasing abilities for self-care, while resulting in paraplegia. All levels of injury will result in varying losses of bowel and bladder functioning. The most common spinal cord injuries are to C1, C2, C4, C6, T11, and T12 because of the increased movement capabilities of those areas.

Types of Fractures Causing SCI

Because the cervical area is the most unstable area of the spinal cord, it is the most vulnerable area for injury. Cervical trauma results from flexion, hyperextension, and compression injuries and fractures. Hyperflexion injuries are the most common types of fractures, often resulting from motor vehicle crashes when a person's head hits the windshield with extreme force. This commonly occurs with a head-on collision of motor vehicles. Because the degree of hyperflexion is limited by the chin reaching the chest, the extent of injury is often not as great as with hyperextension injuries. Diving accidents may also result from hyperflexion injuries, generally causing damage at the level of C4 or C5. These injuries cause hyperflexion and dislocation of the vertebrae, with resulting tearing of the posterior ligament. The most common hyperflexion injuries occur at the level of C5 or C6 because of the greater degree of movement of this area of the c-spine.

Hyperextension injuries result from falls in which the patient strikes the face or chin during the fall resulting in hyperextension of the neck (Figure 36-3). This may also occur in a rear-end motor vehicle collision. In this situation the anterior ligament is torn along with vertebral fractures. Because a greater degree of movement of the neck is possible with this type of injury, complete transection of the spinal cord is more likely to occur in these types of injuries. In such cases, there is loss of movement and sensation below the level of injury. Hyperextension injuries may result in C4, C5, or C6 damage. Compression injuries occur from direct falls on the head, sacrum, or feet. As a result, the vertebrae fractured on impact compress the spinal cord. Diving accidents can be the main culprits in SCIs resulting from compression injuries.

Vertebral Injuries

The different vertebrae are injured in different ways. For example, the rib cage provides stability to the thoracic region of the spinal cord. Therefore, injuries to this region are not as common. Most injuries result from substantial impact to the thoracic spine. Compression injuries resulting from falls to the feet or buttocks may cause thoracic injuries as can a fall on the upper back. Gunshot wounds are also common culprits in thoracic injury. The most common thoracic injuries occur at T12 and L1. Second to cervical injuries, the lumbar area is a common site for SCI, also because it is less protected from injury. Extreme flexion of the spine in this area may cause injury. Sacral injuries are relatively common and are generally a result of falls. A common cause for sacral injuries is falls on the ice. The nerve roots from the lower spinal segments are susceptible to injury; however, the likelihood of permanent damage to this area is less than with vertebral fractures at other levels of the vertebrae.

Types of Incomplete SCI

Complete transection of the spinal cord results in flaccid paralysis and total loss of motor and sensory function below the level of the injury. Incomplete SCI results from partial transection of the spinal cord. With an incomplete lesion, some of the spinal tracts may be intact and loss of motor and sensory function will vary according to the level of the injury and the type of incomplete lesion. Four syndromes are associated with incomplete injury to the spinal cord and are: Central cord syndrome, anterior cord syndrome, Brown-Séquard syndrome, and posterior cord syndrome (Table 36-1).

TABLE 36-1 Syndromes of Incomplete Cord Injury

SYNDROME	TYPE OF INJURY	FUNCTIONAL DEFICIT
Anterior cord	Flexion injury to cervical spinal cord	Motor paralysis below level of injury; decreased sensation, pain and temperature sensation below level of injury
Brown-Séquard	Penetrating injury (gunshot wound or knife wound) causes hemisection of the spinal cord	Ipsilateral motor paralysis and loss of vibration and position sense Contralateral loss of pain and temperature
Central cord	Hyperextension or hyperflexion injury damages cervical central cord; anterior horn is damaged	Weakness in upper extremities greater than weakness in lower extremities
Posterior cord	Cervical hyperextension injury damages posterior cervical spinal cord	Loss of position sense

Adapted from Jones, L., & Bagnall, A. (2004). Spinal injuries centres (SICs) for acute traumatic spinal cord injury. The Cochrane Database of Systematic Reviews (4), *CD:004442.*

Central cord syndrome occurs with hyperextension-hyperflexion injuries and causes damage to the central aspect of the cervical spinal cord. Central cord syndrome is characterized by microhemorrhages and edema in the central cord and compression of the anterior horn cells of the spinal cord. This syndrome causes weakness in the upper extremities to a greater degree than the weakness found in the lower extremities. Weakness is generally caused by edema and hemorrhage in the central area of the spinal cord. At this location of the spinal cord, nerve tracts travel to the hands and arms. Recovery usually depends on the resolution of the edema as early in the postinjury phase as possible. If spinal tracts are intact, the degree of loss of function will be less.

Anterior cord syndrome often results from a flexion injury that causes compression of the anterior two thirds of the spinal cord. A disc or bone fragment is generally the culprit in an anterior cord injury. This results in motor paralysis below the site of the injury. Decreased sensation, including pain and temperature sensation, also occur below the level of the injury. Because the posterior tracts of the spinal cord are not affected, touch, vibration, position, and motion sensation are not affected. Dorsal column function is also intact. Surgical treatment involves removal of bone fragments if the compression of the spinal cord is caused by fracture injury.

Brown-Séquard syndrome is often caused by a penetrating injury, such as a gunshot or knife wound. Ruptured discs may also cause this syndrome. Brown-Séquard syndrome is characterized by transection of half (also known as hemisection) of the spinal cord. As a result, ipsilateral (same side) motor paralysis and loss of vibration and position sense occur. Contralateral (opposite side) loss of pain and temperature also occur. Careful assessment can guide the diagnosis of this syndrome.

Cervical hyperextension injuries may result in posterior cord syndrome. As a result of this type of injury, compression of the posterior portion of the cervical spinal cord occurs. Dorsal columns of the spinal cord are injured resulting in loss of position sense (proprioception). Motor function, pain, and temperature sensation are salvaged with this type of injury.

Categorizing Incomplete SCIs

The American Spinal Injury Association (ASIA) Impairment Scale categorizes the degree of incomplete injury and expectations for functioning with each level of injury. Studies by the Model Spinal Cord Injury Systems (UAB) have gathered data related to neurological recovery from SCI over a 10-year period. The data reveal that improvements in ASIA motor score (and thus functioning) are related to the severity of injury. Patients with better ASIA grades after injury are more likely to have improvements in motor scores. Patients with motor score injuries at Grade B have a mixed prognosis; Grade A injuries have the worst prognosis for improvement (ASIA, 2004). Violent causes for injuries lead to a worse prognosis than nonviolent causes for injuries. Controversy still exists regarding how patients are classified with incomplete injuries, however, and there may be discrepancies in classification of patients. Nurses should be aware of this situation. These classification methods, though, are extremely useful to nurses and other health care providers in understanding the functional abilities of patients with spinal cord injuries and the degree to which improvement can be anticipated and supported.

Specific guidelines are provided by the ASIA to classify the level of SCI. These guidelines can be used by nurses and all health care providers to determine specific impairments related to the injury. Motor and sensory functioning should be tested along each nerve root to determine functioning or absence of functioning.

Damage to the spinal cord occurs as a result of the primary injury, as well as from the secondary effects of cellular and vascular changes that may occur after the primary injury. These secondary changes can occur from hemorrhage, edema, electrolyte imbalances, and release of catecholamines and toxic enzymes. These changes create a cascade of events that further lead to ischemia and hypoxia, and ultimately to further damage to the spinal cord. Consequently, early protective care and treatment are essential to halt this cascade of damaging events. Currently, there are a number of spinal cord centers in the United States meant to provide expert treatment for SCI. While research is considering whether the outcomes at the centers are better, it still is not known if the long-term outcomes are better if patients are immediately taken to one of these centers or cared for in a local hospital (Jones & Bagnall, 2004). Certainly, care within a few hours of injury is absolutely necessary to prevent long-term problems.

Nontraumatic SCIs

Several conditions may contribute to narrowing of the vertebral column and spinal canal thus contributing to the risk for SCI. Ankylosing spondylitis and rheumatoid arthritis may cause vertebral changes leading to SCI. Additionally, spinal tumors (discussed later in this chapter) may create space-occupying lesions, which compress the spinal cord and lead to SCI. In all these cases, traumatic injury to the spine may occur with resulting loss of motor or sensory function (Tierney, et al., 2004).

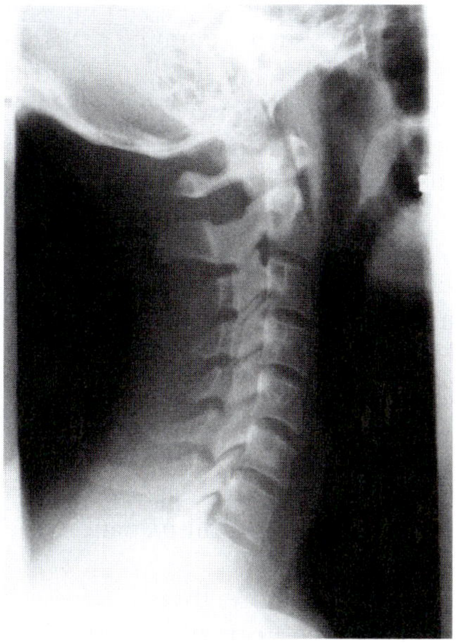

Figure 36-4 Radiological lateral cervical X-ray.

Diagnostic Tests

While there are newer diagnostic capabilities available for diagnosing SCI, the mainstay continues to be the X-ray. Cervical, thoracic, lumbar, and sacral X-rays provide important information about the presence of vertebral fractures. Direct supervision of radiologic tests is necessary to prevent further damage to the spinal cord (Figure 36-4). Protection of the patient from further injury during diagnostic testing is a nursing priority. Some manipulation of positioning under direction of the orthopod or neurologist may be necessary to visualize some cervical fractures and includes pulling the shoulders downward to visualize C7. It may also be difficult to visualize C1 and C2, leading to difficulty in diagnosing the injury.

Computed tomography (CT) and magnetic resonance imaging (MRI) scans may be used in the diagnostic process, but do not provide the essential diagnostic information. MRI scans will provide information about soft tissue injury, and CT scans will provide additional information about fracture and the extent of injury from fracture. Patient support by nurses in the diagnostic process will primarily include teaching about the need for remaining still and not movement. A nurse should be present to reinforce the need for keeping the patient immobile during this process.

Nursing Diagnoses

Based on the information gathered, examples of nursing diagnoses in the patient with SCI in the acute phases may include the following:

- Breathing pattern, ineffective
- Gas exchange, impaired
- Ineffective airway clearance
- Impaired physical mobility
- Elimination, impaired: bowel and bladder
- Risk for injury
- Self-care deficit: all levels
- Anxiety or fear related to the consequences of the SCI
- Ineffective coping related to the SCI

Planning and Implementation

Planning and implementation of nursing care during the acute phases of SCI are primarily related to maintenance of airway and breathing and prevention of further injury. The emergency care of the patient with an SCI must focus on airway, breathing, and circulation and then treatment to facilitate the best recovery from the injury, including pharmacological treatment in the early phase. At the scene of the accident, proper positioning or immobilization and support of ventilation will be the essential treatment modalities. In the emergency department, determination of the need for pharmacological intervention will be a priority, in addition to diagnostic testing to determine level of injury. Support for the patient and family during this crucial time will also be a priority for nursing care.

Acute Management of SCI

Complete spinal cord transection resulting from spinal trauma is always a possibility when injury to the back or neck occurs as in motor vehicle accidents and falls on the head, sacrum, or feet. Emergency treatment at the scene of an accident must take into consideration the possibility of spinal trauma. The likelihood of c-spine injury when a patient has experienced head trauma and is unconscious, is a possibility that must always be a priority assessment consideration. In those cases, immobilization of the head and neck will be essential to prevent further injury. If the patient has normal mental status, including no drug and alcohol impairment, and does not complain of neck pain, significant c-spine injury is unlikely. At the scene of an accident, immobilization of the head and neck and placement of the patient on a backboard for immobilization of the thoracic and lumbar spines is the standard of care. In addition, the patient must be suspected to have potential head injuries, which could also lead to increased intracranial pressure (Figure 36-5). Secondary prevention of further SCI is dependent on careful treatment with immobilization at the scene of the injury. Once a patient arrives at an emergency department, c-spine injury can generally be ruled out if all of the following criteria are met: the patient denies neck pain when asked; no neck tenderness is present on palpation; the patient did not lose consciousness, and there are no alterations in mental status from the injury or from alcohol or drug use. Furthermore, there is no paralysis or sensory changes, which might be indicative of a neck injury, and there are no other injuries, such as fractures in other locations, which could distract health care providers from identifying the presence of neck injury.

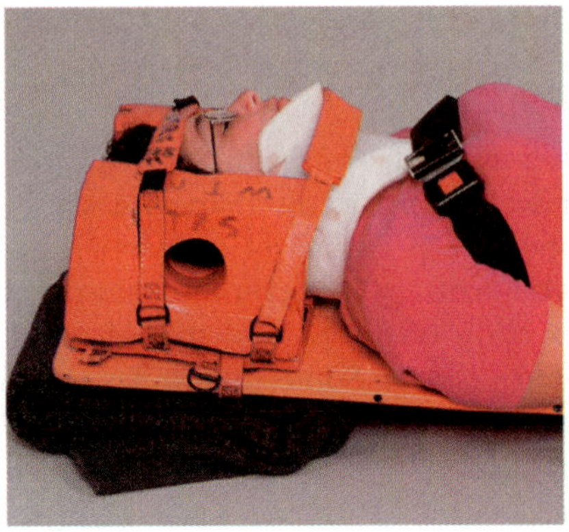

Figure 36-5 Acute management of SCI showing that a slight elevation of the patient's head can help decrease the intracranial pressure.

If any of the above is present, then the physician will order a cervical X-ray to determine if a c-spine injury has occurred. The likelihood of c-spine injury can be determined if there are vertebral fractures, if spinal processes are out of alignment, or if soft tissue swelling is present in the retropharyngeal area. In such cases, immobilization of the head and neck is maintained. It is imperative that nurses pay particular attention to these issues of immobilization of the head and neck to avoid serious and catastrophic consequences for the patient. Patients whose c-spine injuries were initially missed or had delayed diagnosis had a 10 times higher likelihood of serious secondary neurological damage of catastrophic proportions than patients who were initially correctly diagnosed (Jones & Bagnall, 2004).

For thoracic and lumbar spine injuries, complaints of pain and loss of a degree of motor and sensory function are indicators of potential SCIs In all cases, it is imperative that the patient is immobilized and medical care is sought immediately so that care can be taken to prevent further injury to the spinal cord.

It is crucial in the early stage of an SCI to stabilize the spinal cord to prevent further injury, align the spinal cord, and prevent deformities. Movement of the region surrounding the injury may lead to permanent injury, to paralysis, and to loss of function to an even greater degree than the initial injury itself. Patients involved in an accident who attempt to move to get away from a dangerous accident site may cause a worsening of the damage to the injured area leading to permanent damage to the spinal cord.

Controversy continues to exist about immobilization methods at the scene of a motor vehicle accident. Differences in opinion still exist with regard to whether to immobilize the head and neck in neutral position or to immobilize the head and neck in the position in which the patient is found. At the hospital, both surgical and manual techniques are used to stabilize an SCI. For patients who are helmeted, as in football, hockey, and motorcycle accidents, the patient's head and neck are immobilized with the helmet in place, because removal of the helmet may cause extension of spinal cord damage. This has been accepted as the standard of practice in sports medicine, and by the National Collegiate Athletic Association (NCAA). If the patient has arrested, respiratory support should be attempted with the chin-jaw thrust without movement of the head and neck. The safety of removal of the helmet when further airway support is needed has not been documented through research.

At the emergency department, the helmet and shoulder pads of a football player can be removed together at the same time, by a health care provider qualified to remove this equipment. However, football injuries generally do not involve high cervical injuries that produce respiratory arrest. Therefore, removal of the helmet for emergency respiratory support is not generally an issue. Football injuries to the spinal cord occur more often at the level of C5 or C7 because of the type of impact during play. With motorcycle accidents, the concern for additional injuries where there may be bleeding and hemorrhage may be a concern to health care providers and may therefore impair emergency treatment for the SCI. Only experienced and qualified practitioners in the emergency department should remove helmets in patients who potentially have SCI (Waninger, 2004).

Traction may be used as a method of treatment to achieve stability of the spine after SCI, although it is becoming less used with early surgical treatment for stabilization of the injury. Even though currently used in many cases, there is no evidence that spinal immobilization prevents adverse events in patients with spinal cord trauma. In fact, immobilization may lead to further damage to the airway and compromise pulmonary function (Bunn & Roberts, 2004). The debate about the use of traction details benefits and risks associated with each side of this argument. Immobilization is thought to prevent further damage. It is also thought that immobilization will cause airway compromise and lead to a life-threatening situation. Nurses should discuss the patient's treatment plan with the physician and collaborate on a detailed, individualized,

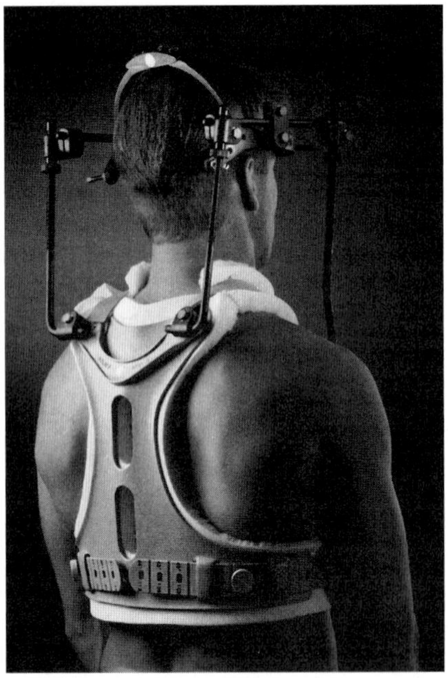

Figure 36-6 Halo vest (Courtesy of DePuy Acromed).

plan for each patient, understanding the specific restrictions and directions for the use of traction.

If used for cervical injuries, traction will support the process of realignment and will prevent mobility of an unstable area of the spinal column. Traction is not generally used for stability in thoracic or lumbar injuries. When used, cervical traction is usually accomplished with the use of Halo traction (described later). Cervical tongs, such as Crutchfield, Gardner-Wells, and Vinke, may be used; however, this type of traction is rapidly becoming obsolete. Tongs are attached by screws implanted in the patient's skull to accomplish reduction of the injury. Initially, five pounds of weight are applied per interspace beginning with C1 to the level of injury. Nurses should be aware of the fear associated with insertion of tongs and screws for attachment of Halo traction. Although not generally painful, the use of the drill for inserting tongs or screws in the skull creates anxiety in an already extremely anxious person. Care must be taken to ensure that weights (if used) hang freely and that tongs are secure as patients are turned in bed.

Currently, halo traction is the standard of care, and more frequently used than the cervical tongs either early in the treatment period or in the postoperative recovery period. The Halo traction brace also uses traction through the attachment of screws in the patient's skull. More movement is possible than with cervical tongs as the vest allows for the patient to be out of bed and contribute to personal care while continuing to stabilize the head and neck and thus the spinal cord (Figure 36-6).

During the period following surgery and if traction is used, the patient may be on bedrest. Sometimes a special bed, such as the Roto-Rest system may be used to promote circulation and prevent decubitus ulcers. However, patients may remain in a regular bed while cervical tongs are in place. Traction leading from the head of the bed must be evaluated periodically to ensure that weights are hanging free. Nurses must turn patients with assistance of additional personnel to prevent the dislodging of pins and prevent improper alignment of the patient.

For less serious injuries, hard and soft cervical collars may be used for head and neck immobilization. These collars allow for even more movement by the patient, however, they do not provide the degree of stability needed for an SCI. Whiplash injuries without damage to the spinal cord or stable c-spine fractures may provide enough stability and restriction of movement to allow for healing of inflammatory responses and strains of muscles in the head and neck area. At the scene of an accident, hard cervical collars along with sandbags may be used for immobilization of the spine for transport to an emergency center.

For thoracic and lumbar injuries, support braces (e.g., Clam-shell brace) may be used in combination with surgery for stabilization of the spine. Use of immobilization beds, such as a Roto-Rest, may be used in some circumstances depending on surgeon preference. These beds provide for stability, while also aimed at the prevention of the development of pressure ulcers. Halo vests may also be used in some circumstances to promote stabilization of the spinal cord and vertebral column.

Familiarity with Christopher Reeves' condition led to increased public awareness of the ventilation needs of patients with high cervical cord injuries. C3 or C5 innervation of the phrenic nerve is necessary for the innervation of the diaphragm, therefore, transection of the cord in high areas of the c-spine cause interruption of phrenic nerve innervation to the diaphragm resulting in the need for ventilatory support. The nurse should be aware that injury at the level of C4 or above will require mechanical ventilation. Patients should be on high-flow oxygen with pulse oximetry when they arrive at the emergency department until there is information about the level of the SCI.

Patients with high cervical injuries are not the only patients who experience respiratory-related problems and issues. Patients with T1 through T12 injuries will experience interruption of innervation of the intercostal muscles leading

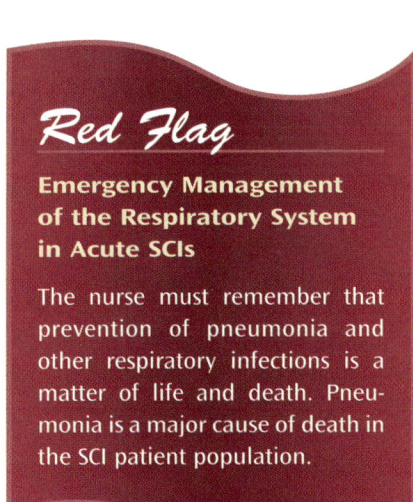

> *Red Flag*
>
> **Emergency Management of the Respiratory System in Acute SCIs**
>
> The nurse must remember that prevention of pneumonia and other respiratory infections is a matter of life and death. Pneumonia is a major cause of death in the SCI patient population.

to inability to cough effectively and difficulty with inspiration and expiration. Additionally, tidal volume and vital capacity may diminish because of the loss of innervation of the intercostals muscles. During the rehabilitation period, tidal volume and vital capacity may increase as patients develop abilities to use accessory muscles.

Because of the interruption in chest muscle innervation, patients, particularly those patients with injuries at T7 and above, will need assistance with removal of secretions, especially during the acute phase of treatment. Attention to careful suctioning along with attention to patient responses to suctioning are crucial to prevent hypoxia and bradycardia. Patients with injuries at or above T12 are at risk for pneumonia and atelectasis. Therefore, vigorous pulmonary toileting is critical in the postinjury care of the SCI patient. Consultation with respiratory therapists will provide for care to decrease the risk of respiratory and pulmonary alterations, while maintaining safety. Careful attention to respiratory status and pulse oximetry readings, staying alert for readings less than 95 percent are necessary to prevent respiratory complications in this vulnerable patient.

Respiratory infections are also probable when compromised respiratory function is present as with these types of injuries. Attention to respiratory assessment, noting adventitious and abnormal breath sounds, will help to prevent the development of pneumonia and atelectasis. The age-old nursing standard of turning, coughing, and deep breathing is no more important in any patient population than in the SCI patient. The mechanics of accomplishing this standard, however, are fundamentally different because of the degree of nursing care assistance needed for the SCI patient during turning, coughing, and deep breathing.

Evidence-Based Care

Research has been ongoing for years to investigate and determine the potential for regeneration or repair of damaged spinal cord tissue. Patients are always extremely interested in current research that leads to hope for repair of the spinal cord for quadriplegia and paraplegia, so it is imperative that nurses who work with SCI patients have knowledge of the current research in this discipline. With today's technology, patients are readily able to access information and may need assistance in interpreting study results and information that is accessed. High-profile patients, like Christopher Reeve, sparked public interest in research to find a cure for SCI, and therefore most patients are informed, especially because of their personal stake in the success of scientific research (Estores, 2003). Therefore, staying aware of cutting-edge research on the nurse's part will engender confidence in nursing care and support for hope, as appropriate, on the part of the patient. It's important for nurses to remember that false hope for the possibility of walking again is different than placing hope in research to find a cure. Sometimes so much emphasis is placed on not supporting false hope that it is at the expense of a hopeful outlook on the part of the patient.

Studies that have focused on removal of myelin-producing cells, growth in the laboratory, and transplantation in injured areas of animals have shown promising results of growth of healthy myelin. Restoration of nerve transmissions in animals has already been shown. Current research is also examining the potential for bone marrow stem cells to repair damaged cells when transplanted into the cerebrospinal fluid (CSF) to migrate to injured areas in animals and is thus showing much promise. Mesenchymal stem cells have been found to migrate to injured thoracic spinal cord tissue, through injection into the subarachnoid space, providing a less invasive way to get stem cells to the site of injury. Stem cells have been shown to be effective in promoting recovery in stroke, through the prevention of cell death, and it is thought that this may be possible with SCIs as well, although this has not been shown yet.

Unfortunately, studies with human subjects have not been replicated yet; therefore, research still has much progress to make. Macrophages hold some interest in promoting axon regeneration, and research on the concept of bridging across glial scar tissue at the site of the injury has also shown promise. The use of cAMP and Schwann cells are being studied to determine if these cells have a positive effect on axon regeneration. Gangliosides are also being studied because of their potentially positive effect on axon growth. Gangliosides have been shown to have promise in Parkinson's disease and for strokes, increasing the belief that they may also be useful in injured spinal cord tissue. Decreasing the damaging effects of chondroitin is also of interest. Chondroitin has an inhibitory effect on axon growth, and the administration of chondroitinase ABC degrades chondroitin promoting regeneration of tissue. Apparently, the make up of scar tissue with glial cells impairs the growth of other potentially useful cells. Developing circuits, which would allow for growth around the scar tissue (or a bridge), is holding much interest at this time too. Much interest exists in finding a successful treatment for SCI, which will lead to regeneration or repair of nerve cells in the spinal cord; this research is occurring around the world (Bunge & Pearse, 2003; Campos, et al., 2004; Chinnock & Roberts, 2004; Satake, Lou, & Lenke, 2004).

Current research has shown initial effectiveness of drug therapy in improving functional ability in SCI patients. Used for long-term treatment, patients with long-standing SCI have been treated with a new drug, 4-AP (4-aminopyridine). Those patients receiving this experimental treatment showed significant improvement in motor and sensory function when treated with the new drug as compared to patients in control groups. This shows promise especially for the potential of new drugs contributing to improvement of function in more than the first few hours post injury (Hinkle, 2004).

Landmark studies changed the standard of care for SCI several years ago when it was noted that secondary injury after the accident could be as much of the culprit for long-term loss of function as the primary injury. From that research came the standard of treatment with methylprednisolone administered intravenously within eight hours of injury (Bracken, 2004; Tierney, et al., 2004). More recently, magnesium sulfate at high doses is being studied for its inhibitory effect on excitotoxicity of the neural cells as a cause for secondary injury and resolution of secondary injury effects. This has shown the promising effects of neuroprotection in animal studies (Kaptanoglu, Beskonakli, Okutan, Surucu, & Taskin, 2003).

Accurate assessment is critical in all stages of care after SCI. In the early stages of injury, it may be difficult to assess motor and sensory function because of spinal shock. Continued assessment, however, provides a picture of effectiveness of medical treatment and nursing intervention. It will also help in determining realistic functional goals for rehabilitation and quality of life. Motor function is assessed as a part of the neurological assessment completed during the nursing assessment. Movement of extremities and movement against resistance should be included in the motor assessment along with flexion and extension of joints. Sensory assessment early in the treatment period after injury includes determination of sensation along dermatomes. Dermatome charts provide an idea of expected sensory function along sections of the body (dermatomes) innervated by spinal or cranial nerves (see dermatome chart). Spinothalamic tract sensation is tested by cotton swab, whereas pain sensation as a determination of posterior column function is tested by pin prick. Sensation alterations are determined as anesthesia, analgesia, hypoesthesia, and hyperesthesia. Proprioception (position sense) is tested by movement of the great toe upward or downward and asking the patient to confirm the direction.

Deep tendon reflexes (DTR) are tested to determine the presence of **spinal shock,** a loss of all motor and sensory function, generally occurring after SCI, or the degree of injury or impairment, complete or incomplete (Figure 36-7). The presence of DTRs indicates incomplete injury or resolution of spinal shock. During the phase of spinal shock, the patient has absent DTRs and a

A B C D

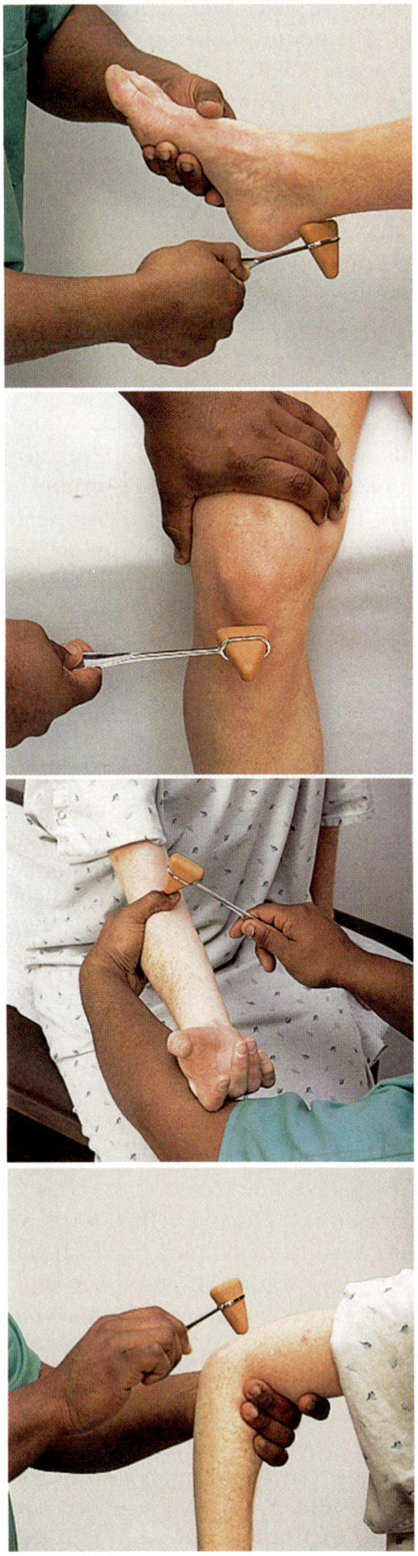

Figure 36-7 Assessment of deep tendon reflexes: A. Achilles, B. Patellar, C. Biceps, D. Triceps.

flaccid paralysis. Presence of perineal reflexes may indicate the possibility that bowel and bladder training can be successful.

Understanding motor, sensory, and reflex activity will be beneficial in determining realistic functional goals with the patient. Rehabilitation, including bowel and bladder training, will depend greatly on the functional status of the patient. Taking into account the meaning of assessment data regarding motor, sensory, and reflex information will be beneficial in understanding the progress that the patient is making.

Pharmacology

Landmark studies just a few years ago were the first studies to really show that improvement could be achieved in neurological status after SCI. The introduction of pharmacological management was implemented. Little ground had been gained in the improvement of neurological status until these studies showed the effectiveness of methylprednisolone. Early treatment of spinal cord trauma with high doses of corticosteroids has been shown to be extremely effective in the prevention of spinal cord damage after trauma occurs. Currently, only treatment with the methylprednisolone protocol has shown effectiveness in the acute phase of SCI. Three clinical trials confirmed the effectiveness of methylprednisolone therapy. This research showed that intravenous (IV) administration of a 30 mg/kg bolus of methylprednisolone followed by 5.4 mg/kg/hr for 23 hours improves neurological recovery of function if administered within eight hours after injury (Tierney, et al., 2004).

Higher or lower doses of methylprednisolone have not been shown to be effective, and studies of doses begun after 8 hours post injury have had mixed results. Research continues to examine the promising effects of methylprednisolone and to identify other steroids that may be useful in the treatment of SCI. A recent study has shown that methylprednisolone given for an additional 24 hours (up to 48 hours) contributes to further improvement in function in those patients whose treatment was started 3 to 8 hours after injury (Bracken, 2004). Nurses must be particularly astute to the crucial need for methylprednisolone in the first hours after injury to provide patients with the best possible opportunity for improvement in motor and sensory function.

The improvement of neurological function after administration of methylprednisolone occurs because of the reduction of edema to the area of injury, but it is also thought to occur because of the effect of the methylprednisolone on the reduction of leukocytes to the area along with a decrease in free fatty acid production. Steroid treatment also inhibits breakdown of phospholipids, improving blood flow to the spinal cord, and stopping the inflammatory response, thereby avoiding further injury to the spinal cord. Methylprednisolone has been shown to counter many of the injury cascades that cause injury to the spinal cord.

When injury occurs, blood flow to the gray matter of the spinal cord is impaired. Several hours later, circulation to the white matter also diminishes. This disturbance of blood flow is related to several factors including edema, thrombi in the microcirculation, vasoconstriction from histamine release, and hypovolemia from spinal shock and hemorrhage. In addition, shifting of electrolytes to the extracellular compartments contributes to tissue damage, leading to necrosis. Movement of sodium in particular contributes to edema leading to further tissue damage. The gray matter is especially sensitive to hypoxia and as hemorrhage, edema, and thrombi accumulate, the cascade of injury sequelae is put into motion.

As the inflammatory response continues, edema begins to exert more pressure on the spinal cord, consequently damaging sensitive tissue. As the spinal edema progresses the swelling moves throughout the spinal cord. Keep in mind that these events are occurring within the immovable vertebral column; therefore, further damage to the spinal cord becomes even more likely. Finally, the release of free radicals exerts their neurotoxic effects. As this process proceeds, secondary injury following the primary injury leads to increasing damage from the initial injury. This cascade of events occurs within the first eight hours after injury. This cascade of events has been shown to be effectively halted by the administration of methylprednisolone, if given in this early stage.

Adverse effects of corticosteroid therapy may include delayed wound healing and hyperglycemia and should be assessed in patients receiving this therapy. This may mean that patients are more at risk for infection. Thus, patients may experience longer than necessary hospitalizations because of this risk for infection. Vigilant attention to assessment will serve to prevent infection or identify early signs of infection that can be treated immediately. Because of the effectiveness of corticosteroid therapy, nurses should be particularly attentive about the need for this treatment remembering that the medication's effectiveness has a small window of opportunity.

Attention to daily measurement of weight and to continuous neurological assessments is necessary to determine the effectiveness of the pharmacological therapy. Treatment after the initial stage of injury may consist of laminectomy and surgical fusion (especially if there is spinal cord compression), followed by traction, and treatment of spasticity, bladder and bowel dysfunction, and skin care for the long-term.

Surgery

Surgical treatment accomplishes stability of the spine through fusion of the vertebrae adjacent to the injury. Surgical instrumentation through the use of rods is used to improve stability of the thoracic spine. Often, cervical fusion will still be followed by traction postoperatively; however, cervical traction is used less frequently currently, depending on the stability after surgery and the potential for use of the more mobile halo traction. Fusion creates a stable spine without mobility after the operative procedure. Therefore, patients will need to be prepared for this change in function and mobility. This lack of potential for movement may require psychological adjustment by patients in the rehabilitation period. The operative procedure is generally performed with a posterior approach laminectomy in which rod instrumentation is used for stability or bone from the iliac crest used for the fusion. An anterior or lateral approach to the laminectomy can also be used for a spinal fusion.

Emergency Management of Complications of SCIs

There are several severe complications of SCIs. Spinal shock and neurogenic shock are forms of distributive shock that have high mortality rates and cause crises in the person with an SCI. The immediate response of the spinal cord to injury is spinal shock. This is a physiological response, as opposed to an anatomical response, which results in flaccid paralysis below the level of injury and a myriad of additional problems. Spinal shock results in complete loss of motor and sensory function including movement, bowel and bladder function, sexual functioning, autonomic responses, and reflex activity.

The pathophysiological response follows the damage of the sympathetic and parasympathetic nervous systems. If the injury is above T6, sympathetic innervation will be lost, and the heart, therefore will not receive input from the sympathetic innervation. At that level of injury, parasympathetic innervation will continue, and as a result bradycardia and vasodilation occur. Release of catecholamines occurs initially, which causes hypertension; but subsequently, hypotension occurs because of the impaired venous return. This situation results in hypotension and pooling of blood in extremities. Control by the hypothalamus will also be lost, resulting in loss of temperature control.

Patients with higher levels of injury (cervical injuries) experience the most life-threatening forms of spinal shock because of the effects on the autonomic nervous system. Because the autonomic response is not affected to the same degree in lower SCIs, patients with thoracic and lumbar injuries are not generally affected by spinal shock.

Spinal shock occurs soon after the injury, within the first week after injury, sometimes within 30 to 60 minutes of the injury and continues for up to six weeks or longer. Resolution of spinal shock is indicated by return of reflexes, replacement of flaccidity with hyperreflexes, and reflex emptying of the bladder. Appearance of Babinski's reflex is an indicator of returning reflexes. The bulbospongiosus reflex (also known as penile reflex) in male patients also appears at the resolution of spinal shock. Because of the effects of spinal shock, it is difficult, if not impossible to determine the level of injury and loss of function until spinal shock has resolved.

During the phase of spinal shock careful attention to fluid volume with administration of IV fluids is essential. Antiembolism stockings will prevent pooling of blood in extremities and will assist with circulation and prevention of formation of thrombi. Fluid overload may quickly cause congestive heart failure; therefore, astute assessment is always a priority.

There has been a tendency to view the prognosis for ambulation as related to the presence of spinal shock and the presence or absence of reflexes on the day of injury. This has been discounted by research, especially with regard to the recovery of reflexes in a caudal to rostral sequence, which has been the traditional view of recovery from spinal shock. Research now shows that reflexes reappear over several days following injury, and the pattern of recovery may be what is more related to the recovery of ambulation abilities (Table 36-2). Most often, the delayed Babinski response is the first reflex to recover followed by the cremasteric reflex. Deep tendon reflexes tend to recover in one to two weeks. Rehabilitation efforts may begin while the patient is still experiencing spinal shock.

As with spinal shock, neurogenic shock occurs more frequently in patients with SCI above the level of T6. Technically, neurogenic shock is included as an aspect of spinal shock, in patients with SCI only. Because of disruption of sympathetic input, decrease in vascular resistance and loss of vascular tone occurs from T1 and L2. Neurogenic shock is manifested by hypotension, bradycardia, and hypothermia. In this situation, the heart rate response to volume depletion or volume overload is lost; therefore, nurses must assess frequently for the signs of fluid overload or fluid volume deficit.

Autonomic dysreflexia, also known as autonomic hyperreflexia, is a life-threatening complication of SCI occurring as a disordered discharge of autonomic responses, which results in massive discharge of sympathetic responses. These sympathetic responses are triggered by input of noxious stimuli occurring below the level of injury. As a result, messages sent to the CNS are blocked at the level of injury. Patients with injuries above the level of T6 are at the greatest risk for this complication. Up to 85 percent of patients with injuries above the level of T6 experience autonomic dysreflexia after spinal shock has resolved. Most commonly, the noxious stimulus that triggers the autonomic response is a distended bladder or bowel or some other abnormality com-

TABLE 36-2 Assessment of Reflexes in Spinal Shock

REFLEX	ASSESSMENT
Babinski reflex	Stimulation of the sole of the foot causes dorsiflexion of the great toe
Bulbospongiosus reflex	Tap to dorsal area of penis causes contraction of the bulbospongiosus muscle
Cremasteric reflex	Stimulation of inner aspect of thigh causes testes to retract on same side
Deep tendon reflex	Percussion and stretching of tendon causes contraction of muscle; includes biceps, triceps, quadriceps, and Achilles tendon reflexes

Adapted from Estes, M. (2006). Health assessment and physical examination *(3rd ed.). New York: Thomson Delmar Learning.*

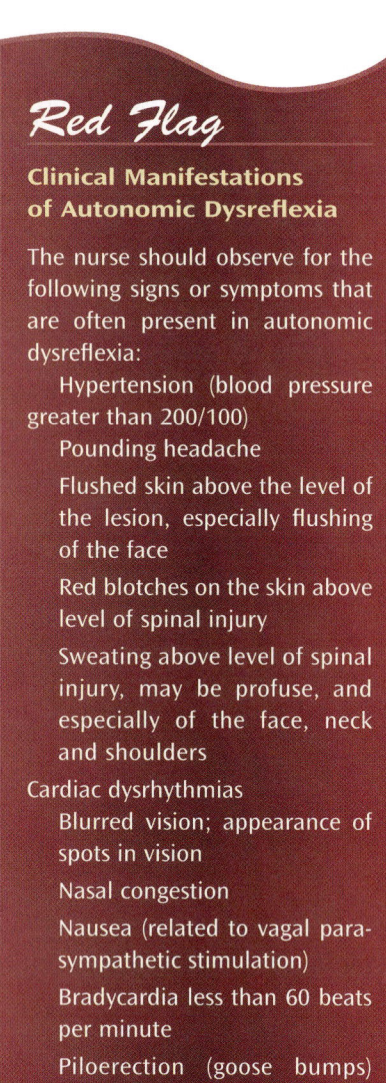

> *Red Flag*
>
> **Clinical Manifestations of Autonomic Dysreflexia**
>
> The nurse should observe for the following signs or symptoms that are often present in autonomic dysreflexia:
>
> - Hypertension (blood pressure greater than 200/100)
>   - Pounding headache
>   - Flushed skin above the level of the lesion, especially flushing of the face
>   - Red blotches on the skin above level of spinal injury
>   - Sweating above level of spinal injury, may be profuse, and especially of the face, neck and shoulders
> - Cardiac dysrhythmias
>   - Blurred vision; appearance of spots in vision
>   - Nasal congestion
>   - Nausea (related to vagal parasympathetic stimulation)
>   - Bradycardia less than 60 beats per minute
>   - Piloerection (goose bumps) above or below level of spinal injury
>   - Feelings of anxiety

monly dealt with by people without injured spinal cords without a second thought. Spasms, abdominal pain, skin irritation, and pressure sores may also precipitate the response. As sympathetic nervous system activation occurs below the level of injury, vasoconstriction occurs along with a number of additional, sometimes life-threatening physiological responses.

Because the signal for a healthy physiological response to the noxious stimulus cannot transcend the level of the SCI and get through to the CNS, the sympathetic response from the level of injury will cause vasoconstriction of vessels below the injury. This ultimately results in severe, life-threatening hypertension. As a compensatory mechanism to lower the blood pressure, the parasympathetic nervous system produces vasodilatation above the level of the lesion. This results in bradycardia, but continued vasoconstriction in the lower body causes blood pressure to persist and ultimately to rise. The blood pressure may rise to 240/120 mm Hg, becoming a life-threatening situation. In this situation the priority for care is to identify and treat the condition immediately. Vasodilation of the vessels in the head and neck occur as well, creating flushing of the head and neck.

Unfortunately, the compensatory parasympathetic responses only occur above the level of injury, whereas, the sympathetic responses affect the entire body, causing the danger and life-threatening situation that arises. Ultimately, this scenario can lead to cerebral vascular accidents, renal failure, seizures, dysrhythmias, and death. Identifying and treating the stimulus for the response will correct these physiological responses to autonomic dysreflexia and is therefore a high priority for nursing care as well as for patient education. Nursing care focuses on assessment, identifying the source of the noxious stimulus, and treating or correcting the stimulus for the autonomic response. For example, a distended bladder can be caused by kinked tubing of the Foley catheter, triggering an autonomic response. Nursing care emphasizes checking the urinary drainage bag and tubing and teaching about the need to keep tubing unrestricted.

The following situations may trigger autonomic responses necessitating immediate treatment. The nurse must first identify the causative factor or triggering stimulus and remove the stimuli shown in Box 36-1. Guidelines for treatment of autonomic dysreflexia are outlined in the Skills 360° feature.

Teaching should emphasize to patients and their caregivers the need for identification of symptoms and assessment and treatment of stimuli for the autonomic responses. For example, if symptoms occur during digital stimulation, the caregiver must stop until the response has subsided. Autonomic dysreflexia as a result of skin irritation is usually alleviated by loosening clothing. This situation is especially dangerous, because the patient generally does not have the sensation to detect the problem; therefore, life-threatening hypertension may occur before it is detected. Caregivers need to pay particular attention to meticulous care, including proper position, proper fitting clothing, attention to bowel and bladder programs, and assessment for the potential for the development of autonomic dysreflexia.

To prevent serious consequences, pharmacological treatment of the physiological hypertension effect of autonomic dysreflexia must occur while the trigger for the response is being investigated. Vasodilators, such as nifedipine and nitrates, may be used to treat the hypertension resulting from autonomic dysreflexia. Phenoxybenzamine may also be used. Nifedipine will cause coronary and peripheral vasodilation; phenoxybenzamine will block catecholamines, while nitrates are coronary vasodilators. Phenoxybenzamine has also been shown to be effective for bladder spasms.

Teaching related to prevention of autonomic dysreflexia should include a discussion about the need to change positions in the wheel chair and bed at least every two hours. Vigilant attention to bowel and bladder programs will also result in prevention of the syndrome. Identification of symptoms of auto-

BOX 36-1

STIMULI THAT TRIGGER AUTONOMIC RESPONSES

The nurse should monitor the patient with an SCI for the following signs that are typical of stimuli for autonomic responses:

- Distended bladder
- Constipation or bowel impaction
- Pain
- Muscle spasms
- Sexual activity
- Labor (in females)
- Decubitus ulcers
- Urinary tract infections
- Tight clothing
- Ingrown toenails

Skills 360°

Management of Autonomic Dysreflexia

The nurse should monitor for the following clinical manifestations of autonomic dysreflexia:

- Recognize the signs and symptoms and continually monitor blood pressure and heart rate. Guidelines suggest every two to five minutes.
- Loosen any restrictive clothing or devices (urinary leg bag may be causing constriction).
- If the patient has an indwelling catheter, check for kinked tubing, and patency of system. Remove any kinks or obstructions. If the catheter is not draining, it should be irrigated with 10 to 15 mL of normal saline instilled at body temperature. Do not put pressure on the bladder. Guard against cold solutions, which may exacerbate the autonomic dysreflexia. If the catheter is still not draining, remove and replace the catheter, and consult the physician.
- Monitor the patient's blood pressure during drainage of urine by a urinary catheter. Drainage of large volumes of urine could cause hypotension.
- If symptoms persist, check for fecal impaction the second most common cause of this condition.
- Expect order for antihypertensive agent (e.g., nifedipine or nitrates) with rapid onset and short duration.
- For a pregnant woman who has signs of autonomic dysreflexia, refer the patient immediately for care by an obstetrical health care provider.
- After stabilization of the patient, provide teaching regarding the signs and symptoms of the disorder, and the need to seek immediate treatment.

nomic dysreflexia must be treated as a medical emergency, and once home, patients should be reminded to call 911 if symptoms occur, especially if not resolved by conventional treatment (removal of kinked catheter tubing, etc.). Patients and caregivers should also be prepared to explain to emergency and hospital personnel the probably nature of their condition, because many health care providers do not typically encounter autonomic dysreflexia.

The Paralyzed Veteran's of America Consortium for Spinal Cord Medicine also provides clinical guidelines for health care providers and for patients and caregivers to use in the identification and treatment of this disorder. These clinical guidelines have been adopted universally at spinal cord centers across the United States.

Nursing Management during the Rehabilitation Phase of Recovery

The patient with an SCI has nursing care and physical care needs for the rest of his or her life. Patients continue to be at risk for alterations in respiratory status: ventilation and gas exchange leading to risk for pneumonia, alterations in skin integrity and mobility, alterations in bowel and bladder elimination, altered circulation, alterations in neurological status, autonomic and spinal sensory and motor function, and numerous psychosocial and family related potential alterations. Essentially, the patient with an SCI has the potential for complications involving all aspects of the body, mind, and spirit.

Bowel and bladder dysfunctions are common complications of SCI, and most patients experience some degree of both bowel and bladder dysfunction because of loss of innervation of the bowel and bladder. During the phase of spinal shock, urinary retention occurs. During this phase, indwelling urinary catheterization is necessary, because the bladder is atonic and will become distended. On resolution of this phase, urinary output may stabilize, because reflex emptying may become possible as a result of decreasing inhibitory responses from the brain. At this time, patients can generally have intermittent catheterization, especially if they can tolerate increases in oral fluid intake. Patients should drink at least 3 liters of fluids per day to offset the potential for urinary tract infections (UTIs), a real risk at this stage and throughout the rest of the patient's life.

Paraplegic patients may be able to accomplish self-catheterization as a goal of the rehabilitation process. Quadriplegic patients will need caregiver support if intermittent catheterization is possible. In both cases, patients and caregivers will need to be taught aseptic technique for bladder and catheter care. Once an indwelling urinary catheter is discontinued, the nurse must assess regularly for urinary retention. Urinary retention will lead to UTI, so diligent assessment of urinary function is essential. Urinary retention will also lead to the development of urinary calculi, a somewhat common occurrence among patients with SCIs. Teaching regarding fluid needs is essential. The inclusion of cranberry juice in the fluid intake is controversial, because it has not been shown to decrease bacteriuria in patients with SCI (Waites, Canupp, Armstrong, & DeVivo, 2004). The use of cranberry juice does provide fluids and important nutrients, so is not detrimental. For patients with indwelling catheters, teaching regarding aseptic technique when changing and cleaning catheter bags, the use of leg bags, and nighttime catheter drainage management is important. Strict attention to proper catheter and urinary drainage bag care will decrease the potential for urinary tract infection.

Bowel elimination will also be affected by impaired reflex activity, which will lead to constipation and the possibility of impaction. It has also been found that colonic motility postprandially is diminished in patients with SCI (Korsten, et al., 2004). This will lead to even more difficulty with bowel elimination. A bowel training program must be implemented as soon as tolerated by the patient. Prevention of constipation and fecal impaction will be essential aspects of this bowel training program. During the rehabilitation phase of recovery, patients and caregivers are taught the digital dilation technique to facilitate bowel elimination. Stool softeners and assurance of dietary roughage and nutrients to support bowel elimination are essential. Adequate fluid intake will also support bowel elimination.

Bowel training is often assisted by consideration of time of day and timing of meals. Assisting the patient to the bathroom or commode soon after the morning meal, if that time is preferable, will promote bowel elimination. Establishing the routine, often with timing in relationship to meals will be beneficial to bowel elimination and to the regaining of a degree of normalcy in the patient's life.

Alterations in temperature regulation in patients with SCIs resulting from impaired autonomic nervous system responses makes the patient vulnerable to changes in environmental temperature. Hypothermia is a risk for patients, especially in the acute phase. Additionally, because of altered sensation that also occurs with the injury, patients should be taught not to use heating pads because of the risk for burns. Patients may also be in danger of frostbite, especially with loss of sensation and the vasodilation that accompanies spinal shock. These dangers may continue according to the level of SCI.

During all phases of the postinjury period and for the rest of the patient's life, the risk for decubitus ulcers is great because of the impact of an SCI on mobility. This was made real as it was identified as the initial culprit in the series of events that led to the death of Christopher Reeve in 2004. In the acute phase of the SCI, nurses must assess skin frequently and turn patients at least every two hours. This is a challenge when patients are in Halo traction or in cervical traction. Turning must be accomplished with at least two nurses, paying close attention to security of tongs if present.

The loss of innervation of the diaphragm and intercostal muscles leads to continued risk for pneumonia for the rest of the patient's life. The patient and family members must always be vigilant to the need for deep breathing, for activity, and for good pulmonary toilet. For many patients, the reality of an SCI is that the person with a c-spine injury will be dependent on a ventilator for the remainder of his or her life. This will require specialized nursing care, with teaching for family members and caregivers, along with home health nursing care. It will also require attention to maintenance of secretions and frequent auscultation of breath sounds to determine the possibility of the development of pneumonia, so that treatment can be instituted. Family members and caregivers will require instruction related to tracheostomy care, as the patient with a c-spine injury will have a tracheostomy for the purposes of ventilatory support and for suctioning to remove secretions.

Current research has identified the benefit of transcutaneous electric nerve stimulation (TENS) for stimulating the diaphragm to promote increased independence in ventilation and breathing. This research has been successful in allowing a degree of independence for short periods of time for patients who are dependent on a ventilator. Implanted TENS electrodes are providing a new source of ventilation support and lessening the risk of pneumonia and other hazards of loss of nerve innervation to the diaphragm and intercostals muscles.

Patients with cervical injuries and higher thoracic injuries who are not dependent on a ventilator will still need careful attention to pulmonary hygiene because of the loss of innervation of intercostal muscles. Paraplegics are not at risk to the degree that quadriplegics are with regard to respiratory status. They must still be aware of the need for respiratory care and the hazards of bedrest during times when they may need increased time in bed. In particular, because of the danger of decubitus ulcers, increased time in bed will bring with it increased risk for pneumonia (Winslow & Rozovsky, 2003).

Both quadriplegics and paraplegics will be confined to a wheelchair for the rest of their lives. Paraplegics and quadriplegics with lower cervical injuries will have the ability to manually power their wheelchairs. Quadriplegics with high injuries will need motorized wheelchairs with high back support and head support. The actuality of wheelchair confinement while out of bed means that patients are always at risk for development of decubitus ulcers at pressure points. Because patients have lost the sensation of pain that able-bodied patients have after sitting for extensive periods of time, they do not sense the need to change positions. Therefore, it is important to vary the times when in the wheelchair and in bed. Additionally, patients may be able to do lifting exercises periodically to relieve pressure on the sacrum. A turning schedule while in bed for quadriplegics is always a necessity for patients and their caregivers.

In reality, complications of decubitus ulcers are a serious threat to patients' well-being. Constant assessment by nurses during the hospitalization and rehabilitation phases and by caregivers in the home environment will help to identify early beginnings of pressure areas. Even with scrupulous nursing care and strict attention to turning and position changes, the chances of patients developing decubitus ulcers is great. Proper nutrition will promote skin integrity, and changing positions regularly will promote circulation in pressure areas. Consultation with Wound, Ostomy, Continence (WOC) nurses is helpful in determining strategies for preventing and for treating decubitus ulcers. Decubitus ulcers are difficult to treat once they are present. The dangers of infection become even higher once a patient has a decubitus ulcer. Currently, the best intervention for decubitus ulcers is prevention. Detailed individualized information regarding the prevention of decubitus ulcers is the best approach (Garber & Rintala, 2003).

A helpful tool for nursing staff and for caregivers of patients with SCI is a turning schedule. It is easy to develop a tool based on the patient's preferences for meals and other needs for supine position. Caregivers should develop some kind of method for remembering the turn schedule so that turning times are not missed. Because of the serious risk for decubitus ulcers, turning during the night is necessary. Caregivers will need support and assistance with turning a patient who is not able to assist. Patients who are paraplegic will be able to assist with turning and may become independent with turning. They will still need a turn schedule. The schedule provided above can be modified based on the patient's preferences, including time slots and being on the back and on a particular side at some times of the day. If, for instance, the patient's television is on the left side of the bed, the patient may have favorite programs that will necessitate turning to the left side at those times of the day. The schedule can be adjusted accordingly.

Patients who are quadriplegic will need complete assistance with transferring to the wheelchair and back to the bed. Nurses will need to be aware of proper transfer techniques and body mechanics to transfer patients. Rehabilitation facilities will assist patients and caregivers to learn the transfer techniques. Caregivers providing care for quadriplegic patients will need support of additional caregivers or family members in some circumstances.

A significant concern with immobility is the degree of atrophy of muscles that occurs. Range of motion exercises of all muscle groups is essential every day to maintain muscle tone, prevent the loss of muscle mass, and prevent contractures. Once patients are discharged from the hospital, caregivers will need to take over this activity and will need detailed teaching about this essential need that patients will have. Significant time is necessary for the level of exercise that patients will need, depending on level of injury.

Bone loss and the development of osteoporosis is also a concern in patients who have SCIs. Attention to calcium needs is necessary, within the specification of the total dietary prescription for the patient. Research has shown that patients with SCIs are more at risk for hip fractures than the general population because of increased bone loss. Bone loss also occurs at a faster rate in the knees. Based on this information, prevention efforts for fractures are a priority.

An upper motor neuron lesion will lead to spasticity, a common and disturbing situation that patients face. Spasticity often occurs on the resolution of spinal shock, which was characterized by complete suppression of reflexes, flaccidity, and loss of muscle tone. In contrast, after spinal shock resolves, a situation of hyperreflex activity often occurs. Spasticity may affect as many as two thirds of patients within the first year after SCI and is characterized by the involuntary uncontrolled movement of extremities associated with lower motor neuron lesions. Spasms interfere with positioning, with activities of daily living, and with most activities that could lead to any degree of independence. Furthermore, spasms can progress to becoming quite painful for patients.

Life for patients with SCIs changes in ways that most able-bodied people can never imagine. If physiological concerns were the only issues for nursing, providing care would certainly not be complicated. Major impacts on independence and body image occur no matter what the level of injury. Richmond and Thompson (2002) described psychosocial concerns for patients with SCIs as "devastating mental health issues with which the patient must deal" (p. 45). Varying degrees of dependence and loss of function create psychosocial responses that nurses must anticipate and support.

Because the SCI involves extreme overwhelming consequences and losses for patients, including losses to independence, to sexuality, to career, to lifestyle, and even to relationships, patients will experience significant grief and will move through the stages of grief for the losses as their recovery progresses. Early in the acute period after the injury, patients may focus on staying alive; but soon, their response may turn to denial and then anger as they experience the grief that accompanies this overwhelming situation. After the initial progression through the high acuity phase, patients realize how dependent they are on other people for the basic activities of daily living including bathing, eating, toileting, and elimination, along with all other activities. Realization of this level of dependence comes as a horrible blow and shock as they realize what has happened.

Initially, patients may emphasize their beliefs that they will be walking again and resuming their previous lifestyle. This may be a healthy outlook as the level of injury is still being determined. Later, this outlook may manifest as a denial of the extent of injury or of the lasting effects of the injury. Working through the grief associated with the injury may be a lifelong process for patients with SCIs.

Patients may be fearful of being dropped or injured while being turned or transferred. With the mechanics of traction and special beds, this is always a possibility and therefore not an unrealistic fear of patients. Furthermore, they may believe that their recovery is dependent on not being further injured. Making sure that two nurses are available for turning will reassure patients about their safety. Allowing the patient to work through the grief at his or her own rate will be necessary and will promote a healthy response to the process, which include viewing one's life in a positive way, a way in which the patient sees methods of contributing in spite of this overwhelming life change. Recent research has shown that some patients, even years after the injury, still mourn the losses associated with the injury and maintain a degree of anger and anxiety. These findings suggest that the process of acceptance and adjustment is a complex process not progressing in the same manner in all patients (Livneh & Martz, 2003). Nurses should not place expectations on patients and their psychosocial behavior at any point in time.

When adjustment or acceptance begins, patients start to look to the future and set goals for care and the future. At this stage, listening to stories from patients with SCI who have achieved levels of independence will be helpful to patients. Patients with similar injuries can have a profound positive effect on patients with more recent injuries. This is one reason that rehabilitation tends to be so successful. The development of camaraderie and friendships support the process of more than rehabilitation but also the movement through the stages of grief. During this stage, patients often start to find meaning in the experience and a purpose in life consistent with their new life experience.

Patients who have experienced an SCI are at more risk for suicide than the general population. Consultation with mental health professionals, including psychiatric mental health advanced practice nurses, will help nurses and family members to understand the patient's psychosocial responses to the injury and to identify meaningful ways to support the patient to progress in a mentally healthy manner while confronting and dealing with the injury, and to finding meaning in this life experience.

Extremes in patients' behavioral responses to the injury ranging from fear to sadness to anger may be seen in different patients. Responses to an SCI are not linear in the way in which they are lived. A caring approach with understanding of the extreme vulnerability and loss that the patient experiences will be effective in these circumstances. Generally, patients' responses to caring, involved nurses are not manipulative but rather appropriate and healing.

Evidence-Based Care

Treatment for spasticity has typically involved medication treatment. Baclofen has been the standard of treatment for years, with modest success. Other medications that may be useful include dantrolene, diazepam, and clonidine. Newer medications have become available, and newer modalities for administration of baclofen through the intrathecal route have become available. Individual studies have reported significant improvement in spasms for patients receiving baclofen by the intrathecal method (Taricco, Adone, Pagliacci, & Telaro, 2004). The use of valium has also been studied, and positive effects noted; however, the drowsiness associated with the use of valium is a limiting factor in its use. The current standard for treatment continues to be baclofen used alone or in combination with valium. In general, treatment for spasticity involves the use of baclofen and then using a decision tree to move upward to the addition of valium and then to intrathecal baclofen if patients become unresponsive to the previous therapy.

> *Red Flag*
>
> **Risk for Disuse Syndrome and Hazards of Immobility**
>
> Vigilant scheduling of range of motion exercises and weight bearing exercises (as possible with assistance of physical therapists) for patients will prevent atrophy of muscles and the possibility of contractures of extremities. This is a real risk in patients with the realities of immobility that patients with SCIs face every day. Nurses and caregivers must pay particular attention to the need for a schedule for exercising the muscle groups every day.

Collaborative Management

SCIs create a nursing intensive situation for patients. It is one of few conditions where the need for nursing care is generally much greater than the medical care needs of patients after the acute phase of recovery. This means that nursing care can potentially have a much greater impact on the outcomes of care than medical care will have for this population of patients. In the acute phase of postinjury care, collaboration by members of the team will contribute to the greater positive outcomes. As the patient progresses, the care becomes much more nursing related while medical and other team members will contribute much less to the care of these patients. Therefore, the nurse has a great responsibility and a great opportunity to contribute to quality of life for patients who have experienced SCIs The challenges for nursing in caring for patients with SCIs relates to the comprehensive needs and the vulnerability of patients who are injured. The primary responsibility of nurses is in caring for the person in a holistic manner during the human response to injury, which epitomizes the core of nursing practice.

Because the effects of an SCI require lifelong adjustments and care, patients must be as knowledgeable as health care providers in the details of their care. This means that the health care team must emphasize inclusion of the patient in care throughout the entire recovery period. A primary nursing model of care will support the care of patients with SCIs in a much more thorough manner than other models of care. This is especially true during the rehabilitation phase of recovery; however, it is also beneficial in all phases of care. Because assignment of a primary nurse to the care of the patient with SCIs throughout the hospital and rehabilitation phases will ensure the development of a thorough nursing care plan with attention to interdisciplinary needs of the patient, this model will provide for the best nursing care outcomes.

An injury with significant consequences, such as an SCI, will result in a spiritual crisis for many patients, especially patients without strong spiritual development prior to the injury. Patients may question why this has happened to them, or why their God would allow something like this to happen. They may even feel like they are being punished for behavior that may have contributed to the event. In those cases, guilt may be a response that patients struggle to overcome. As patients progress through recovery, they may ask themselves questions about their purpose in life and why they are alive after such a horrendous accident. Patients may emerge from their recovery with a renewed sense of purpose in life, finding purpose in their place in life as a person who has an SCI and who can carry the message to others about finding themselves in the face of adversity. Patients are supported by the positive action of patients with SCIs who are role models as they advocate for research and improved care.

Nurses who are uncomfortable in caring for patients experiencing spiritual distress or spiritual crises will have difficulty caring for patients with SCI. Referral to a chaplain or religious leader of the patient's wishes will be helpful in the early stages of the injury and recovery. During this time, the life-threatening aspects of the injury will be more related to the spiritual needs than the questions that patients may have about spirituality. As the recovery progresses, questions of a spiritual nature and the meaning of their life in this new situation become more common. The ability to assess the need for spiritual care as a part of assessment of spiritual distress or spiritual crisis will be essential at this time.

Keeping in mind that a large majority of patients with SCI are young adult males, and the developmental tasks related to intimacy and isolation, sexuality issues are a major concern for recovery and rehabilitation. The nurse who is caring for the patient with SCI must have a thorough knowledge of level of injury and how the injury will affect sexual functioning. Unawareness of specific effects along with a lack of understanding of sexual issues for the patient with SCI will lead to distrust of the nurse and will inhibit the therapeutic relationship. Serious discussions at the request of the patient are necessary to promote understanding of the effects of the injury. The potential for alterations in sexual response, orgasm, erection in males, and fertility may all be possibilities. No matter what the level of lesion, a lack of sensation in the perineal area and thus sensation during intercourse will occur.

If the patient has an upper motor neuron lesion, reflex sexual activity will be possible, and psychogenic erection may be possible for a patient with a lower motor neuron lesion. Reflex erection will not be possible for a patient with a lower motor neuron disorder. If it is possible, ejaculation may be retrograde into the bladder. Men with upper motor neuron lesions may be able to have erections as a result of external stimulation, and they may also have spontaneous erections, although these erections cannot be controlled or maintained.

Women with an SCI will not be able to have an orgasm, but they may remain fertile. Pregnancy and normal vaginal delivery is possible for women with SCIs. Nurses should assess for the presence or absence of menstrual periods since the injury. Generally, a professional with expertise should be available to discuss the details of sexuality after SCI. The nurse will still be asked questions from the patient and the significant other throughout the recovery period and will need to have an understanding of sexuality issues for the patient with an SCI. An honest, open approach is helpful for nursing care in this situation. A primary nursing model of care will enhance the development of a plan that can appropriately address sexuality for patients with SCIs.

Discussions among the nurse and the patient and significant other should emphasize the importance of open communication by partners. Respect for the religious and cultural backgrounds of the patient and significant other is essential during any discussions of sexuality. New families will experience grief over the loss of this aspect of their new lives; patients and spouses with longer term relationships will also experience significant loss, while perhaps being more comfortable with their lives together with this change for the future. Young men and women who have not established significant relationships yet will certainly experience sadness at the change in their sexuality.

Patients often have an indwelling urinary catheter, so teaching must emphasize the need to be mindful of this. For women, birth control methods, as appropriate, should be discussed. Autonomic dysreflexia may complicate what is believed to be a normal delivery if a woman does become pregnant. Sexual counseling may emphasize becoming aware of one's erogenous zones and learning to seek sexual pleasure from the partner's stimulation of these areas. Emphasis on the aspects of sexuality that remain and that can be maximized is important. Inclusion of the partner in discussions, if the patient is open to that, may be helpful.

Recent research has shown that the physical aspects of sexuality were not the most important factors in the quality of a relationship in a couple where one partner has experienced an SCI. Rather, it is the perception that the partner is happy and enjoys the experience. Psychosocial factors were more important than physical factors in contributing to a satisfying sexual relationship in these couples. Studies of the efficacy of sildenafil (Viagra) have also been undertaken in men with erectile dysfunction resulting from SCI. In men with injuries at the level of T6 through L5, a significant positive effect of the medication on satisfaction with the sexual experience was shown. Later studies have shown even more promise for the use of sildenafil in treating erectile dysfunction in men with SCIs. A significant number of patients with complete injuries benefited from the medication. This lends hope to the possibility of improving the quality of the sexual experience in men who have experienced SCIs.

Family members will also experience issues of coping with the injury, coping with changes in life and role changes that the patient experiences and role change for the family members as well. Spouses of patients with SCI will experience fears of the loss of independence, changes in levels of intimacy, and transition to the caregiver role. These changes will have a serious impact on family members, and they may experience the same movement through the stages of mourning as the patient does. Family members may experience denial and anger as the life of the entire family is transformed. Parents may

Respecting Our Differences

Cultural Considerations

Cultural issues will always be a factor to consider when providing care to patients with SCIs. Studies of young Hispanic (American) men who suffered an SCI found that family members, and even the fathers of young Hispanic (American) men, were involved in care, even though there is a degree of pride and a macho aura for males in this culture. Categorizing and stereotyping patients and families should be avoided. Assessment of cultural preferences and approaches to caring for family members must be performed and included in the plan of care. Because intimate care of a patient is a strong part of care of patients with SCI, close attention should be paid to the beliefs about intimate care in a particular culture, and nurses must support family members as they are faced with care that might be unfamiliar in their culture.

> **DOLLARS AND SENSE**
>
> **Costs of SCIs**
>
> SCI is costly in terms of loss of life and functioning and losses to quality of life, notwithstanding the health care costs. First year costs of health care in the United States for paraplegics average $209,000 and for quadriplegics the costs are $470,000. Lifetime health care costs average $730,000 for paraplegics and $1.2 million for quadriplegics. Considering the loss of personal income and the career effects of an SCI, the lifetime costs are staggering. Even beyond those costs, however, are the personal and psychosocial effects of an SCI.

care for adult children who had already left home, and spouses may be providing complete care for husbands and wives with SCI who once played a major role in the financial support of the family.

Nursing support to family members during this time should involve answering questions about the injury and level of function, care requirements, and referral sources. Family members will also need to understand their participation in the activities of daily living and the level of assistance needed. Social workers will be helpful with family members to determine the kinds of assistance with activities of daily living that can be provided when the patient goes home. Some patients may have resources for live-in help while many other families will plan on much more participation by family members in care depending on finances and resources available.

Evaluation of Outcomes

Presented below are the outcomes for care for the patient with an SCI presented according to nursing diagnosis. For alterations in neurological status the outcome of care will depend on the level of injury, and the nurse must look to the positive gains that can be made, such as head and shoulder movement and autonomic function not compromised, not to the outcomes that cannot be achieved, such as return of neurological function.

Because the patient with SCI experiences alterations in all areas of functioning, outcomes presented in Table 36-3 specify the expected outcomes for this patient. For example, it may not be possible to achieve independence in self-care abilities, but the nurse and patient can identify outcomes related to self-care that can be achieved. It is essential that the nurse identify the nursing diagnoses and outcomes that are the highest priority and ensure that the patient can achieve a lack of compromised status in those areas, such as tissue integrity and gas exchange.

SPINAL CORD TUMORS

The causes of spinal cord tumors are unknown. Spinal cord tumors can be classified as primary or metastatic tumors and may also be benign tumors. Most primary spinal cord tumors are benign, including the meningiomas and neurofibromas. The majority of spinal cord tumors are extramedullary (located outside the spinal cord) in origin and are classified as intradural or extradural tumors. Malignant metastatic tumors, lymphomas, and myelomas are generally extradural tumors. Primary extramedullary tumors, including neurofibromas and meningiomas, can be either intradural or extradural tumors.

Because of the location of spinal tumors, injury to the spinal cord occurs that causes spinal cord dysfunction the same as with SCI. The primary difference in effects is the gradualness of the dysfunction that occurs as opposed to the suddenness of SCI. The degree of magnitude of long-term sequelae depends on the extent of the tumor and the degree to which surgery removes the tumor and allows for normal spinal cord function.

Epidemiology

Only about 10 percent of spinal tumors are of the intramedullary type, which are located within the spinal cord itself. Ependymoma is the most common type of intramedullary tumor and occurs most often in the area of C6 through T2. The rest of the intramedullary tumors are gliomas and occur primarily in the cervical area of the spinal cord (Tierney, et al., 2004).

TABLE 36-3 Outcomes of Care for Patient with SCIs

Neurological status: Spinal sensory or motor function

Indicators:

Head and shoulder movement (as capable): Not compromised

Autonomic function: Not compromised

Deep tendon reflexes: Not compromised

Flaccidity: Not present: (as capable according to injury)

Neurological status: autonomic: Patient will be free of autonomic dysreflexia. Patient and family will verbalize signs of AD and appropriate actions to take.

Grief resolution: Patient and family members will exhibit movement through stages of grief.

Family normalization: Family members will verbalize return to preinjury lifestyle with modifications.

Depression: Patient will be free of depression.

Caregiver lifestyle disruption: Caregiver will identify methods for maintaining lifestyle within the new caregiver role.

Mobility level: Patient will achieve mobility with assistive person and device.

Nutritional status: Patient will consume nutrients adequate for body requirements.

Respiratory status: Gas exchange: lungs will be clear AP and laterally.

Self-care: Activities of daily living: Patient will accomplish activities of daily living with assistive person and devices.

Sexual functioning:

Indicators:

Adapts sexual technique as needed

Expresses ability to be intimate

Expresses ability to perform sexually despite physical imperfections

Expresses knowledge of personal sexual capabilities

Tissue integrity: Skin: Patient will be free of alterations in skin integrity. Skin will be pink, without evidence of development of ulcers.

Etiology

Metastatic tumors occur most frequently as a result of metastasis from the breast, kidneys, prostate, colon, and from lymphomas and multiple myeloma. Prostate tumors tend to metastasize to the thoracic region of the spinal cord, most commonly T8 through T10. Ovarian cancer usually metastasizes to the lumbosacral region of the spinal cord. Metastasis from other primary sites usually spread from the organ to the adjacent vertebral body. Multiple sites of the spinal cord may also be involved, especially with metastasis from the breast or prostate.

Pathophysiology

Pathophysiological changes that occur with a spinal cord tumor occur most often as a result of compression of the spinal cord at the level of the lesion. Compression of the spinal cord causes varying losses of motor and sensory function. Compression may also cause ischemia because of obstruction of

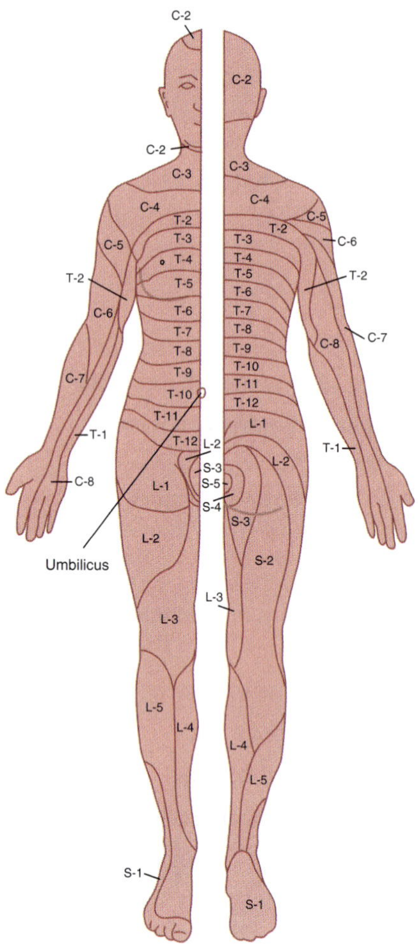

Figure 36-8 Anterior and posterior dermatomal distributions.

circulation. Edema may be present as injury to the spinal cord occurs and may ascend the spinal cord leading to death of tissue above the level of the tumor. Invasion of the spinal cord by tumors will cause loss of impulses and motor and sensory deficits, compression of spinal nerves, and alterations in reflex activity. Therefore, direct compression and ischemia, secondary to compression and culminating in arterial or venous obstruction, are the primary causes of spinal cord dysfunction associated with spinal cord tumors. In more rare circumstances, intramedullary tumors will cause symptoms from infiltration of spinal cord tissue.

The signs and symptoms of the tumor will lead to validation of the location of the spinal tumor, at the cervical, thoracic, lumbar, or sacral levels. It will be possible to map the sensory changes with the use of a **dermatome** (the area of skin innervated by a posterior spinal root) chart, which will show a correlation with the particular dermatome (Figure 36-8).

Assessment with Clinical Manifestations

Because spinal tumors often have gradual growth, symptoms may not be present until there is significant growth of the tumor. On the other hand, metastatic tumors may grow rapidly. Focal signs that may identify the location of the tumor include cranial nerve disturbances, respiratory difficulties, and **paresthesia** (abnormal numbness and tingling sensation). Commonly, pain is the earliest sign of metastasis to the vertebrae. Pain may also occur as a result of compression of a nerve root. Pain along with weakness and sensory changes are often identified. Patients may seek health care because of difficulties with bowel and bladder function, which become difficult to manage.

Motor deficits can occur for several pathophysiological reasons, as a result of upper and lower motor neuron lesions and from compression of spinal nerves. Loss of reflexes, weakness, and muscle wasting occur. An upper motor neuron lesion will result in spasticity and increased DTRs. Lower motor neuron lesions will result in weakness and flaccidity. Brown-Séquard syndrome (discussed previously in the chapter) may also occur. Sensation may be affected according to spinal tracts, which are compressed by the tumor. Unilateral compression by a tumor can cause contralateral and ipsilateral sensory affects because of its effect on the spinal tracts. Alterations in urinary elimination may progress to urinary retention, which signifies the need for urinary catheterization. Bowel elimination alterations may occur initially as constipation followed by increasing difficulty with bowel elimination.

The rate of growth of spinal cord tumors can ultimately be determined by neurological assessment. Patients tend to visit their health care provider as they identify changes in motor function and sensory function. Many spinal cord tumors are slow growing tumors, however, and may develop over a few years, with negligible neurological deficits for a significant period of time. If the tumor is a soft tumor, it may also conform somewhat to the space in the spinal column. However, a hard tumor will not conform as easily and will produce neurological deficits earlier.

Diagnostic Tests

Because progression of symptoms may be gradual, a detailed history and physical examination will be essential. Determining the progression of events through the history will be helpful in ascertaining how symptoms have occurred and increased and spread throughout the spinal cord over time. Additionally, neurological assessment will determine muscle weakness, sensory loss, pain, and altered DTRs.

Diagnosis of a spinal cord tumor will center on results of an MRI, so patients will initially undergo this procedure. Positron emission tomography (PET) images will also be performed to identify cancerous tissue. Physicians will perform an MRI and CT scan when patients seek treatment because of symptoms along with a history of known tumor elsewhere. In these situations, there is thus a potential for metastasis. Sometimes only the complaint of back pain, which is new in a patient with a history of cancer, will be the reason for diagnostic tests for spinal cord tumor. A myelogram will be performed to identify blockage of areas of the spinal cord. CSF analysis will also be performed at the time of myelogram (Daniels, 2003).

Nursing Diagnoses

Nursing diagnoses may be similar to the diagnoses for patients with SCI; however, degree of severity of neurological impairment will depend on progression of the tumor. It is important to identify symptoms early to prevent damage to the spinal cord. Based on the information gathered, examples of nursing diagnoses in the patient with spinal cord tumors may include the following:

- Pain related to compression of the spinal cord by the tumor.
- Neurovascular dysfunction related to growth of tumor compressing the spinal cord.
- Impaired elimination, bowel and bladder related to tumor growth and compression of the spinal cord.

Planning and Implementation

The initial focus of planning for the patient with a suspected spinal cord tumor will be to plan with the patient for the diagnostic tests, which will be performed to determine the etiology for the presenting symptoms. Patients will often arrive at the health care facility experiencing pain and loss of functioning, and if they have previously had a diagnosis of cancer, they may be quite fearful and anxious about the possibility of return of the malignancy. Once diagnosis is made, it is important to provide teaching to support the plan of medical care, which will usually include surgery. Preoperatively and postoperatively the patient will generally be receiving corticosteroid therapy for treatment of any edema related to the growth of the tumor. Postoperatively, the patient will participate in planning related to follow-up with chemotherapy and radiation therapy. Nursing care in all stages of medical and surgical treatment will include teaching related to the treatment modality and expected patient responses to the treatment modality.

Long-term planning and implementation will focus on assessment of neurological status and the potential for the patient to resume self-care activities. Treatment of pain will be a priority for nursing management throughout the course of the illness and treatment.

Pharmacology

There are a variety of pharmacological measures taken in the management of spinal cord tumors. The primary classifications of pharmacological treatments are in the forms of chemotherapy and the corticosteroids that are administered. Chemotherapy has limited application for treatment of spinal cord tumors. Chemotherapy may be useful for gliomas, lymphomas, and some lung and breast cancers. Adjuvant therapy, such as tamoxifen, may also be useful, when there is metastasis from the breast. Intrathecal chemotherapy is showing promise with the direct infusion of chemotherapy into the CSF from an Ommaya reservoir.

Dexamethasone at high doses is useful in treatment to decrease the edema associated with the spinal cord tumor. Ascending edema may be present, and the use of corticosteroids will be quite useful in these cases. This treatment in combination with radiation may provide relief of symptoms in patients with inoperable tumors. Patients must have antacids to protect the gastrointestinal (GI) tract when taking these corticosteroids (Broyles, Reiss, & Evans, 2007).

Surgery

For patients with epidural metastases, irradiation along with high doses of dexamethasone (25 mg four times daily) for three days and then in tapered doses is the usual treatment (Tierney, et al., 2004). This will result in reduction of edema and relief of pain. Surgery to remove the tumor in these patients is not usually performed unless irradiation and medical treatment is not successful, although there is controversy about the decision to do surgery in these patients. Radiation therapy tends to delay progression of symptoms. The prognosis in these patients is generally poor. For patients with most extramedullary intradural tumors, surgical removal of the tumor may be successful. Prognosis depends on the origin of the tumor and severity of compression and symptoms.

Emergency surgery is indicated when there is rapid progression of neurological symptoms. Sudden loss of motor and sensory function, including paralysis or loss of bowel and bladder function indicate a need for immediate surgery. This may maintain bowel and bladder function in patients with metastatic lesions and is an important quality of life consideration. Better neurological outcome is related to the degree of neurological deficit that is present. The greater the degree of neurological impairment, the poorer the prognosis. Paralysis is not reversible.

Extradural tumors often involve a less complicated surgery for removal. Such tumors as meningiomas may be completely removed. Intramedullary tumors are much more complicated and the chances for complete removal by surgery are less likely because of invasion of surrounding tissues. In these situations, surgery to accomplish decompression may be the primary goal.

Postoperative nursing care involves detailed neurological assessment along with treatment of pain and other complications. Motor and sensory function must be frequently assessed to identify the possibility of edema developing postoperatively. Complications that have been identified postoperatively in patients undergoing spinal cord tumor resection include the development of intracranial subdural hematomas, as unusual as this may seem. The development of a headache postoperatively should always be reported to the health care provider because of this possibility. It is thought that a puncture of the dura such as occurs with spinal surgery may cause the brain to be displaced downwardly, causing traction, laceration of vessels, and the collection of blood in the subdural space.

Newer techniques for surgery have become available. Laminectomies may still be performed to remove tumors. These surgeries may also involve spinal fusion. Laser surgery and microneurosurgical techniques are becoming available and improving outcomes in patients with spinal cord tumors. Microsurgical lasers make it possible to cut minute tissue bands and achieve immediate hemostasis, resulting in far fewer complications from bleeding and damage to the spinal cord.

During the surgical procedure, intraoperative monitoring of motor evoked potentials (MEPs) has become available to identify the possibility of motor impairment as a result of the surgical technique. Through the use of electrical stimulation these MEPs will provide information about the functioning of fibers in the spinal cord. These MEPs can be followed to determine functional integrity of the motor fibers, and when identified as lost, will be seen as damage to motor pathways. With these newer surgical techniques, surgery has become successful in treating spinal cord tumors.

Radiation Therapy

Radiation therapy is the primary treatment for metastatic spinal cord tumors. Primary spinal cord tumors may also be treated with irradiation. Because the spinal cord is more sensitive to radiation therapy than the brain, measures must be taken to protect the spinal cord from excess exposure. Radiation complications will cause a radiation damage manifested as sensory impairments occurring after the completion of the radiation treatment. This can progress to increasing neurological impairment, paralysis, and loss of bowel and bladder function.

Evaluation of Outcomes

Potential patient outcomes for each of the example nursing diagnoses for the patient with spinal cord tumors are:

- Pain related to compression of tumor, surgical treatment. The patient should verbalize an adequate relief of pain along with the ability to realistically cope with the pain if it is not completely relieved.
- Neurovascular dysfunction. The patient will demonstrate complete return of neurological functioning depending on prognosis.
- Impaired elimination, bowel and bladder. The patient will resume normal bowel and bladder function depending on prognosis.

PERIPHERAL NERVOUS SYSTEM DYSFUNCTION

Peripheral nervous system dysfunction is generally understood as **neuropathies** (dysfunctions of the peripheral nervous system). Neuropathies affecting the peripheral nervous system affect the cranial nerves, spinal nerves, peripheral nerves, and the autonomic nervous system innervation. Peripheral neuropathy results from altered structure or function of a peripheral nerve and may include motor, sensory, or autonomic impairments. Peripheral nerves innervate the extremities, and when damaged, result in motor and sensory impairments affecting the extremities. Peripheral nerves have motor and sensory components, with motor components originating in the lower motor neurons. Some nerves may be motor nerves, others are sensory nerves, and some are mixed in nature.

Etiology

Several etiologies exist for neuropathies, including disease and metabolic problems, drug induced causes, connective tissue causes, infections, trauma, neoplasms, entrapment syndromes, environmental exposure to toxins, and hereditary conditions. In addition to the above etiologies, injury can also cause neuropathy. Injuries to nerves often involve a plexus or injury to an extremity.

Pathophysiology

A thorough understanding of sensory dermatomes, reflexes, and muscle innervation will aid in understanding the signs and symptoms of neuropathies and nerve injuries. It will be possible to map neuropathies of sensory nerves through the use of a dermatome chart. Decreased or loss of sensation of light touch and pinprick will be noted along a particular dermatome. Patients generally complain of tingling, numbness, paresthesias (described by patients as pins and needles), and **dysesthesias** (described as a burning sensation). Pain is often a symptom accompanying nerve trauma and neuropathies, as is commonly seen in diabetic neuropathies (discussed in chapter 57) and trigeminal **neuralgia** (pain associated with peripheral nerves, and following the course of nerves).

There are many neuropathies; those caused by underlying disease, infections, and disorders, such as diabetes, uremia, alcoholism and nutritional deficiencies, acquired immune deficiency syndrome (AIDS), leprosy, sarcoidosis, are discussed elsewhere in this book. Neuropathies may also be caused by toxicities following exposure to industrial agents, pesticides, metals (mercury, thallium, and lead), and drugs, such as phenytoin, many of the neoplastic agents, and such drugs as isoniazid and pyridoxine used in high doses. Neuropathies may also occur as a complication of malignant disease, may occur before signs of the malignancy are apparent, or may occur after remissions and exacerbations. Careful assessment of occupational and health histories is necessary to reveal the possible etiologies for the onset of neuropathies.

Guillain-Barré Syndrome

An increasingly common peripheral nerve disorder is Guillain-Barré syndrome (GBS), which is characterized by acute neuropathy involving motor and sensory nerves throughout the peripheral nervous system.

Epidemiology

According to the Guillain-Barré Syndrome Foundation, the syndrome affects 1 or 2 people per 100,000 population in the United States. It is the most common cause of rapidly acquired paralysis in the United States (Blumenthal, Pria, Bon-Harlev, & Amir, 2004).

Etiology

GBS is an acute idiopathic polyneuropathy that often follows an infective illness. A flu-like illness caused by a variety of pathogens has been most often implicated as the instigating factor in GBS. Most frequently, *Campylobacter jejuni* has been associated with developed of the illness in adults, followed by cytomegalovirus, Epstein Barr, mycoplasma pneumonia, hepatitis A, and hepatitis B. It has also been associated with inoculations with vaccines for influenza, tetanus, hepatitis A, and hepatitis B, as well as with surgical procedures (Tierney, et al., 2004). Usually the acute infectious illness precedes the development of this syndrome by one to three weeks and is most often respiratory or GI in nature (Blumenthal, et al., 2004). The syndrome is thought to be an autoimmune disorder triggered by the infectious agent or event. Because of their decreased immune function, the elderly are more likely to develop GBS after one of these events (Kuwabara, 2004).

This neuropathy is a rapidly progressing disorder affecting primarily the motor components to the peripheral nerves involved. It is believed that the underlying illness triggers a demyelinization of the nerves leading to development of the neuropathy. This dysfunction is characterized by weakness that is generally proximal and symmetrical in distribution. Severity of the weakness varies widely across patients.

GBS usually begins in the legs and proceeds spreading to the arms, face, and sometimes to the muscles of respiration. Motor involvement is more common than sensory involvement; however, patients may experience peripheral paresthesias. Patients may also complain of neuropathic pain. Autonomic dysfunction is common in these patients and may include life-threatening tachycardias, hypotension hypertension, facial flushing, sweating abnormalities, pulmonary dysfunction, and impairments of sphincter control, similar to the autonomic dysfunction that can occur with SCIs.

Pathophysiology

GBS triggers an immune response, which causes destruction of the myelin sheaths of peripheral nerves. Because of the demyelination process, loss of nerve conduction occurs. This demyelination is generally patchy in its involvement. Edema and inflammation of nerves accompany the process leading to further impairment involving the nerves.

Assessment with Clinical Manifestations

Ascending GBS is the most common form of the disease and is characterized by a weakness that starts in the lower extremities and progresses to the trunk and arms, and finally to the cranial nerves affecting the head and neck. Motor deficits with this form of the disorder are symmetrical. DTRs are weak or absent, and sensory impairments of numbness is worse in the toes. Respiratory involvement occurs in 50 percent of patients with ascending GBS.

Descending GBS progresses from the brainstem downward with motor deficits occurring initially with the cranial nerves with progressing weakness downward. Respiratory involvement occurs rapidly in this form of the disease. DTRs are weak or absent. In most patients, GBS is usually seen as weakness of motor function progressing upward from the legs and involving the respiratory muscles in its progression up the trunk. Respiratory difficulties occur as the diaphragm and intercostal muscles become involved. Of the cranial nerves, the facial nerve (cranial nerve [CN] VII) is most frequently involved, although CN IX, X, XI, and XII may also be affected. Effects of cranial nerve involvement will be seen as dysphagia, paralysis of the vocal cords, and difficulty eating. If the vagus nerve is affected, autonomic nervous system signs will be apparent. Sensory involvement from GBS is characterized by pain and paresthesias affecting the hands and feet. Pain generally occurs in the extremities and more often during the night, which interrupts sleep patterns.

Assessment of occupational, infectious, and other exposure history is essential in the diagnostic phase of the illness. As the illness progresses, assessment of the extension of weakness, involvement of respiratory muscles, and the onset of respiratory dysfunction is essential. Assessment of the onset of autonomic symptoms is also a priority, especially the development of hypotension, which may become an emergency. Because patients may require care in critical care units, ongoing in-depth assessment should be done and recorded to note the progression, if any, of weakness. Neurological assessment should include assessment of paresthesias, dysesthesias, and paresis, along with any complaints of pain. Location and movement and progression of the paresis should be noted with each assessment. Vital signs should include any changes in respiratory status, the presence of hypotension or hypertension, and changes in heart rate, including tachycardia.

Detailed assessment of respiratory function is necessary throughout the stages of the disease. Assessment of respiratory rate, depth, and quality is essential at frequent intervals to detect what may seem to be minor changes in respiratory function. The nurse must also assess for signs of respiratory insufficiency, including signs of decreased oxygenation, such as cyanosis, diaphoresis, dyspnea, and anxiety. Pulse oximetry is necessary to maintain assessment of respiratory function. Oxygen will be administered as ordered.

Diagnostic Tests

Diagnosis is made through confirmation of the history of the patient and CSF analysis, which shows a high protein content. These changes may not occur at the same time as symptoms, because it takes two to three weeks to develop. Medical diagnosis will emphasize differential diagnosis, using a process of excluding other causes for the symptoms, which may include botulism, poliomyelitis, and exposure to heavy metals. The disease progresses over several months, however, most patients make a complete recovery. Ten to 20 percent of patients experience a permanent disability.

Nursing Diagnoses

Based on the information gathered, examples of nursing diagnoses in the patient with GBS may include the following:

- Ineffective breathing pattern
- Impaired gas exchange related to ventilation-perfusion inequality
- Ineffective coping related to anxiety, lower activity level and the inability to perform normal activities of daily living
- Knowledge deficit related to self-care and risk prevention

Planning and Implementation

Treatment of GBS is supportive in nature. Plasmapheresis has been shown to be effective, if instituted within three to four days of onset of the illness. It has also been shown to be effective for exacerbations that occur in chronic forms of the dysfunction. Treatment with prednisone is ineffective and actually has been shown to extend recovery time (Tierney, et al., 2004). Care focuses on support of respiratory function and the monitoring of pulmonary function tests to identify weakness of respiratory muscles and the need for critical care management. Management of hypotension is also a priority of care.

Prevention and treatment of respiratory failure is a priority of management. Common progression of the disease as it becomes more life-threatening and includes decreases in vital capacity, decreased ability to cough, and ineffective airway clearance. As vital capacity decreases, the atelectasis and hypoxemia become problematic. Additionally, increasing weakness occurs of the diaphragm and intercostal muscles occur as innervation decreases. At this point intubation and respiratory support may become necessary.

An additional concern for health care is the potential for autonomic dysfunction. Disturbances in cardiac rate and rhythm can occur, so cardiac monitoring is necessary in the critical stages of the illness. Additionally, paralytic ileus and urinary retention may occur as a result of autonomic dysfunction. A nasogastric tube may be necessary for gastric decompression. Intermittent catheterization or indwelling urinary catheter will be used for urinary retention.

Supportive and caring nursing interventions are essential because of the extremely frightening nature of this illness. Teaching about the effects of the illness and the usual self-limiting nature of the illness will provide realistic reassurance to patients. Providing answers to patient and family questions will be beneficial, as those answers are available. Because of the uncertain nature of the development of the illness, answers to the types of questions that patients have are not always available. The health care provider may provide information about the usual progression of the disease that occurs in a majority of patients.

Alterations in respiratory function comprise the priority nursing diagnoses. Patients may experience ineffective airway clearance and ineffective breathing patterns related to the weakness of respiratory muscles. Supportive respiratory care, along with suctioning if necessary to provide a clear airway, is essential in the critical stages of the illness. Instructions to cough and deep breathe, as the patient is able, will help to prevent the development of pneumonia. If respiratory function continues to decline, ventilatory support is necessary, and respiratory care by the nurse becomes the priority of care.

At this stage, patients may be frightened, fearing that they are dying. Because recovery statistics are currently optimistic, providing optimistic information about recovery potential will be helpful to patients. Caring and comforting presence by the nurses is essential in this stage of the illness. Patients are sometimes on ventilator support for months, so the optimism for positive outcome is difficult to maintain for many patients. Additionally, patients who are receiving ventilatory support will need assistance with communication, provided by the nurse.

Preventing alterations in skin integrity becomes a priority as weakness progresses, and independent movement and mobility is impaired. Turning the patient on a strict schedule is necessary to prevent the development of decubitus ulcers. Assessment of skin integrity is an essential component of nursing care contributing to the outcome of skin integrity for patients with GBS.

Of even greater concern related to immobility is the risk for deep vein thrombosis (DVT) and pulmonary embolism (PE). Prevention of DVT and PE is a priority and is achieved by administration of minidoses of heparin. Compression boots for prevention of DVT are not used because of the risk for damage to peripheral nerves with pressure from the boots (Green, Hartwig, Chen, Soltysik, & Yarnold, 2003).

Additionally, because of immobility, the risk for disuse syndrome is a potential issue. Range of motion to the extremities and all joints will prevent contractures as weakness develops in patients. Assistance with mobility and ambulation in many patients will be necessary as the rehabilitation stage progresses.

The progressing alterations in neurological status in patients with GBS mean that detailed neurological assessments are necessary in frequent intervals. Nurses must assess for progressing weaknesses affecting motor and sensory function as well as cranial nerve function. Neurological assessment is emphasized in early stages of the illness, but when respiratory function is affected, the priority for nursing care shifts to respiratory care, including maintenance of a patent airway and adequate respiration. Alterations in autonomic function frequently occur and can be dangerous in its effects. Nurses should be astutely aware of changes in blood pressure and heart rate. Most patients during this time will have hemodynamic monitoring with continuous electrocardiogram (ECG) monitoring to detect any dysrhythmias. Self-care abilities will vary with different patients and differing degrees of weakness. Support for eating, bathing, dressing, and all aspects of self-care are often necessary at some stages of the illness.

Pain becomes a serious concern as patients are recovering from GBS. This means that patients will need frequent assessment of pain and medications for the relief of pain. This may need to be accomplished by epidural infusions of narcotics, such as morphine. Pain will also interfere with sleep patterns, so relief of pain will also aid with sleep. As recovery progresses, an interdisciplinary approach to rehabilitation is most beneficial. Physical therapy will be necessary to help patients regain function and abilities.

Evaluation of Outcomes

Potential patient outcomes for each of the example nursing diagnoses for the patient with the GBS are:

- Ineffective breathing pattern. The patient's breathing pattern is maintained by eupnea, normal skin color, and regular respiratory rate or pattern.
- Impaired gas exchange related to ventilation-perfusion inequality. The patient maintains optimal gas exchange as evidenced by normal arterial blood gases (ABGs) and alert, responsive mentation or no further reduction in mental status.
- Ineffective coping related to anxiety, lower activity level and the inability to perform normal activities of daily living. The patient identifies own maladaptive coping behaviors, available resources, and support systems, describes or initiates alternative coping strategies and describes positive results from new behaviors.
- Knowledge deficit related to self-care and risk prevention. The patient should demonstrate motivation to learn, identify perceived learning needs, and verbalize an understanding of desired content.

Trigeminal Neuralgia

The cranial nerves are the peripheral nerves that originate from the brain. The 12 pairs of cranial nerves may be especially vulnerable to injury; some are more vulnerable to disease than others. The major cranial nerve dysfunctions discussed in this chapter are trigeminal neuralgia and Bell's palsy. An extremely painful condition, trigeminal neuralgia (also known as **tic douloureux**) affects the trigeminal nerve (CN V). This condition is characterized by extreme, intense pain affecting one or more branches of CN V. Unlike many other peripheral nerve conditions, there are no motor or sensory deficits associated with this condition. Patients describe the pain as sharp, stabbing, burning, and intense. This pain is so intense that it can become disabling. Pain is unilateral in location according to the affected nerve. The term tic refers to facial spasms that accompany episodes of the pain.

CN V is the largest of the cranial nerves and has three divisions: the ophthalmic, maxillary, and mandibular (Figure 36-9). CN V has both motor and sensory components. The motor component innervates the temporal muscles, the muscles used for chewing (masseter), and sensory fibers relay pain, touch, and temperature sensation. The ophthalmic branch innervates the forehead, eyes, nose, temples, paranasal sinuses, and the nasal mucosa. The maxillary branch innervates the upper jaw, teeth, lip, cheeks, hard palate, maxillary sinus, and part of the nasal mucosa. The mandibular branch innervates the lower jaw, teeth, lip, buccal mucosa, tongue, part of the external ear, auditory meatus, and meninges. Trigeminal neuralgia generally affects the maxillary and mandibular branches and only rarely the ophthalmic branch of the nerve.

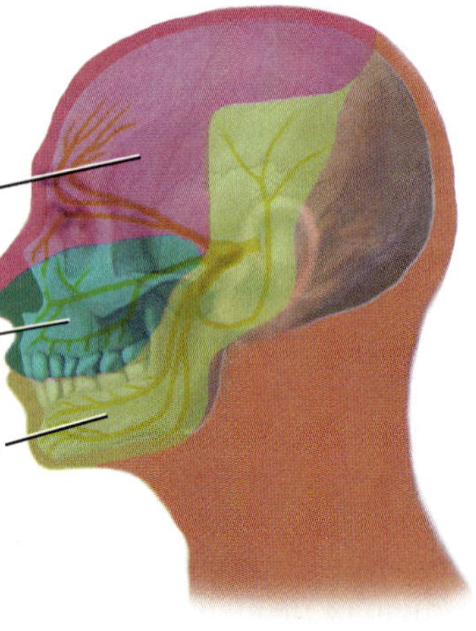

Figure 36-9 Areas of face innervated by the trigeminal nerve (CN-V): A. Ophthalmic, B. Maxillary; C. Mandibular.

Epidemiology

Trigeminal neuralgia affects women more than men and generally occurs in middle and later years of life.

Etiology

Trigeminal neuralgia is believed to occur from pressure exerted by blood vessels on the fifth cranial nerve. This pressure eventually causes demyelination of the nerve resulting in severe pain (Brown, 2003).

Pathophysiology

The course of trigeminal neuralgia often includes remissions and exacerbations. Careful history will reveal periods of pain followed by remissions, which may last from days to years. As patients age, remissions tend to become shorter and less frequent. Characteristic of almost all cases of trigeminal neuralgia is a severe, almost disabling pain. Pain is described as a sudden, **lancinating** (stabbing or piercing) facial pain that originates near one side of the mouth and shoots toward the eye, ear, or nostril on the same side. The pain of trigeminal neuralgia may be triggered by touch, drafts of air, eating, and movement (Tierney, et al., 2004). Patients often try many ways to avoid pain, including not doing things that might trigger the pain, such as eating, talking, washing the face, brushing the teeth, or shaving. Therefore, patients may seek health care already being emaciated and disheveled in appearance. Patients may also attempt to talk without moving their face if this is known to trigger the pain.

The etiology of this disease is not known; however, infection (especially of teeth), and trauma have been associated with development of the disorder. Pressure by an artery next to the trigeminal nerve has been identified in many cases. Pressure may also be associated with a tumor or aneurysm, although intracranial tumor as a cause of trigeminal neuralgia is unlikely (Brown, 2003).

Assessment with Clinical Manifestations

Nurses should assess the location, intensity, quality, and characteristics of pain, including the patterns of occurrence, and aggravating and precipitating factors associated with trigeminal neuralgia. Nurses must assess the frequency of episodes of pain, the use of medications, and monitor lab values for side effects of the carbamazepine that involve liver function.

Diagnostic Tests

Diagnosis of trigeminal neuralgia is generally based on physical examination, which identifies the characteristic features of the pain following the pathway of the trigeminal nerve. CT scan is normal unless an underlying lesion or pathology exists. Multiple sclerosis as an underlying pathology has been identified in some cases, and should always be explored in younger patients with trigeminal neuralgia, even when there are no other neurological dysfunctions indicative of multiple sclerosis (Tierney, et al., 2004). Complaints of bilateral pain may also be associated with multiple sclerosis and should be evaluated (Brown, 2003). Occasionally, even when CT and MRI scans are negative, unsuccessful neurological treatment leads to further exploration, which will reveal structural cause for the dysfunction, such as pressure from an artery or vein on the nerve. In these cases, separation of the vessel from the nerve will lead to relief of symptoms. Trigeminal neuralgia is not generally caused by an intracranial mass. Surgical exploration is not used for patients with multiple sclerosis.

Nursing Diagnoses

Based on the information gathered, examples of nursing diagnoses in the patient with trigeminal neuralgia may include the following:

- Acute pain related to neurological impairment
- Alteration in nutritional status, less than body requirements related to pain associated with eating
- Social isolation related to pain
- Risk for loneliness related to pain and discomfort

Planning and Implementation

Medical treatment of trigeminal neuralgia is currently primarily comprised of pharmacological intervention. Other methods of treatment may include surgery and injections with alcohol, however alcohol injection and surgery are much less frequently recommended currently. The drug most commonly used for the treatment of trigeminal neuralgia is carbamazepine (Tegretol). Carbamazepine can also aid in diagnosis, because patients may respond immediately to this medication (Brown, 2003). Because this drug can be toxic to the liver and can also cause bone marrow depression, patients' laboratory values must be closely monitored while taking this medication. If patients cannot tolerate this medication, other choices include phenytoin (Dilantin), the second choice for pharmacological therapy. Gabapentin, baclofen, capsaicin, and amitriptyline may also be used for relief of symptoms if first-line therapy is not successful.

Medical treatment may become less effective over the long term, and surgical treatment may become necessary in some patients who have chronic trigeminal neuralgia. Neurodestructive procedures may be undertaken if medical treatment is not successful.

The primary concern of patients with trigeminal neuralgia is severe pain radiating along the nerve tract. Nursing care will focus on assisting patients to seek medical treatment for diagnosis, and supporting patients through exacerbation of the nerve dysfunction. This dysfunction becomes a chronic pain syndrome with the exacerbations and remissions associated with it. Even though carbamazepine has been useful in treating the dysfunction, it is not always effective, and its side effects may lead to the need to discontinue the medication. Pain and uncertainty about the medication regimen leads to psychosocial responses, including social isolation and loneliness. Malnutrition may occur because of the guarding by patients to prevent an episode of pain. Because patients do not want to get themselves in a situation where they may experience pain, they may isolate themselves socially, delay self-care activities of washing and brushing their teeth, and experience alterations in nutrition related to this fear of causing pain.

Assisting patients with nutrition, medication administration, assessment for side effects, and pain assessment and management are the primary nursing interventions for this dysfunction. Nursing interventions to assist patients to avoid the aggravating and precipitating factors may be helpful in preventing occurrences of the pain. Nutritional assessment and teaching regarding the necessity of a balanced diet, perhaps with the inclusion of soft foods will be helpful in maintaining nutritional status.

The social isolation that patients may experience because of the dysfunction can become quite severe. Identification of family members who are supportive of the patient in times of severe pain will be helpful in providing a safe and caring environment for the patient. Also, helping family members to understand the severity of the pain will bring a level of support to patients through the difficult painful episodes.

Evaluation of Outcomes

Potential patient outcomes for each of the example nursing diagnoses for the patient with trigeminal neuralgia are:

- Acute pain related to neurological impairment. The patient will report pain free status (0 on scale of 0 to 10). This may need to be adjusted depending on the success of treatment. The goal will be to maintain the patient in a pain-free state.
- Alteration in nutritional status, less than body requirements related to pain associated with eating. The patient will maintain nutritional status for body requirements.
- Social isolation related to pain. The patient will resume social activities once pain free.
- Risk for loneliness related to pain and discomfort. The patient will reconnect with friends and family and report a lower level of loneliness which is specifically related to the condition.

Bell's Palsy

Bell's palsy is a facial neuropathy that is characterized by paresis and pain. Considered an idiopathic neuropathy, patients complain of symptoms of paresis (weakness) initially, which worsen over the next few days. Pain often accompanies the paresis or may precede the symptoms of paresis. Generally the pain is self-limiting and may last for only a few days. Restriction of eye closure, stiffness of the face, and fine movement of the facial muscles occurs. Patients may also complain of alterations in taste.

Epidemiology

Bell's palsy is the most common cause of facial paralysis. Affecting men and women equally, approximately 40,000 people are diagnosed in the United States each year. Pregnant women are disproportionately affected.

Etiology

Bell's palsy is generally considered an inflammatory disorder and may be associated with reactivation of herpes simplex virus. Although this belief is controversial, it does have wide support as the cause (He, Zhou, Wu, Li, & Zhou, 2004). Increased support for the association of the herpes simplex virus and Bell's palsy is being reported (Doganci, Odabasi, & Turn, 2003).

Pathophysiology

Bell's palsy results from a lower motor neuron dysfunction causing a unilateral facial nerve (CN VII) paresis or paralysis on one side of the face.

Assessment with Clinical Manifestations

Characteristic symptoms of Bell's palsy initially include facial weakness (paresis), which begins abruptly and worsens over the following days. Pain accompanies the weakness but usually only lasts a few days. Patients complain of facial stiffness and may have limited eye closure and restricted movement of the facial muscles, which subsequently results in difficulty eating. Alterations in taste have also been known to occur.

Diagnostic Tests

Diagnosis of Bell's palsy is generally made after physical examination and careful assessment of cranial nerve function. The clinical picture of distorted face is a classic sign of Bell's palsy. Electromyography (EMG) may be performed to assess nerve damage, and MRI, CT scan, and X-ray will detect the presence of a tumor applying pressure on the facial nerve.

Nursing Diagnoses

Based on the information gathered, examples of nursing diagnoses in the patient with Bell's palsy may include the following:

- Acute pain
- Alteration in nutritional status, less than body requirements
- Disturbed sensory perception
- Disturbed body image
- Readiness for enhanced self-concept

Planning and Implementation

Because many of the cases recover without treatment, controversy exists regarding treatment of Bell's palsy. Only about 10 percent of patients experience long-term disability or disfigurement. In those patients, treatment is necessary to prevent disfigurement. In other patients, more than 80 percent have reported resolution of symptoms and recovery without treatment (He, et al., 2004). Poor prognosis for recovery is seen in patients who are elderly, who experience severe pain at onset, or who have degeneration of the facial nerve. Treatment for patients with severe pain consists of corticosteroids, generally prednisone 60 to 80 mg in divided doses for 4 to 5 days, with tapering doses over the next 7 to 10 days (Tierney, et al., 2004). Sometimes acyclovir is also prescribed for treatment because of the herpes virus association, although this is controversial. Studies have not shown the efficacy of acyclovir used alone as treatment. There is limited evidence that acyclovir used in combination with prednisone may result in improvement of symptoms.

Acupuncture as a complementary medical treatment has shown great promise in the treatment of Bell's palsy. Preliminary studies show significantly better responses in patients receiving acupuncture versus patients in a control group. However, these results are based on limited studies (He, et al., 2003).

Generally, assessment and teaching regarding the need to seek treatment early are the priority nursing interventions. Treatment should be started early after symptoms occur, within five days of onset to be effective, so early identification and referral for treatment is a necessity. For patients with restricted eyelid closure, instruction should be given to use eye drops to keep the eyes lubricated. If the patient cannot close the eye, an eye patch should be used to protect the eye or the patient should be taught to manually close the eye. Teaching regarding the use of corticosteroids should also be provided to patients.

Nutritional deficits occur with Bell's palsy because of the limitations on movement of the mouth on the affected side of the face. Frequent, small meals with soft foods are best tolerated by most patients. Sipping drinks through a straw and chewing on the affected side are often limited or impossible. Because of the difficulties with eating and the potential for disfigurement, emotional support is necessary during this time. Alterations in body image and self-concept occur because of the change in appearance. Emotional support provided by the nurse is necessary during this time. Reassurance that most patients recover completely is often difficult to understand when looking at oneself in the mirror and seeing a side of the face that sags and an eye that will not close.

Patients suggesting that they are interested in trying complementary or alternative therapy should be referred to their health care provider for further information. Nurses should become aware of the potential beneficial effects of complementary methods, such as acupuncture, and support patients in their attempts to find successful treatment for this condition. Sometimes, facial exercises and electrical nerve stimulation are suggested for treatment of Bell's palsy. Currently, there is no evidence that either treatment modality is efficacious. There is some evidence that electrical nerve stimulation may be helpful in treatment of long-term symptoms of Bell's palsy.

Evidence-Based Care

Recent research has shown that patients receiving the intranasal influenza vaccine used in Switzerland had an increased incidence of Bell's palsy. The intranasal influenza vaccine currently in use in the United States has not shown this association (Mutsch, et al., 2004).

Evaluation of Outcomes

Potential patient outcomes for each of the example nursing diagnoses for the patient with Bell's palsy are:

- Acute pain. The patient should verbalize an adequate relief of pain along with the ability to realistically cope with the pain if it is not completely relieved.
- Alteration in nutritional status, less than body requirements. The patient will maintain nutritional intake for body requirements.
- Disturbed sensory perception. The patient will report no numbness, tingling, or pain.
- Disturbed body image. The patient demonstrates enhanced body image and self-esteem as evidenced by ability to look at, touch, talk about, and care for actual or perceived altered body part or function.
- Readiness for enhanced self-concept. The patient will verbalize acceptance of self.

Ménière's Disease

Ménière's disease is a disorder thought to be caused by a range of inflammatory, traumatic, autoimmune, or idiopathic events leading to eventual dysfunction of the vestibulocochlear nerve (CN VIII) (Dieterich, 2004).

Epidemiology

Higher incidences of Ménière's disease have also been found in patients with herpes simplex virus (Vrabec, 2003). In addition, an association between Ménière's disease and the presence of hypothyroidism has also been investigated to determine if thyroid hormone supplements can be implicated in Ménière's disease (Brenner, Hoistad, & Hain, 2004). Research results indicate that the medication is probably not the underlying association, but rather it is believed that an autoimmune component can contribute to both hypothyroidism and Ménière's disease. This possibility is more likely in patients who are over 60 years of age.

Etiology

The etiology of Ménière's disease is not always certain, although two known infectious and traumatic causes of the disorder are syphilis and head trauma.

Pathophysiology

The events of inflammation, trauma, and autoimmune dysfunction are thought to cause one of the classic vertigo syndromes, which ultimately occur as a result of distension of the compartments in the inner ear leading to endolymphatic hydrops. Eventually rupture of the membranous labyrinth causes paralysis of the CN VIII (Dieterich, 2004).

Assessment with Clinical Manifestations

Ménière's disease is characterized by episodic vertigo along with a low-frequency sensorineural hearing loss, tinnitus, and a sense of pressure or fullness in the ear. Nystagmus is also present. Vertigo lasts from a few to several hours; however, symptoms progress in most patients to include a chronic tinnitus and hearing loss.

Diagnostic Tests

The diagnosis of Ménière's disease is made by the assessment of the several parameters that typically characterize the disease. Specific hearing tests to identify sensory or neural hearing loss will be undertaken initially, as will physical assessment to identify tinnitus and nystagmus. The caloric test will be done to assess for nystagmus, testing the vestibular system, and MRI may be performed to rule out tumor as the cause of symptoms. The caloric test is performed by irrigating the ear with cold water and observing the patient for rapid eye movements as a result. Hearing tests to identify sensory origin of hearing loss indicate an inner ear etiology for the hearing loss. Hearing tests which identify a neural etiology for the hearing loss will indicate CN VIII nerve damage. Electrocochleography may also be done to assess the electrical activity of the inner ear.

Nursing Diagnoses

Based on the information gathered, examples of nursing diagnoses in the patient with Ménière's disease may include the following:

- Risk for injury related to vertigo
- Nausea related to disturbance of the vestibular system
- Disturbed sensory perception, auditory

Planning and Implementation

Treatment for Ménière's disease is aimed at lowering pressure in the inner ear. Diuretics along with a low-sodium diet will relieve symptoms in many patients. Antibiotics may be used if infection is suspected as the underlying cause of symptoms. Ototoxic antibiotics, such as intratympanic gentamicin, may also be instilled in the ear; however, this is controversial as it has been shown to contribute to higher levels of hearing loss than in patients who had surgical section of the vestibular nerve (Hillman, Arriaga, & Chen, 2003; Hillman, Chen, & Arriaga, 2004). Surgical repairs may be performed but less frequently than medical treatment and with more danger of hearing loss.

Treatment of symptoms is important for patients because of the extreme discomfort caused by the vertigo, as well as the nausea and vomiting that often accompany the vertigo. Treatment with antiemetic medications is helpful to most patients. Bedrest may be the most promising and effective treatment for the vertigo associated with Ménière's disease. Medication treatment with antihistamines, using meclizine (Antivert) most commonly, has been successful in most patients. Histamines work by improving microcirculation. Corticosteroids have also been shown to have limited use when given over two to three weeks with tapering doses. Long-term therapy with corticosteroids may be used to maintain hearing and decrease the frequency of attacks (Dieterich, 2004).

Ménière's disease can be extremely disabling to patients because of the vertigo, nausea, and vomiting. The primary concern is the risk for injury from falls because of the vertigo. Teaching regarding safe activity and the need for bedrest should be provided to the patient. The degree of relief as a result of medications should be assessed periodically by the nurse. Additionally, assessment of hearing should also be performed periodically to determine if the disease is progressing and whether it has negative effect on the patient's hearing. Nausea is another disabling symptom of the disease. Assessment of the presence of nausea and teaching regarding the use of antiemetic medications is necessary with these patients.

Because experimental treatments exist for Ménière's disease, the nurse must be aware of current research that examines the different treatment for Ménière's disease and support the patient in talking with the health care provider to determine the best course of action. Emotional support is a primary intervention for patients with Ménière's disease. This can be a disabling disorder and can cause extreme distress. Frequently, the family members of a patient with Ménière's disease will not understand the disabling effect; therefore teaching for the family is essential.

Pharmacology

Recently, intratympanic steroids have been studied to determine their usefulness in the treatment of Ménière's disease. Because it is thought that there could be an autoimmune component to the disease, steroids, such as dexamethasone, could be useful for their anti-inflammatory effects. Current studies have shown promising results in restoring hearing loss in patients with endolymphatic hydrops associated with Ménière's disease (Hillman, Arriaga, & Chen, 2004). Administration of this medication is performed by the physician after anesthetization of the tympanic membrane.

Surgery

In those patients who are refractory to other methods of treatment for Ménière's disease surgery may become necessary. Surgery of the vestibular portion of the CN VIII is effective in these patients. Removal of the semicircle canals is also effective but not appropriate for patients whose hearing is not affected. Removal of semicircle canals is only used in patients with limited hearing in the affected ear.

Evaluation of Outcomes

Potential patient outcomes for each of the example nursing diagnoses for the patient with Ménière's disease are:

- Risk for injury related to vertigo. The patient will be free of fall or injury.
- Nausea related to vertigo. The patient will be free of nausea and vomiting.
- Disturbed sensory perception, auditory. Hearing status will be maintained at predisease level.

Peripheral Nerve Injuries

Injury to peripheral nerves can result from acute trauma or chronic entrapment syndromes. Motor vehicle accidents, falls, sports injuries, and occupational accidents may cause acute injuries. Impact from sharp objects may cause transection and laceration of nerves, and direct blows to nerves may cause injury by contusions to nerves. Traction on nerves through improper application of orthopedic traction or in motor vehicle accidents may also cause peripheral nerve injuries. Shoulder injuries are common nerve injuries resulting in motor vehicle accidents.

Pathophysiology

Trauma and injury often occurs in the plexuses. A plexus comprises a network of axons and may be vulnerable to injury. The brachial plexus is a common area of injury. Downward pressure on the shoulder may lead to upper brachial plexus injury, and a lower plexus injury results from traction and stretching of the arm. An upper plexus injury results in a functioning hand with a weak arm and shoulder, and a lower plexus injury results in a strong arm with a weak hand. Herniated discs and trauma are common causes of sciatic injury.

Assessment with Clinical Manifestations

The type and extent of injury will determine the signs and symptoms associated with the injury. Motor and sensory deficits along with autonomic affects may occur together or alone with injury. Signs and symptoms may include paralysis or paresis if some of the lower motor neurons are intact, muscular atrophy, absent DTRs, sensory losses, warm dry skin and trophic changes including cold, cyanotic skin.

Neurological assessment is an essential aspect of care of the patient with a peripheral nerve injury. Paresthesias, paralysis, paresis, and pain are common results of nerve injuries, and the degree of dysfunction associated with each of these findings will vary and may change according to the injury.

Diagnostic Tests

Most often, diagnosis is based on a history of injury along with a neurological examination. Neurological assessment will establish the motor and sensory components of the dysfunction and injury, including pain associated with the injury. CT, MRI, EMG, and nerve conduction velocity (NCV) studies are most useful in determining the type and extent of injury and nerve damage.

Nursing Diagnoses

Based on the information gathered, examples of nursing diagnoses in the patient with peripheral nerve injuries may include the following:

- Disturbed sensory perception related to nerve injury function
- Acute pain related to nerve injury
- Impaired physical mobility related to nerve injury
- Risk for injury related to casting or splinting
- Risk for altered tissue integrity related to casting or splinting
- Alteration in self-care related to nerve injury

Planning and Implementation

Treatment of peripheral nerve injuries may include surgical anastomosis of severed nerves. This is done soon after the injury to prevent further deformity. As the nerve shortens with surgery, contractions are at risk for occurrence. After surgery the limb is placed in a flexion position to compensate for the contraction. Physical therapy is essential to capitalize on the potential for regaining functionality of the extremities innervated by injured nerves. Pain associated with the injury should be treated with analgesics. It is important to identify and treat the pain, because pain will decrease the success of physical therapy and rehabilitation.

Pain management is essential, so in-depth pain assessment will be an ongoing nursing management issue. Determination and management of losses of motor and sensory function are the priorities for nursing care. Assessment of motor and sensory function along with color, warmth, and trophic changes of extremities are necessary. Because traumatic injuries, such as penetrating injuries, occurring with stab wounds can cause peripheral nerve injuries, it is important to assess neurological status of the peripheral nerves adjacent to the injured area when this type of injury occurs. Delay in treatment can mean significant loss of nerve function (Sunderamoorthy & Chaudhury, 2003).

If immobilization of the affected limb is ordered by the physician, the nurse will need to provide teaching regarding splint or cast care. Assessment by the nurse of circulation in the splinted or casted extremity will be a priority of care. The patient and family members should be taught to look for alterations in warmth, color, and the presence of tingling which are indicators of autonomic dysfunction and should be reported to the physician. The skin may be susceptible to breakdown and should be thoroughly assessed and cared for with lotion for dry skin. Lost sensory function will mean that patients will have disturbed sense of temperatures and should be careful with application of heat and cold because of the potential for injury to the extremity.

> **Safety First 1**
>
> **IV Therapy and Peripheral Nerve Injury**
>
> It is important to note that damage to peripheral nerves can occur from insertion of IV cannulas into the cephalic vein. If patients complain of numbness or tingling on insertion of an IV cannula, the nurse should remove the cannula immediately. Measures to prevent injury to the superficial peripheral nerves, especially the superficial radial nerve include removing the cannula if the patient experiences paresthesias or numbness, and limiting probing when inserting an IV cannula. Peripheral nerve injury can be temporary or it may be permanent.

Evaluation of Outcomes

Potential patient outcomes for each of the example nursing diagnoses for the patient with a peripheral nerve injury are:

- Disturbed sensory perception related to nerve injury. The patient will report complete sensation without numbness or tingling in affected nerve areas, and will demonstrate motor functioning without restriction of movement in affected areas.

- Acute pain related to nerve injury. The patient should verbalize an adequate relief of pain along with the ability to realistically cope with the pain if it is not completely relieved.
- Risk for injury. The patient will identify signs of injury from cast or splinting and report to nurse or health care provider.
- Risk for tissue injury. The patient will identify signs of tissue injury from cast or splinting and report to nurse or health care provider.
- Self-care, activities of daily living, completely independent. The patient will complete activities of daily living without assistance.

Carpal Tunnel Syndrome

Carpal tunnel syndrome is considered an entrapment neuropathy in which compression of the median nerve occurs in the carpal tunnel, most often from pressure of the carpal ligament in the tunnel.

Epidemiology

Occupation-related history reveals the highest risk factors for development of the disorder, including repetitive movement of the wrists for prolonged periods of time. People at risk for development of carpal tunnel syndrome include computer keyboarders, typists, pianist, and construction workers who work with vibrating equipment. Women are affected more than men, perhaps because of the number of women in occupations where word processing is a dominant part of the job. Carpal tunnel syndrome has also been known to exist in athletes who are involved in repetitive digital flexion activities.

Etiology

Entrapment disorders occur from compression on the nerve from the anatomical structure. Ulnar nerve and radial nerve entrapment can also occur, although not as frequently as carpal tunnel syndrome.

Pathophysiology

The combination of a narrow channel along with edema, which may occur with trauma to tissues, results in pressure on the nerve in the structure resulting in entrapment. Carpal tunnel syndrome is characterized by pain of a burning and tingling nature. Patients may also complain of an aching pain that is exacerbated by activity, especially flexion and dorsiflexion of the wrist. The pain usually is worse at night. Distribution of pain along the median nerve is characteristic of the carpal tunnel syndrome and occurs as edema of tissue entraps the median nerve at the wrist a vulnerable area. The median nerve enters the carpal tunnel beneath the transverse carpal ligament. The tunnel comprises the transverse carpal ligaments superiorly and the carpal bones laterally and inferiorly. As the lumen of the tunnel narrows, movement of the nerve is compromised.

The resulting pain may radiate up the forearm and even to the shoulder and chest (Tierney, et al., 2004). Assessment reveals numbness and tingling when invoked by the carpal compression test, which involves pressure applied over the carpal tunnel. Muscle weakness appears later than the sensory disturbances.

Assessment with Clinical Manifestations

Symptoms of carpal tunnel syndrome include sensory and motor losses. Sensory losses follow the nerve track and include the palmar aspect of the first three fingers and half of the fourth fingers, and the dorsal aspects of the terminal phalanges of the second, third, and half of the fourth fingers. Patients complain of wrist pain, especially at night. Most pain is in the wrist and the areas innervated by the median nerve but may also radiate up the forearm. Pain is worse on wrist flexion. The patient also experiences weakness in areas of the hand, including difficulty with abduction of the thumb. As the condition progresses, wasting of the hand muscles can occur.

Diagnostic Tests

Diagnosis of carpal tunnel syndrome is made through the use of EMG and motor and sensory conduction delays determined through these tests. Physical assessment reveals positive Tinel's and Phalen's sign. Tinel's sign is elicited by tapping over the median nerve at the wrist and is positive if pain occurs. Phalen's sign is elicited by flexing the wrists at a right angle for one minute. Phalen's sign is positive if pain and tingling occur on flexion of the wrist.

Nursing Diagnoses

Based on the information gathered, examples of nursing diagnoses in the patient with carpal tunnel syndrome may include the following:
- Disturbed sensory perception related to carpal tunnel syndrome.
- Acute pain related to carpal tunnel syndrome.

Planning and Implementation

Nursing care of the patient with carpal tunnel syndrome primarily involves teaching about the use of the hand and wrist splint through limitation of movement to relieve pressure on the median nerve. Because many cases of carpal tunnel syndrome are occupational in origin, discussion of modifications to occupational activities may be necessary. Patients may have many concerns about work related activities, which should be referred to the health care provider. Physical therapy may be helpful in regaining activity after treatment concludes. Rest is important and limitation of movement is essential to prevent additional pressure on the median nerve.

Currently, the numbers of people affected by carpal tunnel syndrome is increasing because of word processing activities and keyboarding affecting many different types of workers. A thorough occupational history is necessary. Teaching about prevention of the syndrome includes proper positioning of wrists and hands at keyboards with wrists off the surface of the desk, or with support provided through gel type devices. For athletes experiencing symptoms, rest and immobilization will generally result in alleviation of symptoms. Nonsteroidal anti-inflammatory medications will also be of use in these patients. Surgery is usually not necessary for carpal tunnel caused by athletics.

Pharmacology

Treatment of carpal tunnel syndrome consists of relief of pressure on the median nerve through splinting of the hand and wrist for two to six weeks. Patients are taught to modify and limit their hand activities during this time. Nonsteroidal anti-inflammatory drugs may also be administered. Corticosteroid injections are used if there is no improvement with the traditional less invasive treatment.

Surgery

A surgical intervention which frees the median nerve may be a last resort in the treatment of carpal tunnel syndrome.

Evaluation of Outcomes

Potential patient outcomes for each of the example nursing diagnoses for the patient with carpal tunnel syndrome are:
- Disturbed sensory perception related to carpal tunnel syndrome. The patient's sensory motor functioning will not be compromised, as exhibited by freedom of movement and complete sensation in affected extremity. The patient will be free of numbness or tingling in affected extremity.
- Acute pain related to carpal tunnel syndrome. The patient should verbalize an adequate relief of pain along with the ability to realistically cope with the pain if it is not completely relieved.

KEY CONCEPTS

- Complete SCI results in loss of motor and sensory function below the level of injury.
- Spinal shock occurs immediately after injury and includes complete loss of motor and sensory functioning below the level of injury.
- Emergency treatment of SCI is essential to preserve functioning and to provide for improvement in the degree of neurological impairment.
- Understanding the anatomical and physiological effects of an SCI will provide an understanding of the neurological impairments that may be expected.
- Nursing management of the patient with an SCI in the acute phase will include assessment of respiratory and neurological impairment.
- Spinal cord tumors result from benign and metastatic tumors. Surgical removal of tumors is a priority; however, radiation and chemotherapy may be modes of treatment.
- Assessment of neurological status and loss of motor and sensory functioning is a priority for the patient with a spinal cord tumor.
- Peripheral nervous system disorders occur as a result of injury, disease, occupational exposures, infection, medications, as well as a myriad of other stimuli.
- Pain and sensory disturbances along with motor disturbances in some disorders are the primary symptoms of a peripheral nervous system disturbance.
- GBS often results from exposure to infectious organisms and progresses upward from the legs, causing paresis or paralysis of the diaphragm and intercostals muscles.
- Teaching regarding the effects and treatment of peripheral nervous system disorders is a hallmark of nursing care.

REVIEW QUESTIONS

1. The nurse is caring for a patient who has a C6 SCI. She anticipates that the patient understands the teaching about the long-term effects of the injury when the patient says:
   1. I will be able to transfer myself to the wheelchair and bed.
   2. I will be able to feed myself.
   3. I will be on a ventilator to support my breathing for the rest of my life.
   4. I will not need urinary catheterization after I am discharged from the hospital.

2. The patient has experienced an incomplete SCI resulting in Brown-Séquard syndrome. What abnormalities should the nurse expect the patient to experience (select all that apply)?
   1. Loss of pain and temperature sensation on the opposite side
   2. Loss of all motor and sensory function below the level of the injury
   3. Loss of motor function (paralysis) on the same side as the injury
   4. Loss of position sense and vibration on same side as the injury

3. What response would be the best response for a patient with a new SCI who asks if his current paralysis will be permanent?
   1. If there is a loss of function at the accident, it is not possible to regain motor functioning.
   2. There is often a period of spinal shock when it is difficult to determine if the paralysis will be permanent, and when it resolves there can be some regaining of abilities.
   3. You're experiencing spinal shock now; in three weeks you will regain your functioning when the spinal shock resolves.
   4. It's best to start trying to accept your limitations; it's unlikely that any improvement can occur.

4. A patient has been diagnosed with trigeminal neuralgia. Which medication is likely to be prescribed as a first choice for treatment?
   1. Phenytoin (Dilantin)
   2. Gabapentin
   3. Baclofen
   4. Carbamazepine (Tegretol)

5. Which of the following is not generally present in a patient with Ménière's disease?
   1. Hypothyroidism
   2. Nystagmus
   3. Tinnitus
   4. High-frequency hearing loss

6. The nurse is seeing a patient with Ménière's disease in the clinic for the first time; which of the following would the nurse do first:
   1. Assess for a history of taking thyroid supplements
   2. Teach about safety to prevent falls in patients experiencing vertigo

Continued

REVIEW QUESTIONS—cont'd

3. Refer to a health care provider for treatment of tinnitus
4. Instruct the patient about the need for bedrest

7. Which of the following is most indicative of pain associated with carpal tunnel syndrome?
1. Burning, tingling pain, worse during the daytime when the patient is most active
2. Burning, tingling pain that may be worse during the nighttime
3. Throbbing pain that increases with extension of the wrist
4. Throbbing pain that is worst with rest

8. Positive Phalen's sign for carpal tunnel syndrome is indicated by which of the following?
1. Relief of pain on flexion of the wrist at a right angle for one minute
2. Pain and tingling experienced on tapping over the median nerve at the wrist
3. Relief of pain experienced upon tapping over the median nerve at the wrist
4. Pain and tingling experienced on flexion of the wrist at a right angle for one minute

9. Emergency treatment with methylprednisolone for a patient with an SCI must be instituted in what time period?
1. Within the first 8 hours after injury
2. Within the first 24 hours after injury
3. Within the first hour after injury
4. Within 72 hours after injury

10. A patient with a cervical SCI has an upper motor neuron lesion. The nurse can anticipate that care will include which of the following?
1. Administration of baclofen for spasticity
2. Teaching regarding self-catheterization
3. Teaching regarding ability to perform self-care dressing activities, including buttoning one's shirts and tying shoe laces
4. Range of motion for flaccid extremities

11. The priority nursing action for a patient with an SCI experiencing a pounding headache and blood pressure of 220/120 indicating autonomic dysreflexia is to:
1. Call the physician for order for antihypertensive medication
2. Check for distended bladder or kinked catheter tubing
3. Assess heart rate and skin temperature
4. Check for fecal impaction
5. Calcium channel blockers

REVIEW ACTIVITIES

1. Visit a rehabilitation facility and interview a patient with an SCI and family member to try to understand the physical and psychosocial issues faced by patients with SCI and their families. Ask about what changes are needed in the physical environment of the home of a patient with SCI. Ask about how family members have made changes in their lives.

2. Discuss the pathophysiological rationale for the use of methylprednisolone for SCI.

3. Develop a teaching plan for the prevention of carpal tunnel syndrome.

4. Discuss the postoperative care of the patient who has had surgical removal of a spinal cord tumor.

5. Explore the Christopher Reeve Paralysis Foundation Web site, and identify information provided for patients, for family members, and for health care professionals. Identify the newest research that is being reported on the Web site and consider how this research will impact nursing care of SCI patients.

Visit the Contemporary Medical-Surgical Nursing online companion resource at www.delmarhealthcare.com for additional content and study aids. Click on Online Companions then select the Nursing discipline.

Degenerative Neurological Dysfunction: Nursing Management

CHAPTER 37

Doris Denison, MSN, APRN, BC, CCRN

CHAPTER TOPICS

- Headaches
- Seizures
- Multiple Sclerosis
- Parkinson's Disease
- Alzheimer's Disease
- Myasthenia Gravis
- Amyotrophic Lateral Sclerosis
- Huntington's Chorea

KEY TERMS

Akinesia
Aura
Bradykinesia
Cephalalgia
Chorea
Convulsion
Diplopia
Epilepsy
Plasmapheresis
Ptosis
Rhinorrhea
Seizure
Tremor

Chronic and degenerative neurological diseases can be both challenging and frustrating for patients, families, and health care providers. There is no known cure for these diseases. This chapter focuses on the management of chronic headache (cephalalgia), seizures, multiple sclerosis, Parkinson's disease, myasthenia gravis, amyotrophic lateral sclerosis, and Huntington's disease.

These neurological disorders involve either chronic disease or progressive deterioration of mental or physical function and can be devastating to both the patient and his or her family. The patient may become depressed, angry, fearful, or withdrawn when having to deal with the progression of the disease. Changes in body image, self-esteem, and lifestyle can enhance the emotional trauma of dealing with a progressively debilitating process. Families may experience despair, hope, love, resentment, guilt, and empathy for their family member. As the patient's condition continues to deteriorate, the family needs to deal with the emotional conflict precipitated by their sense of duty to the patient and the need to live their own lives. Health care providers are similarly frustrated by their wanting to alleviate the physical symptoms, prevent complications, maximize the patient's self-care abilities, and assist with lifestyle changes.

HEADACHE

Headache **(cephalalgia)** is the most common form of chronic pain and is responsible for an estimated 20 million visits to a health care provider every year. The National Headache Foundation estimates that more than 75 percent of Americans suffer from headaches, and of those, about 9 percent seek medical attention and 80 percent self-medicate. The cost of missed workdays and medical treatment is estimated to be about $50 billion annually. The level of dysfunction from headache varies with each person. For some patients, headache occurs occasionally and is relieved by an over-the-counter (OTC) analgesic. Others experience frequent and debilitating headaches that decrease their ability to work, interfere with personal relationships, alter family life, and decrease their quality of life. Headaches may also be a symptom of a more serious underlying condition that requires immediate intervention by a health care provider.

Headaches are generally classified as primary or secondary in nature. When no organic cause can be identified, it is considered a primary headache. Types of headaches include: tension-type, migraine, and cluster. The majority of headaches (90 to 98 percent) are primary. Secondary headaches have an underlying organic cause, such as aneurysm or tumor. Only primary headaches will be discussed in this chapter. Secondary headaches are discussed with the organic cause.

Tension-Type Headache

Tension-type headache is the most common type, accounting for 90 percent of primary headaches, and is considered the most difficult to treat. Tension-type headache is defined as intermittent with a variable duration.

Uncovering the Evidence

Headache in the Workplace

Discussion: The purpose of this research was to study the impact of headaches on work attendance and its economic impact in two different workplaces. Questionnaires were sent to 800 employees in Sweden. Four hundred were privately employed, and 400 were employed at a public university hospital. The questionnaire addressed a variety of variables: number of headaches in a three-month period, duration of the headaches, decreased ability to work effectively, and number appointments with a health care provider for treatment of headache.

The prevalence of headache was 64 percent in the privately employed group and 78 percent in the hospital. Fifty percent of the subjects reported going to work despite their headache, and the mean number of days was 6.6 for the privately employed group and 6.1 days for the hospital employed group. A 25 percent decrease in work effectiveness was calculated. The economic impact was calculated as approximately 1.4 billion per year.

Implications for Practice: The economic impact of decreased workplace productivity is substantial, and the authors suggest that workplace-based treatment and prevention programs may be both financially and clinically advantageous.

Source: Raak, R., & Raak, A. (2003). Work attendance despite headache and its economic impact: A comparison between two workplaces. Headache, 43, *1097–1101.*

Epidemiology

Prevalence of tension-type headaches has been reported as low as 30 percent and as high as 90 percent on a yearly basis. Lifetime prevalence is 78 percent, 63 percent for men, and 86 percent for women. Prevalence peaks between 40 and 50 years of age (International Headache Society, 2004).

Etiology

Etiology is multifactorial and may include:

- Sustained contraction of the pericranial muscles (muscle contraction headache).
- Referred pain from upper cervical joints, ligaments, and muscles.
- Prolonged peripheral pain may cause central sensitization.
- Physical or psychological stress, lack of sleep, anxiety, and depression.

Pathophysiology

Tension-type headache is caused by irritation of the pain-sensitive structures of the brain. The intracranial structures include portions of the trigeminal (cranial nerve 5 [CN V]), facial (cranial nerve 7 [CN VII]), glossopharyngeal (cranial nerve 9 [CN IX]), vagus (cranial nerve 10 [CN X]), and upper cervical nerves, the large arteries, and the venous sinuses. When the sensory receptors of the muscles, tendons, joints, and skin are stimulated, they transmit pain messages to the pain-sensitive areas of the brain. Tension-type headaches may be episodic or chronic (Table 37-1).

Assessment with Clinical Manifestations

Patients describe their headache as bilateral with a pressure or tightness sensation, becoming worse with physical activity, and a mild to moderately severe discomfort level. The headache does not involve vomiting, but there may be occasional feelings of nausea. Sensitivity to light (photophobia) or sound (phonophobia) may be reported. The headaches may occur over weeks, months, or years, and many patients can experience a combination of migraine and tension-type.

Identification of the headache's cause and its effect on the patient is the focus of collaborative care. A thorough history and physical examination is necessary. The health care provider needs to ask specific questions concerning the headache signs and symptoms (see the Patient Playbook). Diagnostic studies done to rule secondary causes of headache are summarized in Box 37-1. For complete discussion of these diagnostic studies, refer to chapter 34.

Diagnostic Tests

There are a variety of diagnostic tests that can be used in determining the type of headache that a patient suffers. These diagnostic studies could detect the cause of the headache and prevent the headache from progressing to a more severe problem (e.g., space-occupying tumor, malignant brain tumor). See Box 37-1 for a listing of the typical diagnostic studies used in assessing headaches.

BOX 37-1

HEADACHE DIAGNOSTIC STUDIES

Neurological examination (local infection; tenderness; swelling; bruits).

Routine laboratory studies (CBC; electrolytes; urinalysis).

CT (of sinuses).

Special studies (CT; EMG; EEG; MRI; MRA; angiography).

Legend: CBC, complete blood count; CT, computed tomography; EEG, electroencephalography; EMG, electromyography; MRI, magnetic resonance imaging; MRA, magnetic resonance angiography.

TABLE 37-1 Tension-Type Headache Comparison

	EPISODIC	CHRONIC
Duration	30 minutes to 7 days	minutes to hours
Frequency	10 episodes in six months	15 days/month for six months
Nausea or vomiting	none	possible nausea; no vomiting
Photophobia	sometimes	sometimes
Phonophobia	sometimes	sometimes

PATIENT PLAYBOOK

Questions Specific for Headache Assessment

The following are questions to ask patients when assessing their headaches:

Where does the headache hurt, and what were you doing when the headache started?

How long before the pain becomes severe? Slow? Fast?

How long do they usually last, and do the headaches recur (return within 24-hour period)?

How long have you had the headache?

Describe the pain and is the pain mild, moderate, or severe?

Rate your headache on a scale of 1 to 10 (10=worst; 1=least).

Do you have trouble with your vision before or during the headache?

Do you have any other symptoms with the headache?

What makes the headache worse and better?

How do the headaches affect your life?

Do you take any prescription, OTC medications, vitamins, or herbal supplements?

Have you seen doctors in the past concerning your headaches?

Have you been under more stress than usual lately?

Have you been depressed?

Do you have any family members with a history of headaches?

BOX 37-2

NURSING DIAGNOSES FOR HEADACHES

The following is a list of common nursing diagnoses for headaches:

- Acute pain related to headache, visual disturbances, and inability to perform job-related activities.
- Ineffective coping related to severe pain, stress, and changes in lifestyle.
- Disturbed sensory perception related to auditory, visual, and sensory alterations.
- Deficient knowledge related to lack of understanding about headaches and treatment regimen.
- Sleep deprivation related to pain, nausea, vomiting, and medication.
- Ineffective role performance related to pain and medication side effects.

Nursing Diagnoses

The nursing diagnoses for all of the headache types is displayed in Box 37-2.

Planning and Implementation

Nursing management of tension headaches focuses on patient teaching. Teaching should include medication regimen, nonpharmacological management, and stress reduction methods. The application of these management techniques can assist the patient treat their headaches and potentially alleviate the patient's pain (Frazel, 2004).

Pharmacology

Medication regimens commonly used for treatment of tension-type headaches are nonnarcotic analgesics, such as aspirin, acetaminophen, or ibuprofen. These may be combined with narcotics (codeine) or barbiturates (butalbital) for difficult to treat headaches. Patients should be cautioned about long-term use of aspirin because of its connection with gastric bleeding and coagulation alterations in susceptible patients. Long-term use of narcotics or barbiturates may be habit-forming. Chronic use of acetaminophen can lead to kidney damage and liver damage when combined with alcohol (Table 37-2).

Alternative Therapy

Nonpharmacological management includes techniques, such as application of heat or cold, biofeedback, acupuncture, acupressure, and hypnosis. Application of heat or cold reduces muscle tension and decreases pain. The nurse should teach the patient to use heat or cold for no more than 15 to 20 minutes for each application and to remove it from the skin between treatments. Biofeedback involves applying physiological monitoring equipment, teaching the patient about muscle tension and its connection with peripheral blood flow, and training the patient to relax muscles in response to the machines feedback.

Acupuncture involves the insertion of thin needles into specific areas of the body to modify physiological function. A provider trained in this ancient Chinese technique is required. Acupressure is an ancient Japanese and Chinese therapy that applies finger pressure to relieve pain, discomfort, and promote healing. This technique also requires a trained provider. Hypnosis is used to assist the patient to alter the pain perception of their headaches. Many patients who prefer to not take medications may be more comfortable with nonpharmacological treatment of their headaches.

Stress reduction methods may include exercise programs, meditation, yoga, or tai chi. Exercise programs, such as walking, swimming, or riding a bike, are

TABLE 37-2 Medications to Treat Headache

TENSION-TYPE HEADACHE	MIGRAINE HEADACHE	CLUSTER HEADACHE
Nonnarcotic Analgesics	***Nonnarcotic Analgesics***	***100 Percent O_2 Via Face Mask***
Aspirin	Aspirin	Ergot alkaloids
Acetaminophen (Tylenol)	Acetaminophen (Tylenol)	Dihydroergotamine (DHE)
Ibuprofen (Motrin Advil)	Ibuprofen (Motrin, Advil)	Ergotamine (Ergostat)
Caffeine	Naproxen (Aleve, Anaprox)	Triptans
Narcotic Combinations	***Narcotic Analgesics***	***Sumatriptan (Imitrex)***
Butalbital + aspirin (Fiorinal)	Codeine + acetaminophen (Tylenol #3 or #4)	Intranasal
Butalbital + acetaminophen (Fioricet)	Meperidine (Demerol)	Lidocaine
Caffeine + acetaminophen (Midol)	Butorphanol (Stadol)	Capsaicin
Antidepressants	***Triptans***	***Nonnarcotic Analgesics***
Sertraline (Zoloft)	Naratriptan (Amerge)	Indomethacin (Indocin)
Paroxetine (Paxil)	Sumatriptan (Imitrex)	
		Narcotic Analgesics
Amitriptyline (Elavil)	Almotriptan (Axert)	Butorphanol (Stadol)
Nortriptyline (Pamelor)	Frovatriptan (Frova)	Calcium channel blockers
	Rizatriptan (Maxalt)	Verapamil (Calan)
	Zolmitriptan (Zomig)	
	Ergot alkaloids	Lithium (Lithane, Eskalith)
	DHE	
	Ergotamine (Ergomar, Ergostat)	
Beta Blockers	***Beta Blockers***	***Corticosteroids***
Propranolol (Inderal)	Atenolol (Tenormin)	Prednisone
	Metoprolol (Lopressor)	
	Propranolol (Inderal)	Anticonvulsants
	Timolol (Blocadren)	Valproic acid (Depakote)
	Calcium channel blockers	
	Verapamil (Calan)	
	Nifedipine (Procardia)	
	Nimodipine (Nimotop)	
	Antidepressants	
	Amitriptyline (Elavil)	
	Imipramine (Tofranil)	

Adapted from Broyles, B. E., Reiss, B. S., & Evans, M. E. (2007). Pharmacological aspects of nursing care *(7th ed.). New York: Thomson Delmar Learning.*

useful in reducing stress. Meditation involves concentrated attention focused on one's inner state. Yoga is an ancient philosophy of the mind, body, and soul in harmony. Yoga therapy uses specific postures and sequences of postures to stretch or block areas of the body. Tai chi involves almost weightless, fluid movements, with a focus on breathing, balance, and the concepts of empty and full. All of these techniques can be recommended to help patients with life-stress management.

Evaluation of Outcomes

Potential patient outcomes for each of the example nursing diagnoses for the patient with tension-type headaches are:

- Acute pain related to tension-type headache. The patient should verbalize adequate pain relief and the ability to realistically cope with the pain if not completely relieved.
- Ineffective coping related to pain. The patient should verbalize feelings, identify personal strengths, and accept support.
- Disturbed sensory perception related to auditory, visual, and sensory alterations. The patient should verbalize decreased symptoms.
- Deficient knowledge related to lack of understanding. The patient should describe disease process, symptoms, and control measures.
- Sleep deprivation related to pain or medication side effects. The patient will report an optimal balance of rest and activity.
- Ineffective role performance related to pain and medication side effects. The patient should demonstrate healthy adaptation and coping skills.

Migraine Headache

Migraine headaches are common disorders. They are often self-treated; patients have their own interventions that they use, or nothing seems to decrease the headache and they just suffer with the pain. Migraine headaches affect patient's relationships, his or her employment, and often can be frustrating to live with the pain. Migraine headaches, along with cluster headaches, are considered a vascular headache.

Epidemiology

Migraine headache accounts for half of all patients with headache. It is estimated that 23 million Americans suffer from migraines, and more than 11 million experience significant headache related disability. Migraines affect 18 percent of women and 6 percent of men. Headaches may begin as early as 10 years of age with the highest incidence between 35 and 45 years and decreases with advancing age. The incidence of migraine is highest among Caucasians. Up to 65 percent of patients with a family history of headaches will also suffer from headaches. It is estimated that in the United States, $17 billion per year are related to diagnosis, treatment, and lost job productivity.

Etiology

Migraine headaches are the result of the interaction of various factors of varying importance in different individuals. Causative factors include:

- Genetic predisposition.
- Susceptibility to specific stimuli.
- Hormonal activity.
- Environmental triggers.
- Stress.

Pathophysiology

Migraines are characterized by vasodilation of the dural blood vessels, resulting in stimulation of the trigeminal nerve pain pathways. Then neuropeptides, involved in pain transmission, are released. The neuropeptides make the vasodilation worse and sensitize the brainstem, causing the associated symptoms of light, sound, movement, and odor sensitivity.

Assessment with Clinical Manifestations

The focus of care for the patient with a migraine is to identify the specific type of migraine and rule out any secondary causes. A thorough history and physical examination is necessary. The health care provider needs to ask specific questions concerning the headache signs and symptoms. Migraine headaches are characterized as episodic head pain, present on waking or occurring over a few minutes to hours while awake, and lasting from 4 to 72 hours. Approximately 98 percent of migraine patients experience moderate to severe pain during attacks and describe the pain as a steady ache to violent throbbing. They will identify the pain as being on one side of the head. The pain is made worse by physical activity. In addition, many migraine headaches are preceded with an **aura** (sensation that occurs immediately before a disorder, such as a migraine headache or a seizure). Associated aura symptoms include nausea, vomiting, and photophobia, phonophobia, and certain odors (osmophobia).

Diagnostic Tests

Diagnostic studies need to be done to rule out secondary causes of the headaches. They are summarized in Box 37-1.

Nursing Diagnoses

The nursing diagnoses for all of the headache types is displayed in Box 37-2.

Planning and Implementation

Nursing management of migraine headaches also focuses on patient teaching. Teaching should include medication regimen, trigger avoidance, nonpharmacological management, and stress reduction methods. Medication regimens commonly used for treatment of migraine headaches are based on severity of symptoms. For moderate pain relief, nonnarcotic analgesics may be sufficient. Symptom control for more severe headaches may include: alpha-adrenergic blockers, serotonin receptor agonists, vasoconstrictors, or corticosteroids (Glassroth, 2004). The nurse should teach the patient to avoid headache triggers. These triggers are listed in Table 37-3.

TABLE 37-3 Migraine Headache Triggers

Foods Containing Amines

- Cheese
- Chocolate

Foods Containing Nitrates

- Processed lunch meat
- Hot dogs
- Smoked meats

Foods Containing

- Vinegar
- Onions
- Monosodium glutamate (MSG)

Fermented or Marinated Foods

- Caffeine
- Nicotine
- Ice cream
- Alcohol (specifically red wine)
- Emotional stress
- Fatigue

Drugs

- Ergot containing compounds
- Monoamine oxide (MAO) inhibitors

Evaluation of Outcomes

Potential patient outcomes for each of the example nursing diagnoses for the patient with migraine headache are:

- Acute pain related to migraine headache. The patient should verbalize an adequate relief of pain along with the ability to realistically cope with the pain if it is not completely relieved.
- Ineffective coping related to pain. The patient should verbalize feelings, identify personal strengths, and accept support.
- Disturbed sensory perception related to headache. The patient should verbalize decreased symptoms.
- Deficient knowledge related to lack of understanding. The patient should describe disease process, symptoms, and control measures.
- Sleep deprivation related to pain or medication side effects. The patient will report an optimal balance of rest and activity.
- Ineffective role performance related to pain and medication side effects. The patient should demonstrate healthy adaptation and coping skills.

Cluster Headache

Cluster headaches are a relatively uncommon type of headache. They can be as painful as a migraine headache and like the migraine are considered a vascular headache.

Epidemiology

Cluster headaches account for approximately 8 to 10 percent of all headache sufferers. Unlike migraine headaches, they occur more often in men than women. They do not occur in childhood but begin in patients between 30 and 60 years of age. Cluster headaches are not seen in first-degree relatives (parent, child).

Etiology

Cluster headaches are believed to be a variant of migraine headaches. The cause is unknown, but a seasonal relationship is often noted in these patients. Patients are usually awoken at night without warning signs or aura.

Pathophysiology

The pathophysiology of the cluster headache is similar to a migraine headache; however, the triggers are different. The triggers include vasodilating agents (nitroglycerine), histamine, alcohol, and nicotine. Acetylcholine (ACh) is believed to play a role in the parasympathetic symptoms.

Assessment with Clinical Manifestations

The rapid onset of the pain with cluster headaches often wakes the patient from a sound sleep in the middle of the night. The pain is unilateral (one side of head), usually behind the eye, and so severe that the patient is unable to lie still, but paces the floor holding their head. Associated symptoms include nasal congestion, **rhinorrhea** (watery discharge from the nose), tearing, and redness of the eye on the affected side. Cluster headaches do not cause nausea and vomiting. They occur as a series of attacks. Each attack can last from 15 minutes to up to two hours. A cluster of attacks consists of one or more attacks everyday for 4 to 12 weeks. Then the patient usually has an attack free period lasting months to years.

Diagnostic Tests

Diagnostic studies need to be done to rule out secondary causes of the headaches. They are summarized in Box 37-1.

Nursing Diagnoses

The nursing diagnoses for all of the headache types is displayed in Box 37-2.

Planning and Implementation

The focus of collaborative care for the cluster headache patient is to rule out any secondary causes and prevention of attacks. A thorough history and physical examination is necessary. The health care provider needs to ask specific questions concerning the headache signs and symptoms. Diagnostic studies need to be done to rule secondary causes of the headaches. They are summarized in Box 37-1. In research studies, thermography has been used during an attack to demonstrate a cold spot above the eye, indicating reduced blood flow in that area.

Management of cluster headaches focuses on prevention. Teaching should include medication regimen and trigger avoidance. Medication regimens commonly used for treatment of cluster headaches are abortive and prophylactic drugs. Abortive therapy includes oxygen, subcutaneous or nasal sumatriptan, and topical lidocaine. Prophylactic therapy includes steroids, ergotamine preparations, lithium, calcium channel blockers, and anticonvulsants.

Evaluation of Outcomes

Potential patient outcomes for each of the example nursing diagnoses for the patient with cluster headaches are:

- Acute pain related to cluster headache. The patient should verbalize an adequate relief of pain along with the ability to realistically cope with the pain if it is not completely relieved.
- Ineffective coping related to pain. The patient should verbalize feelings, identify personal strengths, and accept support.
- Disturbed sensory perception related to headache pain. The patient should verbalize decreased symptoms.
- Deficient knowledge related to lack of understanding. The patient should describe disease process, symptoms, and control measures.

- Sleep deprivation related to pain or medication side effects. The patient will report an optimal balance of rest and activity.
- Ineffective role performance related to pain and medication side effects. The patient should demonstrate healthy adaptation and coping skills.

SEIZURES

A **seizure** is a sudden, uncontrolled discharge of electricity in the brain. Seizures are frequently a symptom of an underlying pathology. Seizures secondary to systemic or metabolic pathology are not considered epilepsy, if the seizures stop when the pathology is resolved. A **convulsion** is the abnormal motor response or jerking movements that occur during a seizure. **Epilepsy** involves spontaneously recurring seizures caused by chronic pathology. It is one of the most common neurological conditions (Gambrell & Flynn, 2004).

TABLE 37-4 Seizure Causes

Physiological
CNS infections
Inborn errors of metabolism
Congenital malformations
Acquired metabolic disorders
• Hypoglycemia
• Uremia
• Hepatic encephalopathy
• Electrolyte disturbances
• Acid-base disturbances
Structural lesions
• Stroke
• Trauma
• Subarachnoid hemorrhage
• Subdural hematoma
• Tumors
• Scarring from old brain injuries
Iatrogenic
New medications or withdrawal from medications
Drug or alcohol use or withdrawal
Idiopathic
Common seizure triggers
• Fevers
• Menstrual cycle
• Flashing lights
• Fatigue
• Strong emotions
• Intense exercise
• Loud music

Epidemiology

About 2.5 million people in the United States have epilepsy with an increase of approximately 180,000 new patients each year. About 3 percent of people will receive a diagnosis of epilepsy at some time in their lives. The estimated annual cost of the diagnosis, treatment, and disability related to seizures is $12.5 billion. For hundreds of years, a diagnosis of seizures or epilepsy has carried a stigma. In recent years, Congress has allocated $4 million to epilepsy programs to support research, treatment, and public education.

Etiology

Seizures occur when there is an imbalance in the central nervous system (CNS). Individual susceptibility varies patient to patient. The episodic nature of seizures suggests triggers initiate the process. There are multiple causes for seizures (Table 37-4).

Pathophysiology

Seizure generation has two components: a seizure focus and the neuronal connections to that focus. The seizure focus is a group of hyperexcitable neurons. The area of the brain that is connected to the focus will determine the seizure manifestations. For example, a slow growing brain tumor near the in the frontal lobe will eventually cause a seizure to occur. The seizure focus is near the motor cortex, adjacent to the increasing tumor mass. When the hyperexcitable focus discharges, it is transmitted to the motor strip and a clonic seizure is the result. There are three global causes for seizures: physiological, iatrogenic, or idiopathic. Box 37-3 summarizes the causes of seizures. Environmental or physiological factors that can trigger a seizure are listed in Table 37-4.

Assessment with Clinical Manifestations

The clinical manifestations of a seizure are determined by the site of the disturbance (focus). The system of classification that has been used for 25 years is summarized in Table 37-5. In this system seizures are divided into three major classes: partial, generalized, and unclassified.

Phases of a seizure include the prodromal phase, the aural phase, the ictal phase, and the postictal phase. The prodromal phase is the signs or activity before the seizure, for example, a headache or feeling depressed. The aural phase is a sensation or warning that the patient remembers. An aura can be visual, auditory, gustatory, or visceral in nature, for example, an odor or flash-

BOX 37-3

SEIZURE DIAGNOSTIC STUDIES

Neurological Examination

CT scan or MRI of the brain (rule out tumors, hemorrhage)

Routine laboratory studies: (CBC; electrolytes; LFTs, toxicology screen).

Skull X-rays (to rule out fractures, bone erosion, or separated sutures)

EEG (if no seizure activity on standard test, may require 24 hour continuous test).

Other: PET scan; SPECT scan

Legend: CBC, complete blood count; CT, computed tomography; LFTs, liver function tests; EEG, electroencephalography; MRI, magnetic resonance imaging; PET, positron emission tomography; SPECT, single-proton emission computerized tomography.

TABLE 37-5 Seizure Classification

Partial (Local, Focal) Seizures

Simple partial seizures (consciousness not impaired)

- With focal motor symptoms
- With somatosensory or special sensory symptoms
- With autonomic symptoms
- With disturbance of higher cerebral function

Complex Partial Seizures (Impaired Consciousness)

Begin as simple partial and progress to impaired consciousness

- With no other features
- With features of simple partial seizures
- With automatisms

Impairment of consciousness at onset

- With no other features
- With features of simple partial seizures
- With automatisms

Partial Seizures Evolving into Generalized Seizures

- Simple partial evolving to generalized
- Complex partial evolving to generalized
- Simple partial evolving to complex partial to generalized

Generalized Seizures (Bilaterally Symmetric, without Local Onset)

- Absence seizures
- Myoclonic seizures
- Clonic seizures
- Tonic seizures
- Tonic-clonic seizures
- Atonic seizures
- Unclassified epileptic seizures

Adapted from Commission on Classification and Terminology of the International League against Epilepsy. (1981). Proposal for revised clinical and electroencephalographic classification of epileptic seizures. Epilepsia, *22, 489–501.*

ing lights. The ictal phase is the actual seizure. The postictal phase is the period immediately following the seizure. During this phase the patient is usually confused, disoriented, and does not remember the seizure. If left alone the patient may sleep deeply for several hours. A seizure may include some or all of the phases.

Additional clinical manifestations may include automatisms, clonus, autonomic symptoms, or Todd's paralysis. Automatisms are coordinated involuntary motor activities that occur during the seizure. Examples include lip smacking, chewing, fidgeting, and pacing. Clonus is the descriptive term for the pattern of spasm with muscle rigidity followed by muscle relaxation. Autonomic symptoms occur in response to stimulation of the autonomic nervous system. These symptoms include pallor, sweating, epigastric discomfort, flushing, piloerection, or dilation of pupils. Todd's paralysis is a temporary, focal weakness or paralysis following a seizure that can last up to 24 hours.

The focus of collaborative care for the patient with seizures is to obtain a comprehensive and accurate description of the seizures. A thorough health history and physical examination is necessary. The health care provider needs to ask specific questions concerning seizures (Box 37-4). Diagnostic studies need to be done to rule out secondary causes of the seizures. They are summarized in Box 37-3. Discussion of the specific tests can be found in chapter 34. The nurse needs to develop a comprehensive plan to help the patient deal with the psychosocial aspects of having a seizure disorder.

Generalized Seizures

Generalized seizures originate in all of the regions of the brain cortex. There is no aura or warning, but there is loss of consciousness. The seizure may last for a few seconds or several minutes.

- Absence seizures usually occur during childhood and last 5 to 10 seconds. If the seizure last for more than 10 seconds, there may be automatisms, such as eye blinking or lip smacking. They frequently occur in clusters and can occur dozens or even hundreds of times per day. The electroencephalogram (EEG) will show a 3 Hz (cycles per minute) spike and wave pattern, unique to this type of seizure.
- Atypical absence seizures usually begin before age 5 and are associated with mental retardation and a tendency for multiple seizure types. They last longer and are associated with muscle spasms.
- Myoclonic seizures are characterized by sudden, brief arm muscle contractions. Consciousness is usually not impaired.
- Clonic seizures demonstrate rhythmic, repetitive clonic movements of the arms, neck, and face. These movements are bilateral and symmetrical.
- Tonic-clonic (formerly called grand mal) seizures are the most common type of generalized seizure. The seizure will progress through all of the seizure phases and last two to three minutes. Because of the suddenness of this type of seizure, injuries, such as limb fractures, tongue biting, and head trauma, can occur. These seizures can occur any time of the day or night, whether the patient is awake or not. Seizure frequency is highly variable.
- Atonic seizures (drop attacks) are a sudden loss of muscle control, usually the legs, that results in falling to the floor, increasing the possibility of injury.

BOX 37-4

QUESTIONS SPECIFIC FOR SEIZURE ASSESSMENT

Have you ever had seizures before? What age?

Any trauma, tumors, or infections of the CNS?

Do you use nicotine products? How much? For how long?

Do you consume alcohol products? How much? For how long?

Any environmental exposure? Metals? Chemicals? Gases?

Do you use any recreational drugs?

Are you currently taking medication to prevent seizures? If yes, what?

Have you taken seizure medications in the past? If yes, what? Why did you stop?

Do any other members of your family have a history of seizures?

Any nausea, vomiting, or diarrhea recently?

Do you have headaches; muscle or abdominal pain; mood, behavior, or mentation changes before or after a seizure?

Do you have any numbness, tingling, or paralysis after a seizure?

Red Flag

Intranasal Drug Delivery

When an intravenous (IV) line is not available, intranasally administered benzodiazepines (midazolam) are a rapid and effective method to treat an acutely seizing patient. The most concentrated form of the medication must be combined with an atomized drug delivery system to maximize the delivery of the medication. Intranasal delivery is more effective than rectal administration.

Skills 360°

Nursing Assessment of the Seizing Patient

The nurse should evaluate the following activities during the seizure activity:

- Onset—Was it sudden? Was it preceded by an aura?
- Duration—When did it start? When did it stop? Any changes?
- Behaviors—Before, during, and after.
- Type of body movements. Describe in detail.
- Any loss of consciousness? How long?
- Incontinence—Bladder or bowel.
- Amnesia or confusion post seizure?

Partial Seizures

Partial seizures begin in a specific brain region and consciousness is usually not impaired. The clinical manifestations depend on the region of the brain where the seizure focus starts. There may be an aura or warning signs.

- Simple partial seizures are when consciousness is not lost. Depending on the seizure focus there may be motor, sensory, autonomic, or higher level cognitive clinical manifestations.
- Complex partial seizures are the most common type of epileptic seizure in adults. Consciousness and awareness of surroundings is lost. Automatisms may occur. The seizure typically lasts one to three minutes.

Status Epilepticus

Status epilepticus is defined as either continuous seizures lasting more than five minutes or two or more different seizures with incomplete recovery of consciousness between them. The most common cause of status epilepticus is abruptly stopping of antiepileptic drugs (AEDs). Status epilepticus can present clinically with tonic, clonic, or tonic-clonic movements. It is a medical emergency, because it is often accompanied by respiratory distress brought on by hypoxia or anoxia. Morbidity and mortality for status epilepticus is 20 percent. Subclinical status epilepticus is seen with partial seizures but can only be verified by EEG.

Diagnostic Tests

There are a variety of diagnostic tests that can be used in determining the origin and pathology of seizure activity. A list of these tests is shown in Box 37-3.

Nursing Diagnoses

Based on the information gathered, examples of nursing diagnoses in the patient with seizures may include the following:

- Risk for ineffective airway clearance related to obstructed airway during seizure activity.
- Risk for injury related to seizure activity and postictal weakness or paralysis.
- Anxiety related to changes in lifestyle, uncertainty, and changes in self-concept.
- Ineffective therapeutic regimen management related to lack of knowledge of seizure treatment.
- Ineffective coping related to chronic disease, altered self-concept, and social stigma.

Planning and Implementation

Prevention of seizures is the management goal. If the diagnostic testing reveals a treatable cause for the seizures, then it should be resolved. Epilepsy (recurrent seizures) is controlled in 70 percent of patients with antiepileptic medications (Table 37-6). A significant number of the remaining 30 percent may benefit from surgical intervention. Once the diagnosis of epilepsy is established, patient safety and health teaching by the nurse become the primary focus. The patient and their family need accurate information concerning the manifestations, etiology, and treatment of seizures. The nurse needs to educate and support the patient and family as they adjust to the lifestyle changes that are required. Teaching should address the physical, emotional, and social aspects of the disease. Actions and potential side effects of the medication regimen need to be taught, monitored, and adjusted to the desired patient response. Medications can only be effective if taken as prescribed. Seizure activity can be triggered if the patient suddenly stops or takes antiseizure medications sporadically.

The psychosocial affects may be more devastating to the patient and family than the seizures. During the period of adjustment, the patient may experi-

TABLE 37-6 Medications to Treat Seizures

FIRST-LINE DRUGS	SECOND-LINE DRUGS	STATUS EPILEPTICUS DRUGS
Phenytoin (Dilantin)	Ethosuximide (Zarontin)	Lorazepam (Ativan)
Valproate (Depakote	Methsuximide (Celontin)	Phenytoin (Dilantin)
Carbamazepine (Tegretol)	Clonazepam (Klonopin)	Fosphenytoin (Cerebyx)
Lamotrigine (Lamictal)	Topiramate (Topamax)	Phenobarbital (Luminal)
Phenobarbital (Luminal)	Gabapentin (Neurontin)	Midazolam (Versed)
	Primidone (Mysoline)	Propofol (Diprivan)
	Felbamate (Felbatol)	
	Levetiracetam (Keppra)	
	Zonisamide (Zonegran)	
	Oxcarbazepine (Trileptal)	

Adapted from Broyles, B. E., Reiss, B. S., & Evans, M. E. (2007). Pharmacological aspects of nursing care *(7th ed.). New York: Thomson Delmar Learning.*

ence problems at home, work, or with personal relationships. Safety precautions need to be implemented in the home and work environment. Fear of discrimination and social isolation may require counseling for both the patient and their family.

Pharmacology

The primary methods for treating seizure activity are pharmacological interventions. Many patients are treated successfully with their medication regimens, and the patients are able to live normal lives while adhering to the pharmacological interventions. A composite list of the medications commonly used is provided in Table 37-6.

Surgery

Surgical interventions for some patients with seizure activities is also a successful method of management. A surgical method of treatment is normally employed after other more conservative forms of management have been practiced. Table 37-7 provides the major surgical methods used to treat seizures.

Evaluation of Outcomes

Potential patient outcomes for each of the example nursing diagnoses for the patient with seizures:

- Risk for ineffective airway clearance related to seizure activity. The patient should not experience aspiration.
- Risk for injury related to seizure activity. The patient should not experience injury.
- Anxiety related to changes in lifestyle and self-concept. The patient should verbalize increased psychological and physiological comfort.
- Ineffective therapeutic regimen management related to lack of knowledge. The patient will verbalize understanding of disease process, etiology, and treatment measures.
- Ineffective individual coping related to chronic disease. The patient should verbalize feelings, identify personal strengths, and accept support.

TABLE 37-7 Surgical Treatment of Seizures

SURGERY	PROCEDURE
Temporal lobectomy	Removal of all or part of temporal lobe. Elimination of seizure focus.
Focal lesionectomy	Removal of scar tissue that is seizure focus.
Corpus callosotomy	Excision of the corpus callosotomy.
Hemispherectomy	Modified radical excision of temporal lobe in children with intractable seizures.
Vagus nerve stimulation	Placement of bipolar leads on vagus nerve and then attaching a programmable signal generator.

MULTIPLE SCLEROSIS

Multiple sclerosis (MS) is a chronic inflammatory disease of the CNS. MS is a relatively common neurological degenerative disorder and can be debilitating in some who are diagnosed with the disease. MS is known for its combination of remission times and its exacerbations of the disease symptomatology. Many people with multiple sclerosis live well with the disorder and learn to adapt well during the times of disease exacerbation. Typically, when a person is hospitalized for his or her MS disorder, the crisis is related to the secondary complications of the disease. For example, later in the disease process patients can become fatigued and are not able to be as mobile. One result of their fatigue and the degenerative nature of the disease are respiratory complications, which is common in the acute phase of MS.

Epidemiology

MS is the major cause of chronic disability in young adults. Onset of symptoms usually occurs between the ages of 20 and 40. MS occurs more frequently in Caucasian females than males (1.7:1). The ratio of Caucasian to non-Caucasian is 2:1. Geographically it is more common in the temperate and cold climates of the higher latitudes of the northern and southern hemispheres. There is some evidence that MS has a genetic connection. Incidence of MS in first-degree relatives is 20 times higher than in the general population. It is estimated that greater than 400,000 people are diagnosed with MS in the United States (Denis, et al., 2004).

Etiology

The cause of MS is not known. Current theories identify autoimmune-mediated inflammatory demyelination and axonal injury. No virus has been isolated. It is believed that two factors may initiate the inflammation: exposure to an environmental agent and genetic susceptibility. Research has demonstrated that multiple genetic factors are involved. Future research may identify how these genes operate and interact with the environment.

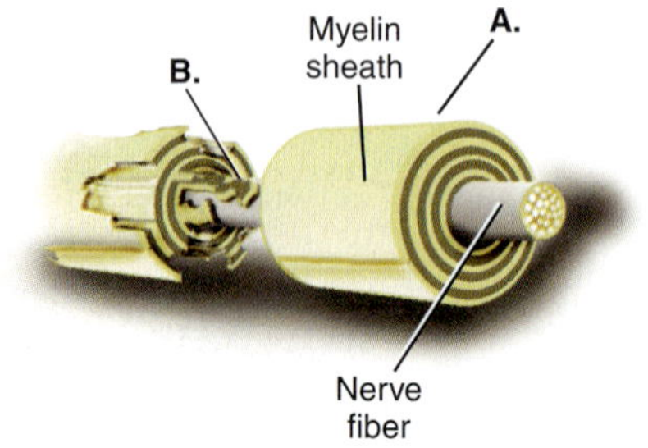

Figure 37-1 A. Normal nerve fiber and myelin sheath, B. MS destruction of myelin sheath.

Pathophysiology

MS involves the white matter of the CNS. Inflammatory cells (activated lymphocytes and monocytes) cross the blood-brain barrier, surround the blood vessels, and destroy the neuronal myelin sheath (Figure 37-1). Neurons and some axons are spared. The individual lesions are called plaques and may be as a few millimeters to as long as several centimeters. Because it acts like an insulator, loss of myelin and the subsequent degeneration and atrophy of the axons interrupts impulse transmission.

Assessment with Clinical Manifestations

The clinical course of MS has four categories: relapsing-remitting, secondary progressive, progressing-relapsing, and primary progressive. Relapsing-remitting disease is the most common form of the disease, seen in 80 percent of all cases. It is characterized by recurrent episodes of neurological dysfunction evolving over days or weeks. Recovery from each episode may be complete, partial, or with residual deficits occurring over weeks to months. Symptoms do not progress during remissions.

Secondary progressive disease is characterized by gradual deterioration with or without relapses, remissions, or plateaus. For many patients this is the second phase of the disease that started as relapsing-remitting. Progressing-relapsing disease starts with a gradual progression of disability without plateaus or remissions. Primary progressive disease is characterized by gradual neurological disability with noted relapses.

The clinical manifestations of MS may vary greatly among patients and can vary over time in the same patient. The most common presenting symptoms are: sensory loss (37 percent), optic neuritis (36 percent), weakness (35 percent), paresthesias (24 percent), diplopia (15 percent), ataxia (11 percent), and vertigo (6 percent). A summary of the clinical manifestations of MS can be found in Table 37-8. The clinical manifestations of MS can be exacerbated by being in a hot, humid environment or taking a hot bath.

TABLE 37-8 Clinical Manifestations of MS

SENSORY	MOTOR	CEREBELLAR	OTHER
Numbness	Paresis	Loss of balance	Fatigue
Paresthesia	Paralysis	Loss of coordination	Optic neuritis
• Burning	Foot dragging	Ataxia	Impotence
• Tingling	Diplopia	Nystagmus	Sexual dysfunction
• Prickling			
Pain	Bowel/Bladder	Speech disturbances	Depression
Decreased perception	• Retention	• Dysarthria	Euphoria
• Position	• Incontinence	• Dystonia	Visual loss
• Temperature		• Scanning speech	Trigeminal neuralgia
• Depth		• Slurred speech	Facial palsy
• Vibration		Tremor (dysmetria)	Heat intolerance
Lhermitte's sign		Vertigo	Nystagmus
			Scotomas

Adapted from Denis, L., Namey, M., Costello, K., Frenette, J., Gagnon, N., Harris, C., et al. (2004). Long term treatment optimization in individuals with multiple sclerosis using disease-modifying therapies: A nursing approach. Journal of Neuroscience Nursing, 36*(1), 10–22.*

Diagnostic Tests

There is no single diagnostic test that confirms or rules out the diagnosis of MS. However, there are some specific tests that may assist with the diagnosis. A magnetic resonance imaging (MRI) of the brain and spinal cord with gadolinium infusion may identify bright lesions (T2-weighted images) in the corpus callosum and periventricular regions. A lesion larger than 5 mm helps to confirm the diagnosis.

Newer neuroimaging techniques such as fluid-attenuated-inversion-recovery (FLAIR) and magnetic resonance spectroscopy (MRS) have increased sensitivity and specificity for white matter abnormalities. FLAIR is able to detect two to three times the number of lesions seen on T2-weighted images. MRS looks at levels of *N*-acetylaspartate (NAA). Decreased NAA levels in MS plaques and apparently unaffected areas of white matter suggest the presence of axonal damage.

Lumbar puncture may be done to obtain cerebrospinal fluid (CSF) for analysis. Discussion of the procedure and CSF analysis is discussed in chapter 34. In MS, elevated immunoglobulin G (IgG) index, presence of oligoclonal bands (OCBs), and increased myelin basic protein in the CSF analysis helps to confirm the diagnosis. Oligoclonal bands are found in 85 to 90 percent of patients with MS but can also be found other inflammatory or infectious diseases.

Evoked potentials are also discussed in depth in chapter 34. Abnormal findings are demonstrated in more than 75 percent of patients with a diagnosis of MS. The test may be repeated to monitor for improvements related to medication regimens or disease progression. Neuropsychological screening also uses standardized tests to identify and quantify the cognitive, emotional, and behavioral abilities of the patient. The results can be used to help the patient

Skills 360°

Questions Specific to MS

The nurse should ask the patient the following questions as related to MS:

Have you experienced any recent of past viral infections? Vaccinations? Recent infections?

Do you live in a cold or temperate climate? Did you live there as a child? Adolescent?

Have you recently experienced increased emotional or physical stress? Pregnancy?

Is there any history of chronic fatigue or malaise in your family?

Have you recently lost or gained weight? How much? Was it a planned weight loss?

Do you have any problems with chewing or swallowing?

Have you experienced any problems with urination? If yes, describe.

Any problems or recent changes with bowel function? If yes, describe.

Have you experienced generalized muscle weakness or fatigue? Tingling? Numbness?

Do you experience tripping or stumbling while walking? If yes, describe episodes.

Have you experienced joint or muscle pain? Muscle spasms? If yes, describe.

Do you ever feel dizzy or like you are spinning? Describe.

Have you experienced any vision changes? Describe.

Do you have a constant ringing in your ears? Does it get better or worse? Describe.

Have you experienced any decrease in desire or performance of sexual activity?

Do you have any feelings of depression, anger, euphoria, or social isolation? Describe.

and their family understand the impact of the disease on the patients functional ability. Serial reassessment can track improvement or lack of progress.

Nursing Diagnoses

Based on the information gathered, examples of nursing diagnoses in the patient with MS may include the following:

- Impaired physical mobility related to muscle weakness, paralysis, or spasticity.
- Self-care deficit related to neuromuscular deficits.
- Impaired urinary elimination related to neuromuscular degeneration.
- Constipation related to inactivity and abdominal muscle weakness.
- Ineffective coping related to feelings of helplessness.
- Risk for impaired skin integrity related to decreased muscle strength and inactivity.
- Risk for ineffective airway clearance related to weak or ineffective cough effort.
- Risk for imbalanced nutrition: less than body requirement related to muscle weakness.

Planning and Implementation

The focus of collaborative care for the patient with MS is multifaceted and involves modification of the disease course, symptom management, prevention of complications, and management of psychosocial issues. A thorough health history and physical examination is necessary. Because there is no diagnostic test that specifically identifies MS, analysis of the history, physical examination, and diagnostic tests findings are needed to confirm the diagnosis.

A program of physical therapy using exercise and assistive devices can help the patient to maintain a high level of functioning. A daily exercise program should include range-of-motion and muscle-strengthening components. If assistive

Uncovering the Evidence

Thalmic Stimulation for Tremor

Discussion: The purpose of this research is to study the long-term effect of deep brain stimulation (DBS) in patients with MS. The methods used are preoperative and postoperative evaluation of the study participants including MRI, the Extended Disability Status Scale (EDSS), the Bain-Finchley tremor scale, neuropsychological testing, and a patient self-assessment of the benefits of surgery.

The findings revealed the EDSS scores averaged 7.2 before surgery, 6.8 at six months postsurgery, and 7.8 at late follow-up. Tremor scores averaged 5.4 before surgery, 1.7 at six months postsurgery, and 2.1 at late follow-up. MRI scans did not show any new MS plaques related to the DBS probe. Neuropsychological testing showed mild to moderate decline in cognitive function related to disease progression.

Implications for Practice: Use of deep brain thalamic stimulation significantly reduced the tremor experienced by patients with MS but did not improve other objective measures of function. Surgical implantation of DBS for relief of tremors should only be considered in patients with stable disease and disabling upper extremity symptoms.

Source: Schulder, M., Sernas, T., & Karimi, R. (2003). Thalamic stimulation in patients with multiple sclerosis: Long-term follow-up. Stereotactic and Functional Neurosurgery, 80*(1–4), 48–55.*

TABLE 37-9 Drugs for Treatment of MS

DRUG	USES	SIDE EFFECTS
Immunomodulating Drugs		
Interferon beta-1a (Avonex)	Slow disease progression Reduce relapse	Flu-like symptoms; mild anemia; elevated enzymes
Glatiramer acetate (Copaxone)	Slow disease progression	Flu-like symptoms; injection site reactions; chest pain; weakness
Immunosuppressant Drugs		
Mitoxantrone (Novantrone)	Slow disease progression Reduce relapse	Nausea; diarrhea; amenorrhea; alopecia; anemia; respiratory or urinary infections
Corticosteroid Drugs		
Corticotropin (ACTH)	Exacerbations	Edema; euphoria; weight gain; insomnia
Methylprednisolone (Solu-Medrol)	Exacerbations	Edema; euphoria; weight gain; insomnia; hypertension; acne
Prednisone (Deltasone)	Mild exacerbations	Edema; euphoria; weight gain; insomnia; hypertension
Muscle Relaxants		
Diazepam (Valium)	Spasticity	Fatigue; ataxia; drowsiness; depression; vertigo; diplopia; confusion
Baclofen (Lioresal)	Spasticity	Drowsiness; vertigo; dizziness; ataxia; insomnia; slurred speech
Antiepileptic Drugs		
Gabapentin (Neurontin)	Neuropathic pain	Somnolence; dizziness; ataxia; fatigue
Carbamazepine (Tegretol)	Neuropathic pain	Sedation; dizziness; fatigue; ataxia; fever; confusion
Antidepressants		
Amitriptyline (Elavil)	Neuropathic pain	Dry mouth; sedation; tachycardia; ataxia; confusion
Fluoxetine (Prozac)	Depression	Insomnia; headache; anxiety; dizziness
Stimulant Drugs		
Amantadine (Symmetrel)	Fatigue	Insomnia; depression; anxiety; ataxia; headache; fatigue; confusion
Modafinil (Provigil)	Fatigue	Headache; dizziness; depression; anxiety; insomnia; fever; confusion; ataxia
Cholinergic Drugs		
Bethanechol (Urecholine)	Urinary retention	Hypotension; bradycardia; drooling; diarrhea; bowel or bladder obstruction
Neostigmine (Prostigmin)	Urinary retention	GI upset; urinary urgency; bradycardia; sweating; increased salivation
Anticholinergic Drugs		
Probanthine (Pro-Banthine)	Urinary frequency	Dry mouth; blurred vision; photophobia; urinary retention; constipation; tachycardia
Oxybutynin (Ditropan)	Urinary frequency	Dry mouth; blurred vision; photophobia; urinary retention; constipation; tachycardia

Adapted from Broyles, B. E., Reiss, B. S., & Evans, M. E. (2007). Pharmacological aspects of nursing care *(7th ed.). New York: Thomson Delmar Learning.*

devices, such as a brace, cane, or walker, are needed to maintain independence, the health care provider needs to teach safe use and maintenance of the device. If mild spasticity develops, physical therapy can help by retraining alternative muscle groups. When there is severe spasticity, medications can be helpful.

Stress reduction methods may include exercise programs, meditation, yoga, or tai chi. All of these techniques can be recommended to help patients with life-stress management.

Pharmacology

The health care provider needs to ask specific questions related to MS and its clinical manifestations. Modification of disease progression can be accomplished by using medications. Symptom management involves a variety of medications and other forms of therapy (Table 37-9). The major disease symptoms include spasticity, tremors, pain, urinary problems, sensory problems, depression, and fatigue.

Surgery

When spasticity can no longer be managed with oral baclofen (Lioresal), the patient may be a candidate for intrathecal (area surrounding the spinal cord) medication delivery. First, the patient is evaluated by physical therapy for baseline functioning level. Then a test dose of Lioresal is given, and the patient is again evaluated for functional improvement. Improvement is a positive indicator for surgical implantation of the catheter (near the spinal cord) and pump. The pump is then programmed (similar to a pacemaker) to deliver the lowest dose of Lioresal needed to manage spasticity. The patient must follow up with the health care provider every three months.

Evaluation of Outcomes

Potential patient outcomes for each of the example nursing diagnoses for the patient with MS are:

- Impaired physical mobility related to neuromuscular degeneration. The patient will verbalize increased strength and endurance.
- Self-care deficit related to neuromuscular deficits. The patient will participate in activities of daily living as much as possible.
- Impaired urinary elimination related to neuromuscular degeneration. The patient will report none or decreased episodes of incontinence.
- Constipation related to inactivity. The patient will report regular bowel movements.
- Ineffective coping related to feelings of helplessness. The patient should verbalize feelings, identify personal strengths, and accept support.
- Risk for impaired skin integrity related to inactivity. The patient will maintain intact skin.
- Risk for ineffective airway clearance related to weak or ineffective cough effort. The patient should not experience aspiration.
- Risk for imbalanced nutrition: less than body requirement related to muscle weakness. The patient should demonstrate methods to increase appetite.

PARKINSON'S DISEASE

Parkinson's disease is a relatively common neurological degenerative disorder that was first discovered by Dr. James Parkinson in the 1800s. Among the several types of Parkinson's disease, the idiopathic or degenerative form is the most common. A wide variety of causes are associated with Parkinson's disease, including genetic, environmental, and medication regimens. Parkinson's disease can be slow in its progression, but it is a disorder that ultimately leads to disability.

Epidemiology

Parkinson's disease occurs worldwide with equal incidence between men and women. Disease symptoms usually begin between the ages of 40 and 70, with peak age at onset occurring in the sixth decade. In North America, there are approximately one million patients with Parkinson's disease. It is estimated that 1 percent of the population over age 65 is afflicted.

Etiology

The etiology of Parkinson's disease is unknown. Several factors may play a part in the causing the disease including hereditary predisposition, environmental toxins, and aging. Several studies have examined the possibility of a gene that can be linked to Parkinson's disease. There have been a few case reports of multiple cases within an extended family. The search for a specific gene responsible for Parkinson's disease continues.

Environmental toxin exposure has been identified as a potential cause. Chemicals such as carbon monoxide, carbon disulfide, cyanide, manganese, and methylphenyltetrahydropyridine (MPTP) have been linked to the development of Parkinson's disease. MPTP is a contaminant often found in illicit street drugs. Another environmental exposure connected to the development of Parkinson's disease is seen in welders, but the age of onset is earlier (30 to 40 years old).

Two theories are being examined concerning aging as a cause of Parkinson's disease. The first theory states that the disease is an accelerated form of aging. The second theory attributes the cause to some acute insult to the substantia nigra, followed by a slow loss of neurons, and development of symptoms in the sixth decade of life. Research continues in hopes of eventually identifying a specific cause for Parkinson's disease.

Pathophysiology

Parkinson's disease is a slowly progressive degenerative neurological disorder caused by the loss of nerve cell function in the basal ganglia. The basal ganglia includes several structures, the substantia nigra, striatum, globus pallidus, subthalamic nucleus, and the red nucleus. Loss of nerve cells in the substantia nigra causes a reduction of dopamine production. Dopamine is the neurotransmitter essential for such functions as control of posture, supporting the body in an upright position, and voluntary motions (Calne & Kumar, 2003).

Assessment with Clinical Manifestations

Parkinson's disease often begins with mild or intermittent symptoms. The patient or his or her family may notice that he or she is feeling more tired than usual, he or she may move slower than previously, or a slight tremor may occur. Often the symptoms are attributed to aging. Because the disease is progressive, eventually the patient's ability to function independently is impaired.

Tremor is defined as a rhythmic, purposeless, fine trembling, or quivering movement resulting from the involuntary alternating contraction and relaxation of opposing groups of skeletal muscles. Resting tremor (also called passive tremor) occurs while at rest. Intention tremor occurs with initiation of movement. Parkinson's disease tremor is most commonly seen in the fingers and hands but may involve the entire arm, lower extremity, or facial musculature. The tremor disappears with complete relaxation and often is reduced during voluntary movements. Hand tremors are often described as pill-rolling (rhythmic movement of the thumb across the palm of the hand).

Muscle rigidity is a stiffness seen with resistance to passive muscle stretching. Lead-pipe rigidity is stiffness and inflexibility that remains uniform through-

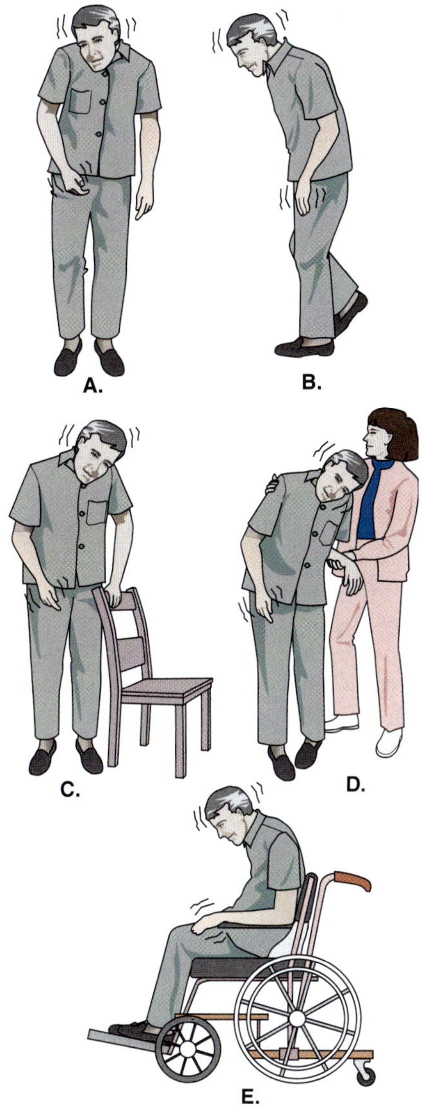

Figure 37-2 Progression of Parkinson's disease: A. Flexion of affected arm, B. Shuffling gait, C. Need for sources of support to prevent falling, D. Progression of weakness to point of needing assistance for ambulation, E. Profound weakness.

out the range of passive movement. Cogwheel rigidity is an abnormal rigor in muscle tissue characterized by jerky, ratchet-like movements when the limb is passively stretched. The rigidity is secondary to the depletion of dopamine causing a sustained contraction of the skeletal muscle groups. A common complaint is muscle soreness, a feeling of fatigue, achiness, and pain.

Akinesia (loss of movement) and **bradykinesia** (slowness of voluntary movement and speech) are responsible for the mask-like expression, difficulty swallowing, monotonous speech, and lack of arm swing. The patient has difficulty initiating movement, turning, or redirecting forward movement. Postural disturbances are secondary to the loss of postural reflexes and are characterized by stooped posture, shuffling gait, and broad-based turns. There is also a loss of the ability to protect oneself from harm. These voluntary movement changes put the patient at risk for injury from falls (Figure 37-2).

Common secondary manifestations of Parkinson's disease include: fine motor deficits, monotonic voice, mask-like face, generalized muscle fatigue, cognitive changes (e.g., impaired memory, visuospatial, depression), drooling, dysphagia, constipation, orthostatic hypotension, and urinary dysfunction. Many of the secondary manifestations can be exaggerated by the medications used to treat Parkinson's disease.

Diagnostic Tests

There are no specific diagnostic tests to confirm the diagnosis of Parkinson's disease. The diagnosis is based on history, physical examination, and presence of the major clinical manifestations. A conclusive diagnosis is possible only after all other potential causes have been ruled out. MRI and EEG may be normal. Magnetic resonance single-photo emission computed tomography (SPECT) has shown some promise in identifying the degeneration of the neurons in the substantia nigra. Positron emission tomography (PET) scanning can be done serially to identify the loss of dopamine producing cells in the brain. A full discussion of these tests can be found in chapter 34.

Nursing Diagnoses

Based on the information gathered, examples of nursing diagnoses in the patient with Parkinson's disease may include the following:

- Impaired physical mobility related to rigidity, bradykinesia, and akinesia.
- Impaired verbal communication related to dysarthria and tremor.
- Imbalanced nutrition: less than body requirements related to dysphagia.
- Self-care deficit related to inability to perform activities of daily living.
- Constipation related to immobility.
- Disturbed thought processes related to hallucinations and decreased cognitive abilities.
- Sleep deprivation related to rigidity and weakness.
- Risk for injury related to postural disturbances.

Planning and Implementation

Because of the chronic progressive nature of Parkinson's disease, the primary concern of the nurse caring for these patients is health teaching. In the early stages, the nurse needs to educate and support the patient and family as they adjust to the lifestyle changes that are required. Teaching should address the physical, emotional, and social aspects of the disease. In the beginning, actions and potential side effects of the medication regimen need to be taught, monitored, and adjusted to the desired patient response (Imke, 2003).

Maintaining a positive attitude can be difficult for both patients and their families. Short-term counseling with a capable psychotherapist can be helpful. Parkinson's disease is sometimes accompanied by depression and anxiety. Dopamine is not the only neurotransmitter that is out of balance. Serotonin is involved in mood, and when serotonin is depleted clinical depression can result. Depression decreases energy levels and productivity and interferes with personal relationships. Treatment with antidepressants can help to improve mood.

Nutrition is often a concern in patients with Parkinson's disease. Muscle weakness, tremor, and rigidity can make ingestion of a healthy diet difficult. Weight needs to be monitored. Serial monitoring of serum albumin and proteins levels can identify patients at risk for malnutrition. Supplemental feedings may be required. For patients with swallowing difficulties strategies, such as smaller, more frequent meals, adding commercial powders to thicken liquids, and upright positioning, may be beneficial.

Exercise and physical therapy can help the patient to maximize function. Regular moderate exercise can reduce stiffness and tremors. Working with a speech therapist can help the patient to maximize language and cognitive function. As the disease progresses, the patient and family will require more assistance with activities of daily living, emotional support, and potential financial concerns. Issues, such as admission to an extended care facility or hospice, need to be introduced early in the disease progression. This allows the patient to participate in the decision-making process. A thorough history and physical examination is necessary. Health care management involves the use of pharmacological therapy or surgical interventions. The goal of Parkinson's disease management is to prevent functional disability; however a cure is not currently possible.

Collaborative Management

Parkinson's disease demands the multidisciplinary approach to care of the patient. The focus of collaborative management for the Parkinson's disease patient is to:

- Decrease the severity of the clinical manifestations (symptomatic).
- Interfere with the pathological mechanisms of the disease (protective).
- Provide new neurons or stimulate growth and function of remaining cells (restorative).

Pharmacology

The goal of treatment is to control tremor and rigidity and to improve the patient's ability to carry out the activities of daily living. Replacing the dopamine deficit in the basal ganglia sounds simple. However, dopamine cannot be given orally as it is metabolized before reaching the brain.

Levodopa, a precursor of dopamine, can be given orally and then is converted to dopamine in the brain. Dopamine replacement is most effective in the first three to five years of use. Long-term use is associated with side effects, such as dyskinesias, hallucinations, and severe orthostatic hypotension. When anticholinergic drugs are given with the dopamine replacement, the effect of the dopamine is extended. The newer drugs, catechol-*O*-methyltransferase (COMT) inhibitors, block the enzyme that inactivates dopamine and increase the effectiveness of levodopa.

There are many medications used to treat Parkinson's disease, and examples of these medications are shown in Table 37-10.

Surgery

Some patients with Parkinson's disease respond differently to the pharmacological methods of treatment. Other patients have the potential for less conservative treatments in the form of surgical interventions. Some of these types of surgical management (Table 37-11) are relatively recent and have varying levels of success.

TABLE 37-10 Pharmacologic Management of Parkinson's Disease

DRUG	INDICATION	SIDE EFFECTS
Dopamine Precursors		
Carbidopa/levodopa (Sinemet)	Decrease rigidity; bradykinesia; tremors	Nausea; vomiting; orthostatic hypotension; dry mouth; constipation; dizziness; cough; sleep disturbances; hallucinations; confusion; dyskinesia
Dopamine Receptor Antagonists		
Bromocriptine (Parlodel)	Activation of dopamine receptors	Nausea; postural hypotension; sleep disturbances; confusion; agitation; hallucinations; dyskinesia
Pergolide (Permax)	Activation of dopamine receptors	Nausea; postural hypotension; sleep disturbances; confusion; agitation; hallucinations
Pramipexole (Mirapex)	Activation of dopamine receptors	Nausea; dizziness; somnolence; weakness; constipation; sleep attacks
Ropinirole (Requip)	Activation of dopamine receptors	Nausea; dizziness; somnolence; syncope; sleep attacks
Antiviral Agents		
Amantadine (Symmetrel)	Decrease rigidity and akinesia	Confusion; lightheadedness; anxiety; blurred vision; dry mouth; urinary retention; constipation
Anticholinergic Agents		
Benztropine (Cogentin)	Decrease tremors and rigidity	Dry mouth; blurred vision; urinary retention; photophobia; constipation; tachycardia; confusion; depression; hallucinations
Biperiden (Akineton)	Decrease tremors and rigidity	Same as Cogentin
Orphenadrine (Disipal)	Decrease tremors and rigidity	Same as Cogentin
Procyclidine (Kemadrin)	Decrease tremors and rigidity	Same as Cogentin
Trihexyphenidyl (Artane)	Decrease tremors and rigidity	Same as Cogentin
Monoamine Oxidase B (MAO-B) Inhibitor		
Selegiline (Eldepryl)	Delays disease progression	Malaise; dizziness; nausea; tremors; restlessness; increased bradykinesia; orthostatic hypotension; arrhythmias
COMT Inhibitors		
Tolcapone (Tasmar)	Improves motor function	Hepatic failure; dyskinesia; nausea; orthostatic hypotension; sleep disturbances; hallucinations
Entacapone (Comtan)	Improves motor function	Vomiting; diarrhea; constipation; dyskinesia; orthostatic hypotension; hallucinations; sleep disturbances

Note: When these drugs are used in combination the side effect profile is enhanced.
Adapted from Broyles, B. E., Reiss, B. S., & Evans, M. E. (2007). Pharmacological aspects of nursing care *(7th ed.). New York: Thomson Delmar Learning.*

TABLE 37-11 Surgical Management of Parkinson's Disease

SURGERY	PROCEDURE	OUTCOME
Thalamotomy	Lesion placed in the thalamus	Relief of tremors
Pallidotomy	Destruction of globus pallidus using electrical stimulation	Improved control of symptoms
Deep-brain stimulation	Placement of electrode(s) in the thalamus, then attaching to a pulse generator implanted in the infraclavicular region.	Relief of tremors
Experimental Treatments		
Adrenal tissue transplant	Provide viable dopamine producing cells into the caudate nucleus.	Long-term results have not been promising
Stem cell transplant	Provide viable dopamine producing cells into the caudate nucleus.	Long-term results have not been promising

Adapted from Lozano, A. (2003). Surgery for Parkinson's disease the five W's: Why, who, what, where, and when. Advances in Neurology, 91, *30–307.*

ETHICS IN PRACTICE

Stem Cell Controversy

Recent controversy has focused on the legal and ethical issues of using fetal tissue or stem cells obtained from cord blood. There is a continuing level of interest from specific research institutions and from specific lobbying groups to pursue the legalizing of stem cell harvesting. The future of this controversy is unfolding in continuing decisions at this time.

Evaluation of Outcomes

Potential patient outcomes for each of the example nursing diagnoses for the patient with Parkinson's disease are:

- Impaired physical mobility related to rigidity, bradykinesia, and akinesia. The patient will demonstrate increased strength and endurance.
- Impaired verbal communication related to dysarthria and tremor. The patient will demonstrate improved ability to express self.
- Imbalanced nutrition: less than body requirement related to dysphagia. The patient will demonstrate methods to assist with food intake.
- Self-care deficit related to inability to perform activities of daily living. The patient will participate in self-care activities as much as possible.
- Constipation related to immobility. The patient will report regular bowel movements.
- Disturbed thought process related to hallucinations. The patient will maintain reality orientation and communicate clearly with others.
- Sleep deprivation related to rigidity and weakness. The patient will report an optimal balance of rest and activity.
- Risk for injury related to postural disturbances. The patient will not experience injury.

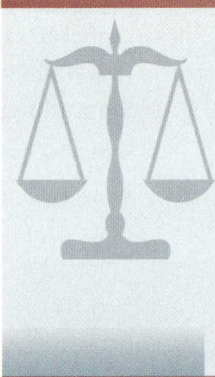

Uncovering the Evidence

Immunization for Parkinson's Disease

Discussion: The purpose of this study was to evaluate the use of vaccine to activate immune cells in ways that are neuroprotective in a mouse model of Parkinson's disease. The methods involved the treatment of mice with Copaxone (copolymer-1), currently used to treat MS. The researchers then took immune cells from the immunized mice and injected them into mice which had received MPTP. MPTP causes Parkinson's-like neuronal degeneration in the brain. The findings revealed that mice treated with the Copaxone-treated immune cells had less degeneration of dopamine-producing neurons, lost fewer dopamine-transmitting nerve fibers, and had only a small decrease in dopamine production when compared to controls.

Implications for Practice: The use of vaccination for Parkinson's disease may serve as a method for arresting disease progression. More basic research needs to be done and to be approved by the Food and Drug Administration (FDA). Clinical trials must demonstrate both effectiveness and a low side effect profile.

Source: Benner, E., Mosley, R., Destache, C., Lewis, T., Jackson-Lewis, V., Gorantla, S., et al. (2004). Therapeutic immunization protects dopaminergic neurons in a mouse model of Parkinson's disease. Proceedings of the National Academy of Sciences of the USA, 101*(25), 9435–9440.*

ALZHEIMER'S DISEASE

Alzheimer's disease is the most common cause of dementia in Western countries, accounting for 70 percent of all cases. Alzheimer's disease is the fourth leading cause of death among the elderly. Alzheimer's disease has an incredible impact on the health care budget because of the chronic nature of the patients and their long-standing health care needs. Recently, the National Institutes of Health (NIH) has contributed greatly to the research funding for the study and interventions related to Alzheimer's disease. And, nursing as a profession has significantly impacted the methods of care for patients with this neurological degenerative disease.

Epidemiology

In the United States, it is estimated that four million people are diagnosed with Alzheimer's disease. And as the population ages, this number is expected to double by 2020. The financial burden on the patient, family, and society is estimated to exceed $100 billion per year. The incidence of Alzheimer's disease is slightly higher in Americans with African and Hispanic heritage. Women and men are affected equally.

Etiology

The exact etiology of Alzheimer's disease is unknown. However, risk factors for Alzheimer's disease include advancing age, family history, and possibly head injury. Advancing age is a major risk factor for developing Alzheimer's disease. It is not a normal part of the aging process. After age 65, the risk of Alzheimer's disease doubles every 10 years. Children of a parent diagnosed

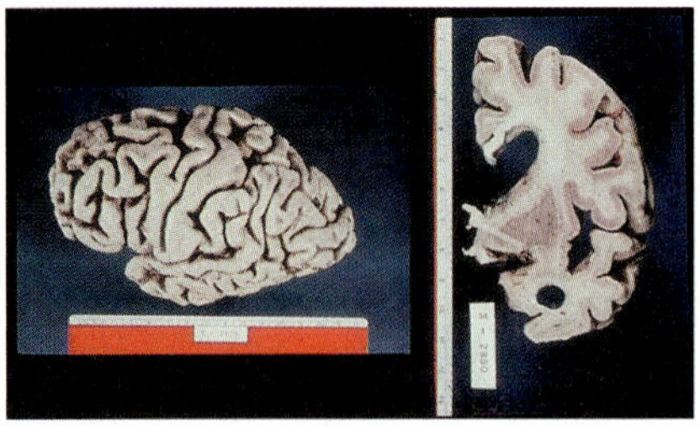

Figure 37-3 At autopsy, the cerebral cortex displays changes (white spots) caused by Alzheimer's disease (photo courtesy of the Alzheimer's Association).

with Alzheimer's disease have a 50 percent risk of developing the disease. Repeated head injury is thought to activate, by some unknown method, preexisting risk factors.

Pathophysiology

While the exact cause of Alzheimer's disease is unknown, there are many pathophysiological findings that are understood. Several important findings are known, but how they are related is not yet understood. These findings include:

- Neuronal degeneration in the hippocampus (causing memory loss) and cerebral cortex (causing speech, reasoning, and higher function loss) (Figure 37-3).
- Neuritic plaques are spherical bodies, composed of protein fragments and remnants of axons and dendrites, which form outside of the neurons. They are considered a hallmark sign of Alzheimer's disease.
- Neurofibrillary tangles occur inside the neurons, when the normal microtubular arrangement become disrupted (tangled). They are considered another diagnostic sign of Alzheimer's disease.

The presence of neurofibrillary tangles and neuritic plaques has been suggested as a possible pathological mechanism. Whether or not the neuronal death is caused by a direct toxic effect or by predisposing the cells to injury remains to be determined. Neurotransmitter systems, such as ACh, serotonin, and norepinephrine, diminish over the course of the disease. Many of the clinical manifestations are related to the reduction or loss of these neurotransmitters in the brain (Eggenberger & Nelms, 2004).

Assessment with Clinical Manifestations

Alzheimer's disease is classified into three stages based on progression of clinical manifestations (Table 37-12). Disease progression is highly variable and may not follow the model exactly. In the early stage, cognitive deficits may not be recognized, family and friends may begin to identify subtle changes in memory and personality, and patients and families may compensate for the deficits. In the middle stage, continuing changes in memory, orientation, speech, and ability to perform the activities of daily living, may put the patient at risk for injury.

In the late stage, the patient is completely dependent on others for care. Common complications of the late stage of Alzheimer's disease include pneumonia, malnutrition, falls, dehydration, depression, delusions, and paranoid reactions.

Diagnostic Tests

Alzheimer's disease is diagnosed by ruling out other possible causes for the patient's symptoms. Currently the only method that can conclusively diagnose Alzheimer's disease is by finding pathological changes in brain tissue obtained by biopsy or autopsy. A dementia workup includes evaluation for delirium, depression, infections, thyroid dysfunction, nutritional deficits, heart failure, chronic pulmonary disease, arrhythmias, pain, and trauma. Laboratory studies should include complete blood count (CBC), electrolytes, renal, thyroid, and liver panels, and urinalysis. EEG, MRI, MRS, computed tomography (CT), SPECT, and PET scans may help to rule out other causes (discussed in chapter 34). Serial testing of memory and cognitive skill can be accomplished by using the Mini-Mental State Examination (MMSE) or other similar testing methods. Final diagnosis requires presence of dementia, disease onset between the ages of 40 and 90 years, and absence of other systemic system or CNS diseases.

TABLE 37-12 Stages of Alzheimer's Disease

STAGE	TIMEFRAME	CLINICAL MANIFESTATIONS
Early	2–4 years	Forgetfulness; poor memory (may compensate by using notes)
		Declining interest in people, environment, and current events
		Impaired acquisition of new information
		Impaired judgment; mild cognitive changes
		Job performance declines; may lose job
		May be apathetic, irritable, or show signs of depression
		Normal EEG and CT
Middle	2–12 years	Progressive memory loss
		Disorientation to time, place, and events
		Impaired ability to follow simple directions or simple math
		Significant impairment of cognitive function and judgment
		Wanders at night due to sleep-wake cycle disturbance
		Neglects personal hygiene and activities of daily living
		Becomes increasingly irritable, evasive, and anxious
		May experience episodes of violent behavior
		EEG—slowing; CT—normal or dilated ventricles
Late	8–12 years	Extreme weight loss secondary to lack of eating
		Severe impairment of all cognitive functions
		Unable to communicate (verbal or written)
		Dependent on others for activities of daily living
		Incontinent of urine and feces
		Pathological reflexes can be elicited
		Motor skills are lost; becomes bedridden
		EEG—diffuse slowing
		CT—dilated ventricles and sulcal enlargement

Adapted from Larson, E., Shadlen, M., Wang, L., McCormick, W., Bowen, J., Teri, L., et al. (2004). Survival after initial diagnosis of Alzheimer's disease. Annals of Internal Medicine, 140*(7), 501–509.*

Nursing Diagnoses

Based on the information gathered, examples of nursing diagnoses in the patient with Alzheimer's disease may include the following:

- Self-care deficit related to inability to perform activities of daily living without assistance.
- Risk for injury related to impaired judgment, poor memory, and gait instability.
- Disturbed thought processes related to memory loss and cognitive deficits.
- Risk for ineffective coping related to disease progression.
- Impaired verbal communication related to cognitive decline.

Planning and Implementation

Because of the chronic progressive nature of Alzheimer's disease, a primary concern of the nurse caring for these patients is health teaching. In the early stages, the nurse needs to educate and support the patient and family as they adjust to the lifestyle changes that are required. Teaching should address the physical, emotional, and social aspects of the disease. In the beginning, actions and potential side effects of the medication regimen need to be taught, monitored, and adjusted to the desired patient response.

Nutrition is often a concern in patients with Alzheimer's disease. Muscle weakness and cognitive dysfunction may make ingestion of a healthy diet difficult. Weight needs to be monitored. Serial monitoring of serum albumin and proteins levels can identify patients at risk for malnutrition. Supplemental feedings may be required. For patients with swallowing difficulties strategies, such as smaller, more frequent meals, adding commercial powders to thicken liquids, and upright positioning, may be beneficial.

Exercise and physical therapy can help the patient to maximize function. Regular moderate exercise can reduce weakness and muscle atrophy. Working with a speech therapist can help the patient to maximize language and cognitive function. As the disease progresses, the patient and family will require more assistance with activities of daily living, emotional support, and potential financial concerns. Issues, such as admission to an extended care facility or hospice, need to be introduced early in the disease progression. This allows the patient to participate in the decision-making process.

Collaborative Management

The goal of collaborative management is to improve or slow the disease progression and maintain independent functioning for as long as possible. The health care team must work together with the patient and his or her caregiver(s) to support, educate, counsel, and provide strategies to assist with controlling the behavioral manifestations of the disease. Teaching for the patient and their family should include disease pathophysiology, medication actions and side effects, safety measures, and signs and symptoms of disease progression.

Pharmacology

Over the course of Alzheimer's disease there are many potential medications that a patient can be given. Cholinesterase inhibitors are given to enhance cognition and have a variety of successes in their treatment. In addition, a number of antidepressants may be given as the patients with Alzheimer's disease are often emotionally upset. There are even patients that have psychotic disturbances that can require medicinal therapy. A variety of medications can be given to patients with Alzheimer's disease. Examples are cholinesterase inhibitors to improve cognition (e.g., tacrine), serotonin reuptake inhibitors (e.g., citalopram, sertraline) to manage depression, tricyclic antidepressants (e.g., desipramine), and antipsychotics (e.g., haloperidol, risperidone) for the management of psychoses and behavioral disturbances.

Evaluation of Outcomes

Potential patient outcomes for each of the example nursing diagnoses for the patient with Alzheimer's disease are:

- Self-care deficit related to inability to perform activities of daily living. The patient will participate in self-care activities as much as possible.
- Risk for injury related to impaired judgment, poor memory, and gait instability. The patient will not experience injury.
- Disturbed thought process related to memory loss and cognitive deficits. The patient will maintain reality orientation and communicate clearly with others.

- Risk for ineffective coping related to disease progression. The family will acknowledge need for assistance.
- Impaired verbal communication related to cognitive decline. The patient will demonstrate improved ability to express self.

MYASTHENIA GRAVIS

Myasthenia gravis is a chronic, autoimmune, progressive neuromuscular disease characterized by abnormal weakness and fatigability of skeletal muscles. It is relatively rare compared to many of the other degenerative neurological disorders but is very affecting to those patients who contract the disease. It is typically a disorder that is not thought of when a patient first presents with clinical manifestations. Other diseases are ruled out, and then myasthenia gravis is confirmed by the history and physical, along with specific diagnostic tests that can be administered.

Epidemiology

Incidence rate is 5 per 100,000 people in the United States. More women than men (3:2) are diagnosed with myasthenia gravis. It can occur at any age but is most commonly seen between 10 and 65 years, with the peak age of onset between 20 and 30 years. Familial incidence is approximately 5 to 7 percent. Tumor of the thymus gland (thymoma) is present in up to 10 percent of myasthenia gravis patients. Thymoma is more common in patients over 30 years of age.

Etiology

Although the exact cause is unknown, it is believed to have an autoimmune etiology. Patients may seek health care providers for their fatigue and other somewhat vague symptoms, without suspecting a neurological disorder.

Pathophysiology

The autoimmune process destroys or blocks some of the ACh receptors at the postsynaptic muscle junction. There is a decrease in the number of available ACh receptor sites and concurrent structural change that diminishes ACh uptake. The end result is decreased strength of muscle contraction and with continued stimulation, profound fatigue. Usually the muscles innervated by the cranial nerves (face, lips, tongue, neck, and throat) are affected, but myasthenia gravis can affect any skeletal muscle group (Wakata, et al., 2004). There are three types of myasthenia gravis:

- Ocular—weakness of the eye and lid muscles only.
- Bulbar—involves breathing, swallowing, and speech (cranial nerves IX and XII) and.
- Generalized—involves the proximal muscles of the limbs and neck, usually with both ocular and bulbar manifestations.

Assessment with Clinical Manifestations

The onset of myasthenia gravis is usually gradual and extremely variable. The manifestations may fluctuate from hour to hour, from day to day, or over longer periods. They are made worse by exertion, exposure to temperature extremes, infections, menses, and excitement. Early findings in most patients are **ptosis** (drooping of eyelids) and **diplopia** (double vision). The ptosis may be unilateral or bilateral and becomes worse when the patient tries to look

> **Red Flag**
>
> **Administering the Tensilon Test**
>
> The Tensilon test is not without risk to the patient. The nurse should monitor the heart rate of all patients undergoing this testing. Special attention must be given to the older patient, especially those with a history of cardiac problems (those taking digoxin or beta blockers). Atropine should be immediately available to treat potential cardiac side effects.

upward. The diplopia may be unilateral or bilateral. Pupillary response to light and accommodation remain normal. This progresses to weakness of other muscles innervated by the cranial nerves results in loss of facial expression, a smile that resembles a snarl, jaw drop, nasal regurgitation of liquids, choking on foods and secretions, and slurred, nasal speech.

Next, the muscles of the neck and extremities are affected. Problems with fine motor movements of the hands may include changes in handwriting patterns, difficulty in combing hair, repetitive movements, climbing stairs, walking, or running. Proximal limb muscles are more often affected than the distal muscles. As the disease continues to progress, weakness and fatigue can affect all muscle groups (Wakata, et al., 2004).

Diagnostic Tests

Diagnostic tests for myasthenia gravis include:

- Serum assay for circulating ACh receptor antibodies. If increased, it is confirmation of myasthenia gravis with a sensitivity of 80 to 90 percent.
- Electromyography (EMG)—there is a reduced response to electrical stimulation when myasthenia gravis is present. Refer to chapter 34 for a full discussion of this test.
- CT or MRI may be ordered to determine if the thymus gland is abnormal. Refer to chapter 34 for a full discussion of these tests.
- Tensilon test—the patient is injected (intravenously) with edrophonium chloride (Tensilon), a short-acting anticholinesterase agent. In patients with myasthenia gravis the response is rapid improvement of manifestations within 15 to 30 seconds and lasting approximately five minutes.

Nursing Diagnoses

Based on the information gathered, examples of nursing diagnoses in the patient with myasthenia gravis may include the following:

- Ineffective breathing pattern related to weakness of chest muscles and fatigue.
- Ineffective airway clearance related to chest muscle weakness and impaired cough and gag.
- Impaired verbal communication related to weakness of lips, mouth, pharynx, jaw, and larynx.
- Imbalanced nutrition: less than body requirements related to muscle weakness and dysphagia.
- Activity intolerance related to muscle weakness and fatigue.

Planning and Implementation

There is no cure for myasthenia gravis. The goal of treatment in patients with myasthenia gravis is to improve their muscle weakness and induce remission with minimal side effects. Treatment modalities include medications, plasmapheresis, and surgery. The most common management technique is the administration of anticholinesterases and immunosuppressive medications.

Once the diagnosis of myasthenia gravis is confirmed, patient safety and health teaching by the nurse become the primary focus. The patient and his or her family need accurate information concerning the manifestations, etiology, and treatment of myasthenia gravis. The nurse needs to educate and support the patient and family as they adjust to the lifestyle changes that are required. Teaching should address the physical, emotional, and social aspects of the disease. Actions and potential side effects of the medication regimen need to be taught, monitored, and adjusted to the desired patient response. Medications that may interfere with neuromuscular function should be avoided.

Activities of daily living are often compromised by the generalized muscle weakness and fatigue in patients with myasthenia gravis. Once the nurse establishes a baseline of functioning level for the patient, frequent monitoring of activities and assisting as needed, helps the patient to maintain as near normal a lifestyle as possible. Rest is critical, and the nurse should teach energy conservation measures to maximize function.

Communication may become difficult for the patient with myasthenia gravis. Dysarthria and nasal speech result from weakness of the muscles involved in speech. The speech dysfunction may make communication with others difficult. Alternative forms of communication, such as using yes or no questions, flash cards, pencil and paper, eye blinking, or communication boards, may reduce the patient's frustration.

Exacerbations of myasthenia gravis may be related to stress, comorbid diseases, hormonal fluctuations, trauma, medications, or extreme temperatures. Frequent assessment of respiratory function is necessary. Increasing muscle weakness often affects swallowing and breathing. This can result in aspiration, inability to clear secretions, or respiratory insufficiency. With severe respiratory dysfunction, the patient may require intubation, ventilatory support, and admission to an intensive care unit. Other causes for respiratory dysfunction are myasthenic crisis (severe muscle weakness due to stress or medicine) and cholinergic crisis (excess ACh).

When patients experience myasthenic crisis, **plasmapheresis** (removal of serum antibodies) may be used to stabilize their disease. It may also be used as a short-term treatment before the patient is scheduled for thymectomy surgery. Plasmapheresis is usually done at the bedside with a blood cell separator machine. The procedure takes approximately three to five hours and is repeated every two to three days for two weeks. Temporary improvement in muscle strength is seen after the first treatment.

Nutrition

Nutrition is often a concern in patients with myasthenia gravis. Muscle weakness and decreased ability to chew or swallow can make ingestion of a healthy diet difficult. Weight needs to be monitored. Serial monitoring of serum albumin and proteins levels can identify patients at risk for malnutrition. For patients with swallowing difficulties, strategies such as smaller, more frequent meals, high calorie snacks, adding commercial powders to thicken liquids, and upright positioning may improve nutritional intake.

Pharmacology

Pharmacological therapies constitute the primary methods of treatment for myasthenia gravis. Anticholinesterase agents (e.g., Mestinon, Prostigmin) are the first medications used to treat myasthenia gravis. Mestinon prevents the inactivation of ACh and enhances the stimulus transmission at the cholinergic junctions. When patients do not respond well to Mestinon, immunosuppressive agents may be tried (e.g., immune globulin, prednisone, Imuran). Prednisone is the drug of choice. Improvement or remission is seen in 70 to 80 percent of patients treated with glucocorticosteroids. Several types of medications (e.g., neuromuscular blocking agents, antiarrhythmic agents, beta blockers, or antibiotics) may increase the weakness experienced in myasthenia gravis, so this should be evaluated by the nurse.

> **Red Flag**
>
> **Administration of Anticholinesterase Agents**
>
> Oral anticholinesterase agents must be administered on time or the patient may be too weak to swallow the pills. Mestinon's effect begins in 30 to 45 minutes, peaks in about two hours, and lasts three to six hours. The dosage schedule is usually individualized to produce maximal muscle strength for the patient.

Surgery

Surgical management for myasthenia gravis involves the removal of the thymus gland. For about 85 percent of patients with myasthenia gravis, surgery improves their clinical manifestations, and approximately 35 percent become drug free. Patients with pronounced respiratory weakness before surgery are at a higher risk for ventilator weaning difficulties after surgery.

Evaluation of Outcomes

Potential patient outcomes for each of the example nursing diagnoses for the patient with myasthenia gravis are:

- Ineffective breathing pattern related to weakness. The patient's breathing pattern is maintained as evidenced by eupnea, normal skin color, and regular respiratory rate and patterns.
- Ineffective airway clearance related to weakness, impaired cough, and impaired gag reflex. The patient will not experience aspiration.
- Impaired verbal communication related to muscle weakness. The patient will demonstrate improved ability to express self.
- Imbalanced nutrition: less than body requirements related to muscle weakness and dysphagia. The patient will ingest adequate nutrition.
- Activity intolerance related to muscle weakness and fatigue. The patient will identify methods to reduce activity intolerance.

AMYOTROPHIC LATERAL SCLEROSIS

Amyotrophic lateral sclerosis (ALS) is also called Lou Gehrig's disease, after the New York Yankee first baseman, who was diagnosed with the disease in 1939. ALS is a similar disorder to MS, but it is much faster in its progression, and its prognosis is much more severe.

Epidemiology

ALS is the most common motor neuron disease. Age of onset for the disease is between 40 and 60 years of age. It is more common in men than women by a ratio of 2:1. In the United States incidence is 5 per 100,000 people. Each year approximately 5,000 patients are diagnosed with the disease. There is an autosomal dominant component in 5 to 10 percent of all cases. ALS is a progressive disease that leads to death from respiratory arrest. Death usually occurs within 2 to 6 years.

Etiology

The exact cause of ALS is unknown. Several potential mechanisms have been suggested: a defect in glutamate metabolism, free radical damage, altered nucleic acid production by nerve fibers, and an autoimmune component. The excitotoxic hypothesis suggests that a defect in the metabolism, transport, and storage of glutamate (a neurotransmitter) may allow the toxic accumulation of glutamate to destroy the neurons. The second hypothesis states that accumulation of excess oxygen free radicals causes oxidative stress that destroys the motor neurons. The cytoskeletal hypothesis proposes that damage to the nerve fibers contributes to the motor neuron death. An autoimmune component has been reported in some patients. Current research focuses on identifying the disease mechanism and developing new treatments or potentially a cure in the future (Attarian, Vedel, Pouget, & Schmied, 2006).

Pathophysiology

ALS progressively demyelinates the motor neurons in the anterior horn of the spinal cord, brainstem, and cerebral cortex. It involves both upper and lower motor neurons. When upper motor function is lost, the affected muscles become spastic and weak, and deep tendon reflexes are increased. The loss of lower motor neuron innervation results in muscle flaccidity, weakness, atrophy, and paralysis. Intellectual ability, vision, hearing, and sensory function are not affected by the disease. Bowel and bladder function are usually spared until late in the disease (Attarian, et al., 2006).

Assessment with Clinical Manifestations

The initial manifestations of ALS can vary among patients, but usually weakness and wasting of the limbs are the first patient complaints. As the disease progresses other manifestations may be seen including:

- Muscle weakness, wasting, and atrophy, first in the hands, then in the shoulder and upper arm, and then in the lower limbs.
- Muscle spasticity and hyperreflexia.
- Muscle fasciculations (fine twitching).
- Atrophy of the tongue causing dysarthria and dysphagia.
- Dyspnea that can progress to respiratory failure.
- Fatigue.

Diagnostic Tests

There are no specific diagnostic studies or laboratory tests for confirmation of the diagnosis of ALS. An EMG may show abnormal electrical activity in the muscles. Nerve conduction studies may demonstrate abnormal responses to electrical stimuli. Muscle or nerve biopsy may demonstrate atrophy. CT, MRI, and EEG may be useful in ruling out other causes for the manifestations. A full discussion of these tests can be found on chapter 34.

Nursing Diagnoses

Based on the information gathered, examples of nursing diagnoses in the patient with ALS may include the following:

- Impaired mobility related to muscle wasting, weakness, and spasticity.
- Impaired communication related to impairment of the muscles of speech.
- High risk for aspiration related to impaired muscles of swallowing.
- Ineffective breathing pattern related to impaired muscles of breathing.

Red Flag

Locked-in Syndrome in ALS

The patient with ALS may develop locked-in syndrome as the disease progresses. Locked-in syndrome refers to a functional state where there is full consciousness and cognition, but severe paralysis makes communication and movement impossible. Lack of movement puts the patient at risk for complications, such as pressure sores, pneumonia, and sepsis. A regular schedule of preventive interventions needs to be implemented. Loss of the ability to speak can be devastating for the patient with intact cognition. A simple method of communication using eye blinking and vertical eye movements should be established. Currently there are computer-assisted methods of communication available. However, they are expensive and may pose a financial burden for the patient and his or her family.

Planning and Implementation

Because of the progressive, degenerative nature of ALS, the primary concern of the nurse caring for these patients is health teaching. In the early stages, the nurse needs to educate and support the patient and family as they adjust to the lifestyle changes that are required. Teaching should address the physical, emotional, and social aspects of the disease. The actions and potential side effects of the medication regimen need to be taught, monitored, and adjusted to the desired patient response.

Exercise and physical therapy can help the patient to maximize function. Regular moderate exercise can reduce stiffness and spasticity. Working with a speech therapist can help the patient to maximize language function. As the disease progresses, the patient and family will require more assistance with activities of daily living, emotional support, and potential financial concerns. Issues, such as admission to an extended care facility or hospice, need to be introduced early in the disease progression. This allows the patient to participate in the decision-making process.

End-of-life issues need to be discussed with the patient and their family, early in the disease progression. When the patient is unable to chew or swallow the insertion of a gastrostomy will help to prevent aspiration pneumonia. Loss of the patient's ability to protect their airway may require the insertion of a tracheostomy and chronic mechanical ventilation that alters the patient's quality of life. These decisions need to be addressed before an emergency situation occurs.

Collaborative Management

Currently there is no cure for this disease. Treatment is supportive and requires a multidisciplinary approach, including medications, therapy (physical, occupational, speech, nutrition), teaching, counseling, and support. Physical therapy should include a regular exercise regimen and supportive or assistive devices as needed. Occupational therapy can assist with adaptive devices to help with activities of daily living. Speech therapy can help the patient with improving or augmentation of altered speech patterns. Nutrition assessment and the eventual use of a gastrostomy tube for feeding may be necessary.

Nutrition

Nutrition is often a concern in patients with ALS. Muscle weakness, and decreased ability to chew or swallow can make ingestion of a healthy diet difficult. Weight needs to be monitored. Serial monitoring of serum albumin and proteins levels can identify patients at risk for malnutrition. Supplemental feedings and insertion of a feeding tube may be required. For patients with swallowing difficulties, strategies such as smaller, more frequent meals, adding commercial powders to thicken liquids, and upright positioning may be beneficial.

Pharmacology

Pharmacological management is used extensively in the treatment of ALS. Medications used for management of ALS include glutamate inhibitors (e.g., riluzole), benzodiazepines (e.g., diazepam), skeletal muscle relaxants (e.g., dantrolene), and antiarrhythmic agents (e.g., quinidine).

Evaluation of Outcomes

Potential patient outcomes for each of the example nursing diagnoses for the patient with ALS are:

- Impaired mobility related to muscle wasting, weakness, and spasticity. The patient will report increased strength and endurance.
- Impaired communication related to impairment of the muscles of speech. The patient will report improved ability to communicate.
- High risk for aspiration related to impaired muscles of swallowing. The patient will not experience aspiration.
- Ineffective breathing pattern related to impaired muscles of breathing. The patient's breathing pattern is maintained as evidenced by eupnea, normal skin color, and regular respiratory rate and patterns.

HUNTINGTON'S DISEASE (HUNTINGTON'S CHOREA)

Huntington's disease (also called Huntington's chorea) is a rare abnormal hereditary disorder of the CNS. It is characterized by chronic progressive **chorea** (involuntary purposeless, rapid movements) and mental deterioration that results in dementia.

Epidemiology

Men and women are affected equally, and the disease is more prevalent in patients of western European ancestry. The prevalence of Huntington's disease is estimated to be 5 to 10 per 100,000 people. In the United States, it is estimated that 30,000 individuals are affected and more than 125,000 at risk for developing the disease. The onset of Huntington's disease is usually between 30 and 50 years of age. Because of the late onset of the disease, transmission of the affected gene has often occurred years before the patient was diagnosed.

Etiology

Huntington's disease is genetic in its causation. This confirmed reason for Huntington's disease makes this a distinguishing characteristic among the other degenerative neurological diseases. More information regarding the genetic influences for Huntington's disease is enumerated in the Genetics section.

Pathophysiology

The pathological process of Huntington's disease is similar to Parkinson's disease. There is destruction of cells in the caudate nucleus and putamen areas of the basal ganglia and extrapyramidal motor system. Other areas of the brain may atrophy. The neurotransmitters, gamma-aminobutyric acid (GABA) and ACh are decreased. Dopamine is not affected, but the decrease of ACh causes a relative increase of dopamine in the basal ganglia. In Parkinson's the decreased dopamine causes slowing or loss of movement, but in Huntington's the excess dopamine causes uncontrolled movement.

Genetics

Huntington's disease is caused by autosomal dominant gene transmission. Offspring of a patient with Huntington's disease have a 50 percent chance of inheriting the gene. Identification of the gene responsible for Huntington's disease, which became available in 1993, allows the family members to be tested. This may be a difficult decision for the patient's family. If the test is positive, they will develop Huntington's disease. Family members who are asymptomatic may not want to know that they will develop the disease as they age (Etchegary, 2006).

Assessment with Clinical Manifestations

The hallmark clinical manifestations are intellectual decline and abnormal movements. Initially the patient may report feelings of restlessness, forgetfulness, clumsiness, frequent falls, and problems with speech, coordination, and balance. As the disease progresses, depression, memory loss, emotional lability, and impulsiveness may impair the patient's ability to work or maintain a normal routine. Motor manifestations include facial grimaces, protrusion of the tongue, jerky movements of the arms and legs, and gait disturbances. The gait changes put the patient at risk for falls. The disease progresses over a 10- to 20-year period until the patient is totally dependent. Death usually occurs because of aspiration pneumonia or sepsis.

Diagnostic Tests

Diagnosis of Huntington's disease involves a thorough history and physical examination. Genetic testing is done to identify the Huntington's trait. PET and SPECT studies may show evidence of decreased glucose metabolism. CT and MRI scans may identify gross wasting of the caudate nucleus and putamen and, in the late stages, atrophy of the lobes of the brain (Daniels, 2003). A full discussion of these tests can be found in chapter 34.

Nursing Diagnoses

Based on the information gathered, examples of nursing diagnoses in the patient with Huntington's disease may include the following:

- Risk for injury related to impaired motor function.
- Disturbed thought process: psychotic episodes related to lack of self-control and depression.
- Impaired nutrition: less than body requirements related to dysphagia.
- Impaired verbal communication related to cognitive deficits.
- Ineffective role performance related to disease process.

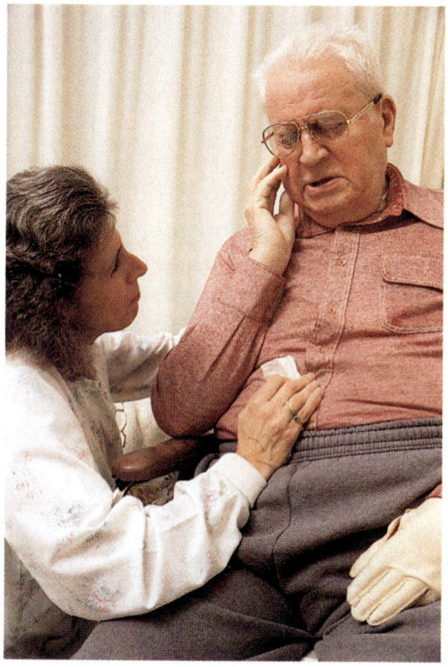

Figure 37-4 Nurse supporting and teaching patient with Huntington's disease in regard to the chronic debilitating nature of the disorder.

Planning and Implementation

There is no known cure for Huntington's disease at this time. Management is manifestation-based, supportive, and protective. Because of the chronic, progressive nature of Huntington's disease, the primary concern of the nursing caring for these patients is health teaching. In the early stages, the nurse needs to educate and support the patient and family as they adjust to the lifestyle changes that are required (Figure 37-4). Teaching should address the physical, emotional, genetic, and social aspects of the disease. The actions and potential side effects of the medication regimen need to be taught, monitored, and adjusted to the desired patient response.

Exercise and physical therapy can help the patient to maximize function. Regular moderate exercise can reduce stiffness and tremors. Working with a speech therapist can help the patient to maximize language and cognitive function. As the disease progresses, the patient and family will require more assistance with activities of daily living, emotional support, and potential financial concerns. Issues, such as admission to an extended care facility or hospice, need to be introduced early in the disease progression. This allows the patient to participate in the decision-making process.

Collaborative Management

Disease management includes rehabilitative therapy, teaching, counseling, and professional legal, financial, and estate planning advice. Support needs will increase as the patient's disease progresses. Families will require physical, emotional, and possible financial support, as a result of the patient's diagnosis.

Nutrition

Nutrition is often a concern in patients with Huntington's disease. Muscle weakness, tremor, and rigidity can make ingestion of a healthy diet difficult. Weight needs to be monitored. Serial monitoring of serum albumin and proteins levels can identify patients at risk for malnutrition. Supplemental feedings may be required. For patients with swallowing difficulties strategies, such as smaller, more frequent meals, adding commercial powders to thicken liquids, and upright positioning, may be beneficial.

Pharmacology

Pharmacological methods of treatment are carefully considered when treating Huntington's disease. Many medications can be used, and it is important to assess the combinations of medications that are used. Due to the organic nature of deterioration of the mental capabilities, there can be a tendency to overmedicate the patient with Huntington's disease. The care provider must assess the rationale for giving the medications and carefully administer these combinations of medication therapy. The common classifications of medications used in the treatment of Huntington's disease are shown in the Box 37-5.

BOX 37-5

MEDICATIONS ADMINISTERED TO MANAGE HUNTINGTON'S DISEASE

- Rilutek (riluzole) is currently being studied to decrease cognitive manifestations.
- Skeletal muscle relaxants to modify the choreiform movements.
- Antipsychotics to block the dopamine receptors in the brain.
- Antidepressants to help control the chorea, behavioral changes, and depression.

Evaluation of Outcomes

Potential patient outcomes for each of the example nursing diagnoses for the patient with Huntington's disease:

- Risk for injury related to impaired motor function. The patient will not experience injury.
- Disturbed thought process related to psychotic episodes. The patient will maintain reality orientation and communicate clearly with others.
- Impaired nutrition: less than body requirements related to dysphagia. The patient will ingest adequate nutrition.
- Impaired verbal communication related to cognitive deficits. The patient will demonstrate improved ability to express self.
- Ineffective role performance related to disease progression. The patient will demonstrate healthy adaptation and coping skills.

KEY CONCEPTS

- There is no known cure for chronic and degenerative neurologic diseases.
- Headache is the most common form of chronic pain.
- Types of headaches include tension-type, migraine, and cluster.
- Tension-type headache is caused by irritation of the pain-sensitive structures of the brain.
- Migraine is characterized by vasodilation of the dural blood vessels, resulting in stimulation of the trigeminal nerve pain pathways.
- Cluster headaches are believed to be a variant of migraine headaches.
- A seizure is a sudden, uncontrolled discharge of electricity in the brain.
- Seizures are divided into three major classes: partial, generalized, and unclassified.
- Generalized seizures originate in all of the regions of the brain cortex. There is no aura or warning, but there is loss of consciousness.
- Partial seizures begin in a specific brain region, and consciousness is usually not impaired.
- Status epilepticus is defined as either continuous seizures lasting more than five minutes on two or more different seizures with incomplete recovery of consciousness between them.
- MS is a chronic inflammatory disease of the CNS.
- There is no single diagnostic test that confirms or rules out the diagnosis of MS.
- Parkinson's disease is a slowly progressive degenerative neurological disorder caused by the loss of nerve cell function in the basal ganglia.
- Many of the secondary manifestations can be exaggerated by the medications used to treat Parkinson's disease.
- Alzheimer's disease is the most common cause of dementia in Western countries.
- Neuronal degeneration in the hippocampus and cerebral cortex, neurofibrillary tangles, and neuritic plaques have been suggested as a possible etiology of Alzheimer's disease.
- Myasthenia gravis is a chronic, autoimmune, progressive neuromuscular disease characterized by abnormal weakness and fatigability of skeletal muscles.
- ALS is a progressive disease that leads to death from respiratory arrest.
- Huntington's disease is characterized by chronic, progressive, involuntary, purposeless, rapid movements, and mental deterioration that results in dementia.
- Huntington's disease is caused by autosomal dominant gene transmission.

REVIEW QUESTIONS

1. A patient who has a migraine headache would be sensitive to:
   1. Touch
   2. Taste
   3. Humidity
   4. Sound

2. Nursing documentation of seizure activity should be:
   1. Brief and concise
   2. Highly descriptive and detailed
   3. In a flow sheet format
   4. Limited to the findings of the neurological examination

3. The teaching plan for a patient with epilepsy should include which of the following precautions?
   1. Warn your coworkers that you have a seizure disorder
   2. Wear a medical alert bracelet
   3. Lose weight to help control your seizures
   4. Avoid situations that are stressful

4. Eating which of the following food products is associated with migraine attacks?
   1. Dairy products
   2. Citrus juice
   3. Decaffeinated tea
   4. Coffee

5. Two distinguishing features of migraine are:
   1. Mood change and sharp pain between eyes
   2. Family history of headaches and headache-related disability
   3. Bilateral headache and rhinorrhea
   4. Insomnia and nausea

6. The most common sign or symptom reported by a patient with myasthenia gravis is:
   1. Early morning fatigability
   2. Pain that gets worse with position changes
   3. Weakness on exertion
   4. Fecal incontinence

Continued

REVIEW QUESTIONS—cont'd

7. Which of the following neurotransmitters is decreased in patients with Parkinson's disease?
   1. Acetylcholine
   2. Norepinephrine
   3. Serotonin
   4. Dopamine
8. Which of the following is the priority safety intervention when protecting the patient having a seizure?
   1. Placing a tongue blade between their teeth
   2. Ensure that the patient is restrained
   3. Position the patient to prevent aspiration of secretions
   4. Determine if the patient is incontinent
9. Which of the following drugs must be kept at the bedside of patient's with myasthenia gravis?
   1. Atropine
   2. Neostigmine
   3. Inderal
   4. Tensilon
10. An abnormal plantar reflex is commonly seen with:
    1. Cerebellar dysfunction
    2. Diffuse cerebral dysfunction
    3. Lower motor neuron lesions
    4. Upper motor neuron lesions
11. The brief sensory experience that occurs prior to the onset of seizure is called the:
    1. Prodromal phase
    2. Aura
    3. Epileptic cry
    4. Ictal phase

REVIEW ACTIVITIES

1. Discuss the differences in pathophysiology and treatment of tension-type, migraine, and cluster headaches.
2. Discuss the ethical issues related to withholding enteral feedings from a patient in a persistent vegetative state.
3. Describe the pathophysiology involved in the development of Parkinson's disease.
4. List four nursing interventions for the patient with myasthenia gravis and impaired swallowing.
5. Compare any three of the neurological degenerative disorders described in the chapter, as related to pathophysiology and clinical manifestations.

Visit the Contemporary Medical-Surgical Nursing online companion resource at www.delmarhealthcare.com for additional content and study aids. Click on Online Companions then select the Nursing discipline.

UNIT

VIII

Alterations in Sensory Function

Chapter 38 Assessment of Sensory Function

Chapter 39 Visual Dysfunction: Nursing Management

Chapter 40 Auditory Dysfunction: Nursing Management

CHAPTER

38

Assessment of Sensory Function

KEY TERMS

Arcus senilis
Auricle (pinna)
Cerumen
Consensual response
Corneal reflex
Direct response
Ectropion
Entropion
Esotropia
Eustachian tube
Exotropia
Labyrinth
Nystagmus
Ossicles
Otalgia
Otorrhea
Palpebrae
Papillary reflex
Ptosis
Strabismus (tropia)
Stye (hordeolum)
Xanthelasma

Crisamar J. Anunciado, MSN, FNP, RN

CHAPTER TOPICS

- Anatomy and Physiology of the Eye
- Assessment of the Eye
- Anatomy and Physiology of the Ear
- Assessment of the Ear

The visual and auditory senses have profound relationships to the function of the human body. The eyes are the windows to the soul is an often-quoted adage. It is through vision that an individual experiences the world around him or her. The ears provide senses for the person to have an awareness of his or her environment and an interpretation of the stimuli surrounding him or her. Both of these sensory organ systems are integral to the function and well-being of a person. When either or both of these organ systems have disorders, the person is affected greatly and can require assistance of many types from his or her health care providers.

In this section of this chapter, there will be a discussion of the anatomy and physiology of the eye, as well as important assessment components for a thorough assessment. This includes (a) review of related history, (b) test for visual acuity, (c) evaluation of visual fields, (d) testing ocular movements, (e) testing of cranial nerve reflexes, (f) external eye examination, and (g) ophthalmoscopic examination.

ANATOMY AND PHYSIOLOGY OF THE EYE

Disorders in vision may interfere with the individual's ability to function independently and affect his or her quality of life. The eyes are sensory organs, which receive visual stimuli that are transmitted to the brain for interpretation through the cranial nerve (optic nerve II). Approximately 70 percent of all sensory information reaches the brain through the eyes (Estes, 2006).

A thorough assessment of the eyes will reveal both local and systemic health, which in many cases may help the clinician identify eye and vision problems. It is important to note that the leading causes of blindness include diabetic retinopathy, glaucoma, cataracts, and age-related macular degeneration (Watkinson, 2005). Routine assessment of the eyes may help detect these and other problems early and prevent progression of these diseases that lead to vision problems and even blindness.

The structures and function of the eye are complex yet well understood. In this section are the identified anatomical structures of the eye. In addition, the physiology of each structural component of the eye is provided.

External Eye

The external eye comprises the orbital cavity, eyelashes, eyelids, extraocular muscles, lacrimal gland, and conjunctiva. The eye is an intricate body part and obviously vital to many functions in life.

Because the eyes are delicate organs, many protective structures surround it. The external parts of the eyes are protected from trauma by the bony structure of the orbital cavity. The eyelashes extend across the eyelids to protect the eyes from dust and foreign bodies. The eyelids **(palpebrae)** protect the eyes by covering the anterior aspect of the eyes, distributing tears and lubricating the eyes, protecting the eyes from foreign bodies, and limiting the amount of light that enters the eyes (Estes, 2006).

There are six extraocular muscles that hold the eyes stably in place and control eye movement (Figure 38-1). This includes two oblique muscles and four rectus muscles. These extraocular muscles are innervated by three cranial nerves, namely, oculomotor (cranial nerve III), trochlear (cranial nerve IV), and abducens (cranial nerve VI).

The lacrimal gland is part of the lacrimal apparatus. It is located in the temporal region of the superior eyelid. It moistens the eyes by producing and distributing tears across the conjunctiva and cornea.

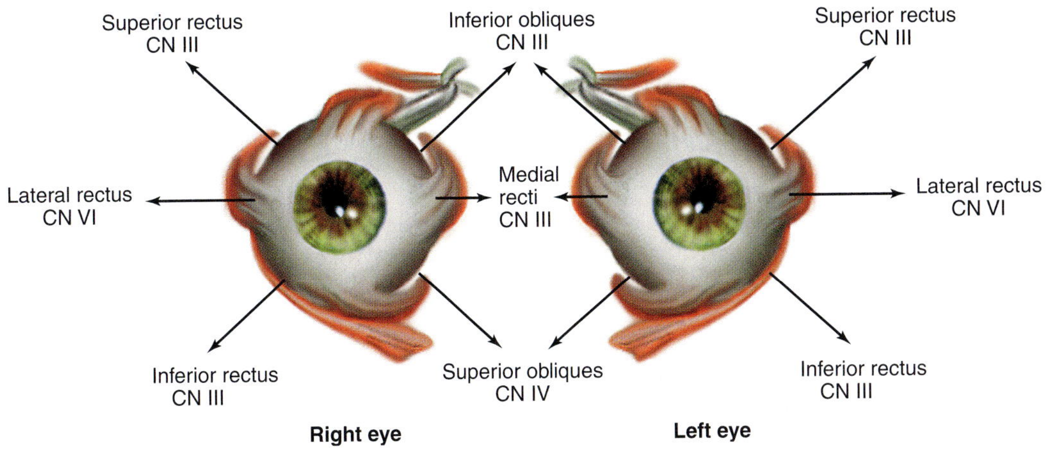

Figure 38-1 Direction of movement of extraocular muscles.

The conjunctiva is the uppermost layer that lines the eyelids and the anterior portion of the eyeball. This is divided into two portions: (a) the palpebral conjunctiva lines the eyelids, and (b) the bulbar conjunctiva covers the sclera. The conjunctiva protects the eyes from injury because of foreign bodies and desiccation.

Internal Eye

There are three coats, or tunics, comprising the internal structures of the eyes: (a) the outer fibrous coat include the sclera and the cornea; (b) the middle tunic includes the choroids, ciliary body, and iris; and (c) the inner nervous tunic is comprised of the retina and its structures.

The sclera appears as the white of the eye. It is a dense, avascular structure that supports the internal structure of the eye, maintaining its size and shape. The cornea is a smooth, avascular, and transparent tissue that is continuous with the sclera, replacing the sclera over the iris and the pupil. It separates the fluid in the aqueous chamber (anterior chamber) from the external environment. It retracts and permits light rays entering the eye through the lens to the retina. It has sensory innervation for pain as it is fed by the trigeminal nerve (cranial nerve V). Stimulation of this nerve causes the **corneal reflex,** a protective blink (Estes, 2006).

The choroids, located posteriorly, and ciliary body, located anteriorly near the iris, comprise the middle layers of the eye. The choroid contains small arteries and veins that provide blood supply to the eye (Estes, 2006). The iris is a circular, pigmented, and contractile muscular disc located at the center of the eye in front of the lens and behind the aqueous humor. The actions of the dilator and sphincter muscles of the iris, through the pupil as its central aperture, control the amount of light reaching the retina. This muscular activity is controlled by the parasympathetic (causes constriction) and sympathetic (causes dilation) nervous system. The **papillary reflex** causing direct and consensual reactions occur because of light stimulation. The optic nerve (cranial nerve II) transmits the stimulation to the brain, and the oculomotor nerve (cranial nerve III) transmits the reflex from the brain to both eyes. The lens is located immediately behind the iris at the papillary opening. It contains no blood vessels, nerves, or connective tissue. It is composed of transparent elastic fibers within the lens capsule. Contraction, or relaxation, of the ciliary bodies attached to the lens changes its thickness, thereby causing the lens to focus and refract light onto the retina (Estes, 2006).

The anterior chamber is located directly behind the cornea. It is filled with a clear, watery substance called aqueous humor, which is continuously produced by the ciliary body and drained through the Schlemm's canal. The movement of fluid in the anterior chamber maintains intraocular pressure of about 15 mm Hg $\pm$ 3 mm Hg. The vitreous humor is a clear gelatinous substance located between the lens and the retina in the posterior chamber of the eye. It maintains the placement of the retina and its structures, as well as the shape of the eyeball (Estes, 2006). The retina is the innermost coat of the eyeball. It is the sensory network of the eye, receiving visual stimuli, and transmitting images to the brain from the optic disc, traveling via the optic nerve, through the optic tract, and then through the optic radiation for processing in the visual cortex (Estes, 2006). Blood circulation is provided by four sets of vessels stemming for the optic disc and extending outward; they are: (a) superior nasal, (b) inferior nasal, (c) superior temporal, and (d) inferior temporal (Estes, 2006). The macula or fovea is the site for central vision and color perception. Other neurosensory elements located in the retina are the rods, which mediate black and white vision, and cones, which mediate color vision.

ASSESSMENT OF THE EYE

Assessment of the eye by necessity includes the need for obtaining a thorough health assessment. This health history will include such things as the present history of the current eye problem, as well as the past history of the eye. In addition, the family history and personal and social history is essential as well.

Present Eye Problem

The nurse should ask the patient a variety of questions that address the current condition of his or her eye disorders or disease (see Patient Playbook).

> PATIENT PLAYBOOK
>
> **Obtaining a History of Eye Disorders**
>
> The nurse can ask the patient the following types of questions:
>
> - Is there any presence of unilateral or bilateral eyelid involvement causing vision impairment (e.g., hordeola or **ptosis** [drooping of the eye])?
> - Is there difficulty with vision with one or both eyes? Use of corrective lenses? Description of what type vision impairment, near or distant vision, presence of halos around lights, diplopia, cataract, and floaters.
> - Are you having any pain? The nurse can use OLDCART as an acronym for assessing pain in the eye. O = Onset (when did the pain start?), L = Location (identify location of pain, e.g., outside or inside the eye), D = Duration (how long has the pain been going on? Is it continuous or intermittent?), C = Characteristics (what type of pain is it, e.g. sharp, dull, superficial, deep, burning itching?) A = Aggravating factors (what makes it worse?), R = Relieving factors (what makes it better?), and T = Treatment (any treatment done? If so, what type?).
> - Do you have any secretions coming from your eye? (e.g., color [clear or yellow], consistency [watery, creamy, or foamy], presence or absence of tears, and conjunctival redness).
>
> *Adapted from Estes, M. (2006).* Health assessment and physical examination *(3rd ed.). New York: Thomson Delmar Learning; Hoyt, K. S., & Haley, R. J. (2005). Innovations in advanced practice: Assessment and management of eye emergencies.* Topics in Emergency Medicine, 27(2), *101–117.*

Past Medical History

In addition, to the current status of the eye, the nurse must gather information regarding the previous medical history specific to the eye. There are several areas of concern as demonstrated in Box 38-1.

Family History

It is important to determine what types of genetic disorders potentially influence the eyes of the patient. Some of these disorders are listed in Box 38-2.

Personal and Social History

A personal and social history may influence the function of the eyes. Therefore, the nurse must gather information specific to these areas of their patient's condition. The following are areas for the nurse to focus on:

- Employment and history of eye exposure to environment irritants.
- Activities that may cause harm to the eye (e.g., smoking, contact sport, fencing, squash, or motorcycle riding).
- Allergies including which type if it is seasonal, perennial, and other associated symptoms.
- Corrective lenses including which type, duration of use, adequacy of correction, and date of late eye exam.
- Use of protective devices at work, sports, or other activities, which may endanger the eye.

Examination and Findings

Systematic eye assessment includes inspecting and palpating the appendages or extraocular structures surrounding the eye to include the eyebrows and surrounding tissues, then moving inward to test for visual acuity, assessing extraocular eye muscle movement, and lastly, performing an ophthalmoscopic examination of the intraocular structures. The equipment the nurse needs to examine the eye is: cotton wisp, eye cover, ophthalmoscope, penlight, Rosenbaum near vision card, and a Snellen chart.

Inspection and palpation of the eye includes the following examination components: (a) testing for visual acuity; (b) inspection and palpation of external ocular structures; (c) testing for visual fields; (d) testing for extraocular muscle function; and (e) ophthalmoscopic examination.

Visual Acuity

Begin eye assessment by testing for visual acuity. Visual acuity testing is the test of central vision assessing the eye's ability to distinguish small and specific details, using the smallest identifiable object that can be seen at a specific distance

> **BOX 38-1**
>
> **HISTORY OF THE EYE**
>
> - History of any trauma or injury to the eye as a whole or specific structure or supporting structure of the eye, description of event surrounding the injury, and attempts at correction and degree of success.
> - History of any eye surgery, when it was done, why it was done, and what was the outcome.
> - Other chronic illness, which may affect vision (e.g., diabetes, glaucoma, or hypertension)
>
> *Adapted from Estes, M. (2006).* Health assessment and physical examination *(3rd ed.). New York: Thomson Delmar Learning; Kuehn, B. M. (2005). Inflammation suspected in eye disorders.* Journal of the American Medical Association, *294(1), 31–32.*

> **BOX 38-2**
>
> **EYE DISORDERS**
>
> - Any type of eye cancer (e.g., retinoblastoma)
> - Cataracts, diabetes, macular degeneration, color blindness, allergies affecting the eye, and other types of illness that may affect vision
> - Strabismus, myopia, and hyperopia, which are disorders of eye refraction

(usually 20 feet using the Snellen's chart or 16 inches using the Rosenbaum near vision card).

Using the Snellen's chart, have the patient stand 20 feet away from the chart. Make sure the room is well-lit. Test each eye individually by covering one eye at a time with gauze or eye cover. Avoid applying pressure to the covered eye. If testing with and without corrective lenses, test without corrective lenses first. With one eye covered, have the patient read the letters on one line moving progressively downward to increasingly smaller lines until the patient could no longer discern all the letters. Record the corresponding visual acuity designated for that line. Repeat test on the second eye and cover the first eye. Record visual acuity findings and analyze results. A measurement of 20/20 vision indicates normal visual acuity. The higher the number to the right of the line, the worse the vision (e.g., 20/100 is worse than 20/60).

If a Snellen's chart is not available, a Rosenbaum near vision chart may be used. Have the patient hold the card at a comfortable distance of about 14 to 16 inches away from his or her face. Test one eye at a time by covering one eye with an eye cover or gauze. Ask the patient to read the letters of the smallest line possible. Record findings and analyze data.

Visual Field Confrontation Test

A visual field confrontation test is used to grossly assess peripheral vision. The nurses uses his or her own normal visual fields to compare with the patient's visual fields. Sit or stand opposite the patient at eye level, about two feet away. Ask the patient to cover the left eye as the nurse covers his or her right eye, which is directly opposite the patient's covered left eye. Then stare at each other's uncovered eye. The nurse extends his or her arm midway between himself or herself and the patient. The nurse holds a small object in his or her hand, such as a pen or penlight, and gradually brings this object centrally from eight different directions: right, left, above, below, and midpoints between these directions. The patient tells the nurse each time when he or she sees the object. The nurse and patient should be able to see the object entering the field of vision at the same time. Repeat this test with the other eye. The confrontation test is crude and imprecise. It can only be considered significant if it is abnormal. For more accurate visual field testing, refer the patient to an eye specialist (Estes, 2006).

Test for Color Vision

Color vision testing of the eyes may be done using color plates or an Ishihara chart, which are available in numerals produced in primary colors (Estes, 2006). When the patient identifies all the colors on six plates, the patient has normal color vision. Red green color blindness is a genetic disease that occurs in men, almost exclusively. Other diseases may also cause color blindness, such as macular degeneration, nutritional deficiency, or pathology of the fovea centralis. For routine color vision testing, check the patient's ability to identify or appreciate primary colors (McCullough, 2005).

Extraocular Eye Examination

The nurse must assess and evaluate the patient's extraocular eye in regard to the location, eyebrows, extraocular structures, eyelids, conjunctiva, cornea, iris, and pupil. Begin the assessment by observing the placement of the eyes in relation to the patient's face. The eyes should be location a third of the way down from the scalp line and approximately one eye's width apart. Inspect the patient's eyebrows. Note their size, shape, extension, and hair texture. If the eyebrow hair is usually coarse or does not extend to the temporal canthus, suspect hypothyroidism. Inspect the surrounding orbital tissue for signs of flakiness, edema (periorbital edema is an abnormal finding possibly due to hypothyroidism or the presence of renal disease), redness (may be a sign of infection or irritation), and puffiness, which may indicate allergies. In addition

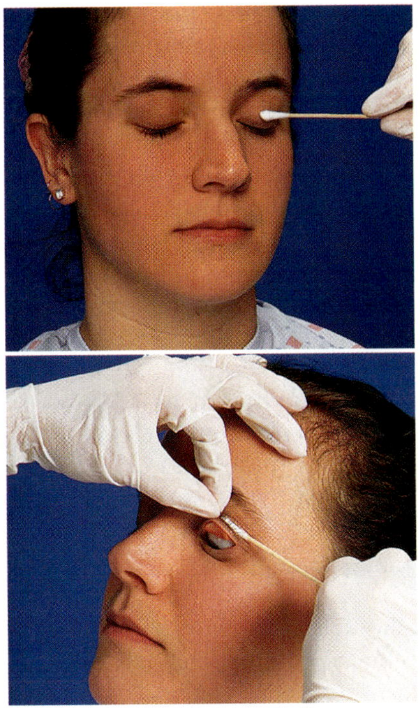

Figure 38-2 Assessing palpebral conjunctiva.

there may be lesions; such as **xanthelasma** (a yellow, lipid-rich plaque present on the eyelids), a **stye** or **hordeolum** (a localized inflammatory swelling of one or more of the glands of the eyelid), or sagging tissue below the orbit, which results from excessive tissue under the eyelid that may cause incomplete eyelid closure. To assess the eyelids, note the position of the globe of the eye (normal, prominent, or sunken). When the eye is open, the upper eyelids should partially cover part of the iris but not the pupil itself. If one eyelid covers the iris more than the other eyelid, consider ptosis, caused by a weakness of the levator muscle or paralysis of the oculomotor nerve (cranial nerve III). Observe the eyelids for excessive tearing or drying. The eyelashes should be turned upward and the eyelid margins should be pink. Also inspect the eyelids for inversion (when the lower lid is turned in toward the globe of the eye), called **entropion** or eversion (when the lower lid is turned away from the globe of the eye called **ectropion**).

Inspect both the bulbar and palpebral conjunctiva. To inspect the bulbar conjunctivae, gently pull the upper and lower eyelids apart without applying pressure to the globe of the eye. Ask the patient to look up, down, and to each side. The bulbar conjunctiva should be clear and free of erythema. Redness or erythema and the presence of cobblestone appearance may indicate allergies or infection (conjunctivitis). A common condition, called pterygium, is an abnormal growth of the conjunctiva extending over the cornea. It may interfere with vision if it crosses over the pupil. Inspect the palpebral conjunctivae (Figure 38-2). Ask the patient to look down. Lift the upper eyelids by holding the eyelashes against the eyebrows. The palpebral conjunctivae should be pink in appearance for Caucasians, red-orange in color for African Americans, and yellow-orange in color for Asian (Americans). Inspect the lid for color changes, erythema, edema, exudates, or foreign bodies (Estes, 2006).

Examine the cornea by shining a penlight tangentially (from both outer sides of the eye) and then directly into the cornea. The cornea should appear clear with no lesions. Test for corneal sensitivity, the trigeminal nerve (cranial nerve V), by touching a wisp of cotton on the cornea. The normal response is a blink, which indicates intact sensory and motor fibers trigeminal and facial nerve (cranial nerve VII), respectively. A condition called **arcus senilis** (lipid deposition on the periphery of the cornea) may be present in patients over the age of 60. This may indicate lipid disorder especially if it appears at a younger age.

Examine the iris pattern (it should be clear and flat), shape (round), size (regular and equal), and color bilaterally. In the presence of excessive pressure caused by acute-angle glaucoma, the iris may be pushed forward, causing the anterior chamber to appear small.

The nurse should test for direct and consensual pupillary response. Dim the lights in the examination room to allow the pupils to dilate. Shine the penlight (20 inches away) directly into one eye. Observe for pupillary constriction on the pupil being tested **(direct response)** and observe for pupillary constriction on the opposite pupil **(consensual response).** Pupillary constriction should be equal and simultaneous in both eyes. Note any inequality and sluggishness of response. Repeat the test on the other pupil. Test the pupils for accommodation by placing your finger approximately four inches from the bridge of the patient's nose. Ask the patient to look at a fixed object in the distance and then look at the nurse's finger. The patient's pupils should constrict when his or her eyes focus on the nurse's finger.

Extraocular Eye Muscle Movement

Assess for intact oculomotor (cranial nerve III), trochlear (cranial nerve IV), abducens (cranial nerve VI) nerves, and the six extraocular muscles (Miller & Newman, 2004). Test for the cardinal fields of gaze (Figure 38-3). Hold the patient's chin to stabilize the head and prevent movement. The nurse asks the patient to watch his or her finger as it moves through the six cardinal fields of gaze. Then he or she asks the patient to look to the extreme lateral or temporal

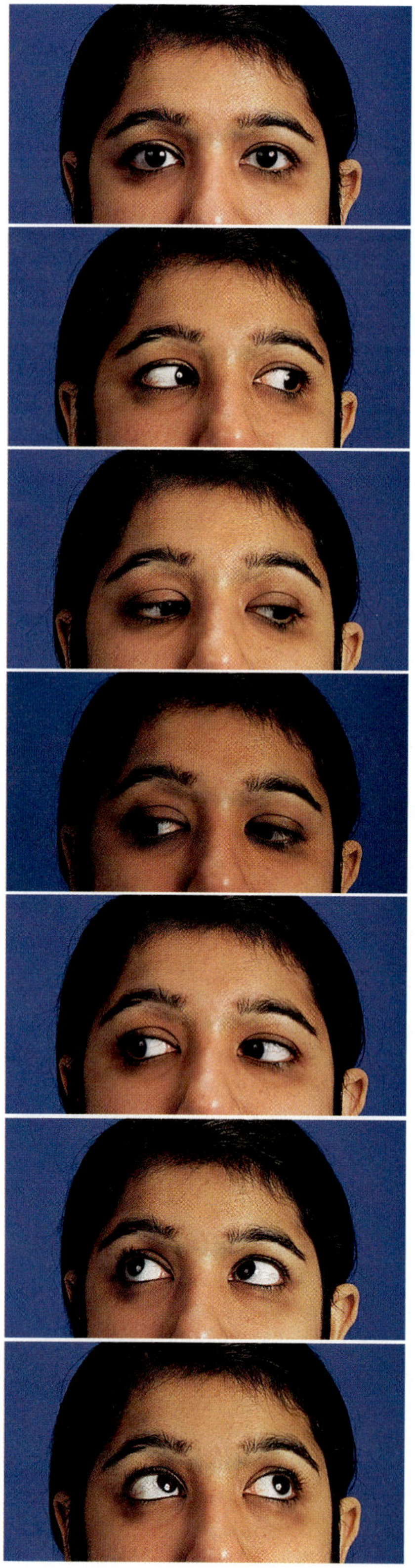

Figure 38-3 Cardinal fields of gaze.

field. Note any oscillating movement or back and forth movements of the eye, which is called **nystagmus.** A slight movement or nystagmus may present in the lateral gaze, but it is abnormal in any other fields of gaze.

Assess for corneal light reflex or Hirschberg test. Ask the patient to focus his or her gaze on a nearby object. Shine a penlight on the bridge of the patient's nose from about one foot away. Light should fall on the same place on the cornea bilaterally. If it does not, the patient may lack extraocular muscle coordination, which may be because of a condition called **strabismus (tropia)** (Estes, 2006).

Perform the cover, uncover test. You only perform this test when an abnormality is detected on one of the two previous tests. Ask the patient to look straight ahead at an object. Cover one eye with the eye cover. Observe the uncovered eye for any movement as it focuses on the object. Then, remove the cover on the other eye and observe any movement on this eye as it focuses on the object. Repeat this test on the other eye. Movement on the covered or uncovered eye may indicate convergent strabismus **(esotropia)** or divergent strabismus **(exotropia).**

Ophthalmoscopic Examination

An ophthalmoscopic examination can be helpful in identifying pathologies of the eye (Figure 38-4). This section describes the specific assessment techniques when using the ophthalmoscope.

Posterior Segment Structures

The funduscopic assessment (CN II) requires the use of a direct ophthalmoscope to assess the structures in the posterior segment of the eye. The ophthalmoscope consists of two parts: the head and the handle. To activate the light source in the head, depress the rheostat button and move it as far as possible. Move the aperture selector to produce the largest beam of light that can be visualized by focusing the beam of light on the palm of the hand. The larger beam is preferred when assessing an average-sized pupil, and the smaller beam makes assessment of a smaller pupil easier. Table 38-1 lists the various apertures of the ophthalmoscope and their uses. The lens selector allows you to choose lenses of varying power for different parts of the assessment. These lenses are marked with red and black numbers, signifying different focal lengths. The 0 lens sits between the red- and black-numbered lenses and has no correction. In some ophthalmoscopes, there is no color designation (red or black) and the lens power is signified by + or − signs in front of the numbers. A + sign is equivalent to black and focuses closer to the ophthalmoscope; a − sign is equivalent to red and focuses further from the instrument. These lenses compensate for the refractive error of both the patient and the nurse.

TABLE 38-1 Apertures of the Ophthalmoscope

○	Small round light	Used to examine eyes with small, undilated pupils
◯	Large round light	Used for routine eye examinations and examination of dilated eyes
▦	Grid	Used to assess size and location of funduscopic lesions
▯	Slit light	Assesses anterior eye and determines elevation of funduscopic lesions
●	Green light (red-free filter)	Used to assess retinal hemorrhages (which appear black) and small vessel changes

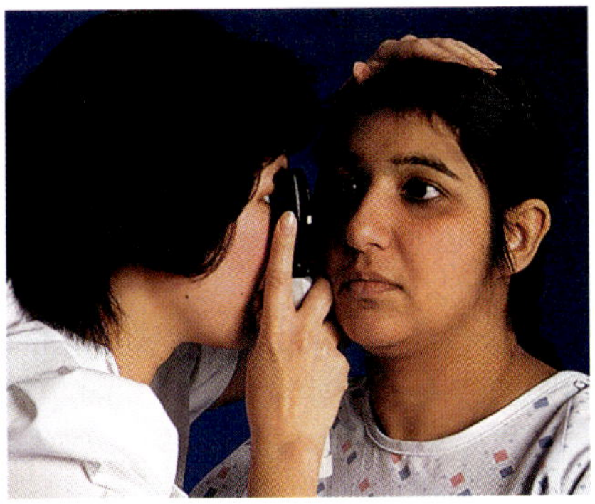

Figure 38-4 Examining with ophthalmoscope.

Retinal Structures

In a darkened room, ask the patient to remove eyeglasses; contact lenses may be left in place.

1. Instruct the patient to look at a distant object across the room. This will help to dilate the eyes.
2. Set the ophthalmoscope on the 0 lens and hold it in front of your right eye with your index finger on the lens selector.
3. From a distance of 8 to 12 inches from the patient and about 15° to the lateral side, shine the light into the patient's right pupil, eliciting a light reflection from the retina; this is called the red reflex.
4. While maintaining the red reflex in view, move closer to the patient and move the lens selector from 0 to the + or black numbers in order to focus on the anterior ocular structures.
5. For optimum visualization, keep the ophthalmoscope within an inch of the patient's eye.
6. At this point, move the lens selector from the + or black numbers, through 0, and into the − or red numbers in order to focus on structures progressively more posterior.
7. Focus on the optic disc at the nasal side of the retina by following any retinal vessels centrally (Figure 38-5).
8. You may need to reverse direction along the vessel if the disc does not appear.
9. Observe the retina for color and lesions, the retinal vessels for configuration and characteristics of their crossing, and the optic disc for color, shape, size, margins, and comparison of cup-to-disc ratio.
10. Describe the size, position, and location of any abnormality. Use the diameter of the disc (DD) as a guide to describe the distance of the abnormality from the optic disc. Use the optic disc as a clock face as a reference point to describe the location of the abnormality. Describe the size of the abnormality in relation to the size of the optic disc.
11. Repeat on the left eye.

Refer to Table 38-2. The red reflex is present. The optic disc is pinkish orange in color, with a yellow-white excavated center known as the physiological cup. The ratio of the cup diameter to that of the entire disc is 1:3. The border of the disc may range from a sharp, round demarcation from the surrounding retina to a more blended border but should be on the same plane as the retina. In general, there are four main vascular branches emanating from the disc, each branch consisting of an arteriole and a venule. The venules are approximately four times the size of the accompanying arterioles and are darker in color. Light

Skills 360°

Developing Skill with an Ophthalmoscope

The nurse practitioner student informs his preceptor that he is having difficulty using an ophthalmoscope. When he shined the light on the last patient's eyes, the appearance was more white than red. He asks you to help him improve his technique. How would you respond to the student?

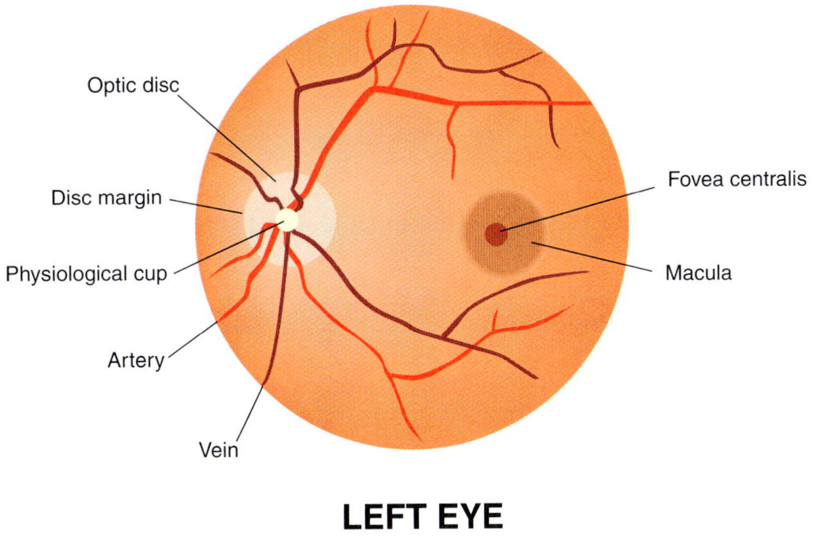

Figure 38-5 Optic disk.

TABLE 38-2 Retinal Color Variations

FINDINGS	CHARACTERISTICS
Fair-skinned individual	Retina appears a lighter red-orange color Tessellated appearance of the fundi (pigment does not obscure the choroid vessels)
Dark-skinned individual	Fundi appear darker in color; grayish purple to brownish (from increased pigment in the choroid and retina) No tessellated appearance Choroidal vessels usually obscured
Aging individual	Vessels are straighter and narrower Choroidal vessels are easily visualized Retinal pigment epithelium atrophies and causes the retinal color to become paler

often produces a glistening "light reflex" from the arteriolar vessel. Normal arterial-to-venous width is a ratio of 2:3 or 4:5.

The red reflex is absent.

The presence of cataracts can prevent the red reflex from being observed due to the opacity of the lens.

The red reflex is absent and the pupil appears white.

Leukocoria, or white reflex, is found in retinoblastoma, congenital cataracts, and retinal detachment. This is often referred to as the cat's eye reflex.

The optic disc is pale.

Pallor is due to optic atrophy caused by increased intracranial pressure or from congenital syphilis; an intracranial space-occupying lesion, for example, meningioma; or end-stage glaucoma.

Optic atrophy is abnormal.

Optic atrophy occurs in retinitis pigmentosa. Arteriole narrowing and "bone spicule" are also noted on the fundus. There is a loss of central or peripheral vision, night blindness, and glare sensitivity in this familial condition.

The physiological cup exceeds the normal 1:3 ratio. The disc appears elevated above the plane of the surrounding retina.

Disc edema and loss of vision are caused by the papillitis resulting from optic neuritis. The disc is hyperemic, the margins are blurred, and the disc surface is elevated.

Disc edema and an elevated disc without loss of vision are found in papilledema, which is caused by increased intracranial pressure obstructing return blood flow from the eye. This is also called a "choked disc."

Glaucomatous cupping occurs due to increased intraocular pressure. The physiological cup is enlarged and may extend to the edge of the optic disc. Blood vessels are displaced nasally.

The normal white stripe of retinal arteries appears instead as a copper-colored stripe.

This is the copper wire appearance of retinal arteries characteristic of hypertensive changes.

At the crossing of retinal arteries over veins, the vein is not seen on either side of the overlying artery.

This finding is arteriovenous (A-V) nicking, a sign of retinal arteriolar sclerosis that occurs as the walls become thickened and obscure portions of the veins that lie underneath. This can also occur in hypertension.

Superficial retinal hemorrhages are flame-shaped hemorrhages found in the fundi or they may appear as red hemorrhages with white centers called Roth's spots. These hemorrhages form a pattern related to the nerve fibers that radiate from the optic disc.

These hemorrhages may be due to severe hypertension, occlusion of the central retinal vein, and papilledema. Roth's spots are sometimes associated with infective endocarditis.

Deep retinal hemorrhages, or dot hemorrhages, appear as small red dots or irregular spots in the deep layer of the retina.

Deep retinal hemorrhages can be associated with diabetes mellitus.

Diffuse preretinal hemorrhages occur in the small space between the vitreous and the retina.

Preretinal hemorrhages may occur in conjunction with a sudden increase in intracranial pressure.

Microaneurysms are tiny, round, red dots that can be seen in peripheral and macular areas of the retina.

These dots are small retinal vessels that dilate in diabetic retinopathy.

Neovascularization is the formation of new vessels that are very narrow and disorderly in appearance and may extend into the vitreous. These vessels may bleed, resulting in a loss of vision.

Neovascularization occurs in proliferative diabetic retinopathy.

Fluffy white or gray slightly irregular areas that appear on the retina and are ovoid in shape are abnormal.

Cotton wool spots represent microscopic infarcts of the nerve fiber layer and are due to diabetic or hypertensive retinopathy.

Drusen are small white dots in the fundus that are arranged in an irregular pattern. They may also occur on the optic disc, and may become shiny with calcification.

Drusen are findings of the normal aging process. They may cause loss of vision if they occur in the macular region.

Hard exudates are yellow with distinct borders, and are small unless they coalesce. They are arranged in round, linear, or star-shaped patterns.

Hard exudates are associated with diabetes mellitus or hypertension.

A cleft defect of the choroid and retina is abnormal. The size ranges from medium to large.

Coloboma is a congenital abnormality.

The red-orange retinal reflex is absent in the area of a retinal detachment. The area appears pearly gray and is elevated and wrinkled.

A detached retina may be associated with severe myopia, cataract surgery, or diabetic retinopathy, or it may be caused by trauma.

Fibrous white bands that obscure the retinal vessels are abnormal. Neovascularization may also be present.

These findings occur in proliferative diabetic retinopathy

Red Flag

Night Driving

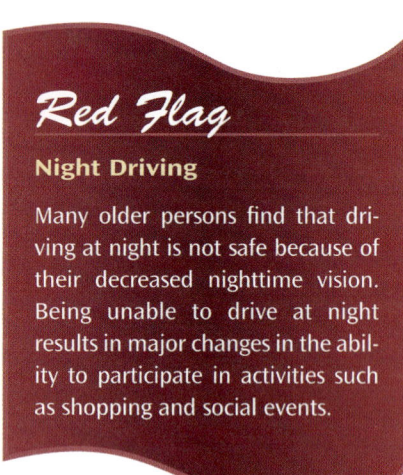

Many older persons find that driving at night is not safe because of their decreased nighttime vision. Being unable to drive at night results in major changes in the ability to participate in activities such as shopping and social events.

Macula

When the retinal structures and the optic disc have been assessed:

1. Move the ophthalmoscope approximately two disc diameters temporally to view the macula or ask the patient to look at the light. The red-free filter lens of the ophthalmoscope may also be helpful in assessing the macula. Because the macula is not clearly demarcated and because it is very light sensitive, you may have difficulty assessing it. The patient tends to turn away when the light strikes the fovea, making it difficult to assess details of the macular area.
2. Note the fovea centralis and observe for color, shape, and lesions.
3. Repeat with the other eye.

The macula is a darker, avascular area with a pinpoint reflective center known as the fovea centralis.

The retina is pale with the macular region appearing as a cherry-red spot.

This finding is central retinal artery occlusion, an indication of Tay-Sachs disease.

An enlarged macula is abnormal.

Respecting Our Differences

Gerontological Variations

Visual impairments are among the most prevalent chronic conditions in the older patient. Sight provides information to enable the patient to function safely in the environment. Prevention of sensory impairment and resulting handicaps are challenges for patients and health care providers.

During the aging process, the eye undergoes significant changes. First, by the age of 42, the lens cortex becomes more dense, compromising its ability to change shape and focus. This condition, presbyopia, is responsible for farsightedness and the need for bifocals. Next, there is a tendency for the lens to yellow and become cloudy. This change impairs a person's ability to discern various colors, especially blues and greens. In addition, pupils become smaller so that the amount of light reaching the retina is reduced. As a consequence, elderly individuals need more light to see and their eyes take longer to accommodate to darkness and glare. Finally, a decrease in tear production predisposes the individual to corneal irritation and conjunctivitis.

Cataracts, age-related macular degeneration, and glaucoma are the most common visual problems among elderly persons. Cataracts involve opacity and yellowing of the lens, which results in dimmed and blurred vision. Cataracts can be surgically removed.

Age-related macular degeneration is loss of central vision. Individuals experiencing this change require the use of magnification to compensate for visual loss. Systemic diseases that aggravate macular degeneration include diabetes mellitus and hypertension.

Glaucoma may cause total blindness if not treated. Increased intraocular pressure and inability of aqueous humor to flow out into collecting channels places pressure on the optic nerve. Early detection of glaucoma is critical; screening is recommended for all adults over age 40.

Inspection of the eyelids of the older individual often reveals slightly drooping upper and lower lids. The globe appears to be deeper in the socket, and the lacrimal gland may be visible because of lost subcutaneous fat around the eye (Watkinson, 2005).

Macular edema is caused by the leakage of fluid from retinal blood vessels. This can occur in diabetes mellitus, hypertension, age-related macular degeneration, and retinal blood vessel obstruction.

Sharply defined, small red spots are found in and around the macula.

These microaneurysms are pathognomonic of diabetes mellitus.

Macular borders are blurred, with a few spots of pigment near the macula; a hole may appear to be present in the center of the region, or a hemorrhage may have occurred.

This finding is characteristic of age-related macular degeneration. Hemorrhages, patches of retina atrophy, and pigmented areas may also be associated with this condition.

ANATOMY AND PHYSIOLOGY OF THE EAR

Ear

The ear has three sections: the external, the middle, and the inner ear.

External Ear

The external ear, which is also called the **auricle** or **pinna,** extends through the auditory canal to the tympanic membrane. The auricle receives sound waves and funnels them through the auditory canal to produce vibrations on the tympanic membrane. The auricle is composed of cartilage.

The external auditory canal is an S-shaped tube approximately 2.5 cm in length, with the outer third made up of cartilage and the remainder of bone covered by a thin layer of skin (Figure 38-6). The canal is lined with tiny hairs and modified sweat glands that secrete a thick, waxlike substance called **cerumen,**

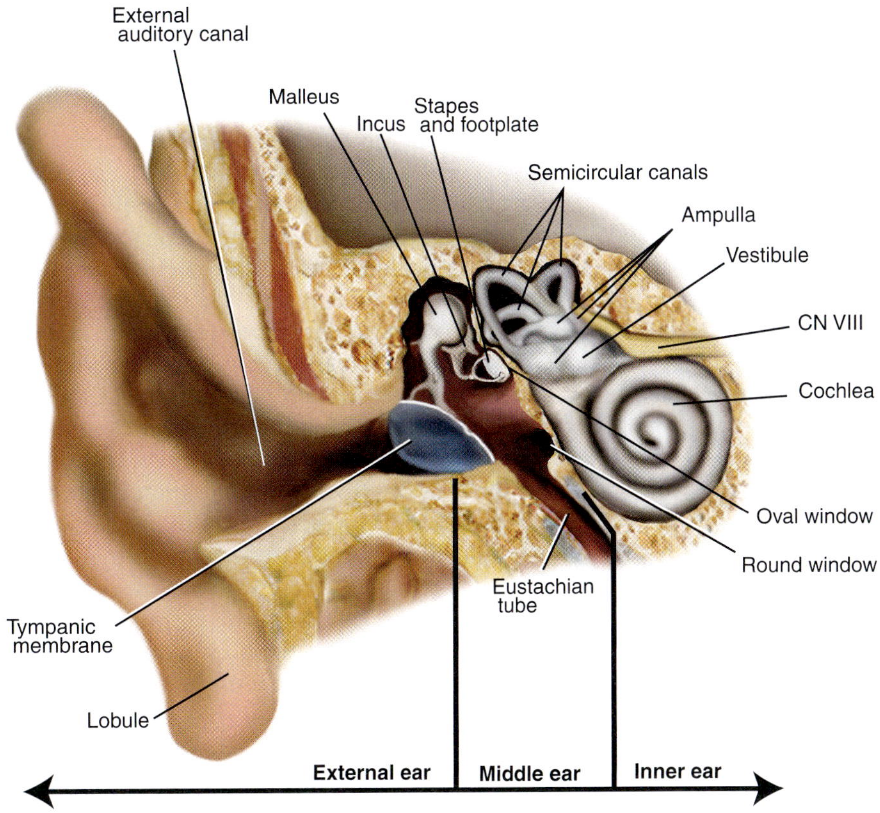

Figure 38-6 Cross-section of the ear.

which can vary in consistency from dry and flaky to wet and waxy. Cerumen ranges from a pale, honey color in light-skinned individuals to dark-brown or black in dark-skinned people.

Middle Ear

The middle ear is composed of the tympanic membrane, the ossicles, and the tympanic cavity. The cavity is an air-filled compartment that separates the external ear from the internal ear. The tympanic membrane, which is circular or oval and is about an inch in diameter, sits in an oblique position in the external canal so that it leans slightly forward. The rim of the tympanic membrane is called the annulus, the superior portion is the pars flaccida, and the tighter, largest area of the drum is the pars tensa.

The **ossicles** are three tiny bones—the malleus (hammer), the incus (anvil), and the stapes (stirrup)—that play a crucial role in the transmission of sound. The long handle, or manubrium, of the malleus extends downward from the short process and meets the tympanic membrane at the umbo. The stapes is held against the wall of the tympanic membrane at the oval window by tiny ligaments. The head of the malleus articulates with the incus, which in turn articulates with the stapes; they work as a unit when the tympanic membrane begins to vibrate. Vibrations set up in the tympanic membrane by sound waves reaching it through the external auditory canal are transmitted to the inner ear by rapid movement of the ossicles.

The tensor tympani and the stapedius are two tiny muscles involved in movement of the ossicles. The tensor tympani maintains the tension of the tympanic membrane and pulls the malleus inward when it contracts. The stapedius works in opposition by pulling the stapes outward. This coordinated movement is an important mechanism in reducing the intensity of loud sounds that might otherwise result in serious damage to hearing receptors in the inner ear.

The middle ear is connected to the nasopharynx by the auditory or **eustachian tube,** which serves as a channel through which air pressure within the cavity can be equalized with air pressure outside to maintain normal hearing. Equalization of pressure is aided by yawning or swallowing, which causes the opening of valve-like flaps that cover the openings of the eustachian tubes.

Inner Ear

The inner ear is a complex, closed, fluid-filled system of interconnecting tubes called the **labyrinth,** which is essential for hearing and equilibrium. The labyrinth has bony and membranous portions. The bony labyrinth is composed of the cochlea, the semicircular canals, and the vestibule. The vestibule is located between the cochlea and the semicircular canals and is important in both hearing and balance. The three semicircular canals located at right angles to each other provide balance and equilibrium for the body. The cochlea is a snail-shaped structure made up of three compartments. The first two compartments contain perilymph, and the third contains endolymph. As sound waves travel through the ear, they cause the perilymph and the endolymph to vibrate, stimulating the thousands of hearing-receptor cells of the organ of Corti. Nearby nerve fibers transmit impulses along the cochlear branch of the vestibulocochlear nerve to the brain, allowing us to hear. The human ear is capable of hearing within a frequency range of 20 to 20,000 Hz, and a decibel range of 0 to 140. Figure 38-7 illustrates the decibel levels of various commonly heard sounds.

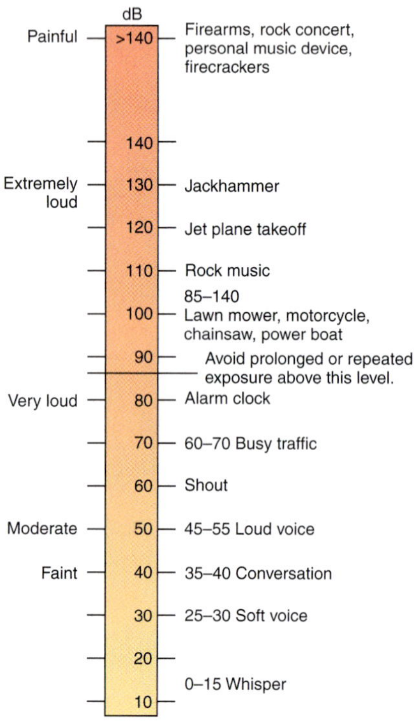

Figure 38-7 Decibel scale of frequently heard sounds. *Courtesy of Singular Publishing Group.*

ASSESSMENT OF THE EAR

Assessment of the ear by necessity includes the need for obtaining a thorough health assessment. This health history will include such things as the past and present history of the current ear problem, as well as, family, personal, and social history.

Present History of Ear Problem

The most common complaints of long-term ear problems are because of hearing loss and tinnitus. Pain, discharge, and dizziness or vertigo are often short-term conditions (Estes, 2006). See the Patient Playbook for an assessment of the ear for potential disorders.

Past Medical History

In addition, to the current status of the ear, the nurse must gather information regarding the previous medical history specific to the ear. There are several areas of concern as demonstrated in Box 38-3.

Family History

It is important to determine what types of genetic disorders potentially influence the ears of the patient. Some of these disorders are hearing loss, Ménière's disease, allergies, or renal disease.

PATIENT PLAYBOOK

Assessing Ear Problems

The nurse can ask the following questions to further examine problems of the ear:

- Dizziness or vertigo

1. Assess for onset and duration of dizziness or vertigo.
2. Describe characteristics of dizziness to include type of motion, movement, changes in position, and body involvement (e.g., head or neck movement).
3. Ask patient if there are any associated symptoms (e.g., nausea, vomiting, ringing in the ears, unsteady gait, loss of balance, falling, vision changes, or hearing loss).
4. Ask patient any alleviating or relieving factors.
5. Note any medications taken, prescription and nonprescription medications, which may cause a side effect of dizziness or vertigo.

- Changes in or loss of hearing

1. Assess for onset and duration (constant hearing loss or intermittent).
2. Ask patient if it is it bilateral or unilateral, if the patient can hear loud or soft sounds, and if hearing loss is partial or complete.
3. Note any associated symptoms (i.e., ear pain, tinnitus, drainage, swelling, or fever).
4. Ask patient if he or she noted any alleviating or aggravating factors.
5. List any medications taken, prescription, and nonprescription medications, which may cause a side effect of changes in hearing or hearing loss.

- **Otorrhea** (liquid discharge or drainage from the ear)

1. Ask patient if the drainage is unilateral or bilateral.
2. Discuss characteristics of secretions (e.g., yellowish, purulent, bloody, foul odor, or watery).
3. Ask if there are any other associated symptoms (e.g., fever, headache, hearing loss, dizziness, or upper respiratory infections).
4. Discuss if any aggravating or alleviating factors.
5. Ask about timing, following trauma, and if it is constant or intermittent draining).

- **Otalgia** or ear pain

1. Ask patient about onset and duration of pain (i.e., constant, intermittent).
2. Note if pain is localized, unilateral or bilateral, and if it is radiating to the jaw or pinna region.
3. Ask about the type of pain (i.e., aching, dull, sharp, or stabbing).
4. Ask patient if there is any associated symptoms (e.g., hearing loss, fever, drainage, tinnitus, sore throat, dizziness, or fever).
5. Discuss any aggravating or relieving factors.

Adapted from: Estes, M. (2006). Health assessment and physical examination *(3rd ed.). New York: Thomson Delmar Learning.*

BOX 38-3

HISTORY OF THE EAR

- History of any trauma or injury to the ear as a whole or specific structure of the ear, description of event surrounding the injury, and attempts at correction and degree of success.
- History of any ear surgery, chronic ear problems in childhood, and use of antibiotics and other medications.
- Other chronic illness, which may affect hearing (e.g., diabetes, hypertension, cardiovascular disease, nephritis, bleeding disorder, gastrointestinal disease, or reflux esophagitis).

Adapted from Estes, M. (2006). Health assessment and physical examination *(3rd ed.). New York: Thomson Delmar Learning.*

Personal and Social History

A personal and social history may influence the function of the ears. Therefore, the nurse must gather information specific to these areas of their patient's condition. In addition, the nurse can focus on employment and history of exposure to environment noise and use or lack of use of protective hearing devices.

Examination and Findings

Physical assessment of the ear consists of three parts:

1. Auditory screening (CN VIII)
2. Inspection and palpation of the external ear
3. Otoscopic assessment

Auditory Screening

Voice-Whisper Test

The following steps are necessary for a voice-whisper test:

1. Instruct the patient to occlude one ear with a finger.
2. Stand 2 feet behind the patient's other ear and whisper a two-syllable word or phrase that is evenly accented.
3. Ask the patient to repeat the word or phrase.
4. Repeat the test with the other ear.

The patient should be able to repeat words whispered from a distance of 2 feet.

The patient is unable to repeat the words correctly or states that he or she was unable to hear anything.

This indicates a hearing loss in the high-frequency range that may be caused by excessive exposure to loud noises (see Skills 360° feature).

Tuning Fork Tests

Weber and Rinne tests help to determine whether the type of hearing loss the patient is experiencing is conductive or sensorineural. In order to understand how these tests are evaluated, it is important to know the difference between air and bone conduction. Air conduction refers to the transmission of sound through the ear canal, tympanic membrane, and ossicular chain to the cochlea and auditory nerve. Bone conduction refers to the transmission of sound through the bones of the skull to the cochlea and auditory nerve.

Weber Test

To do a Weber test:

1. Hold the handle of a 512-Hz (vibrates 512 cycles per second to create a specific frequency) tuning fork and strike the tines on the ulnar border of the palm to activate it.
2. Place the stem of the fork firmly against the middle of the patient's forehead, on the top of the head at the midline, or on the front teeth (Figure 38-8).
3. Ask the patient if the sound is heard centrally or toward one side.

The patient should perceive the sound equally in both ears or "in the middle." No lateralization of sound is known as a negative Weber test.

The sound lateralizes to the affected ear.

This occurs with unilateral conductive hearing loss because the sound is being conducted directly through the bone to the ear. Conductive hearing loss occurs when there are external or middle ear disorders such as impacted cerumen, perforation of the tympanic membrane, serum or pus in the middle ear, or a fusion of the ossicles.

Skills 360°

The Patient with Decreased Hearing

Observe the patient for signs of hearing difficulty and deafness during the health history and physical exam. Turning the head to facilitate hearing, lip reading, speaking in a loud voice, or asking you to write words are signs of hearing difficulty. If the patient is wearing a hearing aid, ask if it is turned on, when the batteries were last changed, and if the device causes any irritation of the ear canal.

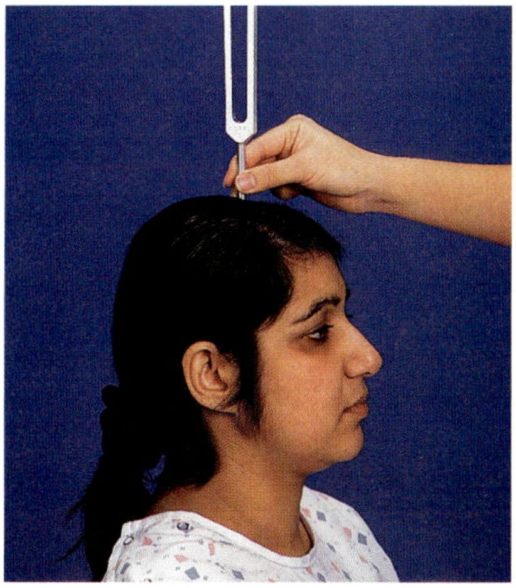

Figure 38-8 Weber test.

The sound lateralizes to the unaffected ear.

This occurs with sensorineural loss related to nerve damage in the impaired ear. Sensorineural hearing loss occurs when there is a disorder in the inner ear, the auditory nerve, or the brain; disorders include congenital defects, effects of ototoxic drugs, and repeated or prolonged exposure to loud noise.

Rinne Test

To do a Rinne test:

1. Stand behind or to the side of the patient and strike the tuning fork.
2. Place the stem of the tuning fork against the patient's right mastoid process to test bone conduction (Figure 38-9A).
3. Instruct the patient to indicate if the sound is heard.
4. Ask the patient to tell you when the sound stops.
5. When the patient says that the sound has stopped, move the tuning fork, with the tines facing forward, in front of the right auditory meatus, and ask the patient if the sound is still heard. Note the length of time the patient hears the sound (testing air conduction) (Figure 38-9B).
6. Repeat the test on the left ear.

Air conduction is heard twice as long as bone conduction when the patient hears the sound through the external auditory canal (air) after it is no longer heard at the mastoid process (bone). This is denoted as AC>BC.

The patient reports hearing the sound longer through bone conduction; that is, bone conduction is equal to or greater than air conduction.

This occurs when there is a conductive hearing loss resulting from disease, obstruction, or damage to the outer or middle ear.

Bone conduction is prolonged in the context of a normal tympanic membrane, patent eustachian tube, and middle ear disease.

These findings are typical of otosclerosis.

A

B

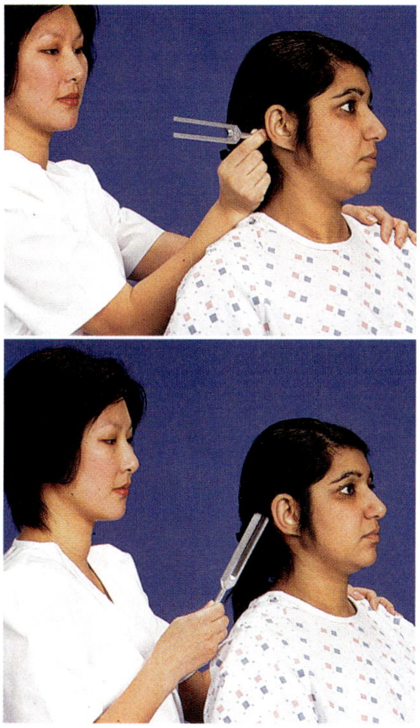

Figure 38-9 Rinne test.

External Ear

Inspection

To perform an inspection of the external ear:

1. Inspect the ears and note their position, color, size, and shape.
2. Note any deformities, nodules, inflammation, or lesions.
3. Note color, consistency, and amount of cerumen.

The ear should match the flesh color of the rest of the patient's skin and should be positioned centrally and in proportion to the head. The top of the ear should cross an imaginary line drawn from the outer canthus of the eye to the occiput. Cerumen should be moist and not obscure the tympanic membrane. There should be no foreign bodies, redness, drainage, deformities, nodules, or lesions.

The ears are pale, red, or cyanotic.

Vasomotor disorders, fevers, hypoxemia, and cold weather can account for various color changes.

The ears are abnormally large or small.

These abnormalities can be congenitally determined or the result of trauma. Frequently, this is accompanied by an absent external ear canal and middle ear, but an intact inner ear.

An ear that is grossly misshapen, damaged, or mutilated is abnormal.

Blunt trauma, such as in contact sports, to the side of the head is usually the cause.

Red Flag

Cerebrospinal Fluid Drainage from the Ear

If the patient has cerebrospinal fluid (clear liquid that tests positive for glucose on Dextrostix) leaking from the ear, be sure to use good hand washing technique and avoid placing any objects into the ear canal in order to prevent the development of meningitis. A patient with this finding needs immediate referral to a qualified specialist.

An external ear that is erythematous, edematous, warm to the touch, and painful is abnormal.

Perichondritis is an inflammation of the fibrous connective tissue that overlies the cartilage of the ear.

A tumor on the external ear is abnormal.

Basal cell and squamous cell carcinoma are the most common external ear tumors. Prolonged sunlight exposure is a predisposing factor for these tumors.

Purulent drainage is abnormal.

Purulent drainage usually indicates an infection.

Clear or bloody drainage is present (see Red Flag feature).

Clear or bloody drainage may be due to cerebrospinal fluid leaking as a result of head trauma or surgery.

A hematoma behind an ear over the mastoid bone is abnormal. This is called Battle's sign and indicates head trauma to the temporal bone of the skull.

A hard, painless, irregular-shaped nodule on the pinna is abnormal.

Tophi are uric acid nodules and may indicate the presence of gout. These are usually located near the helix. Many other nodules are benign fibromas.

Sebaceous cysts are abnormal.

Sebaceous cysts or retention cysts form as a result of the blockage of the ducts to the sebaceous gland.

Lymph nodes anterior to the tragus or overlying the mastoid are abnormal.

Lymph nodes may be enlarged due to a malignancy or an infection such as external otitis.

Palpation

To palpate the external ear:

1. Palpate the auricle between the thumb and the index finger, noting any tenderness or lesions. If the patient has ear pain, assess the unaffected ear first, then cautiously assess the affected ear.
2. Using the tips of the index and middle fingers, palpate the mastoid tip, noting any tenderness.
3. Using the tips of the index and middle fingers, press inward on the tragus, noting any tenderness.
4. Hold the auricle between the thumb and the index finger and gently pull up and down, noting any tenderness.

The patient should not complain of pain or tenderness during palpation.

Auricular pain or tenderness is noted.

Auricular pain is a common finding in external ear infection and is called acute otitis externa.

There is tenderness over the mastoid process.

Mastoid tenderness is associated with middle ear inflammation or mastoiditis.

The tragus is edematous or sensitive.

This finding may indicate inflammation of the external or middle ear.

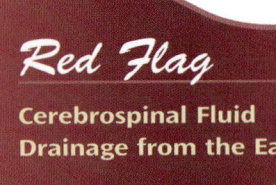

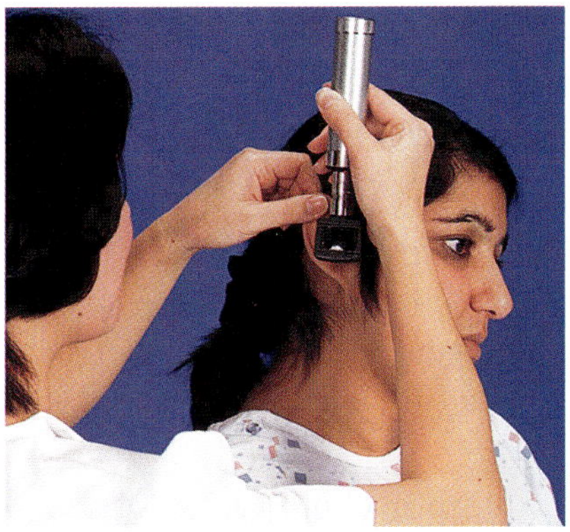

Figure 38-10 Assessment with otoscope.

Otoscopic Assessment

The steps in an otoscopic assessment are:

1. Ask the patient to tip the head away from the ear being assessed.
2. Select the largest speculum that will comfortably fit the patient.
3. Hold the otoscope securely in the dominant hand, with the head held downward and the handle held like a pencil between the thumb and the forefinger.
4. Rest the back of the dominant hand on the right side of the patient's head (Figure 38-10).
5. Use the ulnar aspect of the free hand to pull the right ear in a manner that will straighten the canal. In adults and in children over 3 years old, pull the ear up and back.
6. If hair obstructs visualization, moisten the speculum with water or a water-soluble lubricant.
7. If wax obstructs visualization, it should be removed only by a skilled practitioner, either by curettement (if the cerumen is soft or the tympanic membrane is ruptured) or by irrigation (if the cerumen is dry and hard and the tympanic membrane is intact).
8. Slowly insert the speculum into the canal, looking at the canal as the speculum passes.
9. Assess the canal for inflammation, exudates, lesions, and foreign bodies.
10. Continue to insert the speculum into the canal, following the path of the canal until the tympanic membrane is visualized.
11. If the tympanic membrane is not visible, gently pull the pinna slightly farther in order to straighten the canal to allow adequate visualization.
12. Identify the color, light reflex, umbo, the short process, and the long handle of the malleus. Note the presence of perforations, lesions, bulging or retraction of the tympanic membrane, dilatation of blood vessels, bubbles, or fluid.
13. Ask the patient to close the mouth, pinch the nose closed, and blow gently while you observe for movement of the tympanic membrane. A pneumatic attachment may be used to create this movement if one is available.
14. Gently withdraw the speculum and repeat the process with the left ear.

The ear canal should have no redness, swelling, tenderness, lesions, drainage, foreign bodies, or scaly surface areas. Cerumen varies in amount, consistency, and color. The tympanic membrane should be pearly gray with clearly defined landmarks and a distinct cone-shaped light reflex extending from the umbo toward the anteroinferior aspect of the membrane. This light reflex is seen at 5 o'clock in the right ear and at 7 o'clock in the left ear. Blood vessels should be visible only on the periphery, and the membrane should not bulge, be retracted, or have any evidence of fluid behind it (Figure 38-11). The tympanic membrane should move when the patient blows against resistance.

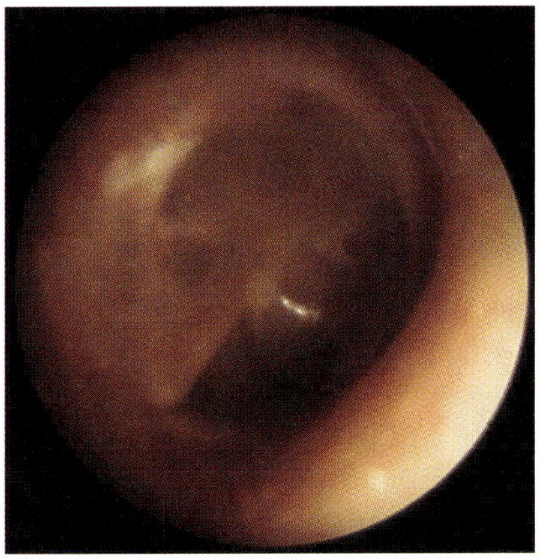

Figure 38-11 Normal tympanic membrane. *Courtesy of Singular Publishing Group, Inc.*

A foreign body in the external auditory canal (EAC) is abnormal.

Both adults and children can have foreign bodies in the EAC. Some objects are more difficult to remove than others; for instance, vegetables in the EAC can swell with time and make removal challenging.

Tympanostomy tubes, or PE tubes (pressure equalization) are surgically placed for prolonged otitis media with effusion (OME). The tubes allow drainage of the effusion, normal vibration of the ossicles, and equalization of pressures across the tympanic membrane. When a myringotomy has been performed with tympanostomy tube placement, the presence of the tubes (or lack of) needs to be documented.

A painful, boil-like pustule in the EAC is abnormal.

Furunculosis is an infection of a hair follicle. EAC edema and otorrhea may also be present.

Skills 360°

Recurrent Acute Otitis Media in a Toddler

Eighteen-month-old Jared is brought to the pediatrician's for a sick child visit. His mother confides in you that she is a single parent and is having a difficult time balancing work and family. This is Jared's sixth ear infection in the past 4 months. His mother is missing work to take him to the pediatrician's office and she cannot always take him back to the daycare center because of his fever. Jared's mother says, "I never knew it would be this hard," and she starts to cry. How should the nurse respond? What anticipatory guidance can be provided?

Red Flag

Risk Factors for Otitis Media

- Less than 2 years of age
- Frequent upper respiratory tract infections
- Cold weather
- Males
- Caucasians, Native Americans, Alaskan natives
- Family history (parents, siblings)
- Pacifier use after 6 months of age
- Smoky environment
- Daycare attendance
- Bottle fed
- Down syndrome
- Craniofacial disorders

Black or brown spores, yellow or orange spores, or white fluffy hyphae in the EAC are abnormal.

Prolonged use of aural antibiotics can cause otomycosis, or a fungal infection, in the ear. Different strains of fungi cause the variations in appearance.

Bony, hard lesions in the deep EAC are abnormal.

These are exostoses. Patients who frequently participate in cold-water activities are at risk for developing them. If an exostosis becomes large enough, it can block the EAC and trap debris between it and the tympanic membrane. This can lead to infection.

Exquisite pain accompanied by erythema deep into the EAC and on the tympanic membrane, along with serous-filled blebs, is abnormal.

This describes viral bullous myringitis. This can easily be mistaken for acute otitis media.

The appearance of chalk patches on the tympanic membrane is abnormal.

These are calcifications found in myringosclerosis, which can occur after tympanic membrane surgery, infection, or inflammation. Myringosclerosis can be associated with a gradual hearing loss. Involvement of the entire tympanic membrane is called tympanosclerosis.

Air bubbles on the tympanic membrane are abnormal.

Conditions such as coryza and influenza and changes in extratympanic pressure (such as in scuba diving, airplane travel) can lead to eustachian tube failure.

The presence of blood in the middle ear is abnormal.

Hemotympanum occurs as a result of trauma to the head. The tympanic membrane can have a bluish hue or can be red in appearance.

A severely retracted tympanic membrane has exaggerated landmarks. Mobility of the tympanic membrane is decreased.

Retraction of the tympanic membrane can occur when the intratympanic membrane pressures are reduced, as in eustachian tube blockage caused by otitis media with effusion or allergies. Repeated negative pressure in the middle ear sucks in the tympanic membrane and leads to retractions. Over time, keratinized epithelial debris deposits itself in these retraction pockets and leads to ossicle fixation. This leads to cholesteatoma. A foul smelling ear discharge, as well as deafness, may accompany cholesteatoma.

There is redness, swelling, narrowing, and pain of the external ear. Drainage may be present.

Acute otitis externa is caused by infectious organisms or allergic reactions. Predisposing factors include excessive moisture in the ear related to swimming, trauma from cleansing the ears with a sharp instrument, or allergies to substances such as hairspray (see Skills 360° feature).

Hard, dry, and very dark yellow-brown cerumen is abnormal.

Old cerumen is harder and drier, and may become impacted if not removed.

The tympanic membrane is red, with decreased mobility and possible bulging (Figure 38-12).

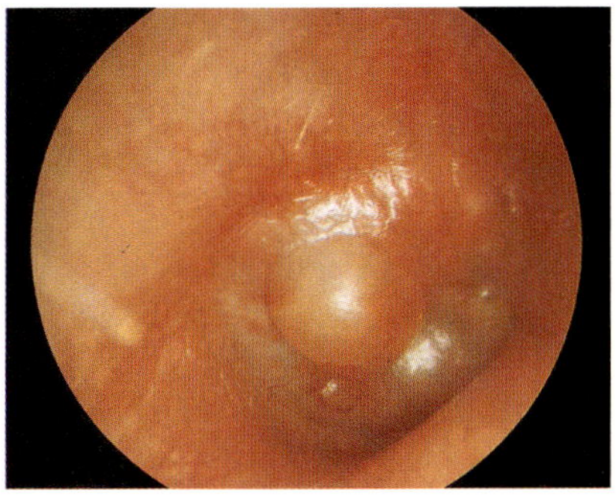

Figure 38-12 Acute otitis media. *Courtesy of Singular Publishing Group, Inc.*

Red Flag

Hearing Loss Risk Factors

- Noise exposure
- Smoking
- Ototoxic drugs
- Congenital or heredity
- Cardiovascular disease
- Aging
- Tumors
- Trauma
- Chronic infection
- Systemic disease
- Tympanic membrane perforation
- Ménière's disease
- Barotrauma

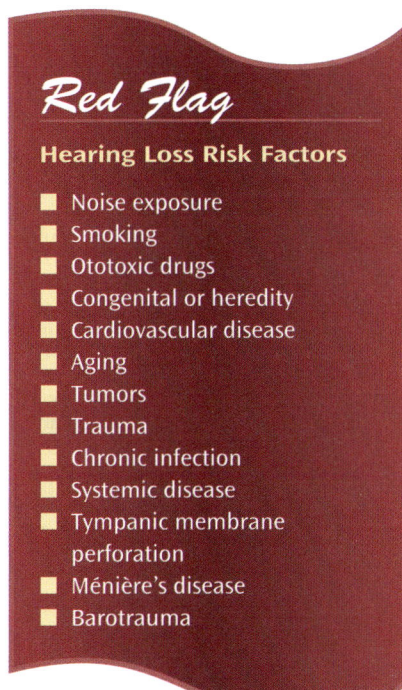

This is acute otitis media (AOM), or an inflammation of the middle ear. Pain and fever may accompany the ear infection. Otalgia, fever, decreased hearing, irritability, disturbed sleep, and otorrhea may accompany the middle ear infection. *Streptococcus pneumoniae, Haemophilus influenzae,* and *Moraxella catarrhalis* are the major pathogens that cause AOM.

Along with a bulging eardrum and decreased mobility, the landmarks are diffuse, displaced, or absent (see Red Flag feature).

The late stage of acute otitis media causes landmarks to become progressively obscured.

Amber-yellow fluid on the tympanic membrane is abnormal. It may be accompanied by a fluid line or bubbles behind the membrane. Bulging may be present and mobility of the eardrum may be decreased. The patient may complain of ear popping, pain, and decreased hearing.

Otitis media with effusion, or serous otitis media, can be caused by allergies, infections, and a blocked eustachian tube. Table 38-3 compares AOM, OME, and otitis externa.

The tympanic membrane appears to have a darkened area or a hole.

A perforated eardrum is caused by untreated ear infection secondary to increasing pressure. Trauma to the ear canal can also cause a perforation (see Red Flag feature).

The tympanic membrane is pearly gray and has dark patches.

These patches are usually old perforations in the tympanic membrane.

The tympanic membrane is pearly gray and has dense white plaques.

These plaques represent calcific deposits of scarring of the tympanic membrane from frequent past episodes of otitis media.

TABLE 38-3 Comparison of AOM, OME, and Otitis Externa

	AOM	OME	OTITIS EXTERNA
TM color	Diffuse red, dilated peripheral vessels	Yellowish	WNL
TM appearance	Bulging	Bubbles, fluid line	WNL
TM landmarks	Decreased	Retracted with prominent malleus	WNL
Movement of tragus	Painless	Painless	Painful
Hearing	WNL/decreased	WNL/decreased	WNL
EAC	WNL	WNL	Erythematous, edematous

KEY CONCEPTS

- The eyes are sensory organs, which receive visual stimuli that are transmitted to the brain for interpretation through the cranial nerve (optic nerve II).
- The external parts of the eyes are protected from trauma by the bony structure of the orbital cavity.
- There are three coats or tunics comprising the internal structures of the eyes.
- The retina is the innermost coat of the eyeball, and it is the sensory network of the eye.
- The health history of the eye includes such things as the present history of the current eye problem, as well as the past history of the eye.
- In an assessment of the eye, it is important to determine what types of genetic disorders potentially influence the eyes of the patient.
- Systematic eye assessment includes inspecting and palpating the appendages or extraocular structures surrounding the eye.
- Visual acuity testing is the test of central vision assessing the eye's ability to distinguish small and specific details.
- A visual field confrontation test is used to grossly assess peripheral vision.
- Assessing extraocular eye muscle movement involves cranial nerves III, IV, and VI.
- An ophthalmoscopic examination can be helpful in identifying pathologies of the eye.
- The most common complaints of long-term ear problems are due to hearing loss and tinnitus. Pain, discharge, and dizziness or vertigo are often short-term conditions of the ear.
- The ossicles are three tiny bones that play a crucial role in the transmission of sound.
- Physical assessment of the ear consists of auditory screening, inspection, and palpation of the external ear and otoscopic assessment.

REVIEW QUESTIONS

1. Mr. Carter has a disorder of his palpebrae, which are his:
   1. Eyelashes
   2. Eyelids
   3. Conjunctiva
   4. Lacrimal glands

2. The extraocular muscles are innervated by which cranial nerves?
   1. Cranial nerves II, III, and VI
   2. Cranial nerves II, IV, and VI
   3. Cranial nerves III, IV, and VI
   4. Cranial nerves II, III, and IV

3. The parasympathetic nervous system causes the pupils to:
   1. Constrict
   2. Dilate
   3. Diverge
   4. Converge

4. Mrs. Johanson has a congenital defect that causes her to have color vision problems. This is due to a dysfunction of her:
   1. Rods
   2. Pupils
   3. Sclera
   4. Cones

5. The Snellen chart is responsible for testing:
   1. Pupil constriction
   2. Sensitivity to light
   3. Visual acuity
   4. Depth perception

6. Mr. Treat has recently experienced a yellow, lipid rich plaque lesion on the eyelid, which is labeled:
   1. Stye
   2. Xanthelasma
   3. Arcus senilis
   4. Entropion

7. After a head injury, Mr. Barnett experiences a left eye that does not constrict when light is shined in the right eye. This is labeled a problem associated with:
   1. Direct response
   2. Indirect response
   3. Consensual response
   4. Accommodation

8. When using the ophthalmoscope, the red numbers indicate:
   1. Anterior eye problems
   2. Posterior eye problems
   3. Glaucoma tendencies
   4. Pupil abnormalities

Continued

REVIEW QUESTIONS—cont'd

9. Mr. Lever has a purulent drainage coming from his left ear. This is described as:
   1. Otalgia
   2. Cerumen
   3. Vertigo
   4. Otorrhea

10. Mrs. Studer has a potential conduction problem of both ears. A test is performed that evaluates whether sounds are heard centrally or on one side. This is what type of test?
    1. Weber test
    2. Rinne test
    3. Voice-whisper test
    4. Otitis media

REVIEW ACTIVITIES

1. Select three to five patients and assess their eyes with an ophthalmoscope.

2. Compare and contrast four patients' pupil responses to both direct and indirect light stimulation.

3. Describe the red light reflex and the shape of the optic disk in an eye exam on a patient.

4. Perform nerve conduction testing with three patients' ears.

5. Describe the shapes of four patients' ears.

Visit the Contemporary Medical-Surgical Nursing online companion resource at www.delmarhealthcare.com for additional content and study aids. Click on Online Companions then select the Nursing discipline.

Visual Dysfunction: Nursing Management

CHAPTER 39

Karen Wikoff, RN, DNS

CHAPTER TOPICS

- Ocular Movement Disorders
- Visual Acuity
- Refraction
- Presbyopia
- Color Perception
- Inflammatory and Infectious Ocular Diseases
- Ocular Disorders Resulting from Neurological Disorders
- Low Vision and Blindness

KEY TERMS

Amblyopia
Aphakic vision
Astigmatism
Blepharitis
Cryopexy
Diplopia
Emmetropia
Entropia
Enucleation
Exotropia (wall eyes)
Hyperopia (farsightedness)
Hypotany
Keratometry
Myopia (nearsightedness)
Nystagmus
Papilledema
Presbyopia
Ptosis
Strabismus

The eyes are complex organic structures and have a variety of intricate physiological elements (Figure 39-1). The visual fields of the eye are normally predictable and exist in specific pathways (Figure 39-2). Visual disturbances can range from minor disturbances easily managed with corrective lens to severe disturbances requiring complex interventions, including surgery. Whether the disturbances are minor, severe, or somewhere in between, the patient must adapt to the visual restrictions in activities of daily living. Dysfunction in vision can be the result of abnormalities in ocular movement, visual acuity, refraction, accommodation, color perception, and inflammatory and infectious diseases. Vision dysfunction may occur secondary to other pathological considerations, such as papilledema in neurological disorders and diabetic retinopathy.

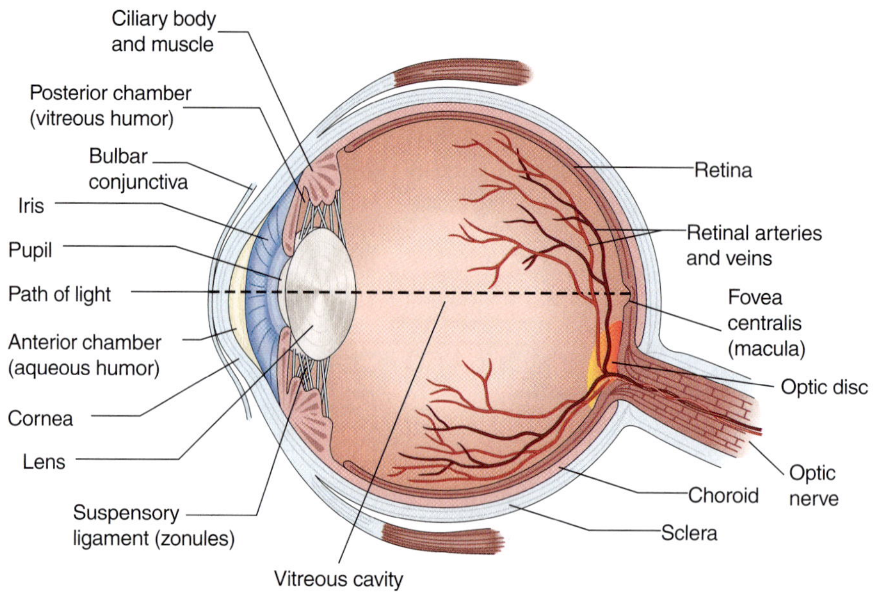

Figure 39-1 Lateral cross section of the interior eye.

OCULAR MOVEMENT DISORDERS

Ocular movement dysfunction can be the result of deviation in muscle movement from normal physiology (Figure 39-3), involuntary eye movement, or paralysis. There are three main ocular movement dysfunctions: (a) strabismus, (b) nystagmus, and (c) ocular muscle paralysis.

Strabismus

Ocular movement is controlled by the six extraocular muscles, four rectus and two oblique muscles (Riordan-Eva & Whitcher, 2004). **Strabismus** occurs when one muscle is weak and result in one eye deviating from the other when the eyes are focused on an object (Estes, 2006). Depending on the muscle or muscles involved the eye may deviate in an inward, upward, outward, or downward pattern. An eye that deviates outward is called **exotropia (wall eyes),** and an eye that deviates inward is known as **entropia. Diplopia,** or double vision, is the primary symptom of strabismus (Druz, 2005). **Amblyopia** is a reduction in visual acuity caused by cerebral blockage of visual stimuli, which can develop in the eye affected by strabismus. Causes of strabismus include weak ocular muscle tone, reduced visual acuity, or an oculomotor nerve lesion (Michelson, 2005).

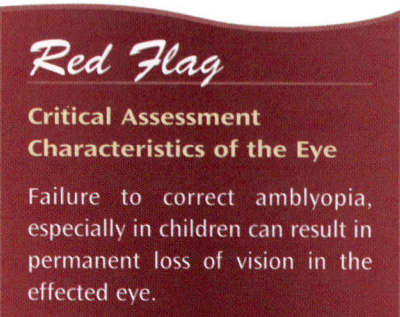

> ***Red Flag***
>
> **Critical Assessment Characteristics of the Eye**
>
> Failure to correct amblyopia, especially in children can result in permanent loss of vision in the effected eye.

Nystagmus

Nystagmus is an involuntary rhythmic movement of the eyes in a back and forth, or cyclical, movement. This can be caused by lesions in the labyrinth, vestibular nerve, cerebellum, and brainstem. Drug toxicities (e.g., phenytoin or alcohol), retinal disease, and diseases involving the cervical cord may, also, produce nystagmus.

Ocular Muscle Paralysis

Paralysis of ocular muscles may occur as a result of trauma or pressure on cranial nerves or diseases, such as diabetes mellitus (DM) or myasthenia gravis. This can result in limited abduction, abnormal closure of the lid, **ptosis** (drooping of the eyelid) or diplopia from unopposed muscle movement.

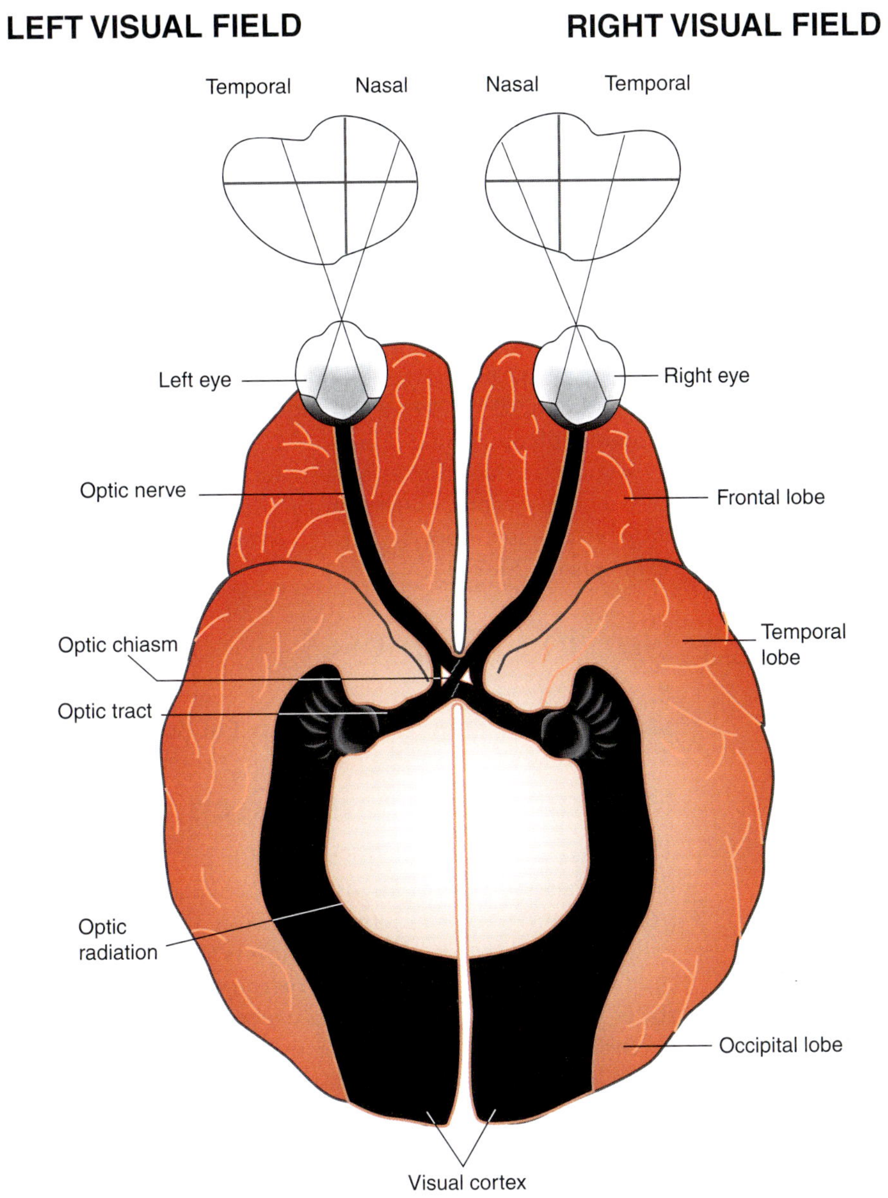

Figure 39-2 Visual pathway.

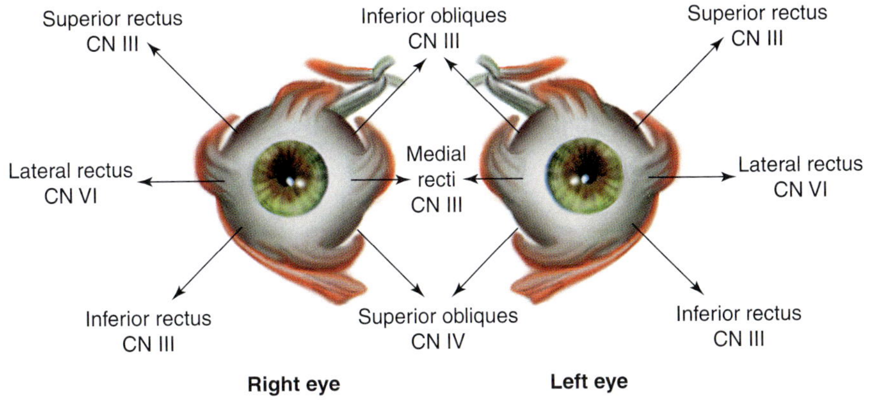

Figure 39-3 Direction of movement of extraocular muscles.

BOX 39-1

NURSING DIAGNOSES FOR EYE DISORDERS

- Acute pain as related to pathophysiology of eye dysfunction.
- Anxiety related to possible vision loss.
- Disturbed sensory perception related to visual impairment.
- Ineffective health maintenance related to knowledge deficit.
- Risk for injury related to impaired vision.
- Self-care deficit related to impaired vision.

Assessment with Clinical Manifestations and Diagnostic Tests

Ocular motor testing is the evaluation of the alignment of the eyes and their movement (Estes, 2006). The nurse assesses the movement of the eyes on a regular basis and associates dysfunction with particular diseases and dysfunction (e.g., head injuries, increased intracranial pressure, or neurological insults). In normal vision each eye generates a visual image separate from the other eye, and the brain then merges the two images together into one image. Failure to merge the two images results in diplopia. To measure the binocular alignment the patient is asked to look at a penlight held several feet away while the nurse observes for location of the light reflection on the cornea. The light should be centered on the cornea, and any deviation suggests dysfunction of the ocular muscles. A second method of evaluating for ocular movement dysfunction is to instruct the patient to follow a target with both eyes as the target is moved in the direction of gaze. The nurse assesses the movement for speed, range, symmetry of movement, and fixation (Michelson, 2005).

Nursing Diagnoses

Based on the information gathered, examples of nursing diagnoses in the patient with eye disorders are included in Box 39-1.

Planning and Implementation

The nurse must carefully plan care for patients with oculomotor problems. Collaborative care for patients with ocular motor dysfunction includes monitoring the patient for changes in vision and correcting the muscle(s) surgically. Generally surgical intervention is a method of treatment used last and only when vision is impaired. Treatment of ocular motor problems usually starts with correction of refractive errors. In some situations the use of occlusion therapy may be effective. The nurse patches the eye to occlude vision either all or some of the time. In addition to adhesive patches, opaque contact lenses or occluders mounted on eyeglasses may be used depending on the individual's age and adherence to the medical regimen. Medical treatment for ptosis can include a pair of eyeglasses with a crutch made to hold up the eyelid; surgical repair can include adjustment of the one or more of the ocular motor muscles. In some situations correction of ptosis may be considered cosmetic and therefore not covered by traditional health insurance.

Evaluation of Outcomes

Potential patient outcomes for each of the example nursing diagnoses for the patient with eye disorders are shown in Box 39-2.

VISUAL ACUITY

Disorders of visual acuity include cataracts, glaucoma, retinal detachment, and macular degeneration. Traumatic injuries can affect visual acuity, as well as other components of eye function, depending on the location of the injury in or around the eye from foreign body, contusions, lacerations, and penetrating injuries. Ocular cancer is also discussed in this section. Corneal disorders that impact visual acuity are corneal abrasions, scarring, and keratoconus and are covered in this section.

BOX 39-2

EVALUATION OF OUTCOMES FOR PATIENTS WITH EYE DISORDERS

- Acute pain as related to pathophysiology of eye dysfunction. The patient should verbalize an adequate relief of pain along with the ability to realistically cope with the pain if it is not completely relieved.
- Anxiety related to possible vision loss. The patient should be able to recognize the signs of anxiety, demonstrate positive coping mechanisms, and describe a reduction in the level of anxiety experienced.
- Disturbed sensory perception related to visual impairment. The patient achieves optimal functioning within limits of visual impairment as evidenced by ability to care for self, to navigate environmental safely, and to engage in meaningful activities.
- Ineffective health maintenance related to knowledge deficit. The patient describes positive health maintenance behaviors, such as keeping scheduled appointments, making diet and exercise changes, improving home environments, and following treatment regimens.
- Self-care deficit related to impaired vision. The patient safely performs (to maximum ability) self-care activities. Resources are identified that are useful in optimizing the autonomy and independence of the patient.

Cataracts

A cataract occurs as a part of the aging process for many individuals. In the United States, by the age of 80, more than half of the population will develop cataracts or have had cataract surgery. Cataracts occur simultaneously in both eyes yet the problem is often more acute in one eye than the other. Risk for the development of cataracts is seen in conjunction with disease (e.g., diabetes), personal behavior (e.g., smoking, alcohol use), medical treatment (e.g., side effect from use of steroids), and environment (e.g., exposure to sunlight).

Pathophysiology

Cataracts occur as the opacity of the lens becomes cloudy or turns a yellowish brown color, distorting the light passing through to the retina. The lens is made of water and protein; when the protein clumps together this produces the cloudiness. When the lens develops the yellowish brown color it often results in color distortion. Symptoms of cataracts include cloudiness or blurriness, reduced night vision, and color distortion or faded colors. Cataracts can also form after traumatic eye injury or secondarily to other eye problems, such as diabetes or surgery for glaucoma. Some children may be born with a congenital cataract that may or may not affect vision (McGwin, Hall, Searcey, Modjarrad, & Owsley, 2005).

Assessment with Clinical Manifestations and Diagnostic Tests

A visual acuity test such as use of the Snellen chart (Figure 39-4) is part of the assessment for vision impairment related to cataracts. A dilated eye examination will be performed to assist with diagnosis. Patients with cataracts usually notice no pain or discomfort (Estes, 2006).

Nursing Diagnoses

Based on the information gathered, examples of nursing diagnoses in the patient with cataracts are shown in Box 39-1.

Planning and Implementation

Management for patients with cataracts starts with adjusting corrective lens as frequently as necessary to ensure optimal vision. Surgical treatment for cataracts begins when vision is sufficiently impaired to interfere with activities of daily living.

A

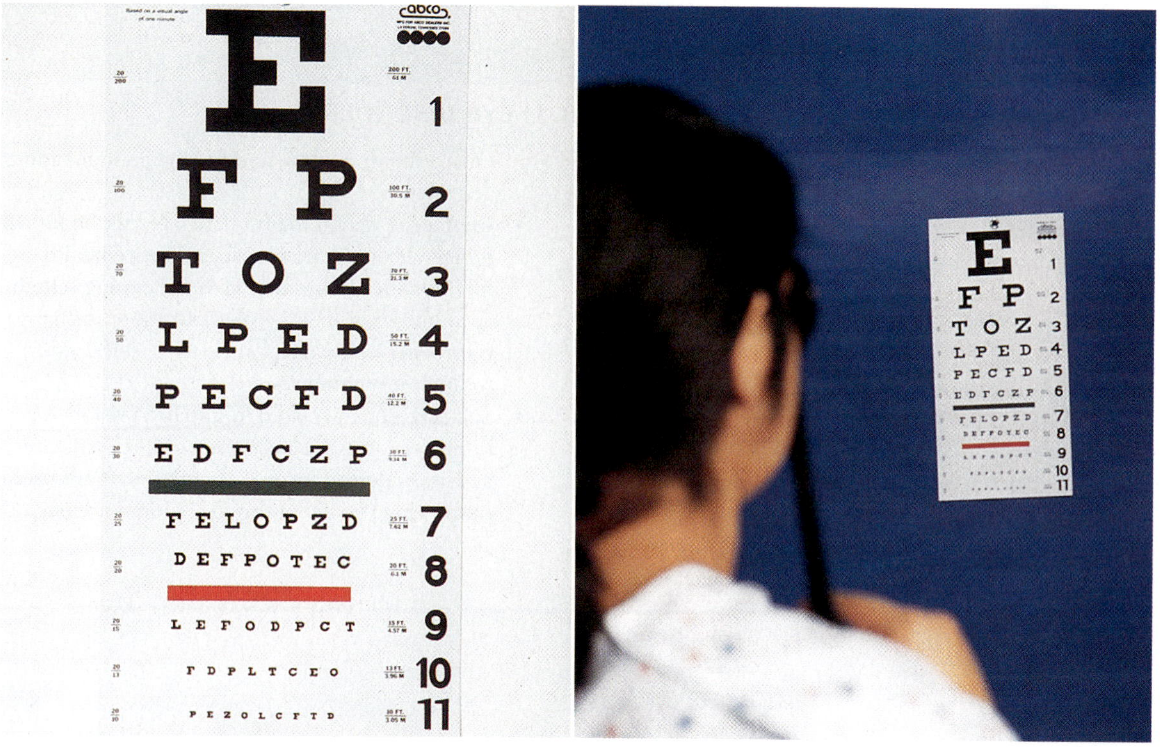

B

Figure 39-4 Visual acuity testing: A. Snellen vision chart, B. Assessing distance vision.

Surgery

There are two types of surgery phacoemulsification (phaco) or extracapsular surgery. In phaco an incision is made in the cornea, and a small probe is inserted into the eye. The device attached to the probe emits ultrasound waves that break up the lens, allowing for suction removal. In extracapsular surgery a slightly larger incision is made, and the lens is removed as a whole. An artificial intraocular lens (IOL) with corrective power is placed in the remaining posterior capsule of the eye. Following either surgery a patient may need glasses only for reading. When an IOL cannot be inserted, the eye is unable to accommodate resulting in **aphakic vision** (absence of the crystalline lens of the eye), which requires special corrective lenses (McGwin, et al., 2005).

Cataract surgery is done almost exclusively as an outpatient procedure. The patient will arrive in the morning and plan to be discharged by the afternoon. Preoperative nursing care includes preoperative history and physical, including medication usage, administration of eye drops to dilate the pupil and cause vasoconstriction, and patient education. Oral medications may be given in the preoperative phase to reduce intraocular pressure, such as acetazolamide (Diamox, Acetazolam). During the intraoperative procedure, the cataract is removed, and an IOL is placed in most patients.

Postoperative care usually includes use of eye drops including a steroid and antibiotic placed subconjunctivally. The eye is usually left unpatched, and the patient is discharged home. Patient education is extremely important in preparation of the patient prior to surgery and in the aftercare. Because many patients having cataract surgery are older, there is a need to emphasize the postoperative care of eye drop instillation. The postoperative period should be relatively free of complications, and pain or swelling are generally not expected. If pain with nausea and vomiting should occur, notify the ophthalmologist.

Evaluation of Outcomes

It is expected the patient will have improved vision from the preoperative assessment. Corrective lenses may or may not be necessary. Refer to Box 39-2 for evaluation of outcomes.

Glaucoma

Glaucoma is a group of diseases related to the amount of intraocular pressure in the eye occurring as a result of neurodegenerative processes. Increasing intraocular pressure can rapidly result in optic nerve damage causing a decrease in vision and blindness. There are two primary forms of glaucoma, closed angle and open angle. In addition, there is congenital, normal tension, and secondary forms, such as pigmentary and neovascular glaucoma. This section will cover the primary forms. After cataracts, glaucoma is the second leading cause of blindness worldwide. As the world population ages this will become an ever-increasing problem, because the blindness it causes is permanent. Open-angle glaucoma is more commonly seen in people of African or European decent, whereas individuals of Asian decent are more likely to develop closed-angle glaucoma (Katz, 2004).

Pathophysiology

In open-angle glaucoma the channels (trabecular meshwork or canal of Schlemm) that drain fluid within the eye become blocked, causing pressure to rise. This increased pressure pushes backward on to the vitreous humor, causing damage to the retina. Normal intraocular pressures (IOP) ranges from 10 to 21 mmHg, and as the pressure begins to rise it causes a gradual loss of vision. Because there are few symptoms, and vision loss is gradual, individuals may not notice for a long time that they are losing their sight. Closed–angle glaucoma occurs when there is a similar increase in IOP, but the onset is sudden, causing headaches, blurred vision, and pain in the eye (Katz, 2004).

Assessment with Clinical Manifestations and Diagnostic Tests

Glaucoma is determined through a comprehensive eye exam including a visual acuity test, visual fields test, dilated eye exam, and tonometry. Tonometry measures the pressure within the eye. Once it becomes apparent that there is a significant increase in IOP, it is important to take more than one measure of it. Several readings need to be taken throughout the day to establish a diurnal curve with the highest reading to be the treated pressure. The thickness or thinness of the cornea may give a false higher or lower IOP (Gray, 2005).

Nursing Diagnoses

Based on the information gathered, examples of nursing diagnoses in the patient with IOP are shown in Box 39-1.

Planning and Implementation

Glaucoma cannot be cured, and the damage is irreversible; nevertheless, the progression of the disease can be controlled with eye drops, oral medications, laser procedures, or surgery. These procedures and surgeries are done on an outpatient basis.

Pharmacology

All medications used to lower the IOP by either reducing aqueous inflow or increasing aqueous outflow with the goal of keeping the pressure in the mid to lower range (12 to 16 mmHg) of normal IOP. These drugs fall in the following categories: sympathomimetics, parasympathomimetics, beta-adrenergic antagonists, carbonic anhydrase inhibitors, and prostaglandin analogues. Each category has its advantages and disadvantages. The current gold standard for treatment of glaucoma is timolol.

Surgery

An increasingly popular choice of treatment is a trabeculoplasty, an argon laser procedure where the laser causes some of the areas of the drainage system to shrink, allowing for stretch opening of adjacent areas for increased outflow. This procedure often allows patients to reduce medications and avoid or delay further surgery.

The conventional surgery of choice is a trabeculectomy (creation of a fistula), where a small area of the trabecular meshwork is removed to allow the aqueous humor to drain. This procedure is done under local anesthetic, often with sedation. Follow-up includes an annual gonioscopy to inspect the anterior chamber of eye and for determining ocular motility and rotation. A gonioscopy is where a special lens with a mirror-like effect is placed on the eye to evaluate the trabecular meshwork through the slit lamp.

An area of increasing interest among ophthalmologists is use of surgically implanted drainage devices for patients with glaucoma resistant to eye drops (Gray, 2005). While these drainage devices are offering new alternatives, they are not without complications. Patients may develop **hypotany** (low intraocular pressure), inflammation, and excessive scar tissue formation.

Evaluation of Outcomes

The patient is followed regularly for progression of disease and changes in vision. With eye drops it is expected that the progression of disease will be greatly slowed, and there will be no loss of vision. Laser and surgical procedures should result in stabilization of vision and intraocular tension. Medications may or may not still be needed following laser or surgical intervention. Refer to Box 39-2 for evaluation of outcomes.

Retinal Detachment

Retinal detachment may also be called a detached retina or retinal tear. This occurs when the retina detaches by lifting or pulling away from its normal position. If not treated promptly, this can cause permanent vision loss. Retinal detachment can occur at any age, but it is more common in individuals over age 40. Other risk factors include extreme nearsightedness, previous history or family history of retinal detachment, previous cataract surgery, or a past eye injury.

Pathophysiology

The retina is composed of two layers; these layers can separate from each other or the wall of the eye. The more inner layer detects light, and the outer layer provides the support and nutrients to the retina. The nerve cells that detect light entering the eye then translate the information into nerve signals about what the eye sees. When the detachment occurs the retina no longer can process what it sees, which results in vision loss in that area. This vision loss can be minimal or severe depending on the size and location of the tear or detachment. There is always some vision loss after a retinal detachment (Wilkinson, 2005).

Assessment with Clinical Manifestations

The clinical manifestations of retinal detachment include floaters in the visual field and flashes of light or sparks when patients move their eyes or head. Floaters are like little cobwebs or specks that float in the visual field. The patient sees small dark shadowy shapes or crooked lines that move as his or her eye moves or drift when the eyes stop moving. They may be more annoying when looking at something bright like the sky or something white. Floaters are

> *Red Flag*
>
> **Retinal Detachment as an Emergency**
>
> The nurse must recognize the initial manifestations of retinal detachment and identify the situation as an emergency. The nurse must immediately refer the patient to an eye care professional (ophthalmologist).

not usually treated unless they impair vision sufficiently to warrant treatment or cause retinal tears or detachment.

While floaters and flashes can occur for other reasons and do not signal retinal detachment, they may be a warning sign. The patient describes a shadow or curtain that has come down in the visual field and will not go away. Side vision is often affected and progresses over time (hours or days) as more of the retina separates from the wall. If the detachment involves the macula, vision loss can be severe or total in the affected eye. Retinal detachments rarely self-repair, and surgery is usually necessary (Wilkinson, 2005).

Diagnostic Tests

Retinal detachment is diagnosed through the medical history and an eye examination specifically through an ophthalmoscope (Figure 39-5). A tear or hole may be seen at the edge of the detachment.

Nursing Diagnoses

Based on the information gathered, examples of nursing diagnoses in the patient with retinal detachments are shown in Box 39-1.

Planning and Implementation

As stated in the Red Flag feature, retinal detachment is a medical emergency, and anyone experiencing the symptoms should see an eye care professional immediately. Retinal tears are evaluated for progression to detachment prior to initiating treatment. The treatment for a tear may be **cryopexy** (freezing of the retinal tear area) or laser photocoagulation performed in an outpatient surgery center or physician's office. The laser makes small burns around the tear to weld the retina back into place, where cryopexy freezes the area around the tear, and scar formation connects the tissues. Both of these procedures are done to keep the vitreous humor from passing through the tear and increasing the size of the detachment, thereby increasing the vision loss.

A

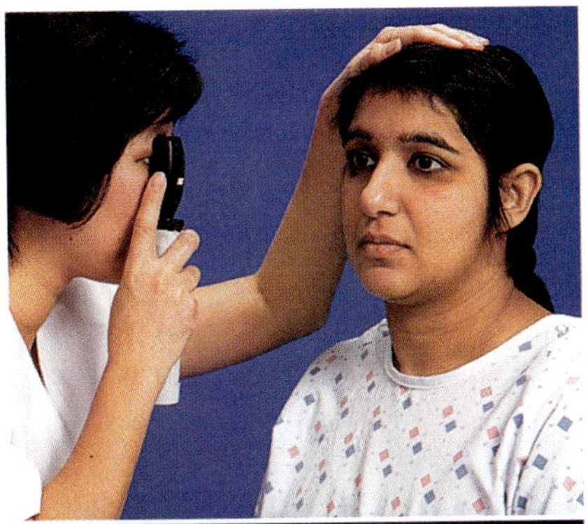

B

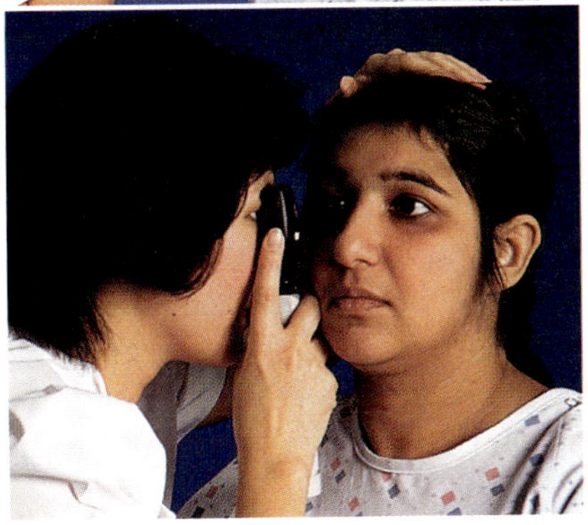

Figure 39-5 Examining retinal structures.

Surgery

Surgical options for retinal detachments include scleral buckling surgery, pneumatic retinopexy, or vitrectomy. A scleral buckle, the most common method of treatment, requires that a piece of silicone, rubber, or semihard plastic be placed against the outer surface of the eye and sutured into place. The piece pushes the sclera toward the middle of the eye, allowing the retina to settle back against the wall of the eye. The buckle may encircle the eye or just cover the area around the detachment. This surgery is usually performed in a hospital or outpatient surgical center under local or general anesthesia. Postoperative care includes monitoring for swelling, redness, tenderness, and pain management. This procedure has an 80 to 90 percent success rate. The scleral buckle can cause an increase in IOP, and the changes in the eye shape from buckle can result in a refractive error, affecting vision (Wilkinson, 2005).

When a pneumatic retinopexy is used to reattach the retina, the physician uses a bubble of gas to push the two layers back together again. This is usually done as an outpatient procedure under local anesthesia. Cryopexy or photocoagulation may be used to then seal the tear. The bubble is gradually absorbed over a week and keeps the tear closed and the retina flattened until a seal forms between the retina and the wall of the eye. This surgery takes about three weeks to achieve optimal healing. The patient may be expected to lie in a specific position for 16 to 21 hours per day to keep the bubble in the right location. Patients with confusion or attention problems would not be candidates for this type of procedure. The success rate is about 73 to 80 percent.

The third possible procedure is a vitrectomy, where the surgeon removes the vitreous fluid from the middle of the eye. The physician may then treat the retina with photocoagulation. At the end of surgery silicone oil or gas is injected into the eye to replace the vitreous fluid. This surgery may require an overnight hospital stay. The postoperative care includes assessment for bleeding into the vitreous area, further retinal detachment, fluid buildup in the clear cover of the eye (corneal edema), and increased IOP.

Evaluation of Outcomes

The expected outcome for a patient postprocedure for retinal detachment is that vision is optimized to its fullest potential. Patients may require new corrective lens after healing throughout the healing process. Refer to Box 39-2 for evaluation of outcomes.

Macular Degeneration

Recent statistics show approximately eight million individuals over the age of 55 have signs of early or intermediate age-related macular degeneration (AMD). Macular degeneration is largely an age-related disease process whereby central vision gradually deteriorates. Women are at greater risk of developing AMD, and Caucasians are more likely to develop the disease than African Americans. Family history and smoking are also significant risk factors.

Pathophysiology

Age-related macular degeneration is a painless disease where the macula gradually breaks down from the development of fatty, yellow, metabolic waste products, which accumulate in the retina. There are two forms of AMD, dry and wet. Dry (atrophic) AMD is the most common cause type, accounting for 90 percent of all people with AMD. This occurs because of a gradual deterioration of the macula from waste product buildup and lack of proper nutrition. The progress is slow and usually results in mild to moderate loss of sight; this usually does not cause a total loss of reading vision. Wet (neovascular) AMD is more devastating, because it can result in severe sight loss within a few short months. This type of AMD is caused by an abnormal growth of blood vessels in the macula, leaving the surface of the retina uneven (Wormald, Evans, Smeeth, & Henshaw, 2005).

Assessment with Clinical Manifestations

The most common early sign of dry AMD is blurred vision. As time progresses and fewer macular cells function, details become less clear with some improvement in brighter light. Continued degeneration can result in a small but growing blind spot in the middle of the visual field. As dry AMD worsens it can deteriorate into wet AMD because of the increased development of blood vessels in the area.

In wet AMD, instead of straight lines the patient sees wavy lines on the Amsler grid. As fluid leaks into the macular area from the increased blood vessels it lifts the macula causing a distorted vision. Central vision can also be lost as small blind spot may also begin to develop into wet AMD.

History of symptoms and complaints is important in the initial diagnosis. Determine whether the visual changes have an onset that was gradual or rapid, what is the duration of the symptoms and the degree of visual impairment, such as mild, moderate, or severe. Diagnosis is largely through the routine eye exam starting with use of the familiar Snellen chart where central vision is tested. Further testing includes dilating the pupil using a mydriatic to visualize the macula. A fundus examination is completed using direct ophthalmoscopy (Wormald, et al., 2005).

Diagnostic Tests

Diagnosis begins with an initial visual exam for specific signs of macular degeneration. Fluorescein angiography and indocyanine green angiography may be used to identify signs of macular degeneration.

Nursing Diagnoses

Based on the information gathered, examples of nursing diagnoses in the patient with AMD are shown in Box 39-1.

Planning and Implementation

Ongoing self-monitoring of vision is important in this disease. Patients can place an Amsler grid on the refrigerator and every morning assess for changes to vision. Diet supplements with vitamins, antioxidants, and zinc can have significant benefit in preventing disease progression. Patients may find the use of low vision aids, such as magnifiers for reading, telescopes to see into the distance, and talking watches supportive in maintaining quality of life.

The wet form of AMD may be treated with use of a laser, which may stop or lessen vision loss in the early stages. The laser destroys existing blood vessels, and the scar formation afterward may result in some permanent vision loss in the area of the retina affected. It is effective in about 50 percent of the cases. Photodynamic therapy using a light-activated drug given intravenously, and a laser beam can close the abnormal vessels while leaving the retina intact. Repeat treatment may be needed because closed vessels can reopen. Vitamins, antioxidants, and zinc are useful in prevention as well as use of sunglasses that block ultraviolet sunrays from sun exposure. Currently there is no treatment for dry AMD (Wormald, et al., 2005).

Evaluation of Outcomes

Patients rarely lose all their vision from macular degeneration. They are generally able to perform many normal daily activities even with poor central vision. Refer to Box 39-2 for evaluation of outcomes.

Traumatic Injuries

Traumatic injuries can occur at any age or at any time. The most common traumatic injuries include damage from penetration by foreign bodies, physical pressure resulting in a contusion, lacerations from sharp objects, and penetrating injuries.

Foreign Bodies

Foreign bodies in the eye are a common problem and can be the result of dust, dirt, eyelashes, or a fingernail. Because the cornea is an extremely sensitive area, a corneal abrasion may result. Corneal abrasions are often painful even when the scratch is relatively minor.

Planning and Implementation

It is important to seek health care immediately for any foreign body that is not removed by blinking. Fast-acting anesthetic agents can numb the area and allow a qualified health care professional to remove the object. Irrigation with normal saline can be used to rinse out loose particles of dust or dirt. Afterward antibiotic ointment may be used to prevent infection, and anti-inflammatory drops may be used to reduce discomfort until the cornea heals. An eye patch may be used to minimize movement of the eyelids during the healing process (Hoyt & Haley, 2005).

Evaluation of Outcomes

Successful removal of the foreign object, as well as return to normal eye function and sight, is the goal of removing an object from the eye. Refer to Box 39-2 for evaluation of outcomes.

Red Flag

Impaled object in the Eye

The health care provider must treat the impaled object found in an eye by doing the following: (a) remember to assess the patient for priority injuries first, (b) leave the object in place and stabilize the patient's head, (c) place a cup over the impaled object and tape in place (Figure 39-6), and (d) transport the patient in a safe and efficient manner remembering to not allow the impaled object to move.

Contusion

A periorbital contusion, or black eye, is a relatively common result of a traumatic injury to the face or head. Bleeding occurs in the area surrounding the eye; however, this may not be the extent of the injury. Often the eye globe is pushed back into the socket, stretching the surrounding muscles and soft tissues. This can result in the ocular muscle conditions and even rupture the globe. Pain and swelling are the most common clinical manifestations. Double

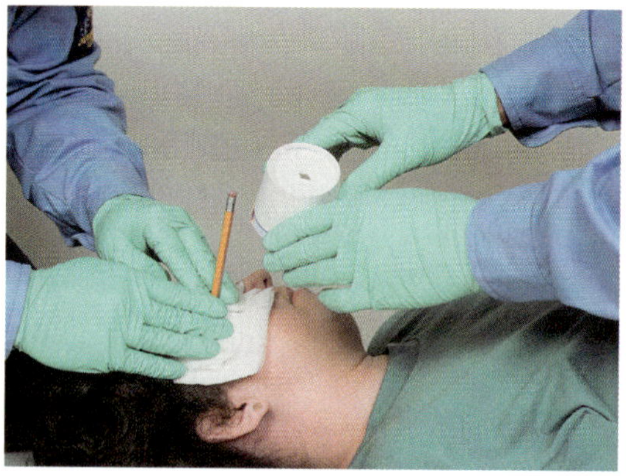

Figure 39-6 A cup helps hold an object impaled into the eye in place.

vision, loss of vision, loss of consciousness, inability to move the eye (look in different directions), and blood on the surface of the eye are signs of a more serious injury.

Planning and Implementation

Immediate health care attention should be sought for the above clinical manifestations. Initial treatment includes testing visual acuity and ophthalmoscopy. Additional testing may be performed depending on what was found, including X-rays to rule out orbital fractures. Rest and ice are the interventions for first aid. The ice should be wrapped in a cloth and applied to the effected area for 20 minutes an hour for every hour while awake for the first 24 hours. Avoid potential causes of injury until the eye has healed. Assessment by an ophthalmologist is necessary for injuries to the eye itself.

Evaluation of Outcomes

Return to normal eye function and sight with resolution of the excess fluid and swelling in the eye area are the desired results when treating a periorbital contusion. Refer to Box 39-2 for evaluation of outcomes.

Laceration and Penetrating Injuries

A full-thickness injury may occur to the cornea in the form of a puncture, or it may occur as a linear or irregular corneal laceration. The initial injury can cause complete or partial vision loss and put the patient is at risk for a secondary infection. Diagnosis is determined through the use of the standard Snellen chart and use of the slit lamp. Pressure on the globe should be avoided, the eye should be patched, and a patient with this condition should be referred to an ophthalmologist for a detailed examination.

Planning and Implementation

Every effort should be made to avoid any further injury by shielding the eye and elevating the head of the bed. The patient should be instructed not to touch the eye area and to rest until seen by the ophthalmologist. If there is a protruding body, do not remove it; the ophthalmologist should remove it. If the patient develops nausea and vomiting, antiemetics and NPO (nothing oral) status may be initiated. Broad-spectrum antibiotics should be started intravenously or orally after nausea and vomiting subside. Frequent eye examinations on follow-up are recommended for patients with lacerations or penetrating injuries because of an increased risk of traumatic cataracts and secondary glaucoma.

Evaluation of Outcomes

Rapid emergency treatment and referral to an ophthalmologist is the best option for minimal complications and vision loss. It is expected that vision loss will be related to the significance of the injury and damage to the cornea and other eye structures. Refer to Box 39-2 for evaluation of outcomes.

Ocular Cancer

Eye cancer can occur in nearly any anatomical structure of the eye, including the eyelid, the orbit, and conjunctiva. The most common ocular cancer is melanoma. A melanoma can develop in the ciliary body, conjunctiva, choroid, iris, and eyelid. A choroidal melanoma is the most common primary intraocular tumor.

Pathophysiology

Choroidal melanoma arises from melanocytes within the choroid. They may range from darkly pigmented to no coloration. As they grow choroidal melanomas can push against the retinal epithelium causing atrophy and decrease in normal choroidal circulation. These melanomas may progress silently until they produce noticeable vision loss. If the melanoma erodes into the blood vessels in adjacent areas, it can lead to vitreous hemorrhage. Metastases to distant locations are the generally the ultimate cause of death rather than local spread. The most common site of choroidal melanoma metastasis is the liver.

Assessment with Clinical Manifestations

Clinical manifestations can include ocular hypotension or hypertension and cataract if the tumor grows anteriorly. Patients may initially complain of blurred visual acuity and floaters. Severe ocular pain is rarely occurs and is related to the melanoma impinging on the posterior ciliary nerves or from increased intraocular pressure. Sunlight exposure is a likely contributor to the development of choroidal melanoma.

Diagnostic Tests

Ultrasound of the globe and orbit areas is useful in detecting tumors more than 2 to 3 mm thick. Computed tomograph (CT) scans and magnetic resonance imaging (MRIs) are less sensitive than ultrasound and more expensive. Other tests may be used to rule out metastases, such as chest radiograph and liver enzymes. Biopsy may be used only in cases in which it is difficult to distinguish whether the tumor is primary or metastatic.

Nursing Diagnoses

Based on the information gathered, examples of nursing diagnoses in the patient with ocular cancer are shown in Box 39-1. See also nursing diagnoses for patients with metastatic cancer in chapter 15.

Planning and Implementation

In the early stages of potential ocular cancer, the nurse must assess for abnormal ocular changes. The nurse must always refer the patient to ophthalmologists for further assessment and treatment plans. The majority of the management for patients with progressive or serious ocular cancers involves surgical interventions.

Surgery

The classic approach for large and complicated choroidal melanomas is the surgical removal of an eye, called **enucleation.** The reason for enucleation over globe sparring is to reduce the risk of metastatic spread. Enucleation may also be done in rare circumstances to relieve intolerable pain in a blind eye.

A medium-sized tumor is treated to plaque brachytherapy using iodine 125 because of its lower energy emission and good tissue penetration. The plaque is temporarily sutured to the sclera and limbus underlying the melanoma. Radioactive plaques are left in place for three to seven days. The goal of treatment is arrest of tumor growth or regression in size of the tumor. Complications of plaque brachytherapy include cataract, scleral necrosis, radiation retinopathy, and optic nerve damage. External beam irradiation using charged particles, such as protons, is an alternative to the brachytherapy.

Small tumors may be treated with a block incision, which is used hoping to salvage the eye, and many of these patients retain some useful vision. A block incision removes the tumor surrounding choroid, retina, sclera, and a 3-mm margin of health tissue. Complications include vitreous hemorrhage, retinal detachment, residual tumor, and cataract.

Postoperative care includes use of antibiotic, steroid, and cycloplegic eye drops. Patients may or may not have to wear and eye patch. In patients with enucleation postoperative care includes preparation for an artificial eye (ocular prosthesis) as a cosmetic substitute for the real eye.

Evaluation of Outcomes

Survival rates are 50 to 70 percent over 10 years for patients with choroidal cancer. The risk for metastases is great because of the often late diagnosis of the problem. Typical areas for metastases after the liver include lung, brain, and bones. Visual prognosis is poor, and patients require frequent follow-up eye examinations. Refer to Box 39-2 for evaluation of outcomes.

Corneal Disorders

Damage to the cornea can be painful and a serious dysfunction of the eye. Corneal disorders include corneal abrasions (one of the most common eye injuries), ulcerations, and keratoconus.

Abrasions

Corneal abrasions are one of the most common eye injuries and probably the most neglected. These injuries may result in permanent scarring and a loss of visual acuity and function. They occur as a disruption in the integrity of the corneal epithelium or because the corneal surface was denuded from physical external forces such as contact lenses or sports injuries. Many of these injuries are minor, but they can lead to blindness. These same injuries can place economic burdens on otherwise healthy people resulting in lost time at work or school. Corneal abrasions usually heal in two to three days without treatment; however, they can result in bacterial keratitis if the epithelium integrity is damaged or deteriorate into a corneal ulceration. Clinical manifestations include pain, watering, foreign body sensation, and photophobia. Treatment includes prophylactic antibiotics after trauma or surgery, cycloplegics for comfort, and an eye patch, which may or may not be worn (Calder, Balasubramanian, & Stiell, 2004).

Ulcerations

A corneal ulceration is considered an ophthalmologic emergency. Bacterial corneal ulcers usually occur from a traumatic break in the corneal epithelium allowing bacteria to enter. Other bacterial causes can include tear insufficiency, malnutrition, and contact lens use. Herpes simplex virus (HSV) is one of the most common causes of corneal ulceration. Visual acuity is affected based on location of the ulcer and whether inflammation is present in the cornea. Clinical manifestations include blurred vision, photophobia, pain, redness, and mucopurulent drainage. Emergent treatment includes an ophthalmologic consultation, cultures, and treatment with an antibiotic ointment to prevent vision loss.

Keratoconus

Keratoconus is a progressive, noninflammatory bilateral disease of the cornea characterized by thinning of the cornea layers leading to corneal surface distortion. The resulting visual loss is from irregular astigmatism, myopia, and secondarily from scarring. Risk factors for developing keratoconus include ocular allergies, rigid contact lens wear, and vigorous eye rubbing. It usually presents at puberty and progresses until the third or fourth decade of life; however, it can occur at any time.

Clinical manifestations include decreasing vision with distortion, glare, and diplopia. Patients often complain of difficulty in achieving satisfactory optimum vision with corrective lenses. Eyeglasses and soft contact lenses may be effective initially; however, as vision deteriorates rigid contact lenses may provide better vision. Diagnosis is determined through refraction, **keratometry** (measurement of the cornea), and use of the slit lamp. Primary treatment is rigid contact lenses. There is no direct pharmacological management of keratoconus; however, anti-inflammatory and antihistamine topical medications are sometimes helpful (Calder, et al., 2004).

Planning and Implementation

Corneal disorders of a serious nature are treated primarily with corneal transplantation. Corneal transplants are possible through the donation of cadaver corneas, letting family know of a person's wish to be a donor may improve the availability to corneas for transplant. Corneal transplants are done most often to treat vision loss as a result of disease, swelling, scarring, infection, or chemical burns. This is an outpatient surgical procedure lasting about an hour. Follow-up care includes the wearing of an eye shield for the prevention of injury during the healing process and antirejection eye drops.

Evaluation of Outcomes

Complete resolution of the corneal disturbances and no loss of visual acuity or function are desired outcomes. Refer to Box 39-2 for evaluation of outcomes.

REFRACTION

In normal vision, **emmetropia,** the light falls onto the retina without any distortion or abnormal bending of the light. In errors of visual refraction, which are the most common vision problems, the light passing through the layers of the eye to the retina is distorted. This can be caused by irregularities in the cornea, the focusing power of the lens, and the length of the eye (Huether, 2004).

Pathophysiology

There are three types of refraction error (Figure 39-7). **Myopia (nearsightedness)** occurs when the light passing through the eye is overbent or overrefracted. As a result the light rays are focused in front of the retina when viewing a distant object. Objects that are viewed up close are clear and distant objects are unclear. Myopia is treated with a corrective lens that redirects the light to the retina by changing the angle of the light. These corrective lenses are cut biconcave. **Hyperopia (farsightedness)** occurs when the light passing through the eye is focused behind the retina when looking a close objects. As a result, images up close are unclear, but images over 20 feet distant are clear. Hyperopia is treated with a convex corrective lens that redirects the light to the retina. The third refractive error is **astigmatism,** in which the light is spread over a diffuse area. Astigmatism occurs when there is an unequal curve of the cornea, and the light rays are bent unevenly. The exact cause of astigmatism is unknown, although there is some familial pattern. Astigmatism is treated with corrective lens in a cylindrical shape. It is not uncommon for refractive errors of myopia or hyperopia to coexist with astigmatism.

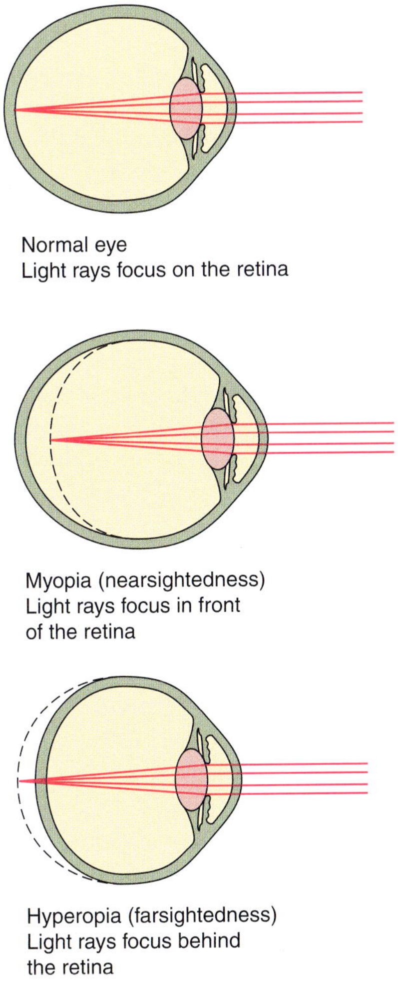

Normal eye
Light rays focus on the retina
Myopia (nearsightedness)
Light rays focus in front of the retina
Hyperopia (farsightedness)
Light rays focus behind the retina

Figure 39-7 Eye refraction.

Nursing Diagnoses

Based on the information gathered, examples of nursing diagnoses in the patient with refraction problems are shown in Box 39-1.

Planning and Implementation

There are a variety of forms of management for refraction disorders. Several treatments are common (e.g., eyeglasses), and other dysfunctions require surgical intervention.

Eyeglasses

Refraction errors are treated with corrective lenses, such as eyeglasses or contact lenses. The strength of a pair of eyeglasses is determined by having a patient view through a number of different strength lenses until the patient identifies the best correction. Eyeglass prescriptions then have the lenses ground to achieve that strength.

Contact Lenses

Contact lenses provide similar vision correction to eyeglasses and are fit to the curvature of the cornea. The contact lenses float on the cornea using the normal eye secretions to maintain adequate moisture content. Dehydration can result in decreased visual acuity and direct contact with the cornea. There are currently two different types of contact lenses, hard and soft. Hard lenses have little flexibility and change the shape of the cornea was well as provide correction. Hard contact lenses require cleaning and can only be worn while awake. Soft contact lenses come in daily wear and extended wear options. The daily wear lenses are worn during the day hours and taken out at night and soaked in a cleaning solution. The extended wear option allows the user to wear the lenses even at night for up to a week without removal. The lenses are then either cleaned or disposed of depending on the type. Contact lenses can cause corneal abrasions and progress into corneal ulcerations if care is not adequate.

Surgery

Surgical treatment for refractive errors includes radial keratotomy (RK), laser vision correction, and Intacs. These procedures are done in physician offices or outpatient surgery centers. RK uses a diamond knife to make several incisions into the cornea in a circular rotation. This alters the mechanical structure of the cornea and changes its shape to correct nearsightedness. Results are rapid and patients see quite well within one to two days. Laser vision correction is done with photorefractive keratotomy (PRK) and laser in situ keratomileusis (LASIK). In PRK an excimer laser is used to reshape the surface of the cornea after the surface epithelial cells are removed. This differs from LASIK, in which a corneal flap is created and the laser is applied beneath. Rapid recovery is expected with PRK and LASIX procedures and a return to near normal vision without further correction. Intacs are a nonlaser procedure in which an intracorneal ring segment is placed under the cornea, which may be helpful for patients with low-level myopia. The benefits are they are removable and adjustable as eye changes occur.

Postoperative care includes use of antibiotic drops and steroid drops immediately after the procedure. Verification of flap placement, smoothness, and absence of debris are assessed. Patients may complain of scratchiness, tearing, burning, and sensitivity to light, which wane as time progresses. Makeup and swimming are contraindicated for the first one to two weeks postoperatively. Complications associated with these surgeries include dislodged flaps and flap folds, infection, refractive complications, such as overcorrection or undercorrection and dry eye syndrome.

Evaluation of Outcomes

It is expected with any of these procedures that optimal vision will be achieved. In most cases vision improvement is evident within one to two days. Refer to Box 39-2 for evaluation of outcomes.

PRESBYOPIA

Older adults begin to experience a loss of near acuity (near vision) as the lens loses its elasticity and accommodation of the lens fails. The condition, **presbyopia,** is evident as a patient will begin to hold reading material at a further and further distance from the eyes to establish focus. Treatment consists of using reading glasses or adjustments to glasses with a bifocal (two foci) or trifocal (three foci) in which the reading correction is in the lower portion of the lens.

COLOR PERCEPTION

Color perception determines much about how the world is perceived. The ability to distinguish color is composed of two stages; the first is through the light-sensitive receptors, and the second is through the neural components of processing, partitioning, and encoding information about wavelength that the photoreceptors collect. Hue is determined by the wavelength of content of colors that allows us to perceive colors. There are two separate and remarkably different systems for determining colors, the blue-yellow system and the red-green system. The blue-yellow system is more likely to be injured through toxic exposure, eye disease, or trauma, whereas the red-green system is more likely to be impaired because of congenital defects. These congenital defects rarely affect the blue-yellow system (Harper, Arsura, Bobba, Reddy, & Sawh, 2005).

Colorblindness

Colorblindness can be an acquired abnormality of color vision, such as with aging, when normal sensitivity to color gradually diminishes. It is thought to result from the progressive yellowing of the lens occurring with aging. While all colors become less intense, the ability to discriminate between blue and green is greatly affected. In patients with DM, color vision deteriorates more rapidly than in the general population (Harper, et al., 2005).

The genetic link to colorblindness is a cross-linked trait and occurs in about 8 percent of the male population. Among females colorblindness occurs in only about 0.5 percent of the population. The genetically linked colorblindness results in the inability to distinguish red from green. Testing for colorblindness is done with an Ishihara chart. There is currently no treatment for this visual dysfunction.

INFLAMMATORY AND INFECTIOUS EYE CONDITIONS

There are a number of intraocular and extraocular inflammatory and infectious conditions. The eye surface is a moist area rich in nutrients and subject to potential inflammation or infection, as are the areas around the eye. Blinking is one of the eye's protective mechanisms, with 12 to 20 blinks per minute the eye effectively brushes away most bacteria; furthermore, the natural tears are nutrient poor and contain antibacterial substances. Thus infectious conditions can occur as a result of the acquisition of a virulent microorganism or uncontrolled growth of an existing organism because of lowered resistance in the patient. The external conditions of hordeolum, chalazion, blepharitis, conjunctivitis, and keratitis are discussed. The internal structures of the eye are almost impenetrable; therefore, most internal infections are the result of trauma or surgical intervention (Kuehn, 2005).

Hordeolum

The sweat glands in and around the eyelid are at risk of inflammation or infection. When these inflamed sweat glands are reddened, swollen, and tender to touch they are called a hordeolum or stye.

Planning and Implementation

Management of inflammatory and infectious eye conditions includes the use of warm moist compresses and antibiotic ointment. In addition, the practice of good medical asepsis and avoiding touching the eye area are highly recommended.

Chalazion

A chalazion is a small benign tumor similar to a sebaceous cyst, hordeolum, or even a sebaceous carcinoma. To obtain a definitive diagnosis a biopsy is often necessary. Clinical manifestations include an initial redness and tenderness that progresses to swollen area without signs or symptoms of infection.

Planning and Implementation

Management of chalazion includes teaching good hand washing and avoiding touching the eye area with unclean hands. Antibiotic ointments may be applied, with warm moist compresses. Drainage and crusts are moistened with a wet cloth prior to removal. Surgical intervention may be indicated for chalazions that interfere with vision or are cosmetically displeasing.

Blepharitis

Inflammation of the hair follicles (cilia) and glands along the edges of the eyelids is called **blepharitis.** The eyelids become sore, red, and tender, with sticky exudates. The patient may complain of itchiness, watering eyes, and loss of eyelashes. Photophobia may also be a complaint. This is the most common infection seen by ophthalmologists (Kuehn, 2005).

Planning and Implementation

Blepharitis is most often a result of a staphylococcal infection and is treated with antibiotic eye ointment. Treatment should be vigorous to prevent development of hordeolum. Eyelid areas should be cleansed gently and patted dry frequently to minimize exudate developing crusts and hardening.

Conjunctivitis

Conjunctivitis, also called pink eye, can be the result of exposure to allergens or irritants and as such is not contagious. However, there is a bacterial or viral form known as infectious conjunctivitis and easily transmitted to others. Clinical manifestations are watery eyes, reddened appearance, itching, and burning-like pain.

Viral conjunctivitis may be caused by adenovirus, HSV, and rubella. In bacterial conjunctivitis the offending organisms include pneumococcus, streptococcus, staphylococcus, and gonococcus.

Parasitic infections can also occur such as *Chlamydia trachoma* or *Onchocerca volvos.* These infections while rarely occurring in the western countries are a leading cause of blindness in the world. Diagnosis is obtained through use of cultures and antigen detection assays (Kuehn, 2005).

Planning and Implementation

The care provided for conjunctivitis is focused on preventing spread and individual treatment. Good hand washing technique prior to touching the eye area and avoiding touching the eye and then handling other objects are good techniques for prevention. Health care workers should wear gloves when treating the eye. Allergen causes are treated with removal of the allergen if possible, rinsing with artificial tears, and use of topical medications, such as antihistamines and corticosteroids. Eye drops that treat the reddened appearance, such as vasoconstrictors may be cosmetically beneficial.

Care for bacterial or viral infections includes application of appropriate antibiotic ointments after a culture of the eye drainage is obtained. Oral antiviral agents, such as acyclovir or ganciclovir, may also be used. During the healing time makeup should be avoided and all old makeup replaced to prevent reinfection.

Patients with parasitic infections are treated with topical antibiotics or oral antibiotics (tetracycline or sulfonamides) depending on their exposure and recurrence.

Keratitis

Keratitis occurs when there is an inflammation and ulceration of the cornea. Because of the involvement of the cornea there is often a loss in visual acuity. The clinical manifestations include watery eyes, pain, and photophobia. Keratitis can be caused by drugs, vitamin A deficiency, sun exposure, trauma, immune-mediated response, or microorganisms. The most common viral cause is HSV and bacterial causes are *Staphylococcus aureus, Streptococcus pneumoniae, pseudomonas,* mycobacterium, and serratia. Patients wearing contact lens are at risk for bacterial infections and in particular those using extended wear contact lens.

Planning and Implementation

Therapy is directed at treating the underlying causes; for the bacterial causes antibiotic ointments are used if the epithelial layer remains intact. Systemic antibiotics maybe required for infections that leak into the cornea. HSV keratitis can result in retinitis or cataract, and if left untreated the virus may travel to the trigeminal ganglion and a latent infection is established.

Keratoconjunctivitis Sicca

Some individuals develop an inflammation of the cornea and conjunctiva known as keratoconjunctivitis sicca or dry eye syndrome. This occurs when the individual produces fewer tears and is more common in women, especially after menopause. Aging is also a risk factor, as people grow older they produce less lipids, which affects the tear film. With less oil to seal the water layer, the tears evaporate more quickly or rundown the cheek instead of staying in the eye to moisten it. Clinical manifestations include a scratchy or sandy feeling as though something was in the eye, irritation, burning, redness, and blurred vision that improves with blinking (Kuehn, 2005).

Planning and Implementation

The care goal is primarily to treat with artificial tears for lubricating the eyes. Closing the eye's drainage ducts with punctual plugs is an option for some patients, thereby keeping more fluid in the eye. One risk group are patients that are critically ill and in an intensive care unit often because of less blinking, potential for dehydration and dry conditions with in the unit. These patients require additional proactive care.

> **PATIENT PLAYBOOK**
>
> **Treatment of "Dry Eyes"**
>
> The nurse should instruct the patient to:
>
> - Drink 8 to 10 glasses of water daily.
> - Make a conscious effort to blink more frequently.
> - Avoid rubbing the eyes.
> - Inform the patient that high altitude, dry or winter climates may make the condition worse.

Iritis and Uveitis

Iritis is the inflammation of the iris, and uveitis is the inflammation of one or all parts of the uveal tract. The uveal tract includes the iris, the ciliary body, and the choroid. Currently uveitis is divided into four components: (a) anterior; (b) confined to the iris and the anterior chamber (iritis); (c) confined to the iris the anterior iris, the anterior chamber, and the ciliary body (iridocyclitis); and (d) posterior uveitis (choroiditis). Posterior uveitis is uncommon except in patients with AIDS that may develop cytomegalovirus retinitis. Uveitis can be acute and chronic (Kuehn, 2005).

Pathophysiology

While the exact pathophysiology is unknown, it is believed that uveitis is caused by an immune reaction. It is postulated the immune reaction is directed against foreign antigens. Uveitis is often associated with infections, such as HSV and autoimmune disorders, such as systemic lupus erythematosus and rheumatoid arthritis. Clinical manifestations include pain, eye redness, blurred vision, photophobia, and tearing. In posterior uveitis there may be floaters or occasional photophobia.

Assessment with Clinical Manifestations

A thorough ophthalmic assessment would include visual acuity, extraocular movement, ophthalmoscopy, measurement of IOP, and slit lamp examination. There is no laboratory or radiographic test that is generally performed except tests associated with the initial diagnosis of systemic disease.

Planning and Implementation

The first line of treatment is cycloplegic and steroidal ophthalmic drops. Patients may also receive oral steroids and immunosuppressive agents. Follow-up with an ophthalmologist is imperative. If vitreous hemorrhage occurs a vitrectomy may be used in patients who cannot take immunosuppressive agents.

OCULAR DISORDERS RESULTING FROM OTHER PHYSIOLOGICAL PROCESSES

While there are many other disorders that have ocular ramifications, this chapter will deal with the following three problems: (a) an ocular disorder occurring as a result of neurological dysfunction (papilledema); (b) diabetes retinitis related to DM; and (c) retinitis pigmentosa (RP) a genetic disorder.

Papilledema

When there is an increase in intracranial pressure as a result of trauma or other disease process a swelling of the optic disc **(papilledema)** may occur. Other causes include any tumors occupying space in the central nervous system, meningitis, and encephalitis. Papilledema usually occurs bilaterally and can develop rapidly or slowly over time depending on the underlying cause.

Pathophysiology

Because the subarachnoid space of the brain is continuous with the optic nerve sheath, as the cerebrospinal fluid pressure increases, the pressure is transmitted to the optic nerve. This results in swelling and inflammation of the optic nerve at the entrance to the retina. Clinical manifestations include headache, nausea, and vomiting. While visual symptoms may not occur, some patients develop graying of vision or transient flickering, blurry vision, and diplopia. Visual acuity is usually unaffected until the condition is quite advanced. In severe cases blindness can occur rapidly unless the pressure is relieved and the swelling decreases.

Planning and Implementation

Care is tailored to treat the underlying cause or causes. Efforts to reduce papilledema include carbonic anhydrase inhibitor diuretics, weight reduction in idiopathic intracranial hypertension, and corticosteroids for inflammatory causes. Surgical treatment may include removing the tumor, a ventriculoperitoneal shunt, or optic nerve sheath decompression.

Diabetic Retinopathy

Patients with DM are at risk of developing many different ophthalmic complications, including corneal abnormalities, glaucoma, cataracts, and neuropathies. However, the most common and potentially most blinding complication is diabetic retinopathy (see chapter 57).

Etiology

Risk factors include duration of diabetes, development of renal complications, systemic hypertension, and elevated serum lipids.

Pathophysiology

The exact mechanism by which diabetes causes retinopathy is unknown, however, there are several hypotheses. The first is that growth hormone may play a causative role, second is hematologic abnormalities in diabetes, such as erythrocyte aggregation, increased platelet aggregation, and sluggish circulation, may be factors. The third is related to the abnormal glucose metabolism where high levels of blood glucose are thought to have an affect on the retinal capillaries causing them to function poorly eventually leading to retinal hypoxia. About 8,000 eyes become blind each year from diabetes (Horowitz, Brennan, & Reinhardt, 2005).

Assessment with Clinical Manifestations and Diagnostic Tests

As with many eye disorders initial diagnosis may come with routine eye examination. To determine the extent of microvascular damage fluorescein angiography or ultrasound of the retina may be done.

Nursing Diagnoses

See Box 39-1. See also nursing diagnoses for patients with DM in chapter 57.

Planning and Implementation

The most important management of patients with DM is the management of glucose levels with the goal of intensive glucose control will decrease the incidence and progression of disease. The goal of the American Diabetic Association (ADA) to maintain a glycosylated hemoglobin level of less than 7 percent can help prevent or at least minimize the long-term complications of DM. Treatment with laser photocoagulation, vitrectomy, or cryotherapy has been successful in some patients in preserving vision. Patient education regarding glucose control, managing other complications well, and cessation of smoking have also proven beneficial.

Retinitis Pigmentosa

RP is the name given to a group of inherited diseases affecting the retina. Currently there are about 70 different genetic defects that have been identified.

Pathophysiology

RP is a progressive disease with a progressive loss of vision due to the loss of viable photoreceptors. In the progressive disease, central vision is spared the longest, with peripheral vision affected first. The individual may have either the rods or the cones affected. When the rods are primarily affected, it results in symptoms of night blindness and slow loss of peripheral vision, whereas the individual with cones primarily affected has decreasing visual acuity, development of color blindness, and day vision problems.

Assessment with Clinical Manifestations

History of loss of night vision and tunnel vision are often reported by patients. A complete history of vision changes is important as well as the adaptation to darkness. A complete ophthalmic examination is used to identify disease development or progression.

Nursing Diagnoses

Based on the information gathered, examples of nursing diagnoses in the patient with RP problems are shown in Box 39-1.

Planning and Implementation

There are multiple studies underway looking at methods of treatment and prevention; however there is no medical treatment currently. Today there is some recommendation for vitamin A supplementation. Treatment of symptoms may be somewhat beneficial, such as cataract removal as cataracts develop; however, vision will still be affected by the development of RP, with possibly only central vision improvement. Future treatments may involve retinal transplants, artificial retinal implants, gene therapy, stem cells, nutritional supplements, and drug therapies.

DOLLARS AND SENSE

Financial Impact of Blindness

The elderly have many problems associated with low vision or legal blindness. Obviously, the ability to drive is impaired, as well as the preparation techniques for meals. However, one of the greatest affects of the visual impairment is on the financial status of the elderly. This group of people (i.e., elderly with low vision) have many difficulties in maintaining financial security and suffer profusely from their dysfunction.

Source: Boyle, E. (2006). Visual impairment reduces functional status of elderly patients. Ocular Surgery News, 24*(1), 73–74.*

LOW VISION AND BLINDNESS

Low vision is a general term used to describe a permanent functional vision loss that is not correctable by medication, surgery, or corrective lenses. Patients classified with low vision may have any one of a wide range of diseases. These individuals may find that their ability to perform activities of daily living, work, and pleasure are impaired. In addition to the traditional assessment for vision and visual acuity, consideration should be given to the individual's ability to cope with their limitations.

Legal blindness is defined as vision of 20/200 on a Snellen chart or less in the better eye with correction. Of the individuals in above classification about 10 percent are fully sightless. The rest have some vision, from light perception alone to relatively good acuity. Those who are not legally blind but have serious visual impairment possess low vision (Estes, 2006).

Epidemiology

The most common causes of blindness around the world, according to the World Health Organization, are shown in Box 39-3. Many of these diseases can be prevented through adequate nutrition and disease treatment, especially if treatment of infections is done in a timely manner.

BOX 39-3

CAUSES OF BLINDNESS

Cataracts 47.8 percent
Glaucoma 12.3 percent
Age-related macular degeneration 8.7 percent
Trachoma 3.6 percent
Corneal opacity 5.1 percent
Diabetic retinopathy 4.8 percent

Planning and Implementation

The care necessary for individuals with low vision and blindness is varied. Mobility is one of the greatest challenges for patients with these dysfunctions. In an era where individual transportation rather public transportation is the norm, the ability to get from place to place is greatly impeded in our social context. Patients can travel using a white cane, an international symbol of blindness, which when swung in a low sweeping motion across the intended path can detect obstacles. Individuals choosing to use guide dogs have been guaranteed access to public places as an individual personal right.

Assistive Devices

Patients with low vision have some options to help improve vision. Reading devices are available with a bifocal power of up to +5.00 diopters (D); however, this may distort vision for walking and other activities. Therefore, the patient may need a second pair of corrective lenses for other activities.

Microscope devices are used when the needed power is greater than 12 D. Because of the greatly reduced focal length, microscopes often are prescribed monocularly. Near telescopes, have a narrow field of view and can be designed for the individuals regular working distance.

Handheld magnifiers provide greater magnification than high-add readers and allow for a greater reading distance than microscopes, but they require good motor control. For this reason, handheld magnifiers are primarily used for short-term activities, such as shopping or using a phonebook. Stand magnifiers require less motor control and allow for a longer working distance. When illuminated, these magnifiers can increase the ease of readability for the patient.

Closed circuit televisions can provide a larger field of view than other forms of magnification. A handheld magnifier or camera is used to scan over the material that is projected onto the television monitor in an enlarged format.

Other adaptive equipment is available through multiple resources listed in the previous chapter. Large print newspapers and magazines are available in some communities. Dial markers can be used to dry gauges on ovens, dishwashers, washers, and dryers. Self-threading needles, books on tape, and talking clocks and watches are just some of the available adjuncts for patients.

HEALTH PROMOTION

It is the charge of health care workers to ensure that patients are educated regarding prevention of eye-related disease. Patients should be encouraged as part of their normal health promotion behaviors to see their eye care specialist on a regular basis. Because malnutrition is a cause of many eye conditions, patient education on adequate nutrition should be considered part of every episode of patient teaching.

Safety

In these same patients, safety should be an ongoing concern with patient education directed to methods to prevent injury to allow a patient the greatest freedoms without possible harm. Patients should be oriented to new environments, how to access care, or taught what to do in emergencies. In the health care setting, patients should be oriented to the individuals caring for them and the location of important items (e.g., call lights or bathrooms). At mealtime, patients need to be oriented to location of various eating utensils and foods on the tray. When ambulating a patient, the nurse should allow the patient to grasp his or her arm below the elbow and walk a half step ahead of the patient. Instruct the patient regarding any obstacles in the path and give notice to changes in direction. Safety precautions will make the patient more comfortable and ease the tradition from the home setting to the health care setting.

KEY CONCEPTS

- There are three main ocular movement dysfunctions: (a) strabismus, (b) nystagmus, and (c) ocular muscle paralysis.
- Ocular motor testing is the evaluation of the alignment of the eyes and their movement.
- Disorders of visual acuity include cataracts, glaucoma, retinal detachment, and macular degeneration.
- Glaucoma is a group of diseases related to the amount of IOP in the eye occurring as a result of neurodegenerative processes.
- Retinal detachment may also be called a detached retina or retinal tear.
- Macular degeneration is largely an age-related disease whereby central vision gradually deteriorates.
- The most common traumatic injuries of the eye include damage from penetration by foreign bodies, physical pressure resulting in a contusion, lacerations from sharp objects, and penetrating injuries.
- Eye cancer can occur in nearly any anatomical structure of the eye including the eyelid, the orbit, and conjunctiva.
- Corneal disorders include corneal abrasions, ulcerations, and keratoconus.
- In errors of visual refraction, which are the most common vision problems, the light passing through the layers of the eye to the retina is distorted.
- Older adults begin to experience a loss of near acuity (near vision) as the lens loses its elasticity and accommodation of the lens fails.
- The ability to distinguish color is composed of two stages, the first is through the light-sensitive receptors and the second is through the neural components of processing, partitioning, and encoding information about wavelength that the photoreceptors collect.
- Infections of the eye can occur as a result of the acquisition of a virulent microorganism or uncontrolled growth of an existing organism because of lowered resistance in the patient.

Continued

KEY CONCEPTS—cont'd

- Conjunctivitis, also called pink eye, can be the result of exposure to allergens or irritants and as such is not contagious.
- An ocular disorder occurring as a result of neurological dysfunction is papilledema.
- RP is the name given to a group of inherited diseases affecting the retina.
- Low vision is a general term used to describe a permanent functional vision loss that is not correctable by medication, surgery, or corrective lenses.
- Patients should be encouraged as part of their normal health promotion behaviors to see their eye care specialist on a regular basis

REVIEW QUESTIONS

1. Which of the following is not one of the three main ocular movement dysfunctions?
   1. Strabismus
   2. Nystagmus
   3. Color blindness
   4. Ocular muscle paralysis

2. Mr. Jones has an abnormality of the eye in which both eyes are affected, yet the problem is often more acute in one eye than the other. This is most likely which condition?
   1. Cataract
   2. Keratoconus
   3. Glaucoma
   4. Retinal detachment

3. Mr. Bears has glaucoma, which was determined by testing the pressure within his eye. The diagnostic test revealing the presence of this eye pressure is:
   1. Intracranial pressure
   2. Ballottement
   3. Tonometry
   4. Trabeculectomy

4. Mrs. Carpenter, 83, has an eye condition where she has blurred vision and states it is better in bright light. In addition, she sees wavy lines on the Amsler grid (diagnostic test). This is most likely which condition?
   1. Glaucoma
   2. Diabetic retinopathy
   3. Age-related macular degeneration
   4. Strabismus

5. A patient is found after an accident with an impaled object in an eye. The nurse remembers to first do what?
   1. Place a cup over the impaled object and tape in place
   2. Remembers to assess the patient for priority injuries
   3. Pull out the object and observe for bleeding
   4. Turn the patient on their side, to prevent aspiration

6. What is the most common cause of ocular cancer?
   1. Melanoma
   2. Diabetes mellitus
   3. Intracranial pressure problems
   4. Hypertension

7. Mary has been rubbing her eye profusely for the past several weeks. Which of the following complications would she most likely be predisposed to from the rubbing action?
   1. Hyperopia
   2. Keratoconus
   3. Corneal ulceration
   4. Refraction

8. Mr. Clark has a visual problem that is correct with convex corrective lens. His problem is most likely what?
   1. Hyperopia
   2. Myopia
   3. Astigmatism
   4. Corneal abrasion

9. Mrs. Thomlin has an eye disorder in which there are inflamed sweat glands that are reddened, swollen, and tender to touch. This is:
   1. Uveitis
   2. Iritis
   3. Hordeolum
   4. Conjunctivitis

10. Mr. Evans has an inflammation of the cornea and conjunctiva known as keratoconjunctivitis sicca or dry eye syndrome. Which of the following is not an appropriate nursing intervention for this condition?
   1. Make a conscious effort to blink more frequently
   2. Avoid rubbing the eyes
   3. Inform the patient that high altitude, dry, or winter climates may make the condition worse
   4. Decrease daily intake of water

REVIEW ACTIVITIES

1. Assess six patients for ocular movement dysfunction by assessing their cranial nerves (CN) III, IV, and VI.
2. Evaluate four patients in regard to their visual acuity by administering a Snellen eye chart examination.
3. Examine three patients with an ophthalmoscope to specifically identify the retina and ask the patient questions specific to the condition of a retinal detachment.
4. Obtain permission to observe several specific eye diagnostic tests in either an acute care facility or clinic that performs eye tests.
5. Describe the emergency care for a patient with an object impaled in his or her eye.
6. Compare and contrast the three main types of refraction.
7. Compare and contrast two inflammatory and infectious eye conditions.
8. List at least five devices that can be used with patients who have low vision.

Visit the Contemporary Medical-Surgical Nursing online companion resource at www.delmarhealthcare.com for additional content and study aids. Click on Online Companions then select the Nursing discipline.

Auditory Dysfunction: Nursing Management

CHAPTER 40

Diane Montgomery, PhD, RN

CHAPTER TOPICS

- Conductive Hearing Loss
- Sensorineural Hearing Loss
- Health Promotion
- Protective Devices
- Auditory Testing
- Communication Adaptation
- Hearing Aids

The ability to hear is one of the basic five senses in the body, which are considered necessary for an individual to communicate and interpret environment cues. With loss of normal hearing, the individual experiences decreased functional ability and social isolation. As an individual gets older, hearing begins to deteriorate. The ability to remain independent and maintain a healthy quality of life depends on the ability to function in society. Some hearing loss can be prevented while others who have already experienced profound loss may be helped with hearing devices.

KEY TERMS

Auditory
Bullous myringitis
Cerumen
Cholesteatoma
Mastoidectomy
Mastoiditis
Myringoplasty
Myringotomy
Ossicles
Otalgia
Otitis media
Otosclerosis
Ototoxic
Schwartze's sign
Stapedectomy
Tinnitus
Tympanometry
Tympanosclerosis
Vertigo

AUDITORY DYSFUNCTION

Auditory (pertains to the sense of hearing) dysfunction affects an individual's ability to hear sounds. The degree and amount of dysfunction is associated with the affected location in the auditory system. This section of the chapter will discuss auditory dysfunction and its nursing management.

Epidemiology

Loss of hearing is the third leading cause of health problems in the United States affecting for the most part the elderly and young. Approximately 28 million Americans or roughly 1:10 have some degree of auditory dysfunction. One in four 65-year-olds and one in two 75-year-olds are hearing impaired. When hearing is diminished or lost, an individual has difficulty communicating with others and therefore must find alternative ways in which to exchange ideas. As the population ages so will the increase of hearing loss related to the aging process and prolonged excessive noise exposure. Research indicates that there is an increasing number of 46- to 64-year-olds with complaints of hearing loss secondary to repeated high noise exposure throughout their lifetimes (Bogardus, Yueh, & Shekelle, 2003; Brors & Bodmer, 2004; Rovig, 2004). Society has become more noise infested with new inventions to make tasks easier. Examples of excessive noise producers would include power tools, appliances, and other electronic devices. Excessive noise exposure has been linked to employment, loud music, high volume traffic, domestic appliances, and toys. The costs related to hearing loss are enormous and approximately $56 billion dollars per year are attributed to lost production, special education, and necessary medical care. Prevention is the first step in preserving hearing. Prevention begins with awareness of the level and type of noises throughout the environment and taking steps to decrease the amount that comes in contact with the inner ear. Depending on the cause and severity of loss, management can range from prevention to assistance with mechanical devices and cochlear implants to aural rehabilitation.

Etiology

Hearing loss can be caused by several factors including noise-induced exposures, disorders in the auditory system, and the normal aging process. The ability to perceive sound differs in degrees from the inability to understand certain words or certain sound's pitch to total deafness. Most people who have a hearing problem may not recognize that there is a problem until others mention the change in mannerisms. Although some are aware that they are experiencing a loss in hearing, they are often unwilling to tell anyone for fear of being stigmatized or being excluded from certain activities. A large number of individuals are too self-conscious and therefore not willing to reveal a weakness to others or show that they are aging. Hearing loss has long been considered an aging disease but can be associated with other factors.

Acquired Hearing Loss

Acquired hearing loss is caused by repeated damage to the auditory system. Besides noise pollution, head trauma, and infectious etiologies, such as otitis media and communicable diseases, can cause damage to the sensitive auditory system. Harm from noise can be related to a single loud blast or gradual repeated abuse throughout one's lifespan.

Ototoxic Medications and Auditory Dysfunction

Auditory dysfunction can also be caused by **ototoxic** (a substance that damages the acoustic nerve or hearing mechanism) medications, which include aminoglycoside antibiotics (gentamicin, tobramycin), loop diuretics (furosemide),

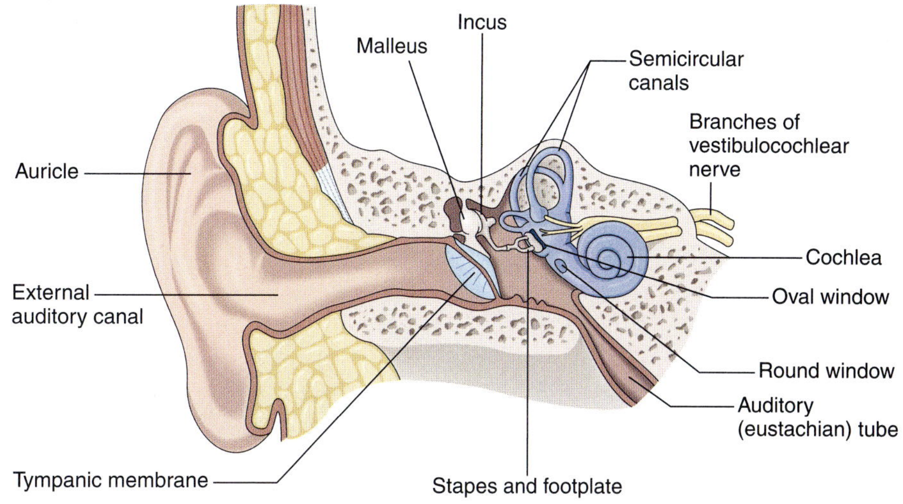

Figure 40-1 Ear structure.

antimalarial drugs (quinine sulfate, mefloquine), chemotherapy (cisplatin, carboplatin), and high-dose salicylates. Some of the medications cause temporary damage to the auditory system, in other words, when the medication is discontinued, the hearing will return to the previous state, while others cause permanent damage. Permanent damage is found to occur with aminoglycosides and chemotherapy drugs (Yueh, Shapiro, MacLean, & Shekelle, 2003). When a known ototoxic medication is prescribed, the risks and benefits to the patient should be considered. A baseline and follow up hearing test is recommended depending on the substance. There are over 200 different medications, which are labeled ototoxic, so the nurse needs to be diligent when administering medications. Being alert to the slightest change in the patient's hearing and investigating likely causes. Common symptoms experienced, include sensorineural hearing loss, tinnitus, and decreased equilibrium.

Head Trauma

Head trauma can also cause hearing loss, specifically injury to the temporal bone. The auditory receptors are located in the temporal region of the skull. Trauma to the area or an abrupt change in air pressure can cause a perforated tympanic membrane leading to the development of scar tissue and eventual hearing loss.

Pathophysiology

To understand the mechanism of hearing, the nurse must know the anatomy of the ear and how sound waves are transmitted, received, and interpreted. The ear has two main functions, hearing and maintaining balance equilibrium. The anatomy of the ear is such that it allows sound waves to be transmitted to the brain for interpretation from the outside world (Figure 40-1). Understanding the mechanism of how the ear functions is essential for the nurse to care for patients who experience hearing dysfunction. The responsibility of the nurse lies with preventing further damage to the auditory system, identifying the hearing loss, assisting the patient in adjusting to the degree of loss, and rehabilitation of auditory function when possible.

The ear is divided into three main sections: external ear, middle ear, and inner ear (Figure 40-2). The external canal extends from the external os or opening to the tympanic membrane. The middle ear is an air filled cavity, which contains the **ossicles** (the tiny bones located in the inner ear chamber: malleus, incus, and stapes), tiny bones that assist with transmitted sounds from the tympanic membrane to the inner ear. The inner ear provides the necessary

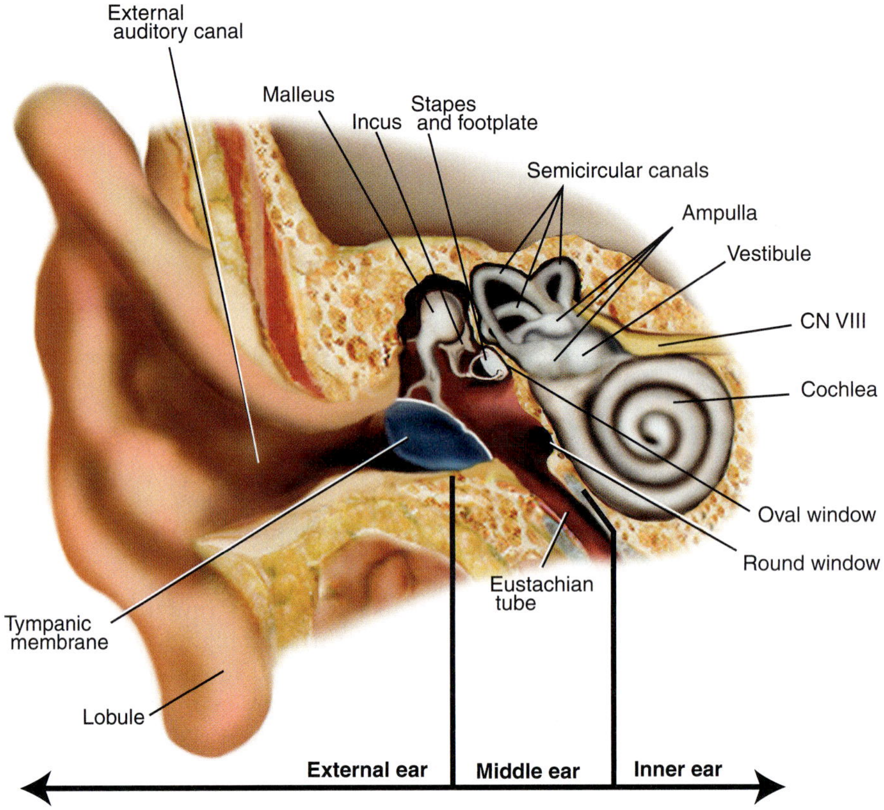

Figure 40-2 Cross-section of the ear showing the external, middle. and inner ear.

components for hearing and maintaining equilibrium, which begins with the oval window and contains the vestibule, semicircular canals, and cochlea. Inside the cochlea is the organ of Corti, responsible for transmitting sound to the acoustic nerve (eighth cranial nerve), which travels to the brain for interpretation. In other words, sound causes the tympanic membrane to vibrate, which results in movement of the ossicles; this movement travels through the oval window into the inner ear and disrupts the fragile hair lining of the Corti (end organ of hearing) located in the cochlea, sending an impulse to the acoustic nerve and then to the brain for interpretation.

The formation of the ear begins during the third week of gestation and continues through the first trimester of pregnancy, therefore any insults incurred during this most critical period of development can result in malformations of the ear. Depending on the extent and location of the abnormality, loss of hearing can occur.

Auditory dysfunction can occur at any age. As discussed above, hearing difficulties are related to several factors, including congenital malformations, noise level, and length of exposure, or acquired through infections or other pathology. The ability to learn speech, communicate and socialize depends on the capability to hear and interpret sounds.

> **Red Flag**
>
> **Prevention of Hearing Loss during Pregnancy**
>
> Women of childbearing age should be tested for rubella immunity before getting pregnant or while pregnant if not tested previously. A titer of greater that 1:8 antibody titer indicates immunity. If the woman does not have adequate titers or is nonimmune, she should be immunized in the postpartum period to avoid acquiring the disease during a subsequent pregnancy. The most susceptible period of pregnancy is the first trimester, and therefore the immunization, which is a live virus, should not be given within three months of the pregnancy or anytime during the pregnancy.

Genetics

Congenital hearing loss can be derived from genetics, natal infections, or physical deformities of the ear. Inherited hearing loss can result from multiple of factors associated with autosomal dominant (50 percent chance), recessive (25 percent chance), or cross-linked (carried on the sex gene, male increased risk) chromosomal abnormalities. Certain conditions, such as

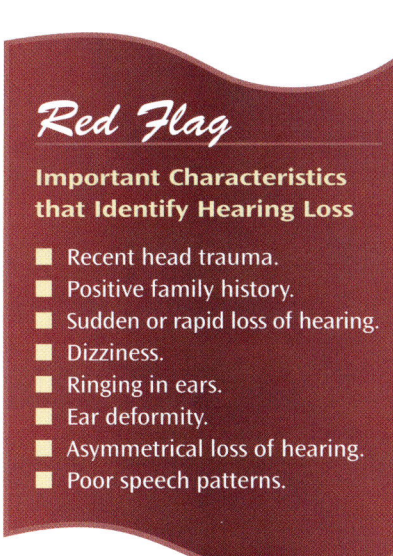

> ***Red Flag***
>
> **Important Characteristics that Identify Hearing Loss**
>
> - Recent head trauma.
> - Positive family history.
> - Sudden or rapid loss of hearing.
> - Dizziness.
> - Ringing in ears.
> - Ear deformity.
> - Asymmetrical loss of hearing.
> - Poor speech patterns.

Down, Usher, and Treacher Collins syndromes, have known associated hearing impairments (Phillips, 2003). Other factors related to congenital hearing loss are ototoxic drugs administered before or after birth or maternal prenatal infections commonly associated with the TORCH infections (a set of infections which affect the growing fetus: toxoplasmosis, rubella, cytomegalovirus, and herpes-virus type 2 and other viruses, such as syphilis, HIV, hepatitis B, and human parvovirus).

Assessment with Clinical Manifestations

The history of a patient is the most important part of assessing a patient with hearing loss. It is necessary for the nurse to observe and assess for warning signs related to a loss of hearing while interviewing the patient. During the health history, the nurse should cover problems with balance, nutrition, such as any foods which affect hearing or cause ear discomfort, sleep disturbance-related to tinnitus or vertigo, functioning level, and allergies, which may affect the eustachian tube functioning.

Ascertaining an accurate health history is the initial way to identify a hearing problem and guide the physical exam to identifying the origin of the problem. Inquiring about any changes in hearing perception, balance, and physical signs of ear disorders are important factors to lead the focus of the physical exam. Included in the history should be items, such as pain or fullness in the ears, dizziness, or tinnitus. Has their communication style changed, are they more attuned to lip reading? Does the patient have any food allergies or taken any medicines that would be ototoxic? Have they had to alter their activities of daily living related to ear discomforts?

When performing a physical exam on a patient, a simple noninvasive way to test hearing would be the whisper test. Standing approximately two feet away from the patient and covering the opposite ear, the nurse whispers a word or phase to the patient and then has the patient repeat what was said. If the patient is unable to hear the word, it is repeated slightly louder until the patient can hear. Failure to repeat the correct word or phase or having to say the word in a normal or loud tone would indicate the need for formal audiometry testing.

Hearing loss is often subtle, and the individual learns to compensation to overcome the deficit. There are various degrees of loss of hearing that the individual can experience. The assortment includes missing some syllables or words, the inability to hear some tones or pitches, or profound deafness. The first clinical signs that emerge are when a person asks to have things repeated, asks others to speak louder, answers questions inappropriately, or does not respond to a question when asked. Common missed sounds are found in numbers, for example, the person misinterprets 50 for 15 or has difficulty distinguishing certain letters, such as th and s. Hearing impaired individuals often tilt their heads to listen or display unusual facies such as frowning when trying to listen to the conversation. Additional signs may include weariness or unexplained irritability. There is a misconception that people get used to the noise and therefore can tolerate higher degrees.

Degrees of hearing impairment are categorized into minimal, moderate, severe, and profound depending on the level of decibels (dB) of sound heard. Decibels are logarithmic units of measurement of sound intensities used to measure a person's hearing capabilities. Normal hearing is 0–15 dB; slight loss 16–25 dB; mild impairment 26–40 dB; moderate 41–55 dB; moderate severe 56–70 dB; severe 71–90 dB; profound greater than or equal to 91 dB (Bogardus, et al., 2003; Punch, Joseph, & Rakerd, 2004). Profound hearing loss is usually characteristic of a congenital abnormality. Individuals who are exposed to intensities greater than 80 dB on a regular basis are at increased risk of gradual irreversible hearing loss.

Three Classifications of Auditory Dysfunction

Auditory dysfunction is classified in three ways, conductive and sensorineural dysfunction and mixed. Loss of auditory function depends on the degree of loss, etiology, and location of damage in the auditory system.

Conductive Hearing Loss

Conductive hearing loss is generally treatable and is associated with an obstruction. Conductive hearing loss affects all pitches of sound waves and is associated with an obstruction in the external and middle sections of the ear. Because the patient appears to have loss of hearing in all frequencies levels, they tend to hear better in noisy situations. Speech patterns are appropriate, although they tend to speak softer because they have a tendency to perceive their own voice louder.

Conductive loss results in a blockage of sound waves in the external or middle portions of the ear. The loss results from insults from obstructions, infections, congenital deformities, and damage. The hearing loss is associated with anything that interferes with air conduction in the outer and middle ear chambers. This includes cerumen, foreign body, otitis externa, middle ear disease (e.g., otitis media with or without effusion), **otosclerosis** (a progressive hearing loss of predominately low tones), and stenosis of external auditory canal. Most of these conditions can be treated by medical or surgical management. Air conduction is decreased in conductive hearing loss, which is necessary for sound waves to be transmitted to the ossicles for vibrations and therefore be transmitted to the brain for interpretation. In conductive loss the sound is perceived as faint or distant but clear. Patients try to compensate by speaking softer because their own voice is perceived as louder. They have no added difficulty with hearing in a noisy environment. Conductive hearing loss can be differentiated from sensorineural by the loss of all frequencies as opposed to loss of the higher frequencies found in sensorineural loss.

Temporary causes of auditory dysfunction result from obstruction in the ear canal, which can be cerumen or foreign bodies lodged in the external canal. These substances obstruct the canal preventing sound from reaching the tympanic membrane, thereby preventing the vibratory movement necessary to initiate the sequence of hearing sound waves. The external canal can be visually inspected with an otoscope. By eliminating the obstruction, the patient can instantly hear as before. Another cause of conductive loss would be an external otitis media, which causes a narrowing of the canal leading to interference of sound waves hitting the tympanic membrane.

The most common cause of intermittent loss of conductive hearing is infections. Otitis infections include otitis media or otitis media with effusion. The infection decreases the vibratory movement of the tympanic membrane necessary for passing sound waves to the acoustic nerve to be interpreted by the brain. Repeated insults from recurrent otitis media may cause permanent hearing loss. Therefore, the nurse must be diligent in recognizing those at risk. Repeated damage to the tympanic membrane can cause scarring and thickening of the membrane, causing the vibratory response to be diminished and thereby affecting the ability to hear.

Conductive loss is also affected by injury to the middle ear, which would include the auditory ossicles. Pathology that would affect this region includes trauma, infections, and scar tissue. Adhesions from chronic otitis media can cause fibrous bands to interfere with movement of the ossicles causing a conductive hearing loss. Other conditions include otosclerosis, which is a progressive disorder that affects the ossicles and the stapes in particular (note: discussed in further detail later in the chapter).

Sensorineural Hearing Loss

Sensorineural hearing loss is caused by defects in the inner ear, in the acoustic nerve (eighth cranial nerve), or in areas of the brain. Congenital anomalies, systemic insults, and environmental factors fall into this category. The loss is noticed more in high-frequency pitches, and the patient appears to have more difficulty hearing in noisy environments, such as restaurants.

Sensorineural loss results from damage or deformities of the inner ear, the area where sound is identified by the cochlea and sent to the brain via the acoustic nerve. Sensorineural hearing loss is permanent and therefore cannot be corrected or treated, just managed. Sound is perceived as distorted. There is a greater loss in the higher frequency ranges, and therefore the patient has difficulty trying to understand conversations in a noisy crowed area. Specific conditions, which cause nerve damage would include noise pollution, presbycusis, congenital, environmental, infections, and various systemic conditions. In sensorineural hearing loss bone conduction is affected, which can be identified using the Rinne test.

Sensorineural hearing loss is the impaired function of the inner ear, which includes the auditory connections to the brain. The patient has the ability to hear sound but cannot understand speech. Causes of sensorineural hearing loss include congenital and hereditary factors, noise trauma, Menière's disease, and ototoxicity. Systemic infections such as tuberculosis, syphilis, Lyme disease, cytomegalovirus, human immunodeficiency virus (HIV), and Paget disease of bone can also lead to sensorineural hearing loss. Smoking has also been linked to sensorineural hearing loss from damage over the years to the fine ciliary hairs of the inner ear from both the smoker and secondhand smoke. Other disorders such as diabetes mellitus, bacterial meningitis, and trauma have been linked to sensorineural hearing loss (Yeuh, Shapiro, MacLean, & Shekelle, 2003).

Menière's Disease

Menière's disease is a degenerative condition of unknown etiology, which leads to progressive hearing loss predominately in middle age. Studies link the disease to excessive accumulation of fluid in the labyrinth or inner ear. Symptoms appear as dizziness, unilateral ringing in the ear, feeling of pressure or fullness in ear, and unilateral hearing loss. The patient experiences episodic attacks, which can render him or her debilitated and confined to bed for extended periods of time during the acute attack. The onset of the acute phase at times is so severe that the patient may drop to the floor. Menière's disease is a progressive chronic condition in which no cure is available. Approximately 50 percent of patients who have unilateral symptoms will develop signs in the unaffected ear over the course of the disease. Menière's disease usually affects patients between the ages of 30 and 60 years and tends to appear in families and is therefore thought to have a genetic component (Perez, Chen, & Nedzelski, 2004). When performing a physical examination, the neurological assessment is found to be within normal limits.

Pharmacology

Pharmacological management during the acute phase includes antihistamines, anticholinergic medications (antiemetic/antivertigo), and sedatives, which include benzodiazepines. Between attacks the patient should be placed on diuretics, medications with vasodilating properties, and antihistamines. Up to 85 percent of patients improve with medical management. Others may require surgical interventions.

Surgery

Surgery is indicated in patients who have frequent incapacitating attacks that interfere with activities of daily living. During surgery the vestibular nerve is resected to help relieve vertigo and stop further hearing loss. In perioperative teaching, the nurse provides safety and ways to minimize vertigo. The patient is instructed to call for assistance with ambulation and avoid sudden head movement and postural changes. Televisions, florescent bulbs, and flickering lights should also be avoided.

Patient and Family Teaching

After ruling out other central nervous system disorders, nurses should offer support, reassurances that Menière's disease is not life-threatening, and education on management, which includes special dietary intervention, the course of disease, and medication administration, which includes possible side effects. Patients are helped by initiating a low-salt diet and the elimination of all caffeine-containing products. These measures have been found to help decrease the symptoms. Patients should also stop smoking and avoid prolonged exposure to smoke. During the acute phase the patients are confined to bed rest and assistance with ambulation to prevent injury.

Labyrinthitis

Labyrinthitis is a rare disorder, which involves the inflammation of the labyrinth section of the inner ear caused by head trauma or various viral or bacterial infections. An organism enters into the inner ear chamber through the oval window causing the patient to experience sudden onset of vertigo, sensorineural hearing loss, horizontal nystagmus, and occasionally nausea and vomiting. The patient experiences a whirling vertigo with movement of the head. This condition generally affects healthy middle-aged adults and has a temporary self-limiting course. The disorder is usually preceded by an upper respiratory infection or an otitis media. Permanent hearing loss may occur if the organism damages the sensitive hairs of the inner ear. Safety of the patient should be a priority. Treatment includes administration of an anticholinergic medication, such as meclizine or prochlorperazine. The short course of the disease is helped by lying in a dark room with decreased stimuli. Antibiotics are prescribed if a bacterium is identified as the suspected organism. Although, many patients experience a single episode in their lifetimes, this can be a recurrent condition.

Vertigo

Vertigo (a sensation or feeling of a loss of equilibrium, sometimes referred spinning or whirling) is a condition that affects the equilibrium of a patient who experiences the feeling of motion while standing still. Vertigo is produced by an injury or lesion to the labyrinth or inner ear caused by various toxic substances, middle ear disease, postural hypotension, or occasionally as a complication to ear surgery. Patient's safety is of utmost importance. Patients are instructed to rise slowly and gradually increase their activity over time (Badke, Shea, Miedaner, & Grove, 2004).

Otalgia

Otalgia (pain in the ear) can occur with a variety of conditions from otitis infections, airplane rides, loud noise, trauma, or referred pain associated with dental conditions. The cause of the pain must be identified to be able to determine the appropriate management.

Mixed Conductive and Sensorineural Hearing Loss

Mixed conductive and sensorineural hearing loss occur when hearing loss results from a combination of both conductive and sensorineural factors. An example of mixed would be presbycusis, a progressive degenerative hearing loss associated with age caused by wear and tear on the inner ear over the years. This deterioration is from loud noise exposure of occupation and recreational environments and the aging process. Other causes would include inherent conditions from disease, dietary habits, and tobacco and alcohol ingestions.

Tinnitus (a ringing, buzzing, or jingling sound in the ear) is a symptom that is frequently reported and can be associated with both a conductive or sensorineural problem. The ringing, which can be disabling to some people, can be caused by something as simple as impacted cerumen or foreign bodies lodged in the external canal to a sign of Menière's disease or other pathology. Exposure in an area where a high level of noise is experienced for an extensive amount of time such as a rock concert can cause a temporary ringing in the ear, which should resolve within 48 hours after exposure (Folmer, Martin, & Shi, 2004).

When a patient presents with a complaint associated with the auditory system, the nurse takes a complete history to get a good picture of the lifestyle, habits, past and present medical history, and occupational and environmental risks. Items that must be included are occupations (current and past), hobbies, environmental living conditions, childhood illnesses, and family history including any genetic disorders known to have associated hearing deficits (Lang, 2004). Common symptoms that the patient presents to the office or clinic with are ear discharge, ear pain, ringing or other sounds in the ears, pressure or fullness, hearing loss, dizziness, or loss of balance. Obtaining the sequence of events will help to focus the physical exam assessment and lead to the diagnosis.

Mixed consists of a combination of both conductive and sensorineural properties. When the patient presents to the health care provider with mixed hearing loss, they exhibit signs and symptoms of both etiologies. A patient will experience properties of both bone and air conduction loss.

Changes with the Aging Process

Changes with the aging process have been associated with both conductive and sensorineural hearing loss. Alterations in the auditory system seen with aging include an increase in cerumen production, which appears to be drier (increasing the tendency to develop an impaction), an increase in the amount of hair growth in the external canal, and loss of elasticity in the lining of the canal leading to collapse. Atropic aging changes in the middle and inner ear lead to degeneration of neurons and decreased vascularity causing increased loss of hearing. The most common condition associated with aging is presbycusis, a degenerative loss of hearing related to constant insults to the fine hair lining of the cochlear over a lifetime. The exact cause is unknown. Loss of hearing associated with higher pitched sounds is most affected (Hietanen, Era, Sorri, & Heikkiness, 2004).

Etiologies of Conductive and Sensorineural Hearing Loss

There are a variety of causes for conductive and sensorineural hearing loss. Each of these etiologies has different clinical manifestations and effects on patients suffering from the different conditions.

Cerumen Production

The most common cause of conductive hearing loss is obstruction, which can be caused by a variety of reasons. The most common is impacted **cerumen** (a wax-like substance formed within the ear). Many people feel that it is necessary to use a cotton applicator to remove the wax or other debris from the canal and do not realize the ear is unique in that it cleans itself. By using the cotton-swab or other object the wax is merely pressed down contributing to impaction. Any object inserted into the canal has the potential to cause damage to both the canal and the tympanic membrane. The amount of cerumen production depends on the individual, and therefore it may be necessary to periodically have the ear canal irrigated to assist in the removal. Various otitic solutions are readily available and can be used to emulsify and disperse excess or impacted cerumen to also assist in removal (Rodgers, 2004).

Foreign Body

Anything that is abnormally found in the external ear canal is a foreign body. Cotton tips, which occasionally dislodge from cotton swab applicators, insects, or other objects, are just a few examples. Insects at times look for dark, moist areas and find their way into ear canals. If the patient presents with a buzzing or scratching sound in the ear, insects should be the first thought. If an insect is alive in the canal, the insect must be first killed before attempting to remove it. By instilling mineral oil or lidocaine, which kills the insect, makes the insect easier to be removed. Avoid placing water into the canal, which only makes the insect swell and thereby become lodged in the canal, making it more difficult to remove. Because the external ear canal is narrow and S-shaped, it makes many foreign bodies difficult to remove, and consequently the patient may need a referral to an otologist for removal.

Trauma

External ear trauma can result in accidental or induced injury, which often results in a perforated tympanic membrane or perichondrial hematoma. Etiologies of trauma range from abuse, sports or recreational injury, and industrial mishaps to accidents. External canal trauma can also be caused by insertion of objects in the canal. With a perforation, the patient experiences excruciating ear pain for a brief period of time and then relief in which they may then encounter a discharge. Any perforation of the tympanic membrane increases the risk of infections and decreases the ability to hear.

Eustachian Tube Dysfunction

For the auditory system to function properly, the eustachian tube must be fully open and functioning. The eustachian tube connects the middle ear with the nasopharynx, and its purpose is to equalize pressure and provide ventilation. When infectious processes cause inflammation or edema in the tube, it increases the risk of developing an otitis media. Common etiologies, which contribute to bilateral inflammation of the eustachian tube, are the common cold or upper respiratory infection and allergic rhinitis. The buildup of secretions and bacteria cause edema and obstruction of the tube. This creates decreased ventilation and the production of secretions leading to otitis media and decreased mobility of the tympanic membrane and thereby a decrease in hearing. When a unilateral eustachian tube obstruction is found, the patient should be evaluated for a tumor, which is a classic indication.

Ear Infections

The external otitis or what is commonly referred to as swimmers' ear affects the external ear canal, causing a narrowing and sometimes an occlusion to the canal. In this event sound waves cannot reach the tympanic membrane or just minimally reach the membrane decreasing the ability to hear sounds. Hearing loss is generally temporary and when the condition resolves hearing returns to normal. Prolonged moisture in the canal is the most common cause. External otitis can also be caused by foreign bodies in the ear, injury to the canal, and cerumen impaction. The most common offending organisms include corynebacterium, *Micrococcus* species, *Staphylococcus aureus,* and *Pseudomonas aeruginosa.* The classic symptom of external otitis is pain on movement of the ear lobe and the feeling of fullness. Prevention is the solution when considering external otitis.

Complications of Auditory Dysfunction

There are a wide variety of complications associated with auditory dysfunction. Among these are the common inflammation of the middle ear, otitis media, as well as perforated tympanic membrane, and other tympanic membrane anomalies, mastoiditis, masses in the external and middle ear, and otosclerosis. Each of these pathologies can cause hearing loss and have varying complications within the auditory system.

Otitis Media

Otitis media, an inflammation of the middle ear, is the most common cause of conductive hearing loss. The patient usually experiences allergies or an upper respiratory infection prior to developing an acute otitis media. Otitis media affects all age-groups but especially the young child. The most common organisms are *Streptococcus pneumoniae, Hemophilus influenzae, Moraxella Catarrhalis, Staphylococcus aureus,* and various other organisms to some degree. Acute otitis media can develop into otitis media with effusion, an accumulation of fluid behind the tympanic membrane with absence of infection. The fluid can be serous or mucoid consistency and can develop into a glue ear, which prevents the movement of the tympanic membrane. Decreased movement of the membrane prevents the ossicles from moving and thereby causes a temporary hearing loss. Once the fluid is dissolved, the hearing should return to normal.

Otitis media is diagnosed by history and physical examination and treated with antibiotics specific to the offending organism. The nurse educates the patient on management in the acute episodes stressing the importance of completing the course of antibiotics, common complications, such as perforation of the tympanic membrane, and when to seek medical care. Patients often experience ear pain, so nurses should evaluate the pain on a pain scale and discuss mild analgesics, which have been found to be helpful. Flying is not recommended until the infection is cleared. Instruct the patient to avoid water sports and to keep the ear dry during the acute phase. At the first sign of excruciating pain, the patient should be advised to seek medical care to rule out perforation of the tympanic membrane or other complications.

Perforated Tympanic Membrane

A complication of recurrent otitis media is a perforated tympanic membrane. Because the membrane is then unable to cause vibration of the ossicles, a conductive hearing loss is noted. The amount of loss is dependent on the size and location of the opening. A larger perforation that appears in the middle section of the membrane tends to cause the most hearing loss. Most perforations resolve spontaneously but can be repaired by grafting if persistent. The nurse needs to stress to the patient that no water or other substances should be placed into an ear that has a perforation unless directed by the health care provider.

When the patient presents frequently with otitis media, it may become unclear as to whether the previous infection had resolved or that a new one is now present. Chronic otitis media can cause persistent damage to the ossicles, which will result in sensorineural loss of hearing over time. Untreated chronic otitis media can lead to the spread of infection into the surrounding areas, such as brain abscess, meningitis, and mastoiditis.

Other Tympanic Membrane Disorders

Other complications of chronic otitis infections cause the tympanic membrane to retract, form adhesions, or develop necrosis of the tympanic membrane or ossicles. Scarring of the tympanic membrane decreases the movement or vibration of sound waves reaching the middle ear causing interference with the movement of the ossicles and thereby causing conductive hearing loss. Another complication of chronic otitis media is perforation of the tympanic membrane, which would also affect the patient's ability to hear sound waves by decreasing the vibratory movement of the ossicles.

Tympanic membrane abnormalities that interfere with the ability to hear include **tympanosclerosis** (formation of fibrous tissue around the ossicles preventing vibratory movement) and **bullous myringitis** (the presence of an infec-

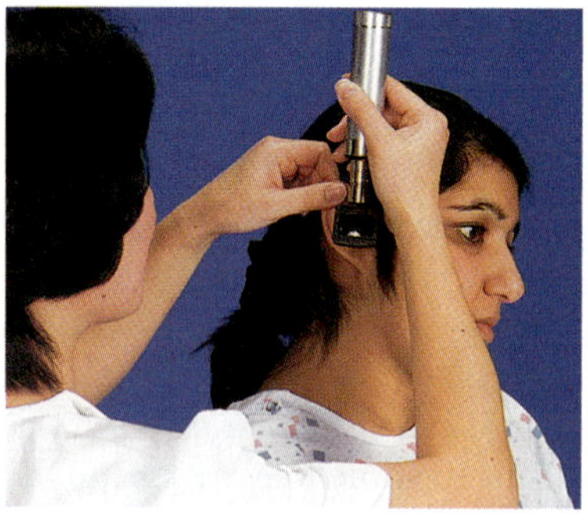

Figure 40-3 Position for otoscopic examination.

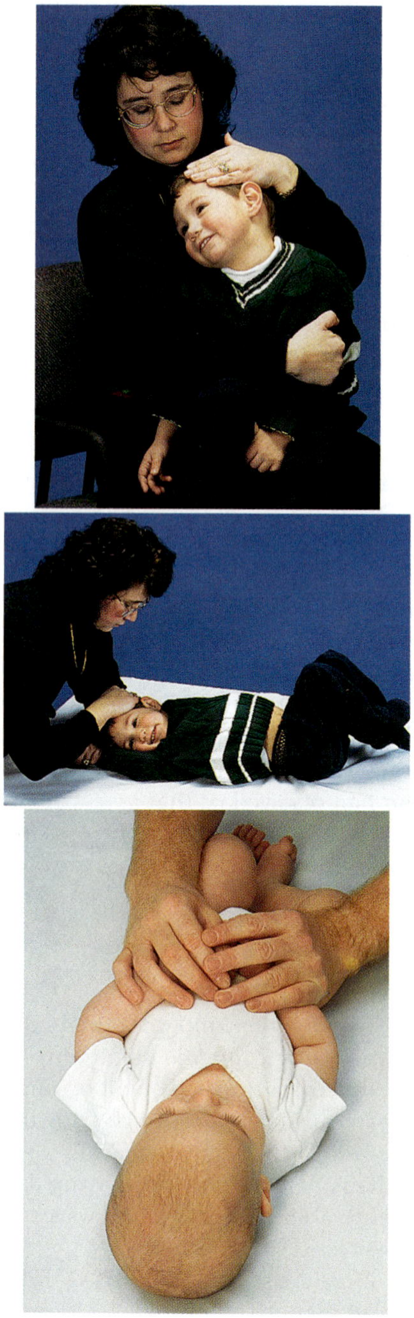

Figure 40-4 Positioning the child for the otoscopic examination.

tious vesicle and inflammation of the tympanic membrane caused by the organism *Mycoplasma pneumoniae*).

Mastoiditis

Mastoiditis (infectious process of the mastoid sinuses) interferes with bone conduction. The mastoid process is located directly behind the ear and connects temporal bone. Inflammation can occur with chronic middle ear infection. Signs and symptoms usually occur two to three weeks after an occurrence of otitis media and include pain and erythema to the site, fever, and protuberance of the auricle. Treatment of mastoiditis is a medical emergency.

Masses in the External and Middle Ear

Cholesteatoma is a cyst that contains an accumulation of squamous epithelium, keratin, and other debris and is associated with chronic otitis. As the lesion grows, it spreads into the middle and inner ear causing damage to the auditory structures and may continue to grow into surrounding areas and the brain tissue if not identified and removed in a timely manner. Damage to other cranial nerves that innervate the face can also lead to facial paralysis. Severe conductive hearing loss can result if damage occurs to the ossicles. Nursing management includes identification and monitoring patients at risk.

Other masses that cause a conductive hearing loss include benign (infectious polyp) or malignant tumors, which interfere with the ability of sound to reach the tympanic membrane or ossicles.

Otosclerosis

Otosclerosis is the most common cause of auditory loss in an individual from the age 15 to 50. Otosclerosis occurs as a result of the formation of spongy bone around the oval window, thus preventing movement of the stapes and causing atrophy of the organ of Corti. The ossicles become fused together and therefore are unable to vibrate and transmit sound waves to the acoustic nerve. Although the etiology is unknown, it has been linked genetically to certain families and is categorized as an autosomal dominant disorder. Otosclerosis generally presents in puberty and is more commonly seen in the Caucasian race, and females tend to be more prone to develop the condition. Pregnancy also appears to aggravate the condition.

Diagnostic Tests

The diagnosis of auditory dysfunctions should be investigated if the patient or the family report behavioral changes (speech too soft or too loud, repeats statements, or asks others to repeat phases frequently). Abnormal reports on hearing handicap inventory for adults and failed auditory testing should also be evaluated further. If the patient presents with a chief complaint of loss of hearing, it is important to ascertain if the condition appeared gradually or suddenly.

Otoscopic Examination and Tympanometry Testing

The use of the otoscope is a basic examination device used by the nurse in examining the inner ear. Correctly positioning the otoscope is essential and involves first placing the patient in a comfortable sitting position. Then the nurse holds the otoscope securely in the dominant hand and uses the other hand to correctly position the ear (Figure 40-3). A child can be allowed to lie down if they provide too much of a challenge to be in a sitting position (Figure 40-4). In addition, the nurse positions the ear differently in the infant than the adult (refer to a physical examination text for specific procedures).

While using the otoscope, **tympanometry** is a test performed (by the nurse) and is used to detect abnormalities in the middle ear such as fluid, eustachian tube dysfunction, or problems with the ossicles. The tip of the instrument is placed in the external os of the ear, a seal is established, and negative or

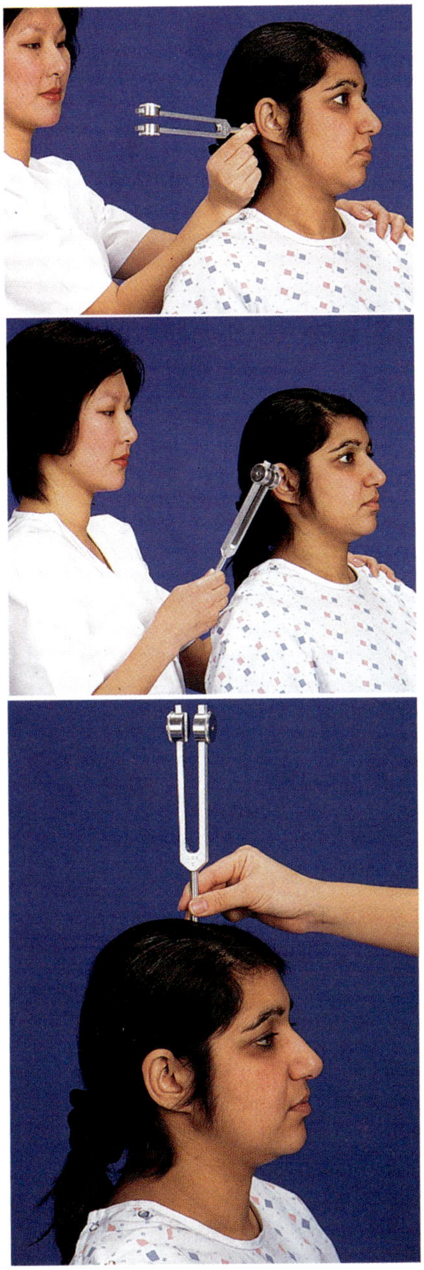
A
B

Figure 40-5 A. Rinne test, B. Weber test.

positive pressure is injected into the air to assess the movement of the tympanic membrane. The degree and direction of the movement will determine normality of the middle ear. The peak or lack of peak on the graph that is produced will indicate if there is an abnormality. Flat lines would indicate a perforated membrane, otitis media, or obstruction in the canal, such as cerumen or probe tip. The most important thing for the nurse to remember is to have a good seal; if there is a leak in the seal, air will escape around the probe tip and the pressure will not be sufficient to get an accurate test finding.

Rinne and Weber Tests

Specific tests performed to assess the patient's hearing would include the Rinne and Weber tests (Figure 40-5). By testing air conduction versus bone conduction of sounds, the examiner will be able to determine an auditory dysfunction. The Rinne test (tests air conduction) and the Weber tests (tests bone conduction) are performed using a tuning fork of 250, 500, or 1,000 Hz. To perform the Weber test, the nurse places the tuning fork on the front midportion of the patient's head and has the patient indicate if he or she hears the sounds equally in both ears testing for a unilateral deficit. The sound will be louder in the affected ear if it is a conductive loss and louder in the good ear if it is a sensorineural loss. The Rinne test, used to compare bone and air conduction, is performed by placing the tuning fork behind the ear on the mastoid process and having the patient say when the sound is no longer heard, the tuning fork is then moved to the front of the ear just outside the os, and the patient is then asked to indicate when sound is no longer heard. The Rinne test is normal is air conduction is twice as long as bone conduction (Estes, 2006).

Audiometer Test

The audiometer is the most common instrument in testing the hearing of individuals of all ages. The younger child who is unable to designate in which ear the sound is heard would not be able to perform this test and therefore other methods should be used. The audiometer emits specific sound pitches at different frequencies ranging from 125 Hz to 8,000 Hz (Punch, et al., 2004; Yueh, et al., 2003). Audiometric testing is performed on the patient by a specially trained nurse or audiologist. The patient is taken to a soundproof room (for best results) and tested on the different sound frequencies. The patient is asked to identify in which ear the tone is heard. A variety of sounds at different pitches is produced by the examiner, which tests the tone intensity of the hearing deficit. A printed audiogram is then obtained that notes the frequencies heard in each ear. Normal ranges are established nationally.

Brainstem Auditory Evoked Response Test

Brainstem auditory evoked responses (BAER or ABR) is another measuring device, which calculates the ability to hear in a patient who is unresponsive or incapable of performing an audiometer. The BAER measures the sound impulse needed to evoke a brain response, which will indicate the patient's ability to hear. This method is used mainly in patients who are unable to cooperate with standardized hearing testing, such as with auditory neuropathy, muscular dystrophy, psychiatric disorders, and abnormal brainstem disorder, such as stroke or other degenerative diseases. It is also widely used in newborns and young children who are unable to perform standard hearing tests. Because this machine utilizes high frequencies, adults over 70 years old are poor candidates for this method of testing because the aging process affects the ability to hear high-frequency sounds. The BAER is a painless test that produces clicks, which are introduced into the ear; on hearing these sounds the brain generates electrical impulses, which are then recorded (Box 40-1). The inability to initiate a brain response will indicate if the patient has a hearing deficit, an abnormality in the inner ear, eighth cranial nerve lesion, or other brainstem lesions. These abnormalities would then have to be further investigated (Johnson, Nicol, & Kraus, 2005; Sismanis, 2005).

BOX 40-1

ASSESSING A PATIENT WITH A HEARING DEFICIT

Questions to include in the history when trying to identify a hearing deficit should include:

- Are you able to hear a conversation in a crowded room or on the telephone?
- Do you have to turn the TV or radio up to hear the programming?
- Do you often get frustrated or argue when speaking with a family member or friend?
- Does hearing interfere with your social life?
- Do you avoid going to church, a movie, concert, or other activities because you cannot hear well?
- Do you have trouble understanding the conversation when in a noisy environment?

Nursing Diagnoses

Based on the information gathered, examples of nursing diagnoses in the patient with auditory dysfunction may include the following:

- Disturbed sensory perception, auditory, related to obstruction of ear canal, damage to inner ear.
- Anxiety related to inability to communicate.
- Knowledge deficit related to self-care and risk prevention.
- Impaired social interaction related to inability to hear others.

Planning and Implementation

Nursing care consists of educating the patient on proper care of the external ear. Avoid cleaning the ear canal with cotton tip applicators or other device, keeping it dry and free of debris. Cleaning increases the risk of tissue damage and interferes with the ear's normal process of cleansing. Once otitis externa develops, keep the patient comfortable with pain medication, treat the infection with topical antibiotics directed toward the most likely organisms (e.g., *Pseudomonas, S. aureus*), and reinforcing prevention.

Congenital and hereditary hearing loss can appear at any time in one's life span. Family patterns can be identified in most cases, but there are isolated cases as well. Hearing screening is now mandatory at birth to identify as many cases as early as possible to initiate interventions. In some cases the loss is gradual and does not present until later in life, or it may be an isolated case where no other family members are affected. Therefore, early identification using hearing screening devices should also be performed yearly at the annual medical maintenance visits.

Pharmacology

The administration of medications is dependent on the disease process and the organism involved. Antibiotics are used to treat infections of the ear specific to the suspected disease. Common organisms found in the ear are *S. pneumoniae, M. catarrhalis,* nontypeable *Haemophilus influenzae,* and *S. aureus.* The first line of treatment for acute otitis media is usually a course of amoxicillin when symptomatic (Broyles, Reiss, & Evans, 2007). Acute otitis media infection affects the pediatric patient more than the adult patient and is usually preceded with symptoms of upper respiratory disease, nasal congestion, cough, and sore throat. Other contributing factors would be environmental smoke, allergens, day care attendance, immune deficiencies, and hereditary factors.

PATIENT PLAYBOOK

Prevention of Otitis Externa

- Keep the ear canal dry.
- Dry the external canal immediately after water sports or bathing.
- Do not put anything into the ear canal.
- Use of drying agents such as 1:1 solutions of 2% boric acid and 70% ethyl alcohol or 1:1 solution of white vinegar and 70% ethyl alcohol helps dry the canal (place two to three drops into the ear canal before and after swimming).
- If otitis external present, stay out of the water until infection resolved.

Otitis media with effusion follows an episode of otitis media and is characteristic by fluid in the middle ear. Prolonged fluid in the middle ear leads to decreased hearing and may cause permanent damage if not resolved in a timely fashion. Chronic otitis media occurs when the individual experiences frequent ear infections that leads to repeated insults to the middle ear. This can lead to loss of hearing but also may lead to other complications such as mastoiditis. Mastoiditis requires immediate attention and initiation of parental antibiotics. Other findings that would affect the hearing would be a cholesteoma or a collection of proliferating epithelial cells, which if not treated would lead to other serious complications as discussed previously.

Menière's disease can be managed with a low-salt diet. Medications found to be helpful are diuretics (such as furosemide and Diazide), vasodilators, antihistamines, anticholinergics, and sedatives (benzodiazepines). While experiencing extreme vertigo, diazepam (valium), and meclizine (Antivert) seem to manage the condition. There is no cure for the disease. The condition waxes and wanes through out the patient's life. Safety is a critical issue in the acute phase. Surgical intervention can be performed in patients with extreme vertigo (endolymphatic decompression) to relieve the pressure in the labyrinth (Perez, et al., 2004).

Surgery

On examination, increased vascularity is seen in tympanic membrane infections, such as otitis media, as indicated by a positive **Schwartze's sign** (rosy or reddish-blue color of the tympanic membrane related to vascular changes). An abnormal Rinne test indicates bone conduction to be equal or greater than air conduction. Surgical management has been found to be successful in improving approximately 90 percent of hearing in these patients. During the procedure a stapedectomy is performed whereby the stapes is removed and replaced with a prosthetic one. During surgery, the labyrinth and perilymph systems are disturbed, which can cause dizziness, nausea, vomiting, and nystagmus of the lateral gaze. Nursing care includes safety measures. The patient should be instructed to keep his or her head movement to a minimal and to avoid sudden head movement, coughing, sneezing, or straining. Nurses can also educate the patient on increasing the ingestion of vitamin D and calcium in his or her diet, which has been found to promote bone calcification in some studies.

Patients may choose to manage otosclerosis in a nonsurgical way, such as using amplifying devices or hearing aids. The nurse is in an ideal position to discuss all of the options with the patient in addition to reinforcing advantages and disadvantages presented by the surgeon, should the patient choose a stapedectomy with reconstruction. The nurse will also assist the patient in the referral process and be the main person to answer questions. Whether surgical repair is performed or not, safety is a concern, because the patient is probably experiencing decreased hearing and vertigo. Patients may also feel compelled to discuss the genetic component, because some patients may fear passing the condition on to the next generation.

Removing Foreign Bodies

Gentle irrigation performed in the medical clinic is effective in removing cerumen. The nurse instructs the patient about the procedure, gathers the equipment, and performs the irrigation. If patient has a perforated tympanic membrane, irrigation is contraindicated. Nausea, dizziness, or pain may be experienced during the procedure and should be reported. Documentation includes type and amount of solution and end results of what is obtained. The uses of cerumen curettes or spoons should only be done by specially trained medical personnel. Removing cerumen sometimes requires a wax emulsifier to dissolve the wax a few days before the irrigation (if the wax is hard and lodged into the canal).

Foreign body removal from ears involves manual removal with alligator forceps or curette. If a live insect is present in the canal, it must be killed before removing to make removal easier. Solutions used to kill the insect include placing a few drops of mineral oil or lidocaine into the canal.

Preoperative Care

Preparing a patient for surgery is an important part of nursing care. Preoperatively the nurse assesses the patient's baseline hearing abilities. If the degree of hearing will be affected during the procedure, the patient and nurse should discuss ways to communicate after surgery to aid in the patient's recovery process. With any surgery of the auditory system, the patient should be instructed not to do anything that will interfere with the eustachian tube function, such as blowing his or her nose, coughing, or sneezing, which may increase pressure in this area, leading to disturbance of the surgical site. It is important to explain this before the surgery, so that the patient understands what to expect after the procedure. This will also assist in communicating the directions to the patient if there is interference with his or her hearing after the procedure.

When preparing the patient for any auditory surgery, the nurse must address the patient's expectations and what he or she perceives are the end results. A complete history is performed reviewing past medical and surgical history. The patient should be assessed for the level of communication skills, so postoperatively the patient will be easier to converse with for postoperative instructions. During the interview, the nurse needs to talk in a slow, deliberate fashion, facing the patient and allowing for extra time if needed for understanding instructions. Try not to give lengthy instructions that the patient will have difficulty understanding. If the patient has hearing aids the nurse might suggest that the patient wear them into the surgical suite. All preoperative evaluations and laboratory testing is reviewed, the patient's functioning ability is evaluated, and the consent form is signed. As part of the preoperative workup, the patient should have baseline studies to compare postoperative hearing ability. The patient is assessed by using an audiogram and tympanometry to determine the etiology of dysfunction and baseline acuity.

Nurses are utilized in a variety of settings. The nurse in the physician's office assists with preparing the patient for surgery and what is expected postoperatively, obtaining a history, performing the auditory exam (if specially trained), and discussing what to expect immediately before and after the procedure. The patient is also prepared psychologically because feelings of grief may be experienced with any degree of hearing loss, and the sense of hearing is vital in communication. The patient also needs to know what the procedure entails.

Most often, local anesthesia is used with conscious sedation so the patient can be guided throughout the delicate process. The fact that the patient may be awake can be frightening to many patients; therefore the nurse needs to reassure the patient. Points to be discussed with patients undergoing any surgery would be steps of the procedure, postoperative expectations, alleviating the fear of unknown, and prevention of complications. The patient's compliance of preoperative and postoperative instructions leads to better patient outcomes.

A major concern of the patient would be complete loss of hearing after the procedure. Understanding and identifying realistic expectations of outcomes will help the patient throughout the surgical process. Postoperative pain management should be ordered for any discomfort the patient may feel. Common side effects of analgesic medications include dizziness or tinnitus, which may also be an effect of manipulating the components of the auditory system. The vertigo or tinnitus needs to be differentiated to identify common postoperative signs and symptoms following auditory procedures as opposed to complications.

Postoperative Care

Postoperative care of a patient who undergoes surgery to the auditory system, besides routine care of all patients having any surgical procedure, is preventing introduction of organisms or infection into the site, observing for excessive bleeding, or other possible complications. Vomiting may be a side effect from anesthesia and needs to be acted on immediately. Vomiting could cause damage to the surgical site. Patients who undergo auditory surgery should have their heads elevated, be monitored for vertigo, and avoid quick movements or turning of the head. The nurse needs to remember that the patient may have hearing loss in the operated ear and therefore should speak clearly in the unaffected ear or have a pad and pencil available for communication. When the patient is discharged from the hospital, instructions should be reiterated, such as avoiding sneezing, blowing nose, or other activities that could cause pressure in the middle ear. If the patient has to sneeze, he or she should do so with his or her mouth open. The patient should avoid showers, shampooing, or dipping head in water for at least one to two weeks or until the surgical site is healed. The surgical dressing should be kept in place, unless otherwise directed, and kept dry and clean. Part of discharge planning would also include the administration of medications, such as analgesics, antiemetics, antivertigo agents, and possibly antihistamines. Instructions on how to take the medications and what side effects to watch for should be included.

Instructions should also include positioning the patient on the opposite side away from the surgery. Lying on the operative side may affect the healing process and disrupt the graft (if one was used). The patient should avoid blowing his or her nose for at least one week, but if he or she finds it necessary to blow his or her nose, have the patient gently blow one nostril at a time. Likewise, if necessary to cough or sneeze, this should be done with the mouth open to avoid pressure on the ear. Physical exercise should be avoided for at least one week, after which time the patient can return to work unless contraindicated. If the patient works in a high noise environment, ear protection should be used.

Initially patients may have some dizziness or tinnitus and should be assisted with ambulation until this has resolved. Hearing may also initially be diminished in the operative ear but should return close to preoperative status depending on the type of procedure performed. After surgery, the patient should be assessed for cranial nerve functioning to note any deficits that might have occurred as a result of the surgical procedure. The cranial nerves most likely affected would be five, seven, eight, and nine, because they innervate many structures in this area. The patient can also exhibit some nystagmus especially when looking to the side.

In addition, care of the operative site would include noting the amount and type of drainage or bleeding, changing the dressing as directed (according to the surgeon), and teaching the patient or family on dressing changes after discharge if indicated. Depending on the procedure, little bleeding is expected after surgery. Some patients may have a small amount of serosanguineous discharge that can be easily absorbed by a cotton ball changed as often as necessary. Common postoperative findings include decreased hearing in the operative ear and various noises, such as snapping or crackling. Outcome goals include pain control, healing in a relatively short time, and as normal ear functioning as possible. A hearing test should be performed after the healing process has completed. Patients should avoid flying, water sports or underwater diving, physical activity, and heavy lifting for one to three weeks following surgery depending on the type of surgical procedure performed and based on the surgeon's recommendations.

Middle Ear and Mastoid Surgery

Myringotomy, or incision into the tympanic membrane, has been performed for years to promote drainage and relieve pressure. Before the invention of the tympanometry tubes, the physician, in the office, would make a small incision into the tympanic membrane if perforation was imminent or to identify the type of organism responsible for the otitis media when the antibiotic was not treating the infection. With any perforation of the tympanic membrane there is a chance of introducing an organism into the middle ear so the patient needs to be watched closely for signs and symptoms of otitis media, such as drainage from the ear canal, otalgia, and fever.

Myringoplasty (plastic surgery of the tympanic membrane) is performed in a patient who has a small perforated tympanic membrane that has failed to resolve or heal. The procedure involves placing a patch over the perforation. Chronic otitis media is a common cause. Following the procedure the patient is instructed to keep the canal dry and follow-up frequently in the office to assess the healing process. If the patch does not solve the problem or the hole gets bigger, a tympanoplasty must be performed. Repairing the tympanic membrane does not always improve the conductive hearing loss.

Stapedectomy or tympanoplasty is performed when reconstruction is necessary in the middle ear to improve conductive hearing loss. With the tympanoplasty a portion of the temporalis fascia is used to graft the affected portion of the middle ear. Care must be taken not to disturb the ossicles from their position. Risk factors that can occur after this type of surgery include increased pressure in the middle ear, displacement of the prosthesis of the ossicles, difficulties with balance, a risk of developing an infection, and postoperative pain.

A **stapedectomy** is a removal of the stapes and replaces the stapes with a prosthetic device, which is performed mainly in a patient with otosclerosis. A similar surgery, which is performed to repair one or more of the ossicles, is an ossiculoplasty. This procedure is also performed in a patient with otosclerosis. When the stapes becomes fused, it becomes necessary for the patient to undergo surgery for the insertion of a prosthetic replacement. This procedure has shown to increase the patient's ability to hear.

Mastoidectomy is an incision of the mastoid sinuses, which are located directly behind the ear. When a radical mastoidectomy is performed it involves the middle ear, and therefore is important to mention. The nurse is responsible for monitoring the patient postoperatively, watching for presence and amount of discharge or bleeding, fever, neck stiffness, limited neck range of motion, vomiting, dizzy, disorientation, headaches, or facial paralysis, all of which are complications that can occur following this type of surgery. When changing the dressing, aseptic technique must be used to avoid any infection. The mastoid bone is in direct contact with brain tissue, and therefore any infection can travel to the brain and cause further complications. Other complications include decreased muscle mass and disruption to hearing.

Other auditory surgery involves the removal of an acoustic neuroma, which is a benign tumor of cranial nerve VIII where the nerve enters the auditory canal or at the temporal bone. Early signs include a gradual unilateral hearing loss, tinnitus, intermittent episodes of mild vertigo, and decreased sensation in the canal. As the tumor grows and extends into the auditory system, the damage and hearing loss cannot be reversed. Treatment includes surgical removal of the tumor with as little damage to the surrounding tissues and cranial nerves. Facial paralysis is commonly coexists. Postoperative nursing management is similar to other auditory surgical procedures as previously discussed.

Repair of Inner Ear Disorders

Cochlear implant is commonly used in young children with congenital hearing loss but recently has also been used in older adults to assist with sensorineural hearing loss. The patient undergoes a surgical procedure to insert the device just behind the ear. The device is divided into three sections: a headpiece, speech processor, and receiver. The headpiece contains a microphone and transmitter, which picks up the sounds in the environment and sends them to the speech processor, which rearranges the sounds and sends them to the receiver, which is implanted behind the ear. The receiver then converts the sound waves to nerve impulses, which are sent to the brain for interpretation. Patients who receive the implant will be able to hear some sounds but will not have normal hearing. Studies have shown that individuals who receive cochlear implants have less depression, anxiety, and quality of life issues than those who chose not to have one (Birgen, Harris, Lindbaek, & Oslo, 2004; Cohen, Labadie, Dietrich, & Haynes, 2004). The best candidates for cochlear implants are patients who have established speech and language skills (Cullen, et al., 2004).

A great deal of controversy exists among the deaf community about the ethics of implanting cochlear implants in young children. The basis for this ethical dilemma stems from the beliefs that American Sign Language is a natural language and should remain as such. Leaders in the deaf community want to protect the deaf culture and therefore feel that children should be reared in that culture. It is believed that deaf individuals communicate and receive cues through visual images and live in a specialized culture similar to other cultures and encompass accepted values and beliefs. By implanting cochlear implants, which give the individual the ability to hear sounds, it alters the culture of the individual, which then contradicts the belief system in the deaf community. To compound the argument, studies show that children who are born deaf or who become deaf at an early age do not fair as well on language acquisition and still need the exposure of the deaf culture to exist. On the other hand, in research by Nicholas and Geers (2006), cochlear implants increased spoken language ability in profoundly hearing impaired children. The benefits of a cochlear implant to a hearing impaired child to achieve both speech and language skills comparable to a normal hearing child appears greater if the implant is placed when the child is a toddler as opposed to a preschooler. Adults and children who have had cochlear implants have been found to successfully integrate and function in a hearing society, but deaf community leaders feel they lose some of their cultural identity by doing so.

Uncovering the Evidence

Cochlear Implants in Children

Discussion: The purpose of this research project was to explore the results of improving hearing loss in 13 infants with profound hearing loss and had cochlear implants between the ages of 6 to 12 months of age. Infants were tested using two behavioral methodologies that have been successful for investigating speech perception and language skills in infants with normal hearing. The research involved using equipment that assessed infants' discrimination of speech sounds. In addition, the study was used to assess infants' ability to learn associations between speech sounds and objects. The findings revealed patterns of hearing associated with visual responses for the early implanted infants were similar to those of normal hearing infants. Also, the mothers' speech to infants with the implants was similar in pitch to infants with normal hearing who had the same duration of experience with sounds.

Implications for Practice: The nursing discipline can explore methods of patient education regarding the early identification of hearing impaired infants. The earlier the disorder is assessed, the potential increasing methods of treatment (e.g., cochlear implants) and the better the results for the patient. In addition, parents can be encouraged to stay in contact with their health care providers as related to questions or suspected concerns that are seen in their children.

Citation: Miyamoto, R., Houston, D., & Bergeson, T. (2005). Cochlear implantation in deaf infants. Laryngoscope, *115(8), 1376–1380.*

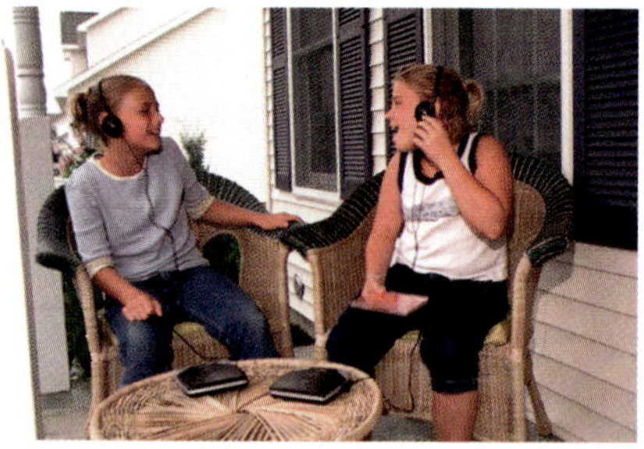

Figure 40-6 Hearing loss has been attributed to listening to loud music through earphones.

Patient and Family Teaching

Part of patient teaching involves preventive measures to assist the patient in maintaining an optimum quality of life. To do this, one looks to the levels of prevention. In caring for the patient, the nurse assists and discusses ways to prevent injury to the auditory system and to identify those at risk of developing an auditory dysfunction in every medical encounter. Other responsibilities include preventing further damage once loss occurs. Identification of patients with the greatest risk factors leads the preventive management.

Primary Prevention

The prevention model directs identification and management incorporating this into the nurse's role. Primary prevention speaks to minimizing risks in the environment. Primary prevention begins with educating and making the public aware of what constitutes dangerous noise. Any noise above 85 dB is considered dangerous, and prolonged exposure can cause damage to the sensitive auditory system. Areas found to be at the highest levels of noise pollution include various occupational and recreational activities. Occupations known to be at high risk include firefighters, police officers, airline personnel, and the military. Recreation also contributes to high noise levels whether as a participant or observer. Examples of high noise producing sports include hunting, car racing, and musicians. The obsession with rock concerts in teens and younger adults places the next generations at an increased risk of hearing loss, supporting recent studies indicating an increased prevalence of hearing loss found in the middle adult years (Figure 40-6). Preventive measures would also include the use of protective head gear, muffs, and hats to guard against head trauma, which inadvertently can cause auditory dysfunction.

Preventive measures should include educating the patient to become more aware of noise in the environment: turning down radio and television volumes; avoiding long periods in noisy surroundings, such as rock concerts; and wearing protective devices when indicated. When loud noise cannot be avoided, ear plugs or ear headphones should be used to decrease the amount of elevated sound levels that reach the inner ear. Included in the patient's education is the fact that the common practice of using plain cotton or cotton balls to decrease noise does not prevent the sound from reaching the inner ear and causing damage.

Environmental noise in the workforce is a serious problem and contributes to the increasing number of individuals who acquire hearing loss. To protect these workers the regulating body of OSHA (Occupational Safety and Health Administration) has specific guidelines that must be adhered to. OSHA supplies regulations associated with high noise levels in the workplace to prevent hearing loss associated with machinery or other equipment. Nurses who work in occupational nursing have stringent guidelines to follow established by OSHA. The occupational health nurse monitors the health status of each worker. As part of the nurse's responsibility he or she is specially trained in audiometric testing. In each clinic, a soundproof room is provided for the most accurate hearing assessment. All new employees are required to have a baseline hearing screening and yearly thereafter. Annual training and educational programs addressing noise pollution in the workplace are mandatory. Monitoring the noise levels in the workplace and keeping documentation of the levels are required to adhere to OSHA recommendations. In any work environment where the sound level measures greater than 90 dB, the employees must wear protective hearing equipment. A worker who is demonstrating changes in his or her hearing status in an environment that measures between 85 and 90 dB must also wear protective devices, because prolonged exposure to greater than 85 dB can cause permanent hearing loss.

Ear protection equipment comes in various forms.

- Ear plug are inserted into the ear canal and block the entire canal. Sound levels can be blocked from entering the ear by 15 to 30 dB if fitted properly. Commonly spongy type plugs, which easily mold to fit most auditory canals, are dispersed in many employee health clinics.
- Ear muffs fit snuggly over the entire external ear. Sound levels are also blocked by 15 to 30 dB.
- A combination of both ear plugs and the ear muff offers the most protection. The combination would be recommended in areas of extremely high noise level, for example airline runway workers.

Nurses have the responsibility to educate patients on the level of noise exposure in the household. Simply performing yard work puts the patient at risk of exposure greater than safe levels. Lawn mowers and leaf blowers emit noise levels greater than 90 dB. Most people are unaware of the level of noise that is produced by common household items. Patients should be instructed to spend shorter periods of time performing household tasks that use equipment that emits high levels of sound.

Secondary Prevention

Secondary prevention refers to the early detection (screening and referral). Everyone should have periodic hearing tests as part of their annual medical visits, especially if they work or live in an environment that has excessive noise levels. People are often unwilling to reveal a problem with their hearing, so this is an ideal time to discuss hearing and identify deficits. The earlier the loss is identified, the more quickly the management can be started.

Tertiary Prevention

Tertiary prevention is aimed at maintaining optimal functioning. Once the damage is done, it is important to maintain what hearing capabilities are left. Prevention of further damage is imperative, and education should be directed to decreasing sound insults by turning radio, television, and stereo volumes down to a safe level and taking breaks when using high level noise producing devices or using protective devices.

Noise Pollution

In the world today we are faced with noise pollution that leads to damage to the auditory system on a daily basis. Being more aware of the amount and type of noise in the environment is the starting point in prevention. The most effective preventive measure is controlling the noise exposure in the environment. Turn radio, television, and movie volume down to a safe level of less than 80 to 85 dB (Box 40-2). Other things that produce high noise emissions

BOX 40-2

COMMON SOUNDS AND ASSOCIATED DECIBELS LEVELS

- 20 dB Whisper
- 60 dB Conversation
- 70 dB Vacuum cleaner, traffic noises
- 90 dB Lawn mower, motorcycle, hair dryer
- 110 dB Model airplane
- 120 dB Chain saw, leaf blower, snowmobile, loud thunder clap
- 130 dB Jack hammer, ambulance siren
- 140 dB Jet engine, fire arms, firecrackers
- 150 dB Rock concert

are firecrackers, machinery, gun shots, children's toys, and traffic. Hearing loss can also be caused by a sudden burst of sound, which causes an acute loss through trauma to the auditory mechanism, or it can be chronic with prolonged exposure to loud noises. Acute loss may be temporary with hearing returning in a couple of weeks.

Work environment provides a sustained high noise environment and protection is necessary. Protection of trauma to the ears can be achieved using various devices. When a worker, such as an air traffic controller, is exposed to extensive noise, ear muffs should be worn. Other devices to decrease sound trauma to the auditory system include ear plugs, which come in form fitting and premolded designed to fit a specific person's external ear canal. OSHA regulates the work environment and recommends that a hearing conservation program be in place for all industry, including monitoring of sound levels; annual hearing tests for all workers, including a baseline for comparison; mandatory annual training of all employees; hearing protective devices worn by every employee exposed to excessive noise levels; and accurate record keeping (Van Campen, et al., 2005).

Along with the workplace, recreational activities provide an enormous amount of sound and require protection. Hunting, skeet shooting, or target practice where a firearm is discharged are a few examples. Often not considered as noise producers, children's toys are found to have in some cases excessive levels of noise with the beeps, whistles, honks, and various other sounds. These are made to be amusing and entertaining for children, without consideration of the long-term consequences of the excessive noise levels and exposures.

Yard work is one of the biggest offenders of excessive noise pollution: the lawn mower, leaf blower, and other outdoor equipment emit a high level of noise at greater than 90 dB. Frequent breaks are recommended to eliminate prolonged exposure. Shorter periods of time spent with high frequency noise and wearing protective gear is less damaging and decreases long-term sequelae.

Studies show that the inability to hear disrupts normal routines, school and work performance, relationships, and activities of daily living. Warning signs of excessive noise exposure include having to raise your voice in normal conversation or the inability to hear a conversation approximately two feet away. After leaving a noisy area voices appear muffled or dull and frequently ringing of the ears is heard, or pain is experienced in the ears for short periods of time.

Skills 360°

Communicating with the Hearing Impaired

- Get the patient's attention.
- Face the individual directly.
- Ensure good lighting behind the patient.
- Can they read lips?
- Use simple clear sentences.
- When rephrasing the statement, change the wording.
- Keep hands or items away from your mouth while talking.
- Do not eat or chew gum when speaking.
- Be cognizant of facial expressions.
- Talk into the good ear (if one).
- Do not yell.
- Write things down for clarification.
- Use sign language.

Adapted from DeLaune, S., & Ladner, P. (2006). Fundamentals of nursing *(3rd ed.). New York: Thomson Delmar Learning.*

Communication Tools

As discussed previously, patients should be screened routinely for a hearing deficit when they present for their annual medical examinations. This gives the patient and medical provider a baseline and a way to monitor the pattern of hearing deficit expected over time. Because hearing loss is part of the aging process, it is expected to have some loss over a life span.

Once identifying a hearing deficit, it is important for the nurse to assist in establishing individual ways for the patient to communicate (see Skills 360° feature). Individuals with hearing loss tend to isolate themselves from others, so encouragement is needed for the patient to continue to be involved in outside activities and to not isolate himself or herself from previous enjoyable events. Understanding that everyone will experience some degree of hearing loss as part of the natural aging process may reassure some individuals. The patient needs to accept the fact that it is expected that some degree of loss will be experienced as he or she grows older. Offering ways for the patient to build confidence in communication and not be excluded in conversations is the responsibility of the nurse.

Individuals who have no hearing have access to various mechanisms in which to alert them to various sounds and therefore are able to function in a hearing world. These devices include items with flashing lights for door bells, telephones, alarms, and baby alerts. Some alarm clocks have flashing lights, and others have a vibratory mechanism to awaken the individual. Closed caption TV assists with keeping up with the latest in programming. Some telephones are set up to print out the message to communicate.

Lip reading is another way of communication that adds the ability to combine facial expressions and gestures to read words. Approximately 40 percent of people who have lost hearing understand spoken words and are able to learn to lip read. This also is found to be one of the first ways to communicate when hearing starts to diminish as compensation for the loss.

For patients who have an existing hearing impairment who use American Sign Language to communicate, learning sign language, as with any other foreign language, will facilitate communication. The nurse has an important role in patient care as the educator, mediator, and advocate. Without good communication the patient will not feel confident to raise questions and concerns for discussion. Also to be considered is the age at which the patient became impaired. If the patient has a congenital hearing loss or became deaf before acquiring language skills, he or she will communicate using both oral and sign language because he or she probably was raised with both. In contrast, a person who became deaf after acquiring spoken language, which is the case in the majority of hearing-impaired individuals, is reliant on verbal cues and will use amplification devices or lip reading for communication. No matter when the person lost his or her hearing, he or she will use other means of understanding what is being said, such as body language and facial expressions. The nurse needs to be cognizant of how he or she is expressing himself or herself so as not to be misinterpreted (Gates, Feeney, & Higdon, 2003)

Respecting Our Differences

Hearing Impairment in Different Ethnic Backgrounds

When the nurse is communicating with a patient who has hearing impairment from a different ethnicity, personal and cultural belief systems should be considered. Every patient comes with his or her own personal values, cultural variables, and cultural rules. Some patients may misinterpret gestures used to emphasize or to communicate a statement. Many gestures often have different meanings in the various cultures. So, the nurse needs to be careful and observant when using gestures in communication with the hearing impaired. Pointing, for example, is considered rude in some cultures.

Touch is also often used when trying to get a patient's attention, but in some cultures that may also be misinterpreted as offensive or a violation on the person. Another misinterpreted offensive act that needs to be kept in mind is closeness or getting too close to the patient to ensure that the patient can see what you are trying to convey. The nurse needs to recognize the patient's personal space and not get too close to communicate.

Another point to consider is direct eye contact; Americans place value on eye contact, while other cultures consider it rude to establish eye contact. The nurse needs to be cognizant of the patient's personal values when communicating and modify communication techniques with hearing impaired individuals from different cultures. Accepted length of silence also varies with different ethnicities. Allotting more time, not interrupting, and being prepared to repeat instructions will help with communication. Interrupting the patient is also often interpreted as rude or a loss of interest in what the patient is trying to convey. Understanding communication styles of different cultures is important but also avoiding stereotyping the patient at the same time.

Adapted from Daniels, R. (2004). Nursing fundamentals: Caring and clinical decision making. *New York: Thomson Delmar Learning; DeLaune, S., & Ladner, P. (2006).* Fundamentals of nursing *(3rd ed.). New York: Thomson Delmar Learning.*

Rehabilitation

In many cases the hearing deficit is permanent, and therefore the nurse must assist the patient in ways to compensate for the deficiency. One of the most important monitoring elements is obtaining a baseline hearing test and performing periodic screening tests throughout the patient's life span. Keeping abreast of the changes in loss of hearing over time will enable the nurse to adjust the patient teaching accordingly. Assisting the patient in accepting the loss and discussing ways to alter communication techniques are part of the nurse's responsibility, as well as providing the patient with preventive measures to avoid further loss. Patients who are computer literate can be given helpful resource Internet sites to obtain more information. Those who are not as computer savvy can be given contact numbers for additional information. Identifying support groups in the community for the patient to share similar characteristics have been helpful.

Patients who have a hearing deficit will isolate themselves from others. Encouraging participation is social activities is important. Patients can be offered activities that do not require a lot of conversation. Family members are a big part of the patient's life and need to be involved in the management and encouraged to include the patient in family gatherings. The focus for patients with hearing deficit should be on safety. Patients who are unable to hear the sounds around them are in danger of injury. The inability to hear a horn or siren puts them in arms way when crossing the street. At the same time, someone calling to them to avoid the dangerous situation is missed.

Hearing Aids

Hearing aids amplify sound, and therefore make it easier for patients with a hearing deficit to participate in conversations and activities. Whether or not a patient will wear a hearing aid depends on several factors. The patient's lifestyle and personality will influence this decision to some degree. A certain stigma is associated with a patient wearing a hearing aid, which prevents some patients from seeking the help they need. Other considerations are cosmetic, especially in the elder patient who does not want to appear old. Some patients are dissatisfied with the results, which stems from unrealistic expectations in the patient who feels the aid will return hearing to normal. Those who seek the assistance of hearing aids are usually motivated by difficulty hearing the television, radio, or other sounds, such as doorbell or telephone. Others seek assistance, because they feel left out of conversations. For stereo effect, hearing aids are fitted for both ears whether one or both ears have a deficiency.

Hearing aids are helpful in patients with auditory dysfunction where sound amplification is required. They all function about the same consisting of a microphone to pick up the sound, an amplifier to increase the intensity of sound, and receiver to deliver the sound to the inner ear. Hearing aids come in various shapes and sizes depending on a multitude of factors. Factors that contribute to the type of aid purchased are personal preference, particular auditory dysfunction, amplification, handling ease, design, and cost. Audiologists fit the patient with the most appropriate one for the patient. A period of adjustment is necessary initially.

At first the patient should try to adjust to the hearing aid by wearing it in a quiet environment with limited noise interference. Many older patients live in quiet households where this can easily be accomplished. Once becoming aware of noises in the home, the patient can venture out and listen to natural outdoor sounds and proceed to noisier environments, such as shopping areas. This gradual adjustment period allows the patient to adapt to the feel of wearing the instrument and learn to operate the controls thereby able to adjust the volume to a comfortable level. There are different types that the patient can purchase, which are described in the accompanying display (Box 40-3).

Some of the problems encountered by patients who are obtaining hearing aids are looks, cost, limited education, unrealistic expectations, difficulty in

BOX 40-3

TYPES OF HEARING AIDS

- In the canal and completely in the canal are the smallest available hearing aids. This type of aid fits completely in the ear canal, which allows the patient confidentiality and is cosmetically aesthetic. A patient with intact dexterity would be a candidate, because it is smaller than the others and more difficult to adjust volume or change batteries. As the patient ages, agility appears to decrease, so this would not be appropriate for an elderly patient who would have difficulty managing the small device.
- In ear hearing aids are fitted in the outer portion of the ear and molded to the patient. A slightly larger size allows the patient easier handling. This type of aid is given to a patient with mild to severe hearing loss.
- Behind the ear aid fits over the lobe of the ear, the mechanism sits in a case behind the ear and is connected to a molded ear piece. This type is more cumbersome but easier to manage in the older population and young children. Some patients do not have the dexterity to manage the in ear type and need one more bulky. Patients who benefit the most from this type would be those individuals with mild to profound hearing loss.

care, and maintenance. A patient must accept the fact that they have a hearing problem and be optimistic about wearing the device to make it a successful venture. Nurses in a medical clinic or office come in contact with patients who wear a hearing aid and have questions about the device and therefore are often used as the resource individual. It is therefore important to know how to care for the apparatus.

There are two available types of hearing aids, analogue and digital, each with its own advantages and disadvantages. Analogue hearing aids come in two different forms. The basic analogue hearing aid is an amplifier of sounds programmed by the audiologist. The programmable analogue hearing aid has a microchip and is programmed to accommodate various environments. The digital hearing aid is more complex. It converts sound waves to digital signals and utilizes similar principles of the programmable analogue also adjusting to various conditions (Cohen, Labadie, Dietrich, & Haynes, 2004).

The patient needs a period of adjustment to be able to ignore background noises and focus on the conversation at hand. The background noise can be distracting and difficult to disregard. Programmable aids can be adjusted according to the deficiency and will filter out background noises to assist the patient in hearing the conversation. The patient must be aware that the hearing aid is just that an aid for participation in social situations where hearing is necessary not a cure for the disability, and it will it restore the patient's hearing to normal.

Although only one in five who would benefit with a hearing aid actually wear one, research has found that wearing hearing aids has positive effects on physical, psychological, and social functioning in patients with profound hearing loss. Patients who had assistance with hearing whether cochlear implants or hearing aids were also found to have better quality of life (Cohen, et al., 2004). Encouraging patients to obtain and utilize hearing aids can help to reduce the social isolation that individuals with hearing loss experience.

When communicating with a patient who has a hearing aid, look for ways to decrease background noises. Hearing aids amplify all sounds, and it is distracting for the patient when various alarms, conversations, and other sounds (e.g., telephones, pagers) are simultaneously heard. Take the patient into a quieter environment or private room if available to decrease as many extraneous noises as possible (Figure 40-7).

PATIENT PLAYBOOK

Care of Hearing Aids

- Change batteries immediately when not working.
  Batteries last approximately one week.
  Do not store batteries more than a month.
  Batteries are small, which makes them difficult to change and easily lost.
- Turn off the appliance when not in use.
  Leave the compartment open to reduce energy usage.
- Remove debris accumulated (directed by manufacturer).
  Clean ear molds at least once a week.
- Avoid hair products.
- Store in a cool dry place.
- Keep away from heat and moisture.
- Keep away from children and pets.

Adapted from Mueller, H., & Hawkins, D. (2006). Troubleshooting hearing aid fitting issues: The case of the missing "ping." Hearing Journal, 59*(1), 10, 12, 14–15.*

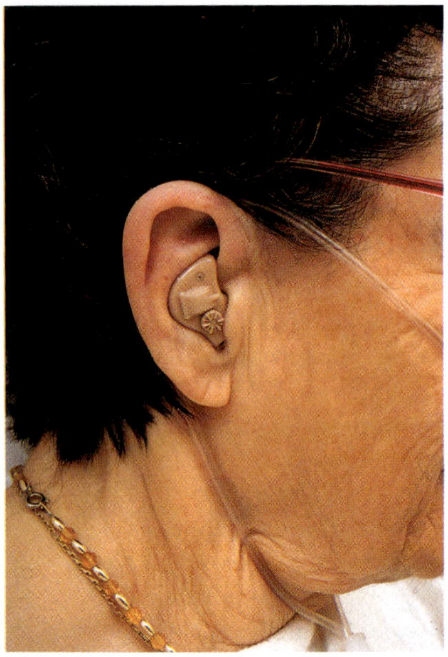

Figure 40-7 If a patient relies on hearing aids, make sure they are functioning before beginning the assessment examinations.

Other amplification devices assist the patient such as telephone amplification or typing machines are also available. These assist the patient in being able to communicate with others via telephone. The TDD (telecommunication device for the deaf) is a machine that allows the patient to type in a message, which is relayed to another individual with a similar piece of equipment or to an operator who then translates the calls. If the medical office sees a lot of patients who are hearing impaired, special telephone access should be available. Also, while in the hospital, the patient with a hearing impairment may need assistive devices on his or her telephones to communicate with family and friends to avoid feeling isolated.

External Otitis

External otitis, inflammation of auditory canal, results from moisture in the canal in most cases. The patient normally complains of pain and fullness in the canal demonstrated by moving the pinna of the ear. It is difficult to examine the canal, because edema is present that occludes or partially occludes the canal. Often a discharge is present. Treatment includes topical medications and mild pain relievers. Patient teaching includes instructions on techniques to maintain the integrity of the canal. Medical management depends on the identification of the organism to differentiate it from bacterial, viral, or fungal.

Often patients clean ear canals with anything that appears to be handy and do not realize that the canal should be left alone. Only the outer portion of the ear should be cleaned. By inserting different objects into the canal, injury to the tissue can occur, leading to a prime area for organisms to attack. Therefore, preventive patient teaching should include putting nothing smaller than your elbow into the ear, drying the canal after water sports or baths, and reporting any signs or symptoms of ear discomfort as soon as experienced.

Once external otitis appears, patient teaching should include instillation of the topical medication. As with all medications, it starts with washing hands. You may warm the drops by rubbing the bottle in your hands for a few minutes; never place it in a microwave because this causes uneven heating and an increased possibility of causing a burn. Have the patient tilt his or her head or lie on his or her side with the infected ear pointing to the ceiling; pull the pinna up and back, instill the drops, and have the patient remain in this position for approximately five minutes to ensure absorption. Until the canal is healed, water should be kept out of the ear. This can be accomplished by placing cotton in the os.

Otitis Media

Otitis media is infection of the middle ear common in children but can occur in any age. Treatment includes observation as well as the administration of appropriate antibiotics. With the increase of antibiotic resistance, if the patient is not acutely ill, it is now recommended to observe the patient for 48 to 72 hours to see if the condition resolves spontaneously. The nurse is important in maintaining contact with the patient and family for follow-up evaluation. If the patient is prescribed an antibiotic, the importance of completing the full course of medication is strongly encouraged. Other teaching topics include avoiding water sports, keeping the ear canal dry while bathing, and watching for changes in the patient's condition that may warrant follow-up before the recommended two to four week reevaluation. Chronic otitis media occurs when the patient has longstanding history of ear infections.

Overview of Nursing Care for Auditory Dysfunction

The nurse working with a patient who has hearing loss must understand the anatomy of the ear and the dynamics that cause the deficit. Loss that is attributed to obstruction is managed by removing or treating the blockage to allow sound waves to penetrate the inner chamber of the ear. The management of permanent loss is to supply the patient with assistive devices, such as hearing aids, telecommunication devices, and other signaling mechanisms. And lastly the patient must be taught communication skills, encouraged to participate in social engagements, and learn sign language or the technique of reading lips. Nurses look for measurable outcomes that indicate the patient is coping with the loss of hearing. A favorable outcome is when the patient has learned effective communication and participates in social activities. Effective communication is essential in patient teaching, to ensure the patient understands the diagnosis, etiology, management, and follow-up at every medical encounter.

Once the patient is diagnosed, the nurse can work with other health care providers to direct the best patient care for that patient. The nurse can assist the patient by educating the patient about the different disease processes, testing procedures, and follow-up expectations. Preparation of the patient aids in the progression of the disorder and the ability to work through the dysfunction. Some patients may require hospitalization until the acute phase is resolved.

Hearing loss is becoming an increasing problem and at a younger age. Loss of hearing is a societal burden that affects all aspects of an individual's life. Nurses need to start by becoming proactive in auditory health and restoration of auditory functioning by becoming sound aware. They need to promote appropriate precautions and protection for the patient's auditory system and promptly identify sudden hearing losses. Ways to decrease the amount of noise in the environment need to be emphasized to preserve as much hearing ability as possible before loss of functioning has occurred affecting the patient's quality of life.

What the future brings is promise in new technology for the hearing impaired, including devices to improve communication, understanding, and interpreting sound either implanted or external. Cochlear devices will be totally implanted with improved hearing and be undetectable to others. Improved oral-auditory educational programs to assist patients with hearing and interpreting cues for enhanced communication need to be developed. Nurses need continuing education in ways to communicate with the hearing impaired and remain strong advocates as the mediators between health care providers, patients, and social services to provide the best care for their patients.

Future research is looking at preserving the fine hair cells of the inner ear from damage received from high-intensity noise, ototoxic drugs, and other insults. Experimentation is being considered in replacing lost hair cells and developing more advanced devices to improve hearing (Brors & Bodmer, 2004). Nurses need to keep abreast of new discoveries to assist patients in decision making and appropriate patient care after the procedure is undertaken. Further research examining the ways to incorporate hearing assessment and ensure effective communication with patients to increase satisfaction and adherence to medical care should be developed. Quality of life should also be considered as new interventions are developed to identify which patients benefit most.

Evaluation of Outcomes

Potential patient outcomes for each of the example nursing diagnoses for the patient with the auditory dysfunction are:

- Disturbed sensory perception, auditory, related to obstruction of ear canal, damage to inner ear. The nurse will be able to assist in impacted cerumen with irrigation if the cause of the obstruction. If damage to the inner ear is present, the nurse gives support and perioperative instructions and assists the patient in obtaining auditory devices appropriate for the source.
- Anxiety related to inability to communicate. The patient should be able to recognize the signs of anxiety, demonstrate positive coping mechanisms, and describe a reduction in the level of anxiety experienced.

- Knowledge deficit related to self-care and risk prevention. The patient will demonstrate and report steps in the proper technique in handling and managing a hearing aid. He or she will have knowledge in volume control, storing when not in use, and cleaning the device appropriately.
- Impaired social interaction related to inability to hear others. The nurse will support and provide alternative ways to communicate and encourage the patient to participate in social activities. The patient will be willing to participate in one social event with family or friends.

KEY CONCEPTS

- The type of hearing loss depends on the affected location of the auditory system.
- The number of individuals with auditory dysfunction increases as environmental noise levels increase and the population ages.
- Permanent hearing loss is multifactorial.
- Prevention is the solution to preserving auditory function.
- Often the family member or friend identifies a hearing problem before the patient.
- Conductive hearing loss is differentiated from sensorineural by loss of all sound frequencies, not just higher frequencies.
- Meniére's disease is a chronic progressive condition for which no cure is currently available.
- A thorough history is necessary to identify causes of auditory complications.
- Insects found in the auditory canal should be killed before extracting. Never use water to kill the insect.
- Audiometer is used to test hearing in all ages and should be preformed annually.
- Nursing care consists of educating the patient on proper care of the external auditory canal.
- It is important to discuss postoperative expectations and communication methods before surgery for better patient understanding.
- Ear protection equipment is mandatory in occupations in which the sound levels measurement is greater than 90 dB.
- Frequent breaks are recommended when working with high noise producing equipment.
- Safety is of utmost importance in patients with hearing impairment.
- Effective communication is essential in patient teaching; poor communication leads to confusion, decreased satisfaction, and compliance.
- Always remember the patient cannot hear what is being said and include the patient in all aspects of care.

REVIEW QUESTIONS

1. A 70-year-old patient complains of difficulty hearing when out to dinner with his family. The type of hearing loss he most likely has is:
   1. Conductive hearing loss
   2. Sensorineural hearing loss
   3. Mixed hearing loss

2. A patient who has conductive hearing loss will have the following characteristics:
   1. Hearing loss is associated with higher pitch tones.
   2. Sound is perceived as distorted.
   3. Patient talks louder to hear better.
   4. Conversation can be heard in noisy environments.

3. You are taking care of a patient who just underwent a tympanoplasty. Which of the following interventions is appropriate?
   1. Place patient lying on operative side
   2. Encourage deep breathing and coughing
   3. Tell patient that hearing will return to normal immediately
   4. Assist patient with ambulation until vertigo resolved

Continued

REVIEW QUESTIONS—cont'd

4. A 65-year-old patient who is on high doses of aspirin to treat rheumatoid arthritis suddenly complains of tinnitus and difficulty hearing telephone conversations. The patient asks what can be done. The nurse responds by:
1. Performing Rinne and Weber tests
2. Informing the patient that tinnitus occurs with aging
3. Instructing the patient that tinnitus is a side effect of aspirin
4. Directing the patient increase the volume on the receiver

5. Signs and symptoms of Meniére's disease include all of the following *except*::
1. Tinnitus
2. Severe vertigo
3. Conductive hearing loss
4. Sensorineural hearing loss

6. An adolescent comes in with complaint of hearing loss in the left ear. On examination with an otoscope the canal is found to be blocked with cerumen. What is the next course of action?
1. Gently irrigate the canal
2. Insert a cotton swab to remove debris
3. Use an ear curette
4. Refer to otologist for removal

7. A 65-year-old patient comes into the clinic with gradual onset of hearing loss. What are some ways to improve communication with the patient who has a hearing deficit?
(select all that apply)
1. Get the patient's attention before speaking
2. Stand with the lighting behind you
3. Speak very loud
4. When asked to repeat, repeat same phase slower
5. Keep hands away mouth while talking

8. A patient is diagnosed with a sensorineural hearing loss and asks if a hearing aid will help return his hearing to normal. Which statement about hearing aids is correct?
1. Hearing aids only help patients with conductive hearing loss.
2. Hearing aids increase volume but not clarity of sounds.
3. Hearing aids will assist patient to hear sounds as normal.
4. Hearing aids will eliminate background noises.

9. Degrees of hearing impairment are categorized according to sound intensity measurements or decibels. Normal hearing is measured at what range?
1. 0–15 dB
2. 16–25 dB
3. 26–40 dB
4. 41–55 dB

10. True or False: A patient who is exposed to a loud blast greater than 120 dB lasting 20 seconds can have permanent hearing loss.
1. True
2. False

11. Some work environments provide a sustained high noise setting and protection of employees hearing is therefore essential. The occupational nurse must follow OSHA guidelines, which include which of the following? (select all that apply)
1. Baseline and annual hearing testing of all workers
2. Monitoring sound levels in the workforce
3. Biannual education and training of noise pollution
4. Mandatory hearing protectors on all employees

12. A patient complains of frequent attacks of vertigo, tinnitus, nausea, vomiting, and intermittent hearing loss. These manifestations are characteristic of:
1. Presbycusis
2. Meniére's disease
3. Otosclerosis
4. Mastoiditis

REVIEW ACTIVITIES

1. You are the nurse taking care of a patient who is scheduled for a tympanoplasty. What are some of the things that you would tell this patient about the procedure to alleviate his or her fears of becoming totally deaf? What patient teaching would be important to include regarding the immediate postoperative period?

2. Identify resources in your clinical facility and community for patients with hearing loss. Choose a specific program and find out what is offered in ways to assist those with a hearing deficit. What does the program offer? Is the program easily accessible? Does the program monitor patient's progress?

3. Using the Internet, locate the different communication devices available for patients with a hearing deficit? Research the cost and available financial resources to assist the patient in obtaining these devices. What requirements or steps does the patient need to complete to obtain the pieces of equipment?

4. Make arrangements to visit an audiologist's office and become more familiar with the various types of hearing aids. Becoming more familiar will provide the students with a better understanding on ways to help the patient better adjust to his or her hearing aid.

5. Experience the sensation of hearing loss by wearing an ear muff and ear plugs. Have the other students practice different types of communication techniques. Discuss what works best and why.

Visit the Contemporary Medical-Surgical Nursing online companion resource at www.delmarhealthcare.com for additional content and study aids. Click on Online Companions then select the Nursing discipline.

UNIT

IX

Alterations in Immunological Function

Chapter 41 Assessment of Immunological Function

Chapter 42 Immunodeficiency and HIV Infection/AIDS: Nursing Management

Chapter 43 Allergic Dysfunction: Nursing Management

CHAPTER 41

Assessment of Immunological Function

Patrick Heyman, PhD, ARNP-BC

KEY TERMS

Acquired immunity
Agglutination
Antibodies
Antigen
Antigen presenting cells (APCs)
Basophils
Cell-mediated immunity
Chemokines
Complement
Cytokines
Cytotoxic (killer) T cells
Dendritic cells
Eosinophils
Extravasation
Granulocytes
Granuloma
Haptens
Helper T cells
Human leukocyte antigens (HLA)
Humoral-mediated immunity
Immunogen
Immunoglobulins (IG)
Inflammation
Innate immunity
Interferons (IFNs)
Interleukins (IL)
Leukocytes
Macrophage
Monocytes
Neutropenia
Neutrophils
Phagocytosis
Toxoid

CHAPTER TOPICS

- Role of the Immune System
- Innate Immunity
- Acquired Immunity
- Inflammation
- Immune Activation and Response
- Assessment of Immune System

The immune system is tasked with three distinct and interrelated duties: (a) defense of the body from external invaders (pathogens and toxins); (b) surveillance in identifying the body's cells that have mutated and may become or have already become neoplasms (tumors); and (c) maintain homeostasis by removing cellular detritus from the system to ensure uniformity of cells and function (Price & Wilson, 2003). Traditionally, immunologists were only concerned with the first duty. It is only recently that the additional tasks of the immune system came to light. In many ways, the immune system can be thought of as the body's policy enforcers. It is responsible for making sure that the body's cells look sharp and do their jobs. Cells that slack or misbehave are destroyed, so not to affect the functioning of other cells. In its role of enforcer, the immune system also makes sure that the functioning of the body's cells is not impaired by foreign invaders. When the body is damaged, the immune system leads the way preparing the injured area for the healing and reparation process. With so much power over the functioning and viability of the body's cells, it is no coincidence that some of our worst diseases come about as a result of immune dysfunction.

Describing the immune system is a difficult task. Although there are relatively clear divisions in immune function, the components that make up these divisions have overlapping roles. Any general statement is sure to have two or three exceptions, and it is practically impossible to describe or define one part of the immune system without using terms that belong in another part and have not yet been defined. After a brief historical introduction, the approach of this text is to describe the overall interaction of the immune system, and then to discuss each of the components in greater detail, and then put the physiology together.

Fast Forward ▶▶▶

Immune Function and Cardiovascular Health

It is known that the inflammatory part of the immune system plays a part in the formation of atherosclerosis (atherogenesis) in arteries for several years. In particular, it is known that macrophages ingested subendothelial cholesterol and became foam cells. In the past four years we have also learned that C-reactive protein (CRP) levels confirm that **inflammation** (a nonspecific response to any foreign invader involving the immune system) plays a part in atherogenesis and myocardial infarction (MI). It is thought that at least part of the antiatherosclerotic benefit of Statin cholesterol-lowering medications is because of their anti-inflammatory properties. But even more recently, it has been discovered that the specific (acquired) immune system plays a part in atherogenesis. Without lymphocytes, progression of an atherosclerotic plaque cannot occur. Natural killer (NK) cells are also implicated in atherogenesis (Linton, Major, & Fazio, 2004; Whitman, Rateri, Szilvassy, Yokoyama, & Daugherty, 2004). Essential enzymes in atherogenesis that interact with immune and inflammatory cells are being identified (Boehm, et al., 2004). Most of the experimental research is currently being conducted in animals because of the ethics involved, but human research is also taking place on a limited scale. In the future, assessing immune function will become part of assessing cardiovascular health.

OVERVIEW OF IMMUNITY

The immune system is generally divided into two large categories, innate and acquired. **Innate immunity** (immunity that is inherent within a species and develops regardless of exposure), also called natural immunity, is present at birth and functions similarly regardless of the pathogen earning it the designation nonspecific. **Acquired immunity** refers to immunity that is not present at birth and develops either as a result of exposure or through an external source, such as colostrum or injection of immunoglobulin. Acquired immunity is also called adaptive or specific, because the immune response develops and changes in response to the specific pathogen. Adaptive immune responses are considered either humoral-mediated or cell-mediated. **Humoral-mediated immunity** refers to immunity that is mediated by B lymphocytes, plasma cells, and antibodies. **Cell-mediated immunity** refers to immunity that is mediated by T lymphocytes.

This simple division between types of immunity is muddied by the interactions between the innate (nonspecific) and adaptive immune systems. The adaptive immune system requires the innate immune system for initial activation. Once activated, however, much of its effector mechanisms (effectors are any cell or chemical that acts to eliminate invaders, as opposed to recognition) involve potentiating innate immune responses. Thus the innate system forms part of the adaptive system's response and vice versa. The innate immune system can eliminate some threats by itself, but many invaders either overwhelm it or evade detection by it. In these cases, the adaptive immune system is required. It takes 4 to 10 days for the adaptive immune system to mount its first response. Once developed, however, the adaptive immune system will retain some of its effector cells as memory cells. On subsequent exposures, the adaptive immune system can mount a response almost immediately.

The vital characteristics of both systems are recognition and effector mechanisms. Recognition mechanisms are the methods by which various immune system cells recognize invading cells and toxins or aberrant host cells. Effector mechanisms are the methods by which the immune system destroys and eliminates these threats.

The nonspecific immune system relies on receptors that detect common pathogenic features, such as bacterial cell wall polysaccharides. Most of these receptors are found on the surface of various white blood cells, but some of them are found on plasma proteins, such as complement C1q and CRP. A complement is a cascade of proteins in serum that, when activated, attract more leukocytes (white blood cells) to the site of activation, encourage phagocytosis, and lyse pathogen cell membranes. When one of the receptors is bound to its substrate, it activates a series of reactions that activates the nonspecific immune system and calls white blood cells to the site of injury. This process is called inflammation and will be discussed later in the chapter. The specific immune system also relies on receptors, but instead of relying on common pathogenic features, the receptors are designed to respond to only one feature, called an antigen. The two main receptors of the adaptive immune system are the T cell receptor (TCR) and antibodies. In a population of lymphocytes, there may be up to one million different receptors represented. When an invader is identified, only those lymphocytes whose receptors match the invader are activated (thus the specificity). Antibodies are released by B lymphocytes and contain the same receptors that the manufacturing cell featured. The B cell receptor is a membrane-bound antibody. The antibodies are plasma borne proteins that serve much the same purpose as the plasma proteins of the innate immune system, except that instead of recognizing common pathogenic features, antibody receptors recognize only their specific antigen.

Antigen

The term **antigen** originally referred to a molecule that caused antibodies to be generated, but it has now been refined to mean any molecule that can bind with a specific antibody. The term **immunogen** refers to any molecule that elicits an immune response. These may include viruses, bacteria, pollen, toxins, foods, transplanted organs, or transfused blood. There is a fine difference between immunogens and antigens, but for most purposes, they can be used interchangeably.

The bulk of an antigen's surface causes no immune response. Only certain portions of the surface are reactive. These reactive portions are called epitope (sometimes also called antigenic determinant). Most antigens have more than one kind of epitope and are called multivalent. Other antigens have repeated arrays of the same epitope. Antibodies are produced in response to epitope, not the antigen as a whole. Thus a multivalent antigen may react with more than one kind of antibody. A given epitope may be present on more than one antigen, so that one antibody may potentially react with more than one antigen.

The difference between immunogens and antigens is that all immunogens are antigens, but some antigens are not immunogens. That is, that some antigens by themselves do not elicit an immune response or antibodies. These are called **haptens.** For a hapten to elicit an immune response, it needs to be bound to carrier molecule at which point it becomes an immunogen. Two factors influence the ability of an antigen to elicit an immune response. One is the size or weight of the molecule. Smaller molecules tend to cause less reaction. The other factor is the concentration. Small quantities of an antigen may not cause an immune response. Haptens are clinically significant, because once bound to their carrier molecule, the immune system will produce three different kinds of antibodies against them. The first kind of antibody will react to the hapten regardless of whether it is bound or not. The second kind of antibody will react to the carrier molecule regardless of whether it is bound to the hapten or not. The third kind of antibody only reacts to the hapten-carrier complex. Hapten antibodies are important in immunology research, but they are also clinically significant as they form the physiological basis for penicillin allergy cross-reactivity with cephalosporins and other antibiotics. In clinical practice, immunogen and antigen are often used interchangeably, but a nurse should know the distinction.

Self versus Nonself

In all three of its roles, the immune system's essential requirement is the ability to distinguish between what is self and what is foreign (nonself). A group of genes responsible for the recognition of self is called major histocompatibility complex (MHC). The MHC manufactures two major types of MHC proteins that are essential in identifying the body's cells as self. Class I MHC proteins are present on the surface of the cell membrane of almost all host cells with a developed nucleus and platelets. They are also called **human leukocyte antigens (HLA),** because they were first identified on leukocytes. Substances lacking HLA are identified as nonself. Each person has an HLA that uniquely identifies him or her. As far as science can tell there are no two persons that have identical HLA, although twins may have similar HLA. MHC class II molecules are found mainly on immune system cells, but can be induced in other cells by interferons (proteins formed when cells are exposed to invaders, such as viruses that are able to activate other components of the immune system). Classes I and II MHC proteins also serve to present antigen to T cells.

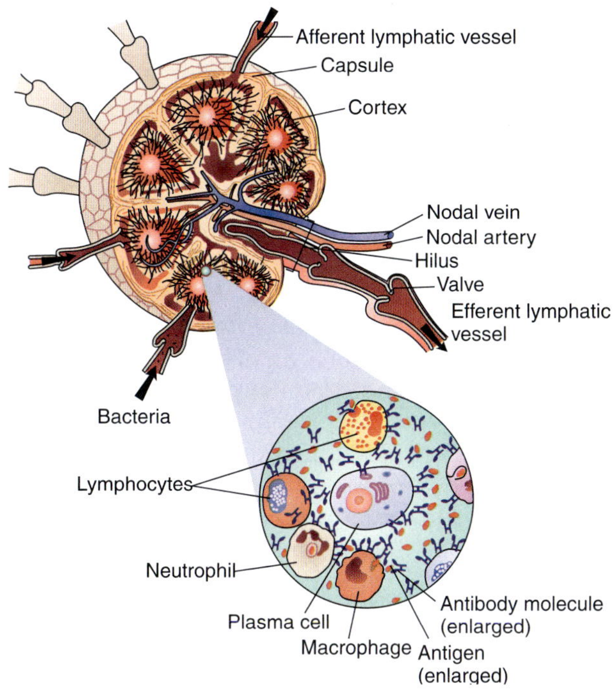

Figure 41-1 Cellular components of the immune system.

ANATOMY OF THE IMMUNE SYSTEM

The anatomy of the immune system is detailed and complex. There are many elements to consider within the immune system, and their interrelationships are complicated in nature. The structures of the immune system have been examined extensively within the field of biology and are well-defined. There are both larger anatomic organs and cellular components of a hematological nature comprising the immune system (Figure 41-1).

Physical Barriers

The human body is constantly surrounded by pathogens in the air, on solid surfaces, and in water. Pathogens are ingested with every meal and inspired with every breath. Before ever encountering an immune system cell, a pathogen must penetrate the body's outer defenses. These consist of barriers (e.g., mechanical, chemical, and microbial) that are considered to be part of the innate immune system. In addition to the barriers themselves, each of these areas is populated with members of the innate immune system and often with lymphoid tissue.

The most obvious physical barrier is the skin. The outermost layer consists of several layers of keratinized, water-resistant squamous cells. But skin is made even more formidable by secretions of lactose that lower the pH of skin, making it a less hospitable environment. Perspiration contains salt, which can be toxic to pathogens by hypertonic mechanism. Sebaceous glands secrete sebum that helps to trap invaders and actually inhibits some type of bacteria.

With regard to the digestive system, saliva in the mouth forms the first chemical barrier. The pH of saliva, combined with several enzymes, make it an unattractive place to live. The hydrochloric acid and pepsin of the stomach form the next inhospitable atmosphere that invaders will encounter. Bile salts, fatty acids, lysolipids, and other digestive enzymes are found in the small intestine. After making it through this gauntlet of digestive enzymes, the large intestines are thoroughly colonized with a wide array of flora, both bacterial and fungal. There are about 400 different kinds of bacteria in the intestines, weighing over a kilogram and outnumbering the body cells 10 to 1. These native flora make the intestines less hospitable to invaders through competition for space and nutrients.

The respiratory system begins with nasal hair and turbinates in combination with mucous secreting membranes, which all serve to trap invading pathogens and may contain immunoglobulin A (IgA) antibodies. Once in the bronchus, mucous secretions in combination with a cilia "elevator" serve to bring foreign particles to the carina, where the cough reflex helps to expel the invaders from the body. The epithelium of the lungs secretes two proteins called surfactants A and D, which coat pathogens making them more easily phagocytosed.

The eyes are protected by lashes and the blink reflex. Tears, which contain antimicrobial factors including IgA antibody, help to wash out pathogens that make it past the lids and lashes. The vagina is colonized with lactobacilli that secrete lactic acid, lowering the pH of the vagina and making it less hospitable. Yeast and lactobacillus compete with potential pathogens for nutrients, further preventing infection.

Leukocytes

The main cells of the immune system are white blood cells collectively referred to as **leukocytes.** Like all blood cells, leukocytes originate from the bone marrow. Stem cells (undifferentiated cells) in the marrow develop into the various white blood cells. In addition to serving as the birthplace for leukocytes, the bone marrow also acts as a reservoir for mature cells that may be needed in event of infection or blood loss. Although most leukocytes originate in the bone marrow along with red blood cells (RBCs), most spend little time in the blood. Leukocytes spend most of their time in storage, in lymphoid tissues, or dispersed throughout the host tissues. Leukocytes use blood mainly as a transport system to travel to areas of the body where they are needed. There are six families of leukocytes that have distinct roles in the body's defense. These are the monocyte-macrophages, dendritic cells, mast cells, granulocytes, lymphocytes, and NK cells. All the leukocytes except the lymphocytes are considered part of the innate immune system. Lymphocytes are the only leukocytes associated with the adaptive immune system. All the leukocyte families originally come from pluripotent stem cells in the bone marrow. The pluripotent stem cell differentiates into common lymphoid and common myeloid progenitors. All lymphocytes as well as NK cells are descended from the common lymphoid progenitor. The common myeloid progenitor differentiates into monocyte, dendritic cells, granulocyte, erythrocyte, and platelet precursors. The common lymphoid progenitor can also give rise to a dendritic cell that is indistinguishable from the dendritic cell derived from the myeloid.

It is imperative to understand progressive differentiation in order to understand leukocytes. The leukocytes found in the blood and lymph tissues are typically not fully differentiated. As a case study, monocytes descend from the common myeloid progenitor as previously discussed. Monocytes circulate in the blood until summoned to the tissues. At this time, they exit the blood vessels through specialized openings in the vessel wall and enter the tissue. Once in the tissue, monocytes differentiate yet again, maturing into macrophages, which usually live in the tissues until their death. Thus the macrophage is the final differentiation of a monocyte, and the monocyte is simply a relatively inert circulation form of the cell. Another way to think of progressive differentiation is to think of the monocyte as an observation form and the macrophage as the functional form. Most other leukocytes also undergo progressive differentiation. The exception is the granulocytes, which circulate in fully differentiated form.

Proliferation is the other concept necessary to understand white blood cells. Although lymphocytes originate in the bone marrow from stem cells, they are also able to reproduce within lymph tissue. When activated, lymphocytes will proliferate (reproduce) first and then differentiate into their final functioning form. This allows the few cells that are able to respond to a given invader to reproduce quickly without a corresponding increase in lymphocytes that are not needed for the present threat.

Monocyte-Macrophages

Monocytes are leukocytes found in relatively small quantities in the blood, because most of them are either in the tissues or stored in the bone marrow. Arising from the common myeloid progenitor, the majority of monocytes remain in the marrow, serving as a reservoir against infection. The immature stage is referred to as monocyte, while the fully differentiated stage is called a **macrophage.** Monocytes are continuously migrating to tissue and differentiating into tissue macrophages. Tissue macrophages are called different names, depending on the tissue in which they have differentiated. Tissue macrophages in the nervous system are called microglial cells, and macrophages in the liver are called Kupffer cells. No matter where they differentiate, tissue macrophages serve the same function, which is to monitor the surrounding tissue for invaders and foreign antigen. Collectively, they are sometimes referred to as mononuclear phagocytes.

Macrophages are one of three phagocytic cells (cells that engulf and destroy foreign pathogens, toxins, or other antigens) in the immune system. Having differentiated in tissues, macrophages are relatively immobile, monitoring the nearby tissue for invaders. Macrophages have receptors for a wide variety of common pathogen features, such as the glucan receptor and mannose receptor, scavenger receptor, which binds to negatively charged ligands that are components of many gram-positive bacterial cell walls, and the CD14 (LPS) receptor, which detects bacterial lipopolysaccharide. On detecting an invader, macrophages attempt to engulf the invader in an amoeboid-like process called **phagocytosis.** The cell membrane distorts and wraps around the particle until the two sides of the cell membrane touch. The cell membrane edges fuse themselves together, and the particle is encased in a vesicle made of membrane that was formerly part of the cell's outer membrane. This vesicle is called a phagosome or endocytic vacuole. Lysosomes containing destructive enzymes are then fused with the phagosome, and the enzymes are released into the phagosome. The phagosome-lysosome complex is called a phagolysome.

Macrophages are **antigen presenting cells (APCs)** and act as one of the first responders in the immune response process. Once activated, a macrophage releases cytokines and chemokines. **Cytokines** affect the way other cells act (*Cyto-* "cell" and –kinein "move"). **Chemokines** attract other leukocytes to the area to battle the invaders in a process called chemotaxis. See Table 41-1 for a list of selected cytokines released by macrophages and their effects. Because macrophage recognition of pathogens is so important, one of the main distinguishing features of pathogenic microbes (as opposed to nonpathogenic microbes) is the ability to overwhelm or evade macrophages and other segments of the innate immune system. For example, some bacteria coat themselves in a thick polysaccharide that is not recognized by macrophage or neutrophil receptors. Other pathogens, such as mycobacteria, can actually live and multiply inside of phagosomes by keeping the lysosomes from fusing with the phagosome.

One unique characteristic of macrophages is the ability to form giant multinucleated cells. When confronted with an overwhelming opponent, several macrophages can join together to form one large cell, the aforementioned giant multinucleated cells. This allows macrophages to engulf invaders that they other wise could not engulf.

Dendritic Cells

Dendritic cells are star-shaped cells that are so called because they resemble a neuron's dendrites. While we have been studying macrophages for more than 100 years, we have only known about dendritic cells for less than 35 years, and

TABLE 41-1 Important Cytokines Released by Macrophages and Their Effects

CYTOKINE	LOCAL EFFECT	SYSTEMIC EFFECT
IL-1β	Activates endothelium Activates lymphocytes Local tissue destruction Increases access of effector cells	Fever Production of IL-6
TNF-α	Activates endothelium and increases vascular permeability, leading to increased entry of IgG, complement, and increased fluid drainage to lymph nodes.	Fever Mobilization of metabolites Shock
IL-6	Lymphocyte activation Increased antibody production	Fever Induces acute-phase protein production
CXCL8	Chemotactic factor recruits neutrophils, basophils, and T cells to site of infection	
IL-12	Activates NK cells Induces the differentiation of CD4 T cells into TH1 cells.	

Adapted from Janeway, C. A., Jr., Travers, P., Walport, M., & Shlomchik, M. J. (2004). Immunobiology, the immune system in health and disease *(6th ed.). New York: Garland Science Publishing.*

there is still much that we do not know about them. Their life cycle is more complicated than that of macrophages. The immature dendritic cells migrate to tissues, particularly the skin, airway, spleen, and lymph nodes. Like tissue macrophages, tissue dendritic cells are called different names depending on the tissue in which they live. Tissue dendritic cells that live in the skin are called Langerhans cells. Immature tissue dendritic cells are both phagocytic and macropinocytic; that is, they can ingest large amounts of surrounding interstitial fluid. Tissue dendritic cells break down proteins and display the ingested antigens on their cell membranes. At the end of their life cycle, they will migrate to lymph nodes and induce tolerance in lymphocytes, because they do not have costimulatory molecules in their immature stage. The signals for maturation are either direct contact with a pathogen or inflammatory cytokines. Pathogens are ingested when they are recognized by their common features as described above. Macropinocytosis allows the dendritic cell to ingest pathogens that have some mechanism to escape detection by phagocytic receptors. As the products are degraded inside the dendritic cell, they are able to recognize bacterial DNA, bacterial heat shock proteins, and viral double stranded RNA. Once activated, they differentiate into mature dendritic cells, develop costimulatory molecules, and migrate to the lymph nodes to activate the lymphocytes that migrate through the nodes (Vuckovic, et al., 2004).

Mature dendritic cells carry high levels of MHC on their cell membranes to present antigen to T lymphocytes. When the T cell with the right receptor recognizes the presented antigen, it proliferates and differentiates. The truly amazing thing about dendritic cells is that they are able to activate only the specific T lymphocytes that are needed to respond to a given invader, whether it is a virus, bacteria, or fungus. In some cases, this may mean activating just 1 in 10,000 or 1 in 1,000,000 T lymphocytes.

Fast Forward ▶▶▶

Dendritic Cell Research

Dendritic cells are seen as the missing key in many immunological disorders. Dendritic cell infection is crucial in defeating the body's defenses against several viruses, including Ebola and HIV (Geisbert, et al., 2003; Janeway, Travers, Walport, & Shlomchik, 2004). Both of these viruses neutralize dendritic cells keeping the body from mounting a defense against them. By the time the immune system is mobilized, it is often too late. It is hoped that understanding dendritic cells will aid in the treatment and possible vaccination against these diseases. Dendritic cells are also implicated in tumor formation, and research is being conducted to see if dendritic cells can be manipulated in a way as to be a kind of vaccine against cancer cells. In a cancer vaccine, dendritic cells would be harvested from the patient's body and cultured. Once a thriving culture has been established, tumor cells from the patient are introduced to the culture. The primed dendritic cells are then injected back into the patient where they initiate the immune response against the cancer. Trials are currently underway testing this technique in melanoma, lymphoma, prostate cancer, and colon cancer. Because of the large expense involved in developing a dendritic culture for each patient, additional research is being done to try and up-regulate dendritic cells in the body. In the opposite direction, research is being done in the areas of immune down-regulation. It is hoped that dendritic cell research will be able to provide effective cures for some autoimmune diseases and transplant rejection (Fecci, et al., 2003).

The dendritic cell's strength is also a vital weakness exploited by several viruses, such as human immunodeficiency virus (HIV) and measles. Instead of activating lymphocytes in lymph nodes against these viruses, the infected dendritic cell acts as a transportation system, allowing the virus to then infect the T lymphocytes.

Much of the extracellular debris that is ingested by dendritic cells is harmless, often by-products of dead body cells. Dendritic cells are essential in inducing and maintaining tolerance to these antigens, keeping the immune system from reacting to the body's antigens (Vuckovic, et.al., 2004). As T lymphocytes exit the thymus gland, dendritic cells are responsible for destroying cells that are reactive to self-antigens. This process is referred to as central tolerance and removes the majority of self-reactive T lymphocytes. Dendritic cells also induce peripheral tolerance, suppressing self-reactive lymphocytes that escaped central tolerance or cells that are reactive to antigens not expressed in the thymus.

Mast Cells

Mast cells are also descended from the common myeloid progenitor and differentiate in the tissues. Their blood borne precursor is currently unknown. Mast cells tend to live near the skin and connective of small blood vessels and contain granules with stored chemicals. When activated, they release substances within the granules (degranulate) that affect vascular permeability, particularly histamine. See Table 41-2 for a list of mast cell products. Mast cells are thought to play an important part in protecting mucosal surfaces from pathogens and help the inflammatory process to begin the process of healing damaged tissue, although they are primarily known for their role in immunoglobulin E (IgE)-mediated allergic reactions. In fact, mice that do not have fully differentiated mast cells cannot produce IgE-mediated inflammatory responses.

TABLE 41-2 Molecules Released by Mast Cells on Activation

CLASS OF PRODUCT	EXAMPLES	BIOLOGICAL EFFECTS
Enzyme	Tryptase, chymase, cathepsin G, carboxypeptidase	Remodel connective tissue matrix
Toxic mediator	Histamine, heparin	Toxic to parasites
		Increase vascular permeability
		Cause smooth muscle contraction
Cytokine	IL-4, IL-13	Stimulate and amplify TH2 cell response
Cytokine	IL-3, IL-5, GM-CSF	Promote eosinophil production and activation
Cytokine	TNF-α	Promotes inflammation, stimulates cytokine production by many cell types, activated endothelium
Chemokine	CCL3 (MIP-1α)	Attracts monocytes, macrophages, and neutrophils
Lipid mediator	Leukotrienes C4, D4, E4	Cause smooth muscle contraction
		Increase vascular permeability
		Stimulate mucous secretion
	Platelet-activating factor	Attracts leukocytes
		Amplifies production of lipid mediators
		Activates neutrophils, eosinophils, and platelets

Adapted from Janeway, C. A., Jr., Travers, P., Walport, M., & Shlomchik, M. J. (2004). Immunobiology, the immune system in health and disease *(6th ed.). New York: Garland Science Publishing.*

Granulocytes

The **granulocytes** are so called because when stained, they have granule-shaped objects visible within their cytoplasm, much like mast cells. They also have lobed irregular nuclei, earning the designation polymorphonuclear leukocytes (PMNs). The granules are lysosomes, which are vesicles filled with destructive enzymes. These enzymes are used to destroy invaders. **Neutrophils** are the most numerous granulocytes and thought to be the most important. Neutrophils are the third and final phagocytic cell in the immune system. On engulfing an invader, the granules are fused to the vesicle, and the enzymes are released into vesicle; where they may destroy the particle. Neutrophils are especially reactive to bacteria, and the number of circulating neutrophils greatly increases during bacterial infections. Neutrophils are the first responders to chemotaxis and are rarely found in healthy tissue. Neutrophils are relatively fragile compared to macrophages. They can only ingest a few bacteria before dying, but macrophages can ingest a hundred bacteria. Pus is mostly made up of bacteria and dead neutrophils. Because of their expendable nature, they appear in the blood in large numbers, with several times that number in reserve in the bone marrow. They are the most numerous granulocyte and often the most numerous leukocyte. Deficiency in neutrophils, called **neutropenia,** can cause overwhelming bacterial infection.

The other two classes of granulocyte cells are exocytic, meaning they produce their effects on outside cells as opposed to phagocytosed cells. **Eosinophils** are found in small quantities in the blood as most of them are distributed in the tissues. Their primary effector function is to release their highly toxic granules that can kill parasites and other microorganisms. They also produce cytokines, leukotrienes, and prostaglandins. Eosinophils are involved in defense against parasites and increase in numbers when the body has a parasitic infection. They are most well-known for their role in IgE-mediated allergic reactions and are often present in mucous secretions during allergic reactions.

Basophils, are the final and most inscrutable granulocyte. Not much is known about them, but they appear to have an effect against fungus and also play a role in inflammation. They behave similarly to eosinophils and are distributed throughout the tissues.

Natural Killer Cells

NK cells arise from the common lymphoid progenitor. They appear as large lymphocytes with cytoplasmic granules and circulate in the blood. Although lacking antigen-specific receptors, they are able to detect and attack a limited number of abnormal cells, such as tumor cells and cells infected with the herpes simplex virus (HSV). They are also able to kill cells that are coated in antibody, a process known as antibody-dependent cell-mediated cytotoxicity (ADCC), and are mediated by the Fc receptor (see antibody discussed later). NK cells are also activated by interferons and macrophage-derived cytokines.

Lymphocytes

There are two major types of lymphocytes, T lymphocytes and B lymphocytes, or simply T cells and B cells. All lymphocytes originally descend from the common lymphoid progenitor but differentiate differently depending on where they mature. Some lymphocytes mature in the bone marrow, while others migrate to the thymus for maturation. B lymphocytes are so called, because they mature to their intermediate stage in the bone marrow. When activated, B lymphocytes complete their differentiation process and become plasma cells, releasing antibodies. T lymphocytes are so called, because they mature in the thymus. T cell development is more complex than that of B cells. The first division of T cells is based on receptor chains. Most T cells have receptors consisting alpha (α) and beta (β) chains, but a second division T cells have receptors made of gamma (γ) and delta (δ) chains. These are called $\alpha{:}\beta$ and $\gamma{:}\delta$ T cells, respectively. The $\alpha{:}\beta$ T cells eventually become CD4 and CD8 T cells.

The function of $\gamma{:}\delta$ T cells is poorly understood, but they appear to function as innate immune cells, rather than adaptive immune cells.

Most inactivated lymphocytes are small and rather featureless with inactive nuclear chromatin. As late as the 1960s, many textbooks described these cells as having no known function. Indeed, lymphocytes do show little activity until activated by the presence of antigen and costimulatory molecules, usually presented by an APC, such as a macrophage or dendritic cell. On activation, lymphocytes differentiate into lymphoblasts, which undergo mitosis and then differentiate into the final activated phase taking on their specialized functions. Once the infection has been eradicated, most of the lymphocytes that were produced as a result of lymphoblast proliferation undergo apoptosis (programmed cell death); however, a few remain as memory cells enabling the body to respond rapidly to subsequent infections by the same pathogen.

The main functional characteristic of lymphocytes is the ability to mount specific immune responses against virtually any foreign antigen. All lymphocytes have a prototype receptor that changes during the intermediate maturation process so that taken as a whole, they are able to react with almost any possible antigen. The B cell and T cell receptors are closely related in structure, but they are different in function and will be discussed in more depth. The B cell receptor (BCR) actually consists of the antibody that the B cell will release when activated and can recognize only one specific antigen. BCRs (and antibodies) are only able to detect antigen that is in the extracellular fluid. The T cell antigen receptor (TCR) is structurally similar to the BCR, but does not recognize whole antigens. Rather it detects fragments of antigen that are displayed by MHC molecules on the surface of host cells. Thus the T cell, detects antigen within the host cells, such as viruses that have commandeered a cell's processes or a parasitic bacteria. Variability in the BCR and TCR is attained by mutation of the genes responsible for their production.

B Lymphocytes and Antibodies

B cells are lymphocytes that develop in the bone marrow. Their primary job on activation is to produce antibodies. B cells develop in the bone marrow until they express the immunoglobulin M (IgM) molecule on their cell surface. Once the IgM molecule is expressed the immature B cell undergoes self-tolerance testing and viability testing. The immature B cell migrates to the secondary lymph tissues, where it develops into a mature B cell, expressing both IgM and immunoglobulin D (IgD) molecules. Mature B cells, also called naïve B cells because they have not encountered their specific antigen yet, recirculate through the lymph tissues waiting to encounter their antigen and become activated. On activation, B cells proliferate and then become plasma cells, secreting antibodies.

The only immune function of the B cell is to release **antibodies** (proteins produced by plasma cells that recognize and bind to a specific antigen) when activated. Unlike T cells, which venture out of the lymph nodes when activated, plasma cells stay in the lymph node, secreting antibodies to be delivered to the systemic circulation. An antibody itself is a molecule composed of two segments, a recognition/binding segment and an effector segment. The recognition segment binds to the antigen, and the effector segment activates other components of the immune system. Thus antibodies may neutralize threats directly by physically binding to them and keeping them from damage. At the same time, antibodies recruit other components of the immune system to attack and destroy the threat.

Antibodies are a category of protein called **immunoglobulins (Ig).** All immunoglobulins share a similar structure. They are generally y-shaped molecules, with two recognition segments and one effector segment. The recognition segment is called the variable region or V region, because it changes from antibody to antibody to ensure that a wide range of antigens can be recognized. The different immunoglobulins perform different effector functions in the body.

B cells will be selected to secrete more of a given immunoglobulin depending on the type of immune response and the location in the body of the activated B cell. Immunoglobulin G (IgG) is the most abundant immunoglobulin in the body and is further divided into four subtypes (IgG1, IgG2, IgG3, and IgG4), where IgG1 is the most abundant in plasma and IgG4 is the least abundant. IgA is divided into two subtypes (IgA1 and IgA2). IgM and IgA can form polymers in the blood. IgM forms a pentameter, a molecule composed of five IgM antibodies joined by their C terminuses. IgA appears in the blood as both a monomer (single antibody) and a dimer (two antibodies joined at the C region).

Naïve B cells express both IgM and IgD on their surface. When activated, the B cell will produce IgM and IgD antibodies. However, later in the immune response, the B cell will change to producing IgG, IgA, or IgE by irreversibly recombining its DNA. At this point the cell can no longer produce IgM or IgD antibodies. The signal to switch antibody production is mediated by cytokines and T cells.

Antibodies work by four basic functions: neutralization, opsonization, activation of inflammation, and activation of complement. Neutralization is accomplished solely by the variable region of the antibody, and its effectiveness is determined by the antibody's affinity for the antigen. Its mechanism is the complete binding of an antigen by the antibody, so that there are no available binding sites, effectively rendering the invader inert. This process is especially important for bacterial toxins and viruses. A special case of neutralization is **agglutination.** This occurs when the arms of the antibody bind to the same epitope on different antigens. For example, the IgM pentameter has 10 binding sites and could theoretically bind 10 different bacteria that share the same epitope. This causes clumping, called agglutination. The second mechanism is called opsonization. When antibodies coat a bacteria or other pathogen, it can induce nearby macrophages to engulf the pathogen. This is especially important against bacteria that have natural defenses to keep macrophages from engulfing them. The third mechanism is the activation of inflammatory processes, including the activation of NK cells. The fourth mechanism is the activation of the complement cascade. Complement is a cascade of lytic proteins that are activated by antibodies. The activation of complement by itself can cause the death of some invaders, but it is always a signal to nearby phagocytic cells to attack the pathogen.

In an immune response IgM is the first antibody to be released. IgM has a fairly low binding affinity for epitope, and it is believed that the 10 binding sites of the pentameter provide a higher effective affinity for repetitive epitope, such as bacterial capsule molecules. Essentially it allows the IgM molecule to stick to an antigen longer until higher affinity antibodies can be manufactured. Although IgM appears in the blood as a flat pinwheel, on binding to an antigen, the other binding sites bend toward the antigen surface like spider legs. The pentameric nature of IgM also makes it a particularly potent activator of the complement cascade. Thus IgM is an excellent first responder.

IgG, IgA, and IgE are produced later in the immune response. They are smaller than IgM and can diffuse relatively easily out of the blood and into the tissues. IgG is the principal antibody found in the blood and tissues, while IgA is principally found in secretions, such as tears and saliva. IgG is an excellent opsonin, but IgA is not. This makes sense, as IgA works on epithelial surfaces that do not normally contain complement or phagocytes. These antibodies are produced and secreted close to where they will function. IgE is found only in low levels, but it has an extremely high affinity for mast cells and binds to mast cells even before it binds to antigen. Antigen binding to this mast cell–associated IgE triggers mast cells to degranulate and release their inflammatory mediators.

T Lymphocytes

T lymphocytes progenitors leave the bone marrow and migrate to the thymus gland, where they develop into T lymphocytes instead of B lymphocytes. Most of the T lymphocyte progenitors die in the thymus by apoptosis. T lymphocytes are divided early in development into α:b and γ:δ T cells. The α:β T cells later develop into CD4 and CD8 T cells. CD4 and CD8 are surface proteins on the membranes of T cells. For years, CD8 has marked **cytotoxic (killer) T cells,** and CD4 has marked **helper T cells,** which further differentiate into two subclasses, TH1 and TH2 cells.

During development, T lymphocytes go through two selection process. Positive selection encourages lymphocytes that bind weakly to self-antigens. While negative selection eliminates lymphocytes that bind strongly to self-proteins. The reason for this twofold process is that lymphocytes must be able to bind with MHC I and II (self-antigens) to generate an immune response, but lymphocytes that bind too strongly could possibly cause autoimmune disease. The MHC antigens that the T lymphocytes recognize as self are determined the by the MHC antigens present in the thymus gland.

Each naïve T lymphocyte can detect only one specific antigen, and it wanders the body's lymph nodes in search of its antigen. If it finds it, it proliferates and then differentiates into its active phase. It takes more than simply meeting its specific antigen to activate the naïve T cell. The T cell must meet its antigen while being displayed by an APC that also displays costimulatory molecules. Naïve CD8 T cells always differentiate into cytotoxic (killer) T cells, but they require more costimulation than CD4 cells to do so.

Primary Lymphoid Organs

Anatomically speaking, the immune system is largely identified with the lymphoid portion of the immune system. The primary lymphoid organs are the bone marrow and thymus gland, because lymphocytes develop and mature within them. The thymus gland is located superior to the heart. The thymus gland also serves as a reservoir for T lymphocytes. It is believed that the major function of the thymus gland is in the development of the immune system. It is larger in children than in adults. Removal of the thymus in children causes a reduction in the number of T lymphocytes and a higher number of granulocytes (Eysteinsdottir, et al., 2004). The effects of removing the thymus gland in adults are not well understood and only recently have begun to be studied. New evidence shows that the thymus is active in adults, and efforts should be made to preserve it during cardiothoracic surgery.

Secondary Lymphoid Tissue

Although lymphocytes are distributed throughout the body, they are concentrated in several tissues. The tissues where they aggregate and function are called secondary lymphoid tissues and include the spleen, lymph nodes, and epithelial lymphoid tissues. Secondary lymphoid tissues are strategically placed in the body so that invading pathogens will encounter them as early as possible, allowing the immune system to be activated before extensive damage can be done.

Spleen

The spleen is a fist-sized organ located on the left side of the body, behind the stomach. It acts as a filter, collecting antigen from the blood and destroying senescent RBCs. Most of the spleen is made up of tissue called red pulp, which primarily serves as the site of RBC destruction and also houses macrophages. Interspersed throughout the red pulp, lymphocytes surround arterioles forming pockets called white pulp. The organization of white pulp consists of two layers, the periarteriolar sheath, consisting mainly of T lymphocytes, and the B-cell corona, consisting of mainly B lymphocytes. The white pulp is responsible for generating immune responses to blood-borne immunogens and plays an important role in preventing septicemia. Removal of the spleen often results in life-threatening infections known as overwhelming postsplenectomy infections (OPSI) (Jirillo, et al., 2003).

Lymph Nodes

The lymph nodes are encapsulated lymphoid structures located throughout the lymphatic vascular system and provide the tissues and lymph with the same function that white pulp of the spleen provides for blood. Ranging in size from 1 to 20 mm, lymph nodes are responsible for generating immune responses to the immunogens in the lymph drainage and interstitial fluid that drains from local tissues into the lymph vessels. Lymph nodes are typically bean-shaped, with two layers, an outer cortex and an inner medulla. Several afferent lymphatic vessels enter into the cortex, which is separated into several compartments called follicles. Each follicle leads to the medulla, where the lymph fluid is consolidated, and one larger efferent lymphatic vessel exits from the medulla. The medulla is also associated with an artery and vein that is used for incoming naïve lymphocytes. The lymph nodes also act as a pump for lymph fluid, activated by random skeletal muscle contraction.

Lymph node follicles are divided into several distinct regions. The outer portion of the follicle is made up mostly of B cells. During an immune response, areas of intense B cell proliferation are called germinal centers. Follicles that do not contain germinal centers are called primary lymphoid follicles. Once a germinal center has been established, it is called a secondary lymphoid follicle. Primary follicles contain inactive B cells surrounding a specialized cell of uncertain origin, called a follicular dendritic cell (FDC). The FDC secretes chemokines that attract both inactive and active B cells. The next section of the cortex is called the paracortical area and is mostly made up of T lymphocytes. The third part of the cortex, which is closest to the medulla, is made up of macrophages and antibody-secreting plasma cells and is called the medullary cords.

Lymph nodes are designed so that APCs from the tissues will come into the lymph node through the afferent lymphatic vessel and encounter B lymphocytes first, then T lymphocytes, and will then take up residence in the medullary cords. This ensures that it will encounter both kinds of lymphocytes, and if the lymphocyte with the specific antigen it is presenting is not present, as that lymphocyte recirculates through the body, it will encounter it in the medullary cords. The recirculating naïve T lymphocytes enter the node through the arteriole using special adhesion molecules, called L-selectin, which allows them to stick to the artery's surface. Activated B cells remain in the lymph node and form germinal centers, but activated T lymphocytes need to travel to the site of infection. When T cells mature, they lose their L-selectin, so that they can no longer enter lymph nodes through the artery.

Epithelial Lymphoid Tissues

In addition to lymph nodes, there are also patches of unencapsulated lymphoid tissue located throughout the body in connective tissue. The gut-associated lymphoid tissues (GALT) include the tonsils, adenoids, Peyer's patches in the small intestine, and the appendix. GALT collects antigen from the surface of epithelial cells in the digestive tract. Peyer's patches are the most organized of the GALT and consist of a B cell center surrounded by smaller numbers of T cells. Specialized epithelial cells called multifenestrated cells collect the antigen from the lumen of the small intestine. Similarly, bronchial-associated lymphoid tissue (BALT) and mucosa-associated lymphoid tissue (MALT) provide the same functions in the bronchial tree and other mucosa.

Chemical Components

In addition to the leukocytes and antibodies, there are also a number of chemicals that make up the immune system. Many of these are secreted by leukocytes, but some are not. Chemical components serve several different functions. Two of these functions have already been discussed briefly in the leukocyte section; attracting cells and changing cell behavior. Chemicals that attract other leukocytes to the area are called chemokines. Chemicals that change the behavior of other cells are called cytokines. Some cytokines may induce vasodilation or increase vascular permeability. Other cytokines may activate leukocytes. The third function of chemical components is opsonization. A fourth function of chemical components is pathogen or toxin neutralization and direct destruction.

Cytokines

Cytokines are small proteins that affect the behavior of cells. The cytokines may act in an autocrine manner (affecting the cell that secreted it), paracrine manner (affecting adjacent cells), or even endocrine manner (affecting distant cells). The ability of a cytokine to act on distant cells depends on its ability to enter the blood and how long it stays in the blood (half-life). An important concept in understanding cytokines is that of kinases and kinase inhibitors. These enzymes destroy cytokine and preserve cytokine, respectively. Each cytokine has its own set of kinases and kinase inhibitors, which are important in the regulation of immune responses. Some diseases may not have anything to do with underproduction or overproduction of cytokines, but rather problems with these regulatory proteins. Too much kinase or too little kinase inhibitor will result in abbreviated immune response, while too little kinase or too much kinase inhibitor will result in prolonged immune response.

When cytokines were first being discovered, they were named **interleukins (IL),** to signify that they were secreted by a leukocyte. Over time, it became apparent that the cytokines are a diverse group of molecules structurally and behaviorally. Newer nomenclatures are being developed that group the cytokines according to their structure or function.

The **interferons (IFNs)** are a class of cytokine that was so named because it interfered with viral replication in cells that were previously uninfected. IFNs bind to nearby cells through an IFN receptor, which induces the cell to produce a variety of proteins that inhibit viral replication. In mice, the ability to manufacture the protein Mx in response to interferon confers immunity to influenza. In addition to this protein production, IFNs also stimulate the immune response to viruses by inducing the synthesis of MHC class I molecules on the surfaces of infected cells. Recall that the specific immune response to viruses depends on presenting antigen bound to MHC to T cells. Finally, IFNs activate NK cells to destroy viruses and virus-infected cells.

Chemokines

Chemokines are a subgroup of cytokines that attract other cells, a process called chemotaxis. They function mainly as chemoattractants, recruiting monocytes, neutrophils, and other leukocytes to the area; however, some chemokines also have roles in lymphocyte development and angiogenesis. Chemokines can be secreted by a wide variety of cells, including endothelial cells and keratinocytes (skin cells). They have been discovered fairly recently and originally shared the interleukin designation with cytokines. More recently, there has been as change in nomenclature to reflect their structure. The two main families of chemokines are called CC and CXC chemokines. The chemokine itself is designated by the letter *l* and a number, while the receptor is designated by the letter *r* and the same number. Thus, IL-8 became CXCL8 and binds to the CXCR8 receptor.

Complement

The **complement** system is a cascade of several lytic proteins that aid in pathogen destruction. They were first observed being activated by antibodies and enhancing the action of antibodies. Hence their discoverer called them antibody-complement proteins, which were later simplified to complement. The complement cascade consists of enzymes that aid in the destruction of pathogen membranes. To keep these enzymes from destroying host cells, they circulate in the blood as zymogens. To be activated, the zymogen is cleaved into two parts, freeing the active enzyme. An example of zymogens elsewhere in the body is pepsinogen, stored in stomach epithelial cells. Once secreted into the stomach, the hydrochloric acid cleaves pepsinogen into pepsin, which breaks down peptide bonds. This mechanism keeps pepsin from digesting the cell that stores it.

Complement proteins are designated by the letter *c* and then a number. The number does not represent the step in the cascade, but the order in which they were discovered. The complement cascade performs all four chemical component functions (cytokine, chemokine, opsonin, and effector). The three pathways for complement cascade activation are (a) the classical pathway, (b) mannose-binding lectin (MB-lectin) pathway, and (c) the alternative pathway. The classical pathway always begins with the binding of C1q to the pathogen surface. The MB-lectin pathway is initiated by the binding of MB-lectin to mannose containing carbohydrates in bacteria and viruses. MB-lectin is a serum protein that increases during inflammation. The alternative pathway can be initiated by the binding of spontaneously activated C3 in plasma to the surface of a pathogen.

PHYSIOLOGY OF THE IMMUNE SYSTEM

The physiology of the immune system is extremely complicated and complex. There continue to be many functions within the immune system that are not well understood and research exploring the immune system is extensive and ongoing.

Innate Immune Response

Innate immunity is dependent largely on the recognition of common pathogenic features, such as mannose and glucan found in bacterial cell walls. Because macrophages live in the tissues, they are usually the first immune system cell to encounter pathogens and typically begin the innate immune system response. When a macrophage recognizes an invader in addition to attempting to phagocytose the invader, it also releases cytokines and chemokines, thus inducing the inflammatory response. Inflammation plays three roles in the innate immune response. First, it brings more effector cells to the site and augments their killing ability. Second, it provides a physical barrier, through capillary coagulation, to keep the pathogens from spreading into the blood. Third, it prepares the tissues for healing. Inflammation is characterized by localized pain, erythema (redness), heat, and edema (swelling).

The first reaction to inflammatory chemokines and cytokines released by activated macrophages is local vasodilation, which causes the erythema and some of the heat. Vasodilation also serves to slow blood flow. The second reaction is the expression of adhesion molecules by the endothelium (inner layer of the arterial wall) to bind to circulating leukocytes. The combination of slowed blood and adhesion molecules allows leukocytes the time to migrate through the arterial wall into the tissues in a process called **extravasation.** The first leukocytes to migrate to the area are neutrophils, followed by monocytes, which differentiate into additional tissue macrophages. Later, eosinophils and basophils will migrate to the site (Janeway, et al., 2004).

The third reaction in the inflammatory process is increased vascular permeability. This allows fluid and plasma proteins to leak into the inflamed tissues, causing edema and pain. The plasma proteins, including complement and clotting factors, aid in the inflammatory process and immune response. For example, once the complement cascade is activated, C5a increases vascular permeability, induces adhesion molecules, and activates phagocytic cells and mast cells. Activated by C5a, the mast cells degranulate, releasing the inflammatory molecules histamine and tumor necrosis factor (TNF)-α.

This triggers the fourth reaction in the inflammatory process, causing blood clots to form, walling off the infected area from the blood supply. This allows the infectious antigens in the edematous fluid, usually inside a dendritic cell, time to travel through the lymph vessels to a lymph node where an adaptive immune response can begin. TNF-α is critical in the isolation of the infection from the rest of the body.

In addition to these local effects of inflammation, systemic effects are also evident. The release of TNF-α, IL-1β, and IL-6 (endogenous pyrogens) raise the body's temperature. Elevated temperature helps the body in a number of ways. It inhibits the growth of most pathogens, which tend to prefer lower temperatures; adaptive responses tend to be more effective; and increased temperature helps to protect the body from the harmful effects of TNF-α.

TNF-α is critical in the innate immune response, because it is so potent in vasodilation, increasing vascular permeability, and inducing clotting. These properties make it ideal for sending leukocytes to the site of infection and then walling it off. Unfortunately, if a pathogen does make it to the systemic circulation, these same qualities make TNF-α release backfire. When sepsis occurs, widespread systemic release of TNF-α occurs by macrophages in the spleen and liver. This systemic release causes systemic vasodilation leading to loss of blood pressure. At the same time, TNF-α also causes increased systemic vascular permeability leading to a loss of oncotic pressure and plasma, aggravating the drop in blood pressure caused by vasodilation. The clotting properties of TNF-α cause disseminated vascular coagulation throughout the systemic circulation, further impeding blood flow, while depleting the body's supply of clotting proteins, putting the patient at risk for hemorrhage. This condition is known as septic shock. It is the spleen's job to minimize systemic TNF-α release by filtering the blood and sequestering any pathogens.

TNF-α, IL-1β, and IL-6 also induce a response known as the acute phase response. The acute phase is characterized by a change in the proteins that the liver produces and secretes into the plasma. The proteins that are produced as a result of TNF-α, IL1β, and IL-6 are called acute-phase proteins. Some of the proteins act similar to antibodies, but rather than binding to specific antigens, they have broad-spectrum binding. Anything that triggers inflammation will trigger all of these proteins, so it is not a targeted response, as are antibodies. The first acute-phase protein is CRP. It has already been mentioned that CRP can activate complement. CRP binds to phosphocholine in bacterial and fungal cell walls and acts as an opsonin in its own right in addition to being able to activate complement. Another acute-phase protein is MB-lectin, which in addition to activating complement acts as an opsonin to monocytes, which unlike fully differentiated tissue macrophages, do not express a mannose receptor. The other two important acute-phase proteins are the lung surfactants SP-A and SP-D. These proteins bind to pathogens in the lung and act as opsonins for phagocytes.

The last systemic effect of inflammatory cytokines is **leukocytosis,** an increase in the numbers of circulating leukocytes, especially neutrophils. Additionally, TNF-α has a role in stimulating dendritic cells to migrate from the tissues in which they reside to lymph nodes. The systemic actions of the endogenous pyrogens (TNF-α, IL-1β, IL-6) are summarized in Table 41-3.

Adaptive Immunity

Adaptive immunity refers to the process whereby lymphocytes are activated against the specific invader that is threatening the body. It is also called specific, because only lymphocytes that are capable of countering the current pathogen are activated. The process of activation, proliferation, and differentiation takes four to seven days to occur. The end result of the process is destruction of the pathogen and the development of lymphocytes that are able to immediately respond to the same invader during subsequent infections.

TABLE 41-3 Systemic Effects of the Endogenous Pyrogens (TNF-α, IL-1β, and IL-6)

TISSUE AFFECTED	ACTION ON TISSUE	NET RESULT
Liver	Acute-phase protein production	Activation of complement
		Opsonization
Bone marrow, endothelium	Leukocytosis	Phagocytosis
Hypothalamus	Increased body temperature	Decreased viral and bacterial replication
Fat, muscle	Protein and energy mobilization to increase body temperature	Increased antigen processing
		Increased specific immune response
Dendritic cells	Migration to lymph nodes	Initiation of adaptive immune response

Adapted from Janeway, C. A., Jr., Travers, P., Walport, M., & Shlomchik, M. J. (2004). Immunobiology, the immune system in health and disease *(6th ed.). New York: Garland Science Publishing.*

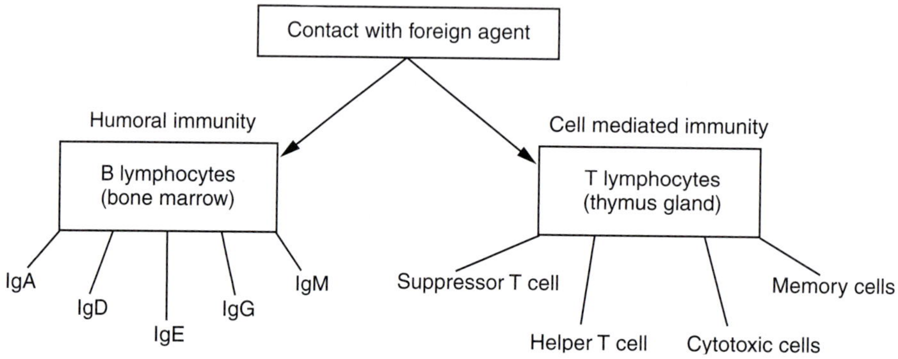

Figure 41-2 Humoral- and cell-mediated immunity in acquired immunity.

There are two basic pathways by which the adaptive immune system functions. These are termed humoral-mediated and cell-mediated immune responses (Figure 41-2). Both forms of immunity involve T cells and antibodies (produced by B cells), but the mechanism of activation is different.

Cell-Mediated Immune Response

Cell-mediated immunity refers to the activation of naïve T lymphocytes to proliferate and mature into armed effector T cells (Cytotoxic, TH1, and TH2 cells). A naïve T cell needs to have antigen presented to it by its appropriate MHC molecule. But this alone does not activate the naïve T cell. The T cell must also simultaneously receive a costimulatory signal. The only cells that are able to produce both classes of MHC and costimulatory molecules are dendritic cells, macrophages, and B cells. These are termed professional APCs and are the only cells that can activate or prime naïve T cells. Priming occurs in lymphoid tissues where naïve T cells are constantly recirculating.

When infection occurs, the innate immune system signals tissue dendritic cells to differentiate into mature dendritic cells that express costimulatory molecules. Cytokines also stimulate the dendritic cells to migrate into the lymph nodes. The vascular changes during inflammation serve to increase lymph drainage, which in turn speeds the dendritic cell's journey to the lymph nodes. There are resident macrophages in all the lymph nodes, and B cells are constantly recirculating through lymph nodes. In response to inflammatory cytokines, both can develop costimulatory molecules and thus be potentially able to prime T cells. Dendritic cells, however, are vastly more potent in priming T cells, and it is believed that in vivo, they are responsible for most if not all T cell activation.

As T cells migrate through lymph nodes, they transiently bind with every APC they meet. If the T cell recognizes its specific antigen in the presence of costimulatory molecules, the bond is strengthened and can last for days while the cell proliferates and differentiates into its active state. Its progeny, so far as space allows will also bind to the APC. The activated T cell will produce IL-2, which stimulates it and its progeny to proliferate and differentiate. Without the IL-2, the activated T cell will not proliferate. If a T cell recognizes its antigen, but costimulatory molecules are not present, the cell will go into an inactive state called anergy. Anergic cells cannot produce IL-2. Many transplant drugs that suppress the immune response to keep the body from rejecting the transplanted organ work by disrupting IL-2 from functioning normally.

After several days of proliferation, the activated T cells differentiate into mature effector cells that are able to produce all the effector molecules required in their roles as helper or cytotoxic T cells. These effector T cells no longer require costimulatory molecules to react to their specific antigen. They lose the adhesion receptors that allow them to recirculate in the lymph tissues and develop receptors that allow them to bind to the endothelium of infected tissue. This change ensures that they will be able to distribute to the infected tissues.

The case with naïve CD4 cells is a bit more complicated. Although, CD4 cells do not need large amounts of costimulation to activate, they must choose whether to become TH1 or TH2 cells. If TH1 cells are preferred, cell-mediated immunity will continue. If TH2 cells are preferred, humoral-mediated immunity will be stimulated. The difference can have profound consequences on the outcome. Bacteria such as *Mycobacterium tuberculosis* and *M. leprae* live inside of macrophages and other phagocytic cells. If TH1 cells are predominantly produced, there will be relatively small amounts of bacteria found, few antibodies, and the patient will most likely live a long time. If TH2 cells are predominantly produced, there will be large amounts of antibody produced, but because the bacteria are sequestered in macrophages, the antibody will not be able to reach them. The bacteria will multiply freely; the disease will be much more severe, and the patient will likely die soon.

Viral and other intracellular parasites cause activation of cytotoxic T cells, which are selective serial killers of other cells expressing the specific antigen. Cytotoxic cells kill host cells that are infected with pathogen. This accomplishes two things. It prevents more pathogen from multiplying inside the infected cell, and it allows the pathogen to be released into the extracellular fluid where it is susceptible to antibodies, macrophages, and other components of the immune system.

TH1 cells' main effector function is to activate macrophages. Most of the time, macrophages need no help from TH1 cells to destroy pathogens, but there are certain pathogens that live inside phagosomes and are able to prevent formation of the phagolysome. In addition to these macrophage parasites, other pathogens are not destroyed by macrophages unless the macrophage is activated. TH1 cells activate such macrophages to induce destruction of the already phagocytosed pathogen and to phagocytose extracellular pathogens. TH1 cells also activate B cells to produce certain classes of antibody.

The study of TH1 cells and macrophages has led to the conclusion that macrophages are naturally in an inactivated state and require two signals for activation. One of these signals is IFN-γ; the other signal can take a variety of forms. In TH1 cells, that second signal is provided by CD40 ligand (a membrane-associated protein). The IFN-γ can be produced by CD8 T cells, the TH1 cell itself, or NK cells. Activated macrophages also use a positive feedback mechanism, secreting IL-12, which induces the selective production of more TH1 cells. These mechanisms make activated macrophages extremely effective effector cells, but in addition to consuming large amounts of energy, their activation is associated with local tissue destruction because the proteases and oxides they release are equally destructive to host tissue.

In addition to the activation of macrophages, TH1 cells also express CD40 ligand and can kill infected macrophages. This may need to occur if the pathogens escape from the phagosome and enter the macrophage's cytoplasm. Both CD8 and TH1 cells can kill macrophages in this case. When the pathogens are released from the dead macrophages they can be killed directly by the TH1 cell or by CD8 T cells and are then susceptible to the antibody.

TH1 cells are also critical in recruitment of phagocytic cells to the site of infection. They produce IL-3 and granulocyte-macrophage colony-stimulating factor (GM-CSF), which stimulate neutrophil and macrophage production. They also produce the TNF-α and TNF-β, which continue the inflammatory process. They produce the chemokine CCL2, which attracts other T cells and macrophages to the site. Thus, although inflammation is considered part of the innate immune response, in its later stages, it is promulgated by the adaptive immune system. When pathogens are able to resist the efforts of the activated macrophages, chronic infection with inflammation occurs. This is often accompanied by a characteristic pattern in which macrophages envelop the area, T cells are present around the perimeter, and it is called a **granuloma.** Giant cells, previously described under the macrophages section, form in the center of the granuloma and attempt to sequester the pathogens. The purpose of a granuloma is to wall off the infection from the rest of the body, and it is sometimes surrounded with collagen tissue to aid in this purpose. The tissue in the center of the granuloma will die secondary to hypoxia and the effects of activated macrophages and is called caseation necrosis. If nothing else happens, eventually the infection will take over the entire body, but will take a fairly long time to do so. Acquired immunodeficiency syndrome (AIDS) patients are unable to form granulomas to sequester local infections and are susceptible to rapid fulminant forms of infections that would usually take years to kill most patients.

TH2 cell–mediated immunity will be discussed, because their primary function is to activate B cells, thus making them part of humoral immunity.

Humoral-Mediated Immune Response

Humoral-mediated immunity is the adaptive immunity pathway that was first discovered in the form of "antitoxins" in the blood against tetanus and diphtheria. Body fluids were once called humors, thus the term humoral immunity. All antibodies are produced by plasma cells that arise from the proliferation and differentiation of activated B lymphocytes. B lymphocytes typically require the help of a CD4 T lymphocyte, hence the designation helper T cells. Both TH1 and TH2 cells can activate B cells, but TH2 cells are more associated with humoral immunity.

The BCR has two functions in the naïve B cells; it serves to activate internal signals when bound to its specific antigen and also serves to bring the antigen inside the cell, where it is degraded and displayed on MHC class II molecules. The B cell does not typically proliferate until activated by a CD4 cell. Some pathogens, however, can directly induce B cell activation without T cell help, but the antibodies secreted will be limited in nature. Thus, just like the naïve T cell, the naïve B cell also requires costimulation. Protein antigens always require a T cell's costimulation, but many microbial constituents, such as bacterial polysaccharides and certain cell wall components, do not require T cell costimulation. This may be an added defense mechanism against autoimmunity, because bacteria do not produce protein, but host cells do. This relaxing of the costimulation requirement ensures quicker responses against bacterial antigens, while still protecting host cells from accidental activation against self-antigens.

Antibodies serve a variety of effector functions as described in B lymphocytes section, but the production of specific antibody classes is directed by T cells. IgM is the antibody class that will naturally be secreted by plasma cells, but makes up less than 10 percent of circulating antibody. CD4 T cells direct the change in antibody class production, a process called isotype switching. Cytokines are the driving factor in isotype switching, which involves recombining the DNA of the B cells, a usually irreversible process. Thus, a B cell that has switched from IgM production to IgA, IgG, or IgE cannot go back to making IgM.

Naïve B cells are continuously recirculating through the lymph nodes, much like naïve T cells. When they encounter their specific antigen, they are arrested in the lymph node at the B cell-T cell border by the development of adhesion molecules. Because they are trapped at the border or the T cell zone, it is likely that the APCs will also activate nearby specific T cells that can activate the B cell. Once activated, B cells travel to the medullary cords to proliferate and differentiate.

Next, B cell activation occurs, which is the formation of the germinal center as the proliferating T and B cells move to a primary follicle. B cells undergo somatic hypermutation with the goal of producing antibodies that have even more affinity for their specific antigen. Affinity maturation is the process whereby the B cells with the highest affinity are selected for survival. This process of affinity maturation also allows for progressively higher affinity antibodies to be produced over time. It will not be long, however, before T cells are activated and migrate to germinal centers to direct the humoral response. Non–T cell activation is important for immunity against encapsulated bacteria, such as *Haemophilus influenza* B (HIB), which can escape detection by phagocytic cells and hence activation of T cells.

The Total Immune Response

For a pathogen to invade the body, it must first pass the epithelial surfaces of the body (e.g., skin, mucous membranes, lungs) that have their own antimicrobial properties. Once past the epithelial surface, the pathogen will soon encounter tissue phagocytes (i.e., tissue macrophages, dendritic cells), which initiate the innate immune response and inflammation. It is unknown how many infections are cleared by the innate immune system alone, because such infections are likely to cause few if any symptoms. Moreover, deficiencies in innate immunity are rare, and when they are present, individuals succumb quickly to infection, unable to mount either an innate or an adaptive immune response.

Inflammation causes tissue dendritic cells to migrate to the lymph nodes, where it will activate the specific T lymphocytes that recognize its presented antigen. CD8 and CD4 T cells proliferate and differentiate into cytotoxic T cells and helper T cells. The helper T cells differentiate into TH1 and TH2 subclasses. The exact stimulus for preference of TH1 or TH2 is currently unknown but involves the nature of the presented antigen and cytokines. Cytotoxic cells destroy parasites and host cells infected with parasites. They also release cytokines that prevent uninfected cells from becoming infected and potentiate inflammation. TH1 cells activate macrophages and B cells. TH2 cells activate B cells to produce antibodies. Both TH1 and TH2 cells produce cytokines that affect inflammation. Effector cells of both the innate and adaptive immune system are guided to the site of infection by chemokines and adhesion molecules on the vascular endothelium. Antibody production takes place in the lymph nodes and are secreted into the blood. Memory T and B cells are produced and are ready to mount an accelerated immune response upon subsequent infection with the same pathogen (Fecci, et. al., 2003).

Immunological Memory

One of the main characteristics of the adaptive immune system is memory, the ability to remember past pathogens and mount an accelerated and heightened immune response against them. Memory responses are called secondary, tertiary, and so on. Memory is the property of the immune response that is exploited by immunization. Most memory cells are in a resting state, but a few are dividing at any given time. It is not known what the signal for memory cell division is. It is known that IL-7 maintains all memory T cells, and IL-15 maintains CD8 memory T cells. When an animal protein is injected, primed T cells are available almost immediately and are at maximum strength within five days. It takes a month before B cell and antibody production is at maximum capacity.

The responses of memory cells are different than primary immune responses. Memory T cells do not require costimulation, but on recognizing their antigen, they immediately begin proliferating. Memory B cells, already having been selected for their antibodies, produce primarily high-affinity IgG, IgA, and IgE as opposed to IgM. Memory B cells do not express IgM on their cell membranes, but whichever of the high-affinity isotopes they will produce, IgG, IgA, or IgE. The increased affinity of their receptor combined with increased ability to bind to T cells allows them to respond much quicker to infection than during the primary response. Memory cells also suppress the activation of naïve B and T cells. This effect is used therapeutically in mothers who are Rh− with Rh+ babies. Rh+ antibodies can be injected into the mother, which will suppress the production of Rh+ immune response.

Mechanisms of Immunization

The effector mechanisms of the immune response will depend on the infectious agent. The primary (initial) immune response is usually sufficient to clear the infection from the body, although some pathogens can evade the immune system and live in the body as long as the host lives. In some of these cases, protective immunity may be induced against the pathogens, preventing them from establishing a persistent presence in the first place. In the case of other pathogens, such as polio, even though the primary immune response clears the infection, the tissue damage is debilitating. Protective immunity involves two components. The first is antibodies, and the second is effector cells, such as primed T cells that can counter the infection. IgA antibodies are present in mucosal secretions and can keep some pathogens from ever entering the body, much less establishing a primary infection. This is the goal of immunization.

Immunization refers to the process first discovered by Edward Jenner 200 years ago. It involves the stimulation of the adaptive immune system so that when a person is exposed to the pathogen, his or her body has already developed immunity against it. In some cases, it is the toxin that a pathogen produces that is the true threat. This is the case with tetanus and diphtheria. In some cases, the toxic receptor-binding functions are located on separate portions of the toxin. In this case, it is possible to cleave the binding site from the toxin. This is called a **toxoid** and produces antibodies against the toxin but cannot harm the person. Toxoid immunizations can also take advantage of linked recognition of antigens. For example, once a baby has been immunized against the tetanus toxoid, it can be linked to HIB polysaccharides (Burns, Carroll, Drayson, Whitham, & Ring, 2003).

In cases where the toxin is extremely toxic or unusual, it may not be practical or possible to develop an immunization for human protection. Snake venom is an example of such a toxin. Snake toxin works too quickly for the adaptive immune system to be effective. Instead of immunizing a human, horses are immunized with the toxin. The horses produce antibodies against the venom, which are then separated and stored. These antivenom antibodies (antivenin) can then be injected into a snake bite victim. When the antibodies are against an organism, such as rabies or malaria, they are not called antivenin, but generically immunoglobulins. Antibodies have a limited half-life and confer immunity only for a limited time. Use of antibodies in this manner is called passive immunization (injection of antibodies to confer immunity rather than stimulating the body to produce its own antibodies).

Immunization against actual pathogens can be accomplished in one of four ways. First, a small amount of the pathogen, enough to cause an immune response but not enough to cause disease, can be inoculated. This depends on the virulence of the pathogen. Cholera needs several thousand cells to be ingested to cause disease, while Shigella can cause disease by ingesting as few as a dozen. The second option is for attenuated pathogen to be used; that is, using pathogen whose potency has somehow been altered so that it produces no or less severe disease. The oral polio vaccine is a live vaccine and occasionally caused polio instead of preventing it. The third option is to use dead pathogens that will produce an immune response despite not being alive. Some pathogens will not cause an immune response when inoculated in dead form. This could possibly be because of clearance of the dead pathogen by the innate immune system before activation of the adaptive immune system is possible. The fourth method is to use a surrogate nonpathogen. This is the technique used by Jenner for his first vaccine. The cowpox virus does not cause disease in humans, but it is close enough antigenically speaking to the smallpox virus to induce immunity to it.

Some immunizations are given as a series, usually about a month apart. This technique takes advantage of the germinal center's hypermutation. It takes about a month for germinal centers to become fully operational. Reimmunizing at this point, causes hypermutation to increase, causing a jump in the affinity of the antibodies produced. This is necessary for some dead pathogen vaccines, because it mimics what would naturally happen if there were dividing pathogens in the body. Without being able to reproduce, dead pathogens or antigens will be cleared relatively quickly, even by low-affinity antibody. Thus, reimmunization serves to boost the affinity as well as the amount of antibody produced against the antigen.

ASSESSMENT

Assessment of the immune system begins with a health history and physical exam, much like any other assessment. However, lab values play a larger part in immune assessment than some other areas. There is a tendency among some health care providers to focus only on the lab values, but the whole patient should be assessed, not only the lab tests. The history should include both past and present indicators and determinants of immune status. Areas to be considered include age; gender; infections and immunizations; allergies; disease states that affect immune status, such as autoimmune disorders, cancer, transplants, and diabetes; nutrition; surgeries; medications, and blood transfusions. The physical exam should include examination of skin and mucous membranes, lymph nodes and tonsils, respiratory, cardiovascular, genitourinary, and neurological systems.

Age and Developmental Considerations

Babies do not have a developed adaptive immune system. They receive much of their initial acquired immunity from their mothers in the form of colostrum during the first few days of breastfeeding and from immunizations. A health history of an infant or young child should include a breastfeeding history. As children develop and grow, their relatively naïve immune systems incline them to having more infections than adults. This is because of the relative lack of memory cells, which means that any infection that overwhelms the innate immune system will cause 4 to 10 days of illness, while the adaptive immune system is activated and mounts a response. As children grow older, the amount of infections should begin to plateau and level off as their repertoire of memory cells grows.

Young adulthood is typically a time of good health, but there are some areas of concern that should always be in the back of the nurse's mind. Many autoimmune diseases, including systemic lupus erythematosus (SLE) and multiple sclerosis (MS), tend to manifest in early adulthood. As the patient passes onto middle age and older, a variety of changes in the immune system make

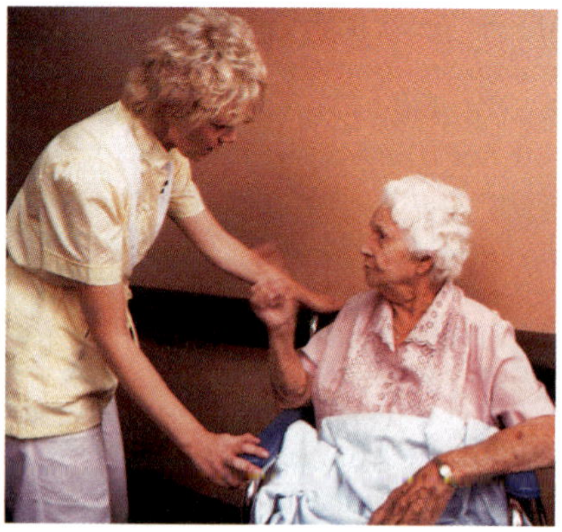

Figure 41-3 The aging process is a variable in this elderly woman's susceptibility to immune-related disease.

the body more susceptible to infections. Production and function of lymphocytes tends to decline. Response to APCs may also decrease, with fewer lymphocytes becoming activated in response to the innate immune system's activation. Autoimmune diseases continue to increase, although the exact etiology is unknown, because of decreased immune function and increased mutation, cancer incidence also increases.

Other physiological changes in combination with environmental factors and comorbidities also make older adults more susceptible to pathogens (Figure 41-3 and Table 41-4). As adults age, glomerular filtration tends to slow, causing a decrease in total urine production. At the same time, the bladder becomes less sensitive, even neurogenic, causing urine retention. In men, prostate hypertrophy can amplify this effect. The combination of less urine production and increased urine retention makes the bladder more susceptible to bacterial colonization, because ascending bacteria are not adequately

TABLE 41-4 Age-Related Changes in Immunological Function

BODY SYSTEM	CHANGES	CONSEQUENCES
Immune system	Impaired function of B and T lymphocytes	Suppressed responses to pathogenic organisms with increased risk for infection
	Failure of lymphocytes to recognize mutant or abnormal cells	Increased incidence of cancers
	Decreased antibody production	Anergy (lack of response to antigens applied to skin such as PPD)
	Failure of immune system to differentiate self from nonself	Increased incidence of autoimmune diseases
	Suppressed phagocytic immune response.	Absence of typical signs and symptoms of infection and inflammation
		Dissemination of organisms usually destroyed or suppressed by phagocytes (reactivation or spread of TB)
GI system	Decreased gastric secretions and motility	Proliferation of intestinal organisms resulting in gastroenteritis and diarrhea
	Decreased phagocytosis by liver Kupffer cells	Increased incidence and severity of hepatitis B, increased incidence of liver abscesses
	Altered nutritional intake with inadequate protein intake	Suppressed immune system
Urinary system	Decreased kidney function, hematuria, proteinuria, enlargement of prostate gland, neurogenic bladder, altered genitourinary tract flora	Urinary stasis and increased incidence of UTIs
Pulmonary system	Impaired ciliary action because of exposure to smoke and environmental toxins, reduced cough reflex	Impaired clearance of pulmonary secretions; increase incidence of respiratory infections
Integumentary system	Thinning of skin, loss of elasticity, loss of adipose tissue	Increased risk of injury, breakdown and infection
Circulatory system	Impaired microcirculation	Stasis and pressure ulcers; reduced healing of wounds
Neurologic function	Decreased sensation and slowing of reflexes	Increased risk of injury (ulcers, abrasions, burns, falls)

Adapted from DeLaune, S., & Ladner, P. (2006). Fundamentals of nursing *(3rd ed.). New York: Thomson Delmar Learning; Martins, P., Pratschke, J., Pascher, A., Fritsche, L., Frei, U., Neuhaus, P., et al. (2005). Age and immune response in organ transplantation.* Transplantation, *79(2), 127–132.*

cleared on urination. Proteinuria and hematuria also increase with age, providing additional growth medium for bacteria in the bladder.

As skin ages, it begins to lose elasticity and subdermal fat, decreasing its strength. Concomitantly, many older adults have nutritional deficits, whether caused by diet or by malabsorption. Deficits in protein, vitamins, and minerals can cause delayed wound healing. The combination of thinner, brittle skin with impaired wound healing makes older adults more susceptible to infections. Peripheral neuropathies and peripheral arterial disease impair sensation and circulation, causing injuries to go unnoticed, and delaying healing further. Decreased mobility can lead to venous stasis ulcers and pressure ulcers.

Smoke and other particulate pollutants, which are omnipresent in industrial society, impair pulmonary function by damaging tissues. This results in increased mucous production and decreased elasticity secondary to scar tissue and can also lead to metaplasm and neoplasm. Concurrently, the cilia elevator and cough reflex decline in older adults, impairing their ability to clear the excess mucus. The mucus provides a growth medium for bacteria and enables inhaled toxins to remain in the lung, where they continue to damage lung tissue and may lead to cancer, fibrotic lung diseases, or emphysema.

Decreased gastric secretions and decreased gastric motility allow ingested and normal intestinal flora to proliferate, causing infections and opportunistic infections. Decreased motility also keeps pathogens in contact with the digestive mucosa longer, giving them more opportunity to penetrate the mucosa. Ulcers and colon polyps may cause gaps in healthy epithelial tissue, serving as an avenue for pathogen penetration.

Immunizations and Infections

Immunization is the most efficient way to prevent infectious diseases, but it is not without disadvantages. Immunization usually confers immunity only for a limited period of time. With newer immunizations, such as hepatitis B and varicella, the period of immunity is not well established. Vaccinations with live pathogens may potentially cause the disease they are meant to prevent. For example, the oral polio vaccine is no longer administered in the United States, because the virus is shed in the feces and a child in the house may contract polio. Moreover, many immunizations are produced using egg as a growth medium, and people with allergy to eggs may not tolerate many immunizations. Many immunizations need multiple inoculations to be effective, meaning the patient or the patient's parents must be responsible enough to return for the full immunization series. The childhood immunizations against tetanus, diphtheria, and pertussis (DPT) as well as the immunizations against polio and HIB require three to four inoculations. Additionally, tetanus and diphtheria require booster inoculations every 5 years (note: tetanus is sometimes given on a 10-year schedule; but if any puncture or impaling wounds are experienced, a booster should be given if the last tetanus immunization was more than 5 years ago).

The type and date of immunization should be documented as well as any booster immunizations. The time from immunization is important, as discussed previously. Recommended immunization schedules for childhood and adolescent immunizations can be obtained from the U. S. Centers for Disease Control and Prevention (CDC) either downloaded from their Web site (www.cdc.gov) or ordered by mail.

It is important to assess whether a patient has had an illness before administering an immunization. A patient who has had mumps or rubella does not need to be immunized against them. However, a patient who had unilateral mumps would benefit from immunization, as it may recur in the other salivary gland. Known exposures to diseases for which the patient has been immunized are important. Tuberculosis exposure history and risk level assessment are important. People living in institutions, such as prisoners and hospital patients, are especially at risk. The last purified-protein derivative (PPD) tuberculosis test should be documented. A special case is the bacille Calmette-Guérin (BCG) vaccine against tuberculosis. This immunization was frequently given in third world countries, but its efficacy and duration are limited. However, patients who have received the BCG immunization will often show false-positives on PPD tuberculosis skin tests. Additionally, immunosuppression or immunodeficiency may cause PPDs to show false-negatives. In patients with history of BCG or with depressed immune systems, documentation of a chest X-ray (CXR), in addition to or lieu of the PPD, may be necessary.

Documenting past illness and infections is also important, especially for blood-borne pathogens, sexually transmitted diseases (STDs), and any treatments the patient may have undergone. The major blood-borne pathogens are hepatitis A, B, C, D, and E and HIV. Some blood-borne pathogens, particularly, hepatitis B and HIV, are also STDs and are often transmitted along with other STDs, such as HSV, humanpapilloma virus (HPV), syphilis, gonorrhea, and chlamydia. Many STDs also cause lesions that can serve as an entry point for other pathogens.

Patterns of illness may reveal either immune system dysfunction or an anatomic abnormality that predisposes the patient to a certain kind of infection. For example, patients with cystic fibrosis will have recurrent pulmonary infections as a result of inadequate mucous clearance, not because of immunosuppression. A thorough history will help to distinguish between causes of infections. History about persistent or recurrent infections and sores and lesions should be obtained.

Allergies

Ask the patient about any allergies that he or she may have to medications, food, or environmental factors. For all three causes of allergies, the source of the allergy, type and severity of reaction, the duration, treatment, resolution, and recurrence should be documented. If there have been recurrences, it should be noted whether the severity is increasing or decreasing. For severe allergies, or allergies that are increasing in severity, the nurse should inquire whether the patient has an emergency epinephrine injection system. Also document whether the patient has a Medicalert bracelet or necklace. The allergies should be documented on the history and placed on the front of the chart.

Allergies are inappropriate hypersensitivity immune reactions, and it is important to distinguish between true allergic reactions and other kinds of adverse drug reactions or unpleasant side effects. Amoxicillin can cause an amoxicillin rash in small children, which is harmless, transient, and does not indicate an allergy. This kind of rash should not be documented as an allergy to amoxicillin or penicillin. Nor should gastrointestinal (GI) bleeding secondary to nonsteroidal anti-inflammatory drug (NSAID) medications be documented as an allergy. True, it may be life-threatening, and is most likely a contraindication to future NSAID use, but it is not an allergy. Likewise, GI distress with erythromycin ethylstearate is not an allergy. Many patients will say they have allergies to medications simply because they do not like the side effects of the medication. However, there is a vast difference between having an allergy to a medication and simply, not tolerating the medication well. Being able to distinguish between the two is important in taking an allergic history. This is not to say that nonallergic adverse drug reactions are not significant, but mislabeling them as allergies is a significant error.

Food allergies are important to document, especially if the patient will be staying in a hospital, long-term care facility, or other overnight health care institution. Environmental allergies, such as to mold, dust, cosmetics, metals, or latex, are also important. If a patient has a latex allergy, care must be taken to ensure that all latex instruments, such as stethoscopes, are appropriately covered and that nonlatex gloves, dressings, and catheters are used. Allergies to adhesives can sometimes be worked around by using paper tape or skin prep, but sometimes reactions will still occur. In these cases, it should be considered as to how essential the adhesive is in the patient's treatment, how long the adhesive will be applied, and whether any antihistamines or other immunoactive medications will be administered.

The patient should also be asked about any history of atopic diseases, such as urticaria (hives), asthma, and atopic dermatitis. These diseases often accompany one another and are an indication of a hyperactive immune system. Patients with atopy are more likely to have other allergic problems.

Autoimmune Disorders

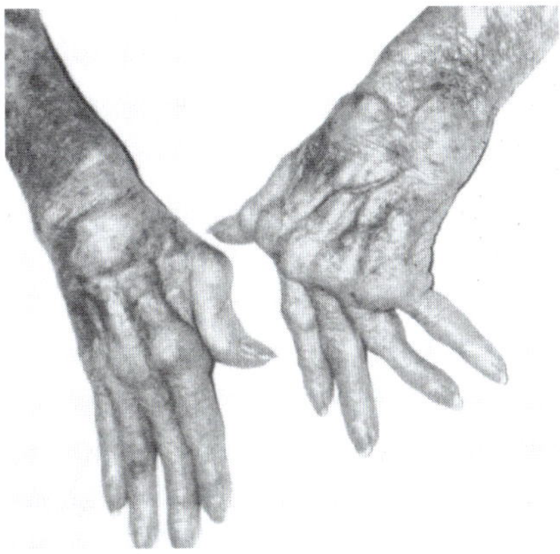

Figure 41-4 RA, an autoimmune disorder, may cause severe ulnar deformity.

Ask the patient about any autoimmune diseases such as SLE, rheumatoid arthritis (RA), MS, and psoriasis (Figure 41-4). The onset, severity, duration, and treatments should be assessed. If the patient does not have any autoimmune disorders, the patient should be asked about family history. Family history of autoimmune disease strongly suggests a genetic predisposition to these kinds of disorders. Although autoimmune diseases are rare individually, collectively, they account for 5 percent of the U.S. population.

Generally speaking, autoimmune diseases affect more women than men. This difference is currently attributed to differences in sex hormones between men and women. Estrogen has shown an up-regulatory effect on immune function, while androgens have shown a suppressive effect on immune function. Estrogen increases the effects of T lymphocytes and decreases suppressors, while androgens preserve IL-2 and suppressor function. Estrogen also has an affect on the B-cell population expressing CD5 antigen that is associated with autoimmune disease.

> *Red Flag*
>
> **Alcohol Consumption and Corticosteroids**
>
> If a patient has an autoimmune disorder, documenting alcohol consumption is important. High doses of corticosteroids and autoimmune diseases are associated with a condition called avascular necrosis (also called osteonecrosis ischemic necrosis) in which the marrow and eventually the trabecular bone die, leaving the bone weak and brittle. Corticosteroid use in patients who drink large amounts of alcohol is associated with an increased risk of avascular necrosis over corticosteroids alone. Patients who complain of bone pain may need to be referred for diagnostic magnetic resonance imaging (MRI) (Assouline-Dayan, Chang, Greenspan, Shoenfeld, & Gershwin, 2002).

Cancer

Personal and family history of cancer is obtained, including details of the date of diagnosis, type of cancer, method of diagnosis, and any treatments. Depending on the age, gender, and family history it may be appropriate to inquire about cancer screening, such as visual surveillance for skin cancer, testicular self-exam, last prostate exam, breast self-exam, last Pap smear, and colon cancer screening, such as hemoccult blood, sigmoidoscopy, barium enema, and colonoscopy. The patient should also be asked about any changes in their health. The acrostic caution is often used as a mnemonic:

C change in bowel or bladder habits.

A area (or sore) that does not heal.

U unusual bleeding or discharge.

T thickening or a lump in the breast, testicles, or elsewhere.

I indigestion or difficulty swallowing.

O obvious change in a wart or a mole.

N nagging cough or hoarseness.

Chronic Illnesses

Assessment of chronic illnesses may also provide information about immune status. Many chronic diseases generate or depend on chronic states of inflammation for their progression. Atherosclerotic disease needs inflammation to progress, while osteoarthritis generates chronic local inflammation. Other diseases may depress the immune system. Chronic renal disease is associated with lower levels of erythropoietin and fewer numbers of all blood cells, including leukocytes. Additionally, remaining leukocytes may have altered function because of changes in blood pH and build up of uremic waste toxins.

Hyperglycemia in diabetes is associated with increased infections primarily because of neuropathy and arterial insufficiency, which in turn cause decreased awareness of injury and decreased wound healing. Additionally, glycosylation of leukocytes impairs their functions. Chronic obstructive pulmonary disease (COPD) can cause recurrent infections because increased secretions and decreased cilia elevator activity.

Surgery

Surgery can have an impact on immune function. Splenectomy in particular results in immunosuppression and leads to overwhelming postsplenectomy infections (see Spleen section). Removal of lymph nodes has a local effect on immune function, allowing pathogens to colonize longer before encountering the adaptive immune system. Removal of the thymus affects the maturation and function of T lymphocytes. Organ transplantation can affect immune function in several ways. Most transplanted organs will be attacked as nonself by the adaptive immune system. Immunosuppressive drugs are usually indicated throughout the rest of the patient's life, putting the patient at risk for both acquired infections and opportunistic infections. A transplanted kidney may actually aid immune function by increasing erythropoiesis, but this effect will most likely be negated by immunosuppressive therapy. Heart transplant patients receive a double hit to the immune system, because the thymus is usually removed along with the dysfunctional heart, and they receive immunosuppressive therapy. A special case is blood transfusion and use of other blood products, such as platelets and fresh frozen plasma. Transfused blood usually has antigens foreign to the patient's blood and may put them at risk for altered immune function. Moreover, there is a small chance that the patient may have been exposed to a blood-borne pathogen, such as HIV or hepatitis C. It is important to remember that although the blood supply is tested well for these common pathogens, lab errors do occur, and there may be new developing diseases that we have not yet identified (El-Alfy & El-Sayed, 2004).

TABLE 41-5 Selected Stressful Life Events and Their Corresponding Life Change Units (LCU) from the Social Readjustment Rating Scale (SRRS)

LIFE EVENT	LCU
Death of spouse	100
Divorce	73
Marriage	63
Being fired from work	47
Reconciliation with spouse	45
Retirement	45
Outstanding personal achievement	28
Starting or ending school	26
Change in sleeping habits	16
Vacation	13

Adapted from Scully, J. A. (2000). Life event checklists: Revisiting the social readjustment rating scale after 30 years. Educational and Psychological Measurement, 60*(6)*, *864–876.*

Stress and Social Support

Stress, both real and perceived, can have a negative effect on immune function (Isowa, Ohira, & Murashima, 2004). Meanwhile, exercise, although stressful to the body, reduces perceived stress and in moderation can improve immune function (Glass, et al., 2004). It is currently unknown whether real or perceived stress has more influence on immune function, as studies often show conflicting results. It is currently believed that the brain influences the immune system via the limbic hypothalamus-pituitary-adrenal (HPA) cortex axis (Reiche, Nunes, & Morimoto, 2004). The limbic system is responsible for somatic effects of emotions. It is also believed that the immune system influences the HPA axis, a concept called bidirectional communication. This area is undergoing intense research at the moment in everything from exercise to biofeedback and prayer to meditation.

Patients should be asked about perceived stress in their lives as well as potentially stressful life events. Table 41-5 shows selected common life events and the average rank of how much stress they cause according the social readjustment rating scale (SRRS) (Holmes & Rahe, 1967). The patient is asked if any of the listed life events have occurred in the past 12 months. The associated scores are tabulated, and the sum is indicative of how much stress the patient is experiencing based on life events. Scores under 149 are considered low; scores of 150 to 200 are mild; scores of 201 to 299 are moderate; and scores above 300 are high. It is important to note that the SRRS was not developed simply as an indicator of stress but as an indicator of disease risk. It is important to keep in mind that the life events listed in the table are averages, and the actual stress caused by any one event may be greater or less than the

Uncovering the Evidence

Stress and Aging

Discussion: This study's purpose was to explore the effects of telomeres, which shorten as a person ages and then contribute to age-related dysfunction. The findings from this research study were that telomeres of monocytes in women who report the highest levels of stress showed an average of 10 years of aging when compared to women who reported low levels of stress. The important aspect to this study is that the cells assayed were immune cells, indicating the persons with higher levels of stress are more likely to experience age-related immune dysfunction. It is important to note that telomere length was affected by perceived stress regardless of actual stressful events.

Implications for Practice: The results of this study prompt the nurse to always remember to assess the stress levels of patients. And, to identify the amount of stress that patients are experiencing. In addition, this is extremely important for patients who are experiencing immunological disorders.

Source: Epel, E. S., Blackburn, E. H., Lin, J., Dhabhar, F. S., Adler, N. E., Morrow, J. D., et al. (2004). Accelerated telomere shortening in response to life stress. Proceedings of the National Academy of Science USA, 101*(49), 17312–17315.*

average. The nurse should also note that positive life events, such as a vacation, may be as stressful as negative life events.

Another area related to stress is social interaction. There are several studies that show that social isolation is associated with decreased immune functioning (Hawkley & Cacioppo, 2003). It is important to note that it is perceived social isolation (loneliness) that is associated with morbidity and mortality. Patients should be asked whether they feel lonely, isolated, or disconnected. In addition to stress and loneliness, sleep, energy level, and exercise should be assessed. The more normal a patient feels in daily life, the more likely he or she is to have a normally functioning immune system.

Pharmacology

A comprehensive list of medications should be obtained. The nurse should ask how long the patient has taken each medication and whether he or she is taking more or less than the prescribed dose. Many common medications, including NSAIDS, corticosteroids, cytotoxic agents, and anesthetics, can cause immune suppression in a variety of ways. Patients should also be asked if they have had an adverse event, such as leukopenia, in response to any medications.

In addition to medications, the nurse should also inquire about any herbal medications and over-the-counter (OTC) medications the patient is using. Tobacco, alcohol, and recreational drugs should be documented, as they can all have immune effects.

Lifestyle and Environmental Factors

The nurse should ask about any behaviors that may put the patient at risk for infections or altered immune function. These may include sexual behavior, travel history, and nutritional status. Occupational hazards may include inhaled toxins, such as coal dust or chemicals in factories. Other hazards may include being near radioactive substances or X-rays. Living near farms, factories, shipyards, and mines can put the patient at risk for decreased immune function. Exposure to sun and use of sunscreen is important in assessing risk for skin cancer.

Physical Examination

Vital signs should include age, temperature, blood pressure, and respirations. Temperature elevations may be suppressed in elderly patients and patients with immunodeficiency. The patient should be assessed for chills and perspiration. Examination of the skin and mucous membranes should include inspection for lesions, dermatitis, urticaria (hives), erythema, edema, discharge, and subcutaneous bleeding. The tonsils should be inspected, and the lymph nodes palpated in the face and neck, axilla, and groin. Nodes should be assessed for size, shape, consistency, and tenderness. The patient's respiratory cardiovascular, GI, genitourinary, and neural status should be evaluated, particularly paying attention to signs indicative of infection or signs that indicate increase risk of immune dysfunction. Hygiene and functional limitations should also be noted. Box 41-1 shows common physical signs associated with impaired immune function.

BOX 41-1

COMMON PHYSICAL SIGNS ASSOCIATED WITH IMPAIRED IMMUNE FUNCTION

Vital Signs

Elevated temperature
Changes in blood pressure
Changes in pulse
Changes in respiratory rate
Changes in weight

Constitutional

Chills
Night sweats

Respiratory System

Rhinitis
Cough (dry or productive)
Adventitious lung sounds (wheezing, crackles, rhonchi)
Bronchospasm

Cardiovascular System

Dysrhythmia
Vasculitis
Decreased peripheral pulses
Anemia

GI System

Hepatomegaly
Cirrhosis
Splenomegaly
Colitis
Vomiting
Diarrhea

Genitourinary System

Frequency and burning on urination
Hematuria
Proteinuria
Discharge

Skin

Dermatitis
Discharge
Lesions
Rashes
Hematoma or purpura
Edema
Urticaria (hives)
Inflammation

Neurosensory System

Cognitive dysfunction
Hearing loss
Visual loss or disturbance
Headaches
Ataxia
Tremor
Tetany
Decreased peripheral sensation

Adapted from Estes, M. (2006). Health assessment and physical examination *(3rd ed.). New York: Thomson Delmar Learning.*

Integumentary System

Skin should be examined for color, turgor, moisture, and temperature. Skin changes can often be indicators of immune dysfunction. Psoriasis manifests as scaly plaques. Patients with Sjögren's disease tend to have scaly skin and excessive perspiration. Patients with scleroderma have thick smooth skin. Patients with Grave's disease may have pretibial myxedema (thickening of the shin skin), fine, brittle hair, increased perspiration, and exophthalmus (bulging eyes). Elevated skin temperature may indicate inflammation, and cool skin temperature may indicate arterial insufficiency.

Skin lesions may also indicate immune status. Lesions and rashes should be characterized regarding their shape, configuration, and distribution. Any exudates or vesicles should also be noted. Rashes and lesions may indicate allergic disorders, such as urticaria (hives) or atopic dermatitis. Local maculopapular rashes with or without vesiculation are more indicative of a contact dermatitis or localized infection. Full body rashes are usually indicative of a systemic reaction. Dermographism is common in patients with chronic urticaria; dermographism means skin drawing and refers to an inflammatory response after lightly drawing on a patient's skin with a finger or other blunt instrument (note: dermographism should not be confused with the scratch test; see diagnostic tests). Moles should be carefully screened using the ABCD approach (asymmetry, border, color, and diameter). Suspicious lesions should be referred for biopsy. Kaposi's sarcoma is a usually rare skin cancer that occurs naturally but is fairly common in patients with HIV. Kaposi's sarcoma manifests as maculopapular lesions that range in color from pink to bluish-purple. Various infectious diseases cause rashes and lesions, including measles, herpes-zoster (chickenpox and shingles), HSV, and syphilis. Skin eruptions associated with viral infections are called viral exanthems. SLE is often associated with a malar rash, which is a red rash in the shape of a butterfly across the cheeks and nose. Patients with RA may have nodules and bony spurs in their finger joints. Their hands may become deformed from the disease. Many autoimmune diseases may cause alopecia. Alopecia is also associated with chemotherapy and radiation therapy.

Eyes, Ears, Nose, and Throat

Patients with allergies often have inflamed nasal turbinates and may have tender sinuses. They also tend to exhibit serous otitis media, visible as small air bubbles behind the tympanic membrane. Serous otitis media is caused by Eustachian tube inflammation, which does not allow mucosal secretions to drain. Patients may complain of headache, earache, vertigo, or lightheadedness associated with head movements. They may report exacerbation of any or all these symptoms when lowering the head such as when bending over.

The eyes may have dark circles underneath them, sometimes called allergic shiners, because of venous stasis. Patients with immune disorders or chronic allergies may have periorbital edema secondary to increased vascular permeability. The conjunctiva may be inflamed and can mimic infectious conjunctivitis.

The mouth may be dry from mouth-breathing because of chronic nasal obstruction. The throat may be inflamed from postnasal drip, and the tonsils may be enlarged. Patients with enlarged tonsils should be asked if that is a usual finding for them or a new finding. Exudates and lesions should be noted. Patients with immunosuppression may have thrush, an opportunistic candida infection, which appears as white patches throughout the mouth, throat, and tongue.

Lymph Nodes

Assessment of the lymph nodes includes inspection and palpation. The nodes of the head and neck and axillary and femoral nodes should be examined.

The location, size, shape, consistency, tenderness, and mobility should be noted. Having a few nontender, mobile, palpable nodes is usually a normal finding. Thinner patients tend to have more palpable nodes. Palpable supraclavicular nodes should always be considered an abnormal finding and should be referred for further evaluation.

Respiratory System

Patients with allergies may also have respiratory symptoms. Recent studies have shown a link between allergic rhinitis in children and asthma. Patients with suppressed immune systems are at risk for pneumonia. Careful examination of the respiratory system is indicated. The skin and nails should be inspected for signs of cyanosis or clubbing. The chest should be observed for shape, breathing pattern, respiratory effort, and thoracic expansion. The lungs should be auscultated with attention paid to the breath sounds. Patients with allergies and acute bronchitis may wheeze. The nature of cough should be noted, and any sputum produced examined. Patients with comorbid conditions such as cancer or COPD should be evaluated in relation to their baseline.

Cardiovascular System

Much of the cardiovascular system can be evaluated while examining the skin. The temperature of extremities and the presence of hair on extremities give clues to peripheral arterial circulation. The nature of the pulses should be evaluated at least in the arms and feet. Weak or thready pulse may be associated with infections. Blood pressure may rise or fall in conjunction with infection. Absent foot pulses may also be a sign of arterial insufficiency. The heart sounds should be carefully noted. Murmurs may signify valve damage that makes the valves more susceptible to certain infections.

Neurological System

Many autoimmune diseases attack nervous tissue causing demyelination or other nerve damage. Nerves contain the CD4 antigen that HIV targets, making neurological dysfunction common in HIV and AIDS patients. Other diseases that decrease sensation such as Hansen's disease (leprosy) and diabetes mellitus increase the incidence of infections simply because the patient is not aware of any injury. Mental status, reflexes, sensation, deep tendon reflexes, and balance should be tested. Other signs of neurological dysfunction, such as tremor should also be noted.

DIAGNOSTIC TESTS

Most diagnostic tests for the immune system are blood tests. These hematological tests are identified and described in the section that follows. Other tests involve either biopsy of tissue or nuclear medicine tests.

Complete Blood Count with Differential

The most common laboratory test is the complete blood count (CBC) with differential. A normal CBC includes a gross leukocyte count, often abbreviated as WBCs (white blood cells). The differential breaks the WBCs into categories that usually include neutrophils, basophils, eosinophils, monocytes, and lymphocytes. Dendritic cells are not part of the CBC with differential (Box 41-2), and the differential does not distinguish between subtypes of lymphocytes.

To date, there has been no test to determine the status of dendritic cells. However, Vuckovic, et al. (2004) discovered a simple assay that allows for blood dendritic cell counts. In addition to total dendritic cells, it also allows for precise counting of five dendritic cell subsets. The researchers were able to use the new assay method to show that dendritic cells decrease in healthy individ-

BOX 41-2

CBC WITH DIFFERENTIAL

Differential values are usually reported as percentages of the total WBC count. Neutrophils are usually divided into two classes. Mature neutrophils are usually designated as segs (segmented cells). Immature neutrophils are designated bands, because their nuclei appear to have bands across them. Some labs will also report a value abbreviated as ANC (absolute neutrophil count). If the ANC is absent, it may be calculated by the nurse by adding the percentages of segs and bands and multiplying the sum by the WBC total. This number will give the total number of neutrophils in a cubic millimeter of blood. If the number is less than 1,000, the patient is considered to have immunosuppression. If the number is less than 500, the patient is considered to have severe immunosuppression. In addition to the segs and bands, occasionally, a patient may have a third category called blasts. Blasts are immature cells and should never be in circulation under normal circumstances. The most common reasons for blasts to appear are leukemia, rheumatic disease, or severe bone injury.

uals with age. They were also able to observe changes in various cell subsets with different cancers. It will take a few years for normal values to become established, but it is most likely that within the next 5 years dendritic cell testing will become common in immunological testing. In the next 10 to 15 years, it may become as routine as the CBC with differential.

Interpretation of CBC with differential can be straightforward or difficult. It is important that the nurse assess the whole patient and not simply the lab values. Nurses must always check the laboratory's normal ranges when interpreting a patient's lab tests. In general, neutrophil counts will increase during bacterial infections as the bone marrow releases some of its stores. If the percentage of segs increases more than the percentage of bands, it is called a shift to the right. If the bands increase more than segs, it is called a shift to the left and is usually indicative of either a more severe infection or an infection that has been going on longer.

Basophils typically do not increase or decrease in number in response to infections. However, they do increase in response to some inflammation and inflammatory diseases, such as Crohn's disease. They also increase in response to disorders involving the common myeloid precursor, such as polycythemia vera, myelofibrosis, and chronic myeloid leukemia. Hypothyroidism can also cause increases in basophils, and hyperthyroidism can cause decreases in basophils. Eosinophils typically increase during parasitic infections and during allergic reactions. Decreased eosinophils are usually not a cause for concern.

Mononuclear cells are relatively low in number, because most of them simply use the blood as a transport system before migrating to the tissues to differentiate into macrophages. As one of the first inflammatory responders, monocytes may increase or decrease in response to various conditions depending on the severity of the reaction, the duration of reaction, and the number of monocytes in the marrow reservoir.

Lymphocytes are the second most populous leukocyte in the blood. Increased lymphocytes may occur as an increase of absolute numbers lymphocytes or simply as a percentage of total leukocytes. There are a variety of disorders (Box 41-3) and medications that cause neutropenia. The most common medications that cause neutropenia are chemotherapeutic, thyroid inhibitors, and trimethoprim-sulfamethoxazole (Septra, Bactrim). In addition, many other medications cause neutropenia, such as antibiotics (e.g., penicillins,

BOX 41-3

ETIOLOGY FOR VARIOUS INFECTIONS THAT CAUSE NEUTROPENIA

Severe Neutropenia

Bacterial sepsis (especially gram-negative bacteria)
Infectious mononucleosis
Hepatitis B virus
HIV

Viral Infections

Infectious mononucleosis
Hepatitis B virus
HIV
Measles
Mumps
Rubella
Roseola
Malaria
Leishmaniasis
Cytomegalovirus
Colorado tick fever
Influenza
Dengue fever
Viral hepatitis
HSV
Parvovirus
Respiratory syncytial virus
Small pox
Varicella
Yellow fever

Bacterial Infections

Tuberculosis
Typhoid fever
Brucellosis
Tularemia
Rocky Mountain spotted fever

Fungal Infections

Histoplasmosis

Adapted from Janeway, C. A., Jr., Travers, P., Walport, M., & Shlomchik, M. J. (2004). Immunobiology, the immune system in health and disease *(6th ed.). New York: Garland Science Publishing.*

cephalosporins, and sulfonamides), cardiovascular medications (e.g., antiarrhythmics, antihypertensives), analgesics (e.g., NSAIDs, aspirin), antithyroids, antihistamines, and heavy metals (Broyles, Reiss, & Evans, 2007).

Radiological Tests

Radiological tests can also provide information about immune status. CXRs are often used to determine tuberculosis status and confirm pneumonia. MRIs, computed tomography (CT), and numerous nuclear medicine tests are used to screen for neoplasm.

Erythrocyte Sedimentation Rate

Blood is made up of RBCs and plasma. When still, the RBCs will settle to the bottom, and the plasma will float to the top. The erythrocyte sedimentation rate (ESR), sometimes called sed. rate, is simply a measure of how quickly the settling occurs. It is expressed in milliliters/hour. The normal ESR values change with age and gender and pregnancy. Elevated ESR is caused by acute inflammation phase reactants binding to red blood cells. ESR is used as a marker of tissue inflammation and is highly sensitive, but nonspecific (Daniels, 2003).

C-Reactive Protein

CRP is an acute-phase protein that is produced by the liver. It is one of the three binding mechanisms for C1q in the classical pathway for complement activation. It can be used to determine whether a disease is inflammatory or not. Examples include distinguishing type 1 from type 2 diabetes and distinguishing osteoarthritis from RA. CRP is nonspecific and is often ordered in conjunction with ESR. In recent years, subtypes of CRP have been discovered. Highly sensitive CRP (hsCRP) has been implicated as a marker for MI. The caveat is that hsCRP can help determine short-term risk for MI, but not long-term risk. In other words hsCRP is an indicator of atherosclerotic plaque rupture, but a link with atherosclerotic plaque formation has not been established.

Total Complement (CH50)

CH50 is a marker for the function of the entire complement cascade. It measures the ability of the sample to lyse IgG-coated RBCs. False readings can be obtained by delaying the test after obtaining the sample, so care must be taken to ensure that the sample is tested as soon as possible. Low complement levels indicate depletion or lack of production by the liver. The most common causes of depletion are the rheumatic diseases (e.g., SLE, vasculitis), septic shock, pancreatitis, severe burns. Lack of production may be caused by liver failure or severe malnutrition. Total complement is most useful in tracking the course of rheumatic diseases where a value of 20 percent below baseline indicates an exacerbation.

Complement C3

Because C3 convertase is the common link between all three complement activation pathways, it can serve as a marker for complement activation. The protein is measured by immunochemical assay. The interpretation is similar to total complement.

Complement C4

The C4 protein is involved only in the classical (intrinsic) pathway and can be used as an indicator of classical pathway complement activation. The protein is measured by immunochemical assay. The interpretation is similar to total complement.

Phagocytic Cell Function Tests

Despite the name, only the function of neutrophils and macrophages are tested, as dendritic cells are not found in high enough concentrations. The most basic phagocytic cell function test does not involve function at all, but is simply the sum of neutrophils and monocytes from the CBC with differential. The function assay evaluates the ability of phagocytic cells to recognize, ingest, degranulate (as appropriate), and otherwise destroy various pathogens.

Protein Electrophoresis

Electrophoresis takes two forms, but both involve putting a protein sample onto a gel and passing electrical current through the gel. The proteins will migrate to the other side of the gel. The distance various proteins travel is dependent on their size and electrical affinity. Some gels are uniform in their density, and protein distance will depend only on electrical affinity of the protein. Other gels are graded from less dense to more dense. These gradient gels will trap larger proteins, so that smaller proteins travel farther. Electrophoresis allows a sample of several kinds of proteins, such as serum, to be separated so that each kind of protein can be studied individually. Electrophoresis is used most commonly in immunological management of patients to evaluate serum proteins, such as albumin and globulins (alpha-, beta-, and gamma-globulins). They can also be used to screen for certain tumor proteins that are not secreted by normally functioning cells.

Immunoglobulin Electrophoresis

Immunoglobulin electrophoresis uses the same process as above, but in this case, the immunoglobulins are being separated and measured individually. Measuring the various immunoglobulins can aid in the diagnosis and management of several immunological and inflammatory disorders (Table 41-6).

Radioallergosorbent Test

IgE is usually present in serum in such small quantities that electrophoresis cannot accurately measure it. Radioallergosorbent test (RAST) is used to measure serum IgE. RAST is most often used in diagnosing allergies in combination with skin tests.

Antibody Screening Tests

Numerous tests are available that test for specific antibodies. Each antibody test is ordered individually and may test for antibodies against various bacteria, viruses, fungi, parasites, or cancers. Presence of the antibodies does not necessarily indicate that a patient has that particular disease.

Autoantibody Tests

Autoantibodies are antibodies that are produced against self and are always an abnormal finding. Autoantibodies attack and damage normal tissue and are responsible for some of the pathology of autoimmune diseases. One of the most common autoantibodies tested for are antinuclear antibodies (ANA), which attack the nuclei of cells. ANA is most commonly associated with SLE and other autoimmune disorders, but it can also be associated with various medications (Box 41-4). Another common autoantibody is rheumatoid factor (RF), which is commonly found in patients with rheumatoid diseases such as SLE and RA. Although usually an abnormal finding, both ANA and RF can be found in healthy older adults.

TABLE 41-6 Diseases Commonly Associated with Abnormal Immunoglobulin Levels

IMMUNOGLOBULIN	NORMAL RANGE	INCREASED LEVEL	DECREASED LEVEL
IgA	50–350 mg/dL	Lymphoproliferative disorders (e.g., multiple myeloma) Berger's disease (IgA nephropathy) Chronic infection Autoimmune disorders SLE Rheumatoid arthritis Liver disease (e.g., portal cirrhosis) Henoch Schonlein Purpura	IgA Hypogammaglobulinemia Protein losing enteropathy Hereditary ataxia and telangiectasia Nephrotic syndrome
IgE	less than 25 g/dL	Allergic disorders Asthma Allergic rhinitis or hay fever Inhalant allergy Atopic rhinitis or sinusitis Atopic dermatitis Urticaria Bronchopulmonary *Aspergillus* Hypersensitivity pneumonitis Drug allergy Food allergy Parasitic infection Ascariasis Visceral larva Migrans Toxocara Capillariasis Echinococcosis Hookworm (Necator) Amebiasis Immunological disorders Hyper-IgE, recurrent pyoderma (Job-Buckley syndrome) Thymic dysplasia or deficiency Wiskott-Aldrich syndrome Pemphigoid Periarteritis nodosa Hypereosinophilic syndrome Neoplasm (i.e., IgE myeloma)	Congenital Hypogammaglobulinemia Acquired hypogammaglobulinemia Sex-linked hypogammaglobulinemia Ataxia-telangiectasia IgE deficiency

Continued

TABLE 41-6 Diseases Commonly Associated with Abnormal Immunoglobulin Levels—cont'd

IMMUNOGLOBULIN	NORMAL RANGE	INCREASED LEVEL	DECREASED LEVEL
IgG	800–1,500 mg/dL	Chronic granulomatous infection	Hypo-IgG
		Inflammation	Protein-losing enteropathy
		Multiple myeloma	Nephrotic syndrome
		Liver disease	
		Infections	
		Autoimmune disease	
IgM	45–150 mg/dL	Liver disease	Hypo-IgM
		Primary biliary	Protein-losing enteropathy
		Cirrhosis	
		Early hepatitis	
		Waldenstrom's macroglobulinemia	
		Infection	
		Brucellosis	
		Malaria	
		Trypanosomiasis	
		Toxoplasmosis	

Adapted from Boehm, M., Olive, M., True, A. L., Crook, M. F., San, H., Qu, X., et al. (2004). Bone marrow-derived immune cells regulate vascular disease through a p27Kip1-dependent mechanism. Journal of Clinical Investigation, 114*(3), 419-426; Janeway, C. A., Jr., Travers, P., Walport, M., & Shlomchik, M. J. (2004).* Immunobiology, the immune system in health and disease *(6th ed.). New York: Garland Science Publishing.*

Antigen Tests

Antigen tests look for the presence of a specific antigen in the body. Commonly, antigen tests are used to determine the presence of a pathogen. Hepatitis B surface antigen (HBsAg) and Hepatitis B core antigen (HBcAg) tests can be used to determine whether a patient with hepatitis B antibodies has a chronic infection, has a latent infection, or has cleared the infection.

Other antigen tests look for antigens that the patient's body manufactures normally or abnormally. CD4 antigen can be used to measure the status of helper T cells in patients with HIV. Other CD4 antigens can be used to detect T cell leukemias and lymphomas or B cell tumors. Abnormal antigens include lupus erythematosus (LE) cell tests. LE cells are abnormal neutrophils that contain abnormal DNA and are present in two thirds of SLE patients. The indirect Coombs' test is used to determine erythrocyte antigens and help to determine blood type. The direct Coombs' test detects antibodies against RBCs and can help to diagnose hemolytic and autoimmune disorders.

Biopsy

A biopsy is simply a sample of living tissue. The biopsy is then examined for abnormalities. Examination may be histological (microscopic examination) or use a variety of previously described tests. Biopsies may be complete or partial. A complete biopsy completely removes the tissue being tested. Moles are often completely biopsied. Complete biopsies are sometimes considered curative if they remove all diseased tissue. Partial biopsies take only a portion of

BOX 41-4

DISEASES ASSOCIATED WITH ANTINUCLEAR ANTIBODIES (ANA)

Normal patient without underlying abnormality: 3–30% (More common in older women)

Rheumatoid Conditions

SLE
RA
Mixed connective tissue disease
Sjögren's syndrome
Necrotizing vasculitis

Infection

Tuberculosis
Chronic active hepatitis
Subacute bacterial endocarditis
HIV

Miscellaneous Conditions

Type 1 diabetes mellitus
MS
Pulmonary fibrosis
Silicone gel implants
Pregnant women
Elderly patients

Medications (Drug-Induced LE)

Phenytoin
Ethosuximide
Primidone
Methyldopa
Hydralazine
Penicillamine
Carbamazepine
Procainamide
Thiazides
Griseofulvin
Chlorpromazine
Isoniazid
Quinidine
Gold salts
Minocycline

Adapted from Broyles, B. E., Reiss, B. S., & Evans, M. E. (2007). Pharmacological aspects of nursing care *(7th ed.). New York: Thomson Delmar Learning; Janeway, C. A., Jr., Travers, P., Walport, M., & Shlomchik, M. J. (2004).* Immunobiology, the immune system in health and disease *(6th ed.). New York: Garland Science Publishing.*

the tissue and are considered diagnostic. Skin biopsies are used to screen and remove cancers or potentially cancerous lesions. Common biopsies of the skin include punch biopsy, incisional biopsy, excisional biopsy, and shave biopsy. Aspiration biopsy uses a needle to remove a portion of the tissue or fluid. Fine needle aspiration (FNA) biopsy is used to biopsy delicate internal organs. Liver, bone, and muscle biopsies all carry significant risk of infection and hemorrhage; all three usually require anesthesia.

Skin Tests

Skin tests test for an IgE-mediated hypersensitivity reaction to a specific substance. Skin tests usually take the form of patch tests, scratch tests, prick tests, or intradermal injection. In each case, the patient is exposed to a small amount of the substance to be tested. The exposed area is observed for reaction. In the patch test, the substance is simply placed against the skin. In the prick test, a needle with a small amount of the substance is used to prick the patient's skin. The scratch test is similar to the prick test, except that the patient's skin is scratched instead of pricked. The scratch test should not be confused with dermographism. A small amount of the substance is injected in the intradermal space in the intradermal test. The patch test is the least sensitive, while the intradermal test is the most sensitive. However, the more sensitive tests carry more risk of anaphylaxis and false-positives. The scratch test is the most likely to cause these adverse reactions and has been largely superseded by the prick test. The results of the prick test can be distorted by bleeding or by placing pricks to close together.

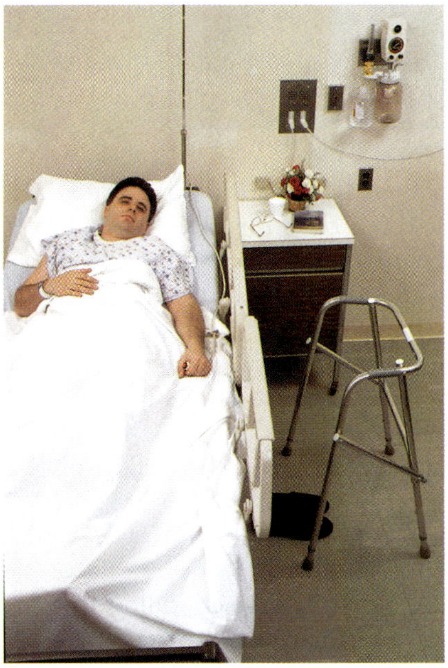

Figure 41-5 Stress management techniques will be important in the nursing considerations for this patient newly diagnosed with an STD.

Anergy Tests

Anergy tests inject a small amount of antigen into the intradermal space and the area is measured for induration at 48 to 72 hours. An induration of 5 mm or more is considered positive. The PPD used to screen for tuberculosis is an anergy test. Lack of induration is usually a sign that a patient has not contracted tuberculosis; however, false-negatives are common in patients with HIV, because their immune system is too suppressed to mount a reaction. This is referred to as anergy.

Anergy tests can also be used to screen for T cell immunodeficiency. A variety of antigens are injected in the intradermal space. Most healthy persons will display reaction to at least one of the antigens. Lack of reaction after 48 hours is considered a sign of immunodeficiency.

Nursing Management

Because so many immune function tests are blood tests, it is important that the nurse ensure that aseptic technique and appropriate wound care are maintained. This is especially important in patients who are or may be potentially immunosuppressed.

The primary nursing consideration in immune assessment is stress management (Figure 41-5). Patients who are hospitalized may benefit from stress reduction techniques, such as music, wearing their own clothes, exercise, and laughter. While assessment of immune function may occur as a routine procedure, such as determining whether a sore throat is streptococcus infection related, it is often associated with high stress situations. The fear of possibly having contracted an infectious disease such as HIV or herpes simplex virus can be more stressful than actual dealing with the disease (see Patient Playbook feature). The disease itself is bad enough, but social stigma that is carried for life can be worse in the patient's mind. Care must be taken to alleviate undue stress and fear when assessing the immune system. Because of the stressful nature of these kinds of assessments, patients may not understand instructions they are being given or may not remember. It is important not only to educate patients verbally, but to give them additional written education and instructions. One particular example is HIV testing. Because of the large social stigma and negative associations, federal law mandates that HIV test results can not be given out over the phone or mailed. Although patients sign a form stating that they understand this at the time they have blood drawn, many of them become upset when they call for their results and are told that they must come back into the clinic. Written instructions can help to allay this kind of situation.

It is also important not to prediagnose patients. Although a high ANA test is strongly associated with SLE, there are more than 15 other causes of elevated ANA, including various medications. In addition to fear of contracting a disease the uncertainty associated with not knowing what is wrong with one's body is also considerable. Many patients may be relieved to find out they have a disease, because it validates what they already suspected, which is that something was wrong with them. Some patients may actually become angry when they find out that diagnostic tests have returned negative. It is important to empathize with patients no matter which way their tests return.

Finally, patients should be educated on primary and secondary prevention of immune-related diseases. Immunizations, good hygiene, exercise, and stress management are all part of maintaining a healthy immune system. Patients should be educated about appropriate screening measures and symptom recognition for conditions they may be at risk for. This includes HIV and other STD tests for patients who engage in risky sex, regular PPDs for patients at risk for tuberculosis, and CBCs for patients with high risk for agranulocytosis or aplastic anemia.

PATIENT PLAYBOOK

Stress Reduction in Immunocompromised Patient

The following are suggestions for the nurse providing patient education for patients who are immunocompromised:

- Instruct family to wear isolation masks when visiting their family member.
- Open curtains in the patient room to let in sunlight, which decreases isolation.
- Explain to the patient that sunlight also has ultraviolet (UV) rays, which act as a microbicide (tuberculosis is particularly susceptible to sunlight).
- Explain to the patient and family that the reason the health care providers leave equipment in the room, including items like stethoscopes, is to control the contamination of the patient room.

KEY CONCEPTS

- The immune system is responsible not only for protecting the body against invading pathogens and toxins, but it is also responsible for removing extracellular detritus, protecting against cancer, and preparing damaged tissue for repair.
- The immune system is divided into two interacting systems called the innate and acquired immune system.
- Recognition of self and nonself is the most important aspect of the immune system's role, or else pathogens will be welcomed, and host cells will be destroyed.
- Antigens are substances that can bind with antibodies, and most antigens can bond with more than one kind of antibody.
- The sites where lymphocytes mature, bone marrow and thymus gland, are called primary lymphoid organs. The sites where lymphocytes aggregate to function are called secondary lymphoid tissues.
- B lymphocytes mature into plasma cells that secrete antibodies. There are five classes of antibodies that have distinct functions.
- IgM is the first antibody released. It forms a pentameter to effectively increase its affinity to antigen.
- B lymphocytes undergo mutations so that later antibodies have much higher affinity for their antigens.
- T lymphocytes mature into cytotoxic T cells and helper T cells, which further differentiate into TH1 and TH2 cells.
- The dendritic cell is the key to the activation of the immune system.
- The chemical components of the immune system act as cytokines, chemokines, opsonins, and effectors.
- The same properties that make TNF-α in isolating infections and activating the immune system make it deadly during sepsis.
- When the immune system is overwhelmed locally, it forms a granuloma to sequester the infection from the rest of the body.
- Active immunization creates memory B cells, which will quickly produce antibodies if the body is later infected with the pathogen.
- Passive immunization provides an infusion of antibodies that allow the body a reprieve to allow the body's own immune system a chance to activate.
- Vital assessment findings include age, gender, immunizations, medications, allergies, and past illnesses.
- Stress and social support can have a dramatic impact on immune function.
- Physical examination for immune assessment covers the entire body. The skin, mouth, and lymph nodes particularly tend to show early signs of immune changes.
- Laboratory tests should always be interpreted in light of the health history and physical examination.
- Aseptic technique and universal precautions should always be used when obtaining immune laboratory or diagnostic tests.
- Empathy and therapeutic listening can mitigate the stress of testing.

REVIEW QUESTIONS

1. Which of the following is not a role of the immune system?
   1. Defense of the body from external invaders
   2. Signal the body that bone marrow is suppressed
   3. Destruction of senescent erythrocytes and other cellular debris
   4. Surveillance against cancer

2. Which of the following are APCs? More than one answer may be possible.
   1. Neutrophils
   2. Dendritic cells
   3. Macrophages
   4. NK cells

3. What is the term for a substance that binds to a specific antibody? More than one answer may be correct.
   1. Hapten
   2. Antigen
   3. Immunogen
   4. Complement

4. Which of the following is a phagocytic cell?
   1. Neutrophils
   2. Basophils
   3. NK cells
   4. Plasma cells

Continued

REVIEW QUESTIONS—cont'd

5. What cell is the most potent activator of lymphocytes?
1. Macrophages
2. Neutrophils
3. Mast cells
4. Dendritic cells

6. Which of the following are primary lymphoid organs?
1. Bone marrow
2. Lymph nodes
3. Spleen
4. Thymus gland

7. Which of the following is a characteristic of innate immunity?
1. Developed by colostrum
2. Mediated T cells
3. Has memory
4. Initiates inflammation

8. When giving immunizations, which of the following assessments is not necessary?
1. Allergy to eggs
2. Family history of measles
3. History of past immunizations
4. History of past illnesses.

9. Which of the following reactions indicates a medication allergy?
1. GI bleed with aspirin
2. Nausea with azithromycin
3. Diarrhea with tegaserod
4. Angioedema with ramipril

10. Which surgery usually results in the destruction of a primary lymphoid organ?
1. Cholecystectomy
2. Splenectomy
3. Tonsillectomy
4. Heart transplant

11. Increased neutrophil count may be indicative of (more than one answer may be correct):
1. Bacterial infection
2. MI
3. Inflammatory bowel disease
4. Allergy

12. When assessing the immune system, which of the following provides the lens for interpretation of the assessment?
1. Health history
2. Physical examination
3. Laboratory values
4. Horoscope

REVIEW ACTIVITIES

1. Your patient, a 24-year-old Caucasian woman has been hospitalized with fever, fatigue, and weight loss and is awaiting results of diagnostic tests. She is afraid that she has SLE. What would you tell her regarding her lab tests?

2. Your patient is a 60-year-old Caucasian male who has been having increasing urinary tract infections (UTIs). What changes would put him at risk for increased UTIs? What additional things should be assessed?

Continued

REVIEW ACTIVITIES—cont'd

3. Your newly admitted patient has a latex allergy. What steps should be taken in their care?

4. Your patient is a 19-year-old student about to enter a nursing program. What immunizations should she need?

5. Your patient is a 32-year-old male and has come into the clinic for STD testing. What issues should you address with the patient regarding STD testing?

Visit the Contemporary Medical-Surgical Nursing online companion resource at www.delmarhealthcare.com for additional content and study aids. Click on Online Companions then select the Nursing discipline.

CHAPTER

42

Immunodeficiency and HIV Infection/AIDS: Nursing Management

Ruth Grendell, MSN, RN

CHAPTER TOPICS

- The Protective Immune Response
- Immune Deficiency Disorders
- Hypersensitivity Disorders
- Autoimmune Disorders
- Collaborative Management of Patients with Immune Disorders
- Immunosuppressive Therapies

The immune system is vital to the human body as related to its processes for recognizing and protecting the body. There are many complex and intricate components to the immune system, which continue to be researched and understood. Recently, immunologists have recognized the immune system as a core control mechanism that is of equal importance as the neurological and endocrine control systems. It is important for the nurse to understand the numerous communication networks among these three systems and what happens when dysfunctions occur. In addition, the nurse must be knowledgeable about the guidelines and strategies developed by the health care system for a wide variety of immune system disorders that specifically involve nursing management. The focus of this chapter is to provide an overview of the immune response and its function in protecting the body and to discuss the collaborative and nursing management of individuals with immune deficiency disorders.

KEY TERMS

Allograft or homograft transplant
Antigen
Apheresis
Autoimmunity
Autologous transplant
Histocompatibility leukocyte antigens (HLA)
Immune response
Immunity
Immunodeficiency
Monoclonal antibodies
Plasmapheresis (plasma exchange)
Primary immune response
Secondary or specific antibody response
Syngeneic transplant

IMMUNODEFICIENCY

Immunodeficiency is the inability to produce a normal complement of antibodies or immunologically sensitized T cells (cell-mediated immunity) especially in response to specific antigens. The clinical hallmark is a propensity to unusual or recurrent severe infections. Most common infections from defects in the cell-mediated response are fungal and viral. Most common infections from defects in the humoral-mediated response are bacteria initiated. **Immunity** is the quality or state of being immune; a condition of being able to resist a particular disease through preventing development of a pathogenic microorganism or by counteracting the effects of its products. The **primary immune response** occurs when an antigen is initially introduced into the system. It involves both mast cell degranulation and activation of plasma proteins, i.e., complement, clotting factors, and kinin—polypeptides that increase blood flow and permeability of small blood capillaries. The **secondary or specific antibody response** includes the activation of B cells and the memory cells (IgG, IgM, IgA, and IgE); and activation of T cells, cytotoxic (killer) cells, lymphokine-producing cells, helper cells, and suppressor cells (humoral immunity) to a specific antigen. Common diagnostic studies related to the immunological disorders are listed in Box 42-1.

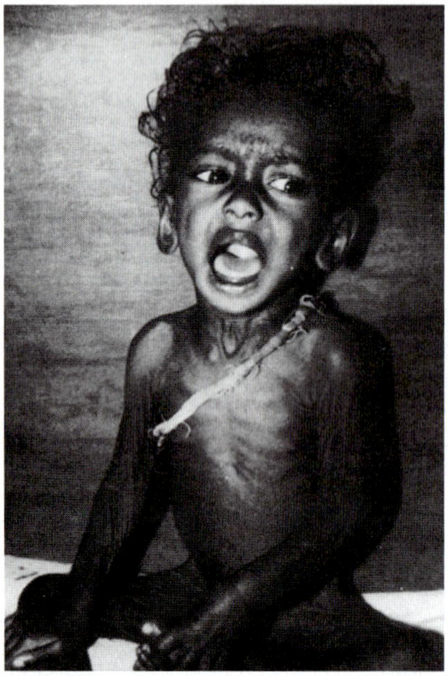

Figure 42-1 Child with HIV suffering with marasmus.

HUMAN IMMUNODEFICIENCY VIRUS INFECTION

One of the most recognized immunodeficiency diseases is human immunodeficiency virus (HIV) and the resulting acquired immunodeficiency syndrome (AIDS) diagnosis. By 2004, approximately 37.8 million people were documented as infected with HIV. This number included 35.7 million adults and 2.1 million children younger than 15 years of age known to be living with HIV/AIDS. The Centers for Disease Control and Prevention (CDC, 2005b) estimate that 850,000 to 950,000 U.S. residents are living with HIV infection; one fourth of these are unaware of their infection. Half of young people under 25 years of age acquired the infection through heterosexual sex; approximately two thirds of pediatric cases were acquired in utero from the infected mother. In 2003, the number of documented AIDS cases in the United States was 43,171 including 59 children under 13 (CDC, 2005b) (Figure 42-1). There is no cure or vaccine; however, technological advances in drug therapy have slowed the progression of the disease and increased life expectancy.

Epidemiology

HIV has become a worldwide disease with incredible negative affects on certain populations. The disorder was first named lymphadenopathy-associated virus (LAV) by French scientists in 1983. Later an American scientist labeled the virus as the human T cell lymphotropic virus. Three years later a different strain was discovered in Africa. This was the first clue that the virus could mutate quickly. There are two related but distinct types of HIV, HIV-1 and HIV-2. HIV-2, which is found primarily in Western Africa, comprises six distinct phylogenetic lineages designated as subtypes, or clades. Three groups of HIV-1 are currently recognized: M (major group), N (new or non-M, non-O), and O (outlier). The 11 subtypes of HIV-1 group M are identified as A–K. HIV-1 subtype B is primarily responsible for the epidemic in North America and Western Europe. Other subtypes, or clades, have been discovered in India, Africa, and Asia (Figure 42-2). This poses the great concern that new infections caused by these mutations will be evident worldwide as infected people travel from country to country (Bunnel, et. al., 2005).

BOX 42-1

CLASSIFICATION OF IMMUNOLOGICAL DISORDERS

Immunodeficient (Type I)

Acquired immunodeficiency syndrome (AIDS)
DiGeorge's syndrome—or anomaly: (Congenital absence of the thymus and parathyroids with loss of cellular immunity. Immunoglobulins are normal. Individual has facial abnormalities, congestive heart disease, decreased calcium, and increased susceptibility to infections—due to defect on chromosome 22.)

Autoimmune (Type II)

Myasthenia gravis
Ankylosing spondylitis (Marie-Strümpell disease)
Fibromyalgia
Polymyositis and dermatomyositis
RA* (classified as connective tissue disorder)
SLE* (vascular and connective tissue disorder)
Sjögren's syndrome
Vasculitis
Reiter's syndrome
Polymyalgia rheumatica and cranial arteritis.
Grave's disease* (unknown etiology, but autoimmune basis is suspected).
Hyperthyroidism with goiter (gland enlargement) and ophthalmopathy
Progressive systemic sclerosis (scleroderma)
*Includes disorders involving both the autoimmune and hypersensitive responses

Mixed Connective Tissue Disease

Lyme disease (rheumatic joint disease with a known cause, a tickborne spirochete).
Secondary arthritis (Whipple's disease)

Immunoproliferative (Type III)

a. Leukemia

Hypersensitive (Type IV)

Allergies
Asthma
Contact dermatitis
Note: List is not all inclusive.

Adapted from Porth, C. (2004). Pathophysiology: Concepts of altered health status *(6th ed.). Philadelphia: Lippincott, Williams & Wilkins.*

Etiology

Risk factors for HIV include unsafe sexual practices, rape, prostitution and multiple sexual partners, exposure to contaminated blood and contaminated needles, occupational exposure, and perinatal exposure (Jones, 2004). Perinatal exposure can occur during the pregnancy, during vaginal delivery, and through breastfeeding. Approximately 23 percent of babies born to HIV-infected women are infected. Additional contributing factors include genital lesions associated with other sexually transmitted diseases (STDs), unprotected anal intercourse, and sexual intercourse during menstruation. The risk

Uncovering the Evidence

HIV Transmission from Africa to the United States

Discussion: Increasing numbers of African immigrants have come to the United States in recent years. Several HIV-positive pregnant women from various African countries are seeking health care in city clinics. Health care personnel are unfamiliar with their particular needs and the cultural and structural barriers that African women encounter related to HIV prevention. A qualitative study conducted in a Philadelphia clinic identified barriers such as legal status, language problems, fear of the American health system, misunderstanding about HIV transmission, and lack of information about available antiretroviral treatment. Many of the infections are diagnosed later in their own countries, and because of the lack of knowledge about the disease they are slower to accept treatment. Other findings revealed that the male partner is excluded from treatment because of denial, refusal to be tested, or abandoning the family. Women are afraid to reveal their HIV positive status to family and friends; they hide their medications and use them inconsistently; they have little decision-making power about safe sexual practices (see Figure 42-2). Immigrants are ineligible for some of the health care benefits, because they cannot provide proof of residence and are unable to navigate the U. S. system, and many are too poor to afford medications.

Implications for Practice: There is a great need for developing culturally appropriate education about HIV prevention and treatment. Health care personnel need to know and understand the fears, experiences, and concerns of these populations.

Source: Foley, E. (2005). HIV/AIDS and African immigrant women in Philadelphia: Structural and cultural barriers to care. AIDS Care, *17(8), 1030–1043.*

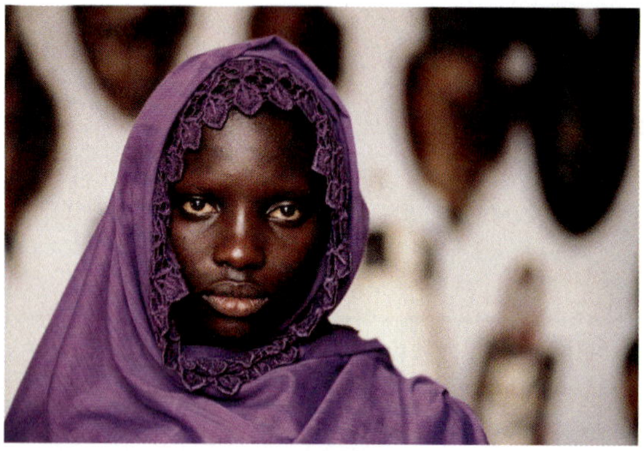

Figure 42-2 AIDS is continuing to rise in African women at alarming rates.

for infection is greater for the receiving partner because of the prolonged contact with the semen; however, the inserting partner may also be at risk. A recent survey indicated that young people are having casual sex at an earlier age and feel less guilt about it than previous generations (Figure 42-3). Sexual activity by teenagers is considered the norm. The availability of birth control, the acceptance of satisfying individual needs, and gender equality were cited as reasons for the cultural shift in behaviors. Oral sex has also become mainstream (Baker, 2005). HIV infection can be transmitted by blood, semen, vaginal or cervical secretions, and breast milk. The sero-conversion (the presence of antibodies in the blood) usually occurs in one to three months or up to six months after exposure. The infected individual is still infectious when no symptoms are present, and the ability to transmit infection is lifelong.

Occupational exposure as a risk factor is a concern for health care workers and for other service occupations, such as police and correction officers. Exposure to HIV infected blood via contaminated needle stick or sharp object, contact with infected breast milk, mucous secretions (vaginal, semen), and exposure to blood in the laboratory are the common sources. The actual risk is quite low; however the exposure risk increases (a) when there is visual blood on the instrument that causes the injury to the worker and (b) when the patient diagnosed with AIDS dies within 60 days of the worker's exposure because it is presumed that HIV concentrations were high at the time of the

Skills 360°

Transmission of HIV

The nurse should be aware of the following information. HIV is a fragile virus, which can be transmitted only under specific conditions that permit contact with infected body fluids. Transmission of HIV is similar to transmission of infection by other pathogenic microorganisms. Transmission of the HIV can then occur (a) within a short time frame after a person becomes infected with the HIV; (b) transmission is also dependent on a large amount of the virus entering the receiving body (host); (c) transmission is dependent on the potency, or virulence, and concentration of the virus; and (d) transmission is dependent on the immune status of the new host. HIV cannot be transmitted through casual contact, such as shaking hands, sharing eating utensils, using toilet seats, or working along side an HIV infected worker. The HIV is not transmitted through tears, saliva, urine, emesis, sputum, feces, or sweat.

Adapted from DeLaune, S., & Ladner, P. (2006). Fundamentals of nursing *(3rd ed.). New York: Thomson Delmar Learning.*

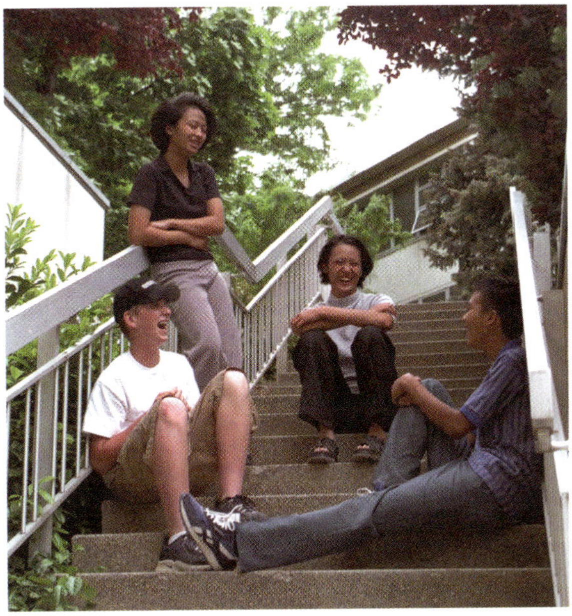

Figure 42-3 HIV in adolescents remains a risk because of the unsafe sexual practices in this population.

exposure. Workers at risk should follow the standard precautions when handling any body fluids and blood, and when performing procedures that place them at risk. Recommendations from the U.S. Public Health Service include at least a four-week prophylactic therapy with a combination of retroviral drugs. Transmission of HIV from an HIV-infected health care worker to a patient is also possible. Following standard precautions in all contacts with patients and administering prophylactic therapy to the patients should be followed.

Pathophysiology

The pathophysiology of HIV begins with several alterations of a limited number of cells that have CD4 receptors on their surfaces. Primary targets for the development of HIV because of these receptor sites are the CD4+ T cells (helper cells) that have more CD4 receptors. Other cells that have CD4 receptor sites include lymphocytes, monocytes, macrophages, astrocytes, and oligodendrocytes. The HIV retrovirus interacts specifically with the host cell receptors and uses the host cells for viral replication. HIV then interacts with the CD4 glycoprotein, which resides on the cell membranes, fuses itself to the cell, and injects itself into the cytoplasm where the viral ribonucleic acid (RNA) genome is then translated into deoxyribonucleic acid (DNA) by a retroviral enzyme-reverse transcriptase. The next step of the interaction involves a second DNA strand that is then formed as the cell's genetic material becomes partially viral. Normally, CD4+ T cells orchestrate the immune system process in responding to foreign antigens. An adult has approximately 800 to 1,200 of the T helper cells per μL of blood that have a lifespan of about 100 days; however an infected cell may die within 2 days, thus releasing the viral content (virions) into the blood stream to infect other cells. HIV replicates rapidly; sometimes more than 10 million virions are produced daily.

Significant loss of the CD4+ T cells results in the inability for the body to maintain homeostasis and increases susceptibility to opportunistic infections, or it can reactivate a latent disease process the individual previously experienced, such as the varicella zoster virus of chickenpox in childhood that can reemerge as shingles. Individual responses to the disease are varied; some individuals remain symptom free for many years; others succumb quickly. Even though an individual has no noticeable symptoms, the viral replication process continues.

In addition to damaging the immune system, HIV infection can cause damage to other parts of the body. Cranial and peripheral neuropathy, cardiomyopathy, pneumonitis, malabsorption in the small intestine, nephritis, cervicitis, arthritis, psoriasis, and gonad dysfunctions have all been directly associated with HIV infection. The results of damage to the hematological system are several types of anemia. It is sometimes categorized as a multisystem disease.

The criteria used to establish the diagnosis of AIDS are at least one of the following conditions: a CD4+ below 200 cells/μL; the development of one or more of fungal, viral, protozoal, or bacterial opportunistic infection(s); development of opportunistic cancers, such as invasive cervical cancer, Kaposi's sarcoma, Burkitt's lymphoma, immunoblastic lymphoma, or primary lymphoma of the brain; wasting syndrome defined by a loss of 10 percent or more of body mass; development of dementia.

Preexisting comorbidities, such as alcoholism, drug dependence, liver and kidney and other organ diseases, history of sexually transmitted diseases and psychiatric illnesses are additional influencing factors associated with the transmission and progress of HIV/AIDS. Early diagnosis, appropriate treatment with antiretroviral medications and medications to prevent opportunistic infections has increased survival rates.

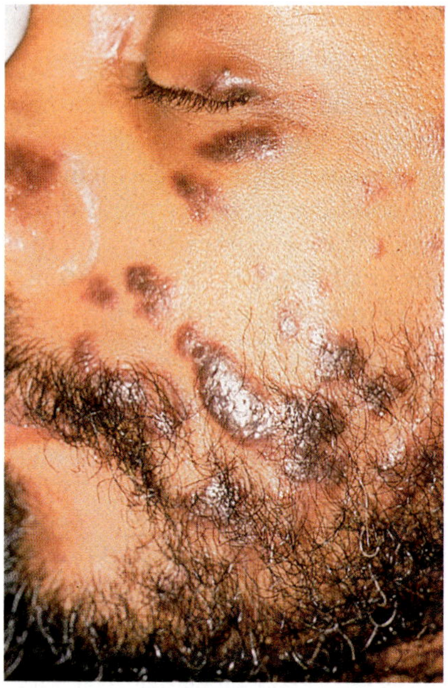

Figure 42-4 Kaposi's sarcoma. Courtesy of Robert A. Silverman, M.D., Clinical Associate Professor, Department of Pediatrics, Georgetown University.

Assessment with Clinical Manifestations

Early clinical manifestations of HIV disease resemble an acute mononucleosis-like syndrome, including chills and fever, myalgia, malaise, sort throat, nausea, photophobia, lymphadenopathy, maculopapular rash, and headache. Sometimes, there is a latent period of 10 years or more before other symptoms occur. Later clinical manifestations include chills and fever, night sweats, dry productive cough, dyspnea, lethargy, confusion, stiff neck, seizures, headache, malaise, fatigue, oral lesions, skin rash, abdominal discomfort, diarrhea, weight loss, sustained lymphadenopathy, and a wide variety of emotional responses, such as anger, fear, guilt, denial, depression, and suicidal tendencies.

As the immune system becomes overpowered, opportunistic infections or malignancy can occur. The most common infection is *Pneumocystis carinii* pneumonia (PCP). Additional respiratory infections include *Mycobacterium* tuberculosis, cytomegalovirus (CMV) infection, *Streptococcus* pneumonia, or pneumonias caused by multiple organisms. Kaposi's sarcoma (Figure 42-4), a vascular malignancy first noticed on the skin or mucous membranes, can also invade the lungs (Porth, 2004). Other systems that can be involved include vision disturbances or blindness because of CMV and herpes type 1 virus or varicella-zoster virus infections; adrenal insufficiency; gastrointestinal (GI) disturbances because of virus, yeast, protozoa, and bacteria infections or invasion of cancers; neurological disorders because of infection and the AIDS dementia complex; musculoskeletal arthralgia (joint pain) and weakness; and fluid and electrolyte imbalances.

Diagnostic Tests

During the initial infection, testing may reveal a high viral load and a dramatic drop in the CD4+ cell count. At this time antibodies are beginning to form and can be detected in approximately 4 to 12 weeks. However, the disease may not be detected in the early stages, because the person does not seek attention or inadequate history information is taken by the health care provider. If testing is performed too early, the report may be a false-negative result. Some HIV antibody tests such as the enzyme-linked immunosorbent assay (ELISA) results provide an indeterminate report. The Western blot test may not confirm the original immunoassay test. Repeated testing is recommended. Other testing methods include home test kits, salivary tests, and urine tests. However, the individual should not rely on the results without follow-up care with a health care provider. The current emphasis for monitoring is on evaluating the CD4+ cell counts (Daniels, 2003). The CDC has developed a classification system for HIV-infected adolescents and adults that emphasizes the importance of CD4+ testing in managing clinical manifestations.

A list of diagnostic tests and procedures is depicted in Box 42-2. Periodic testing is conducted to determine the patient's status and progress of the disease. Additional diagnostic tests would be performed to identify opportunistic infections. The individual may also have preexisting chronic disease conditions that require monitoring. The diagnostic findings are used to prescribe therapy. As new therapies are developed and individuals live longer with the disease, treatment will be required for many of the diseases that normally

BOX 42-2

DIAGNOSTIC STUDIES RELATED TO IMMUNOLOGICAL RESPONSE

Standard Blood Studies

- RBC count, hemoglobin/hematocrit, and reticulocyte count
- Sedimentation rate: The speed for RBCs to settle in a column of citrated blood per hour. Used in diagnosing progress of several abnormal conditions (such as chronic infections).
- WBC with differential count: Elevated in presence of infection.
- Lymphocytes: Cell markers: T cell, B cell, and so on.
- Platelet count: Involved in coagulation process.
- Proteins: Albumen, globulins, fibrinogen levels.
- C-reactive protein: Synthesized in liver; is a natural inhibitor of coagulation; deficiency in liver disease.
- Complement activity: System of 25 plasma proteins. When activated, a cascade of events mediates the defense against infection; facilitates phagocytosis, eliminates antigen-antibody complexes and destroys cell membrane of bacteria.

Additional Tests of Immunological Status

HIV Antibody Tests

- CD4 count: The hallmark of HIV infection—diminished or depleted T helper lymphocytes.
- CD4/CD8+ ratio: CD4+ lymphocytes are the primary target of the virus; therefore they decline, and there is a greater risk to develop opportunistic infections. The ratio to CD8+ lymphocytes is also low. CD8+ lymphocytes are suppressor-cytotoxic T lymphocytes.
- HIV-RNA concentration: Measures the amount of HIV in the blood—the viral load. The virus can be detected in the early stage of infection. The concentration level can be used as a baseline value. Changes in the virus count are important and are used to guide treatment strategies.
- ELISA: Detects HIV antibodies.
- Western blot test: Detects antibodies to specific viral proteins. This test is expensive and is often used as confirmation of a positive ELISA test.
- HIV antigen tests: Used for diagnosis in early stage of acute infection.
- DNA-PCR amplification: Detects the proviral DNA molecules in the infected nuclei of lymphocytes from the peripheral blood.

Immune Deficiency Disorders

- T and B lymphocyte assays: Increase in T lymphocytes is associated with acute lymphocytic leukemia, infectious mononucleosis, and multiple myeloma. Reduced levels may be due to AIDS, chronic lymphocytic leukemia, severe combined immunodeficiency disease (SCID) or long-term immunosuppressive therapy.
- Immunoglobulin assays: (Measures levels of IgG, IgA, IgM, IgD, and IgE. Increased levels of IgA and IgE may be seen in autoimmune and allergic disorders. Reduced levels of IgG, IgA, and IgM may be seen in lymphocytic leukemia.
- Bone marrow: Used to diagnose most blood dyscrasias, e.g., aplastic anemia, leukemias, pernicious anemia, thrombocytopenia.
- Lymphangiography: Visualization of the lymphatic system to detect primary malignancy (lymphoma) or metastatic disease. An oil-based dye is injected into the lymphatic system. X-ray studies are done.
- Allergy and autoimmune disorder testing: Includes skin testing for sensitivity to specific antigens and food allergies. Elimination diets are also used.

Note: The list is not inclusive.

Adapted from Daniels, R. (2003). Delmar's manual of laboratory and diagnostic tests. *New York: Thomson Delmar Learning.*

PATIENT PLAYBOOK

Patient, Family, and Caregiver Education

Patients, family, and personal caregivers should:

- Know the drugs being taken and how to take them (whether they should be taken with food or on an empty stomach; what time of day, and so on).
- The goal of retroviral therapy and importance of adhering to the prescribed regimen.
- Understand the interactions that can occur with other medications and herbal therapies.
- The importance of repeated testing and ongoing contact with the health care system.
- Recognize the potential side effects from the antiretroviral drugs and how to manage them (diarrhea, nausea, vomiting, gastric distress, headache, and so on).
- Know what social support and counseling services are available and how to access and use them.
- The changes in symptoms that should be reported immediately to the health care provider (fever, persistent shortness of breath, chest pain, dehydration, pain, watery diarrhea and abdominal pain, rectal bleeding, vision changes, onset of weakness, seizures, new oral lesions, rashes, severe depression, anxiety, hallucinations, exhibiting dangerous behavior toward self or others).

Adapted from DeLaune, S., & Ladner, P. (2006). Fundamentals of nursing *(3rd ed.). New York: Thomson Delmar Learning.*

occur in the aging population such as coronary artery disease, chronic obstructive lung disease, hypertension, and diabetes.

Nursing Diagnoses

A number of diagnoses related to HIV infection are used according to the stage of the disease, problems of the body system(s) involved and psycho-social factors. Based on the information gathered, examples of nursing diagnoses in the patient with HIV may include the following:

- Acute pain related to HIV.
- Fear in response to the diagnosis of HIV.
- Risk for infection related to HIV.
- Ineffective coping related to anxiety, lower activity level and the inability to perform normal activities of daily living related to HIV.
- Knowledge deficit related to self-care and risk prevention for HIV.

Planning and Implementation

The goals of nursing interventions are to improve the quality and quantity of the patient's life. Nurses use a holistic and individualized approach directed toward health promotion, prevention of infection, providing education related to safe sexual practices, identifying the risks of drug use, and decreasing the risk of perinatal transmission of HIV (Jones, 2004). Additional interventions include helping the patient to participate in self-care and to improve nutrition, to learn how to decrease fatigue, and to promote communication with the health care system and support network. Some of the greatest challenges are to assist the individual in coping with a chronic or life-threatening disease, overcoming fear, and minimizing spiritual distress.

In the advanced stages of the disease the goal of nursing care is to address the physical and emotional responses of the patient, whether potential or actual, which are related to the AIDS diagnosis. In many cases, the patient continues to receive care in the home except for crisis events. Home health care nurses must be alert for changes within the family structure as living with a chronic disease poses many stresses on the family unit including social isolation because of stigma associated with the disease, dependence, anger, frustration, economic concerns, feelings of powerlessness, and loss of control. Patients and families often need assistance in making treatment decisions and dealing with all the changes that transpire.

Terminal care can be especially stressful if the patient develops AIDS-dementia complex (ADC) because of HIV infection in the brain or by HIV associated central nervous system (CNS) problems. Cognitive, behavioral, and motor dysfunctions that occur include decreased concentration, depression, forgetfulness, social withdrawal, progression to dementia, paraplegia, incontinence, and coma. The focus of interventions is on maintaining a safe environment. Frequent reorientation and stress reduction methods assist in preventing confusion and disorientation. Support is given to the family and caregivers as they provide end-of-life care. Despite the many advances in HIV therapy, there still is no miracle cure. Nurses are a pivotal part in providing terminal care.

Collaborative Management

The goals of collaborative management are to initiate an effective antiretroviral treatment regimen, to promote health, and to prevent or treat opportunistic infections. The patient must assume a partnership role in the plan of care through making lifestyle changes, and adherence to the prescribed regimen. Education about the disease, modes of transmission, and how to improve personal health is of prime importance. The family and significant others who pro-

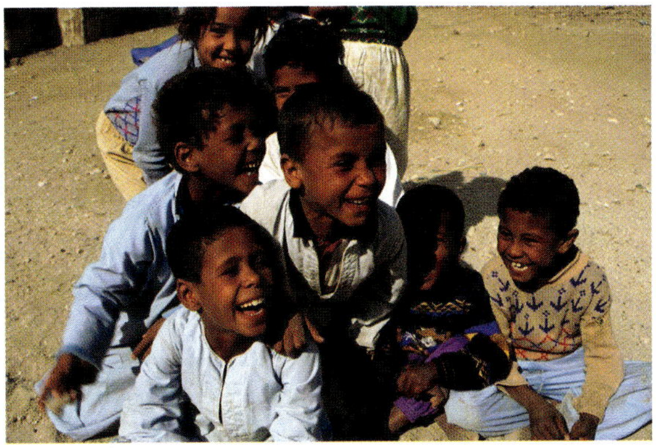

Figure 42-5 Organizations like UNICEF have initiated maternal and child health programs for diseases like AIDS to control the spread of the disease in countries like Africa.

vide social support should also be included in counseling and the plan of care. Collaborative management of the disease primarily takes place in the outpatient and community settings. The patient may be hospitalized for crisis events.

Pharmacology

Drug therapy is initiated as early as possible to reduce the HIV RNA (virion) levels in the blood and to maintain or increase the CD4+ levels to greater than 200 cells/μL and to delay the development of HIV-related symptoms and opportunistic infections. Highly active antiretroviral therapy (HAART) refers to a combination of antiretroviral drugs and is currently the preferred method to avoid development of viral resistance to the drugs. Resistance can also develop if the patient does not to adhere to the dose schedule for each drug. Each of the prescribed drugs is designed to target a specific phase of the viral cycle; therefore a missed or delayed dose permits the virus to continue to replicate itself. Several new drugs have been introduced that provide the opportunity to use more than one combination for individuals who do not respond to a specific group (Stenson, et. al., 2005).

Side effects include nausea and vomiting, anemia, leucopenia, myopathy, fatigue, headache, dizziness, and nasal congestion; dose-related peripheral neuropathy, hypersensitivity reaction, sore throat, rash, pruritus, cough, shortness of breath, and hepatitis. These drugs can also produce potentially lethal interactions with other drugs including over-the-counter (OTC) drugs and herbal therapies. The drugs are expensive, and many patients are not able to afford them, tolerate the side effects, or cannot adhere to the necessary scheduling and dietary changes. Children, especially, have difficulty with adherence to the therapy because of the numerous reactions, the aftertaste, and interactions with foods. Facilitating adherence requires educated and committed health care providers to work with the children and their caregivers (Pontali, 2005).

Long-term effects of HAART include hypertension, diabetes, osteopenia, and hyperlipidemia. Recent studies have indicated that suspending antiretroviral therapy for short intervals did lower triglycerides and blood pressure levels without decreasing the CD4+ blood levels. However, several of the study participants and health care providers opted to return to the antiretroviral therapy rather than risk further HIV complications (Casseb, Da Silva, & Alberto, 2005; Jacobs, Neil, & Aboulafia, 2005).

Three groups of drugs are currently approved as antiretroviral therapy: (Group 1) nucleoside reverse transcriptase inhibitors (NRTIs), nonnucleoside reverse transcriptase inhibitors (NNRTIs), and nucleotide reverse transcriptase inhibitors; (Group 2) protease inhibitors (PIs); and (Group 3) fusion inhibitors (Box 42-3). Scientists are continuing to research the possibility of developing a vaccine against HIV; however, one vaccine is not effective against the variety of HIV strains.

Fast Forward ▶▶▶

New Drug Therapy for HIV-Associated Tuberculosis (Tb)

It is estimated that 12 million people worldwide are currently infected with HIV and Tb, and the numbers are increasing. Both are killer diseases and can progress rapidly in the developing world where health care is minimal. The World Health Organization (WHO) has set a goal for limiting the growth in Tb cases by 2015. A recent release by the Associated Press described a new antibiotic therapy for treating Tb. Approximately 2,500 people will participate in clinical trials using a combination therapy consisting of moxifloxacin and the traditional Tb drugs in South Africa (Figure 42-5), Uganda, Brazil, the United States, Canada, Spain, Tanzania and Zambia. Moxifloxacin has been approved in 104 countries for treatment of bacterial respiratory and skin infections. The trials are sponsored by Global AIDS Alliance, a Washington, D.C.–based organization and Bayer Pharmaceuticals. Scientists believe the combination therapy will shorten the therapy to two or three months, lower the risk of developing resistant strains, provide therapy for more patients, and save many lives. The shorter therapy time will also improve adherence to the treatment program. If the clinical trials reveal significant effectiveness, the therapy could be approved within five years. The sponsors have agreed to make the therapy available at affordable prices to most of the poorer income countries.

Adapted from Leonard, T. (2005, October 18). New tuberculosis drug therapy could cut treatment time. Associated Press news release. In San Diego Union Tribune, *p. A8.*

BOX 42-3

ANTIRETROVIRAL DRUG CLASSIFICATIONS

Nucleoside Reverse Transcriptase Inhibitors (NRTIs)

Zidovudine (AZT, ZDV, Retrovir)—the first developed drug
Didanosine (ddl, Videx)
Stavudine (d4T, Zerit)
Lamivudine (3TC, Epivir)
Abacavir (Ziagen)

Nucleotide Reverse Transcriptase Inhibitor

Tenofovir DF (Viread)

Nonnucleoside Reverse Transcriptase Inhibitors (NNRTIs)

Nevirapine (Viramune)
Delavirdine (Rescriptor)
Efavirenz (Sustival)

Protease Inhibitors (PIs)

Saquinavir (Fortovase
Indinavir (Crixivan
Ritonavir (Norvir)
Nelfinavir (Viracept
Amprenavir (Agenerase)
Kaletra (combination of lopinavir and ritonvir)

Fusion Inhibitor (Entry Inhibitor)

Enfuvirtide (Fuzeon)

Adapted from Broyles, B. E., Reiss, B. S., & Evans, M. E. (2007). Pharmacological aspects of nursing care *(7th ed.). New York: Thomson Delmar Learning.*

Evaluation of Outcomes

Potential patient outcomes for each of the example nursing diagnoses for the patient with HIV are:

- Acute pain related to HIV. The patient should verbalize an adequate relief of pain along with the ability to realistically cope with the pain if it is not completely relieved.
- Fear in response to the diagnosis of HIV. The patient should manifest positive coping behaviors and verbalize a reduction in the amount of fear of the having this disease.
- Risk for infection related to HIV. The patient remains free of infection, as evidenced by normal vital signs and absence of purulent drainage from wounds, incisions, and tubes. Infection is recognized early to allow for prompt treatment.
- Ineffective coping related to anxiety, lower activity level, and the inability to perform normal activities of daily living related to HIV. The patient identifies own maladaptive coping behaviors, available resources, and support systems, describes or initiates alternative coping strategies, and describes positive results from new behaviors.
- Knowledge deficit related to self-care and risk prevention for HIV. The patient should demonstrate motivation to learn, identify perceived learning needs, and verbalize an understanding of desired content.

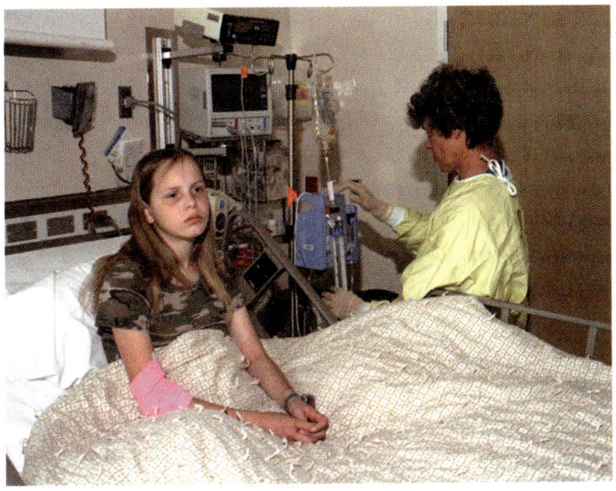

Figure 42-6 A child who is immunosuppressed from chemotherapy.

IMMUNODEFICIENCY DISORDERS

Immunodeficiency disorders are due to dysfunction or impairment of one or more of the **immune response** (a body response to an antigen that occurs when lymphocytes identify the antigenic molecule as foreign and induce the formation of antibodies and lymphocytes capable of reacting with it and rendering it harmless) mechanisms. The mechanisms include phagocytosis, humoral response, B cell- and T cell-mediated response or combination, the complement system, and a combined cell and humoral response. The primary immunodeficiency disorders are associated with the various cell-mediated deficiencies. Examples of disorders include chronic granulomatous disease, DiGeorge syndrome, ataxia telangiectasia, selective IgA, IgM, or IgG deficiency, and graft-versus-host disease. Secondary immunodeficiency disorders can be treatment-related, such as radiation or surgery; drug-induced, such as chemotherapy and corticosteroids; infectious diseases including AIDS, chronic liver or renal disease, diabetes mellitus, malignancies, and systemic lupus erythematosus (SLE); and stress. SLE is also classified as an autoimmune disease.

Young children and older people have suppressed immune systems and are more susceptible to infections than young and middle-aged adults because of a lack of sufficient immune resources (Figure 42-6). The destruction of lymphocytes by radiation or removal of lymph nodes, thymus, or spleen places the individual at high risk. Splenectomy is especially harmful for children. Cell-mediated immunity is greatly reduced in persons with Hodgkin's disease. Malnutrition also adversely affects cell-mediated immunity.

Graft-versus-Host Disease

Graft-versus-host (GVH) disease is the result of a transfusion of blood or a tissue transplant with cells that are incompatible with the host. It is hypothesized that lymphocyte T cells from the donor product attack and destroy the vulnerable cells of the host. The acute rejection response occurs approximately 7 to 30 days after the transplant. Target organs are the skin, lungs, the GI tract, and the liver. Clinical manifestations include maculopapular rash, pruritus, or pain; mild jaundice may be seen in liver disease along with elevated liver enzymes and possible hepatic coma; GI bleeding and malabsorption may occur in GI system disease. Bacterial and fungal infections are the greatest concern immediately after the transplant when granulocytopenia (great reduction in granulocytes) occurs. Interstitial pneumonitis is a common problem later in the rejection process. Corticosteroids are used to halt the rejection process; however, they, too, increase the individual's risk for infection.

Chronic GVH disease can appear approximately 100 days after the transplantation. Clinical manifestations resemble those of SLE. The skin has a scleroderma-like appearance, which is a taut, firm, hard, and edematous state; the lacrimal ducts and oral mucosa are dry.

Allograft or homograft transplant refers to cells and tissue obtained from the same species, as from a close relative or unrelated donor, who has a similar type of cell compatibility. The greatest success is with tissues from the cornea, bone marrow, artery, and cartilage. Sources for stem cells are peripheral blood, bone marrow, and umbilical cord blood. Histocompatibility testing is done to determine the similarities and differences in the complex set of proteins (**histocompatibility leukocyte antigens [HLA]** markers) on the surface membranes of all human nucleated cells, tissues, and blood cells, except red blood cells (RBCs). If the tissues of two people are histocompatible, there is less chance for the graft to be rejected. However, major incompatibility will trigger the immune response against the graft, and there is a greater chance for rejection. HLA gene markers on a cell to an antigen provide a biochemical profile unique as a fingerprint that is primarily determined by genetic factors. HLA genes take many forms and many combinations occur. Antigens located on a chromosome are inherited from each parent and the frequencies of HLAs vary considerably among the different races. There is a great need for donors from racial and ethnic groups (National Marrow Donor Program, 2005).

Bone marrow transplant (BMT) is currently used as treatment for a variety of hematological, malignant, and nonmalignant disorders, including immunodeficiency diseases and severe autoimmune diseases. A **syngeneic transplant** uses bone marrow cells donated by an identical twin with no detectable tissue incompatibility. An **autologous transplant** is the removal of bone marrow cells from the individual—treated and stored—then returned after the individual receives intensive chemotherapy or radiation. This process eliminates the GVHD response; however, a relapse may occur either because of contamination of the cells by malignant cells or failure of the chemotherapy or radiation to eradicate the malignant cells.

Immunosuppressive Therapy

Several immunosuppressive drugs have been designed to target specific phases of the immune response. Drugs are used in combination to permit lower doses of each drug and to minimize side effects. It is also important to use adequate drug doses that will suppress the immune response, yet retain enough immunity to prevent opportunistic infections and to prevent rejection of the transplant. The traditional therapy usually includes a calcineurin inhibitor (cyclosporine), a corticosteroid (prednisone; methylprednisolone), and mycophenolate mofetil (CellCept).

Monoclonal antibodies, genetically engineered immunosuppressive agents, are also used in combination with other drugs to prevent graft rejection. These agents hold great promise in the treatment of cancer, transplant rejection, and diagnosis of disease. Recombinant DNA technology, another form of genetic engineering, uses segments of DNA from one type of organism (e.g., *Escherichia coli,* yeast, or mammalian tissue) and combines it with genes of another organism to create large amounts of human proteins. The proteins include human insulin and cytokines, substances produced by white blood cells (WBCs) that assist in immunological cell growth, i.e., interlukin-2 and α-interferon. The cytokines function in both inflammation and the immune response (Janeway, Travers, Walport, & Shlomchik, 2004).

Apheresis is sometimes used for treating autoimmune diseases and other disorders. The procedure consists of withdrawal of blood from a donor, removal of one or more components (as plasma, blood platelets, or WBCs) from the blood, and transfusion into patients with low platelet or WBC counts; the remaining blood is transfused back into the donor. **Plasmapheresis,** or **plasma exchange,** is a process for removing plasma that contains components that are thought to be the cause of a disease, such as autoantibodies or antigen-antibody complexes. The plasma is usually replaced by normal saline, lactated Ringer's solution, frozen plasma, or albumen. The procedure involves removing whole blood through a needle inserted into one arm, circulating the blood through a cell separator where the blood is separated into plasma and the cellular components; the destructive components are removed, and the remainder of the contents is returned via a needle inserted in the opposite arm. The platelets, plasma proteins, WBCs, and RBCs can be selected separately. Side effects associated with the procedure are hypotension, probably because a vasovagal response or transitory volume changes, and citrate toxicity. Citrate, an anticoagulant, may cause hypocalcemia and result in headache, dizziness, and paresthesias (Broyles, Reiss, & Evans, 2007).

Hypersensitivity Disorders

Hypersensitivity to an allergen, or **antigen,** is because of a heightened immune response. The sensitization begins as an individual develops IgE antibodies to an antigen. The IgE antibodies adhere to the basophils and mast cells on the mucosal surfaces, the respiratory tract, and the GI tract. Reexposure to the antigen, or allergen, results in the hypersensitive responses, such as sneezing, asthma symptoms, and potential anaphylaxis. The responses are dependent on the host's defense mechanisms, the characteristics and concentration of the allergen, the route of entry, the amount of exposure, and the organ that is affected. Hypersensitivity disorders are more thoroughly discussed in chapter 43.

AUTOIMMUNE DISORDERS

Organs and tissues commonly affected by autoimmune disorders include blood components, such as RBCs, blood vessels, connective tissues, endocrine glands, such as the thyroid or pancreas, muscles, joints, and skin. Most of the autoimmune disorders are associated with the connective tissues of the body. Among the most common disorders are osteoarthritis, rheumatoid arthritis (RA), gout, SLE, progressive systemic sclerosis (scleroderma), and ankylosing spondylitis, which are all diseases that have common clinical manifestations of pain and impaired mobility.

Many factors are involved that cause the immune system to fail to recognize the body's normal tissue as self. Basically, these self-killing cells begin to break down normal cells in a particular area of the body resulting in the autoimmune disorder. Several theories have been proposed including genetic predisposition, infections, interaction of T and B cells, introduction of foreign tissue such as a blood transfusion or transplant tissue, and environmental factors. Viral infections have been linked to development of multiple sclerosis (MS) and type I diabetes mellitus. Rheumatic fever, caused by a streptococcal infection, has been linked to rheumatic heart disease. Drugs can be precipitating factors. Hormones have an effect on autoimmune diseases and more women have autoimmune disease than men. Autoimmune disorders and allergy are both caused by hypersensitivity reactions. It is believed that a history of allergies indicates increased risk of autoimmune disorders. Age is considered a factor because there is an increase of autoantibodies.

Much research has been conducted over the past 10 years to understand how the immune system works and to discover how the immune system may be enhanced to prevent these disorders or to promote healing. We do know that the immune system is sensitive to internal and external environmental factors. Nutrition has been found to play a vital role in the body's ability to fight infection and disease. Obesity may be a contributing factor to immune dysfunction. Depression has been identified as a factor that interferes with recovery, motivation, and compliance as well as decreasing energy and immune function.

Autoimmune disorders can involve a single organ or tissue that can result in local tissue damage, such as in Hashimoto's thyroiditis. The thyroid becomes enlarged and symptoms of hypothyroidism are present. Treatment is lifelong thyroid hormone replacement. Crohn's disease affects the GI system; MS affects the CNS. System-wide autoimmune disorders, such as SLE, involve the reaction of autoantibodies to almost every cell in the body. Goodpasture's syndrome is a disorder in which autoantibodies destroy the basement membrane of the lungs and kidneys. A person may experience a cluster of autoimmune diseases, e.g., RA and Addison's disease. As a result many outcomes may occur and encompass a multitude of autoimmune disorders. Some disorders have multiple interrelated causes.

Hormones or other substances normally produced by the affected organ may need to be supplemented. This may include thyroid supplements, vitamins, insulin injections, or other supplements. Disorders that affect the blood components may require blood transfusions. Measures to assist mobility or other function may be needed for disorders that affect the bones, joints, or muscles. **Autoimmunity** is controlled through balanced suppression of the immune system. The goal is to reduce the immune response against normal body tissue while leaving the immune response intact against microorganisms and abnormal tissues.

Rheumatoid Arthritis

RA is one of several inflammatory joint diseases that plague patients. The disease causes chronic inflammation in the connective tissue in the joints. RA can also cause systemic symptoms, such as "fever, malaise, rash, lymph node or spleen enlargement, and Raynaud phenomenon (transient lack of circulation to the fingertips and toes)" (Crowther & McCance, 2004, p. 1094). This is a debilitating chronic autoimmune disease that can be controlled and treated, but to date there is no known cure.

Epidemiology

Once thought of as an old person's disease, RA affects people from the young to the old. In the adult population the first symptoms of RA appear generally between the ages of 20 and 40, but can occur at any age (Hellman & Stone, 2004). RA occurs in 1 to 2 percent of adults and develops more in women to men (three to one ratio).

After the age of 55 it is estimated that RA occurs in 2 percent of men and 5 percent of women. A higher incidence is seen in North American Indians and Eskimos, which supports a genetic link. The onset of symptoms and speed with which the disease progresses, appears to also be linked to age and stressors. When RA develops at a younger age, the progress appears to be slow and insidious. In contrast, when the onset is after the age of 60, the patients develop symptoms that are acute and widespread but have a shorter duration and a better prognosis. On the other hand, with pregnancy, most women report an improvement in symptoms, but up to one third of women report no change in symptoms. Statistics related to RA include that 10 percent of patients will experience remission, 15 percent develop severe progressive and destructive symptoms, and 75 percent experience a slow progressing and gradually worsening course of symptoms.

Etiology

Despite years of research, the exact cause of RA remains elusive. It is thought to be a combination of genetic hormonal, environmental, and reproductive factors that lead to the development of the disease. Research has determined that most patients with RA have a Class Two HLA with an identified five amino acid sequence (Hellman & Stone, 2004).

Bacteria, mycoplasmas, and viruses may also be contributors to RA occurrences. The Epstein-Barr virus has been of particular interest to researchers in the cause of RA. Rheumatoid factors (RFs) develop as a result of prolonged or concentrated exposure to the organisms (an antigen-antibody response). RFs are immunoglobulins (Ig) that have become autoantibodies (IgG, IgM, and, occasionally IgA). The RF attacks the host tissue (self-antigens), specifically the synovial membrane, forming immune complexes (Crowther & McCance, 2004).

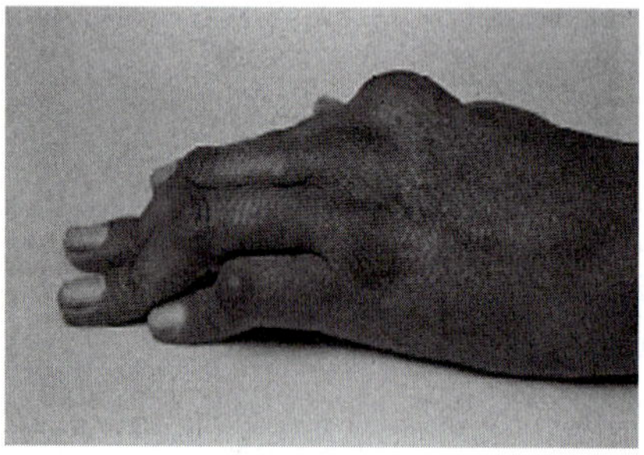

Figure 42-7 Arthritis is considered a chronic health problem. Courtesy of Arthritis Foundation.

Pathophysiology

Joint deformity in RA is the result of repeated inflammation episodes (Figure 42-7). Damage occurs in four phases. (a) Initiation phase: some changes in the synovial lining of the joint are evident. (b) Immune response phase: A cascade of events begins as CD4 T cells stimulate the immune response; many leukocytes, macrophages, and fibroblasts migrate to the synovial fluid; B lymphocytes arrive and release the IgM antibody that can be measured as rheumatoid factor (RF). Proinflammatory cytokines and enzymes begin the erosive tissue damage process; complement and other chemotaxins help to increase the inflammation; and the cytokines tumor necrosis factor-alpha (TNF-α) and interleukin-1 (IL-1) perpetuate the inflammatory process. (c) Inflammatory phase: Swelling caused by inflammation damages tiny blood vessels that contain the synovial fluid; the body releases arachidonic acid and lysosomal enzymes. Oxygen radicals develop. As the inflammation continues, the cells increase in size and become hyperactive stromal cells that thicken the synovial membrane. (d) The destruction phase: A thickened fibrous scar tissue (pannus) is formed and adheres to the articular (joint) surface of the cartilage. The fibrous tissue may become calcified; the joint becomes fused and results in permanent deformity. Joints commonly affected are the knees, ankles, shoulders, wrists, and proximal interphalangeal and metacarpophalangeal joints.

Assessment with Clinical Manifestations

Common early clinical manifestations include diffuse musculoskeletal pain, low-grade fever, possible anorexia, and loss of weight. Later, articular (within the joint) manifestations include synovitis (inflammation of the synovial capsule causing escape of synovial fluid into the synovial capsule). Subsequent hypertrophy and symmetrical joint deformity (particularly wrists, hands, or knees) occur. Pain; muscle spasm; and weakness, because of contractures of muscles, tendons, and ligaments; and muscle and soft tissue damage greatly impact the person's daily activities. Many times the shoulders are affected. Extra-articular manifestations that can occur at any time during the course of the disease include Sjögren's syndrome (chronic inflammatory eye disorder), pulmonary fibrosis, pericarditis, nerve compression, and vasculitis. Development of nontender rheumatoid nodules that are made up of granulation tissue surrounding a core of fibrous debris can occur in the subcutaneous tissue and even in visceral organs, such as the lungs and the heart. Sleep disturbances are common (Capriotti, 2004).

Stiffness and diminished function after prolonged activity especially on arising in the morning are hallmarks of the progressive severity of the disease (Figure 42-8). The person self-limits motion, usually by holding the extremity in a flexed position, which may result in contractures that further contribute to decreased joint function. At times, the individual may have a remission of symptoms for several months or years; however, remission seldom occurs if the joint damage extends beyond two years. Early diagnosis is important to prevent joint damage; however, erosion damage can be evident for 30 percent of those with an early diagnosis, and 60 percent have definite joint damage by two years. Diagnosis can be challenging because of the many clinical manifestations that mimic other syndromes (Capriotti, 2004).

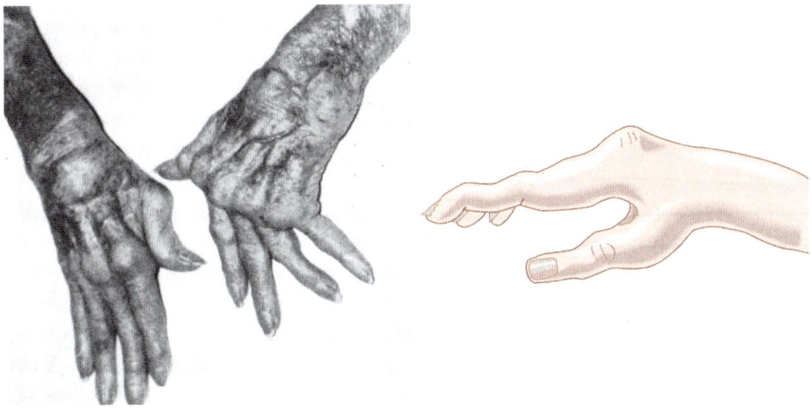

Figure 42-8 RA often results in ulnar deviation and swan neck deformity of the hand.

Skills 360°

Assessment of JRA

In 1975 a mysterious disease outbreak primarily affecting young people in Lyme, Connecticut, was misdiagnosed as JRA. Scientists discovered the disease was caused by the *Borrelia burgdorferi* (Bd), a spirochete bacteria. Lyme disease is usually transmitted by the deer tick, but a variety of other insects can be hosts. The disease can also be transmitted through sexual contact. The spirochete often embeds into multiple organs, tendons, muscles, the heart, and brain; it may lie dormant in cysts, and then reemerge at a later time. It is often resistant to drug therapy. Clinical manifestations mimic symptoms of several other diseases including Lou Gehrig's disease, chronic fatigue and fibromyalgia syndromes, irritable bowel syndrome, SLE, RA, and syphilis. ELISA and Western blot antibody test results may be inconclusive. Careful assessment and monitoring are essential.

Initial clinical manifestations include flu-like symptoms (headache, fever, and muscle aches); later manifestations include neck rigidity, jaw discomfort, muscle pain and stiffness, lymphadenopathy, burning sensations in lower extremities, and red eyes. Initial skin assessment may reveal a bull's eye mark and rash; however, different skin marks have been noted. Check for ticks on patients, especially on the lower extremities, who have been outside in high grassy areas, hiking, hunting, or camping in remote places. Ticks should be removed with tweezers without twisting. Provide education on preventive measures. The disease can also be transmitted through the placenta from mother to fetus and by blood transfusion.

Adapted from Sellman, S. (2005). Disease of disguise: Learning about Lyme. Canadian Journal of Health and Nutrition, *275(15), 76–78.*

Juvenile Rheumatoid Arthritis

Juvenile idiopathic rheumatoid arthritis (JRA) is the most prevalent chronic disease in children under 16 years of age. Approximately 30,000 to 50,000 children in the United States have been diagnosed with the disease, and several cases have been reported worldwide. Onset usually occurs around 8 years of age with a later peak during puberty. Disease symptoms frequently mimic those of other diseases, and diagnostic tests can be inconclusive, resulting in misdiagnosis and a missed opportunity for early treatment. Initial symptoms are frequently called growing pains; however, enlarged knuckles that are warm to the touch complaints of pain in ankles, feet, or knees; and decreased range of motion should receive prompt attention (Myer, Brunner, Melson, Paterno, & Ford, 2005).

The chronic recurrent systemic and joint inflammation episodes restricts the child's ability to participate in physical activities, limits interaction with peers, frequently subjects them to taunting by other children, and affects the quality of life. Growth development is slowed, and because of the long-term articular and systemic effects of the disease and side affects of the immunosuppressive drugs, the child and family must face lifelong challenges. Children often have a better response to the drug methotrexate (MTX) than adults. Thalidomide, a drug once used as a sedative and antinauseate in the 1950s and 1960s, has been used in a six-month clinical trial with 13 children in the United States and Brazil. There was a positive response from 11 of the participants permitting a decreased use of steroids. Six individuals were able to discontinue steroid therapy. The participants agreed to use birth control precautions because of the teratogen side affects of the drug. Thalidomide is also

Uncovering the Evidence

Surgical Interventions for JRA

Discussion: To evaluate the outcome of surgery for children and adolescents who were followed for a minimum of 12 years postarthroplasty. Eight patients diagnosed with refractory JRA were evaluated preoperatively and postoperatively related to amount of pain, range of motion, walking ability, and radiological evaluation of alignment and component loosening (a total of 15 knees were evaluated).

Preoperatively, seven participants were in wheelchairs, and others had mobility dysfunction; postoperatively, six were able to walk and had a mean arc of motion from 36° to 79°. Twelve knees were pain free; radiographic evaluation indicated 13 of the 15 knees were in natural alignment and 2 were in valgus (bent outward). Three knees required further revision. All the participants were employed; all could function independently; four were married; and three had children.

Implications for Practice: Arthroplasty is a reasonable procedure for those who do not respond to the nonoperative procedures.

Source: Palmer, D., Mulhall, K., Thomson, C., Severson, E., Santos, E., & Saleh, K. (2005). Total knee arthroplasty in juvenile rheumatoid arthritis. Journal of Bone and Joint Surgery (Am), *87(7), 1510–1514.*

used the cancer complications of HIV/AIDS in adults. Use of the drug must be carefully monitored (Pediatric Alert, 2004).

BOX 42-4

THE AMERICAN COLLEGE OF RHEUMATOLOGY CRITERIA FOR DIAGNOSIS OF RA

- Morning stiffness lasting more than one hour
- Arthritis of three or more joint areas
- Arthritis of hand joints
- Symmetrical arthritis
- Rheumatoid nodules over extensor surfaces or bony prominences
- Serum rheumatoid factors
- Radiographic changes

Source: Janeway, C. A., Jr., Travers, P., Walport, M., & Shlomchik, M. J. (2004). Immunobiology: The immune system in health and disease *(6th ed.). New York: Garland Science Publishing.*

Diagnostic Tests

The most commonly used laboratory diagnostic test is that of serum RF. This factor is positive in approximately 80 percent of all patients with RA. Other laboratory findings (Box 42-4) that will show an elevation or be positive when RA is present are antimitochondrial antibody (AMA); antinuclear antibodies (ANA); antistreptolysin O (ASO); complement C3; C-reactive protein; lupus erythematosus cell preparation (LE prep); thyroid antibody (TA), and erythrocyte sedimentation rate (ESR). Slight anemia may be present. X-rays are useful when a series of films over time can be obtained. Comparison films allow monitoring of changes in the bony structure. Bone scans can detect early joint changes and confirm diagnosis of RA.

Samples of synovial fluid are assistive when confirming RA or differentiating diagnoses. Synovial fluid in early disease is straw-colored, slightly cloudy, and with many flecks of fibrin. The WBC count will be 3,500 to 25,000/mm^3.

Nursing Diagnoses

Based on the information gathered, examples of nursing diagnoses in the patient with RA may include those found in Table 42-1.

Planning and Implementation

Expected outcomes include preserving the individual's participation in daily activities, maintaining pain at a level that permits participation in self-care; to be able to balance rest and activity; to adhere to the therapeutic regimen; and to cope effectively with the numerous psycho-social-spiritual impact of the disease. The nurse is an integral part of the multidisciplinary team in coordinating the various activities that promote optimal outcomes. The nurse must, also, be knowledgeable of the latest drug safety information. Vigilant assessment of the patient's

TABLE 42-1 Nursing Diagnoses, Nursing Interventions Classifications and Nursing Outcomes for RA

NURSING DIAGNOSIS	NURSING INTERVENTION CLASSIFICATIONS (NIC)	NURSING OUTCOMES CLASSIFICATIONS (NOC)
Pain, acute	Analgesic administration	Comfort level
	Pain management	Pain control
	Heat/cold application	Pain level
	Medication management	
	Transcutaneous	
	Electrical nerve stimulation (TENS)	
Pain, chronic	Analgesic administration	Comfort level
	Pain management	Pain control
	Heat/cold application	Pain: disruptive effects
	Medication management	Pain level
	Progressive muscle	
	Relaxation	
	Simple massage	
	Transcutaneous	
	Electrical nerve stimulation (TENS)	
Impaired physical mobility	Bed rest care	Coordinated movement
	Energy management	Joint movement: Active
	Exercise therapy: Ambulation	Mobility
	Exercise therapy: Joint mobility	Self-care: Activities of daily living
	Self-care assistance	Transfer performance
	Teaching: Prescribed activity/exercise	Knowledge: Prescribed activity
		Motivation
Activity intolerance	Activity therapy	Activity tolerance
	Energy management	Endurance
	Exercise promotion: Strength training	Energy conservation
	Teaching: Prescribed activity/exercise	
Self-care deficit:	Self-care assistance: Bathing/hygiene	Self-care: ADL
Bath/hygiene	Self-care assistance: Dressing/grooming	Self-care: Bathing
Dressing/grooming	Self-care assistance: Toileting	Self-care: Hygiene
		Self-care: Dressing
		Self-care: Grooming
		Self-care: Toileting

Adapted from DeLaune, S., & Ladner, P. (2006). Fundamentals of nursing *(3rd ed.). New York: Thomson Delmar Learning; Janeway, C. A., Jr., Travers, P., Walport, M., & Shlomchik, M. J. (2004).* Immunobiology, the immune system in health and disease *(6th ed.). New York: Garland Science Publishing.*

increased susceptibility to infections and toxic effects of immunosuppressive therapy to organs and tissues is essential. The nurse must be able to provide appropriate preoperative and postoperative care and participate in discharge education procedures to aid the patient and caregiver with skills and coping strategies to effectively manage living with a chronic disease. Particular attention should be given to social support and prevention of feelings of isolation.

The goals of treatment focus on pain management and reduction of inflammation, promoting remission, and increasing function abilities, and helping individuals to cope with the disabilities. Progression of the disease can be slowed with early aggressive treatment. Multidisciplinary approaches are used, including muscle strengthening, range of motion, and activities to prevent imbalance and the risk of further injury because of falls. Many people derive benefits from water exercise. Applications of heat or cold and use of analgesic ointments to the affected areas often provide pain relief; however actual massage can aggravate the inflammation in the acute inflamed joints. Immersion of the hands in warm paraffin baths followed by hand exercises has also been beneficial in relieving pain and stiffness. Transcutaneous electrical nerve stimulation (TENS) is commonly used for pain relief. Complementary or alternative therapy is a popular method with patients to integrate with the traditional medical methods. Acupuncture, yoga, massage, guided imagery, and therapeutic touch are examples. Surgeries, such as tendon transfer, surgical removal of the synovia in the affected joints, fusion of a joint, arthroplasty, and joint replacement have provided many individuals with freedom from pain, increased mobility, increased independence and quality of life (Price, 2004).

Nutrition

Although there is no specific nutritional therapy for the treatment of RA, it is important to employ the services of a dietitian. Weight loss is often associated with RA related to several factors: loss or change of appetite because of the stress of the disease or prescribed medications, inability to prepare meals secondary to loss of strength in hands or decreased stamina to prepare the meals; and depression because of the impact of a chronic and debilitating disease. Recommended nutritional intake is high in calories and vitamins (Crowther & McCance, 2004).

Pharmacology

Medications to manage RA include (a) selective and nonselective nonsteroidal anti-inflammatory drugs (NSAIDs); (b) synthetic and biological disease-modifying antirheumatic drugs (DMARDs); and (c) corticosteroids. Usually first-line nonselective NSAIDs that are available as OTC drugs and prescription NSAIDs are used to alleviate the symptoms of RA; however, they do not prevent the progress of the disease (OTC drugs are usually prescribed until a definite diagnosis of RA is made). Long-term use of NSAIDs can cause GI distress and bleeding and impaired renal function. Often a combination of drugs is used along with the NSAIDs. Prostaglandin analogues or proton pump inhibitors are used to protect the stomach mucosa. Until recently, COX-2 inhibitors (selective NSAIDs) were mainline drugs to reduce inflammation and to alleviate the pain and of arthritic disorders. However, FDA approval of Vioxx and Bextra has been withdrawn, and precautions have been issued for the use of Celebrex.

Aurothioglucose (goldthioglucose, Solganal) has sometimes been given intramuscularly to relieve the joint inflammation and to slow the progress of RA and JRA. It has been an adjunctive medication when symptoms have not responded to NSAIDs. There are several side affects, such as allergic reactions, skin rashes, nausea and vomiting, abdominal cramps, diarrhea, anorexia, and metallic taste. Currently the drug is rarely used (Spratto & Woods, 2007).

Currently, most individuals diagnosed with RA receive a combination therapy of MTX and a biological DMARD. Synthetic DMARDs include MTX, which has a potent immunosuppressant and anti-inflammatory effect. Infliximab (mAb) is a monoclonal antibody, which binds directly to the TNF-α and impairs its ability to bind to receptors on cell surfaces. It, also, has anti-inflammatory effects. Adalimumab, another genetically engineered IgG antibody drug, attaches to the TNF and impairs its ability to bind to cell surface receptors (Table 42-2).

TABLE 42-2 Examples of Drugs Used for RA Therapy

DRUG CLASSIFICATION	CHARACTERISTICS	SIDE EFFECTS	PRECAUTIONS/INTERVENTIONS
Nonselective NSAIDs Motrin, Advil (ibuprofen) Aleve (naproxen) Indocin (indomethacin Relafen (nabumetone) Feldene (piroxicam)	Provide pain and stiffness relief. Inhibit the cyclooxygenase pathways, which produce prostaglandins during inflammation cascade.	Esophagitis, gastritis, gastroduodenal ulceration.	Misoprostol (Cytotec) a prostaglandin analogue to protect gastric mucosa; Caution: not to be used in pregnant women, nursing mothers, and women planning pregnancy Prilosec (omeprazole) and other proton pump inhibitors to protect gastric mucosa
Selective NSAIDs COX-2 inhibitors	Reduce pain and inflammation. Most effective in combination with DMARDs	Gastric irritation (reduced in comparison to NSAIDs)	Proton pump inhibitors to reduce gastric side effects Some removed from market because of cardiovascular problems
Synthetic DMARDS Methotrexate (MTX) Infliximab Adalimumab	Diminish progression of RA	Bone marrow suppression, hepatotoxicity, pulmonary fibrosis, pneumonitis Hypersensitivity reactions	Vigilant monitoring of liver and renal function and symptoms of immunosuppression. CBC, CXRs. Teratogenic effects: not for pregnant women or women planning pregnancy. Alcohol abstinence.
Biological DMARDs TNF-α antagonists—Enbrel (etanercept) Remicade (infliximab) Humira (adalimumab) Adalimumab	Diminish cytokine response to inflammation; reduces damaging effects (erosion of bone) Safe for children over 4 years old with juvenile RA	Immunosuppression infliximab: Greater chance for developing lymphoma	Discontinue drug if infection occurs. Pregnancy safety is unknown. Children to have immunizations up to date.
Costimulatory blockers Abatacept (CTLA4Ig)	Inhibits stimulation of antigen-presenting cells in activation of T lymphocytes. Best results in combination with MTX.	Upper respiratory infection, GI distress, rash, dizziness	Monitor for adverse side effects.
Interleukin antagonists Kineret (anakinra)	Reduces erosive damage due to cytokines released by monocytes and macrophages.	Injection site reactions, headache, GI distress.	Not to be used in combination with TNF antagonists—increased risk of infection. Contraindicated for persons with active or chronic infections. No live vaccines to be given. Has not been tested in children, or for pregnancy safety.
Drugs under investigation Rituxan (rituximab) Genetically engineered monoclonal antibody.	Targets specific surface antigens on circulating B lymphocytes. Shows promise alone and in combination with MTX to reduce progress of RA	Immunosuppressant	

Adapted from Capriotti, T. (2004). The "alphabet" of rheumatoid arthritis therapy. Nursing, 13*(6), 920–928.*

"Abatacept (CTLA4Ig) is the first in a new class of biologic DMARDs known as co-stimulatory or second-signal blockers" (Capriotti, 2004, p. 425). Clinical trials have shown diminished inflammation and reduction in symptoms over a 12-month period. Kineret (anakinra), an interleukin antagonist, interferes with the proinflammatory effects of the body's cytokines.

Drugs under investigation include Rituxan (rituximab), a genetically engineered monoclonal antibody that targets specific surface antigens on circulating B lymphocytes. The drug has been used in treating lymphoma. A recent large investigation was conducted by the Arthritis Foundation to determine the effects of the rituximab in combination with MTX and cyclophosphamide. Findings demonstrated marked improvement in RA symptoms, but further research is needed (Capriotti, 2004; Chambers & Isenberg, 2005). Rituximab has also been used in combination with thalidomide for treatment of lymphoma and used alone or combination with other drugs to treat dermatomyositis, IgM-mediated neuropathies, Wegener's granulomatosis, Goodpasture's syndrome, myasthenia gravis, refractory pemphigus vulgaris, and idiopathic thrombocytopenia. The safety profile of rituximab indicates there are fewer adverse affects than other immunosuppressive agents. However, more research is needed because many of the studies have been small (Chambers & Isenberg, 2005).

Surgery

Most of the surgeries performed to correct the damage done by RA are joint replacements (arthroplasty). Most joints can be replaced with some degree of normal mobility returning to the joints. The most common joint replacements done are total hip and total knee replacements. These will be discussed in detail in the section on osteoarthritis. Finger, shoulder, elbow, and ankle joints can also be replaced.

Other surgeries done to repair RA damage are synovectomies (removal of the synovial membrane) joint fusions (total immobility of the affected joint), and tendon transfers to prevent deformities or relieve contractions.

Evaluation of Outcomes

Refer to Table 42-1 for the nursing diagnoses, nursing interventions classifications, and nursing outcomes displayed for RA.

Sjögrens's Syndrome

Sjögren's syndrome is a chronic inflammatory disorder involving the eyes that is primary problem or secondary to RA. There is a decrease in lacrimation and salivation due to obstruction of the secretory ducts by the immune complexes. Dry eyes (keratoconjunctivitis sicca) and dry mouth (xerostomia) are hallmarks of the disorder.

Manifestations include swelling of the lacrimal ducts and parotid glands and fatigue. The presence of RF, ANAs, and antiextractable nuclear antigen are revealed through diagnostic tests. Instillation of artificial tears helps to keep the eyes moist and to prevent corneal abrasions. Artificial saliva can also be used for the xerostomia. Untreated, the syndrome can result in visual problems, oral ulcerations, dental caries, and dysphagia. The presurgical procedure, nothing by mouth (NPO), is an uncomfortable experience for patients with this disorder. Artificial saliva should be used and ocular lubricants should also be instilled preoperatively.

Systemic Lupus Erythematosus

SLE is the most severe form of this autoimmune disorder and is classified as a multisystem disease. The discoid type is a milder form that affects the skin, primarily the face, neck, and upper chest. A third type of this disorder is a reversible form due to reactions to various medications, such as oral contraceptives, isoniazid, procainamide, and methyldopa, and others that are known to bind with the person's DNA. Another possibility is because of the correlation of the patient's genetic predisposition to SLE and how the medication is metabolized. SLE is a relatively rare condition that affects younger women between the ages of 15 and 40 years; therefore, this suggests a hormonal influence is involved. It is more commonly seen in African American, Hispanic (American), and Asian (American) women than in Caucasians. The incidence is higher in some families than in others. Pregnant women with SLE are more prone to spontaneous abortion and premature delivery. Close monitoring is needed (Alarcon-Segovia, et al., 2005).

Epidemiology

SLE is most prevalent among women and, in particular, those of African American, Asian (American), or Native American descent. The onset of SLE generally occurs between the ages of 15 and 45, with 80 percent of cases affecting women during their childbearing years. The incidence of SLE in the African American population is 1:250 versus 1:1000 in the Caucasian population (Trethewey, 2004).

Etiology

The etiology is unknown. Genetic predisposition, infection, environmental irritants, physical and emotional stress, and exposure to ultraviolet (UV) B radiation have been suggested as potential contributing factors.

Pathophysiology

A combination of factors is involved in the development of ANAs. The hyperactivity of B cells and a defect in the body's T suppressor cell that normally protects the body from developing ANAs triggers the inflammatory cascade of events that result in systemic tissue damage. The basement membrane of the kidneys is particularly vulnerable; deposits of the antibody complex can lead to glomerulonephritis. The ANAs that are produced in SLE are specifically directed at the cell nuclei (the cell command centers). When the cells die, the nuclei are released into the blood stream and bind with the ANAs and form a large complex that is deposited in the tissues. SLE complexes can affect any organ system, including the musculoskeletal system, the CNS, the heart, and blood vessels, causing vasculitis that results in a diminished supply of oxygen to the organs and tissues (Porth, 2004).

Assessment with Clinical Manifestations

Polyarthritis (involving many joints) and polyarthralgia (pain in many joints) are present in a majority of the cases. Pain is present in the small joints of the hands, feet, wrists, and knees. Extraarticular manifestations include lethargy, malaise, fever, and loss of weight. In the acute stages the patient may have a butterfly rash on the face that resembles the face of a wolf (Figure 42-9). The person may also develop pleural effusion and basilar pneumonia, generalized lymphadenopathy, pericarditis, hepatosplenomegaly. In severe cases delirium convulsions, psychosis, and coma may occur.

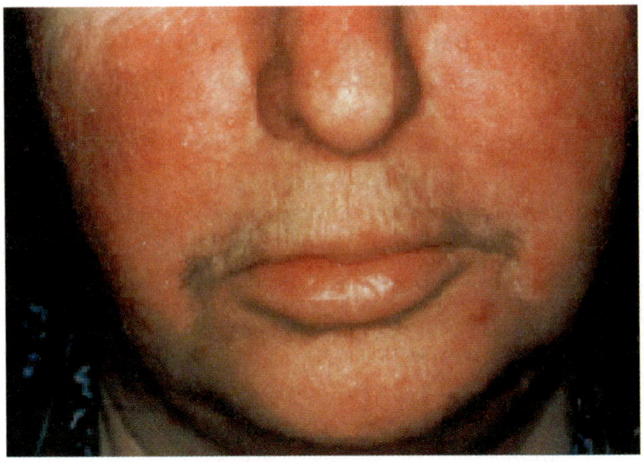

Figure 42-9 Butterfly rash seen in SLE. Courtesy of the American Academy of Dermatology.

Manifestations of the chronic form are related to the organ or tissues involved. Fever, malaise, and weight loss may continue. The cutaneous lesions of the discoid type are evident as well as erythematosus (diffused redness) of exposed skin. Additional symptoms include generalized lymphadenopathy, severe hemolytic anemia, thrombocytopenic purpura, enlargement of the spleen, and cardiopulmonary problems, including pleural effusion, tachycardia, and peripheral vascular syndromes, i.e., Raynaud's phenomenon and gangrene. Ulcerative mucous membrane lesions; GI disturbances, such as nausea, vomiting, bloody stools, and hepatic dysfunction; myalgia; and multiple neurological symptoms can occur. The disease is often called the great imitator and can be confused with RA because of the symmetrical joint involvement.

The course of the disease is variable. An acute episode can progress rapidly; however, the disease commonly develops into a chronic phase with remissions and exacerbations. The disease seems to be more severe when the onset occurs at a young age. Glomerulonephritis is the common cause of death. Cardiac and CNS problems are also major causes of morbidity. Recent developments in scientific technology has greatly improved survival rates and contributed to a better quality of life. However, the long-term survival rate is still unpredictable (NIAMS, 2005).

Diagnostic Tests

SLE should be suspected in patients with glomerulonephritis, photosensitivity, characteristic skin rashes, CNS disease, and various cytopenias, such as the Coombs'-positive anemia, hemolytic anemia, leukopenia, and thrombocytopenia. The ANA titer represents the most sensitive American College of Rheumatology (ACR) criteria (Gill, Quisel, Rocca, & Walters, 2003). More than 99 percent of patients with SLE demonstrate an elevated ANA titer at some point, although other situations, such as advancing age, infections, RA, and certain drugs, produce positive results. Testing for antibody to double-stranded DNA antigen (anti-dsDNA) and antibody to Sm nuclear antigen (anti-Sm) are specific to SLE and are therefore useful in differential diagnosis. Particularly in high titers, these tests demonstrate a high specificity for SLE, although their sensitivity is low, indicating that while these tests are useful in establishing a diagnosis of SLE, they should not be used to rule out SLE in the presence of a negative test result. A decrease in the complement factors C3 and C4, as well as an increase in their degradation products C3d/C4d, can be seen in active disease as a result of circulating immune complex disposition in tissues and activation of complement and are therefore useful in measuring disease activity.

Additional diagnostic tests may be warranted to rule out the presence of associated systemic complications. A kidney biopsy may be required if blood and urine evaluations indicate evidence of renal disease. In the presence of possible neuropsychiatric complications, a lumbar puncture may be performed to rule out infection. Magnetic resonance imaging (MRI) is the modality of choice for the identification of white matter lesions but may lack clarity in its ability to distinguish lesions from cerebral vasculitis. Psychometric testing may also be used. The presence of antiphospholipid antibodies and lupus anticoagulant are constitutive for antiphospholipid syndrome (Daniels, 2003).

Nursing Diagnoses

Refer to Table 42-1 for the nursing diagnoses, nursing interventions classifications, and nursing outcomes displayed for RA.

Planning and Implementation

A multidisciplinary approach is used to address the acute and chronic disease symptoms. The patient must be a partner in making treatment decision and in providing the health care team about the patterns of disease activity. The goals include prevention in progressive loss of organ function, reducing the possibility of exacerbation events, minimizing disability, and preventing complications of medication therapy. Medications include NSAIDs to reduce pain, inflammation, and fever. An antimalarial drug, such as hydroxychloroquine sulfate (Plaquenil), is sometimes used to control the fatigue, rash, cutaneous and musculoskeletal symptoms, and lung inflammation. Corticosteroids are used for initial symptoms and may be used periodically in low doses. Immunosuppressive drugs, such as cyclophosphamide, can be used.

A combination of rituximab, cyclophosphamide, and prednisolone was used in a study of five female patients with refractory SLE. All of the participants responded well to the therapy. Several small studies reported similar results. Consistent improvement in clinical manifestations and laboratory findings were reported (Chambers & Isenberg, 2005). Allogenic stem cell transplantation for patients with acute forms of SLE who have not responded to three or more months of medication therapy and immunosuppressive agents may prove to be a preferred treatment in the future. Current research activities are investigating the interaction between genes and environmental triggers and development of new drugs (NIAMS, 2005).

Nursing interventions will depend on the stage of the disease, the patient's response to the condition, and the severity and type of disease. Patient education is of prime importance throughout the course of the disease, including appropriate skin care, nutrition, and minimizing the risk of opportunistic infections. Because exposure to UV rays seems to exacerbate the disease process, it is imperative that the individual avoid sun exposure. The patient and caregiver must also be knowledgeable about the diagnosis and prognosis of the disease, the medication regimen, interactive effects with food and other medications, and the importance of communicating with the health care providers. Learning to cope with the disease, exacerbations, and prognosis involves psycho-social-spiritual support systems.

Evaluation of Outcomes

Refer to Table 42-1 for the nursing diagnoses, nursing interventions classifications, and nursing outcomes displayed for RA.

Progressive Systemic Sclerosis (Scleroderma)

Progressive systemic sclerosis is a rare connective tissue disease that involves excessive collagen deposition and changes in both the humoral and cellular immunity. Etiology is unknown. The localized form is less severe and primarily affects the skin. The morphea type skin lesions are hard, oval, and white with a purple ring surrounding them. Linear scleroderma has a lesion that is similar to a thick line of skin on the arms, legs, or forehead. That can become fixated to the subdermal structures, including the fascia that covers tendon sheaths and muscles.

Assessment with Clinical Manifestations

The generalized form involves the skin and many internal organs. Organs involved include the skin, the synovium, digital arteries, and parenchyma and small arteries in internal organs in the limited subcutaneous scleroderma form. The skin, muscles, joints, lungs, esophagus, heart, digestive system, and kidneys are often affected in the diffuse subcutaneous form, often termed as CREST. Clinical manifestations include:

- **C**alcinosis: The development of small white calcium deposits under the skin. A chalky fluid drains when the lumps break open.
- **R**aynaud's syndrome is prevalent in most patients with scleroderma. Spasms of arteries and arterioles occur spontaneously usually due to exposure to cold or emotional stress.
- **E**sophageal movement is decreased because of deposits of collagen and muscle atrophy.
- **S**clerodactyly of the fingers and toes.
- **T**elangiectasia: A permanent dilation of the capillaries, arterioles, and venules.

The localized form usually has a slow onset and clinical manifestations may not occur for 10 to 20 years. Clinical manifestations include pain, edema, calcification, and muscular atrophy. When the heart, lung, or kidney involvement is severe, it tends to occur early in the disease and often leads to high mortality.

Treatment is supportive and tailored to the clinical manifestations. The primary goal is to promote remission. Steroids and immunosuppressants in high doses are used. Nursing interventions include prevention of skin breakdown and ulceration. Patient education is directed toward proper skin care using gentle soaps and nonalchohol astringent lotions, and educating the patient how to manage the polyarthralgia and polyarthritis associated with Raynaud's phenomenon. Additional information includes avoiding activities that trigger pain, using protective joint strategies, avoiding extremes of cold, eliminating smoking, and resting the painful part during acute pain. Patients with esophageal dysfunction may require diet modifications. Ensuring that the patient continues follow-up care, and psycho-social-spiritual support is an important measure.

Case Study

Nursing Care Plan

Mrs. Donovan, has been HIV positive for nine years. She is in her primary health care provider's clinic complaining of intermittent nonbloody diarrhea and abdominal cramping that she has had for four weeks. In addition, she has a small burn wound on her right forearm that she states has not been healing well. She has lost 10 percent of her body weight in the past three weeks. She states, "I do not have the energy to eat or get dressed." On further questioning she said she has eaten primarily bread, cereal, milk, and potatoes.

Mrs. Donovan's vital signs are: blood pressure: 132/76; pulse: 78; respiration: 16; and temperature: 36.9° C (98.4° F). While at the clinic, Mrs. Donovan produces a stool specimen, and testing is performed for ova parasites, bacterial pathogens, *Clostridium difficile*, leukocytes, fecal fat, and D-xylose. Mrs. Donovan is educated as to appropriate nutritional habits and evaluated for dehydration symptomatology.

Assessment

Mrs. Donovan is a female patient with diarrhea, abdominal cramping, and a recent weight loss of 10 percent of her body weight. She has dry, scaly skin; pale conjunctiva; decreased hemoglobin, hematocrit, and mean corpuscular volume (MCV); decreased sodium, potassium, iron, and zinc; decreased serum albumin and transferrin; and a specific gravity of 1.028.

Nursing Diagnosis #1: Imbalanced Nutrition: Less than Body Requirements, related to inability to absorb nutrients because of HIV enteropathy.

NOC: Nutritional status; Nutritional status: Food and fluid intake; Nutritional status: Nutrient intake

NIC: Nutrition management; Electrolyte management; Enteral tube feeding; Nutrition therapy; Nutritional counseling; Nutritional monitoring; Weight gain assistance

Expected Outcomes

The patient will:

1. Receive adequate nutrients to meet metabolic needs.
2. Stabilize weight within 48 hours after initiation of nutrition support.

Case Study

3. Gain 0.25to 0.5 kg/wk.
4. Select a diet high in calcium, iron, protein, and calories.

Planning/Interventions/Rationale

1. Weigh daily; record hourly intake and output (I & O); monitor blood pressure, pulse, and respiration rate every hour, breath sounds, edema. *Monitors overall health status for changes, balance of fluid intake and output, and signs of deterioration.*
2. Utilize a nocturnal tube feeding to deliver formula. *Antidiarrheal agents (antimotility drugs) can be very effective in reducing most diarrhea within 24 to 48 hours when administered correctly.*
3. Obtain food preferences from patient and offer smaller frequent meals. *Facilitates digestion and improves energy levels.*
4. Record percentage of meals consumed. *Monitors accurate consumption of nutrients.*
5. Coordinate medication administration with their absorptive characteristics. *To decrease malabsorption.*

Evaluation

1. Fluid intake and output balanced; diarrhea subsided in 24 hours; and afebrile.
2. Laboratory values within normal limits 48 hours postadmission.
3. Weight stabilized within 48 hours and patient tolerating small frequent meals.
4. The patient was able to select food items as prescribed by the nutritional support team and gained 0.45 kg in eight days.

Nursing Diagnosis #2: Diarrhea related to opportunistic enteric pathogens secondary to HIV.

NOC: Bowel elimination; Electrolyte and acid-base balance; Fluid balance; Hydration

NIC: Diarrhea management

Expected Outcomes:

The patient will:

1. Report less diarrhea within 24 to 48 hours.
2. Describe contributing factors to the diarrhea episodes.
3. Increase signs of rehydration within 24 to 48 hours (e.g., moist mucous membranes and skin turgor).

Planning/Interventions/Rationale

1. Monitor vital signs every four hours. *Severe dehydration causes a febrile response, and decreased fluids can cause hypotension.*
2. Increase oral intake to maintain a normal urine specific gravity or to approximate volume of diarrhea losses. *Good indicator of renal function and severity of dehydration.*
3. Encourage liquids (water, apple juice, or flat ginger ale) and discontinue solids.
4. Gradually add semisolids and solids (crackers, yogurt, rice, bananas, or applesauce) as diarrhea improves. *Absorption increases as diarrhea subsides.*

Evaluation

Patient will begin to show increased signs of hydration as diarrhea episodes decrease.

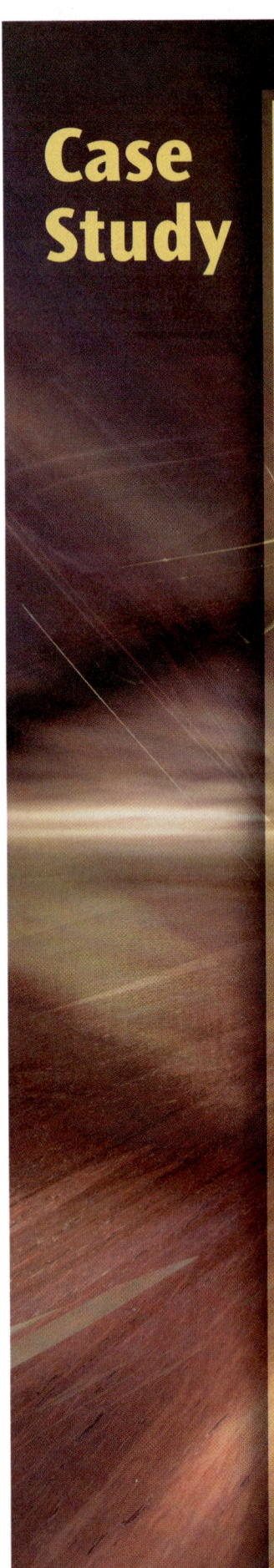

KEY CONCEPTS

- The immune system is vital to the human body as related to its processes for recognizing and protecting the body.
- The immune system provides the body with surveillance methods of protection against external threats to the body, such as viruses, bacteria, and other foreign substances, and to internal threats including abnormal tumor cells that develop.
- Normally, CD4+ T cells orchestrate the immune system process in responding to foreign antigens.
- The immune system may also have undesirable effects when the body recognizes allergens or self-tissue as abnormal or nonself.
- Immunodeficiency disorders are due to dysfunction or impairment of one or more of the immune response mechanisms. The mechanisms include phagocytosis, humoral response, B cell- and T cell-mediated response or combination, the complement system, and a combined cell and humoral response.
- The clinical hallmark of immune deficiency is a propensity to unusual or recurrent severe infections.
- The etiology of many of the immune disorders is unknown. A complete history and physical examination are important components of the diagnostic process. A definitive diagnosis may take months to years as new symptoms appear.
- Many factors are involved that cause the immune system to fail to recognize the body's normal tissue as self, including genetic predisposition, infections, interaction of T and B cells, introduction of foreign tissue, such as a blood transfusion or transplant tissue, and environmental factors.
- Organs and tissues commonly affected by autoimmune disorders include blood components, such as RBCs, blood vessels, connective tissues, endocrine glands such as the thyroid or pancreas, muscles, joints, and skin. Most of the autoimmune disorders are associated with the connective tissues of the body.
- The patient plays an important role in planning and adhering to the treatment regimen.
- The goals in managing a chronic disease are to prevent or slow disease progression, managing existing comorbidity symptoms and complications, undergoing therapeutic procedures, rehabilitation activities, managing medications, and all the activities of daily living.
- Some of the greatest challenges are to assist the individual in coping with a chronic and life-threatening disease, overcoming fear, and minimizing spiritual distress.

REVIEW QUESTIONS

1. During the early stages of a chronic disease, patients tend to focus on:
   1. Medication schedule
   2. Interpretation of symptoms
   3. Impact of lifestyle changes
   4. Understanding the disease process

2. The goal of HAART is to:
   1. Minimize side affects of the drugs
   2. Encourage patient compliance to the medication schedule
   3. Lower the CD4 cell levels
   4. Avoid viral resistance for each drug

3. Early clinical manifestations of GVHD include:
   1. Respiratory problems, i.e., interstitial pneumonitis
   2. Skin rash and pruritus
   3. Taut, firm, leather-like skin
   4. Dry lacrimal ducts and oral mucosa

4. Monoclonal antibodies are:
   1. B-cell antibodies developed against a foreign antigen
   2. Defective T-cell antibodies that do not recognize self tissue
   3. Genetically engineered immunosuppressant drugs
   4. Used in vaccines to assist in preventing infections

5. Hypersensitivity disorders are due to a (an):
   1. Immune deficiency disorder, such as HIV
   2. Autoimmune disorder, such as RA
   3. Heightened immune response to an antigen
   4. Desensitization of humoral immune components

Continued

REVIEW QUESTIONS—cont'd

6. The reversible form of SLE is due to reaction to drugs that are known to bind with the individual's DNA, such as:
   1. Beta blockers, such as Inderal
   2. Oral contraceptives, such as Levora
   3. Antibiotics, such as tetracycline
   4. Antimalarials, such as Plaquenil
7. Cell-mediated immunity is initiated by:
   1. Specific antigen recognition by T cells
   2. Nonspecific antigen recognition by B cells
   3. Release of complement cells into the blood stream
   4. Release of cytokines from white blood cells
8. Passive immunity involves:
   1. Transfer of antibodies through the heart of the mother to fetus
   2. Inoculation with vaccine containing live or killed infectious organisms
   3. Development of sensitized lymphocytes within the host body
   4. Response of memory cells to entry of an infectious organism
9. Sero-conversion is the presence of antibodies of HIV in the blood are detected by diagnostic studies with in:
   1. One to two weeks after exposure to HIV
   2. One to three months or more after exposure to HIV
   3. One month following the start of antiretroviral drug therapy
   4. Six months when immune-antibody complexes are formed
10. Criteria used to diagnose AIDS in an individual with HIV include at least one of the following conditions:
   1. CD4+ cell count above 200 cells/μL
   2. Anemia due to diminished RBC count
   3. Dysfunction of one or more organs
   4. Development of an opportunistic cancer

REVIEW ACTIVITIES

1. Review a case study related to HIV/AIDS. Role-play how you would assess a patient who is HIV positive on your assigned clinical unit. Formulate a nursing care plan and teaching plan for the patient in the case study.
2. Divide into small groups. Using a diagnostic studies text, research information and provide a report to entire group on the following tests: ELISA, Western blot technique, and T4 helper lymphocytes (CD4 cells). Include information that should be given to the patient and caregiver. Discuss the nurse's role regarding preparation for the procedure, in patient education, and in discussions with the health care team in planning interventions related to the diagnostic report.
3. Access the CDC National Prevention Information Network (NPIN) at: http://www.cdcnpin.org.

   Review the guidelines and recommendations for NIV/AIDS listed by category (community, counseling and testing, evaluation, patient care, prevention, surveillance, treatment and traveler's health). Write a report indicating what you see as the nurse's role in each of these categories.
4. Many patients with chronic immune diseases are perceived as demanding and manipulative. Consider some of the alternative measures (in addition to ones mentioned in the chapter) that can be used to help them cope with chronic pain and the disruption to their lives. Provide the rationale for their use.
5. Many persons diagnosed with an immune disorder continue to work, manage the household, care for children, or participate in social activities.
   a. Prepare information that contains guidelines for protection from infectious diseases.
   b. Locate the policy at your clinical facility regarding the procedures to follow when an employee is accidentally exposed to blood and other fluids of a person with HIV or AIDS diagnosis.
6. Research at least two immune disorders listed in Table 43-2 that have not been discussed in this chapter. Prepare a report that includes the etiology, clinical manifestations, collaborative, and nursing management. Document anticipated outcomes using the NOC classification system.

CHAPTER 43

Allergic Dysfunction: Nursing Management

Linda Meuleveld, BA, RN, COHN-S, CCM, DABFN, VPS

CHAPTER TOPICS

- Immune System
- Allergic Dysfunction
- Pathophysiology of Allergic Reactions
- Types of Hypersensitivity
- Management of Patients with Allergic Disorders
- Atopic Asthma
- Prevention and Management of Anaphylaxis
- Allergic Disorders According to Type and Character

KEY TERMS

Allergen
Anaphylaxis
Angioneurotic edema
Antigen
Atopic dermatitis (AD)
Atopy
Autoantibody
Contact dermatitis
Hereditary angioedema (HAE)
Histamine
Hypersensitive response
Latex allergy
Pruritus
Serum sickness
Stridor
Urticaria
Wheezing

Diseases related to allergic dysfunction affect more than 50 million Americans. Common allergic diseases include allergic rhinitis, latex allergy, atopic dermatitis, food allergy, drug allergy, and allergy to venom of stinging insects. According to the National Institute of Allergy and Infectious diseases, allergies are the sixth leading cause of chronic disease in the United States, costing the health care system $18 billion annually. While the true number of deaths from drug reactions is unknown, anaphylactic reactions to penicillin occur in 32 of every 100,000 patients (American Academy of Allergy, Asthma, and Immunology, 2006).

ALLERGIC DYSFUNCTION

Allergic dysfunction is an altered response of the human body's natural defense against attack by microorganisms. When unfamiliar substances are identified and destroyed or inactivated, the body is performing a normal adaptive immune response. These immune responses fall into three categories shown in Table 43-1.

Immune responses are triggered when foreign substances called **antigens,** substances capable of stimulating an immune response, are identified by the immune system. The immune system has the ability to remember antigens from a primary immune response and respond quickly with a secondary response when the antigen is reintroduced. The immune system must also be able to distinguish between body proteins and foreign proteins to direct its attack toward the invading organism. The ability to recognize self from nonself is an important. Recognition is one of the four R's of immune response:

- Recognize self from nonself and triggering a response only when threatened by foreign invaders.
- Respond to nonself invaders by producing antibodies.
- Remember the invader so that there can be a quicker response if a subsequent invasion is detected.
- Regulate its action by turning on for the invader and turning off when the invader is destroyed.

Genetics

Genetics play a role in the way a person responds to invading organisms. **Atopy** is a personal or familial tendency to become sensitized and produce immunoglobulin E (IgE) antibodies in response to ordinary exposure to allergens. As a consequence, atopic individuals can be said to have a genetic predisposition to produce a prolonged IgE antibody response to allergens that are found in the general environment, such as pollens, dust mites, and molds. Atopy is a clinical definition that describes an IgE antibody high responder.

Red Flag

Emphasize History of Allergies

When a patient mentions that he or she has allergies, the comment is a significant contribution to the medical history. It would be appropriate to discuss family history of allergies. Atopic individuals may have multiple allergies.

Pathophysiology

Most antigens are composed of proteins. All body cells have antigens on their surface. These antigens are unique to the individual and help the immune system differentiate between self and invader.

When a person is exposed to an **allergen,** a substance that induces an allergic reaction, for the first time, the immune system reacts protectively. The immune system initiates a series of biochemical and cellular events that translate into clinical symptoms. These events involve antigens, antibodies, release of **histamine** (a hormone that causes vasodilation and an increase in permeability of blood vessel walls), and varying response times, depending on the

TABLE 43-1 Immune Responses

IMMUNE CATEGORY	RESPONSE/ACTION
Defense	Resisting invasion by foreign microorganisms
Homeostasis	Removing damaged cells
Surveillance	Recognizing and removing mutated cells

Adapted from Janeway, C. A., Jr., Travers, P., Walport, M., & Shlomchik, M. J. (2004). Immunobiology, the immune system in health and disease *(6th ed.). New York: Garland Science Publishing.*

person and the exposure. Histamine is a chemical produced by the body during allergic reactions (Janeway, Travers, Walport, & Shlomchik, 2004).

Antibodies circulate in the bloodstream and are present in almost all body fluids. When allergens first enter the body of a person predisposed to allergies, a series of reactions will occur that produce allergen-specific IgE antibodies. The IgE antibodies travel to cells, called mast cells, soon after they are produced. Large quantities of mast cells are found in the connective tissue of the nose, eyes, lungs, and gastrointestinal (GI) tract. IgE antibodies attach themselves to the mast cells and wait for their particular antigen to appear.

Primary and Second Response

The response to an allergen may be immediate or delayed. These responses are called the primary and secondary immune response (Figure 43-1). These two responses are immunoglobulin M (IgM) and immunoglobulin G (IgG). They are two classes of immunoglobulin the body produces in response to an antigen. IgM predominates in the primary phase, with IgG appearing later. On a subsequent exposure to the same antigen, in a secondary response, some IgM and large amounts of IgG are produced.

Antibodies are members of a class of proteins known as immunoglobulins, which are produced by B lymphocytes in response to an antigen. They are used by the immune system to neutralize foreign objects. Each antibody recognizes a specific antigen unique to its target. An antibody is specific to an antigen and is a primary immune defense.

IgE Response

After repeated low-dose exposure to allergens, atopic individuals develop specific IgE antibodies to the allergens. Subsequent exposure initiates a secondary humoral response. IgE molecules specific to an antigen attach to cell surface receptors on mast cells. The mast cell's response includes the release of histamine. The release of histamine creates the clinical manifestations of an allergic reaction.

Early Response

Within minutes after exposure of an allergic subject to antigen, an immediate (early) response follows. In the upper airway, the allergic individual begins to sneeze, which is followed closely by an increase in nasal secretions. After about five minutes mucosal swelling begins, leading to reduced airflow. These physiological changes are associated with increases in histamine, leukotrienes, prostaglandins, tryptase, and other proinflammatory mediators.

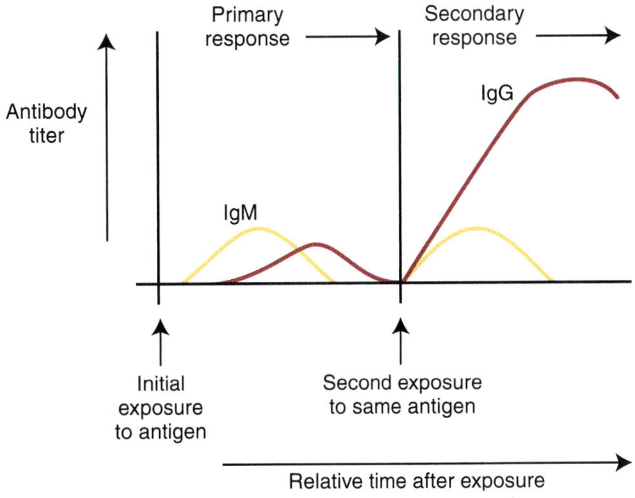

Figure 43-1 Primary and secondary immune responses. Following the initial exposure to a foreign antigen, the primary immune response, IgM, develops gradually. When the antigen is encountered a second time, it triggers a secondary response. In the secondary response large amounts of IgG are rapidly produced.

Late Response

Other than the immediate response to antigen, another response begins hours later. The late response does not occur in everyone. It appears to be dose related. The primary manifestation is airway obstruction.

Diagnostic Tests

The physicians most qualified to treat allergic diseases are allergists and immunologists. Diagnosis begins with a detailed medical history and physical examination. If indicated, a skin allergy test will be done, and blood testing may be done to determine the allergen causing the reaction. When the triggers are identified, a treatment program can be established. The first step in treatment is to minimize exposure to the identified allergen. Medications may be prescribed to reduce allergic symptoms and inflammation.

Nursing Diagnoses

This chapter will examine a variety of allergic disorders, and the specific treatment strategies for each will be presented. These sections will also include nursing diagnoses. However, the following are examples of general nursing diagnoses that are examples in the patient with allergic dysfunction and may include the following. (Note: the evaluation of outcomes will be presented as they apply in the diseases that follow in this chapter):

- Ineffective breathing pattern.
- Ineffective coping related to anxiety, lower activity level, and the inability to perform normal activities of daily living.
- Activity intolerance related to fatigue.
- Fear and anxiety related to actual or potential lifestyle changes.

TYPES OF HYPERSENSITIVITY

The immune system will normally react to protect people in the presence of a foreign antigen. The person with a hypersensitive reaction will have one of four types of reaction, as shown in Table 43-2.

An exaggerated or misdirected immune response to an allergen that results in tissue injury is called a **hypersensitive response.** These are classified in the Gell-Coombs spectrum of human hypersensitivity.

Type 1 Hypersensitivity

The type 1 hypersensitive reaction is an immediate type of hypersensitivity reaction. This reaction occurs when a specific antigen induces an allergic reaction, provoked by reexposure to the same antigen. The contact, inhalation,

TABLE 43-2 Hypersensitive Reactions: Gell Coombs Classification

TYPE	NAME	REACTION
Type 1	Anaphylactic	Allergic rhinitis, asthma
Type 2	Cytotoxic	Transfusion reaction
Type 3	Immune complex	Systemic lupus erythematosus Rheumatoid arthritis
Type 4	Delayed hypersensitive	Transplant rejection reaction

Adapted from Janeway, C. A., Jr., Travers, P., Walport, M., Shlomchik, M. J. (2004). Immunobiology, the immune system in health and disease *(6th ed.). New York: Garland Science Publishing.*

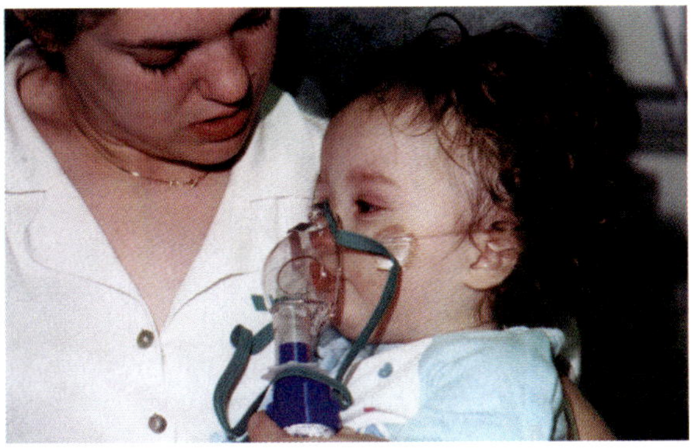

Figure 43-2 A child has experienced an allergenic crisis and is continuing to be treated with nebulizer medications via a mask to deliver the inhalants.

ingestion, or injection of the allergen creates an allergic reaction mediated by specific IgE antibodies, the cellular release of histamine, and other vasoactive mediators, resulting in an immediate local or systemic reaction **(anaphylaxis)**.

The immediate type of hypersensitivity reaction may occur locally or systemically. The symptoms may range from mild to sudden death due to anaphylactic shock. Clinical examples include allergic rhinitis, allergic asthma, atopic dermatitis, and systemic anaphylaxis. When the patient has respiratory symptoms, there is a higher incidence of morbidity and mortality (Figure 43-2). Fatal and near fatal anaphylactic reactions can be traced to reexposure to foods, such as peanuts and drugs, such as penicillin or insulin. Hypersensitivity usually appears on repeated contact with the allergen (Box 43-1).

Type 2 Hypersensitivity

Type 2 hypersensitivity reactions are cytotoxic reactions where the antibody (IgG or IgM) is directed against antigen on an individual's own cells or against foreign antibody, such as that acquired after blood transfusion. This may lead to cytotoxic action by killer cells or to lysis mediated by the complement system. Cytotoxic reactions are serious and potentially life-threatening (Box 43-2).

Type 3 Hypersensitivity

Type 3 hypersensitivity reactions are immune complex reactions where immune complexes (antigen and usually IgG or IgM) are deposited in the tissue. The complement is activated causing local tissue damage and inflammation. The types of disease encountered are classified into acute and chronic serum sickness and local inflammatory response due to deposition of immune complexes in tissues (the Arthus reaction) (Box 43-3).

Type 4 Hypersensitivity

Type 4 hypersensitivity reactions are cell-mediated reactions, which are also called delayed hypersensitivity. Allergic contact dermatitis after exposure to ointments containing active drugs is the most frequent form of drug-mediated delayed hypersensitivity. Various forms of type 4 hypersensitivity are recognized: contact hypersensitivity, tuberculin-type hypersensitivity, and granulomatous hypersensitivity. Examples of diseases manifesting type 4 granulomatous hypersensitivity are Crohn's disease, leprosy, tuberculosis, sarcoidosis, and schistosomiasis.

Autoantibodies can also cause disease. An **autoantibody** is an antibody that reacts against a person's own tissue. They are organ specific. Systemic lupus erythematosus is an example of an autoimmune disease that is non–organ specific in that it is characterized by damage to multiple organs. Examples of diseases in humans caused by autoantibodies are autoimmune hemolytic anemia, autoimmune thrombocytopenic purpura, bulbous pemphigoid, glomerulonephritis (Goodpasture's syndrome), Graves' disease (hyperthyroidism), insulin-resistant diabetes mellitus, myasthenia gravis, pemphigus vulgaris, and pernicious anemia.

Atopy and allergy are not interchangeable terms. Atopy refers to an individual being prone to develop allergies because of a genetic state of hyperresponsiveness to sensitizing agents. It is associated with conditions such as asthma, allergic rhinitis (hay fever), and atopic dermatitis (allergic dermatitis). Allergy refers to the hypersensitivity that occurs on reexposure to a sensitizing allergen, causing the release of histamine and other inflammatory mediators.

Sensitizing agents can enter the body through various routes. They may be airborne and are breathed in; they may come in contact with the skin or

BOX 43-1

EXAMPLES OF TYPE 1 ALLERGIC REACTIONS

Anaphylaxis
Atopic asthma
Atopic eczema
Drug allergy
Hay fever

Adapted from Guillet, G., Guillet, M., & Dagregorio, G. (2005). Allergic contact dermatitis from natural rubber latex in atopic dermatitis and the risk of later type I allergy. Contact Dermatitis, 53*(1), 46–51.*

BOX 43-2

DISEASES MANIFESTING TYPE 2 HYPERSENSITIVITY

Autoimmune hemolytic anemia
Goodpasture's syndrome
Hemolytic disease of the newborn
Myasthenia gravis
Pemphigus

Adapted from Heidary, N., & Cohen, D. Hypersensitivity reactions to vaccine components. Dermatitis, 16*(3), 115–120.*

LAW IN PRACTICE

A Drug Side Effect or Hypersensitivity Reaction?

A 14-year-old girl was admitted for observation with the diagnosis of a rash related to antibiotic (amoxicillin) use. Three days earlier her parents had taken her to the doctor with complaints of a sore throat, cervical lymphadenopathy, and general malaise. The physician noted that the patient had a temperature elevation of 100.2° F (37.9°C). The patient was concerned that she would be too ill to take a trip a week away with her class during spring break. The physician responded to parental pressure by ordering amoxicillin. After three days, the parents brought their daughter to the emergency department with a rash covering most of her body. They were sure she was having a reaction to the oral penicillin she had been taking. The last dose of amoxicillin had been taken that morning.

The patient was diagnosed with mononucleosis (Epstein-Barr virus). The amoxicillin had been ordered to diminish the effects of a presumed bacterial infection. The patient was actually suffering from a viral infection that would not respond to an antibiotic.

The rash was not a symptom of penicillin allergy and did not indicate a future adverse reaction to penicillin. This fact was related to the patient by both the physician and the nurse assigned to the patient.

At a later date the patient was treated with penicillin for an infection and experienced an anaphylactic (type 1) reaction. She recovered, but her family sued the physician for prescribing penicillin when the patient had a previous allergic reaction to penicillin. Because the nurse had explained to the family that the patient's rash was a side effect of amoxicillin, and not an allergic reaction to penicillin, she was also named in the suit. The case was settled out of court.

The earlier rash and the new penicillin allergy were not related. It is unfortunate for the patient that she developed an allergy to penicillin. The new drug allergy was not a consequence of the earlier rash. It is possible, however, for an atopic individual to be more prone to the development of allergies.

The nurse in this case delivered appropriate information to the patient and her family regarding the earlier rash and the amoxicillin. Nurses must be 100 percent confident of their knowledge when relaying information to patients and their families. Appropriate documentation of the conversation with the family by the nurse provided the only source of information regarding relay of information to the family and validated the nurses' comments.

Adapted from Janeway, C. A., Jr., Travers, P., Walport, M., & Shlomchik, M. J. (2004). Immunobiology, the immune system in health and disease *(6th ed.). New York: Garland Science Publishing.*

BOX 43-3

EXAMPLES OF HUMAN IMMUNE COMPLEX DISEASES

Polyarteritis nodosa

Poststreptococcal glomerulonephritis

Systemic lupus erythematosus

Adapted from Janeway, C. A., Jr., Travers, P., Walport, M., & Shlomchik, M. J. (2004). Immunobiology, the immune system in health and disease *(6th ed.). New York: Garland Science Publishing.*

mucous membranes. They may be swallowed and enter the GI system. They may enter the skin through injection or other means (Table 43-3).

Assessment with Clinical Manifestations

There are many elements of the nursing assessment in patients with allergic disorders. In addition, these patients also have many clinical manifestations. The nursing assessment is primarily divided into objective and subjective data as shown in Box 43-4.

Planning and Implementation

An altered immune system can manifest itself in many ways, but allergic, type 1 hypersensitive reactions (allergies), are the most common. Most of these allergies are chronic and are distinguished by remissions and exacerbations. Allergy treatment for chronic allergies focuses on a variety of issues. Initially, the nurse can help the patient make lifestyle changes to help the patient adjust to minimal allergen exposures. Next, the nurse should also reinforce the thought that medication and desensitization will only reduce the immune

TABLE 43-3 Categories of Sensitizing Agents (Allergens)

AIRBORNE (RESPIRATORY)	CONTACT (SKIN, MUCOUS MEMBRANE)	INGESTED (GI)	INJECTED (PERCUTANEOUS)
Pollens: plants, grasses, trees	Plants	Foods: egg, milk, peanut, shellfish, soy wheat, and nuts	Drugs
Pollens: plants, grasses, trees	Plants	Foods: soy wheat, and nuts	Drugs
Mold: fungal spores	Drugs	Drugs	Vaccines
Dust mites	Metals		Insect stings
Animal dander	Cosmetics		
House dust	Fibers, latex, chemicals		

Adapted from Janeway, C. A., Jr., Travers, P., Walport, M., & Shlomchik, M. J. (2004). Immunobiology, the immune system in health and disease *(6th ed.). New York: Garland Science Publishing; Mohapatra, S., Lockey, R., & Shirley, S. (2005). Immunobiology of grass pollen allergens.* Current Allergy and Asthma Reports, 5*(5), 381–387.*

Skills 360°

Prevention and Asthma

Asthma is a serious and growing health problem. An estimated 14.9 million people in the United States have asthma and are at risk for serious chronic or immediate illness. Asthma is responsible for about 500,000 hospitalizations, 5,000 deaths, and 134 million days of restricted activity a year. Yet most of the problems caused by asthma could be averted if people with asthma and their health care providers managed the disease according to established guidelines. These prevention efforts are essential to interrupt the progression from disease to functional limitation and disability and to improve the quality of life for people with asthma.

Adapted from Ait-Khaled, N., & Enarson, D. (2006). Management of asthma: The essentials of good clinical practice. International Journal of Tuberculosis and Lung Disease, 10*(2), 133–137.*

BOX 43-4

ASSESSMENT OF ALLERGIC DISORDERS

Objective Data

- Rash: location, symmetry, skin dryness, irritation, scratches, scaly skin, and urticaria (hives)
- Respiratory: wheezing or strider and shortness of breath
- Eyes: conjunctivitis, lacrimation, excessive rubbing, and blinking
- Ears: diminished hearing, immobile, or scarred tympanic membrane
- Nose: rhinitis, sniffling, sneezing, and swollen nasal passages
- Throat: continual throat clearing, red throat, swollen lips or tongue, or palpable lymph nodes in neck

Subjective Data

- Health information, health history, respiratory problems, seasonal exacerbations, and past allergies
- Medications: unusual reactions and OTC medications for allergies

Adapted from Estes, M. (2006). Health assessment and physical examination *(3rd ed.). New York: Thomson Delmar Learning.*

response to the allergen and help moderate the expectation of a symptom-free future. In addition, management of hypersensitivity reactions can include skin testing, and exploration of food allergies can also be identified though an elimination diet. Last, emotional stress and fatigue can intensify an allergic reaction. The nurse can be influential in helping the patient learn stress management and relaxation techniques, such as imagery and deep breathing.

ATOPIC ASTHMA

Asthma is a common inflammatory disease of the airways that causes airway hyperresponsiveness, mucous production, and mucosal edema. Asthma leads to recurrent episodes of clinical manifestations, such as cough, chest tightness, respiratory wheezing, and dyspnea. Asthma differs from other obstructive disorders in that it is largely reversible, either with management or spontaneously.

Epidemiology

Atopic asthma is the most common form of asthma. According to the National Institute of Environmental Health Sciences, of the 17 million asthma sufferers in the United States, 10 million (approximately 60 percent) have atopic asthma. Three million are children, and 7 million are adults.

Etiology

Most patients with asthma also suffer from other allergic disorders. In fact, research from the World Health Organization shows that at least 70 percent of asthmatics also suffer from allergic rhinitis or hay fever. Nasal allergies and allergic asthma are both triggered by exposure to allergens, initiating a series of events that result in tightening of the airways, swelling of the lining of the airways, nose and eyes, and mucous production.

Atopic (extrinsic) asthma typically develops in childhood. Eighty percent of children with asthma have other allergies. Typically there is a family history of allergies. Other conditions, such as hay fever or eczema, are also present. Atopic asthma experienced in childhood often goes into remission in early adulthood, only to appear at a later age.

Pathophysiology

IgE plays a critical role in the allergic process. When an individual is sensitized to an allergen, such as pollen or animal dander, he or she produces an IgE antibody directed against that allergen. The IgE antibody attaches to mast cells. When the individual is exposed to that same allergen again, the allergen binds to the IgE on the mast cell causing it to release substances, such as histamine, prostaglandins, and leukotrienes, which cause symptoms, such as chest tightness, coughing and **wheezing** (a whistling sound when breathing out related to airway constriction).

Deaths from asthma have been declining in all categories but children younger than age 5. In this age range the asthma death rate has increased from 1.7 per million in 1999 to 2.1 per million in 2003.

Assessment with Clinical Manifestations

The clinical manifestations of atopic asthma include wheezing (rhinorrhea and rash [urticaria]). There will be a drop in the peak flow expiratory rate. When asthma symptoms are under control, the airways are open, and it is possible to force more air into the peak flow meter. When the airways are inflamed and constricted, it is not possible to blow as hard into the meter, making the peak flow rate lower.

Patients with allergic asthma may experience:

- Shortness of breath (SOB) with exertion or late at night.
- Coughing that may become chronic. It is usually worse at night, after exercise, or when breathing is exposed to cold, dry air.
- Chest tightness.

Prolonged attacks that don't respond to treatment with bronchodilators are a medical emergency and require emergency care. The nurse plays a vital role in evaluating patients for potential allergic reaction. A thorough nursing assessment should include discussion of subjective data such as:

Health information that discusses health history.

Respiratory problems, past allergies, and seasonal exacerbations.

Respecting Our Differences

Ethnicity and Asthma Acute Care Admissions

Studies have shown that minority children (defined as African American and Hispanic [American]) have more hospitalizations and have more frequent emergency department visits than other groups. The study confirms that emergency departments serve as a safety net for children with asthma during exacerbations, particularly disadvantaged minorities. Evidence suggests that education and supportive programs can help improve outcomes for these children of different ethnic backgrounds.

Adapted from Ait-Khaled, N., & Enarson, D. (2006). Management of asthma: The essentials of good clinical practice. International Journal of Tuberculosis and Lung Disease, *10(2), 133–137; Boudreaus, E., Edmond, S., & Race (2003). Ethnicity and asthma among children presenting to the emergency department.* Pediatrics III, *(5), e615–e621.*

PATIENT PLAYBOOK

Triggers for Asthma

The nurse can instruct the patient to avoid triggers for asthma in the following ways:

- Pollen: Keep windows and doors closed, and use air conditioning to keep pollen out.
- Dust mites: Use special coverings for mattresses and pillows. Remove carpets, rugs and drapery in bedrooms. Wash bedding in hot water.
- Toys should not include stuffed animals.
- Keep humidity between 30 and 40 percent.
- Use a vacuum cleaner with a filter. Change filter and bag often.
- Animal hair and dander: Pet removal is best. If around pets, keep them out of bedrooms and off furniture.
- Mold: Try to eliminate mold in the environment. Dehumidifiers can help. Avoid freshly cut grass.
- Environment: Avoid cigarette smoke and all other types of smoke. When outdoor air quality is poor, stay indoors. Cover the nose and mouth during cold weather.
- Exercise: Perform slow warm-ups and cool-downs and be sure to use asthma medication approximately 10 minutes before beginning an exercise routine.

Adapted from Broyles, B. E., Reiss, B. S., & Evans, M. E. (2007). Pharmacological aspects of nursing care *(7th ed.). New York: Thomson Delmar Learning; DeLaune, S., & Ladner, P. (2006).* Fundamentals of Nursing *(3rd ed.). New York: Thomson Delmar Learning.*

Skin rashes, past or present.

Unusual reactions to medications: OTC, medications for allergies and medications, vitamins, and health remedies taken over the previous two weeks.

Perceptions of health and family history.

Difficulties with malaise, fatigue, food intolerances, itching, or vomiting.

The physical exam with suspected allergic dysfunction should include observation of:

Skin: The presence of a rash should be noted, with a description that includes location, symmetry, skin dryness, irritation, scratches, scaly skin, urticaria (hives), or **pruritus** (itching).

Breathing: Listen for wheezing or stridor. Wheezing is the expiratory sound produced by the turbulent flow of air through constricted small airways (bronchioles). **Stridor** is the audible symptom produced by the rapid turbulent flow of air through a narrowed segment of the respiratory tract.

Eyes: Conjunctivitis, excessive rubbing and blinking, or lacrimation.

Ears: There may be complaints of diminished hearing and immobile or scarred tympanic membranes.

Nose: Rhinitis (inflammation of the mucous membrane that lines the nose) sneezing, sniffling, or swollen nasal passages.

Throat: Constant throat clearing, red throat, swollen lips or tongue, or palpable lymph nodes in the neck.

Diagnostic Tests

To determine presence of asthma, the clinician must determine that periodic problems with airway obstruction are present, that airflow is at least partially reversible, and that other etiologies have been ruled out. Family history, potential environmental factors (e.g., air pollution, high pollen counts, or molds) and comorbid factors (drug-induced asthma or gastroesophageal reflux) may accompany asthma. In addition the presence of various allergic reactions can be tied to asthma (eczema, rashes, or temporary edema). Any of the aforementioned variables may be used as diagnostic criteria for the presence of asthma.

Identification of the specific allergen provoking the reaction is pursued at some future point, when the allergic reaction is in remission. The gold standard for establishing allergen specific IgE antibodies is the skin-prick test (SPT). With this test a drop of allergen is applied to an intradermal prick. Positive results are indicated by a characteristic "wheal and flare" response. Use of certain medications can interfere with the validity of a skin-prick response. These include antihistamines, benzodiazepines, theophylline, and antidepressants. Corticosteroids have no effect on the SPT.

Nursing Diagnoses

Based on the information gathered, examples of nursing diagnoses in the patient with asthma may include the following:

- Ineffective breathing pattern related to SOB, mucus, and airway irritants.
- Impaired gas exchange related to ventilation-perfusion inequality.
- Ineffective coping related to anxiety, lower activity level, and the inability to perform normal activities of daily living.

Planning and Implementation

The management for asthma is heavily focused on patient education. Patient and family teaching is related to the prevention of asthmatic attacks through patient and family communication. The patient education includes a discussion of learning to anticipate triggers and practicing avoidance. Asthma triggers irritate the lungs and produce mucus, inflammation, and tightening of the bronchial tubes. Common triggers for asthma are shown in the patient playbook. In addition, there continue to be numerous research studies for the management of atopic asthma, and the future is promising for the continued advancement of the treatment of this condition (see Fast Forward feature).

The therapeutic management of asthma utilizes a balance among the diagnostic variables, the acute therapies for asthma, and the prevention or maintenance care of the patient (Table 43-4; Skills 360° feature).

Fast Forward ▶▶▶

Future Management of Atopic Asthma

Researchers are targeting new forms of treatment for atopic asthma. Future therapies may focus on cytokines, substances that maintain the chronic inflammation responsible for asthma. Other research may also lead to the development of new anti-inflammatory drugs, which may retain the anti-inflammatory effects of corticosteroids but cause fewer systemic side effects.

Adapted from Broyles, B. E., Reiss, B. S., & Evans, M. E. (2007). Pharmacological aspects of nursing care *(7th ed.). New York: Thomson Delmar Learning.*

TABLE 43-4 Therapeutic Management of Asthma

Diagnostic	Health history and physical exam Pulmonary function studies Bronchodilator therapy response Chest X-ray Pin prick test when indicated Sputum specimen (r/o bacterial infection) Blood level IgE, eosinophils
Treatment: Acute asthma	Inhaled beta-adrenergic drugs O_2 per mask or nasal prongs IV medications (e.g., corticosteroids, aminophylline) Nebulized or inhaled anticholinergic agents Increased fluid intake (oral plus IV to 3,000 mL Intubation and assisted ventilation, as indicated
Prevention and maintenance	Eliminate triggers Desensitization (if indicated) Follow prescribed drug regimen Trigger assessment of home and work Progressive plan for exercise

Adapted from Broyles, B. E., Reiss, B. S., & Evans, M. E. (2007). Pharmacological aspects of nursing care *(7th ed.). New York: Thomson Delmar Learning.*

PATIENT PLAYBOOK

Prevention of Serious Allergen Responses

The nurse can instruct the patient to prevent allergen responses by the following:

- The type of allergen influences the method of management needed.
- The nurse can help the patient, and other family members, to explore ways of avoiding allergen exposure by altering contact with specific allergens, such as pets, pollens, foods, or medications.
- The nurse can recommend the wearing of a medical alert bracelet.
- The nurse can make sure the allergen is listed prominently in all medical and dental records. The patient should also be encouraged to notify any other medical providers of the allergy

Adapted from Amado, M., & Portnoy, J. (2006). Recent advances in asthma management. Missouri Medicine, *103(1), 60–64.*

Skills 360°

Health Promotion for Patients with Asthma

Health care management of illnesses focuses on diagnosis and treatment. This is an important component of the care plan for the patient experiencing an allergic reaction, such as allergic asthma. Treatment is directed toward reducing symptoms and regaining normal activities of daily living. This approach is necessary, but there is a new interest in creating and implementing effective health management and disease prevention programs, that would enable the patient with asthma to avoid becoming symptomatic. Research done by the Centers for Disease Control (CDC) indicates that an estimated 50 percent of an individual's health status is governed by lifestyle behaviors. Nurses play an important role in communicating to their patients' ways of pursuing healthy behaviors that will keep the patient's allergies from becoming symptomatic.

Adapted from Ait-Khaled, N., & Enarson, D. Management of asthma: The essentials of good clinical practice. International Journal of Tuberculosis and Lung Disease, *10(2), 133–137; Amado, M., & Portnoy, J. Recent advances in asthma management.* Missouri Medicine, *103(1), 60–64.*

Pharmacology

Medications are effective in managing asthma by reversing and treating bronchospasm, inflammation, and mucous clearance. A wide variety of medications are used to treat asthma and are shown in Tables 43-5 and 43-6.

Drug therapy is an effective treatment for symptom relief. The major categories of drugs for symptom relief of chronic allergies include antihistamines, decongestants, multidose inhalants (Figure 43-3), corticosteroids, antipyretics, and mast cell stabilizers. The nurse can caution the patient about the many side effects associated with their use (Box 43-5).

Hyposensitization

When the allergen cannot be avoided and drug therapy is not effective, immunotherapy is recommended to reduce the level of sensitivity. It is a process in which small amounts of an allergen extract is administered in increasing dosages until hyposensitivity is achieved. Hyposensitization is indicated for individuals with anaphylactic reactions to insect venom (hymenoptera). Complete desensitization is not possible, and the nurse should instruct the patient to continue to avoid the offending allergen (Muller & Golden, 2004).

TABLE 43-5 Pharmacology Facts: Pharmaceutical Therapy for Asthma

CLASSIFICATION	DRUG	REACTION	COMMENT
Beta-adrenergic agonist Inhaled bronchodilator Systemic bronchodilator	Albuterol (Proventil, Ventolin), Metaproterenol (Alupent, Metaprel).	Relax bronchospasm bronchodilation Increases mucociliary clearance	Contraindicated with cardiac disorders Slow reaction
Corticosteroid Anti-inflammatory medications	Hydrocortisone (Solu-Cortef), Methylprednisolone (Medrol and Solu-Medrol), Prednisone	Reduce inflammation Decreases edema in bronchi Decrease mucous secretions	Side effects; skin changes, obesity, muscle weakness
Leukotriene modifier (a new class of anti-inflammatory recently FDA approved)	Zafirlukast (Accolate) Zileuton (Zyflo)	Inhibit the allergic process	Throat irritation Possible bronchospasm

Adapted from Broyles, B. E., Reiss, B. S., & Evans, M. E. (2007). Pharmacological aspects of nursing care *(7th ed.). New York: Thomson Delmar Learning.*

TABLE 43-6 Pharmacology Facts: Pharmaceutical Therapy for Symptom Relief of Chronic Allergies

CLASSIFICATION	DRUGS	INDICATIONS
Antihistamine	Coricidin, Seldane, Claritin	Allergic rhinitis, urticaria
Decongestant	Pseudoephedrine, Sudafed, Neo-Synephrine, Dristan	Nasal congestion
Corticosteroid	Flunisolide, Beconase, and Nasalide	
Antipruritic	Calamine Lotion, and Tacaryl	Urticaria, pruritus
Mast cell stabilizer	Intal, NasalCrom, and Tilade	Allergic rhinitis and asthma symptoms

Adapted from Broyles, B. E., Reiss, B. S., & Evans, M. E. (2007). Pharmacological aspects of nursing care *(7th ed.). New York: Thomson Delmar Learning.*

BOX 43-5

PHARMACOLOGICAL MANAGEMENT FOR SYMPTOM RELIEF

Antihistamines, such as Coricidin, Seldane, and Claritin, are used for treatment of allergic rhinitis and urticaria. Their side effects include drowsiness, sedation, and poor coordination that could be hazardous when driving or operating machinery. These drugs can also cause GI upset, mouth dryness, blurred vision, and vertigo.

Decongestant (sympathomimetic) drugs such as pseudoephedrine, Sudafed, Neo-Synephrine, and Dristan are used in the management of chronic allergy patients. Because they are available OTC, they have a potential for misuse, resulting in the patient becoming overmedicated.

Corticosteroids are found in nasal inhalers such as Flunisolide, Beconase, and Nasalide.

Antipyretic drugs are applied topically in the form of Calamine lotion and Tacaryl.

Mast cell stabilizing drugs, such as Intal, NasalCrom, and Tilade, inhibit the release of histamines after antigen IgE interaction. They are available as a nasal spray, inhalant nebulizer solution, or oral tablet. They are often used to treat allergic rhinitis and asthma symptoms and have a low incidence of side effects.

Adapted from Ait-Khaled, N., & Enarson D. (2006). Management of asthma: The essentials of good clinical practice. International Journal of Tuberculosis and Lung Disease, *10(2), 133–137; Broyles, B. E., Reiss, B. S., & Evans, M. E. (2007).* Pharmacological aspects of nursing care *(7th ed.). New York: Thomson Delmar Learning.*

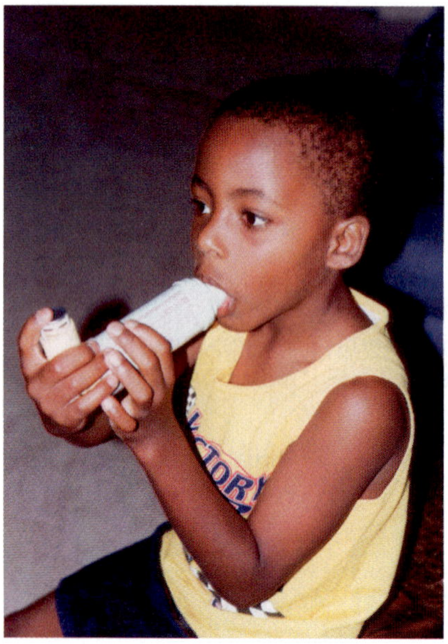

Figure 43-3 A child with an asthma attack using a metered-dose inhaler with a spacer and mouthpiece.

Evaluation of Outcomes

Potential patient outcomes for each of the example nursing diagnoses for the patient with asthma are:

- Ineffective breathing pattern related to SOB, mucus, and airway irritants. The patient's breathing pattern is maintained by eupnea, normal skin color, and regular respiratory rate or pattern.
- Impaired gas exchange related to ventilation-perfusion inequality. The patient maintains optimal gas exchange as evidenced by normal arterial blood gases (ABGs) and alert responsive mentation or no further reduction in mental status.
- Ineffective coping related to anxiety, lower activity level, and the inability to perform normal activities of daily living. The patient identifies own maladaptive coping behaviors, available resources, and support systems, describes or initiates alternative coping strategies, and describes positive results from new behaviors.

ANAPHYLAXIS

Anaphylaxis is an immediate, life-threatening hypersensitive allergic reaction (Gell and Coombs Type I: Immediate hypersensitivity reaction). This sudden and severe allergic reaction occurs within minutes of exposure in hypersensitive patients. It progresses rapidly and can result in anaphylactic shock and death within 15 minutes if medical intervention is not immediately pursued. Speed is the cardinal principal in therapeutic management of anaphylaxis. Anaphylaxis can be triggered by exposure to food (e.g., peanuts, wheat germ), medications (e.g., penicillin, morphine sulfate), insect venom (e.g., bee stings, spider bites), latex (e.g., gloves, equipment), exercise, or other diagnostic agents.

Epidemiology

Nearly 41 million people in the United States have sensitivities that put them at risk for anaphylaxis. It is estimated that 500 to 1,000 fatalities each year are related to anaphylaxis (Centers for Disease Control, 2002). The frequency of anaphylaxis is increasing, and this has been attributed to the increased number of potential allergens to which people are exposed. Unfortunately, in many patients being evaluated for anaphylaxis, no specific trigger can be identified.

Etiology

There are numerous risk factors associated with the incidence and prevalence of anaphylaxis. The nonmodifiable risk factors include age, gender, and race. Modifiable risk factors include the allergens route of entry, atopy, and exposure history (Box 43-6).

BOX 43-6

MODIFIABLE RISK FACTORS FOR ANAPHYLAXIS

Age

Adults have a higher reported rate of reactions to antibiotics, contrast media, anesthetic agents, and insect stings, whereas children have a higher rate of reported reactions to food antigens.

Gender

Anaphylaxis is more frequent in boys than girls under age 15, but among adults, women are more frequently affected than men. Women have a higher incidence of reactions to aspirin, muscle relaxants, contrast material, and latex, and men have a higher recorded incidence of anaphylaxis to insect sting venom. Women are also at higher risk for idiopathic anaphylaxis.

Race

No differences have been noted with race.

Route of Entry

Anaphylaxis can occur with all routes of administration, with episodes more frequent and severe if the offending antigen enters through the skin, (parenterally) rather than orally.

Atopy

The incidence of anaphylaxis to latex and foods is higher in atopic individuals. The data are conflicting regarding antibiotic reactions, with some studies finding anaphylaxis to penicillin more common in atopic patients and others finding no correlation between atopy and penicillin allergy, or even a lower risk for penicillin hypersensitivity with atopic individuals. Atopic people may be predisposed to anaphylactic or anaphylactoid reactions in general and atopy have been implicated as a risk factor for idiopathic anaphylaxis and exercise-induced anaphylaxis.

Exposure History

The likelihood of a repeat episode of anaphylaxis occurring decreases as the time interval between the original episode and subsequent reexposure increases. In addition, medications administered continuously are less likely to trigger a reaction than those given intermittently.

Adapted from Lebovidge, J., Stone, K., Twarog, F., Raiselis, S., Kalish, L., Bailey, E., et al. (2006). Development of a preliminary questionnaire to assess parental response to children's food allergies. Annals of Allergy, Asthma, and Immunology, *96(3), 472–477; Murphy, K., Hopp, R., Kittelson, E., Hansen, G., Windle, M., & Walburn J. (2006). Life-threatening asthma and anaphylaxis in schools: A treatment model for school-based programs.* Annals of Allergy, Asthma, and Immunology, *96(3), 398–405.*

BOX 43-7

DEATHS FROM ANAPHYLACTIC SHOCK

- Bee stings (hymenoptera): 40 to 100 deaths
- Food allergy: 150 to 200 deaths. (Tree nuts and peanuts are the most common food allergens.)
- Latex allergy: 2.7 million to 16 million people allergic.
- Drug allergy: up to 27 million people are allergic to penicillin. An estimated 75 percent of U.S. anaphylactic deaths are related to penicillin allergy.
- Asthma: asthmatics are at particular risk for experiencing life-threatening anaphylaxis.

Adapted from Lebovidge, J., Stone, K., Twarog, F., Raiselis, S., Kalish, L., Bailey, E., et al. (2006). Development of a preliminary questionnaire to assess parental response to children's food allergies. Annals of Allergy, Asthma, and Immunology, 96*(3), 472–477; Murphy, K., Hopp, R., Kittelson, E., Hansen, G., Windle, M., & Walburn, J. (2006). Life-threatening asthma and anaphylaxis in schools: A treatment model for school-based programs.* Annals of Allergy, Asthma, and Immunology, 96*(3), 398–405.*

Statistics issued by the CDC indicate that each year in the United States allergic reactions to bee stings, food allergy, latex allergy, drug allergy, and asthma result in anaphylactic reactions. Many of these reactions result in death due to anaphylactic shock, as illustrated in Box 43-7.

Pathophysiology

Anaphylaxis can be induced or aggravated by exercise, and some patients have recurrent symptoms for no identifiable reason. Histamine and other substances are generated or released when the antigen reacts with IgE on basophils and mast cells. These substances cause smooth muscle contraction (responsible for wheezing and GI symptoms) and vascular dilation and characterize anaphylaxis. Vasodilation and escape of plasma into the tissues causes urticaria and angioedema and result in a decrease in effective plasma volume, which is the major cause of shock. Fluid escapes into the lung alveoli and may produce pulmonary edema. Obstructive angioedema of the upper airway may also occur. Arrhythmias and cardiogenic shock may develop if the reaction is prolonged. Fluid escapes into the lung alveoli and may produce pulmonary edema. Obstructive angioedema of the upper airway may also occur. Arrhythmias and cardiogenic shock may develop if the reaction is prolonged.

Assessment with Clinical Manifestations

Patients with anaphylaxis have a wide variety of both local and systemic clinical manifestations. These reactions are depicted both in Figure 43-4 and Table 43-7.

Planning and Implementation

Anaphylactic reactions occur suddenly in hypersensitive patients following exposure to an offending allergen. The speed of response is the cardinal principal in therapeutic management of anaphylaxis. The following are four areas

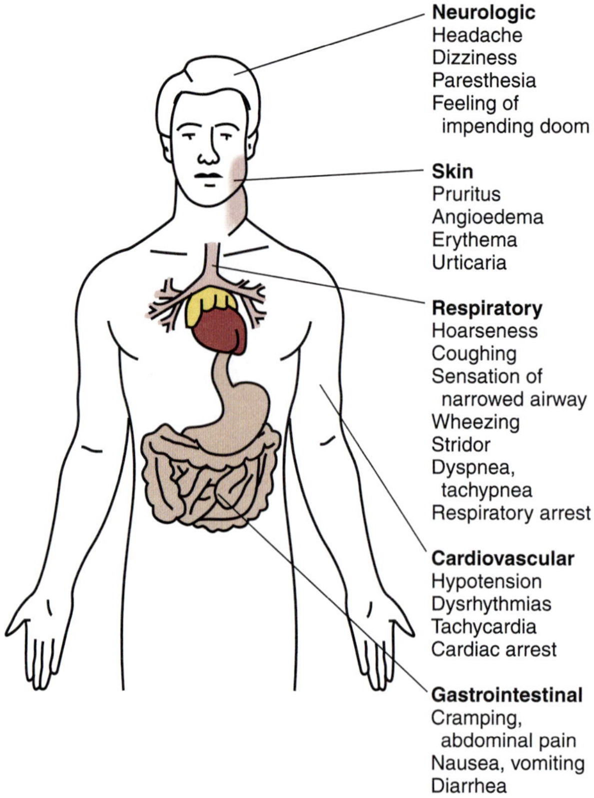

Figure 43-4 Clinical manifestations of a systemic anaphylactic reaction.

Red Flag

Potential Allergens That Cause Anaphylaxis

There are numerous potential allergens that can cause anaphylaxis in hypersensitive (atopic) patients:

- Drugs: penicillins, insulin, tetracycline, cephalosporin, insulin, tetracycline, nonsteroidal anti-inflammatory drugs (NSAIDS), or chemotherapeutic agents.
- Insect venoms: wasps, hornets, yellow jackets, ants, or bumblebees.
- Foods: eggs, nuts, shellfish, chocolate, milk, peanuts, fish, or strawberries.
- Animal serums: tetanus antitoxin, diphtheria antitoxin, rabies antitoxin, or snake venom antitoxin.
- Treatment: blood products, iodine contrast media, or allergenic extracts in hyposensitizing therapy.

Adapted from Battais, F., Mothes, T., Moneret-Vautrin, D., Pineau, F., Kanny, G., Popineau, Y., et al. (2005). Identification of IgE-binding epitopes on gliadins for patients with food allergy to wheat. Allergy, *60(6), 815–821; Scarlet, C. (2006). Anaphylaxis.* Journal of Infusion Nursing, *29(1), 39–44.*

TABLE 43-7 Clinical Manifestations of Anaphylaxis

SYSTEM	SYMPTOM
Skin	Urticaria and angioedema, flushing, and pruritus
Respiratory	Dyspnea, wheezing, airway angioedema, and rhinitis
GI	Nausea, vomiting, diarrhea, cramping, and pain
Cardiovascular	Tachycardia, hypotension, cardiac arrest, and chest pain
Neurological	Headaches, dizziness, seizures, and sense of impending doom

Adapted from Lebovidge, J., Stone, K., Twarog, F., Raiselis, S., Kalish, L., Bailey, E., et al. (2006). Development of a preliminary questionnaire to assess parental response to children's food allergies. Annals of Allergy, Asthma, and Immunology, *96(3), 472–477.*

TABLE 43-8 Treatment of the Patient with Anaphylaxis

INITIAL MEDICAL MANAGEMENT	MEDICAL THERAPY
Recumbent positioning	Epinephrine
Airway management Intubate if necessary	IV fluids
IV access	Histamine H_1 antagonists Histamine H_2 antagonists Steroids Inhaled/aerosolized beta-agonists

Adapted from Broyles, B. E., Reiss, B. S., & Evans, M. E. (2007). Pharmacological aspects of nursing care *(7th ed.). New York: Thomson Delmar Learning; Murphy, K., Hopp, R., Kittelson, E., Hansen, G., Windle, M., & Walburn, J. (2006). Life-threatening asthma and anaphylaxis in schools: A treatment model for school-based programs.* Annals of Allergy, Asthma, and Immunology, *96(3), 398–405.*

of primary concern for the crisis management: (a) recognize the signs and symptoms, (b) maintain a patent airway, (c) prevent spread of the allergen by using a tourniquet when appropriate, and (d) administer appropriate drugs. In addition, the nurse must place the patient in a recumbent position, elevate the legs, keep the patient warm, and provide support for respirations with oxygen. The patient must have a maintained blood pressure with intravenous (IV) fluids. Hypovolemic shock may occur because of fluid moving from intravascular to interstitial spaces. Hypovolemic shock, if not treated early, leads to irreversible tissue damage and death (Pumphrey, 2003).

When an allergic disorder is diagnosed, treatment is aimed at reducing exposure, treating symptoms, and desensitizing the person through immunotherapy (Table 43-8). Adjuncts to therapy include medical alert bracelets, bee sting kits with an EpiPen, and education in emergency self-administration.

Pharmacology

Pharmaceutical management of anaphylaxis is necessary as an immediate treatment. Epinephrine is the most common medication given in acute care setting during the crisis of anaphylaxis, and Benadryl is likely the most typical nonprescription medication given to prevent anaphylaxis or to treat the early clinical manifestations of an allergenic reaction (Table 43-9).

TABLE 43-9 Pharmacology Facts: Pharmaceutical Therapy for Anaphylaxis

CLASSIFICATIONS	DRUGS	INDICATIONS
Parental adrenergic agents	Epinephrine (EpiPen, adrenalin)	Urticaria, angioedema, airway obstruction Bronchospasm
Inhaled beta-antagonists	Albuterol (Proventil, Ventolin)	Bronchospasm
H_1 receptor blockers (antihistamines)	Diphenhydramine (Benadryl)	Cutaneous lesions
H_2 receptor blockers (antihistamines)	Cimetidine (Tagamet)	Cutaneous lesions
Corticosteroids	Methylprednisone (Solu-Medrol, Depo-Medrol)	Bronchospasm, cutaneous lesions

Adapted from Broyles, B. E., Reiss, B. S., & Evans, M. E. (2007). Pharmacological aspects of nursing care *(7th ed.). New York: Thomson Delmar Learning.*

ALLERGIC CONDITIONS

An allergy is a specific immunological reaction to a normally harmless substance, one that does not bother most people. People who have allergies often are sensitive to more than one substance. Types of allergens that cause allergic reactions include pollens, dust particles, mold spores, food, latex, insect venom, or medicines.

Allergic Rhinitis (Hay Fever)

Pollen allergy, or hay fever, is one of the most common chronic diseases in the United States, with allergy to ragweed being the most common source of allergic rhinitis. Rhinitis is an inflammation of the nasal membranes and is characterized by a complex of symptoms that include sneezing, a stuffy or runny nose, itchy eyes, nose, and throat, and watery eyes. Allergic rhinitis symptoms are generated when the immune system encounters an allergen (pollen, mold, or dust) and a hypersensitive reaction causes the body to produce antibodies. Those antibodies combine with the allergen and produce histamine. The allergen is inhaled and causes a local inflammation or irritation of the mucous membranes that line the nose. Allergic rhinitis may be seasonal, reflecting an allergy to tree, grass, or weed pollens. Perennial allergic rhinitis can be the result of indoor allergens, such as feathers, mold spores, animal dander, or dust mites. Avoiding the allergen is the best treatment. Other treatments include treating the symptoms with antihistamines, decongestants, eye cleansing medications (Figure 43-5), and corticosteroids applied by nasal spray. Secondary infections indicated by facial pain or a greenish-yellow discharge may require antibiotic therapy.

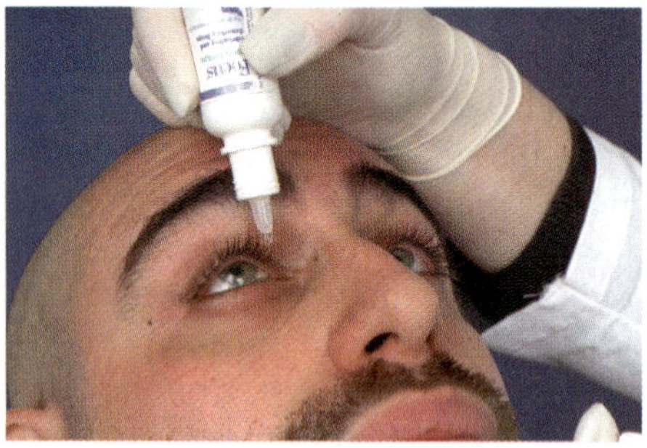

Figure 43-5 An eye cleansing medication being instilled via eye droplet.

Nursing Diagnoses

Based on the information gathered, examples of nursing diagnoses in the patient with allergic rhinitis may include the following:

- Risk for impaired membrane integrity related to inflamed mucous membranes.
- Deficient knowledge related to self-care and risk prevention.
- Fear and anxiety related to actual or potential lifestyle changes.
- Anxiety related to allergen avoidance.

Evaluation of Outcomes

Potential patient outcomes for each of the example nursing diagnoses for the patient with allergic rhinitis are:

- Risk for impaired membrane integrity related to irritation of the mucous membranes that line the nose. The patient has a resolution of the irritation of the nasal membranes.
- Deficient knowledge related to self-care and risk prevention. The patient should demonstrate motivation to learn, identify perceived learning needs, and verbalize an understanding of desired content. Knowledge of avoidance techniques should help avoid the risks and decrease anxiety.
- Fear and anxiety related to actual or potential lifestyle changes. The patient will be able to recognize the signs of anxiety, demonstrate positive coping mechanisms, and describe a reduction in the level of anxiety experienced.

Allergic Contact Dermatitis

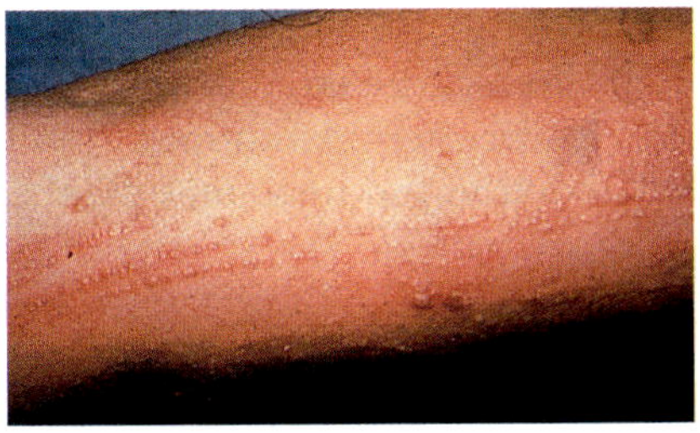

Figure 43-6 ACD note linear pattern to lesions. Courtesy of CDC.

Allergic contact dermatitis (ACD) is an inflammation of the skin caused by direct contact with an allergy causing substance. It is a type 4 allergic reaction, or delayed hypersensitivity reaction. The skin inflammation varies from mild irritation and redness to open sores, depending on the type of irritant, the body part affected, and the sensitivity of the individual. Irritants include water, soaps, detergents, solvents, acids, and alkalis. The rash is generally confined to the site of contact, but may be transmitted by the fingers to other sites (e.g., eyelids and genitals). Patients with atopic dermitis are particularly susceptible to developing ACD. There is typically a delay between the time of exposure and the onset of symptoms. Mild symptoms include itching, redness, swelling, and small blisters that may break, ooze, and crust over (Figure 43-6). More acute symptoms can occur with reexposure. These symptoms may involve respiratory symptoms, and rarely, symptoms may lead to respiratory collapse or shock. Latex allergy is a well-known example of ACD. Chemicals used in the harvesting and manufacture of latex can cause a cutaneous inflammatory condition similar to other sources of ACD reactions, such as poison ivy and nickel. A person wearing latex gloves may experience ACD. Treatment includes identification and avoidance of the allergen, moisturizing creams, topical steroid ointments, and antibiotics for secondary infection. Severe cases may require a short course of oral steroids.

Nursing Diagnoses

Based on the information gathered, examples of nursing diagnoses in the patient with ACD may include the following:

- Risk for impaired skin integrity related to urticaria and puritus.
- Deficient knowledge related to self-care and risk prevention.
- Fear and anxiety related to actual or potential lifestyle changes.

Evaluation of Outcomes

Potential patient outcomes for each of the example nursing diagnoses for the patient with ACD are:

- Risk for impaired skin integrity related to urticaria and pruritus. The patient's skin condition should be improved by decreased inflammation, urticaria, and pruritus.
- Deficient knowledge related to self-care and risk prevention. The patient should demonstrate motivation to learn, identify perceived learning needs, and verbalize an understanding of desired content.
- Fear and anxiety related to actual or potential lifestyle changes. The patient will be able to recognize the signs of anxiety, demonstrate positive coping mechanisms, and describe a reduction in the level of anxiety experienced.

Atopic Dermatitis

Atopic dermatitis (AD), also called atopic eczema or endogenous eczema, is a chronic disease that affects the dermis (skin). AD is linked to an exaggerated immune and inflammatory response that triggers elevated levels of (IgE. Studies done by the National Institute of Health indicate that 15 million people in the United States have symptoms of atopic dermatitis and that AD may develop at any age, but most often begins before the age of 5. AD is characterized by rashes and intense itching that may be accompanied by swelling, redness, blistering, oozing, crusting, and scales. The rashes are most commonly located on the face, inside the elbows, behind the knees, and on the hands and feet. The appearance of the skin depends on the amount of scratching and degree of secondary skin infection. The condition has periods of flare when symptoms exacerbate, and periods when the skin clears, and AD is in remission. Irritants found to be linked to flares of AD include wool and synthetic fibers in contact with the skin, certain soaps and detergents, solvents, dust, sand, and intermittent wetting and drying of the skin. The intense itching that is characteristic of AD provides a focus for nursing intervention. Scratching and rubbing in response to itching increases the inflammation and the possibility of secondary skin infections. Corticosteroid ointments and creams are used to treat AD. Antibiotics are added to the treatment plan as indicated.

Nursing Diagnoses

Based on the information gathered, examples of nursing diagnoses in the patient with AD may include the following:

- Risk for impaired skin integrity related to urticaria and pruritus.
- Deficient knowledge related to self-care and risk prevention.
- Fear and anxiety related to actual or potential lifestyle changes.

Evaluation of Outcomes

Potential patient outcomes for each of the example nursing diagnoses for the patient with AD are:

- Risk for impaired skin integrity related to urticaria and pruritus. The patient's skin condition should be improved by decreased inflammation, urticaria, and pruritus.
- Deficient knowledge related to self-care and risk prevention. The patient should demonstrate motivation to learn, identify perceived learning needs, and verbalize an understanding of desired content.
- Fear and anxiety related to actual or potential lifestyle changes. The patient will be able to recognize the signs of anxiety, demonstrate positive coping mechanisms, and describe a reduction in the level of anxiety experienced.

Urticaria

Urticaria (nettle-rash, hives, or wheals) is a hypersensitive dermatological manifestation in response to the release of histamine in an antigen-antibody reaction. This immune reaction causes vasodilation, skin eruptions, profound itching, and pain. The rash is composed of red circular, slightly elevated, or irregularly shaped eruptions and can appear on any part of the body. Each individual hive (or wheal) lasts a few hours and then fades away without a trace, as new hives appear. Urticaria may be localized in some patients, while others may have widespread eruptions. Many substances can trigger urticaria through an immediate hypersensitivity reaction (type 1). Urticaria is a symptom that can develop through exposure to a variety of things: viruses, medications, foods (most commonly nuts, chocolate, and fruits), parasites, chemicals (latex), physical stimulants (cold or pressure), and insect bites. In some cases the allergen

TABLE 43-10 Pharmacology Facts: Pharmaceutical Therapy for Urticaria

CLASSIFICATIONS	DRUGS	INDICATIONS
Topical steroids	Triamcininolone (Aristocort)	Ointment used on dry or cracked skin, creams are used on inflamed skin or weeping lesions
Systemic steroids	Prednisone (Deltasone)	Severe cases involving more than 20 percent of total body surface (TBSA)
Antihistamines	Diphenhydramine (Benadryl) Hydroxyzine HCL (Atarax, Vistaril)	Used to relieve pruritus associated with contact dermatitis

Adapted from Broyles, B. E., Reiss, B. S., & Evans, M. E. (2007). Pharmacological aspects of nursing care *(7th ed.). New York: Thomson Delmar Learning.*

is idiopathic (no discernible cause). The acute form of urticaria lasts less than four to six weeks. Chronic hives is a case of hives that lasts longer than six weeks. Antihistamine medications are the primary treatment for urticaria (Table 43-10).

Nursing Diagnoses

Based on the information gathered, examples of nursing diagnoses in the patient with urticaria may include the following:

- Risk for impaired skin integrity related to urticaria and pruritus.
- Deficient knowledge related to self-care and risk prevention.
- Fear and anxiety related to actual or potential lifestyle changes.

Evaluation of Outcomes

Potential patient outcomes for each of the example nursing diagnoses for the patient with urticaria are:

- Risk for impaired skin integrity related to rash and itching. The patient's skin condition should be improved by decreased inflammation.
- Deficient knowledge related to self-care and risk prevention. The patient should demonstrate motivation to learn, identify perceived learning needs, and verbalize an understanding of desired content.
- Fear and anxiety related to actual or potential lifestyle changes. The patient will be able to recognize the signs of anxiety, demonstrate positive coping mechanisms, and describe a reduction in the level of anxiety experienced.

Angioneurotic Edema

Angioneurotic edema (also known as angioedema) is a condition that results from an allergic type reaction that involves histamine and the blood vessels in subdermal tissue. It is similar to hives, only the welts are larger, and it originates in a deeper layer of tissue. Angioedema may be caused by an allergic reaction to pollens, foods, medications, bee stings, cold, light, or exercise. Other types may be inherited or occur for idiopathic reasons. It is characterized by the appearance of large welts, usually appearing around the eyes and lips, but the welts may also occur on the hands, feet, and throat. Subdermal or submucosal edema may occur in other areas of the body, but when it occurs in the ear-nose-throat area, serious laryngeal swelling can be a hazard. Airway patency is a primary concern when a patient exhibits obvious edema of soft tissues of the face and neck. Airway intervention may be necessary. Angioedema may be progressive in nature and can be a prelude to anaphylaxis. Medications, such as epinephrine (EpiPen, Adrenaline), and antihistamines are directed toward blocking histamine that is producing the reaction.

> ### *Red Flag*
> **Food Allergy and the Impact of Ingredients**
>
> It is important for the nurse and the patient with a food allergy to become familiar with the composition of ingredients listed on food labels. A small amount of one ingredient has the ability to induce an allergic reaction. Here's an example:
>
> Have you heard of casein? Casein is found in milk protein. It is an inactive ingredient sometimes added to products, like creamers and cheese, and may cause allergic reactions in patients with allergies to dairy products.
>
> The Food and Drug Administration (FDA) received a report in which a child with a preexisting allergy to dairy products suffered a severe allergic reaction following ingestion of a chewable vitamin. The child was taken to the emergency department and recovered with treatment. The label on the vitamin indicated that the vitamin was free of starch, yeast, soy, wheat, dairy, gluten, egg, fragrance, artificial colors, and preservatives. However, the other ingredients section of the label listed sodium caseinate as an ingredient. The small amount of casein in one vitamin was sufficient to trigger child's allergic reaction.
>
> *Adapted from Janeway, C. A., Jr., Travers, P., Walport, M., & Shlomchik, M. J. (2004).* Immunobiology, the immune system in health and disease *(6th ed.). New York: Garland Science Publishing; Parker, E., Donato, L., Dalgleish, D. (2005). Effects of added sodium caseinate on the formation of particles in heated milk.* Journal of Agricultural and Food Chemistry, *53(21), 8265–8272.*

Nursing Diagnoses

Based on the information gathered, examples of nursing diagnoses in the patient with angioneurotic edema may include the following:

- Ineffective airway clearance related to soft tissue edema.
- Ineffective breathing pattern related to bronchospasm.
- Anxiety and agitation related to air hunger.
- Pain related to swelling of abdominal organs.
- Risk for impaired skin integrity related to urticaria and pruritus.
- Fear and anxiety related to the inability to control body response.

Evaluation of Outcomes

Potential patient outcomes for each of the example nursing diagnoses for the patient with angioedema are:

- Ineffective airway clearance related to soft tissue edema. The patient will maintain a patent airway as evidenced by unrestricted respirations.
- Ineffective breathing pattern related to bronchospasm. The patient will resume normal breathing patterns as evidenced by chest observation and auscultative chest sounds.
- Anxiety and agitation related to air hunger. The patient will demonstrate more relaxed postures as oxygen perfusion of tissues improves.
- Pain related to swelling of abdominal organs. The patient should verbalize an adequate relief of pain along with the ability to realistically cope with the pain if it is not completely relieved.
- Risk for impaired skin integrity related to urticaria and pruritus. The patient's skin condition should be improved by decreased inflammation, urticaria, and pruritus.
- Fear and anxiety related to the inability to control body response. The patient should be able to recognize the signs of anxiety and stress, demonstrate positive coping mechanisms, and describe a reduction in the level of anxiety experienced.

Food Allergy

A food allergy, or hypersensitivity, is an abnormal response to a food triggered by the body's immune system. The reaction to the food allergen may be either immediate or delayed. The patient may experience symptoms that range from GI distress to anaphylaxis. In adults, the foods that most often cause allergic reactions include shellfish, peanuts, walnuts, fish, and eggs. Children are often allergic to eggs, milk, and peanuts.

Some foods can cause severe illness and, in some cases, a life-threatening allergic reaction (anaphylaxis) that can constrict airways in the lungs, severely lower blood pressure, and cause suffocation by the swelling of the tongue or throat. Food allergens are proteins in a food that enters the bloodstream when the food is digested. The immune system produces IgE, a food specific antibody in people with inherited allergic tendencies.

- The first time a person with a specific food allergy eats the specific food, IgE specific to that food is released by the immune system.
- The second time that specific food is eaten, it interacts with the food-specific IgE and triggers the cells to release histamine.
- An allergic reaction to food can occur within minutes of eating the food. In other situations the allergic response may not occur for an hour.

When a person is allergic to a particular food, itching of the mouth may occur as they eat the food. If the food is digested, GI symptoms, such as vomiting, diarrhea, and cramping, may occur. When the allergens reach the bloodstream, there may be a drop in blood pressure. Hives and atopic eczema develop when the allergens reach the skin. As the reaction reaches the lungs, asthma may develop. A mild symptom such as a tingling in the mouth can progress rapidly to anaphylaxis requiring immediate assistance.

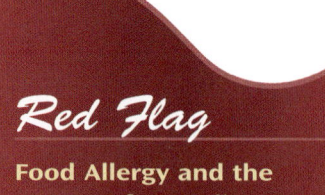

Eliminating foods that trigger an allergic reaction are identified through a process that eliminates suspect foods from the diet. The food is then reintroduced, and the result is evaluated. Treatment of food allergy consists of avoiding foods that trigger a reaction and treating symptoms during a reaction. Patients with known food allergies should wear a medical alert bracelet stating the food allergy. Many of these individuals also carry a syringe of epinephrine (EpiPen) and are prepared to inject themselves if they feel they are having an allergic reaction.

Nursing Diagnoses

Based on the information gathered, examples of nursing diagnoses in the patient with food allergies may include the following:

- Ineffective airway clearance related to soft tissue edema.
- Ineffective breathing pattern related to bronchospasm.
- Anxiety and agitation related to air hunger.
- Risk for impaired skin integrity related to urticaria and pruritus.
- Deficient knowledge related to self-care and risk prevention.
- Fear and anxiety related to actual or potential lifestyle changes.

Evaluation of Outcomes

Potential patient outcomes for each of the example nursing diagnoses for the patient with food allergies are:

- Ineffective airway clearance related to soft tissue edema. The patient will maintain a patent airway as evidenced by unrestricted respirations.
- Ineffective breathing pattern related to bronchospasm. The patient will resume normal breathing patterns as evidenced by chest observation and auscultative chest sounds.
- Anxiety and agitation related to air hunger. The patient will demonstrate more relaxed postures as oxygen perfusion of tissues improves.
- Risk for impaired skin integrity related to urticaria and pruritus. The patient's skin condition should be improved by decreased inflammation, urticaria, and pruritus.
- Deficient knowledge related to self-care and risk prevention. The patient should demonstrate motivation to learn, identify perceived learning needs, and verbalize an understanding of desired content
- Fear and anxiety related to actual or potential lifestyle changes. The patient will be able to recognize the signs of anxiety, demonstrate positive coping mechanisms, and describe a reduction in the level of anxiety experienced.

Latex Allergy

Latex allergy is a reaction to certain proteins in latex rubber. The amount of latex exposure needed to produce sensitization or an allergic reaction is unknown. Increasing the exposure to latex proteins increases the risk of developing allergic symptoms. In sensitized persons, symptoms usually begin within minutes of exposure, but they can occur hours later and can be quite varied. Mild reactions to latex involve skin redness, rash, hives, or itching. More severe reactions may involve respiratory symptoms, such as runny nose, sneezing, itchy eyes, scratchy throat, and wheezing. Anaphylaxis is a possibility. Health care providers wear latex gloves on a frequent basis and can become susceptible to latex allergy conditions.

Nursing Diagnoses

Based on the information gathered, examples of nursing diagnoses in the patient with latex allergies may include the following:

- Ineffective airway clearance related to soft tissue edema.
- Risk for impaired skin integrity related to urticaria and pruritus.

- Deficient knowledge related to self-care and prevention.
- Fear and anxiety related to actual or potential lifestyle changes.

Evaluation of Outcomes

Potential patient outcomes for each of the example nursing diagnoses for the patient with latex allergies are:

- Ineffective airway clearance related to soft tissue edema. The patient will maintain a patent airway as evidenced by unrestricted respirations.
- Risk for impaired skin integrity related to urticaria and pruritus. The patient's skin condition should be improved by decreased inflammation, urticaria, and pruritus.
- Deficient knowledge related to self-care and prevention. The patient should demonstrate motivation to learn, identify perceived learning needs, and verbalize an understanding of desired content.
- Fear and anxiety related to actual or potential lifestyle changes. The patient should be able to recognize the signs of anxiety, demonstrate positive coping mechanisms, and describe a reduction in the level of anxiety experienced.

Serum Sickness

Serum sickness is a type 3 hypersensitivity reaction that results from the injection of foreign protein or serum. The incidence of serum sickness is declining in the United States because of public health programs that have decreased the need for specific antitoxins, such as rabies and tetanus antitoxin. Primary serum sickness occurs 6 to 21 days after the administration of the antitoxin. Classic symptoms of serum sickness include pain and swelling at the injection site, followed by temperature elevation of 101 to 104° F (38.3 to 40° C), arthralgia, lymphadenopathy, and skin eruptions. Because it takes time for the body to produce antibodies to a new antigen, symptoms do not develop until 7 to 21 days after initial exposure to the antiserum. However, patients may develop symptoms in 1 to 3 days if they have previously been exposed to the offending agent. Exposure to certain medications (particularly penicillin) can cause a similar process. Unlike other drug allergies, which occur soon after receiving the medication for the second (or subsequent) time, serum sickness can develop 7 to 21 days after the first exposure to a medication. Blood products may also induce serum sickness. Other causes of serum sickness include serum used in the prophylaxis or treatment of botulism, diphtheria, gas gangrene, transplant rejection, and snake and spider bites. Treatment includes stopping the therapy that involves the suspected antigen and providing supportive therapy for the symptoms. Medications used to treat serum sickness include antihistamines and antipyretics. Corticosteroids agents help modify the immune response.

Nursing Diagnoses

Based on the information gathered, examples of nursing diagnoses in the patient with serum sickness may include the following:

- Risk for impaired skin integrity related to urticaria and pruritus.
- Risk for imbalanced body temperature. Fear and anxiety related to actual or potential health decline.
- Impaired physical mobility related to serum sickness.

Evaluation of Outcomes

Potential patient outcomes for each of the example nursing diagnoses for the patient with serum sickness are:

- Risk for impaired skin integrity related to urticaria and pruritus. The patient's skin condition should be improved by decreased inflammation, urticaria, and pruritus.

- Risk for imbalanced body temperature. The patient maintains body temperature within a normal range.
- Fear and anxiety related to actual or potential health decline. The patient should be able to recognize the signs of anxiety, demonstrate coping mechanisms, and describe a reduction in the level of anxiety experienced.
- Impaired physical mobility related to serum sickness. The patient should perform physical activity independently or with assistive devices as needed. In addition, the patient should be free of complication of immobility, as evidenced by intact skin, absence of thrombophlebitis, and normal bowel patterns.

Contact Dermatitis (Dermatitis Medicamentosa)

Contact dermatitis is an acute or chronic skin inflammation triggered in the epidermis by contact with a specific antigen or irritant. Primary irritant dermatitis results from direct allergen contact with the skin and usually produces discomfort immediately following exposure. ACD is a delayed hypersensitivity reaction requiring several hours for the reaction to become apparent. The skin inflammation and rash appear the same for both primary irritant dermatitis and allergic contact dermatitis. Affected individuals have abnormal redness of the skin (erythema) or itching (pruritus) following contact with various metal alloys (e.g., nickel), cements, and household cleaners. Strong irritants (e.g., acids, alkalis) can produce an immediate reaction that has the appearance of a thermal burn. The most common agents for allergic contact dermatitis are plants, such as poison ivy, poison oak, and poison sumac. Treatment of contact dermatitis depends on the type, extent, and area of skin lesions. Wet compresses, topical steroids, and systemic steroids (e.g., Prednisone) are used to treat severe cases involving 20 percent of total body surface.

Nursing Diagnoses

Based on the information gathered, examples of nursing diagnoses in the patient with contact dermatitis may include the following:

- Risk for impaired skin integrity related to urticaria and pruritus.
- Deficient knowledge related to self-care and risk prevention.
- Fear and anxiety related to actual or potential lifestyle changes.

Evaluation of Outcomes

Potential patient outcomes for each of the example nursing diagnoses for the patient with contact dermatitis are:

- Risk for impaired skin integrity related to urticaria and pruritus. The patient's skin condition should be improved by decreased inflammation, urticaria, and pruritus.
- Deficient knowledge related to self-care and risk prevention. The patient should demonstrate motivation to learn, identify perceived learning needs, and verbalize an understanding of desired content.
- Fear and anxiety related to actual or potential lifestyle changes. The patient will be able to recognize the signs of anxiety, demonstrate positive coping mechanisms, and describe a reduction in the level of anxiety experienced.

Hereditary Angioedema

Hereditary angioedema (HAE) is an inherited disorder of the immune system that causes painless swelling, particularly of the face, and abdominal cramping. HAE is a lifelong affliction that usually becomes apparent in adulthood. It is caused by low levels or improper function of a protein called C1 inhibitor. Patients with HAE are often found to be depleted of C1 inhibitor. This, in turn, affects blood vessels. People with HAE can develop rapid swelling in several prominent sites: subdermal tissues (face, hands, arms, legs, genitals, and buttocks); abdominal organs (stomach, intestines, and bladder), with a colicky pain in the abdomen that can mimic a surgical emergency; and the upper airway (larynx), which may result in laryngeal edema. Occasionally, erythema or mild urticarial eruptions may precede the edema. Precipitating factors of attacks may include trauma (particularly dental trauma), anxiety, and stress. Depending on the symptoms and the sites of the angioedema, intensive support may be necessary, including IV fluids. Intubation may be necessary in cases that are complicated by laryngeal edema.

Nursing Diagnoses

Based on the information gathered, examples of nursing diagnoses in the patient with HAE may include the following:

- Ineffective airway clearance related to soft tissue edema.
- Ineffective breathing pattern related to bronchospasm.
- Anxiety and agitation related to air hunger.
- Pain related to swelling of abdominal organs.
- Risk for impaired skin integrity related to urticaria and pruritus.
- Fear and anxiety related to the inability to control body response.

Evaluation of Outcomes

Potential patient outcomes for each of the example nursing diagnoses for the patient with HAE are:

- Ineffective airway clearance related to soft tissue edema. The patient will maintain a patent airway as evidenced by unrestricted respirations.
- Ineffective breathing pattern related to bronchospasm. The patient will resume normal breathing patterns as evidenced by chest observation and auscultative chest sounds.
- Anxiety and agitation related to air hunger. The patient will demonstrate more relaxed postures as oxygen perfusion of tissues improves.
- Pain related to swelling of abdominal organs. The patient should verbalize an adequate relief of pain along with the ability to realistically cope with the pain if it is not completely relieved.
- Risk for impaired skin integrity related to urticaria and pruritus. The patient's skin condition should be improved by decreased inflammation, urticaria, and pruritus.
- Fear and anxiety related to the inability to control body response. The patient should be able to recognize the signs of anxiety and stress, demonstrate positive coping mechanisms, and describe a reduction in the level of anxiety experienced.

KEY CONCEPTS

- Allergic diseases are common, affecting about 15 to 20 percent if the population.
- Immune response is triggered when the body recognizes and defends itself against allergens (microorganisms, viruses, and substances) recognized by the body as foreign and potentially harmful.
- Hyperresponsiveness is an overreaction of the body's immune response to allergens.
- Gell and Coombs classifications are categories of immune response.
- Atopy is an inherited tendency for hyperproduction of IgE antibodies to common environmental allergens.
- Anaphylactic reactions are severe, life-threatening allergic reactions.
- Atopic asthma (allergic asthma) is a type 1 immune response to allergens.
- Hypersensitive reaction include other diseases and conditions, including food allergy, drug allergy, urticaria, latex allergy, drug allergy, and serum sickness.

REVIEW QUESTIONS

1. Your patient has a history of abdominal bloating, cramping, and loose stools and thinks that she has a food allergy. As a nurse, you know:
1. Elimination and challenge diets form the basis for the diagnosis of food allergy.
2. An SPT will help locate the problem.
3. Blood testing will identify the food allergy.
4. Hair sample testing will identify the food allergy.

2. A patient being treated for anaphylaxis will be given what drug by intramuscular injection?
1. Hydrocortisone
2. Epinephrine
3. Theophylline
4. Captopril

3. Your patient with a newly diagnosed latex allergy is being discharged from the hospital today. As part of your discharge teaching plan, you inform the patient that he needs to seek immediate medical attention if the following occurs:
1. His medical alert bracelet falls off.
2. He accidentally ingests sunflower seeds.
3. He experiences swelling around the lips or eyes.
4. He feels his heart pounding after strenuous exercise.

4. Atopic individuals have an inherited tendency to hyperproduce what type of antibodies in response to common environmental allergens?
1. IgE
2. Mast cells
3. Histamine
4. Prostaglandin

5. Hyposensitization (immunotherapy for a specific allergen) has been proven a benefit in which of the following conditions?
1. Dust mite allergy
2. Peanut allergy
3. Wasp venom hypersensitivity
4. Urticaria

6. A patient with an immediate type 1 hypersensitivity will respond to a SPT with the appropriate antigen by:
1. A wheal and flare response immediately
2. A wheal and flare response 48 hours later
3. An increased susceptibility to herpes zoster
4. A wheal and flare response within 5 to 10 minutes

7. You are covering for another nurse during lunch. You answer a call light for one of her patients. The patient is restless and complains of itching. The patient has an IV piggyback running. What first step should you take?
1. Tell him you will get his nurse
2. Take his blood pressure
3. Shut off the IV piggyback and slow the IV to a keep open rate
4. Give him a drink of water and turn on the call light

8. Which of the following signs and symptoms would be consistent with a diagnosis of atopic eczema in a 10-month-old infant?
1. Webbing between the fingers and toes
2. Lactose intolerance
3. Dermatitis on face and flexural aspects of arms and legs
4. Swollen eyes

9. Severe reactions to penicillin are more likely to happen when the medication is given by what route?
1. Orally
2. Intramuscular
3. Through a nebulizer
4. Parentally

10. Your patient is diagnosed with asthma. Which of the following nursing diagnoses would be most appropriate for this patient?
1. High risk for infections
2. Sexual dysfunction
3. Ineffective airway clearance
4. Fluid volume deficit

REVIEW ACTIVITIES

1. List four examples of hypersensitivity type 1 allergic reactions.

2. Develop a teaching plan for the family of a 14-month-old patient with newly diagnosed atopic asthma.

3. Name four categories of potential allergens that may cause anaphylaxis in hypersensitive patients.

4. Describe the best manner of diagnosing a food allergy.

5. What is the relationship of IgE and histamine in an allergic reaction?

6. What is the best treatment for hay fever (allergic rhinitis)?

7. Define atopy and discuss the impact it has on allergic reactions.

Visit the Contemporary Medical-Surgical Nursing online companion resource at www.delmarhealthcare.com for additional content and study aids. Click on Online Companions then select the Nursing discipline.

UNIT

X

Alterations in Integumentary Function

Chapter 44 Assessment of Integumentary Function

Chapter 45 Dermatological Dysfunction: Nursing Management

Chapter 46 Burns: Nursing Management

CHAPTER

44

Assessment of Integumentary Function

Cynthia A. Worley, BSN, RN, WOCN

KEY TERMS

Actinic keratoses
Anasarca
Annular
Bullae
Burrows
Comedones
Dermatomal
Diaphoresis
Differentiation
Eczematoid
Edema
Keratinization
Lentigines
Lesions
Macules
Neoangiogenesis
Nodules
Papules
Pigmentation
Plaques
Pruritus
Pustules
Regeneration
Telangiectasia
Tumors
Turgor
Vesicles
Wheals
Xerosis

CHAPTER TOPICS

- Anatomy and Physiology of the Integumentary System
- Skin Changes throughout the Life Span
- Factors Regulating Skin and Wound Repair
- Assessment of the Integumentary System

The skin is the largest organ of the body and is capable of regeneration and repair. If stretched flat, it wound measure about 3,000 square inches or almost two square meters. The skin weighs about six pounds, receives one third of the body's circulating blood volume and undergoes a seven-fold growth from birth to death. Its thickness ranges from 0.04 mm on the eyelids to 1.6 mm in soles of feet and palms of hands. The variations in thickness are also related to underlying structures and their protection (e.g., bones, muscles, or internal organs). Maintaining skin integrity is a complex process, and the skin is constantly exposed to a changing environment. The skin forms a protective barrier, assists in maintaining a homeostatic environment, and can resist limited physical, mechanical, and chemical assaults. The epidermal appendages, hair, nails, sweat, and sebaceous glands, which are also lined with epidermal cells, aid in repair and resurfacing in the event of skin injury (Johnstone, Farly & Henley, 2005).

ANATOMY AND PHYSIOLOGY

Human skin is divided into two layers, the epidermis (the outermost layer) and the dermis (the innermost layer) (Figure 44-1). Subcutaneous tissue lies below the dermis of the skin. Table 44-1 provides an overview of the structure, function, and clinical presentations of problems related to abnormal function of skin.

Epidermis

The epidermis is comprised of five layers of stratified squamous epithelial cells named (outer to inner) the stratum corneum, stratum lucidum, stratum granulosum, stratum spinosum, and stratum germinativum (Figure 44-2). Each layer has its own functions within the differentiation process. The epidermis is the thin, stratified outer skin layer that is in contact with the environment. It is avascular and without lymphatic channels or connective tissue. Therefore, the epidermis must derive its nourishment and blood supply from the underlying dermis (Johnstone, et al., 2005).

Epidermal tissue replenishes itself through a process called **keratinization.** Keratin is a highly insoluble, fibrous protein. During its lifecycle, the keratinocyte is first formed in the basal layer (stratum germinativum) and undergoes biochemical and morphological changes as it migrates from the innermost epidermal layer to the outermost epidermal layer. The epidermis is undergoing a constant turnover of new cells averaging every 26 to 42 days with complete renewal about every two months, a process called **differentiation.** The layers of the epidermis are named to reflect the changes occurring in the keratinocyte during differentiation. All layers of the epidermis consist of these types of peaks and valleys.

Cells in the Epidermis

Melanocytes are also present within the epidermis and are responsible for skin color or **pigmentation.** The normal number of melanocytes is nearly the same from person to person, regardless of skin color. It is the size and distribution of

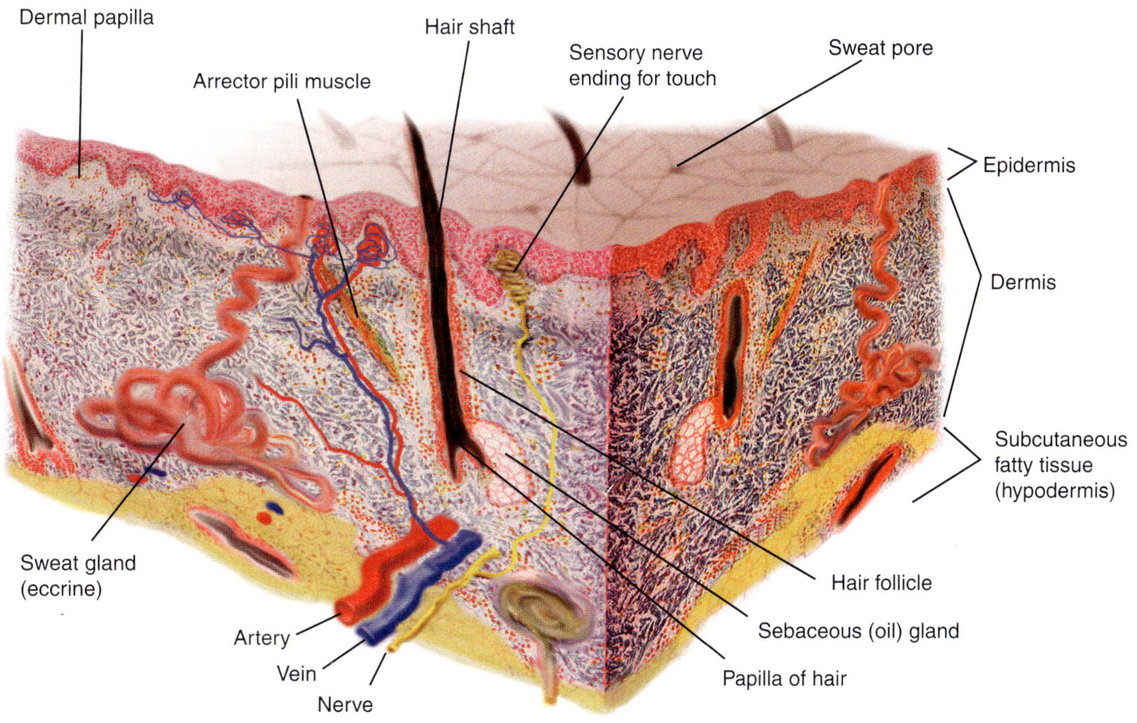

Figure 44-1 Structures of the skin.

TABLE 44-1 Structures and Functions of the Skin

STRUCTURE	NORMAL FUNCTION	RESULT OF ABNORMAL FUNCTION	ABNORMAL CLINICAL PRESENTATIONS
Epidermis			
Stratum corneum	Protective barrier	Dryness, scaling, reduced barrier function	Psoriasis, eczema, pressure ulcers, burns (thermal or chemical)
Keratinocytes	Keratin synthesis, replenish stratum corneum	Reduced or impaired barrier function, abnormal transformation	Ichthyosis, actinic keratosis, skin cancers
Melanocytes	Skin pigmentation, melanin production	Increased or decreased skin color, malignant changes	Hyperpigmentation or hypopigmentation, suntan, malignant melanoma
Langerhans' cells	Immune response	Contact dermatitis	Rash, psoriasis
Basal cells	Replenish epidermal layers	Increased production, abnormal transformation	Basal cell carcinoma
Epidermal Appendages			
Apocrine gland	Apocrine sweat production	Odor, staining	Chromidrosis
Eccrine gland	Perspiration, thermoregulation	Fluid and electrolyte loss; reduced heat dissipation	Arrhythmia, heat stroke, heat exhaustion, anhidrosis
Sebaceous gland	Sebum production, lubrication, antimicrobial barrier	Obstruction of flow of sebum	Oily skin, acne
Hair follicle	Protection, appearance	Poor self-image	Alopecia, folliculitis, hirsutism
Nails	Protection, mechanical	Exposed nail bed, nail changes	Fungal infections, subungual problems, psoriasis
Dermis			
Macrophage	Immune response, chemotactic response	Poor inflammatory response, delay in healing	Job's syndrome
Mast cell	Histamine response, chemotactic response	Abnormal histamine release	Allergic responses, urticaria
Fibroblasts	Synthesis of collagen scaffold	Abnormal skin and wound tensile strength	Poor quality granulation tissue, fragile skin, scurvy, scleroderma, systemic lupus erythematosus
Endothelial cells	Neoangiogenesis: new vasculature (blood vessels)	Decreased blood flow, necrosis of tissue	Peripheral arterial and vascular disease
Lymphatic vessels	Removal of cellular debris and microorganisms	Poor interstitial fluid regulation	Edema, acute and chronic
Nerve fibers	Sensory perception	Inadequate tissue enervation, **pruritus** (itching)	Pruritus, atopic dermatitis, excoriation of skin
Subcutaneous tissue (below dermis-attaches skin to underlying tissues)	Protection of underlying structures, storage of energy and hormones	Atrophic changes, inadequate protection, malignant changes	Emaciation, obesity, malignant lipomatous tumors

Adapted from Johnstone, C., Farley, A., & Hendry, C. (2005). The physiological basis of wound healing. Nursing Standard, 19*(43), 59–65.*

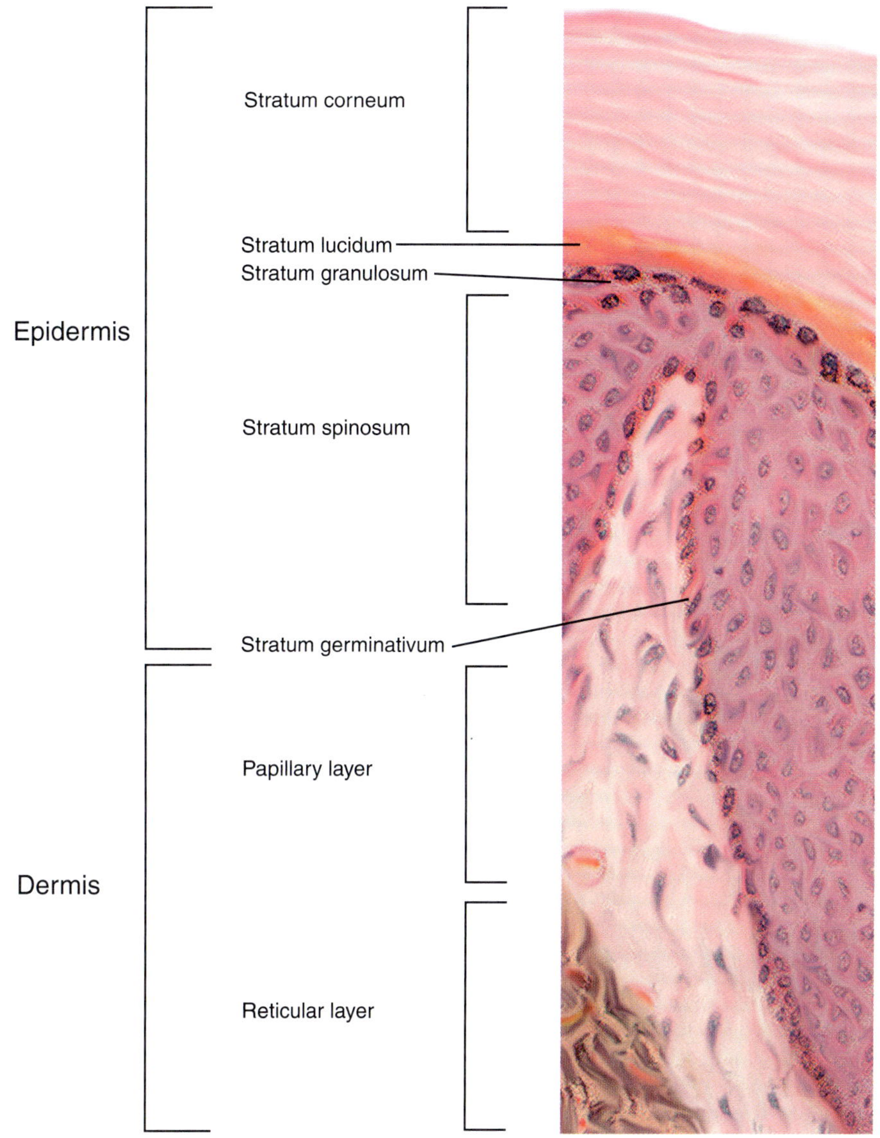

Figure 44-2 Epidermal and dermal layers of skin.

melanosomes, the structures within melanocytes containing the melanin pigment, which differentiates lighter-skinned from darker-skinned individuals. Carotenoids are responsible for the yellow tone of the skin in some individuals.

Langerhans' cells originate in bone marrow and are antigen-presenting cells (APCs). They are responsible for foreign antigen recognition and provide immune protection. Langerhans' cells are found in several layers of the epidermis and are impaired by ultraviolet (UV) radiation. It is believed that Langerhans' cells are directly involved with allergic contact hypersensitivity.

Epidermal Appendages

The epidermal appendages are down-growths of the epidermis and extend into the dermis. They consist of exocrine, apocrine, and sebaceous glands, hair and hair follicles, and nails. The exocrine sweat glands play a role in thermoregulation; apocrine glands are located primarily in the axillae, breast areolae, and the anogenital area. These glands enlarge and become active because of reproductive hormones at puberty. Sebaceous glands are found throughout the skin except in the palms of the hands and soles and dorsum of the feet. Most sebaceous glands are associated with hair follicles (pilosebaceous unit). Sebaceous gland development is regulated by androgens and is the earliest sign of puberty. Testicular androgen regulates sebaceous gland secretions in the male and ovarian androgen regulates secretion in the female.

Hair serves physiological functions, such as insulation and prevention of heat loss, protection from UV light, tactile perception, and acts as social and sexual ornamentation. Most of the body is covered with fine or faint hair called vellus hair. Terminal hair is the coarser, darker hair of the scalp, eyebrows, and eyelashes.

The nails are layers of keratinized cells cemented together. The nail plate serves as a protective covering for the distal tips of the fingers and toes. The nail root lies posterior to the cuticle and is attached to the matrix. The matrix is undifferentiated epithelial tissue from which the nails arise and is located in the proximal nail bed. The nail bed is the vascular bed of the nail and lies under the nail plate. The periungual tissue surrounds the nail plate and the free edge of the nail. The pale, crescent-shaped area at the proximal end of each nail is the lunula. A damaged nail matrix produces a distorted nail. Nails are sensitive to physiological changes and will grow more slowly in cold weather and during illness (Doughty, 2004).

Dermis

The dermis provides the principle mass of the skin and mainly comprises collagen bundles usually 1 to 4 mm thick. Functions of the dermis include prevention of mechanical trauma, water storage, sensory enervation, and thermoregulation. The dermis contains macrophages, mast cells, fibroblasts, and lymphocytes, all of which play vital roles in wound healing.

Dermal Proteins

The essential proteins produced in the dermis are collagen, reticular fibers, and elastin. Collagen constitutes the majority of fibers in the dermis and is the major structural protein of the body. This protein is the most stress-resistant fiber of the dermis and provides tensile strength to the layer. Vitamin C is essential for production of collagen.

Components of the Dermis

The cells found within the dermis are important to tissue regeneration and repair. The macrophage is responsible for ingestion of bacteria and other substances and is the principle mediator of wound healing. Macrophages arise from the bone marrow and initially circulate in the blood as a monocyte. In the dermis the macrophage functions as part of the immune response and along with the Langerhans' cells, are capable of processing and presenting antigens to immuno-competent lymphocytes.

Endothelial cells are responsible for the formation of new blood vessel generation or **neoangiogenesis.** They reside in the lining of blood vessels and are activated shortly after injury to the vessel. Mast cells are responsible for histamine release in response to tissue injury and trigger the body's reaction to allergens. Fibroblasts are responsible for synthesis of collagen, elastin, reticular fibers, and ground substance (a viscoelastic substance that has the ability to mold to irregular objects and bind water). Fibroblasts are the principle cells of the dermis. Collagenase and gelatinase, the two enzymes produced by fibroblasts, also degrade collagen bundles. The dermis protects the epidermal appendages and supports a nerve and vascular network.

Lymphatic glands play a role in immune response by removing excess interstitial fluid and microbes. Blood vessels are responsible for perfusion and metabolic skin requirements and play a role in thermoregulation. Nerve fibers are responsible for perception of heat, cold, pain, itching, and pressure and also regulate vasoconstriction, vasodilation, and sweat secretion (Johnstone, et al., 2005).

Subcutaneous Tissue

The subcutaneous tissue consists of adipose or fat cells and lies below the dermis; however, it is not actually part of the skin. Collagen is also found in the subcutaneous layer. Thickness of this tissue varies throughout the body; it is nearly nonexistent in the eyelid, areolae, penis, scrotum, and anterior tibial region and is thickest in the waist area. The distribution of subcutaneous tissue is mediated by hormones, age, heredity, and eating habits. Subcutaneous tissue provides padding over bony prominences, joints, muscle, and internal organs, and serves as a shock absorber.

Protection

The skin provides an effective barrier against many forms of trauma, including mechanical, thermal, microbial, chemical, and radiant insults. The intact epidermis provides a physical barrier against microbial and chemical invasion. The natural biochemical barrier of the skin is called the acid mantle. The acid mantle consists of a mixture of lipoproteins (sebum) secreted by appendages in the epidermis and the acidity of this layer resists bacterial growth and invasion. Sebum has natural antibacterial substances that retard growth of microorganisms. Sebum and keratin also act as barriers against aqueous and chemical solutions. The mechanical strength of the skin comes from bonding of the structures in the epidermis and dermis. Subcutaneous tissue acts as a shock absorber, protecting underlying structures. Melanocytes, the pigment-producing cells of the epidermis screen and absorb UV radiation.

Homeostasis

Homeostasis refers to the fluid and electrolyte regulation function of the skin. Normal human skin breathes water off by the moisture vapor transport mechanism. Normal skin fluid loss is usually 200 g of water within 24 hours. The barrier properties of the skin prevent dehydration by controlled evaporation of internal fluids. The sweat glands open and close in response to external stimuli and to any changes in internal core temperature. The skin also limits absorption of external fluids and gases.

Excretion

The skin functions in the release of urea, bile, sweat, lactic acid, carbon dioxide, and sodium chloride. These functions are excretory in nature and eliminate substances that otherwise would be debilitating and toxic to the body. The renal and respiratory systems also excrete many of these substances.

Thermoregulation

Thermoregulation is the control of body temperature. The skin acts to control body temperature by conduction of heat through the skin for evaporation or absorption by other objects, radiation of heat from body surfaces, convection of heat by air currents, and evaporation of sweat. When the skin senses a warm external environment, the blood vessels dilate in response to promote heat loss. Conversely, the vessels constrict in a cool or cold environment to conserve the body's core temperature.

Synthesis

The skin synthesizes vitamin D by using UV light to convert 7-dehydrocholesterol in the epidermis. Vitamin D is important to calcium and phosphate metabolism and in the mineralization of bone.

Sensory Perception

The skin receptors function primarily in sensation of heat, cold, pain, light touch, itch, and pressure. Different nerves are responsible for each different stimulus and the concentration of nerve endings varies anatomically. Skin sensation is an integrated protective response to the external environment and an important protective mechanism of the skin. For example when a hand comes in contact with a hot object, one immediately pulls away from the heat source.

Psychosocial Function

The skin serves as an organ of communication and identification. The skin presents who we are to our external environment. Healthy skin provides a general sense of well-being and influences self-image. The increase in sebum production experienced during adolescence can trigger changes in the skin, such as acne. Severe cases of acne or cutaneous diseases will significantly alter a person's perception of self. Skin reactions to anger, anxiety, or fear may be manifested as sweating, pallor, or flushing. Reactions to a person's appearance indicate that the skin also serves the function of sexual attraction (Saunders & Edwards, 2004).

Healing

The skin can heal damage to its integrity by either a process of repair or regeneration. **Regeneration** is achieved by replacing damaged cells with the same cell type. Superficial damage to the epidermis is healed by resurfacing the wound with epidermal cells. Only the epidermis and superficial dermis are capable of regeneration, because epithelial, endothelial, and certain tissue substances can be reproduced. The skin repairs a dermal injury by filling the defect with dissimilar tissue because the dermis cannot be regenerated by the body (Johnstone, et al., 2005).

SKIN CHANGES THROUGHOUT THE LIFE SPAN

The skin undergoes numerous changes throughout the human lifecycle. Most of these changes are normal, harmless, and unchangeable. Changes, such as the damage caused by UV light exposure, can be minimized by appropriate preventive treatment (American Academy of Dermatology (AAD), 2006; Weil, 2005).

Newborn and infant skin is porous and easily damaged. The barrier function is not fully developed, the immune system immature, and the skin readily absorbs substances. Most dermatological products, with the exception of a few sun protection products, cannot be used on this age-group. During childhood the barrier and immunological functions of the skin mature. By 2 years of age barrier capability and immune functions are fully developed.

In the adolescent group hormonal secretion stimulates changes in hair follicles and sebaceous, eccrine, and apocrine glands. Hair follicle stimulation produces hair growth on the face in males and in the axilla and genital areas of both genders. This age-group is highly conscious of physical appearance, and the changes wrought by increased sebum production from the facial sebaceous glands resulting in acne can make teenagers self-conscious. Many dermatological pharmaceutical and over-the-counter preparation manufacturers target this audience with products designed to improve appearance (Frith, 2006).

During adulthood the evidence of sun exposure in younger years is seen as wrinkles; weathered-looking skin; age spots; **actinic keratoses** (premalignant lesions); and **telangiectasias** (dilatation of small blood vessels) (Figure 44-3) on the cheeks, nose, and ears, as well as pigmental changes, such as freckles

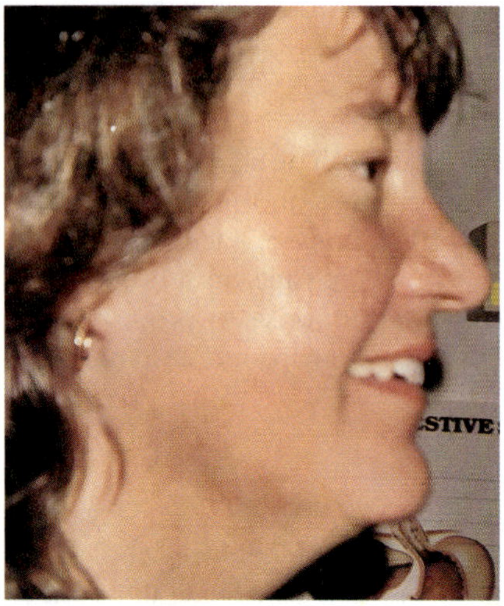

Figure 44-3 Telangiectasias.

and **lentigines** (flat brown spots seen on aged exposed skin). Non–sun-related changes include decreasing elasticity and immune responses and decreased healing rates. In the older adult there is a further decrease in the skin immune response, decreased rate of cellular repair, thinning skin, and a thinning and flattening of basement membrane resulting in an increased risk of skin damage from mechanical trauma. There is also a gradual loss of blood vessels resulting in decreased tissue perfusion and nourishment. Decreased vascularity in the skin of older adults results in diminished capacity to clear potent topical steroids, and therefore the use of such drugs ought to be avoided (AAD, 2006; Centers for Disease Control and Prevention [CDC], 2006d; Olson, 2004).

Cellular Effects of Aging on the Skin

Normal skin begins to show signs of aging by age 30 to 35 years. Sun exposure and burning in childhood, adolescence, and adulthood increases risk for malignant skin changes as people age. Continued sun exposure causes the skin to age more rapidly. Aged skin is thin, inelastic, and fragile. Normal aging should not be confused with photo-aging, because the two processes are biologically different. The difference can best be demonstrated by comparing the skin under the arm with the sun-exposed surface of the lower arm.

Changes in Epidermis

The epidermis becomes thin, and the rate of epidermal rejuvenation by keratinocytes in the basal layer decreases. Hair loss does not increase, but the hair follicles become less active and less dense. Decreased number of Langerhans' cells means a reduced immune response. Melanocytes in the hair bulb decrease production of melanin resulting in the loss of hair pigmentation. There is also a reduction in the density of sweat and sebaceous glands and blood vessels, which result in a decrease in skin hydration. Nails become more brittle and thicker. The number of mast cells decreases, resulting in a reduction in histamine release and inflammatory response. Macrophage differentiation rates are slower, and their functional capacity is diminished resulting in fewer available macrophages to marshal an immune response (Olson, 2004).

Changes in Dermis

The decrease in the number of elastin fiber bundles means that the skin becomes less tolerant of mechanical stressors and more prone to injury. Lymphatic glands decrease their efficiency at managing interstitial fluid levels. The number of blood vessels around glands and hair follicles decreases. Older patients experience a change in their degree of sensory perception and have a diminished capacity to sense pain, itching, heat, and cold. Fibroblasts produce less collagen, elastin, and reticular fibers, resulting in a decreased rate of granulation tissue formation and wound healing.

Changes in Subcutaneous Tissue

The skin becomes atrophic and fragile when subcutaneous tissue is lost. With this loss comes a decrease in the protective padding provided by this tissue layer, and the shock absorber function is reduced. Bony prominences, joints, bones, and internal organs are at increased risk for damage.

FACTORS REGULATING SKIN AND WOUND REPAIR

Many cellular substances control the healing pathway, because healing is a complex interaction between growth factors, cytokines, enzymes produced by cells throughout all phases of healing, and hormones. Growth factors are multichain protein molecules that control the proliferation and differentiation of

Uncovering the Evidence

Efficacy and Safety of Emollient Cream on Photo-Damaged Skin

Discussion: A two-year controlled study was conducted with 240 older adult participants to determine the efficacy and safety of Tretinoin emollient cream in the treatment of photo-damaged skin on the face. Tretinoin or a placebo product was applied once a day. Scheduled assessments were conducted over the study period. Findings indicated a significant improvement in the rough appearance, fine and coarse wrinkling, mottled hyperpigmentation, lentigines and sallowness of participants treated with tretinoin emollient. These findings suggest that tretinoin is an appropriate therapeutic treatment to use and test with a larger group of people with photo-damaged skin.

Implications for Practice: Health care providers can intervene in people at risk for potential photo-aging problems. The tretinoin medication can continue to be tested for its positive effects and application of it as a viable option for intervention.

Source: Kang, S., Bergfeld, W. Gottlieb, A., Hickman, J., Humeniuk, J., Kempers, S., et al. (2005). Long-term efficacy and safety of Tretinoin emollient cream 0.05% in treatment of photodamaged skin. American Journal of Clinical Dermatology, 6*(4), 245–253.*

cells. Growth factors function much like hormones in that they bind to certain sites on the membranes of cells and stimulate changes within those cells. Matrixmetalloproteases (MMPs) are collagenase, gelatinase, and stromelysin and are the most well-known MMPs. Hormones also participate in the regulation of wound healing. Metabolic conditions affecting regulation of hormones also contribute to problems in wound healing, particularly deficiencies in estrogen and insulin secretion and excess secretion of cortisol.

Healing is the restoration of structure and function of the skin after tissue damage. Injury precipitates a complex cascade of processes that are interdependent and interactive, the natural sequencing of which results in normal repair. Wounds that proceed normally through the repair process to healing are referred to as acute wounds. Recalcitrant or indolent wounds are wounds that fail to heal in the normal process and are referred to as chronic wounds. The understanding of wound repair is based on the acute wound model. The phases of wound healing are inflammation, proliferation, and maturation, and many factors are associated with impaired wound healing (Olsen, 2004).

ASSESSMENT

A thorough history will assist the health care provider to determine a correct diagnosis of skin and wound problems. The components of an adequate assessment are the history, chief complaint, past medical history, current medications, allergies, family history, psychosocial, and lifestyle history, including travel and occupational history and a review of systems. A thorough medication history is important to help determine if the skin disorder is related to drug side effects, such as vitamins, corticosteroids, antibiotics, hormones, and antimetabolites (antineoplastics used in cancer therapy).Chronic skin problems can affect an individual's self-image and confidence. People often spend large sums of money on products and cosmetic procedures to help erase the physical and psychosocial effects of their troubling skin conditions. People often must consider how much can be reasonably spent to improve skin appearance if it means that some basic necessities must be sacrificed (Doughty, 2004).

Dollars and Sense

Improving Appearance and Self-Image

Regardless of age or gender our self-image and, thus, our self-worth is linked to the visual image we present to ourselves and others. Our appearance generates the initial and long-term perception on which others base their judgments about our intelligence, physical ability, general attitude, and value as a human being. Initial judgments are made rapidly and may take a long time to overcome. Therefore when a physical abnormality, such as a skin disease, scarring, or even a skin blemish, threatens our self-image we tend to seek ways to overcome or alter our appearance because to do nothing threatens our emotional and perhaps eventually, our physical health. Achieving a personally and socially acceptable appearance through cosmetics, medications, or surgery can be costly. When choices must be made about whether to spend limited resources on shelter, food, clothing, health care, or appearance, a decision about what constitutes a reasonable return on investment must be made.

Review of Systems

The screening procedure includes a review of systems designed to identify problems of which the patient might have been unaware or did not previously mention in the history. Documentation of the general skin condition should be made. Specific problems of the skin should be described and noted with the appropriate biological system. The review of systems can be accomplished by means of a personal questionnaire or data can be collected through a direct interview as part of the history taking process. Refer to Table 44-2 for examples of information to include.

Assessment of the Skin

Overall skin color is noted. A generalized alteration in total body skin color and tone may indicate a systemic problem. Normal skin tone should be congruent with the patient's stated race (see Respecting Our Differences). Presence of a jaundiced skin tone indicates a hepatic or biliary pathology. Decreased generalized skin turgor suggests dehydration. Cyanosis and a cool temperature in an extremity suggest circulatory and vascular problems. There is a normal color vari-

TABLE 44-2 Review of Systems Related to Skin Disorders

Personal perception of the skin problem	Description of daily hygiene practices
	Self-treatment or prescribed skin products for current or previous skin disorder.
	Description of onset, course, and treatment of current skin problem
	Contact with pets
Nutrition patterns	Recent changes in diet and food supplements
	Description of any changes in skin, hair, nails, mucous membranes, and healing of sores or lesions
Elimination patterns	Excessive sweating or dryness of skin
	Location of any swelling
Activities and exercise patterns	Use of protective skin preparations (some may be toxic)
	Fluid replacement practices
Sleep and rest patterns	Effects of skin problem on sleep and rest patterns.
Environmental changes	Change in laundry products, cosmetics, or other personal skin products
	Change in climate (heat, cold, or geographical changes because of travel)
	Stressful events
Self-concept Self-image	Emotional response and perception related to effects of skin problem on self-concept and self-image
	Impact on interrelationships
Coping strategies	Usual response to stress (effective or ineffective)
Cultural influences	Factors that may influence choice of treatment options.
	Beliefs or values that may influence feelings about the skin disorder

Adapted from Estes, M. (2006). Health assessment and physical examination *(3rd ed.). New York: Thomson Delmar Learning.*

ation between sun-exposed areas and areas that generally remain covered or protected from the sun. However, the color should be uniform. Hyperpigmentation may indicate sun damaged areas (liver spots on the hands), and hypopigmented areas may indicate abnormal pigment or infectious processes.

> **Respecting Our Differences**
>
> **Skin of People of Color**
>
> Some skin conditions are misdiagnosed, such as psoriasis, eczema and atopic dermatitis. Darker spots may remain after a primary lesion heals. The skin is also prone to developing keloid scarring (a scar that continues to grow after healing takes place and invades normal tissue). It is also important to protect the darker skin from UV light.

Moisture

Moisture refers to the skin's level of hydration. The skin should feel supple and moist but not wet or clammy. Dryness, ichthyosis (dry, scaly skin), or **xerosis** (abnormal dryness of skin, mucous membranes, or conjunctiva) indicate a decreased level of naturally produced skin lubricants (sebaceous gland secretions). Relate findings of the examination to the patient's age to determine normal level of moisture. Skin that feels overly moist or cool is abnormal. **Diaphoresis** (profuse sweating) is abnormal and may indicate certain types of poisoning (e.g., alcohol), neurological problems, or endocrine problems.

Temperature

The temperature of the normal skin is uniformly warm and is a reflection of normal circulation. Excessive warmth indicates a higher core body temperature and is abnormal, possibly indicating an infectious process. Conversely, cooler skin temperatures usually indicate a circulatory problem (e.g., in emergent situations, cool skin indicates shock). Compare areas of temperature differences with the same area on the opposite side.

Texture

Texture refers to the general feel of the skin. Stroke the skin with the fingertips. Normal skin should feel smooth and resilient. Lumps or areas of unusual thickening or thinning (atrophy) are abnormal. Any raised or depressed areas should be noted and further evaluation is necessary.

Turgor

Turgor is the skin's elasticity, resilience, and hydration. It is measured by examining the amount of time required to return to normal after pinching the skin upward (Figure 44-4). The nurse gently pinches a fold of skin between thumb and forefinger; then releases the tented skin fold. If the skin remains elevated or tented for more than three seconds, turgor is decreased. Normal skin should return to its' usual contours within three seconds. As elasticity decreases with age, so does skin turgor.

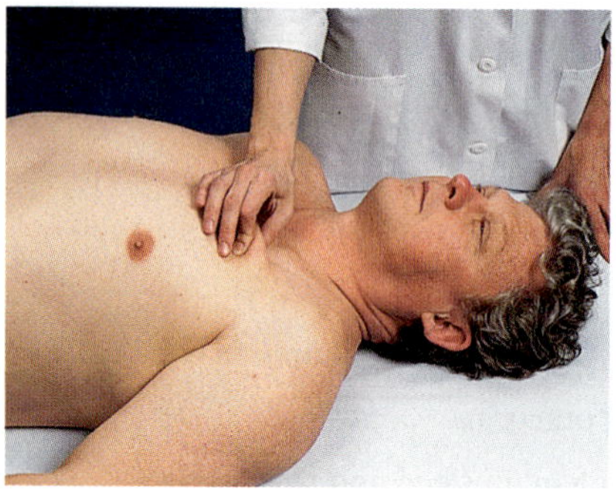

Figure 44-4 Nurse assessing skin turgor.

Edema

Edema is an abnormal collection of fluid in the interstitial spaces between cells resulting in a lifting and separating of the layers of the skin. The nurse should assess for edema in any shiny, tight area of the skin noted on inspection. Severe edema can result in a blanching of the skin because of the pressure of the accumulated fluid. Palpate any edematous area for temperature changes, tenderness, and mobility. Press on the area for five seconds then release the area to assess for pitting edema. Depth of the residual indentation is measured in either millimeters or centimeters. Generalized edema or **anasarca** is associated with malnutrition, terminal illness, and metabolic fluid overload problems.

Tenderness

Tenderness is assessed by palpation and is an abnormal finding. Healthy skin palpation should not elicit any pain response unless injury is evident. Tenderness in a skin area may be indicative of infection, or related to a deep tissue problem. A classic symptom of tenderness is guarding, in which the patient protects the area from palpation by the health care provider.

Odor

Odor is a symptom of an underlying problem in healthy skin, with the exception of the axillae. Odor from open wounds usually represents bacterial or fungus colonization or may represent hygiene problems in skin folds or other areas of the body. Greenish-blue drainage with a musty odor indicates a possible *Pseudomonas* infection. Odor may also be indicative of a metabolic problem. A fruity odor of breath may indicate a serious metabolic disturbance of type 1 diabetes, called diabetic ketoacidosis, an emergent situation of overproduction of ketone bodies that results in metabolic acidosis.

Lesions

Lesions (altered areas of tissue) or wounds should be treated as abnormal findings and assessed and described in an orderly fashion. Location, distribution, size, arrangement, color, configuration, secondary changes, presence of drainage, contours, consistency, mobility, and tenderness must be documented (Figure 44-5). The names and descriptions of primary lesions (Figure 44-6) are summarized in Box 44-1.

Secondary lesions are the result of primary lesions, and include crusts, scales, fissures, erosions, excoriations, ulcerations, atrophy, scars, keloids, umbilicated (depressed like the umbilicus), and zosteriform, which is a linear arrangement such as seen in herpes zoster and keratosis follicularis (Figure 44-7).

Mobile lesions move freely when palpated; immobile lesions do not, indicating attachment to underlying tissue. Locations of lesions are described using position relative to anatomic landmarks. Size is measured in millimeters or centimeters. Distribution refers to the pattern of occurrence on the skin. Lesions may be localized, regional, or generalized. Arrangement refers to the pattern of nearby lesions (i.e., linear or satellite). Configuration relates to the shape of the lesion. Box 44-2 defines typical terminology used to describe the distribution and configuration of lesions.

Fast Forward ▶▶▶

Safety Measures to Prevent Untoward Events

For the past 10 years the Joint Commission on Accreditation of Healthcare Organizations (JCAHO) has required health care enterprises that seek JCAHO accreditation to provide written reports of untoward events and the actions being taken to prevent recurrence of such events. Accreditation can be withheld and monetary penalties can be incurred for failure to prevent such events. Increasing pressure to reduce health care costs and improve the quality of health care outcomes is beginning to generate closer examination of preventable conditions that are costly to treat. In the near future incidence of hospital-acquired skin problems; such as pressure ulcers, could result in denial of payment for care rendered.

BOX 44-1

PRIMARY LESIONS

- **Macules:** Flat circumscribed changes of the skin (flat nevi, café au lait spots, vitiligo, telangiectases, or capillary hemangiomas).
- **Papules:** Elevated circumscribed lesions (elevated nevi, verrucae, molluscum contagiosum, or individual lesions of lichen planus).
- **Nodules:** Circumscribed elevated, usually solid lesions (fibromas, neurofibromas, xanthomas, erythema nodosum, and various benign or malignant growths).
- **Plaques:** Elevated disc-shaped lesions (psoriasis, lichen simplex or chronicus neurodermatitis).
- **Tumors**: Larger and deeper circumscribed solid lesions—benign or malignant (lipomas, strawberry or cavernous hemangiomas, neoplasms).
- **Wheals:** Solid superficial elevations usually in response to pruritus conditions (insect bites, urticaria, or allergic reactions).
- **Vesicles:** Sharply circumscribed, elevated fluid-contain Vesicle lesions (herpes, dyshidrosis, pompholyx, varicella, or contact dermatitis).
- **Bullae:** Larger circumscribed, elevated fluid-containing lesions (burns, contact dermatitis, pemphigus, or epidermolysis bullosa).
- **Pustules:** Circumscribed elevations containing purulent exudates (pustular psoriasis, bromoderma, or smallpox)
- **Comedones:** Plugged secretions of horny material retain within a pilosebaceous follicle.
- **Burrows:** Linear lesions produced by tunneling of animal parasite (scabies).
- Telangiectasia: relatively permanent dilatation of superficial venules, capillaries, or arterioles (lupus erythematosus, dermatomyositis, or scleroderma).

Adapted from Estes, M. (2006). Health assessment and physical examination *(3rd ed.). New York: Thomson Delmar Learning.*

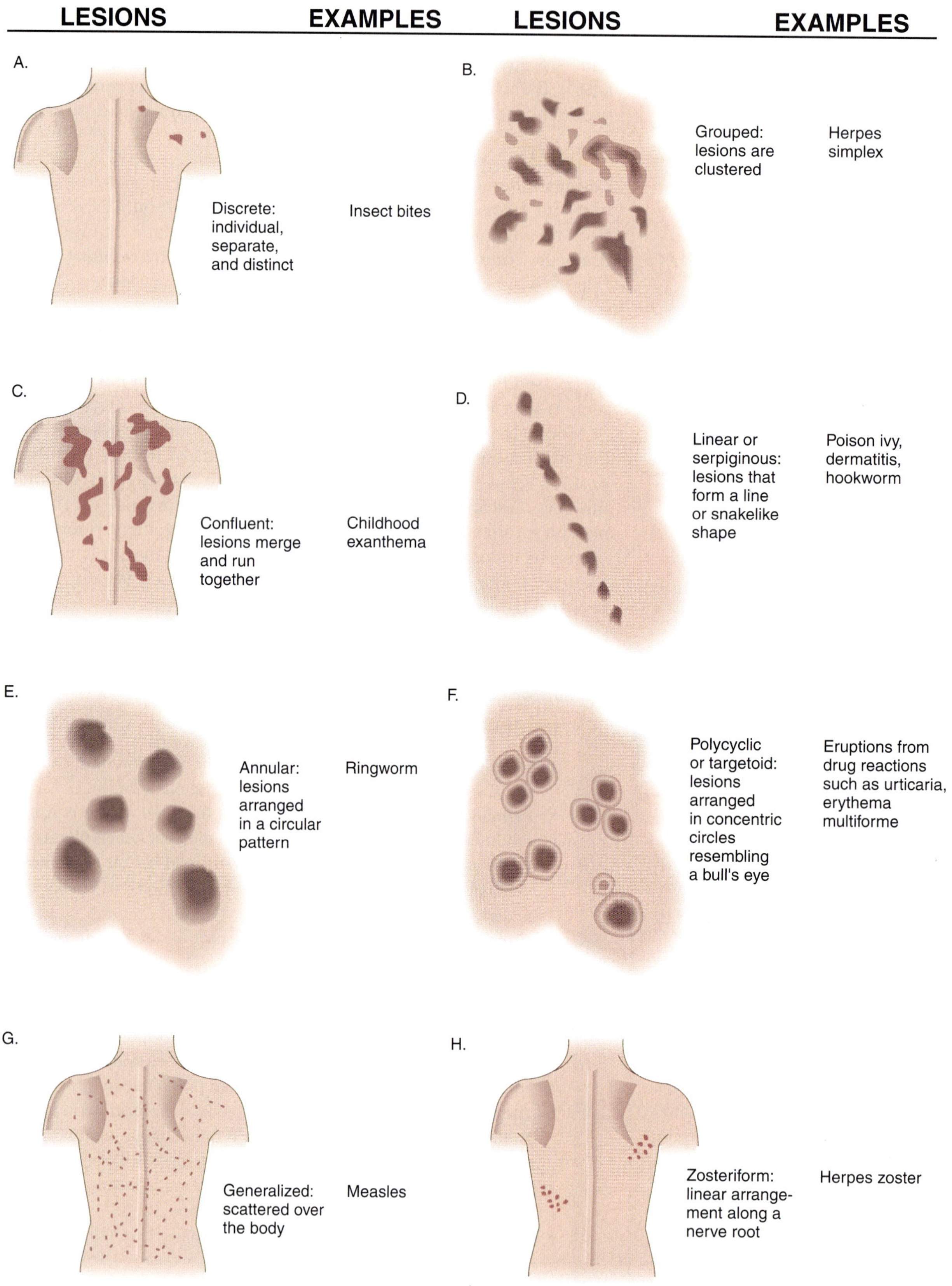

Figure 44-5 Arrangement of lesions.

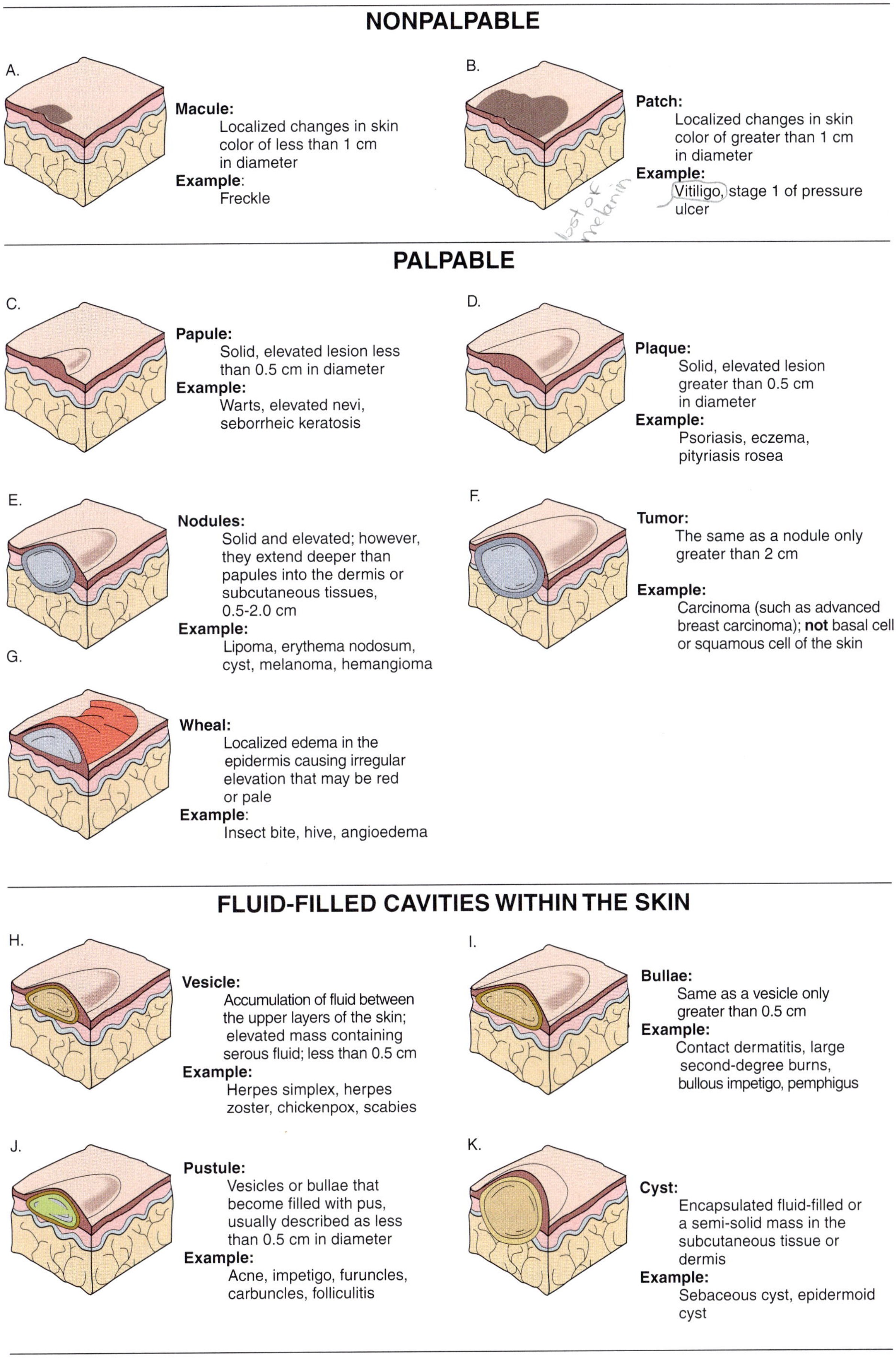
NONPALPABLE
A.
Macule:
Localized changes in skin color of less than 1 cm in diameter
Example:
Freckle
B.
Patch:
Localized changes in skin color of greater than 1 cm in diameter
Example:
Vitiligo, stage 1 of pressure ulcer
PALPABLE
C.
Papule:
Solid, elevated lesion less than 0.5 cm in diameter
Example:
Warts, elevated nevi, seborrheic keratosis
D.
Plaque:
Solid, elevated lesion greater than 0.5 cm in diameter
Example:
Psoriasis, eczema, pityriasis rosea
E.
Nodules:
Solid and elevated; however, they extend deeper than papules into the dermis or subcutaneous tissues, 0.5-2.0 cm
Example:
Lipoma, erythema nodosum, cyst, melanoma, hemangioma
F.
Tumor:
The same as a nodule only greater than 2 cm
Example:
Carcinoma (such as advanced breast carcinoma); not basal cell or squamous cell of the skin
G.
Wheal:
Localized edema in the epidermis causing irregular elevation that may be red or pale
Example:
Insect bite, hive, angioedema
FLUID-FILLED CAVITIES WITHIN THE SKIN
H.
Vesicle:
Accumulation of fluid between the upper layers of the skin; elevated mass containing serous fluid; less than 0.5 cm
Example:
Herpes simplex, herpes zoster, chickenpox, scabies
I.
Bullae:
Same as a vesicle only greater than 0.5 cm
Example:
Contact dermatitis, large second-degree burns, bullous impetigo, pemphigus
J.
Pustule:
Vesicles or bullae that become filled with pus, usually described as less than 0.5 cm in diameter
Example:
Acne, impetigo, furuncles, carbuncles, folliculitis
K.
Cyst:
Encapsulated fluid-filled or a semi-solid mass in the subcutaneous tissue or dermis
Example:
Sebaceous cyst, epidermoid cyst

Figure 44-6 Morphology of primary lesions.

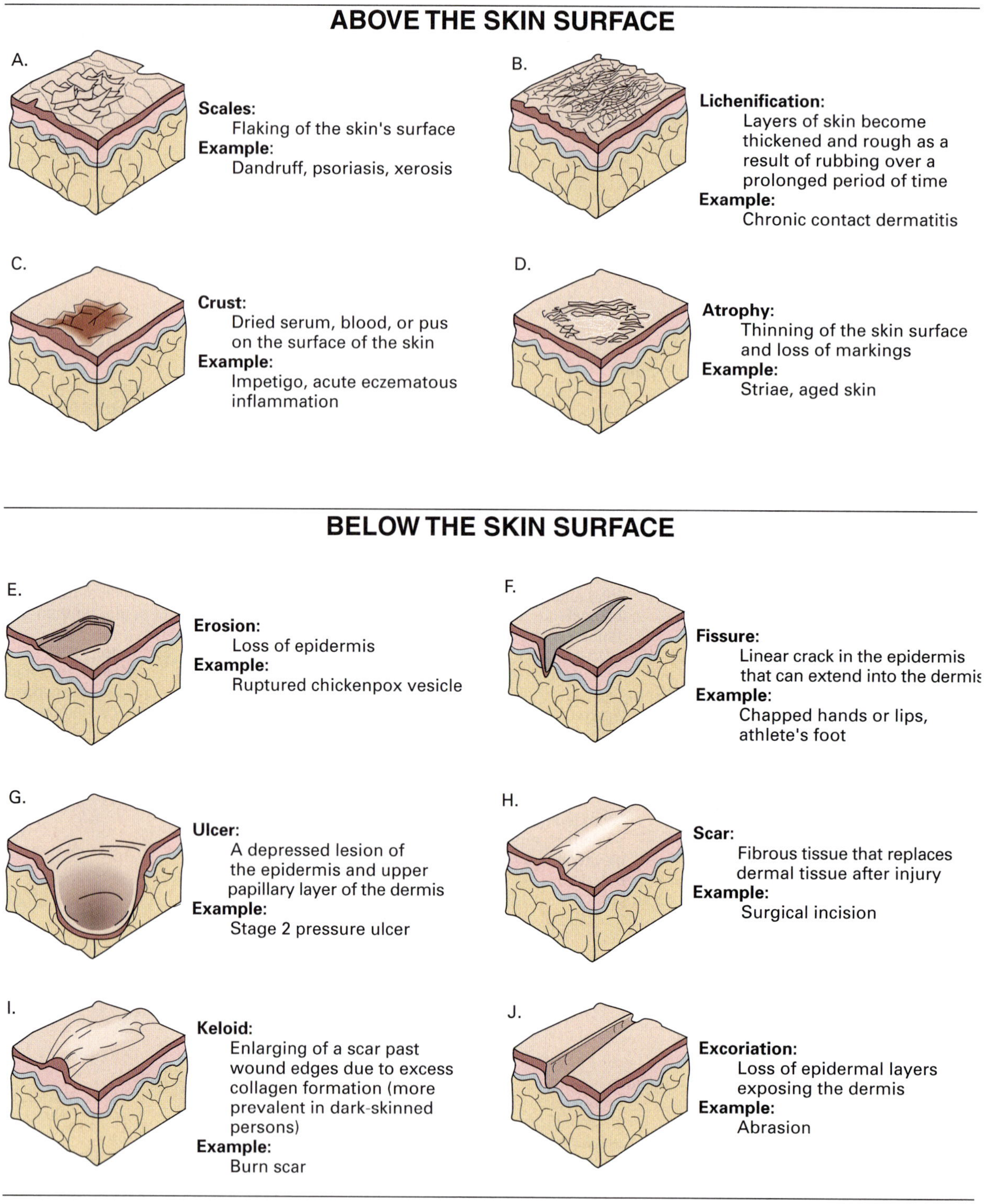

Figure 44-7 Morphology of secondary lesions.

DIAGNOSTIC TESTS

Diagnostic tests for skin and wound care problems are based on a thorough assessment and documentation of the findings. The nurse should explain the procedure prior to starting the test and allow time for questions from the patient and any caregivers. A biopsy is usually taken from fresh, well-developed

BOX 44-2

DESCRIPTION AND CONFIGURATION OF SELECTED GROUP OF LESIONS

- **Annular:** Ring shaped (superficial fungal infections such as ring-worm, pityriasis rosea, seborrheic dermatitis, psoriasis, and others).
- **Dermatomal:** Localized into a dermatome supplied by one or more dorsal ganglia (herpes zoster and segmental vitiligo).
- **Eczematoid:** Suggest inflammation with tendency to thickening, oozing, vesiculation, or crusting (related to eczema).
- Iris lesions: Target-like concentric ringed lesions (erythema multiforme-Steven Johnson varieties).
- Keratosis: Circumscribed patches of horny thickening (seborrheic or actinic keratoses, chronic dermatitis and callus formation).
- Linear: Band-like configuration (nevi or scleroderma lichen striatus).
- Serpiginous: Serpent-shaped (lesions of cutaneous larva).

Adapted from Estes, M. (2006). Health assessment and physical examination *(3rd ed.). New York: Thomson Delmar Learning.*

lesions. The nurse should teach appropriate wound care of biopsy sites, possible side effects of tests, such as bleeding from sites or evidence of infection, and follow-up instructions. Mohs' micrographic surgery is a tissue-sparing method used to map tumors during frozen section (Daniels, 2003). For example, basal cell carcinomas spread finger-like projections into surrounding tissue that are not readily visible. Tissue is removed in thin layers and the edges are mapped to determine if the tumor has been completely removed or residual tumor still exists in the surgical site. Many of the skin disorders can result in additional hospital admissions and could be prevented with appropriate nursing management. There are many additional expenses to the health care system for continued skin breakdown issues (e.g., pressure ulcers or radiation burns).

Nursing Diagnoses

Based on the information gathered, examples of nursing diagnoses in the patient with disorders of the integument may include the following:

- Activity intolerance related to pain (or risk for activity intolerance)
- Anxiety related to the appearance of the integumentary disorder and its impact on interpersonal relationships
- Risk for infection related to a barrier break in the skin
- Disturbed sensory perception related to sensory nerve damage

The Health Care Team

A team of health care providers brings integrated expertise from multiple disciplines to the care of patients with integumentary system diagnoses. Both general practice and advance practice nurses, such as certified wound, ostomy, and continence therapists, may manage or provide the care. As appropriate, general and specialist health care providers, pharmacists, physical and occupational therapists, nutritionists, clergy, psychologists, and social workers may also collaborate on an integrated health care team. Some team members may provide care at community health care sites, and others may provide hospital-site care.

KEY CONCEPTS

- The epidermis is comprised of layers with unique functions and made up of stratified epithelial cells.
- The dermis provides the principle mass of the skin, and its functions include water storage, sensory enervation and thermoregulation and prevention of mechanical trauma.
- Functions of the skin include protection, homeostasis, regulation of fluid and electrolytes, excretion, thermoregulation, synthesis, sensory perception, psychosocial impression, and healing.
- Many of the skin changes that occur throughout the lifespan are normal, harmless and unchangeable. Normal skin begins to show signs of aging by ages 30 to 35.
- Acute wounds heal in an orderly manner in the healthy individual.
- Delayed healing occurs in chronic wounds to repeated or prolonged insults to tissues.
- A thorough history will assist the health care provider to determine a correct diagnosis of skin and wound problems.
- Assessment of the skin includes observation of color variations, moisture, temperature, texture, turgor, presence of edema, tenderness, odor, scars, and lesions.

REVIEW QUESTIONS

1. The epidermis replenishes itself by a process labeled as:
1. Colonization
2. Reconstruction
3. Keratinization
4. Differentiation

2. Cells that are responsible for skin pigmentation are:
1. Langerhans' cells
2. Fibroblasts
3. Macrophages
4. Melanocytes

3. Neoangiogenesis, a process during the wound healing process is the responsibility of:
1. Mast cells
2. Endothelial cells
3. Fibroblasts
4. Carotenoids

4. The major function of the subcutaneous tissue is to provide:
1. Nutrients to the dermis and epidermis
2. Padding over body joints and other internal structures
3. Regulation of diffusion of oxygenation to tissues
4. Maintenance of homeostasis and fluid and electrolyte balance.

5. Regeneration of skin is accomplished by replacing damaged tissue with:
1. Dissimilar cell tissue
2. A network of growth factor cells
3. The same cell type
4. Scar tissue

6. Repeated or prolonged insults to tissues can result in development of:
1. Telangiectasia
2. Capillary hemangiomas
3. Dermatomal lesions
4. Pressure sores.

7. The substances that control the proliferation and differentiation of cells are known as:
1. Growth factors
2. Tumors
3. Burrows
4. Bullae

8. In assessment of an edematous area, the nurse should palpate for:
1. Hard nodules
2. Temperature changes, tenderness, and mobility
3. Keratosis
4. Hypopigmentations and macular lesions

9. A teenager with severe acne decides that he does not want to participate in the swimming exercises that are part of the physical education course at his school. The nursing diagnosis that best describes this person's behavior is:
1. Ineffective coping related to lack of social support
2. Impaired skin integrity related to the skin lesions
3. Social isolation related to anticipatory fear of rejection
4. Anxiety related to lack of knowledge about his disease

Continued

REVIEW QUESTIONS—cont'd

10. Patient teaching for older adults should include information about avoiding the use of potent topical steroids because:
    1. Decreased vascularity in the skin decreases capacity to clear medications from the system.
    2. Thinning of skin increases risk of skin damage and bleeding when medication is applied.
    3. Lentigines (flat brown spots) can become darker and increase absorption of skin products.
    4. Presence of telangiectasias on the head and face delays absorption of topical skin products.

REVIEW ACTIVITIES

1. Develop an interview guide of questions to ask about skin problems. Interview at least three individuals from different cultures regarding their cultural beliefs about the etiology of skin disorders and the traditional remedies used. Compare your findings and provide a written report.
2. Develop a case study scenario for a 35-year-old person of color with psoriasis. Design a concept map outlining the various problems associated with the skin disorder. Develop a list of nursing diagnoses that can be applied in developing a plan of care for this person. (This may be a small group activity.)
3. Develop a teaching or learning plan for explaining how specific occupations (health care professionals, factory workers, plumbers, electricians,) and hobbies place persons at risk of contact dermatitis.
4. Design a check list for assessing the sun damage (photo damage) on an older person's skin. Which areas are at greatest risk of damage? Examine an older family member or a friend using this check list. Prepare an informational brochure for that individual.
5. Access the American Academy of Dermatology Web site at: http://www.aad.org and click on Public Resource Center. Click on Skincarephysicians.com. Select one of the skin disorder links (acne, actinic keratosis, aging skin, eczema, psoriasis, rosea, or skin cancer). Review the information and develop an instruction pamphlet based on the answers to questions posed on the specific skin disorder.
6. Access the American Academy of Dermatology Web site at: http://www.aad.org and click on Public Resource Center. Click on Kids Connection. This is a special section for children age 8 to 12. Review the list of various skin disorders, such as relationship of diet to skin problem, or what causes hives or warts. Prepare a poster describing information about a selected skin disorder and share it with your class or share it with a group of children accompanied by a brief presentation.

Visit the Contemporary Medical-Surgical Nursing online companion resource at www.delmarhealthcare.com for additional content and study aids. Click on Online Companions then select the Nursing discipline.

Dermatological Dysfunction: Nursing Management

Cynthia A. Worley, BSN, RN, WOCN

CHAPTER 45

CHAPTER TOPICS

- Guidelines for Nursing Management of Patients with Dermatological Dysfunction
- Debridement
- Methods of Treatment
- Common Skin Disorders
- Precancerous and Cancerous Conditions

KEY TERMS

Abscess
Acne
Anthropophilic
Atopic dermatitis
Autolytic debridement
Carbuncles
Cellulitis
Comedones
Contact dermatitis
Debridement
Enzymatic debridement
Folliculitis
Furuncles (boils)
Humectants
Lichenification
Mechanical debridement
Pediculosis
Pediculosis pubis
Photoaging
Photoallergic
Photochemotherapy
Phototherapy
Phototoxic
Pruritus
Psoriasis
Sycosis
Sycosis barbae
Tineas
Xerosis
Zoophilic

The care of people with dermatological problems can be complex. In Western societies a person's physical appearance is highly valued, and a visible dermatological condition can be devastating psychologically and financially. Assessment of any skin condition requires knowledge of the anatomy and physiology of the skin, ability to determine the etiology of the problem, and critical thinking skills to determine the best of many effective methods of treatment. Some treatments are applicable across a wide variety of conditions; others are specific to certain conditions only. Before determining the appropriate treatment options for a variety of common dermatological conditions, the general guidelines for treatment must be considered.

GENERAL GUIDELINES FOR MANAGEMENT OF PATIENTS WITH DERMATOLOGICAL DYSFUNCTION

Health care providers agree that the fundamental principles of wound healing and skin repair, must guide the health care provider assessing and diagnosing any skin problem or condition. The health care providers must first determine the etiology of the problem by taking a thorough history as discussed in chapter 44. Onset, duration, exacerbation, alleviation, and previous treatment must be examined. Without an accurate diagnosis of the cause of the skin or wound problem, appropriate treatment cannot be initiated. A patient with diabetes and a neuropathic ulcer on the plantar surface of the foot cannot be successfully treated without addressing the issue of glycemic control. Patients with a lower extremity ulcer must first be evaluated to determine if the ulcer is venous, arterial, or mixed before the appropriate medical or surgical intervention can be initiated.

On examination of the skin or wound problem the health care provider must eliminate or control infectious processes and remove any necrotic or devitalized tissue impeding healing. Initiating any treatment without first addressing these two critical issues may have disastrous consequences. Wound and skin lesions will not heal in the presence of heavy bacterial contamination. The body's immune response is concentrated on controlling the microbial burden rather than on initiating inflammation in the presence of infection or colonization. Necrotic tissue has been shown to harbor bacteria and interfere with wound healing and therefore must be removed for healing to begin. Infection is defined as the presence of 10^5 colony forming units (CFUs) identified on microscopic examination (Estes, 2006).

Next, the health care provider should identify any barriers to healing and correct those issues. The patient who is malnourished and trying to heal a large surface area burn or other type of skin condition will find that healing is frustrated by the nutritional problem. Adequate protein, vitamin, and mineral intake, as well as hydration are essential for healing. Patients with untreated or poorly controlled comorbidities, such as poor circulation or an impaired immune status, are at risk for impaired wound and skin healing by virtue of their chronic illness. The patient with an allogenic or matched-unrelated donor bone marrow transplant is immunologically at risk for any type of opportunistic infection as well as for graft-versus-host disease (GVHD), a risk factor in this type of transplant patient. The patient with GVHD of the skin is treated using steroids, and healing is impaired by the use of steroids. Therefore, during the GVHD treatment, breakdown of the patient's skin will be slow to resolve.

A moist wound environment must be provided and maintained for the wound to heal properly with a minimum of complications. Research has shown that wounds heal best in a moist environment; in other words, under some sort of dressing that prevents drying of the wound bed. If the wound is allowed to dry out, healing is delayed or halted, because the wound microenvironment is not conducive to cell proliferation and optimal cellular activity. White blood cells (WBCs), fibroblasts, macrophages, and endothelial cells all require moisture to migrate, divide, and perform their specific functions that facilitate healing. Finally, the health care provider knows that all of these guidelines for healing require that the patient understands the condition and participates fully in the treatment (Sheffield, Smith, & Fife, 2004).

DEBRIDEMENT

Debridement is the removal of necrotic tissue from a wound. Necrotic tissue is an impediment to wound and skin healing, and the necrotic tissue does not have to occur in large amounts to interfere with repair. A scab is not nature's

Real World, Real Choices

Sacral Pressure Lesion

Scenario

You are asked to evaluate the skin problem of an 89-year-old man with a history of a cerebrovascular accident (CVA) that has left him with right-sided weakness, dysphasia (difficulty swallowing), and aphasia (inability to speak). He is unable to provide you with a health history, but he is accompanied by a family member who is familiar with the patient's health history. Through your interview of this family member you learn that the patient has a history of hypertension and chronic atrial fibrillation. The patient resides in a skilled nursing facility and must rely on the nursing staff for all of his care. He is able to transfer from the bed to a wheelchair with assistance. The skin problem is a partial-thickness wound on the patient's sacrum that was discovered one week ago. There is an erythematous border around the wound and some bruising at the right edges. The base is pink and moist without odor. The family member reports that the facility's staff has been using a barrier ointment on the area. The patient is alert, cooperative, and afebrile.

Guideline 1: What is the etiology of the problem?
Guideline 2: How would you remove the necrotic tissue and what clinical manifestations would indicate an infection?
Guideline 3: What would be barriers and concerns for this patient?
Guideline 4: How and why would you maintain a moist wound dressing?

protective dressing; instead, a scab simply indicates that the wound bed has been allowed to dry. Even a paper cut will heal more rapidly with a topical antibiotic ointment and a cover dressing than when it is left open to dry.

There are four methods of debridement used to remove necrotic tissue from wounds. **Mechanical debridement** primarily makes use primarily of gauze dressings to remove necrotic or devitalized tissue from wounds. The gauze is moistened with saline or another solution, packed into the wound, and allowed to dry. Removal of the dry gauze mechanically lifts necrotic tissue from the wound. This is an inexpensive method of debridement. It is also painful to the patient and disruptive to both the new tissue bed being formed and to existing healthy tissue, which also adheres to the gauze and is torn away when the gauze is removed. It is not unusual for the wound bed to bleed when the gauze is removed, indicating a disruption of the new vascular network (Worley, 2004).

Enzymatic debridement is accomplished using a chemical debriding agent, usually an enzyme. Papain urea, either as a single ingredient or used in conjunction with a chlorophyll and copper complex and collagenase-based products are effective in liquefying necrotic tissue over time. Any enzymatic debriding agent requires a prescription and careful adherence to the directions for application. Most are rendered inactive in the presence of heavy metal ions, such as silver, or when the wound is treated with an antibiotic solution.

Autolytic debridement makes use of the normal phagocytic action of macrophages and leukocytes present in the wound. Moist wound dressings help the wound bed maintain a natural level of moisture, facilitating a normal inflammatory response. It is during inflammation that the macrophages and leukocytes establish control over bacteria present in the wound and provide the clean up service that removes cellular debris and devitalized or necrotic tissue. Debridement by autolysis is slower than enzymatic or sharp debridement,

> **DOLLARS AND SENSE**
>
> **The Finances Involved in Treatment Choices**
>
> Treatment decisions that were once perceived as the best choices are now given close scrutiny to arrive at the most efficient use of the financial and human resources of the hospital while attaining the highest quality clinical outcome for the patient. The decision about whether a procedure can be safely and effectively accomplished in an outpatient setting using local or regional anesthesia or conscious sedation is based on published research of cost versus benefit studies that are reviewed by peers. In addition, issues of access and postoperative care and support for the patient are taken into consideration. The risk of postoperative complications that require professional monitoring and critical clinical judgment with timely intervention also influences the decision about how to proceed with the debridement. No longer is there just one way to provide treatment. Treatment decisions are made by cost, as well as by the effectiveness of the outcome.

but it is the preferred method when the patient is immunocompromised or at risk for bleeding problems.

Sharp debridement is usually performed by a physician or specially trained nurse or other treatment team member. It can be done at the patient's bedside or take place in an operating room. Debridement is usually performed on deeper, chronic wounds, such as pressure ulcers and necrotic surgical wounds. The necrotic tissue is cut away from the wound using a cautery or scalpel. Sharp debridement is the quickest method used to remove devitalized tissue, but it is more costly when it must be done in the operating room under general anesthesia.

Conservative sharp debridement can be performed without anesthesia outside of the operating room when only superficial or loosely adherent tissue is removed. This method is rarely used alone, because not all the necrotic tissue can be readily removed. Usually an enzyme is used in conjunction with conservative debridement, especially if a series of debridements are required to remove all the necrotic tissue. The patient's condition must be thoroughly assessed prior to determining the most appropriate method of debridement (Worley, 2005).

METHODS OF TREATMENT

Topical therapy is used to perform a variety of functions in the treatment of dermatological problems. Lotions, solutions, and creams are used to restore normal skin hydration levels, reduce inflammation, relieve dermatological symptoms, act as a delivery system for other medications, reduce dryness and flaking, provide antimicrobial action, and cleanse and protect the skin. These types of medications are chosen for their active ingredient, the primary agent in the formula that treats the condition, or as a delivery system for the active ingredient to ensure that the active agent stays in contact with the skin. Table 45-1 lists common agents that are used to treat various skin conditions.

Topical vehicles used to deliver medications range from creams and ointments to aerosols and powders. Vehicles discussed in this section include creams, ointments, gels, aerosols, lotions, powders, and pastes. Most creams, by definition, are primarily water-based or oil-in-water-based emulsions with the water content 60 percent or less. The cream vehicle has the ability to provide lubrication to the skin and can be used almost anywhere on the body. They also are less occlusive and may increase dryness in some patients. Creams usually contain preservatives and can contain alcohol or propylene glycol, which can also cause dryness.

Ointments are similar to creams in that they are usually an oil-in-water emulsion, but the water content is 40 percent or less. Ointments are more occlusive and provide a better delivery vehicle because of their ability to trap the medication next to the affected area and increase absorption. Ointment preparations should not be used in situations of severe eczematous inflammation or in areas containing dense hair.

Gels are semisolid preparations, usually a combination of propylene glycol and water, which are most effectively used with inflammatory conditions that produce exudates. They make a good vehicle for medications effective for pruritic lesions, like poison ivy, because they have a drying and cooling effect. Some gels contain alcohol and can cause discomfort when used in dry, cracked, or eroded areas. Aerosols suspend the active ingredient in a base and deliver that ingredient under pressure. They are more drying and can be used to deliver medications to wet or hairy areas.

Lotions are powders suspended in a liquid, usually water, alcohol, or oil. The medications are delivered in a uniform residual film and have a cooling effect. Lotions can be used in hairy areas, such as the scalp, and have the

TABLE 45-1 Agents to Treat Skin Conditions

Topical Medications

MEDICATION	INGREDIENT OR TRADE NAME	NURSING MANAGEMENT
Antifungals	Nystatin (Mycostatin) Clotrimazole (Lotrimin) Terbinafine HCL (Lamisil) Ketoconazole (Nizoral) Miconazole (Micatin)	Drug chosen based on species of dermatophyte and severity and duration of infection Review application and preapplication instructions Possible side effects include skin irritation and overgrowth of fungus when occlusion is used
Antineoplastics	Imiquimod (Aldara) Fluorouracil (Carac and Efudex)	Depending on whether lotion, cream, or solution usually applied once or twice daily Drug causes considerable inflammation and discomfort if large areas are treated
Antiparasitics	Permethrin (Nix and Elimite) Lindane (Kwell) Pyrethrin (RID) Malathion (Ovide) Ivermectin (Stromectol)	Infestations in home require entire family be treated as well as bedding, clothing, and carpets Combs, brushes, curlers, head scarves or coverings, and hair clips must be washed in hot, soapy water
Antipruritics	Lotions: Menthol (Eucerin itch relief) Camphor (Neutrogena anti-itch moisturizer) Calamine lotion Oatmeal suspensions (Aveeno) Wraps: Boric acid (1 tbs/1 L H_2O) Burrow's solution Potassium permanganate Alumen acetate	May be applied frequently to relieve symptoms and discomfort unless contains an analgesic agent Solutions containing analgesic agents should be applied as prescribed (two to four times daily) Observe for contact sensitivity
Antiseptics	Chlorhexidine gluconate (Hibiclens) Iodine solutions Hydrogen peroxide Acetic acid Buffered sodium hypochlorite (Dakin's solution)	May be used for irrigating and cleansing wounds but should not be used to moisten packing materials Should not be used in healing well-granulated wounds Protect periwound skin from solutions
Antivirals	Docosanol (Abreva) Penciclovir (Denavir) Famciclovir (Famvir) Valacyclovir (Valtrex) Acyclovir (Zovirax)	Apply as prescribed May be oral medication or topical medication or both modalities may be used
Corticosteroids	Hydrocortisone (Westcort, Hydrocort, Hytone, etc) Triamcinolone (Kenalog and Aristocort) Clobetasol dipropionate (Temovate) Fluocinonide (Lidex) Desonide (DesOwen)	Avoid use of strong formulation in treating face, neck, and intertriginous areas because increased side effects may result Should be applied evenly over affected areas Should be applied only for prescribed time limit and monitored for side effects

Continued

TABLE 45-1 Agents to Treat Skin Conditions—cont'd

Topical Medications

MEDICATION	INGREDIENT OR TRADE NAME	NURSING MANAGEMENT
Immunomodulators (topical)	Pimecrolimus (Elidel)	Used to treat atopic dermatitis
	Protopic ointment (Tacrolimus)	May safely be used on face and around eyes
		Side effects are burning and stinging, increased risk of secondary infection and some risk of systemic absorption
Lubricating agents	Urea (Carmol)	Apply evenly and best applied immediately after bathing
	Lactic acid (Amlactin and Lac-Hydrin)	
	Petrolatum (Aquaphor and Eucerin)	
	Zinc oxide	
Psoriatic and seborrheic dermatitis shampoos	Chloroxine (Capitrol)	Side effects include skin irritation and dryness
	Pyrithione (Nizoral and Head & Shoulders)	
	Selenium (Selsun and Selsun Blue)	
	Tar solutions: Denorex, Ional T, Neutrogena T, and Tegrin Medicated	
	Sulfur/Salicylic acid: Ional Plus and Sebulex	
Psoriasis	Orals: Psoralens (Oxsoralen Ultra, 8-MOP, Trisoralen)	Side effects include nausea, insomnia, dizziness, headache, depression, and malaise
	Acitretin (Soriatane)	
	Methotrexate	Immunosuppressive, hepatic fibrosis
	Topical: Anthralin (Drithocreme, Psoriatec, ad Curastain)	Skin irritation and skin staining are primary side effects
	Tazorac	Mild irritant dermatitis
	Vitamin D_3 analogue (Dovonex)	Strong preparations should be washed out every morning with strong detergent (like Dawn liquid)
	Tars: Ichthyol, Mazon, PolyTar soap, Tegrin Medicated, and Fototar	
Rosacea medications	Metronidazole (Metro-Gel)	Preparations may sting or burn on application
	Sulfur/Na sulfacetamides (Avar, Clenia, and Sulfacet-R, Plexion)	Avoid triggers (sunlight, alcohol, and spicy foods)
	Azelaic acid (Finacea)	
Wart preparations	Cantharidin (Cantharone)	Protect normal skin from preparation
	Silver nitrate	Side effects include blister formation, skin irritation, pain, and dryness
	Salicylic acid (Compound W, etc.)	
	Podophyllin/podofilox (Condylox, Podocon, and Pododerm)	
	Interferon	
	Dichloroacetic acid	

Adapted from Broyles, B., Reiss, B., & Evans, M. (2007). Pharmacological aspects of nursing care *(7th ed.). New York: Thomson Delmar Learning.*

potential to absorb some moisture. They can cause drying because of the alcohol content, and the medication can wear off easily.

Powders are finely ground solid substances. They can be absorptive and can be used in hairy areas but can become caked in high-moisture areas, like the groin or perineum. Pastes are usually powders in ointments with water content of 50 percent or greater. They provide protection and decrease absorption. Zinc oxide is a commonly used paste. Most patients object to paste preparations, because they are messy and unsightly.

Both the active ingredient and the vehicle must be appropriate for the condition being treated. If the condition produces weeping blisters, a water-based preparation can provide a soothing, cooling, and drying effect. An ointment-based preparation provides the opposite effect; it increases the amount of moisture in the area and promotes lubrication. Inflamed skin absorbs substances more readily than noninflamed skin. When absorption of a medication needs to be increased, covering the area to be medicated with an occlusive dressing enhances the absorption rate (Broyles, Reiss, & Evans, 2007).

Topical Corticosteroids

Corticosteroids are the most commonly prescribed topical medications used to treat dermatological conditions. Steroids are used to decrease inflammation, relieve pruritus, and induce remission of certain cutaneous disorders. These drugs have a potency ranking of from I to VII. The least potent steroids, such as Hytone, fall into group VII and the most potent steroids, such as Cormax, fall into group I. Most dermatoses can be treated with steroids with a low to moderate potency. The best results are achieved when preparations of adequate strength are used for a specified length of time. Most of the group I steroids should never be used under occlusive dressings (Rudy & Parham-Vetter, 2003).

Side effects of steroids include atrophy of the treated area, telangiectasia, acneiform eruptions, burning and dryness, and bruising. It is rarely beneficial to apply a steroid cream more than twice daily, and the patient should be instructed to either follow-up with their health care provider or contact the office if and when the condition improves. As the condition improves, the frequency of application may be changed or the patient may be switched to a lower strength of steroid, another tar preparation, a moisturizer, or another topical preparation may be recommended. Table 45-2 provides information that is important for patients to understand. It is critical for the nurse to provide detailed patient education on the proper use and application of these potent drugs.

Topical Soaks and Wraps

Some dermatological conditions require soaks and wraps as standard treatment. Soaks and wraps can be performed in a variety of ways with a variety of solutions, the use of which will depend on the condition and goal of treatment. A wet environment will soften and loosen cellular skin debris, relieve pruritus, promote drying of moist dermatoses, decrease discomfort, and provide a cooling and soothing environment. Gradual evaporation of water provides the cooling effect to irritated or burning skin.

Soaks can be accomplished by either soaking or bathing the affected area in the solution or by moistening gauze and applying the gauze to the affected area as a dressing. The usual length of exposure is 15 to 20 minutes. Colloidal oatmeal (Aveeno) added to bath water is temporarily soothing but does nothing to increase skin hydration. Tar preparations will reduce inflammation and are helpful in scaling conditions, such as psoriasis or eczema.

Aluminum acetate solutions, such as Burrow's solution or Domeboro solution, a combination of aluminum sulfate and calcium acetate solution, have antimicrobial properties, but can be drying. A 1:40 Burrow's solution obtained

TABLE 45-2 What Every Patient Needs to Know About Topical Medications

PRINCIPLE	ACTION	RATIONAL
Accurate and appropriate use of product		
1. Review preapplication instructions.	1. Patients must clearly understand how to apply the medication, when to apply it, and where to apply it	1. Creams or ointments should be applied evenly and sparingly once or twice daily and only to the affected areas. Correct application will eliminate many potential problems
2. Instruct the patient in regard to appropriate application technique	2. Apply after bathing or cleansing the area.	2. Hydration of the area increases absorption of drug
3. Emphasize that medication is only to be used for the prescribed length of time and only on the area for which it is prescribed	3. Do not apply to face, perineal area or axillae unless otherwise directed by health care provider	3. Monitor areas closely if steroid is applied to these areas. Perineal and axillary areas are high-moisture areas, which will increase absorption.
4. Emphasize that overuse or misuse can result in serious cutaneous and systemic complications	4. Do not apply to broken or irritated skin	4. Absorption of the drug is increased in areas where skin is not intact.
5. Caution patient against lending medication to friends or relatives		
6. Instruct patient about who to call if any problems occur.		

Adapted from Broyles, B., Reiss, B., & Evans, M. (2007). Pharmacological aspects of nursing care *(7th ed.). New York: Thomson Delmar Learning.*

by mixing one packet in one pint of water can be used to moisten gauze dressings. The moistened gauze is then placed over the affected area and wrapped with dry gauze. Both tap water and saline can also be used in soaks and wraps. Potassium permanganate ($KMnO_4$) in a solution ranging from 0.25% to 0.5% has a cooling effect useful in relieving pruritus and removing cellular debris while providing an antimicrobial effect against *Pseudomonas aeruginosa*. Aluminum acetate solutions are useful in treating allergic conditions involving open, weeping blisters such as poison ivy, poison oak, or poison sumac.

Boric acid solutions can be used as mild bacteriostatic and fungistatic soaks to treat mild infectious processes. Bath oils are not recommended, because they provide a false lubricity to the skin and increase fall risk in the bathtub. As with any drug, patient education is critical to successful treatment.

Wraps are another method of delivering a solution to a target area. Wet wraps can be used immediately after soaking and will increase hydration and prolong the contact time of the solution with the affected area while providing a cooling and soothing effect. The location and severity of the condition will dictate how the wraps need to be applied.

In isolated areas such as forearms or lower extremities, a rolled gauze dressing, such as Kerlix or Kling, may be impregnated with the solution and wrapped around the affected area followed by a dry layer. When whole body treatments are required, wet pajamas or long underwear saturated with the solution and covered by a dry plastic sweat suit will accomplish the desired effect. Cotton gloves and socks can be used to deliver the solution to the hands and feet. The face can be dressed with a wet, then dry, layer of gauze with holes cut for the eyes, nose, and mouth. Moistening the dressings prior to removal reduces discomfort and tissue damage. As with any medication, the patient must be educated about the proper application techniques.

Moisture Retentive Dressings

Moisture retentive dressings are designed to maintain a moist wound environment. They are chosen based on the amount of drainage produced by the wound and the frequency with which they need to be changed. These dressings allow control of the affected skin's environment and provide a protective layer over wounds, ulcers, and refractory dermatoses. Modern-day wound dressings provide a protective barrier against dirt, added trauma, bacteria, and irritants. Moisture retentive dressings decrease discomfort, provide an optimal environment for healing and tissue regeneration, enhance absorption of topical medications, and have a longer wear time than more traditional treatment methods, such as Telfa or other types of gauze dressings (Altman, 2004).

Ranging from impregnated gauze wraps (Unna's boot or Vaseline gauze) to the more technologically advanced hydro fibers (Aquacel) and alginates (Sorbsan and Kaltostat), these dressings are usually easily applied and removed. Moisture retentive dressings can be used in a wide variety of dermatological conditions, from venous stasis ulcers and pressure ulcers to surgical and traumatic wounds. Selection of the most appropriate dressing is dependent on accurate diagnosis and wound assessment. For example, a hydrocolloid dressing will manage light to moderate drainage and has a wear time of up to seven days. However, a moderately draining lesion may overwhelm a hydrocolloid dressing before that seven-day period expires. A calcium alginate dressing is most appropriate for a heavily draining wound but requires a secondary or cover dressing to prevent desiccation of the dressing and the wound. Types of moisture retentive dressings include, but are not limited to, hydrocolloids, foams, hydro fibers, and transparent films.

Moisturizers and Lubricants

Products designed to hydrate the skin play an important role in the treatment of many pruritic, inflammatory, and zerotic skin conditions. In these conditions the goal is to eliminate drying agents from the treatment regimen. Perfumed soaps, lotions, and oils usually contain alcohol as the delivery vehicle for the fragrance and therefore should not be used in the treatment of dermatological conditions.

Skin is not dry because of a lack of oil but from a lack of water. Thus, the primary goal is to apply water to the skin and prevent its evaporation by occlusion. In other words, sealing the moisture into the skin allows hydration of the epidermis and retention of the moisture. Moisturizers and lubricants are designed to hydrate the epidermal layers of the skin. The excellent barrier properties of the skin prevent moisturizers and lubricants from penetrating beyond the epidermis. Regular usage of body moisturizers, particularly within three to five minutes of bathing or showering will aid in prevention of dry, flaking and itching skin.

If emollient products do not succeed in hydrating the skin, it may be necessary to prescribe more potent agents. **Humectants,** such as Aquacare/HP and Carmolare, are substances that promote moisture in skin. Urea and alpha-hydroxy acid are examples of humectants. Urea is a topical keratolytic, functioning to remove excess keratin and to soften and hydrate skin. Alpha-hydroxy acid products hold in skin moisture and decrease rough scale that creates the sensation of dryness. The most common alpha-hydroxy acids are lactic acid (LactiCare) and ammonium lactate (LacHydrin) (Broyles, et al., 2007).

Moisturizers and lotions containing aloe, vitamin E, jojoba, collagen, and elastin are also popular. Many people who use products containing these ingredients achieve the same results as if they used prescription-strength products containing urea or alpha-hydroxy acid. However, there is no scientific evidence showing that these ingredients have any intrinsic benefit beyond their minimal lubricating properties.

Phototherapy and Photochemotherapy

Sunlight has a profound effect on the skin and is associated with a variety of diseases. The skin of a person who has spent a significant amount of time outdoors or who has spent years achieving a healthy tan is thickened, wrinkled, and usually has darker pigmentation (Goldberg, 2004). Ultraviolet (UV) light from the sun causes the most skin reactions and conditions and is classified by the wavelength of the light: ultraviolet A (UVA), ultraviolet B (UVB), or ultraviolet C (UVC). UV light is beyond the spectrum of human vision, in the portion of the electromagnetic spectrum measuring 10 to 400 nanometers (nm) (Note: A nanometer is $1/10^7$ of a meter).

UVA light causes immediate and delayed skin pigment changes and does not contribute to burning and redness. However, the longer the light wavelength, the deeper the penetration into the skin and substructures. UVA can penetrate beyond the epidermis into the dermis and subcutaneous tissue. Chronic exposure to UVA results in the degenerative changes in connective tissue seen in **photoaging** (degenerative changes in connective tissue caused by chronic exposure to UVA), skin cancers, and immunosuppression. UVA can penetrate window glass and has **phototoxic** (rapidly developing nonimmunological skin reaction when exposed to light) and **photoallergic** (sensitivity to light that causes allergic reactions) effects. This type of light is consistent throughout the day and the year.

UVB light is far more damaging and produces the most harmful effects to the skin. This type of radiation is strongest in the summer when the earth is closest to the sun and is most intense between the hours of 10 am and 2 pm. Water, snow, and shiny surfaces reflect UVB radiation. The high amounts of radiation delivered by UVB produces the immediate skin changes associated with sun exposure: sunburn, tanning, inflammation, delayed erythema, and blistering and pigmentation changes. Chronic exposure to UVB also produces photoaging, photocarcinogenesis, and immunosuppression. Window glass absorbs UVB, and prior exposure to UVA enhances the sunburn reaction to UVB. UVC light is almost completely absorbed by the ozone layer and is transmitted only by artificial sources, such as germicidal lamps and mercury arc lamps.

Normal Aging versus Photoaging

Normal signs of aging begin to appear around age 30 to 35. However, unprotected, chronically exposed children can acquire significant sun-related skin changes by the time they reach the age of 15, and the effects of sun damage become apparent after the age of 20. Sun-damaged skin is characterized by thickened, yellowed, coarsening of the epidermis, irregular pigmentation, atrophy of subcutaneous tissue, telangiectasias, deep wrinkling, and other changes, including premalignant changes. UV light, produced naturally by the sun and artificially by other light sources, inhibits deoxyribonucleic acid (DNA) mitosis. UVA and UVB light are used in the treatment of dermatological diseases. UV light is also used to control pathogenic bacteria and viruses and is used in clean room technology where the sterility of the enclosed environment is critical. The differences between the normal aging process and aging related to sun damage are summarized in Table 45-3.

Phototherapy

Phototherapy is the treatment of certain dermatological conditions with artificially produced, nonionizing UV light. This type of therapy is useful in treating certain photobiological conditions, such as psoriasis, vitiligo, eczema, and

TABLE 45-3 Normal Aging versus Photoaging Skin

NORMAL AGING SKIN	PHOTOAGING SKIN
Thin, fragile, and inelastic	Thickened, wrinkled, yellowish skin (solar elastose)
Thinning of epidermis	Thinning of skin, fine wrinkling (atrophy)
Gradual loss of blood vessels, dermal collagen, fat, and elastic fibers	Prominent blood vessels with easy bruising and tearing
Fine, shallow wrinkles that disappear with skin stretching	Deep wrinkles that do not disappear with skin stretching
Decrease in density of hair follicles, sebaceous glands, sweat ducts, fine dryness of skin	Diffuse erythema in fair-skinned persons
Loss of subcutaneous tissue causes skin to become atrophic and fragile	Bleeding into skin following minor trauma (usually in sun exposed areas only—back of the neck, hands, arms), telangiectasias on cheeks, nose, and ears
Reduced elastin fibers result in decreased resilience of skin	Freckles on face
	Lentigo (large brown macules) on face, back of hands, arms, chest, upper back
	Other pigmentation changes such as guttate hypermelanosis (discrete round, white macules) and irregular deep brown pigmented areas
	Seborrheic keratosis (superficial stuck on lesions, more numerous on sun-exposed areas)
	Actinic keratosis (localized thickening of epidermis)
	Comedones and cysts around the eyes

Adapted from Goldberg, D. (2004). Photodamaged skin. *New York: Marcel Dekker.*

cutaneous T cell lymphoma. UVB light is used in the treatment of photosensitive dermatoses and is contraindicated in patients with a history of previous nonmelanoma skin cancers or a family history of melanoma. Dosing of UVB is based on an estimation of the patient's ability to tolerate the treatment based on skin types I through VI and the minimal erythema dose, the smallest amount of UVB required to produce erythema. For example, patients with skin type I have a poor ability to tan, burn easily and severely, and then peel, whereas people with skin type VI are darkly pigmented and never burn. A genetic history is associated with each skin type. Skin type I people have fair skin; freckles; blue, green, or gray eye color; blonde, red, or light brown hair; and a northern European heritage. Skin type VI people have black skin and an African, American Indian, East Indian, or Hispanic (American) heritage (Goldberg, 2004).

A thorough history should be taken by the health care provider prior to initiation of any phototherapeutic regimen that includes skin malignancies, current medications, previous history of radiation exposure or therapy for cancer, and any medical conditions that can be stimulated by UV light, such as herpes simplex, cataracts, or lupus erythematosus. Ophthalmological assessment should be performed on any person displaying early cataract changes, a possible contraindication for photochemotherapeutic ultraviolet A light (PUVA). A variation of standard phototherapy, called the Goeckerman regimen, incorporates photosensitization with keratolytic agents and antipruritic properties of tar preparations. This therapy is used primarily for psoriasis vulgaris and atopic dermatitis. It is a labor-intensive process, requiring the patient to take tar preparation baths and after-bath topical tar medications followed several hours later by phototherapy.

Photochemotherapy

Photochemotherapy is UVA therapy combined with oral or topical 8-methoxypsoralen. This type of UV therapy is used to treat severe and unresponsive forms of psoriasis, atopic dermatitis, and cutaneous T cell lymphoma

(CTCL). The concept is that photosensitizing medications increase the skin sensitivity to the long-wave UVA light (Broyles, et al., 2007). These medications also induce repigmentation of skin in patients with vitiligo and have an antimitotic effect on psoriasis and CTCL. Dosage is established based on body weight, and the medication is taken with food one-and-a-half to two hours prior to treatment to minimize nausea. Topical preparations can be used to treat smaller areas or in patients for whom systemic administration is contraindicated. Phototherapy and photochemotherapy are long and sometimes complicated processes. Patients must be able to understand the treatment process and be willing to comply with the treatment regimen. A summary of important patient information can be found in the Patient Playbook.

COMMON SKIN DISORDERS

This section is by no means inclusive of the many types of dermatological problems encountered by patients and health care professionals. It will, however, serve as a framework with which to gain insight into the diagnosis and treatment of such conditions.

Acne

Acne is a papulopustular disorder of the pilosebaceous unit in which abnormally adherent keratinocytes cause plugging of the follicular duct, causing accumulation of sebum and keratinous debris. Onset can be from 8 to 10 years of age and continue until the late 20s or early 30s. It is the most common

PATIENT PLAYBOOK

Strategies for Management of Phototherapy and Photochemotherapy

The nurse should encourage the following as related to strategies for managing phototherapy and photochemotherapy:

- The nurse reviews pretreatment instructions with the patient, including when to take pretreatment medications.
- The patient and nurse should review the treatment schedule. Initial treatments are scheduled three times per week with rest periods.
- Psoralens should be taken with food one-and-a-half to two hours prior to photochemotherapy treatment to minimize nausea and ensure system absorption.
- Topical psoralens must be applied 30 minutes prior to beginning treatment.
- Assess patient prior to beginning treatment sessions. Ask patient about photosensitizing medications, over-the-counter (OTC) preparations, or other prescriptions.
- Skin needs to rest in between treatments, because erythema will manifest six to eight hours after exposure.
- Severe erythema that continues between rest periods may require a delay in treatment for a short time until erythema lessens and do not increase dosage if a treatment has been missed.
- Provide protective goggles to prevent eye damage from the light source.
- Arms and legs may require extra dosing; all other areas must be shielded.
- There is higher risk of burning with topical psoralens than with systemic medication. Absorption of drug is increased in areas where skin is not intact.
- Inform the patient that treatments will be delayed or stopped at their request.
- Caution patient against lending medication to friends or relatives
- Instruct patient about who to call if any problems occur.

Adapted from Altman, G. (2004). Delmar's fundamental and advanced nursing skills *(2nd ed.). New York: Thomson Delmar Learning; Broyles, B., Reiss, B., & Evans, M. (2007).* Pharmacological aspects of nursing care *(7th ed.). New York: Thomson Delmar Learning.*

dermatological problem in the pediatric and adolescent populations but can be seen in newborns (related to maternal androgens). Severity can range from mild to the severely scarring acne conglobata. About one in four people has acne significant enough to seek professional treatment. Acne is more prevalent in Western cultures and occurs in males and females equally, with the exception of acne conglobata, which occurs more in males (Liao, 2003).

Acne lesions can be inflammatory or noninflammatory and present as **comedones** (blackheads), papules, pustules, or nodules. Noninflammatory lesions are closed comedones and open comedones. Inflammatory papules, pustules, and nodules are classified as mild, moderate, or severe as shown in Table 45-4. Acne can have a profound psychological effect on people, yet it is often dismissed as merely a phase of the normal growth process and a minor affliction not worthy of treatment. Diagnosis is based on the physical appearance of the lesions.

Treatment of acne is based on the severity of the disease and includes cleansing with gentle surfactant products without abrasive soaps or other ingredients. Suppression of inflammation is important in the prevention of scarring. Benzoyl peroxide has a potent antimicrobial effect and will reduce the size and number of comedones and inhibit secretion of sebum. Topical antibiotics may also be prescribed to reduce bacteria associated with acne. Failure to respond to topical treatments indicates the need to evaluate the patient for systemic antibiotics, usually given over an extended period of time. Long-term usage of antibiotics may result in monilial vaginitis, thrush, and gastrointestinal (GI) symptoms (Spratto & Woods, 2007).

Hormone therapy may be indicated for severe cystic acne. Topical estrogens suppress sebaceous gland activity; estrogen therapy may need to be continued for three to four menstrual cycles. Severe disease may require the use of isotretinoin to inhibit inflammation. The dosage is determined by body weight, in divided doses, usually taken over several months. Comedonal acne responds slowly and several months of treatment are needed.

Mild inflammatory acne (defined as fewer than 20 pustules) is treated with benzoyl peroxide products, beginning with the lowest concentrations. Moderate to severe inflammatory acne is usually treated twice daily with benzoyl peroxide products, topical antibiotics, or a combination therapy of benzoyl peroxide, and sulfacetamide/sulfur products. Severe nodulocystic acne requires aggressive treatment, because the scarring can be severe. Oral antibiotics, conventional topical therapy, and periodic intralesional injections of Kenalog can keep this problem under control.

Atopic Dermatitis

Atopic dermatitis is a chronic, pruritic skin condition characterized by inflammation of the skin. The exact cause is unknown, but it does have a hereditary tendency. There is a cyclic pattern of exacerbation and remission that can continue throughout the patient's lifetime and a seasonal pattern may be demonstrated as

TABLE 45-4 Severity Grading of Inflammatory Lesions

SEVERITY	PAPULES/PUSTULES	NODULES
Mild	Few to several	None
Moderate	Several to many	Few to several
Severe	Numerous or extensive	Many

Adapted from Estes, M. (2006). Health assessment and physical examination *(3rd ed.). New York: Thomson Delmar Learning.*

well. Health care providers believe that atopic dermatitis is a complex relationship between genetic, environmental, immunological, and pharmacological factors. Flares of the disease can be precipitated by stress, infection, seasonal climate changes, irritants, and allergens.

The disease usually begins in childhood and may stabilize as the patient ages. The prevalence of atopic dermatitis in children is currently estimated to be 7 to 17 percent having increased greatly since the 1960s. It is an increase that cannot be explained by genetics alone. Changes in lifestyle and environmental factors, as well as increased recognition, may be contributing to the increase. Diagnosis is based on the basic features of the disease and requires that patients exhibit three or more of these features: pruritus, typical morphology and distribution, chronic or chronically relapsing dermatitis, family history (asthma, allergic rhinitis, or atopic dermatitis), **lichenification** (thickening of the epidermis) in flexural areas in adults, and facial and extensor involvement in children.

Atopic dermatitis starts with itching that becomes a habitual itch-scratch cycle. Chronic dermatitis is the result of scratching over a long period of time that causes thickening of the skin. Acute inflammation begins with erythematous papules and erythema and may coalesce into dry, scaly patches. Distribution of the dermatitis tends to be symmetrical and is more pronounced in areas not covered by clothing. Patients with atopic dermatitis are susceptible to bacterial, viral, and fungal skin infections due primarily to a break in the integrity of the natural barrier properties of the skin. Secondary infections involving *S. aureus* are common.

Treatment of atopic dermatitis is aimed at relief of the dryness and pruritus and decreasing inflammation. The goal is to break the inflammatory cycles causing excess drying and cracking of the skin and the itching and scratching associated with the disease. Hydration of the skin is critical, and it is important to identify and control the triggers that cause the disease to flare. Occlusives, moisturizers, topical steroids, and tar preparations are used to control atopic dermatitis and are frequently used in combination. Occasionally, systemic antihistamines and antibiotics may be required. Systemic steroids are rarely used.

Cellulitis

Cellulitis is an infection of the skin characterized most commonly by redness, heat, pain, swelling and, occasionally, fever, malaise, chills, and headache (Figure 45-1). Abscess formation and tissue destruction usually follow if cellulitis is left untreated. Most health care professionals view cellulitis as a symptom rather than a disease and agree that the need to determine the cause is important. Typically, systemic antibiotics are used to treat cellulitis, but sometimes silver sulfadiazine creams are used. The patient is encouraged to refrain from weight bearing if the cellulitis is located in the lower extremities or foot because weight bearing can encourage more rapid spread of the infection either locally or to the bloodstream, causing septicemia. It is not uncommon to observe a generalized sloughing of epidermis in the involved area after resolution of the infection.

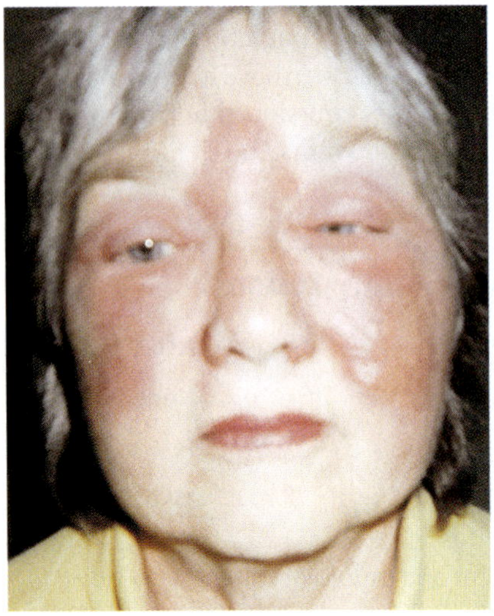

Figure 45-1 Cellulitis.

Contact Dermatitis

Contact dermatitis is categorized into two groups, irritant and allergic. Irritant contact dermatitis results when the skin comes in contact with a substance in the environment that acts as an irritant. It is a nonimmunological response to the irritant that is dependent on the person's ability to maintain the normal epidermal barrier. The extent of the dermatitis is related to the exposure time and concentration of the irritant. Characterized by erythema, blister formation, erosions, scaling, and drying and crusting of skin, irritant contact dermatitis damages the barrier component of the skin and can be either acute or

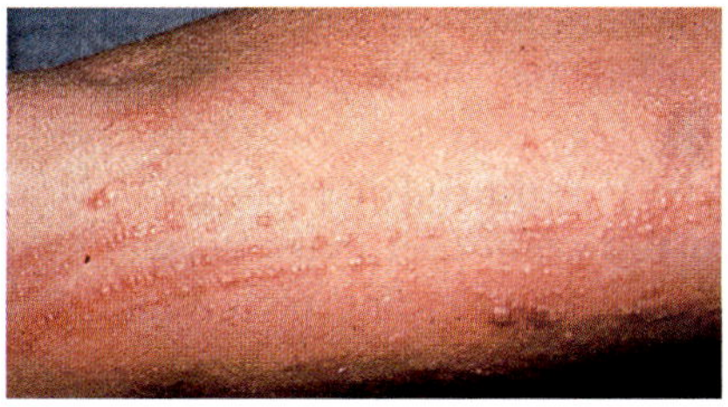

Figure 45-2 Allergic contact dermatitis. Courtesy of the Centers for Disease Control and Prevention.

chronic. Mild irritants cause drying, erythema, and fissuring. Chronic exposure to the irritant causes thickening of the epidermis and eczematous inflammation. Identification of the irritant is critical to treatment. Since the advent of universal precautions, many health care providers have developed this type of dermatitis in response to the latex in the gloves used for patient care or to the powder used inside the gloves to facilitate easy donning (Altman, 2004).

Allergic contact dermatitis is an inflammatory response to an antigen that follows absorption of that antigen into the skin; in other words, allergic contact dermatitis is a delayed hypersensitivity reaction (Figure 45-2). The person will not have a reaction with the first exposure, but their immune system will recognize the antigen during the sensitization phase and mark, or recruit, T lymphocytes within the body that will recognize the antigen with the next exposure. Reexposure to the antigen during the elicitation phase results in a skin response characterized by erythema, wheals and welt formation, blister formation, inflammation, papules, vesicles, scaling, fissures, and crusting. Examples of allergic contact dermatitis include adhesives allergies, cosmetics allergies (particularly around the eyes), plant allergies, such as poison ivy, poison oak or poison sumac, and metal allergies. Anyone can be allergic to any substance from skin care products, from deodorants to dyes used in shoemaking and the plastic earpieces on eyeglasses. Diagnosis is made through a careful history and examination of the skin condition, including any occupational or causal exposure to chemicals. Biopsy of the area is usually not helpful.

Treatment of irritant and contact dermatitis is dependent on identification of the sensitizing substance and controlling the symptoms. Patch testing is helpful in determining the cause of allergic contact dermatitis, but the health care professional needs to also test the patient's consumer products, such as soap, shampoo, and deodorant, as well as look for other possible causes. Patients need to read labels carefully, because many products contain sensitizing agents, such as lanolin, parabens, and fragrance.

It is important to minimize topical treatments and instruct the patient how to appropriately apply topical medications. Wet compresses can be used with solutions that provide a cooling effect. Topical corticosteroids are usually prescribed for application one to two times daily in chronic or recalcitrant cases. Usually removal of the causative substance will cause the condition to resolve. Antihistamines can be prescribed for pruritus. Severe plant reactions may require a short course of prednisone.

Folliculitis

Folliculitis is an acute inflammation of the hair follicle caused by physical irritation, infection, or chemical irritation. It is common and can be an associated symptom of a variety of inflammatory skin diseases. Removal of adhesive dressings, ostomy pouches and other adherent materials may trigger a follicular skin reaction. Superficial folliculitis is confined to the upper part of the hair follicle and presents as a nontender or tender pustule. Inflammation of the entire hair follicle, called **sycosis,** presents as a red, swollen mass that eventually turns into larger pustules. Deep, painful lesions may heal with scarring. The most common causes of folliculitis are bacterial *(S. aureus). Staphylococcus* folliculitis may occur on any body surface where the skin has been abraded or traumatized. **Sycosis barbae** is the inflammation of the entire hair follicle in an area that is traumatized through shaving it and begins with the development of papules or pustules that rapidly evolve into a more diffuse problem as shaving continues. Most infections are treated with oral antibiotics. Localized inflammations are treated topically with mupirocin (Bactroban). Extensive disease is treated with oral antibiotics (dicloxacillin or cephalexin) for at least two weeks until inflammation has cleared.

Shaving can also cause pseudofolliculitis barbae, a foreign body reaction to hair in individuals with a genetic inclination for curly, spiral shaped hair. This condition is commonly referred to as ingrown hair. In some instances, loops of hair can be seen imbedded in the skin and can be released by washing the beard for several minutes using a circular motion with a washcloth or toothbrush or using a syringe needle under the loop and firmly elevating the hair. Prevention requires that patients prone to this condition make certain that whiskers are softened prior to shaving, use a hair releasing technique, and avoid close shaving. Using a double or triple-bladed shaving system, alternately shaving with an electric razor, and avoiding the closest shave setting, helps to decrease the production of sharply-angled hair tips.

Fungal Infections

Fungal infections are also known as **tineas** and are perhaps the most common dermatological problems encountered by health care professionals. Dermatophytes comprise a large group of fungi that have the ability to invade and infect the skin, surviving on the dead keratinocytes found in the stratum. They can also survive on mucosal surfaces, such as mouth and vaginal areas where the keratin layer does not form, and can, in rare instances, invade deeper tissues. Normally, the acid mantle of the skin protects the epidermis from bacterial and dermatophyte invasion. Patients who are immunosuppressed, have a genetic susceptibility to dermatophyte infection, taking courses of antibiotics or chemotherapy, or engage in any activity that would cause a change in pH of the acid mantle including washing with harsh soaps or frequent showering are at risk for development for fungal infections.

Classification of dermatophytes occurs in several ways. Dermatophytes are classified by place of origin, type of inflammation and type of hair invasion. The origin may be an animal or **zoophilic** source; it may be a human or **anthropophilic** source; or it may emanate from an environmental or geophilic source. Anthropophilic dermatophytes are only found on human skin, hair, or nails. Zoophilic dermatophytes originate from animals but can be transferred to humans. Geophilic dermatophytes live in the soil but can infect humans.

Differences in types of fungal inflammations are evident in the severity of the inflammatory response. Animal and human infections result in a brisk inflammatory response. Environmentally sourced fungal infections usually produce a milder inflammation. Some species of dermatophytes invade the hair shaft. Microscopic examination of infected hair reveals spores either inside the shaft, or both inside the hair shaft and on the hair surface.

The most common fungal infections include tinea versicolor, candidiasis, tinea pedis, tinea cruris, tinea capitis, and tinea corporis. Tinea versicolor is a chronic infection seen on the trunk, arms, and neck. The organism causing this infection is the *Pityrosporum* species found in the normal flora of the skin in highest concentration in areas of increased oil production. Factors contributing to any fungal proliferation include heat and humidity, malnutrition, pregnancy, burns, steroid therapy, immunosuppression, and oral contraception. Lesions are circular and scaly, often appearing as white patches on tan skin. Diagnosis of tinea versicolor is made using a Wood's lamp and potassium hydroxide (KOH) stain (Figure 45-3). Cultures are rarely necessary. Treatment is selenium shampoos when the infection involves the scalp and hair. Other areas are treated with topical antifungal preparations and keratolytic soaps.

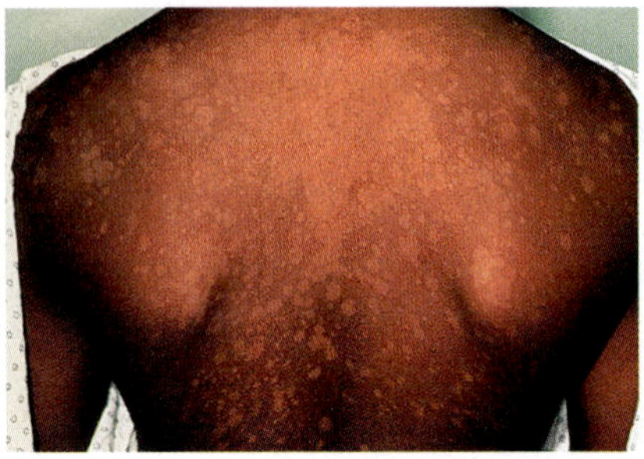

Figure 45-3 Tinea versicolor. Courtesy of Robert A. Silverman, M.D., Clinical Associate Professor, Department of Pediatrics, Georgetown University.

Candidiasis is perhaps the most common of all fungal infections and is caused by a proliferation of the normal yeast flora in the mouth, intestinal tract, or vaginal tract. Yeasts proliferate best in a warm, dark, and moist environment. Therefore yeast infections are usually confined to skin folds and creases or mucous membranes. Predisposing factors include immunosuppression, diabetes, oral contraceptives, antibiotic therapy, skin maceration, and topical steroid therapy. This form of yeast only affects the outer layers of epidermis and mucous membranes.

Monilial vulvovaginitis is the most common cause of vaginal discharge, itching, and odor. KOH wet mount examinations are routinely used to diagnosis this infection. Vaginal antifungals are effective in treating this type of yeast infection. However, the disease is considered recurrent if three or more episodes occur within one year.

Oral candidiasis is usually seen in infants resulting from passage through the birth canal, but it is also seen in adults. The infection involves the tongue and cheek lining causing a red, painful, fissured tongue surface with a white coating. The infection may then extend to the esophagus and trachea. An oral antifungal suspension is used to treat this infection in adults, and systemic antifungals may also be required. The solution is swished around in the mouth, then either spit out or swallowed, depending on whether there is esophageal involvement.

Tinea pedis is the most common infection of the feet. Like skin creases and folds, shoes provide a warm, moist environment for yeast growth. Tinea pedis is common in men, uncommon in women and, though uncommon, should be differentially diagnosed in prepubertal children with foot dermatitis. The locker room and communal bath areas of sports facilities is a prime source of this infection, hence the term "athlete's foot." Infections are found most commonly in the toe webs and soles of the foot. Toe webs can become macerated with scale, and the infection can spread out from the toe web if left untreated. Tinea pedis infections consist of erythematous, red macules, and pustules that become crusted. Itching is the most common complaint along with burning. Scratching the itch can result in secondary infections that compound treatment challenges (Carter, Dufour, & Ballard, 2004). Diagnosis is based on visual assessment of the lesions. OTC or prescription medications may be used to treat tinea pedis depending on the severity of the infection and whether it is acute or chronic.

Tinea cruris occurs in the groin and inner thigh areas, primarily during the summer months. Sweating and wearing wet clothing contribute to the development of the disease, again providing the warm, moist environment needed for yeast to proliferate. Men are affected far more frequently than women. The skin irritation caused either by skin or by clothing rubbing on the inner thigh surfaces can be misdiagnosed as a yeast rash. Also known as "jock itch" or "jock rot," tinea cruris lesions present in half-moon shapes and are usually bilateral with itching, burning, odor, and maceration of epidermis. As with most tinea infections, diagnosis is made based on presentation of rash and treatment can be either an OTC or a prescription antifungal.

Tinea capitis is a fungal infection involving the scalp that can extend onto the neck. The *Trichophyton* species is responsible for this infection that usually begins with several round patches of dryness or scale. Tinea capitis is common in urban areas, but it is also seen in impoverished areas where living conditions are crowded. Spores are shed in the area of people infected, and direct contact is not required for spread of the disease. Infection of the hair shaft is preceded by scalp infection, with the fungus growing through the stratum corneum and into the hair follicle below the area where the hair follicle is formed. The dermatophyte cannot cross the perifollicular stratum corneum into the hair but must burrow deep into the follicle to avoid the cuticle. This explains why topical antifungal agents are ineffective in treating this form of tinea.

Diagnosis of tinea capitis is based on the clinical presentation of lesions called kerions and patterns of hair loss. Clinically, these lesions present as boggy, indurated, tumor-like masses that are palpable in the scalp and exude pus. Four patterns of inflammation have been identified: (a) noninflammatory black dot pattern, a well-defined pattern of hair loss where the hair shafts are broken at the point where they exit the stratum corneum causing the appearance of a black dot; (b) inflammatory with a positive test for the presence of the *Trichophyton* antigen; (c) seborrheic with white flakes that resemble dandruff;

and (d) pustular with discrete pustules or scabbed areas without scaling or significant hair loss.

Occipital or cervical lymphadenopathy is usually present and lack thereof ought to cause the health care professional to question a tinea capitis diagnosis. Treatment includes oral antifungal medications and topical shampoos to reduce or control spore loads and treat asymptomatic carriers.

Tinea corporis involves the face, excluding the area of a beard in men, trunk, and limbs. This form of fungal infection has many manifestations with lesions varying in inflammation and depth of involvement. The classic presentation is a distinct, circular lesion with an advancing red, scaly border. Papules may be present. Itching, erythema, and follicular involvement are also common characteristics of the disease, which is also known as ringworm. Diagnosis and treatment is the same as for other tinea infections. It is important to minimize exposure of other people to the infection and begin treatment as soon as possible. Fortunately, treatment for fungal infections is readily available and effective.

Furuncles and Carbuncles

Localized bacterial infections can manifest as painful, indurated, or fluctuant, fluid-filled masses called **furuncles (boils).** Cellulitis can be prodromal or concurrent with the infection. An **abscess** is a cavity containing pus surrounded by inflamed tissue, the healing of which only begins after incision and drainage. *S. aureus* is the most common pathogen and furuncles occur primarily in areas of friction or minor trauma, such as beltlines, anterior thighs, neck area, axillae, and waistline. Deep red, firm, tender papules enlarge rapidly into a deep-seated nodule that remains stable and erythematous for days and then becomes fluid-filled. These painful lesions are most uncomfortable in constricted areas, such as the neck. The abscess either remains deep, is eventually reabsorbed, or it ruptures through the epidermis. Scarring is common when rupture occurs.

Carbuncles are aggregates of infected follicles originating deep in the dermis and subcutaneous tissue. Unlike furuncles, carbuncles form an erythematous, swollen, broad, and slowly evolving mass that can ulcerate and drain from multiple openings. This process is called pointing. Malaise, chills, and fevers, either precede or occur simultaneously with the infection. Sloughing and scarring are common. Several diseases can produce furuncles, the most common being a ruptured epidermal cyst or pilar cyst of the scalp. Warm compresses are used to provide comfort and draw the infection to the surface. Incision and drainage is the most rapid form of treatment. Once drained, the area should be packed to prevent closure of the skin before the abscess cavity heals outward. Oral antibiotics are prescribed for 5 to 10 days.

Herpes Infections

Herpes simplex viral infections are caused by two different viral types: herpes simplex virus-1 (HSV-1) and herpes simplex virus-2 (HSV-2). HSV-1 is generally associated with oral cold sores and fever blisters, and HSV-2 is associated with genital infections. Both types of infections are becoming more common and may be related to oral-genital sexual contact. Many of these infections are asymptomatic, and evidence of previous infection is determined by an immunoglobulin G (IgG) antibody titer.

HSV infections have two phases: the primary infection during which the virus becomes imbedded in the nerve ganglion and the secondary phase characterized by recurrent infections at the same site. Recurrence of genital herpes is six times more frequent than oral-labial occurrence. Infection can occur at any site on the skin, and infection in one area does not preclude subsequent infection at another site. The primary infection is usually asymptomatic. The severity of the disease increases with age and the virus can be spread through respiratory droplets, direct contact with infected people with active lesions, or contact with virus-containing fluid, such as saliva or cervical secretions.

Symptoms of primary infection occur three to seven days after exposure, beginning with sensitivity in the area; pain, tenderness, or burning. The lesions are grouped vesicles that are uniform in size on an erythematous base that heals as a tissue depression referred to as umbilicated. Crusts then form and usually heal without scarring. Secondary infection can be activated by local skin trauma, such as chapping or abrasion, or by a systemic response, such as fever or fatigue. The activated virus travels down the peripheral nerve to the site of the initial infection and causes the classic focal, recurrent infection. Prodromal symptoms last 2 to 24 hours, then the vesicles rapidly form on an erythematous base, becoming large, dome-shaped, fluid-filled lesions. They rupture and form erosions in the mouth or vaginal area or crusts on the lips and skin. The crusts are usually shed in about one week leaving pink, reepitheliazed skin. Secondary infections are less severe than primary infections. Diagnosis of HSV is done by assessment of the lesions and laboratory tests that depend on the stage of the disease for their sensitivity. Tzanck smear, Pap smear, viral culture, and serology for IgG antibody titer are common diagnostic tools. Treatment of HSV consists of cool, moist compresses of Burrow's solution, controlling secondary infections, and systemic or topical antivirals that may include Acyclovir, Famvir, or Valtrex.

Cutaneous Herpes Simplex

Cutaneous herpes simplex is a manifestation of HSV and mimics other vesicular eruptions. The most common forms are herpes whitlow, HSV of the buttocks or trunk, and herpes gladiatorum. Herpes whitlow usually occurs on the fingertips and can resemble a bacterial infection or warts. Health care professionals with frequent contact with oral secretions are particularly at risk. HSV of the buttocks is more common in women and the cause has not been identified. HSV of the trunk appears similar to herpes zoster, and diagnosis may only become apparent at the time of recurrence. Herpes gladiatorum is most frequently found in athletes who participate in contact sports. It is disseminated by direct skin-to-skin contact and early diagnosis is important to prevent further transmission.

Herpes Zoster

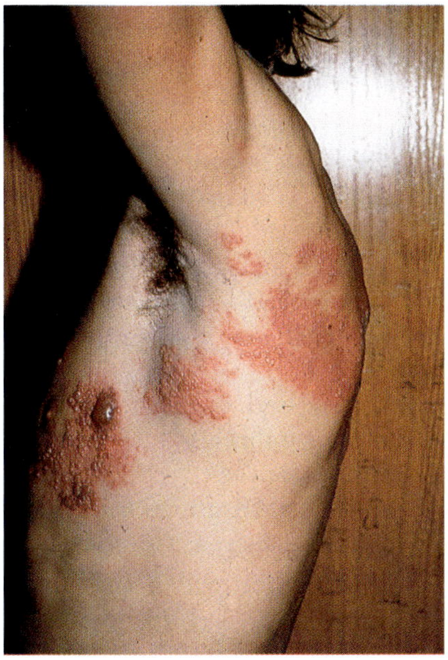

Figure 45-4 Herpes zoster. Courtesy of Robert A. Silverman, M.D., Clinical Associate Professor, Department of Pediatrics, Georgetown University.

Herpes zoster, more commonly referred to as shingles, is a cutaneous infection caused by reactivation of the varicella chickenpox virus. As with HSV, the virus can become dormant along the skin of a dermatome, or nerve root ganglion, until conditions such as immunosuppression, emotional upsets, radiation, or lymphoma cause the virus to become active. The reactivated virus travels down the nerve, infecting the skin and giving this disease its classic asymmetrical appearance. Most commonly seen on the face, chest, and buttocks, any dermatome area of the body can be affected (Figure 45-4). Herpes zoster is less communicable than varicella, but people who have not had varicella may develop the disease after exposure to varicella. Prodromal symptoms include pain known as preherpetic neuralgia, itching, and burning generally localized to the dermatome area, and may precede eruption by four to five days.

The eruptions begin with red, swollen plaques that spread through the affected dermatome. Vesicles of varying sizes arise in the plaque and quickly become engorged with a milky fluid, usually three to four days following erythematous plaque formation. The disease is extremely painful, requiring significant amounts of narcotics and sometimes hospitalization. The patient has great difficulty tolerating dressings and clothing coming in contact with the affected area. Pain is neuropathic and results from altered central nervous system signal processing.

Diagnosis of herpes zoster is made by history and physical examination of the pattern and the character of the vesicles and surrounding skin. Treatment of herpes zoster centers on pain control and antiviral therapy. Antiviral medications must be started within 72 hours of the onset of the rash or pain. Pain can be severe enough to require nerve blocks. Selection and dosage of medications is determined according to the needs of the individual patient. The same antiviral drugs used to treat HSV are used to treat herpes zoster.

Impetigo

Impetigo is a common, superficial skin infection beginning as a focal erythema and progressing to pruritic vesicles, erosions, and honey-colored crusts. Caused by staphylococci, streptococci, or both, these lesions can resemble infections, such as poison ivy. Clinical presentation begins with vesicle formation affecting only the stratum corneum. Diagnosis is based on history and appearance. Children in close physical contact with each other in school or in daycare have a higher rate of infection than the adult population. The disease is self-limiting but can last weeks without treatment. Lesions are usually confined in one area but can develop satellite lesions. The thin-roofed bullae collapse but may retain fluid for several days. A thin, varnish-like, honey-colored crust appears in the center of ruptured bullae. If the crust is removed a bright red, inflamed, moist base that oozes clear fluid is revealed. Serious secondary infections, including osteomyelitis, arthritis, and pneumonia, can follow seemingly superficial infections in infants. The skin around the nose, mouth, and limbs are the most common sites. Regional lymphadenopathy is common. Acute nephritis can occur when whole families are infected, usually developing one to three weeks after infection. Cultures are not routinely performed to confirm the diagnosis because its unique presentation confirms the diagnosis. Treatment of impetigo consists of oral antibiotics and topical mupirocin ointment (Carter, et al., 2004).

Pediculosis

Infestation with lice is called **pediculosis.** The louse, which is visible to the naked eye, is endemic all over the world and is estimated to cause 10 million cases in the United States annually. There are two species of lice that infect humans: the body louse, or *Pediculus humanus,* is the largest and infests the body and scalp; the smaller crab louse, or *Phthirus pubis,* infests the hair in the pubic area. Head lice can be found in all social and economic levels but are far more prevalent in people living in crowded conditions, and those living with poor hygiene conditions or practices.

The female louse lays eggs called nits each day for up to one month and then dies. The nits are firmly cemented to the base of a hair shaft close to the skin where adequate warmth will incubate them for 8 to 10 days and then they hatch. The louse will fully mature in 18 days. Nits are difficult to remove from the hair shaft. Head lice produce pruritic red papules and are most common in children. More girls than boys are affected, and head lice are found primarily at the back of the head and neck and behind the ears. The pruritus is worse at night.

Pediculosis pubis is a contagious, sexually transmitted disease (STD) and 30 percent of those persons infected with pediculosis pubis also have another STD. Pubic hair is the most common site, but the lice frequently spread to the perianal hair. The most common complaint is pruritus. Diagnosis is made by the presence of nits and pruritic rashes in a localized area. Combing will detect and remove live lice, both of which are easily visible under the microscope. Treatment of head lice consists of application of 1% permethrin lotion after a pretreatment shampoo. The lotion is allowed to remain on the hair for 10 minutes and then rinsed. Gamma benzene hexachloride available as 1% lindane or Kwell shampoo may be used, but it is less effective. Gloves must be worn when using Kwell shampoo, and the patient should avoid getting the shampoo on other body parts.

Pyrethrin, or RID, can be used for any type of pediculosis infection, but is less effective than other treatments. Treatment for pubic or body lice consists of lindane lotions or creams. Any treatment usually requires multiple applications. Bedding, head coverings, brushes, and combs must be dry cleaned or washed in hot, soapy water. Clothing of people with body lice may need to be ironed along each seam to remove oviposits.

Pemphigus

Pemphigus is a chronic problem resulting in the development of blisters. It is fairly uncommon in the general public, but incidence is increased in Mediterranean regions and Jewish peoples. Pemphigus is an epidermal autoimmune disease caused by circulating IgG autoantibodies that react with the intracellular cement that binds cells together. Bullae and blisters form, then rupture with crusting of the erosions. The bullae are flaccid, and the fluid released at the time of rupture smells foul. Treatment involves oral corticosteroids and other immunosuppressive medications, which controls but does not cure.

Pruritus

Itching, or **pruritus,** is one of the most common manifestations of dermatological problems. Even patients with normally healing wounds experience itching as part of the healing process. Most health care professionals involved in treating patients with dermatological problems agree that pruritus is a symptom not a disease. The cause of the itching needs to be determined and treated. In addition, the pruritus must be treated because the irritation leads to excoriation of the skin from scratching, and it is known that any break in the skin is an entrance for contaminants.

Pruritus can be a secondary symptom of conditions ranging from dry skin to cancer. Systemic diseases, such as herpes zoster, kidney failure resulting in uremia, drug reactions, hematological cancers, such as leukemia and lymphoma, liver diseases that increase bilirubin levels, and diabetes, can all have a pruritic component. Pruritus can also be caused by contact with chemical irritants, adhesives, plants, household chemicals, such as laundry products and other cleaning solutions, lawn care products, dyes, and fabric protection products. In other words, anything can cause a patient to itch. Skin tends to dry out more in the cold weather months than in warm weather months. Nonhummidified heat causes an increase in evaporation rates of the skin's natural water content. Perfumed soaps and lotions use alcohol as the vehicle for the fragrance and thus are drying agents. Universal precautions require health care professionals to wash their hands frequently and to wear gloves for patient care, contributing to drying the skin of their hands. Pruritus is also associated with allergic reactions to a variety of substances. People with hay fever or other environmental allergies complain of itching eyes. The determination of the cause of the pruritus is important to the treatment of the condition and alleviation of the itching.

Appropriate management of any skin condition requires accurate assessment and diagnosis of the problem. Dry skin may be the source of the pruritus or a contributing factor. Topical antihistamine creams and anesthetics are generally ineffective and should be avoided, because they can be potent sensitizers, particularly if used on inflamed skin. Elderly patients may have trouble following a regimen of frequent bathing or showering because of decreased mobility and increased fall risk. Application of more hydrating products is better in this situation but may require the assistance of other people. Antihistamine therapy should be used with caution in elderly patients, because these patients have a low tolerance and may experience enhancement of the usual side effects of antihistamine therapy.

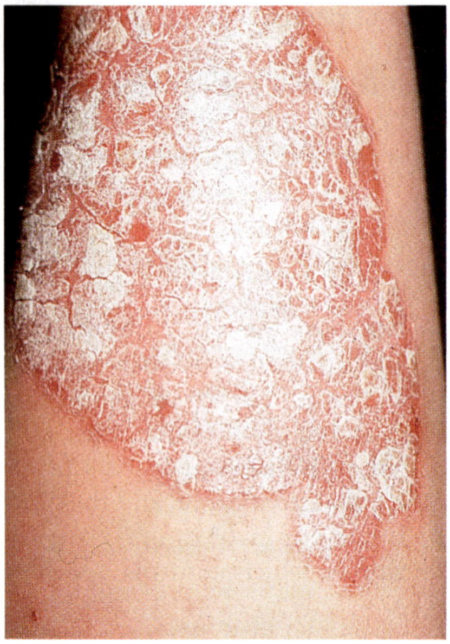

Figure 45-5 Psoriasis. Courtesy of Robert A. Silverman, M.D., Clinical Associate Professor, Department of Pediatrics, Georgetown University.

Psoriasis

Health care professionals estimate that 1 to 3 percent of the population has this genetically transmitted disease that crosses all racial groups. The origin is unknown, and the disease is lifelong, characterized by exacerbations and remissions that can be physically and emotionally debilitating. **Psoriasis** is a T cell mediated inflammatory disease characterized by epidermal hyperplasia (overproduction of epidermal tissue) usually localized in certain regions of the body. The prevalence of arthritis with psoriasis is higher than in the general population. Arthritis occurs in 5 to 42 percent of people with psoriasis. There have been several types of psoriasis identified. The most common forms are psoriasis vulgaris or classic plaque psoriasis, guttate psoriasis, and pustular psoriasis. Less frequently seen types include erythrodermic psoriasis, light-sensitive psoriasis, human immunodeficiency virus (HIV)-induced psoriasis, and Reiter's syndrome (Young, 2003).

Classic plaque psoriasis appears as well-defined plaques with a whitish or silvery appearance on a pink, violaceous or blue background (Figure 45-5). The borders or margins are raised and well-defined. The predominant locations of classic lesions are the scalp, elbows, knees, and lumbosacral areas. Smaller plaques tend to coalesce into larger ones.

Guttate psoriasis is less common comprising less than 2 percent of the psoriatic population. The onset of guttate psoriasis usually follows an upper respiratory infection caused by group-A B hemolytic streptococci *(Streptococcus pyogenes)* or a viral upper respiratory infection. This form usually presents two to three weeks after the infection and has a distinctive presentation. Scattered 1 to 10 mm drop-like papules appear suddenly on the trunk and extremities, sparing the soles of the feet and palms of the hands. About 30 percent of people developing guttate psoriasis have their first episode before the age of 20; the disease may resolve spontaneously, is more responsive to treatment than the classic form, or it may evolve into chronic plaque psoriasis.

Generalized pustular psoriasis, also called von Zumbusch psoriasis, is the most common form of this version of psoriasis. Characterized by an explosive onset of burning erythema, it is a serious and sometimes fatal disease. Pustules form in an erythematous bed and coalesce into lakes of pus, appearing on the elbows, anal region, genitalia, and fleural areas of the axillae and knees. The patient is febrile, toxic, tachycardic, tachypneic, and has leukocytosis. Mortality rates can be as high as 30 percent without adequate treatment and relapses are common.

The diagnosis of psoriasis is made based on its visual presentation. The lesions of each of the three previously described types of psoriasis are distinctive, and biopsy is usually not necessary. In as high as 35 percent of cases other family members also have psoriasis, but the disease can skip generations. Pruritus is common in most forms of psoriasis. The severity of the disease is rated using the psoriasis activity and severity index (PASI). There are three steps involved when using the PASI to calculate the disease severity and the percentage of body involvement: (a) the overall severity of the lesion, (b) the psoriatic lesion signs, and (c) calculate the PASI (Young, 2003).

When using the PASI, the health care provider must first determine the degree of inflammation. Psoriatic plaques are successfully treated when the induration disappears. Residual skin that appears erythematous with hyperpigmentation or brown pigmentation is common when the plaque disappears and is often seen as a need to continue treatment when, in fact, use of the prescribed treatment should halt. When the plaque cannot be palpated, the treatment may be stopped. Treatment of psoriasis includes biological therapies, topical corticosteroids, UVB, and topical tar and anthralin preparations and is based on the percentage of the body surface involved. Topical and intralesional steroids, vitamin D analogues, tar and anthralin preparations, and UVB are recommended treatment options when less than 20 percent of the body surface is involved. Combination UVB and tar preparations, PUVA, methotrexate, cyclosporine, and the biological therapies are reserved for patients with more than 20 percent of body surface affected by the disease or the disease is recalcitrant. Patients often tell the health care provider that their mild psoriasis improves with exposure to natural sunlight. Steroids can be applied topically, administered by intralesional injection or taken orally. The treatment for psoriasis is usually lengthy and the cycle of exacerbation and remissions can last throughout the patient's lifetime.

Many topical and systemic treatments exist for psoriasis. Steroids can provide a rapid response and are usually given in pulse doses. UUV light therapy is used only on classic and guttate psoriasis. Tar and anthralin preparations are relatively inexpensive, but the staining effect is viewed negatively by many patients. Intralesional steroids can be used in limited areas only, because atrophy and telangiectasias occur at injection sites.

Rosacea

Rosacea is a chronic, inflammatory condition characterized by erythema, papules, pustules, and telangiectasis. Its etiology is unknown. The erythema is caused by atrophy of the papillary dermis and dilation of the superficial vasculature of the face. Commonly referred to as the rosacea mask, this condition affects the face and nose but can occur centrally in the T zone that includes the forehead. Blackhead formation is unusual. The condition has an insidious onset, usually developing between 30 and 50 years of age and affecting more women than men. It is more common in fair-skinned persons, predominantly of Celtic origin, with a history of flushing referred to as flushers and blushers. Factors affecting this condition include familial genetic predisposition, sun exposure, alcohol consumption, consumption of caffeine-containing products, extremes of temperature, spicy foods or beverages, and emotional stress. Sebaceous hyperplasia of the nose, termed rhinophyma, is seen more frequently in men and is associated with chronic rosacea. Commonly known as a W. C. Fields nose, sebaceous hyperplasia is often mistaken as an indication of excessive alcohol consumption. Eyelid inflammation and conjunctivitis can also occur.

Diagnosis of rosacea is based on the patient's history and clinical presentation. Treatment involves topical and sometimes systemic regimens. Avoidance of triggers, such as sunlight, alcohol, and spicy foods, may be enough to control mild rosacea. More severe cases require more persistent treatment. Topical retinoids, benzoyl peroxide, and topical antibiotics assist in controlling the severity of outbreaks.

Systemic therapy consists of oral antibiotics and retinoids. Oral contraceptives may also be used as adjunctive treatment and steroids may be required to treat severe, refractory cases. Patients should be cautioned not to over wash the face and to use only gentle cleansers. Avoid washcloths and sponges when cleansing the face, because fabrics can be abrasive. Prescribed medications should be applied to the entire face not just the affected areas, waiting 15 to 20 minutes after washing to apply medications.

Scabies

Scabies is a highly contagious, pruritic skin infection caused by a mite *(Sarcoptes scabiei)*. Social and economic status has no bearing on the distribution of the disease, and it is prevalent throughout the world. Outbreaks usually occur in situations of close personal contact with the mite, gained through the sharing of inanimate objects, such as clothing or bedding with resultant transmission of the mite. Schools and skilled nursing facilities are common sites of infestation secondary to close contact and crowded sleeping areas.

Only the female mite causes the disease, burrowing under the stratum corneum to the stratum granulosum to lay eggs that hatch in 3 to 10 days. Both mites and eggs can exist outside the body. Either straight or serpentine burrows are visible on the skin and are anywhere from 5 to 20 mm in length. The burrows are pink-white and slightly elevated. Mites can often be seen at the end of the burrow, appearing in a vesicle or as a black dot. Vesicles are isolated and filled with a clear fluid rather than purulent material. These discrete lesions are a vital point in diagnosis. The most common areas of occurrence are the finger webs, buttocks, scrotum, penis, axillae, breasts, and the hands and soles of the feet in infants. Infants may have more widespread involvement. Severe itching is the most common complaint. Scratching will destroy the burrow and may make diagnosis difficult initially. Extensive involvement will result in erythema, scaling, and infection.

Diagnosis is based on the clinical presentation and the microscopic examination of scrapings of the involved areas. Mineral oil and potassium hydroxide wet mounts are used for diagnosis. A drop of mineral oil is placed over the suspected lesion then a scalpel blade is used to scrape off a sample of the affected area for examination under low power magnification. In the oil the skin scrapings adhere together while the mite moves freely and is readily identifiable. Potassium hydroxide mounts are performed in the same manner. Biopsy is rarely used.

The treatment of scabies is topical. Permethrin cream (Elimite) is the most effective medication. The cream is applied nightly for three nights, massaging the cream into the skin from the neck down. The cream is washed off in the morning. The patient needs to be cautioned that the product can stain clothing and bedding and that the odor can be objectionable. Gamma benzene hexachloride (Lindane and Kwell) may also be used, but it is not as effective as permethrin. All other people in the household or facility must also be treated to avoid recurrence. Clothing must be laundered in hot water or dry cleaned. All hard surfaces must be vacuumed, and the debris collected must be sealed in a plastic bag for disposal. Fabric articles that cannot be washed or dry cleaned should be placed in plastic bags and completely sealed for several weeks to avoid reinfestation.

Low dose steroids or antihistamines can be used to treat the pruritus. Hyperkeratotic plaques may form with continued scratching. Repetitive scratching causes excoriations in the skin, allowing entry of bacteria into the epidermis. If the bacteria enter the bloodstream, bacteremia and sepsis can result and be life-threatening.

The normal immune system will not affect the mite bio-burden. Immunosuppressed patients will not present with normal symptoms, will not have the normal itch-scratch cycle, and therefore may not seek early treatment. In this population the concentration of mites will be higher and such infestations may require prolonged treatment. Caregivers for these patients are also at risk for developing scabies because of the large numbers of mites.

Stasis Dermatitis

Stasis dermatitis is a condition that occurs on the lower extremities of patients with venous insufficiency and is exclusive to that disease. Cycles of inflammation, ulceration, and scarring result in brown-staining of the epidermis, induration, and sclerosing of the skin. Patients with stasis dermatitis have an increased propensity for developing allergies to topical agents. Inflammation may be chronic or acute. Pruritus, scaling, fissuring, weeping, and maceration are characteristics of stasis dermatitis. The scaling can become thick in chronic conditions, and fibrosis of the skin is common.

Diagnosis of stasis dermatitis is based on the clinical presentation, a careful history, and the other diagnostic methods for venous insufficiency previously discussed in chapter 27. Treatment of stasis dermatitis involves determining the etiology and hydrating the skin using topical steroids and wet dressings. Petrolatum products are usually contraindicated, because they will damage the rubber in compression wraps and stockings. Oral antibiotics may be given if the cellulitis is severe or bacterial overload is suspected. Wet dressings and compresses will soothe the area and suppress inflammation. Topical steroids should not be placed directly on ulcers, because they will stop the healing process.

Warts

Warts are benign epidermal growths caused by human papilloma virus (HPV). They are most common in children but can occur at any age. They are transmitted by touch; it is not uncommon to see additional lesions called kissing lesions in adjacent areas. The most common sites are the hands, fingers, periungual areas, and plantar surfaces. They can resolve spontaneously or require years of treatment. Warts obscure the normal lines in the skin and can be unsightly. Large collections can cause emotional problems in children when the perceptions of self-image are forming. They can also be erroneously perceived as a hygiene issue. Common warts *(Verruca vulgaris)* are elevated, well-circumscribed, irregularly shaped plaque-like projections with hyperkeratosis areas. Verruca plana, also known as plane warts, flat warts, or juvenile warts, are slightly raised, irregularly shaped, slightly keratotic lesions usually found on the dorsum of the hands and on the face. This type of wart is prevalent in patients with compromised immunity.

Diagnosis is based on the patient's history and visual inspection of the affected areas. Treatment of common warts includes topical salicylic acid preparations, liquid nitrogen, electrocautery, and blunt dissection for large lesions. Intralesional bleomycin sulfate is prescribed when other treatments fail. Treatment for plane warts includes retinoids, liquid nitrogen, cautery, and 5-fluorouracil cream.

Xerosis

Xerosis or severe dry skin can be either a result of dehydrated epidermis or be associated with a variety of dermatological conditions. Age-related xerosis results from a decrease in sebum production and water loss. Xerosis is more common in the winter months when it is referred to as winter itch and in dehumidified environments. The most severely affected skin appears criss-crossed with shallow, red fissures and that itch or burn, initiating an itch-scratch cycle. Xerosis may be treated by hydrating with an appropriate topical lotion after bathing. Severe cases may require a lactic acid lotion. As with other pruritic conditions, bathing or showering should be done with warm water and without scrubbing. Application of the lotion or cream should take place within three to five minutes after patting the skin dry.

PRECANCEROUS AND CANCEROUS CONDITIONS

Light-induced changes in the skin are dependent on the intensity and exposure of the skin to light as well as genetic factors. Tanning has a preventive aspect but by definition tanning is a sun-induced darkening of the pigment in the skin. The skin tans following moderate to intense exposure to the UVA of the sun. Research demonstrates that alternate UV light sources produce the same damage and photoaging as exposure to natural UV sources. In fact, the large amounts of UV radiation delivered to the skin from tanning bed sources can actually accelerate photoaging.

Sunburn

Sunburn is an overexposure to UVA that causes an inflammatory reaction of the skin. UV radiation changes skin cells histologically and has a cumulative effect over the lifespan. As with other burn classifications, sunburn is classified as first-, second-, or third-degree. First-degree sunburn produces mild, tender erythematous skin followed by desquamation. The skin heals without scarring. Second-degree sunburn is characterized by more tenderness and extreme erythema with edema and blister formation. The patient may peel more than once. There are no immediate curative treatments for sunburn. Topical aloe vera gels have gained favor in the last decade but only provide temporary relief from the burning or heat sensations. Topical anesthetics, such as Solarcaine, provide only temporary pain relief. Deep or third-degree sunburns are uncommon. They are induced by artificial means, such as sunlamps, tanning booths, or tanning lamps, that produce effects similar to third-degree thermal burns. Hospitalization is usually required for treatment of third-degree sunburn.

Sun Protection

Prevention of UV-induced skin damage to the dermal collagen and elastin fibers is best achieved by avoidance or at the least, the use of protective clothing and products with high sun protective factor (SPF). Remember, UV exposure has a cumulative effect. Approximately 43 percent of all Caucasian children in the United States experience one or more sunburns annually. Protection and good sun education needs to begin early. Unfortunately, many cultures view tanned skin as appealing and erroneously view the healthy tan as an indication of a more youthful mentality and physical appearance. In actuality, the more sun exposure people receive as children, adolescents and young adults, the faster signs of aging appear.

There are many methods for sun protection. To some extent the stratum corneum and melanin provide natural protection. Because sunburn is particularly harmful to the skin, causing precancerous and cancerous lesions, emphasis should be placed on prevention of the burn. Individuals who burn easily need to use sunscreens with an SPF of between 12 and 30. The more fair-skinned the person, the higher the SPF needs to be. It is safer to avoid exposure between the peak sunlight hours of 10 am to 3 pm. Even waterproof sunscreens should be reapplied every two hours and after exposure to water. For persons working out of doors, wearing dark, loose dry clothing with a tight weave will provide good protection. Long-sleeved shirts, hats, and long pants rather than shorts are best for individuals whose work requires exposure to the sun during peak hours. There is some evidence that antioxidant vitamin supplements will reduce sunburn erythema.

Sunscreens are designed to absorb, scatter, or diffuse UV radiation and visible light. Sunscreens should never be used as a means to lengthen the time an individual spends in the sun; this negates the beneficial action of the sunscreen. Titanium dioxide is an inorganic or nonchemical sunscreen that effectively blocks a wide spectrum of light. These products are thick pastes, some of which have colorful tints that children like for application to the nose and lips. Chemical sunscreens (PABA) absorb radiation, but can cause allergic reactions.

Malignant Skin Lesions

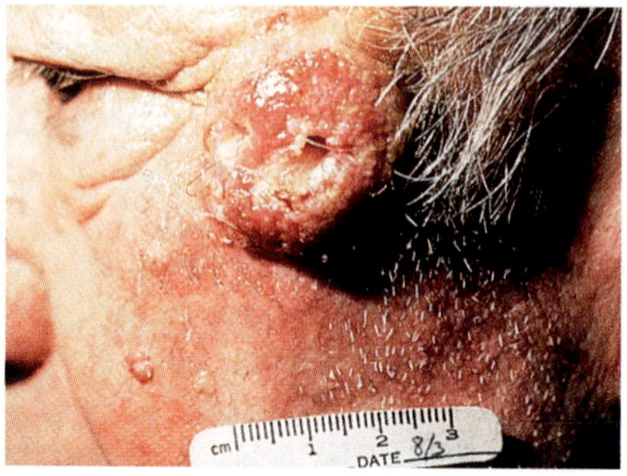

Figure 45-6 Squamous cell carcinoma. Courtesy of Robert A. Silverman, M.D., Clinical Associate Professor, Department of Pediatrics, Georgetown University.

The most common form of photodermatosis is actinic keratosis (AK), an intraepidermal form of squamous cell skin cancer (Figure 45-6). It is more common in Caucasians and affects nearly 100 percent of elderly white persons. AK lesions appear in areas of chronic, high-intensity sun exposure and consist of aggregates of anaplastic keratinocytes that have undergone histological or morphological cell changes. Most actinic keratoses are seen on the face, scalp, and ears of men and on the arms. They can appear to spontaneously resolve, but new lesions frequently appear in the area. Left untreated, 10 to 20 percent of these lesions will invade the basement membrane of the epidermal-dermal junction and become invasive, more serious skin cancers.

Diagnosis is based on palpation and biopsy. The lesions are usually only a few millimeters to 1 to 2 centimeters in diameter and may range in number from a few to hundreds. AKs range in color from a tan to a reddish tone but can also be the patient's normal skin color. The lesions are better recognized by palpation than by visualization. The epidermis is generally hyperkeratotic; the thicker the lesion, the more carefully it must be watched by the health care professional (American Academy of Dermatology, 2002).

Thickened AK lesions can progress to squamous cell cancer and be histologically indistinguishable from primary squamous cell skin cancer. Induration, inflammation, and oozing are suggestive of invasive malignant changes. Immunosuppression is a risk factor. Treatment of actinic keratoses can vary; cryotherapy, surgery, topical chemotherapy, and topical steroids are all methods to contain and control the disease.

Nonmelanoma Skin Cancers

The nonmelanoma skin cancers are the most common types of skin cancer in the United States. Over one million new cases were diagnosed in 2002, 70 percent of which were nonmelanoma cancers. The nonmelanoma skin cancers include basal cell carcinoma (BCC) and squamous cell carcinoma (SCC).

Basal Cell Carcinoma

Basal cell carcinoma (BCC) arises from the basement membrane at the epidermal-dermal junction. BCC results when basal cells fail to mature into the keratinocytes that normally become the stratum corneum and continue their mitotic activity beyond the basal layer. These growths result in bulky tumors that displace epidermis and dermis, eventually extending finger-like projections into other tissues including fascia, cartilage, and bone. BCC rarely metastasizes beyond the skin and, if present, is usually seen in patients with large primary tumors and tumors resistant to surgery and radiotherapy.

There are four types of BCC: nodular (most common); superficial (seen most frequently on the trunk and actinically damaged skin); morpheaform or sclerotic (more aggressive form producing more extension into surrounding tissue); and pigmented (seen in dark-complexioned persons). Each classification has distinctive characteristics:

- Nodular BCC appears as a pearly, translucent bump that bleeds easily and has telangiectasias within the lesion.
- Superficial BCC appears as a well-demarcated, erythematous, scaly patch that may form multiple sites with pearly, raised borders.
- Sclerotic BCC appears as pale yellow or white, flat or depressed, scar-like plaques that may remain undetected because of their appearance.
- Pigmented BCC lesions may appear blue, black, or brown with telangiectasias and a raised pearly border.

Diagnosis of BCC is determined by its appearance and also by biopsy. The pearly raised border is common in all types and is a valuable diagnostic tool for skin cancer.

Squamous Cell Carcinoma

Squamous cell carcinoma (SCC) is the most common skin cancer in the United States, comprising about 80 percent of all nonmelanoma skin cancers. This is a tumor consisting of keratinizing cells that can arise in the epidermis and proliferate indefinitely. SCC can occur anywhere on the skin and on mucous membranes. UVB in the form of exposure to sunlight during childhood, sunburns, ionizing radiation, outdoor occupations, freckling, facial telangiectasias, light skin, hazel or blue eyes, blonde or red hair, living in the southern parts of the United States and psoralen/PUVA treatment for psoriasis are all important in development of SCC.

SCC can spread by expansion and infiltration into surrounding tissues, shelving or skating, conduit, and infiltration and metastasis. Unlike BCC, SCC can initially spread to local lymph nodes and then on to the more distal lymph nodes via the lymphatic system. Metastasis occurs late in the course of the disease and only after the initial spread to subcutaneous and deeper facial lymph nodes. The rate of metastasis can be as high as 10 percent depending upon type, location, size, and underlying medical conditions. The lesions arising from AK will have a thick, adherent scale. The tumor is soft and easily movable within the skin and may have an inflamed, red base. The lesions are most commonly seen on the bald scalp, ears, forehead, and backs of the hands. SCCs not arising directly from AKs but from sun-damaged areas appear as firm, moveable, elevated masses with sharply defined borders and little surface scale.

Diagnosis is by the clinical presentation of the lesion and by biopsy. The health care provider needs to clearly differentiate between SCC and other processes producing similar lesions, such as Bowen's disease, leucoplakia, lichen sclerosis, atrophicus of the vulva, and cutaneous horn. Examples of treatment options are: cryotherapy (AK) liquid nitrogen, electrosurgery, surgical excision, topical chemotherapy, interferon, and biological modifiers.

Melanoma

Malignant melanoma is a serious tumor arising from abnormal melanocytes. Tumor cells grow rapidly and melanocytes are present in the skin, eyes, ears, GI tract, leptomeninges, and oral and genital mucous membranes. Melanoma has the ability to spread to any organ or tissue, including the brain and heart. Risk factors for the development of melanoma include UVB skin damage from sunburn, UVA radiation from tanning beds, a history of atypical moles, a family history of melanoma, and a previous history of nonmelanoma skin cancers, congenital giant nevus, immunosuppression or repeated blistering sunburns. Once a melanoma breaks through the basement membrane, the tumor has the ability to spread horizontally along the epidermal-dermal junction. Continued growth results in invasion of the dermis and substructures, signifying a vertical growth phase. Vertical growth carries a poorer prognosis (Ayers, 2004).

Recognition of melanoma in its early stages is important for treatment. The ABCDEs of melanoma are: *A*symmetry, *B*order irregularity, *C*olor variation, *D*iameter enlargement, and *E*levation. Changes in color and shape are always suspicious, because they are early signs of differentiation between nevi and melanomas. There are four subtypes of melanoma and each has a slightly differing presentation: Lentigo maligna melanoma is characterized by macular lesions with varied coloration and convoluted borders with notching; superficial spreading melanoma arises with a preexisting melanotic nevus and is 2.5 cm or less in size; nodular melanoma is elevated throughout the lesion resembling a blueberry and is associated with vertical growth; acral-lentiginous melanoma occurs on palms, soles, nail beds, mucocutaneous and mucosal surfaces, and varies in color from tan or brown to darkly pigmented lesions.

There are differing opinions as to whether melanoma in situ and amelanotic melanoma fit into these subtypes. Melanoma in situ presents with flat or raised lesions with histological features of melanoma but is confined to the dermis. Amelanotic melanoma is commonly nodular in nature and usually has an unpigmented pink color. Local recurrence is related to tumor depth and is defined as tumor growth near an original scar. Satellite lesions consist of small cutaneous tumors present in the dermis and subdermis located between the primary site and the lymphatic basin. Regional lymph node metastasis is predictive of visceral spread, and distant metastasis is more frequently to nonvisceral sites such as the skin, subcutaneous tissue, and distant lymph nodes. Late recurrence occurs 10 plus years after initial diagnosis and treatment. In about 2 to 6 percent of metastatic melanoma cases arise from an unknown primary site. Such melanomas are identified in lymph nodes. Survival rates are highest with cutaneous metastases and lowest with visceral metastases.

Diagnosis of the initial disease is based on its clinical presentation and biopsy. Ulceration is associated with tumor thickness and is significant.

Complaints of pruritus are also of concern. Lymphatic mapping with sentinel lymph node biopsy (SNB) is recommended for patients with regional lymph node metastases and is indicated in newly diagnosed invasive melanoma, for medium-thickness lesions or in thin lesions with a history of ulceration. Staging of disease is based on the TNM system (T, tumor; N, nodes; M, metastasis) used for most types of cancer staging. The treatment of malignant melanoma is summarized in Table 45-5.

Treatment consists of primary lesion excision for in situ disease and for lesions with a depth of 2 mm or less and margins of 2 cm margins or less. There

TABLE 45-5 Treatment of Malignant Melanoma

STAGE OF DISEASE	MEDICAL TREATMENT
Melanoma in situ	May have elective regional lymph node dissection (ERLND)
Excision with 0.5 cm margins	Some clinicians believe ERLND improves survival by removing occult nodal metastases before spreading to distant sites
<2 mm thick: 1 cm margins	Allows for adequate staging
≥2 mm thick: 2 cm margins	
Regional metastasis	Therapeutic lymph node dissection
	Possible adjuvant therapy
	Interferon
	Interferon alfa-2b and other trials
	Immunotherapy—parvum *(C. Parvum)*, transfer factor, immunomodulators
	Adjuvant chemotherapy and chemoimmunotherapy
	Excision of in-transit metastases
	Hyperthermic regional limb perfusion
	Adjuvant radiation therapy
	Adjuvant hormonal therapy
Stage III	Therapeutic lymph node dissection
	Other therapies as outlined above
Stage IV	Surgical management of isolated metastases
	Radiation therapy for palliation
	Hyperthermic perfusion
	Intralesional BCG
	Chemotherapy
	Dacarbazine (DTIC)
	Nitroureas
	Temozolomide
	Immunotherapy
	Interleukin 2 (experimental)
	Interferon (experimental)
	Monoclonal antibodies—immune response booster (experimental)
	Vaccine (experimental)—stimulate immune response to melanoma-associated antigens

Adapted from Broyles, B., Reiss, B., & Evans, M. (2007). Pharmacological aspects of nursing care *(7th ed.). New York: Thomson Delmar Learning; Spratto, G., & Woods, A. (2007).* 2007 PDR nurse's drug handbook. *New York: Thomson Delmar Learning.*

is some controversy among health care providers regarding elective regional lymph node dissection (ERLND) and its efficacy in treating localized disease. ERLND is the surgical excision of regional lymph nodes around the primary melanoma site when no nodes are palpable. The theory is based on the belief that disease will spread to the nodes initially before going to distant sites. ERLND does allow for adequate staging of the disease. Disease with regional lymph node involvement may be treated with multiple therapies including dissection, hyperthermic limb perfusion and possible adjuvant therapy in the form of biological response modifiers, such as interferon, chemotherapy, radiation therapy, and hormonal therapy. Adjuvant therapy is always recommended for patients who are free of disease but at high risk for recurrence and to complement excision in the management of metastasis to lymph nodes.

Limb isolation using a bypass circuit is used to deliver high-dose chemotherapy to an affected limb without risking systemic toxicity. Limb isolation is performed under general anesthesia. The main artery and vein of the affected extremity are connected to a bypass circuit to completely isolate the blood flow to and from the limb and a high dose of chemotherapy agent is administered into the perfusion circuit. Hyperthermic isolated limb perfusion is still used for intransient metastasis. The difference between these two isolated limb procedures is that in hyperthermic treatments the blood in the limb is heated prior to chemotherapy administration, because the heat is thought to increase effectiveness of the chemotherapy in advanced disease. Stage IV disease is not curable at this time, but several promising treatment regimens and experimental protocols are ongoing.

Nursing Management

Because of the advances in cancer treatment, cancer is now considered a chronic rather than fatal illness (see chapter 15). Patients are living for many years following cancer treatment. Patients with any cancer diagnosis may face psychological issues that are different from those experienced by the non–cancer population. For many years, the C word has struck fear into hearts and minds. Even in major cancer centers in this country some patients are concerned about their diagnosis becoming common knowledge. Family members ask health care professionals to not tell Mother or Dad about their cancer for fear of how the diagnosis might affect the patient. Others are deeply concerned about how a cancer diagnosis will affect their personal relationships with family, coworkers, and friends. In some cultures, a cancer diagnosis carries a social and economic stigma that results in isolation and shunning of the patient.

Skin cancers are visible, as is the treatment. A nurse may be in a unique position of being the first person to whom a patient voices fears about the diagnosis, treatment, and prognosis of the disease. The vast majority of patients want to know how the disease progresses, what to expect from treatment, how to prevent recurrence, and various other aspects of care and treatment. Nurses must implement strategies that help the patient maintain a healthy, natural skin barrier, if possible.

Cancer care is multidimensional, incorporating the skills and knowledge of a variety of health care professionals including social workers, nutritionists, chaplains, psychologists and other nursing and medical disciplines. Support groups, both hospital-based and national organizations, exist to provide information and a common experiential framework for patients and caregivers. The psychological impact of any disease has profound effects on the patient's life. Changes in body image, possible lifestyle changes because of time-consuming skin care regimens; concerns about disease progression, treatment failure or recurrence; and financial concerns will color the patient's perceptions and attitudes from the time of diagnosis forward. The nurse is often the first member of the health care team to whom the patient turns for information and support.

KEY CONCEPTS

- Care of persons with dermatological problems can be complex.
- Fundamental principles of wound healing and skin repair must guide the health care provider assessing and diagnosing any skin problem or condition.
- The health care provider should identify any barriers to healing and correct those issues.
- A moist wound environment must be provided and maintained for the wound to heal properly with a minimum of complications.
- Necrotic tissue is an impediment to wound and skin healing.
- Topical therapy is used to perform a variety of functions in the treatment of dermatological problems.
- Steroids are used to decrease inflammation, pruritus, and induce remission of certain cutaneous disorders.
- Moisture retentive dressings are designed to maintain a moist wound environment.
- Products designed to hydrate the skin play an important role in the treatment of many pruritic, inflammatory, and zerotic skin conditions.
- Sunlight has a profound effect on the skin and is associated with a variety of diseases and the effects of sun damage become apparent after the age of 20.
- Phototherapy is the treatment of certain dermatological conditions with artificially produced nonionizing UV light.
- There are many types of dermatological problems encountered by patients and health care professionals including acne, dermatitis, cellulitis, folliculitis, fungal infections, furuncles and carbuncles, herpes infections, impetigo, pediculosis, psoriasis, rosacea, scabies, warts, and xerosis.
- Sunburn is an overexposure to UVA that causes an inflammatory reaction of the skin.
- Prevention of UV-induced skin damage to the dermal collagen and elastin fibers is best achieved by avoidance.
- The most common form of malignant skin lesions are AK.
- Nonmelanoma skin cancers are the most common types of skin cancer in the United States, including BCC and SCC.
- Malignant melanoma is a serious tumor arising from abnormal melanocytes.
- Advances in cancer treatment in the last decade cancer, it is now considered a chronic rather than fatal illness.
- Radiation therapy is the prescribed treatment in greater than 50 percent of patients diagnosed with cancer and produces permanent skin changes in the irradiated area.

REVIEW QUESTIONS

1. The fundamental principles of wound healing and skin repair include:
   1. Clean the wound with an antibacterial substance, protect it with a dressing
   2. Clean the wound with an antiseptic substance, cover it with a sterile dressing
   3. Clean the wound with an antiseptic substance, leave it open to the air to heal
   4. Clean the wound, remove devitalized tissue, and apply moist sterile dressings

2. Commonly, treatments for dermatological dysfunctions are:
   1. Managed pharmacologically
   2. Managed with topical applications
   3. Managed by combining topical and systemic therapies
   4. Managed by removing the causative agent

3. Dermatological disorders are visually evident, therefore:
   1. Lesions are difficult to differentiate without microscopic diagnostic analysis.
   2. Lesions are readily identifiable.
   3. Lesions must be covered so as not to attract attention.
   4. Lesions can often be self-treated with OTC medications.

4. The etiology of dermatological dysfunctions may be:
   1. Bacterial, chemical, or endocrine
   2. Bacterial, viral, or fungal
   3. Allergenic, vascular, or genetic
   4. All of the above

Continued

REVIEW QUESTIONS—cont'd

5. Photoaging refers to:
   1. The facial age lines, which are evident in close-up photographs
   2. The facial age lines caused by prolonged exposure to ultraviolet B radiation
   3. The patches of discoloration caused by prolonged use of tanning beds
   4. The erythema caused by prolonged exposure to the sun
6. Which of the following is true concerning contact dermatitis?
   1. It is an infection of the skin characterized by redness, heat, pain, and swelling.
   2. It is usually diagnosed by biopsy.
   3. It is an acute inflammation of the hair follicle.
   4. It is treated on identification of the sensitizing substance and controlling the symptoms.
7. Most common dermatological problems encountered by health care professionals are:
   1. Tineas
   2. Staphylococcal infections
   3. Sexually transmitted infections
   4. Malignancies
8. Which of the following is true concerning rosacea?
   1. It is a highly contagious, pruritic skin infection caused by a mite.
   2. It has an insidious onset, develops between 30 and 50 years of age, affects more women than men, and is more common in fair-skinned persons.
   3. It is classified and evaluated by using the PASI method.
   4. It is a T cell-mediated inflammatory disease characterized by epidermal hyperplasia.
9. The ABCDEs of melanoma include:
   1. Altitude, brownness, circularity, diameter, and evolution
   2. Always, be, careful, to diagnose, early
   3. Asymmetry, border irregularity, color variation, diameter increase, and elevation
   4. Age, black coloration, dryness, and erythema
10. Pruritus:
    1. Is one of the most common dermatological diseases
    2. Is usually a sign that healing is underway
    3. Should alert the health care provider to change the wound dressing
    4. Can accompany malignant dermatological conditions

REVIEW ACTIVITIES

1. Arrange to spend a day observing patient care in a dermatology practice and note in a journal:
   - Types of complaints that motivate patients to seek care.
   - Questions that the health care providers usually asks the patient.
   - Diagnostic procedures, which are undertaken.
   - Length of time patients has been under care, for the same condition.
   - Types of treatment prescribed.
   - Questions that the patients usually ask the health care providers.
   - Extent to which the principles of wound healing and skin care are practiced.
   - Your impression of dermatological practice.
2. List three nursing diagnoses commonly associated with dermatological dysfunction. Identify two nursing interventions for each of your three nursing diagnoses.

Continued

REVIEW ACTIVITIES—cont'd

3. Discuss appropriate nursing interventions for the care of the patient with herpetic infections.
4. Evaluate the reasons that your peers believe that when they were adolescents they could have chosen to not protect themselves well from sunburn and develop strategies to encourage self-protection.
5. Examine warts that are present on your peers or patients and interview them regarding how they feel about having this condition. Explain the pathophysiology and strategies for treatment.

Visit the Contemporary Medical-Surgical Nursing online companion resource at www.delmarhealthcare.com for additional content and study aids. Click on Online Companions then select the Nursing discipline.

CHAPTER 46

Burns: Nursing Management

Tanya D. Williams, RN, BSN, MSN, CCNS, APRN-BC

Tammy Coffee, MSN, RN, ACNP

Lynne Yurko, RN, BSN, CNA-BC

CHAPTER TOPICS

- Epidemiology, Etiology, and Pathophysiology of Burns
- Emergent Phase of Burns
- Acute Phase of Burns
- Rehabilitative Phase of Burns

KEY TERMS

Allograft
Autograft
Burn shock
Deep partial-thickness burn
Eschar
Escharotomy
Full-thickness burn
Heterograft (xenograft)
Homograft
Superficial burn
Superficial partial-thickness burn
Tumor necrosis factor
Zone of coagulation
Zone of hyperemia
Zone of stasis

Both physical and psychological healing subsequent to a major burn are prolonged processes. Both are accompanied by pain and drain energy. It is therefore easy for those recovering from a major burn to exist within a limited monotonous environment, slipping first into boredom, then into depression and desperation. Florence Nightingale recognized the critical responsibility nurses have for managing not only a patient's treatment regimen but also that patient's environment. Nightingale (1860) stated that fresh air, direct sunlight, elimination of unnecessary noise, variety of form, and brilliance of color are actual means of recovery, and what nurses must do is manage these aspects of the patient's environment so as to put the patient in the best condition for nature to act upon him or her.

BURNS

Burns are injuries to the skin and its underlying tissues caused by heat, chemicals, or electricity. Burn injuries are the second leading cause of accidental death in the United States. Approximately 80 percent of all burn injuries occur in the home with the remaining 20 percent occurring in industrial settings. Approximately 2.5 million people seek medical treatment for burns each year with 150,000 resulting in hospitalization and 10,000 resulting in death. When death occurs, it is either immediately after the injury or weeks later as a result of multisystem organ dysfunction (Stocking, 2005). The physical, psychological, and financial impact of the burn injury can be catastrophic and devastating to the patient and the patient's family.

Epidemiology

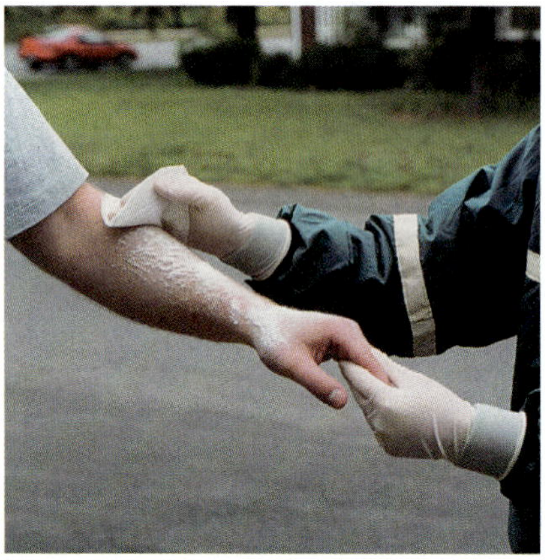

Figure 46-1 Dry chemicals should be brushed off first, and then large volumes of water used to rinse the residue off the patient.

The skin is the largest human organ. A burn injury occurs when skin tissue is damaged. Causative agents include flame, scald, direct contact, chemicals, electrical current, and radiation (Figure 46-1). Commonly, burn events are associated with improper use of space heaters, fireplaces, and matches, as well as with ignition of clothing during cooking or smoking (Doe Report, 2005). Flame injuries are the most complicated and fatal burns with average hospital cost ranging from $36,000 to $117,000 (O'Conner & Besner, 2004). The larger the burn, the higher the cost, with additional expenses resulting from lost wages, property loss, and long-term care.

Etiology

Approximately 90 percent of burns are caused by household accidents. Scald burns occur more often in children age three and younger, and flame burns are more common with older children and adults (O'Conner & Besner, 2004). Over the past 40 years morbidity and mortality from burn injuries have decreased by 50 percent in the United States. During the 1960s burns covering

DOLLARS AND SENSE

Blood Transfusion in Burns

Blood transfusions are a common practice for treating burn patients during the emergent and acute phases of recovery. Overall, approximately 11 million units of blood are transfused yearly in the United States. On average, each unit of blood costs $150. There are limited data to guide appropriate use of transfusions. In an effort to identify current burn center health care provider blood transfusion practices, a survey delineating transfusion practices was distributed to burn center directors across the country. They were asked to list factors affecting their blood transfusion thresholds and to provide their blood transfusion threshold based on patient age and percent of burn. The 2004 results of the survey reveal variable values in a variety of areas. For instance, one health care provider may interpret a hematocrit of 27 percent as need for blood, and a second health care provider may see no need for transfusion until the hematocrit falls to 22 percent. This 5 percent variability can have a significant impact on the cost of care. Without a standard practice guideline, cost of transfusions cannot be predicted or controlled. Prospective studies to establish safe, clinically effective, and cost effective guidelines are needed.

half the body were fatal. Today patients with burns covering 90 percent of the body can survive. This decline is because of successful prevention efforts and improved clinical management of people who sustain severe burns. Advances in treatment include an improved understanding of burn resuscitation, enhanced wound care treatments, appropriate infection control, improved treatment of inhalation injuries, and an improved approach to the hypermetabolic response to burn injuries.

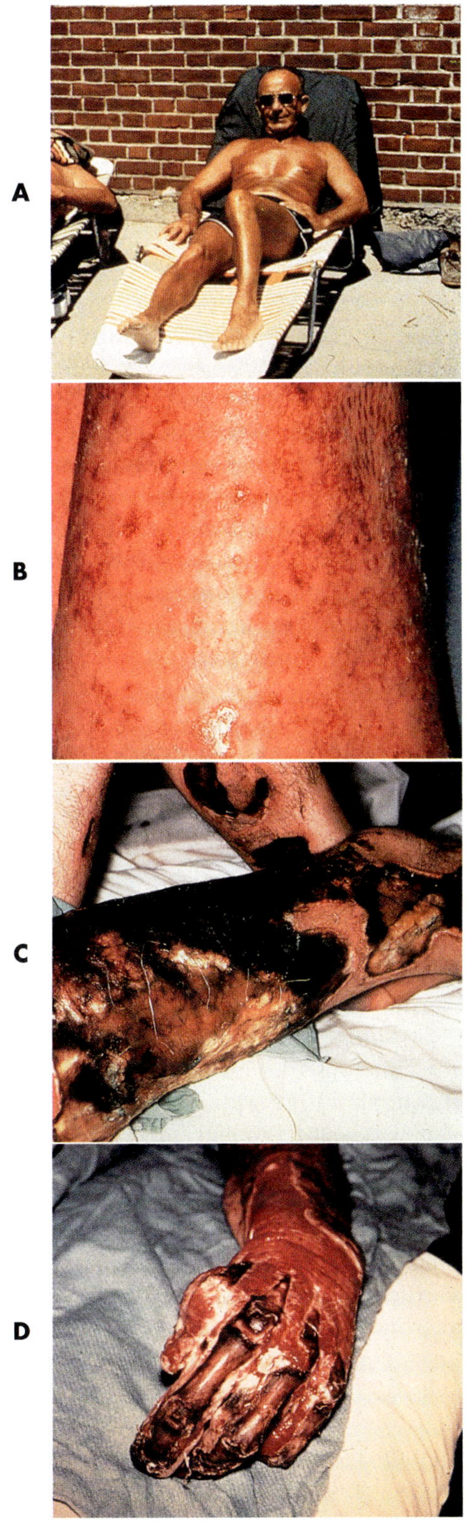

Figure 46-2 Types of burns. Courtesy of the Phoenix Society for Burn Survivors.

Pathophysiology

The depth of a burn is dependent on the temperature of the burning agent and the length of time in which the agent is in contact with the skin. Early tissue damage may occur at temperatures of 104° F (40° C). Irreversible damage to the dermis occurs at temperatures of 158° F (70° C). Burn injuries are described as **superficial** (first-degree burns), **superficial partial-thickness** or **deep partial-thickness** (second-degree burns), and **full-thickness** (third- and fourth-degree burns). All are based on the degree of destruction of the epidermal and dermal layers of the skin (Figure 46-2).

Superficial burns involve only the protective outer epidermal layer of the skin that helps prevent injury, minimizes water loss, and regulates temperature. Sunburns are commonly superficial burns. Patients may have some areas of superficial burns surrounded by deeper burns. Partial-thickness burns are characterized by destruction of the epidermis and varying depths of the dermis, the second layer of skin that lies below the epidermis and above subcutaneous tissue. These burns are likely to be painful because nerve endings have been injured and exposed; but they have the ability to heal because portions of the epithelial cells are not destroyed. The presence of blisters often indicates a more superficial partial-thickness injury. Blisters may increase in size as the result of continuous exudation and collection of tissue fluid. During the healing phase of a partial-thickness burn, dryness and itching are common and are caused by increased vascularization of sebaceous glands, reduction of secretions, and decreased perspiration.

Full-thickness burns include destruction of the epidermis and the entire dermis, as well as possible damage to the subcutaneous layer, muscle, and bone. Nerve endings are destroyed, resulting in a painless wound. **Eschar,** is burned skin that is dead (denatured protein) and appears leathery that may form as the result of surface dehydration. Black networks of coagulated capillaries may be seen. Full-thickness burns require removal of the burned skin and grafting, because the destroyed tissue is unable to epithelialize. Often a deep partial-thickness burn may convert to a full-thickness burn because of infection, trauma, or decreased blood supply.

As a result of burns normal skin function is diminished, resulting in physiological alterations, including loss of protective barriers, escape of body fluids, lack of temperature control, destroyed sweat and sebaceous glands, and a diminished number of sensory receptors. The severity of these alterations depends on the extent of the burn and the depth of the damage.

Local Tissue Response

Damage to the skin from a thermal injury can result in immediate tissue changes. These changes, known as the zones of injury, were first described by Jackson in 1953. If the heat damage is severe enough, a **zone of coagulation** is formed. This is the area of the burn that has the most contact with the causative agent, causing the protein to coagulate. The damage is irreversible. Surrounding this area the blood vessels are damaged resulting in decreased perfusion to the area, or a **zone of stasis.** The cells in this area are still viable but because of poor blood flow and tissue edema are at risk for death over the next few hours or days. Other factors, such as dehydration and infection, may lead to further tissue necrosis in this area of stasis. Meticulous wound care, hydration, and prevention of infection are essential in limiting further destruction of this area. At the outer edge of the burn is a **zone of hyperemia,** or inflammation, characterized by viable cells with minimal injury. Blood flow is increased because of vasodilation from the release of vasoactive substances. This increased blood flow brings leukocytes and nutrients necessary to promote wound healing.

Systemic Tissue Response

A major burn injury is one of the most serious forms of trauma an individual can experience. Virtually every organ system is affected. Physiological changes are both local and systemic in nature. Systemic changes develop in a burn of greater than 25 percent of the total body surface area (TBSA). A shock state, known as **burn shock,** develops that is both a hypovolemic and a cellular shock. Burn shock involves massive fluid shifts of plasma, electrolytes, and proteins into the burn wound. This inflammatory response to the injury is necessary for healing, but excessive production causes cell damage. Tissue damage results from the release of many cellular mediators and vasoactive substances, such as histamine, serotonin, prostaglandins, and interleukin-1. These substances cause a systemic inflammatory response that affects multiple organ systems and causes increased vascular permeability, resulting in significant hypovolemia, an insufficient amount of circulating vascular volume, and edema. This phase begins at the time of burn injury, peaks in 12 to 24 hours, and lasts for 48 to 72 hours.

During the burn shock phase intravascular fluid is lost via evaporation through the wound and by edema formation. Vasodilation and increased capillary permeability results in the movement of fluid, electrolytes, and protein from the intravascular space to the interstitial space. Fluid movement is caused by both oncotic and osmotic forces. When capillary permeability reestablishes, this protein will be unable to move back into the intravascular space. The lymphatic system becomes overloaded and is unable to recirculate the protein. A significant hypoproteinemia, an abnormally low level of protein, ensues. The sodium level within the damaged tissue increases causing further movement of water from the intravascular space that potentiates wound edema and hypovolemia. Edema may be severe in highly vascular areas, such as the face. Patients with large surface area burns experience edema throughout the body that can impair peripheral circulation by compressing circulatory vessels in an extremity.

A generalized physiological response develops immediately after a burn injury. Initially a release of catecholamines (e.g., epinephrine and norepinephrine), vasopressin (antidiuretic hormone), and angiotensin II causes intense vasoconstriction and increased systemic vascular resistance. The blood pressure may be elevated, and the patient is tachycardic. This physiological response assists in the initial attempt to conserve fluid, but its increased capillary force also promotes burn edema. Cardiac output is decreased because of the release of these vasoconstrictive agents and its subsequent increased system vascular resistance and increased cardiac workload. Cardiac function continues to be depressed even after adequate fluid resuscitation pointing to the myocardial depressant effects of inflammatory mediators, such as **tumor necrosis factor** (an inflammatory biochemical), is released from the burn wound.

Pulmonary function may be affected even in the absence of an inhalation injury. More effort is required to breathe because of edema formation and from an increased pulmonary vascular resistance that develops from the release of mediators, such as serotonin. Also, the patient may be at risk for airway obstruction because of oropharyngeal swelling that increases once fluid resuscitation begins.

The kidneys, liver, and intestines are also affected during a major burn. Decreased blood flow to the kidneys as a result of hypovolemia and vasoconstriction and a significant release of antidiuretic hormone places the patient at risk for renal failure. Patients at greatest risk for renal failure have had a delay in their initial fluid resuscitation or develop sepsis. Hepatic perfusion is also compromised contributing to liver ischemia. Finally, the decreased bowel perfusion makes the patient prone to a paralytic ileus. Breakdown of the small intestine may occur, causing bacteria to move or translocate across the intestinal wall into the blood vessels, promoting the development of sepsis, an overwhelming bacterial infection of the blood and body organs.

Compromise of the immune system is the last significant effect of a burn injury. The break in skin integrity destroys the body's first line of defense. A complex change in the body's immune system results in bone marrow depression, immunosuppression, and a shorter life span of red blood cells. Damaged tissue triggers the release of the inflammatory cytokine cascade. The cascade is an inflammatory response designed to destroy microbes and potentiate tissue repair. Release of these cytokines (tumor necrosis factor and interleukins) impairs the function of lymphocytes, macrophages, and neutrophils, increasing the risk of infection. The nutritional deficit that occurs also decreases the burn patient's ability to fight infection. For the patient with a major burn injury, an infection that progresses to sepsis and multisystem organ dysfunction has serious consequences.

After the period of burn shock the patient remains acutely ill. This period is characterized by hypermetabolism (a higher than normal metabolic rate) and impaired nutrition. A negative nitrogen balance begins at the onset of the burn and is the result of tissue destruction, protein loss, and the stress response. It continues throughout the acute period and is secondary to continued loss of protein from the wound, tissue catabolism resulting from immobility, and an increased metabolic rate. Special attention to the nutritional needs of the patient is an integral part of the comprehensive care during this time. The patient is vulnerable to significant weight loss because of fluid evaporation from the wound and loss of solid body mass because of increased metabolism.

Complications of the gastrointestinal (GI) system occur frequently after thermal injury. Gastric and duodenal ulceration has been reported in severely burned patients. Bleeding is the major clinical problem for patients with these lesions. Treatment is aimed at prevention and is best accomplished by antacids, histamine-2 (H_2) blockers, and enteral feedings. Cholecystitis, pancreatitis, and hepatic dysfunction may also be seen as the result of tissue ischemia from hypoperfusion.

Planning and Implementation

Management of a person with a burn injury is extensive and costly. Discharge planning begins on admission using a multidisciplinary approach to ensure that quality and cost-effective care are provided. Three periods of treatment can be identified in the care of the seriously burned patient: the emergent, acute, and rehabilitation periods. The emergent period refers to the first 24 to 48 hours post-burn when the patient is admitted, the severity of the injury is determined, first aid and wound care are given, and burn shock is treated. The acute period of treatment begins at the end of the emergent period and lasts until all of the full-thickness wounds are covered with skin grafts or partial-thickness wounds are healed. The physical healing time is determined by the patient's medical condition, nutritional status, and ability to heal. A 40 percent injury requires approximately 40 days to heal. The rehabilitation period focuses on the patient returning to a useful place in society. Two areas of concern during the rehabilitation phase are (a) the restoration of function over joint surfaces that were scarred and (b) the emotional assistance that the patient and family will need.

The rehabilitation of the patient actually begins during early hospitalization and is addressed throughout the hospital stay. After the initial discharge, the patient may require emotional assistance and counseling, and many readmissions

BOX 46-1

PREHOSPITAL CARE OF MAJOR BURNS

- Remove victim form source of burn.
- Douse with water and remove nonadherent smoldering clothing to stop the burning process.
- If chemical burn, carefully remove clothing and flush wound with large amounts of water.
- If electrical burn and victim is still in contact with source, do not touch victim. Remove electrical source with dry nonconductive object.
- Establish patent airway and assess for inhalation injury. Give oxygen if available.
- Check peripheral pulse to assess circulatory status.
- Assess and initiate treatment for injuries requiring immediate attention.
- Remove tight-fitting jewelry and clothing.
- Cover burn with moist sterile or clean cover.
- Cover victim with warm, dry cover to prevent heat loss.
- Transport victim to nearest acute care facility.

Adapted from American Burn Association. (2005). Advanced burn life support course: Provider's manual. *Chicago: Author; Stocking, J. (2005).* Initial assessment and resuscitation. *Retrieved March 5, 2006, from http://www.astna.org.*

may be necessary for reconstructive procedures. Emotional and social healing depends on each patient's ability to cope with a new body image and society's acceptance of the change in the patient's physical appearance. Each of the three periods and the management required is discussed.

EMERGENT PHASE

The goals of management during the emergent period, the first 24 to 48 hours after a burn, are to secure the airway, support circulation by fluid replacement, keep the patient comfortable with analgesics, prevent infection through careful wound care, maintain body temperature, and provide emotional support. The nurse and physician work collaboratively to achieve these goals. The specific details of treatment are discussed under Nursing Management.

Prehospital Care and First Aid

At the scene of a burn injury, the first action should be to remove the victim from the hazardous environment. Removal may be accomplished by untrained witnesses to the injury or by trained emergency personnel. Length of exposure to the causative agent is directly related to the severity of the injury. Box 46-1 lists prehospital care priorities.

The most common causative agents for burn injury are scalding fluids, fire, chemicals, and electricity. Other types of injuries result from contact with hot surfaces. Regardless of the cause, the burning process must be stopped. Scald burns are the most common burn injury, particularly in children. Scald injury may be caused by steam or hot fluids and may affect a widespread area. Scald injury is related to the temperature of the liquid and length of exposure. Initial care consists of cooling the skin with cool water. First aid follows the same treatment plan as for all burns, that is, to stop the burning process.

Flame and flash injuries are the second most common types of burn injury and are commonly associated with an inhalation injury. These injuries may occur from house fires (caused by smoking in bed or children playing with matches) or ignited gasoline or propane. Injuries may be combined partial- and full-thickness burns. Duration of contact with the flame source will determine the depth of the injury. In the case of fire, flames should be extinguished, flammable or hot material removed from the victim, and the victim and rescuer removed from the unventilated or hazardous surroundings. If clothing is on fire, the victim's first reaction is to run, which only fans the flames. The best intervention is to stop the person, wrap him or her in a blanket, coat, sheet, or towel, and roll him or her on the ground to exclude oxygen and thereby put out the fire. The rule is stop, drop, and roll.

People who are confined to a wheelchair or limited in their movement because of a disability should learn to use a blanket or rug to smother a fire. The victim should drop to the ground and roll to smother all flames. The victim should never stand, because this will cause the flames and smoke to engulf the facial area, possibly igniting the hair and causing an inhalation injury. Any water source can be used to extinguish flames, cool the burn, or dilute the chemical unless the victim is still in contact with an electrical source. Once all the flame is extinguished, clothing (excepting clothing that adheres to the burned area), jewelry, and debris are carefully removed. Any clothing removed should be saved for possible analysis of flammability. Contact burns occur from direct contact with a hot substance, such as hot metal, stoves, tar, or irons. The area of burn is usually confined to the area where the substance came into contact with the skin. The treatment goal is to stop the burning process.

Currently there are more than 30,000 chemicals that are considered hazardous by regulatory agencies, and 2 percent of all burn unit admissions are chemical-related (American Burn Association, 2005). When chemical burns

Red Flag

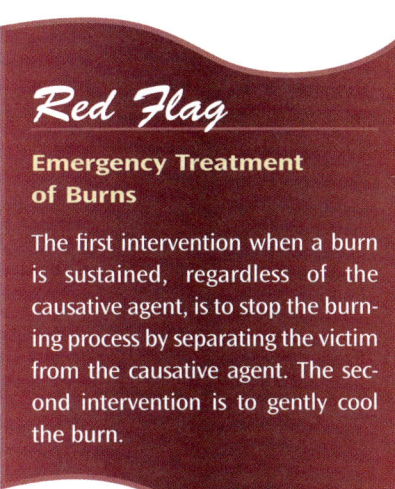

Emergency Treatment of Burns

The first intervention when a burn is sustained, regardless of the causative agent, is to stop the burning process by separating the victim from the causative agent. The second intervention is to gently cool the burn.

occur, they are usually acquired as a result of accidents in the home or an industrial setting. Household chemical burns may be caused by drain cleaners, disinfectants, and other chemicals used in the home. Industrial chemicals such as strong acids (hydrochloric), alkali and organic compounds, such as phenol, and petroleum products (gasoline) are common causes of chemical burns.

The severity of the injury is related to the chemical involved, its concentration, length of exposure, and the immediate treatment. Extent of penetration depends on the agent. Alkalis produce more tissue damage by a liquefaction necrosis process that loosens cellular tissue and allows deeper penetration. Acids cause protein coagulation necrosis that forms eschar that limits penetration (Collemer, 2004). Treatment should include irrigation of the area with copious amounts of water or saline, which will decrease the concentration, volume, duration of contact, and the mechanism of action.

Ocular chemical burns can occur from a ruptured airbag or whenever a chemical splashes onto the face. Treatment includes careful irrigation of the eye with water. Adequacy of the irrigation is determined by testing a sample of the irrigated fluid with litmus paper to test for the presence of acid or alkali. Ingestion of noxious chemicals may burn the upper GI tract. These burns are difficult to treat and frequently cause complications. If the chemical is a powder, the powder should be brushed off the skin prior to flushing the area (American Burn Association, 2005).

Hydrofluoric acid is used regularly in industrial settings. When skin comes into direct contact with the chemical, local tissue injury, systemic hypocalcemia, and potential arrhythmias can occur. Traditionally, treatment has been centered on the application of topical calcium gels or calcium gluconate injections, with intra-arterial infusions of calcium gluconate reserved for distal extremities and digits. New research indicates that facial hydrofluoric acid burns can be treated with a calcium gluconate infusion through the external carotid artery; a new option that has reportedly increased patient satisfaction when compared to the alternative forms of treatment (Nguyen, Mohr, Ahrenholz, & Solem, 2004).

Electrical burns account for approximately 3 percent of all burn unit admissions and approximately 1,000 deaths per year (American Burn Association, 2005). Electrical burns usually result from accidental contact with an exposed object that conducts electricity. Examples include electrical wiring, power transmission lines, and lighting. Damage depends on the intensity of the current. Voltage determines whether the current can enter the body or not. Low voltage cannot enter the body unless the skin is broken or moist. High voltage can enter the body and easily overcomes resistance. Electrical burns pose a special hazard to the victim because the total body surface area of the burn is not always apparent and is often internal. Dysrhythmias and neurological dysfunction are common. Extreme care must be taken when removing the victim from the electrical source to prevent a similar injury to the rescuer.

Initial management of all burn injuries follows the completion of the primary survey: airway, breathing, circulation, and presence of a neurological deficit. All are assessed and initial management begins. This includes the removal of the patient's clothing and a brief neurological exam. A secondary assessment is completed as long as the patient has no life-endangering injuries. The secondary assessment includes a more thorough head-to-toe assessment. A history is obtained, which includes the mechanism of injury, medical history (including allergies), and medications the patient is taking. During this assessment, the burn wound is evaluated and treated. Life-threatening conditions are always cared for before the burn wound. Standard precautions should be followed whenever there is a possibility of exposure to blood or other body fluids. This includes the wearing of gown, gloves, mask, and eye protection.

Burn wounds are covered with dressings dampened with normal saline or water, which eases the pain, reduces edema, and prevents evaporation of body water. The patient's entire body is wrapped in a dry cover to prevent heat loss.

> **BOX 46-2**
>
> **BURN CENTER REFERRAL CRITERIA**
>
> A burn unit may treat adults or children or both. Burn injuries that should be referred to a burn unit include the following:
>
> - Partial-thickness burns greater than 10 percent TBSA
> - Burns that involve the face, hands, feet, genitalia, perineum, or major joints
> - Third-degree burns in any group
> - Electrical burns, including lightning injury
> - Chemical burns
> - Inhalation injury
> - Burn injury in patients with preexisting medical disorders that could complicate management, prolong recovery, or affect mortality
> - Any patient with burns and concomitant trauma (such as fractures) in which the burn injury poses the greatest risk of morbidity or mortality
> - Burned children in hospitals without qualified personnel or equipment for the care of children
> - Burn injury in patients who will require special social, emotional, or long-term rehabilitative intervention
>
> *Adapted from American Burn Association. (2005).* Advanced burn life support course: Provider's manual. *Chicago: Author; Stocking, J. (2005).* Initial assessment and resuscitation. *Retrieved March 5, 2006, from http://www.astna.org.*

Ice should never be used, because sudden vasoconstriction causes severe shifting of body fluids and may increase the depth of injury. Although sterile dressings are preferred, clean dressings may be used because all dressings will be removed when the patient arrives at the medical facility. Oils, salves, and ointments should never be used on burns prior to evaluation at the hospital.

In the prehospital period pain in extensive burns is best controlled by gentle and minimal handling and by application of dressings to exclude air from burned surfaces. The degree of pain is usually inversely proportional to the depth of the burn injury. As mentioned earlier, full-thickness burns are usually painless, because nerve endings have been destroyed.

Burns are often more severe than they first appear to be; therefore even patients with burns that appear to be superficial should be seen by a health care provider. Patients with major burns should be transported to a regional burn center. According to the last recorded statistics developed by the Organization and Delivery of American Burn Association, there are 139 hospitals in the United States that have burn centers (Doe Report, 2005). These burn units are located throughout the country, and most are found in major medical centers in urban areas. Canada has 17 burn care centers. A hospital or burn center should be notified before a burn victim is transported so that they have time to prepare for the patient's arrival. Box 46-2 lists criteria for referral to a burn center.

Transfer of the patient should not be delayed because of difficulty in establishing an intravenous (IV) line. The American Burn Association teaches that an IV line is not necessary if the patient is less than 60 minutes from the hospital. When an IV line is established the recommended solution is Ringer's lactate infused at 500 mL/hour for an adult and 250 mL/hour for a child age 5 years or older.

For obviously small burns, fluids may be given by mouth with caution. Large burns may cause decreased peristalsis, and therefore nothing should be given by mouth. Patients with large burns, or who have inhaled smoke, may vomit and attention is needed to prevent them from aspirating vomitus.

To optimize burn care, the American Burn Association has created a national standard for voluntary review of burn centers according to a systematic approach to burn care. The verification is granted for a three-year period by the American Burn Association and the American College of Surgeons. Because of potential management problems, they recommend transfer of patients to a burn center based on burn size, depth, mechanism, and comorbid factors.

Emergency Department Management

Rapid and efficient care is essential in the emergency department management of the victim with a major burn. If any respiratory distress is present, an airway is established. Prophylactic intubation may be initiated if any heat or smoke has been inhaled, or if the head, neck, or face is involved. Inhalation injuries are best managed with controlled ventilation, because swelling of the upper airway can progress to obstruction. Endotracheal intubation is preferred over a tracheostomy. Edema of the respiratory passages frequently subsides within a few days after the initial injury; therefore surgery of the airway should be avoided. Depending on the severity of symptoms, emergency treatment may include oxygen, suctioning, and postural drainage.

After an airway has been established, circulatory support is addressed. Fluid is best replaced through two large caliber peripheral IV catheters. Placement of these catheters is preferred through an unburned site to prevent the introduction of infection. An indwelling urinary catheter is inserted to adequately monitor urine output. Hourly urine output measurements are used as a guide to the adequacy of fluid (plasma volume) replacement. Patients with burns more than 20 percent of TBSA are more prone to nausea, vomiting, and an ileus. Oral fluids are not recommended, because they create a threat of vomiting and aspiration. A nasogastric tube is inserted and attached to suction to prevent gastric distension (Doe Report, 2005).

Assessment with Clinical Manifestations

The professional burn care nurse understands the concepts that make the specialty of burn care unique. They develop a specialized knowledge base that accommodates every aspect of the patient's being and complements clinical nursing practice. Burn care nurses also participate in the advancement of burn care practice.

The assessment of the person who has sustained a severe burn focuses on the severity of the burn injury. Knowledge of circumstances surrounding the burn injury is extremely valuable in the management of a burn victim. This information can be obtained from either the burn victim or witnesses to the event. Data should include: (a) how the burn injury occurred; (b) when the burn injury occurred; (c) duration of contact with the burning agent; (d) location (enclosed area suggests possibility of smoke inhalation or carbon monoxide poisoning); and (e) presence of an explosion (suggests possibility of other injuries).

The burn victim's age and general health may modify treatment. Elderly patients and young patients have a higher mortality rate than a young adult with the same percentage of burn. Preexisting endocrine, pulmonary, cardiovascular, or renal disease or a history of drug abuse will decrease a victim's ability to cope with severe burns. Because most burn patients will require topical and systemic therapy with a number of drugs, allergies, and drug sensitivities must be determined and documented.

Many factors are considered in evaluating the severity of burn injury, including size and depth of the burn, the cause of the injury, and the patient's preinjury health status. Identification of known and unknown disorders may prevent fatal complications in the burn victim. A prior illness, such as diabetes or renal failure, may become acute during the postburn phase. The physiological stress of the burn experience may exacerbate a latent disease process or worsen an already active process and thus increase mortality. Diabetes and chronic obstructive pulmonary disease may be aggravated, or patients with atherosclerotic heart disease may develop a myocardial infarction.

For adults, the rule of nines is a tool used to estimate the percentage of the TBSA burned (Figure 46-3). The percentage of TBSA burned is estimated with the use of charts that depict anterior and posterior drawings of the body. In adults, the body is divided into areas equal to the multiples of 9 percent. In clinical practice the burned area is shaded in on the drawings and the amount of body surface burned is calculated from the shaded areas. Calculations are modified for infants and children younger than 10 years of age because of their relatively larger head and smaller body (consult a pediatric textbook for these figures).

The depth of the burn injury is evaluated on the basis of appearance, color, and sensation as shown in Table 46-1. The burn is classified as superficial (first-degree), superficial partial-thickness, or deep partial-thickness (second-degree), or full-thickness (third-degree). A laser Doppler is being used more frequently to evaluate the blood flow in the injured tissue to assist in definitive diagnosis of depth of injury.

The severity of a burn also depends on the age of the victim. Infants younger than 2 years of age and adults older than 60 years have a higher mortality rate than people in other age-groups with a similar size injury. The infant has a weak antibody response to infection, and in older victims the serious burn may aggravate the degenerative processes or exacerbate a preexisting health problem.

The body part involved is an important factor in evaluating the severity of a burn. The part of the body burned must be considered when the severity

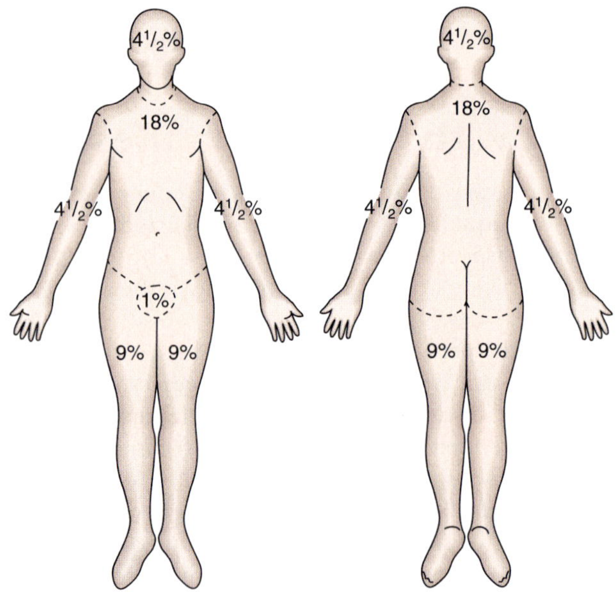

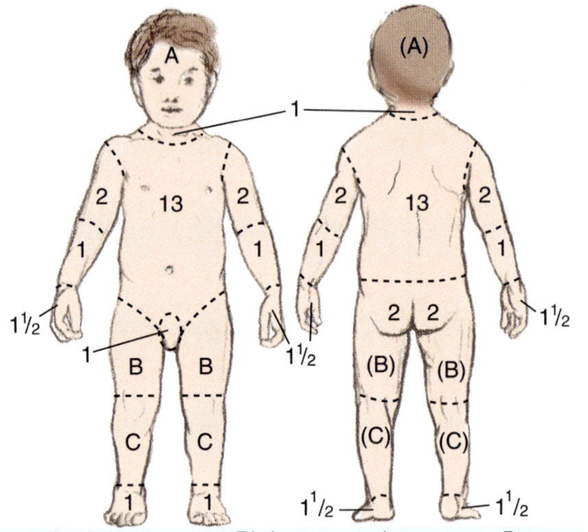

Area	Birth	1 yr	5 yr
A (head)	19	17	14
B (one thigh)	6 ½	7 ½	9
C (one leg)	6	6	6

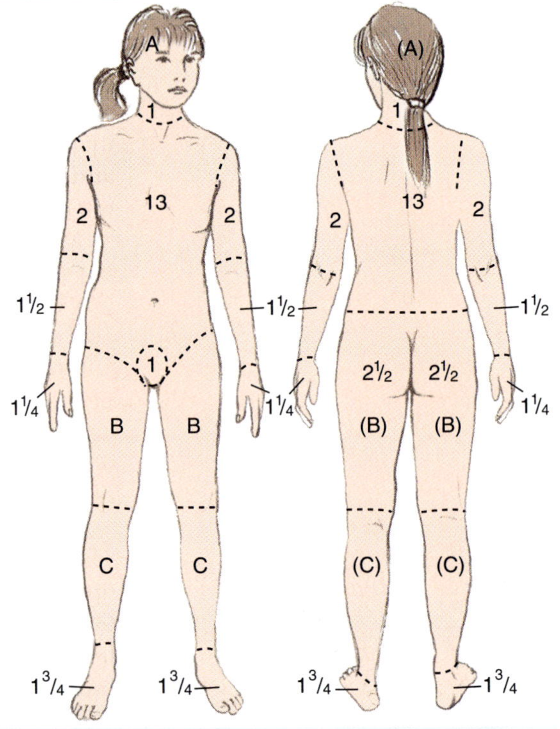

Area	10 yr	15 yr	Adult
A (head)	11	9	8
B (one thigh)	8 ½	9	9
C (one leg)	6	6 ½	7

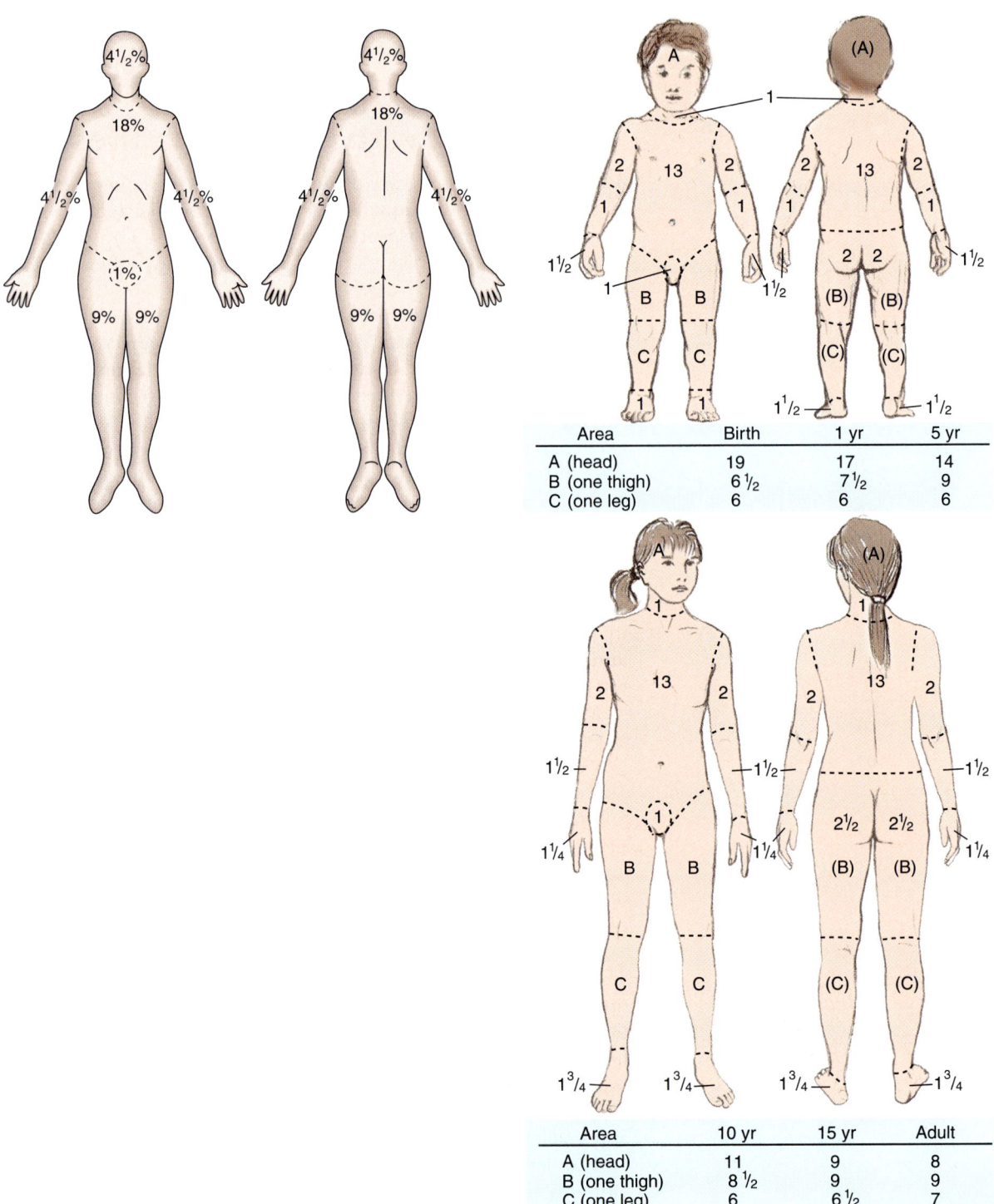

Figure 46-3 The rule of nines is used to estimate the percentage of body surface area burned.

of the burn is estimated. For example a 3 percent burn of the anterior surface of the thigh is not as serious as a 3 percent burn to the neck, face, or perineal area. Injuries that involve cosmetic and functional areas of the body require a longer period of recovery because of both physical and emotional reactions to the burn injury. A burn of the face, hands, and feet requires extensive, meticulous care, with extensive physical and occupational therapy. A burn of the head, neck, and chest may also involve injury to the respiratory tract and result in severe respiratory distress. Burns of the perineum are difficult to manage

TABLE 46-1 Characteristics the of Depth of a Burn Injury

	SUPERFICIAL (FIRST-DEGREE)	PARTIAL-THICKNESS (SECOND-DEGREE)	FULL-THICKNESS (THIRD-DEGREE)
Skin depth	Epidermis	Entire epidermis; partial dermis; sweat glands; hair follicles intact	Epidermis, dermis; extends to subcutaneous tissue, possibly muscle and bone
Cause	Flash flame; ultraviolet light; sunburn	Contact with hot liquids or solids; flash flame to clothing; direct flames; chemicals; ultraviolet light	Contact with hot liquids or solids; flame; chemicals; electrical contact
Appearance	Dry, no blisters Minimal or no edema Blanches with fingertip pressure and color returns when pressure removed	Superficial partial injury Blisters that will increase in size; blanches with fingertip pressure and color returns when pressure returns; moist Deep partial injury Blisters present slower to increase in size; blanching decreased; less moisture	Dry with leathery eschar; charred vessels visible under eschar; blisters rare but thin-walled blisters that do not increase in size may be present; no blanching with pressure
Color	Increased redness	Superficial partial injury Pink Deep partial injury Pale, mottled with dull, white, tan, cherry red areas	White, charred, dark tan, black, dark red
Sensation	Painful	Painful	No pain; deep throbbing; nerve endings dead
Healing time	2 to 5 days with peeling; no scarring; may discolor	Superficial partial injury 5 to 21 days, no grafting Deep partial injury 21 to 35 days with out complications; may convert to full-thickness and require grafting	No healing potential; requires excision and grafting

Adapted from Doe Report. (2005). Burn injuries. The Doe report medical reference library. *Retrieved March 1, 2006, from http://www.doeroport.com; O'Conner, A., & Besner, G. (2004).* Burns a surgical perspective. *Retrieved April 8, 2006, from www.emedicine.com.*

because of the potential for contamination and infection. The circumferential or encircling burn of a limb, the neck, or the chest has serious consequences. This type of burn will cause constrictive contraction of the skin and produce a tourniquet effect that may impair breathing or circulation.

Identifying the causative agent is of prime importance, because the nature of the agent has a direct effect on prognosis and treatment. As mentioned previously, mechanisms of burn injury are flame and flash, contact, scald, chemical, and electric. The factors determining the severity of burns are: Size of burn, depth of burn, age of victim, body part involved, mechanism of injury, history of cardiac, pulmonary, renal, or hepatic disease, and injuries sustained at time of burn.

LAW IN PRACTICE

Burns as a Result of Abuse

Burns obtained as a result of child abuse are found in pediatric burn admissions. Common occurrences involve children 3 years of age and younger with either scald or contact burns. Socioeconomic status and single parent homes with more than two children have the highest incidences. Hospitalization is lengthy with a high rate of morbidity and mortality. When a child survives, the length of stay may be extended beyond recovery while a social worker, psychologist, and a child life specialist prepare the child for placement with other family members, or foster care. The Child Abuse Prevention and Treatment Act of 1974, requires all professionals to report suspected abuse or neglect (DeLaune & Ladner, 2006). Similarly, all professionals are required to report suspected abuse of elderly patients who may present with burns. Typical signs of abuse include: 12 or more hours delay in seeking treatment without a plausible reason, treatment sought by a nonrelation, parent of a pediatric patient or child of an elderly patient appears to be under the influence of drugs or alcohol, parent of a pediatric patient or child of an elderly patient is inattentive or lacks empathy, injury is inconsistent with description of the circumstances leading to the injury, and elderly patient sustains injuries ordinarily covered by clothing.

Nursing Diagnoses

Based on the information gathered, examples of nursing diagnoses in the patient in the emergent phase of burns may include the following:

- Ineffective airway clearance related to secretions, tracheobronchial edema, and obstruction.
- Deficient fluid volume related to intravascular fluid shift and evaporation.
- Hypothermia related to impaired temperature regulation and wound exposure.
- Risk for infection related to impaired skin integrity.
- Impaired skin integrity related to impaired perfusion and burn injured skin.
- Acute pain related to exposed nerve endings and associated trauma.
- Anxiety related to situational crises and threat of death.

Planning and Implementation

Nursing interventions include maintenance of a patent airway, adequate fluid volume, normothermia, initial wound care, comfort, emotional support, and patient and family education. People who are burned on the face and neck or those who have inhaled flame, steam, or smoke are observed closely for signs of laryngeal edema and airway obstruction. Data indicating potential or existing inhalation injury that is incurred from breathing in harmful gases, vapors, or particulate matter include: burns to face and neck, singed hairs (nasal, beard, or eyelashes), intraoral charcoal, especially on teeth and gums, brassy cough, hoarseness, copious sputum production, carbonaceous sputum, burn injury that has occurred in a closed space, smell of smoke on victim's clothes or on victim, and respiratory distress.

Adequate ventilation and oxygenation may be possible with the victim breathing room air; however, when any inhalation injury has occurred, it is best to give oxygen. When smoke is inhaled, carbon monoxide, which has an affinity for hemoglobin over 200 times as strong as that of oxygen, binds with hemoglobin, displacing oxygen. High carboxyhemoglobin (hemoglobin bound to carbon monoxide) levels impair tissue oxygenation resulting in tissue asphyxia. Providing the victim with 100 percent oxygen by mask will reverse this condition. If the victim is in respiratory distress or has a suspected inhalation injury endotracheal intubation may be necessary.

During fluid resuscitation, adequate volume is assessed by monitoring mental status, vital signs, peripheral perfusion, body weight, and urine output. A 15 to 20 percent weight gain in the first 72 hours of resuscitation is anticipated. Significant laboratory measurements include serum and urine electrolytes, serum and urine osmolality, and hematocrit. Hourly urine output is commonly used as a gauge for adequate fluid replacement. Fluid should be titrated to ensure an output of 0.5 mL/kg/hr or 30 to 50 mL/hour. The most common reasons for a urine output below 30 mL/hour, indicating insufficient fluid replacement, are that the calculated fluid replacement is behind schedule, and the patient's fluid requirements are greater than predicted. The urine is observed for color and analyzed for the presence of blood. The health care provider is notified if hematuria is present.

Other clinical criteria that indicate adequate resuscitation are pulse rate of 120 beats per minute or less, central venous pressure in the low to normal range, pulmonary artery end-diastolic pressure in the low to normal range, and mental lucidity. Signs of adequate fluid resuscitation include: pulse of 70 to 120 beats per minute; urine output of 30 to 50 mL/hour (adult); systolic blood pressure of 100 mm Hg; central venous pressure: 5 to 10 mm Hg; pulmonary capillary wedge pressure (PCWP): 5 to 15 mm Hg; and blood pH normal range: 7.35 to 7.45 and Base deficit greater than −6.

Acidosis indicates that fluids have not been given in sufficient quantities to maximize tissue perfusion. Anaerobic metabolism ensues when the metabolic tissue requirements are not met during resuscitation. Recent studies have indicated that presence of a base deficit, particularly less than −6 is a good indicator of the patient not having adequate fluid resuscitation.

After the first 48 to 72 hours, edema reabsorption begins. The urinary output increases dramatically and is no longer a reliable guide to fluid needs. Fluid needs are assessed by measuring serum and urine electrolyte levels. Fluid replacement, using 5 percent dextrose and water, is based on individual patient assessment. If dehydration occurs from diuresis, fluid replacement therapy is continued until blood volume is stabilized. Potassium may be added to the IV fluid because of potassium losses in the urine. The patient is monitored closely for signs of water intoxication pulmonary edema or congestive heart failure.

Patients may complain of moderate to severe thirst during this period. Aggressive oral hygiene may alleviate patient discomfort. If oral fluids are permitted, accurate recording of ingested fluids is important. Unlimited oral intake and failure to measure it may provide too much fluid in the circulating blood, resulting in water intoxication.

The loss of skin greatly decreases the severely burned patient's ability to regulate body temperature. The environment must be heat controlled and kept warmer than usual. Room temperature is maintained at 80 to 85° F (26.6 to 29.4° C) with humidity of 40 to 50 percent. Drafts must be eliminated. Fluid warmers, heat lamps, and warming blankets are used during burn shock. Prolonged exposure to air is avoided. Exposed areas of the body are covered with sterile sheets and blankets to decrease the loss of body heat through the open wounds while other areas of the burn are being cleansed.

Care of the burn wound can be delayed until all first aid measures have been initiated. Wound care should be carried out carefully and with as little discomfort to the patient as possible. One of the most important factors to be considered in wound care is that the patient has lost the ability to withstand infection in the area where the skin is damaged or destroyed. The goals of the initial wound care are as follows: (a) cleanse the wound to eliminate or decrease the dead tissue and debris that serve as the media for bacterial growth, (b) prevent further destruction of viable skin, and (c) provide for patient comfort.

During the admission procedure, the burn wound and the entire body are washed to remove dirt and debris as well as loose dead tissue on the burned areas. Detergents or antiseptic preparations are effective cleansing agents. Gentle cleansing with gauze is effective in removing dead tissue without causing further tissue damage. All hair in and around the burn wound is shaved and wiped off the skin, because hair attracts and shelters bacteria. Singed hair is clipped short to avoid bacterial contamination of the wound. Firm, intact blisters can remain undisturbed, because they are a natural protective and pain-free dressing. If the blisters are broken and the epidermis is separated, loose tissue must be debrided.

After the wound is cleaned and before a dressing is applied, cultures of the wound are obtained. Baseline cultures provide information about organisms present in the wounds at the time of admission. Prophylactic antibiotics are usually not indicated. Photographs are taken on admission and at intervals during the patient's hospitalization. These pictures provide a record of the appearance of the burn wound on admission, before the application of topical therapy, and during the healing process.

The constricting effect of nonviable tissue (eschar) from a full-thickness injury to the chest, neck, or extremities is an early complication. Edema forming rapidly under the constricting eschar will produce a tourniquet effect that causes occlusion of venous and arterial circulation and may result in ischemic necrosis, especially with unburned areas distal to the constrictive eschar. Frequent monitoring of distal pulses is part of an ongoing assessment to ensure uninterrupted vascular flow to all extremities. Extremities should be monitored for signs and symptoms of circulatory compromise, including diminished peripheral pulses, decreased capillary refill, paleness or cyanosis, temperature decrease, and increase in pain or paresthesia. It may be necessary to monitor circulation every 15 minutes.

Circumferential burns that go all the way around the neck or chest can lead to constriction of chest wall expansion and airway compromise, resulting in respiratory distress. Part of the respiratory assessment is monitoring chest excursions, respiratory rate, and ventilator settings, if the person is intubated, for high pressures and low tidal volume.

Pharmacology

Morphine sulfate is the drug of choice for pain relief and is given intravenously, in small increments (2 to 4 mg). A morphine drip can be used and titrated to the patient's pain. No medication of any kind should be given intramuscularly or subcutaneously, because it may pool and be absorbed later when cardiac output and blood pressure improve. Large doses of sedatives and analgesics are avoided because of the danger of respiratory depression and the potential for masking other symptoms (Broyles, Reiss, & Evans, 2007).

Tetanus prophylaxis is recommended by the American College of Surgeons. It is administered in the emergency department after determining the patient's immunization status. If the patient has been previously immunized but has not received tetanus toxoid in the preceding five years, the vaccine can be administered. If information about prior tetanus immunization is not known, treatment can be delayed for 72 hours until the status is determined or until a dose of human tetanus-immune globulin hormone can be administered with the initiation of an active tetanus immunization program.

BOX 46-3

INDICATIONS FOR FLUID RESUSCITATION

- Burns greater than 20 percent TBSA in adults
- Burns greater than 10 percent TBSA in children
- Patient older than 65 or younger than 2 years of age
- Patient with preexisting disease that would reduce normal compensatory responses to minor hypovolemia (i.e., cardiac or pulmonary disease or diabetes)

Adapted from American Burn Association. (2005). Advanced burn life support course: Provider's manual. *Chicago: Author.*

Replacing fluids and electrolytes (fluid resuscitation) is an essential part of the treatment of burn victims and is instituted as soon as the severity of the burn based on the parameters in Box 46-3 and the patient's condition are known. Ideally, fluid therapy is started within an hour after a severe burn to prevent the onset of hypovolemic shock. Insertion of two large-caliber peripheral catheters permits the rapid administration of fluids and electrolytes.

Fluids administered during the first 48 hours are given to maintain circulating blood volume. Traditional treatment of large burns includes blood transfusion. Whole blood is commonly administered during initial treatment. Additional fluids and electrolytes are added to replace losses from vomiting or from nasogastric drainage.

Two types of fluids are considered when calculating the needs of the patient: crystalloids and colloids. Crystalloids may be isotonic or hypertonic. Isotonic solutions, such as lactated Ringer's or physiological (0.9%) sodium chloride, do not generate a difference in osmotic pressure between the intravascular and interstitial spaces. Thus, large amounts of fluids are required to restore and maintain the intravascular volume. Hypertonic salt solutions have a milliosmolal content of 400 to 600 (280 to 300 mOsm is isotonic), thus creating an osmotic pull of fluid from the interstitial space back to the depleted intravascular space. The use of hypertonic solutions decreases the amount of fluid a patient needs during resuscitation, which helps decrease burn tissue edema and minimizes cardiopulmonary complications (pulmonary edema and congestive heart failure).

The consensus formula used to calculate the volume of IV fluid required for fluid resuscitation is based on the Parkland Formula (American Burn Association, 2005). Using this formula, the patient's fluid requirements for the first 24 hours post-injury are estimated. For adults the formula is: 2 to 4 mL of lactated Ringer's solution × body weight (in kg) × percent burn. Because blood volume falls rapidly, the first 48 hours is crucial as edema increases significantly. As edema increases, additional fluid is lost through the burn and the loss may be increased as high as 15 times normal. IV replacement is a must and is accomplished at a rapid rate. The time is calculated from the time of injury and not from the time the emergency care was initiated. The first one half of the total amount calculated is given in the first 8 hours after the injury. The second half is administered over the next subsequent 16 hours. For example, if a patient weighing 75 kg has a 70 percent TBSA burn, the fluid requirements are:

- 4 mL lactated Ringer's × 75 kg × 70 percent = 21,000 mL needed over the first 24 hours
- One half is needed in the first 8 hours, one half × 21,000 = 10, 500 mL in 8 hours, or 1,312 mL/hour.
- One half is needed in the next 16 hours, one half × 21,000 = 10, 500 mL in 16 hours, or 656 mL/hour.

Colloids may also be used to replace body fluids. The use of colloids is avoided in the first 12 hours post-burn. The capillary permeability caused by the burn injury begins to close at 12 hours. At this time patients may receive colloids, such as fresh frozen plasma, albumin, or dextran. The oncotic pressure generated by the colloids also helps pull fluid back into the intravascular space. In addition, fresh frozen plasma is beneficial in restoring lost clotting factors. Red blood cells are used only if the patient has had a significant loss or destruction of red cells. During the second 24 hours post-burn, one half to two thirds of the initial 24-hour volume is generally required. Also during this second 24-hour period, colloid solutions are used to replace intravascular volume once capillary permeability significantly decreases (Doe Report, 2005).

Surgery

Treatment of the constricting effects of the eschar by incising it is an **escharotomy,** which is performed on the burn unit. An escharotomy is a linear surgical incision through the burn eschar that releases the constriction

Respecting Our Differences

Refusal of Blood Products

Patient autonomy and the right to refuse treatment have long been subjects of controversy. Personal beliefs and lifestyles must be fully respected as treatment plans are developed and implemented, even when refusal of treatment puts the patient at risk for survival. The Jehovah's Witnesses religious community refuses transfusion of blood or blood components to remain faithful and obedient to God's law, as they perceive it (Karcioglu, Oskara, Civancr, & Ozucclik, 2003). The removal of such a critical and traditionally effective treatment is a challenge, particularly when the patient is fully competent and fully informed about the need to maintain circulating blood volume.

> **Safety First** 1
>
> **Burn Prevention in the Community**
>
> Burn prevention informational health and safety fairs do not target audiences that involve children. Traditionally, trinkets, handouts, and posters are given away or are on display. To address this gap, the Central Ohio Burn Education Coalition, developed a television media Safety Day to provide a fun way for families to learn various child safety topics (DeLaune & Ladner, 2006). A wheel of safety similar to the Wheel of Fortune was used and each participant was asked to spin the wheel. Depending on what color the wheel stopped on, the player was asked an age-appropriate question about burn prevention. The youngest player was 3 years old. A correctly answered question afforded the player a visor imprinted with "Practice Your Plan." Incorrectly answered questions afforded the player an educational session that included information about home fire drills, before they received a visor. The wheel is mobile and has been used on college campuses and at the Ohio state fairs.

caused by the full-thickness injury. Patients have limited pain during an escharotomy, because the nerve endings have been damaged by the burn.

The patient is kept as comfortable as possible by gentle handling of the burn areas and by keeping the wounds covered so that air does not reach them. Small doses of morphine are given intravenously. Patients with significant burn injury receive a profound insult to their body and self-image. They are aware that they may not survive, which causes fear and helplessness. The shock and pain of the accident, the chaos and rush to the hospital, and the unknown surroundings and people all intensify the emotional stress. The nurse spends the most time with the patient and has a considerable influence on the patient's psychological adjustment.

Patient and Family Teaching

Nurses can help prevent accidental burns by participating in health education programs that stress fire prevention and the consequences of fires, such as burns, deformities, and death. Nurses also can promote legislation that would control hazardous practices and make working and living environments safer. Community health nurses are in an unusually advantageous position to recognize unsafe practices in the home and to help families develop safe habits of living. Nurses can raise the awareness of patients and the community to the burn problem with education and burn awareness campaigns.

Prevention programs can be developed to highlight seasonal activities that result in burn injuries. Approximately 80 percent of all accidental burns occur in the home and are caused primarily by ignorance, carelessness, and the curiosity of children. More than 35 percent of all fires and burn injuries involve children playing with matches and cigarette lighters. Prevention focuses on teaching parents and others caring for children to keep matches and cigarette lighters out of the reach of children. Some causes of seasonal burn injuries are barbecuing in the spring, sun exposure in the summer, yard clean-up in the fall, and holiday activities in the winter.

Smoke detectors are present in 13 of 14 homes. Data suggest that half of the home fires and three fifths of fire-related deaths occur in homes without smoke detectors. About one third of the homes with smoke detectors have hundreds of fire-related deaths, because the smoke detector does not work. Working smoke detectors wake people to the fire and allow them time to escape to safety. Prevention includes teaching the following: all homes should have working smoke detectors on each level of the home and in the hallway outside of the bedrooms, and batteries should be tested periodically and changed twice yearly in the spring and the fall.

In states and countries with time changes, such as the change between Eastern Standard and Daylight Savings times in the United States, battery changes can be timed to coordinate with these time changes. Batteries should never be removed for the reason that they go off during cooking as it is easy to forget to replace them. In most cities in the United States, the fire department will install smoke detectors free of charge to the elderly and others unable to do so for themselves. Fire departments in many communities have free smoke detectors for those unable to afford them. People who use home oxygen therapy should not smoke or be around flames. The oxygen should be at least 10 feet from an open flame (e.g., cigarettes, lighters, pilot lights, and candles). The high risk of burn injury can be reduced with patient and family education.

Burn injuries to adults are most often related to accidents while they are cooking, using microwave ovens, or smoking or otherwise using matches. Burns commonly occur when a person is distracted while cooking or falls asleep while smoking. Prevention centers on teaching persons of all ages to be especially careful of scald burns when using microwave ovens. Scald burns can occur when the power of the microwave is underestimated. All users need to be educated about the safe use of these ovens. Smokers need to be reminded to never smoke in bed, to be particularly careful about falling asleep while

Fast Forward ▶▶▶

Burns and Dementia

New diagnostic and treatment regimens are resulting in prolonged life for both males and females. Longer life spans are associated with an increased incidence of dementia. More elderly patients with dementia are being admitted to burn units. The literature about dementia patients focuses on comorbid diseases and the association between dementia and incidence of burns in the elderly has not been studied in depth. Alden, Rabbits, and Yurt (2005) published a retrospective study of patients with dementia at a large urban burn center. Their data revealed that 22 percent of the study group required ventilatory support, 75 percent required intensive care, and 25 percent did not survive their burn. These staggering statistics suggest that a burn prevention program adapted to the elderly demented population is already overdue.

smoking and sitting in overstuffed furniture, and to be sure that cigarettes are completely extinguished, especially before going to bed. Elderly patients with dementia are at uniquely increased risk for severe burns.

The government's role in fire prevention centers around laws designed to protect the public. For example, rigid enforcement of laws requiring that industrial products be labeled when they are known to be flammable and that new products be tested carefully for their flammable qualities before being placed on the market is evidence of government efforts to protect the public from accident by fire. The surgeon general's report on goals to be achieved by 2010, include an increase in functioning residential smoke alarms and a reduction in residential fire deaths (Box 46-4) (USDHHS, 2000). These goals are particularly focused at high-risk groups: American Indian/Alaska natives and African Americans.

Industry can be made safer by constant vigilance of management in cooperation with fire safety officers and health care professionals to identify hazards and implement a safety program. All chemicals should be labeled, and antidotes should be identified and available. A core group of every workforce should be versed in emergency treatment of all types of burns for the protection of every employee.

Evaluation of Outcomes

Potential patient outcomes for each of the example nursing diagnoses for the patient in the emergent phase of burns are:

- Ineffective airway clearance related to secretions, tracheobronchial edema, and obstruction. The patient maintains a patent airway, adequate oxygenation, and ventilation and is free from strider and adventitious breath sounds.
- Deficient fluid volume related to intravascular fluid shift and evaporation. The patient experiences adequate fluid volume and electrolyte balance as evidenced by urine output greater than 30 mL/hour, normotensive blood pressure, heart rate 100 beats/minute, consistency of weight, and normal skin turgor.

BOX 46-4

HEALTHY PEOPLE 2010

The Surgeon General's goals for 2010 related to burn injury are focused on decreasing residential fire deaths through the presence of a functioning smoke alarm on every floor.

Goal # 1: Reduce the incidence of residential fires

1998 baseline: 1.2 per 100,000 people
2010 target: 0.2 per 100,000 people

Goal # 2: Increase total population living in residences with functioning smoke alarms on every floor

1998 baseline: 88 percent
2010 target: 100 percent

Goal #3: (Developmental) Increase the proportion of people who have access to responding prehospital emergency medical services

Adapted from United States Department of Health and Human Services (USDHHS). (2000). Healthy People 2010: Understanding and improving health. *Retrieved May 5, 2006, from http://www.healthpeople.gov.*

- Hypothermia related to impaired temperature regulation and wound exposure. The patient remains normothermic without clinical manifestations of infection.
- Risk for infection related to impaired skin integrity. The patient remains free of infection, as evidenced by normal vital signs and absence of purulent drainage from wounds, incisions, and tubes. Infection is recognized early to allow for prompt treatment.
- Impaired skin integrity related to impaired perfusion and burn-injured skin. The patient's skin condition should be improved as evidenced by decreased redness, swelling, and pain.
- Acute pain related to exposed nerve endings and associated trauma. The patient should verbalize an adequate relief of pain along with the ability to realistically cope with the pain if it is not completely relieved.
- Anxiety related to situational crises and threat of death. The patient should be able to recognize the signs of anxiety, demonstrate positive coping mechanisms, and describe a reduction in the level of anxiety experienced.

ACUTE PHASE

The acute period of treatment begins at the end of the emergent period and lasts until the burn wound is healed. The length of this period varies. If the burn is a partial-thickness injury, the acute period extends for 7 to 21 days; if the burn is a full-thickness injury over a large percentage of the body requiring surgery for skin grafting, the acute period may last for months. During this phase, a multidisciplinary approach to care is needed. During the acute period the two main principles of management are treatment of the burn wound and avoidance, detection, and treatment of complications. The most common complications are infection (septicemia and pneumonia), renal disease, and heart failure.

Diagnostic Tests

Laboratory testing during the acute period focuses on monitoring the patient's fluid and electrolyte balance. Chemistry profiles may be obtained once or twice daily during the patient's critical phase while fluid resuscitation is in progress. Complete blood counts are monitored to assess the patient's white blood cell count and hemoglobin and hematocrit values. Wound cultures are obtained once or twice weekly to track the bacterial colonization of the wounds. Ongoing surveillance of wound cultures is essential for early treatment of infection.

Evaluation of nutritional status is monitored through prealbumin levels and urine urea nitrogen. Patients who are intubated or have inhalation injuries require periodic chest X-rays. In addition, bronchoscopy is performed on patients with inhalation injuries to assess the degree of injury to the lungs.

Assessment with Clinical Manifestations

Burn patients are often frightened and anxious about their injury and the associated treatments. These responses can be compounded by the intensive care unit environment. Burn patients experience both physical and psychological pain. Physical pain is usually focused on specific activities, such as wound cleansing and debridement, dressing changes, and physical therapy. The nurse must assess the patient's reaction to pain and intervene appropriately.

A thorough head-to-toe assessment of the burn patient is performed every eight hours. Data includes mental status; vital signs; breath sounds; bowel sounds; dietary intake; motor ability; intake and output; weight pattern; circulatory assessment; and observation of burn wounds, grafts, and donor site. Purulent drainage, abnormal color, foul odor, redness or swelling in surrounding normal skin, or presence of healing should be noted. Changes in these parameters from shift to shift or from day to day make further investigation necessary.

Nursing Diagnoses

Based on the information gathered, examples of nursing diagnoses in the patient during the acute phase of burns may include the following:

- Impaired skin integrity related to burn injury and nutritional deficits.
- Risk for infection related to impaired skin integrity and altered immune response.
- Imbalanced nutrition: less than body requirements related to increased metabolic needs, protein loss, and decreased appetite.
- Acute pain related to exposed nerve endings and immobility.
- Deficient fluid volume related to increased insensible loss and evaporation.
- Impaired physical mobility related to decreased strength and endurance, activity intolerance, and depression.
- Disturbed body image related to altered body appearance or function.

Planning and Implementation

Nursing interventions for the care of the patient in the acute phase include promoting skin integrity, prevention of infection, providing nutrition, comfort and pain management, maintaining fluid balance, relieving anxiety, promoting activity, supporting and encouraging coping and self-care, and prevention of hypothermia. Healing of the burn wound is an essential component of care of the patient. Expert assessment skills are required to monitor the wound during healing and to detect any signs of infection. Wound care may be needed one to three times daily. Wound cleansing, debridement, and dressing application is accomplished during these treatments. The patient is adequately medicated prior to the procedure. Strict barrier precautions are maintained. Caregivers wear gowns, masks, eye protection, and gloves. The goals of wound care include prevention of infection, removal of devitalized tissue, prevention of further destruction of healthy tissue, and minimization of pain.

Hydrotherapy using a shower, tub, or spray table facilitates the removal of topical medications and loosens debris, sloughing eschar, and exudate. Wound care in a tub permits immersion of the patient into water or antimicrobial solutions. Soaking helps in the removal of topical agents and eschar and helps facilitate range of motion. Generally, tub therapy is limited to 30-minute intervals to prevent heat loss. Tub therapy is avoided in critically ill patients and those with a wound infection, because the infection may be transmitted to other areas of the body through the tub water. A spray table may be used for patients who are poorly mobile, have wound infections, or during their more critical phase. This method of hydrotherapy allows the patient to be recumbent, and water is provided through the use of temperature-controlled hoses. For patients who are mobile, a regular shower can be used. This method helps the patient resume activities of daily living.

Nonsurgical burn wound management involves removing exudates and necrotic tissue, cleaning the area, stimulating granulation and revascularization, and applying dressings. Restoring skin, whether by natural healing or grafting, starts with the removal of eschar and other cellular debris from the burn wound. This removal is called debridement and is an important part of wound healing. After removal of the gauze dressings, the wound is cleansed with a mild soap or noncytotoxic wound cleansing agent. Nonadherent exudate or debris is removed.

The burn patient is at tremendous risk for infection. Measures to prevent infection begin at the time the patient is admitted to the hospital and continue until healing is complete. Burn wound infection occurs through auto contamination, in which the patient's own normal flora overgrows and penetrates the internal environment. Burn wound infection also occurs through cross-contamination, in which organisms from elsewhere are transferred to the patient. Sources of infection may be endogenous or exogenous. Bacteria that survive in the hair follicles and glands are a source of endogenous infection. In addition, after burn injury, bacteria that normally live in the intestinal tract migrate or translocate across the intestinal wall and spread to the general circulation by way of the lymphatic system. Local and systemic infections (septicemia) are the most common complications of burns and are the major cause of death, particularly in burns covering more than 25 percent of the body. Therefore thorough wound cleansing is necessary to remove the debris that acts as a media for bacterial growth.

Organisms commonly causing burn wound infection include *Pseudomonas aeruginosa, Acinetobacter, enterococci,* and *Staphylococcus aureus (S. aureus)*. These organisms are normally found on the skin or in the intestine and become a source of infection. Treatment of antimicrobial resistant organisms, such as methicillin-resistant *S. aureus,* vancomycin-resistant *enterococci,* and *aspergillosis,* is an increasingly difficult problem in burn centers (Havener, Roth, Arakere, and Barenfanger, 2005).

Fungal infections have an increased incidence in burn patients because of the use of broad-spectrum antibiotics. *Candida albicans,* which normally is found in the GI tract, accounts for the majority of the fungal infections. Cultures of the patient's wound may be taken on admission and at biweekly intervals to determine the presence of bacteria and their sensitivity to antibiotics.

Infection is commonly the cause of deterioration in the condition of a burn patient. Signs of infection include erythema and edema at the wound edges, increasing pain, odor, drainage, and decreasing function. The wound may show changes in color from red to violet, dark brown, or black and tissue necrosis may occur. Signs of sepsis in the burn patient are change in sensorium, fever, tachypnea, tachycardia, paralytic ileus (decreased tolerance of feedings), abdominal distension, and oliguria.

Drug therapy, isolation therapy, and environmental manipulation are strategies for preventing the introduction of exogenous organisms into the wound. Systemic antibiotics are used when burn patients have symptoms of an actual infection, including septicemia. Broad-spectrum antibiotics are given until the results of blood cultures and sensitivity status are available. At that time, more specific antibiotics, including the aminoglycosides, such as amikacin (Amikin) or gentamicin (Garamycin or Alcomicin) and cephalosporins, such as cephalothin (Keflin) or ceftriaxone (Rocephin), are used. Because of increased metabolism, burn patients generally require a larger than normal dose of these drugs to maintain therapeutic blood levels. If aminoglycosides are used, serial peak and trough blood levels are monitored to determine the efficacy of treatment and evaluate potential ear and kidney toxicity (Broyles, et al., 2007).

Placing the severely burned patient in a special burn unit can decrease the possibility of infection, because the unit environment is specifically equipped for infection control. If the patient is cared for in a general hospital unit, a private room is essential, and all equipment needed by the patient remains in the room. Some burn care philosophies state that isolation therapy effectively reduces cross-contamination. However, methods of isolation are varied and controversial. Some burn centers practice virtually no isolation, whereas others use near-total sterile conditions.

All isolation methods emphasize proper and consistent hand washing as the most effective technique for preventing infection transmission. All health care personnel wear gloves during all contact with open wounds. The use of sterile versus clean gloves for routine wound care varies by agency and is a matter of debate. Regardless of sterility, change gloves when handling wounds on different areas of the body and between handling old and new dressings.

The equipment on burn units is not shared among patients. Disposable items (e.g., pillows, syringes, and dishes) are used as much as possible. Assign any equipment used in daily routine care (e.g., thermometer, blood pressure cuff, and stethoscope) to that patient. Daily cleaning of the equipment and general housekeeping are essential for infection control. All equipment must be cleaned after use for one patient before it is used for another patient.

Because *Pseudomonas,* a gram-negative bacterium, has been shown to sequester in plants, the presence of plants and flowers is prohibited. Some burn units do not permit patients to eat raw foods (such as salads, fruit, and pepper) to reduce exposure to *Pseudomonas* organisms. Rugs and upholstered articles are difficult to clean and may harbor organisms, and their use is also restricted.

Visitors are restricted when the patient is immunosuppressed. People with upper respiratory infections or other illnesses and small children should not come into direct contact with the burn patient. Some burn units recommend that all visitors wear protective clothing (gowns, gloves, masks, and shoe and hair covers) in the room of the burn patient, but no data support the effectiveness of this approach.

Collaborative Care Management

Patients who suffer burn injuries require specialized care, which is best obtained in a burn unit. A multidisciplinary team including surgeons, nurses, physical and occupational therapists, social workers, microbiologists, clergy, child life workers, psychologists, volunteers, and other disciplines is involved in the approach to care. Referrals to other services are determined by the needs of the patient. For example, patients with other conditions, such as diabetes, may require consultation from an expert to assist in managing the diabetes during the acute period of their burn. Consultation with a psychiatrist may be indicated for patients whose burns were self-inflicted or for those who are having difficulty adjusting to their postburn appearance.

Nutrition

Metabolism can be increased by two or three times normal after moderate to severe burns because of stress, fluid loss, hypercatabolism, and immobility. Shivering and elevated levels of catecholamines, cortisol, and glucagon present after thermal injury increase oxygen consumption and heat production. In addition, there is depletion of liver and muscle glycogen and fat deposits, resulting in negative nitrogen balance and weight loss. Protein is broken down to provide amino acids for gluconeogenesis, preventing amino acids from incorporating into protein. This decreased rate of protein production prolongs wound healing and increases the patient's susceptibility to infection (Roth, 2007).

A burn patient remains catabolic until caloric intake exceeds caloric expenditure. This catabolic state may last for days or months depending on the severity of the burn. The patient's energy and protein requirements become those needed for normal homeostasis plus those required to offset the catabolic state and repair the burn injury.

Maintenance of a nutritional support program is critical to survival and is initiated on admission. The goals of the nutritional support program are to establish oral intake as soon as possible and to maintain sufficient caloric and protein intake to restore tissue loss. A team approach provides comprehensive input and integrates the efforts of the patient, health care provider, nurse, pharmacist, dietitian, and occupational and physical therapists.

A nutritional assessment is made during the first days of the burn injury and includes anthropometric measurements (to determine actual weight loss compared with ideal weight), indirect calorimetry, and laboratory studies (electrolytes, liver function tests, and urine). The admission assessment provides a baseline against which progress can be evaluated. Twenty-four-hour urine specimens and urea nitrogen tests may be obtained two to three times a week to evaluate the patient's nitrogen balance. Transferrin or prealbumin levels provide sensitive indicators of visceral protein status. Urinary nitrogen and serum albumin levels can be affected by insensible protein loss and hydration status.

Albumin's half-life of 20 days makes day-to-day evaluation of albumin difficult to interpret. On the other hand, prealbumin, which has a short half-life of 20 to 25 hours, provides a sensitive indicator of nutritional status and the patient's response to feeding.

Nutritional requirements for the burn patient are highly variable, depending on the extent and depth of injury and the patient's age, gender, preburn nutritional status, and preexisting diseases. Total caloric needs may be as high as 3,500 to 5,000 calories per day. Calories are provided to the patient as 20 percent protein, 50 percent carbohydrate, and 30 percent fat. Dietitians in burn centers most commonly use the Curreri formula and variations of the Harris-Benedict equation. These formulae are used as a guide to begin nutritional support (Roth, 2007).

Protein is essential to replace nitrogen loss through the wound and in urine and to promote tissue repair and healing. Protein needs in the adult increase from a normal of 0.8 g/kg of body weight to 1.5 to 3 g/kg. Protein calories must be dedicated to the wound and not used for energy needs. This is accomplished by providing the patient with sufficient carbohydrate and fat for energy use.

Increased carbohydrate and fat intake is provided to avoid protein catabolism and meet the patient's energy needs. Approximately 5 mg/kg/min of glucose are provided. Excessive carbohydrate administration is avoided to prevent increased carbon dioxide production and hyperglycemia. In addition to calories, fat provides fat-soluble vitamins and essential fatty acids. Calories provided by fat are limited to 30 percent because of the adverse effect that high fat levels have on the immune system.

Vitamin and mineral supplements are essential for optimal wound healing. Vitamins C and A, zinc, and iron are provided at doses higher than the recommended daily allowances. Vitamins A and C have roles as cellular antioxidants and are required for collagen synthesis. Patients may receive as much as 1,000 mg of vitamin C and 5,000 to 10,000 IU of vitamin A per day. Zinc levels decrease because of increased nitrogen excretion in the urine during the acute phase. Zinc is essential for wound healing and has a vital role in immune function. Patients receive supplementation of up to 220 mg/day. Iron may be supplied to treat anemia caused from blood loss after skin grafting. The use of anabolic steroids in combination with increased protein intake for the restoration of weight gain can be significantly increased post-burn (Demling, 2005).

Enteral feeding (oral or tube feeding) is the preferred method for the burn patient. A paralytic ileus or gastric dilation is frequently seen in the severely burned patient because of shock, stress, or sepsis. This may limit the patient's ability to tolerate gastric feedings for the first few weeks. Commonly, small-bore feeding tubes are inserted into the duodenum or endoscopically into the jejunum so that feedings may be initiated within the first 24 hours of injury. Early feeding decreases hypermetabolism, improves nitrogen balance, minimizes bacterial translocation from the gut secondary to muscle atrophy, and decreases diarrhea and hospital length of stay. Total parenteral nutrition is generally reserved for patients who are unable to tolerate enteral feeding.

Oral feeding is encouraged whenever possible. However, it is difficult for the patient to consume the number of calories needed from food alone because of pain and decreased gastric motility. Therefore, a combination of food by mouth, with supplements, such as milk shakes or commercially prepared products, and tube feedings may be necessary to meet the patient's nutritional requirements. The patient's food preferences are determined and the family is encouraged to bring favorite foods from home. Care is coordinated so that meal times are relaxed and not associated with other procedures, such as wound care. A social situation can be created by having burn patients eat together or with family members. Pain medication is provided so that the patient is comfortable at mealtime. Coordination with occupational therapy staff is essential if the patient needs assistive devices to hold utensils and cups.

Monitoring the patient's nutritional status is an ongoing process. Weight loss and gain are monitored daily during the critical phase and biweekly as the wounds heal. Initially, weight gain occurs because of fluid retention. As diuresis occurs, the patient's weight decreases because of fluid loss. Significant weight loss reflects protein loss and loss of fat reserves, as well as muscle mass. Prealbumin, urine urea nitrogen balance, and cholesterol levels are obtained to track nutritional status.

The patient's tolerance of feeding is monitored by evaluating bowel function. Diarrhea may be a problem for patients receiving antibiotics or tube feedings. Often burn patients have difficulties with constipation because of administration of opioids and decreased activity. Stool softeners, laxatives, and increased fluid intake may need to be provided.

Pharmacology

Administration of medications for the burn patient is supportive in nature. Analgesia is essential for pain control. The most commonly used agents are opioids, such as morphine sulfate, fentanyl, and codeine. Patients with major burns may require agents, such as ranitidine, famotidine, or sucralfate to prevent stress ulcers. Systemic antimicrobial agents are used only when evidence of infection is present. Topical antimicrobial agents are applied to the burn wounds based on depth of injury and wound culture results. Anabolic steroids, such as oxandrolone, have had positive effects in the recovery phase of a major burn. Anabolic steroids are used to attenuate the catabolic state, restore lean body mass, and promote wound healing (Demling, 2005). Current research is focused on the benefits of administration during the acute phase of injury. In addition, many burn patients have preexisting illnesses and require ongoing medication management of their current health problems.

There are a variety of topical medications that are used in the acute phase of burn therapy. For example, petroleum based antimicrobial ointments (bacitracin or Neosporin) are used for partial-thickness burns. Silver sulfadiazine (Silvadene) is a broad-spectrum cream which is used for deep partial- to full-thickness burns. Silvadene protects against gram-negative, gram-positive, and candida organisms. Mafenide acetate (Sulfamylon) is used to medicate deep partial- to full-thickness burns. It penetrates thick eschar and cartilage and inhibits epithelial tissue development. Silver nitrate is used to medicate deep partial- to full-thickness burns but penetrates eschar poorly. Other topical medications are collagenase, Acticoat, Xeroform, and Mepitel.

There are a variety of wound coverings used in the management of acute burns. For example, biosynthetic coverings are used for partial-thickness burns and wounds (e.g., Biobrane, TransCyte, and calcium alginate). Biological wound coverings for partial-thickness or excised wounds, flaps, or grafts are cadaver allograft, vacuum assisted closure dressings ([VAC] a negative-pressure wound dressing that promotes formation of granulation in tissue), pig skin (heterograft, xenograft), and PolyMem (Gottlieb & Furman, 2004; O'Conner & Besner, 2004).

Pain control is a major part of the burn patient's care. Uncontrolled pain affects all aspects of recovery, including tolerance of wound care, ability to eat, mobility, wound healing, and psychological adjustment. Acute pain is most successfully managed with narcotics. The methods and routes of administration are carefully evaluated on an individual basis. Attention is paid to pain management needs during dressing changes and other daily activities. During dressing changes, parenteral narcotics are given to achieve rapid onset of action. The use of agents such as ketamine, fentanyl, and self-administered nitrous oxide may be beneficial for some patients. Some methods for minimizing pain during dressing changes are to provide analgesic medications before dressing change, provide clear explanation to gain patient's cooperation, handle burned areas gently, encourage patient to participate in treatment whenever possible, and the use of distraction (DeLaune & Ladner, 2006).

Organization and planning for patient comfort from pain, itching, or general discomfort includes a plan for procedural, background, and breakthrough pain. The nursing assessment and plan of care and assessment include pain assessment with vital signs. An around-the-clock approach to pain management is essential for the burn patient. Undermedication may occur if the patient fears becoming addicted and fails to report pain or if the nurse fails to adequately evaluate the degree of pain. The use of a numerical analogue scale in which the patient rates the pain helps determine whether the pain is being adequately controlled. Providing medication at frequent intervals helps to maintain ongoing comfort. Time-released opioids and patient-controlled analgesia are also viable options. In addition, alternative methods of pain management can be used (e.g., music therapy, meditation, and diversional activities).

Surgery

Surgical management of burn wounds focuses on excision and wound covering. Skin grafts are applied to cover the burn wound and speed healing, to control contractures, and to shorten convalescence. Successful grafting reduces the patient's vulnerability to infection and prevents the loss of body heat and water vapor from the open wound. Grafting may be performed for cosmetic or functional purposes during the rehabilitative period. Procedures may be performed throughout the acute phase as burn wounds are made ready and donor sites are available.

Grafts may be permanent or only provide temporary coverage. An **autograft** is a permanent graft. The surgeon removes a piece of skin from a remote unburned area of the body and transplants it to cover the burn wound. A **homograft,** or cryo-preserved cadaveric **allograft** (skin graft), is a graft of skin obtained from a cadaver 6 to 24 hours after death that is used as a temporary graft. It can be used as fresh donor skin (stored in the refrigerator) or frozen donor skin obtained from a tissue bank. Disadvantages to the use of homografts are the high costs ($750 to $1,000 per square foot) and the risk of transmitting a blood-borne infection.

A **heterograft (xenograft)** is a graft of skin obtained from another species, such as a pig. Homografts and heterografts are both temporary skin coverings. Homografts, heterografts, synthetic substitutes, and biosynthetic dressings (Biobrane) are intended to provide temporary coverage while the burn wound heals. As the wound heals, these temporary coverings are gradually rejected and are easily removed from the newly healed skin. The advantage of a temporary graft is to reduce water, electrolyte, and protein losses at the burn surface. The covered wound is less painful and allows the patient freedom of movement. Temporary grafts act like human skin and may be used until the patient is ready for an autograft. Often, autografting is delayed as a result of complications, such as infection, pneumonia, or the critical status of the patient.

Dermal replacements or synthetic substitutes for skin are currently being developed and used in burn units throughout the United States. Integra, AlloDerm, and cultured epithelium are new products currently available. All of these products are expensive. The product alone may cost $20,000 or more per patient. Cost effectiveness is being evaluated, comparing costs and patient outcomes. The ultimate skin substitute should include the following properties: it would be inexpensive, nonantigenic, flexible and durable, prevent fluid loss, serve as a barrier to infection, adjust to the wound surface, grow with a child, not cause hypertrophic scarring, store easily with a long shelf-life, and be applied in one operation. There currently is not a perfect substitute for skin (Gottlieb & Furman, 2004).

Before the graft is placed on the wound, the surgical procedure of tangential excision or fascial excision is performed. In the tangential technique, the surgeon excises thin layers of the necrotic burn surface until bleeding tissue is encountered. Bleeding indicates that a bed of healthy dermis or subcutaneous fat has been reached.

In the fascial technique the surgeon excises the burn wound to the level of superficial fascia. Fascial excision usually is reserved for deep and extensive burns. Blood loss is minimal and grafting is usually successful. It is then covered with an autograft or skin substitute. The procedure is best performed between the second and fifth burn day.

Split-thickness skin grafts, full-thickness skin grafts, and primary closure are surgical techniques used to cover the burn wounds. Skin grafts are generally of split-thickness and include the upper layers of skin (epidermis) and part of the middle layer (dermis) causing a partial-thickness injury at the site of surgical removal (donor site). The grafts are removed with a dermatome blade from almost any unburned part of the body. The sizes of these grafts are determined by the sites available and the area to be covered.

Grafts may be used as sheets or are meshed. Meshing of the graft involves taking the sheet of skin after it is removed from the donor and feeding it into a meshing instrument that perforates the sheet with tiny slits. The meshing of the graft makes it more expandable so that it can be stretched to cover wider areas of the body surface. Healing time is slower for a meshed graft, because the skin must fill in open meshed areas (interstices), as well as attach to the granulation bed.

Sheet grafts are applied directly to the burn wound without meshing. They result in better functional and cosmetic outcomes and are used on the face, neck, hands, or around joints. Full-thickness grafts are composed of layers of skin down to the subcutaneous tissue. They are used if there is a well-defined area of a full-thickness burn, and it provides a better cosmetic appearance than split-thickness grafts when healed. Areas that benefit from full-thickness grafts are the hands, neck, and face. Full-thickness grafts can also be used in rehabilitative stages to restore body function and to release skin contractures.

Primary closure is another method of burn wound closure. It is used to close small burns by pulling the skin together and suturing the burn area together or by closing the area with local skin flaps. Graft sites require skilled nursing management. Autografts are secured in surgery with staples, dressings, and splints. Special precautions are taken to prevent sliding, slipping, or movement of the graft. The grafted area may be covered with a large, occlusive, bulky dressing to hold new skin securely in place. VAC dressings can be utilized during this time period. Splints applied in the operating room help to provide immobilization and maintain the position of the grafted areas.

The VAC device helps control wound drainage and enhances healing via a negative pressure dressing. Patients with compromised venous circulation or diabetic neuropathy sustaining a burn have been shown to benefit from use of this device. In addition, review of the literature suggests that this device has a positive impact on the length of hospital stay and thus on cost containment.

The dressing remains intact for 48 to 72 hours. Sheet grafts and full-thickness grafts are examined every 24 hours, because drainage or blood can accumulate under the graft. This fluid can be removed by aspiration with a needle, rolling the fluid with a cotton tip, or by cutting a small slit in the graft to drain the fluid. The graft dressings are removed slowly and carefully so that the graft is not disturbed.

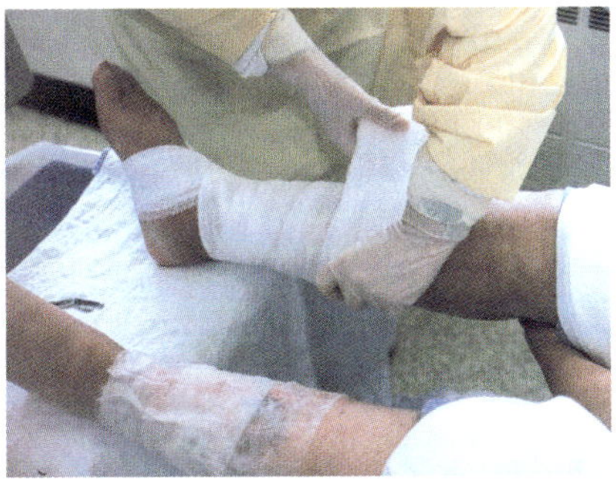

Figure 46-4 Nurse wrapping wet gauze with an external dressing of dry gauze bandages for a donor for burn tissue.

The donor site represents a wound similar to that of a partial-thickness injury. Care of the donor site is as important as care of the graft itself, because donor sites that fail to heal result in an enlargement of the patient's open wound surface. Donor sites may be treated by a variety of methods. One method is covering the exposed surface with Xeroform and leaving it exposed to the air. Exposing the donor site to a heat lamp also promotes healing, because, as the drainage from the wound dries, it serves as a protective covering. The site usually heals within two weeks. Other methods include the use of Op-Site or Biobrane to the donor site. The area is kept wrapped and checked daily for drainage and healing (Figure 46-4). Many patients complain of severe pain in the donor site, and the nurse should not hesitate to give medications for pain. The pain should subside in 24 to 48 hours as the wound dries. The

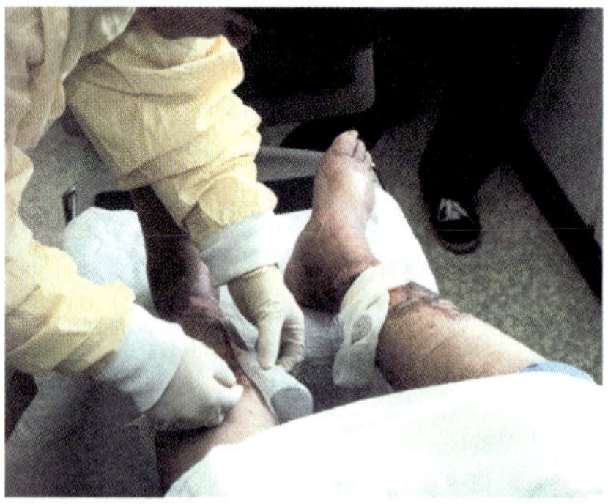

Figure 46-5 Nurse participating in mechanical debridement with burn patient.

wound is inspected daily for any signs of infection (erythema, purulent drainage, or foul odor). If infection develops, antibiotics may be administered, and the wound may be treated with wet dressings.

In deeper wounds in which eschar, or devitalized tissue, is present debridement may be required. Debridement may be surgical, enzymatic, or mechanical. Surgical debridement involves cutting the dead tissue away and is performed in the operating room with the patient under anesthesia. Enzymatic debridement involves the use of a topical enzyme that promotes separation of the eschar from the wound bed. During mechanical debridement, manual removal of eschar using gauze sponges, tweezers, scissors or other instruments is performed (Figure 46-5). As this is a painful procedure for patients, they must be adequately medicated. During this cleansing procedure, the wound is carefully assessed for signs of healing or infection.

Patient and Family Teaching

There are wide variety of patient and family teaching needs for the patient in the acute phase of burns. To begin, patients are taught the importance of maintaining fluid and electrolyte balance after discharge and the need to notify their health care provider immediately if they experience weight loss accompanied by headache, lightheadedness, fatigue, decreased urinary output, irritability, or rapid pulse, which are signs of fluid deficit. Patients also need to report signs of electrolyte imbalance, such as an increase in fatigue, abdominal distension, anorexia, vomiting, constipation, muscle cramps, paresthesia, or confusion. Patients are also taught to eat a well-balanced diet with sufficient fluid intake.

As the patient's wounds heal and pain is controlled, the patient needs to regain and maintain an optimal ability to move purposefully. Range-of-motion exercises are taught and performed actively at least three times a day. If the patient cannot move a joint actively, perform passive range-of-motion exercises. Burned hands require special attention. Encourage the patient to perform active range-of-motion exercises for the hand, thumb, and fingers every hour while awake. Ambulation is started as soon as possible after the fluid shifts have resolved. Patients with a variety of attached equipment (IV catheters, nasogastric tubes, electrocardiographic leads, and extensive dressings) can ambulate with preparation and assistance. Ambulation is performed two or three times a day and progresses in length each time. Regular physical activity inhibits the loss of bone density, strengthens muscles, stimulates immune function, promotes ventilation, and prevents many complications.

A burn injury is a sudden, unexpected event. Its impact on psychological well-being is enormous and promoting mental health is a major area of the burn patient's care. The psychological responses in the acute burn phase are related to the threat of survival. During the acute period, a variety of behaviors may be seen. The six most common reactions are withdrawal, denial, regression, anger and hostility, depression, and anxiety (Doe Report, 2005; Swartz, 2004). As the patient becomes aware of the extent of the injury and begins to evaluate its implications on his or her life, many problems may occur that affect the ability of both the patient and family to cope with the situation. During each of the psychological reactions, the patient may change their interactions with other people and exhibit a variety of behaviors that are somewhat dysfunctional. The nurse must adapt the care to accommodate these changes in behavior. The nurse plays a major role in maintaining and restoring the patient's mental health. Pain plays a significant role in the patient's level of anxiety and is commonly identified by patients as the worst part of their hospital stay. Controlling pain assists in decreasing anxiety. Ongoing education is imperative to assist the patient to understand the care given and to make realistic plans for the future. It is important for the patient to maintain a sense of hope for the future so that he or she can resume a normal life. Without hope, the patient will have less ability to cope, a sense of failure, and less gratifying interpersonal relationships. Emotional recovery from a burn injury is slower than physical recovery. Symptoms of psychological distress are present in a large number of patients up to one year after a burn injury. These symptoms include intrusive and distressing memories of the burn injury and avoidances of thoughts and feelings related to the burn. In addition, patients may experience increased irritability, anxiety, and sleep disturbances.

People with burn injuries are also at risk for the development of posttraumatic stress disorder (PTSD). In this condition symptoms occur after a psychologically traumatic event that would be considered outside the range of normal human experience (Swartz, 2004). The size and severity of burn and degree of disfigurement does not consistently predict the patient who will develop PTSD. Patients are more likely to develop PTSD if there is an actual or perceived lack of social support, the presence of a maladaptive coping style, or high emotional distress. Patients may be nonsymptomatic during hospitalization but develop PTSD after discharge. Therefore, ongoing psychological evaluation and intervention is necessary during hospitalization and during the months that follow.

The nurse needs to explore with the patient how she or he coped with stressful events in the past. It is important to remember that some patients were raised to be stoic when in pain or distress. Other patients were encouraged to express their feelings openly. Nurses should support the patient's coping style unless the patient indicates that he or she would be interested in exploring new methods of coping. Relaxation exercises, meditation, and music therapy may be useful in helping the patient cope with pain and other stressors. In some situations, hypnosis may be used with the goal of having the patient develop the ability to induce self-hypnosis during dressing changes and other stressful events. Patients are usually helped to cope if they are kept fully informed about what is planned for their care and what will be expected of them during various treatments. Then they are not forced to cope with unexpected events that can be upsetting, especially when they have had to give up most of their independence.

Families, like patients, cope best when they are kept fully informed and have a realistic understanding of what lies ahead for the patient. The family can be deeply disrupted by a serious burn to a family member. Initially, they are concerned about the patient's survival and need careful explanations of what is being done for the patient and why. The explanations may need to be repeated more than once, because the family members may be too distressed to comprehend what they are being told.

Social workers are helpful in exploring the family's concerns about role disruptions, plans for child care, financial concerns, and their own feelings of distress. Often the family members require considerable support from health professionals to work through their own feelings before they can be supportive to the patient. The burn team members meet to decide who will provide what support to the family. The family can best provide realistic support to the patient when they have accurate knowledge about what the patient will experience at each step in the recovery process. The family also needs information about community resources available to them and to the patient.

The patient is encouraged to express how he or she feels about the change in appearance. Individual counseling may be necessary for some patients as they integrate the change in their appearance into their self-concept. Other patients will benefit from being referred to a patient support group where they meet other patients in various stages of recovery. The patient is encouraged to participate as much as possible in his or her own care. Independence in the activities of daily living is supported. Some patients will require more encouragement than others in assisting with tasks, such as wound care. It is important that the patient be involved in developing a daily plan of care including meal selection, time of treatments, rest periods, therapy, and socialization.

Evaluation of Outcomes

Potential patient outcomes for each of the example nursing diagnoses for the patient with the acute phase of burns are:

- Impaired skin integrity related to burn injury and nutritional deficits. The patient's skin condition should be improved as evidenced by decreased redness, swelling, and pain.
- Risk for infection related to impaired skin integrity and altered immune response. The patient remains free of infection, as evidenced by normal vital signs and absence of purulent drainage from wounds, incisions, and tubes. Infection is recognized early to allow for prompt treatment.
- Imbalanced nutrition: less than body requirements related to increased metabolic needs, protein loss, and decreased appetite. The patient verbalizes and demonstrates selection of foods or meals that will achieve a cessation of weight loss and weighs within 10 percent of ideal body weight.
- Acute pain related to exposed nerve endings and immobility. The patient should verbalize an adequate relief of pain along with the ability to realistically cope with the pain if it is not completely relieved.
- Deficient fluid volume related to increased insensible loss and evaporation. The patient experiences adequate fluid volume and electrolyte balance as evidenced by urine output greater than 30 mL/hour, normotensive blood pressure, heart rate 100 beats/minute, consistency of weight, and normal skin turgor.
- Impaired physical mobility related to decreased strength and endurance, activity intolerance, and depression. The patient should perform physical activity independently or with assistive devices as needed. In addition, the patient should be free of complications of immobility, as evidenced by intact skin, absence of thrombophlebitis, and normal bowel patterns.
- Disturbed body image related to altered body appearance or function. The patient demonstrates enhanced body image and self-esteem as evidenced by ability to look at, touch, talk about, and care for actual or perceived altered body part or function.

REHABILITATION PHASE

Although rehabilitation efforts are started from the time of admission, the technical rehabilitative third stage begins with wound closure and ends when the patient returns to the highest possible level of functioning. The emphasis during this phase is the psychosocial adjustment of the patient, the prevention of scars and contractures, and the resumption of preburn activity, including work, family, and social roles. This phase may take years or even last a lifetime as patients adjust to permanent limitations that may not be apparent until long after the initial injury.

Diagnostic Tests

Specific diagnostic testing during the rehabilitation period depends on the patient's condition and progress toward goals. Overall, limited testing is required. Evaluation of nutritional status (prealbumin and urine urea nitrogen measurements) and the presence of infection (complete blood counts and wound or blood cultures) may be necessary (Daniels, 2003).

Assessment with Clinical Manifestations

Nursing management of the patient with burns during the rehabilitative phase includes continuous patient assessment, identification of nursing diagnoses, implementation of patient care interventions, and the evaluation of outcomes.

The patient must be helped to maintain range of joint motion to prevent scars from healing in positions that will result in deformity. Complaints of pain and pressure should not be overlooked, because neurological or circulatory damage may occur from an improperly applied splint or poor positioning. It is important that patients understand why ambulation or motion is necessary even though it may be painful.

The emotional impact of a severe burn is enormous. The psychological scars last forever and affect the victim and family for the rest of their lives. The extent to which the family unit adapts affects how the patient reacts to his or her new body image and feelings of self-worth. The hospital environment and hospital personnel influence the adaptation process. In the immediate post-burn period the nurse is primarily concerned with physiological survival of the patient. At the same time, the nurse must be able to identify psychological problems and coping mechanisms of the patient and family.

The nurse is responsible for assessing the patient's response to positioning, splinting, and exercise and the ability of the patient and family to perform daily wound care after discharge. Correct positioning must be maintained to avoid the development of contractures. The splinted limb is assessed for adequate circulation, cyanosis, and temperature, as well as the presence of adequate pulses. Exercise, activities of daily living, and ambulation must be continuously assessed for patient tolerance, both physically and emotionally. Complete and comprehensive instructions of wound and dressing care followed by return demonstrations are necessary before discharge.

Nursing Diagnoses

Based on the information gathered, examples of nursing diagnoses in the patient in the rehabilitative phase of burns may include the following:

- Impaired physical mobility related to pain, decreased strength and endurance, and contractures.
- Disturbed body image related to altered body function and visualization.
- Risk for impaired skin integrity related to nutritional deficit and fragile new tissue.
- Chronic pain related to joint and tissue contractures.
- Ineffective coping related to situational crises and ineffective support systems.

Planning and Implementation

Nursing interventions during rehabilitation of burns includes the promotion of mobility, self-care, a positive body image, skin integrity, comfort, and facilitation of patient and family coping through teaching. As the survival rate of patients with large and deeper burns increases, so does the challenge to maintain optimal functioning and cosmetic results. The percentage of patients with joint limitations increases as the degree and extent of burns increases. Although these patients may be critically ill, their rehabilitative needs must be addressed immediately. A comprehensive program of positioning, splinting, exercise, ambulation, and activities of daily living must begin on the first or second day post-burn and be carried through until after discharge. Any delays in initiating treatment will be detrimental to the patient's ultimate functional outcome.

Contractures are among the most serious long-term complications of burns. They result from muscle and joint stiffening, skin grafting, and prolonged bedrest. Although occupational and physical therapists are primarily responsible for addressing the patient's rehabilitation needs during all phases of the patient's recovery, the nurse is responsible for ensuring that all the recommendations of allied care providers are followed.

Therapeutic positioning is critical for patients with burn injuries, because the position of comfort for the patient is often one of joint flexion, which predisposes him or her to contracture development. Maintain the patient in a neutral body position with minimal flexion. Therapeutic positioning, placing body parts in antideformity positions, is vital to the prevention of burn contractures. The patient must be repositioned in bed (side-lying, supine, or prone) frequently and regularly around the clock. Correct positioning varies, depending on the area of the body burned. Maintaining appropriate positioning helps to maintain extremities and joints in the position of normal function and decrease contractures. Beds with pressure-reducing capability or low air loss may be necessary to limit skin pressure.

Prolonged rest in a semi-Fowler's position or with the pillow pushing the head forward must be avoided, even though many patients like this position, because it enables them to see about the room better. The bed can often be turned so that the patient can look about without having to assume positions that may lead to the formation of contractures. The bedside table may be changed from one side of the bed to the other at intervals to stimulate other body positions.

Splints prevent or correct contractures and immobilize joints after grafting. They are custom made and are often molded directly on the patient to ensure optimal conformity. It is the responsibility of the nurse to apply the splint properly and according to an established schedule. An improperly applied splint can promote contractures and lead to additional complications. The nurse assesses the splinted limb for adequate circulation, cyanosis, temperature, and the presence of pulses. Complaints of pain and pressure should be assessed, because damage may occur with an improperly applied splint. Some health care providers prefer to use the open method of treatment and use frequent exercise instead of splinting to prevent contractures.

Exercises and ambulation for prevention and correction of contractures are begun as soon as the patient is stable. Active exercises are preferred, although active assistance and gentle pressure exercises may be more realistic. Supervision by a physical or occupational therapist is desirable. Exercises may be performed more easily in water and may be done concurrently with dressing changes if the patient is able to tolerate the activity. Continuous passive pressure motion devices may be used to prevent contractures of affected joints. When burns are completely covered (by healing or by graft), exercises may be performed more easily in an occupational therapy or physical therapy department where the patient may also benefit from a change in environment.

Ambulation decreases the risk of thromboembolia and renal calculi, promotes optimal ventilation, helps maintain range of motion and strength in the lower extremities, orients the patient to the environment, and provides a sense of functional independence. Patients who have large burns have less ability to tolerate activity and will require a progressive approach to mobilization. Initially, the patient may need to be transferred with maximal assistance onto a stretcher chair and progress to a sitting position. Gradually, the patient may progress to a standing pivot transfer into a nearby chair and eventually ambulate with minimal assistance. Before getting out of bed, an elastic bandage support must be applied to the lower extremities to prevent venous stasis, edema, and orthostatic hypotension.

One of the ultimate goals in the rehabilitation of the burned patient is to maintain or restore the patient's independence in performing the activities of daily living. The occupational therapist aids in this process by selecting activities appropriate to the patient's medical, physical, and mental status. Activities that the nurse can encourage are self-feeding, communicating by telephone, reading mail, and assisting with grooming or burn wound management. The nurse supports the information taught by the physical and occupational therapists so that progress can be continued on the nursing unit, in the clinic, or in the home.

Regardless of its size, a burn injury represents a change in the individual's perception of self. As the burn heals, the patient must deal with a new appearance.

One specific area to address with the patient is the reaction of others to the sight of healing wounds and disfiguring scars. Patients with facial burns are especially subjected to stares and other reactions from the general public. Visits from friends and short public appearances before discharge may help the patient begin adjusting to this problem. Community reintegration programs can assist the psychosocial and physical recovery of the patient with serious burns.

The patient must have the opportunity to talk about concerns or fears. Some patients may be unable to discuss these with their family or significant others. The nurse must be prepared to listen actively and help the patient accept changes in appearance. The patient must be allowed to grieve for the loss of the former self. However, the patient should be encouraged to focus on the positive aspects of self.

To the adolescent, the thought of being different or conspicuous may be unbearable. If possible, the patient should see facial burns only after being prepared for the experience. The patient will need support and understanding to cope with his or her image in the mirror. The patient will exhibit readiness by asking to look in the mirror. Interaction with other burn patients who are further along in the healing process may help the patient feel that recovery is possible. In some cases, the recovery is good and although differences in skin pigmentation remain, the redness that accompanies healed burn wounds often fades considerably within a few months. Pigmentation problems are more acute for persons with brown or black skin. Their healed skin may be a different shade, freckled, or whitish. Commercial makeup products that help blend skin tones are available.

Whenever a wound of connective tissue heals, hypertrophic scarring will occur unless the skin adheres to the underlying structure. Hypertrophic scarring results from the overgrowth and overproduction of tissue. This occurs especially in areas of stress and movement, such as the hands, legs, and chest. The thickened rigid scar that results may later cause contractures. The application of controlled constant pressure to the surface of an immature scar will reduce the scar and leave smooth pliable tissue. If this pressure is applied to new healthy tissue, hypertrophic scarring decreases. These dressings also inhibit venous stasis and edema formation in areas with decreased lymphatic outflow. The pressure garments are constructed of a specially designed elastic woven material that provides tridimensional control. It is fitted to each patient individually and then custom made. Until the garment is completed, bandages can be used for a pressure dressing.

Even though pressure garments help decrease the formation of thick, disfiguring scars, patient acceptance is a problem. The garments are uncomfortable and make the patient warm, especially during hot weather. They must be tight enough to produce the 24 mm Hg of pressure required to exceed capillary pressure to be effective in reducing edema and scar formation. The patient must wear the garments 23 hours a day for six months to a year. A plan for exercise and splinting must be established before discharge. To prevent scar contracture, daily therapy sessions may be necessary for several weeks or months. The occupational therapist can develop aids to help with the activities of daily living.

Although less severe, pain remains a problem during the rehabilitation phase. Small areas of skin may remain open and continue to require dressing changes. In addition, newly healed skin is sensitive. Physical and occupational therapy and increasing activity may result in discomfort. Interventions are focused on administration of analgesics, diversional activities, relaxation techniques, and providing information about what the patient can expect. Daily hydrotherapy helps the patient relax tense muscles.

After discharge, the patient continues to adjust to temporary or permanent loss of function, cosmetic disfigurement, and the reactions of others. The ability to manage depends on coping mechanisms before the burn, the severity and site of the burn, and the reaction of others. The patient's adaptation to these changes can be evaluated during outpatient visits when the burn team and appropriate personnel are available.

Job retraining may be necessary if the burn injury caused loss of joint function or other physical limitations that prevent the patient from returning to former employment. The local office of the state labor and industry board can assign a vocational counselor to help the patient return to the workforce. Even if retraining cannot begin for several months, the contact with the vocational counselor and anticipation of retraining may help the patient look beyond immediate problems and think of the future.

Collaborative Care Management

Patients who are recovering from burn injuries require specialized rehabilitation care. A multidisciplinary team including physicians, nurses, physical and occupational therapists, social workers, clergy, child life workers, psychologists, volunteers, and other disciplines is involved in this approach to care. Nurses working in the rehabilitation unit need to provide care for patients of all age-groups and they must understand the rehabilitation requirements of burn patients. Community-based support services for patients are provided through rehabilitative and outpatient services. With patients being discharged earlier, education and wound care are generally completed after discharge. Treatment and teaching plans begin at admission and continue throughout the course of healing, regardless of the site for care. A multidisciplinary team of advanced burn care professionals is available and resources are provided to patients and families at different levels of healing. Support groups are available to assist patients with resocialization and coping with their burn injury for many years after discharge.

Nutrition

In the rehabilitative phase of burns, nutritional requirements continue to decrease. There is no longer the need for fluid resuscitation as an example. In addition, there is not the need for vitamin supplements. However, there is still a need to have a well-balanced diet with adequate fluid intake.

Pharmacology

The number of medications prescribed decreases as the patient progresses through the rehabilitation period. As wounds heal, less analgesia is required, and antimicrobial agents are prescribed only for documented infections. During the rehabilitative phase, the medications are needed primarily in a supportive fashion.

Surgery

Initial skin grafting is completed during the acute period. However, the patient may require reconstructive surgery to improve function and plastic surgery to reform ears, noses, or eyelids during the rehabilitation period. Scar tissue and contractures commonly occur one to two years post-burn and may require additional skin grafting. Therefore, surgical management continues to be a form of management as necessitated by the patient's condition as they recover.

Patient and Family Teaching

Before discharge, burn patients and their families have a great need for education so that they may take increasing responsibility for their own care. Discharge teaching involves the entire burn team, who work together to prepare the patient and family for discharge. Early discharge planning accomplishes two goals. First, it helps solve problems early. For example, if the

Fast Forward ▶▶▶

Discharge Instructions using CD-ROM

Patient and family discharge instructions using a CD-ROM as adjuvant to written information is the wave of the future. Content of the CD-ROM can include:

- Description of the skin
- Depth of the burn
- Procedure for cleansing the burn
- Application of therapeutic garments
- Description and discussion of grafts and donor sites
- Care of healed skin
- Expectations as healing progresses

patient's house burned and needs to be repaired, the family may need to relocate. This could be done before discharge, thus preventing the added stress of moving after discharge. Second, early discharge planning emphasizes the future. If discharge is discussed, the patient and his or her family may realize more quickly that recovery and return to home are possible.

An effective, yet inexpensive, discharge education strategy is provision of written instructions. However, not all patients and their family members can read and complex procedures may be difficult to adequately illustrate in two dimensions. A CD-ROM can be inexpensively used and readily updated for individual or group viewing on home computers, DVD players, and some game systems.

Complete and comprehensive instructions followed by return demonstrations contribute to learning the necessary skills to be independent in self-care activities after discharge. Patients with a major burn should not be discharged from the hospital until they can care for themselves physically, with assistance if necessary, and are prepared to meet the stresses involved in returning to their former living patterns.

A major goal in discharge teaching is to prevent excessive scar formation by exercising, splinting, and applying pressure dressings. If these methods are not effective, reconstructive surgery may be necessary. A patient recovering from a major burn may need 12 to 18 months to achieve complete wound healing. Instructions should include how to care for the healed graft and nongrafted areas. Signs and symptoms of complications, including areas that may blister and break down, and signs of infection are also addressed. Written discharge instructions should include the name and phone number of a health care provider or nurse who the patient may call with questions or problems concerning follow-up care. A referral may be made to a home health agency that may be of assistance in dressing the patient's wounds at home.

Evaluation of Outcomes

Potential patient outcomes for each of the example nursing diagnoses for the patient in the rehabilitative phase of burns are:

- Impaired physical mobility related to pain, decreased strength and endurance, and contractures. The patient should perform physical activity independently or with assistive devices as needed. In addition, the patient should be free of complications of immobility, as evidenced by intact skin, absence of thrombophlebitis, and normal bowel patterns.
- Disturbed body image related to altered body function and visualization. The patient demonstrates enhanced body image and self-esteem as evidenced by ability to look at, touch, talk about, and care for actual or perceived altered body part or function.
- Risk for impaired skin integrity related to nutritional deficit and fragile new tissue. The patient's skin condition is improved as evidenced by decreased redness, swelling, and pain.
- Chronic pain related to joint and tissue contractures. The patient should verbalize an adequate relief of pain along with the ability to realistically cope with the pain if it is not completely relieved.
- Ineffective coping related to situational crises and ineffective support systems. The patient identifies own maladaptive coping behaviors, available resources and support systems, describes or initiates alternative coping strategies, and describes positive results from new behaviors.

Case Study

Nursing Care Plan

Gary Bradburn, age 34, was admitted to the emergency department following a fire at a plywood mill where he worked. He had been exposed to the fumes from the burning materials and to the extreme heat and smoke of the fire. His face and surrounding hair, lower arms, and hands have first-, second-, and third-degree burns. His eyebrows and nasal hairs are singed, and his teeth have deposits of soot on them. To escape from the rear of the building, he had to make his way through the smoke and flames before reaching the outside. He rolled on the ground to extinguish the flames from his clothing. Gary is alert enough to answer questions.

One hundred percent oxygen is administered by mask. His neck is stabilized, and blood is drawn for baseline hematocrit, electrolyte, blood urea nitrogen (BUN), cyanide, and carboxyhemoglobin levels. Lactated Ringer's solution is started through a large-bore cannula in a peripheral vein. Pain medication is administered. The physician requests close monitoring for signs of impaired oxygenation (e.g., tachypnea, agitation or anxiety, and symptoms of upper airway obstruction, such as hoarseness, wheezing, or stridor). The emergency department nurse mentions that burns can result in multisystem damage; therefore, assessment of neurological and cardiovascular changes and symptoms of shock are also of prime importance. She comments that the first 24 to 36 hours are critical for burn patients and that early intubation may be necessary to avoid later difficulty because of edema of the larynx.

Assessment

According to the rule of nines assessment tool, a 34-year-old male suffering from first-, second-, and third-degree burns on approximately 27 percent of his body. The majority of the burns are superficial and first-degree in nature, but there is a potential of damage to the upper airway as evidenced by the nasal hairs and eyebrows being singed. In addition, the patient's oxygen saturation level is 92 percent, which is somewhat low for a man of this patient's age. The blood pressure, 138/86; pulse, 90; and respirations, 22. The patient's breath sounds are clear to auscultation and not diminished in the bases.

Nursing Diagnosis 1: Impaired gas exchange due to exposure to smoke poisoning and heat damage to lungs

NOC: Respiratory status: Impaired gas exchange and Impaired spontaneous ventilation; Ineffective tissue perfusion: Cardiopulmonary

NIC: Airway management; Oxygen therapy; Respiratory monitoring

Expected Outcomes

The patient will:

1. Demonstrate improved ventilation, adequate oxygenation as evidenced by an oxygen saturation level of at least 95 percent during his hospitalization.
2. Maintain clear lung fields and remain free of signs of respiratory distress during his hospitalization.

Planning, Interventions, Rationales

1. Monitor respiratory rate, depth, and effort including use of accessory muscles, nasal flaring, and abnormal breathing patterns. *These behaviors and a look of panic in the patient's expression may be indicators of hypoxia.*

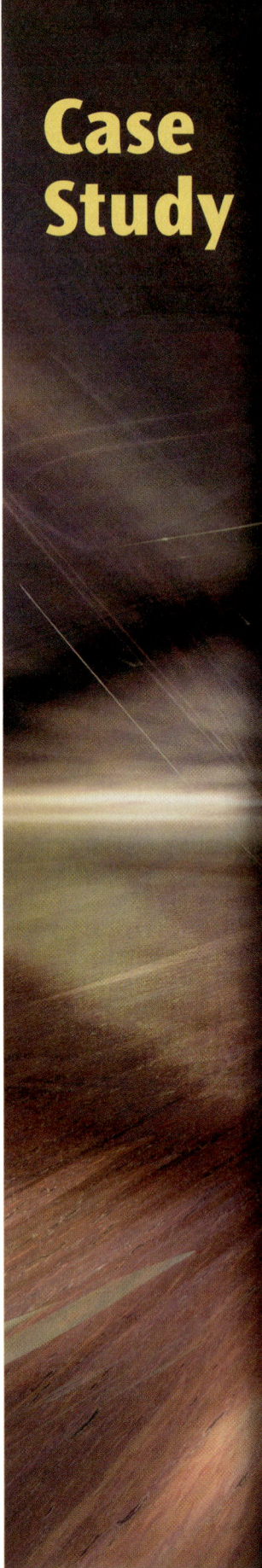

Case Study

2. Auscultate breath sounds every hour or more frequently as needed. *Crackles and wheezes may signify airway obstruction that can lead to or exacerbate existing hypoxia.*
3. Administer humidified oxygen through appropriate device. Monitor patient's behavior and mental status for onset of restlessness, agitation, or confusion. *Behavioral changes and mental status can be early signs of hypoventilation and impaired gas exchange.*
4. Monitor oxygen saturation continuously. Note blood gas results as available. *O_2 saturation of less than 90 percent or a partial pressure of O_2 of less than 80 indicates significant oxygenation problems.*
5. Position patient in semi-Fowler. Turn patient every two hours. Observe patient closely *following position changes. Turning critically ill patients with low hemoglobin levels or decreased cardiac output on either side can result in desaturation. Turn carefully and watch closely.*

Evaluation

Patient's oxygen saturation levels increased to 94 percent within 24 hours and to 96 percent and above within 48 hours. In addition, the patient's respiratory rate slowed to 16 to 20 breaths per minute within 24 hours, and the lungs were clear on auscultation throughout the acute hospitalization.

Nursing Diagnosis 2: Ineffective breathing pattern due to compensatory tachypnea

NOC: Respiratory status: Impaired spontaneous ventilation and Ineffective airway clearance

NIC: Airway management; Respiratory monitoring

Expected Outcomes

The patient will:

1. Return to a normal (regular) or effective breathing pattern.
2. Demonstrate an absence of cyanosis and other signs or symptoms of hypoxia.
3. Maintain arterial blood gases (ABGs) within an acceptable range.
4. Demonstrate appropriate coping behaviors related to breath control.

Planning, Interventions, Rationales

1. Observe rate and depth of respirations and breathing patterns and signs of cyanosis. Auscultate chest for presence of breath sounds and secretions. Monitor diagnostic test results. *Ongoing assessment provides basis for interventions to aid in restoring adequate breathing patterns and oxygenation.*
2. Observe for changes in emotional responses. *Dyspnea can have physiological or psychogenic causes. Fear, anger, and anxiety adversely influence breathing patterns (hyperventilation) and loss of sense of control.*
3. Medicate with analgesics as appropriate. *Promotes deeper respiration and ability to cough if necessary to clear airway (pain may be cause of hyperventilation).*
4. Suction airway as needed. *Removes obstructing secretions, clears airway for patient's who are unable to cough.*
5. Administer oxygen at lowest concentration prescribed. *Higher levels can inhibit patient's respiratory drive.*

Evaluation

Patient maintained a respiratory rate of 16 to 20 breaths per minute without any signs of cyanosis. He did not have any uncontrolled anxiety and was able to breathe in a controlled manner throughout this time of crisis. Analgesics were given periodically without affecting his rate and breathing pattern.

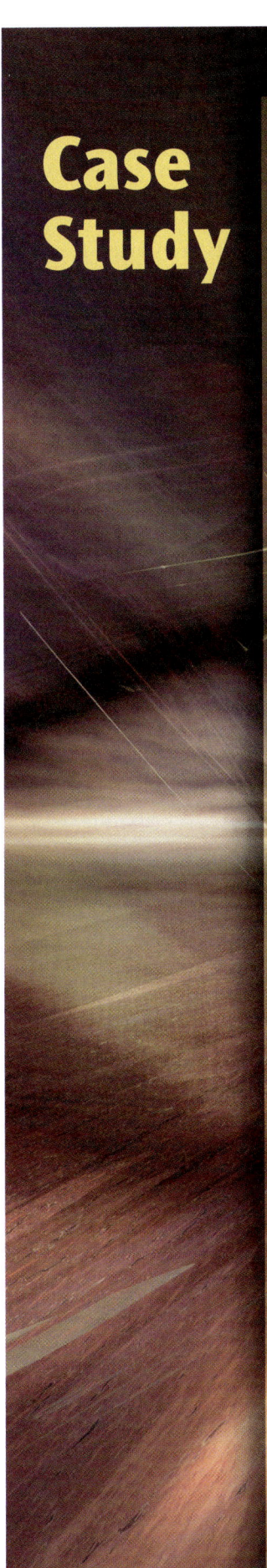

KEY CONCEPTS

- Burn injuries can be traumatic, life-altering experiences for patients and their families.
- Patient and family responses to a burn injury depend on age, culture, socioeconomic status, coping mechanisms, body image, family support, and previous experiences with pain.
- The goals of management during the emergent period, the first 24 to 48 hours after a burn, are to secure the airway, support circulation by fluid replacement, keep the patient comfortable with analgesics, prevent infection through careful wound care, maintain body temperature, and provide emotional support.
- The acute period of treatment begins at the end of the emergent period and lasts until the burn wound is healed.
- Although rehabilitation efforts are started from the time of admission, the technical rehabilitative third stage begins with wound closure and ends when the patient returns to the highest possible level of functioning.

REVIEW QUESTIONS

1. Increased capillary permeability:
   1. Resolves within 12 hours
   2. Causes fluid to shift from the interstitial space to the intravascular space
   3. Only occurs with chemical burns to the skin
   4. May cause hypovolemic shock in large total body surface area burns

2. The rule of nines refers to a method:
   1. Used to estimate the total body surface burned
   2. Used to calculate fluid requirements
   3. Used to determine oxygen needs
   4. Used to estimate the depth of a burn

3. A superficial partial-thickness burn includes:
   1. Color pink, small thin-walled blisters
   2. Color pink, area moist, blisters large, pain sensation intact
   3. Color pink, area moist, will not blanch or refill, texture leathery
   4. Color pink, area moist, blanches with slow capillary refills no blisters

4. Factors that may contribute to insensible fluid loss in the burned patient include:
   1. Loss of protective covering of the skin
   2. Increased temperature
   3. Increased respirations
   4. All of the above

5. Wounds that appear moist and pale with sluggish capillary refill and white in color can be classified as:
   1. Deep partial
   2. Full-thickness
   3. Superficial-partial
   4. Partial

6. The fluid shift in burn shock is primarily:
   1. Water, electrolytes, and albumin
   2. Red blood cells, white blood cells, and water
   3. White blood cells, electrolytes, and globulin
   4. Water electrolytes and white blood cells

7. A 70-kg male patient sustains a full-thickness burn to his face, anterior trunk, and bilateral forearms. What is the total body surface area (TBSA) burned?
   1. 36 percent
   2. 32 percent
   3. 28 percent
   4. 24 percent

8. Calculate the fluid resuscitation requirement using the Parkland formula for the above patient.

9. What is the volume to be infused during the first eight hours (include hourly rate)?

10. What is the volume to be infused during the next 16 hours (include hourly rate)?

REVIEW ACTIVITIES

1. A married couple, both 30 years old is brought to the emergency department after burns from a house fire. The husband has a partial-thickness burn, and the wife has a full-thickness burn. What subjective data would help differentiate these two types of burns?

2. Incorporating general principles of psychological care, develop one nursing approach for each of the following patient responses to a severe burn: withdrawal; denial; regression; anger or hostility; and depression.

3. Describe the burn prevention teaching for a physically disabled 60-year-old man that lives alone?

4. Discuss the differences in priorities of care during the emergent and rehabilitative phases of burn injury.

5. You are caring for a 28-year-old male patient that does not understand why second-degree burns are categorized as superficial partial and deep partial. Describe how you would explain the categorized difference to him.

Visit the Contemporary Medical-Surgical Nursing online companion resource at www.delmarhealthcare.com for additional content and study aids. Click on Online Companions then select the Nursing discipline.

UNIT

XI

Alterations in Gastrointestinal Function

Chapter 47 Assessment of Gastrointestinal Function

Chapter 48 Nutrition, Malnutrition, and Obesity: Nursing Management

Chapter 49 Upper Gastrointestinal Tract Dysfunction: Nursing Management

Chapter 50 Lower Gastrointestinal Tract Dysfunction: Nursing Management

Chapter 51 Hepatic, Biliary Tract, and Pancreatic Dysfunction: Nursing Management

CHAPTER

47

Assessment of Gastrointestinal Function

Elizabeth Torrence, RN, MN, EdD

KEY TERMS

Achalasia
Aerophagia
Barium
Barium enema
Borborygmus
Chyme
Constipation
Diarrhea
Dyspepsia
Dysphagia
Enterokinase
Flatulence
Heartburn (pyrosis)
Laparoscopy
Lavage
Murphy's sign
Odynophagia
Paracentesis
Trocar

CHAPTER TOPICS

- GI Tract Anatomy and Physiology
- Assessment of the GI Tract
- Clinical Manifestations of Pathology of the GI Tract
- Diarrhea
- Constipation
- Diagnostic Tests for the GI Tract

The gastrointestinal (GI) system functions in a fascinating relationship of various organs and biochemical systems working synergistically to provide nutrition to every cell in the body while assisting the body to rid itself of solid and semisolid waste and undigested food. When the learner studies the GI system, it is necessary to have knowledge of all other systems, because the GI system cannot be viewed unitarily as merely a hollow tube whose motility might change secondary to increased, decreased, or obstructive barriers. GI system dysfunction might be outside of the intestinal system yet influence GI function. GI dysfunction often presents as a complex of clinical signs and symptoms. The learner should approach the study of the GI system much as one would approach any ill individual. The patient must be viewed holistically and not as an isolated system. This chapter will detail selected problems associated with deregulation or dysfunction that might occur in the GI system regardless of etiology.

ANATOMY AND PHYSIOLOGY

The major organs of the GI tract include the intestinal tract (the hollow organs from the mouth to the anus) (Figure 47-1), the pancreas that through its exocrine function produces digestive enzymes, and the liver and biliary systems, which achieve important metabolic, digestive, and absorption functions. For this chapter, it is important to remember that the liver produces bile that aids in digestion and absorption of dietary fats and fat-soluble vitamins. Chapter 51 on liver dysfunction will detail other activities of the liver.

The GI tract has been called an integrated system in that its function is prescribed by neuronal control and endocrine functions. These controllers, aid in motility, digestion, absorption, and adjustment of nutrition intake (Keshav, 2004).

Mouth, Lips, Cheeks, Tongue, and Pharynx

The mouth, lips, cheeks, tongue, and pharynx aid in chewing, mastication, and moving food and fluid into the esophagus. Saliva, a product of exocrine glands in the oral cavity, lubricates the mouth and begins the digestive process. Approximately 1 to 2 liters of saliva are produced daily. Saliva serves to lubricate food in transit from the mouth, dissolves food in the mouth to enhance taste, contains alpha amylase (salivary amylase), which begins the digestion of carbohydrates, as well as antibacterial enzymes and immunoglobulins that are believed to protect an individual from serious infection.

The pharynx, controlled by the brainstem cranial nerves (glossopharyngeal and trigeminal nerves), participates with the tongue and other muscles of swal-

A

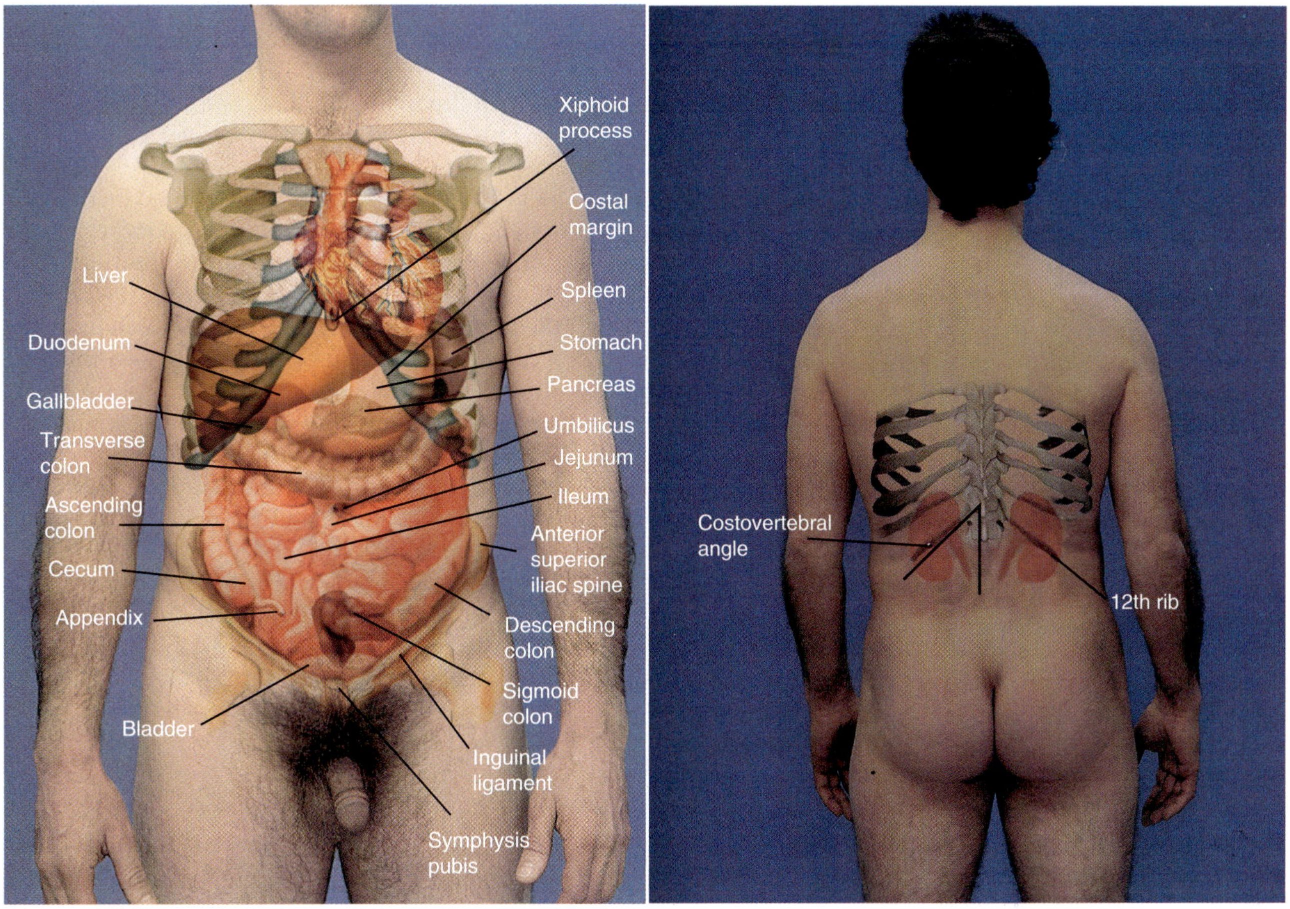

B

Figure 47-1 Digestive tract and structures of the abdomen: A. Anterior view, B. Posterior view.

lowing (pharyngeal, laryngeal, and esophageal). The process of swallowing, actively innervated, allows a bolus of food or fluids to enter through a relaxed esophageal sphincter into the esophagus.

Esophagus

The esophagus is a muscular hollow tube that moves food and fluid via peristaltic action toward the stomach. The esophagus is highly vascular and when compromised (e.g., ulceration or infection) can cause great irritation to the patient.

Stomach

Food enters the stomach, is mixed by the churning muscles of the stomach, and is moved along via the peristaltic activity of the stomach called the gastric slow wave. The gastric slow wave is three peristaltic waves per minute. When the contents of the stomach are semiliquid **(chyme),** the pyloric valve opens, and the chyme enters the duodenum of the small intestine.

When there is anticipation of food entering the stomach, the first phase of gastric secretion occurs (cephalic phase). Once food reaches the stomach, the gastric phase begins. The parietal cells under the influence of acetylcholine and histamine secrete HCl (hydrochloric acid). Gastrin produced by gastric G cells stimulates the parietal cells to secrete in response to food in the stomach. HCl in the stomach triggers pepsinogen, which generates pepsin. Pepsin begins the digestion of proteins in the food substrate. Within the stomach, intrinsic factor binds to vitamin B_{12}. This protects B_{12} from destruction as it is transported to the terminal ileum and absorbed. Gastroferrin in the stomach binds iron so that it can later be absorbed in the duodenum (Keshav, 2004).

Duodenum

The duodenum is the first part of the small intestine. The small intestine (duodenum, jejunum, and ileum) functions as the major digestive and absorptive area of the intestine. The duodenum collects pancreatic enzymes and alkaline bile via the ampulla of Vater. This serves to neutralize the acid environment from the stomach. The duodenal enterocytes release **enterokinase,** an enzyme that hastens effective digestion. Enterocytes from the brush border cells elaborate disaccharidases and peptidases that continue the digestive process. Because of the alkalinity, the bile salts emulsify fatty foods, which enhance the action of the digestive process. Fatty acids and cholesterol diffuse through the lipid membrane of the enterocytes, undergo complex transformation with apolipoproteins to produce chylomicrons, and are released. Transport proteins aid in absorption of sugars, amino acids, and electrolytes into the enterocytes. The duodenum selectively absorbs iron and calcium. Gallbladder contraction and pancreatic secretion are stimulated in response to duodenal secretion of cholecystokinin and secretin.

Interestingly, the small intestine is comparatively free of bacteria. Gastric acid, Brunner's glands, and Paneth cells in the small intestine aid the antimicrobial environment. Secretory dimeric immunoglobulins A (sIgA) also participate in maintaining the minimal antimicrobial setting (Keshav, 2004).

Pancreas

The pancreas is an essential organ of digestion. It produces copious amounts of the digestive enzymes trypsinogen, chymotrypsinogen, procarboxypeptidase A and B, pro-elastase, phospholipid A, pancreatic lipase, pancreatic amylase, ribonuclease, and deoxyribonuclease. The pancreas secretes these enzymes in response to the production of cholecystokinin. Additionally the pancreas produces 2 liters/day of a bicarbonate-rich alkaline liquid. This liquid neutralizes the acidic chyme entering the head of the duodenum. The alkaline environment thus enhances the action of the pancreatic enzymes.

Liver and Biliary Systems

The liver and biliary systems will be fully reviewed in chapter 51. Both systems are interrelated to the function of the GI system.

Jejunum and Ileum

The jejunum and ileum are the main areas for absorption of nutrients, vitamins, amino acids, sugars, and triglycerides. The jejunum and ileum together measure approximately 6 meters (19.5 feet) in length. Enzymes, such as disaccharidases and peptidases, are released from the mucosal cells. The jejunum acts on jejunal contents to absorb dietary folic acid.

Intrinsic factor is removed from vitamin B_{12} and absorbed in the terminal ileum. As fat is digested and absorbed in the terminal ileum, bile salts are reabsorbed and then recycled via entero-hepatic circulation. Another important difference in the ileum is the increase in lymphoid cells in the distal ileum. The distal ileum maintains a higher bacterial load. The lymphoid cells protect the terminal ileum in cases of Crohn's disease and bacterial infection.

Cecum and Appendix

The cecum is the first part of the large intestine. The appendix is a blind-ended tube-like structure exiting from the cecum. These structures have no function in the human. They are mentioned because of disorders that affect them, such as appendicitis and colorectal cancer.

Colon

The colon is the large intestine. It is approximately 1.5 meters in length. Its major function is to reabsorb liquid. The colon is rich in bacterial species. The majority of the bacteria are anaerobic bacteria. These bacteria are potentially pathogenic. The goblet cells of the large intestine generate large amounts of mucus. This coats and protects the epithelium from bacterial incursion.

Rectum and Anus

The rectum and anus act as a reservoirs and controllers of defecation. When the rectum is distended, the increased pressure stimulates peristalsis in the sigmoid colon and relaxation of the internal anal sphincter. The abdominal muscles contract and intra-abdominal pressure increases; if the external anal sphincter (under voluntary control) is relaxed, feces is expelled.

ASSESSMENT

The abdominal health history provides the nurse with important subjective information that assists in the physical assessment of the abdomen. Areas that the nurse needs to collect information from the patient in regards to GI abdominal health history are:

1. Family history. Does anyone in the family now have or have had GI problems, e.g., gallbladder disease, gall stones, liver dysfunction, jaundice, irritable bowel disorder, ulcerative colitis or Crohn's disease, stomach ulcers, hemorrhoids, any cancers of the GI tract (pancreas, liver, esophageal, stomach, colon, or rectal), gastroesophageal reflux disease (GERD), pancreatitis,

hernias (inguinal or other) hiatal, tubal pregnancy, ovarian cyst, uterine dysfunction, diarrheal conditions, or other chronic conditions that affected the GI system?

2. Past abdominal history and current problems. Has the patient ever experienced any of the conditions listed in number 1 or had any GI dysfunction? Does the patient have any current GI dysfunction? Has there been any recent weight gain or weight loss? Elicit details. Any GI surgery or other GI procedures? For what? Results? Has the patient been out of the country recently, if so, where?
3. Eating habits. Recall previous 24 hours; unusual eating requirements
   a. Appetite
   b. Food intolerance
   c. Bowel habits
4. Nutritional assessment. This is an excellent time to discuss health promotion activities, such as the food pyramid. The USDA Center for Nutrition Policy and Promotion released the latest food pyramid (Roth, 2007). It allows the consumer to select foods from various categories of the pyramid and monitor their own dietary and nutritional needs. Professionals are directed to explore this site to monitor dietary intake. Often during this part of the history, the nurse can ask about exercise and activity patterns.
5. Dysphagia or heartburn (pyrosis). Has the patient experienced any difficulty in swallowing? If so when did it begin? Have patient describe how often and circumstances when it occurs. Has the patient ever experienced burning in the throat or stomach? A feeling of fullness? At this point the nurse can ask about a chronic cough or recurrent upper respiratory infections. If the patient experiences any of these symptoms, what has the patient done to relieve these symptoms? What makes these symptoms worse?
6. Nausea/vomiting. How often? Describe the events before, during, and after the symptoms? Was there anything unusual about the vomitus, e.g., smell, color, presence of blood? Hematemesis caused from vomiting can occur with irritation or tears of esophagus, with stomach or duodenal ulcerations, and with esophageal varices. Careful questioning about the presence, amount, and circumstance is essential.
7. Abdominal pain. This is a vital symptom and can herald a variety of disorders. Acute pain in the abdomen is referred to as the acute abdomen. This requires urgency in assessment; early surgical intervention may be lifesaving.
   a. Ask the patient to point (with one finger) to the area that is painful.
   b. Is the pain just in this area or does it radiate (move around)? If so, where does it move? Is there anything that makes the pain better or worse?
   c. How long has the patient had the pain? Is the pain constant?
   d. Describe the character of the pain, e.g., dull, cramping, burning, stabbing, aching, or bloating type pain? On a scale of 1 to 10, with 10 as the worst pain the patient may have ever experienced, have the patient categorize the intensity of the pain.
   e. Is pain changed by food? Better or worse?
   f. What makes the pain worse (aggravating factors)?
   g. What things has the patient done to get pain relief (alleviating factors), e.g., antacids or other medications, rest, ice, heat, walking, lying still, other position(s)?
8. Medications. Because most medications are taken orally, it is essential to have the most up-to-date summary of all medications the patient takes. This includes all over-the-counter (OTC) medications and supplements. Included in this assessment should be the amount of alcohol the patient consumes. Skill in asking questions about medications is important, because patients often do not consider the nonsteroidal anti-inflammatory

drugs (NSAIDs), such as aspirin, acetaminophen, naproxen, ibuprofen, or any type of vitamin supplements as medications or that these may influence the GI system (Broyles, Reiss, & Evans, 2007).

GI Symptom Assessment

Because the GI system is responsible for the processing of ingested foods and fluids and the removal of waste products of digestion, any disruption in the processes that are responsible for these functions can lead to various symptoms. Nurses care for patients with GI dysfunction in the inpatient setting and in the clinic and outpatient or home environment. More than 50 percent of individuals with GI complaints have no physical findings, anatomical abnormality, or abnormal lab work (Giles, et al., 2005). This creates a conundrum when helping the individual understand the diagnostic and treatment parameters of a GI disorder.

Leading symptoms and complaints from patients with GI disorders include heartburn, **dysphagia** (difficulty in swallowing), dyspepsia, nausea and vomiting, gas, diarrhea, constipation, pain, and bleeding. Interestingly these symptoms may be associated with a GI problem but may also be associated with a separate and unconnected system disorder. Sometimes symptoms are minor and may require patient education in terms of diet change or lifestyle modification, but sometimes symptoms are indicative of a serious GI disorder.

In general, nurses should be familiar with GI symptoms and the approach needed for the patient. The nurse must know the inclusive history of the patient's symptom and listen carefully to how this symptom occurs in the patient's life. This will be valuable information as the diagnostic problem is differentiated, and a treatment protocol is put into place. The symptoms described are common GI symptoms that are important to know. These will be referred to in future chapters discussing various GI disorders.

Heartburn

Heartburn occurs daily in 7 to 10 percent of all Americans. **Heartburn (pyrosis)** is a substernal burning sensation often radiating to the neck experienced within one hour of eating or one to two hours after reclining. Ingesting foods that irritate the esophagus or decrease the esophageal sphincter pressure causes heartburn. Activities that increase intra-abdominal pressure (e.g., bending, lifting, exercise, straining at stool, or Valsalva maneuver) may also be related to heartburn. When assessing the patient for heartburn, the nurse should assess if the discomfort of heartburn changes with position, food, stress, or exercise.

When a patient describes this symptom, it is described as a burning in the throat, neck, and suprasternal or substernal area. Because of the current focus on GERD in the lay media, patients will often indicate that they have indigestion or acid reflux. Many times patients will have self-medicated with OTC preparations, such as antacids, acid blockers, or other similar available medications. It is important to elicit from the patient when this symptom is experienced. Because the cause of this symptom can be acid contents regurgitated into the esophagus, antacids improve the symptom. There are things that make heartburn worse—a late meal or snack, foods that are directly irritating to the mucosal surface of the esophagus or that lower esophageal sphincter tone, activity that raises intra-abdominal pressure (bending, lifting, and straining). If a patient has a chronic complaint of heartburn, the provider will do a workup for reflux disorder.

Painful Swallowing (Odynophagia)

Odynophagia (pain experienced when a person swallows) is associated with erosion of the esophagus. There are many cause of this pain. It is often linked with infections of the esophagus and subsequent inflammation (esophagitis) or esophageal erosion. Immunocompromised patients who have *Candida,* herpes, and cytomegalovirus infections (patients undergoing cancer chemotherapy or those with acquired immunodeficiency syndrome [AIDS] or human immunodeficiency virus [HIV]) may also develop painful swallowing. This can occur from esophagitis associated with certain medications, some antibiotics, tetracycline, doxycycline, and some antiviral agents.

Difficulty Swallowing (Dysphagia)

The patient will describe dysphagia as the food gets stuck or as a lump (globus) in his or her throat. Dysphagia is either oropharyngeal or esophageal (it is important to review the swallowing process and the afferent and efferent motor function provided by the cranial nerves [CN]). Oropharyngeal dysphagia is important to determine, especially if the patient is older or may have sustained a recent cerebrovascular accident. In addition, when a patient is in the hospital, it is important for the nurse to have any swallowing deficit assessed to determine interventions needed to prevent the patient from aspirating. Other neurological causes that interfere with motor control of the tongue or other oral structures are those that interrupt myoneural function. Afferent input to the swallowing center is through CN V, X, and XI; efferent motor response is mediated by CN V, VII, IX, X, and XII. Some examples of afferent input disorders are myasthenia gravis, certain neuropathies, multiple sclerosis, and Parkinson's disease. Structural abnormalities can also inhibit swallowing, such as oropharyngeal tumors, extrinsic pressure from an enlarged thyroid gland, or Zenker's diverticulum. Zenker's, or cricopharyngeal, diverticulum occurs from an abnormal cricopharyngeal sphincter. Upper esophageal sphincter (UES) dysfunction (cricopharyngeal achalasia) also contributes to oropharyngeal dysphagia. Either a motility disorder or a structural or mechanical process that impairs food moving through the esophageal lumen causes esophageal dysphagia. The patient will describe this sensation as food getting stuck.

The nurse should assess to determine if the dysphagia occurs with solids or liquids or both; whether the difficulty in swallowing is intermittent or getting progressively worse. This may be because of a mechanical or a motility disorder. Dysphagia associated with only solid food is suggestive of mechanical obstruction, (e.g., an esophageal ring—Schatzki's ring, which is a mucosal ring at the lower esophagus). The symptoms associated with an esophageal ring are often intermittent and long-standing. Progressive symptoms may be because of strictures from chronic reflux disease or carcinoma. If the patient is older, has a history of smoking, and ethel alcohol (ETOH) use, and has experienced weight loss, the patient may have an esophageal growth. Dysphagia associated with solids and liquids is suggestive of a problem with esophageal motility. Causes of this type of dysphagia may be esophageal spasms, achalasia, or scleroderma. If solid food is regurgitated, especially with coughing, **achalasia** (a motility disorder from failure of smooth muscle to relax or absence of muscular contraction of the lower esophagus) should be suspect.

Indigestion (Dyspepsia)

Indigestion, or **dyspepsia,** is an uncomfortable feeling in the upper abdominal region. This term is used to describe several imprecise complaints, such as epigastric pain, gnawing, bloating, fullness, early satiety, belching, heartburn, burning, and nausea. Dyspepsia is the most common symptom that patients complain about to their provider. It accounts for 70 percent of visits to a primary care provider. Twenty-five percent of adults have experienced some type of dyspepsia. Of those individuals who have undergone a diagnostic endoscopy for dyspepsia, about half will have normal results. Fifteen to 25 percent will be diagnosed with reflux disorder, and about 29 percent will have peptic ulcer disease. Patients over the age of 45 with dyspepsia often have weight loss, dysphagia, and recurrent vomiting. Alarm symptoms associated with dyspepsia include weight loss, anemia, bleeding, persistent vomiting, and dysphagia. One to 2 percent will have gastric cancer.

Dyspepsia is divided into nonulcer dyspepsia and dyspepsia secondary to peptic ulcer disease. Nonulcer dyspepsia is associated with GERD, problems with motility, gallbladder, liver, pancreatic dysfunction, medication-induced dyspepsia, dietary causes, ETOH ingestion, and endocrine or metabolic disorders, e.g., diabetes. Gallstones can cause severe indigestion, but the dyspepsia associated with gallstones or chronic cholecystitis is described as episodic. The dyspepsia and pain last a few hours and subside. *Helicobacter pylori* gastritis has been implicated in nonulcer dyspepsia but can lead to duodenal and gastric ulceration. *H. pylori* has been implicated in gastric cancer (Butcher, 2003).

Queasiness, Nausea, Regurgitation, and Vomiting

Nausea is a vague, unpleasant sensation of queasiness or feeling sick to the stomach, which may be accompanied by pallor, sweating, and increased saliva production. There is usually distaste for food, and the urge to vomit. Vomiting (emesis) or retching is the forceful expulsion (reverse peristalsis) of stomach contents through the mouth that involves the muscles of the chest and stomach (Table 47-1). Regurgitation is an effortless return of gastric contents into the mouth. Regurgitation can occur in the absence of vomiting and as a part reflux. Vomiting is centrally controlled and may be stimulated by afferent vagal fibers, the vestibular system, and the chemoreceptor trigger zone (CTZ). The causes of nausea and vomiting derive from various pathways and can be categorized into neurogenic, chemical, mechanical, infection, or irritation of the GI tract. More specifically, nausea and vomiting can be from medication, GI infection, food poisoning, intestinal obstruction, appendicitis, cholecystitis, systemic illnesses, pregnancy, or motion sickness or be self-induced. Mechanical complications can include rupture of the esophagus with subsequent mediastinitis (Boerhaave syndrome) or a Mallory-Weiss tear, which occurs at the esophagogastric junction.

Hiccups (Hiccoughs)

Hiccups are caused by sudden contraction of the diaphragm. Gastric distension can cause self-limiting hiccups. These occur from gastric distension with carbonated beverages, aerophagia (air swallowing), extreme hot or cold

TABLE 47-1 Act of Vomiting

Afferent Input		
Afferent vagal fibers Splanchnic autonomic fibers from GI viscera	Serotonin 5-hydroxytryptamine (5-HT_3) receptors	*Stimulated by biliary or GI distension, mucosal or peritoneal irritation*
Vestibular system (CN VII)	Histamine H_1 and muscarinic cholinergic receptors	*Stimulated by motion, infection, vestibular neuronitis, acute labyrinthitis, Ménière's disease*
CNS centers—Vomiting center dorsal part of the medulla oblongata (main site of neural control of vomiting)		*Stimulated by sights, smells, or emotional (psychic) experiences*
Chemoreceptor trigger zone (CTZ) located in the floor of the 4th ventricle (outside of the blood-brain barrier)	Serotonin 5-HT_3 receptors Dopamine D_2 receptors	*Stimulated by drugs and chemotherapeutic agents, toxins, hypoxia, uremia, acidosis, and radiation*

Adapted from Rizzo, D. (2006). Fundamentals of anatomy and physiology *(2nd ed.). New York: Thomson Delmar Learning.*

liquids, or ETOH ingestion. Certain central nervous system disorders, psychogenic disorders, metabolic disorders, involvement or irritation of the vagus or phrenic nerve, and general anesthesia can also cause hiccups.

GI Gas

This is a general category of symptoms associated with belching, bloating, **borborygmus** (hyperactive bowel sounds), abdominal pain, cramps, and **flatulence** (gas formed within the GI tract and expelled via the rectum). The average adult swallows air into the upper GI tract, and most of the gas in the stomach is from this source. Air swallowing occurs after meals because of gastric distension and lower esophageal sphincter relaxation. Oxygen extracted from air is readily absorbed, but more than 78 percent of air is nitrogen that is only minimally absorbed. If excessive amounts of air are swallowed **(aerophagia),** abdominal distension and pain, belching, and flatulence may be experienced. Belching can be normal, but excessive belching is related to aerophagia. Minor behavioral modification can resolve this problem. Patients who experience severe belching from aerophagia can reduce this by eating slowly, not using a straw when drinking, not drinking carbonated beverages, not smoking, and not chewing gum. If belching is associated with other GI symptoms, more assessment that is complete must be done.

Normally between 500 and 1,500 mL of gas are expelled by the rectum per day. Flatus is produced from a combination of fermentation gases of carbohydrates and swallowed air. If flatulence is associated with a malabsorption disorder, that is, the patient is losing weight, has diarrhea, or may be anemic, a diagnostic workup may be necessary. Lactase deficiency is a cause of increased intestinal gas production. Reducing lactulose in the diet reduces these symptoms. Additionally, counseling the patient to reduce foods that produce gas during digestion is helpful. A trial eliminating or reducing various foodstuffs (e.g., beans, brussels sprouts, broccoli, cabbage, onions, foodstuffs containing high amounts of fructose, maltose, or lactulose) known to produce large amounts of gas during digestion should be recommended. If excessive flatulence persists, the patient may need further workup for a functional GI disorder; other causes of increased gas production are malabsorption syndromes or ingesting poorly absorbed carbohydrates (e.g., sorbitol, lactose, or lactulose).

Diarrhea

Diarrhea can be acute, self-limiting, a life-threatening event, or chronic. By definition **diarrhea** is an increase in the liquid state of the stool. There may also be an increase in frequency. Diarrhea is differentiated into acute and chronic. The World Gastroenterology Organization has practice guidelines for management of the patient with diarrhea. The causes of diarrhea are categorized into osmotic, secretory, mucosal injury, or normal volume.

Acute Diarrhea

Acute diarrhea is less than three weeks in duration and is divided into noninflammatory and inflammatory. In noninflammatory diarrhea, there is an absence of fever, blood in the stool, or fecal leukocytes; whereas in inflammatory diarrhea there are systemic aspects that include fever. An infectious or irritating agent in the bowel usually causes acute diarrhea, except in inflammatory bowel disease and radiation diarrhea. A good history is important in understanding the link of acute diarrhea with a cause.

Noninflammatory Diarrhea

Noninflammatory diarrhea is linked with cramps, bloating, nausea, or vomiting. Noninflammatory diarrhea may be from small intestinal enteritis that is produced by bacteria that produce toxins (e.g., *Staphylococcus aureus, Escherichia coli,* or *Clostridium*). These types of bacterial agents interfere with normal absorption in the small intestine.

Inflammatory Diarrhea

Inflammatory diarrhea is marked by fever and bloody diarrhea, and a health care provider should suspect tissue damage to the colon caused by invasion of an infectious agent. Examples are *Shigella, Salmonella, Campylobacter,* amoebic dysentery, or from a toxin produced by the invading organism (e.g., *Clostridium difficile, E. coli*).

The difference between these diarrheal disorders and inflammatory diarrhea, is that there is usually a smaller amount of diarrheal stool; the symptoms are left lower quadrant (LLQ) cramping, urgency, and tenesmus. Fecal leukocytes are present in infections with invasive organisms. *E. coli* is acquired from eating contaminated, improperly prepared meat. It results in severe, hemorrhagic colitis. It is the most common cause of bloody diarrhea in adults and hemolytic uremic syndrome in children (Friedman, McQuaid, & Grendell, 2003).

Chronic Diarrhea

Chronic diarrhea is greater than three weeks in duration. The causes of chronic diarrhea include osmotic, malabsorption syndromes, secretory and inflammatory conditions, and motility disorders, and chronic infections.

Constipation

Constipation is marked by straining at stool with the production of hard stools, decreased frequency, and a feeling of not completely evacuating the colon. The number of bowel movements a patient has is individual, but if a patient has fewer than three bowel movements per week or must vigorously strain, the patient is considered to have constipation. Constipation is a common complaint. Idiopathic constipation results from colonic inertia, which is a delay in transit time in the large bowel, pelvic floor dysfunction (e.g., dyschezia, anismus, or outlet obstruction), or constipation with normal transit time due to irritable bowel syndrome (Friedman, et al., 2003). It is an increasing complaint of patients as they age. It affects women more than men. It is due to sedentary lifestyle, poor diets (low in dietary fiber and fluid),and medications. In general, the causes of constipation can be categorized into lifestyle, medications, structural abnormalities, systemic diseases, and refractory constipation.

> **Skills 360°**
>
> **Pneumonic for the Nurse Assessing Pain: PQRST**
>
> **P**rovokes: What provokes the pain?
>
> **Q**uality—What makes it better/ worse? What does it feel like?
>
> **R**adiation: Where is it? Where does it radiate?
>
> **S**everity—Rate the pain on a scale of 1–10.
>
> **T**ime and **T**reatment: How long have you had it? What has been done already?
>
> *Adapted from Estes, M. (2006).* Health assessment and physical examination *(3rd ed.). New York: Thomson Delmar Learning.*

Abdominal Pain

Abdominal pain is separated into acute and chronic. Acute abdominal pain, often described as acute abdomen, can be a life-threatening problem. Most of the pain fibers supplying the abdominal viscera are C fibers; C nerve fibers generate dull, poorly localized pain. Abdominal pain is dull, gnawing, or burning and poorly localized. Pain fibers supplying the parietal peritoneum are both A-delta fibers (A-delta fibers generate distinct and localized pain response), and C fibers so that pain is more distinct and localized. A patient will experience abdominal pain when nerve fibers in the serosal, muscular, and mucosal layers are either mechanically (stretched or spasm) or chemically (inflammation, irritation, or ischemic) stimulated. In solid organs of the abdomen, pain is noted only when the capsule of the organ is stretched or invaded, e.g. obstruction, congestion, or a space-occupying lesion (Yamada, 2005). During the assessment of pain (see Skills 360° feature), the nurse should establish the location, quality (e.g., burning, throbbing, twisting, sharp, stabbing, knife-like, colicky, cramping, constricting, penetrating, boring, brief, or constant), intensity, onset, duration, chronology, alleviating and aggravating factors, such as position, movement, food, or liquids, associated symptoms, radiation sites, and behaviors that put the patient at risk (e.g., heavy ETOH intake, NSAIDs use).

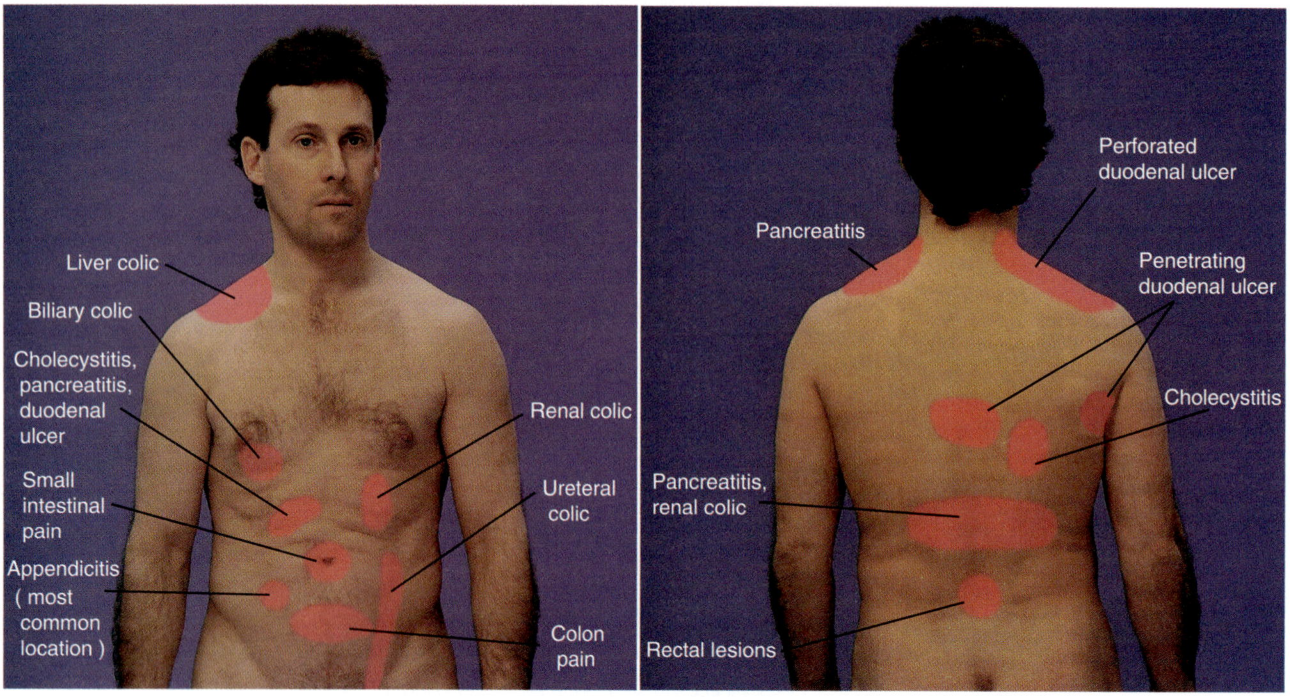

Figure 47-2 Areas of referred pain.

Referred Pain

Referred pain is noted in abdominal and GI disorders because of neuroanatomic features (Figure 47-2) (Table 47-2). A single splanchnic nerve may provide sensory input from several abdominal organs and enter the spinal column at more than one level. Cutaneous and visceral afferent nerves end on the same secondary neuron in the dorsal horn of the spinal cord. This results in confusion by the brain of the place of the original stimulus (Friedman, et al., 2003).

Red Flag

Serious Symptoms to Assess in an Abdominal Assessment

As an emergent condition associated with abdominal assessment, the nurse should observe how the patient is lying in the bed. If there is any guarding of the abdomen, there are serious conditions that should be considered (e.g., peritonitis, appendicitis). In addition, the nurse should note if the patient is lying still because of pain or if the patient is unable to find a position of comfort because of pain, which generally indicates a more serious condition.

Assessment

Although the GI tract begins in the mouth, the mouth and throat assessment is found in the chapters related to disorders of the head, eyes, ears, nose, and throat. When performing a GI assessment, the nurse uses all of the skills used in other types of assessments (Table 47-3).

Observation

When the nurse is looking, listening, thinking, and feeling, (those skills needed for good assessment) divide the abdomen into four quadrants and remember which organs are in each quadrant (Table 47-4). The four quadrants are right upper (RUQ), left upper (LUQ), right lower (RLQ), and left lower quadrant (LLQ).

As the nurse is performing the abdominal assessment, an organized approach to the patient is important. To perform the assessment, the patient should be lying supine. The abdomen should be exposed, the patient's head should be resting on a pillow (if the neck is flexed, the abdominal musculature may be contracted), and the knees should be bent to relax the abdomen. The room should be warm, and there should be suitable lighting. The nurse must note the appearance of the abdomen and describe whether it is flat, distended, enlarged, pulsatile, or symmetrical. The nurse can ask the patient to bear down to note any protrusion through weakened areas of the abdominal wall indicating potential ventral hernias. In addition, the nurse should note skin abnormalities and scars or the presence of jaundice, and cutaneous angiomas

Skills 360°

Skills the Nurse Demonstrates in Abdominal Assessment

Observation and inspection: looking with a careful eye in concert with cognitive thinking skills at the abdomen region.

Auscultation: occurs prior to palpation or percussion, because these techniques may alter normal bowel sounds. Auscultation uses a stethoscope to hear the sounds created by GI function.

Percussion: of the various structures to locate the organs beneath the abdominal wall, to establish the density of the various structures, and to check for swelling, fluid levels, or masses in the abdomen.

Palpation: When palpating the abdomen, the nurse must know both light and deep palpation. Palpation is performed to assess the size, location, and consistency of various structures in the abdomen (Figure 47-3).

Palpation and percussion: are also used to determine pain, tenderness, or masses in the abdominal cavity.

Adapted from Estes, M. (2006). Health assessment and physical examination *(3rd ed.). New York: Thomson Delmar Learning.*

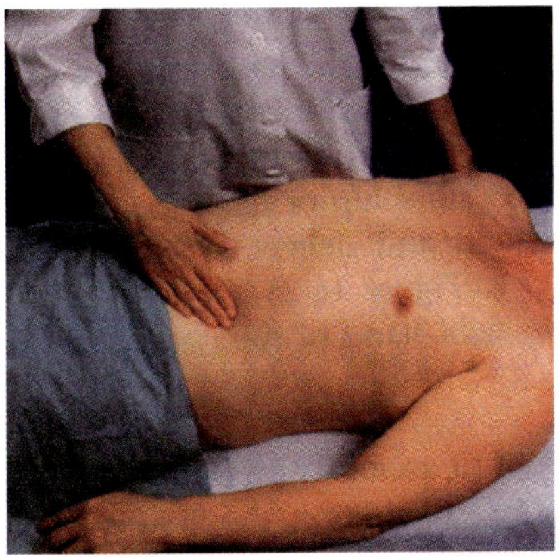

Figure 47-3 Light palpation of abdomen.

TABLE 47-2 Etiologies of Abdominal Pain: Anatomical Regions Where They Are Perceived

Right Upper Quadrant	***Epigastrium***	***Left Upper Quadrant***
Biliary stone	Abdominal aortic aneurysm	Gastric ulcer
Cholecystitis	Appendicitis (early)	Gastritis
Cholelithiasis	Biliary stone	Myocardial infarction
Duodenal ulcer	Cholecystitis	Pneumonia
Gastric ulcer	Diverticulitis	Splenic enlargement
Hepatic abscess	Gastroesophageal reflux disease	Splenic rupture
Hepatitis	Hiatal hernia	
Hepatomegaly		
Pancreatitis		
Pneumonia		
	Periumbilical	
	Abdominal aortic aneurysm	
	Appendicitis (early)	
	Diverticulitis	
	Intestinal obstruction	
	Irritable bowel syndrome	
	Pancreatitis	
	Peptic ulcer	
	Recurrent abdominal pain (in children)	
	Volvulus	
Right Lower Quadrant		***Left Lower Quadrant***
Appendicitis		Diverticulitis
Crohn's disease		Ectopic pregnancy (ruptured)
Diverticulitis		Endometriosis
Ectopic pregnancy (ruptured)		Hernia (strangulated)
Endometriosis		Irritable bowel syndrome
Hernia (strangulated)		Mittelschmerz
Irritable bowel syndrome		Ovarian cyst
Mittelschmerz		Pelvic inflammatory disease
Ovarian cyst		Renal calculi
Pelvic inflammatory disease		Salpingitis
Renal calculi		Ulcerative colitis
Salpingitis		
	Diffuse	
	Gastroenteritis	
	Peritonitis	

Adapted from Estes, M. (2006). Health assessment and physical examination *(3rd ed.). New York: Thomson Delmar Learning.*

(spider angiomas occur with portal hypertension). The nurse should note the umbilicus as to whether it is midline, inverted, or everted and whether there is any discoloration or inflammation or the presence of a hernia (note: Cullen's sign is a faint bluish color around the umbilicus secondary to hemoperitoneum [intra-abdominal bleeding]).

Auscultation

Auscultation is performed prior to palpation or percussion because touching the abdomen may change the tone of the bowel. The diaphragm of the stethoscope is used, and the nurse should warm the hands assessing the diaphragm

TABLE 47-3 Assessment of Abdomen: Normal and Key Findings

AREA OF ASSESSMENT/*NORMAL FINDINGS*	KEY FINDINGS
Abdomen: Inspect, Auscultate, Percuss, and Palpate	
Place patient in a supine position with knees flexed over a pillow, hands at sides or across chest. Undrape patient from xiphoid process to symphysis pubis to expose the abdomen.	Promotes relaxation of the abdominal muscles.
1. Stand at right side of patient. a. Inspect abdomen from rib margin to pubic bone. Note contour and symmetry (observing for peristalsis, pulsations, scars, striae, or masses). b. Inspect umbilicus for contour, location, signs of inflammation, or hernia. c. Observe for smooth, even respiratory movement. d. Observe for surface motion (visible peristalsis). e. Inspect epigastric area for pulsations. *Contour is flat or rounded and bilaterally symmetrical. Umbilicus is depressed and beneath the abdominal surface. Abdomen rises with inspirations and falls with expirations, free from respiratory retractions. Visible peristalsis slowly traverses the abdomen in a slanting downward movement as observed in thin patients. Pulsations of the abdominal aorta are visible in the epigastric area in thin patients.*	1. A convex symmetrical profile reveals either a protuberant abdomen (results of poor muscle tone from inadequate exercise or obesity) or distension (taut stretching of skin across abdominal wall). Asymmetry may indicate a mass, bowel obstruction, enlargement of abdominal organs, or scoliosis. Umbilicus bulging may indicate a hernia. Old scars are flat with a shiny appearance, blending with patient's pigmentation; new scars are raised and reddened. Atrophic lines or streaks reveal linea albicantes (striae) that occur with tumors, obesity, ascites, and pregnancy. Engorged or dilated veins around the umbilicus are associated with circulatory obstruction of superior or inferior vena cava. Uneven respiratory movement with retractions may indicate appendicitis. Strong peristaltic movement may indicate intestinal obstruction. Marked pulsations in epigastric area may indicate an aortic aneurysm.
2. Auscultate the abdominal quadrants for bowel sounds (high-pitched) using the diaphragm of the stethoscope. a. Begin by placing the diaphragm on the RLQ. Listen for a full minute to the frequency and character of the bowel sounds. b. Repeat Step a, proceeding in sequence to RUQ, LUQ, and LLQ. c. Listen at least 5 minutes before concluding the absence of bowel sounds. *High-pitched sounds, heard every 5 to 15 seconds as intermittent gurgling sounds in all four quadrants as a result of air and fluid movement in the gastrointestinal tract. Bowel sounds should always be heard at the ileocecal valve area.*	2. Hypoactive or diminished bowel sounds are soft and low and widely separated so that only one or two are heard in a 2-minute interval. Hypoactive is normal the first few hours after general anesthesia. Hypoactive sounds may indicate decreased motility of the bowel, such as occurs with peritoneal irritation or paralytic ileus. Absent bowels sounds (none heard for 3 to 5 minutes) may signal paralytic ileus, peritonitis, or an obstruction. Hyperactive (loud, audible, gurgling sounds similar to stomach growling; sounds also called borborygmi) may occur with diarrhea or hunger. Rushed, high-pitched, or tingling sounds suggest air or fluid under pressure; this may occur in the early stages of an intestinal blockage when heard in the portion of the bowel that precedes the obstruction (Estes, 2002).
3. Auscultate with bell of stethoscope over the aorta, epigastric area, renal arteries, and femoral arteries. Note bruits over each area. *Free from audible bruits.*	3. A bruit over an abdominal vessel reveals turbulent blood flow suggestive of an aortic aneurysm or partial obstruction (e.g., renal or femoral stenosis).
4. Percuss all quadrants in a systematic fashion. Begin percussion in RLQ, move upward to RUQ, cross over to LUQ, and down to LLQ. Note when tympany changes to dullness. *Tympany is heard because of air in the stomach and intestines. Dullness is heard over organs (e.g., the liver).*	4. Dullness over the stomach or intestines may indicate a mass or tumor, **ascites** (excessive fluid accumulation in the abdominal cavity), or full intestines.
5. Perform light palpation. Never palpate over areas where bruits are auscultated. a. Instruct patient to cough. If patient experiences a sharp twinge of pain in a quadrant, palpate that area last. b. With patient's hands and forearms on a horizontal plane, use fingerpads to depress the abdominal wall 1 cm in all four quadrants. Begin palpation in RLQ, move upward to RUQ, cross over to LUQ, and down to LLQ. Note texture and consistency of underlying tissue. *Should feel smooth with consistent softness.*	5. Tenderness and increased skin temperature may indicate inflammation. Large masses may be due to tumors, feces, or enlarged organs.

Adapted from Estes, M. (2006). Health assessment and physical examination *(3rd ed.). New York: Thomson Delmar Learning.*

Red Flag

Assessments for Acute Appendicitis

Rebound tenderness (Blumberg's sign): is a positive response, which may mean peritoneal irritation. The tips of the fingers are pressed gently into the abdominal wall and then suddenly withdrawn. A painful response is positive. Cutaneous hyperesthesia is elicited in the area of the skin over an appendix that is inflamed. Rebound tenderness is a classic sign of appendicitis (Figure 47-4).

Iliopsoas muscle test: The patient is asked to flex the right thigh (raises the right leg) against resistance (pushing down over the lower part of the thigh). The patient will experience pain in the pelvis because of irritation of the Iliopsoas muscle (Figure 47-5).

Obturator muscle test: The patient flexes the right thigh (raises the right leg) to 90 degrees. Holding the ankle, the leg is rotated internally and externally. If pelvic pain is produced is the muscle is inflamed (Figure 47-6).

TABLE 47-4 The Four Quadrants of the Abdomen

RUQ	LUQ
Liver	Stomach
Gallbladder	Spleen
Head of pancreas	Left lobe of liver
Right kidney and adrenal gland 1	Pancreas
Duodenum	Left kidney and adrenal gland
Hepatic flexure of colon	Splenic flexure of colon
Part of ascending and transverse colon	Part of transverse and descending colon
RLQ	**LLQ**
Cecum	Part of descending colon
Appendix	Sigmoid colon
Right ovary	Left ovary
Right ureter	Left ureter
Right spermatic cord	Left spermatic cord

Adapted from Estes, M. (2006). Health assessment and physical examination *(3rd ed.). New York: Thomson Delmar Learning.*

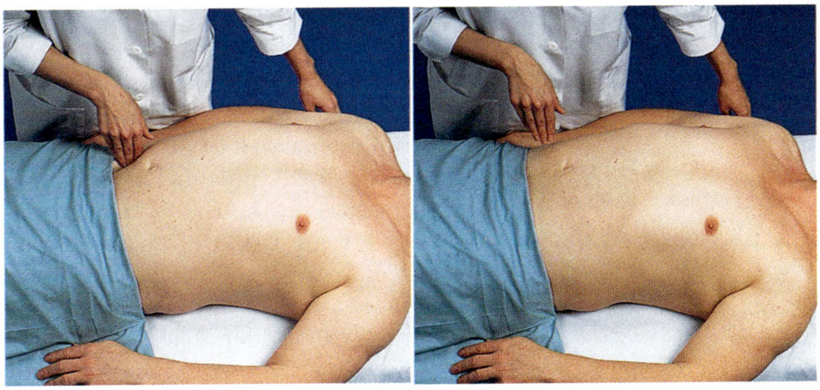

Figure 47-4 Rebound tenderness.

prior to placing on the abdomen. Then, the nurse listens in each of the four quadrants of the abdomen for approximately 20 seconds. Are bowel sounds (peristalsis) present? Describe the frequency and the quality of the sounds. Normally bowel sounds are usually heard every 2 to 5 seconds. Hyperactive bowel sounds are termed borborygmus; to declare absent bowel sound, then a nurse must listen for three to five minutes. In addition, the nurse must listen for vascular sounds; normally no vascular sounds or bruits are heard unless the patient has hypertension.

Percussion

The purpose of percussing the abdomen is to elicit either of two sounds: (a) tympanic (drum-like): this sound is produced over air filled structures; and (b) dull sounds: these sounds are produced over a solid structure (e.g., liver or a mass) or fluid (ascites or a full bladder). During percussion, notice if the patient experiences any pain as this may be a sign of peritoneal inflammation. Ordinarily you may not be able to percuss the liver, because it is not below the costal margin, although it may normally be 1 or 2 centimeters below the costal margin. In an individual with liver disease, you would be able to percuss as well as palpate the liver margins. The spleen is not normally percussed unless there is significant

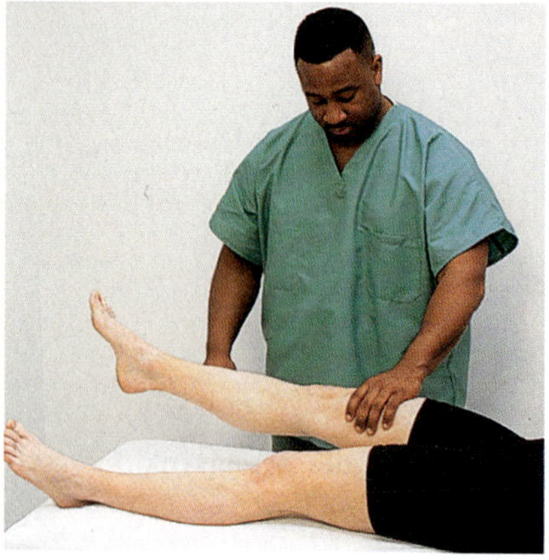

Figure 47-5 Iliopsoas muscle test.

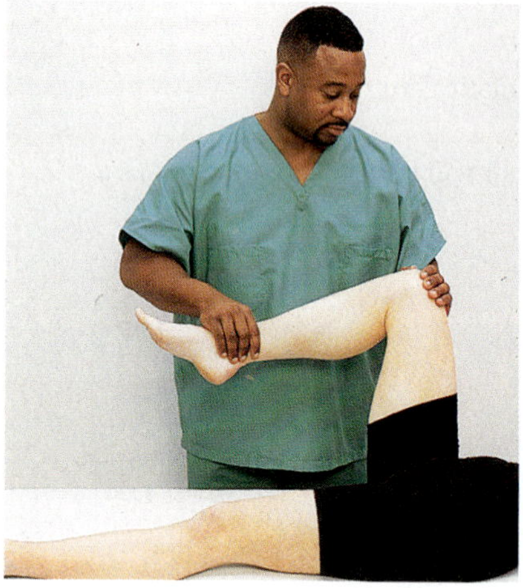

Figure 47-6 Obturator muscle test.

enlargement. Stomach contents often conceal the dull sound produced when percussing the spleen.

If the patient is suspected of having abdominal ascites, there are special maneuvers that the nurse can use to determine fluid in the abdomen. The first is the fluid wave. Shifting dullness is the second maneuver to test for ascites. With the patient lying supine, percuss over the top of the abdomen, this should elicit a tympany; moving down the side to the area of fluid should elicit a dull sound. Turn the patient onto his or her right side, the fluid will shift right. Percuss the upper left side of the abdomen, and tympany should be elicited; continue downward and the sound should change to dull at the level of the fluid shift.

Palpation

To assess the abdomen with palpation, first use light or gentle palpation. Assess each quadrant of the abdomen. This first pass is a scouting expedition that provides the nurse with information about any areas of tenderness or increased resistance.

Light Palpation

To perform light (gentle) palpation, place the palm of the hand lightly and firmly on the abdomen, gently press the fingers into the abdominal wall about 1 cm. If the patient is ticklish, have the patient place his or her fingers on top of your fingers. Often this reduces the ticklishness. Note any areas of tenderness. Areas of tenderness will require more careful assessment once the gentle palpation is completed.

Deep Palpation

Deep palpation involves using the pads and tips (most sensitive areas) of the index, middle, and ring fingers. The motion should be downward (depth of 4 to 5 cm), and the finger pads should move backward and forward to cause the abdominal wall to glide over the structures under the targeted area. To palpate the liver, bimanual palpitation is recommended. The right hand is inserted under the right rib margin. The left hand is placed under the right lower thorax. While the patient is taking a deep breath, the right hand is moved upward and inward. With the left hand move the right thorax upward. The lower margin of the liver will be palpated. It is unusual to be able to palpate the gallbladder. It lies on the posterior surface of the liver just right of the midclavicular line. When the gallbladder is inflamed, it is exquisitely tender. It is important to assess for Murphy's sign, where the patient is asked to breathe in while the examiners fingers are held under the liver border. This allows the gallbladder to descend. **Murphy's sign** is when the patient will guard the movement by an inspiratory arrest secondary to painful contact with the fingers, which confirms cholecystitis (inflamed gallbladder).

During the deep palpation, if any mass or enlargement is noted, the nurse should collect the following information: location, size, shape, surface, consistency (soft, hard, firm, spongy, or nodular), movement, pulsatile, pain, tenderness, and whether the mass is reducible.

Liver

Normally the liver does not descend beyond 1 to 2 cm of the costal margin and is not palpable. There are two methods to assess the liver. The nurse must use deep bimanual palpation to determine liver size. With the patient taking a deep breath, the nurse holds his or her fingers pointing up and parallel to the rectus muscles. The nurse pushes in and up toward the costal margin. The second method is for the nurse to place the right hand under the patient at about the 12th rib. With this hand, the nurse pushes upward. At the same time, the left hand is placed parallel to the rectus muscles with fingers pointing up toward the costal margin. The patient is asked to take a deep breath, and the nurse presses upward and inward. If the liver is palpable, the nurse will feel the liver roll (slip) under the palpating fingers.

Gallbladder

The gallbladder sits posterior to the liver. It is not palpable. Assessment of the gallbladder will be more appropriate taking an accurate history of the potential symptoms the patient has with dysfunction. For example, patients with gallbladder dysfunction may have upper epigastric pain, fatty food intolerance, and nausea.

Spleen

The spleen is not normally palpable. If the spleen is felt, it is softer than the liver. If it is enlarged, it must be measured in centimeters below the costal margin. Because a spleen can be damaged, especially if enlarged, the palpation should be done carefully. The nurse stands on the right side of the patient. With the left hand around the back of the patient, the nurse lifts the left rib cage to push the spleen forward. With the right hand, the nurse asks the patient to take in a deep breath and gently pushes in and up toward the left costal margin.

Pancreas

The pancreas is not palpable. Patients with dysfunction of the pancreas will likely have a supporting history of clinical manifestations related to the etiology of the disorder (e.g., alcoholism or cancer).

Kidneys and Urinary Bladder

To palpate the right kidney, the nurse places his or her left hand under the right flank while lifting forward in an attempt to push the kidney toward the anterior wall. With the right hand, the nurse deeply palpates the anterior wall just below the right costal margin while the patient takes a deep breath. The left kidney is rarely palpable but is palpated the same as the right kidney.

To assess the bladder, the patient should be asked to empty the bladder prior to the assessment. In addition, palpation is light in nature, and the nurse must pay attention to privacy and instruct the patient to relax during the assessment.

Real World, Real Choices

Abdominal Pain, Unknown Etiology

Mrs. Cynthia Reyes is a 56-year-old female, who is admitted to the medical floor due to blood in the stool and abdominal pain for three days. She is primarily going to be assessed with a variety of laboratory and diagnostic tests. A review of systems reveals bowel habit changes, loss of appetite, weight loss greater than 10 pounds, and fatigue for two months. Mrs. Reyes past medical history includes primary hypertension, obesity, GERD, and constipation. The patient's medications include hydrochlorothiazide (HCTZ) 25 mg by mouth every day, omeprazole 20 mg by mouth every day as needed, and Metamucil as needed. The patient's nutritional intake is usually high in fat, low in fiber, and less than two servings of fruits and vegetables per day. Her fluid intake consists primarily of sodas, tea or coffee, and possibly two cups of water per day. Mrs. Reyes' activity is sedentary, and her social history includes working as a clerical assistant for 25 years. She has been smoking cigarettes for 20 years, has an occasional alcohol intake of two to three drinks per week, and denies the use of illicit drugs.

An assessment of Mrs. Reyes reveals that she has GI bleeding and recent history of abdominal pain. Her vital signs are: temperature 36.8° C (98.2° F), pulse 69, respiration 18, and blood pressure 112/56. Bowel sounds normal on four quadrants; tympanic to percussion; no costovertebral angle (CVA) tenderness; pain elicited on palpation of left lower quadrant; palpable mass noted on left lower quadrant area. Patient's skin color is pink and has good turgor. Rectal exam reveals 3-by-4-cm palpable lesion with stool positive for occult blood. Neurological system shows patient to be awake, alert, and oriented for three hours. A psychosocial assessment reveals her to appear nervous, crying, and fearful; patient states she has not been in the hospital since her husband died 10 years ago.

What would your nursing care plan be for Mrs. Reyes?

Umbilicus

Normally the umbilicus is midway between the xyphoid process and the pubis. During the assessment, the nurse should note the shape of the umbilicus. It can be round, oval, recessed, or protruding. An umbilical hernia will be noted during the assessment. With the patient lying supine, the nurse should ask him or her to raise his or her head and shoulder off the examining table. This maneuver contracts the rectus muscles. Normally the abdomen remains symmetrical. If a bulge appears in the midline, the patient may have diastasis recti, a separation of the layers of the muscle.

Referred Pain from Abdominal Structures

There is often pain that is referred from abdominal structures (see Figure 47-2). An assessment of the perianal area (anus and rectosigmoid structures) can reveal such pain. With the patient in a lateral position, a lithotomy (knee-chest) position, or standing position, the nurse visually inspects the area. Both the right and left buttocks are spread to observe the area. The skin around the anus is a dark reddish brown. Note if the skin is intact. Any abnormalities can be described using the face of a clock for location. The anal canal is 2.5 to 4 cm. long. It is surrounded by an external sphincter and internal sphincter. Visually inspect for any external hemorrhoids. Have the patient bear down. There should be no prolapse of any rectal tissue during this maneuver. The pilonidal area (sacrococcygeal) should be carefully inspected and palpated. There should be no edema, induration, or dimpling. With a gloved hand the nurse should place the lubricated finger against the anal verge. Apply firm pressure until you feel the rectal sphincter begin to relax. Slowly insert one finger in the direction of the umbilicus. Insert the pad of the finger first and rotate to introduce the tip of the finger. Continue to rotate the finger to assess the muscular ring of the anal canal. The mucosal surface should feel smooth. Palpate the anal canal and rectum up to about 8 to 10 cm. The nurse should explain to the patient that he or she may feel as if having a bowel movement.

DIAGNOSTIC TESTS

There are a wide variety of diagnostic tests performed for GI disorders. A wide variety of hematological blood tests can be used to confirm areas within the GI tract or accessory organs. These labs can be referred to in laboratory and diagnostic texts, such as that by Daniels (2003). The more common procedures will be covered, such as bowel preparations, nasogastric intubations, feeding tubes, and barium studies. Ensuring quality nursing care, following good nursing education principles, and applying therapeutic communication skills is essential for the patient undergoing diagnostic tests for the GI system (see Ethics in Practice feature).

In addition, when performing many GI procedures, it is standard that the patient is sedated. The technique used today is conscious sedation and is often managed by the nurse in the gastroenterology procedures lab. The nurse who manages conscious sedation has received additional education to manage the patient receiving these agents. These patients are at risk for cardiorespiratory complications from sedation that depresses the central cardiorespiratory center. Patients receiving conscious sedation are usually able to respond to verbal commands throughout the procedure. They can communicate discomfort, and they respond to light tactile stimulation. Airway patency is maintained, and spontaneous ventilation must be satisfactory to maintain adequate oxygenation. To ensure this patients are monitored with pulse oximetry (SpO_2—arterial oxyhemoglobin saturation), a necessary vital sign. The National Guidelines Clearinghouse has established guidelines for patients undergoing conscious sedation. A brief period of amnesia that erases any memory of the

Red Flag

Enema Administration

Patients with severe abdominal pain, ulcerative colitis, or a history of megacolon should have a written order before enemas can be administered, because these conditions would normally prohibit the use of standard bowel preparation procedures, such as administration of laxatives and cleansing enemas.

ETHICS IN PRACTICE

Hepatitis Risks

A 29-year-old man who recently emigrated from a third world country is seeking follow-up care for abdominal pain. On the first visit, you completed his health history and physical examination and obtained laboratory data. Your clinical suspicion is confirmed; the results of the lab tests show that he has hepatitis B. This man is sexually active with his wife. You inform him that it is important that his wife be clinically evaluated. He tells you that he will not have health care insurance for her through his job until next year, and it is too expensive for her to be seen until then. How would you respond? What information would you give to him?

procedure occurs with the use of conscious sedation. Patients should be made aware of this prior to the procedure.

Colonoscopy

Bowel cleansing is necessary for all colonoscopy procedures. The bowel preparation selected depends on the reasons for the procedure. It is important for the nurse to reinforce the importance of following the preparation as ordered by the provider. An adequate procedure cannot be done without adequate preparation of the bowel. The preparation procedure is rigorous, and the patient may have difficulty drinking the large amount of liquids necessary for a complete preparation, but it is essential.

If a clear view of the bowel mucosa is necessary, polyethylene glycol, an electrolyte solution (PEG-ES) is used. The patient is placed on a clear liquid diet for 24 hours prior to the procedure. The polyethylene glycol solution (GoLYTELY and CoLyte) is administered the day before the procedure. It is mixed in a one gallon container and refrigerated. An 8-ounce glass of the preparation is ingested rapidly every 10 minutes until the patient has taken the entire amount. Within about one hour of beginning the preparation, the patient will begin to have bowel movements. The stool will become watery, clear, and free of any solid material.

A second preparation material used is Fleet's phospho-soda. This preparation is also used for colonoscopy. The patient takes two 1.5-ounce doses of the laxative. The first dose is taken in the afternoon before the procedure, followed by 10 ounces of clear liquid and then three to five additional glasses of clear liquids prior to going to bed. Before bedtime, the patient should take the second 1.5 ounces of the Fleet's phospho-soda with the same amount of clear liquid or as directed.

Small-volume enemas may be necessary in the bowel preparation prior to the colonoscopy (or other diagnostic procedures of the bowel). The enema may be self-administered and is available OTC. Advise the patient to use the enema as the instructions on the package indicate.

A pill-based enema preparation is also available. Visicol (sodium phosphate monobasic monohydrate, USP; sodium phosphate dibasic anhydrous, USP). It is a laxative that is used for bowel preparation. Twenty pills are taken over a one-hour period the afternoon before the procedure. At bedtime, the physician may order up to eight more tablets, four at a time every 15 minutes with 8 ounces of water. Dulcolax (bisacodyl USP) tablets, a laxative, may be added to complcte this regimen.

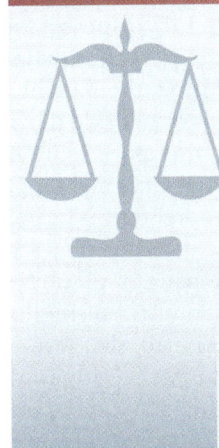

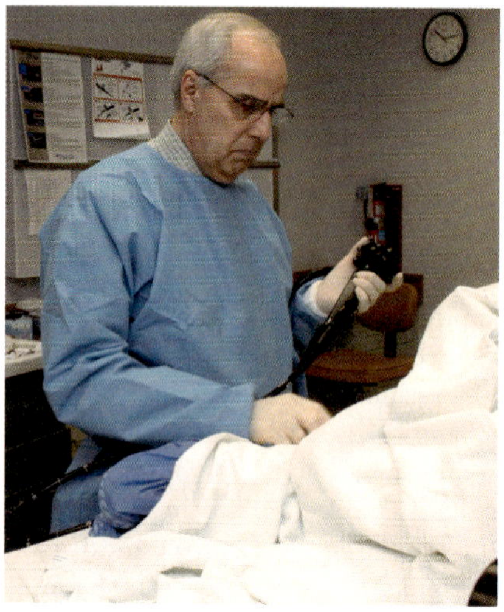

Figure 47-7 A colonoscopy in use to examine the bowel.

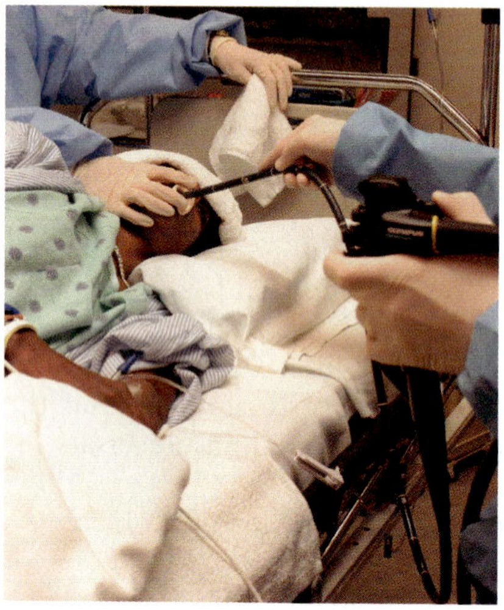

Figure 47-8 An upper endoscopy.

Continuing with bowel preparation, the patient should take nothing by mouth (NPO) for six hours prior to the actual procedure. Some medications may be taken with a sip of water, but the patient must confirm this with the provider. During the procedure itself, the patient may be consciously sedated. In addition, the patient is kept on his or her side during the procedure or positioned in a manner to keep the scope inserted (Figure 47-7). After the procedure, the patient is monitored for a return to a normal LOC and the ability to be discharged.

Patients may not have to undergo bowel preparation if they are being worked-up for chronic diarrhea. For an upper endoscopy, esophagogastroduodenoscopy (EGD), the patient will be NPO. If a patient is undergoing a 24-hour pH study of gastric contents, all medications that suppress gastric secretions would be stopped prior to the test. A patient who is undergoing capsule endoscopy is kept NPO just as with an EGD. During the procedure, the patient is usually managed with conscious sedation until it is finished (Figure 47-8). After the procedure, the patient is usually allowed liquids and food as tolerated.

Laparoscopy

Laparoscopy is a diagnostic procedure where the peritoneal cavity, pelvis and abdomen, is examined. This test is used to detect cysts, adhesions, fibroids, infections of the uterus, fallopian tubes, and ovaries; ectopic pregnancies, liver lacerations, and cirrhosis. The test may also be used for lysis of adhesions, ovarian biopsy, tubal sterilization, foreign body removal, and fulguration of endometriotic implants.

The patient is instructed on fast for eight hours before the surgery; the test is performed either with a local or general anesthetic agent, and the patient is placed in a lithotomy position. Then the patient is catheterized to ensure the bladder is empty, which avoids puncture of the bladder during the test with the laparoscope.

Proctosigmoidoscopy

This is a diagnostic test that takes three steps: (a) digital examination to dilate the anal sphincters to detect obstruction that might hinder passage of the endoscope, (b) a sigmoidoscope to examine the distal sigmoid colon and rectum, and (c) a proctoscope to examine the lower rectum and anal canal. The proctosigmoidoscopy is used to identify internal hemorrhoids, hypertrophic anal papillae, polyps, fissures, fistulae, and rectal and anal abscesses.

The patient is instructed on dietary restrictions and bowel preparations on an individual basis. If the patient has rectal inflammation, a local anesthetic agent is applied to decrease discomfort. Conscious sedation is often used. The patient is secured to a tilting table that rotates into horizontal and vertical positions.

Paracentesis

Paracentesis is the aspiration of fluid from the abdominal cavity. This test can either be diagnostic, therapeutic, or both. For instance, with end-stage liver or renal disease there is ascites (an accumulation of fluid in the abdomen). Pressure caused from the ascites can interfere with breathing and GI functioning. Aspiration in this instance is therapeutic. If a culture specimen is obtained, it is also diagnostic.

Have the patient void and obtain a body weight before the procedure. Place the patient in a high Fowler's position in a chair or sitting on the side of the bed. The skin is prepared, anesthetized, and punctured with a **trocar** (a large bored abdominal paracentesis needle). The trocar is held perpendicular to the abdominal wall and advanced into the peritoneal cavity. When fluid appears, the trocar is removed, leaving the inner catheter in place to drain the fluid. Observe the patient for pressure changes that can result from the rapid removal of fluid.

Postprocedure apply a sterile dressing to the puncture site. Monitor the patient for changes in vital signs and electrolytes. Instruct the patient to record the color, amount, and consistency of drainage on the dressing after discharge.

Nasogastric Tubes

A nasogastric tube can be inserted orally but is most often inserted nasally into the stomach. The size and type of tube selected is dependent on the indication. The tube is used for feeding or administration of medications, especially if the patient has impaired swallowing or is not able to ingest sufficient calories, secondary to neurological or other deficits impairing ability to ingest sufficient nutrition. A feeding tube may be placed distal to the pylorus or the ligament of Treitz (nasoduodenal or nasojejunal) if there is risk of gastroesophageal reflux, aspiration, gastroparesis, or other reasons to bypass the stomach.

In addition, a nasogastric tube provides a method for performing a **lavage** (the irrigation or washing out of the stomach contents). Patients may need to have this procedure performed after swallowing poisons, medications, and toxic substances.

Decompression of the stomach is performed to prevent vomiting or reduction of pancreatic or biliary stimulation especially if the patient has acute pancreatitis or if the patient persistently has gastric residual volumes greater 400 mL.

Esophageal Manometry

Esophageal manometry is a test that measures the pressure and activity of the esophagus in patients who exhibit esophageal motility problems. It is done with patients who have dysphagia, achalasia (cardiospasm), GERD, to exclude scleroderma, or for placement of a pH probe for 24-hour esophageal pH monitoring.

Secretin Testing

Secretin testing is used to determine if a patient has incipient chronic pancreatitis. It is indicated for patients with abdominal pain, weight loss, steatorrhea, or recurrent pancreatitis. The tube used is a Dreiling tube. It is a double-lumen tube with ports in the gastric and duodenal regions. The tube is inserted into the stomach and positioned so that the distal portion is past the ligament of Treitz. Once in place, aspirate is obtained from both the duodenal and gastric port. The pH of the gastric aspirate is checked. The gastric port is aspirated until there is no return of gastric contents. The duodenal aspirate is sent to the lab for cytology and HCO^{-}_{3} levels. A test dose of secretin is administered intravenously to rule out an allergic response. If the allergic response is negative, the full dose is administered. Once the dose is administered, a duodenal aspirate is collected every 20 minutes for a total of four samples. A portion of the sample is placed into a collection tube for HCO^{-}_{3} levels and placed on ice. The remaining fluid is pooled and sent for cytology.

The diagnostic results reveal cytology that should be negative. If positive, pancreatic cancer is suspected. If the HCO^{-}_{3} is less than 90 mEq/L in all samples and the total volume is greater than or equal to 2 mL/kg the diagnosis is chronic pancreatitis.

Equipment for Gastric and Intestinal Intubation

The selection of the tube to use for oral and nasal gastric and intestinal intubation depends on the reason the patient needs the tube to be inserted. Other items needed are water and a straw to drink, emesis basin and towel, tongue blade, water-soluble lubricant and sometimes lidocaine jelly or atomized lidocaine to reduce pain during insertion, irrigating syringe, scissors, tape (Hy-

Tape, the original Pink Tape is recommended) or appropriate dressing to secure tube, and stethoscope to check for gastric insufflation.

Gastric decompression tubes (e.g., Salem Sump tube) are polyvinyl chloride tubes in both adult and pediatric sizes; measured in French diameters (10-, 12-, 14-, 16-Fr diameter). This tube has a double lumen; one is for suction of the gastric contents while the other is for the sump vent. The purpose of the sump vent is to allow air to prevent the main suction tube from adhering to the gastric mucosa or irritating the mucosal wall. This tube has a radiopaque line that allows for visualization of placement with a postplacement X-ray.

Gastric lavage tubes (e.g., Ewald) are large-bore 34-Fr outer diameter tubes used to irrigate the esophagus or the stomach with large volumes of irrigant solution. This tube is used when the aim is to remove particulate matter, e.g., bezoars, clots, or ingested toxins.

Intestinal decompression tubes (e.g., Andersen, Miller-Abbott) are tubes used to decompress the small intestine in the early management of mechanical obstruction without strangulation (Gowen, 2003). These tubes have a tungsten weighted inflatable latex balloon tip. The tubes have 24 aspiration ports designed to screen out material that could block the tubes. The tubes advance via peristaltic movement. Enough slack must be allowed so the tubes can advance. The tubes should not be fixed to the nostril until they have reached their placement point. There may be an order for a prokinetic medication, like metoclopramide or erythromycin, to enhance peristalsis. Distension of the stomach with injection of 350 to 1,000 mL of air can also enhance movement of the tubes.

Potentially these tubes can cause necrosis to the mucosal wall if they are not allowed to move with the peristaltic wave. These tubes are removed at 30-minute intervals, 30 cm at a time. Additionally the weighted tip can pass through the rectum. The capsule section is cut off, and the tube is removed according to instructions. Endoscopic placement is useful in any patient that has any problem that might obstruct easy access through the nasopharynx and esophagus into the stomach.

Wire-guided tube placement enhances the advancement of a nasogastric, nasoduodenal, or nasojejunal tube. A hazard of the wire-guided tube less than 4 mm is that it could potentially penetrate the trachea, perforate a bronchus, and enter the pleural space with minimal resistance. Feeding tubes with weighted tips have been used to enhance movement through the pylorus into the duodenum; however, evidence now indicates that a weighted tip is unnecessary (Marik & Zaloga, 2003).

Patient Preparation for Nasogastric and Nasointestinal Intubation

The nurse explains the procedure to the patient, why the tube is to be inserted, and how long it is anticipated that the tube will remain in place. The patient is kept NPO prior to the procedure (see Patient Playbook feature).

Contraindications and Complications

Contraindications for placement of nasogastric tubes are seen in patients with trauma to the maxillofacial structures or those suspected of possible basal skull fracture.

Complications for placement of nasogastric tubes include trauma that could occur during insertion or removal of the tube. This might be nasal, pharyngeal, laryngeal, esophageal, or gastric trauma or perforation. In the event a tube was inserted in a patient with maxillofacial trauma, intracranial penetration might occur.

In addition, while a nasogastric tube is in place patients might experience pulmonary aspiration, mucosal ulceration or irritation, and fluid and electrolyte imbalance.

PATIENT PLAYBOOK

Insertion of a Nasogastric Tube

- Ask the patient if he has ever had a nasogastric tube inserted before.
- Determine if there is any nasal obstruction or maxillofacial trauma.
- While holding closed one nostril, ask patient to inhale strongly through each nostril. Use the nostril that appears more patent.
- Check the gag reflex. A patient without a gag reflex is at risk for pulmonary aspiration.
- Procedure:
  - Have the patient sit upright (raise the head of the bed). If the patient is not able to cooperate, place the patient in a left lateral position. (This position decreases the risk of pulmonary aspiration.)
  - Placement of the tube depends on the purpose for the tube and the destination.
  - Estimate the length of tube to be inserted One formula suggested for determining length of insertion is the following formula which is (NEX − 50)/2 + 50 cm, where N is the shortest distance from the nose (N) to the earlobe (E) to the xyphoid (X) process. The insertion should be halfway between 50 cm and the xyphoid mark.
  - Lubricate the tube, have patient hold head down, insert tube horizontally to avoid abrading the turbinates. When the tip is at the pharyngeal wall, have patient sip water (dry swallow if NPO) as the tube is advanced. For the patient, this is the most uncomfortable part of the procedure. If the nurse meets resistance, withdraw the tube and retry. Do *not* force the tube. If the patient coughs, becomes cyanotic, or is unable to speak, remove the tube as it may have entered the trachea.
  - Steps to prevent the tube from entering the trachea must be taken in any situation where the patient cannot swallow on request, has an endotracheal tube in place, or a tracheostomy. These patients are at greater risk for inadvertent tracheal placement of the nasogastric tube. It has been reported that 2 percent of patients who have small-bore feeding tubes placed, enter the trachea with major complications occurring in 0.7 percent and death in 0.2 percent (Angus & Burakoff, 2003).
  - While advancing the tube the nurse must observe for cough or hoarseness.
  - Advance the tube to the predetermined length, checking periodically to see if the tube has coiled in the pharynx or mouth.
  - To determine if the tube may have entered the trachea, place the end of the tube under water to observe for air bubbles. Another technique is to inject air into the port and auscultate the stomach to listen for the rush of air (gastric insufflation) into the stomach. A technique not often used is to sample for CO_2 from the tube. Unfortunately, these techniques are not as sensitive as endoscopic placement or radiographic guidance. If the tube is in the trachea, advancing the tube for proper stomach length 40 to 45 cm will cause lung injury.
  - Confirm proper placement of the tube with a postinsertion X-ray. Aspirate the stomach contents and assess pH. A pH less than 4 indicates the aspirate is from stomach contents unless the patient is receiving proton-pump inhibitors.
  - If the tube is to advance into the duodenum, the patient should be placed in the right decubitus position for several hours. Tape the tube with 20 to 30 cm of slack to allow for the tube to advance via peristalsis. If the tube is to advance to the jejunum, after the slack is gone, have patient lie on his or her back and then left decubitus position to encourage movement of the tube into the jejunum.
  - If the position of the tube is assessed fluoroscopically, irrigate the tube to remove any contrast material and to maintain patency of the tube.

Adapted from Estes, M. (2006). Health assessment and physical examination *(3rd ed.). New York: Thomson Delmar Learning.*

Esophageal Dilation

Esophageal dilation is performed when a patient experiences peptic strictures often related to GERD. Another cause of esophageal stricture can be radiation, which is labeled Schatzki's ring. Treatment of these esophageal conditions is often an esophageal dilation procedure, which entails widening of the stricture with dilators, called bougies, of graded sizes (Price, 2004).

Preprocedure preparation includes NPO for six to eight hours. The patient may have conscious sedation, but most often only the pharynx is anesthetized with a topical agent. The procedure is usually done with three sequential dilators. The goal of the procedure is to relieve the difficulty the patient has with swallowing.

Feeding Tubes: Gastrostomy and Jejunostomy

Feeding tubes are placed when a patient is unable to manage his or her needed nutritional intake. Patients require 25 to 30 kcal/kg/day and 30 mL free water/kg/day. The American Society of Parenteral and Enteral Nutrition (ASPEN) maintains guidelines for the indications and use of feeding tubes. The National Guideline Clearinghouse maintains guidelines for the administration of specialized nutrition support as developed by ASPEN. The American Gastroenterological Association (AGA) endorses the use of percutaneous endoscopic gastrostomy tubes for prolonged tube feeding (more than 30 days) and nasogastric feeding when enteral feeding is needed for shorter time periods. The decision to use a nasoduodenal or nasojejunal tube is made if there is a risk of aspiration, GERD, or other reasons to bypass the stomach, e.g., acute pancreatitis. The route to use for enteral nutrition is based on the length of therapy as well as patient comfort.

Patient Preparation

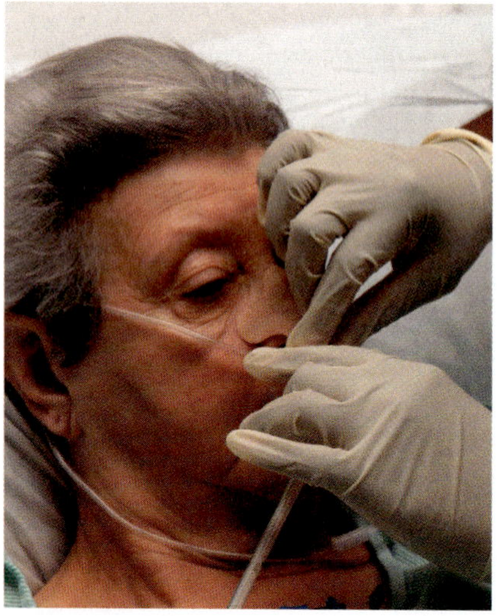
Figure 47-9 A nurse taping a nasogastric tube in place.

If the feeding tube will be used for less than 30 days, select a nasogastric tube in the range of 8-Fr to 18-Fr. A larger bore nasogastric tube allows for suction if needed. Smaller tubes, 8-Fr to 12-Fr, are used for intestinal feeding (duodenal and jejunal). Whatever feeding tube is used, the nurse should read the package insert for the tube used and keep the insert in the patient's chart for reference for others. Complete documentation of time of placement and the length of tube inserted should be done. If the tube is advanced with peristalsis, each time the patient is assessed, the nurse should note the length of tube that is in the patient. A follow-up X-ray is done to check placement of the film and at 12-hour intervals to check for progression. The patient should be prepared by describing the reasons for the tube to be placed as well as the procedure for the intubation. There are times when the insertion of the tube must be done fluoroscopically. Once the tube is in place, it must be carefully taped, and the tube marked with a permanent marker in the event the tube slips out, it will be noted visually (Figure 47-9). Evidence has demonstrated that Hy-Tape, The Original Pink Tape, a unique water-resistant and washable tape is especially suited for securing feeding tubes.

Patients with feeding tubes are at high risk for regurgitation and aspiration of gastric contents as well as oropharyngeal secretions. Other complications include bronchopulmonary injury from inadvertent placement of the feeding tube in the lung, perforation of the GI tract, erosion of the mucosal surface of the nasopharynx, and vocal cord paralysis. A small-bore tube tip can penetrate the brain, especially if the patient has a maxillofacial injury. These small-bore tubes can also knot in the stomach. When the tube is removed, the knot can damage the esophagus or nasopharynx (Noble, 2003).

Feeding tubes can become clogged. This occurs with the use of small-bore tubes, tubes made of silicone, medication that is not crushed sufficiently, medication and tube feeding formula incompatibility, formula and gastric acid precipitation, microbial contamination, and inadequate flushing of the tube. Evidence indicates the most effective method of maintaining patency of a feeding tube is routine flushing with water. To restore patency to a clogged tube it is recommended that pancreatic enzyme solutions be used (Keithley & Swanson, 2004).

Nasopharyngeal discomfort in patients with nasogastric or nasoenteric tubes can be mitigated by allowing the patient an occasional ice chip or using artificial saliva. If the patient needs a nasal tube for longer than 6 weeks, the tube should be replaced and the opposite nostril should be utilized for the replacement tube. To reduce mucosal damage and potential scarring and stricture, the smallest bore tube should be selected for the purpose.

Percutaneous Endoscopic Gastrostomy and Percutaneous Endoscopic Jejunostomy Tubes

A most important decision in determining whether a percutaneous endoscopic gastrostomy (PEG) or percutaneous endoscopic jejunostomy (PEJ) tube is inserted is to evaluate whether there is outcome data related to the underlying illness of the patient. Providers, other health care professionals, patients, and families should be knowledgeable of the benefits as well as the burdens associated with long-term enteral feeding (Calgary Health Region, 2004; Stroud, Duncan, & Nightingale, 2003). PEG tubes have become the procedure of choice for enteral nutrition in the United States. Recent recommendations are that PEG tubes should only be placed in conditions in which the patient can benefit (Plonk, 2005). These are limited and include early head and neck cancer, amyotrophic lateral sclerosis, malignant bowel obstruction with intractable vomiting, and acute stroke with dysphagia persisting for 30 days after hospital discharge.

Complications from the use of PEG or PEJ tubes include infection at the insertion site, fistula formation, peritonitis, sepsis, and necrotizing fasciitis. Of great concern is the high mortality rate, 20 to 40 percent, within one month of PEG or PEJ insertion (Stroud, et al., 2003).

With all enteral feeding, patients may experience nausea, abdominal bloating, and cramps from delayed gastric emptying. It is recommended that patients receive continuous feeding rather than bolus feedings. If needed, prokinetic agents (e.g., erythromycin or metoclopramide) are used to hasten gastric emptying and reduce GI discomfort.

Skills 360°

Communication Regarding Ingestion of the Barium Sulfate

The oral solution of barium sulfate comes in flavored forms, and these have been improved as to their tastes over the past several years. The nurse must learn to communicate carefully that the solution is not as distasteful as it once was. However, the barium sulfate is still somewhat disliked by patients, but the nurse must learn to communicate the reality of the solution, while at the same time not being too negative about its taste.

Adapted from Daniels, R. (2003). Delmar's manual of laboratory and diagnostic tests. *New York: Thomson Delmar Learning.*

Barium Studies

Barium (chalky white contrast medium) is an oral preparation that allows roentgenographic visualization of the internal structures of the digestive tract. The results of barium studies can reveal congenital abnormalities; lesions; spasm; reflux, stricture, and obstruction; inflammation; and ulceration; varices; and fistula. General patient preparation for barium studies should include:

- Placing the patient on NPO status after midnight.
- Administering a laxative the evening before and enemas the morning of the test.
- Forcing fluid postprocedure.
- Follow-up two to three days postprocedure to ensure the patient has had a normal brown stool.

Postprocedure barium will be expelled in the stool, making it milky white. Fluids are forced to help with the excretion of barium. If the barium is not completely excreted, it can cause intestinal obstruction.

Barium Swallow

Barium swallow (esophagraphy) is a fluoroscopic visualization of the esophagus following the ingestion of barium sulfate. Implement the nursing care discussed above for a patient with a barium study.

PATIENT PLAYBOOK

Instructions for a Barium Enema

The nurse instructs the patient:

- To eat a low-residue diet two days prior to the test.
- That during the procedure various positions will need to be assumed on the table to facilitate movement of the barium in the intestines.
- That the test will take about one hour.
- That the postprocedure cleansing enemas will be given to help remove the barium.

Adapted from Estes, M. (2006). Health assessment and physical examination *(3rd ed.). New York: Thomson Delmar Learning.*

Upper GI Study

Upper GI (UGI) is a fluoroscopic visualization of the stomach and small bowel following the ingestion of barium sulfate. In addition to the general preparation of the patient for a barium study, also instruct the patient that:

- He or she should not smoke for 24 hours prior to the procedure (smoking causes an increased production of gastric juices).
- During the procedure (which will last approximately two hours), pictures will be taken at 30-minute intervals with the patient in different positions.

Barium Enema

Barium enema (a rectal infusion of barium sulfate) is the roentgenographic study of the lower intestinal tract. The colon should be free of all fecal material to allow for maximum visualization (see Patient Playbook feature).

KEY CONCEPTS

- The major organs of the GI tract include the intestinal tract, the hollow organs from the mouth to the anus.
- The mouth, lips, cheeks, tongue, and pharynx aid in chewing, mastication and moving food and fluid into the esophagus.
- The abdominal health history provides the nurse with important subjective information that assists in the physical assessment of the abdomen.
- Leading symptoms and complaints from patients with GI disorders include heartburn, dysphagia (difficulty in swallowing), dyspepsia, nausea and vomiting, gas, diarrhea, constipation, pain, and bleeding.
- Dyspepsia is the most common symptom that patients complain about to their health care provider.
- Diarrhea can be acute, self-limiting, a life-threatening event, or chronic.
- Constipation is marked by straining at stool with the production of hard stools, decreased frequency, and a feeling of not completely evacuating the colon.
- Abdominal pain is separated into acute and chronic.
- There is often pain that is referred from abdominal structures and an assessment of the perianal area can reveal such pain.
- There are a wide variety of diagnostic tests performed for GI disorders.
- Adequate bowel preparation is necessary for all GI procedures.
- The laparoscopy is a diagnostic procedure in which the peritoneal cavity, pelvis and abdomen, is examined.
- Paracentesis is the aspiration of fluid from the abdominal cavity.
- Esophageal dilation is performed when a patient experiences peptic strictures often related to GERD.
- Barium (chalky white contrast medium) is an oral preparation that allows roentgenographic visualization of the internal structures of the digestive tract.

REVIEW QUESTIONS

1. What is a product of exocrine glands in the oral cavity that lubricates the mouth and begins the digestive process?
   1. Sweat
   2. Saliva
   3. Tears
   4. Stool

2. Which of the following organs would you expect to find in the left upper quadrant?
   1. Head of the pancreas
   2. Portions of the ascending and transverse colon
   3 Duodenum
   4. Spleen

3. What is acute pain in the abdomen labeled as?
   1. Hematoma
   2. Hypovolemic shock
   3. Acute abdomen
   4. Referred abdominal pain

4. The reason that auscultation is performed first when performing an abdominal assessment is:
   1. It is the quickest part of the assessment process.
   2. It is more convenient and causes less pain for the patient.

Continued

REVIEW QUESTIONS—cont'd

3. It is the easiest skill for the nurse to remember to perform.
4. It does not allow the sounds produced from percussion and palpation to alter what is auscultated.

5. Which of the following is true when assessing the liver?
1. Normally the liver is easily palpated in adults.
2. Normally the liver is percussed 4 to 6 cm above the costal margin.
3. Normally the liver does not descend beyond 1 to 2 cm of the costal margin and is not palpable.
4. Normally the liver sounds hollow on percussion.

6. Which of the following is true of conscious sedation?
1. It is normally only performed for oral surgery.
2. It is difficult to give to a majority of adults, due to the tremendous number of allergic reactions to the anesthesia.
3. It allows patients to respond to verbal commands throughout the procedure.
4. It is best delivered via the rectal route of administration to enhance its absorption.

7. Which of the following assessment techniques is not used to asses for ascites?
1. Fluid wave
2. Murphy's sign
3. Shifting dullness
4. Puddle sign

8. A positive Murphy's sign indicates an inflammatory process associated with:
1. Ascites
2. Appendicitis
3. Cholecystitis
4. Pelvic abscess

9. You have flexed the patient's right leg at the hip and the knee is at a right angle. You then internally and externally rotate the patient's leg and observe the patient's reaction. What is this assessment technique called?
1. Iliopsoas muscle test
2. Obturator muscle test
3. Rovsing's sign
4. Ballottement

10. What is the low-pitched sound that is auscultated in the abdomen and caused by turbulent blood flow?
1. Borborygmi
2. Venous hum
3. Peritoneal friction rub
4. Bruit

11. Secretin testing is used to determine if a patient has:
1. Cholecystitis
2. Gastritis
3. Esophagitis
4. Incipient chronic pancreatitis

REVIEW ACTIVITIES

1. State and describe the organs of the GI tract.

2. Perform a concise GI health history on an adult patient.

3. Describe the physiological processes involved during the act of vomiting.

4. Perform the physical assessment tests to determine if a patient has acute appendicitis.

5. Describe any two of the diagnostic tests used for the abdominal system.

Visit the Contemporary Medical-Surgical Nursing online companion resource at www.delmarhealthcare.com for additional content and study aids. Click on Online Companions then select the Nursing discipline.

Nutrition, Malnutrition, and Obesity: Nursing Management

Ellen K. Fleischman, MBA, RD, RN

CHAPTER 48

KEY TERMS

Anabolism
Catabolism
Chyme
Direct calorimetry
Disaccharides
Indirect calorimetry
Joint Commission on Accreditation of Hospitals (JCAHO)
Macronutrients
Metabolism
Monosaccharides
Peristalsis
Resting energy expenditure

CHAPTER TOPICS

- Normal Nutrition
- Nutrition Support
- Malnutrition
- Obesity

During the 20th century, a shift occurred in the leading cause of death in the United States from infection to chronic disease. Chronic diseases are now responsible for 7 of 10 of the leading causes of death in the United States. The 3 leading causes of *preventable* death according to the Centers for Disease Control are tobacco use, improper diet, and physical inactivity. At least 70 percent of health care spending is on chronic diseases (MMWR, 2004). Nutrition plays a vital role in the prevention and management of chronic diseases, such as diabetes, cardiovascular disease, and cancer, as well as in the prevention of overweight and obesity. According to the American Cancer Society, one third of all cancer deaths in the United States could be prevented by eating a healthy, plant-based diet and maintaining a healthy weight. Nursing care of the medical-surgical patient requires a basic understanding of the physiology involved with nutrition and knowledge of an adequate diet and the interactions between foods and medications, as well as an understanding of the impact of proper nutrition and malnutrition on the health of the patient.

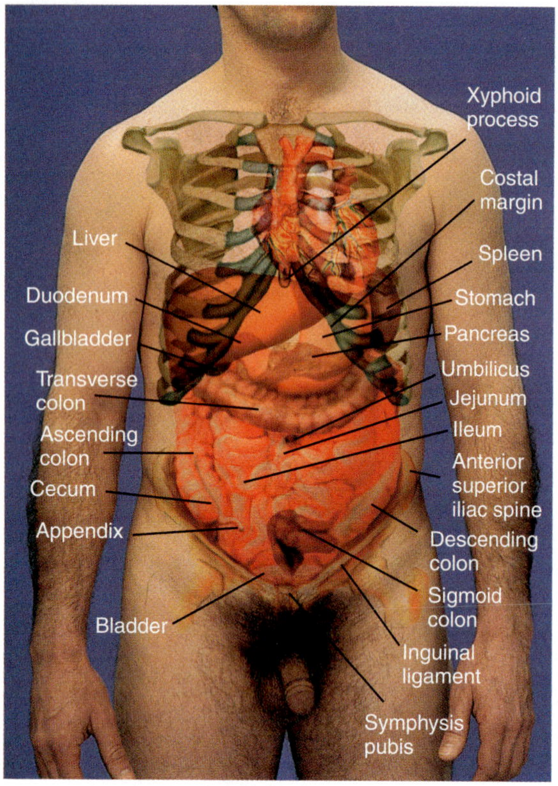

Figure 48-1 The gastrointestinal tract.

THE GASTROINTESTINAL TRACT AND NUTRITIONAL PROCESSES

The gastrointestinal (GI) tract plays a vital role in the nutritional aspects of a person's physiology. Anatomically, the GI tract begins with the mouth and ends with the anus. It includes the oropharyngeal structures, esophagus, stomach, pancreas, liver and gallbladder, small intestine, and large intestine (Figure 48-1). The GI tract is one of the largest organs in the body (Ganong, 2003).

The main functions of the GI tract are to extract and absorb nutrients from foods and beverages people consume, serve as a barrier to microorganisms, and excrete waste products. In addition, the GI tract participates in regulatory, immunological, and metabolic functions.

Processes of Digestion, Absorption, and Metabolism

To digest food and absorb the nutrients the body needs, a person must first process the food eaten. The GI tract converts large particles and molecules into smaller and more easily absorbed components and converts insoluble molecules into soluble ones. The resulting components plus vitamins, minerals, and water cross the intestinal mucosa and are absorbed into the lymph or blood, then delivered to the tissues. Food products end up being broken down into lipids (fats), carbohydrates, and protein. These nutrients are then utilized by the body through **metabolism,** meaning change, in which chemical and energy transformations occur. Nutrition is the source of exogenous compounds needed for metabolism (Ganong, 2003).

Digestion and Absorption

The process of digestion begins in the mouth. The chewing process reduces the size of food particles and saliva moistens the chewed food, preparing it for swallowing. Food and liquid travel from the mouth (oral cavity) down the esophagus to the stomach. In the stomach, food is mixed with acids and enzymes and, as a result, is converted into a liquid substance called **chyme,** as the process of digestion continues. The stomach mixes and churns food, releasing small amounts into the small intestine, where the majority of digestion takes place. The small intestine is divided into the duodenum, jejunum, and ileum. Most digestive processes take place in the duodenum and the upper jejunum, and by the time the food material reaches the middle of the jejunum, absorption of most nutrients has taken place. Starches are broken down to simple sugars by enzymes from the pancreas. Proteins are converted into amino acid chains and single amino acids. Fats are reduced to emulsions that are further broken down into smaller molecules. Secretions from the mouth, stomach, pancreas, small intestine, and gallbladder contribute fluid to the digested material. The majority of this fluid is reabsorbed by the small intestine, along with the remaining **macronutrients,** vitamins, minerals, and trace elements. Most of the remaining fluid is reabsorbed by the large intestine, along with electrolytes and vitamins produced by intestinal bacteria.

Digestion results from mechanical processes, such as teeth grinding and crushing food into small particles, as well as through chemical breakdown of food into molecules that can be absorbed. The process of **peristalsis** moves the food through the GI tract for further digestion and absorption. Absorption of nutrients is a highly complex process involving several mechanisms, including diffusion and active transport.

Carbohydrates

Carbohydrates are consumed in the form of starches; **monosaccharides** (simple sugar molecules) and **disaccharides** (two monosaccharides). The process of starch digestion begins in the mouth, where salivary amylase breaks small amounts of starch into smaller particles. Amylase is deactivated when it reaches the acidic environment of the stomach, and most carbohydrate digestion is completed in the small intestine. Pancreatic amylase breaks large starch molecules into smaller ones, and eventually starch is converted to glucose. Enzymes in the small intestine break down sugar molecules, such as disaccharides into monosaccharides. Monosaccharides are carried through the cells in the intestinal mucosa and into the bloodstream to the liver. Some glucose, a monosaccharide, is stored in the liver and muscles as glycogen, and the rest is carried from the liver to the tissues. Some carbohydrates, pectin, cellulose, hemicellulose, and fiber cannot be digested by the human body, because people are unable to break down certain linkages. These indigestible compounds provide bulk to the stool and assist in the process of elimination.

Proteins

Protein digestion begins in the stomach, where it is broken into smaller molecules called peptides. Further digestion of protein takes place in the small intestine, where peptides are hydrolyzed by enzymes into amino acids. Amino acids are absorbed via active transport and are carried to the liver for metabolism, then released into the circulation.

Lipids (Fats)

Lipids are consumed in the form of triglycerides, phospholipids, and cholesterol. Small amounts of lipids are digested in the mouth by an enzyme, called lingual lipase, and in the stomach by an enzyme, called gastric lipase. Most fat digestion takes place in the small intestine through the action of pancreatic lipase. Fat stimulates the release of hormones, such as cholecystokinin and enterogastrone, which inhibit gastric secretions and slow the motility of food from the stomach to the small intestine. In the small intestine peristalsis breaks large fat molecules into smaller ones, and bile, released by the gallbladder, helps to separate the fat molecules. Lipid molecules in various forms are transported by carrier proteins through the bloodstream to the adipose (fat) tissue, liver, and muscle.

Metabolism

Carbohydrates are transported to the liver in the form of glucose via the portal vein. This process stimulates insulin secretion from the pancreas. In a nondiabetic patient, insulin secretion is adequate to facilitate the process of glucose uptake into tissue cells. If carbohydrate intake is higher than what is needed for energy and storage in the liver and muscle, it is converted to fat for storage in the adipose tissue.

In healthy people, proteins in muscle and throughout the body are kept in balance as they are broken down and synthesized. Amino acids obtained through the digestion of protein intake replace protein stores, provide energy, and what is not needed is excreted in the urine, feces, and through the skin.

Fat is taken to the liver from various sources. The liver repackages the fat onto a carrier protein for transport. Cholesterol is used by cells as part of their cell membrane and by the liver to make bile acids. Fat is used to help hold body organs in place and protect them from trauma and also to insulate the body and thereby maintain body temperature. Fat is also used to transport digesting substances and fat-soluble vitamins, to aid absorption, and for energy. It is stored in the adipose tissue (Ganong, 2003).

COMPONENTS OF A NUTRITIONALLY ADEQUATE DIET

A nutritionally adequate diet is one that meets the needs of the individual at any particular stage of his or her life cycle. For example, a growing child will require more calories and different nutrients than an elderly person. In addition, a nutritionally adequate diet will support vital body systems, support a healthy weight and body composition, and help prevent chronic disease. According to the American Dietetic Association all foods can fit in a healthful diet if the portion sizes are appropriate, foods are consumed in moderation, and regular physical activity is maintained.

The first recommendations for nutrition were established by the Food and Nutrition Board of the National Academies in 1941. The recommended dietary allowances (RDAs) for vitamins, minerals, protein, and energy were developed because of wartime concern for adequate nutrition in military troops. Since that time, the RDAs have been used as a guide on which federal and state nutrition programs have been continually revised (Institute of Medicine [IOM], 2002). The U.S. Department of Health and Human Services (USDHHS) and the U.S. Department of Agriculture (USDA) publish dietary guidelines for Americans every five years. These guidelines were first published in 1980 and provide advice regarding dietary habits to promote health and prevent chronic disease for individuals two years old and older (U.S. Department of Health and Human Services, 2005; USDA, 2005).

The intent of the guidelines is to summarize current knowledge about nutrition into recommendations for the public. An example of an eating pattern that follows the dietary guidelines is the USDA food guide, called *My Pyramid,* displayed in Figure 48-2, which can be used as a teaching tool for patients. In 2004, My Pyramid replaced the former Food Guide Pyramid. The new pyramid symbolizes a personalized approach to healthy eating and physical activity, as well as the benefits of taking small steps toward a healthier lifestyle.

The body of current evidence regarding nutrition and chronic disease prevention led to the formation of a multidisciplinary expert panel from the National Institutes of Health (NIH), Health Canada, and the National Academy of Sciences IOM Food and Nutrition board. This panel was appointed by the USDHHS to review the scientific literature on macronutrients and energy and establish guidelines for intake to promote good nutrition and decrease the risk of chronic disease (Brooks, Butte, Rand, Flatt, & Caballero, 2004).

The panel published a report entitled *Dietary reference intakes for energy, carbohydrate, fiber, fat, fatty acids, cholesterol, protein, and amino acids* (IOM, 2002). This report is the sixth in a series, replacing and expanding the former RDAs with Dietary Reference Intakes (DRIs). This report focuses on carbohydrates, fat, protein, fiber, fatty acids, and cholesterol, as well as on calorie needs and physical activity.

To meet the body's nutritional needs while decreasing the risk for developing chronic disease, adults should get 45 to 65 percent of their calories from carbohydrates, 20 to 35 percent of calories from fat, and 10 to 35 percent of calories from protein. The guidelines for children are similar, except that infants and younger children need a higher proportion of fat, 25 to 40 percent.

Because exercise and nutrition go hand-in-hand to prevent chronic disease, the IOM panel found in their 2002 report that it would be necessary for most adults and children to participate in moderate physical activity for 60 minutes per day to make the transition from a sedentary lifestyle to an active one (Table 48-1). Although this exercise goal is higher than recommendations made in 1996 by the United States Surgeon General, the panel considered moderate physical activity to include routine daily activities, such

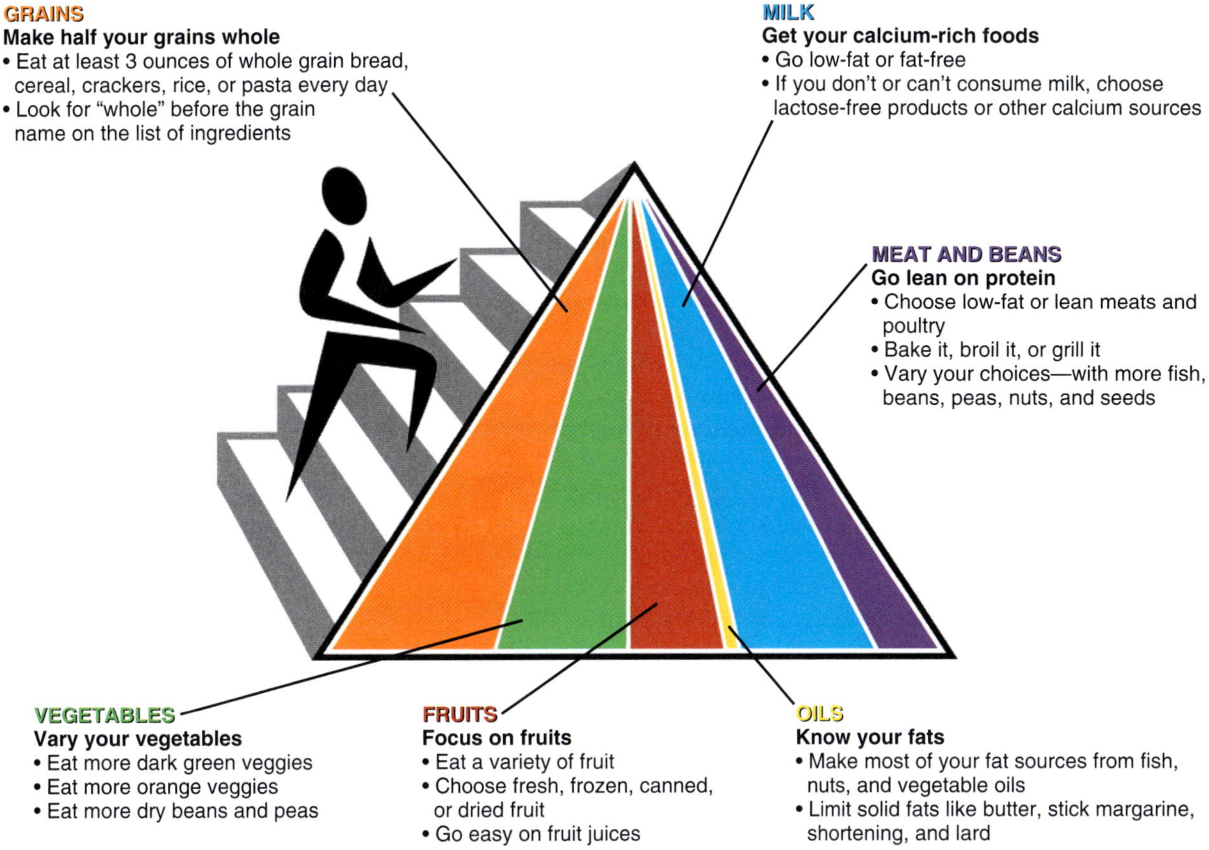

Figure 48-2 *My Pyramid* USDA Food Guide. (From Inside My Pyramid, by the U.S. Department of Agriculture, 2005.)

TABLE 48-1 Macronutrient Recommendations

CALORIE LEVEL	GRAMS PER DAY OF CARBOHYDRATES (45–65 PERCENT OF CALORIES)	GRAMS PER DAY OF FAT (20–35 PERCENT OF CALORIES)	GRAMS PER DAY FROM PROTEIN (10–35 PERCENT OF CALORIES)
1,000	130–163[a]	22–39	25–88
1,200	135–195	27–47	30–105
1,500	168–243	33–58	38–131
1,800	202–292	40–70	45–157
2,000	225–325	44–78	50–175
2,200	247–357	49–86	55–192

[a] *Minimum number of daily carbohydrate grams*

Source: Institute of Medicine. (2002). Dietary reference intakes for energy, carbohydrate, fiber, fat, fatty acids, cholesterol, protein, and amino acids. *Washington, DC: National Academy Press.*

as housekeeping, taking the stairs instead of the elevator, and walking the dog (Brooks, Butte, Rand, Flatt, & Caballero, 2004; IOM, 2002).

Metabolic Rate

In the normal human body, the processes of **anabolism** and **catabolism** are constantly taking place. Anabolic processes take up energy, and catabolic processes release energy. Energy released by catabolic processes supports functions of the body, such as digesting and metabolizing food and physical activity. Metabolic rate is the amount of energy released by the body per unit of time.

An individual's daily energy expenditure is determined by his or her basal metabolic rate, the energy requirement to process food, and the energy expended through physical activity. Energy expenditure can also be affected by extreme climate conditions. Basal metabolic rate (BMR) is the largest component of daily energy expenditure. BMR is the minimum work performed by the body to maintain body tissue integrity and a normal body temperature. BMR is determined by body size, composition, gender, and age.

The energy required to process food is estimated to be approximately 10 percent of daily energy expenditure. Energy expenditure through physical activity varies. Energy balance is achieved when there is a balance between caloric intake and energy expenditure. When an individual is in energy balance, body weight is maintained.

Energy can be defined as the force driving and sustaining mental activity or the capacity for doing work (Medline Plus, 2005a). The standard unit for measuring energy is the calorie, which is the amount of heat energy required to raise the temperature of 1 mL of water at 15° C by 1° C. Because the amount of calories used by the human body is large, the kilocalorie (kcal), equivalent to 1,000 calories, is used. Therefore, if an individual is in energy balance, kilocalories consumed are equal to kilocalories expended (Ganong, 2003).

Part of chronic disease prevention is maintaining energy balance so that energy consumption matches energy expenditure. With this balance, overweight or underweight can be avoided. The IOM Food and Nutrition board published a report in 2002, which included targets for calorie intake and recommended that energy expenditure be 1.6 to 1.7 times an individual's **resting energy expenditure** to maintain a healthy weight. Factors affecting resting energy expenditure include body size, composition, age, and gender (IOM, 2002).

In a research setting, **direct calorimetry** may be used to measure energy expenditure. The subject is enclosed in a chamber, and changes in the temperature of circulating air and water measure heat released by the subject. Heat released by the subject is a direct measure of energy expenditure. Because the subject is enclosed in a chamber and is isolated from caregivers, this method does not work well in the hospital setting.

Indirect calorimetry is therefore conducted in some hospital settings. There are many different methods of indirect calorimetry. Portable indirect calorimeters can be taken to the patient's bedside. They may be attached to the patient's ventilator, or a mask may be used for more stable patients. The machine measures the oxygen and carbon dioxide content of inspired and expired breath, as well as the volume expired by the lungs. Through measurements of gas exchange, energy expenditure is measured. In addition, because carbohydrate, protein, and fat metabolism each require a specific amount of oxygen and release a specific amount of carbon dioxide, this test can measure the amount of carbohydrate, protein, and fat utilized by the body. Because indirect calorimetry equipment is expensive, and the testing is labor intensive, not all facilities offer this service.

There are many methods of measuring and calculating energy expenditure or energy needs. Most calculations utilize factors such as height, weight, and age. In the hospital setting the guidelines and policies of the specific enterprise determine the calculations used. A consult for the clinical dietitian to assess a patient's nutritional needs can be ordered. The registered dietitian (RD) may estimate the patient's intake using the patient's 24-hour food recall or by asking the patient, family members, and health care providers about the amounts and types of foods consumed by the patient over the previous 24 hours. A calorie count may be ordered to compare the patient's intake to the individual's estimated needs. This usually involves recording the percentage intake of each item on the patient's menu for one to three days. A dietetic technician or RD will then summarize the results. This method of assessing a patient's intake is not precise in the hospital setting, however, because it relies on the consistent observation and recording by staff of actual foods eaten at all meals.

NUTRITION AND DRUG INTERACTIONS

The absorption, effectiveness, safety, and elimination of medications can be affected by food, and medications can have an impact on nutritional status. Foods can affect the absorption of medications and alter the pharmacokinetics of a medication. In the hospital setting, nurses need to be aware of potential food-drug interactions to avoid adverse drug events and to reinforce patient teaching (Figure 48-3). Although policies and practices vary, many health care enterprises have a process in place for identifying and monitoring potential food-drug interactions, as well as for teaching patients in preparation for discharge.

Although there are many potential food and drug interactions with which nurses need to be familiar, the interaction between grapefruit juice and certain medications is an interesting one. This interaction was identified accidentally in a study on alcohol consumption and a drug to lower blood pressure. When grapefruit juice was used to mask the taste of alcohol, more of the drug was absorbed than was expected. It was determined that compounds in grapefruit juice affect drug absorption in the small intestine.

Cytochrome P450

A group of enzymes called the cytochrome P450s are found in the liver and are involved with drug metabolism. The interaction between drugs and grapefruit juice involves cytochrome P450 3A and a protein in the small intestine, called P-glycoprotein, which affects the absorption of drugs. Cytochrome P450 3A metabolizes drugs so that they are more easily eliminated. Grapefruit juice can block P-glycoprotein and inactivate cytochrome P450 3A for up to 24 hours. Some of the medications affected by grapefruit juice are cyclosporine and felodipine. A total of 65 drug interactions were identified in the Thomson

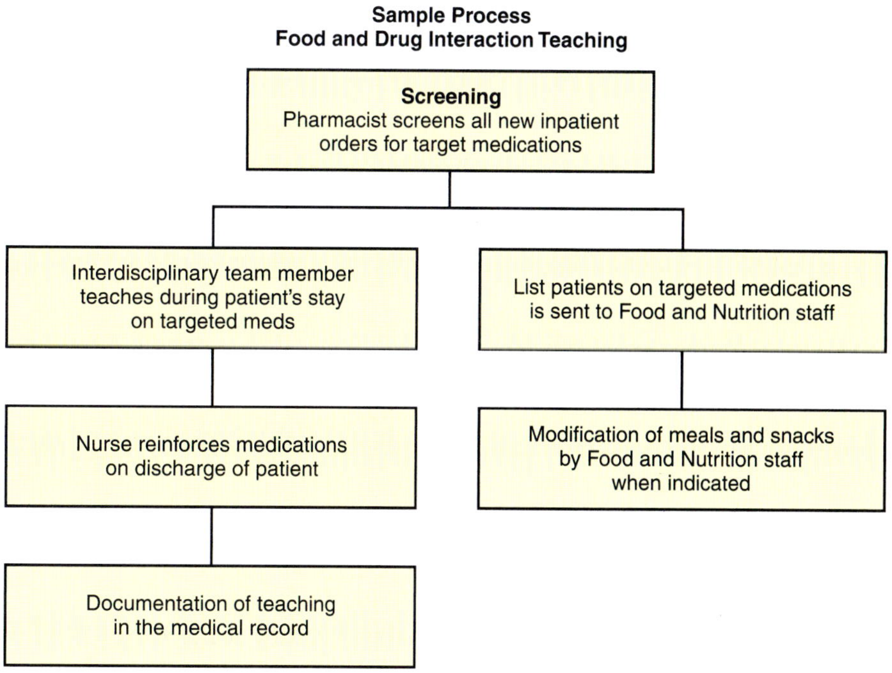

Figure 48-3 Sample process: Food and drug interaction teaching.

Micromedex database when grapefruit was entered as a search topic (Thomson Micromedex Healthcare Series, 2004).

BOX 48-1

FOODS HIGH IN VITAMIN K

Broccoli

Green leafy vegetables, e.g., spinach, Swiss chard, and kale

Liver

Source: Medline Plus. (2005a). Energy preservation. *Retrieved July 20, 2005, from www.nlm.nih.gov/medlineplus.gov.*

Warfarin

Warfarin is a commonly used anticoagulant. Warfarin levels are measured through the international normalization ratio test (INR). Significant variation in the intake of foods high in vitamin K can disrupt the anticoagulation effect of warfarin. Foods high in vitamin K content include bananas, celery, and many other varieties of vegetables and fruits (Box 48-1). Therefore, nurses should advise their patients on warfarin to maintain a *consistent* intake of foods high in vitamin K after discharge to maximize the safety of warfarin therapy.

Natural Products

One area of potential food drug interactions has to do with so-called natural products. Herbal products and dietary supplements are considered by the general public to be safe and beneficial (Bailey & Dresser, 2004). In the 1999 to 2000 National Health and Nutrition Examination Study (NHANES), 52 percent of adults reported taking a dietary supplement in the previous month (Radimer, et al., 2004). Because herbal products and dietary supplements are classified as food supplements rather than medications, they are not regulated by the Food and Drug Administration (FDA). Patients often do not realize the importance of telling health care practitioners about the use of herbal products and dietary supplements, and significant interactions with medications have been documented.

Herbal products can mimic the actions, intensify, or oppose the effects of drugs. St. John's wort, an herbal product used to treat depression, increases the activity of cytochrome P350 A4 and, as a result, more of a drug is oxidized and is therefore less bioavailable. Patients should not mix St. John's wort with medications such as digoxin, theophylline, cyclosporin, and phenprocoumon, because the herb decreases the bioavailability of the medications. When St. John's wort is combined with cyclosporin it can result in organ rejection in post-transplant patients and increased human immunodeficiency virus (HIV) viral load in HIV-positive patients (Bailey & Dresser, 2004). The herb gingko biloba can interfere with warfarin and cause bleeding. Because of the potential interactions of herbal products and dietary supplements with other medications, the nurse needs to ask patients about the use of these herbal products, dietary supplements, and other OTC remedies when obtaining a medical history.

PATIENT PLAYBOOK

Teaching Points for Patients Taking Herbal Remedies

- Be aware that the word *natural* on a product label does not mean that a product is safe.
- Herbal products may interact with both over-the-counter (OTC) and prescription medications.
- Notify the health care provider and pharmacist of herbal products the patient is taking.

NUTRITION SUPPORT: ALTERNATIVE METHODS OF FEEDING PATIENTS

In an ideal situation an individual's nutrient needs would be met and energy balance would be achieved through eating a healthful diet. However, as a result of many different disease states and medical conditions, feeding patients via an alternate route may be indicated.

Enteral Feedings

Enteral nutrition is the term used when feeding a patient occurs through a feeding tube directly into the GI tract. It can be used either as an adjunct to a patient's oral intake or to provide a patient's complete nutrition. Enteral nutrition is normally used when the patient has a functioning GI tract but is unable to meet nutritional requirements by eating. The patient's medical condition may prevent him or her from taking in adequate food by mouth, or his or her intake may be inadequate as a result of acute illness or an inability to take in adequate nutrition due to mechanical problems, such as dysphagia.

LAW IN PRACTICE

The Legal Implications of End-of-life Care

End-of-life medical treatment has been the subject of public debate since the case of Karen Ann Quinlan in 1975. Ms. Quinlan suffered respiratory arrest after drinking alcohol and possibly consuming the prescription medication, Valium. Karen suffered brain damage and was in a persistent vegetative state. After three months in the vegetative state, and with a poor prognosis, her family requested that she be taken off artificial life support. A legal battle ensued, and the Quinlans lost in a New Jersey Superior Court case. The decision was overturned by the New Jersey Supreme Court in January 1976. Karen was taken off the ventilator, but she continued to live in a persistent vegetative state until she died June 11, 1985. She had been unconscious for more than 10 years.

State laws and hospital policies related to end-of-life care vary; however, providing artificial fluids and nutrition via enteral feedings in patients can be considered medical treatment. The ideal situation is when a patient has expressed his or her wishes regarding end-of-life medical treatments (including providing artificial fluids and nutrition) in the form of an advanced directive. Hospitals accredited by the **Joint Commission on Accreditation of Hospitals (JCAHO)** are required to meet standard RI 2.80 on individual rights, which states that the hospital addresses the wishes of the patient regarding end-of-life decisions. Part of this standard requires providing patients with written information about their right to accept or refuse medical or surgical treatment, including forgoing or withdrawing life-sustaining treatment or withholding resuscitative services (2004).

Early enteral feeding has been demonstrated to improve wound healing, improve immune function, and reduce the length of hospital stay in the critically ill (Marik & Zaloga, 2003). When enteral nutrition is indicated the health care provider will order the enteral feeding product, the flow rate for the product to run on an enteral infusion device, and the route of enteral access. RDs in the hospital are an excellent resource to the health care provider and nurse for guidance about enteral feedings. They can assess the patient's nutritional needs, determine the optimal type of feeding and the flow rate to initiate and progress the feeding, establish the goal rate of enteral feeding, and monitor the patient's response to the feeding and ongoing nutrition status.

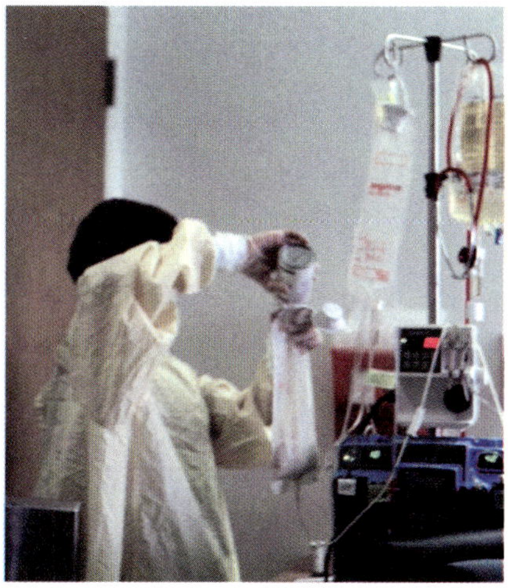

Figure 48-4 Open system gastrostomy feeding.

Before commercial enteral formulas were available, food was blenderized and thinned so that it could be passed down a tube. This practice is discouraged in the hospital setting because of the potential for bacterial contamination and the need to have the proper consistency of feeding. Enteral formulas can be delivered using an open or closed system. Canned enteral feeding products are emptied into a bag with the open system. The open system shown in Figure 48-4 is more labor-intensive for the nurse than the closed system and provides more opportunity for bacterial contamination. Closed system enteral formulas come in prefilled bottles. The formula bottle is spiked using a spike set, and the feeding flows through tubing to the patient. Hang-time of enteral feedings will vary based on hospital guidelines and policy. However, because closed system products are sealed in the manufacturing process, they are sterile and can be hung over a longer period of time than open system products.

The choice of enteral feeding product is usually guided by the facility's enteral formulary (Table 48-2). The formulary normally includes a standard or house formula that is most commonly used. Specialty products, used for selected conditions, such as critically ill or immune-compromised patients, may also be available. Feedings vary in the amount and types of carbohydrate, protein or amino acids, fat, fiber, vitamins, minerals, and other components they contain. In addition, the osmolality of feedings will vary. Isotonic formulas simulate the osmolality of plasma (280–300 mOsm/kg) while hypertonic formulas have an osmolality higher than 300 mOsm/kg.

TABLE 48-2 Enteral Nutrition Formulary

CATEGORY	CAL/L	PRO (G/L)	FAT (G/L)	CHO (G/L)	INDICATIONS FOR USE
Group 1: Enteral Products That Meet the Needs of Most Patients					
Isotonic with Fiber	1,060	44 (17%)	35 (29%)	155 (54%)	Standard house with fiber formula for patients requiring fiber to maintain gut function
High Protein with Fiber	1,000	62 (25%)	29 (25%)	130 (50%)	Patients with protein losses from wounds, fistulas, trauma and hypercatabolic patients
CATEGORY	**CAL/L**	**PRO (G/L)**	**FAT (G/L)**	**CHO (G/L)**	**INDICATIONS FOR USE**
Group 2: Enteral Products with Specific Indications					
Isotonic, No Fiber	1,060	37 (14%)	35 (29%)	151 (57%)	Patients unable to tolerate fiber. Patients requiring restricted protein and/or electrolytes
1.2 Calorie/mL	1,200	53 (18%)	39 (29%)	160 (53%)	To provide adequate kcal without substantially increasing volume, such as with bolus and cyclic feedings
1.5 Calorie/mL	1,500	68 (18%)	65 (38%)	170 (44%)	Patients requiring fluid restricted, nutritionally dense formulas or with high caloric needs
2.0 Calorie/mL	2,000	84 (17%)	89 (40%)	216 (43%)	As above
Renal Failure	2,000	70 (14%)	96 (43%)	223 (44%)	Renal patients with electrolyte imbalances or requiring fluid restrictions. **Note other products may be more appropriate for patients on CRRT or dialysis with stable electrolytes
Hepatic Failure	1,500	40 (11%)	21 (12%)	290 (77%)	Protein-intolerant patients with hepatic encephalopathy
Uncontrolled Diabetes	1,060	45 (17%)	51 (43%)	119 (40%)	Patients unable to obtain glucose control on Group I formulas despite adequate glycemic management
Semi-Elemental, Low Fat, 1.0 Calorie/mL	1,000	63 (25%)	39 (33%)	105 (42%)	Patients requiring semi-elemental/low-fat formula due to GI dysfunction, pancreatitis, or intolerance to intact formulas
Semi-Elemental, High Protein, 1.5 Calorie/mL	1,500	94 (25%)	68 (39%)	135 (36%)	May be beneficial for patients with atypical non-healing wounds or those needing semi-elemental product with caloric density and high protein
Immune-Modulator	1,000	56 (22%)	28 (25%)	130 (53%)	May be useful for some patients needing immune-enhancing nutrients

Source: Used with permission by Sharp Healthcare, which retains all rights thereto.

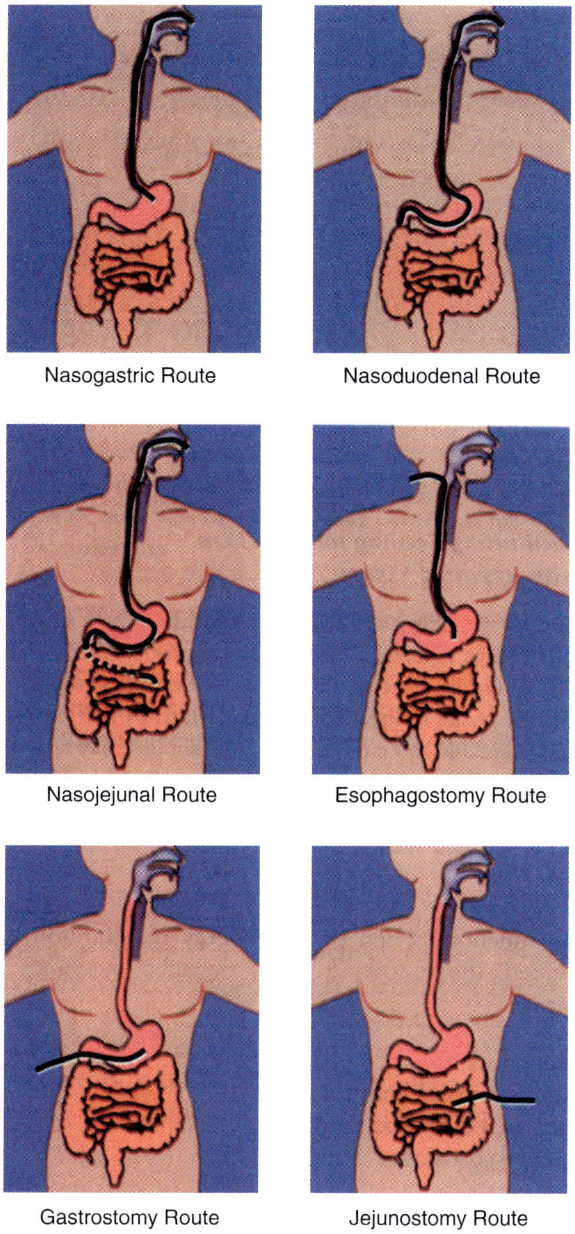

Figure 48-5 Enteral feeding routes.

Enteral feedings may be administered continuously or intermittently. Continuous feeding is provided for most acute hospital patients using an enteral infusion device or pump running 24 hours a day. Feedings can be safely initiated in stable patients at a rate of 50 to 60 mL/hour and advanced by 10 to 25 mL/hour every four to six hours until the goal rate is achieved. Intermittent feedings are provided with different frequencies and volumes, depending on the needs of the patient. These feedings may be especially beneficial for patients receiving lengthy physical therapy or to mimic more normal eating patterns.

Enteral feeding tubes are made out of different types of material, such as silicone or polyurethane, and come in different sizes and lengths. The outer diameter is measured in French (F) units; one French unit is equal to 0.33 mL. The size of feeding tube selected depends on factors such as the product to be infused, location of the tube, and patient comfort. Feeding tubes generally have at least one port for feeding and one for flushing and will range in size from 5 F to 28 F. Feeding tube placement should be verified according to facility guidelines by air auscultation, chest x-ray (CXR), or through aspirating gastric secretions.

If a tube feeding is needed for less than six to eight weeks, it may be placed nasogastrically (NG) through the nose to the stomach or nasojejunally (NJ) through the nose to the small intestine. Placing a feeding tube into the stomach rather than the small intestine allows for easier tube placement and the use of larger bore tubes. Feeding tubes may also be placed into the distal duodenum or proximal jejunum and are referred to as postpyloric tubes. Nasogastric or nasoenteric feeding tubes may be contraindicated in patients with structural pathology in the head and neck or with facial fractures. In some cases an orogastric feeding tube may be used instead (Figure 48-5).

Gastrostomy Feedings

For longer term enteral feedings or when nasogastric or orogastric feedings are contraindicated, a more permanent feeding gastrostomy tube may be placed endoscopically or surgically through the abdominal wall. Various enteral feeding routes are shown in Figure 48-6. Although there are potential complications, such as infection or adverse reaction to anesthesia from the procedure of placing a gastrostomy tube, gastrostomy tubes are easier to maintain and replace than nasogastric or nasoenteric tubes and are more comfortable for the patient.

When a patient is receiving an enteral feeding, the nurse should pay careful attention to signs of possible complications and follow strict infection control practices. Signs of complications include nausea and vomiting, malabsorption, aspiration, abdominal distension, tube obstruction, diarrhea, and constipation. The head of the bed needs to be elevated 30 degrees during feedings and for one hour after a feeding has been discontinued to prevent aspiration. The nurse must ensure that the patient's medications can be safely passed through the feeding tube. Feeding tubes must be flushed before and after feeding and before and after medication administration to avoid tube obstruction. Because complications, such as nausea, vomiting, and diarrhea, can have other causes, it is important to assess for possible causes and notify the health care provider before assuming that the feeding is the cause.

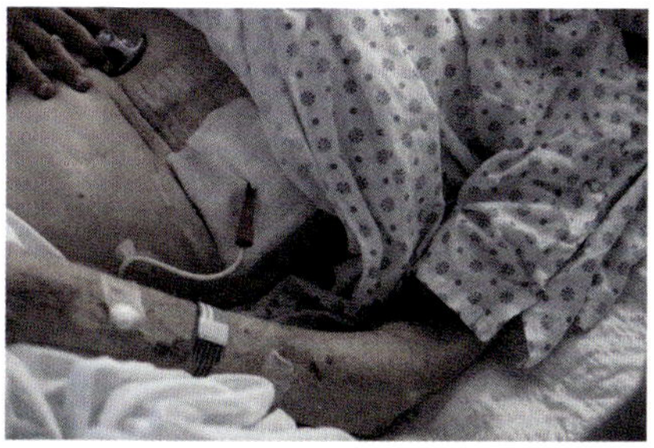

Figure 48-6 Gastrostomy feeding.

Parenteral Nutrition

Parenteral nutrition (PN) is providing nutrients to a patient in an intravenous (IV) solution. This form of nutrition support is indicated when the patient is malnourished, has the potential for becoming malnourished, and is not a candidate for enteral feeding. PN can be provided through a peripheral vein at a low concentration or centrally through a large diameter vein, usually the superior vena cava.

PN formulations usually contain dextrose, amino acids, lipids, vitamins, minerals, and medications. Formulations must be carefully compounded under strict conditions in the pharmacy to prevent dangerous precipitation or infection. Complications of PN can be life-threatening and include GI atrophy, fluid overload, and sepsis.

Patients on PN should be monitored frequently. Some facilities have a nutrition support team for the daily management of enteral and PN. This team may include a health care provider, pharmacist, RD, and registered nurse (RN). This team can assist with the assessment and reassessment of patients on nutritional support.

MALNUTRITION

Malnutrition is a term that is used to describe an altered state of nutrition resulting from a deficiency, or excess, of one or more nutrients. Overnutrition is when a patient's intake is in excess of their need for one or more nutrients and undernutrition occurs when nutritional intake is insufficient. Malnutrition in hospitalized patients is generally a situation of undernutrition. When nutritional status declines in hospitalized patients it is usually associated with higher medical costs and increased likelihood of complications.

Epidemiology

Hospital personnel have been aware of the widespread presence of malnutrition in hospitalized patients since the 1970s when Butterworth published the famous article, "Skeletons in the Hospital Closet" in *Nutrition Today* (1974). Subsequent studies continue to highlight the prevalence and impact of malnutrition in hospitalized patients. The cost of hospital stays for patients who suffer declines in nutritional status, regardless of nutrition status on admission, is higher compared to patients who do not suffer declines in nutrition status.

Etiology

The etiology of malnutrition globally can be multifactorial and may include inadequate food intake because of poverty or isolation or frequent infections that lead to an inadequate intake of calories, protein, vitamins, and minerals. In the hospital setting the patient may be undernourished prior to admission or suffer a decline in nutritional status during the hospital stay. Causes of malnutrition prior to admission include financial constraints to consuming an adequate diet, pain from acute or chronic disease, inadequate intake resulting from medication side effects, and psychological factors, such as isolation and depression. During a hospital stay malnutrition may develop as a result of factors, such as disease state or inadequate food intake because of pain, nausea, and the difference of hospital food from their food preferences at home. The elderly are at high risk for malnutrition because of chronic medical problems, changes in taste and appetite, and social isolation. Other groups at risk for malnutrition include patients with cancer and acquired immunodeficiency syndrome (AIDS) because of the impact of the disease process and treatments on appetite and nutrient intake.

Assessment with Clinical Manifestations

Long-term undernutrition of protein and calories may be reflected in the form of marasmus, a condition resulting from inadequate intake of calories and protein to meet the body's needs. Severe tissue wasting, a decrease in lean body mass and subcutaneous fat stores, dehydration, and weight loss may be observed. The patient with marasmus has a cachectic appearance and may exhibit generalized weakness and a decrease in functioning (Hark & Morrison, 2003). Kwashiorkor is a state of protein depletion that may develop over a shorter period of time. Patients with kwashiorkor may appear weak, lethargic, edematous, and irritable (Hart & Morrison, 2003).

Diagnostic Tests

Laboratory diagnostic tests can be useful in the nutrition screening process to identify patients at risk, identify changes in nutrition status, and monitor the effectiveness of nutrition interventions. Nutrition-related laboratory tests include measures of visceral protein status, including the serum proteins, albumin, transferrin, prealbumin, and retinol binding protein shown in Table 48-3. Although albumin can be used to measure long-term changes in nutritional status, it is not the best indicator of nutritional status in hospitalized patients, because it has a half-life of approximately 21 days and is slow to respond to changes in nutritional status. Levels of less than 3 g/dL may indicate a problem. However, albumin levels in hospitalized patients may be decreased by factors other than malnutrition, such as fluid retention, liver damage, or renal disease.

Serum Transferrin

Serum transferrin can also be used to assess visceral protein stores, but its levels are not specific to nutritional status. Transferrin levels less than 100 mg/dL, 100 to 150 mg/dL, and 150 to 200 mg/dL may be an indicator of severely, moderately, and mildly depleted visceral protein stores, respectively, in patients with normal renal and hepatic function. The half-life of transferrin is eight days, so it is more sensitive than albumin, but not sensitive enough to use in daily monitoring of nutritional status. In addition, transferrin levels can be decreased by medications and medical conditions.

TABLE 48-3 Laboratory Values Related to Nutrition Screening

TEST NAME	NORMAL VALUES FOR ADULTS
Albumin	3.5–5 g/dL
Transferrin	Adult male 215–365 mg/dL Adult female 250–380 mg/dL
Prealbumin	15–36 mg/dL or 150–360 mg/
Retinol binding protein	3–6 mg/dL

Adapted from Halas, M. (2004). Nutrition. In R. Daniels (Ed.), Nursing fundamentals: Caring and clinical decision making. *New York: Thomson Delmar Learning.*

Prealbumin (Transthyretin)

Prealbumin, or transthyretin, has a half-life of 1.9 days and is a more sensitive indicator of nutritional status. It can be used to identify a decline in nutritional status as well as be used to monitor the effectiveness of nutrition interventions. Monitoring daily increases of 1 mg/dL may indicate a positive response to nutrition support; whereas increase of less than 2 mg/dL per week may indicate that nutrition support is inadequate or ineffective. Some medical conditions may alter prealbumin levels, but it is still a useful laboratory value for nutritional status.

Retinol Binding Protein

Retinol binding protein (RBP) has a half-life of 12 hours and can be used to monitor short term changes in nutritional status. RBP levels can be elevated by conditions such as renal disease.

Hemoglobin and Hematocrit

Anemia may occur in hospitalized patients and is defined as a decrease in red cell mass. Hemoglobin and hematocrit are the main measures used to indicate anemia. Iron deficiency may occur as a result of inadequate iron intake or a decrease in iron stores. Although some medical conditions may cause iron deficiency, the main cause of anemia is chronic blood loss. Once the cause of the iron deficiency anemia is identified, iron stores need to be replenished through iron supplementation. Improvement of iron deficiency through supplementation will take several weeks to appear in hemoglobin and hematocrit tests. Therefore, these tests are generally not useful measures of nutritional status.

Nursing Diagnoses

Based on the information gathered, examples of nursing diagnoses in the patient with malnutrition may include the following (Ackley & Ladwig, 2004):

- Adult failure to thrive.
- Deficient knowledge related to: Information misinterpretation or lack of exposure.
- Imbalanced nutrition: Less than body requirements.

Planning and Implementation

There are many interventions that can be employed for patients with malnutrition. The entire health care team must be utilized in both the planning and implementation phases of care.

Goals

The goal for the patient with malnutrition is to restore nutritional status as much as is possible given the patient's comorbid medical problems. This may involve supplementing the regular diet with high protein, providing high-calorie foods and beverages, adding vitamin and mineral supplements, or providing the patient with enteral or PN if he or she is unable to meet his or her nutritional needs with food.

Collaborative Management

The multidisciplinary team approach to improving nutritional status should include the physician, RN, nursing assistant, clinical dietitian, and may also include a pharmacist, social worker, discharge planner, occupational therapist, and other health care team members. The causes of inadequate food intake must be identified through history and physical examination. Modifiable factors must be corrected. This may include obtaining dentures from home for patients unable to chew hospital food, modifying diet textures, or making changes to medications that cause decreased appetite. Members of the multidisciplinary team need to review factors affecting the patient's nutritional status and modify the patient's treatment plan accordingly.

Pharmacology

Malnutrition may be related to medications that cause nausea, vomiting, diarrhea, or anorexia. Attempts must be made to identify the medications causing such side effects and either modify the doses or find a suitable substitute.

Health Care Resources

Malnourished patients who live alone or have limited incomes may benefit from obtaining meals from community services. Senior centers may offer meals at a reduced price. Agencies, such as Meals on Wheels, are available to deliver meals to those in need.

Patient and Family Teaching

Hospital-based RDs and the RN are excellent resources to educate the patient and family members about how to improve the patient's nutritional status. This education may include evaluating the patient's resources at home, referring them to appropriate community resources for meals at home, and reviewing general nutrition principles.

Evaluation of Outcomes

Potential patient outcomes for each of the example nursing diagnoses for the patient with malnutrition are:

- Adult failure to thrive. Patient will consume adequate fluid intake with no signs of dehydration.

- Deficient knowledge related to information misinterpretation or lack of exposure. Patient will list resources that can be used for support after discharge.
- Imbalanced nutrition: less than body requirements. Patient will consume adequate food and fluids to meet nutritional needs and be free of signs of malnutrition.

JCAHO Provision of Care, Treatment, and Services standards require that hospitals have written criteria for when a more in-depth assessment is completed (2004). JCAHO accredited hospitals have a process in place to screen patients for nutrition risk and refer at-risk patients for further assessment.

The Level II nutritional screening tool shown in Table 48-4 uses a point system to identify a patient's level of risk for malnutrition. Nutrition risk triggers

TABLE 48-4 Level II Nutrition Screening

Height: _______ cm/in Weight: ______ kg/lb BMI: ______ IBW: ______ UBW: ______
Diet Order: ____ Age _____ Male/Female
Food allergies/sensitivities noted: Y/N Cultural/religious preferences noted: Y/N

RISK FACTOR	EVALUATION	POINT VALUE	TOTAL POINTS
Weight Status	Unintentional wt loss of 5% or more in past month	1 point	
	≤ 85% IBW	1 point	
	BMI ≥ 30 (obese)	1 point	
Medical Status/Condition	Comatose/unresponsive	1 point	
	Geriatric surgical (≥ 75 years old)	1 point	
	Nausea, vomiting, diarrhea, constipation for 3 days or more	1 point	
Eating Difficulties	Sore mouth	1 point	
	Chewing/Swallowing	1 point	
	Unable to feed self	1 point	
Recent Intake/Appetite (over past month)	Good (≥ 75%)	0 points	
	Fair (50-75%)	1 point	
	Poor (25-50%)	2 points	
	Minimal (< 25%)	3 points	
Skin	Pressure ulcer stage I	1 point	
	Pressure ulcer stage II, III, or IV	Automatic RD referral	
Labs	Albumin level _______	1 point if ≤ 3.0	
Education	If on a modified diet, does pt request or need a diet instruction? Y/N	Automatic RD referral for education if yes	
Risk Determination	CHOOSE ONE: 0-4 Low Nutritional Risk > 4 High Nutritional Risk (RD to follow)		TOTAL POINTS: _______ RD to follow: Y/N

COMMENTS:

____

____

____

Signature ______________________ Date/time ________

This form is used with permission of Sharp HealthCare, which retains all rights thereto.

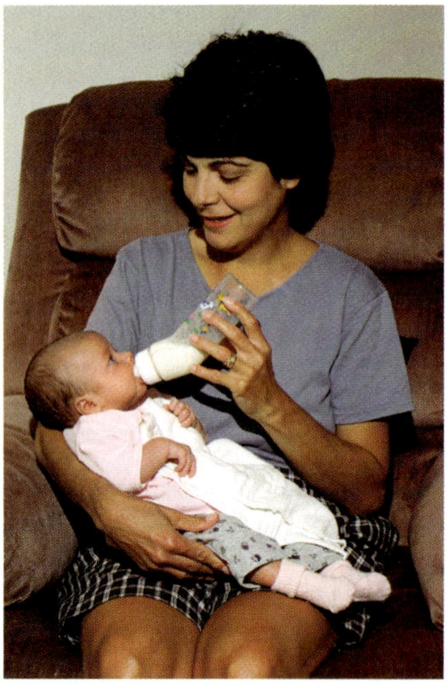

Figure 48-7 Visual assessment for nutritional risk.

may include factors, such as decreased food intake, weight loss, advanced age, and high risk medical diagnoses. Patients at nutrition risk are referred to an RD for further assessment and reassessment.

Taking a verbal diet history provides an opportunity to better assess knowledge and cultural impacts on the patient's nutritional habits. The probes, or questions, on the diet history form provided in Table 48-5 helps ensure that broad areas related to nutritional status are assessed. Yet, it is flexible enough to facilitate deeper exploration of troubling responses from the patient.

The nurse plays a vital role in the identification of patients at nutrition risk and in assisting family members to assess and meet the patient's nutritional needs (Figure 48-7) (Table 48-6). Patients may not initially meet nutrition risk criteria but may experience a decline in nutrition status during the hospital stay. Referring patients to dietetic technicians and dietitians when new nutrition risk factors, such as difficulty swallowing, decreased appetite, weight loss, and skin breakdown, develop can facilitate nutrition interventions. In addition, by ensuring that intake and output records and intake analysis or calorie counts are accurate, the nurse provides important data for the nutrition assessment.

TABLE 48-5 Diet History

Part 1: General Diet Information

Do you follow a particular diet?

What are your food likes and dislikes?

Do you have any especially strong cravings?

How often do you eat fast foods?

How often do you eat at restaurants?

Do you have adequate financial resources to purchase your food?

How do you obtain, store, and prepare your food?

Do you eat alone or with a family member or other person?

In the last 12 months have you

- experienced any change in weight?
- had a change in your appetite?
- had a change in your diet?
- experienced nausea, vomiting, or diarrhea from your diet?
- changed your diet because of difficulty in feeding yourself, eating, chewing, or swallowing?

Part 2: Food Intake History
(24-Hour Recall, 3-Day Diary, Direct Observation)

Time	Food/Drink	Amount	Method of Preparation	Eating Location

TABLE 48-6 Comprehensive Nutrition History

Nutritional History

Physical Assessment

1. General appearance
2. Skin
3. Nails
4. Hair
5. Eyes
6. Mouth
7. Head and neck
8. Heart and peripheral vasculature
9. Abdomen
10. Musculoskeletal system
11. Neurological system
12. Female genitalia

Anthropometric Measurements

Height: ________________ in or cm   % Weight Change: ________________

Weight: ________________ lbs or kg   Body Mass Index: ________________

% Ideal Body Weight: ______________   Waist/Hip Ratio: ________________

% Usual Body Weight: ______________   Triceps Skinfold: ________________

Mid-Arm Circumference: ______________ cm

Mid-Arm Muscle Circumference: ______________ cm

Laboratory Data

Hematocrit (HCT): ______________%   Hemoglobin (HGB): ____________ g/dL

Cholesterol: ______ mg/dL   HDL: ______ mg/dL   LDL: ______ mg/dL

Triglycerides: ______________ mg/dL

TIBC: ______________ μg/dL

Transferrin: ______________ mg/dL

Iron: ______________ μg/dL

Total Lymphocyte Count: ______________ cells/mm^3

Antigen Skin Testing: ______________

Albumin: ______________ g/dL

Glucose: ______________ mg/dL

CHI: ______________

Nitrogen Balance: ______________ g

Diagnostic Data

X-rays ______________

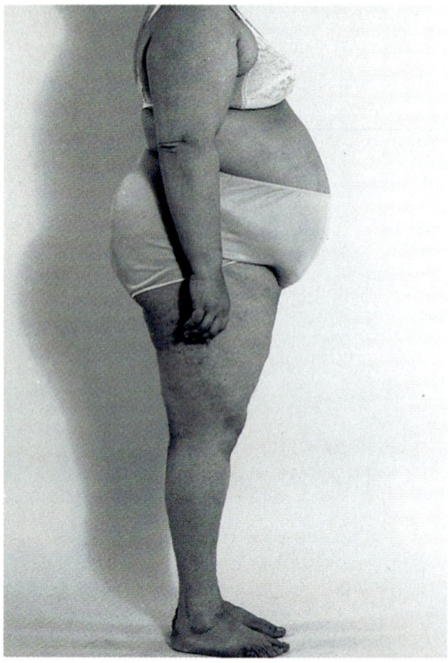

Figure 48-8 Obese adult. *Courtesy of the Armed Forces Institute of Pathology.*

OBESITY

Obesity, as shown in Figure 48-8, continues to be a public health concern in the United States. In 2002 about 65.7 percent of Americans were overweight compared to 55.9 percent between 1988 and1994 (Headley, Ogden, Johnson, Carroll, Curtain, & Flegal, 2004). The causes of obesity appear to be multifactorial, including increased caloric consumption along with inadequate exercise (Goldberg, et al., 2004).

The body mass index (BMI) is a weight-stature index used as a measure of obesity and of malnutrition. The formula for determining BMI appears in Box 48-2. It is calculated using the body weight in kilograms divided by the square of the height in meters. Healthy weight is based on a BMI of 18.5–25. When a BMI reaches 25 to 29.9, it is considered overweight. The BMI of 25 was selected because research reveals increased mortality with BMIs above this level. Obesity is defined as a BMI greater than 30 (National Institutes of Health National Heart, Lung, and Blood Institute, 1998). The BMI categories are presented in Box 48-3.

BOX 48-2

CALCULATION OF BMI

The formula for calculating BMI is as follows:

$$\text{BMI} = \frac{\text{Weight (kg)}}{\text{Height (m}^2\text{)}}$$

BOX 48-3

BMI CATEGORIES

Underweight = less than 18.5

Normal weight = 18.5–24.9

Overweight = 25–29.9

Obesity = BMI of 30 or greater

Source: National Institutes of Health National Heart, Lung, and Blood Institute. (1998). Clinical guidelines on the identification, evaluation, and treatment of overweight and obesity in adults. The evidence report. *NIH Publication No. 98-4083, Bethesda, MD: Author.*

Epidemiology

The incidence of overweight children and teenagers is on the rise. The rate of childhood obesity has tripled over the last 30 years in children ages 6–11, and doubled for ages 2 to 5 and 12 to 19. In a study of 11- to 13-year-old school children it was found that 35.3 percent had a BMI at or above the 85th percentile; and 17.4 percent of them had a BMI at or above the 95th percentile. BMI at or above 85 percent and less than 95 percent is considered at risk for overweight. Overweight is at or above the 95th percentile for gender-specific BMI charts for children. (Hedley, et al., 2004). A significant correlation between BMI, hours of television watched in the evening, and the amount of soft drinks consumed has been noted (Giammattei, Blix, Marshak, Wollitzer, & Pettitt, et al., 2003).

Etiology

Overweight children are at high risk for becoming overweight adults and are at risk for developing chronic diseases normally seen later in life. Overweight and obese adults are at increased risk for developing many serious health conditions, including hypertension, elevated blood lipid levels, type 2 diabetes, gallbladder disease, coronary artery disease, and certain types of cancer (Watkins, 2004).

The cause of type 1 diabetes is not known, but it is proposed that the body's immune system attacks itself, destroying the cells in the pancreas that produce insulin. As a result, type 1 diabetics must monitor their blood glucose regularly and use insulin. The incidence of type 2 diabetes mellitus is increasing significantly, not only in the United States but also in other industrialized societies. This increase is because of a sedentary lifestyle, increasing rates of obesity, and an aging population. Diabetes is the cause of many complications, such as end-stage renal disease and cardiovascular disease, both of which impact the patient's length of hospital stay, hospital costs, and mortality (MMWR, 2004; Winer & Sowers, 2004).

Assessment with Clinical Manifestations

There are many aspects to assessing patients who are obese. The first federal guidelines for identification, evaluation, and treatment of overweight and obesity were released in 1998 by the National Heart, Lung, and Blood Institute (NHLBI) in conjunction with the National Institute of Diabetes and Digestive

Kidney Diseases (NIDDKD). The guidelines were based on an extensive review of the research on overweight and obesity and were established for health care professionals to use in their practice.

The guidelines recommend that health care professionals measure the patient's BMI, evaluate the patient's risk factors, and measure waist circumference. Waist circumference of over 40 inches in men and over 35 inches in women indicates increased risk in patients with a BMI of 25 to 34.9.

Because it has been established that patients may enter the hospital in a state of poor nutrition and that the nutritional status of a well-nourished patient with acute medical problems may deteriorate during the hospital stay, it is critical that nutrition status be monitored throughout hospitalization. Changes in nutrition status may occur more slowly and be less noticeable than changes in medical status. Malnutrition may be identified via physical assessment and laboratory tests.

Physical assessment may be performed by the health care provider and other trained health professionals. A general survey may reveal muscle wasting and lethargy, which may indicate inadequate caloric intake. Increased temperature and respirations may indicate increased fluid and caloric needs. Signs of poor wound healing may indicate the need for increased protein and vitamins. Poor dental health may indicate an obstacle to adequate oral intake.

Nursing Diagnoses

Based on the information gathered, examples of nursing diagnoses in the patient with obesity may include the following (Ackley & Ladwig, 2004):

- Imbalanced nutrition: More than body requirements related to excessive intake in relation to metabolic need.
- Risk for imbalanced nutrition: More than body requirements.
- Disturbed body image.
- Anxiety related to change in lifestyle.

Planning and Implementation

The nurse is responsible for implementing a wide variety of nursing interventions for patients with obesity. Obesity causes many health problems. Therefore, weight loss is recommended to lower blood pressure, improve blood lipid levels, and lower elevated blood glucose. Strategies for successful weight loss include reducing caloric intake, increasing physical activity, and modifying behaviors to improve eating and exercise habits. The initial goal is to reduce body weight by 10 percent of baseline within six months of treatment through the loss of 1 to 2 pounds per week. A 10 percent weight loss in six months can be achieved by decreasing caloric intake by 300 to 500 calories per day for those with BMI between 27 and 35. For those with BMI greater than 35, it will require decreasing caloric intake by 500 to 1,000 calories per day to achieve a 10 percent decrease in weight in six months.

> **PATIENT PLAYBOOK**
>
> **Patient and Family Teaching Related to the Management of Body Weight**
>
> The patient should be taught to decrease food intake through monitoring portion sizes:
>
> - Read labels and serve a standard portion on a plate, rather than serving food out of a box or bag.
> - Eat slowly so that the brain gets the message that the stomach is full.
> - Take seconds of vegetables and salads instead of higher calorie foods.
> - Try to eat three balanced meals at regular times.

Collaborative Management with Multidisciplinary Team Approach

The nurse can play an important role in the nutritional status of the hospitalized patient by referring malnourished patients to the RD, alerting the health care provider regarding patients with swallowing difficulty or changes in nutritional and functional status, addressing the causes of mouth pain, and offering the patient supplemental foods and fluids allowed by the health care provider.

Pharmacology

Medications may be used to assist patients in their weight loss efforts; however, patients should try to modify their diet and lifestyle for at least six months before trying drug therapy prescribed by a health care provider. Weight loss medications can then be included in a weight loss program that includes dietary changes and physical activity. Patients should have BMI greater than or equal to 30 without additional risk factors, such as diabetes.

Surgery

Bariatric surgery for obesity has increased in popularity. The number of bariatric procedures has increased from 6,868 in 1996 to 45,473 in 2001 (Livingston, 2004). Weight loss surgery may be recommended for severely obese patients with BMI greater than or equal to 40 or BMI greater than or equal to 35 with comorbid conditions (i.e., diabetes, heart disease, or sleep apnea) when other methods of treatment have failed. Extremely obese patients are at high risk for premature death and do benefit from the conservative treatment of diet and lifestyle modification compared to patients who are less obese.

There are several types of bariatric surgical procedures. Some limit food intake but do not interfere with the digestive process. In adjustable gastric banding, a band of silicone rubber is placed around the upper part of the stomach creating a pouch and a narrow passage into the rest of the stomach. Vertical banded gastroplasty involves using a band and staples to create a stomach pouch. Although these procedures are easier to perform and may be safer than the procedures which impact the digestive process, the patients may lose less weight, they may suffer from vomiting as a result of the narrow passage into the stomach, and the band may break down.

Procedures that are used more commonly today restrict food intake and alter the digestive process. The Roux-en-Y gastric bypass is the most commonly performed procedure in the United States. A stomach pouch is created and connected to a Y-shaped section of the small intestine, thus bypassing absorption that would take place in the stomach and upper small intestine. Patients lose more weight and at a faster pace than with procedures, such as the adjustable gastric banding and the vertical banded gastroplasty. A disadvantage is that because of the altered digestion, long-term nutritional deficiencies may develop. To avoid nutritional problems, patients need to take vitamin and mineral supplements and ensure adequate protein intake. In addition, patients may suffer from dumping syndrome after consuming high-carbohydrate foods that result in stomach contents moving to the small intestine too quickly. The patient may suffer from nausea, abdominal pain, bloating, weakness, and diarrhea. Bariatric surgical procedures may be performed laparoscopically in some patients, and as a result will have smaller incisions (NIH, 2004).

Nursing care for patients on restricted diets in the hospital setting should be supportive. When conservative weight management is indicated, the nurse can help by gently reinforcing the rationale for weight reduction and assisting the patient with activity. The postoperative diets (Box 48-4) for bariatric surgery patients will be limited initially to facilitate digestion and prevent dumping syndrome.

BOX 48-4

POSTBARIATRIC SURGERY DIET PROGRESSION

First 1 to 2 Days While in the Hospital

- Ice chips
- Water or sugar-free, noncarbonated beverage, about 4 oz per hour

First Postoperative Visit with Surgeon, 5 to 12 Days Postoperatively

- Water
- Sugar-free, noncarbonated beverages
- Sugar free popsicles
- Diet Jell-O
- Decaffeinated coffee or tea
- Chicken or beef broth

Evaluation of Outcomes

Potential patient outcomes for each of the example nursing diagnoses for the patient with obesity are (Ackley & Ladwig, 2004):

- Imbalanced nutrition: More than body requirements. The patient will voice feelings about present weight. The patient will identify internal and external cues that increase food consumption.
- Risk for imbalanced nutrition: More than body requirements. The patient will compare current eating pattern with recommended eating patterns. The patient will explain the concept of a balanced diet.
- Disturbed body image. The patient will correctly estimate the relationship of body to environment.
- Anxiety related to change in lifestyle. The patient should be able to recognize the signs of anxiety, demonstrate positive coping mechanisms, and describe a reduction in the level of anxiety experienced.

NUTRITION AND AGING

There are many physical changes as a result of the aging process, as well as changes in nutrient needs. Older adults generally require fewer calories as they get older based on changes in body composition and decreased activity level. Older adults are more prone to dehydration, because they have decreased total body water as compared to younger people. In addition, their thirst mechanism may be altered and they may have inadequate fluid intake at home due to factors, such as difficulty obtaining groceries or GI problems. Older adults may have more indigestion or food intolerance than younger adults because of a decrease in gastric motility and gastric secretions, as well as delayed gastric emptying. In addition, constipation is a common problem as a result of medications, inactivity, and inadequate fluid and fiber intake.

Research on older individuals with healthy diets and active lifestyles indicates that many of the declines associated with aging can be counteracted by a healthy lifestyle. In a study of men and women 70 to 90 years old who followed a Mediterranean diet, did not smoke, were moderately active, and had moderate alcohol consumption, one third had lower mortality than individuals who had less healthful behaviors (Knoops, deGroot, Kromhout, et al., 2004). Although there are many countries bordering the Mediterranean Sea, common components of the Mediterranean diet include a high intake of fruits, vegetables, nuts, seeds, olive oil as a fat source, poultry, fish, minimal intake of red meat, and low to moderate intake of dairy products and wine (American Heart Association, 2001).

KEY CONCEPTS

- A nutritionally adequate diet plays a vital role in the prevention of chronic disease.
- There are many potential food and drug interactions with which the nurse must be familiar.
- Enteral or PN may be provided to patients unable to meet their nutritional needs through diet.
- Malnutrition in hospitalized patients increases complications, costs, and length of hospital stay.
- Obesity and type 2 diabetes are on the rise.
- The half-life of laboratory tests of nutrition status vary. Laboratory tests with a shorter half-life may be more valuable in the hospital setting.

REVIEW QUESTIONS

1. Nutrition research published in a report by the IOM Food and Nutrition Board recommended an ideal percentage intake of carbohydrates, protein, and fat to prevent chronic disease for adults. These percentages are:
   1. 20 to 30 percent of calories from carbohydrate, 30 to 40 percent from fat, and 40 percent from protein
   2. 45 to 65 percent of calories from carbohydrate, 20 to 35 percent from fat, and 10 to 35 percent of calories from protein
   3. 60 to 70 percent of calories from carbohydrate, 15 to 20 percent from fat, and 15 to 20 percent from protein
   4. None of the above
2. The nurse receives an order from the health care provider for indirect calorimetry. She knows that this is an order to:
   1. Record the patient's calorie count for three days
   2. Measure the amount of calories burned through a blood assay
   3. Estimate energy expenditure by measuring oxygen consumption and carbon dioxide production
   4. Collect accurate intake and output records

Continued

REVIEW QUESTIONS—cont'd

3. BMI is a weight-stature index used to classify obesity. You know your patient is considered obese if his or her BMI is greater than:
    1. 25
    2. 18
    3. 50
    4. 30
4. Your patient is being discharged on a medication called warfarin. In the discharge teaching for this patient, you should emphasize which of the following?
    1. Avoid food sources high in vitamin K to maintain INR levels
    2. Avoid foods high in vitamin C and iron because they will decrease the absorption of warfarin
    3. Maintain a consistent intake of foods high in vitamin K, such as dark leafy greens
    4. Increase your intake of foods high in vitamin K to reduce the dose of warfarin needed
5. Your patient's health care provider has just written an order for "NG" feeding. You know that this means the patient will be having:
    1. A feeding of special medicines for a nuclear gout study
    2. A nasogastric tube for feeding
    3. Oral medicines to prepare for a Niacin-globulin test
    4. A diet high in non-gas producing foods
6. Hospitalized patients may be fed enterally via a tube feeding. Which of the following statements about tube feedings is true?
    1. Because enteral feeding tubes can be uncomfortable for the patient, feeding via the parenteral route is a good alternative with less complications.
    2. To decrease the risk of aspiration, patients receiving continuous feedings should have the head of the bed elevated 30 degrees.
    3. Blenderizing foods and putting them through the patient's tube feeding is as beneficial as using commercial products and is much less expensive.
    4. When a patient has diarrhea, the tube feeding is always the cause.
7. The nurse should be alert to new nutrition risk factors, which can develop during the patient's hospital stay. These risk factors include:
    1. Chewing and swallowing difficulties
    2. Healing of skin breakdown
    3. Increased appetite
    4. Improved mental status
8. Which of the following lab results indications that your patient has decreased visceral protein stores and may be malnourished?
    1. Prealbumin 10 mg/dL
    2. Fasting blood glucose 135 mg/dL
    3. Total cholesterol 249
    4. Hemoglobin 5.2
9. In caring for an elderly patient, the nurse should be aware of the following aspects of aging on hydration:
    1. A decrease in total body fluids, increasing the risk for dehydration
    2. Elderly people are thirstier than younger people and may have fluid overload as a result of increased thirst.
    3. Adequate hydration is not a problem because the elderly usually have access to plenty of fluids.
10. Which of the following statements is true regarding nutrition and chronic disease?
    1. The incidence of obesity is stable; however, diabetes is on the rise.
    2. Poor nutrition is related to chronic disease, and chronic diseases are responsible for 7 of 10 leading causes of death.
    3. Nutrition plays less of a role in the development of type 2 diabetes than type 1 diabetes.
    4. Chronic diseases, such as diabetes, are caused by genetics rather than diet and lifestyle.

REVIEW ACTIVITIES

1. Your patient wants to know how to improve his diet. He is currently overweight and is concerned about getting diabetes because he has a positive family history. What general comments about an optimal diet would you offer and to which resources would you refer him?

2. Determine the BMI for a few friends or family members. Where do their results fall in the classification of normal versus overweight?

3. Review the list of sample tube feedings. Why would a patient need a formula higher in protein?

4. Ask nurses you know in your nearby hospital about their hospital's process for nutrition screening. What kinds of forms do they use, what nutrition risk factors are included, and what is their process?

5. What lifestyle factors are correlated with the rise in childhood obesity? What changes have you noticed during your lifetime regarding childhood obesity and the lifestyles of children today?

6. What are some interventions you can take with your elderly patients to help maintain their nutritional status?

Visit the Contemporary Medical-Surgical Nursing online companion resource at www.delmarhealthcare.com for additional content and study aids. Click on Online Companions then select the Nursing discipline.

Upper Gastrointestinal Tract Dysfunction: Nursing Management

CHAPTER 49

Elizabeth Torrence, RN, MN, EdD

CHAPTER TOPICS

- Oral and Esophageal Disorders
- Nausea and Vomiting
- Gastroesophageal Reflux Disease
- Hiatal Hernia
- Dyspepsia
- Gastritis
- Stomach Cancer

KEY TERMS

Achalasia
Aphthous stomatitis
Apoptosis
Borborygmi sounds
Brash water
Dyspepsia
Dysphagia
Presbyphagia
Pyrosis
Sarcopenia

All illness results from the connection of genetics, environment, biology, and psychosocial variables. Especially in the approach to a patient with an upper gastrointestinal (GI) tract disorder the nurse must consider all of these variables. The degree of symptomatology associated with GI problems is not always explained by the diagnostic findings of endoscopy, manometry, or radiography. Emotional distress can influence individuals who have no history of GI dysfunction. During times of emotional upheaval, individuals may experience intense autonomic responses that can alter motility, vascularity, secretion, and pain perception. Likewise, GI dysfunction can affect areas of the brain, especially areas of the limbic system. This area of the brain is associated with the sleep-wake cycle, arousal, anxiety, and fear.

As with care for all patients, individuals with GI disorders should be listened to with empathy and be given reassurance and education. The nurse should ascertain the patient and family's expectations and concerns, ensure continuity of care through a collaborative care pathway, and support and encourage follow-up for health promotion activities.

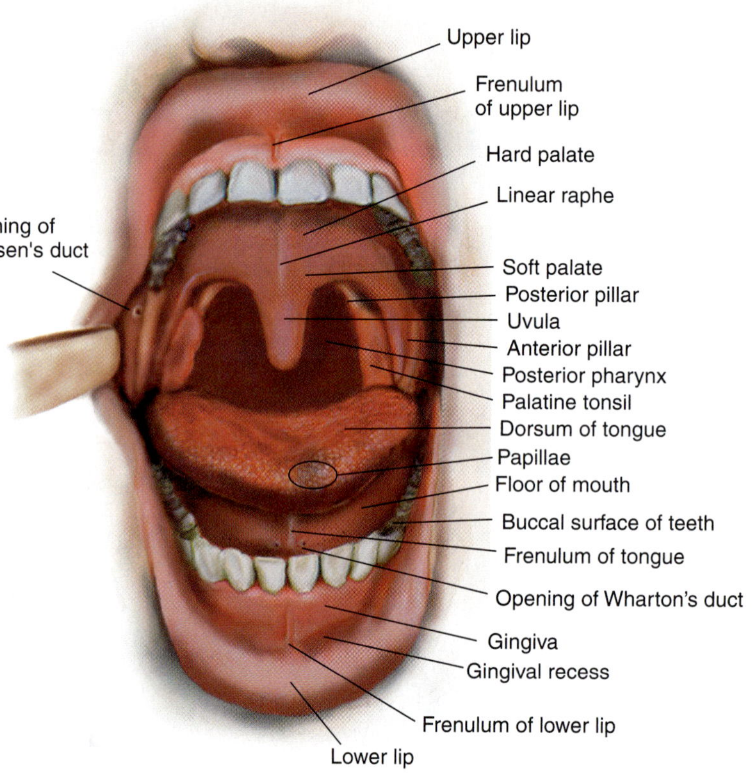

Figure 49-1 Structure of the mouth.

DISORDERS OF THE ORAL CAVITY

Ulcerative conditions of the gums and mucous membranes are labeled mouth ulcers **(aphthous stomatitis)** and occur in 20 percent of the population (Figure 49-1). Most mouth ulcers are minor and heal within 7 to 14 days. Herpetiform ulcers may take up to one month to heal. The causes of oral ulcerations can be found in the Table 49-1.

Etiology

More than 400,000 cancer patients experience oral problems, such as painful mouth ulcers, impaired taste, and dry mouth from salivary gland dysfunction. These individuals should receive dental assessment prior to beginning chemo or radiation therapy. If preexisting oral problems are resolved prior to cancer treatment, it may ameliorate complications and tissue damage. Patients who smoke have seven times the risk of developing gum disease. Nevertheless, any type of tobacco use, cigarettes, pipes, and smokeless tobacco raises the risk for gum disease, oral and throat cancers, as well as fungal infections (candidiasis). Heavy alcohol use also increases the risk of oral and throat cancer, especially if the individual also uses tobacco.

Planning and Implementation

Management of patients who have oral ulcers depends on the cause. Nurses must assess the mouth regularly, particularly when there are suspected complications associated with specific causes or problems (Figure 49-2). Rinsing the mouth with chlorhexidine may relieve the symptoms and reduce the healing time. Topical corticosteroids are also used to resolve these ulcers. Because eating may aggravate the discomfort the patient has with oral ulcer-

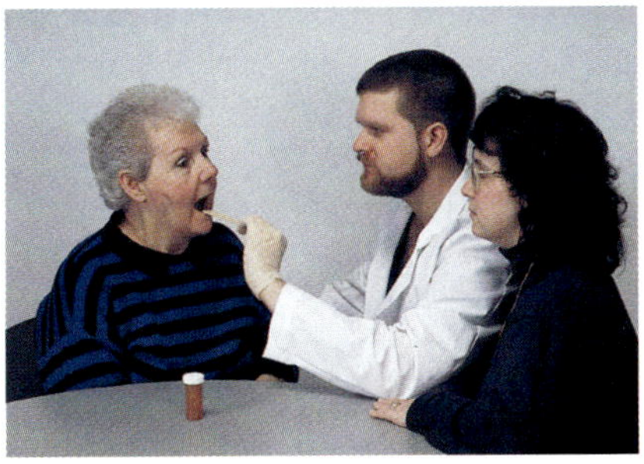

Figure 49-2 A nurse assessing the mouth of this patient with stomatitis with a concerned family member observing.

TABLE 49-1 Main Systemic and Iatrogenic Causes of Oral Ulcers

Microbial Diseases

- Herpetic stomatitis
- Chickenpox
- Herpes zoster
- Hand, foot, and mouth disease
- Herpangina
- Infectious mononucleosis
- HIV infection
- Acute necrotizing gingivitis
- Tuberculosis
- Syphilis
- Fungal infections

Cutaneous Disease

- Lichen planus
- Pemphigus
- Pemphigoid
- Erythema multiforme
- Dermatitis herpetiformis
- Linear IgA disease
- Epidermolysis bullosa

Chronic Ulcerative Stomatitis

- Other dermatoses

Malignant Neoplasms

Blood Disorders

- Anemia
- Leukemia
- Neutropenia
- Other white cell dyscrasias

GI Disease

- Coeliac disease
- Crohn's disease
- Ulcerative colitis

Rheumatoid Diseases

- Lupus erythematosus
- Behçet's syndrome
- Sweet's syndrome
- Reiter's disease

Drugs

- Cytotoxic agents
- Nicorandil

Radiotherapy

Adapted from Furlanetto, D., Crighton, A., & Topping, G. (2006). Differences in methodologies of measuring the prevalence of oral mucosal lesions in children and adolescents. International Journal of Pediatric Dentistry, 16*(1), 31–39; Talhari, C., Angerstein, W., Becker, J., Ruzicka, T., & Megahed, M. (2005). Long-standing oral ulcers.* Lancet, 365*(9463), 1002.*

ations, they may need mouth rinses that contain topical analgesics, such as viscous Xylocaine.

Nonulcerative Causes of Mouth Pain

Erythema migrans (benign migratory glossitis) is a nonulcerative inflammatory and sometimes painful condition of the tongue. It is characterized by multiple areas of erythema surrounded by yellowish-white borders. These lesions may be asymptomatic but often are painful. Because there is no effective treatment for this disorder, symptomatic relief is provided. Patients with particular systemic disorders may also experience oral glossitis. These include anemia, vitamin B deficiencies, oral lichen planus, aphthous ulcers, pemphigus, and syphilis.

Etiology

Causes of nonulcerative mouth pain can include:

- Infections, such as viral herpes simplex or bacterial infections;
- Mechanical injury from eating or drinking hot or spicy food or fluid.
- Irritants, such as alcohol, smoking and chewing tobacco.
- Trauma to the tongue, irregular areas of the teeth or dental appliances.
- Allergies and exposure to certain substances in toothpaste, mouthwash, breath fresheners, certain dyes in food, plastics in certain dental appliances (dentures or retainers), and some medications have been indicated, such as angiotensin-converting enzyme (ACE) inhibitors.

PATIENT PLAYBOOK

Oral Cancer Self-Assessment

The nurse should teach the patient the following as prevention of oral care of his or her face, lips, and oral cavity:

1. Look in the mirror at your face. Check for symmetry. Are there any lumps, swelling, or bumps that you notice on only one side of your face?
2. Assess the skin on you face. Is the texture the same throughout? Are there any moles, sores, or growths that have changed in size or color?
3. Check your neck and under your chin. Can you feel any lumps, tenderness or any area of swelling?
4. Assess your lips. Pull the lips up and down and look for any sores or color changes. Feel for any lumps, bumps, or change in the texture of normal mucous membrane.
5. With a flashlight, pull your cheek out so that you can look inside. Note any area of discoloration—extreme redness, white areas, or other discoloration. Check to see if there are any lumps, swelling, or bumps in either cheek. Is there any area of tenderness?
6. Are there any changes in the upper roof of your mouth, in texture, swelling, or color?
7. Look at all sides of your tongue. Are there any changes?
8. If you find anything that appears different or if you have any sores or areas in your mouth that do not heal within two weeks, call your dentist for follow-up.

Adapted from Estes, M. (2006). Health assessment and physical examination *(3rd ed.). New York: Thomson Delmar Learning.*

Nursing Diagnoses

Based on the information gathered, examples of nursing diagnoses in the patient with mouth pain may include the following:

- Impaired oral mucous membrane related to oral pain.
- Health-seeking behaviors related to oral pain.
- Risk for infection related to mouth pain.
- Risk for imbalanced nutrition, less than body requirements, related to oral pain.
- Impaired tissue integrity related to mouth pain.

Planning and Implementation

Once the cause of the disorder is determined, the plan of care can be formalized. During the diagnostic assessment, comfort measures and removal of known irritants should be initiated. Predisposing and contributing factors should be identified, and interventions to alter these factors should be part of the plan of care. Ulcerations should resolve in one week to 10 days once the contributing factors have been removed. Good oral hygiene is essential. Chlorhexidine 2% aqueous mouthwash is recommended. Topical pain relief can be provided with the use of oral mouthwash. Products such as benzydamine hydrochloride (Difflam) can be used. Topical corticosteroids can promote resolution of the ulcers. Products such as triamcinolone acetonide in cellulose paste are used. Any patient who has a mouth ulcer that lasts longer than three weeks should receive follow-up.

Evaluation of Outcomes

Potential patient outcomes for each of the example nursing diagnoses for the patient with mouth pain are:

- Impaired oral mucous membrane related to oral pain. The patient has intact oral mucosa.
- Health-seeking behaviors related to oral pain. The patient demonstrates appropriate oral hygiene.
- Risk for infection related to mouth pain. The patient remains free of infection, as evidenced by normal vital signs and absence of purulent drainage from wounds, incisions, and tubes. Infection is recognized early to allow for prompt treatment.
- Risk for imbalanced nutrition, less than body requirements, related to oral pain. The patient verbalizes and demonstrates selection of foods or meals that will achieve a cessation of weight loss and weighs within 10 percent of ideal body weight.
- Impaired tissue integrity related to mouth pain. The patient's skin condition should be improved as evidenced by decreased redness, swelling and pain.

Burning Mouth Syndrome

Burning mouth syndrome (oral dysesthesia, glossopyrosis, and glossodynia) is a constant burning sensation of the tongue seen in patients past middle age. It is thought to be a type of neuropathy. The discomfort is relieved by eating and drinking. There are many organic causes of this disorder, which include candidiasis, lichen planus, diabetes, xerostomia, ill-fitting denture, certain medications, and glossitis related to nutritional deficiencies such as vitamin B, folate, and iron. Patients with this syndrome should also be assessed for psychological dysfunction such as depression, cancer fears, or anxiety.

Planning and Implementation

In addition to gingival health, it is essential to assess the condition of the teeth. The nurse should determine if the patient has the ability to clean their teeth properly, note when the patient last visited a dentist for oral care, and determine if their dentition interferes with eating and nutritional intake. Oral care for the patient while hospitalized is essential (see Patient Playbook).

Dysphagia

Swallowing is a complex activity that begins in the mouth with adequate wetting and mastication of food and fluid. This requires good dentition, a healthy oropharynx, adequate salivation, and muscular strength. Because of the increasing numbers of older patients and limitations caused by age-related decreases in muscle mass **(sarcopenia),** dysphagia in the elderly **(presbyphagia)** is underestimated. **Dysphagia** (difficulty swallowing) represents a major problem in the older adult and needs special attention to prevent aspiration pneumonitis or pneumonia, airway obstruction, malnutrition, and dehydration. Aspiration normally involves solid and liquid material entering the larynx below the true vocal cords. In addition, there is silent aspiration, which occurs without a cough response or voice change. Dysphagia must be recognized and assessed. Swallowing changes must be differentiated from age-related primary presbyphagia or secondary presbyphagia from other disorders (e.g., stroke, neuromuscular disorders). More than half of patients who experience a stroke demonstrate dysphagia dependent on when they are screened (Box 49-1).

> **BOX 49-1**
>
> **DYSPHAGIA**
>
> Nurses are often the first health care provider who notices that the patient is experiencing chewing or swallowing problems. The estimates of dysphagia in health care facilities range from 25 to 45 percent. By the year 2010, the Agency for Health Care Research and Quality (AHRQ) predicts that because of our aging population more than 16,500,000 people will experience dysphagia and need care or intervention. Many disciplines are interested in the problem of swallowing. These include nurses, speech pathologist, occupational therapists, physical therapists, pulmonologists, respiratory therapists, otolaryngologists, and neurologists. Hence the nurse will be actively involved with the health care team in the assessment and management of patients with this disorder.

Assessment with Clinical Manifestations

To prevent or decrease aspiration risk, screening must be done for all patients suspected of having swallowing problems or dysphagia especially patients who are at risk or have had a stroke (Box 49-2). Bedside assessment of aspiration risk is variable because of the increase in false-positive results. Interrater and intrarater reli-

> **BOX 49-2**
>
> **NORMAL SWALLOWING**
>
> **Normal Swallowing Requires:**
>
> - Intact and integrated functioning of cranial nerves V, VII, IX, X, XI, and XII, nucleus of the medulla, and sensorimotor cortical system
> - Coordination of sensory stimuli, motor function, and coordinated movements during the swallow.
>
> **Stages of Swallowing:**
>
> - Oral prep.
> - Food and liquids placed in the mouth.
> - Thorough biting, sucking, and sealing ingested material between lips and jaw.
> - Oral contents are chewed and mixed with saliva, forming a bolus because of voluntary movements of the tongue, jaw, and floor of the mouth.
> - Oral.
> - Food or liquid directed posteriorly toward oropharynx via movement of tongue, palate, and facial muscles.
> - Pharyngeal—swallowing.
> - Bolus of oral contents moved through the faucial arches and squeezed through the pharynx via muscles of the pharynx and the base of the tongue.
> - Nasopharynx closed by soft palate, larynx moves upward, the epiglottis tilts, the glottis, and supraglottis closes off using the true and false vocal cords.
> - Cricopharyngeal sphincter relaxes and opens to allow the bolus to enter esophagus.
> - Esophageal.
> - Involuntary peristalsis advances the bolus through the esophagus into the stomach—sequential waves of muscular contractions.
>
> *Adapted from Estes, M. (2006).* Health assessment and physical examination *(3rd ed.). New York: Thomson Delmar Learning; Payton, C. (2005). Referral diagnosis and management of dysphagia.* Pulse, *65(8), 64–65.*

ability studies demonstrate inconsistency in assessment results. Nonetheless this assessment should be done, and if dysphagia is suspected, nursing measures to prevent aspiration should be put into place. Cervical auscultation is one method of determining if a patient is aspirating during swallowing. Cervical auscultation by a skilled clinician has produced significantly high false-positive results. Cervical auscultation is performed by listening with the bell of the stethoscope over the lateral area of thyroid cartilage produced during swallowing (Estes, 2006). Eighty percent of the time, people exhale after swallowing. In the elderly and dysphagic patients, inspiration was found to be more common (Smith & Connolly, 2003). It is not recommended as a stand alone method to determine aspiration.

Diagnostic Tests

Patients who have difficulty swallowing will often be scheduled for a barium swallow exam, an endoscopic evaluation, esophageal manometry, and possibly esophageal transit scintigraphy. The presence of a gag reflex has been used as an indicator of the patient's ability to prevent a silent aspiration, although studies with videofluoroscopy demonstrated aspiration in patients with an intact gag reflex (Higo, Tayama, Nitou, Watanabe, & Ugawa, 2003). Bedside water swallow tests produce subjective results and though done may not detect dysphagia. Despite overdiagnosing swallowing disorders, a most important part of the assessment of dysphagia remains a careful bedside assessment. The nurse should perform an in-depth history with careful questioning of the patient and the caregiver concerning problems associated with swallowing (Box 49-3). Investigators have suggested the use of a dysphagia checklist as a screening tool for all patients.

BOX 49-3

ASSESSMENT OF A PATIENT WHO IS EXPERIENCING DIFFICULTY SWALLOWING

Is the patient exhibiting any of the following symptoms?

- Difficulty swallowing liquids—may indicate a neurological disorder.
- Difficulty with voice (dysphonia) or speech (dysarthria, abnormal speech articulation)—may indicate motor dysfunction.
- Difficulty swallowing solids—may indicate a structural abnormality.
- Regurgitation—may indicate pharyngeal pouch.
- Progressive dysphagia—may indicate hypopharyngeal tumor. (Are there any indications of aspiration?)
- Wet voice quality, coughing after eating or drinking, recurrent pulmonary infections. (Is there pain or discomfort when swallowing?)
- Have patient describe what happens when he or she swallows.
- Does the patient have problems managing oral secretions? Do you assess that the patient drools?
- Are mealtimes prolonged? Is there difficulty with chewing? Does food feel like it sticks in the throat or chest?
- Has the patient lost any weight?
- How much is the patient drinking daily?
- Does the patient drink fluids during the meal?
- Has the patient noticed a change in eating habits?
- Are there any problems with the patient's dentition?
- When was the last time the patient had a dental check-up?
- With all of the questions related to symptoms the nurse should ask about the onset, duration, severity of the problem, and relieving or aggravating factors.

Adapted from Estes, M. (2006). Health assessment and physical examination *(3rd ed.). New York: Thomson Delmar Learning.*

Fiberoptic endoscopic examination of swallowing can be used but is poorly tolerated in frail elderly. The contraction of the pharynx blocks the view of the food or liquid in the pharynx and esophagus but after the swallow, what remains in the pharynx can be identified. Some investigators have proposed that the use of pulse oximetry with the water swallow screening test can be a sensitive predictor of dysphagia with aspiration (Smith & Connolly, 2003). With the water swallow screening test a 2 percent drop in baseline SaO_2 was able to demonstrate aspiration in over 81 percent of patients with dysphagia. This is an important assessment skill for the nurse to develop. In many institutions this assessment is performed by specially trained speech and language therapists.

Currently the gold standard for evaluation of dysphagia is videofluoroscopy (also known as modified barium swallow) with or without manometric evaluation. This assessment demonstrates the swallowing mechanism. It also provides information about maneuvers and positions that facilitate and improve swallowing, e.g., tucking the chin (neck flexion) or holding the breath before swallowing. This maneuver may decrease aspiration. Turning the patient's head to the weak side (affected side if the patient has had a stroke) may force the bolus of food toward the unaffected side of the pharynx and augment the swallowing effort. Videofluoroscopy can be poorly tolerated and unsuitable for patients who are frail, unable to follow instructions, or not able to sit. Equipment and trained personnel may not be available to provide the assessment.

Nursing Diagnoses

Based on the information gathered, examples of nursing diagnoses in the patient with dysphagia may include the following:

- Impaired swallowing.
- Risk for aspiration.
- Health-seeking behaviors.
- Risk for injury.
- Risk for nutrition imbalanced, less than body requirements, or readiness for enhanced nutrition.
- Chronic pain.
- Disturbed sensory perception.
- Impaired tissue integrity.

Planning and Implementation

Patients who are experiencing swallowing difficulties have as their primary problems risk for aspiration, impaired swallowing, nutritional imbalance, altered comfort, a need for therapeutic regimen management, and knowledge deficit. Because patients perceive that they experience difficulty in consuming swallowed material, solid or liquid, they are at high risk for many nutritional problems. The problems the patient experiences may be related to oropharyngeal dysfunction from cerebrovascular accidents, neuromuscular disorders, mucosal diseases like gastroesophageal reflux disease (GERD), radiation injury, or mediastinal diseases, such as tumors. Patients must be involved in the collaborative management and planning of their care as the diagnosis and treatment plan is put into place.

Presently there are many recommendations for managing patients with dysphagia, but the evidence for the most effective management of these patients is largely anecdotal. Results have been mixed in that the patient population has not been homogeneous, the protocols and interventions have not been consistent, and differing outcomes have been measured. Functional severity scales are subjective; hence it is difficult to objectively quantify the measurements. Investigators and practitioners draw conclusions that cannot statistically be generalized to larger populations (Hill, Hughes, & Milford, 2005). The first goal of treatment is to ensure treatment of any underlying disorders. The nurse must ensure that aspiration is reduced, and nutritional status must be optimized. Concurrently, individualized plans of care are devised. Interventions that become part of everyday practice and recommendations include dietary manipulation; altered swallowing techniques, referred to as compensatory maneuvers in the rehabilitation literature; surgery; and in some cases enteral feeding. The best therapy for an impaired functional activity is the activity itself.

Nutrition

Once aspiration status is assessed in relation to liquids and solids, a plan for dietary management should be established and the consistency of the food established. Some patients may be restricted to thickened foods (i.e., they cannot swallow liquids). Foods that are tough are difficult to swallow so a mechanical soft diet is ordered for the patient. Some patients may need a pureed diet, especially if their swallowing difficulty is with the oral phase. The dietician or nutritionist should be part of the team who is helping the patient and the family understand the nutritional and food preparation needs. For individuals who experience aspiration or regurgitation, there should be no eating at bedtime. Patients should be instructed to remain upright after eating and reduce the amount of liquid that they drink with meals.

Enteral feeding may be needed for some patients. The general guideline is any patient who cannot take in adequate nutrients and hydration by mouth or who has a functional bowel, must receive nutrients enterally. Patients who are initiated on early enteral nutrition have shorter hospital stays and better outcomes (Hildebrandt, Fracchia, Driscoll, & Giroux, 2003). The nasogastric feeding tube, the percutaneous endoscopic gastrostomy (PEG) tube, or the surgical gastrostomy are the choices available. Nasogastric tubes must be carefully selected for size and comfort as well as ease of insertion. Patients find these tubes uncomfortable. There is a high rate of these tubes being pulled out. Placement of these tubes must be checked radiographically prior to beginning the tube feeding. These tubes can be inadvertently inserted into the lung rather than the stomach or duodenum. The PEG is initially inserted by the physician or an advanced practitioner prepared to insert these tubes. These tubes are sutured in place or have a balloon inflated that prevents their removal. Complications associated with these tubes include bleeding or infection at the insertion site, peritonitis, and the potential for ascites, chest infections, and puncture of other abdominal organs during insertion. PEG feedings are associated with improved outcomes on measures of nutrition, weight, midarm circumference, and serum albumin as well as less treatment failures and fewer deaths.

Difficulty swallowing can be managed by speech pathologists and encouraged by nursing personnel. There are three types of swallowing therapy, compensatory, indirect, and direct therapy (Box 49-4).

BOX 49-4

TECHNIQUES OF SWALLOWING THERAPY

1. Compensatory techniques—postural maneuvers such as proper positioning.
2. Indirect therapy—strengthening exercises to improve the swallowing muscles, such as lip, and tongue mobility exercises, active resistive exercise, vibratory inhibition, ice application, and stretching of oral structural muscles, repetitive head lift exercise to improve anterior excursion of the larynx and the cross-sectional area of the upper esophageal sphincter.
3. Direct therapy—exercises to strengthen the muscles while swallowing liquids and solids.

Adapted from Robbins, J., Gangnon, R., Theis, S., Kays, S., Hewitt, A., & Hind, J. (2005). The effects of lingual exercise on swallowing in older adults. Journal of American Geriatric Society, *53(9), 1483–1489.*

Surgery

Tactile-thermal stimulation and electrical stimulation have been used. Results have shown that most patients responded to electrical stimulation. Swallowing function improved, and the treatment appeared to be safe. In addition, endoscopy can also be used to treat swallowing difficulties, as shown in Figure 49-3. Also, there are some patients that may need surgery. Surgery is needed when there is manometric evidence of obstruction to a bolus at the cricopharyngeal segment. The most common type of surgery is cricopharyngeal myotomy (CPM). The cricopharyngeus muscle is incised to reduce resistance to pharyngeal outflow. This surgery is accompanied by suspension of the thyroid cartilage. Alternatively some patients may be candidates for botulinum toxin injection into the pharyngoesophageal sphincter (PES). This procedure replaces the CPM. Other surgeries are available to patients dependent on the type of dysphagia the patient is experiencing.

ESOPHAGEAL DISORDERS

The lining of the esophagus is extremely vascular, and the esophagus itself is vital to nutritional balance. The more common disorders are elaborated on in this section, including achalasia, GERD, hiatal hernia, and esophageal cancer.

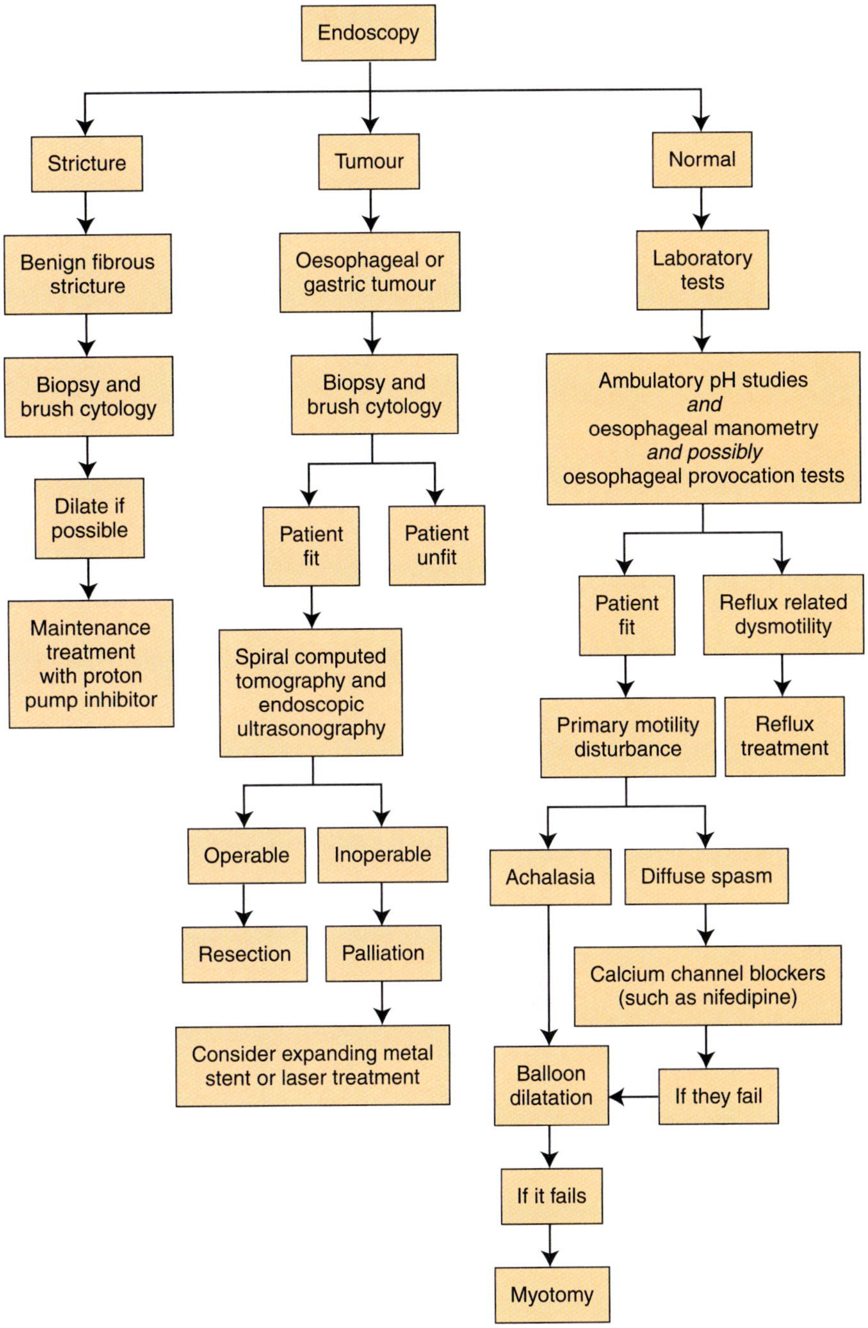

Figure 49-3 Algorithm for endoscopic management of dysphagia. Adapted from Hill, M., Hughes T., & Milford C. (2005). Treatment for swallowing difficulties (dysphagia) in chronic muscle disease. *The Cochrane Database of Systematic Reviews (Oxford)* (2), CD004303.

Esophageal Pain and Achalasia

Esophageal pain can be associated with dysphagia. It can be a result of irritation to the mucosal lining of the esophagus or mechanical distension of the esophagus. Because the pain associated with esophageal disorders is often the same as pain from cardiac origin, it is important to provide the patient reassurance as the diagnostic workup is performed. Esophageal pain is described as burning in the anterior chest. It is sensed in the throat and may radiate to the neck, back, or upper arms. This is similar to cardiac pain. Approximately 20 percent of the time that patients experience pain in the chest, shoulders, arms, neck, and back; it is impossible to differentiate the origin of the pain between cardiac or esophageal. **Achalasia** is a loss of peristalsis in the muscle of the esophagus secondary to a degeneration of neurons in the wall of the esophagus (Estes, 2006).

Nursing Diagnoses

Based on the information gathered, examples of nursing diagnoses in the patient with esophageal pain and achalasia may include the following:

- Acute pain related to esophageal pathology.
- Impaired tissue integrity related to achalasia.
- Imbalanced nutrition, less than body requirements, related to achalasia.

Planning and Implementation

Important in the management and plan of care for patients with esophageal pain is empathetic consideration during the medical workup. This includes explanation, reassurance, information sharing, teaching, and if necessary, collaborative management with psychotherapy. If the patient does have reflux disease, a plan of care should be established to manage this. If the patient is found to have achalasia as a cause of the esophageal pain, particular care will be provided. There is no treatment for peristaltic loss in the esophagus. If it is found on manometry that the lower esophageal sphincter (LES) fails to relax, the aim will be to relax or dilate the LES.

Pharmacology

The first line of treatment for esophageal pain and achalasia is often the same medications used to treat angina of cardiac origin. These include vasodilators, such as nitroglycerin, calcium channel blockers, such as verapamil, and isosorbide dinitrate (Isordil). Unfortunately the effect of these medications is not lasting and surgery is often the necessary next step of management for these patients (Broyles, Reiss, & Evans, 2007).

Surgery

The mainstay of treatment for achalasia is surgery or balloon dilation. This intervention is best for patients over 45 years of age. It is effective between 60 to 95 percent. Patients who have balloon dilatation (pneumatic dilation) are at risk for esophageal damage, tearing, or even rupture during the procedure (2 to 5 percent). The major complications of esophageal dilatation are perforation, bleeding, and bacteremia. Surgical intervention or esophageal myotomy may be selected in younger patients. The muscle fibers of LES are severed during this procedure. Ninety percent of patients experience an effective outcome, but they may also develop reflux disease. Another option to relax the LES and to reduce the symptoms is to inject the muscle with toxin (Botox). Currently the effectiveness of Botox injection is reported to be about 60 percent for about six months. At one year, only 32 percent continued to be symptom free. Although the patient undergoes endoscopy for this procedure, it is useful in patients who are at high risk for surgical intervention.

Evaluation of Outcomes

Potential patient outcomes for each of the example nursing diagnoses for the patient with esophageal pain and achalasia are:

- Acute pain related to esophageal pathology. The patient should verbalize an adequate relief of pain along with the ability to realistically cope with the pain if it is not completely relieved.
- Impaired tissue integrity related to achalasia. The patient will improve the condition of his or her impaired tissue integrity as evidenced by decreased redness, swelling, and pain.
- Imbalanced nutrition, less than body requirements, related to achalasia. The patient verbalizes and demonstrates selection of foods or meals that will achieve a cessation of weight loss and weighs within 10 percent of ideal body weight.

Gastroesophageal Reflux Disease

GERD refers to the backing up of gastric contents into the esophagus. As this happens, the patient experiences **pyrosis,** a substernal burning sensation often radiating to the neck, commonly called heartburn.

Epidemiology

GERD occurs in 15 to 20 percent of all adults. For many of these people, daily symptoms are common.

Etiology

There are several common problems that result in GERD. Causes of GERD are an incompetent LES, a motility disorder of the esophagus as previously described, and pyloric stenosis. In addition, the aging process correlates with an increased incidence of GERD.

Pathophysiology

During the swallowing process, the LES is normally closed. The backflow of gastric juices up into the esophagus is consequently prevented because of the difference in the pressure between the lower esophagus and the stomach. In GERD, the LES relaxes or is incompetent and the gastric contents are allowed to move upward during times of increased pressure. Examples of the pressure changes are when the stomach volume is increased, as after a meal or when the patient bends down.

The gastric contents are acidic and are made of pepsin and bile. These substances are irritating and over time the mucosa of the esophagus is affected by GERD, leading to esophagitis. Ulcerations may develop, which can result in bleeding, scarring, and strictures.

Assessment with Clinical Manifestations

The most common manifestation of GERD is pyrosis, particularly after eating when either bending over or lying down. The patient will experience a regurgitation of a bitter tasting solution in the mouth. This may lead to difficulty swallowing and pain from the irritation of the gastric juices. The patient may develop esophagitis, pharyngitis, or hoarseness. The complication of Barrett's esophagus can even lead to esophageal cancer, described in the next section.

Barrett's Esophagus

Barrett's esophagus was first identified in 1950 by Norman Barrett in a patient who had esophagitis with a peptic ulcer. Barrett's esophagus develops because of chronic reflux esophagitis (GERD), even though 25 percent of the population with Barrett's does not experience GERD. Current research is underway to consider the potential role of prostaglandins and leukotrienes in inducing inflammatory mediators that produce symptoms and promote disease advancement. As the disorder is progressing, chronic exposure of the esophagus to stomach acid damages the esophageal epithelium. Approximately 1 in 200 patients with Barrett's esophagus will develop adenocarcinoma. Even considering this information, there is no current evidence that screening the population for the presence of Barrett's esophagus will decrease the rate of adenocarcinoma of the esophagus. Nonetheless, the American Gastroenterology Association (AGA) recommends upper endoscopy with histological examination of esophageal biopsy for those individuals who have GERD symptoms. Additionally the patient may have a radiological exam, the barium swallow. The barium swallow may show thickening of the esophageal folds, ulcerations, and strictures as well as reflux of barium. Twenty-four hour ambulatory pH monitoring of the esophagus may also be performed as part of the assessment of the patient. Several variables are monitored with this procedure. The most clinically applicable result is the percent of time the pH remains below 4. Normally the pH is below 4 and less than 4.5% in a 24-hour period (1.1 hours out of 24).

Red Flag

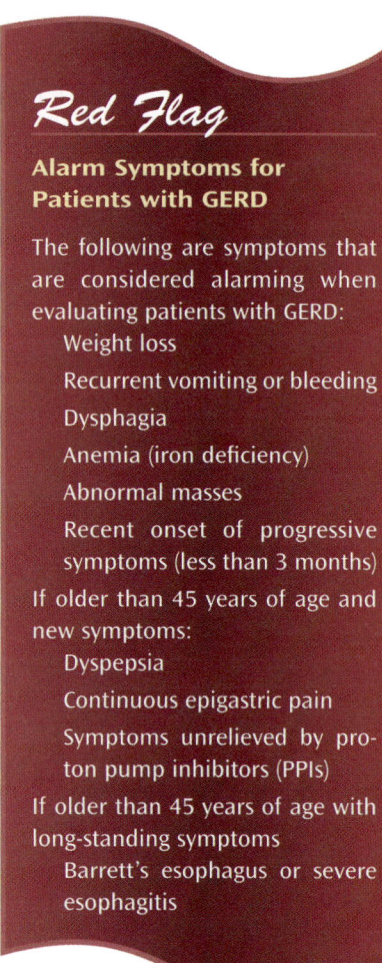

Alarm Symptoms for Patients with GERD

The following are symptoms that are considered alarming when evaluating patients with GERD:

- Weight loss
- Recurrent vomiting or bleeding
- Dysphagia
- Anemia (iron deficiency)
- Abnormal masses
- Recent onset of progressive symptoms (less than 3 months)

If older than 45 years of age and new symptoms:

- Dyspepsia
- Continuous epigastric pain
- Symptoms unrelieved by proton pump inhibitors (PPIs)

If older than 45 years of age with long-standing symptoms

- Barrett's esophagus or severe esophagitis

Patients with Barrett's esophagus present with the symptoms of reflux esophagitis because of the exposure of the esophagus to acidic gastric contents. The patient may describe heartburn or a burning taste in the back of the throat. At times patients may describe a sensation of saliva filling the mouth. This symptom is **brash water.** It occurs when the mouth suddenly fills with saliva secondary to reflex salivary secretion stimulated by acid back flow into the esophagus. Certain foods will also stimulate heartburn.

The aim of treatment for Barrett's esophagus is to decrease the reflux of acid into the esophagus until the symptoms of esophagitis are no longer evident. The American College of Gastroenterology updated their original guidelines for surveillance of individuals with Barrett's esophagus (DeVault & Castell, 2005; Inadomi, et al., 2003). These include two surveillance endoscopies with biopsies showing no dysplasia followed by surveillance every three years; treatment of GERD to reduce inflammation; and if dysplasia is present, confirmation by a second expert pathologist is needed. When a patient has low-grade dysplasia, annual surveillance endoscopies should be done; with high-grade dysplasia, the interval between endoscopies should be shortened, and surgical intervention should be planned. Antireflux surgery is controversial because outcomes of medication therapy (drugs to suppress acid release) when similarly stratified with surgical repair are the same. The management of patients with Barrett's esophagus is the same as for GERD.

Diagnostic Tests

The patient history is a primary method of suspecting GERD. After seeking health care, an upper endoscopy can reveal a reddened esophageal lining, which is indicative of GERD. Further tests can be a barium swallow, a 24-hour ambulatory pH monitoring, which detects the lowered pH levels commensurate with an acid environment, and esophageal manometry, which evaluates the pressures of the esophageal sphincters and esophageal peristalsis (Daniels, 2003).

Nursing Diagnoses

Based on the information gathered, examples of nursing diagnoses in the patient with GERD may include the following:

- Acute pain related to the gastric juices irritating the esophagus.
- Deficient knowledge related to self-care and risk prevention.
- Imbalanced nutrition, less than body requirements, related to the irritation of the esophagus.

Planning and Implementation

The management plan for GERD involves patient education regarding the noninvasive techniques for care (see Patient Playbook feature) and then common medication therapy. If the dysfunction is not able to be arrested, and the disorder continues, surgery may be indicated.

Pharmacology

The patient may initially self-administer antacids to decrease the esophageal pain. The antacids neutralize the gastric juices. If prescription medications are indicated, the patient may then be given histamine receptor blockers (e.g., Pepcid, Tagamet, or Zantac). These reduce the acid nature of the gastric fluids by blocking the histamine, which normally stimulates acid secretion. As GERD becomes more serious PPIs, medications that decrease release of acid may be given. The PPI (e.g., Prevacid, Prilosec) inhibit the hydrogen potassium pump, which reduces gastric acids. PPI allow the esophagus time to heal, as well as create a lesser acid environment.

Surgery

If medication strategies are not effective, surgery may be indicated as the GERD condition persists. Antireflux surgeries change the ability of the LES to inhibit gastric juices from reflux. There are laparoscopic surgeries, which can

PATIENT PLAYBOOK

Patient Education for GERD

The nurse should instruct the patient with GERD to:

- Eat small meals at any given setting and avoid eating two to three hours before sleeping.
- Wash the throat with water after each meal, as this neutralizes the esophagus and cleanses the esophagus from the gastric juices.
- Sit in a semifowler's position if lying down after eating.
- Avoid irritating food substances (caffeine, alcohol, or acidic foods).
- Cease smoking, as it increases gastric acidity and interferes with healing of the esophagus.

tighten the LES, and there is an open, more invasive surgery (Nissen fundoplication) which may be performed.

Evaluation of Outcomes

Potential patient outcomes for each of the example nursing diagnoses for the patient with GERD are:

- Acute pain related to the gastric juices irritating the esophagus. The patient should verbalize an adequate relief of pain along with the ability to realistically cope with the pain if it is not completely relieved.
- Deficient knowledge related to self-care and risk prevention. The patient should demonstrate motivation to learn, identify perceived learning needs, and verbalize an understanding of desired content.
- Imbalanced nutrition, less than body requirements, related to the irritation of the esophagus. The patient verbalizes and demonstrates selection of foods or meals that will achieve a cessation of weight loss and weighs within 10 percent of ideal body weight.

Hiatal Hernia

A hiatal hernia develops when there is a part of the stomach that protrudes through the esophageal hiatus. There are often no symptoms, but when it is evidenced the manifestations are similar to those in GERD.

Etiology

There is a correlation with age and hiatal hernia formation. Other causes are weakened esophageal diaphragm areas, increased intra-abdominal pressure (e.g., pregnancy), and shortening of the esophagus.

Pathophysiology

There are two primary types of hiatal hernias: (a) sliding hiatal hernia (type I), and (b) paraesophageal hiatal hernia (type II). In addition, there are types III, IV, and V, which are less common, and are differentiated by the amount of herniation. In a sliding hiatal hernia the upper stomach slides upward through the gastroesophageal junction. This type of hiatal hernia is often asymptomatic. The paraesophageal hiatal hernia results when a part of the stomach herniates through the esophageal hiatus. In this type of hiatal hernia blood flow can be constricted and patients can develop chronic or acute GI bleeding or gastritis.

Assessment with Clinical Manifestations

The symptomatology for hiatal hernias is similar to GERD, and many are asymptomatic. The manifestations are pyrosis, reflux, a feeling of satiation, dysphagia, bleeding, and substernal chest pain. The reflux symptoms are more common with a sliding hiatal hernia and fullness is more typical in the type II hiatal hernia. Potential complications of hiatal hernias are hemorrhaging, obstruction, and strangulation.

Diagnostic Tests

The presentation of the patient and their history often confirms the diagnosis. More definitive tests to diagnose a hiatal hernia are a barium swallow and an upper endoscopy.

Nursing Diagnoses

Based on the information gathered, examples of nursing diagnoses in the patient with hiatal hernia may include the following:

- Acute pain related to the gastric juices irritating the esophagus.
- Deficient knowledge related to self-care and risk prevention.
- Imbalanced nutrition, less than body requirements, related to the irritation of the esophagus.

Planning and Implementation

The nursing interventions and plan of care is similar for hiatal hernias as for GERD. This includes the potential surgeries and medications that are prescribed.

Evaluation of Outcomes

Potential patient outcomes for each of the example nursing diagnoses for the patient with hiatal hernia are:

- Acute pain related to the gastric juices irritating the esophagus. The patient should verbalize an adequate relief of pain along with the ability to realistically cope with the pain if it is not completely relieved.
- Deficient knowledge related to self-care care and risk prevention. The patient should demonstrate motivation to learn, identify perceived learning needs, and verbalize an understanding of desired content.
- Imbalanced nutrition, less than body requirements, related to the irritation of the esophagus. The patient verbalizes and demonstrates selection of foods or meals that will achieve a cessation of weight loss and weighs within 10 percent of ideal body weight.

Esophageal Cancer

Esophageal cancer, associated with the highest cancer mortality rate (five-year survival rate of 15 percent) is also one of the most rapidly increasing malignancies. This is a disease of older Caucasian males. The peak incidence is in patients 65 to 74 years old. Mortality rates are higher in patients from minority populations. Early detection through screening and surveillance is essential for any GI malignancy and even more so with cancers of the esophagus.

Epidemiology

There are two primary types of esophageal cancer: adenocarcinoma and squamous cell carcinoma. The risk factors for these types of cancer are listed in Table 49-2.

Lifestyle modification and chemoprevention for those individuals at high risk for the development of esophageal cancer is important. The nurse should assist patients to modify riskier behavior and select healthier lifestyles. It is imperative that nurses be involved in smoking cessation programs. Obesity is an important contributing factor in the epidemiology of esophageal cancer. Even though esophageal cancer rates are increasing, there is insufficient evi-

TABLE 49-2 Primary Known Risk Factors for Esophageal Cancer

ADENOCARCINOMA	SQUAMOUS CELL CARCINOMA
Smoking	Smoking
Chronic GERD	Alcohol ingestion
Barrett's esophagus	Exposure to nitrosamines
	Ingestion of lye
	Fanconi's anemia
	Achalasia
	Plummer-Vincent webs
	Tylosis

Adapted from Yang, C., Wang, H., Wang, Z., Du, H. Z., Tao, D., Mu, X., et al. (2005). Risk factors for esophageal cancer: A case-control study in South-western China. Asian Pacific Journal of Cancer Prevention, *6(1), 48–53.*

dence that screening for esophageal cancer is effective except for those individuals with Barrett's esophagus (patients with Barrett's esophagus who have dysplasia are considered at risk and should be on a regular screening regimen dependent on the grade of the dysplasia), those with familial occurrence of adenocarcinoma, patients with tylosis, lye-induced strictures, and Fanconi's anemia (level III evidence). Respected experts suggest screening for patients who have been long-term tobacco users, alcoholics, and those diagnosed with achalasia. The degree of dysplasia found on the first screening will also dictate the screening endoscopy interval the patient will be asked to follow. Screening endoscopy may be recommended every three months for high-grade esophageal dysplasia or as infrequently as every five years if there is no dysplasia. Patients who have mucosal abnormalities should have biopsies and mucosal resection to determine if there is any malignancy present. Chemoprevention for patients at high risk should be implemented. This would include drugs to reduce acid—PPIs and nonsteroidal anti-inflammatory drugs (NSAIDs). NSAIDs seem to inhibit prostaglandin E_2 that decreases the production of the Barrett's epithelial cells (Homs, Steyerberg, Eijkenboom, & Siersema, 2006).

Pathophysiology

Cancer of the esophagus obviously is caused by malignant advancement into the esophageal areas. Once the malignancy penetrates the submucosa, the risk of metastasis as well as increase in mortality are substantial (Wang, Wongkeesong, & Buttar, 2005). Fifteen percent of esophageal cancers are in the upper one third of the esophagus; 50 percent in the middle one third of the esophagus, and 35 percent in the lower third at the gastroesophageal junction (GEJ). The major types of esophageal cancer are adenocarcinoma and squamous cell, as shown in the risk factor table. Identification of the stage of the esophageal cancer (by tissue examination) is necessary for the management of the cancer. Determining the stage of the disease is usually done with endoscopy and computed tomography (CT). Endoscopic ultrasound with fine needle aspiration may also be used. Also, refer to chapter 15 for more information on the theories of cancer cell development.

Assessment with Clinical Manifestations

Patients with esophageal cancer usually present with difficulty in swallowing. At this point, the esophagus is often 50 to 60 percent obstructed. This difficulty is progressive and leads to the second most common presentation pain, odynophagia (Friedman, McQuaid, & Grendell, 2003). Other symptoms often associated with esophageal cancer include anorexia, weight loss, hoarseness and voice change, aspiration, cough, and recurrent upper respiratory infections. Often the patient is anemic without over GI bleeding. As with all GI cancers, systematic staging of the disease is necessary to plan the most effective treatment.

Nursing Diagnoses

Based on the information gathered, examples of nursing diagnoses in the patient with esophageal cancer may include the following:

- Acute pain related to esophageal cancer.
- Anxiety related to diagnosis of esophageal cancer.
- Ineffective coping related to diagnosis of esophageal cancer.
- Imbalanced nutrition, less than body requirements.
- Anticipatory grieving related to diagnosis of esophageal cancer.
- Spiritual distress related to diagnosis of esophageal cancer.

Planning and Implementation

The aim of treatment will be palliative or curative based on the stage of the disease and the patient's health status. The collaborative team managing the patient's care should individualize the options and determine the most appropriate plan. General approaches to caring for patients with cancer are provided in chapter 15.

If the tumor is confined to the mucosa, the patient will undergo either an esophagectomy or endoscopic mucosal resection (Verschuur, et al., 2006). If the tumor penetrates through the submucosa, an esophagectomy is the treatment of choice. If the patient has evidence of metastasis to lymph nodes, chemotherapy and radiation are done prior to any surgical procedure (neoadjuvant therapy). If the cancer is advanced, palliative procedures may be done. The goals of palliative care are to alleviate pain and discomfort by alleviating difficulty in swallowing, to receive adequate nutrition, and to improve the quality of life. Prior to selection of any chemo or radiation therapy treatments, the patient should receive enteral nutritional support. It is recommended that esophageal stenting be selected to relieve symptomatology from tumor load. When a patient with esophageal cancer presents with persistent swallowing problems, anorexia, and weight loss, the cancer is at an advanced and often incurable stage. Hence, the plan for palliation is essential.

Evaluation of Outcomes

Potential patient outcomes for each of the example nursing diagnoses for the patient with esophageal cancer are:

- Acute pain related to esophageal cancer. The patient should verbalize an adequate relief of pain along with the ability to realistically cope with the pain if it is not completely relieved.
- Anxiety related to diagnosis of esophageal cancer. The patient should be able to recognize the signs of anxiety, demonstrate positive coping mechanisms, and describe a reduction in the level of anxiety experienced.
- Ineffective coping related to diagnosis of esophageal cancer. The patient identifies their own maladaptive coping behaviors and available resources and support systems. The patient also describes and initiates alternative coping strategies and the positive results from new behaviors.
- Imbalanced nutrition, less than body requirements. The patient verbalizes and demonstrates selection of foods or meals that will achieve a cessation of weight loss and weighs within 10 percent of ideal body weight.
- Anticipatory grieving related to diagnosis of esophageal cancer. The patient verbalizes feelings and establishes and maintains functional support systems.
- Spiritual distress related to diagnosis of esophageal cancer. The patient expresses hope in and value of his or her belief system and inner resources and expresses a sense of well-being.

Even though there have been significant improvements in diagnosis, surgical techniques, and neoadjuvant chemoradiation therapy, the overall five-year survival rate is less than 15 percent. Patients with a T1 or T2 disease stage have a five-year survival of 40 percent. Care of these patients and their families is a particular challenge to the entire health care team.

GI TRACT PAIN OF NONCARDIAC AND NONPHYSIOLOGICAL ORIGINS

There are several conditions seen in the upper GI tract that are somewhat different from the normal physiological causes. These conditions are noncardiac chest pain, which may have its etiology in the GI tract, panic disorders, and functional GI disorders (FGID).

Noncardiac Chest Pain

It is essential to discuss all patients who might experience noncardiac chest pain. The causes of this type of pain include patients with cardiac, GI, psychiatric, or musculoskeletal disorders. Accurately determining what the cause derives from may be challenging. Many patients have more than one disorder that can lead to chest pain, so decisional pathways (algorithms) have been used to assist in the diagnostic process.

GERD and esophageal motility disorders are discussed in this text, but it is important to discuss visceral hypersensitivity. Increased visceral hypersensitivity (heightened visceral nociception) is linked to patients with chest pain of unknown cause. It is seen with patients who have marked pain response to various visceral stimuli (e.g., distension, acid reflux, motility disorders). These patients must be managed so that any life-threatening disorder is ruled out secondary to cardiac ischemia. The common causes of this type of chest pain must be evaluated. This includes GERD and panic disorder while unusual causes of chest pain must also be examined. These unusual causes include costochondritis (inflammation of the costochondral cartilage), biliary colic, aortic aneurysm, and peptic ulcer disorder.

Panic Disorder

Panic disorder occurs in the same percentage of patients with chest pain as with GERD, 30 to 50 percent. If the diagnosis of panic disorder is suspected, a first step might be to use a panic assessment instrument to further assess the patient. Management of patients with panic disorder can be a challenge. Providing the patient and family with educational materials is important. This includes assisting the patient to understand that this disorder exists in 5 percent of the U.S. populace. Patients can be treated for this disorder with several types of medications and therapy. The most commonly used medications include antianxiety agents and antidepressants. Beta blocking agents are useful for those who also have autonomic symptoms, e.g., palpitations and tachyarrhythmias. Cognitive behavioral therapy that focuses on stress management and improving coping skills may be equal to pharmacotherapy for this disorder.

Functional Gastrointestinal Disorders

Before discussing those GI disorders, which are from organic or physiological changes, it is important for the nurse to be aware that many patients may have no physiological cause of their GI symptoms. Because of the brain-gut connection, patients who have FGID need a biopsychosocial approach. This includes an understanding of the patient's early life, life stress, physiology, and symptom control. As patients are being assessed for their GI symptoms, the workup will include a thorough history of the patient's background. This includes information related to whether the patient has ever experienced any previous psychiatric problems. Evidence demonstrates a high incidence of patients who present with dyspepsia and irritable bowel syndrome have previously experienced sexual abuse. Many patients with FGID have undue stress related to fear of a serious disorder, such as cancer. These patients need reassurance about the effect of stress on the GI tract. These patients experience more anxiety, depression, neuroticism, and somatic complaints. They need an understanding that stress releases neuro-hormones from the brain that have a direct effect on GI function. The question of whether the emotional response is a result of the symptoms must be assessed. Many of these patients are managed by primary care providers so the nurse may encounter these patients in outpatient clinics. These patients need a confident approach, a diagnosis that is realistic, and psychotherapy of the cognitive behavioral type. Placebo trials demonstrate the usual GI medications are not effective for these individuals (Yamada, 2005).

NONULCER DYSPEPSIA

Dyspepsia (indigestion) is a term is used to describe several complaints (e.g., epigastric pain, bloating, fullness, early satiety, belching, heartburn, and nausea). Dyspepsia is divided into nonulcer dyspepsia (NUD) or dyspepsia secondary to peptic ulcer disease (PUD). NUD is responsible for about 40 percent of all patients who complain of recurrent pain or discomfort in the epigastric region of the abdomen or retrosternal region. NUD can be caused by GERD, problems with motility, gallbladder, liver, and pancreatic dysfunction as well as medication-induced dyspepsia, dietary causes, and endocrine or metabolic disorders (e.g., diabetes). The symptoms of dyspepsia have been divided into ulcer-like, dysmotility-like, and unspecified (Logan & Delaney, 2005). Heartburn secondary to reflux (GERD) will not be discussed in this section.

Epidemiology

The health belief model supports the option patients choose to seek care when there is an assessment of a serious illness and the likelihood of cure. Studies have shown that patients with dyspepsia seek health care when there is a belief that lifestyle and stresses are related to the symptoms they are experiencing. Additionally there is a fear that the symptoms are a sign of a serious problem. Historically, a review of 36 studies in 1998 that looked at the results of esophagogastroduodenoscopy (EGD) in patients with dyspepsia, only 1.6 percent of the patients had cancer. In a later review of 17,792 patients who had an EGD, only 1.4 percent were diagnosed with a malignancy (Vakil, Talley, Moayyedi, & Fennerty, 2005).

Pathophysiology

The pathophysiology of dyspepsia is focused in several areas. These include medication side effects, some foods, and gastric sensory and motility dysfunction. Medication side effects are a major contribution to dyspepsia. The major drug groups associated with dyspepsia are NSAIDs, especially in individuals with arthritis, aspirin, potassium supplements, iron, antibiotics, steroids, ACE inhibitors, nitrates, levodopa, estrogen, and quinidine. There is evidence to demonstrate that if patients have to take NSAIDs, they should also take PPIs to protect the gastric mucosa. At times patients must be taken off of the offending medication to relieve the symptoms.

The link between gastric emptying and dyspepsia is controversial; the link between gastric hypersensitivity may be the dominant dysfunction (Talley, 2005). Gastric epithelium may be responsive to gastric acid. The data suggest that PPI therapy is helpful in functional dyspepsia. An older study demonstrated that gastric sensory and motor dysfunction may be linked to a central limbic processing abnormality associated with childhood abuse. A more recent study of patients with functional dyspepsia showed an association between childhood sexual abuse and gastroparesis and an association between adult psychological abuse and gastric hypersensitivity. Although a cause-and-effect relationship cannot be concluded, it continues to be an important relationship.

Assessment with Clinical Manifestations

Patients who present with NUD describe a variety of symptoms. These symptoms include epigastric pain, bloating, fullness, early satiety, belching, heartburn, and nausea.

Diagnostic Tests

Separating the clinical history and distinguishing organic dyspepsia from functional dyspepsia continues to be problematic. Nonetheless, patients worry about unexplained symptoms. The quality of life for individuals who have dyspepsia is compromised. Symptom relief could improve the quality of life and is an aim of care. Because there is a strong relationship between dyspepsia, PUD, and *Helicobacter pylori,* a controversy exists over the decision to evaluate the patient for *H. pylori* or to treat empirically. If PUD is diagnosed, the gastroscopist will obtain a biopsy for histology and urease testing.

Nursing Diagnoses

Based on the information gathered, examples of nursing diagnoses in the patient with NUD may include the following:

- Acute pain related to upper epigastric irritation.
- Imbalanced nutrition, less than body requirements, related to anorexia.
- Deficient knowledge deficit related to self-care and risk prevention.

Planning and Implementation

The approach to patients with NUD is complex. It is based on the dysfunction that causes the dyspepsia. Different studies predict different results. Nurses must be aware of the latest evidence and the recommendations for treatment. There are many questions that impact the management and prognosis of NUD. Gastroparesis continues to be looked at as part of the dysfunction. Gastric hypersensitivity remains under study and treatment for a certain set of patients. Because the association between symptoms and organic or functional causes of NUD are unclear, more assessment of causal relationship is needed. The American College of Gastroenterology endorses that in patients 45 to 50 years of age empiric treatment with acid suppressing agents are appropriate. For patients greater than 50 years of age, EGD is recommended.

Nurses need to be aware of the journey of patients who have dyspepsia. The pain, the uncertainty in diagnosis, the disease burden, the decisional conflict, and the therapeutic regimen cause continuous ambiguity for the patient. Patients need support and knowledge related to the selection of workup as well as the treatment selection.

Pharmacology

There management of NUD is often dependent on pharmacological therapies. For example, placebo response can be demonstrated but is not conclusive as an approach to the management of dyspepsia. Also, prokinetic agents can be useful because 5-hydroxytryptamine $(HT)_4$ receptors can relax the gastric fundus. Currently there are no substantive data to support its use in NUD. Gastric motility can also be addressed with erythromycin or azithromycin (motilin agonist). Stimulation of motilin receptors will hasten stomach emptying. Unfortunately these medications have side effects, which may prevent their use. Erythromycin is a powerful stimulant of motility in the antrum and fundus of the stomach. Fundal stimulation may worsen the dyspepsia. Additionally erythromycin produces conduction problems in the heart. It prolongs the Q-T interval and may cause sudden cardiac death. Azithromycin does not effect cardiac conduction time. Last, visceral analgesics are given, which include 5-HT_3 antagonists (e.g., alosetron) and 5-HT_4 agonists (e.g., octreotide) (Broyles, et al., 2007). The studies done using these agents did not have a placebo control, and therefore randomized controlled studies are needed.

Evaluation of Outcomes

Potential patient outcomes for each of the example nursing diagnoses for the patient with NUD are:

- Acute pain related to upper epigastric irritation. The patient should verbalize an adequate relief of pain along with the ability to realistically cope with the pain if it is not completely relieved.
- Imbalanced nutrition, less than body requirements, related to anorexia. The patient verbalizes and demonstrates selection of foods or meals that will achieve a cessation of weight loss and weighs within 10 percent of ideal body weight.
- Deficient knowledge related to self-care and risk prevention. The patient should demonstrate motivation to learn, identify perceived learning needs, and verbalize an understanding of desired content.

The outcome for patients with dyspepsia is not clear. Patients with dyspepsia must be followed up. Symptomatic treatment of these patients is appropriate when organic disease is ruled out. If the patient also has depression as a comorbidity, the outcome for improvement is poor. All relevant disorders must be considered and treated to optimize patient outcomes.

PEPTIC-ULCER DYSPEPSIA

PUD is one of the two types of dyspepsia. PUD is characterized by a loss of the mucosal lining of the stomach or duodenum. PUD has had a variety of therapies and strategies for treatment over the past several decades. There used to be an emphasis on bland diet medications and stress management to decrease the symptomology of PUD. More recently, recognition of the role of *H. pylori* in PUD greatly changed the management of this disorder.

Etiology

PUD is characterized by persistent pain, weight loss, poor appetite, bloating, nausea, and vomiting. The most common causative link to PUD is *H. pylori.* In the elderly, the prevalence of PUD is linked to the use of NSAIDs (e.g., aspirin, ibuprofen).

Epidemiology

There is also a familial link with the prevalence of PUD in first-degree relatives and monozygotic twins. Tobacco smokers are two times more likely to develop PUD than nonsmokers. *H. pylori* is a leading cause of gastritis, PUD, gastric cancer, and gastric lymphomas. The infection is transmitted by the fecal oral route, saliva, food, and water. If a patient is infected with *H. pylori,* it progresses from superficial chronic gastritis to atrophic gastritis. NSAIDs cause mucosal damage both by direct effect as well as systemic effects. NSAIDs damage epithelial cells and inhibit prostaglandin secretion, specifically COX inhibition, which reduces mucus and bicarbonate secretion, and hampers cell turnover because of reduced blood flow. Individuals with cystic fibrosis have an increased for PUD because of decrease in bicarbonate secretion.

Gastric epithelial cellular metaplasia leads to duodenal ulcer disease. The disease burden for PUD is high. The total direct cost of gastric and duodenal ulcers is estimated to be 3.3 billion dollars with a loss in productivity valued at 6.2 billion dollars (Yamada, 2005).

BOX 49-5

TYPES OF GASTRIC ULCERS

Type I—Ulcers in the gastric body (corpus) not associated with gastroduodenal disease.

Type II—Ulcers in the body (corpus) of the stomach but associated with gastroduodenal disease.

Type III—Ulcers in the prepyloric area.

Adapted from Yamada, Y. (2005). Handbook of gastroenterology *(2nd ed.). Philadelphia: Lippincott, Williams & Wilkins.*

Pathophysiology

Most gastric ulcers are linked to *H. pylori* infection or NSAIDs. Three types develop as shown in Box 49-5.

Assessment with Clinical Manifestations

Abdominal pain is the major presenting symptom. The pain is described as burning, usually in the epigastric region, and is often relieved by food or antacids. A distinguishing symptom is that the patient will relate that the pain awaken them in the middle of the night. If the patient is less than 45 to 50 years of age, empiric antisecretory or acid suppression agents should be initiated unless there are red flag signs. If the patient is over the age of 50, they typically have warning signs or fail to respond to antisecretory or acid suppressing agents.

Diagnostic Tests

When the history of the patient suggests PUD, patients should be tested for *H. pylori*. Then radiographic and endoscopic studies should be performed. And, if the patient demonstrates gastric ulceration on endoscopy, the exam should be repeated two months after medication therapy is initiated.

Nursing Diagnoses

Based on the information gathered, examples of nursing diagnoses in the patient with PUD may include the following:

- Acute pain related to upper epigastric irritation.
- Nutrition imbalance, less than body requirements, related to anorexia.
- Knowledge deficit related to self-care and risk prevention.

Planning and Implementation

Patients who are diagnosed with gastric or duodenal ulcers are treated in a similar manner as for nondyspepsia disorder. In addition, there are specific strategies using both pharmacological and surgical therapies.

About 10 percent of the time, patients are not responsive to ulcer treatment. If a patient has not responded to treatment in 12 weeks, a reevaluation of his or her treatment regimen should occur. It is sometimes found that the patient has not followed the regimen prescribed, has not discontinued the risk factors, such as smoking or the use of NSAIDs. If after evaluation, it is found that the patient has been conforming to his or her regimen, but ulcer disease persists, further endoscopic follow-up with multiple biopsies is required. Zollinger-Ellison syndrome (ZES) should be considered. This syndrome results from a gastric acid–secreting tumor, a gastrinoma. Approximately 90 percent of patients with ZES will develop PUD. The symptoms are refractory PUD, PUD with diarrhea, obstruction, perforation, or hemorrhage. ZES is diagnosed if fasting gastrin levels are greater than 1,000 pg/mL (normal is less than 150 pg/mL). Both medical and surgical treatment of ZES are available. Control of acid hypersecretion is important. PPIs are the most effective medication in the treatment of ZES. These medications inhibit acid secretion and promote ulcer healing. If the tumor has not metastasized, the gastrinoma should be resected. If curative resection is not an option, chemotherapy can be selected.

Pharmacology

There are specific medication categories with which PUD is managed. Overall, the types of medications that are used are: antacids, H_2 receptor antagonists, PPIs, and cytoprotective agents.

Over-the-counter (OTC) antacids are useful for the dyspepsia associated with PUD. The expected effects of these agents are to neutralize acid by cytoprotective activity (e.g., increased prostaglandin release, mucous production, and bicarbonate release), inhibition of pepsin, and binding of bile salts. Adverse effects may include hypercalcemia, metabolic alkalosis, renal problems, diarrhea or constipation, and sodium overload. These adverse effects depend on the formulation that is used (Broyles, et. al., 2007).

H_2 receptor antagonists are those medications that reduce acid secretion. Those that are approved for use are cimetidine, famotidine, nizatidine, and ranitidine. Once daily dosing of these agents is used to treat PUD.

PPIs are those agents that inhibit both basal and stimulated acid secretion. They are more effective in managing day time acid secretion than H_2 receptor antagonists. Patients should take these medications 30 minutes to one hour prior to meals.

Cytoprotective agents are those medications that bind to tissue proteins and form a protective barrier for the gastroduodenal epithelium. This protects from any erosive effects of acid, bile salts, and pepsin. Sucralfate is an example. Misoprostol is a cytoprotective agent that is a prostaglandin E_1 analogue. It inhibits gastric acid secretion and stimulates bicarbonate and mucous secretion. The limiting factors to all of these agents are the side effects. The nurse should be aware of other medications that the patient is receiving and knowledgeable of any untoward interaction. Patients need to know what side effects to be aware of and report these to their provider.

Complications of PUD and the Subsequent Therapy

Even though *H. pylori* causes PUD, the elimination of *H. pylori* is controversial for patients who have NUD. For patients who have *H. pylori*–related PUD, therapy to eliminate the infection is indicated. Because single-agent treatment regimens are ineffective, triple or quadruple therapy with antibiotics and PPIs is practiced. Additionally there is evidence that in *H. pylori* is eliminated in 80 to 95 percent of patients who receive two weeks of bismuth subsalicylate, metronidazole, and tetracycline plus an antisecretory agent. Follow-up is not necessary if the patient becomes asymptomatic although a one month follow-up to confirm *H. pylori* elimination should be considered. The rationale for treatment of patients with *H. pylori* infection is stunning. If *H. pylori* is eliminated, the recurrence rate of PUD is less than 10 percent; if *H. pylori* infection is not treated, the PUD recurrence rate is 50 to 100 percent.

For patients who have PUD that is linked to NSAIDs, the anti-inflammatory agent should be discontinued. Treatment would include the same regimen as for PUD secondary to *H. pylori* except for the antibiotic regimen. If NSAIDs must be continued, the use of PPIs have shown to heal both gastric and duodenal ulcers.

Surgery

Pharmacological management of PUD has been so effective that surgical management of PUD is infrequent. Whenever a patient has refractory PUD, gastric carcinoma must be ruled out. The operative solutions to the management of PUD are used only when the ulcer disease is intractable and the patient has persistent and severe symptoms (e.g., pain, blood loss). The procedures include vagotomy and drainage, highly selective vagotomy, vagotomy and antrectomy, and laparoscopic surgery. Highly selective vagotomy is the most widely used procedure for patients with duodenal ulcer. The vagal branches that serve the proximal stomach are ligated, which leaves the antral and pyloric portions of the vagus innervation to the stomach intact. This produces a 50 to 79 percent reduction in acid production. Antral resection of the stomach with a selective vagotomy and has the lowest ulcer recurrence rate. The type of surgery selected is dependent on the condition of the duodenum and the amount of stomach that must be resected. In the Billroth I anastomosis the duodenum is sewn to the stomach; in the Billroth II anastomosis, a gastrojejunostomy is performed and a blind duodenal limb is created.

If a patient experiences a perforated ulcer emergent surgery is indicated. If surgery is delayed, peritonitis and sepsis will result. Often the patient will have a gastric resection, which includes the ulcer. If the patient also experiences a hemorrhage with the perforation, the ulcer bed must be ligated or resected.

A complication seen after surgery for PUD is the dumping syndrome and accelerated gastric emptying occurs with truncal vagotomy and gastric drainage procedures. With the advent of highly selective vagotomy procedures the prevalence of dumping syndrome has declined. Early dumping syndrome occurs when hyperosmolar gastric contents rapidly pass into the intestines. This produces fluid shifts and the release of vasoactive hormones. Within 15 minutes to one hour the patient experiences diarrhea, pain, borborygmi, nausea, and vomiting as well as flushing, weakness, palpitations, diaphoresis, lightheadedness, and syncope. Late dumping syndrome occurs between two to four hours after a meal, and it is believed to be a result of excessive postprandial insulin release. The patient experiences reactive hypoglycemia. Management of dumping syndrome requires dietary modification. Patients should be instructed to eat low-carbohydrate meals and to limit fluid intake during meal time. Patients may also benefit from lying supine after a meal to delay gastric emptying.

Evaluation of Outcomes

Potential patient outcomes for each of the example nursing diagnoses for the patient with PUD are:

- Acute pain related to upper epigastric irritation. The patient should verbalize an adequate relief of pain along with the ability to realistically cope with the pain if it is not completely relieved.
- Nutrition imbalance, less than body requirements, related to anorexia. The patient verbalizes and demonstrates selection of foods or meals that will achieve a cessation of weight loss and weighs within 10 percent of ideal body weight.
- Knowledge deficit related to self-care and risk prevention. The patient should demonstrate motivation to learn, identify perceived learning needs, and verbalize an understanding of desired content.

In addition, medical management of PUD is extremely effective. Ninety to ninety-five percent of patients with PUD are treated successfully and do not require surgery. When surgery is needed, highly selective vagotomy and truncal vagotomy with antrectomy is preferred. The selection of Billroth I and II is dependent on the condition of the duodenum.

GASTRITIS, DUODENITIS, AND ASSOCIATED ULCERATIVE LESIONS

These conditions are not diseases. Gastritis has been classified into nonatrophic, atrophic, and special forms (note: the classification system for gastritis is the Updated Sydney System). Nonatrophic gastritis is caused by *H. pylori.* Atrophic gastritis is associated with *H. pylori* and with environmental factors, and special forms of gastritis include chemical, radiation, lymphocytic, noninfectious, and infections other than *H. pylori.* Gastritis can be acute or chronic. Acute gastritis presents as an acute upper GI blood loss, either a hemorrhagic blood loss or erosive. Chronic gastritis can be due to *H. pylori* without ulceration but with chronic superficial inflammation. Chemical gastritis is most often caused by NSAIDs and reflux of bile into the stomach. Atrophic gastritis is asymptomatic unless complications occur. Patients with autoimmune gastritis often present with anemia, either iron deficiency or pernicious. The patient will have the symptoms of vitamin B_{12} deficiency, which include red, smooth, sore tongue; anorexia; and numbness, paresthesia, weakness, and ataxia. Patients with gastritis are treated both symptomatically and as related to the causative factor. Peptic duodenitis is a direct result of chronic exposure to gastric acid. The epithelium of the duodenum is replaced with gastric mucous-secreting cells as an adaptive response to the acid exposure. These patients may have the same symptoms as patients with PUD. Patients with gastritis and duodenitis will require nursing management based on nursing diagnoses similar to most of the other GI disorders (Box 49-6).

BOX 49-6

NURSING DIAGNOSES FOR GASTRITIS, DUODENITIS, AND ASSOCIATED ULCERATIVE LESIONS

- Acute or chronic pain
- Fear
- Anxiety in response to an uncertain diagnosis
- Ineffective coping related to disease burden
- Deficient knowledge
- Decisional conflict
- Risk for injury, irritation to mucosa or muscular wall
- Imbalanced nutrition, less than body requirements
- Impaired tissue integrity

STOMACH CANCER

Stomach cancer, also called gastric cancer, refers to the growth of a cancerous tumor in the stomach. It can develop in any part of the stomach and grow along the stomach wall into the esophagus or small intestine. Stomach cancer may extend through the stomach wall and spread to nearby lymph nodes and to organs, such as the liver, pancreas, and colon. Stomach cancer also may spread to distant organs, such as the lungs, the lymph nodes above the collar bone, and the ovaries. When stomach cancer spreads to an ovary, the tumor in the ovary is called a Krukenberg tumor. Stomach cancer is the second leading cause of cancer in the world.

Epidemiology

The American Cancer Society (2006a) estimates that 13,510 men and 8,350 women will be diagnosed with stomach cancer, and 11,550 men and women will die of cancer of the stomach in 2005. From 1998 to 2002, the median age at diagnosis for cancer of the stomach was 72 years of age. Approximately 0.1 percent were diagnosed under age 20; 1.6 percent between the ages of 20 and 34; 4.6 percent between the ages of 35 and 44; 10.3 percent between the ages of 45 and 54; 16.3 percent between the ages of 55 and 64; 26.3 percent between the ages of 65 and 74; 28.2 percent between the ages of 75 and 84; and 12.7 percent 85 and older.

Stomach cancer affects men twice as often as women, and is more common in African American people than in Caucasian people. Stomach cancer is more common in Japan, Korea, parts of Eastern Europe, and Latin America than in the United States. People in these areas eat many foods that are preserved by drying, smoking, salting, or pickling. Scientists believe that eating foods preserved in these ways may play a role in the development of stomach cancer. On the other hand, fresh foods (especially fresh fruits and vegetables and properly frozen or refrigerated fresh foods) may protect against this disease.

The overall five-year survival rate for people with stomach cancer in the United States is 22 percent. One reason for this is that most stomach cancers are found at an advanced stage. The outlook for survival is worse if the cancer is in the upper part of the stomach.

Etiology

Evidence is growing that in addition to genetic disposition, nutritional imbalance, consumption of certain foods, such as smoked foods, among other eating habits, hormonal and psychological factors, along with other immune suppressive factors play an important part in the development of GI cancer. Some studies suggest that a type of bacterium called *H. pylori,* which may cause stomach inflammation and ulcers, may be an important risk factor for this disease.

Pathophysiology

Stomach cancers are primarily adenocarcinomas and can be found in any part of the stomach. In stomach cancer patients, as in all cancer patients, the body's regulatory, repair, and immune mechanisms fail to prevent formation of a cancerous tumor. Some researchers call this failure a regulatory freeze or tolerance, which is because of a combination of causal factors that vary from one individual patient to another.

Cancer cells develop in every human being; however, not every newly produced cancer cell leads to a tumor. And, the body possesses a natural defense system in its intact immune system. In addition, an intact regulation of physiological cell death, called **apoptosis,** protects the organism from the development of a cancerous tumor. Therefore, it is of great importance to restore the natural regulatory, repair, and immune mechanisms, as a part of the healing strategy, or as prevention from the outbreak or progression of the disease.

Gastric Lymphoma

Gastric lymphoma is the second most common malignancy of the stomach. More than 90 percent of gastric B cell tumors (mucosa-associated lymphoid tissue or MALT) are associated with *H. pylori* infection. The nonspecific presentation of gastric lymphoma is similar to that of gastric adenocarcinoma. The physical assessment may demonstrate an abdominal mass or adenopathy. To stage this disease, laparotomy is needed. The Ann Arbor staging system is used to stage gastric lymphoma, and the treatment regimen is based on the stage. The prognosis for gastric lymphoma is encouraging. The five-year survival rate is 50 percent. Whereas the overall survival rate for gastric adenocarcinoma is less than 15 percent. Patients with the diagnosis of gastric cancer or lymphoma face a particularly uncertain future. Patients and families need a comprehensive plan of treatment.

Assessment with Clinical Manifestations

As with other forms of cancer, gastric cancer has a wide variety of symptoms. In the beginnings of the disorder, the patient may be asymptomatic. And, when manifestations do occur, they are usually not that specific in nature. The patient may have some mild abdominal pain, anorexia, indigestion, and other ulcer-like symptoms. As the disease progresses, later clinical manifestations are malnourishment, fatigue, and anemia problems associated with GI bleeding, and may have palpable masses. Patients may have referred pain from the stomach area to other body areas.

Diagnostic Tests

The patient history and physical examination are not that helpful in the diagnosis of stomach cancer, because gastric tumors are not palpable and manifestations not specific. The potential bleeding tendencies might show anemia as an indicator, and hematocrit and hemoglobin verify the severity of the anemic condition. Endoscopy, barium swallow, and cytologic washings are typical for more specific confirmation of the cancer. A tissue biopsy reveals the most definitive diagnosis of the cancer typology.

Nursing Diagnoses

Based on the information gathered, examples of nursing diagnoses in the patient with stomach cancer may include the following:

- Acute pain related to the pressure from tumor development.
- Risk for infection related to the immunosuppression of the chemotherapy and radiation.
- Fear.
- Anxiety related to the diagnosis of cancer.
- Imbalanced nutrition, less than body requirements, related to nausea from the administration of chemotherapy or surgical interventions.

Planning and Implementation

Patients with cancer of the stomach do not have one specific therapy that is a cure, except for surgical removal of the stomach. And, even then, the cancer may be metastatic in nature and other body systems may be affected. If there is metastasis, the goals for this patient become palliation and supportive management strategies.

Pharmacology

If surgery is not indicated or does not cure cancer of the stomach, then chemotherapeutic agents are recommended. In addition, chemotherapy may be used prior to surgery and there are positive correlations with this strategy.

BOX 49-7

EXAMPLES OF COMBINATION CHEMOTHERAPY USED IN TREATING STOMACH CANCER

FAM (5-FU, Adriamycin, mitomycin C)

5-FU plus methyl CCNU

5-FU plus Adriamycin

EAP (etoposide, Adriamycin, cisplatin)

FAP (5-FU, Adriamycin, cisplatin)

FAB (5-FU, Adriamycin, carmustine

Source: National Institute of Cancer. (2006). Stomach cancer: NIC drug dictionary. *Retrieved June 25, 2006, from www.cancer.gov.*

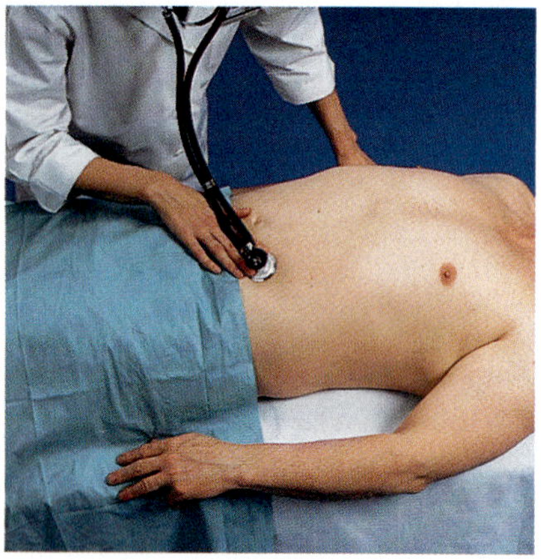

Figure 49-4 Nurse auscultating abdomen in presence of borborygmi sounds from dumping syndrome.

Commonly used chemotherapy for stomach cancer are combinations using 5-FU, Adriamycin, mitomycin C, cisplatin, and nitrosoureas (BCNU, CCNU) (Box 49-7).

Surgery

Surgery is the treatment of choice for stomach cancer, as long as adequate margins (5 to 6 cm) around the tumor can be obtained and regional lymph nodes are removed. Compared to subtotal or partial gastrectomy, total gastrectomy does not improve survival. There are a wide variety of surgical approaches to the treatment of stomach cancer. For example, a partial gastrectomy (e.g., Bilroth I, Bilroth II) may be performed. This surgery removes half to two thirds of the stomach. A total gastrectomy may be performed when there is cancer spread through the gastric tissue. There can also be a total gastrectomy accompanied with an esophagojejunostomy (construction of the esophagus to the duodenum or jejunum). In addition, an antrectomy can be performed, which is a partial resection of the stomach that may include part of the duodenum.

After gastric surgery, the patient may have a variety of complications and manifestations, which require specific nursing care. The management of pain, anxiety, patient education, restoration of general nutrition, and general nursing care for an abdominal surgery are indicated. The patient can have a problem with dumping syndrome, which occurs when there is too rapid filling of the small intestine. The patient has small gastric remains, which are connected to a larger opening into the intestine. The hypertonic intestinal contents draw fluid from the circulating plasma into the jejunum to dilute the high concentration of the fluid at that location. This causes the patient to have GI disorders (e.g., diarrhea, nausea or vomiting, epigastric pain, cramping, stimulated peristalsis, and increased motility). The patient may have unusual abdominal sounds with **borborygmi sounds** (loud, hyperactive bowel tones) (Figure 49-4). Dumping syndrome is treated with feeding with small, more frequent meals, taking liquids and solids at different times, and increasing proteins and fats, because they are eliminated more slowly than carbohydrates. After eating, the patient is encouraged to sit up to prevent reflux problems. Medications that can be prescribed are antacids, anticholinergics, sedatives, and antispasmodics.

The patient also may experience reflux of bile after the removal of the pylorus, which has similar treatments as those described in GERD situations. Also, patients may experience anemia from the lack of iron absorption (iron is normally absorbed in the duodenum and jejunum). In addition, intrinsic factor is decreased due to its production normally occurring in the stomach cells. Consequently, the patient may develop pernicious anemia, which is described in chapter 29.

Other malnutrition problems are somewhat common in gastric surgeries. Patients can develop folic acid deficiencies (refer to chapter 29), calcium absorption problems, and poor absorption of other nutrients from the removal of the stomach. And, the patient may continue to have problems of anorexia, which compromises his or her ability to consume normal meals and food intake. Nursing management is challenged with these types of nutritional problems, and referral to dietitians and counselors is often recommended.

Evaluations of Outcomes

Potential patient outcomes for each of the example nursing diagnoses for the patient with stomach cancer are:

- Acute pain related to the pressure from tumor development. The patient should verbalize an adequate relief of pain along with the ability to realistically cope with the pain if it is not completely relieved.
- Risk for infection related to the immunosuppression of the chemotherapy and radiation. The patient remains free of infection, as evidenced by nor-

mal vital signs and absence of purulent drainage from wounds, incisions, and tubes. Infection is recognized early to allow for prompt treatment.

- Fear related to the diagnosis of cancer; anxiety related to the diagnosis of cancer. The patient should be able to recognize the signs of anxiety, demonstrate positive coping mechanisms, and describe a reduction in the level of anxiety experienced.
- Imbalanced nutrition, less than body requirements, related to nausea from the administration of chemotherapy or surgical interventions. The patient verbalizes and demonstrates selection of foods or meals that will achieve a cessation of weight loss and weighs within 10 percent of ideal body weight.

KEY CONCEPTS

- Nurses are often the first health care provider who notices that the patient is experiencing chewing or dysphagia problems.
- Dyspepsia is the most common symptom that patients complain about to their provider.
- Ulcerative conditions of the gums and mucous membranes are labeled aphthous stomatitis and occur in 20 percent of the population.
- More than 400,000 cancer patients experience oral problems, such as painful mouth ulcers, impaired taste, and dry mouth from salivary gland dysfunction.
- Burning mouth syndrome is a constant burning sensation of the tongue seen in patients past middle age.
- Dysphagia represents a major problem in the older adult and needs special attention to prevent aspiration pneumonitis or pneumonia, airway obstruction, malnutrition, and dehydration.
- The more common esophageal disorders are achalasia, GERD, hiatal hernia, and esophageal cancer.
- The first line of treatment for esophageal pain and achalasia is often the same medications used to treat angina of cardiac origin.
- GERD occurs in 15 to 20 percent of all adults and daily symptoms are common.
- A hiatal hernia develops when there is a part of the stomach that protrudes through the esophageal hiatus, and there are often no symptoms.
- Esophageal cancer, associated with the highest cancer mortality rate, is also one of the most rapidly increasing malignancies.
- Stomach cancer may extend through the stomach wall and spread to nearby lymph nodes, the liver, pancreas, and colon, as well as spreading to distant organs (e.g., lungs, lymph nodes, ovaries).

REVIEW QUESTIONS

1. Mr. Jones has symptoms related to erosion of the esophagus. Which of the following is the correct label for his painful swallowing?
   1. Pyrosis
   2. Dysphagia
   3. Odynophagia
   4. Esophagitis
2. Mrs. Inez is having GI pain, which is specific to a region of her body. This is:
   1. Visceral pain
   2. Somatic pain
   3. Referred pain
   4. Abdominal pain
3. Mr. Steinway has burning mouth syndrome from candidiasis. Which of the following is true of this disorder?
   1. It is seldom seen in middle-aged adults.
   2. It is considered a mental health condition, often resulting from excessive anger.
   3. It is a constant burning sensation of the tongue.
   4. It is the most common GI disorder.
4. A PEG tube is:
   1. Synonymous with a nasogastric feeding tube
   2. Usually not used in the elderly population
   3. Typically inserted by a nurse in the patient's acute care room
   4. Sutured in place and has complications such as bleeding, infection, or peritonitis

Continued

REVIEW QUESTIONS—cont'd

5. Mr. Barnett has pain in the esophagus from esophagitis. This pain can be confused as:
   1. Dental disorders of the teeth
   2. Cardiac pain
   3. Appendicitis
   4. Acute bronchitis
6. Mrs. Tinen has been experiencing heartburn after meals and some regurgitation of fluids that taste foul when she is full, and she is often is not able to lie down comfortably just after eating. This is most likely:
   1. GERD
   2. Stomach cancer
   3. Achalasia
   4. Peptic ulceration
7. Mrs. Johanan is pregnant and experiencing pyrosis and regurgitation after eating her meals. This is most likely:
   1. Esophagitis
   2. Gastritis
   3. Hiatal hernia
   4. Aphagia
8. Mrs. Niyaki has a family history of stomach cancer. Which foods should her nurse instruct her to eat?
   1. Fresh fruits and vegetables
   2. Salted nuts
   3. Dried fish
   4. Smoked meats
9. Mrs. Garcia has recently has a gastric surgery. She is experiencing acute episodes of diarrhea that are sudden in occurrence, which is most likely:
   1. Borborygmi
   2. Flatus
   3. Dumping syndrome
   4. Apoptosis

REVIEW ACTIVITIES

1. Describe how you would instruct a patient to assess his or her oral cavity to detect early manifestations of cancer?
2. Observe a speech pathologist as he or she examines a patient in regard to his or her swallowing evaluation.
3. Ask for permission to observe an endoscopy performed in a special studies laboratory where you are enrolled in your clinical practicums.
4. Describe the patient education for GERD.
5. Describe the clinical manifestations experienced by a patient with peptic ulcer syndrome.
6. Describe how you would approach a patient with a new diagnosis of cancer of the stomach.

Visit the Contemporary Medical-Surgical Nursing online companion resource at www.delmarhealthcare.com for additional content and study aids. Click on Online Companions then select the Nursing discipline.

CHAPTER 50

Lower Gastrointestinal Tract Dysfunction: Nursing Management

Milena Segatore, MScN, MNI-PG, CNRN

CHAPTER TOPICS

- Mal-absorption Conditions
- Acute Abdominal Pain
- Appendicitis
- Diverticulitis
- Bowel Obstructions
- Colorectal Cancer
- Irritable Bowel Syndrome
- Crohn's Disease
- Ulcerative Colitis

KEY TERMS

Acute abdomen
Adjuvant therapy
Anastomosis
Atresia
Borborygmi
Chyme
Colectomy
Diverticula
Diverticulosis
Fecalith
Fulguration
Hematochezia
Ileus
Intussusception
Laparoscopy
Laparotomy
Malrotation
Ostomy
Proctocolectomy
Referred pain
Somatic (parietal) pain
Steatorrhea
Tenesmus
Visceral pain
Volvulus

There are many disorders of the lower gastrointestinal (GI) tract, and patients in acute care settings have a wide variety of dysfunctions in the lower GI tract. The pathologies that exist within each organ are relatively common, and there are both medical and surgical approaches to providing treatment of the conditions of the lower GI tract. Nursing management carefully considers the disorders in the lower GI system and offers treatment and care that is essential to the patient. The types of conditions affect the patients and include, but are not limited to, acute inflammatory disorders, obstructive conditions, cancer within the region, and inflammatory bowel conditions.

SMALL INTESTINE

The small intestine, which is divided into the duodenum, the jejunum, and the ileum, is approximately 600 cm (6 meters, 240 inches, 20 feet, or approximately 6 yards) in length and 1 to 1.5 inches in diameter. The major role of the small intestine is the digestion and absorption of nutrients from the food and fluids ingested. The action of the columnar cells in the small intestine enhances the distribution of the products of digestion via the lymphatics and vascular system. Activity of the small intestine is a function of whether the intestine is in the fed state or the fasting state. **Chyme** (the semiliquid and partially digested stomach contents mixed with acids that enter the small intestine from the stomach) enters the duodenum. The motility of the small intestine mixes food with digestive enzymes. Transport and absorption of nutrients and electrolytes in the small intestine is dependent on nutrient status. Glucose and some amino acids (neutral) absorption are sodium dependent. The sodium/potassium (Na^+/K^+) pump enhances the movement and absorption of these nutrients into the blood. Lower in the colon and ileum, the Na^+/K^+-adenosinetriphosphatase (ATPase) pump enhances nutrient independent absorption of fluids and electrolytes. The hormone aldosterone also plays a role in this function.

Absorption of Nutrients

There are certain nutrients (i.e., vitamins, minerals, and electrolytes) that are absorbed in the GI tract that must be considered as a nurse is assessing the nutritional status of the patient when considering problems with digestion and absorption. During hydrolysis proteins are broken down into amino acids; polysaccharides into simple sugars; triglycerides into glycerol; and fatty acids and nucleic acids into substances more readily available for metabolism.

Folic Acid

Folic acid (folate) is an important water soluble B vitamin. It is essential in the production of red blood cells (RBCs), production of DNA, tissue growth, and cell function. Folic acid is needed for the production of certain digestive acids and to enhance the appetite. Folic acid is required by all childbearing women, as it is known to prevent neural-tube defect in the developing fetus. High total intake of folate has also been found to be inversely related to colon cancer. Usual food sources are beans, bananas, legumes, whole grains, dark green and leafy vegetables, poultry, pork, some shellfish, and liver. Only small amounts of folate are stored in the body so malnutrition can rapidly deplete body stores. Folic acid is absorbed via a Na^+-dependent carrier. Certain medications, like phenytoin (Dilantin) and sulfasalazine (Azulfidine), interfere with folic acid absorption. Folic acid deficiency can change the ability of the small intestine epithelium to absorb folic acid, hence the importance of a well-balanced diet high in folic acid as well as supplementation. Folic acid and B_{12} deficiency can lead to a megaloblastic anemia (Roth, 2007).

Cobalamin

Cobalamin (vitamin B_{12}) is essential to prevent pernicious anemia. Vitamin B_{12} is replaced in the diet by eating meat. Strict vegetarians will develop vitamin B_{12} deficiency unless they eat meat containing this vitamin or take a vitamin supplement. Because the body stores large amounts of B_{12} in the liver, the deficiency may not be readily seen for several years. In the duodenum, cobalamin combines with intrinsic factor (IF), which protects it from proteolysis, until it transits to the ileum where it is absorbed. Additionally pancreatic enzymes are necessary in this process. In summary, a functioning pancreas, the presence of IF, and a functional ileum are necessary to prevent cobalamin (vitamin B_{12})

deficiency. Mal-assimilation of iron may result in folate or vitamin B_{12} deficiency, which produces a megaloblastic red cell. Vitamin B_{12} deficiency produces neurological abnormalities, such as symmetrical paresthesias in the hands and feet, diminished vibratory and proprioceptive sense, ataxia, and spinal cord degeneration.

Iron

Iron (Fe) is essential to prevent anemia. Iron is present in both meat (heme iron) and vegetable (nonheme) sources. Heme iron is more readily absorbed than nonheme iron. Both types of iron are absorbed to a greater degree in the duodenum. Men need less dietary intake of iron (1 to 2 mg) than women (3 to 4 mg), especially menstruating women. The amount of iron absorbed is dependent on the total body iron content as well as the source of the iron. The absorption of nonheme iron can be reduced by the presence of certain food substances—plant phytates (soy beans), polyphenols (tea leaves, red wine), tea tannates, and even bran. Ascorbic acid (vitamin C) enhances the absorption of nonheme iron. Iron deficiency leads to hypochromic microcytic anemia. The patient with iron deficiency presents with pallor, atrophic tongue, koilonychias (spoon-shaped fingernails), cheilosis, or angular stomatitis (reddened lips with angular fissures).

Fat Soluble Vitamins

The fat soluble vitamins (A, D, E, and K) exist in large amounts, because there are large stores of these vitamins in the adipose tissue. Deficiencies are not apparent until there is long-standing mal-absorption or inadequate ingestion of these vitamins. Vitamin D deficiency can lead to many kinds of bone problems, i.e., osteomalacia, osteopenia, bone pain, cramps, and tetany. Vitamin K deficiency may lead to ecchymosis and easy bruising. Night blindness can be caused by a deficiency in vitamin A. Deficiency of vitamin E may lead to progressive demyelination in the central nervous system (CNS).

Hormones and Neurotransmitters

There are several hormones and neurotransmitters that enhance intestinal secretion. These include vasoactive intestinal peptides, bradykinin, prostaglandins, acetylcholine, serotonin, substance P (increases intestinal motility and vasodilatation), neurotensin, histamine, vasopressin, thyrocalcitonin, and others of which the mechanisms of action are unclear. These substances arise from the blood, nerve endings, endocrine cells in the intestinal epithelium, and intact enterocytes.

Substances that prevent secretion and promote absorption are the adrenal corticosteroids, somatostatins, the enkephalins, dopamine, and norepinephrine. The adrenal corticosteroids particularly the glucocorticoids increase absorption of electrolytes. Aldosterone also enhances intestinal absorption of electrolytes, especially sodium through the inhibition of the arachidonic acid cascade. Because the epithelium enterocytes are predominantly sympathetic sites, norepinephrine is the neurohormone elaborated. The effect is to inhibit electrolyte secretion and stimulate absorption. If a sympathectomy is performed, the individual will experience diarrhea. Patients with long-standing diabetes may also experience autonomic neuropathy and develop transient or persistent diarrhea.

Absorption of Fat

Absorption of fat occurs in stages. These are dependent on the function of the pancreas, liver, intestinal mucosa, and lymphatics. Dietary triglycerides must be broken down into glycerol and fatty acids. Disorders that impair lipolysis or fat solubilization could be rapid gastric emptying time with poor mixing of GI contents. This can result from a vagotomy or as part of the postgastrectomy syndrome. In Zollinger-Ellison syndrome, the pH of the duodenum is altered, which moderates the enzyme lipase. Decreased pancreatic function, cholestasis—liver disease, biliary obstruction, or alteration in enterohepatic circulation—may also inhibit fat absorption. Other disorders that will reduce fat absorption are celiac disease, Whipple's disease (chronic bacterial infection with *Tropheryma whippelii*), and lymphatic disorders, including lymphoma, short bowel syndrome (due to surgical removal or bypass of a large portion of the intestine, resulting in inadequate absorption of nutrients), and genetic defects that impair chylomicron formation. In fat mal-absorption, fatty acids bind calcium instead of oxalate. This leads to absorption of oxalate and may cause oxaluria and calcium oxalate kidney stones. Fat mal-assimilation results in diarrhea secondary to the irritant effect of fatty acids on the colon, weight loss, and malnutrition. A quantitative fecal fat determination is necessary to determine if the patient has **steatorrhea,** pale-yellow, greasy, fatty toll, or chronic watery diarrhea.

Absorption of Carbohydrates

Absorption of carbohydrates (CHO) is dependent on the action of enzymatic activity in the GI tract. Humans ingest CHOs in the form of starch, sucrose, and lactose. Digestion begins in the mouth with the action of ptyalin in saliva, which begins the digestive action of starch, an oligosaccharide. Sucrose and lactose are both disaccharides. Pancreatic enzymes and enzymes in the brush border of the intestine break down the oligosaccharides into disaccharides and further into monosaccharides for absorption into the mucosal cells and then into portal circulation.

Disorders that impair digestion and absorption of CHOs include pancreatic insufficiency, a deficiency of the enzymes along the brush border of the intestine, damage to the brush border, or enterocyte function secondary to disorders, such as gastroenteritis, celiac disease, sprue, or short bowel syndrome. These disorders injure the mucosal surface of the small intestine. If disaccharides reach the colon, increased intestinal gas is formed through colonic salvage of mal-absorbed CHOs in the small intestine. This has a salutary (beneficial) effect, because of the reduction in osmoles of the CHO, the fluid loss in feces is reduced. The intraluminal gases produced from the fermentation of the CHOs are carbon-dioxide (CO_2), hydrogen (H_2), and (CH_4) alkane/methane. The absorption of H_2 and then its subsequent exhalation through the lungs is the basis for the hydrogen breath test.

Of the types of enzyme deficiency that can occur, lactase deficiency is common. Lactase is located on the tip of the intestinal villi and is abundant in the jejunum. Intestinal disorders that damage enterocytes will increase symptomatology associated with lactase deficiency. Lactase is highest at birth and declines during the toddler years (three-and-a-half to five years of age). It decreases with age except in the Northern European population. An interesting cultural hypothesis has been proposed. Lactase persistence is common in regions where dairy farming prevails, but interestingly lactase is not induced with increased lactose intake (Box 50-1). Ingestion of small amounts of lactose usually does not produce symptoms even in individuals who are lactase deficient.

> **BOX 50-1**
>
> **EPIDEMIOLOGY OF LACTASE DEFICIENCY**
>
> It is important to emphasize with your patients that lactase deficiency is not a milk allergy. Lactase deficiency causes lactose mal-absorption. Lactase deficiency causes water to be drawn into the small bowel with a resulting osmotic diarrhea as well as the production of gas production causing flatulence, bloating, and cramping. The most common cause is idiopathic (without a recognizable cause). The incidence by ethnic group is as follows:
>
> - Northern European: 2 to 15 percent
> - Latino patients: 50 to 80 percent
> - Ashkenazi Jews: 60 to 80 percent
> - African American patients: 60 to 80 percent
> - American Indians: 80 to 100 percent
> - Asian (American): 95 to 100 percent

If CHO mal-assimilation persists, oxidative metabolism (catabolism) occurs, and fat and muscle (protein) are catabolized. The patient is weakened, with loss of muscle mass and mental slowing. The metabolic rate decreases because of decreased conversion of thyroid hormone, T_4 to T_3.

Absorption of Proteins

Most of protein digestion and absorption commences after pepsin acts on proteins in the stomach secondary to mixing in the stomach. Dietary protein is hydrolyzed by pancreatic protease action in the duodenum once enterokinase and trypsin catalyze (activate) the protease. This occurs in the first two thirds of the duodenum. Digestion occurs in the latter half of the duodenal lumen during sequential action of pancreatic endopeptidases and exopeptidases. The protein is further broken into peptides and amino acids. Cellular digestion of the peptides occurs at the brush border of the intestine. Considering this mechanism, mal-absorption of proteins can occur if there are any disorders that cause pancreatic insufficiency; enterocyte dysfunction, e.g., celiac disease, or loss of mucosal surface, short bowel syndrome. Protein mal-assimilation results in edema. Fluid leaks from the capillaries because of the drop in colloid osmotic pressure. The patient presents with diminished muscle because of the lack of protein. The absorption and assimilation of protein is necessary for most metabolic functions. The immune system is compromised in protein deficiency, which results in recurrent infections. Protein-calorie malnutrition is marasmus whereas protein energy malnutrition is kwashiorkor.

MAL-ASSIMILATION SYNDROMES

Optimal intake, digestion, absorption, and metabolism are necessary for healthy living. Because of the size (length, therefore surface area) of the GI tract there are many diseases that can impact nutrient digestion and absorption. Mal-assimilation occurs either by mal-digestion or mal-absorption.

Epidemiology

The epidemiology of mal-assimilation disorders as a single category is difficult to ascertain. It is important to know that specific risk factors associated with the GI system place individuals, groups, and even countries at risk for disease, disability, and death. In the poorest countries these include underweight, unsafe water and sanitation, diarrheal diseases, zinc deficiency, iron deficiency, vitamin A deficiency, and high serum cholesterol. In developed countries risk factors leading to disease, disability, or death related to the GI system are alcohol consumption, high serum cholesterol, high BMI, low fruit and vegetable intake, and iron deficiency. There are several systemic disorders associated with mal-absorption of nutrients shown in Table 50-1.

Pathophysiology

The two primary pathologies for mal-assimilation disorders are mal-digestion and mal-absorption. A brief description of each is presented.

Mal-Digestion Disorders

Mal-digestion disorders are intraluminal disorders often from impaired hydrolysis of intestinal contents. The major causes of mal-digestion include postgastrectomy dysfunction often referred to as a mixing disorder (see discussion on protein absorption), pancreatic insufficiency, a reduction in bile salt concentration

TABLE 50-1 Systemic Disorders Associated with Mal-absorption of Nutrients

ENDOCRINE DISEASES	DIABETES, THYROID DISORDERS, ADDISON'S DISEASE, AND HYPOPARATHYROIDISM
Collagen-vascular diseases	Scleroderma, vasculitis, systemic lupus erythematosus, polyarteritis nodosa
Amyloidosis	Abnormal production of immunoglobulins leading to inadequate absorption of nutrients from the gastrointestinal tract and gastroesophageal reflux disease
AIDS	Can lead to protein losing enteropathy especially albumin

Adapted from Roth, R. (2007). Nutrition and diet therapy *(9th ed.). New York: Thomson Delmar Learning.*

in the intestine, interruption in the entero-hepatic circulation of bile salts, and certain medications, e.g., neomycin, calcium carbonate, and cholestyramine.

Mal-Absorption Disorders

Mal-absorption disorders are those that impair transport of intestinal contents across the mucosal membrane of the lumen. The major causes of mal-absorption are a reduction in absorptive surface of the intestine secondary to resection or bypass; biochemical or genetic abnormalities, e.g., celiac disease, disaccharidase deficiency, hypogammaglobulinemia, or Hartnup disease (an inherited disorder that prevents the absorption of certain proteins leading to a deficiency of niacin and tryptophan, cystinuria, or monosaccharide mal-absorption); inflammatory or infiltrative disorders; and lymphatic obstruction.

Assessment with Clinical Manifestations

Assessment of mal-assimilation disorders is detailed as there are many changes that potentially can occur throughout much of the body. In general, it is important to assess the patient for weight loss, signs of vitamin and mineral deficiency (e.g., anemia, easy bruising), cheilosis (reddened lips and fissures at lip angles) or glossitis, various dermatitides, tetany, osteoporosis, ecchymosis, paresthesias, fatigue, weakness, muscle wasting, borborygmi and increased flatus (gas production), edema, and change in stools, especially steatorrhea.

Patients with pan-mal-absorption often complain of steatorrhea. Abdominal distension or bloating is caused by a fermentation process that occurs in the colon secondary to unabsorbed carbohydrates by colon bacteria. Anemia is noted as part of a broad array of abnormalities associated with vitamin and mineral deficiencies.

Diagnostic Tests

The patient who has a mal-assimilation disorder will present with a classic symptom array that may include a history of weight loss, change in eating and bowel habits, e.g., polyphagia, diarrhea, foul-smelling stools that float because of increased water and gas content, stools that may have a rancid odor and greasy character (occurs later), abdominal bloating, muscle wasting, bone pain, weakness, tetany, paresthesias, bleeding gums, and dermatological conditions, such as eczema. See Box 50-2 for routine lab tests for mal-assimilation disorders.

To further assess for intraluminal mal-digestion, assessment of biliary function is done. This includes liver biochemistry, abdominal ultrasound, and endoscopic cholangiography. Bile salts may fail to be reabsorbed if the patient has ileal disease. The patient will be evaluated for bacterial overgrowth syndrome (BOS), especially if the patient has a history of gastric or upper intestinal tract surgery. Twenty to 43 percent of diarrhea in patients with diabetes has BOS (Frye, Tamer, & Kunha, 2005).

Nursing Diagnoses

Based on the information gathered, examples of nursing diagnoses in the patient with mal-assimilation disorders may include the following:

- Imbalanced nutrition, less than body requirements secondary to mal-assimilation disorders.
- Risk for impaired skin integrity.
- Deficient knowledge related to diagnosis of mal-assimilation disorders.
- Diarrhea related to mal-assimilation disorders.

Planning and Implementation

Patients who have mal-assimilation disorders present with a variety of symptoms, diagnostic findings, and abnormal laboratory results. Once the site of the defect is established, treatment is instituted. If the problem (e.g., biliary obstruction) is

BOX 50-2

ROUTINE LAB TESTS FOR MAL-ASSIMILATION DISORDERS

CBC with a peripheral smear to distinguish between a microcytic or microcytic anemia

Chemistry Screen:

Serum calcium, phosphorus, and alkaline phosphatase to detect osteopenia

Serum electrolytes: Na^+, K^+, Cl^-, CO_2, Ca^{++}, and Mg^+.

Serum albumin and total proteins to assess protein stores

Serum cholesterol, carotene, and prothrombin time (vitamin K) indirectly gauges fat assimilation

Liver profile AST (aspartate aminotransferase), ALT (alanine aminotransferase), and bilirubin

Serum iron, total iron binding capacity (TIBC), and ferritin to evaluate proximal intestinal function

Serum B_{12} level is indicative of the integrity of ileal function

Red cell folate measures folate stores

Shilling test with intrinsic factor suggests ileal dysfunction

Stool pH tends to be low with CHO mal-absorption (less than 5.5)

D-xylose test measures whether CHO is absorbed. If serum xylose levels are low after a test dose it is indicative of CHO mal-absorption.

H_2 breath test assists in the evaluation of CHO absorption.

Fecal fat measurement: fecal fat loss is about less than 5 percent of dietary intake. Elevation of fecal fat (steatorrhea) is an important diagnostic measurement to determine the presence of generalized mal-assimilation.

Source: Daniels, R. (2003). Delmar's manual of laboratory and diagnostic tests. *New York: Thomson Delmar Learning.*

structural, surgery may be necessary. If the patient has pancreatic insufficiency, enzyme supplements will be administered, or if there is an obstructive lesion or neoplasm, insulin, dietary counseling, lifestyle modification, and surgery are options. If the intestinal mucosa is defective dietary modifications will be necessary (e.g., gluten withdrawal, nutritional supplements, antibiotics for BOS or Whipple's disease). If the lymphatics are the site of the problem, a low-fat diet will be suggested; the health care provider will perhaps suggest medium-chain triglycerides (MCTs), because these are more water soluble and as a result can be absorbed across the small intestinal wall into the blood more easily.

Replacement and or supplement therapy is instituted. This will include minerals, targeted vitamins and multiple vitamin therapy, folic acid, pancreatic supplements, bile salt binding agents, caloric supplements, and enteral supplements if needed.

Patient and Family Teaching

For patients with mal-assimilation disorders, lifestyle and nutritional management are essential. Patients and families will need to understand the basic pathology inherent in the disorder and management principles to maintain a normal adaptive life style.

Evaluation of Outcomes

Potential patient outcomes for each of the example nursing diagnoses for the patient with mal-assimilation disorders are:

- Imbalanced nutrition, less than body requirements secondary to mal-assimilation disorders. The patient verbalizes and demonstrates selection of foods or meals that will achieve a cessation of weight loss and weighs within 10 percent of ideal body weight.
- Risk for impaired skin integrity. The patient's skin condition should be improved as evidenced by decreased redness, swelling, and pain.
- Deficient knowledge related to diagnosis of mal-assimilation disorders. The patient should demonstrate motivation to learn, identify perceived learning needs, and verbalize an understanding of desired content.
- Diarrhea related to mal-assimilation disorders. The patient will pass formed stool no more than three times per day.

ACUTE ABDOMEN

Acute abdomen refers to a constellation of clinical signs and symptoms usually best treated by surgery. The term is nonetiologically specific and connotes a high degree of urgency and acuity. Acute abdomen has also been defined by its consequence, namely, the need for surgery. That is, it has been referred to as a surgical abdomen. Although the severity and pathology may mandate a surgical cure in some, a variety of medical emergencies may also cause acute abdomen, and medical remedies may be curative. By convention, acute abdomen caused by trauma is considered separately.

Epidemiology

Acute abdomen encompasses a spectrum of surgical, medical, and gynecological conditions, ranging from the mild to life-threatening, which require hospital admissions, investigation, and treatment, whereby the primary clinical symptom is abdominal pain. As such, it is seen in patients of every age and socioeconomic group. Acute abdominal pain is a ubiquitous disorder, accounting for 5 to 10 million patient encounters per year in the United States, and 5 to 10 percent of all emergency department (ED) visits. Ten percent of these patients require surgery, and the diagnosis is associated with 10 percent malpractice claims filed annually. The most commonly missed diagnoses are appendicitis and small bowel obstruction. It is estimated that at least half of general surgical admissions are emergent, and half of the admissions are for complaints of acute abdominal pain. In one pediatric study, one third of the children required surgery and in 90 percent of those cases, the diagnosis was appendicitis. Thirty-day mortality is estimated at 4 percent in those admitted with acute abdominal pain, and of those operated on, the rate rises to 8 percent. The highest mortality is associated with patients who require laparotomy for unresectable cancer, ruptured abdominal aortic aneurysm (AAA), and perforated peptic ulcer (Persiani, Biondi, Buccelletti, Rausei, & Silveri, 2006). Among patients 65 years and older, the fastest growing sector is 85 years and older, and the elderly have the highest mortality rates in the adult surgical population.

Generally morbidity, mortality, and diagnostic accuracy are worse for elderly patients with acute abdomen. This has been attributed to delays in diagnosis and treatment and the existence comorbidities Coexisting disease threatens physiological reserve and reduces the ability to cope with the stress of intercurrent acute events and its treatments. Atypical presentations are often related to the physiological effects of aging: For example diminished immunity impairs the ability to generate a febrile response to disease, and reduced neural sensitivity in the elderly may blunt their appreciation of pain, producing delays in presentation. Absence of typical signs and symptoms can be devastating. In acute appendicitis, it is thought to produce a higher rate of perforation. Biliary tract disease, the most common disorder requiring abdominal surgery in the elderly, typically produces right upper quadrant pain, but 25 percent have no significant pain, and fewer than one half will have a fever, leukocytosis, or vomiting. The situation is similar for diverticulitis and perforating ulcer disease. Rebound tenderness, classically the most reliable clinical sign of peritonitis, is normally absent in a large number of elderly. Meticulous perioperative management, use of minimally invasive surgical approaches, and percutaneous drainage of gallbladder and abscesses may help avoid major anesthetic and surgical stresses (Stain, 2005).

Etiology

Virtually all organs within the abdominal cavity are pain sensitive, and the etiology of abdominal pain is as varied as the contents of the abdominal cavity: Disorders affecting respiratory (e.g., pneumonia), vascular (e.g., myocardial infarction, aortic dissection), GI (e.g., appendicitis, cholecystitis), endocrine (e.g., pancreatitis), renal-urinary (e.g., renal lithiasis, pyelonephritis, ureteral obstruction), and reproductive organs (e.g., ectopic pregnancy, spermatic cord torsion, ovarian cyst rupture) can all cause acute abdomen. Common etiologies vary by age and cause can arise over again, or can arise as acute exacerbations of formerly stable chronic problem, e.g. bowel perforation during an exacerbation of inflammatory bowel disease.

Causes can be preliminarily organized as medical or surgical. Medical causes may arise from intra- or extra-abdominal pathology. For example, in the pediatric population, common nonsurgical diagnoses include constipation and pneumonia. Surgical causes can be organized by organ(s) involved and by the underlying pathology. An alternative classification categorizes etiologies into three general groups: vascular (e.g., ischemia, infarction, hemorrhage), obstruction of a lumen (e.g., adhesions, ectopic pregnancy, malignant bowel obstruction; ureteral or common bile duct stone), or perforation of a viscus (e.g., duodenal ulcer, gravid uterus). The most common cause of acute abdomen is appendicitis. In up to one third of cases, a clear diagnosis is never determined; a nonspecific pain is common in children.

Pathophysiology

Regardless of etiology, two major pathological processes, inflammation and obstruction, are implicated in acute abdomen. Inflammation may be infectious or noninfectious, but regardless of cause, the chain of pathological events is the same. Affected structures demonstrate reactive hyperemic, with exudation of fluid into tissues due to increased vascular permeability and an increase of filtration pressure.

Peritonitis is a general term denoting peritoneal inflammation; some authors use this term interchangeably with acute abdomen. Peritonitis can be generalized, or affect selected portions of visceral or parietal peritoneum (Estes, 2006). Consequences of peritoneal inflammation vary by the severity and duration of the underlying condition, the organ involved, patient age (physiological reserve), and comorbidities. Primary or spontaneous peritonitis occurs as a diffuse bacterial infection without an obvious intra-abdominal source of contamination. More common is secondary peritonitis, which occurs as a result of a primary event such as perforation, infection, or gangrene of an intra-abdominal organ. Leakage of GI and pancreatic secretions, bile, blood, urine, or meconium cause chemical peritonitis when they come into contact with the peritoneum. The inflammatory response increases blood supply and edema formation within the peritoneum. There is transudation of fluid into the peritoneal cavity and accumulation of protein rich exudates. Ongoing inflammation glues omentum lying over the affected structure to that structure and inhibits peristalsis, which limits the spread of infection or inflammation. Fluid accumulates within the lumen, causing the intravascular volume to fall and producing clinical signs of hypovolemia.

Intra-abdominal infection and peritonitis result in profound sepsis due to the bacterial content of the viscera and the huge surface area of the peritoneum. There is vast fluid loss, rapid bacterial absorption and endotoxin, and a marked systemic inflammatory response to the release of inflammatory mediators. This course of events sets off a complex septic cascade, which includes intravascular coagulation, circulatory failure, inadequate tissue oxygenation, and finally multiple organ dysfunctions. In the surgical setting, the most common cause of generalized peritonitis is perforation of an intra-abdominal viscus. Ischemia and infarction are potent triggers of inflammation; leakage of blood into the abdominal cavity from any sources tends to produce relatively few signs of inflammation.

Obstruction is the second pathological process. The colon normally generates intermittent contractions of low and high amplitude. Low amplitude, short duration bursts move luminal contents anterograde (frontward) and retrograde (backward), delaying colonic transit time, thus providing time for water and electrolyte absorption. High amplitude contractions create mass movement. In general colonic activation increases colonic motility (Bullard & Rothenberger, 2005). Vomiting develops early and in greater volumes when the level of obstruction in the gut is high, as swallowed air, food, secretions, and bile accumulate behind the site of obstruction and continue to distend the bowel lumen. When propulsive activity in the gut is impeded or blocked, a vicious cycle of distension and secretion is set in motion as the bowel continues to contract with increased, uncoordinated peristaltic activity (Ripamonte & Mercadante, 2004). Ischemia and increasing intraluminal pressures caused by unrelieved obstruction predispose the bowel to rupture.

Assessment with Clinical Manifestations

Given the spectrum of possible causes, a systematic approach is required for assessment and diagnosis. Efficient history taking and focused physical assessment require an appreciation of how pain is produced within the abdomen. Pain is of three types: somatic, visceral, or referred. **Somatic** or **parietal pain** is sharp or knife-like in character, usually precisely localized to the affected area. When visceral inflammation involves richly innervated parietal peritoneum, which is sensitive to mechanical, thermal, and chemical stimuli, sharp pain is felt at the site. In addition, there is reflex contraction of the corresponding segmental area of muscle, which causes rigidity of the abdominal wall (guarding) and hyperesthesia of the overlying skin.

Structurally, visceral peritoneum, which partially or totally invests the intra-abdominal viscera, is insensitive to mechanical, thermal, or chemical stimuli. **Visceral pain,** activated by traction on bowel mesentery, inflammation, ischemia, or distension of hollow or solid viscus is typically described as dull and deep-seated. Usually, it is vaguely localized to area occupied by the viscus during development. It is often associated with restless, diaphoresis, and nausea. Colic is considered a type of visceral pain, arises from hollow viscus with muscle in its walls (gut, gallbladder, or ureter), and results from excessive muscle contraction against an obstruction. Patients may be unable to remain still during the bout of colic but be pain free between attacks. The complex sensory innervation of abdominal cavity produces classical pain syndromes. For example, acute appendicitis typically begins with generalized periumbilical pain, which over time migrates to the right lower quadrant (RLQ).

Referred pain is pain perceived distant from its source. For example, small bowel distension radiates to the back and cholecystitis radiates to the inferior scapular border, reflecting embryological or dermatomal origins.

> **Skills 360°**
>
> **History of Acute Abdominal Pain**
>
> A chief complaint of acute abdominal pain requires immediate focused evaluation: targeted history taking and a focused physical assessment. Physical exam lies at the heart of diagnosis and must be conducted to economically address the following questions:
>
> - How severe is the physiological compromise?
> - Is there a need for immediate resuscitation, urgent surgical consultation, and intervention?
> - What diagnostic modalities will be most efficient and effective in determining the probable cause?

Pain assessment is the focus of the history; elements of the comprehensive pain history are summarized in Table 50-2. Beginning practitioners should be aware that even if they are unfamiliar with classical histories associated with specific pathological events, a comprehensive, systematic, and detailed history is invaluable to the consultants involved later in the care. Individual elements of the history can suggest a possible etiology or influence the degree of urgency appropriate to evaluating the problem. For example, the onset of pain suggests problem acuity: sudden, generalized, excruciating pain, with an onset under one hour suggests an intra-abdominal catastrophe, such as perforation of a viscus (e.g., ruptured ectopic pregnancy) or vascular catastrophe (e.g., bowel infarction or dissection) that may produce shock and require resuscitation and immediate, often life-saving surgery. Gradual onset suggests an inflammatory process.

Pain quality, or character, including any periodicity, is also suggestive. For example, colicky pain suggests an obstructive etiology, such as biliary, ureteric or intestinal colic and may be intense and severe. If colicky pain becomes continuous, significant inflammation should be suspected. Location is possibly the most valuable variable to the underlying diagnosis. For example, blood or pus below the left diaphragm can cause left shoulder pain. Migratory details are important to note; for example, if leaking duodenal contents reach the right paracolic gutter, the patient may complain of RLQ as well as epigastric pain. Late in the evolution of acute abdomen, pain may be generalized due to diffuse peritonitis.

Radiation away from the initial site signifies involvement of other structures: For example, pain from a duodenal ulcer radiating to the back suggests that inflammation has breached the wall and reached structures on the posterior abdominal wall. Radiation to the right scapula should raise the suspicion of gallbladder pathology; radiation into the ipsilateral groin and flank is suggestive of ureteral obstruction (e.g., kidney stones). A temporal course of the acute abdominal pain can further narrow the likely pathology and influence trajectory of care. Severe pain, lasting more than six hours and worsening over

TABLE 50-2 Pain Checklist

Onset	Sudden versus duration (hours or days)
Character	Burning, cutting, boring, crampy, or colicky
Severity	0–10 scale
Location	Consider referred pain patterns
Radiation	Does the pain extend over a wide area?
Duration	Minutes to hours to days
Temporal course	Intermittent (waxing and waning) or continuous; is it getting better or worse?
Ameliorating factors	Is pain improved by changing positioning, food intake, or by medications?
Exacerbating factors	Is pain worse with movement?
Associated manifestations	Nausea, vomiting, changes in bowel habits or patterns; anorexia, rigors, shaking chills, fever, pulmonary, urinary, obstetric and gynecological symptoms (i.e., menstrual history; possible pregnancy), unintended recent weight loss, or drug use (e.g., steroids).

Adapted from Estes, M. (2006). Health assessment and physical examination *(3rd ed.). New York: Thomson Delmar Learning.*

time, increases the likelihood of surgery. If pain is subsiding, the probability of surgical disease falls.

Associated findings are more difficult to interpret. For example, vomiting may be attributable to pain severity or disease in the GI tract or self-induced, and can be bilious (small bowel obstruction) or nonbilious. Generally pain precedes vomiting in a surgical abdomen. This can be seen in appendicitis, cholecystitis, and small bowel obstruction. Vomiting followed by pain is suggestive of a medical cause. Diarrhea with pain is usually due to medical causes, with a few important exceptions. Obstruction causes classical clinical signs and symptoms; obstruction of a muscular viscus causes colicky pain, cresting and receding in waves, rather than the constant pain of inflammation, and tends to be worsened by general disturbance.

Focused history taking should occur simultaneously with inspection of the body habitus (physical appearance) and patient demeanor. It should be noted that the elderly and patients being treated with steroids may not report the same severity of pain as patients not on steroids or younger patients. The patient's overall appearance should be noted; for example, is the patient lying motionless or restless. A patient lying completely still is characteristic of peritonitis and should suggest serious intra-abdominal disease. Restlessness is associated with colicky pain. Dry mucous membranes might suggest dehydration.

The presence of tachypnea, tachycardia, hypotension, cold and clammy skin, altered mentation, low urine output, and fever suggest complicated disease with peritonitis and shock (Estes, 2006). If clinical signs suggestive of shock coexist with abdominal swelling or the patient is prostrate with board-like abdomen, the priority is immediate resuscitation and surgical consultation. Further deterioration may be averted if the patient is taken directly to surgery, where resuscitation and assessment can continue in conjunction with laparotomy.

Severe intravascular volume depletion or electrolyte abnormalities should be addressed immediately to preserve and support the vital functions and restore hemodynamic stability. Compromised renal perfusion raises the need for close monitoring of urinary output as volume resuscitation proceeds. High fever may be seen in abscess, pyelonephritis, septic cholangitis, or gynecological infections, such as salpingitis. However, absence of fever, particularly in the elderly, should never be relied on to exclude infectious intra-abdominal catastrophes. Abnormalities in cardiorespiratory parameters should raise questions about the need for enhanced monitoring and support—from continuous electrocardiographic and pulse oximetry to invasive hemodynamic monitoring, inotropic support, endotracheal intubation or mechanical ventilation. Adequate opioid analgesia should not be withheld during evaluation of the abdomen for fear of masking important clinical signs and delaying diagnosis. These strategies have been shown to be unfounded (Shabbir, et. al., 2004). Effective analgesia also facilitates patient cooperation during the examination.

Inspection should note the contour and color of the abdomen. Distension can suggest the presence of air, blood, or ascites, jaundice, or common bile duct obstruction (Estes, 2006). Cullen's sign, a bluish periumbilical discoloration, can occur with intra-abdominal bleeding; Grey Turner (tenderness) or Fox signs should be sought in the flank and inguinal area respectively. The location of hernia, mass, defects, and visible peristalsis and pulsatile masses should also be noted. Scars should be tested for the presence of herniation. Auscultation for bowel and vascular sounds (bruits, venous hums, or peristalsis) follows inspection. Absence of bowel sounds more than 30 minutes suggests peristalsis has ceased. Gurgles are produced by fluid-gas mixtures. A possibility of obstruction can be detected with absent bowel sounds, and **borborygmi** (a gurgling, splashing sound normally heard over large intestine). Palpation for masses, organomegaly (abnormal enlargement), and pain, and to confirm inspection and auscultatory findings should follow and should begin in areas distant from the pain (Estes, 2006). Every effort should be made to relax the patient. Guarding, or increased abdominal tone, is voluntary or involuntary, local or generalized. Involuntary guarding that fails to disappear during deep inhalation suggests underlying peritonitis.

The triad of generalized pain, board-like abdominal rigidity and rebound suggest peritonitis. Associated signs should be sought, such as Murphy's sign in acute cholecystitis or Rovsing's sign in appendicitis. Percussion concludes the exam, and is useful detecting the presence of air (tympanic) or fluid (fluid waves). Rebound tenderness is more accurately identified by percussion of the abdomen than by palpation with quick release (Estes, 2006). That is, rebound tenderness should be elicited by gently tapping the belly with the percussing finger. Maneuvers, such as the obturator and iliopsoas muscle tests, may be useful in detecting inflamed or perforated appendix. The examination should conclude with examination of the hernia orifices, genital, rectal, or vaginal examinations.

Diagnostic Tests

Laboratory, radiologic, and endoscopic diagnostics should not interfere with resuscitation and restoration of hemodynamic stability. They should complement the details of history and physical exam and are useful in supporting the diagnosis or narrowing the differential (Daniels, 2003). Laboratory findings, like signs and symptoms of shock, are nonspecific but can help focus attention on likely causes. Selection should be driven by historical and physical findings. Hematological investigations should minimally include CBC, with a differential and related tests, such as blood smear. Useful findings include leukocytosis, which suggest an infectious process (may be primary or secondary). Persistent elevation or rising white count suggests underlying inflammation or infection; a leukocytosis of 15,000 to 20,000 per mm^3 suggests bowel necrosis (Daniels, 2003). There can be a poor correlation with white blood cells (WBC) and intra-abdominal inflammation, so exclusions should not be made on the base of a normal WBC count. Abnormalities suggestive of a primary medical cause, such as sickling (sickle-shaped RBCs) that might have led to mesenteric ischemia or infarction may confirm clinical impression. Blood should also be sent for typing and cross-matching for patients who might require surgery or transfusion. A coagulation screen is required for any patient who might require surgery and to eliminate the presence of coagulopathy. Prolongations in international normalized ratio (INR) may require rapid correction prior to operation. Bleeding time may be requested by surgical consultants in specific instances. Prolonged clotting time or thrombocytopenia may suggest the possibility of hemorrhage as a primary or secondary etiology. Biochemistry studies should minimally include serum electrolytes, blood urea nitrogen (BUN), and creatinine as indices of renal function. Other assays should be selected on the basis of history or physical findings. For example, beta-hCG (human chorionic gonadotropin) in suspected pregnancy-related acute abdomen; liver function studies in acute hepatobiliary disease; and bilirubin, amylase, lipase, and calcium in acute pancreatitis; serum phosphate can be increased in mesenteric ischemia. Toxicology may be useful in selected cases (e.g., cocaine related). Microbiological testing (e.g., urine or blood cultures) ought to be considered in the presence of rigors and shaking chills, peritoneal signs, or history or clinical findings suggestive of an infectious etiology (e.g., pelvic inflammatory disease or septic ascending cholangitis) and dipstick-positive urine (for blood or WBC).

A 12 lead electrocardiogram (ECG) should be done in all surgical candidates to exclude acute myocardial ischemia or infarction and arrhythmias as cause of the pain. Presence of abnormalities may suggest the etiology of pain: For example, atrial fibrillation, in conjunction with abdominal pain may be indicative of mesenteric ischemia. Arterial blood gas analysis may be useful in ventilated patients, to assess the need for or adequacy of metabolic correction. Imaging should be selected for maximum yield in the shortest time; its purpose is pathological diagnosis. Common modalities are summarized in Table 50-3.

An upright chest X-ray (CXR) is the most appropriate means of detecting free intraperitoneal (pneumoperitoneum) gas under the diaphragm and should be done in cases of suspected perforation. It may also exclude respiratory causes of acute abdominal pain. The two most appropriate selections in a patient

TABLE 50-3 Imaging Modalities: Acute Abdomen

	ADVANTAGE	DISADVANTAGE	COMMENTS
CXR	Excludes some cardiorespiratory processes.	None.	Identifies 50–90 percent of perforated viscus with pneumoperitoneum.
	Fast, inexpensive, noninvasive, minimal radiation exposure, portable.		Increased sensitivity with left lateral decubitus view.
Abdominal films	Fast, inexpensive, noninvasive, minimal radiation exposure, portable. Cross table lateral in left lateral position can detect as little 5–10 mL free air (e.g., air fluid levels in dilated loops of bowel [obstruction]); distended bowel (paralytic ileus), abnormal calcifica tions (gallstones, kidney stones, and some appendicoliths).	None.	75 percent of perforated duodenal ulcers have free air; colon, and stomach perforation can liberate large amounts of air.
Abdominal or pelvic ultrasound, (transabdominal or intravaginal)	Portable, safe, rapid, low cost, no radiation exposure. Visualizes gallbladder, biliary tree, liver, spleen, pancreas, appendix, ovaries, adnexa, and uterus.	Blind to many areas, especially in presence of large amounts bowel gas or free air. CT outperforms in combination of clinical evaluation and other modalities.	Yield high in those with palpable mass and suspected acute diverticulitis; Less useful if lab results are normal and clinical signs are nonspecific Routine use not associated with shorter LOS.
CT—abdomen and pelvis + IV or oral contrast	Gold standard for identifying disease processes. Work horse of acute abdomen evaluation.	Requires transport and support out of intensive care unit, ED, or operating room. Not as useful with hollow viscera pathology.	For patients who do not go to surgery, CT superior to clinical exam (90 percent versus 76 percent sensitivity) in diagnosing cause. Especially useful in patients without prior known abdominal disease.
Tc99m HMPAO [technetium-99m-hexamethyl propylene amin oxime] white cell labeled scanning	High sensitivity for IBD (91–96 percent).	Not as accurate as CT for abscess and fistulae (abnormal passage leading from an abscess to body surface).	Some role in elderly and appendicitis.

Adapted from Persiani, R., Biondi, A., Buccelletti, F., Rausei, S., & Silveri, N. (2006). Unusual acute abdomen: To operate or not to operate? Lancet, 367*(9521), 1548; Raman, S., Somasekar, K., Winter, R. K., & Lewis, M. H. (2004). Are we overusing ultrasound in non-traumatic abdominal pain?* Postgraduate Medical Journal, 80, *177–179.*

with acute abdomen are plain films of the abdomen (two views) and computed tomography (CT) of the abdomen or pelvis, with or without intravenous (IV) and oral contrast. Rectal contrast may be indicated in selected patients. CT, which provides images with a high degree of anatomic detail, leads to pathological diagnosis in most cases. In one study, clinical examination accurately identified the anatomical lesion in 17.5 percent, and CT achieved (57.5 percent) greater than a threefold improvement. Ultrasound is particularly useful in gynecological and hepatobiliary disease. Angiography may be used when vascular etiologies are suspected (e.g., mesenteric ischemia, hemorrhage).

Consideration must be given to acute medical and surgical causes and prioritized by age. For example, among premature infants necrotizing enterocolitis is a not uncommon occurrence; but it is virtually unheard of among adults. Medical causes frequently produce a clinical picture that lacks specific localization and guarding. The broad differential reflects contents of abdomen represent every body system and can be intra- or extra-abdominal. Psychiatric discords, such as Munchausen's syndrome (fabrication of symptoms or self-mutilation to gain medical attention) or Munchausen's by proxy (faking another person's illness), should remain diagnoses of exclusion. Different classification schemes have been proposed; the variety includes genetic or developmental, infectious, vascular, neoplastic, infectious or inflammatory, and toxic or metabolic causes.

Nursing Diagnoses

Based on the information gathered, examples of nursing diagnoses in the patient with acute abdomen may include the following:

- Fear related to perioperative events.
- Deficient fluid volume related to intake less than body requirements.
- Acute pain related to acute abdomen.
- Risk of infection related to intra-abdominal processes and procedures.

Planning and Implementation

Goals of management are supportive and definitive. Definitive management of the underlying problem is as varied as the potential etiologies of acute abdomen. Supportive care runs the gamut from aggressive symptom palliative to resuscitation. Either may require immediate or delayed surgical intervention. Indications for admission to the hospital include surgical candidates, those who cannot eat or drink, febrile patients from infection, and those who have uncontrolled pain or require IV antibiotics.

Collaborative Management

Indications for adopting a nonsurgical approach include diagnostic uncertainty and equivocal physical findings. These patients should be admitted and closely monitored. Special attention should be paid to immunocompromised patients who may present atypically, and individuals who are unable to communicate. A period of close observation provides an opportunity to stabilize the vital functions, explore potential medical causes, and correct abnormalities. Patients with intra-abdominal sepsis may benefit from short-term, aggressive volume resuscitation and antibiotic therapy. Recent reviews of different antibiotic course of therapy (morbidity, mortality, cost, resource use) for the treatment of secondary peritonitis of GI origin suggested no specific benefit associated with any particular regimen (Wong, et al., 2005). Some potential surgical lesions might be managed initially by watchful waiting, such as a ruptured but contained duodenal ulcer.

Acute abdomen caused by medical conditions (e.g., sickle cell crisis, spontaneous bacterial peritonitis, *Clostridium difficile* pseudomembranous colitis, acute pancreatitis, acute hepatitis, acute salpingitis) require pathology specific management and involvement of appropriate consultants. Discovery of an abscess is not an automatic indication for open surgical management. Depending on location and patient status, percutaneous, fluoroscopy guided percutaneous drainage is often a viable option, sparing the patient urgent operation. For example, acute diverticulitis can often be managed medically with percutaneous drainage of abscesses, followed by elective surgery.

Surgery

There are a variety of potential surgical management strategies for patients with acute abdominal conditions. Surgical consultation should be sought for patients with severe or progressive pain, fecal vomiting, abdominal rigidity or guarding, rebound tenderness, hypertympanic (air-filled) abdomens, unclear etiology, or intra-abdominal fluid accumulation. Indications for operation include uncontrolled intra-abdominal hemorrhage (e.g., AAA in a viable patient), presence of peritoneal signs, pain with signs of sepsis without an obvious source, acute intestinal ischemia, and pneumo-peritoneum. An attitude of watchful waiting may be at adopted to give medical interventions an opportunity to create improvement, but this approach requires frequent and careful clinical monitoring. Surgical decision making about the approach, extent, whether or not to exteriorize the bowel, and how to close the wound are tailored to the specific cause (Golash & Willson, 2005).

Classically operative candidates undergo open **laparotomy,** a surgical incision into the wall of the abdomen, for definitive diagnosis and management. However, over the last decade, minimally invasive surgery, specifically, **laparoscopy,** a visual examination of the interior of the abdominal cavity, has played a growing role. A variety of operations are possible including diagnostic laparoscopy for critical patients with equivocal findings and definitive therapy for obstruction, diverticulitis, and acute appendix. When acute abdomen is caused by a medical problem, laparoscopy allows the surgeon to visualize large surface areas within pelvic and abdominal cavities, to biopsy suspicious areas, aspirate, culture, and ultrasound suspicious structures. Contraindications include hemodynamic instability, mechanical or paralytic ileus, coagulopathy, generalized peritonitis, severe cardiovascular disease, abdominal wall infection or marked distension, and multiple prior abdominal surgeries. Application is also limited by the availability of minimal invasive surgery (MIS) specialist general surgeons.

Laparoscopy is generally safe and well tolerated and can be performed under local anesthesia. Complications can occur during gas insufflation, trocar insertion, and the diagnostic exam; they include arrhythmias, bleeding, bile leak, perforation, laceration, vascular injury, and gas embolism. Postoperative concerns are the same as those associated with open procedures and include surveillance for hemorrhage and infection. Benefits are several; when CT and ultrasound findings are not definitive, laparoscopy provides a better evaluation of peritoneal cavity, paracolic gutters, and pelvic cavity than the standard laparotomy incision and improves diagnostic accuracy. Corrective surgery is often possible immediately following diagnosis. Patients report less pain, faster recovery, shorter stay, and fewer complications. The actual recovery period is related to the cause of the acute abdomen. Laparoscopic findings may necessitate open laparotomy for definitive correction (Majewski, 2005).

Preoperative management is directed at optimizing physical and psychosocial status of the patient. The vital functions require stabilization: systolic blood pressure should be restored to at least 100 mm Hg systolic, heart rate to under 100 beats per minute and adequate oxygenation. In the absence of central venous access, two large-bore IV catheters should be placed. Patients should be fasting (NPO) and may require antiemetics and a steroid bolus if the patient is steroid dependent, in addition to maintenance doses. Attention to glycemic control is indicated in diabetics. Nasogastric tube placement is invaluable for gastric decompression and provides some protection against macroaspiration. A bladder catheter should be placed to facilitate assessment of the adequacy of

> **Skills 360°**
>
> **Adequate Analgesia**
>
> Adequate analgesia remains a significant problem in patients with acute abdominal pain. A recent review of 100 patients in EDs revealed the following disturbing findings. Overall wait time for analgesia ranged from 2 minutes to 14 hours. Patients with mild complaints waited longer than patients with severe pain (mean of 82 minutes). Females waited longer than men (mean 129 minutes versus 69 minutes). Patients transferred to wards fared far worse than those medicated in the ED (mean 5 hours versus ½ hour) (Shabbir, et. al., 2004).

intravascular volume replacement and hourly monitoring of output. Minimal urinary output is 0.5 mL/kg/hr. Preoperative antibiotic coverage is also indicated.

Pregnancy Considerations

Management of gravid women should be similar to that of nonpregnant patients. Like in the elderly, clinical presentation may be atypical, including the lack of peritoneal signs due to the distortion of the anterior abdominal wall and underlying organs. Laboratory findings may also be uncharacteristic. Severe disease, for example, can occur in the absence of leukocytosis. Both factors may delay diagnosis and definitive treatment. The diagnostic process is inherently more complex given the fact that it inescapably involves two patients, evaluation of the fetus, with at least fetal heart tone occurring simultaneously with evaluation of the mother. Evidence suggests that management of gravid women should include obstetrical consultation if surgery contemplated.

The two most common surgical emergencies in gravid women are acute appendicitis and cholecystitis requiring appendectomy in 1:200 to 1:6,000 pregnancies and cholecystectomy in 1:1,130 and 1:12,890 pregnancies. Obstetrical risks to the fetus are greatest in the first (fetal loss, spontaneous abortion) and third trimesters (premature labor, but not fetal loss). Despite improvements in surgical anesthesia, perinatal and perioperative care risks attend surgical intervention in pregnancy. The rate of fetal loss in gallstone pancreatitis is estimated at between 10 to 20 percent and as high as 20 to 30 percent in maternal intestinal obstruction. Ultrasonography is a safe and effective diagnostic modality, and exposure to radiation from a single diagnostic procedure does not result in harmful fetal effects. Magnetic resonance imaging (MRI) is to be avoided if at all possible during the first trimester. If possible, surgery should be deferred to the second trimester, the period of least risk. Laparoscopy, once contraindicated in this group, appears to be a safe alternative to open procedures in experienced hands. Advantages include less fetal depression. However, there is some concern that gas insufflations may elevate fetal risk. Pregnancy-specific recommendations should be incorporated into routine surgical care, such as the use of pneumatic compression devices, fetal monitoring, and careful positioning to relieve the vena cava of the pressure of the gravid uterus.

Evaluation of Outcomes

Potential patient outcomes for each of the example nursing diagnoses for the patient with acute abdomen are:

- Fear related to perioperative events. The patient should manifest positive coping behaviors and verbalize a reduction in the amount of fear of the having this disease.
- Deficient fluid volume related to intake less than body requirements. The patient experiences adequate fluid volume and electrolyte balance as evidenced by urine output greater than 30 mL/hr, normotensive blood pressure, heart rate 100 beats/min, consistency of weight, and normal skin turgor.
- Acute pain related to acute abdomen. The patient should verbalize an adequate relief of pain along with the ability to realistically cope with the pain if it is not completely relieved.
- Risk of infection related to intra-abdominal processes and procedures. The patient remains free of infection, as evidenced by normal vital signs and absence of purulent drainage from wounds, incisions, and tubes. Infection is recognized early to allow for prompt treatment.

Given the criticality of the pain history to the diagnosis of acute abdomen, inability to communicate, whether due to developmental level or diseases of mind and brain, elevates the degree of diagnostic difficulty. This may result in unnecessary hospitalizations and greater reliance on serial laboratory or imaging

Dollars and Sense

Costs of Diagnostics for Acute Abdominal Emergencies

Advances in imaging and widespread use American College of Radiology (ACR) guidelines appear to be influencing resource use. Use of CT imaging in one study improved diagnosis of appendicitis, and the authors estimated a net savings of $4,731 due to improved diagnostic accuracy. Use of CT is also thought to be financially valuable, reducing cost by reducing unnecessary admissions. The use of contrast highly increases spectrum of detectable pathology. Surgical approaches to the management of acute abdomen are believed to have profound impact on resource utilization. Currently, it is estimated that in acute abdominal emergencies, diagnosis is incorrect or too late in 5 to 20 percent of cases, resulting in increased morbidity, mortality, and costs. Laparoscopy may be one of the means of reducing delayed or inaccurate diagnosis (Daniels, 2003; Majewski, 2005).

testing; it may also have a direct impact on morbidity: Young children, unable to relate a detailed history are prey to nonspecific signs and symptoms and have a perforation rate as high as 50 percent.

Morbidity and mortality, readmission rates, and 30-day mortality rates are as varied as the causes of acute abdomen. The presence of comorbid conditions influences physiological reserve and response to stress of disease and trauma of medical, endoscopic, surgical, and anesthetic events.

The care of critically ill patients is labor-intensive, frequently requiring prolonged stays in the intensive care unit, participation of multiple consultants, and individualized nursing care. Pharmacological management of severe sepsis with recombinant activated protein C in early sepsis is expensive but shown to reduce 28-day mortality if used early (Broyles, Reiss, & Evans, 2007).

ACUTE INFLAMMATORY DISORDERS

There are two primary acute inflammatory disorders of the lower GI tract: (a) appendicitis and (b) diverticulitis. Each of these conditions involve inflammatory processes, which can be severe and have important ramifications as acute care pathologies.

Appendicitis

Appendicitis is an inflammation of the appendix organ, which is a small finger-like appendage just below the ileocecal valve. This is the most common emergency abdominal surgery in the United States.

Epidemiology

Appendicitis occurs in approximately 7 percent of the population and affects males more than females. It occurs more in teenagers than adults and most commonly between the ages of 10 and 30 years.

Pathophysiology

The function of the appendix is not completely known, but it does regularly fill with and empty digested food. When the appendix becomes inflamed, it often is obstructed in its proximal lumen, which is labeled **fecalith** (hard mass of fecal material). In addition, the inflamed appendix also includes such things as for-

TABLE 50-4 Classifications of Appendicitis

TYPE	DESCRIPTION
Simple	Appendix is inflamed but still intact.
Gangrenous	There is tissue necrosis and microscopic areas of perforation.
Perforation	There is large perforation, which involves contents flowing into the peritoneal cavity.

BOX 50-3

ROVSING'S SIGN FOR APPENDICITIS

The nurse can assess for appendicitis by first testing for McBurney's point (pain elicited in the RLQ when firm pressure is applied. Then, the nurse can further differentiate the diagnosis by assessing for Rovsing's sign as follows:

- Press deeply and evenly in the LLQ for five seconds.
- Note the patient's response.
- Abdominal pain when felt in the RLQ is a positive Rovsing's sign.

The Rovsing's sign is based on the concept that changes in the intraluminal pressure will be transmitted through the intestine when the ileocecal valve is competent. Pressing on the LLQ traps air within the large intestine and increases the pressure in the cecum. When the appendix is inflamed, this increase in pressure causes pain.

Adapted from Estes, M. (2006). Health assessment and physical examination *(3rd ed.). New York: Thomson Delmar Learning.*

eign bodies, tumors, calculi, and edema of lymph tissue. Appendicitis is classified into three different categories as shown in Table 50-4.

Assessment with Clinical Manifestations

The patient with appendicitis has relatively predictable clinical manifestations. There is periumbilical pain that may initially be vague and generally spread over the lower abdominal region. In time, the pain localizes to the RLQ and is often accompanied with a low-grade fever. During these beginning symptoms, the patient will also become nauseated and local tenderness can be stimulated at McBurney's point as shown chapter 47. In addition, an advanced technique for assessment is labeled Rovsing's sign (Box 50-3).

The different types of pain during appendicitis are somewhat dependent on the location of the inflammation. For example, pain on defecation likely means that the tip of the inflamed appendix is in the pelvis and is located against the rectum. Pain on urination probably means that the inflamed appendix is near the bladder. In addition, there may be some rigidity of the rectus muscles in the region. As the appendicitis condition worsens, and even perforates, the pain will become more acute, even with the patient remaining still. The patient often will draw their knees upward toward their chest in an attempt to decrease pressure from the tension of the abdominal muscles (see Red Flag Feature).

Red Flag

Peritonitis

The nurse must be aware of the potential complication of peritonitis in the patient with appendicitis, which may be fatal. Clinical manifestations for peritonitis are elevated WBC, high fever, severe and acute pain, drawing the knees up to the chest, tachycardia, and diaphoresis. These symptoms should be reported immediately to prevent untreated peritonitis.

Diagnostic Tests

The patient's presenting symptomatology and history are the initial methods of diagnosing the condition of appendicitis. Then, the laboratory and X-ray diagnostics confirm the diagnosis. A CBC is obtained which reveals an elevated WBC (10,000/mm^3 to 20,000/mm^3). In addition, abdominal X-rays, an abdominal ultrasound, and CT scans can be performed to detect the RLQ density of the inflamed area (Daniels, 2003). A urinalysis can be performed to rule out a urinary tract infection, and a pelvic examination on females is performed to rule out gynecological disorders.

Nursing Diagnoses

Based on the information gathered, examples of nursing diagnoses in the patient with appendicitis may include the following:
- Acute pain related to the appendicitis.
- Fear in response to the diagnosis of appendicitis.

Planning and Implementation

The care of the patient with appendicitis is focused first on supporting the patient during the acute pain and diagnosis of the condition. Then the nursing care turns to preparing the patient for the likely surgical management of the disorder. The goals are relieving the pain, reducing the anxiety and fears of the patient, preventing infection, decreasing the chances of dehydration, and preventing postoperative complications.

Pharmacology

Before the surgery, the patient will be started on IV fluids to maintain an adequate vascular volume. Antibiotic therapy is initiated prophylactically (e.g., third-generation cephalosporins) to prevent infection complications. Analgesics can be administered once the diagnosis is confirmed.

Surgery

An appendectomy (surgical removal of the appendix) is performed either with a laparoscopic approach or an open appendectomy. The former is less invasive, made through a smaller incision, and has fewer postoperative complications. During the surgery, there can be a removal of any contaminants from the region with an irrigation of the area with sterile normal saline. After the surgery, the patient is managed with normal postoperative care measures (e.g., ensuring good respiratory effort free of lung consolidation, frequent vital signs, maintaining IV fluids, assessing the wound, treatment for pain, preventing infection). The patient is placed in a semifowler's position to reduce the tension and pulling of tissue on the wound area. The patient will be given a diet as tolerated as they recover and are able to have a normal fluid intake. Discharge will likely occur within 24 hours, and the patient will be instructed to return for a follow-up visit to their surgeon for removal of the sutures within a week. The patient will also be advised to monitor their general activity level and to rest as needed. In addition, potential symptoms of infection and complications related to wound healing will be instructed with the patient education.

Evaluation of Outcomes

Potential patient outcomes for each of the example nursing diagnoses for the patient with appendicitis are:
- Acute pain related to the appendicitis. The patient should verbalize an adequate relief of pain along with the ability to realistically cope with the pain if it is not completely relieved.
- Fear in response to the diagnosis of appendicitis. The patient should manifest positive coping behaviors and verbalize a reduction in the amount of fear of the having this disease and the upcoming expected surgery.

Diverticulitis

Diverticula are sac-like outpouches of mucosa through the muscular layer of the bowel and may occur anywhere along the GI tract. The largest percentage, 90 to 95 percent are found in the sigmoid colon. When there are multiple diverticula and resulting pathology, the process is termed **diverticulosis.** And, diverticulitis results in disorders that progress to an inflammatory process of the diverticular sacs.

Epidemiology

Diverticula disorders increase with age, with only 5 percent having the disorder before age 40 and more than 50 percent of persons over age 80 develop this pathology. Higher incidences are seen in Australia, the United Kingdom, and the United States, and the disease is relatively rare in Africa and Asia.

Etiology

Diet is thought to play the most important role in the causation of diverticular disease. Specifically, diets that are high in fiber deficiencies and highly refined foods are more correlated with diverticular disease. In addition, other correlates with the disorder are decreased activity levels and constipation. The suggestion is that people with decreased blood supply or nutrients in the bowel are more susceptible to diverticular disease.

Pathophysiology

The formation of diverticula within the bowel is what eventually leads to diverticulitis. The muscles where there are diverticular areas thicken, and the lumen is narrowed, which increases intraluminal pressure. With a deficient fiber intake seen in diverticular disease, the bowel develops a higher pressure, and the mucosa herniates through the muscle wall, which forms the diverticulum. As the diverticulum increases in size, it obstructs the bowel area and causes irritability of the colon. Abscesses can form along with perforations, and the further complications of peritonitis and bleeding can occur.

Assessment with Clinical Manifestations

In diverticulosis, there may be a chronic asymptomatic condition with two thirds of the time. If there are manifestations, they would likely be constipation or diarrhea, lower abdominal pain in the left lower quadrant, irritable bowel syndrome (IBS) development, abdominal cramping, generalized fatigue, and low-grade fever. The patient with diverticulosis may have complications of bleeding and inflammation.

As diverticulitis develops, the patient has more acute symptomatology caused by the inflammatory processes in the colon. The most common manifestation is increasing pain levels that are on the left-side quadrant (LSQ) of the abdomen. During this condition, there is more likelihood of perforation of a diverticulum (Figure 50-1). The continued complications that are seen are bowel obstruction, hemorrhage, peritonitis, fistula formation, and adhesions of the inflamed tissue to the small bowel.

Diagnostic Tests

There are a variety of diagnostic tests that are used in diverticular disease. A CT scan is the best method of detecting abscesses and complications evidenced in diverticulitis. Serum studies, such as those in a CBC, will show increased infectious processes (e.g., leukocytosis, elevated sedimentation rate). In addition, bleeding can be evidenced by hemoccult testing and hemoglobin or hematocrit levels. A lower GI series (barium enema) can also confirm diverticular disease and would be contraindicated in acute diverticulitis due to the risk of contamination if there is an existing perforation. Last, abdominal X-rays can detect free abdominal air that is seen in diverticulitis and in perforations.

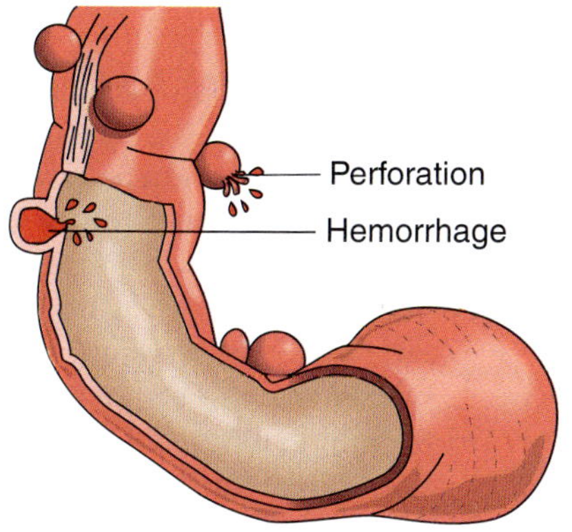

Figure 50-1 Diverticula in the sigmoid colon.

Nursing Diagnoses

Based on the information gathered, examples of nursing diagnoses in the patient with diverticular disease may include the following:

- Acute pain related to the diverticular disease.
- Fear in response to the diagnosis of diverticular disease.

Planning and Implementation

The prevention measures are of high priority for the diverticular disease processes. Nurses can perform patient education in the community related to the necessary dietary changes to include an increased fiber intake and teaching the early symptoms of diverticular disease. The elderly are more predisposed to this disorder, and therefore nurses must remember to address this population for the presence of diverticular disease.

As patients have acute diverticular disease, then their care strategies are dependent on whether they are treated with medications or surgery. Pain levels, anxiety, infections, and postoperative complications are the areas of greatest concern for the nurse. Continued dietary management strategies are employed.

Pharmacology

Broad-spectrum antibiotics are typically administered because of the inflammatory nature of diverticular disease, and specifically diverticulitis. Opioids are usually the analgesics of choice with severe pain; however, morphine is not the drug of choice as it causes increased intraluminal pressure. Stool softeners (Colace) and bulk-forming medications (Metamucil) are used to decreases the aggravation to the bowel area. In addition, antispasmodics (e.g., Pro-Banthine, Daricon) are administered for relief of abdominal cramping (Broyles, et al., 2007).

Surgery

When diverticulitis requires surgery, it is usually for peritonitis, an abscess, or continued hemorrhaging. The diseased portion of the bowel is resected and the remaining bowel is reanastomosed. There may also be a temporary ostomy (see ostomy section in this chapter) required to allow the area of the bowel to heal. The perioperative care is described in the colon cancer section described later in this chapter.

Evaluation of Outcomes

Potential patient outcomes for each of the example nursing diagnoses for the patient with diverticular disease are:

- Acute pain related to the diverticular disease. The patient should verbalize an adequate relief of pain along with the ability to realistically cope with the pain if it is not completely relieved.
- Fear in response to the diagnosis of diverticular disease. The patient should manifest positive coping behaviors and verbalize a reduction in the amount of fear of the having this disease and the upcoming expected surgery.

OBSTRUCTION

The GI tract, extending from mouth to anus, is a hollow food tube, specialized in structure and function for processing food, extracting nutrients, and passing wastes. Structurally, it is designed to generate movement of contents in a rostral (front) to caudal (back/tail) direction. Under the serosa or connective tissue lies a longitudinal layer of smooth muscle that is needed for propulsion. Beneath it lies a circular muscle layer, which alters lumen diameter, including the sphincters. Between them lies the myenteric plexus, which innervates both muscle layers. Lying beneath the muscle layers are submucosa and epithelium. Mucosa forms the lumen surface. Motility is principally generated by autonomic innervation, enteric nervous system, and smooth muscle activity. Stimulatory parasympathetic activity is opposed by inhibitory sympathetic outflow. Neural structures are accompanied on their course by parallel arteries and veins. Functionally, motility varies by region; for example, the colon lacks cyclic motor activity, but it generates low- and high-amplitude intermittent contractions. Low-amplitude, short-duration contractions delay colonic transit, allowing time for water and electrolyte absorption. Coordinated, high-amplitude contractions create mass movement. In general colonic activation increases colonic motility (Bullard & Rothenberger, 2005). Obstruction refers to the partial or complete impairment of the meandering course, innervation, structure, and the pathology involved. GI obstruction can be either mechanical (physical or structural) or functional. Most obstructions occur in the small intestine.

Ileus refers to intestinal obstruction due to partial or complete arrest of intestinal peristalsis and is also known as paralytic or adynamic ileus (Estes, 2006). In ileus, one or more nonmechanical factors interfere with the neuromuscular function of the bowel so as to impede the movement of the intraluminal contents. Acute colonic pseudo-obstruction (ACPO), also known as acute colonic ileus or Ogilvie's syndrome, is defined as a "functional disorder in which the colon becomes massively dilated in the absence of mechanical obstruction (Bullard, & Rothenberger, 2005, p. 1089).

Hindrance of the movement of intestinal contents may be due to physical or mechanical obstruction arising from within the lumen (e.g., malignant bowel obstruction) or bowel wall or by a lesion external to the bowel that compresses it externally. Interference may be partial or complete. Given that nutrient arteries and draining veins travel with neural elements to bowel segments, mechanical obstruction may also compromise supporting neurovascular structures. Obstruction can also be classified as simple or strangulated. Simple obstruction describes an obstruction in one site; closed loop obstructions are characterized by two sites of blockage. Strangulated obstruction is accompanied by vascular compromise of the segmental arterial supply and venous drainage. Strangulating obstruction occurs in nearly 25 percent of cases of small bowel obstruction and can progress to gangrene in as little as six hours. Although strangulation of the large bowel is rare, cecal perforation due to massive distension, or perforation of the bowel wall by tumor, or diverticulum may occur. Should these intra-abdominal catastrophes occur, signs of shock, often accompanied by signs of severe intravascular depletion, dominate the clinical picture and require prompt attention. The patient should be resuscitated and stabilized as described in acute abdomen. If not promptly recognized and relieved, these problems lead to significant morbidity and mortality.

Epidemiology

Patients who develop paralytic or mechanical obstruction span all ages and socioeconomic groups. The incidence of mechanical obstruction is related to the underlying cause. For example, malignant bowel obstruction is a common complication in patients with advanced abdominal or pelvic malignancies, notably colorectal, ovarian, and gastric cancers. Incidence in colorectal cancer (CRC) ranges from 4 to 24 percent and from 5 to 42 percent in ovarian cancer (Ripamonti & Mercadante, 2004). Other cancers (e.g., lung, breast) may also metastasize to the bowel. Small bowel obstruction (SBO) accounts for 20 percent of all acute surgical admissions. It is most commonly (60 percent) due to postoperative adhesions, fibrous bands within the peritoneum, which may compress bowel and cause obstruction, or be a focus for a **volvulus** (a twisting of the bowel on itself that causes obstruction). Prior abdominal surgery or sepsis (e.g., pelvic inflammatory disease, appendicitis) may cause adhesions. Surgeries most commonly associated with SBO are appendectomy, colorectal, and gynecological. Risk appears to be cumulative; gynecological surgery is associated with particularly high rates of adhesions and carries a mortality of 10 to 20 percent. Adhesions can produce SBO in as little as one month following surgery. SBO is associated with a mortality of 5.5 percent.

Ileus is common in medical and surgical populations, especially in bedridden patients, those with multiple comorbidities, and those being treated with opiates. In the intensive care setting, ileus is common in critically ill patients with sepsis, shock, respiratory pathology, and severe electrolyte abnormalities, especially hypokalemia (Bullard & Rothenberger, 2005).

Etiology

Paralytic ileus reflects altered neuromuscular function that impairs gut motility and has multiple potential causes. Ileus may reflect an imbalance between sympathetic and parasympathetic tone, disordered myenteric plexus activity (e.g., postoperative or a myopathy affecting gut muscular function). Medication use (e.g., some anesthetic agents, opiates) may contribute to this state of localized paralysis. Intraperitoneal and retroperitoneal infection, arterial or venous injury and metabolic derangements (e.g., hypokalemia) may also be associated with ileus.

Acute colonic pseudo-obstruction (ACPO) is most commonly associated with intra- or extra-peritoneal surgery. Multiple case reports and case series have linked this obstruction to adhesions that account for most postoperative instances. It is also associated with trauma (e.g., spinal cord injury) and medical conditions (age, sepsis, hypothyroidism; cardiorespiratory disorders, electrolyte abnormalities, i.e., hypocalcemia, hypokalemia, or hypomagnesemia) and medications (e.g., opioids, tricyclic antidepressant, and anesthetics. In the pediatric population large bowel obstruction may be congenital (Hirschsprung disease, aganglionic segment). Non-GI disease, e.g. diabetes mellitus or scleroderma, or idiopathic cases have been described as related causes (Bullard & Rothenberger, 2005).

Postoperative ileus (POI) is a common occurrence and has long been considered a potential and somewhat unavoidable consequence of surgical anesthesia. It prolongs hospitalization and increases costs. It typically leaves the small bowel largely unaffected, with function returning to normal within a few hours. Motility tends to return first to the cecum, then the sigmoid. The colon may remain inert for up to three days. There is no evidence that prophylactic nasogastric decompression after abdominal surgery hastens the return of bowel motility, prevents pulmonary complications, i.e., aspiration, reduces anastomotic leaks, increases patient comfort, or shortens length of stay (LOS). In this setting, nasogastric intubation should be selective rather than routine (Nelson, Edwards, & Tse, 2004). There is some evidence that use of thoracic epidural local anesthesia for patients undergoing laparotomy reduces GI paralysis compared with systemic or epidural opioids and achieves comparable pain relief. Nonsteroidal anti-inflammatory analgesia and laparoscopic procedures (versus open laparotomy) may similarly reduce the occurrence of POI.

Currently under review by the FDA is a novel agent, Alvimopan, (ADL 8-2698; Entereg), a peripherally selective opioid mu receptor antagonist, designed specifically to treat postoperative ileus. Concurrent administration of this GI-specific agent decreased the duration of POI without antagonizing the analgesic effectiveness of systemically administered opioids used ubiquitously to treat major surgical pain. It appears to be safe and well-tolerated when used for up to one week postoperatively. It has a relative contraindication in use with chronic opioid users, in whom it has precipitated local GI adverse effects. Due to minimal systemic absorption, dosage adjustments for renal, hepatic, and age–related impairment are not expected. Common side effects included nausea, vomiting, and hypotension. A detailed review of clinical trials and pharmacology are available elsewhere (Udeh, 2005). Common mechanical causes of SBO and large bowel obstruction (LBO) are summarized in Table 50-5.

The cecum, the widest part of colon with the thinnest muscular wall, is most vulnerable to perforation and least vulnerable to obstruction. By contrast, the sigmoid colon, though mobile, is the narrowest part of the large intestine and therefore, most susceptible to obstruction. Not surprisingly, diseases affecting the sigmoid are common causes of obstruction. In some cases, paralytic and

TABLE 50-5 Bowel Obstruction: Common Mechanical Causes

LOCATION	COMMON CAUSES (IN DEVELOPED NATIONS)
Small bowel	Adhesions (49–74 percent), tumors (~20 percent), hernia (~10 percent)
	Infants: **atresia** (absence or closure of a natural passage of the body, i.e., jejunoileal; duodenal, esophageal, or colonic), **malrotation** (failure during embryonic development of normal rotation of all or part of an organ or system), meconium ileus, volvulus, or **intussusception** (invagination, or telescoping, of one part of the intestine into itself).
Duodenum	Cancer (head of pancreas, duodenum)
Large bowel	Tumors (especially left sided lesions, e.g., CRC, ovarian cancer, diverticulitis (especially sigmoid), volvulus (especially sigmoid or cecum), or impaction.

Adapted from Bullard, K. M., & Rothenberger, D. A. (2005). Colon, rectum and anus. In F. C. Brunicardi (Ed.), Schwartz's principles of surgery *(8th ed., pp. 1055–1117). New York: McGraw Hill; Shatnawi, N., & Bani-Hani, K. (2005). Unusual causes of mechanical small bowel obstruction.* Saudi Medical Journal, 26*(10), 1546–1550.*

mechanical causes may coexist, i.e., in advanced colorectal cancer (Bullard & Rothenberger, 2005; Ripamonte & Mercadante, 2004).

Pathophysiology

In simple obstruction, ingested fluids, food, swallowed air, digestive juices or secretions, and gas accumulate behind the blockage. Distal bowel collapses and proximal loops dilate. Distension stimulates secretory activity, and the absorptive functions of mucous membranes fail. With increasing intraluminal pressures, mucosal veins and lymphatics become compressed, and the bowel wall becomes boggy and edematous. Active secretion and reduced absorption increase intraluminal fluid accumulation. Laplace's law proposes that increasing diameters accelerate the rise in tension experienced by the colon wall. That is, despite impeded or arrested forward transit of bowel contents, the bowel continues to contract with increased, uncoordinated peristaltic activity, leading to a vicious cycle of distension and secretion. Distension intensifies peristalsis and secretory derangements and increases the risks of dehydration, ischemia, perforation, peritonitis, and death. Bacteria content in stagnant bowel segments increases, and as obstruction progresses, may escape into the peritoneal cavity (Ripamonte & Mercadante, 2004).

Strangulation occurs when a loop of bowel is ensnared in a way that catches its vascular supply. Typically, strangulation begins with venous obstruction followed by arterial occlusion, resulting in rapid ischemia, infarction, gangrene and, ultimately, perforation. Treatment outcome reflects the interaction of a variety of factors, including the anatomic location and degree (partial or complete) of obstruction and whether or not the vascular supply is compromised. Whether or not decompression is accomplished before perforation and spillage of luminal contents into the peritoneal cavity occur and the prognosis of the underlying cause also affect outcome. Untreated, the mortality in strangulated SBO approaches 100 percent. Mortality falls dramatically with early surgical intervention.

Assessment with Clinical Manifestations

Assessment and clinical management vary by putative (supposed) cause, and location of the obstruction. SBO produces colicky, midabdominal pain often over a period of days. Vomiting occurs early in the course, especially with proximal simple obstruction. A change in the character of the pain (continuous, increasing severity) suggests the development of more ominous ischemic complications. Pain lasting several days, with progressive distension, suggests a more distal obstruction. Patients may also report constipation and the absence of flatus. A careful past medical history should note prior abdominal or pelvic surgery, history of malignancy (e.g., CRC), Crohn's disease, and drug exposure. LBO is unusual in patients under 50 years of age. Because the most common mechanical cause is CRC, enquiry about changes in bowel habits, stool caliber, unintended weight loss, and blood per rectum is essential. The history is one of gradual, then marked, distension, with lower colicky abdominal pain. Symptoms tend to develop more gradually than in SBO, and an acute onset should suggest an acute obstructive event, such as volvulus. Patients may report reduced to absent flatus for days preceding presentation and distension. If ileocecal valve incompetence allows reflux into small bowel, vomiting may occur.

Careful abdominal examination is necessary in suspected obstruction. Inspection may reveal scarring, which should suggest the possibility of adhesions. Distension, particularly in the flanks, may be prominent especially in LBO due to the distensibility of the colon. In combination with marked visible peristalsis, these findings should suggest intestinal obstruction. Auscultation typically reveals increased bowel sounds and high-pitched tinkling in early obstruction (Estes, 2006). Rushes of high-pitched peristalsis that coincide with cramping are typical. Hypoactive or decreased bowel sounds occur late in the clinical course. Should strangulation, infarction, and perforation occur, the belly may be silent. Auscultation is required for at least two minutes in a quiet abdomen. Paralytic ileus, intestinal obstruction due to partial or complete arrest of intestinal peristalsis, involving large and small bowel may produce abdominal distension, nausea, and vomiting. However, crampy pain is rare and bowel sounds may be preserved.

Percussion should follow auscultation: Gaseous distension typically produces tympanic percussion notes and is more marked in LBO (Estes, 2006). Palpation should follow percussion, and severe pain is unusual unless strangulation, ischemia or infarction, or perforation have occurred. In that case, there may be signs suggestive of peritonitis and acute abdomen, including guarding and rebound tenderness. A careful search for inguinal hernias, a rectal exam for masses (e.g., obturator hernia, CRC), and analysis of stool for occult blood conclude the abdominal assessment.

Diagnostic Tests

Diagnosis of obstruction is usually made on the basis of history and exam findings. However, electrolyte balance and CBC should be minimally assessed; the presence of fluid and electrolyte disorders is more common and more marked and SBO. Leukocytosis and the presence of metabolic acidosis should suggest ischemia or strangulation (Daniels, 2003).

Radiographic studies are intended to confirm diagnosis, distinguish between strangulating and simple obstruction, differentiate the causes, estimate the degree of obstruction, and exclude the possibility of colonic obstruction. Plain films of the chest and abdomen, supine and upright, are the primary studies used to demonstrate the presence of pneumo-peritoneum and air-fluid levels in loops of distended bowel respectively. Plain radiographs are diagnostically more accurate in cases of simple SBO. Cardinal signs of obstruction include absence of distal gas and air fluid levels, i.e. long air-fluid levels, classical step ladder pattern within a loop of bowel or an inverted U. ACPO classically reveals massive colon dilation in the absence of mechanical obstruction. Paralytic ileus produces distension of isolated segments of small and large bowel.

Evidence suggests that regional bowel distension that exceeds critical threshold diameters is positively correlated with the risk of perforation: Those critical diameters include 9 cm for the transverse colon (it is 9 cm), and 12 to 13 cm for the cecum. Should a watchful waiting approach be taken to management, successive measurements should be undertaken to track changes in lumen caliber.

Ultrasonography may reliably exclude SBO in up to 89 percent of patients and has a specificity of reportedly 100 percent. Enteroclysis (barium small bowel enema) or the intubation infusion method has improved preoperative diagnosis of lower grade SBO, but it requires naso-intestinal intubation that often requires conscious sedation and infusing the small bowel with barium liquid. CT enteroclysis, may be more reliable than CT alone in SBO. Enteroclysis is able to differentiate partial from complete obstruction, especially when clinical findings are nonspecific and plain films are normal. Enteroclysis should be avoided if perforation or ischemia are suspected. CT of abdomen and pelvis are indicated in symptomatic patients with indeterminate plain films, and is capable of visualizing varying diameters of bowel proximal and distal to the obstruction.

CT imaging is of growing importance when strangulated obstruction is suspected and demonstrated 81 percent sensitivity for high-grade obstruction. CT, with or without rectal contrast, is both more sensitive and specific for the obstruction than plain films (Aufort, Charra, Lesnik, Bruel, & Taourel, 2005). Contrast studies are secondarily indicated in suspected obstruction; although barium enema may rule out distal large bowel lesions, it should be preceded by endoscopic evaluation. Upper GI studies are contraindicated, because they may transform partial to complete obstruction or further complicate total obstruction.

Nursing Diagnoses

Based on the information gathered, examples of nursing diagnoses in the patient with obstruction may include the following:

- Fear related to perioperative events.
- Deficient fluid volume related to intake less than body requirements.
- Acute pain related to obstruction.
- Risk of infection related to intra-abdominal processes and procedures.

Planning and Implementation

Patients with suspected obstruction require hospitalization for diagnosis and treatment. Resuscitation and stabilization remain the first priorities of care and include reestablishment or support of hemodynamic stability, correction of fluid, electrolyte, and acid-base abnormalities, and transfusion support if indicated in the context of careful and frequent serial clinical and radiological examinations. Once stabilized, or concurrent with stabilization, decompression of the obstruction and definitive treatment of the underlying cause should be undertaken. Generally, mechanical causes should be excluded prior to medical or endoscopic intervention.

Pharmacology

In nonmechanical ileus with potentially reversible cause, the preferred initial management is conservative. Serial assessments to detect signs of peritonitis are recommended. Initially, radiographic evaluation should occur daily or more frequently. Monitoring should occur concurrently with the identification and correction or removal of contributory elements. Consultation with a pharmacist to review the patient's medication profile is often invaluable in identifying contributory drugs and recommending alternatives. Offending medications should be removed (e.g., opiates, anticholinergics). It should be noted that randomized clinical trial (RCT) evidence supports the efficacy of neostigmine use in ACPO; however, it has not been evaluated against endoscopic decompression. Strict bowel rest and careful attention to fluid replacement for loss as well as maintenance, with appropriate laboratory guided electrolyte supplementation (especially potassium), are indicated.

Commonly prescribed medications are: anticholinesterases (e.g., neostigmine), anticholinergics (e.g., scopolamine), antiemetics (e.g., chlorpromazine), antibiotics, and antisecretory medications (e.g., octreotide) (Broyles, et al., 2007). In addition, prokinetic agents should be avoided in mechanical obstruction, and unfortunately they have shown inconsistent results in ACPO. Antibiotics, typically second- or third-generation cephalosporins or broad-spectrum agents (e.g., meropenem), may be used to cover gram-negative bacteria and anaerobes. Selection varies with suspected diagnosis, clinical status of the patient, and institutional resistance patterns. Suspected sepsis should prompt appropriate microbiological cultures and parenteral antibiotic use. Pharmacological management of malignant obstruction often includes the use of analgesics, antispasmodics, anticholinergics, and possibly steroids.

Gastric Decompression

Decompression of SBO is intended to reduce or eliminate vomiting, protect the airway from macroaspiration, the bowel from perforation, and relieve pain. However, the means of decompression remains controversial; that is, whether to use nasogastric or naso-intestinal tubes. The effectiveness of decompression varies inversely with the distance between the tip of the tube and the site of blockage; thus in obstruction, a naso-intestinal, rather than a nasogastric, tube is considered the optimal method of decompression of the distended small bowel. Passage beyond the pylorus has the added advantage of relieving the colicky pain. The higher cost of a longer multipurpose tube, lack of familiarity, and need for two-stage use with initial gastric decompression, followed by advancement under fluoroscopic guidance into the proximal jejunum has been limited in use. In postoperative obstruction due to adhesions following gynecological surgery, gastric decompression successfully relieved SBO in approximately 80 percent of patients. Once bowel function returns, the nasogastric tube should be put to gravity drainage and then removed. Attempts to achieve decompression using a rectal tube are rarely effective, because obstruction is upstream from the site of decompression. However, it may be used with tap water enemas in ACPO in circumstances that cecal distension is not dangerously high or the pain severe. Patients are required to lie prone with hips elevated on pillow or knee chest with hips up, alternating right and elevated lateral decubitus positions hourly. This may be attempted for 24 to 48 hours depending on patient tolerance; failure should be followed by endoscopic intervention. The reported success of conservative management is highly variable, ranging from 20 to 92 percent.

Endoscopic Therapy

Endoscopic options may be appropriate for patients deteriorating with conservative management, who are continuing to progress in their symptomology or are considered inappropriate for a neostigmine trial. Although technically difficult and associated with risk of perforation, colonoscopic decompression may be attempted in ACPO. Success in experienced hands varies between 61 and 78 percent, with recurrence ranging from 18 to 33 percent. Perforation rate in colonoscopic decompression is as high as 3 percent (Bullard & Rothenberger, 2005).

Endoscopy is emerging as a useful modality for managing malignant obstruction. It may serve as a bridge to surgery when successful, providing an opportunity to stabilize the patient and evaluate the extent of disease. In operative candidates, it may avoid the need for diverting colostomy and a second operation for reanastomosis. **Anastomosis** is the surgical joining of the hollow tubular parts. Endoscopic laser therapy in malignant inoperable obstruction has been reported as a safe surgical alternative. Success been related to tumor size; treatment may require several sessions. Common complications include perforation, bleeding fistula, abscess, and pain (Davila, et al., 2005).

For patients with extensive tumor and multiple partial obstructions, endoscopic placement of self-expandable metal stents (SEMS) may be attempted. Location can be esophageal, gastroduodenal, or colorectal, and placement has a lower morbidity than surgery. Success rates are variable. Davila, et al. (2005) reported success in cancer palliation in 90 percent of 336 cases. Complications include perforation, bleeding, tumor ingrowth, overgrowth, and migration. Long-term outcomes, especially if stent placement is followed by chemotherapy or radiation, have not been studied well. Patients have been advised to follow a low-residue diet and use laxatives, stool softeners, or mineral oil to void impaction after SEMS placement. Endoscopic placement of a gastrostomy tube in a patient with malignant obstruction who is not a SEMS candidate may be used to reduce unabsorbed secretions, nausea, and vomiting. The patient may then be able to eat and drink because food drains directly out of the stomach.

Surgery

Definitive management of mechanical obstruction is surgical in most instances, typically by laparotomy or laparoscopic means. Surgery tends to be associated with a higher morbidity and mortality than medical or endoscopic procedures. Indications for urgent surgical consultation and management include a diagnosis of strangulated obstruction, or signs and symptoms of peritonitis, perforation, increasing leukocytosis, respiratory compromise, and fever. Elective laparotomy or laparoscopy should be considered in those whose ileus persists beyond a week, because in these instances the cause is usually mechanical. Patients with SBO who are managed with an initial nonoperative trial (usually a 48- to 72-hour trial) but fail the trial and proceed to surgery experience no apparent disadvantage. In malignant obstruction, contraindications include surgical evidence from past procedures of futility, reobstruction, presence of intra-abdominal carcinomatosis, diffuse intra-abdominal tumor burden or multiple palpable masses, poor performance status, large volume ascites, and patient refusal (Ripamonti & Mercadante, 2004). The choice of procedure is influenced by location and likely cause of obstruction; for example, a procedure by hernia repair might utilize a adhesiolysis in SBO, resection of CRC with anastomosis, or a diverting colostomy. In LBO, common procedures include right hemicolectomy for right-sided lesions and extended right hemicolectomy for lesions in the transverse colon. Other approaches may be diagnostic and palliative, such as the discovery of disseminated intraperitoneal cancer.

Laparoscopic approaches to obstruction, both diagnostic and definitive, are becoming more common and feasible. Evidence from small studies suggests that the minimally invasive approach is associated with more rapid return of GI function and shorter hospital LOS. Laparoscopy may not only be less likely to produce adhesions than laparotomy, but also feasible for lysing (release of) adhesions causing obstruction. However, some authors argue that laparoscopic adhesiolysis carries an unacceptably high risk of perforation and injury to organs caught in the adhesion bands; there is no clear evidence that minimal invasive surgery is superior to open surgical lysis of adhesions in terms of reforming of adhesions and subsequent obstruction (Golash & Willson, 2005).

Evaluation of Outcomes

Potential patient outcomes for each of the example nursing diagnoses for the patient with obstruction are:

- Fear related to perioperative events. The patient should manifest positive coping behaviors and verbalize a reduction in the amount of fear of the having this disease.
- Deficient fluid volume related to intake less than body requirements. The patient experiences adequate fluid volume and electrolyte balance as evidenced by urine output greater than 30 mL/hr, normotensive blood pressure, heart rate 100 beats/min, consistency of weight, and normal skin turgor.

- Acute pain related to obstruction. The patient should verbalize an adequate relief of pain along with the ability to realistically cope with the pain if it is not completely relieved.
- Risk of infection related to intra-abdominal processes and procedures. The patient remains free of infection, as evidenced by normal vital signs and absence of purulent drainage from wounds, incisions, and tubes. Infection is recognized early to allow for prompt treatment.

COLORECTAL CANCER

As life expectancy across the globe continues to lengthen, and as other causes of mortality fall, cancer has become the second overall leading cause of death. Currently, it is the leading cause in women between the ages of 40 and 79 and men between the ages of 60 and 79 (Meric-Bernstam & Pollock, 2005) (Box 50-4). In part due to heightened understanding of etiology of many cancers, widespread public appreciation of preventive strategies (e.g., smoking cessation), increasing sensitivity of screening for early detection (e.g., mammography, colonoscopy), and advances in therapeutics, from 1992 to 1999 cancer death rates overall decreased by 1.5 percent in males and 0.6 percent in women. CRC refers to predominantly epithelial-derived tumors (e.g., adenomas and adenocarcinomas). Other colorectal tumors include carcinoid, lipoma, lymphoma, and leiomyoma (Bullard & Rothenberger, 2005).

BOX 50-4

COLORECTAL CANCER (CRC)

CRC is the fourth most common cancer worldwide; 1,025,152 new cases and 528,978 deaths a year are attributed to CRC. Fifty percent develop liver metastasis sometime in their course. On the European continent, there are 150,000 new cases annually, and 95,000 deaths. In the United States, CRC is the most common malignancy of the GI tract, with annual incidence of 145,000). Estimates for 2005 were 104,950 new cases (United States), with 56,290 dying from the disease. Approximately 40,000 patients will be diagnosed with rectal cancer in 2005. CRC is the fourth most common cancer in both men and women with a lifetime risk that approaches 6 percent (Leonard, Brenner, & Kemeny, 2005).

Epidemiology

Over the past decade, incidence and mortality rates have remained stable or modestly decreased; likely due to improved screening, endoscopic removal of polyps, and modification of environmental factors (e.g., diet). Though highly treatable and often curative if found early, CRC is the second most lethal, accounting for about 55,000 to 56,000 deaths annually. Survival varies widely in the Western world and differences likely reflect different stage at diagnosis and therapy used to treat CRC. If diagnosed early, a five-year survival rate is approximately 90 percent; that percentage falls to 8 percent if diagnosed late. Racial differences in overall survival have been observed, without differences in disease-free survival. For example, mortality among African Americans remains higher than other ethnic and racial groups. More affluent patients appear to fare better than less affluent.

Etiology

One widely held opinion is that cancer "is a genetic disease that arises from an accumulation of mutations that leads to the selection of cells with increasingly aggressive behavior" (Bullard & Rothenberger, 2005, p. 260). Growing understanding of the human genome and its protein products and pathways suggest that virtually hundreds of genes and proteins are involved in the process of cell division and DNA replication. Gene mutations, which appear to be numerous and not uncommon, may activate oncogenes, inhibit tumor suppressor genes (e.g., APC gene), or disable mismatch repair genes. It appears that accumulation of mutations of various genes or proteins can sometimes lead to uncontrolled cancerous growth. A number of genes are being studied in CRC and are summarized in Table 50-6.

Seventy-five to 80 percent of CRC is sporadic or affects individuals of average risk. The remaining 20 to 25 percent report known risk factors. Hereditary CRC has two well-described forms and affects about 6 percent of the CRC population. Hereditary nonpolyposis colon cancer (HNPCC), or Lynch's syndrome, is a rare autosomal dominant disease, accounting for fewer than 5 percent of all CRC. As the most common hereditary CRC syndrome, it arises from

TABLE 50-6 Genetics and Colon Cancer

SUPPRESSOR GENES (LOSS OF FUNCTION)	ONCOGENES (AMPLIFIES FUNCTION)	FUNCTION AND ASSOCIATION
	K-ras (proto-oncogene)	Perturbation of one allele disturbs cell cycle
		Induces cellular proliferation and inhibits apoptosis
DCC gene ("deleted" in colorectal carcinoma)		Loss of both required for malignant degradation
		May involve differentiation
p53 gene		Normally required for initiating apoptosis in cells with genetic damage
		Present in 75 percent of CRCs; present in multiple other cancers
DNA mismatch repair genes (e.g., *hMLH1, hMSH2*)		Normally identify and repair mismatched nucleotides in DNA or small insertion or deletion loops during DNA replication
		Nonrepaired replication errors lead to a damaged DNA
		HNPCC—defect in mismatch repair [caretaker] genes hMLH1, hMSH2, HPMS1-2

Adapted from Bullard, K. M., & Rothenberger, D. A. (2005). Colon, rectum and anus. In F. C. Brunicardi (Ed.), Schwartz's principles of surgery *(8th ed., pp. 1055–1117). New York: McGraw Hill; Meric-Berstam, F., & Pollock, R. E. (2005). Oncology. In F. C. Brunicardi (Ed.),* Schwartz's principles of surgery *(8th ed., pp. 249–294). New York: McGraw Hill.*

errors in mismatch repair. Type I confers a 50 percent risk in first-degree relatives; type 2 is associated with extracolonic malignancies, especially endometrial, ovarian, and cholangiocarcinoma. It is characterized by the development of early cancer (40 to 45 years of age) and is usually in proximal colon. It tends to have a favorable clinical course and respond better to 5-fluorouracil (5-FU) (Bullard & Rothenberger, 2005).

Familial adenomatous polyposis (FAP) is a rare autosomal dominant disorder, genetically related to mutations on the APC gene. Clinically, it is characterized by the development of hundreds, often, thousands of adenomatous polyps throughout the large bowel after puberty. Evolution to CRC is a certainty, occurring in the teens, most sometime during the 30's and inevitably by age 50. In 20 percent of patients, it is a new mutation. Patients may also develop cancers of the thyroid, gallbladder, adrenal glands, and brain (Bullard & Rothenberger, 2005). Individuals with a family history of CRC, but lacking identifiable hereditary syndromes or specific genetic abnormalities, are said to have familial colorectal cancer (FCC). FCC occurs in about 10 to 15 percent of patients; lifetime risk appears to increase with family history (FH). Diagnosis before age 50 is associated with higher incidence (Meric-Bernstam & Pollock, 2005).

Ethnic, racial, and migrant studies suggest important environmental influences in CRC. For example, Israel-, European-, and American-born male Jews are at a higher risk than those born in Africa and Asia; Japanese immigrants to America have a much higher rate than Japanese in Japan. CRC may be related then to a range of cultural, social, and lifestyle practices, and these may account for up to 70 to 80 percent of the cases. The implication is clearly that in many patients, CRC may be linked to modifiable risk factors and that management of risk behavior may have an impact on occurrence.

Validated nonmodifiable risk factors for CRC include age greater than 50 years, male, African American, history of adenomatous polyps, ulcerative colitis, or Crohn's disease, and first-degree relative with FAP, HNPCC, or history of breast, ovarian, or endometrial cancer. Genetics appear to affect the age of onset of CRC. Risk awareness is useful when it is useful in disease prevention, and the following factors have been linked to CRC.

Diet has a complex and poorly understood role in etiology of CRC. Numerous studies have often yielded contradictory results due to methodological limitations and the complexity of the subject itself. However, there appears to be weak but consistent evidence that dietary fat and meat (especially processed) intake is positively correlated with risk. Tumorigenesis appears to be enhanced as fat content increases, possibly by increasing bile acid concentration and altering interactions to amplify cell replication signals, and direct toxicity to gut mucosa, which may induce early changes (Bullard & Rothenberger, 2005). The interaction of dietary fat, protein, and caloric intake is also associated with CRC.

Fiber refers to a range of compounds (e.g., wheat, bran, cellulose, dried beans), and it appears that intake of foods rich in fiber is inversely related to CRC. Risk reduction may be selective for fiber source and may modify carcinogenesis by a number of mechanisms, including binding to bile acids, increasing fecal water, and diluting carcinogens. The selective value of fruit and vegetable fiber over cereal may reflect an association with other factors. There is no RCT evidence that increased dietary fiber intake reduces the incidence or recurrence of adenomatous polyps within a two-to-four-year period. The protective benefits of diets high in fruit and vegetables are equivocal at this time (Delaune & Ladner, 2006).

A recent meta-analysis (14 RCT) found no evidence that antioxidant vitamins confer protection against development CRC adenomas or cancer. The value of folic acid supplementation is being evaluated for its protective effects. There appears to be an inverse relationship between calcium intake and CRC risk. Calcium may bind to bile acids, thereby blocking their access to luminal epithelium or possess other protective effects.

Obesity and sedentary lifestyle increase cancer-related deaths, and in some studies obesity is associated with a twofold increase in CRC risk. The risk appears to increase with increasing body mass index (BMI) (Bullard & Rothenberger, 2005). Absence of a strong or consistent relationship of obesity and CRC may reflect differences in metabolic efficiency rather than simple overeating. Maintenance of a BMI of 18.5 to 25 kg/m^2 throughout life and 30 minutes of physical activity most days is intuitively sensible, though not associated with evidence of reduced risk. Moderate intensity activity (e.g., walking) may have an inverse association with large adenomas.

There is weak evidence that prolonged cigarette smoking (more than 35 years) increases the risk of adenomas and adenoma recurrence after polypectomy. There is only weak suggestion that in average risk individuals, use of NSAIDS, estrogen, folic acid, and calcium may be preventive.

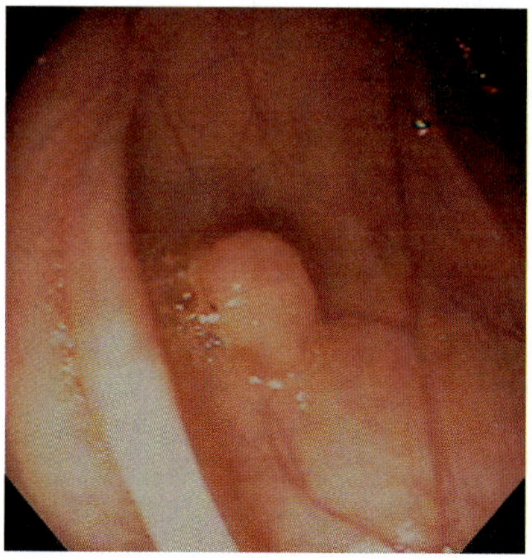

Figure 50-2 Colon polyp.

Pathophysiology

Transformation from normal gut lumen epithelium to adenomatous polyp to carcinoma is a sequence of events is known as the adenoma-carcinoma sequence. A polyp is defined as any projection that protrudes from the surface of the intestinal mucosa into the lumen, regardless of histology (Figure 50-2). Pedunculated polyps have a stalk; sessile polyps lack years and, by definition, are dysplastic. The risk of transformation rises with lesion size. Inflammatory, hamartomatous, postsurgical, and other polyps are not associated with CRC. However, those that arise from abnormal mucosal maturation, due to proliferation or dysplasia, are recognized as cancer precursors. Although most polyps do not evolve to CRC, the fact that most CRC originates as polyp provides the

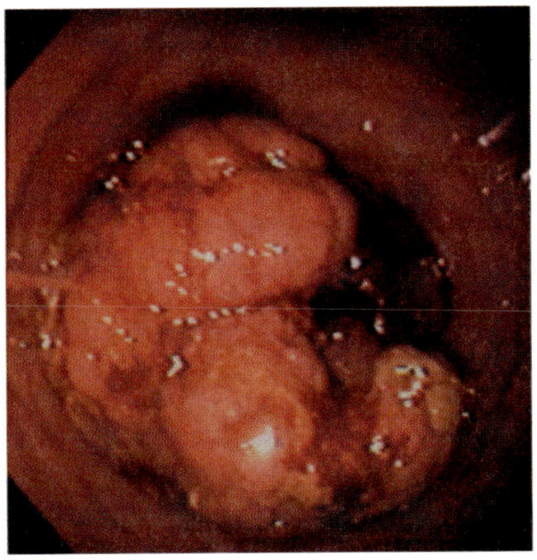

Figure 50-3 Colon cancer.

rationale for secondary prevention strategies and polypectomy before the lesion evolves into a CRC (Bullard & Rothenberger, 2005). Mutational events (activated oncogenes, deactivated suppressors) facilitate cell proliferation, and failure of repair lead to selection of growth advantage and progression to malignancy.

The lesion begins in mucosa and invades the bowel wall, involving adjacent viscera as it grows (Figure 50-3). It can grow to a size large enough to obstruct the gut lumen. Draining lymph nodes are the most common route of spread, and lymph node involvement precedes distant metastases or carcinomatosis. Depth of tumor invasion is the most significant predictor of lymph node spread; carcinoma in situ or high-grade dysplasia carries no risk of lymph node metastasis. The number of positive nodes found at operation correlates with the presence of distant disease and inversely with survival; four or more predict poor prognosis (Otchy, et. al., 2004).

Assessment with Clinical Manifestations

The history should include a detailed family history, including the number, degree of separation, age of onset, and presence of associated cancers that might suggest a familial syndrome. Questioning should address nonspecific complaints, such as fatigue, unintended weight loss, and anorexia. GI specific complaints, such as change in bowel habits, **tenesmus** (distressing, but ineffectual urge to evacuate the rectum), bloody stool, melena, and colicky abdominal pain should be noted (Estes, 2006). Alternating constipation and diarrhea in adults (older than 40 years of age) may be early signs of obstruction; and complaints or findings of blood in stool should never be dismissed as local disease (e.g., hemorrhoids), without excluding more proximal.

Findings are related to site of the lesion and the presence of complications (e.g., obstruction, perforation). Tumors in the cecum and ascending colon may become quite large without producing symptoms, because stool is liquid. Patients with lesions in the ascending colon often bleed chronically from ulcerations and present with anemia rather than prominent GI complaints. Development of microcytic anemia should prompt consideration for colonoscopy. Lesions in the transverse colon can produce cramping, occasional obstruction, and even perforation. Rectosigmoid masses are associated with tenesmus, narrow stools, and **hematochezia,** the passing of stools containing red blood rather than tarry stools. Abdominal exam may reveal visible or palpable masses, dull to percussion.

Diagnostic Tests

Screening for CRC lags far behind screening for other cancers. Screening may be practiced by about 20 percent of U.S. adults. In 1999, only 44 percent of adults underwent sigmoidoscopy or colonoscopy for screening or diagnosis; 40 percent had used fecal occult blood testing (FOBT) kits. Women more often had FOBT; more men had sigmoidoscopy. The most frequent reason for not being screened in one study was lack of recommendation by primary care physicians; other factors include fear or embarrassment, cost and reimbursement issues, and lack of access. There appears to be a real need to increase awareness and promote the use of regular screening as recommended. Current recommendations are summarized here and in Table 50-7. Screening is recommended to commence at age 50 in men and women, but no similar guidance is offered for when screening should cease; the impact of newer technologies, such as virtual colonoscopy is unclear at this time. Although the frequency and duration of screening has not been definitely established, all of the available methods reduce, to some degree, the risk of death from CRC.

TABLE 50-7 Screening and Detection: CRC

Average Risk Individuals

MODALITY	RECOMMENDATION	EVIDENCE
Digital rectal exam	None	Not recommended as an adequate screen, fewer 10 percent lesions within reach.
Fecal occult blood test (FOBT)	Annual Individuals older than 50 years of age.	Pros—Strong evidence for reduction in death ~16–23 percent (Levin, 2005) and incidence of CRC Sensitivity: 25–90 percent Rationale: most tumors and large polyps bleed intermittently. Trigger for other diagnostic testing. Cons—Large no. false positives
Flexible sigmoidoscopy	Every 5 years older than 50 years of age	Pro—Evidence decrease in deaths from CRC within reach; with FOBT increase sensitivity; detects 70–85 percent advanced lesions. Low-risk significant complications. Optimal screening interval not determined.
Barium enema (BE)—Air contrast	Every 5–10 years	No RCT evidence as screening test; less sensitive than colonoscopy detecting polyps. Perforation rare.
Colonoscopy	Every 10 years older than 50 years of age	Pro—Most sensitive and specific Con—Risk increases with diagnostic maneuvers; inconvenient, small risk complications including perforation (0.2–0.3 percent); costly. Frequency based on natural history of the adenoma-carcinoma sequence.
CT colonography Virtual colonoscopy	None	Pro—Noninvasive, short duration (10–15 minutes), requires mechanical bowel prep and air installation. High sensitivity and specificity in experienced hands: polyp detection (greater than 10 mm) approaches 90 percent Con—Clinical outcomes unknown; indirect evidence supports use of this modality; may be less cost-effective than colonoscopy.
CT	None	No screening indications Modality of choice for evaluation of distant metastases or synchronous lesions
Genetic screening	None	Not recommended for screening: rare incidence Con—Limited sensitivity, potentially misleading, not cost effective. Research context only
Carcino-embryonic antigen (CEA)	None	Origin—Embryonic endodermal epithelium. Not indicated for routine screening Nonspecific elevation in variety of malignant and nonmalignant conditions
High-risk groups		Depending on risk factor(s), begin at younger age, and occur more frequently
Genetic testing	Research and clinical decision making	Clinical application led to presymptomatic diagnosis in FAP and HNPCC; technically able to detect APC, *K-ras* mutations; studies in progress to compare these techniques with colonoscopy. Expensive; cost-effectiveness unproven FAP standard of care with genetic counseling, DNA testing for APC gene mutations: specificity is 100 percent; sensitivity 70–90 percent HNPCC tests not as sensitive; sequencing very expensive.

Continued

TABLE 50-7 Screening and Detection: CRC—*cont'd*

Average Risk Individuals

MODALITY	RECOMMENDATION	EVIDENCE
On the horizon	n/a	n/a
Stool based DNA		Screening effectiveness unknown
		Used in patients with known polyps or cancer
Positron emission tomography (PET)	Uses fluor-deoxyglucose (FDG)	Accuracy delineating metastatic from postoperative change; superior to CT for liver, intra-abdominal, and pelvic disease

Adapted from Daniels, R. (2003). Delmar's manual of laboratory and diagnostic tests. *New York: Thomson Delmar Learning; Otchy, D., Hyman, N. H., Simmang, C., Anthony, T., Buie, W. D., & Cataldo P. (2004). Practice parameters for colon cancer.* Diseases of the Colon and Rectum, 47*(8), 1269–1284.*

Nursing Diagnoses

Based on the information gathered, examples of nursing diagnoses in the patient with CRC may include the following:

- Chronic pain related to CRC.
- Fear in response to the diagnosis of CRC.
- Ineffective coping related to anxiety, lower activity level and the inability to perform normal activities of daily living.

Planning and Implementation

CRC has many implications for management strategies. There are a wide variety of manifestations that the patients will have and therefore many types of treatments. For slow development of the disease, less invasive therapies are encouraged, and surgeries are used for patients with more problematic cancer proliferation. See chapter 15 for further nursing implications when caring for patients with CRC.

Pharmacology

Cancer recurs in half of operated patients and is the most common cause of death. There is clear consensus that patients with metastatic CRC should be offered adjunctive chemotherapy (see chapter 15). The standard regimen for adjuvant therapy for CRC is not clear, but 5-FU, the sole agent with proven efficacy, has been joined by an array of new agents, combinations, schedules, and delivery modes. At the forefront of research are biological therapies, also known as immunotherapy, biotherapy, or biological response modifier therapy. Interacting with the body's immune system, they include interferons, interleukins, colony-stimulating factors, monoclonal antibodies (MOAB), vaccines, gene therapy, and nonspecific immunomodulating agents. MOAB antibodies can be designed to react with specific cancer cells, programmed to act against cell growth factors, and may be linked to anticancer radioisotopes to deliver these poisons direct to the tumor (Broyles, et al., 2007).

Radiation Therapy

Radiation therapy (RT) has little role in the treatment of colon cancer of any stage; its potential to injure abdominal viscera limits its usefulness. However RT has usefulness in preoperative and postoperative management of rectal cancer. Most trials of preoperative and postoperative monotherapy have shown a decrease in local recurrence, without a parallel improvement in survival.

Preoperative RT may convert a locally unresectable lesion to one amenable to operation; it favors preservation of the anal sphincter and may delay need for colostomy. The largest trial (Swedish) of preoperative RT reported a 61 percent decrease in local recurrence and overall improvement in survival; others have confirmed this finding in patients with advanced locoregional disease. Preoperative RT appears to be an acceptable alternative to standard practice of postoperative RT for patients with stage II and II resectable rectal cancer. RT followed by surgery has been shown to be more effective than operation alone in preventing local recurrence in patient with respectable rectal cancer and may improve survival. Patients who select preoperative RT should be aware that because staging is not definitive until after operation, they may derive little to no benefit from the intervention and at risk for the related morbidity.

Postoperative RT appears to be less effective, possibly because of rapid repopulation of tumor cells after surgery or relative hypoxia around the healing wound. Postoperative RT causes transient cystitis, diarrhea, and skin irradiation. Patients should be encouraged to consider participating in RCT to help define optimum treatment.

Combination Therapy: Chemotherapy and Radiation Therapy

The intent of preoperative combination therapy in rectal cancer is to maximize the likelihood of resection with clear margins and convert inoperable rectal cancer to an operable lesion. Regimens include 5-FU/leucovorin (LV) infusions, continuous 5-FU, or bolus. Capecitabine is being used. Fluorouracil may prime tumor cells and increase the cytotoxicity of RT, but its effect is unknown at this time.

Combination therapy is considered standard for patients with resected stages II and III rectal cancer. Evidence suggests that in this population, RT alone was superior to watchful waiting in local control of disease but there was no significant survival benefit. Chemotherapy produced a significant survival benefit over watchful waiting but no benefit in local control (Ozer & Diasio, 2004).

Surgery

Once a cancer has been found the major treatment is surgical resection. Endoscopic management at the time of diagnostic colonoscopy can be curative with polypectomy and is estimated to lower the incidence of CRC by 50 to 90 percent. Snare polypectomy is possible for pedunculated lesions; sessile polyps spreading over the mucosa present a greater technical challenge. Endoscopic mucosal resection (EMR) removes potentially malignant lesions or high-grade dysplasia by excising through mid-to-deep submucosa. Polypectomy is not benign and includes risks of perforation and bleeding. However, patients may heal and avoid surgery with bowel rest, close observation, and antibiotics. Every effort should be made to obtain tissue for pathological testing when polyps, masses, or strictures are seen. The optimal number of biopsies when removing polyps is undetermined. Highly suspicious but nondiagnostic lesions should be reviewed with a pathologist. Colonoscopy also allows marking malignant lesions (tattooing or metal clip placement) for subsequent identification during an open procedure and estimation of depth of invasion using endoscopic ultrasound (EUS) before EMR to determine depth of invasion and lymph node involvement. The inability to remove suspicious or cancerous polyps or confirmation of invasive CRC is indications for open or laparoscopic resections (Davila, et al., 2005).

There is weak RCT evidence for the benefit of preoperative mechanical bowel preparation of the bowel, but this practice remains a universal practice in North America. It may be easier to handle a prepared colon; the procedure is inexpensive and relatively safe. Patients can perform the prep at home the day before surgery; however, many present for operation dehydrated and require preoperative rehydration (Otchy, et al., 2004).

Prophylactic preoperative antibiotic coverage against anaerobes and aerobes decrease infection rate, mortality, and costs. Oral-parenteral combinations are common and need not be continued for longer than 24 hours when operation is elective. One large clinical trial demonstrated that a single preoperative dose of cefotaxime and metronidazole is as effective as three doses. Deep vein thrombosis (DVT) prophylaxis, using unfractionated heparin, low molecular weight heparin, or pneumatic calf compression has strong evidence of efficacy. Some surgeons use combinations of medication and mechanical prophylaxis in high-risk patients (Otchy, et al., 2004).

Patients should be screened for nutritional status, but routine supplementation is not indicated. Supplemental nutritional support is appropriate if the patient undergoing active treatment is malnourished or anticipated to be unable to ingest or absorb adequate nutrients for a prolonged period. Every effort should be made to obtain a fully informed consent prior to operation, including the purpose and extent of resection, outcomes, complications, alternatives to surgery proposed, and the prognosis (Ozer & Diasio, 2004).

Prior to definitive resection, it is imperative to visualize the entire colon and rectum to detect synchronous polyps or neoplasms. Preoperative evaluation should be prompt and include the elements in the following section. Preoperative identification of metastatic disease, especially in the lung and abdomen (liver) is not an absolute contraindication for surgery, but it may modify the approach. CT is the diagnostic modality of choice. The liver is the most common site of metastases via portal venous system. Patients with liver lesions who are surgical candidates have a chance of prolonged survival and cure (Leonard, Brenner, & Kemeny, 2005). Intraoperative ultrasound can be used if patients are taken to the operating room urgently. Alternatively, the liver can be scanned postoperatively. Preoperative CXR is common, but it has a yield as low as its cost and risk.

Patients with rectal lesions require preoperative endorectal ultrasonography (EUS) to evaluate lesion size and depth of invasion. This procedure has an accuracy of 82 to 93 percent; its ability to evaluate lymph node involvement is less accurate. Abdominal CT and EUS are the most cost-effective way of staging rectal cancer; pelvic CT and MRI are recommended to evaluate contiguous structures in the presence of large rectal tumors. The value of EUS after preoperative radiation therapy is not clear; accuracy falls due to inflammatory changes and its role is similarly unclear in postoperative surveillance for recurrence, which affects 10 to 30 percent of patients depending on stage and treatment (Davila, et al., 2005).

Carcinoembryonic antigen (CEA) can be used in preoperative elevation (more than 5 ng/mL) and is an independent predictor of poor outcome and increased risk of recurrence regardless of stage. Return to normal after surgery is associated with complete tumor resection and if it remains high, is associated with visible or residual disease (Otchy, et al., 2004). Periodic CEA assay is a cost-effective way of detecting recurrence or metastases and a means of monitoring treatment response in patients with metastatic disease. CEA testing is recommended every two to three months for two or more years (Meric-Bernstam & Pollock, 2005).

Resection of the Colon

Curative resection offers the greatest potential for cure in CRC. It results in 45 percent cure in rectal cancer. Surgery can be prophylactic, elective, or emergent depending on indication and patient presentation. It is usually offered to all new diagnosed patients unless life expectancy is short. Palliative resection in metastatic disease is advisable to halt further bleeding and avert eventual obstruction. A range of options are available for patients who by choice or by comorbidity are not surgical candidates. These options include laser photoablation or colonic stenting of malignant obstruction. In rectal cancer, **fulguration** (destruction of tissue using high-frequency electric sparks), laser photocoagulation, radiation therapy, and endostenting are possibilities. Aggressive preventive resection is advocated in some familial syndromes (Meric-Bernstam & Pollock, 2005). Total **proctocolectomy** (surgical removal of the rectum together with all or part of the colon) with J-pouch ileoanal anastomosis to prevent malignant transformation of the polyps has been advocated in FAP in patients as young as 20 to 25 years and creates the necessity to monitor the rectal stump if left behind. Others recommend abdominal **colectomy** (surgical operation to remove all or part of the colon) with ileorectal anastomosis. For patients with HNPCC found to be harboring adenoma or adenocarcinoma, total abdominal colectomy with ileorectal anastomosis is recommended. Women should consider total abdominal hysterectomy with bilateral salpingo-oophorectomy to avoid cancers of the reproductive organs.

Urgent or emergent surgery is required for CRC-related acute abdomen, suggested by signs of perforation, malignant obstruction or significant hemorrhage. LBO of the right or transverse colon requires right or extended right colectomy; left LBO has multiple options. Perforation requires resection, and peritonitis may be best managed with ileostomy. Management of CRC hemorrhage follows the same principles as elective resection, and failure to locate a site of bleeding should prompt a subtotal colectomy.

Surgical goals for CRC include complete tumor removal with its lymphovascular supply leaving margins of at least 5 cm; extended resections have not been shown to confer added survival benefit. Cancer attached to contiguous organs is technically challenging and requires en bloc resection (removal in a lump as a whole) to achieve a resection free of tumors. Use of no touch surgical technique, avoiding intraoperative manipulation that might shed tumor cells into portal circulation, though intuitively appealing, has no proven benefit to survival. Careful palpation of abdominal contents, with ultrasound examination of the liver during surgery is indicated: Presence of synchronous tumor (incidence 2 to 9 percent) may require total or subtotal colectomy; whether one or two procedures are required appears to make no difference in outcome or complication rates. Ten to twenty percent have liver metastasis at resection, and if the lesion(s) is amenable to resection, a single operation may suffice with a 25 to 40 percent five-year survival rate. Metastases to the ovary occur in 2 to 8 percent of the cases, and bilateral involvement may require bilateral oophorectomy (BSO). In postmenopausal women, consideration should be given due to combined risks of mircrometases and primary ovarian cancer. However, there is no proven benefit for prophylactic oophorectomy.

Palliative approaches usually involve placement of a proximal stoma, or a bypass colonic wall stenting may safely relieve acute malignant obstruction and permit subsequent resection. The comparative effectiveness of immediate resection versus stenting followed by surgery has not been determined.

Rectal Surgeries

Surgical goals in rectal cancer are to preserve the sphincter and avoid colostomy if at all possible; options are stage specific. Trans-anal local excision is possible in some instances with small, early stage tumor. The use of staples now allows end-to-end anastomoses by experienced surgeons with midrectal lesions and preservation of the sphincter with trans-anal or trans-coccygeal resection in some cases. The ideal margin in rectal cancer is 2 cm or more distal and 5 cm or more proximal. Abdomino-perineal resection (APR) with permanent sigmoid colostomy is the traditional operation for distal cancers and considered by most to be unavoidable if the cancer is within 5 to 6 cm of anal verge. Recurrence generally has a bad prognosis; patients may require pelvic exenteration.

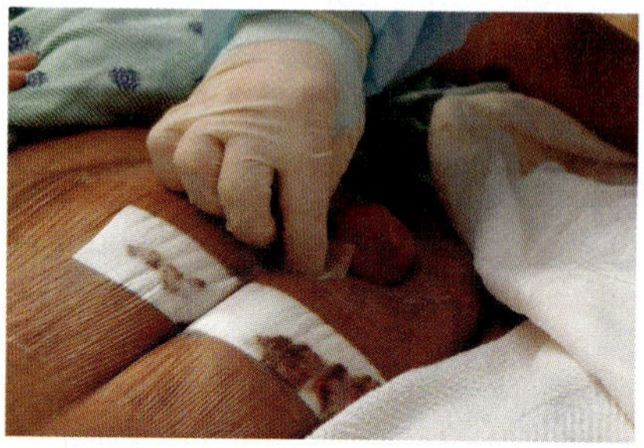

Figure 50-4 Sometimes a colon surgery results in an ostomy.

Ostomy Conditions

As mentioned, the colorectal surgeries often result in the need for an ostomy. An intestinal ostomy is when a surgically created opening is made between the intestine and the abdominal wall (Figure 50-4). The opening at the skin surface exits is labeled the stoma. The actual name of the **ostomy** is individualized to the location of the stoma. Virtually any portion of the large and small intestine can be diverted or used to form a fecal reservoir. For example, an ileostomy is an ostomy made in the ileum. An ileostomy usually requires the

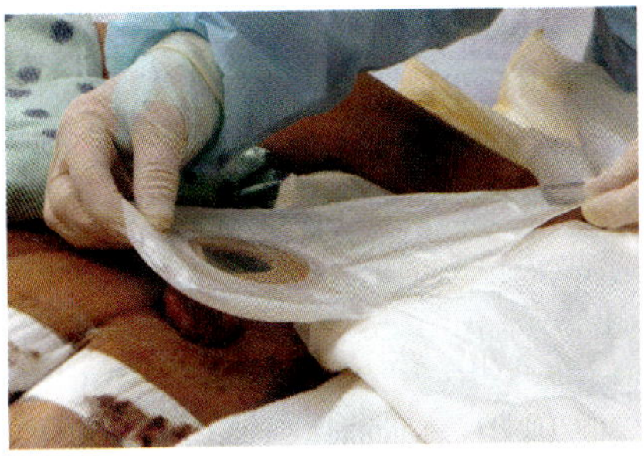

Figure 50-5 Providing ostomy care and applying new ostomy bag.

complete removal of the colon, rectum, and anus. The anus is closed, and the end of the ileum is attached to the skin surface of the abdominal region to form the stoma. There are occasions where the ostomy is temporary (e.g., loop ostomy) to allow the tissues to heal in the area that is dysfunctional; such as diverticulitis or trauma. When the temporary ostomy is not needed, a follow-up surgery reattaches the bowel and restores fecal elimination. Another ostomy is a continent ileostomy (Kock's), whereby an intra-abdominal reservoir is made, and a valve is formed from the terminal ileum on its way to the abdominal wall. The feces collects in the internal pouch device, and the valve keeps fecal material from leaking through the stoma. In addition, a catheter is inserted into the pouch to drain the stool.

The fecal stream is diverted at the most distal point possible to maximize the absorption of the food, fluid, and electrolytes and to preserve continence. The ileostomy is more uncommon than it was during recent decades. A permanent ileostomy is typically reserved for patients with severe Crohn's colitis, familial adenomatous polyposis, or chronic ulcerative colitis. The temporary ileostomy may be created as one stage in an ileoanal reservoir procedure or as a staged procedure for the relief of obstruction of the ascending colon.

The nursing care for patients with ostomies begins preoperatively and follows the patient throughout the acute care experience. In addition, there are specific management strategies for the patient with an ostomy as he or she is discharged from the acute care setting and is going home or to another care facility. Preoperatively, the ostomy patient can be referred to an enterostomal therapist for patient education and thorough explanations of their upcoming surgery and ostomy appliance. In addition, the patient can be given information on the local chapter of the United Ostomy Association organization. This organization provides the patient the opportunity to meet members with ostomies and who can show the patient their ostomy and answer questions. Allowing the patient to ask questions and verbalize their fears and anxiety during this time is important. After the surgery, the postoperative care will include the mechanics of the application of the ostomy bag and devices (Figure 50-5). The patient should be encouraged to observe the nurses when the ostomy appliances are put on the stoma area. Specific instructions will be provided by the enterostomal therapist and as the patient condition improves, the patient and family will participate in the self-care of the ostomy device. An ongoing assessment of the stoma and the surrounding skin surfaces is necessary. The tape or application devices may cause sensitivity reactions or irritation and must be handled for with meticulous care (Estes, 2006). Complications of the ostomy are provided in the Red Flag feature.

As the patient continues to heal, they should be evaluated for continued positive adaptation to their ostomy. Nutrition imbalances, dehydration, electrolyte imbalances, and emotional disturbances, including body image difficulties, are all potential problems that the new ostomy patient may develop. Each of these problems needs to be recognized and then referred to the enterostomal therapist for resolution.

Red Flag

Stoma Complications

The nurse and patient can observe the stoma for the following complications:

- Narrowing of the stoma that may indicate that the stoma is interfering with fecal elimination.
- Stoma separation from the abdominal wall may necessitate the need for surgical repair.
- A stoma that is bulging might indicate a hernia is developing in the stoma area.
- Contact dermatitis as evidenced by a rash or redness around the stomal region. This may be due to the type of tape being used or the specific ostomal appliance.
- Lack of outflow may reveal an obstructed or impacted ostomy, which could require surgical revision.
- Unusual drainage either in color, amount, or odor should be noted and reported as potential manifestations of infection and inflammation.

Staging and Prognosis

CRC prognosis is related to depth of tumor penetration (into bowel wall), presence or absence of lymph node involvement, and distant metastases. Staging systems are used to describe the anatomic extent of malignant process, and their accuracy is crucial to designing appropriate therapy. Postoperative staging is recommended for estimating prognosis and shaping decision making about **adjuvant therapy** (treatment given after the primary treatment) to increase the chances of a cure. Adjuvant therapy may include chemotherapy, radiation therapy, hormone therapy, or biological therapy (Germond, Figueredo, Taylor, Micucci, & Zwaal, 2004). The oldest and most frequently used system after resection is the DUKES, which has undergone several modifications. More recently, the Dukes scheme has been applied to the TNM classification (see chapter 15). The new, parallel scheme subdivides CRC into stages A through D, and because most recurrences are within the first three to four years, five-year survival rates are calculated. Five-year survival has improved for almost every stage over several decades. The reasons are early detection, more careful staging, and improvements in adjuvant therapy. The obvious limited success of surgery, chemotherapy, and radiation in advanced disease (stages C and D) underscore the criticality of early detection. In addition to stage, other indicators of poor prognosis include histology (poorly differentiated), high histologic grade, infiltration at margins, the young and old, males, persistently elevated serum CEA, tumor adherence to adjacent organs, bowel perforation, or colonic obstruction at time of diagnosis. In the future, DNA analysis may be used routinely to assess prognosis.

Evaluation of Outcomes

Potential patient outcomes for each of the example nursing diagnoses for the patient with CRC are:

- Chronic pain related to CRC. The patient should verbalize an adequate relief of pain along with the ability to realistically cope with the pain if it is not completely relieved.
- Fear in response to the diagnosis of CRC. The patient should manifest positive coping behaviors and verbalize a reduction in the amount of fear of the having this disease.
- Ineffective coping related to anxiety, lower activity level and the inability to perform normal activities of daily living. The patient identifies own maladaptive coping behaviors, available resources, and support systems, describes or initiates alternative coping strategies, and describes positive results from new behaviors.

IRRITABLE BOWEL SYNDROME

IBS is relatively common and is a motility disorder of the GI tract. IBS occurs in approximately one in six people, and is characterized with abdominal pain, diarrhea, constipation, or both. The cause of IBS is unknown, although there seems to be a genetic propensity to the disorder. In addition, stress exacerbates the manifestations, as does a diet high in fat, irritating foods, alcohol, and smoking.

Epidemiology

IBS occurs in up to 20 percent of the populations of regions in the Western hemisphere. It presents itself at a ratio of 3:1 women to men and occurs first in the second or third decade of life.

Pathophysiology

IBS is a disorder of intestinal motility. The changes seen are theorized to be caused by CNS alterations to the motor and sensory functions of the bowel. IBS caused an increased motor response in the small bowel and colon with heightened peristaltic intensity. There is also increased secretion of mucus in the colon, but there is not an inflammation of the tissue.

Assessment with Clinical Manifestations

Patients may initially seek health care for their symptomatology of increased abdominal pain or bouts of diarrhea or constipation. The patients may notice they have abdominal bloating and distension. The primary manifestations are the changes in bowel patterns, but otherwise there is a wide variety in the severity and symptoms of the disorder. Often, patients will describe their condition being stimulated when they eat certain foods (e.g., salads, fatty foods).

Diagnostic Tests

Diagnosis is not made with one single test. Usually, other GI tract disorders are also considered and eliminated with a variety of tests to allow the confirmation of the IBS diagnosis. Stool studies, visualization of the lower GI system (e.g., proctoscopy, sigmoidoscopy), manometry, and electromyography are performed. Also, serum studies, such as a CBC and erythrocyte sedimentation rate (ESR), are evaluated. An anemic condition can result from the potential blood loss and an elevated WBC, and ESR may result from a bacterial infection (Daniels, 2003).

Nursing Diagnoses

Based on the information gathered, examples of nursing diagnoses in the patient with IBS may include the following:

- Acute pain related to the IBS.
- Ineffective coping related to anxiety, lower activity level and the inability to perform normal activities of daily living.
- Diarrhea related to the altered GI motility.
- Constipation related to the altered GI motility.

Planning and Implementation

Patients with IBS are going to adapt to their disorder as they have compliance with the management of their disease. A careful assessment of what stimulates the condition is necessary to inform the patient in identifying these risk factors. A general assessment of the patient condition to detect complications, such as dehydration and stress, is important. Avoiding the irritating substances (e.g., alcohol, gas-forming foods, or sugars) is encouraged and referral to a dietitian may be indicated. A bulk-forming diet (e.g., bran) and water can reduce the occurrence of both diarrhea and constipation.

Pharmacology

There is no cure for the IBS condition, but there are several medications and herbal substances that can benefit the patient. Bulk-forming laxatives may reduce the pain and motility symptoms. Anticholinergics can interfere with parasympathetic nervous system innervation and decrease GI motility. Antidiarrheal agents (e.g., Imodium, Lomotil) can be given prophylactically or symptomatically on an as needed basis. Antidepressant drugs can assist in relieving the abdominal pain (Broyles, et al., 2007). There are herbal remedies with antispasmodic effects that can have benefits to the patient with IBS (e.g., anisc, peppermint, sage).

Evaluation of Outcomes

Potential patient outcomes for each of the example nursing diagnoses for the patient with IBS are:

- Acute pain related to the IBS. The patient should verbalize an adequate relief of pain along with the ability to realistically cope with the pain if it is not completely relieved.
- Ineffective coping related to anxiety, lower activity level, and the inability to perform normal activities of daily living. The patient identifies own maladaptive coping behaviors, available resources, and support systems, describes or initiates alternative coping strategies, and describes positive results from new behaviors.

- Diarrhea related to the altered GI motility. The patient passes soft, formed stool no more than three times per day.
- Constipation related to the altered GI motility. The patient passes soft, formed stool at a frequency perceived as normal by the patient. The patient or caregiver verbalizes measures that will prevent recurrence of the constipation.

INFLAMMATORY BOWEL DISORDERS

There are two chronic inflammatory bowel disorders (IBD) that are similar but also have several differences: (a) Crohn's disease, and (b) ulcerative colitis. The cause of both diseases is unknown, but both have a hereditary implication and a geographical distribution. There may be autoimmune relationships to these disorders, but conclusive information has not been ascertained at this time.

Epidemiology

In general, IBD has a higher incidence in Caucasians and African Americans. In addition, there is a less incidence in Jewish populations on a percentage basis. Women are slightly more at risk for these disorders than men. And, persons from ages 10 to 30 are higher at risk. Patients with these pathologies have chronic conditions, typically managed with diet, medications, and even surgery.

Diagnostic Tests

In the early stages of IBD, making a definitive diagnosis can be challenging and difficult. The symptoms are nonspecific and may mimic other conditions. When a patient presents with symptoms, such as diarrhea, abdominal pain, or weight loss, IBD disease may be suspected. A thorough history is obtained, and a physical exam is completed. Initially, a proctosigmoidoscopy is performed to identify whether the bowel area is inflamed. A barium study will demonstrate the string sign, which reveals the constriction of a small intestine segment. The following blood and diagnostic tests are ordered: CBC, albumin, IBD serology panel (ANCA, IgG, ASCA IgG, and ASCA IgA), stool cultures, endoscopy (including video wireless capsule endoscopy), abdominal X-rays, small bowel series, and enteroclysis (Daniels, 2003; Jungles, 2004).

Nursing Diagnoses

Based on the information gathered, examples of nursing diagnoses in the patient with IBD may include the following:

- Chronic pain related to IBD.
- Diarrhea related to IBD.
- Nutrition imbalance, less than body requirements, related to IBD.
- Ineffective coping related to anxiety, lower activity level, and the inability to perform normal activities of daily living.
- Risk for impaired skin integrity related to compromised tissue perfusion.
- Fear and anxiety related to actual or potential lifestyle changes.

Planning and Implementation

There are varied care strategies for patients with IBD. There is not a cure for the disorder, and therefore supportive measures are the objective of care. A variety of medical treatments, surgeries, and nursing care is employed with an obvious need to involve the entire health care team in the care of patients with IBD.

> **Fast Forward ▶▶▶**
>
> **Emerging Therapeutic Options for IBD**
>
> With the considerable advances in our understanding of the immunological mechanisms responsible for mucosal inflammation in IBD, an increasing number of therapeutic agents are being developed. These agents can be broadly divided into biological and nonbiological therapies. Of the nonbiological therapeutic agents, promising results have been offered by dietary manipulation, probiotics, and the newer immunomodulators. However, it is more difficult to discuss the maintenance role of some of the experimental biological therapies, as most trials in humans have concentrated initially on their role in active IBD.

The need for adequate nutrition in any chronic disease state is obvious, and even more so in IBD, in which patients are often malnourished and often highly catabolic, particularly during active disease stages. In children, exclusive nutritional therapy has been shown to be as efficacious as corticosteroids in induction of remission. The role of nutritional therapy in maintenance of remission in adult patients is less clear cut but nevertheless is still vital to the health of the patient.

Perhaps one of the simplest and most successful current therapeutic options in the maintenance of IBD is smoking cessation. Active smoking increases the risk of a disease flare by more than 50 percent compared with nonsmokers. There is a dose-dependent association between smoking and IBD activity, and this is particularly significant above 15 cigarettes smoked per day. Smoking is also associated with increased complication rates and lower scores about quality of life.

Pharmacology

The primary goals of medical therapy for IBD are to provide symptomatic relief, to reduce inflammation in the intestine, and to reduce the incidence of recurrent flares. Despite the variety of agents available for the treatment of IBD, none is ideal or accepted universally (Estiarte, Colome, Artes, & Jimenez, 2003). A combination of sedatives, antidiarrheal agents, and antiperistaltic medications are administered with a palliative goal. The use of corticosteroids in induction of remission of IBD has been shown to be highly effective and is well-established. Despite this, corticosteroids are ineffective in maintaining remission. The corticosteroids can be taken orally or parenterally in patients with acute exacerbations of IBD. Rectal corticosteroids are also given for patients to treat the distal colon disease.

Azathioprine (Imuran), an immunosuppressant and a thioguanine derivative, has become increasingly popular over the past 20 years and is now standard therapy in maintenance of IBD. Methotrexate has an established role in the treatment of active IBD and will induce remission in a significant proportion of patients with corticosteroid- and thiopurine-resistant IBD.

The role of antibacterials in IBD has mainly concentrated on treating active disease, but there is limited evidence for their use in maintenance of remission. Active IBD has been treated with oral metronidazole 200 to 400 mg three times daily, but this regimen is only marginally more effective than placebo. In addition, metronidazole appears to have an acceptable safety profile for use during pregnancy, although the efficacy of this agent in maintenance therapy of IBD has yet to be confirmed.

Surgery

When the nonsurgical methods of management fail, surgery is often recommended. More than half of the patients with IBD will have surgery during the course of their disease. A resection of the diseased portion of the colon is surgically removed, and because of the chronic nature of the disease, the patient may have multiple surgeries in their lifetime. Refer to the section on colon resection for specifics of the care of these surgical interventions. In addition, refer to the ostomy section in this chapter, as patients with IBD often require an ostomy intervention.

Evaluation of Outcomes

Potential patient outcomes for each of the example nursing diagnoses for the patient with IBD are:

- Chronic pain related to IBD. The patient should verbalize an adequate relief of pain along with the ability to realistically cope with the pain if it is not completely relieved.

- Diarrhea related to IBD. The patient passes soft, formed stool no more than three times per day.
- Nutrition imbalance, less than body requirements, related to IBD. The patient verbalizes and demonstrates selection of foods or meals that will achieve a cessation of weight loss and weighs within 10 percent of ideal body weight.
- Ineffective coping related to anxiety, lower activity level, and inability to perform normal activities of daily living. The patient identifies own maladaptive coping behaviors, available resources and support systems, describes or initiates alternative coping strategies, and describes positive results from new behaviors.
- Risk for impaired skin integrity related to compromised tissue perfusion. The patient's skin condition should be improved as evidenced by decreased redness, swelling, and pain.
- Fear and anxiety related to actual or potential lifestyle changes. The patient should be able to recognize the signs of anxiety, demonstrate positive coping mechanisms, and describe a reduction in the level of anxiety experienced.

Crohn's Disease

Crohn's disease is a chronic inflammatory bowel disorder with a relapsing and remitting course. Once remission is achieved, the main aim of the management of Crohn's disease is maintenance of that remission. Significant advances have been made into understanding the etiology and pathogenesis of inflammatory bowel disease. With these advances in understanding come increasing numbers of new agents and therapies, aimed both at active disease and the subsequent maintenance of remission in Crohn's disease.

Pathophysiology

Crohn's disease is a subacute and chronic inflammatory condition that usually begins with a small inflammatory lesion of the intestinal mucosa. Eventually, the inflammation continues and progression through all layers of tissue is seen. The deeper ulcerations, fissures, and granulomatous lesions persist into the deeper layers of the bowel wall. On examination, the affected bowel lumen has a cobblestone appearance with the inflamed areas surrounded by intact mucosa. These lesions are not continuous and are separated with normal tissue. As the disease progresses, the inflammation caused the bowel wall to thicken and become fibrotic and a narrowing of the intestinal lumen occurs. Fistulas are common between loops of bowel, as are adhesions of the diseased bowel areas. The absorption of nutrients is impaired as the jejunum and ileum are affected (Brookes & Green, 2004).

Assessment with Clinical Manifestations

The individual nature of the Crohn's disease allows for a wide variety of clinical manifestations. There is typically abdominal pain and tenderness that accompanies the disorder. Often the pain is relieved temporarily with defecation. In addition, eating can initiate the abdominal discomfort, and patients may consequently limit their food intake. This lends them to have nutritional deficits, weight loss, and experience malnutrition and even secondary conditions (e.g., anemia). Diarrhea is common and not necessarily positive for occult bleeding. There may be a palpable mass in the RLQ. Complications from Crohn's disease include ulcers, abscesses, fistulas, and intestinal obstruction. It can also affect other areas of the body including the joints, eyes, skin, and liver. A significant number of Crohn's patients undergo one or more surgical resections of the GI tract, causing disabilities and lifestyle changes.

Ulcerative Colitis

Ulcerative colitis is a chronic inflammatory bowel disorder that affects both the mucosa and submucosa of the colon and rectum. The patients with this disorder have exacerbations and remissions and have similar clinical presentation to Crohn's disease. The focus of care is supportive in nature; there is not a cure for ulcerative colitis.

Pathophysiology

The inflammatory process of ulcerative colitis begins at the rectosigmoid area of the anal canal. The disease destruction usually moves in a proximal direction but is often contained within the sigmoid and rectal areas. It is recurrent in its ulcerative and inflammatory nature, with abscesses in the submucosa, which spread and can lead to necrosis. Unlike Crohn's disease, the tissue inflammation and disease is continuous in nature as it affects the bowel. Eventually, the disease narrows the bowel with its inflammatory nature and shortens and thickens the bowel. The mucosa becomes reddened and ulcerated, bleeding easily and causing a loss of normal haustral movement (Brookes & Green, 2004).

Assessment with Clinical Manifestations

Ulcerative colitis is replete with exacerbations and remissions. The primary manifestations are diarrhea, abdominal pain in the left lower quadrant, and rectal bleeding. In mild cases, the diarrheal episodes may be fewer than five stools each day. As the disorder is more severe, the diarrhea may increase to as many as 10 to 20 bloody stools each day. The patient then is susceptible to a variety of complications that are secondary to bleeding and the nature of the inflammation. The chronic manifestations result in anemic symptoms, dehydration, fatigue, anorexia, weight loss, and generalized weakness.

Patients with continued ulcerative colitis may develop systemic manifestations, such as arthritis, skin and mucous membrane integrity debilitation, and uveitis or inflammation of the uvea. Patients may have problems with chronic clotting difficulties, which lead to thromboemboli formation.

The chronic loss of blood makes the patient at risk for chronic blood loss anemia (see chapter 29 for further descriptions of anemia). Therefore, the patient is monitored for tachycardia, hypotension, pallor, and follow-up on the level of serum indicators of blood loss (e.g., hemoglobin, hematocrit, or albumin).

The more severe complications of ulcerative colitis also include toxic megacolon and colon perforation. The toxic megacolon is a complication in which there is sudden motor paralysis and swelling of the colon that may affect all of the colon. The symptoms of toxic megacolon are fever, abdominal pain, nausea and vomiting, dehydration, and tachycardia. Perforation is associated with toxic megacolon and has a relatively high mortality rate from resulting peritonitis. In addition, there is an increased risk for CRC in patients with ulcerative colitis (refer to CRC section).

Case Study

Nursing Care Plan

Mr. Tony Gilliam is a 61-year-old old male who is admitted to the medical floor because of blood in the stool and abdominal pain for four days. He is going to be assessed primarily with a variety of laboratory and diagnostic tests. A review of systems reveals bowel habit changes, loss of appetite, weight loss greater than 10 pounds, and fatigue for nine weeks. Mr. Gilliam's past medical history includes primary hypertension, obesity, gastroesophageal reflux disease (GERD), and constipation. The patient's medications include HCTZ 25 mg by mouth every day, Omeprazole 20 mg by mouth every day as needed, and Metamucil as needed. The patient's nutritional intake is usually high in fat, low in fiber, and less than two servings of fruits and vegetables per day. His fluid intake consists primarily of sodas, tea, or coffee, and possibly two cups of water per day. Mr. Gilliam's activity is sedentary, and his social history includes working as a automotive mechanic for 31 years. He has been smoking cigarettes for 36 years, has an alcohol intake of four to six drinks per week, and denies the use of illicit drugs.

Assessment

Patient has gastrointestinal (GI) bleeding and recent history of abdominal pain. His vital signs are: temperature 36.9° C (98.4° F), pulse 74, respiration 18, and blood pressure 122/76. Bowel sounds normal on four quadrants; tympanic to percussion; no costovertebral angle (CVA) tenderness; pain elicited on palpation of left lower quadrant; palpable mass noted on left lower quadrant area. Patient's skin color is pink and has good turgor. Rectal exam reveals three-by-four-cm palpable lesion with stool positive for occult blood. Neurological system shows patient to be awake, alert, and oriented for three hours. A psychosocial assessment reveals him to appear nervous, quiet, and irritable; patient states he has not been in the hospital since his wife died 10 years ago.

Nursing Diagnosis: Acute pain related to colorectal mass.

NOC: Comfort level; medication response; pain control

NIC: Analgesic administration; conscious sedation; pain management; patient-controlled analgesia assistance

Expected Outcomes

The patient will:

1. Decrease pain level from 7 to 3 (on scale of 1 to 10) within 24 hours.
2. Relate an improvement of pain as evidenced by an increase in daily activities within 48 hours.

Planning/Interventions/Rationale

1. Evaluate pain frequently by asking patient to rate pain on scale of 1 to 10. *Provides ongoing assessment of pain that is measurable.*
2. Reduce or eliminate the factors that increase the pain experience. *Decreases overall pain response.*
3. Collaborate with patient to initiate noninvasive pain relief measures. *Broadens measures to decrease pain and incorporates nonmedication approaches to pain relief.*
4. Administer pain medications and assess response to the medications. *Provide optimal pain relief and reduces side effects.*

Evaluation

The patient verbalized that his pain was a 2 (scale of 1 to 10) within 24 hours. He took analgesics every four hours as ordered and had no side effects.

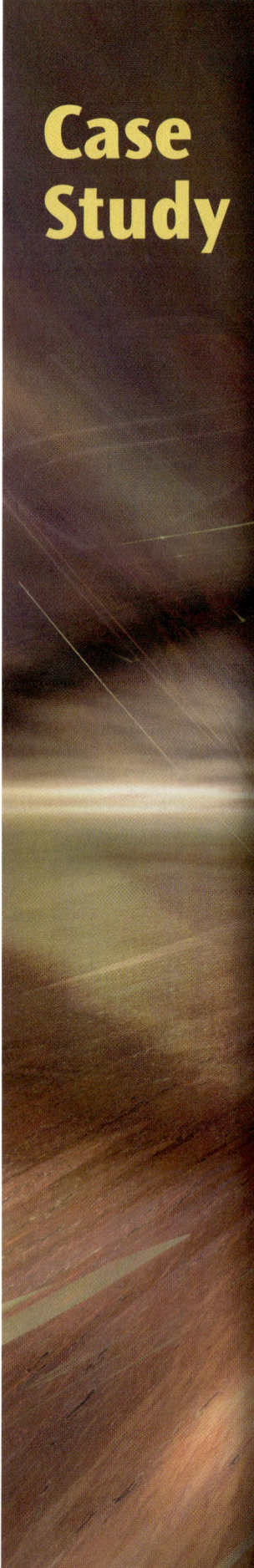

KEY CONCEPTS

- The small intestine (duodenum, jejunum, and ileum) functions as the major digestive and absorptive area of the intestine.
- The pancreas is an essential organ of digestion and produces copious amounts of digestive enzymes.
- The jejunum and ileum are the vital areas for absorption of nutrients: vitamins, amino acids, sugars, and triglycerides.
- The small intestine, which is divided into the duodenum, the jejunum, and the ileum, is approximately 600 cm in length and 1 to 1.5 inches in diameter.
- There are certain nutrients that are absorbed in the GI tract that must be considered as one is assessing the nutritional status of the patient when considering problems with digestion and absorption.
- The two primary pathologies for mal-assimilation disorders are mal-digestion and mal-absorption.
- Mal-digestion disorders are intraluminal disorders often from impaired hydrolysis of intestinal contents.
- Mal-absorption disorders are those which impair transport of intestinal contents across the mucosal membrane of the lumen.
- Describe the nursing management for a patient with an acute abdomen.
- Compare/contrast the acute inflammatory disorders of appendicitis and diverticulitis.
- Evaluate the management strategies of an obstruction of the lower GI system.
- Identify the interventions for patients with colorectal cancer.
- Describe the clinical manifestations of a patient with irritable bowel syndrome, and the associated treatments.
- Compare/contrast the inflammatory bowel disorders of Crohn's disease and ulcerative colitis.

REVIEW QUESTIONS

1. Intussusception that can lead to bowel obstruction is due to:
   1. Twisting of the bowel on itself
   2. A band of connective tissue compressing the bowel
   3. Telescoping of a loop of bowel into a lower loop of bowel
   4. Temporary paralysis of the bowel

2. Crohn's disease impairs the digestive process. Your assessment would include evidence of:
   1. Nausea and vomiting
   2. Weight loss and anemia
   3. Absence of bowel sounds
   4. Constipation and abdominal distension

3. Your teaching strategies for patients who have IBS would focus on:
   1. Lifestyle changes
   2. Bowel hygiene
   3. Dietary modifications
   4. Response to medications

4. IBS is best described as:
   1. A syndrome involving multisystems and many complaints.
   2. A cluster of vague abdominal complaints with no remission times.
   3. A functional bowel disorder with no signs of pathology present.
   4. The presence of diarrhea as the most prominent symptom.

5. Modifications in the daily diet to alleviate IBS symptoms include:
   1. A high soluble fiber diet.
   2. A diet low in fat.
   3. An increase in water intake.
   4. A high-protein diet.

6. An important change in lifestyle to aid in minimizing IBS symptoms is:
   1. Taking sips of cold drinks.
   2. Eating regular snacks.
   3. Drinking water with meals.
   4. Eating slowly.

7. The acidic chime from the stomach that flows into the duodenum is neutralized by the alkaline liquid secreted from the:
   1. Gallbladder
   2. Pancreas
   3. Jejunum cells
   4. Ileum cells

Continued

REVIEW QUESTIONS—cont'd

8. Which of the following neurochemical mediators has been implicated in the transmission of pain in the GI tract?
   1. Monoamine
   2. Epinephrine
   3. Serotonin
   4. Norepinephrine
9. In the United States and other developed countries, IBS is more prevalent in:
   1. Children
   2. Women
   3. Men
   4. The elderly
10. IBS symptoms can exacerbate following which of the events below?
    1. Anticholeric medications
    2. Weather changes
    3. Sexual activity
    4. Dietary intolerances

REVIEW ACTIVITIES

1. IBD has been linked to other illnesses such as multiple sclerosis, asthma, bronchitis, arthritis, and psoriasis. Access the MedicineNet.com at: http://www.medicinenet.com. (a) Review the information regarding the link of IBD to other illnesses; (b) review information on rectal bleeding, potential causes, location, and characteristics; and (c) prepare a brief patient teaching brochure.
2. Interview a nutritionist. Inquire what strategies are used to assist the individual diagnosed with Crohn's disease or IBS to modify the diet. Obtain a menu plan that outlines a typical daily diet. Use a cookbook to determine what recipes would be appropriate for the diet. Prepare a recipe pamphlet for the patient.
3. Develop a self-care teaching plan for a patient with a new colostomy. Discuss the various barriers that would affect the patient's and family members' learning to care for the colostomy. How would you determine whether they are coping with the changes in body function? What strategies can the nurse use to facilitate learning?
4. Research the etiology associated with peritonitis. Discuss the potential severe systemic effects and the usual clinical manifestations.
5. Research the etiology and risk factors for the development of herniations of the bowel. Develop a nursing care plan for a patient who has a surgical inguinal hernia repair.
6. Research information on the etiology and risk factors for development of hemorrhoids. What are the clinical manifestations?

Visit the Contemporary Medical-Surgical Nursing online companion resource at www.delmarhealthcare.com for additional content and study aids. Click on Online Companions then select the Nursing discipline.

Hepatic, Biliary Tract, and Pancreatic Dysfunction: Nursing Management

CHAPTER 51

Valerie Lindquist Stalsbroten, RN, MC

CHAPTER TOPICS

- Hepatic System
- Hepatitis
- Hereditary Diseases of the Liver
- Cirrhosis
- Hepatic Abscesses
- Liver Trauma
- Cancer of the Liver
- Liver Transplantation
- Diseases of the Biliary Tract
- Pancreatitis

The hepatic, biliary tract, and pancreas are organ systems that have tremendous implications on the body. Each of these different organs has physiological functions that are vital to the body's health. If any of these organ structures is compromised, there are many consequences to the health of the individual.

KEY TERMS

Adducts
Ascending cholangitis
Ascites
Chemoembolization
Cholangitis
Cholecystitis
Cholelithiasis
Cholestasis
Gluconeogenesis
Glycogen hydrolysis
Glycogen synthesis
Gynecomastia
Hepatomegaly
Icterus
Jaundice
Kernicterus
Kupffer cells
Laparoscopic cholecystectomy
Liver lobule
Liver sweats
Refractory ascites
Sinusoids
Steatorrhea
Suppurative cholangitis

HEPATIC SYSTEM

The liver is the largest organ in the body. It is located directly beneath the diaphragm and is divided into the right and left lobes. The right lobe is the larger of the two. Directly below the liver are the stomach, pancreas, gallbladder, kidneys, and intestines. The liver is able to repair itself and regenerate damaged tissue to a certain extent. Although the liver is primarily considered when discussing the digestive tract, it is involved with over 400 metabolic functions necessary to a variety of pathways and is essential for life. Some of the vital processes of the liver are metabolism of proteins, carbohydrates, and fats; detoxification and filtering of foreign bodies, bacteria, and antigens; removal of old circulating red blood cells; synthesis of many substances (e.g., clotting factors, bilirubin, and cholesterol); and storage of substances (e.g., vitamins, minerals, and cholesterol).

The liver receives its blood supply from two sources. About 1,500 mL of blood travels through the liver each minute. The hepatic artery provides about one third of the incoming blood directly from the heart. This blood is well oxygenated. The portal vein supplies about two thirds of the incoming blood, carrying nutrient-rich but oxygen poor blood directly from the digestive tract. Blood in the portal vein is collected from the capillary beds, which drain the digestive organs (stomach, intestines, esophagus, spleen, and pancreas) and flows into the esophageal, splenic, pancreatic, mesenteric, epigastric, hemorrhoidal, and rectal veins. These veins are tributaries to the portal vein, which delivers the blood to the liver. Consequently, if blood flow is obstructed through the liver, these tributaries could also be congested. The portal vein is unique in its position between two capillary systems, collecting blood from the digestive organs and delivering it to the liver. If there is dysfunction of the portal vein, scarring or dysfunction of the liver or other impediments to blood flow, then the veins feeding into the portal vein can be affected.

The **liver lobule** is the functional unit of the liver. Each lobule consists of hepatocytes (liver cells) that are arranged in a hexagonal pattern around a central vein. Each hepatocyte has three surfaces: one faces the sinusoid or space of Disse, one faces the canaliculi, and one faces the other hepatocytes. **Sinusoids** are specialized capillaries found only in the liver and are identified by specific types of cells located there (Kupffer cells, hepatic stellate cells, and pit cells). Both the hepatic artery and the portal vein terminate in these sinusoid capillaries. **Kupffer cells** are specialized reticulo-endothelial cells of the liver and belong to the monocyte-macrophage system. They line the sinusoids, and their major responsibility is to phagocytize and filter bacteria, parasites, toxins, antigens, old blood cells, cellular debris, tumor cells, and foreign particles from the blood. As blood flows through the sinusoids, plasma moves into the space (space of Disse) between the sinusoids and the hepatocytes, generating significant portion of the body's lymph. The hepatic stellate cells, found in the space of Disse between the hepatocytes and the sinusoidal endothelial cells, are also known as Ito cells, lipocytes, and fat storing cells. Their major function is to process lipid molecules, especially retinoids. With injury, the hepatic stellate cells can relinquish their lipids and begin producing collagen. Blood flow and portal hypertension can be affected. Pit cells are highly mobile killer lymphocytes attached to the sinusoidal surface. They primarily eliminate tumor cells and virus-infected hepatocytes.

The liver is drained by two systems. A central vein carries blood from the liver lobules into increasingly larger veins. Blood that flows back to the heart from the liver is carried in the right and left hepatic veins. These veins join directly with the inferior vena cava (Figure 51-1).

The body needs available energy for biological processes and normal functioning. Carbohydrates in the form of glucose provide usable high-energy bonds for the liver and other organs. During the time of eating, nutrients can be distributed directly to the areas in the body requiring glucose. Some tissues,

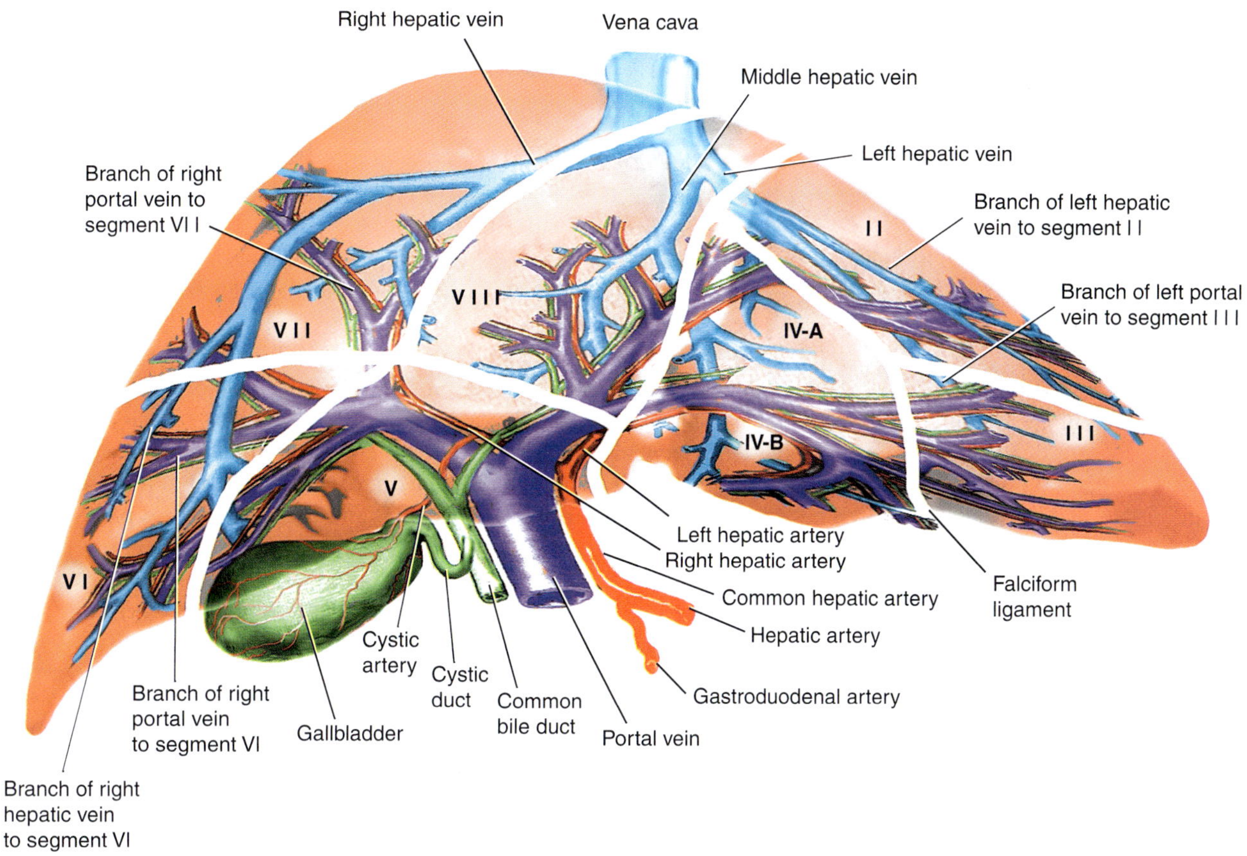

Figure 51-1 Segmental blood supply and ductal system of the liver.

such as muscle, can store limited supplies of fuel in the form of glycogen but only for future use by that organ. However, in the postabsorptive state and the fasting state, it is imperative that tissues have nutrients available for normal functioning. In particular, red blood cells and cells in the central nervous system require a constant level of glucose to function properly because these tissues are unable to store even small amounts of available energy supply.

When there is an abundance of glucose after a meal, the liver converts glucose to glycogen, which is stored in the liver, or to fatty acids, which are stored primarily in adipose tissue. A limited amount of fatty acids can be stored in the liver. During fasting this process is reversed, and the liver mobilizes the fatty acids, rendering them available as high-energy bonds in the form of glucose. **Gluconeogenesis** is the process of the liver converting predominant amino acids to glucose in the fasting state. Regulation of glucose metabolism in the liver is dependent on the concentration of glucose in blood coming into the sinusoids and the levels of insulin, catecholamines, and glucagons in the bloodstream. **Glycogen synthesis** is the conversion of glucose to glycogen, which can be stored in preparation of times of fasting, and **glycogen hydrolysis** is the conversion of stored glycogen into usable glucose to meet the immediate energy needs of the body.

There are a variety of substances that are metabolized in the liver. Each of these products has different effects on the body and is essential for their different functions. Bilirubin is a waste product of the breakdown of the hemoglobin molecule. Old red blood cells (senescent erythroid cells) are catabolized in the spleen, bone marrow, and liver. The hemoglobin molecule is further degraded, and the heme portion of the molecule is converted into bilirubin. Bilirubin binds loosely with albumin and is transported in the bloodstream to the liver, where the bilirubin is removed from the plasma. In the liver, the bilirubin is attached (conjugated) with another substance (glucuronide) so that it

Red Flag

High Bilirubin Levels

Bilirubin is an important indicator for liver and blood disorders (Box 51-1). High values of bilirubin cause jaundice, a yellowing of the skin and corneas. It is potentially damaging to neurological tissue and can cause encephalopathy and irreversible brain damage particularly in newborn infants with severe unconjugated hyperbilirubinemia (Daniels, 2003).

BOX 51-1

BILIRUBIN LABELS

- **Jaundice:** Yellow pigmentation of the skin and sclera.
- **Icterus:** Yellow coloration in the sclera of the eye. It can be used synonymously with jaundice.
- **Kernicterus:** Yellow discoloration and degenerative lesions in the central nervous system (CNS) causing brain damage. Newborns with untreated jaundice may develop kernicterus.
- Phototherapy: Causes some of the H-bonds in the bilirubin molecule to become excited and this renders the molecule more water-soluble and able to be excreted.
- Encephalopathy: Can occur in newborns with unconjugated bilirubin of 20 mg/dL. The onset may be dramatic with refusal to feed, high-pitched cry, and hypertonicity. Survivors can suffer hearing loss, paralysis of upward gaze, mental retardation, and cerebral palsy.
- Crigler-Najjar disease: Recessive inherited disorder characterized by the inability to conjugate bilirubin. Patients display severe neurological impairments and have a life expectance of one year or less.

Adapted from Townes, D. A. (2004). Biliary tract disease. Emergency Medicine, *36(2), 17–19.*

can be excreted in the bile. It can be stored in the gallbladder or directly transported to the small intestine. Bacteria in the intestines breakdown the bilirubin into urobilin and is excreted in the feces. It is not uncommon for newborns to exhibit high bilirubin levels, because they lack the intestinal bacteria to adequately process the bilirubin in the gut or because of blood type incompatibilities and subsequent increased red blood cell destruction.

Conjugated bilirubin is also called direct bilirubin. Unconjugated bilirubin is not bound to another molecule and is referred to as indirect bilirubin. Total bilirubin lab tests reflect the amount of conjugated plus unconjugated bilirubin in the blood. In addition, bilirubin levels are particularly important when assessing newborns.

Bile contains bile salts, fatty acids, cholesterol, bilirubin, and other compounds. Albumin is a protein synthesized in the liver. It is the most abundant protein in the blood plasma and is responsible for transporting molecules, like bilirubin, and maintaining oncotic pressure in the intravascular space. Decreases in serum albumin indicate impaired liver activity or kidney disease, if the kidneys allow the protein to leak into the urine. Decreases in albumin could also reflect malnutrition or low protein intake, which may occur simultaneously with liver or kidney disease. When the oncotic pressure in the intravascular space in decreased, ascites and edema result. Cholesterol is a steroid that is primarily made in the liver, although some cholesterol is absorbed from the diet. It is important in the manufacture of estrogen and other hormones, cortisol, bile acids, and vitamin D. It is essential for the proper functioning of cell membranes. Estrogen is metabolized in the liver. When liver functioning is impaired, estrogen may not be removed from the bloodstream, exposing the body tissues to higher levels of this hormone. **Gynecomastia** (breast enlargement in men) can be a side effect of the buildup of estrogen.

Biliary Tract

The biliary tract is the other system serving the liver and is designed to drain bile. The production of bile is a major function of the hepatocytes. Bile is a fluid consisting of water, electrolytes, cholesterol, phospholipids, bile salts, and bilirubin. Bile is essential for fat emulsification and absorption. It is necessary for the digestion of fats and fat-soluble vitamins. Waste products may also be excreted in the bile fluid. Canaliculi are small, capillary-like structures that drain bile directly from the hepatocytes into increasingly larger bile ducts. Specialized cells lining the bile ducts are called cholangiocytes. The cholangiocytes can modify and reabsorb bile as well as secrete bicarbonate. Bile may be stored and concentrated in the gallbladder, which holds about 40 to 70 mL of bile. The gallbladder is drained by the cystic duct, which feeds into the common hepatic duct (which drains bile directly from the liver, bypassing the gallbladder). Together the cystic duct (from the gallbladder) and the common hepatic duct (from the liver) form the common bile duct, which carries bile that enters the small intestine at the sphincter of Oddi. Most of the bile salts are reabsorbed in the ileum and are, in turn, recirculated to the hepatocytes in the liver.

Pancreas

The pancreas is a long, thin glandular organ that is essential for digestion and metabolism. Two major types of cells are located in the pancreas: acini (exocrine cells) and islets of Langerhans (endocrine cells). Acini cells produce pancreatic enzymes that empty into ducts that feed into the duct of Wirsung. A second duct, the duct of Santorini may also be present. These pancreatic exocrine enzymes empty into the common bile duct through the ampulla of Vater, allowing them to enter the duodenum to aid in digestion. These enzymes are responsible for breaking down carbohydrates, fats, and proteins into smaller substances for absorption. The islets of Langerhans produce insulin (from the beta cells) and glucagon (from the alpha cells) and release these hormones directly into the bloodstream. These hormones are essential for regulating glucose metabolism (see chapter 57 for a discussion of insulin and glucagon). A third endocrine hormone has been identified. This is vasoactive intestinal polypeptide (VIP), and it affects gastrointestinal (GI) functioning.

The acinar cells of the pancreas produce enzymes that aid in the breakdown and absorption of proteins (proteases), lipids (lipase), and carbohydrates (amylase). Nucleases work on DNA and RNA. These enzymes are transported to the duodenum through the pancreatic duct. Because the primary goal is to break down tissues that are essentially the same as body tissues, protective measures are in place to protect the body from its own digestive juices. The acini package the proteases in an inactive precursor form (trypsinogen and chymotrypsinogen) and are activated by enzymes (enterokinase) in the intestinal mucosa. In addition, secretory vesicles in the pancreas have a trypsin inhibitor in case any digestive enzymes get prematurely converted to the active state and epithelial cells in the pancreatic duct secrete bicarbonate.

Diagnostic Tests

There are several ways to assess liver functioning. The nurse can physically palpate and percuss the liver as one method of assessing the size and location of the liver boundaries. In addition, serum tests are performed to screen patients with no symptoms (may be required for some insurance policy qualifications or prior to some procedures), detect disease, direct treatment, and monitor progress. Often liver enzyme assessments will be ordered before a patient is placed on certain medications that could be hepatotoxic. In addition to blood serum tests, bile fluid examinations, endoscopy, liver biopsies, ultrasound, computed tomography (CT), magnetic resonance imaging (MRI), nuclear medicine, angiography, and radiological tests can be performed (Nietsch & Kowdley, 2004).

Liver function tests (LFTs) are often ordered as a group. Usually these include albumin, total and direct bilirubin, alkaline phosphatase, aspartate transaminase (also known as AST or serum glutamic oxaloacetic transaminase [SGOT]), and

BOX 51-2

DISORDERS IDENTIFIED WITH A LIVER BIOPSY

- Hepatitis
- Cirrhosis
- Abscesses, cysts, and benign and malignant tumors
- Infiltrative diseases (hemochromatosis or amyloidosis)
- Metabolic disorders
- Wilson's disease
- Sarcoidosis
- Parasitic and fungal diseases

Adapted from Daniels, R. (2003). Delmar's manual of laboratory and diagnostic tests. *New York: Thomson Delmar Learning.*

Skills 360°

Complications of a Liver Biopsy

Complications of a liver biopsy for the nurse to be aware of:
- Bleeding problems.
- Puncture of the kidney or intestines
- Puncture of lung with subsequent pneumothorax
- Puncture of the gallbladder
- Peritonitis

alanine transaminase (also known as ALT, glutamic pyruvate transaminase [GPT], or serum glutamic pyruvate transaminase [SGPT]). Further testing could include prothrombin time (PT) after receiving vitamin K, gamma glutamyl transpeptidase (GGT), ammonia (NH_3), amylase, viral studies for hepatitis antigens, isocitrate dehydrogenase (ICD), copper, and iron. Specific tests for genetic diseases may be available.

Liver enzymes can be elevated with conditions such as diabetes, obesity, autoimmune disorders, some viral infections (especially hepatitis), and some genetic diseases. Nonsteroidal anti-inflammatory drugs (NSAIDs), antibiotics, cholesterol-lowering medications, systemic acne medications, and antiseizure medications are some of the drugs that can alter liver enzymes. Alcohol is toxic to the liver and can initiate changes in the liver. The most helpful tests for the work-up of jaundice are alkaline phosphatase, AST, and ALT (Lam & Mobarhan, 2004).

The liver biopsy is used to procure a small sample of liver tissue to diagnose liver pathology. It is an invasive sterile procedure performed under local anesthetic. Ultrasound or CT scan may also be utilized at the same time to guide the practitioner in sampling the area of concern. A variety of disorders can be diagnosed, evaluated, or monitored with a liver biopsy, as identified in Box 51-2.

Nursing responsibilities require explaining the procedure to the patient, making sure that the patient has nothing by mouth (NPO) for 12 hours prior to the examination and making sure prothrombin and hemoglobin results are preformed and available before the test. Potential complications for the nurse to be aware of are listed in the Skills 360° feature.

The endoscopic retrograde cholangiopancreatography (ERCP) inspects the liver, gallbladder, and pancreas visually and radioscopically. A fiberoptic duodenoscope is inserted orally under general anesthesia into the duodenum. A small catheter is inserted into the common bile duct and pancreatic duct, and radiographic dye is introduced to visualize the liver, gallbladder, pancreas, and the different ducts. Bile sampling and interventions to remove stones from the ducts may be able to be performed at the time of the test. Potential complications of ERCP are perforation of the stomach, duodenum, and other ducts, pancreatitis, anaphylactic reaction to the contrast dye, aspiration of gastric contents, and reaction to anesthesia (Nietsch & Kowdley, 2004).

Nursing responsibilities include ensuring that the consent form, patent intravenous (IV) line, preoperative labs, and X-rays are available and instructing the patient to be NPO for 12 hours prior to the procedure. After the test, the patient remains NPO until the gag reflex returns. The nurse must continue to assess for signs of peritonitis, abdominal pain, nausea and vomiting, and septicemia.

Bile fluid can be procured by orally inserting a gastroduodenal tube into the duodenum. Fluoroscopic examination is used to confirm placement. Cholecystokinin is administered intravenously to make the gallbladder contract and release the bile, which is then sucked into a specimen trap. This test is done to assess cholecystitis, pancreatitis, parasites, and pancreatic carcinoma. Nursing care is similar to that for ERCP.

Bile salt absorption is a test that identifies unabsorbed bile salts in the feces and exhaled radioactive carbon dioxide in the breath after ingesting C-14 triolein. Presence of abnormal amounts of fecal fat indicates malabsorption of bile salts as well as diseases of the ileum or bacterial colonization in the gut.

Hepatobiliary scan utilizes radionucleotides, which are injected intravenously that are taken up in the bile. Sequential delayed imaging is necessary for 6 to 48 hours after initial injection. The patency of bile ducts is assessed as well as hepatocyte functioning. Acute and chronic cholecystitis, biliary obstruction, bile leak, and biliary atresia can be diagnosed.

The liver scan is a noninvasive test that utilizes IV radionucleotides and ultrasound. The ultrasound passes over the liver and spleen in the upper right quadrant, providing a three-dimensional picture. Hepatitis, cirrhosis, cysts, tumors, abscesses, trauma, and Hodgkin disease are some of the conditions that can be monitored by this technique.

A cholangiogram is an X-ray utilizing IV contrast materials to visualize the biliary ducts. IV cholangiography is being replaced by the ERCP. CT of the liver and biliary tracts may be used to visualize the ducts. Tumors, abscesses, iron overload, hepatitis, cirrhosis, radiation injury, and obstruction can be diagnosed.

Oral cholecystography is an X-ray that utilizes oral contrast material followed by X-ray. Gallstones and cystic duct patency can be assessed. This test has been replaced in some institutions by ultrasound.

Ultrasound of the gallbladder and biliary system is a noninvasive test to identify cholelithiasis and cholecystitis. If stones are seen, the patient may be asked to turn in various positions to ascertain if the stones are free-floating or obstructing ducts. Greater visualization is achieved with the patient fasting for 8 to 12 hours before the examination.

HEPATITIS

Hepatitis is inflammation of the liver. The most common cause of hepatitis is viral infection. Liver injury and subsequent inflammation can also occur from exposure to alcohol, drugs, toxins, and autoimmune conditions. Fatty liver can progress to hepatitis because of congestion creating inflammation (Ship, 2005).

Pathophysiology

There are three phases of hepatitis, which include preicteric, icteric, and posticteric (Box 51-3). The labels for these three phases are describing the level of jaundice seen in the patient.

> **BOX 51-3**
>
> **PHASES OF HEPATITIS**
>
> - Preicteric (prodromal) phase is from the time of infection until the start of signs and symptoms, such as malaise, fever, nausea, and vomiting. Some smokers have an aversion to smoking as an initial sign. Joint pain and itching might also occur.
> - Icteric phase is when jaundice sets in. Urine can be dark from increased bilirubin. Cholestasis may develop.
> - Posticteric phase is the recovery phase when jaundice resolves and the liver starts to repair itself.

Hepatitis can be either acute or chronic. Acute viral hepatitis occurs in the initial period after infection and symptoms are clinically similar for all viral types. Symptoms can range from subclinical asymptomatic infections to fatal acute infections. Traditionally chronic hepatitis has been considered to last greater than six months. Chronic hepatitis is identified by etiology, histology, and location. Only hepatitis B, C, and D are viruses responsible for chronic disease. It is not associated with hepatitis A or E. Other causes of chronic hepatitis include alcohol, liver-toxic substances (like carbon tetrachloride), prescribed medications (drug-induced), autoimmune diseases, and some hereditary diseases, such as Wilson's disease. Chronic active hepatitis (or chronic aggressive hepatitis) might occur after the acute viral hepatitis infection. Liver damage, patchy necrosis, and fibrosis contribute to liver failure and cirrhosis, and death often occurs within five years of onset. Fulminant hepatitis occurs in about 1 percent of infected people, mostly with hepatitis B virus (HBV) or HBV/hepatitis D virus (HDV) infection. This complication is characterized by aggressive progression of the disease, rapid deterioration, and marked liver necrosis. Acute liver failure ensues as the liver is unable to regenerate, and about 60 to 80 percent of these cases end in death (Soriano-Sarabia, et al., 2005).

Viral hepatitis is usually caused by RNA or DNA viruses identified as A to E. Other viruses that can cause hepatitis include non–A to E. Hepatitis F and G have been identified, but not much is known about them at this time. Hepatitis can also be caused by other viruses such as Epstein-Barr, yellow fever, herpes-simplex, varicella-zoster, and cytomegalovirus, although these are rare and are generally considered separate disorders. Table 51-1 offers information on the epidemiology and etiology of hepatitis.

Assessment with Clinical Manifestations

Nursing assessment should include extensive history taking. This would include asking about high risk behaviors, such as drug use, sexual behavior, sharing personal items, and living conditions. Other information should be ascertained, such as travel, exposure to possibly contaminated shellfish, restaurant patronage,

Text continues on p. 1708

TABLE 51-1 Comparison of the Types of Hepatitis

VIRUS NAME TYPE OF VIRUS	SPREAD	PREVENTION/ VACCINATION/ GOOD HEALTH PRACTICES	WHO IS AT RISK	REPORTING PROCEDURES AND FOLLOW-UP	INCUBATION PERIOD AFTER EXPOSURE	SIGNS/SYMPTOMS AND DIAGNOSTIC TESTS	TREATMENT
Hepatitis A (HAV) RNA virus (picornavirus) of the entero-virus family	Fecal-oral route Close personal contact, including sex or sharing a household. Eating food or drinking water contaminated with HAV. Often shellfish caught in contaminated water could be the source. This is particularly possible when eating raw shellfish. HAV can be spread by food handlers infected with the virus.	Hepatitis A vaccine is available usually for people age 2 years and older. Always wash hands with soap and water after using the bathroom, after changing a diaper, before preparing food, and before eating. If hand washing facilities are not available, hand sanitizer should be used. Once infected with HAV, the person will be immune.	People living with infected people. Sex partners of infected persons. People traveling to other countries where HAV is common (everywhere except United States, Canada, Western Europe, Australia, New Zealand, and Japan).	Cases of acute HAV are reported to the public health authorities. Possible follow-up and screening can be done to prevent further infections from occurring.	15–50 days Average is 28 days	Usually the signs and symptoms are mild, viral flu-like symptoms. Some HAV can go undetected because the symptoms may be mild. Rare occasions, HAV can develop into fulminant hepatitis. People with chronic liver disease have a greater possibility of developing fulminating hepatitis. Jaundice is usually not evident. Anti-HAV is detected in serum to confirm diagnosis.	Immediately after exposure treatment is with immune globulin (IG). This is effective in about 85 percent of people if given within two weeks after exposure. After diagnosis, care is supportive, treating fever and flu-like symptoms. The disease usually resolves on its own. Avoiding alcohol is helpful because it can worsen liver disease. HAV has no known chronic carrier state and plays no role in the production of chronic hepatitis or cirrhosis.

Hepatitis B (HBV) or serum hepatitis Double-shelled DNA virus. Virus has a core antigen (HBcAg) and a surface antigen (HBsAg).	HBV is transmitted through blood and body fluids (semen, saliva, or vaginal secretions) via skin and mucous membranes. Unprotected sex. Sharing needles and other drug paraphernalia. Mothers can inoculate the baby during the birth process. Accidental needle sticks.	United States strategy to prevent HBV infection is four-pronged: Prevent perinatal infection of infants born to HBsAg positive mothers. (This would require testing of mothers. This is recommended at the time that the pregnancy is confirmed. If this is not possible, then testing should be done at the time of delivery.) In addition, women who have clinically apparent hepatitis, multiple sexual partners, partners who are HBsAg positive, and women who have been treated for sexually transmitted diseases (STDs) or those who live in areas where there are high rates of HBV should also have	Health care workers and other persons in occupational groups that could be exposed to blood or body fluids. Inmates of long-term correctional facilities. Injection drug users. Sexually active men who have sex with men (MSM). Men and women who have more than one sexual partner in the last six months, have a history of sexually transmitted disease, or who have been treated in a STD clinic. Hemodialysis patients. Recipients of clotting factor concentrates. Long-term travelers. Patients and staff in institutions for the developmentally disabled.	Report all cases to the local health department. Partners of infected persons could be contacted and offered testing and treatment.	48–180 days The average incubation is 120 days HBV is 100 times more infectious than human immunodeficiency virus (HIV) and 10 times more infectious that hepatitis C virus (HCV). Only about 30–50 percent develop acute HBV at the time of infection	Anorexia, nausea, vomiting, jaundice, fatigue, low-grade fever, arthralgias, rashes, light-colored stools, and dark urine are common. Infants often will have low birth weight, jaundice, lethargy, failure to thrive, abdominal distension, and clay-colored stools. Acute HBV may be mild or severe. About 15 percent of HBV infections progress to the chronic state. Liver biopsy may be done. Elevated aspartate aminotransferase (AST), alanine aminotransferase (ALT), bilirubin, PT, and LFTs are usually present. Usually HBsAg, Total anti-HBc, IgM anti-HBc, and Anti-HBs are tested to ascertain previous exposure to the virus or effective antibody	Immediate postexposure treatment Postexposure prevention with the HBV vaccine can be initiated within 12 to 24 hours with 70–90 percent success. Hepatitis B immune globulin (HBIG) can be administered within seven days of percutaneous exposure and two weeks after sexual exposure. Infants born to HBV-positive mothers should be given HBIG within 12 hours of birth, and hepatitis B vaccine should be administered before the child leaves the hospital and at one and six months after delivery. Testing for HBsAg and

Continued

TABLE 51-1 Comparison of the Types of Hepatitis—cont'd

VIRUS NAME TYPE OF VIRUS	SPREAD	PREVENTION/ VACCINATION/ GOOD HEALTH PRACTICES	WHO IS AT RISK	REPORTING PROCEDURES AND FOLLOW-UP	INCUBATION PERIOD AFTER EXPOSURE	SIGNS/SYMPTOMS AND DIAGNOSTIC TESTS	TREATMENT
Hepatitis B (HBV) or serum hepatitis Double-shelled DNA virus. Virus has a core antigen (HBcAg) and a surface antigen (HBsAg). —cont'd		their infants treated prophylactically. Vaccination of all newborns. Vaccination of all adolescents not previously vaccinated (usually required at the state level for all incoming middle-school–aged children). Vaccination of adults and adolescents in high-risk categories.	Babies born to HBsAg-positive mothers. Usually this happens during the birth process when the baby comes in contact with maternal secretions in the birth canal. Transmission across the placenta is unusual. Postpartum transmissions could occur through exposure to maternal blood, saliva, stool, urine, or breast milk. If a nursing mother has cracked nipples or other lesions on her breast, then HBV could be more likely to be transmitted.			response to vaccination. Another antigen, HBeAg, can reflect increased viral activity and subsequent increased infectivity. The presence of anti-HBe can indicate lower infectivity.	anti-HBs should be done between 12 and 15 months. In HBV endemic areas, prevention with HB vaccine should be standard practice for all newborns. After Diagnosis Interferon-alpha (injection three times a week) can decrease inflammation in 35–40 percent of patients. Lamivudine (orally daily) or adefovir dipivoxil (orally daily) may also be helpful, but further study is needed. Corticosteroids are contraindicated since viral replication is enhanced.

Hepatitis C (HCV) RNA virus.	Blood and plasma to skin and mucous membranes. Rarely it is spread by sexual contact. Rarely spread from HCV-positive mother to baby during the birth process.	No vaccine exists for HCV. Prevention efforts concentrate on standard precautions and infection control. Donor screening and product inactivation for blood and tissue products.	Intravenous (IV) drug users are at highest risk. People who received blood products or tissue transplants before 1992. Recipients of clotting factors before 1987. Tattoos and body piercings may be associated with increased infection, depending on sterilization practices of the practitioner.	All cases should be reported to the local health department.	14–180 days. Chronic infection occurs in about 85 percent of HCV-positive people. Chronic liver disease can develop in 70 percent of chronically infected people and can lead to cirrhosis, liver failure, and liver cancer.	Anti-HCV antibodies in serum. Influenza-type symptoms may be more severe than HAV.	Immune globulin is not proven effective immediately after exposure. After diagnosis, interferon, pegylated interferon, and ribavirin in combination are most effective. Hepatitis C patients with liver failure account for approximately 50 percent of all liver transplants.
Hepatitis D (HDV) RNA virus that needs the helper function of HBV to infect new hosts and replicate	Similar to HBV. IV drug users. Sexual partners of infected persons. People who have received blood products before July 1992 or clotting factors before 1987. It is possible for a mother to infect her baby during the birth process.	Preventing HBV also will prevent HDV. It is recommended that all persons be vaccinated. Standard precautions for all patients in the health care setting. Avoid contact with infected blood, contaminated needles, and an infected person's personal items.	See HBV list.	Report cases to the local health department.	14–56 days. Chronic hepatitis usually develops.	Coinfection symptoms are more severe than solitary HBV infection. Some patients are asymptomatic. Anti-HDV antibodies in serum.	Hepatitis preexposure or post-exposure with hepatitis B immune globulin (HBIG) can be used. Chronic HDV is treated with alpha-interferon

Continued

TABLE 51-1 Comparison of the Types of Hepatitis—cont'd

VIRUS NAME TYPE OF VIRUS	SPREAD	PREVENTION/ VACCINATION/ GOOD HEALTH PRACTICES	WHO IS AT RISK	REPORTING PROCEDURES AND FOLLOW-UP	INCUBATION PERIOD AFTER EXPOSURE	SIGNS/SYMPTOMS AND DIAGNOSTIC TESTS	TREATMENT
Hepatitis D (HDV) RNA virus that needs the helper function of HBV to infect new hosts and replicate—cont'd	Coinfection is when HDV is acquired at the same time as the HBV. Super-infection is when chronic HBV patients acquire a subsequent HDV infection at a later date.						
Hepatitis E (HEV) RNA virus	Fecal-oral route. Most often associated with waterborne epidemics, especially in Asia, Middle East, Africa, and Central and South America. Eating food or drinking water contaminated with HEV. Often shellfish caught in contaminated water could be the source.	Hepatitis E vaccine is available usually for people age 2 years and older. Always wash hands with soap and water after using the bathroom, after changing a diaper, before preparing food, and before eating. If hand washing facilities are not available, hand sanitizer should be used. Once infected with HEV, the person will be immune.	People traveling to other countries where HEV is endemic (everywhere except United States, Canada, Western Europe, Australia, New Zealand, and Japan).	Cases of acute HEV are reported to the public health authorities. Possible follow-up and screening can be done to prevent further infections from occurring.	15–64 days.	The clinical course resembles that of HAV. Usually the signs and symptoms are mild, viral flu-like symptoms but can include jaundice, fatigue, abdominal pain, decreased appetite, nausea, vomiting, and dark urine. Some HEV can go undetected because the symptoms may be mild. Anti-HEV is detected in serum to confirm diagnosis.	Immediately after exposure treatment is with immune globulin (IG). This is effective in about 85 percent of people if given within two weeks after exposure. After diagnosis, care is supportive, treating fever and flu-like symptoms. Avoiding alcohol is helpful, because it can worsen liver disease.

	This is particularly possible when eating raw shellfish. HEV can spread by food handlers infected with the virus.						HEV has no known chronic carrier state and plays no role in the production of chronic hepatitis or cirrhosis. HEV is more severe in pregnant women, especially in the third trimester.
Hepatitis F (HCV) Hepatitis F (HFV) is possibly a variant of the HBV virus. Not much is known about the virus.							
Hepatitis G (HGV) or non-A-E hepatitis RNA flavivirus-like agent	Blood and plasma to skin and mucous membranes.	No vaccine exists for HGV. Prevention efforts concentrate on standard precautions and infection control.	IV drug users. Health care professionals and people who come in contact with infected blood products.	All cases should be reported to the local health department.	Chronic infection can occur.	Anti-HGV antibodies in serum. Influenza-type symptoms.	Supportive care after diagnosis Avoid alcohol because it exacerbates liver disease

recent body piercings and tattoos, occupational hazards, and alcohol consumption. Common diagnostic tests appear in Table 51-1.

Nursing Diagnoses

Based on the information gathered, examples of nursing diagnoses in the patient with hepatitis may include the following:

- Activity intolerance related to fatigue.
- Disturbed body image related to jaundice.
- Imbalanced nutrition: less than body requirements related to nausea.

Planning and Implementation

Many practices are in place to protect health care workers from various infections. Standard precautions must be practiced at all times. The ready availability of hand sanitizer in many settings helps decrease infection. The advent of needleless systems for administering IVs and medications has decreased needle sticks in hospitals and clinics. Requirements to have people vaccinated who have a high probability of being exposed to viral infection with hepatitis A (HAV) and HBV also prevent infection (Saldanha, Heath, Lelie, Pisani, & Yu, 2005).

Good health practices should be included in all patient education to prevent viral infection that could lead to the various types of hepatitis. This would include good hand washing after using the bathroom, before meal preparation, and before eating. Avoid raw shellfish. Avoid using anyone else's personal items like toothbrushes, razors, dental floss, nail clippers. Use condoms during sexual intercourse. Be sure of sterile practices before obtaining tattoos or piercings. If traveling, drink only water that is purified or treated. Peel fruits and vegetables before eating. Choose cooked food over raw vegetables. Be sure milk products are pasteurized. The patient should be encouraged to brush his or her teeth with bottled or purified water.

Treatment and nursing interventions focus on reducing the causative agent and addressing bothersome symptoms. For some virus-induced hepatitis, immune globulin or vaccination can be offered after immediate exposure. Other antivirals medications may be available. Promoting adequate physical and psychological rest is important. Diet therapy could limit fats and proteins. Often small, frequent meals are tolerated better than large meals, because hepatomegaly can reduce the capacity of the stomach. Increasing naturally occurring antioxidants in the diet is recommended. Vitamins and dietary supplements can improve nutrition. Often alcoholics eat sporadically, and their nutrition might be more compromised than people with nonalcohol-related hepatitis. Specific drug therapy is mentioned with the individual types of hepatitis. However supportive care can include antiemetics (however, prochlorperazine [Compazine] is avoided because of potential hepatotoxic effects). In all types of hepatitis, regardless of the cause, avoidance of alcohol is always helpful.

Evaluation of Outcomes

Potential patient outcomes for each of the example nursing diagnoses for the patient with hepatitis are:

- Activity intolerance related to fatigue. The patient maintains activity level within capabilities, as evidenced by normal heart rate and blood pressure during activity, as well as absence of shortness of breath, weakness, and fatigue.
- Disturbed body image related to jaundice. The patient demonstrates enhanced body image and self-esteem as evidenced by ability to look at, touch, talk about, and care for actual or perceived altered body part or function.

- Imbalanced nutrition: less than body requirements related to nausea. The patient verbalizes and demonstrates selection of foods or meals that will achieve a cessation of weight loss and weighs within 10 percent of ideal body weight.

Alcoholic Hepatitis

Inflammation of the liver can be caused by agents other than viruses. The most common nonviral source of inflammation is alcohol. Many factors work together in the presence of alcohol that can directly or indirectly cause inflammation to the liver.

Pathophysiology

The pathological factors that contribute to the development of alcoholic hepatitis are shown in Box 51-4.

Planning and Implementation

Treatment of alcoholic hepatitis can include corticosteroids to reduce inflammation; antioxidants to lessen the negative effects of free radicals; antibiotics to combat the increased permeability to intestinal bacteria; and vitamins and minerals to supplement the compromised functioning of the liver to synthesize and store needed materials.

BOX 51-4

PATHOLOGY OF ALCOHOLIC HEPATITIS

- Alcohol interferes with lipid metabolism, creating hyperlipidemia and fatty liver. This in turn can cause congestion and hypoxia, especially around the central veins.
- Long-term alcohol ingestion stimulates liver storage cells (stellate cells) to produce collagen, the protein that forms scar tissue, predisposing the person to fibrosis and resultant cirrhosis.
- Alcohol impairs the integrity of membranes surrounding the hepatocytes as well as membranes around organelles within the cells.
- In the presence of alcohol, prostaglandin and prostacyclin production is reduced. These molecules provide cell-protective functions in the healthy liver tissue, so cell defenses are decreased with alcohol.
- Production of thromboxane B_2 and leukotriene B_4 can increase. These molecules cause constriction of hepatic blood vessels and result in congestion and hypoxia, which leads to inflammation.
- Alcohol can cause an increase of cytokines, including tumor necrosis factor (TNF), which can cause damage to tissues directly and indirectly.
- Alcohol directly increases the permeability of bacteria and endotoxins in the intestine. Endotoxins are found on the outer membrane surface of some bacteria. Kupffer cells are activated by the endotoxins and in turn promote an inflammatory response, congestion, and hypoxia.
- Alcohol can increase the formation of free radicals, such as acetaldehyde. Some free radicals can bind closely with the patient's healthy tissues and create hybrid molecules called **adducts.** The body's own immune system might identify these newly formed molecules as foreign and subsequently launch an immune response to normal healthy tissue. These new hybrid molecules can also interfere with the normal functioning of hepatocytes. Normally, antioxidants in the body help to absorb or deactivate the free radicals, but antioxidants are reduced in the presence of alcohol.

Toxic and Drug-Induced Hepatitis

Inflammation of the liver can be caused by toxic substances and prescribed medications. Most hepatotoxins produce a dose-related effect of the liver, although other organs (especially the kidneys) might also be damaged. Substances that are toxic to the liver include carbon tetrachloride and other hydrocarbons and phosphorus. Amanita (psychotropic) mushrooms can be damaging. Medications that can have a negative impact on liver functioning are isoniazid, methyldopa, amiodarone, monoamine oxidase inhibitors, indomethacin, propylthiouracil, phenytoin, diclofenac, halothane (gas anesthetic), acetaminophen, and tetracycline (Broyles, Reiss, & Evans, 2007).

Autoimmune Hepatitis

Autoimmune hepatitis occurs when the body's natural immune defenses become sensitized to its own liver cells and start attacking hepatocytes and causing inflammation. This happens more to women (70 percent) than to men (30 percent). About half of those affected have other autoimmune disorders occurring, such as Grave's disease, ulcerative colitis, thyroiditis, proliferative glomerulonephritis, and autoimmune anemia.

Diagnosis can be with blood tests for antinuclear antibodies (ANA), antibodies against smooth muscle cells (SMA), and antiliver and antikidney microsomes (anti-LKM). Liver biopsy is definitive for autoimmune hepatitis.

Treatment focuses on slowing down the immune response with corticosteroids or azathioprine (Imuran). Other medications include mycophenolate mofetil, cyclosporine, or tacrolimus.

HEREDITARY DISEASES OF THE LIVER

Often, the many functions of the liver were identified when people presented with hereditary disorders that were traced to a defect or deficiency in liver metabolism. The following are some of the genetic disorders that emphasize the importance of the liver in bilirubin metabolism, copper and iron storage, enzyme production, and lipoprotein metabolism.

Crigler-Najjar disease, type I is a rare, recessive disorder characterized by the total inability to conjugate bilirubin. Most patients die within the first year of life.

Wilson's disease is an autosomal recessive disorder related to copper metabolism. Usually copper is secreted in the bile, but this is prevented in people with this disease. The copper accumulates over many years and is often diagnosed between the ages of 6 and 40. Excess copper can damage brain, eyes, kidneys, and red blood cells. Symptoms can include tremors, rigidity, inappropriate behavior, difficulty with speech, deterioration of work, and personality changes. Cirrhosis results from scarring of the liver. Those with this disease are at a greater risk for developing bone fractures, infection, and impaired kidney function. Some people may be diagnosed during an optical exam, if the examiner notices Kayser-Fleischer rings (brown, ring-shaped pigmentation) in the cornea. Blood and urine can be tested for ceruloplasmin, a protein that binds copper and is usually low in people with Wilson's disease. Liver biopsy would allow examination of liver tissue for copper accumulation.

Most people with Wilson's disease can be treated by avoiding foods high in copper (Box 51-5) and by taking metal-binding drugs (chelating agents). These include penicillamine (Cuprimine or Depen), and trientine (Syprine). Zinc acetate (Gatzin) helps interfere with copper absorption in the stomach and intestines. Liver transplantation is sometimes the only option left for treatment.

Hemochromatosis is the inherited tendency to extract excessive amounts of iron from food. The gene HFE is identified with this disorder. Eventually iron accumulates in the liver, heart, joints, testicles, and thyroid, creating problems such as cirrhosis, liver failure, liver cancer, congestive heart failure, cardiac arrhythmias, impotence, hypothyroidism, and diabetes. Initial complaints are vague, such as fatigue, decreased libido, amenorrhea, abdominal pain, and joint pain. Skin can become bronze or even grayish from the increased iron deposits in the skin. The iron can stimulate skin cells to produce more melanin.

A diagnosis of hemochromatosis can be made by assessing LFTs. When the LFTs are abnormal, the serum transferrin saturation (iron binds to the protein, transferring, in the blood) and serum ferritin (measures the amount of iron stored in the body) can be assayed. Liver biopsy can be used effectively for diagnosis. Several genes could be responsible for this disorder, although the presence of the defective gene is not a guarantee that the disease would be expressed. Genetic testing for the gene HFE is possible to identify the adult version of hemochromatosis. Juvenile hemochromatosis is caused by the gene called hemojuvelin. The cause of neonatal hemochromatosis is not yet known.

Treatment involves decreasing the iron load in the body by phlebotomy. Women often do not experience the effects of the disease until menopause sets in and the regular loss of blood stops. People should avoid foods high in iron, such as red meat, dried peas and lentils, and iron-enriched breads and pastas. Supplements with iron or vitamin C (this increases iron absorption) should be avoided. Discourage use of raw shellfish (increased possibility for infection) and alcohol (toxic to the liver).

Alpha-antitrypsin deficiency is an example of a genetic disorder that shed light on one of the many metabolic functions of the liver. This disorder affects the production of alpha-1 protein, which is produced in the liver and is then transported to the lungs. Its function is to neutralize enzymes that are released by white blood cells after pulmonary infection. If these enzymes are not neutralized, white blood cells continue to attack healthy tissue and destroy lung tissue after the infection is resolved. The alpha-1 antitrypsin deficiency creates problems in the liver, because the alpha protein is not utilized in the production of the alpha-trypsin. It then accumulates in the liver, causing congestion and can eventually lead to cirrhosis. Treatment is with alpha-1 proteinase inhibitor replacement therapy, Prolastin, which is administered intravenously on a weekly basis. However, the liver problems are still concerning, and patients need to practice good liver care by getting vaccinated for HBV and avoiding alcohol. In addition, they should avoid smoking to preserve lung integrity.

Abetalipoproteinemia is an autosomal recessive disorder of lipoprotein metabolism. People with this disease have difficulties absorbing fat from the gut, blood tests show absent low-density lipoproteins (LDL) and very low-density lipoproteins (VLDL) results, and triglycerides are almost undetectable. Total cholesterol is usually below 70 mg/dL. This presents problems with the utilization of fat-soluble vitamins but especially vitamin E, which is necessary for adequate neurological functioning. Red blood cells are deformed. Symptoms involve fatty stools, diarrhea, neurological dysfunction (ataxia, neuropathies, and other disorders), and failure to thrive in infants.

BOX 51-5

DIETARY RECOMMENDATIONS FOR PEOPLE WITH WILSON'S DISEASE

Avoid foods high in copper including:

- Liver
- Shellfish
- Mushrooms
- Nuts
- Chocolate
- Dried fruit
- Dried peas, beans, and lentils
- Soy products
- Avocados
- Barley
- Bran products
- Nectarines

Test tap water for copper. If it contains greater that 100 μg/L, use bottled (demineralized) water or procure a filter that would effectively reduce copper traces.

- Avoid vitamins and supplements with copper.
- Restrict the use of alcohol because of the toxic effects of alcohol on the liver.

Adapted from Roth, R. (2007). Nutrition and diet therapy *(9th ed.). New York: Thomson Delmar Learning.*

CIRRHOSIS

Cirrhosis of the liver is a chronic, progressive condition characterized by destruction of the liver cells and subsequent formation of fibrotic tissue that reconfigures normal, healthy liver tissue. This lack of elasticity causes blood, bile, and lymphatic systems to become congested and obstructed, and further damage is incurred. There are four major types of cirrhosis, which are differentiated by the underlying pathology. These include alcoholic cirrhosis (Laënnec's cirrhosis), postnecrotic cirrhosis (reflecting damage done by hepatitis infections in addition to toxic exposure), biliary cirrhosis, and cardiac cirrhosis. Alcoholic and postnecrotic cirrhosis account for the majority of people diagnosed with this disease.

Respecting Our Differences

Women develop alcoholic hepatitis and cirrhosis at much lower cumulative doses than men and remain at a higher risk of prolonged damage, even after abstinence. Two things may contribute to this observation. First, women have lower amounts of gastric ADH. Therefore, even though they may ingest smaller amounts of alcohol, a larger proportion of the total dose gets absorbed in the intestine and goes directly to the liver. Second, women metabolize fats differently and utilize fats in different proportions than men because of their hormonal makeup. In addition, women may experience a wide variety of manifestations related to the condition of alcoholism (Figure 51-2).

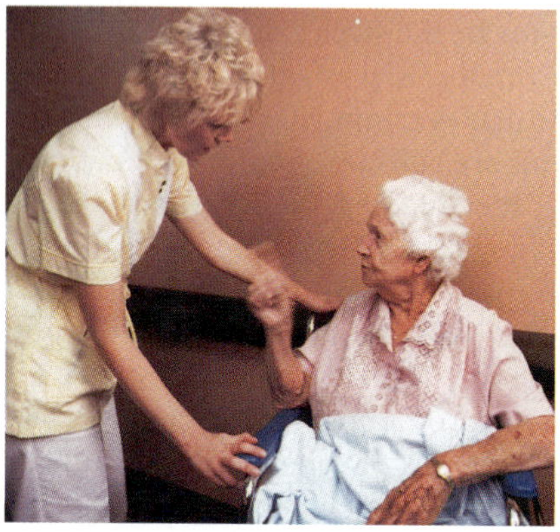

Figure 51-2 An elderly female is expressing hostility during a hallucination caused by alcohol withdrawal.

Alcoholic Cirrhosis

The destruction to the liver from alcohol often progresses from fatty liver to alcoholic hepatitis and culminates in alcoholic cirrhosis. However, some people develop cirrhosis without experiencing the other conditions. The effect of alcohol on the liver was outlined previously in this chapter. It should be noted that hypoxia, congestion, and inflammation provide conditions for fibrosis to occur. With infiltration by fat, leukocytes and lymphocytes, tumor necrosing factors, free radicals, and adducts further destruction is achieved (Kim, Wang, Jeong, Ahn, & Kim, 2005).

Epidemiology

Only about 50 percent of alcoholics develop cirrhosis. Hereditary, gender, and environmental factors influence development of serious disease (see Respecting Our Differences). Variations in different enzymes, such as alcohol dehydrogenase (ADH) and (ALDH), are implicated in some liver disease. ADH is primarily found in the liver, however, gastric ADH is also present to begin the digestion of alcohol when it is still in the stomach instead of absorbing the whole dose when it reaches the intestines. Genetic disorders coupled with heavy drinking can accelerate liver destruction.

Alcoholics with hepatitis C virus (HCV) develop alcoholic cirrhosis and liver problems at a younger age. Alcoholics who smoke greater than one pack per day have three times the rate of alcoholic cirrhosis. Interestingly, alcoholics who drink more than four cups of coffee per day have a fivefold lower incidence of alcoholic cirrhosis (Box 51-6). This is not because of the caffeine, because the same apparent protection does not hold true for equivalent forms of caffeine, such as tea (Rambaldi & Gluud, 2005). People suffering from alcoholism may experience a variety of mental health disturbances, such as clinical depression (Figure 51-3).

Postnecrotic Cirrhosis

Postnecrotic cirrhosis occurs most frequently in the wake of hepatitis infections. Hepatitis C is the predominant cause of viral-related cirrhosis, but often it takes several decades to develop. Chronic HBV and HDV can also cause cirrhosis. Autoimmune hepatitis, inherited diseases, and toxic or drug-induced liver damage can become necrotic and cause cirrhosis to develop.

Biliary Cirrhosis

Blocked bile ducts cause congestion, inflammation, and damage to the tissue in the liver. Some babies are born with biliary atresia, in which the bile ducts are absent or improperly formed, depriving the bile of avenues of exit from the liver and ultimately causing tissue damage. In adults, inflamed or blocked bile ducts can occur and scarring results. This can happen as a complication of surgery or trauma if the ducts are inadvertently injured.

Cardiac Cirrhosis

Cardiac or vascular cirrhosis occurs when blood flow out of the liver is restricted by severe right sided-sided failure. Tricuspid regurgitation can be associated with cardiac cirrhosis. Large amounts of blood are delivered to the liver each minute. When that blood is not able to exit at a predictable rate, liver engorgement occurs and the pressure in the liver vasculature increases, causing venous congestion, anoxia or hypoxia, and hepatic cell necrosis and subsequent fibrosis.

BOX 51-6

QUANTITY OF ALCOHOL CONSUMPTION

One drink is equivalent to:

- 12 oz beer
- 5 oz wine
- 1.5 oz distilled spirits or hard liquor

A heavy drinker would be one who consumes:

- 72 oz beer per day
- 1 liter of wine per day
- 8 oz distilled spirits per day

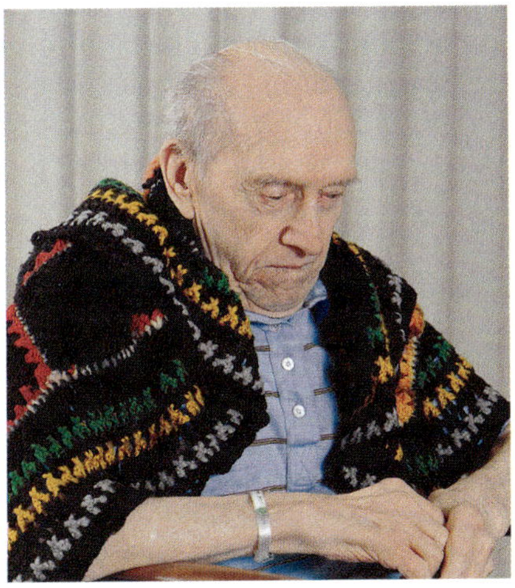

Figure 51-3 An elderly male suffering from alcoholism is clinically depressed.

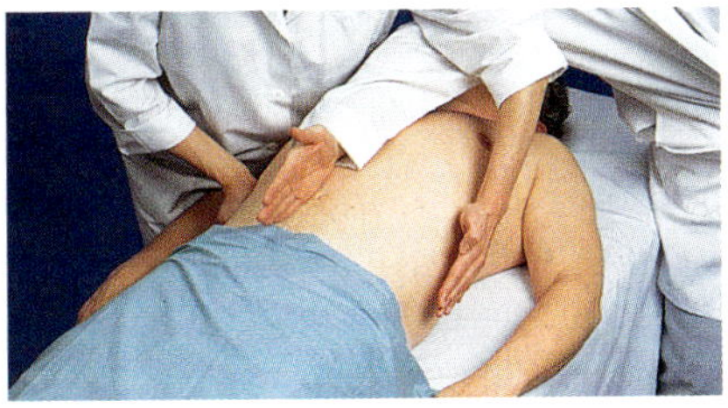

Figure 51-4 Assessing for ascites.

Pathophysiology

The pathophysiology of cirrhosis is multisystemic in its dysfunction. There are many complications evidenced in patients with cirrhosis. Some of the signs and symptoms that a patient has are irreversible, while other changes are reversible. The common complications of cirrhosis are discussed in the following section.

Ascites is the accumulation of fluid in the peritoneal cavity (Figure 51-4) and is seen as a common complication of cirrhosis. With the congestion of blood and lymph in the fibrotic liver, plasma can seep from the liver vasculature into the peritoneum. The term **liver sweats** refers to the movement of plasma from the lymphatic system into this potential space in the abdomen. When volume is decreased in the intravascular space because of plasma moving out, the body perceives this as low blood volume with the need to conserve water and sodium and makes the problem worse by increasing efforts to conserve blood volume (O'Brien, Chennubhotla, & Chennubhotla, (2005). **Refractory ascites** is that which cannot be effectively managed with normal therapies. Patients with refractory ascites are unresponsive to 400 mg of spironolactone (or 30 mg of amiloride) plus 120 mg of furosemide daily for two weeks. Refractory ascites could be caused by lack of compliance with the fluid or sodium restriction, spontaneous bacterial peritonitis, hepatocellular carcinoma, and renal failure.

When ascitic fluid becomes infected with bacteria in the absence of an obvious precipitating event, it is called spontaneous bacterial peritonitis (SBP). Increased fever or abdominal pain are typical, and polymorphonuclear (PMN) body count is greater than 250 cells/μL. It is possible for the peritoneal fluid to have negative bacterial cultures, and this is termed culture-negative neutrocytic ascites. Cefotaxime (Cefizox) is the antibiotic of choice.

With the destruction of liver tissue comes the impairment of the many metabolic functions performed by the liver. Some of the most important functions affected include:

- Storage of fat soluble vitamins. Vitamins A, D, E, and K are essential for many metabolic process that are compromised by decreased liver function.
- Synthesis of clotting factors (factors II, VII, IX, and X are all dependent of the fat-soluble vitamin K, which is not available with decreased liver function).
- Metabolism and transport of bilirubin is impaired. This negatively impacts digestion of fats.
- Regulation of gluconeogenesis, glycogen synthesis, and glycogen hydrolysis is compromised. Hypoglycemia and hyperglycemia can be serious.
- Cirrhosis causes resistance to insulin, and people develop type 2, insulin resistant diabetes.
- Ammonia metabolism where high levels of ammonia can have neurological symptoms. Portal-systemic encephalopathy can result.
- Lipid metabolism is impaired lipid and has a negative effect on cell membranes and organelle membranes. In particular, this can damage nerve cells.
- Albumin, the dominant plasma protein, is not adequately manufactured and can lead to fluid shifts and changes in oncotic pressure throughout the body and lead to renal vasoconstriction. Activation of the renin-angiotensin system causes more sodium and water retention, increasing general hypertension, exacerbating the original problem of portal hypertension and congestion. The problem of decreased plasma in the intravascular space can be a combined effect of mechanical issues. Blood is not able to move through the liver vasculature and squeezes plasma proteins into the peritoneal space. In addition, there are metabolic issues in which damaged liver cells have the decreased ability to synthesis albumin, the primary protein in blood responsible for maintaining oncotic pressure.

Assessment with Clinical Manifestations

Assessment is critical when caring for the person with liver disease. A constellation of signs and symptoms are listed in Box 51-7.

Planning and Implementation

Cirrhosis, along with the resulting ascites, can be treated with the following interventions: fluid restriction of 1,000 to1,500 mL per day, sodium restriction (limited to 200 to 500 mg per day), and diuretic therapy. Spironolactone (Aldactone) is the diuretic of choice because of its potassium-sparing properties. However, amiloride (Moduretic) or triamterene (Dyazide or Maxzide) may also be used. If the patient is compliant with the sodium and fluid restriction, furosemide (Lasix) may be added. Further management can be a paracentesis, peritoneovenous shunt, and transjugular intrahepatic portosystemic shunt. Paracentesis is the limited removal of fluid from the peritoneal cavity for diagnostic or therapeutic purposes. This can be performed at the bedside. It is most often used palliatively to reduce abdominal pressure, which can cause respiratory distress and abdominal pain. Fluid is removed slowly to avoid hypovolemic shock. The peritoneal fluid contains plasma proteins and electrolytes. Usually only 750 to 1,000 mL are removed at a time; however, larger volumes of 3 to 5 liters or more have been reported in the literature. Before the procedure, the nurse has the patient empty their bladder to decrease the

BOX 51-7

CLINICAL MANIFESTATIONS OF LIVER DISEASE

- Gastrointestinal (GI) findings include
  1. Abdominal discomfort, pain secondary to portal hypertension and ascites
  2. Anorexia and malnutrition
  3. Nausea and vomiting
  4. Clay-colored stools secondary to decreased bile formation or transportation
  5. Esophageal varices, hemorrhoids, and GI bleeding
  6. Fetor hepaticus (fruity-smelling breath)
  7. Gastritis
  8. Hepatomegaly
- Neurological findings include
  1. Asterixis
  2. Behavioral changes
  3. Changes in level of consciousness (LOC)
  4. Peripheral paresthesias
  5. Disturbed sleep patterns
- Cardiovascular findings include
  1. Cardiac arrhythmias
  2. Collateral circulation
- Pulmonary findings endocrine findings include
  1. Dyspnea
  2. Hyperventilation
  3. Hypoxemia
- Blood and immune system findings include
  1. Anemia
  2. Thrombocytopenia
  3. Splenomegaly
  4. Impaired coagulation
  5. Leukopenia
  6. Disseminated intravascular coagulation (DIC)
- Skin findings include
  1. Telangiectasias, spider angiomas on nose, cheeks, or torso
  2. Jaundice
  3. Palmar erythema
  4. Pruritus
  5. Caput medusae
  6. Increased skin pigmentation
  7. Petechiae
- Fluid and electrolytes findings include
  1. Ascites
  2. Edema
  3. Hypokalemia
  4. Hypocalcemia
  5. Hyponatremia
- Endocrine findings include
  1. Suppression of secondary sex characteristics in males, such as pectoral alopecia, changes in distribution of pubic and axillary hair
  2. Gynecomastia (in males)

possibility of injury to the bladder. Baseline vital signs, regularity of heartbeat (or electrocardiogram [ECG]), weight, level of consciousness (LOC), and abdominal girth need to be recorded. A consent form is required, so the nurse should allow for patient questions and ascertain the understanding of the procedure. During and after the procedure, the nurse needs to monitor the patient for hemodynamic changes, acid-base imbalances, and signs of electrolyte depletion. Cardiac arrhythmias may result from depletion of potassium or hypovolemia. Temperature is monitored to assess for infection, dressings are assessed for leakage, and urine is measured to ensure adequate output. The head of the bed can be kept at 30 degrees to allow for maximal respiratory expansion and minimize shortness of breath.

Surgery

When ascites continues to be a problem, a surgical shunt to divert excessive peritoneal fluid into the venous system may be attempted. A LeVeen peritoneovenous shunt (LPVS) diverts ascitic fluid via a pressure-sensitive one-way valve from the peritoneum to the internal jugular vein and ultimately into the superior vena cava. The movement of respiration helps to pump fluid through the valve. On inspiration, the diaphragm descends and increases pressure in the abdomen, allowing fluid to move toward the heart and reenter the vascular system. With the plasma proteins and electrolytes circulating, perfusion of the kidneys is improved, urinary output can increase, and there can be an increase in renal sodium excretion. Clinical improvements could include decreased abdominal girth, weight loss, and increased respiratory comfort.

The Denver peritoneovenous shunt (DPVS) is a variation of the LPVS in that it has a pump implanted subcutaneously, which can be manually compressed to open the unidirectional valve and allow for flushing of the tube connecting the peritoneum and jugular vein. This type of shunt did not improve the patency of the intrahepatic tubing. Unfortunately, patients with advanced liver disease and ascites are poor surgical candidates because of their increased abdominal pressure, potential to bleed, increased difficulties in metabolizing medications used in anesthesia, and their susceptibility for infection. Perioperatively, the patient may need antibiotics, blood products, vitamin K, and electrolytes.

Portal Hypertension

Portal hypertension is the constant pressure of the blood, bile, and lymphatics within the liver. This congestion can occur at the incoming sinusoid area (periportal or zone 1 of the liver), around the central vein that drains the blood from the hepatocytes (centrolobular area or Zone 3) or as it leaves the liver on the way to the inferior vena cava. When the blood meets with resistance, it tries to find other routes around the obstruction (collateral circulation). If this is not possible, all the vessels that bring blood to the liver are at risk for becoming engorged as well. It is this phenomenon that is responsible for other complications of cirrhosis such as:

- Esophageal varices—When the blood backs up, the vessels become distended, and in stretching, the walls become thinner and more friable. Varices can become life-threatening when these distended areas rupture and cause severe bleeding. Bleeding is usually caused by irritants (e.g., alcohol, gastric reflux, and some medications), mechanical insults (e.g., food, insertion of nasogastric tubes, or vomiting), and increased pressure or stretching caused by sneezing, vomiting, or physical exercise. It is possible for the patient to lose impressive amounts of blood when esophageal varices bleed. Hypovolemic shock is possible and constitutes a medical emergency.
- Splenomegaly.
- Hemorrhoids.

- Prominent abdominal veins (caput medusae).
- Bacterial translocation—When the veins serving the intestines become congested, there can be increased permeability of the membranes and bacteria may pass more freely into the bloodstream.

Nursing Diagnoses

Based on the information gathered, examples of nursing diagnoses in the patient with portal hypertension may include the following:

- Risk for infection related to portal hypertension.
- Activity intolerance related to portal hypertension.
- Risk for imbalanced fluid volume related to portal hypertension.

Planning and Implementation

There are many interventions for portal hypertension. In many instances, there is a need for surgical intervention as shown in the following section. Shunts to relieve the pressure in the portal vein created by cirrhosis were introduced as early as 1945. These original shunts diverted blood from the portal vein to the inferior vena cava, thus bypassing the fibrotic blockage that caused congestion in the liver. The portal tension was relieved, simultaneously relieving the pressure in the esophageal and gastric veins delivering blood to the portal vein. This was the first definitive surgical treatment for esophageal varices. The procedure fell out of favor in the 1970s because of an associated risk of encephalopathy and lack of clinical data that proved that survival rates were improved over nonsurgical therapy.

However, there were merits in relieving the pressure in the esophageal varices to prevent bleeding. The distal splenorenal shunt (DSRS) was designed to reroute blood only from the veins coming from the esophagus and stomach, while preserving the blood flow through the portal vein. The splenic vein was joined to the left kidney vein thereby selectively decompressing the esophageal and gastric varices. DSRS had a higher surgical mortality but less encephalopathy postoperatively. Patients with alcoholic cirrhosis do not do as well as those with nonalcoholic cirrhosis (Kim, et al., 2005).

A different shunting procedure is the transjugular intrahepatic portosystemic shunt (TIPS). A catheter is introduced by a radiologist into the jugular vein and advanced to the hepatic vein. The catheter is threaded into a large branch of the portal vein, and a stent is placed connecting the portal vein (bringing blood to the liver from the digestive tract) with the hepatic vein (returning blood from the liver to the heart). Advantages to this procedure include:

- Only a local anesthetic and mild sedation are used. (Many people with cirrhosis are unable to tolerate general anesthetics.)
- Major surgery is avoided. The TIPS procedure is tolerated better.
- TIPS reduces ascites in addition to relieving portal hypertension, but DSRS does not.

However, there are some disadvantages with this procedure as well.

- Encephalopathy is a postprocedure complication in about 25 percent of patients.
- If the patient is a candidate for liver transplant, this type of shunt can make transplant more difficult.

Sclerotherapy is the technique of injecting sclerosing drugs into the varices, causing a narrowing of the swollen veins, thus preventing bleeding and reducing swelling. This procedure is done endoscopically. If variceal bleeding reoccurs, the patient can still be offered a shunting procedure.

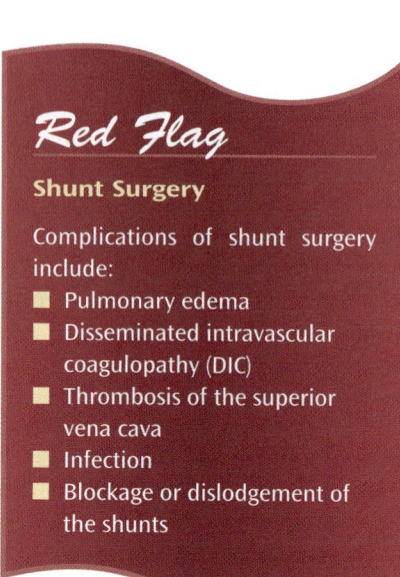

> **Red Flag**
>
> **Shunt Surgery**
>
> Complications of shunt surgery include:
>
> - Pulmonary edema
> - Disseminated intravascular coagulopathy (DIC)
> - Thrombosis of the superior vena cava
> - Infection
> - Blockage or dislodgement of the shunts

Evaluation of Outcomes

Potential patient outcomes for each of the example nursing diagnoses for the patient with portal hypertension are:

- Risk for infection. The patient remains free of infection, as evidenced by normal vital signs and absence of purulent drainage from wounds, incisions, and tubes. Infection is recognized early to allow for prompt treatment.

- Activity intolerance. The patient maintains activity level within capabilities, as evidenced by normal heart rate and blood pressure during activity, as well as absence of shortness of breath, weakness, and fatigue.
- Risk for excess fluid volume. The patient maintains adequate fluid volume and electrolyte balance as evidenced by vital signs within normal limits, clear lung sounds, pulmonary congestion absent on X-ray, and resolution of edema.

Hepatic Encephalopathy

Hepatic encephalopathy is also known as portal-systemic encephalopathy (PSE) or hepatic coma. This is a potentially reversible condition. Neurological symptoms include changes in LOC, slurred speech, behavioral changes and emotional lability, drowsiness, confusion, sleep disturbances, muscle twitching, progressing to rigidity, asterixis, and seizures.

Etiology

The causes of hepatic encephalopathy are from a combination of factors. Conditions that can precipitate hepatic encephalopathy include high levels of protein in the gut (both dietary and inadvertently through GI bleeding), hypovolemia, hypokalemia, constipation, and hepatotoxic medications.

Pathophysiology

It is already seen that impaired liver function can have a negative impact on the central nervous system by affecting the structure and functioning of cell membranes and glucose metabolism (with the consequences of interfering with cerebral energy utilization). When the liver is unable to perform its filtering and detoxifying functions, toxins can accumulate in the blood and eventually have an effect on the brain. However, hepatic encephalopathy is primarily linked to impaired metabolism of ammonia and other products of protein digestion. Protein is absorbed in the gut and intestines and transported to the liver, where it is catabolized into glutamine and ammonia. Ammonia is then used to form urea to be excreted by the kidneys. In addition, bacteria in the gut also produce ammonia. Increased membrane permeability makes it easier for products of digestion and bacterial endotoxins to cross into the portal vasculature. With compromised liver functioning, ammonia is not adequately converted to urea, and the levels of ammonia build up. Elevated ammonia levels are toxic to nerve tissue and cause the constellation of symptoms.

Planning and Implementation

Treatment for hepatic encephalopathy is focused on correcting the precipitating cause and reducing or eliminating dietary protein, preventing GI bleeding, and removing toxic enteric products in the intestines. Lactulose is a synthetic sugar that is used as a laxative. It works by pulling water into the gut to soften stool and increase peristalsis. It also helps to pull ammonia from the blood into the colon for expulsion. A range of two to four stools per day is recommended to treat high levels of ammonia. Oral neomycin can be administered to reduce the amounts of ammonia-producing bacteria in the intestines. IV antibiotics do not seem to have the same positive effect as the enteral route.

Hepatorenal Syndrome

Hepatorenal syndrome (HRS) is the evidence of progressive, irreversible renal failure in the presence of liver failure. Usually this is characterized by renal vasoconstriction and activation of the renin-angiotensin-aldosterone system (RAAS). In addition, there is a sudden decrease in perfusion of the kidneys and accompanying oliguria. The blood urea nitrogen (BUN) and creatinine levels can be elevated. It is not uncommon for serum ammonia and bilirubin to also be elevated. Two types of HRS have been identified. Type 1 is aggressive with rapid impairment of renal flow. Often this is associated with spontaneous bacterial peritonitis (SBP), even after infections appear to be resolved. Life expectancy after diagnosis is about 10 weeks. Type 2 HRS exhibits moderate, more predictable reduction of glomerular filtration. This condition has about a three- to six-month survival time (Gines, Guevara, Arroyo, & Rodes, 2003).

LECITHIN-CHOLESTEROL ACYLTRANSFERASE DEFICIENCIES

Lecithin-cholesterol acyltransferase (LCAT) is an enzyme that is synthesized only in the liver and is essential for cholesterol transport in the serum, lipoprotein metabolism, and lipoprotein structure. This enzyme has an influence on high-density lipoprotein (HDL), LDL, and VLDL levels, which impact cardiovascular functioning and subsequent disease. Diseases that affect the amounts of LCAT in the body have a profound influence on processes requiring lipoproteins. Hereditary disorders that caused the absence of LCAT helped to understand some pathways of lipid metabolism. People with familial LCAT deficiency are mostly of Norwegian descent and owe this condition to a recessive gene that, when expressed, manifests hypercholesterolemia, hyperphospholipidemia (high free cholesterol and phospholipids), and hypertriglyceridemia. Liver failure, renal failure, anemia corneal opacities, and atherosclerosis are common. Treatment is with fat-restricted diets.

FATTY LIVER (HEPATIC STEATOSIS)

The liver is the major organ for processing and storing fats (lipids). The three major types of lipids in the body are cholesterol, triglycerides, and phospholipids (the principle serum phospholipid is phosphatidylcholine, commonly known as lecithin). Lipids are usually hydrophobic (insoluble in water). The liver helps the lipids become modified with proteins to be more water-soluble for transportation in the blood. These new compounds are called lipoproteins. Lipoproteins are necessary for energy, membrane integrity, and synthesis of a variety of molecules needed in metabolic processes throughout the body.

There is a constant cycling of fatty acids between the liver and adipose tissue. As free fatty acid (FFA) concentrations in the blood increase, there is a similar increase of triglycerides synthesized in the liver. However, the liver has a limited capacity to oxidize and reesterify the fatty acids into triglycerides and VLDL, and when the capacity is exceeded and lipids account for more than 5 percent of liver weight, fatty liver results (Ristig, Drechsler, & Powderly, 2005).

Etiology

Certain conditions that can increase circulating fatty acids include obesity, pregnancy, poorly controlled diabetes, malnutrition or kwashiorkor, corticosteroids, prolonged treatment with total parenteral nutrition (TPN), as a side effect of some bariatric surgeries, and exposure to liver-toxic chemicals, such as carbon tetrachloride and yellow phosphorus. However, the most common cause of fatty liver is chronic alcohol ingestion.

Pathophysiology

Alcohol interferes with fat metabolism by causing lipidemia (especially triglycerides), stimulating lipolysis, and increasing the output of VLDL. Alcohol also can cause further damage through lipid peroxidation, which releases free radicals thereby impairing membrane integrity of organelles within the hepatocytes as well as the membrane surrounding the cell (Rambaldi & Gluud, 2005).

Assessment with Clinical Manifestations

Fatty liver can be categorized into two types, depending on the histology. Macrovesicular fatty liver exhibits large fat droplets that balloon the liver cell and push the nucleus to the periphery of the cell. The liver does not limit the amount of FFA it stores from the breakdown (lipolysis) of adipose tissue. Alcoholism, diabetes, and obesity are the most common causes of this type of fatty liver. In microvesicular fatty liver cells, small fat droplets fill the cells, the nuclei are not displaced, and the cells have a foamy appearance. Organelles (mitochondria, lysosomes, and endoplasmic reticulum) within the cells are negatively affected. This is most often seen with pregnancy, Reye's syndrome, and certain drug toxicities such as with valproic acid, tetracycline, and salicylate (Cua & George, 2005).

Macrovesicular fatty liver does not necessarily impair the overall functioning of the liver. It can be a reversible condition, if the cause can be eliminated. The most common finding of fatty liver is **hepatomegaly** (enlarged liver, palpated below the level of the ribs). Many people with this condition are asymptomatic, although some might experience right upper quadrant pain, tenderness, jaundice, and fatigue. Microvesicular fatty liver can be much more concerning clinically. In the early stages, patients can exhibit fatigue, nausea, and vomiting. Jaundice, hypoglycemia, coma, and DIC can result (Ristig, et al., 2005).

Diagnostic Tests

Diagnosis is confirmed by liver biopsy. In addition to specific serum tests, CT and ultrasound can also be ordered.

Planning and Implementation

Nursing care is supportive, depending on the symptoms. In addition, the patients should be taught to:

- Avoid alcohol.
- Follow low fat diet or the diet that is prescribed.
- Monitor signs and symptoms for new medications that might be ordered in place of medications that could exacerbate the fatty liver condition.

HEPATIC ABSCESSES

Hepatic abscess is an area of infection in the liver caused by bacteria, amoeba, or protozoa. This liver complication is relatively common, particularly in undeveloped countries.

Epidemiology

In the United States, Canada, and other developed Western countries the incidence is low, occurring in 8 to 16 people out of 100,000 and in men more than women by a ratio of 2:1. The vast majority of these cases is caused by bacterial infection and is referred to as pyogenic hepatic abscess. In the developing world, hepatic abscesses are much more common and are usually caused by amoeba and protozoa. Incidence is difficult to determine because of lack of access to health care and lack of systematic reporting and recordkeeping.

Etiology

The introduction of pyogenic bacteria into the liver is often (30 percent) secondary to extrahepatic biliary obstruction, such as cholangitis, choledocholithiasis, or biliary-enteric anastomosis, causing an ascending infection into the liver. Sometimes the infection can originate somewhere in the abdomen, with seeding of bacteria (e.g., *Escherichia coli, Klebsiella pneumoniae,* and streptococcal species) into the portal vein, which delivers blood from the digestive organs to the liver. Conditions predisposing to this include appendicitis, diverticulitis, inflammatory bowel disease, and proctitis. Systemic septicemia may be responsible for transporting an infectious agent to the liver via the hepatic artery (as in bacterial endocarditis), although this is rare. Injuries, such as stab wounds, blunt trauma or biopsies, can introduce infective agents directly into the liver. Even neonates have been known to develop hepatic abscesses following umbilical venous cannulation (Aggarwal, 2003).

Reports of hepatic abscesses attributable to *Mycobacterium tuberculosis* are rare. This type of infection probably occurs where milk is unpasteurized or if a tuberculosis patient swallows infected sputum into the GI tract. Infection by ameba and protozoa can present after amoebic dysentery. The causative agent is usually *Entamoeba histolytica.*

Pathophysiology

Obstructive liver disease and portal hypertension can increase the permeability of the membranes in the intestines, allowing infecting agents to enter the portal vein. Bacteria and amoeba enter the capillary system in the liver, where a local infection or abscess can flourish. Once established in the liver tissue, the infecting agent destroys liver tissue, creating a necrotic cavity filled with pus, leukocytes, and products of cell destruction.

Assessment with Clinical Manifestations

Signs and symptoms include fever and right upper quadrant pain. In addition, the patient may experience chills, malaise, pleuritic chest pain, right shoulder pain, anorexia, weight loss, hepatomegaly, and jaundice.

Diagnostic Tests

Lab work would include LFTs, complete blood count (CBC), PT, and blood cultures. Stool cultures identify amebic dysentery. Chest and abdominal X-rays can indicate the presence of gas and can help rule out other diagnoses. Radionucleotide (liver scan) studies can identify abscesses greater than 2 mm. Ultrasound and CT scans are helpful not only in initial diagnoses, but also with guided percutaneous drainage. Percutaneous drainage removes the fluid from the abscess. This fluid can be used to analyze the offending agent so more specific anti-infective treatment can be initiated.

Nursing Diagnoses

Based on the information gathered, examples of nursing diagnoses in the patient with hepatic abscesses may include the following:

- Acute pain related to hepatic abscesses.
- Hyperthermia to hepatic abscesses related to hepatic abscesses.
- Ineffective breathing pattern related to hepatic abscesses.
- Impaired gas exchange related to hepatic abscesses.

Planning and Implementation

Treatment employs anti-infective therapy and drainage of the abscess, either by percutaneous catheter (guided by CT or ultrasound) or surgery (which carries greater risk). Before blood and drainage cultures come back, patients may be started on metronidazole and clindamycin or Cipro. Third generation cephalosporins or aminoglycosides might be used. Percutaneous drainage works best when only one abscess exists. Multiple abscesses are more difficult to drain percutaneously. Left untreated, abscesses can rupture, causing 100 percent mortality rates. Surgical drainage would be performed if other abdominal surgery is required (such as appendectomy or cholecystectomy) or if the location of the abscess in inaccessible any other way.

Poor prognosis is associated with the patient being over 70 years old, having multiple abscesses, having more than one offending infective agent responsible for the abscesses, having malignant disease, and immunosuppression.

Nursing care focuses on ascertaining an accurate history from the patient, including travel history and alcohol use. Because the percutaneous drainage procedure can predispose the patient to pneumothorax, hemorrhage, and leakage into the abdominal cavity, the nurse must be alert to changes in the patient's condition that would indicate evolving problems. This would include changes in vital signs, difficulty breathing, and increased abdominal or chest pain.

Evaluation of Outcomes

Potential patient outcomes for each of the example nursing diagnoses for the patient with hepatic abscesses are:

- Acute pain related to hepatic abscesses. The patient should verbalize an adequate relief of pain along with the ability to realistically cope with the pain if it is not completely relieved.
- Hyperthermia to hepatic abscesses. The patient maintains body temperature below 39° C (102.2° F).
- Ineffective breathing pattern related to hepatic abscesses. The patient's breathing pattern is maintained by eupnea, normal skin color, and regular respiratory rate or pattern.
- Impaired gas exchange related to hepatic abscesses. The patient maintains optimal gas exchange as evidenced by normal arterial blood gases (ABGs) and alert responsive mentation or no further reduction in mental status.

LIVER TRAUMA

The liver is a large, solid organ fixed under the diaphragm. Because of its size, location, and vascularity damage can occur during blunt or penetrating trauma. It is second only to the spleen in being injured in blunt trauma to the abdomen. Most liver trauma in the United States is attributable to motor vehicle crashes and fighting. More men than women are affected.

Etiology

Liver trauma should be suspected if there is a history of the patient receiving an impact from the eighth rib to the middle of the abdomen. Steering wheels and seat belts can cause pressure on the abdomen during a motor vehicle accident (MVA). Often liver trauma occurs in conjunction with other abdominal trauma. About 45 percent of people with blunt liver trauma also have injury to the spleen, and rib fractures occur with 33 percent. Gunshots, stab wounds, shrapnel, and broken ribs can cause penetrating trauma.

Pathophysiology

The pathophysiology of liver trauma is that damage to the liver causes it to not function in its normal fashion. Consequently, liver trauma causes such things as changes in its metabolic functions, coagulation capabilities, and potential changes in the processes of gluconeogenesis. In addition, blunt the liver is so vascular, blunt and penetrating injuries can cause significant bleeding. It is possible for bile to leak into the peritoneal cavity and cause bile peritonitis.

Assessment with Clinical Manifestations

The patient will often feel right upper quadrant tenderness, pain, and nonspecific rebound tenderness. Clinical signs of blood loss and hypovolemic shock should be assessed at regular intervals. These signs include tachycardia, hypotension, tachypnea, diaphoresis, guarding of the abdomen, distension, rigidity, confusion, pallor, and cool, clammy skin. Some of these signs could also be seen with kidney or spleen trauma.

Diagnostic Tests

Lab tests may be nonspecific. Although LFTs could indicate liver damage, increased levels may just be indicative of previously undetected disease, such as fatty liver or alcoholic cirrhosis. An X-ray of the chest and abdomen could be ordered to assess for skeletal trauma, which could indicate associated liver trauma. CT scanning is extremely helpful in localizing site and extent of injury. It is possible to assess active bleeding and avoid unnecessary surgery. The iminodiacetic acid (IDA) radionucleotide study can assess for bile leaks. Angiography can also aid in evaluating vascular integrity.

Nursing Diagnoses

Based on the information gathered, examples of nursing diagnoses in the patient with liver trauma may include the following:
- Ineffective breathing pattern related to liver trauma.
- Acute pain as related to liver trauma.
- Deficient fluid volume as related to liver trauma.
- Ineffective tissue perfusion as related to liver trauma.

Planning and Implementation

Interventions for liver trauma include such things as IV fluid replacement and blood products. Bleeding may be stopped by introducing a catheter into the jugular vein, threading it to the liver, and placing a stent. Transcatheter embolization may also stem the bleeding. An exploratory laparotomy, suture placement, and liver resection might be necessary to stop bleeding. However, recent studies show that 86 percent of liver injuries have stopped bleeding by the time the patient reaches surgery. Treatment tends toward conservative clinical evaluation of hemodynamic status. Most people with liver trauma (80 percent in adults and 97 percent in children) are treated nonoperatively. Recovery may take 3 months for mild trauma to 15 months for more severe trauma.

Evaluation of Outcomes

Potential patient outcomes for each of the example nursing diagnoses for the patient with liver trauma are:
- Ineffective breathing pattern related to liver trauma. The patient's breathing pattern is maintained by eupnea, normal skin color, and regular respiratory rate or pattern.
- Acute pain as related to liver trauma. The patient should verbalize an adequate relief of pain along with the ability to realistically cope with the pain if it is not completely relieved.
- Deficient fluid volume as related to liver trauma. The patient experiences adequate fluid volume and electrolyte balance as evidenced by urine output greater than 30 mL/hour, normotensive blood pressure (BP), heart rate (HR) 100 beats/minute, consistency of weight, and normal skin turgor.
- Ineffective tissue perfusion as related to liver trauma. The patient should maintain optimal tissue perfusion to the periphery, as evidenced by strong peripheral pulses, good capillary refill, and good movement.

CANCER OF THE LIVER

Both benign and malignant tumors can form in the liver. The tumor is named based on the type of tissue from which it originates. In general, men experience more primary liver cancer than women. There is an increased incidence with chronic infections of HBV and HCV, cirrhosis, hemochromatosis, smoking, obesity, aflatoxins (fungal carcinogens found in peanuts, soy, wheat, corn, and rice), and inherited diseases, such as Wilson's disease and alpha-antitrypsin deficiency. Anabolic steroids also carry a risk of hepatocellular carcinoma.

Benign tumors do not metastasize. However, they may require surgical intervention, because they can compress other surrounding tissue or have the potential to burst and bleed. Hemangiomas begin in the blood vessels and hepatoadenomas start in the hepatocytes. Abdominal tenderness, liver mass, and bleeding can be evident. Focal nodular hyperplasia (FNH) can originate in bile duct cells, connective tissue, and hepatocytes.

Pathophysiology

There are two basic types of liver cancer: primary and secondary. These two type of cancer of the liver are described in the following section. Further specifics regarding the pathophysiology of cancer are provided in chapter 15.

Primary Liver Cancer

The most common type (75 percent) of malignant tumors in adults is hepatocellular carcinoma (HCC), also called hepatoma, because it originates in the hepatocytes. This is usually seen with multiple nodules in people with cirrhosis. People with cirrhosis have a 40 times greater risk of developing primary liver cancer than others without cirrhosis. HBV and HCV are also associated with increased incidence. Cholangiocarcinomas, or intrahepatic cholangiocarcinomas, account for 10 to 20 percent of primary liver cancers and begin in the small bile ducts located within the liver. Ascending inflammation from the gallbladder, ulcerative colitis, or chronic parasitic infection can predispose a person to this type of cancer. Angiosarcomas and hemangiosarcomas are the malignant cancers that form in the intrahepatic blood vessels, often as a result of the person being exposed to environmental carcinogens, such as vinyl chloride or Thorotrast. They grow rapidly and are frequently discovered at a point where therapy is ineffective. Hepatoblastoma is a cancer found in children under the age of 4. About 70 percent can be treated with surgery and chemotherapy with good results (90 percent survival with early diagnosis and treatment) (Toyoda, et al., 2005).

Secondary Liver Cancer

The liver is a major site for metastases, harboring and growing cancerous cells that originated in some other part of the body, such as the breast or colon. In most developed countries, this secondary type of liver cancer is more common than cancer that originates in the liver itself. This is not necessarily true for developing countries, where people may be more exposed to nutritional deficiencies, fungal infections, parasites, pesticides, and other carcinogenic agents (Kim, et al, 2005).

Assessment with Clinical Manifestations

Often patients present with epigastric pain, fatigue, anorexia, weight loss, and right upper quadrant pain. Jaundice, ascites, bleeding, and PSE can follow. Diagnosis can be made with ultrasound guided needle biopsy. A liver scan may be done first.

Nursing Diagnoses

Based on the information gathered, examples of nursing diagnoses in the patient with cancer of the liver may include the following:

- Anticipatory grieving related to the diagnosis of cancer.
- Caregiver role strain related to the disability associated with the liver cancer.
- Acute pain related to abdominal pressure.
- Imbalanced nutrition, less than body requirements related to anorexia, faulty absorption, and metabolism.

Planning and Implementation

Unfortunately, many primary liver cancers are fairly resistant to treatment. Often the disease has progressed far enough at the time of diagnosis that surgical resection is not helpful. However, techniques of ablation try to destroy the tumor without removing it. Usually, a thin catheter guided by ultrasound or CT is introduced into the tumor. Radiofrequency ablation (RFA) uses high energy radio waves and high-frequency alternating current to heat and destroy cancer cells. Percutaneous ethanol injection uses ethanol or alcohol to kill tumor cells. Cryosurgery freezes the tumors with liquid nitrogen and kills the cells.

Another technique to treat tumors that cannot be removed is to cut them off from their blood supply by injecting materials into the hepatic artery that causes it to block off. The hepatic artery apparently feeds most of the cancer sites. The healthy liver gets one third of its blood supply from the hepatic artery and two thirds from the portal vein. The catheter is introduced in the groin and threaded up to the hepatic artery via angiography. This procedure can be risky if infection or cirrhosis has already compromised liver circulation. Sometimes the embolizing drugs will be impregnated with chemotherapy drugs to deliver a concentrated dose directly to the area close to the tumor **(chemoembolization)** (Toyoda, et al., 2005).

Radiation

External beam radiation can be used to shrink the cancer, but this is often used palliatively to relieve pressure. More specific information regarding radiation therapy can be found in chapter 15.

Pharmacology

Doxorubicin (Adriamycin, Doxil, or Rubex) is the single most effective drug. Cisplatin (Platinol) and 5-fluorouracil (5FU) may also be added. Researchers are looking for more drugs that could be more targeted against liver cancer. Direct hepatic artery infusion (HAI) can deliver chemotherapy directly to the hepatic artery, allowing for the most concentrated doses to reach the tumor before the drug is detoxified by the liver.

Evaluation of Outcomes

Potential patient outcomes for each of the example nursing diagnoses for the patient with liver cancer are:

- Anticipatory grieving related to the diagnosis of cancer. The patient or family verbalizes feelings and establishes and maintains functional support systems.
- Caregiver role strain related to the disability associated with the liver cancer. The caregiver demonstrates competence and confidence in performing the caregiver role by meeting care recipient's physical and psychosocial needs.
- Acute pain related to abdominal pressure. The patient should verbalize an adequate relief of pain along with the ability to realistically cope with the pain if it is not completely relieved.

- Imbalanced nutrition, less than body requirements related to anorexia, faulty absorption, and metabolism. The patient verbalizes and demonstrates selection of foods or meals that will achieve a cessation of weight loss and weighs within 10 percent of ideal body weight.

LIVER TRANSPLANTATION

The first human liver transplant was performed in 1963, but the first successful liver transplant was done in 1967. With the development of newer immunosuppressive drugs to fight rejection of the implanted organ, liver transplantation has been considered standard practice since 1983. Liver survival rates depend on whether the recipient had an acute or chronic condition prior to the implant. Current survival rates for one year following surgery are 90 percent and for 5 years are 85 percent.

Etiology

There are many diseases and conditions that could be treated with a liver transplant, but the most common cause in the United States is cirrhosis due to hepatitis C. The most common reason for children to have a liver transplant is biliary atresia. In addition, reasons for treatment using liver transplantation are such things as alcoholic cirrhosis, cancer of the liver, ulcerative colitis, Crohn's disease, and various metabolic diseases. Over 17,000 people are on the waiting list to receive liver transplants at any one time.

Types of Liver Transplants

Two types of liver transplants can be performed, orthotopic and auxiliary. Orthotopic liver transplant, where the patient's own liver is removed entirely, is the most common type of transplant. This actually involves three operations:

- The removal of the donor liver, or in the case of a live donor, part of the liver. In the case of a cadaveric liver, the organ is usually removed at the institution where the donor died and is transported to the transplant center. For a living donor, the donor is usually in an adjacent operating suite. It is imperative to preserve the blood vessels and bile ducts to connect with the recipient's blood vessels and bile ducts. After removal, the liver is cooled, the blood is flushed out, and a preservative solution is instilled to replace the donor's blood. There can be ischemic damage to the donated liver during the cooling process.
- The removal of the recipient's liver is the most difficult operation of the three operations. People with liver disease needing transplant have difficulty with clotting, so they have a tendency to bleed. The portal hypertension and cirrhotic scarring makes dissection difficult.
- The implantation of the donated liver into the recipient. Once the blood vessels and bile ducts are connected the new liver should begin functioning. However, it is not unusual for there to be continued bleeding follow ing surgery, and about 20 percent of patients need to be taken back to surgery to remove blood that has oozed into the abdominal cavity.

Auxiliary transplantation is a procedure that was developed in the 1980s and involves leaving part or all of the patient's liver in place and grafting in a healthy whole or partial liver, either from a cadaver or live donor. The auxiliary liver or liver segment regenerates and begins functioning. This type of surgery is used for patients who have genetic defects such as Crigler-Najjar syndrome and only one gene is unable to perform adequately, but that defect compromises the whole liver. In a syndrome such as this, the patient's own liver is able to function normally except for manufacturing the bilirubin gluconate, so problems with clotting factors and fibrosis are not present. The recipient is not totally dependent on the donated liver. Auxiliary transplantation can also be done in the event of major trauma to the liver, drug reactions, and fulminant liver failure, where there is a possibility for the patient's own liver to eventually recover. If the patient's own liver begins to work again, the transplant would not be necessary, and the patient would be able to stop the immunosuppressant drugs. It is technically difficult to attach the new liver to the patient's blood supply. And most postsurgical complications occur at the points of anastomosis.

Liver Donors

The live donor transplant program was developed in the late 1980s. There are several advantages. First it provides an organ for a specific individual. The operation can be planned for a time when both the donor and the recipient are in best health. The progression of liver disease and consequent deterioration may be avoided. The stress of waiting for an organ and living with the anticipation of sudden surgery is relieved. However, there are risks to being a living organ donor. The primary risks include the complications of surgery (Pierie, Muzikansky, Tanabe, & Ott, 2005).

Donor organs can be procured in one of two ways: (a) cadaveric organ, and (b) live donor. The specifics of both types of donor organs are provided in Box 51-8.

BOX 51-8

CADAVERIC AND LIVE DONOR METHODS OF PROCUREMENT

- Cadaveric organs come from people who have been declared brain dead, but other vital organs are healthy and have been adequately perfused. Sometimes the whole liver is transplanted into the recipient. However, the donor liver can be split, and the smaller left lobe implanted into a smaller person or child, and the larger right lobe would go to the larger recipient. Only about 4,000 cadaveric livers are available each year, so splitting the liver is beneficial for more patients but may be technically more difficult surgically.
- Live donor (living donor liver transplants [LDLT]) organs are usually donated to related family members (parents, siblings, or other relatives); however, organs can be donated by people who are not related, provided that the recipient is an appropriate match. The ability of the liver to regenerate makes it possible for the donor's and recipient's livers to grow to normal size after the transplantation surgery.

Liver Recipients

Criteria for receiving a donated liver is rigorously defined by the United Network for Organ Sharing (UNOS). This organization developed an online database, keeping track of all individuals waiting for any kind of transplant, matching donated organs to the list of waiting recipients, and managing time sensitive data. UNOS is a nationwide database that assists in the procurement of organs as well as the prioritization of patients around the United States. This prioritization utilizes the model for end-stage liver disease (MELD) and the pediatric end-stage liver disease (PELD) scores, which have replaced the older Child-Pugh score for predicting outcomes for survival after surgical procedures for end-stage liver disease (Ship, 2005). The conditions for prioritizing organ recipients are provided in Box 51-9.

When an appropriate match has been identified and offered to the institution where the transplant will take place, the institution has only one hour to accept the organ before it is offered to the next appropriate candidate on the waiting list. There is a great deal of stress and anticipation to being on the waiting list, and the nurse can assist the patient and family to deal with these issues during this time.

BOX 51-9

CONDITIONS TO PRIORITIZE ORGAN RECIPIENTS

- Appropriate parameters are met regarding size of the liver, ABO compatibility and MELD or PELD score.
- The amount of time spent on the waiting list.
- The degree of medical urgency.
  1. Candidates who have a life expectancy of less than seven days would include patients with fulminant liver failure.
  2. A person who has received a liver transplant in the last seven days, but the transplanted liver is nonfunctioning (defined as an aspartate aminotransferase (AST) greater than or equal to 5,000 and an international normalized ratio (INR) greater than 2.5 or acidosis with pH less than 7.3 or lactate of two times normal.
  3. Hepatic artery thrombosis in the first seven days of liver implant.
  4. Decompensated Wilson's disease.

Patients are asked to submit a complete list of pagers and telephone numbers to the transplant center so that individual can be notified in the event that a cadaveric liver becomes available. Patients also need to have travel plans worked out in advance in addition to how to pay for transportation. It is also important to keep as healthy as possible before transplant. This includes avoiding alcohol, eating a healthy diet, taking appropriate medications, avoiding recreational drugs, and following medical advice (Box 51-10). In addition, patients need to avoid other people with illnesses. Stress reduction and physical activity are also important (Pierie, et al., 2005).

Diagnostic Tests

All potential recipients and live donors undergo many tests, including psychological assessment to evaluate the decision to proceed with the transplant process. The living donor is evaluated for good general health, compatible blood type, and an altruistic motive for donating this gift of life. Tests for the donor include an abdominal ultrasound, MRI, blood tests, pulmonary function tests, ECG, and an exercise test.

Nursing Diagnoses

Based on the information gathered, examples of nursing diagnoses in the patient with liver transplantation may include the following:

- Risk for imbalanced body temperature related to complications of liver transplantation.
- Fear and anxiety related to actual or potential lifestyle changes.
- Knowledge deficit related to self-care and risk prevention.
- Ineffective coping related to anxiety, lower activity level and the inability to perform normal activities of daily living.

Planning and Implementation

The patient is notified when a liver becomes available. Usually the recipient carries a pager at all times so that the transplant center can notify the recipient of the new liver immediately. If the donated liver is from a live donor, both the donor and the recipient are in surgery at the same time. Usually the patient is in the hospital from one to three weeks.

Usually, the donor's first night after surgery is spent in the intensive care unit (ICU), then the donor is transferred to a specialized unit for recovery.

BOX 51-10

DISQUALIFICATION OF A TRANSPLANT RECIPIENT

Several conditions would eliminate or disqualify a person from being a transplant recipient. These include:

- Continuing to use alcohol or illegal drugs prior to surgery or being at high risk to begin engaging in these behaviors after surgery.
- Demonstrated noncompliance with previous medical care.
- Lack of support people to care for the patient after the operation.
- Advanced cancer of the liver or cancer that has metastasized to the liver. However, early discovery of primary liver cancer that is localized in the liver may be treated with transplantation.
- Advanced disease of the kidney, heart, vasculature, or lungs.
- Human immunodeficiency virus (HIV) or acquired immune deficiency syndrome (AIDS)

The usual hospital stay is four to seven days. Donors are usually recovered enough to go back to work in three to six weeks and are fully recovered in six to eight weeks. Expenses for the donor should be covered by the recipient's health insurance. Some complications that can occur after donation include unregulated proliferation of liver tissue and failure to regenerate new liver tissue, resulting in small for size syndrome.

Postoperative Care

In the postoperative period after transplantation, the most common problems include temporary decreased liver function, bleeding and hemorrhage, acute renal failure, bile leakage, hepatic artery thrombosis (HAT), fluid and electrolyte imbalances, infection and abscess formation, hepatitis recurrence, and acute graft rejection of the newly implanted organ.

Monitoring in the immediate postoperative period includes strict intake and output, paying special attention to measuring output from all drains placed during surgery. Abdominal ultrasound is performed often to assess for HAT, where a clot forms in the hepatic artery. These can be treated with medications or possibly surgery. A drainage catheter may be placed to manage bile drainage. Bacterial infection and the recurrence of HBV or HCV are other possible complications. While in the hospital, particular attention must be paid to vital signs for early signs of infection or rejection.

There is a high-risk period after transplantation that lasts for about three months. During this time it is important to avoid situations where the patient could be exposed to infection. This would include avoiding swimming in lakes and pools, avoid closed conditions, such as being in a movie theater, and avoiding adults and children who are sick or who have been immunized with live vaccine. The liver recipient is especially susceptible to infection because of the antirejections medications and because the liver is still establishing itself in the body. Throughout the rest of the recipient's life, the liver will be assessed for symptoms of graft rejection and the use of immunosuppressants will be continuous. It is imperative to abstain from alcohol. Recreational drug use should likewise be avoided. The patient should not self-medicate with over-the-counter drugs, because some of these could be hepatotoxic. Other long range problems can include diabetes, hypertension, and hypercholesterolemia. Usually the patient has monthly blood tests and assessment for organ rejection. Signs and symptoms of rejection include nausea, pain, fever, and jaundice.

Blood tests (serum bilirubin, transaminases, alkaline phosphatase, and prolonged PT) are usually ordered to assess liver function. A liver biopsy is necessary to determine if the liver is actively being rejected. If the liver was previously damaged from HCV or HBV, it is possible for the new liver to develop hepatitis C or B after the transplant. However, the HCV damage to the liver develops over a long period of time, and there are great benefits of having a transplanted liver (Pierie, et al., 2005).

Most patients can resume normal activity in 6 to 12 months. Women who have received liver transplants can become pregnant, but must be monitored closely, and the risk for premature birth is higher. Usually breast feeding is discouraged because the immunosuppressant medications can be transmitted to the baby through the breast milk.

Pharmacology

Immunosuppressive drugs used to decrease rejection of the new liver have problems with long-term use. In addition to the omnipresent threat of infection, these complications can include:

- Corticosteroids (prednisone) can predispose to osteoporosis, hyperglycemia, edema, and fluid and electrolyte problems.
- Cyclosporin (Neoral, Sandimmune, or Gengraf) can increase hypertension, growth of body hair, and kidney damage.
- FK-506 can produce headaches, tremors, diarrhea, nausea, kidney dysfunction, hyperglycemia, and hyperkalemia.

- Tacrolimus (Prograf) can cause seizures, GI bleeding, and anaphylaxis in addition to the side effects of ascites, hypertension, urinary tract infection, pruritus, rash, anemias, and generalized pain.
- Sirolimus (Rapamune) can cause leukopenia, thrombocytopenia, hyperlipidemia, arthralgias, and tremors.
- Mycophenolate mofetil (CellCept) can cause GI bleeding, diarrhea, vomiting, leukopenia, and sepsis.
- Basiliximab (Simulect) problems include heart failure, anaphylaxis, and wound complications.
- Daclizumab (Zenapax) can cause pulmonary edema.
- Azathioprine (Imuran) is related to serum sickness and can cause the patient to experience fever and chills, nausea, vomiting, anorexia, and pancreatitis.

Evaluation of Outcomes

Potential patient outcomes for each of the example nursing diagnoses for the patient with liver transplantation are:

- Risk for imbalanced body temperature related to complications of liver transplantation. The patient maintains body temperature within a normal range.
- Fear and anxiety related to actual or potential lifestyle changes. The patient should be able to recognize the signs of anxiety, demonstrate positive coping mechanisms, and describe a reduction in the level of anxiety experienced.
- Knowledge deficit related to self-care and risk prevention. The patient should demonstrate motivation to learn, identify perceived learning needs, and verbalize an understanding of desired content.
- Ineffective coping related to anxiety, lower activity level and the inability to perform normal activities of daily living. Patient identifies own maladaptive coping behaviors, available resources, and support systems, describes or initiates alternative coping strategies, and describes positive results from new behaviors.

DISEASES OF THE BILIARY TRACT

The biliary tract is devoted to transporting bile through the liver into the gallbladder and continuing on into the digestive tract. **Cholestasis** is any condition that impedes bile flowing freely through the bile ducts. This failure of bile flow can originate within the liver (intrahepatic) or beyond the liver (extrahepatic). When the bile is not flowing normally, patients usually exhibit:

- Clay-colored stools (because the bile does not reach the intestines where it is converted to urobilinogen, which normally gives feces the typical brown color).
- Dark urine (because an excess of bilirubin is in the circulation and is excreted through the kidneys).
- Jaundice (yellow skin and mucous membranes) and icterus (yellow sclera) also result from the increase in serum bilirubin.

Cholelithiasis

Cholelithiasis or gallstones, is a common problem, affecting about 16 to 20 million people in the United States, or 20 percent of the population. At least one million are diagnosed each year.

Epidemiology

Cholelithiasis is more common in people of northern European descent. Interestingly, 75 percent of elderly Pima Indians have evidence of gallstones.

Etiology

Cholelithiasis is more common in women, and the incidence is related to levels of estrogen. There are more reports of this condition with women on hormone (estrogen) replacement therapy (HRT or ERT) and those who are pregnant. The older, higher dose estrogen birth control pill had a higher incidence of gallstones associated with it. Medications that lower serum cholesterol can increase the occurrence of cholelithiasis. There can be familial tendencies for this condition, but this could also reflect a common diet, lifestyle, and genetics. Obesity is also related to cholelithiasis (Townes, 2004).

Pathophysiology

The most common gallstones are formed from cholesterol, which is a major component of bile. Stones may also be attributed to the calcification of bile pigments, but this is not as common. Stones can block or partially block the outlet of the gallbladder or move through the cystic duct into the common bile duct. **Cholangitis** is the inflammation of the bile duct and is usually attributable to the presence of gallstones. When the bile ducts become inflamed, there is increased edema, which, in turn, affects the circulation to the gallbladder by putting mechanical pressure on the capillaries. Increased edema can increase the permeability of the cell membranes and predispose the tissues to infection from bacteria from the gut. When intestinal bacteria infiltrates the gallbladder and ducts, an infection can be established. If the infection moves in the direction of the liver, it is called **ascending cholangitis.** If pus is produced in the biliary tract, it is called **suppurative cholangitis** (Townes, 2004).

Assessment with Clinical Manifestations

Most often the patient presents with complaints of pain in the midepigastric area, which can radiate to the right scapular region, anorexia, nausea, and vomiting. However, many people are asymptomatic, and the diagnosis of cholelithiasis is made incidentally when the patient has other tests performed. Fever, tachycardia, and hypotension can indicate the presence of infection, which can make the condition more serious.

Diagnostic Tests

The LFTs are often normal. Stones do show up on X-rays. Ultrasound is the most useful diagnostic test because the presence of stones, the motility of the stones, and the thickness of the gallbladder wall can all be assessed. This helps to determine if there is blockage in the biliary tract and if there is inflammation of the gallbladder secondary to the irritation of the stones.

Nursing Diagnoses

Based on the information gathered, examples of nursing diagnoses in the patient with cholelithiasis may include the following:

- Acute pain secondary to biliary obstruction.
- Ineffective coping related to nausea.
- Deficient knowledge related to diagnosis of cholelithiasis.

Planning and Implementation

The primary methods of treating cholelithiasis are surgery and medications. In addition, recommended nutritional programs with a low-fat diet, exercise, and follow-up with patients who have biliary tract manifestations are implemented.

Surgery

The treatment of choice is **laparoscopic cholecystectomy,** which is a surgical procedure using laparoscopy to remove the gallbladder. This operation was introduced in 1988, has a faster recovery time, fewer complications, and fewer bile duct injuries than the open cholecystectomy. In this operation, a small incision is made at the umbilicus plus three other puncture sites. Carbon dioxide gas may be pumped into the abdominal cavity to help to separate the organs, or there may be lifting and spreading devices that achieve the same effect without the gas. A laparoscope with video camera and laser technology is introduced. The gallbladder is dissected from the surrounding organs, drained of fluid and stones, and removed through the incision at the umbilicus. Only about 5 percent of laparoscopic attempts fail and culminate in open cholecystectomy. This happens when the gallbladder is anatomically inaccessible, the dissection to separate it from the surrounding organs is unsuccessful, or the surgeon is unable to remove the stones from the biliary tract. It should be noted that even after cholecystectomy, gallstones can still form in the biliary tree (Lledo, et al., 2005).

The open cholecystectomy can be performed when the laparoscopic technique fails, there are stones that are inaccessible to the laparoscope (Figure 51-5), or other surgeries are required at the same time (as in treating trauma). The surgeon makes an incision in the upper right quadrant beneath the ribs. Often the bile ducts and other abdominal organs will be explored. The gallbladder is dissected and removed, the cystic duct is ligated and a T-tube is inserted into the common bile duct to keep it patent. A Jackson-Pratt (JP) tube can be left in at the surgical site to drain fluid from around the area that housed the gallbladder.

Pharmacology

Nonsurgical treatment is possible utilizing bile salts, which help to dissolve the stones and get them back in circulation. This option is not popular, because it takes a long time to dissolve the stones, and there is more of a possibility that the problem will return. The drugs used in bile acid therapy are ursodeoxycholic acid (URSO, ursodiol, or Actigall) alone or in combination with chenodeoxycholic

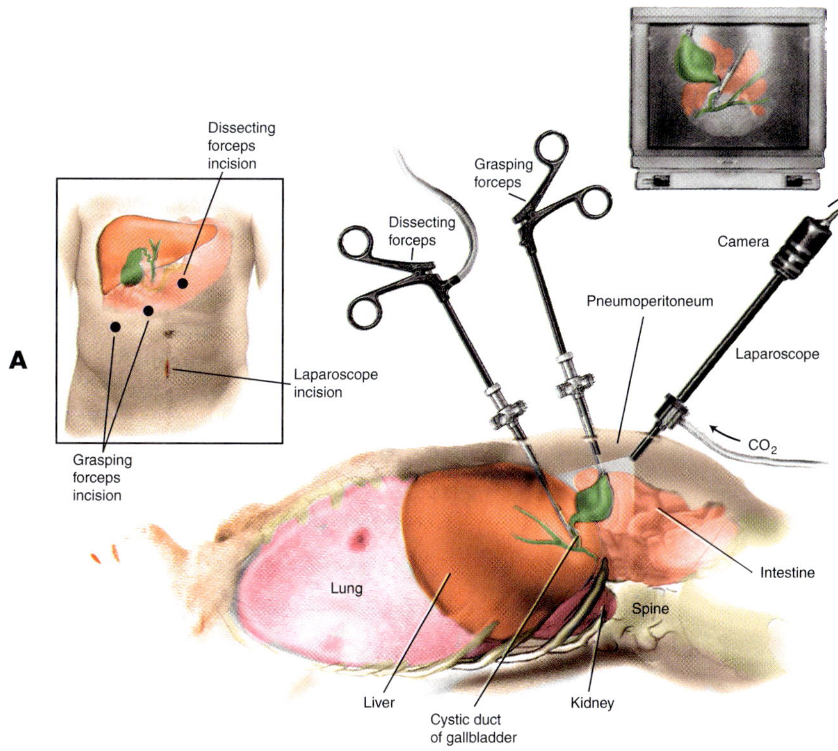

Figure 51-5 Laparoscopic cholecystectomy: A. Lateral view.

Continued

B

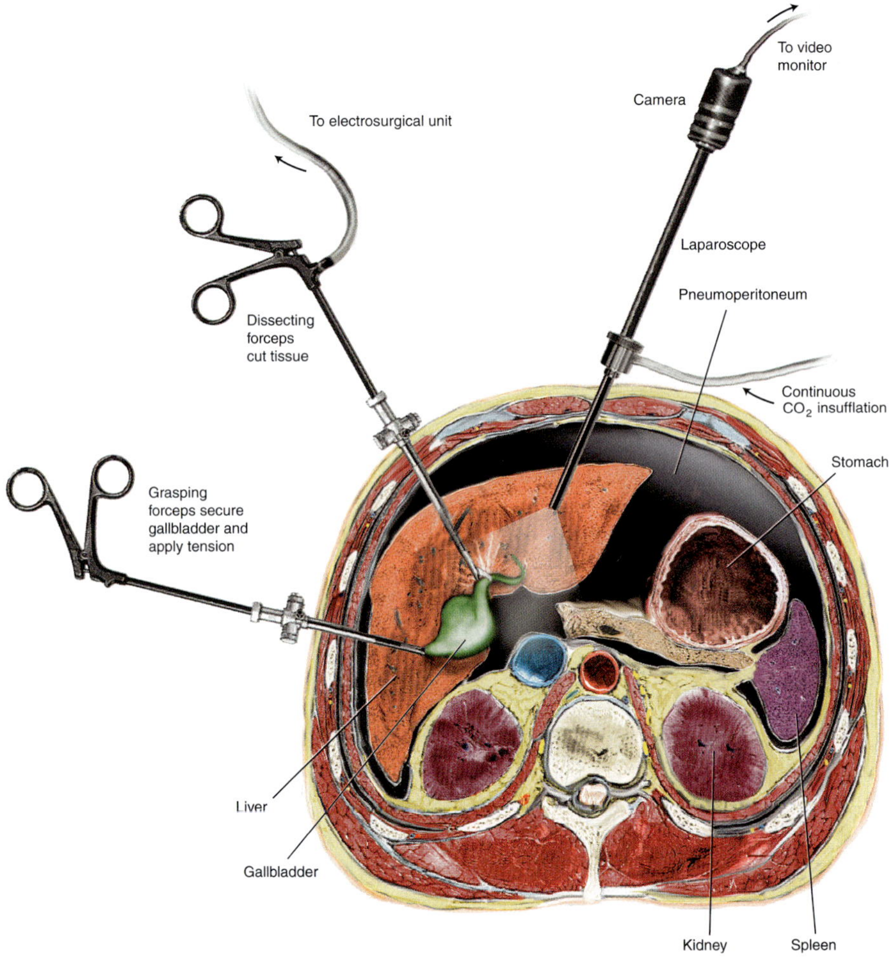

Figure 51-5—cont'd Laparoscopic cholecystectomy: B. Cross-sectional view.

acid (chenodiol, Chenix, or CDCA). Ursodiol may be used to prevent gallstones in people with a higher propensity for developing the condition.

Evaluation of Outcomes

Potential patient outcomes for each of the example nursing diagnoses for the patient with cholelithiasis are:

- Acute pain secondary to biliary obstruction. The patient should verbalize an adequate relief of pain along with the ability to realistically cope with the pain if it is not completely relieved.
- Ineffective coping related to nausea. The patient identifies own maladaptive coping behaviors, available resources and support systems, describes or initiates alternative coping strategies, and describes positive results from new behaviors.
- Deficient knowledge related to diagnosis of cholelithiasis. The patient should demonstrate motivation to learn, identify perceived learning needs, and verbalize an understanding of desired content.

Cholecystitis

Cholecystitis is the inflammation of the gallbladder. This can be acute or chronic and occurs in about 20 million people in the United States. In acute cholecystitis, gallstones are most commonly implicated, but bacteria can also cause the gallbladder wall to become irritated, a condition that is exacerbated by the increased presence of bile. Swelling and edema restricts the outflow of bile, which causes the distension of the gallbladder. Increased distension can alter the integrity and microcirculation of the gallbladder wall, causing sloughing, and possibly necrosis and gangrene. Perforation, rupture and peritonitis are possibilities. Chronic cholecystitis advances from the acute phase where the gallbladder is irritated and inflamed to the establishment of fibrotic tissue and contracted, inflexible capacity of the organ. This can be attributed to:

- Stones causing irritation and obstruction.
- Bacterial infection.
- Circulatory problems secondary to trauma, tumor impingement, shock, surgery, or dehydration.
- Pancreatitis (inflammation of the pancreas) can result if the biliary tract becomes inflamed, and the circulation or emptying of the pancreas is affected.

The epidemiology, etiology, pathophysiology, diagnostic tests, and nursing diagnoses are the same for cholecystitis as for cholelethiasis.

Assessment with Clinical Manifestations

Acute cholecystitis usually presents with pain and abdominal discomfort, which may be referred to the right shoulder. Because bile obstruction is not common, jaundice is not usually present. With chronic cholecystitis, inflammation of the organ is followed by fibrosis. Bile obstruction is more common and can result in inflammation of the bile ducts (cholangitis), the pancreas (pancreatitis), and jaundice. Increased bile salts lead to pruritus (itching).

The nurse should assess for history of pain and dietary discomforts, sleep patterns, and exercise routines. ERT and other medicines need to be assessed. The physical examination often reveals abdominal tenderness on palpation with rebound tenderness. **Steatorrhea** (fatty stools that float) may also be present along with the other classic cholestatic signs. In addition, nursing measures and evaluation of outcomes are the same as for cholelithiasis.

> **Skills 360°**
>
> **Clinical Manifestations of Primary Biliary Cirrhosis**
>
> The nurse should observe the patient with complications of primary biliary cirrhosis for the following manifestations:
>
> - Cholangitis with fever, chills, and pain.
> - Ascending bacterial cholangitis.
> - Septic shock is possible.
> - Cholelithiasis is frequent.
> - Problems related to fat metabolism and fat soluble vitamin deficiencies. Osteopenia and osteoporosis may occur, possibly due to vitamin D deficiency. About 12 percent of patients have vitamin D deficiency. Increased bleeding problems are associated with decreased vitamin K. Vitamin A may also be low, but overreplacement can also lead to problems with liver toxicity.
>
> *Adapted from Townes, D. A. (2004). Biliary tract disease.* Emergency Medicine, *36(2), 17–19.*

Primary Sclerosing Cholangitis

Primary sclerosing cholangitis (PSC) is of autoimmune etiology. Bile ducts within and outside the liver become inflamed and develop scar tissue. This results in the obstruction of bile flow. PSC is associated with ulcerative colitis and Crohn's disease and may share a common autoimmune mechanism. The incidence is greater with men than women. PSC often develops the fibrotic changes characteristic of cirrhosis. In addition to autoimmune causes, toxins and viruses are also being researched. Initial presentation of the problem includes jaundice and itching. Malabsorption of fats is evident by steatorrhea and a decrease in fat-soluble vitamins. Infection can set in from bacteria ascending the bile ducts from the intestines. Diagnosis is primarily by ERCP. MRI can also be helpful. LFTs, renal panel, and electrolytes would be ordered. The fat content in feces may be assessed. Medical treatment usually includes ursodiol, antipruritics, antibiotics, and fat-soluble vitamin supplements. Liver transplant is the only surgical option.

Primary Biliary Cirrhosis

Primary biliary cirrhosis (PBC) is characterized by inflammation and subsequent destruction of the bile ducts. Nine out of 10 cases are middle-aged women, although the incidence is low (10 to 12 cases in one million diagnosed per year). Effects of hereditary factors, hormones, and the immune system are implicated in the incidence of PBC, because the occurrence of PBC is greater with people who have osteoporosis, arthritis, or thyroid problems. Although the disease is rare, it is more likely to occur in families where one relative has already been diagnosed (Prince, Christensen, & Gluud, 2005).

Pathophysiology

Pathology of primary biliary cirrhosis seems to involve the immune system, although the exact mechanism is unknown. Autoimmune factors can cause progressive inflammation. Destruction of the bile ducts predisposes to impaired transportation of bile from the liver. This congestion of bile creates cholestasis (decreased or inability for bile to flow through the bile ducts in the liver), which causes further hepatic injury and fibrosis.

Assessment with Clinical Manifestations

Patients are often asymptomatic in the early stages, but can exhibit increased alkaline phosphatase levels during routine screening tests for physicals. The most common complaints are fatigue and pruritus. Fever, abdominal pain, hepatomegaly, splenomegaly, and hyperpigmentation may also be present. Jaundice, variceal bleeding ascites, and encephalopathy are possible in the later course of the disease. At the time of diagnosis, many people do not have disease that has progressed to the cirrhosis stage, although untreated, destruction of the cells in the bile ducts will progress to fibrosis, and cirrhosis is evident.

Diagnostic Tests

Diagnostic tests include LFTs (especially alkaline phosphatase), PT, and antimitochondrial antibodies (AMA), all of which can be increased. Ultrasound and or CT scan are done to rule out biliary obstruction, and liver biopsy can be done to confirm the diagnosis. Magnetic resonance cholangiography may be employed. The ERCP is more definitive in diagnosing this condition, but it may be technically difficult to perform this test because of the sclerosing of the biliary ducts. Nursing diagnoses and evaluation of outcomes are the same as cholangitis.

Planning and Implementation

Complications include cholangitis with accompanying fever, chills, and pain. Septic shock could result. Aggressive antibiotic therapy would be required to treat this condition. Biliary tree strictures can be treated with cholangiography with balloon dilation of the narrowed duct. Biliary stone disease is possible. If the stones are only found in the gallbladder, the gallbladder can be removed. It may be necessary to remove the stone through sphincterotomy. Cholangiocarcinoma develops in about 10 to 15 percent of people with primary sclerosing cholangitis.

Pharmacology

Even if a patient is asymptomatic, it is important to treat the condition so that disease progression is arrested. Drug treatment focuses on reducing the immune response, modifying cholestasis, treating bacterial infections, controlling symptoms, and decreasing fibrogenesis. The medications to manage primary biliary cirrhosis are ursodeoxycholic acid (URSO, Ursodiol, or Actigall), which is a naturally occurring bile acid that can help to decrease the amounts of other more toxic bile acids; corticosteroids, which can be helpful in decreasing the autoimmune activity; cyclosporin, which is an antirejection drug, but can cause hypertension and kidney dysfunction; immunosuppressants (e.g., methotrexate, chlorambucil), which may be offered, but these can be damaging to the bone marrow; colchicine, an antigout agent, which interferes with white blood cells in initiating and perpetuating the immune response; aggressive antibiotic therapy; cholestyramine (Questran), which is usually recommended to control itching; and antiretroviral therapy (lamivudine or Combivir), which may be effective in arresting the disease (Broyles, et al., 2007).

Surgery

Surgical treatment for primary biliary cirrhosis could include:

- Cholangiography with balloon dilation of narrowed ducts
- Cholecystectomy
- Removal of gallstones through sphincterectomy
- Liver transplantation, which may be the only option for definitive treatment of end-stage disease (Allen, 2005)

Alternative Therapy

Alternative therapy for PBC can include treatment with silymarin. Silymarin is the active ingredient in milk thistle *(Silybum marianum)*. It is thought to protect the liver from toxic substances.

Cancer of the Gallbladder and Bile Ducts

Cancer of the gallbladder is rare. Incidence is higher with people who experience cholelithiasis, which is higher in Native American and Hispanic populations.

Epidemiology

Risk factors for cancer of the gallbladder include age (usually people are over age 60 when diagnosed with gallbladder cancer), bile duct abnormalities (this can predispose to increased irritation of the organs that come in contact with the toxins from the liver), cigarette smoke, chemicals (especially asbestos and azotoluene), and obesity. Women are twice as likely as men to get gallbladder cancer.

Cancer of the biliary ducts is also rare. Risk factors include primary sclerosing cholangitis (cholangiocarcinoma develops in about 10 to 15 percent of people with primary sclerosing cholangitis), ulcerative colitis, congenital abnormalities of the biliary tract (such as biliary atresia), gallstones in the bile ducts, parasitic infections, and toxic materials. In contrast to gallbladder cancer, men are slightly more likely to develop cancer of the bile ducts than women.

Assessment with Clinical Manifestations

Clinical manifestations for cancer of the gallbladder are varied. In addition, the symptomatology may be minimal to severe. Some of the manifestations may be: abdominal pain, especially in the upper right quadrant, anorexia, weight loss, nausea and vomiting, jaundice, pruritus, and an enlarged gallbladder.

Pathophysiology

Cancers within the gallbladder usually begin in the lining of the wall and are adenocarcinomas. Cancers that start in the bile ducts are cholangiocarcinomas. It is thought that the cells in the gallbladder and bile ducts can be damaged by toxins that come from the liver. Cholelithiasis and cholestasis may establish conditions that make these toxins more irritating, progressing to cancer.

Diagnostic Tests

Diagnostic tests include LFTs, ultrasound, CT scan, MRI, and ERCP. Laparoscopy and biopsies may be performed. However, many cancers are diagnosed after the gallbladder has already been removed for treatment of cholelithiasis. The nursing diagnoses and evaluation of outcomes is the same as those for cholangitis.

If the gallbladder has not been removed prior to diagnosing, the cancer may be designated as:

- Resectable, which means that the cancer is contained within the walls of the organ and has not invaded surrounding organs or traveled in the lymph to the nodes.
- Unresectable, which indicates that the cancer has spread to other organs, such as the liver stomach, pancreas, or intestines, and surgical removal would not be beneficial. The cancer could also invade the lymph system.
- Recurrent, which refers to cancer that has been treated or resected but reoccurs at a later time in other tissue.

Planning and Implementation

Treatment is generally by surgery. In addition to removing the areas of cancerous growth, stents can be placed as a palliative measure to keep the biliary tract open. When the tumor is too close to other blood vessels or vital organs, bypass surgeries may help to alleviate some symptoms but are not curative. Radiation and chemotherapy do not have a lot to offer at this time (Allen, 2005).

PANCREATITIS

Pancreatitis is the inflammation of the pancreas, a specialized digestive gland that has both endocrine and exocrine functions. Pancreatitis can take two forms, acute and chronic. Both disorders of the pancreas can be complicating to patients who have these conditions. There are complications for both anomalies of the pancreas and can provide a challenge to the health care providers as management strategies are performed.

Acute Pancreatitis

Acute pancreatitis is a serious but reversible condition that may become chronic if permanent scarring and damage to the pancreatic tissue occurs. It affects about 80,000 people each year in the United States. Mild cases of acute pancreatitis can resolve with resting the gut (NPO), IV hydration and electrolyte replacement, pain control, and bed rest. However, in about 20 percent of cases, serious problems can develop and involve local and systemic damage to tissues. There is a 5 to 10 percent mortality rate in hospitalized patients.

Etiology

Pancreatitis has many causes and a wide variety of resulting complications. The major causes of pancreatitis include: gallstone disease, alcoholism, infections (e.g., ascariasis, clonorchiasis, mumps, toxoplasmosis, coxsackievirus, cytomegalovirus, or tuberculosis), medications (e.g., azathioprine, mercaptopurine, sulfonamides, salicylates, furosemide, or methyldopa), trauma, obstruction, duodenal diseases, toxins, and genetic diseases that predispose the patient to cholelithiasis and obstruction of the biliary ducts, and cystic fibrosis.

Pathophysiology

The pathophysiology for pancreatitis relates to either the presence of gallstones or alcoholism. However, in about 10 to 30 percent of cases, no cause can be identified and is considered idiopathic. Whatever the initial cause of the inflammation, the exocrine enzymes that are produced in the acinar cells of the pancreas and help with digesting protein, carbohydrates, and fats can be prematurely activated, exacerbating the process leading to autodigestion of the surrounding tissues and more inflammation, edema, and ultimately necrosis. The edema compromises the microcirculation of the pancreas and initiates the release of cytokines, such as tumor necrosis factor (TNF), interleukin-1, and platelet-activating factor, all of which contribute to further damage in the pancreas and in other tissues.

Assessment with Clinical Manifestations

With the release of these cytokines and the exocrine and endocrine (insulin, glucagon, and VIP) enzymes into the bloodstream, systemic complications can quickly escalate. Some systemic complications include atelectasis, pleural effusion, acute respiratory distress syndrome (ARDS), respiratory failure, cardiovascular problems with hypovolemia, hypotension and shock, renal failure, coagulation complications, metabolic complications (e.g., hypocalcemia or hyperglycemia), GI problems, encephalopathy, and peripheral fat necrosis.

Clinical manifestations of pancreatitis include abdominal pain that radiates to the back, guarding and rebound tenderness, nausea and vomiting, and abdominal distension. Depending on some of the underlying problems, fever, tachycardia, tachypnea, and hypotension may also be present.

Diagnostic Tests

Laboratory tests include serum amylase and lipase. Both of these are increased with acute pancreatitis. An increased ALT can be indicative of gallstones, which could be associated with pancreatitis. CT scanning is the most useful test for determining the presence of pancreatitis as differentiated from other abdominal issues. Ultrasound can help diagnose the presence of gallstones.

Nursing Diagnoses

Based on the information gathered, examples of nursing diagnoses in the patient with acute pancreatitis may include the following:

- Activity intolerance related to fatigue.
- Acute pain as related to pancreatitis.
- Fear in response to the diagnosis of pancreatitis.
- Ineffective coping related to the diagnosis of pancreatitis.

Planning and Implementation

The goals for mild acute pancreatitis is to rest the gut, provide supportive care to treat symptoms, identify systemic complications early, and decrease pancreatic inflammation. Treatment includes bed rest, vigorous intravenous hydration, electrolyte replacement, pain control, and keeping the patient NPO. Patient controlled analgesia is effective, however morphine potentially causes the sphincter of Oddi to constrict and create more pain, so Demerol is recommended, but hydromorphone (Dilaudid) or other analgesics may be used. Decompression of the stomach by nasal gastric suction can relieve some of the nausea, vomiting, and abdominal distension. Patients may be treated conservatively until they are stable enough to have surgery to remove the gallstones. If a patient requires prolonged IV intervention, total parenteral nutrition (TPN) would be required. If infection is evident, aggressive antibiotic therapy would be used. Surgery may also be needed to treat extensive infections. It is possible for the autodigestion process to involve the circulation to the pancreas. This is a crisis situation that would necessitate surgery to stop the bleeding. Complications with kidney failure are possible and dialysis may be required. Acute pancreatitis can resolve with medical treatment. When the patients are released to home, they are instructed to refrain from drinking alcohol, because of its toxic effects on the pancreas and surrounding organs. Eating smaller, more frequent meals is also advisable.

Evaluation of Outcomes

Potential patient outcomes for each of the example nursing diagnoses for the patient with acute pancreatitis are:

- Activity intolerance related to fatigue. The patient maintains activity level within capabilities, as evidenced by normal heart rate and blood pressure during activity, as well as absence of shortness of breath, weakness, and fatigue.

Skills 360°

Nursing Care for Acute Pancreatitis

The nurse should perform the following measures in the management of acute pancreatitis:

- Strict intake and output and being alert for signs and symptoms of kidney failure.
- Monitor vital signs and be aware of early signs of internal bleeding, infection, and respiratory distress.
- Pain control.
- Assessment of all systems, but especially GI, respiratory, and cardiovascular.
- Blood glucose monitoring.
- Providing information about disease, diagnostic tests, and treatment.
- Provide information concerning alcohol reduction and elimination.

- Acute pain as related to pancreatitis. The patient should verbalize an adequate relief of pain along with the ability to realistically cope with the pain if it is not completely relieved.
- Fear in response to the diagnosis of pancreatitis. The patient should manifest positive coping behaviors and verbalize a reduction in the amount of fear of the having this disease.
- Ineffective coping related to the diagnosis of pancreatitis. Patient identifies own maladaptive coping behaviors, available resources, and support systems, describes or initiates alternative coping strategies, and describes positive results from new behaviors.

Chronic Pancreatitis

Chronic pancreatitis occurs when there is irreversible damage to the pancreatic acini, ducts, nerves, and islet cells because of continued irritation and injury. Pancreatic calcifications or dilated pancreatic ducts may be present. Digestive enzymes from the pancreas can irritate nearby tissue and cause scarring and further impede flow of enzymes, blood, and bile. Patients may present with the typical picture for acute pancreatitis or complain of diabetes symptoms or steatorrhea.

Epidemiology

Chronic alcoholism is implicated in about 70 percent of all chronic pancreatitis cases. Men between the ages of 30 and 40 are more likely affected than women. People may not seek treatment for pancreatitis, but on autopsy, pancreatitis is 50 times more prevalent in alcoholics than nondrinkers. In other cases, flow of exocrine enzymes can be affected by trauma, tumor, or pseudocysts. In 10 to 30 percent of patients, there may be no identifiable cause for the pancreatitis and is considered idiopathic.

Etiology

Chronic pancreatitis has a variety of causes. Hyperlipidemia and hypertriglyceridemia can be implicated. Autoimmune factors could also be at fault. Tropical pancreatitis is associated with people who live within 30 degrees of the equator. Symptoms can begin in childhood. Diabetes, malnutrition, and pancreatic calcifications are present. Environmental toxins, pathogenic agents, and toxic products that could be in the diet (cassava or sorghum) are all being investigated.

Pathophysiology

Chronic pancreatitis can be caused by alcoholism. In addition, chronic pancreatitis can be caused by actual physical trauma or cancer of the organ.

Genetics

The congenital abnormality pancreas divisum is the failure of the pancreatic ducts to fuse during embryonic development, leaving two separate (the dorsal and ventral ducts) to drain the different parts of the pancreas. Pancreas divisum may occur in 7 percent of the population, although those who go on to develop pancreatitis are few. Hereditary illnesses, such as cystic fibrosis and familial pancreatitis (mutations for the trypsinogen and the trypsin-inactivating genes), can illuminate other mechanisms at work. Cystic fibrosis is the most common cause of pancreatitis in children, because of the protein plugs within the ducts, causing reduced flow of pancreatic enzymes. In hereditary (familial) pancreatitis, the patient usually has two or more close relatives in the same generation with the same affliction. It is thought to be autosomal dominant and can be associated with increased pancreatic cancer.

Assessment with Clinical Manifestations

Chronic pancreatitis is characterized by pain, malabsorption, and diabetes mellitus. Pain can be acute or dull and constant. It may be referred to the back and be exacerbated with eating. Chronic irritation over many years may cause the pain to subside. In about 15 percent of patients, pain never develops. Pancreatitis affects digestion and absorption by decreasing the delivery of digestive enzymes to the gut and reducing the secretion of bicarbonate from the pancreatic ducts, lowering the duodenal pH. Weight loss and vitamin deficiency may be evident. Osteopenia and osteoporosis may occur because of decreased vitamin D. Diabetes mellitus occurs in 30 percent of patients with chronic pancreatitis. The inability to mobilize glucagons to maintain blood glucose levels can also be evident.

Diagnostic Tests

Diagnosis of chronic pancreatitis is divided into big duct disease and small duct disease. Big duct chronic pancreatitis indicates a dilation of the main pancreatic ducts and is common in alcoholic pancreatitis. Interventions for big duct disease can include endoscopic or surgical intervention. Small duct disease is more likely to be idiopathic and less responsive to surgical treatment, so emphasis would be on aggressive medical intervention.

Serum lipase and amylase are often normal in chronic pancreatitis. Serum glucose is helpful in diagnosing diabetes, but not in identifying the cause. Decreased serum trypsin, below 20 mg/dL in the presence of steatorrhea, is specific for chronic pancreatitis. Measuring fecal fat and fecal elastase could be important in diagnosing advanced disease (Daniels, 2003).

Abdominal X-ray and ultrasound can indicate pancreatic calcification. Diffuse calcification is seen in advanced pancreatic disease. This can help to differentiate chronic pancreatitis from tumors and focal trauma. Ultrasound can identify pancreatic atrophy or dilated pancreatic ducts. Gas in the bowel can obstruct the view. CT scan is most sensitive for identifying diffuse calcification and the dilation of ducts in big duct and small duct disease. Endoscopic ultrasonography (EUS) combines an ultrasound probe on the end of an endoscope and can contribute a clearer picture of the problem. Another endoscopic examination uses a collection tube in the duodenum, which collects pancreatic secretions when the pancreas is stimulated by the hormones secretin and secretin-cholecystokinin. This test is not available in all treatment centers. MRI and magnetic resonance cholangiopancreatography (MRCP) is useful in diagnosing biliary tract disease and less advanced chronic pancreatitis. The ERCP is probably the most sensitive test, but it carries the most risk and financial burden of all the tests. The ERCP can identify dilation or strictures in ducts, pseudocysts, and anatomical abnormalities. Biopsies can be taken at the time of ERCP to help differentiate between chronic pancreatitis and carcinoma of the pancreas. ERCP is most accurate in advanced disease, but less advanced disease remains much more difficult to diagnose.

Nursing Diagnoses

Based on the information gathered, examples of nursing diagnoses in the patient with chronic pancreatitis may include the following:

- Chronic pain related to chronic pancreatitis.
- Nutrition imbalance, less than body requirements, related to chronic pancreatitis.
- Knowledge deficit related to chronic pancreatitis.

Planning and Implementation

Digestive enzymes can be given orally. Lipase is the most variable enzyme, because it is dependent on the amount of fat in the meal. Lipase preparations need a higher pH than what is found in the stomach to have the most efficacy.

With pancreatitis, the bicarbonate is not secreted from the ducts, and the pH may be lower than usual in the intestine because of the bicarbonate deficiency. Diet should contain a moderate amount of fat (30 percent), high protein (24 percent), and low carbohydrates (24 percent). Diabetic diets can be helpful. Abstaining from alcohol is important, because the alcohol can cause more irritation, pain, and other problems. In addition, patients with chronic pancreatitis have difficulty in regulating blood glucose, because insulin and glucagons may be in short supply. Tight control of blood sugar can predispose the patient to hypoglycemia.

Pharmacology

Pain control often starts with the least potent medication, such as Darvocet-N or tramadol. Narcotic addiction can occur in 20 percent of patients. Tricyclic antidepressants can potentiate the effect of narcotics. Selective serotonin reuptake inhibitors (SSRIs) may also be helpful to treat pain and assist with rest. Pancreatic enzymes can provide some pain relief for people primarily with small duct pancreatitis by addressing some of the causes behind the pain. Gastric acid suppressors can also be used to decrease stomach acid. Antidiarrheals, such as octreotide (Sandostatin), have been beneficial in treating GI endocrine tumors, such as VIP tumors (VIPomas), and controlling the flushing and diarrhea that accompanies them. Antioxidants may also contribute to pain reduction.

Surgery

Surgical interventions for pain reduction can include ablation of the celiac plexus by analgesics guided by radiological means, laparoscopic stenting to keep the ducts open, dilation of strictures, removal of calculi, and drainage of pseudocysts. Open surgeries (nonlaparoscopic) may be used to visualize the pancreas, resect what is necessary, and ablate the nerves, which leads to the organ that conveys so much pain (Figure 51-6).

Evaluation of Outcomes

Potential patient outcomes for each of the example nursing diagnoses for the patient with chronic pancreatitis are:

- Chronic pain related to chronic pancreatitis. The patient should verbalize an adequate relief of pain along with the ability to realistically cope with the pain if it is not completely relieved.

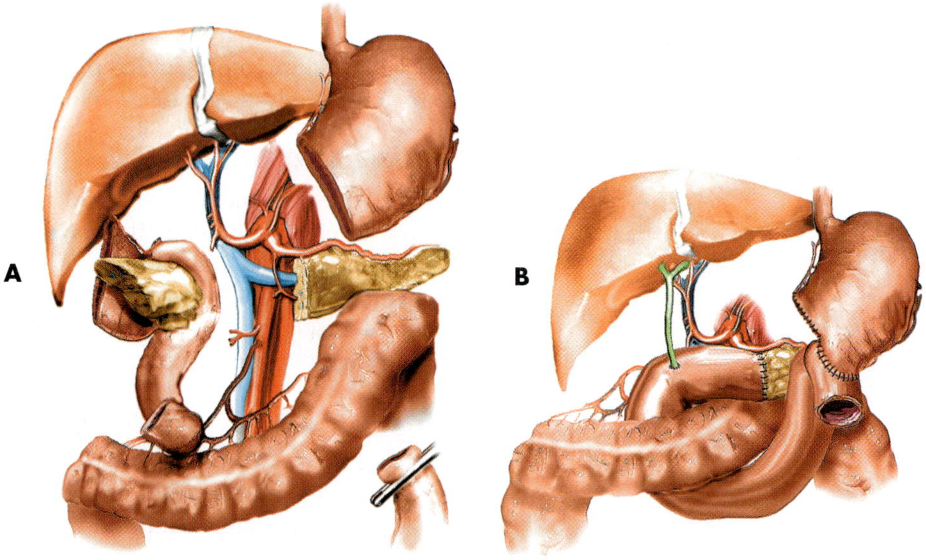

Figure 51-6 Whipple procedure (pancreatectomy): A. Resection, B. Reconstruction.

- Nutrition imbalance, less than body requirements, related to chronic pancreatitis. The patient verbalizes and demonstrates selection of foods or meals that will achieve a cessation of weight loss and weighs within 10 percent of ideal body weight.
- Knowledge deficit related to chronic pancreatitis. The patient should demonstrate motivation to learn, identify perceived learning needs, and verbalize an understanding of desired content.

KEY CONCEPTS

- Bilirubin is an important indicator for liver and blood disorders.
- The biliary tract serves the liver and is designed to drain bile.
- The most common cause of hepatitis is viral infection.
- HAV is transmitted by the fecal-oral route, and HBV is transmitted via blood and body fluids.
- The genetic disorders of the liver involve bilirubin metabolism, copper and iron storage, enzyme production, and lipoprotein metabolism.
- The destruction to the liver from alcohol often progresses from fatty liver to alcoholic hepatitis and culminates in alcoholic cirrhosis.
- Hepatic abscess is an area of infection in the liver caused by bacteria, amoebas, or protozoas.
- The liver is large and because of its size, location, and vascularity damage can occur during blunt or penetrating trauma.
- Liver cancer is named based on the type of tissue from which it originates and in general, men experience more primary liver cancer than women.
- Liver transplantation has been considered standard practice since 1983, with the development of newer immunosuppressive drugs to fight rejection of the implanted organ.
- Cholelithiasis (gallstones) is a common problem, affecting about 16 to 20 million people in the United States.
- The treatment of choice for an inflamed gallbladder is laparoscopic cholecystectomy, which is a surgical procedure using laparoscopy to remove the gallbladder.

REVIEW QUESTIONS

1. The liver has many complicated functions. Which of the following is the definition of gluconeogenesis?
   1. It is the conversion of glucose to glycogen, which can be stored in preparation of times of fasting.
   2. It is the conversion of stored glycogen into usable glucose to meet the immediate energy needs of the body.
   3. It is the synthesis of glucose from amino acids during times of fasting.
   4. It is the production of amino acids and bile.

2. Mr. Portier has an endoscopic retrograde cholangiopancreatography (ERCP). Which of the following organs does this diagnostic test not inspect?
   1. The liver
   2. The thymus
   3. The gallbladder
   4. The pancreas

3. Mr. Victorini has hepatitis A. Which of the following are true of this disorder?
   1. It is blood borne, causes fatigue, and has an incubation time of two to three weeks.
   2. It is life-threatening, irreversible, and debilitating.
   3. It is an RNA virus, spread often by food handlers infected with the virus, and has an incubation time of 15 to 50 days.
   4. It usually is not associated with jaundice, is a DNA virus, is transmitted through blood and body fluids, and often caused by sharing needles in illicit drug use.

4. Mr. Abernathy has a hereditary disease of the liver which is an autosomal recessive disorder related to copper metabolism. Which of the following disorders is this?
   1. Wilson's disease
   2. Crigler-Najjar disease
   3. Alpha-antitrypsin deficiency
   4. Hemochromatosis

Continued

REVIEW QUESTIONS—cont'd

5. Mr. Parker has ascites as a result of his cirrhosis condition. Which of the following is true of this condition?
   1. Refractory ascites is that which can only be treated with a splenectomy.
   2. Ascites is the accumulation of fluid in the pelvis area.
   3. A surgical shunt to divert excessive peritoneal fluid into the venous system may be attempted.
   4. Esophageal varices often result in the abdominal area specific to the ascites condition.
6. Mr. Barnes has a hepatic abscess. Which of the following is true concerning this condition?
   1. It is caused by a decrease in lecithin-cholesterol acyltransferase.
   2. It is categorized into either a macrovesicular and microvesicular disorder.
   3. It is usually caused by bacterial infection and is referred to as pyogenic hepatic abscess.
   4. It is also labeled hepatic steatosis.
7. Mrs. Williams has cancer of the liver. There are two basic types of liver cancer and they are labeled:
   1. Primary and secondary
   2. Type I and type II
   3. Stage A and stage B
   4. Organic and inorganic
8. What is the most common reason for children to have a liver transplant?
   1. Congenital hepatitis B virus
   2. Biliary atresia
   3. Cholangitis
   4. Congenital human immunodeficiency virus
9. Mrs. Adams has acute pancreatitis. Which of the following is true regarding its diagnosis?
   1. The serum laboratory tests of serum amylase and lipase are the best method of confirming acute pancreatitis.
   2. An increased alanine aminotransferase (ALT) is the best indicator for acute pancreatitis.
   3. Computed tomography (CT) scanning is the most useful test for determining the presence of pancreatitis as differentiated from other abdominal issues.
   4. Ultrasound is the most definitive manner in which to diagnose the severity of pancreatitis.
10. Mr. Hines is going to have a liver transplantation. Which of the following is true concerning this management strategy?
    1. Living donor liver transplants seldom come from parents or siblings.
    2. Cadaveric livers come from people who have been declared brain dead and have few other vital organs that are healthy.
    3. When an appropriate match has been identified, the institution has 24 hours to accept the organ.
    4. Criteria for receiving a donated liver is rigorously defined by the United Network for Organ Sharing.

REVIEW ACTIVITIES

1. Compare and contrast conjugated and unconjugated bilirubin.

2. Describe methods of assessing liver functioning.

3. Compare and contrast hepatitis A and hepatitis B.

4. Compare and contrast biliary and cardiac cirrhosis.

5. Describe your emotional feeling regarding providing care for patients who are alcoholics.

6. Describe how you would feel if you were asked to donate your liver to a relative.

7. Compare and contrast an open cholecystectomy and a laparoscopic cholecystectomy.

Visit the Contemporary Medical-Surgical Nursing online companion resource at www.delmarhealthcare.com for additional content and study aids. Click on Online Companions then select the Nursing discipline.

UNIT XII

Alterations in Renal Function

Chapter 52 Assessment of Renal Function

Chapter 53 Urinary Dysfunction: Nursing Management

Chapter 54 Renal Dysfunction: Nursing Management

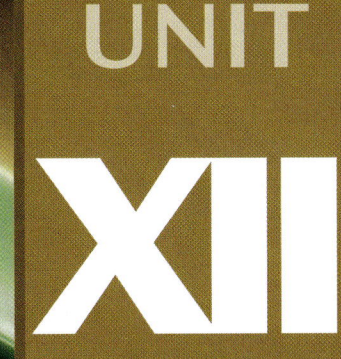

CHAPTER

52

Assessment of Renal Function

Irene Eaton-Bancroft, RN, MSN, CS

KEY TERMS

Calculi
Dysuria
Erythropoietin (EPO)
Hematuria
Homeostasis
Hydronephrosis
Interstitial space
Native kidney
Nephritis
Nephrotoxic
Peristalsis
Polycystic cysts
Pyelonephritis
Radioisotope
Renal
Renal parenchyma
Retroperitoneal space
Uremia
Vesicoureteral reflux

CHAPTER TOPICS

- Anatomy and Physiology of the Renal System
- Assessment Strategies Implemented in the Renal System
- Diagnostic Tests of the Renal System

The urinary system is critically important to the **homeostasis** (maintenance of an optimal and constant state of all body substances) of all body systems. Prevention and early recognition of system dysfunction are critical to the goal of maintaining optimal health status. The objective of this chapter is to equip the learner to assess normal renal system attributes and identify deviations from normal urinary system function.

The **renal** (pertaining to the kidney) component of the urinary system is often considered complex to understand, and its signals of dysfunction are difficult to recognize in a routine patient assessment. The learner is referred to a text on human physiology for a complete understanding of renal function. An anatomy and physiology text will supplement this chapter on renal assessment. The goal of this assessment chapter is to present anatomy and physiology from a system assessment perspective.

ANATOMY AND PHYSIOLOGY

The renal system is vital to the functioning of the human body. It is responsible for a wide variety of activities within the body and is integrated with the function of the other body systems. The renal system controls the fluid balance of the body, controls many of the metabolic processes within the body, and provides stabilization for the human body circulation. At the macrovascular level, the renal system consists of two kidneys, ureters, bladder, and urethra. In addition, the microvascular components of the renal system, such as the nephron, are presented in this chapter. The female and male urinary systems are illustrated Figure 52-1.

Kidneys

The kidneys are amazing organs with a computer-like capability to simultaneously perform multiple and complex functions. Normally, a person is born with two kidneys, though on occasion, a person is found to have a single or even a third kidney. The adult kidney is about the size of one's fist. It measures approximately 12 cm (4.5 inches) long, 6 cm (2.4 inches) wide and weighs 120–170 grams.

The kidneys are positioned in the **retroperitoneal space** (the space between the peritoneum [the membranous sac that surrounds the organs of the abdominal cavity] and the posterior abdominal wall that contains the kidneys and associated structures, the pancreas, and part of the aorta and inferior vena cava) at the level of the 12th thoracic vertebra to the 3rd lumbar vertebra with one on each side of the vertebral column. Positioned advantageously within an intact rib cage, the kidneys are offered protection from blunt trauma. The costovertebral angle (CVA), the point at which the base of the rib cage and the

A

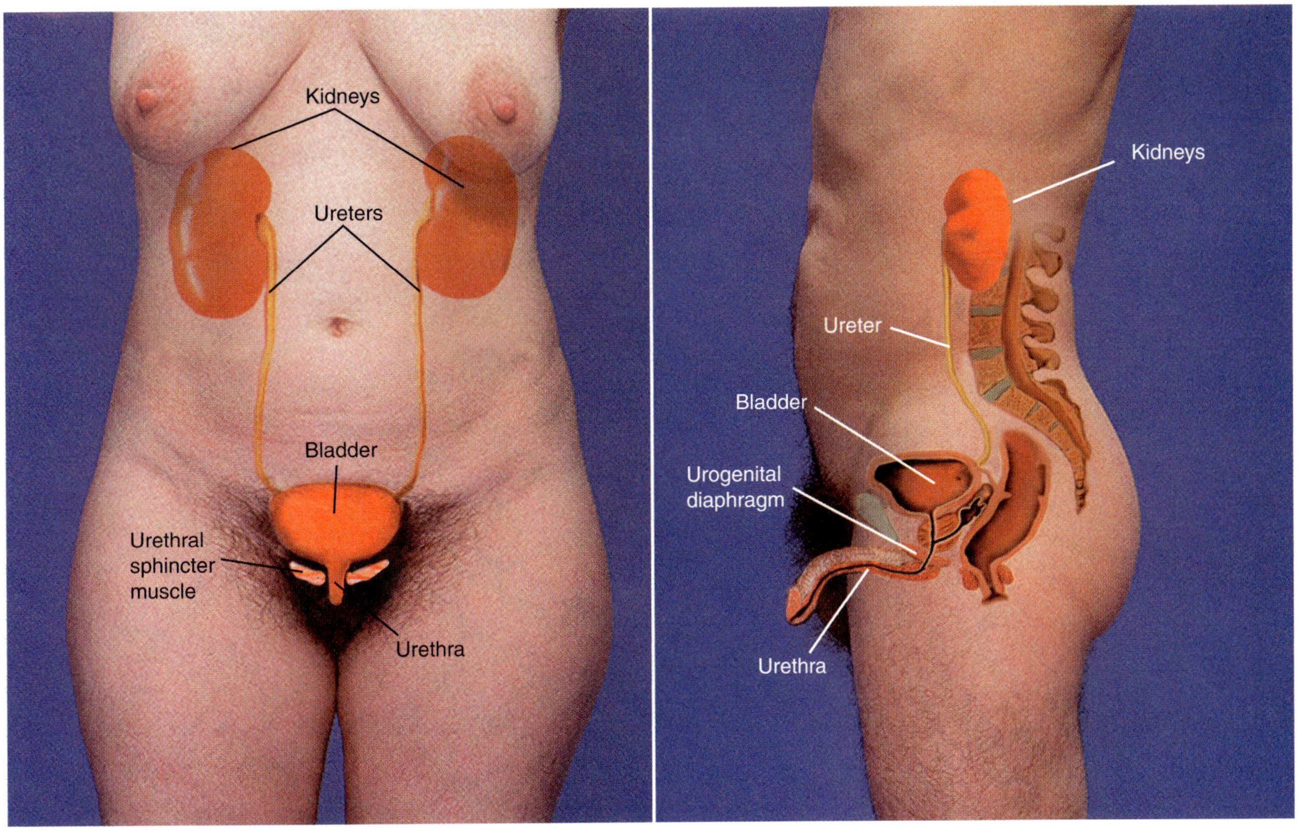

B

Figure 52-1 Urinary Tract: A. Female, B. Male.

spine meet, provides a landmark to locate kidney position during the physical exam. Be aware that the right kidney is positioned slightly lower than the left as it lies just under the larger right lobe of the liver. Under normal circumstance, one may not be able to palpate either kidney (Perkins & Kisiel, 2005).

A tough fibrous capsule covers and contains the kidney. Together with surrounding muscle, fascia, and fatty tissue, it offers protection to these mobile organs during times of vigorous and bouncing-type of activity. Though it is protective of the **renal parenchyma** (the cortex and medulla of the kidney, which contain the functioning units and collecting ducts of the kidney) under normal circumstances, renal capsule rigidity offers little accommodation to events such as **hydronephrosis** (dilation of the renal pelvis due to obstruction of urine flow or from ureteral reflux) secondary to postrenal obstruction. In such cases, the capsule's inability to expand increases potential for injury to the renal parenchyma due to increased intracapsular pressure and circulatory compromise to the nephrons. Acute pain in this area should prompt an expedient and thorough urological exam. The internal anatomy of the kidney is illustrated in Figure 52-2.

Blood supply to the kidney is critical from the perspective of producing hydrostatic pressure adequate for maintaining homeostasis and for the purpose of supplying oxygen and nutrients crucial to organ survival. The renal arteries branch directly from the aorta and deliver approximately 20 percent of the cardiac output to the kidneys.

The kidneys have one to two million nephrons. Microscopic in size, these functioning units produce and excrete urine to maintain homeostasis, as well as regulate or influence many physiological processes. The primary functions of the renal system are shown in Box 52-1.

Renal efficiency is amazing in that one can lose nearly 65 percent of their total kidney function before presenting symptoms of dysfunction. A person can survive easily with a single kidney. Relying on the sufficiency of one healthy

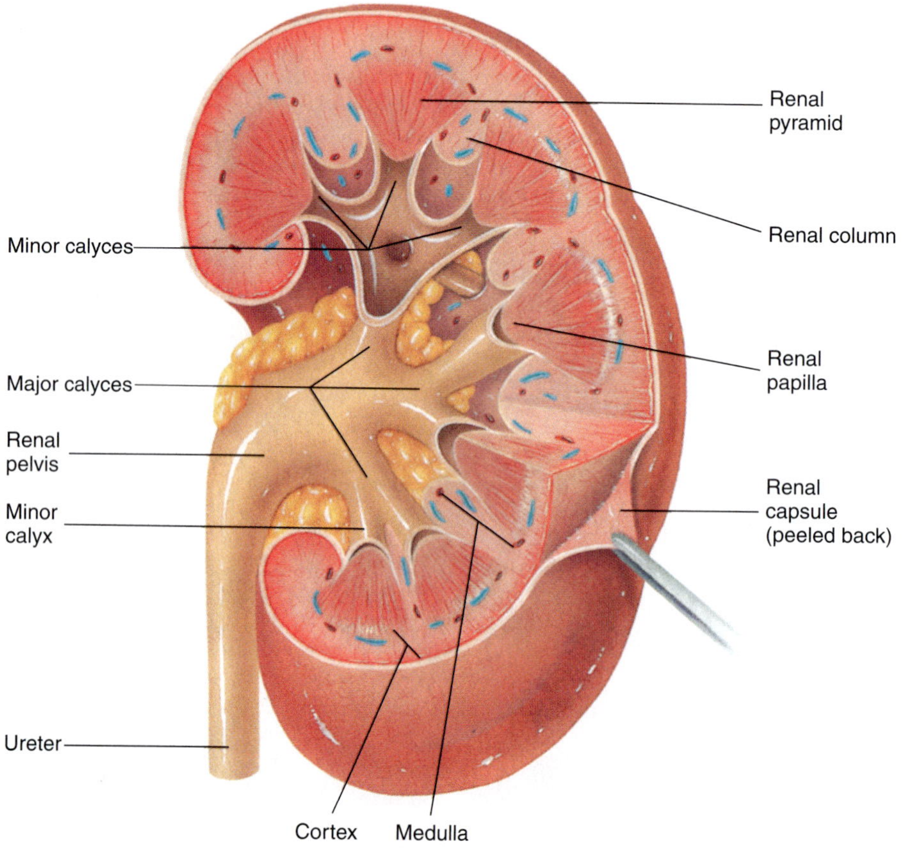

Figure 52-2 The internal anatomy of the kidney.

BOX 52-1

FUNCTIONS OF THE KIDNEY

The primary functions of the kidney are:

- Maintain fluid and electrolyte balance through excretion and reabsorption.
- Assist in blood pressure regulation through the renin-angiotensin system. A lifesaver in situations of fluid loss, this function can accelerate harm to the kidneys as they begin to fail. The mechanism of harm is release of renin by the juxtaglomerular apparatus. Timely nursing intervention in hypertensive episodes of acute renal failure are critical to recovery potential.
- Maintain chemical balance. This function is critical to maintain predictable blood levels of medication calculated on normal urinary excretion levels. The health care provider must stay alert to the potential for toxic blood levels in the event of renal function compromise.
- Maintain mineral balance. Consideration of this function is especially critical to bone health in chronic renal failure.
- Produce erythropoietin in response to low oxygen states.
- Convert vitamin D to its active enzyme form and thus influence calcium metabolism.
- Excrete waste products of protein metabolism.
- Contribute to acid-base balance. Secretion of hydrogen ions, reabsorption of bicarbonate, or generation of new bicarbonate by the kidney serve to counter acidosis and to maintain acid-base equilibrium. Adjusted renal excretion of bicarbonate ions corrects for alkalosis.

kidney, many have chosen to donate their second kidney. Kidney donation from living donors has expanded to include nonrelated recipients. Further information concerning kidney donation is shown in chapter 54.

Ureters

The ureter is a narrow fibromuscular tube that extends from the distal end of the renal pelvis and to the bladder. Composed of smooth muscle, the ureter propels urine toward the bladder by **peristalsis** (smooth muscle involuntary contractions that propel substances along a pathway, such as when the ureters propel urine from the kidneys to the bladder by peristaltic action). Peristaltic strength is sufficient to overcome the resistance offered by the detrusor muscle of the bladder allowing urine to pass into the bladder. Conversely, the 1 to 2 cm the ureters traverse through the detrusor muscle before emptying into the bladder prevents retrograde reflux of urine back toward the kidneys as the bladder fills.

The small diameter of the ureters contributes to easy obstruction during the passage of renal **calculi** (a substance of abnormal concretion composed of mineral salts commonly produced within the renal system) or from the external pressure of masses. Pressure receptors in the ureters and renal pelvis generate the extreme pain experienced during the passage of calculi. In addition, these receptors slow glomerular filtration when sensing high intraurethal pressures (Schafer, 2003). Slowing filtration offers a protective effect toward limiting hydronephrosis.

Urinary Bladder

The urinary bladder is a muscular sac that narrows at the base to form the bladder neck. The bladder is made up of cross-hatched smooth muscle with exceptional stretch capacity. This specific smooth muscle is referred to as detrusor muscle. Distinctively, it has tremendous capacity to stretch and then to contract in response to nervous stimuli. Normal detrusor stretch will allow as much as 500 mL bladder fill volume. Flaccid during the filling phase, the bladder contracts in response to stretch receptors and seeks to expel urine though the internal sphincter. It is at this point that both voluntary and involuntary action is needed to complete the voiding process in the continent adult (Newman, 2005).

The muscle tone of the detrusor muscle surrounding the ureter serves to occlude the ureteral orifice preventing reflux of urine toward the kidney as the bladder fills. Peristaltic pressure overcomes detrusor strength and propels urine through the detrusor area and on into the bladder. The section of the detrusor muscle involved in preventing reflux of urine into the ureter is called the ureterovesicular valve and is normally 1 to 2 cm long. Those with a shorter valve section are susceptible to reflux with subsequent enlarged ureters and intrarenal problems as a result of increased fluid pressures.

The trigone of the bladder is the triangular-shaped section of the posterior wall of the bladder just above and adjacent to the bladder neck. The trigone accommodates the orifices of the ureters at its uppermost borders while the base of this triangular area forms the bladder neck and transitions to the urethra (O'Hara, 2005). The anatomy of the urinary bladder is illustrated in Figure 52-3.

Bladder Neck (Posterior Urethra)

The bladder neck, also considered the posterior portion of the urethra, plays a critical role in continence and in dysfunctions of bladder emptying. Elastic tissue is interwoven into the detrusor muscle of this bladder/urethral section to form the internal sphincter. Smooth muscle places the internal sphincter under involuntary control via a nerve plexus originating at the second and third segment of the sacral spine. Striated muscles of the pelvic floor innervated by the pudendal nerve keep the external sphincter under voluntary control. The act of voiding in the healthy adult requires the active participation of the individual. Good muscle tone and intact innervation to the sphincters can resist the

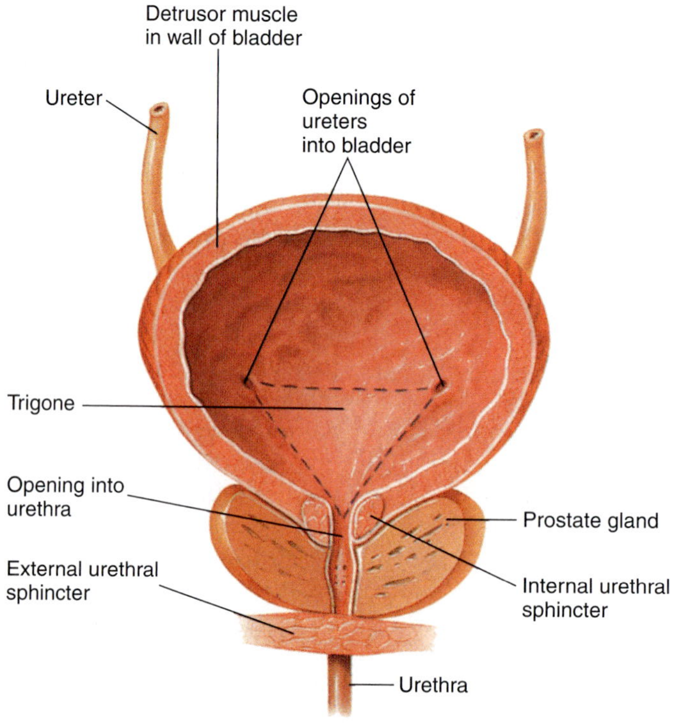

Figure 52-3 The anatomy of the urinary bladder.

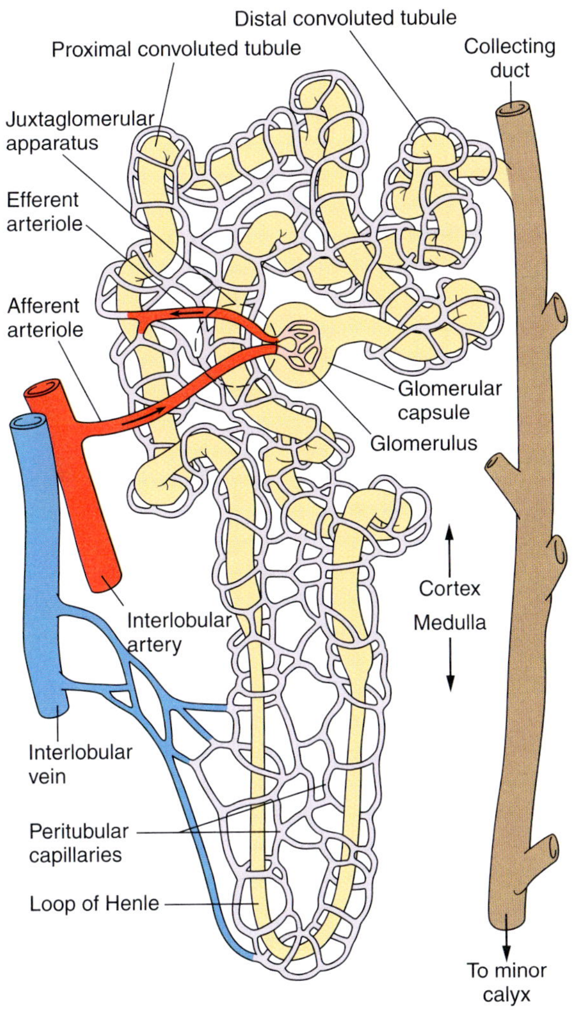

Figure 52-4 The anatomy of a nephron.

contracting detrusor and inhibit bladder emptying for a period of time, though not without discomfort as a reminder of a full bladder (O'Hara, 2005).

Commonly, problems can develop causing interference with bladder functions of urine storage or expulsion. A weak pelvic floor, particularly in cases involving the short urethra of females, can lead to incontinence. In the male, an enlarged prostate gland is the most common cause of urethral obstruction with resulting retention. Benign prostatic hypertrophy, or prostate cancer, is the most common causes of urinary retention in the male. In the female, close proximity of the urethral orifice to the vagina contributes to bacterial invasion of the urinary tract through the urethra with potential for ascending infection traveling by way of the ureter and ultimately into the kidney. These infections are labeled according to anatomic region of infection (e.g., urethritis, cystitis, **pyelonephritis,** or **nephritis**). (Note: Pyelonephritis is an infection of the ureters, and nephritis is an infection contained to the kidney.) These will be discussed in depth in chapter 54.

Nephron

The nephron is the functioning unit of the kidney. The anatomy of a nephron is illustrated in Figure 52-4. They number more than a million with cellular structure differing from section to section to accomplish the multiple and complex tasks. Each unit would seem to have two primary systems with both separate and interrelated functions. Simply stated, the tubular system collects the filtrate of water and solutes then secretes, excretes, or reabsorbs substances as necessary to maintain an internal environment in equilibrium and rid of waste products.

The vascular system of the nephron includes two capillary beds: (a) the glomerular capillary bed is shaped in the form of a tuft and sits in the first segment of the tubule, and (b) the peritubular capillary bed surrounds all portions of the tubule. Both capillary networks are vested in critical and cooperative function with the tubule. Critical to the function of both of these systems is the interstitium with functional solute concentration gradients that support the processes of both the tubule and the peritubular capillary network. The processes and structures of the nephron are presented in Figure 52-5.

Renal Tubule

The renal tubule is a complex component of the kidney. Anatomic sections of the tubule include Bowman's capsule, the proximal tubule, loop of Henle, distal tubule, and the collecting duct. Bowman's capsule, the first segment, is configured somewhat as a funnel. Bowman's capsule cradles the glomerular capillary tuft and receives the approximate 180 L/day of filtered fluids and solutes. Impermeable to protein by both size and negative charge, healthy glomerular capillaries inhibit passage of protein or blood cells into the filtrate. Interestingly, the negative charge present on each of the three glomerular capillary membranes repels the negatively charged and molecularly larger cells. Due to their negative charge or large molecular size, the presence of protein or blood cells in the urine signals problems with filtration.

The proximal and distal tubules are similarly convoluted in shape though structurally quite different. Cell structure of the proximal tubule accommodates greater reabsorption sodium, chloride, glucose, amino acids, bile salts, oxalate, urate, and catecholamines. This begins the process of creating a

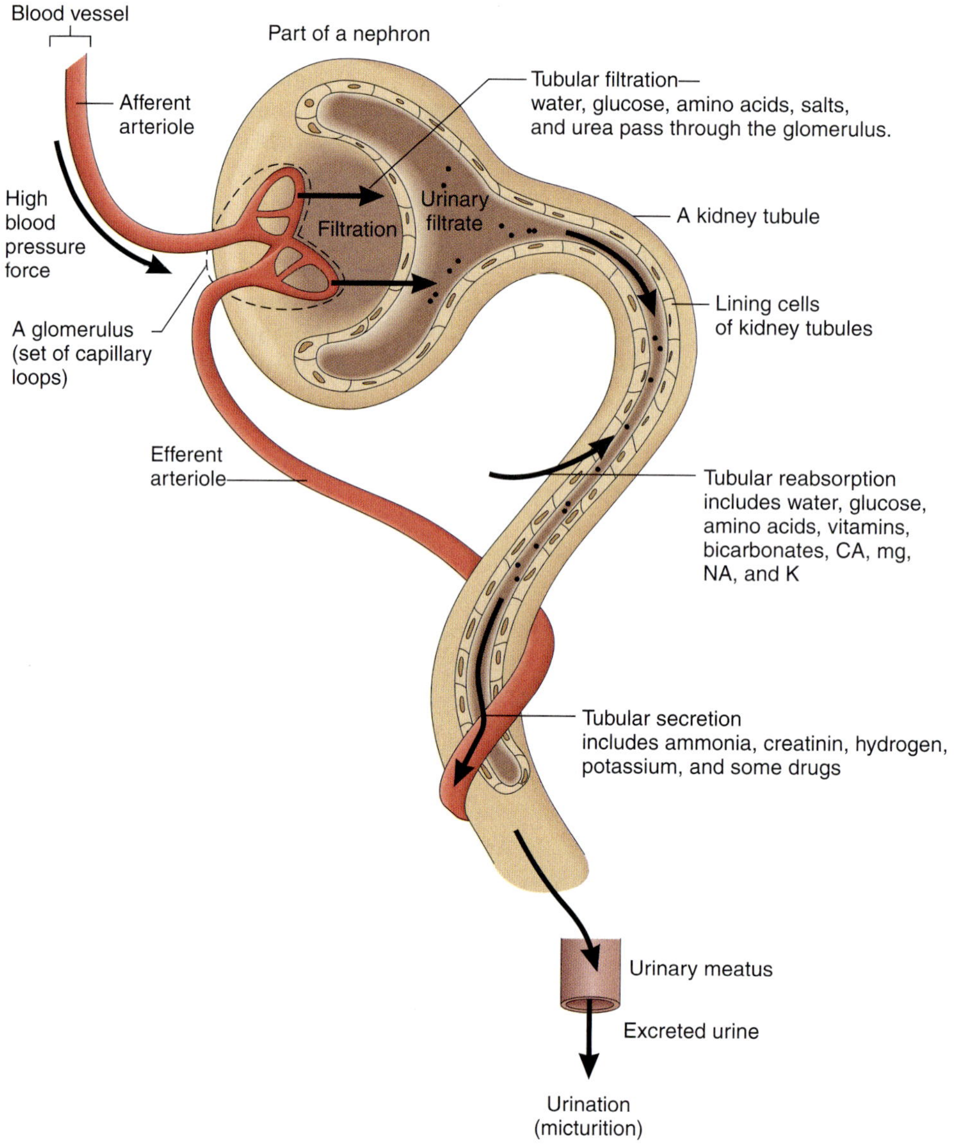

Figure 52-5 Processes and structures of the nephron.

highly concentrated renal **interstitial space,** that area surrounding the nephron loops and the peritubular capillaries, which has a high osmotic pressure due to extremely high levels of sodium. The renal interstitial space facilitates the massive volume water reabsorption required to maintain fluid balance. The interstitial space fluid environment is equipped with osmotic pressures capable of reabsorbing the approximate 165 L/day of the water filtered by the glomerular capillaries.

The loop of Henle changes cellular structure along its descending and ascending paths to create three functionally different sections. The thinner descending section facilitates large quantities of water absorption by osmosis and moderate reabsorption of solutes. Important to urine concentration, the ascending limb is highly impermeable to water. As the ascending limb of the loop of Henle thickens due to cellular structure change, the sodium pump actively moves sodium, chloride, and potassium out of the tubular fluid into the interstitial space. Large amounts of calcium, magnesium, and bicarbonate are also reabsorbed from the thick ascending limb. This solute loss creates a dilute solution in the tubule as the filtrate approaches the distal tubule. The achieved dilution is significant in setting the stage for the significant adjustments needed to accommodate the high variability of individual fluid and solute intake.

Juxtaglomerular Apparatus

The first segment of the distal tubule forms a portion of the juxtaglomerular apparatus. This is a complex of cells made up of those in the distal tubule (macula densa cells) and related cellular structure within the arterioles on either end of the glomerular capillary tuft (juxtaglomerular cells). Though often depicted as distant from one another to demonstrate the configuration of the nephron, in reality these two groups of cells are in intimate contact with one another. Macula densa cells are capable of detecting pressure or sodium solute changes and signaling the juxtaglomerular cells of the afferent arterioles to decrease resistance toward the goal of a greater filtration rate. In addition, macula densa cells stimulate renin release from the juxtaglomerular cells of the arterioles entering and exiting the glomerular tuft. Released renin initiates the angiotensin system thereby increasing the arterial blood pressure. The net result of both actions is increased glomerular filtration rate.

Blood supply to the kidney is critical from the perspective of producing hydrostatic pressure adequate for maintaining glomerular filtration and for the purpose of supplying oxygen and nutrients crucial to nephron function and survival. A renal artery branches directly from the aorta to each kidney. The artery then subdivides courses through the lobules of the kidney and ultimately forms the glomerular and peritubular capillary networks of the nephrons. The efferent arteriole separates these two capillary beds and facilitates the higher hydrostatic pressure gradients necessary for filtration in the glomerulus and the lower hydrostatic pressures in the peritubular capillaries that promote reabsorption to maintain homeostasis.

The afferent arteriole is the short vascular segment between the interlobular arteries and the glomerular capillary network in Bowman's capsule. The afferent arteriole plays a critical role in conjunction with the efferent arteriole in regulating filtering pressures and ultimately influencing systemic blood pressure through constriction, dilation or renin release. These functions are most often referred to as the autoregulatory function of the kidney.

Homeostatic balancing mechanisms are easily disturbed by events producing changes in renal perfusion, such as hypertension or vasoactive drugs, and from renin generated from within the kidney in pathological states. **Nephrotoxic** (having the ability to harm the kidney) agents, such as nonsteroidal anti-inflammatory medications and cyclosporine, are capable of compromising afferent arteriole function with the potential to impose acute renal failure by diminishing glomerular filtration and reducing the blood supply to the nephron.

Renin-Angiotensin System

It is important to understand the renin-angiotensin system and the importance of intervention in pathological states. Basic to the renin-angiotensin cycle is an understanding that renin has the capability of activating critical events. For example, when sensing low volumes of distal tubular filtrate, regardless of the cause, renin release by the juxtaglomerular cells will initiate the formation of angiotensin I, which converts to angiotensin II. Angiotensin-converting enzyme (ACE) is the catalyst in the conversion of angiotensin I to angiotensin II. The cumulative action of these three potent chemicals causes vasoconstriction and yields an increase in blood pressure. Often times, renin release is a direct result of pathology that would be further complicated by its release. One example of a pathology that activates the renin angiotensin cycle is congestive heart failure with associated decrease in renal perfusion or glomerular filtration. Another example of a condition that activates the release of renin is hypertension associated decreased glomerular filtrate. In either case, renin release is detrimental and obliges timely intervention with agents such as diuretics, ACE inhibitors, or other antihypertensive medications. The nurse is given a significant role in reversing acute renal failure when implementing protocol orders in such instances. Prudent and ethical nursing practice

Respecting Our Differences

Age-Related Changes in the Renal System

The following are age-related changes in the renal system. The nurse should be aware of these conditions as they have implications for care of the elderly.

- Decreased muscle tone and elasticity in the ureters, bladder, urinary sphincter, and surrounding structures resulting in problems of incontinence.
- Prostatic hyperplasia in the male resulting in urinary retention.
- Decreased functioning nephrons and glomerular filtration rate. This may be reflected in slightly higher blood levels of urea nitrogen and creatinine.
- Nocturia may become result from problems of retention or from decreases in renal concentration.

attends the clinical observations of urine output patterns, blood pressure parameters, and medication protocols (Hobbs, Irwin, & Rubner, 2005).

ASSESSMENT

The renal system is complex and vital to the human body. There are many disorders that affect the function of the renal system. The nurse must be familiar with the variety of pathologies that affect the renal system and be able to accurately assess the changes in the renal system as they occur. Initially, the health history and physical exam are the primary components of the assessment of the renal system.

Health History

Urinary tract and renal assessment must begin with a thorough health history. The nurse must gather complete information on past illnesses and family history. Hypertension, extensive cardiovascular disease, diabetes, gout, and autoimmune disease are among the more common causes of renal problems. The nurse must query for such disorders as urinary calculi, frequent urinary tract infections, congenital disorders, and stroke. In addition, the nurse must search for a history of cancer with radiation or chemotherapy. The nurse must also include the history of any hospitalizations and surgical history. General health questions should include current health status, nutrition, and work history. Be alert to symptoms suggestive of decreased kidney function. These include significantly reduced energy level, metallic taste in the mouth, anorexia, nausea, pruritus, decreased ability to concentrate, decreased urine output, and related weight gain from fluid retention (Lipman, 2005).

The nurse should ask the patient if he or she smokes and thus be more susceptible to bladder cancer. Also, the patient should be asked if he or she has an extended history of high-nitrogen and low-carbohydrate diets. This could impose abnormally high blood urea nitrogen (BUN). Also, the patient should be asked if his or her diet is excessively high in dairy products and if he or she is taking mineral supplements that may predispose him or her to calculi. And, lastly, the nurse should determine if the patient is generally well hydrated.

Assessment of Urination Patterns

Potential questions for the nurse to ask the patient when assessing renal urination are exemplified in Box 52-2.

BOX 52-2

ASSESSMENT OF URINATION PATTERNS: QUESTIONS TO ASK

Questions to ask the patient when assessing the urination patterns of the renal system

The nurse can ask the following questions when assessing the renal system:

- Is there a change in voiding patterns?
- Is there a history of incontinence, urgency, or frequency of urination?
- Does the patient have difficulty with starting the voiding process?
- Is there burning when urinating?
- What is the color of the urine?
- Has there ever been any indication of **hematuria** (blood in the urine)?
- Is there a feeling of fullness after the patient has voided?
- Is the urinary stream full or are they only able to void in dribbles?

Medication History

One important aspect of the health history for a patient with renal system dysfunction is his or her medication history. The renal system has a direct relationship in the metabolism of many medications, and the health of the renal system is vital to the use of medications for patients. The nurse should assess the medication history by asking questions regarding over-the-counter medications and any alternative therapies. It is especially important to quantify the amount and duration of nonsteroidal anti-inflammatory medication usage. This group of drugs can be especially harmful to the kidneys. Potential for damage increases in the presence of hypertension or exposure to other nephrotoxic drugs as shown in Box 52-3 (Campoy & Elwell, 2005).

Red Flag

Fluid Volume Excess

The nurse must remember that a sudden increase of daily weight can indicate a sudden increase of body fluids. A weight gain of 1 kilogram would indicate retention of 1 liter of fluid. This sudden increase in body fluids could present severe cardiovascular and respiratory problems.

Physical Examination

The physical examination of the renal examination is presented as it relates to each of the anatomic areas (e.g., skin, mouth, or abdomen). In general, weighing the patient establishes changes in weight as well as a baseline weight for further evaluation. Daily weights are critical assessment components for a patient with renal failure.

Skin

Note skin turgor for an indication of hydration state. The patient's skin could be dry and lack turgor or grossly edematous depending on the etiology within the urinary system. Observe for signs of persistent scratching as often occurs with the phosphorus or calcium imbalances of renal failure. Look for pallor or the yellow-gray cast sometimes seen in renal failure. Check the female vulva and perineum for signs of irritation from urinary incontinence or vaginal discharge. Similarly check the penis, scrotum, and perineum of the male for signs of infection or drainage.

Mouth

Check mucous membranes for signs of irritation or dryness and note breath smell. The smell of ammonia is common with **uremia** (accumulation of end-products of protein metabolism in the blood stream due to renal failure).

Abdomen

Inspect and palpate for bladder distension, masses, or enlarged kidneys as is found with renal cell cancer or **polycystic cysts** (cysts with closed sacs that develop abnormally within an organ and have a distinct enclosing membrane).

Kidneys

Palpate the kidneys at the CVA. Normally, the left kidney is not palpable. A normal right kidney may be palpable during deep inhalation. To palpate for the kidneys, place one hand under the posterior flank at the CVA and the other hand in the corresponding anterior position. Palpate deeply during

Skills 360°

Urinary Incontinence

Can you remember that last time that you sneezed or coughed and experienced come loss of bladder control? How did that make you feel? Did you soil your clothes? Now imagine what it must be like for a patient who has urinary incontinence on a regular basis. Interview a patient with urinary incontinence and ask him or her how it affects his or her life. Does the patient perform bathroom mapping when out in public?

BOX 52-3

POTENTIALLY NEPHROTOXIC DRUGS AND OTHER AGENTS

Potentially Nephrotoxic Drugs and Other Agents Include:

Amikacin	Chemotherapeutic agents
Gentamicin	Contrast medium
Amphotericin B	Ethylene glycol
Gentamicin	Gold and other heavy metals
Sulfonamides	Nonsteroidal anti-inflammatory drugs

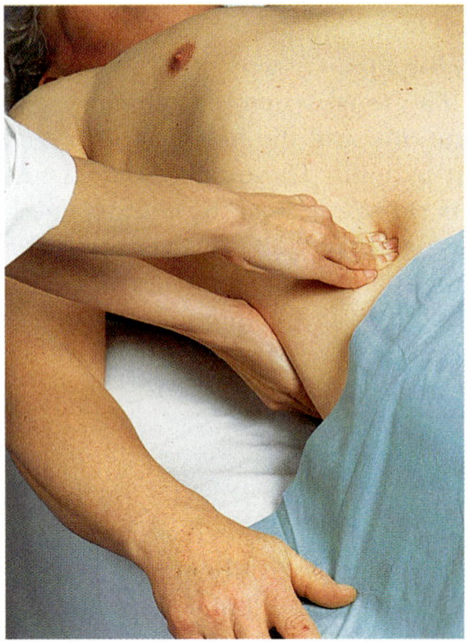

Figure 52-6 Palpation of the right kidney.

patient inspiration noting any tenderness or enlargement. To further check for tenderness in the kidney area, place one hand over the flank and strike it firmly with the fist of the other hand. Tenderness is a common finding in kidney infection as with pyelonephritis or polycystic kidneys. Palpation and percussion are illustrated in Figures 52-6 and 52-7A and B (Estes, 2006).

Lungs

Auscultate all lung fields and check for shortness of breath with rest or activity. A fluid-overloaded pulmonary capillary bed easily infiltrates the lungs with fluid as evidenced by crackles on auscultation and wet lung fields on chest X-ray. Weight, blood pressure, and lung auscultation are readily accessible nursing tools to identify and monitor fluid overload.

Bladder

Using deep palpation, the nurse can assess the bladder. First, palpate the abdomen at the midline, starting at the symphysis pubis and progressing upward to the umbilicus. If the bladder is located, palpate the shape, size, and consistency. It must be noted that an empty bladder is not usually palpable. A moderately full bladder is smooth and round, and it is palpable above the symphysis pubis. A full bladder is palpated above the symphysis pubis, and it may be close to the umbilicus. There are a variety of dysfunctions seen in bladder palpation, which are depicted in Box 52-5.

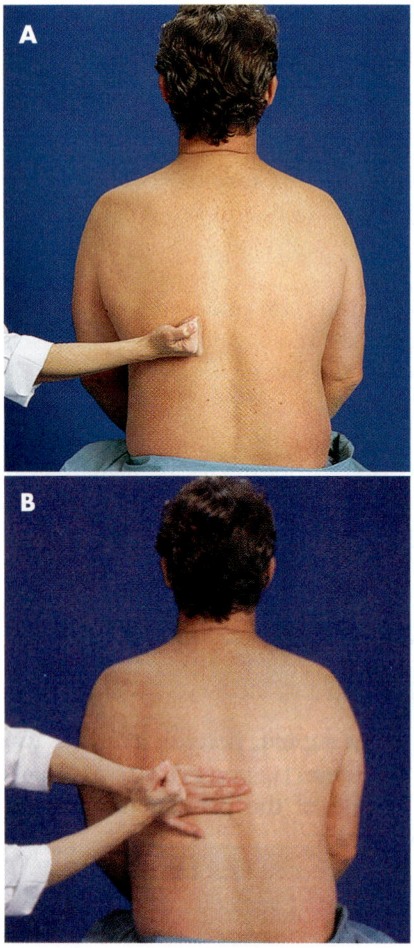

Figure 52-7 A. Direct fist percussion of the left kidney, B. Indirect fist percussion of the left kidney.

BOX 52-4

DIFFERENTIATING KIDNEY PALPATION

The distinguishing features between an enlarged liver and an enlarged kidney include:

1. The edge of the liver tends to be sharper and to extend medially and laterally, whereas the pole of the kidney is more rounded.
2. In addition, the edge of the liver cannot be captured, whereas an enlarged kidney can be.

Distinguishing features between an enlarged kidney and an enlarged spleen include:

1. A palpable notch on the medial edge of the organ favors the spleen.
2. Percussion of the spleen produces dullness, because the bowel is displaced downward; however, resonance is heard over the left kidney because of the intervening bowel.

BOX 52-5

BLADDER ABNORMALITIES

The following are the more common bladder abnormalities:

- A bladder that is nodular or asymmetrical to palpation is abnormal. A nodular bladder may indicate a malignancy. An asymmetrical bladder may result from a tumor in the bladder or an abdominal tumor that is compressing the bladder.
- Men with benign prostatic hyperplasia may be unable to completely empty their bladder because of the pressure that the enlarged prostate places on the bladder.
- Various types of urinary incontinence, due to altered mental status, muscle function, medications, and other causes can lead to incomplete bladder emptying.

DIAGNOSTIC TESTS

Adherence to specimen collection and test preparation protocols are critically important to accurately diagnose and treat urinary system disorders. In addition, patient cooperation during many of the studies is crucial. Patients must be thoroughly informed in advance of the test or assisted through the steps when they are mentally or physically dependent.

> ***Red Flag***
>
> **Using Contrast Agents in Renal Diagnostics**
>
> Protection of renal function for patients receiving a nephrotoxic contrast agent is provided through hydration preprocedure and post-procedure. Patients with fluid restrictions or needing added protection may be given one of the following agents. (Note: expedient administration is imperative.)
>
> 1. Acetylcysteine given in doses of 600 mg by mouth twice daily starting the day before the procedure. A total of four doses are given.
> 2. Sodium bicarbonate is given intravenously. An alkaline environment diminishes contrast media potential for nephrotoxicity.

Urine Studies

Urine studies are valuable diagnostic tests to evaluate renal system function, as shown in Table 52-1.

Blood Studies

Blood studies are valuable diagnostic tests to evaluate renal system function, as shown in Tables 52-2 and 52-3.

Urinary Retention Studies

Postvoid residual of urine is obtained by either of two methods. Catheterization immediately after voiding will give an exact accounting for the volume of urine left in the bladder following voiding. As with any catheterization, there is a potential for infection. Bladder scan is a noninvasive method using ultrasound and achieves comparable results without imposing risk of infection. It is convenient and can be performed at the bedside by the nurse.

Catheterization postvoid must be done immediately after the patient voids to assess for urinary retention (Table 52-4). Sterile technique is imperative. Bladder scanning reliability requires attention to three main points: (a) Follow the operator's manual instructions. This usually requires the selection of an icon representing a male or female patient. Select the male icon for the posthysterectomy female patient. Rationale: ultrasonic adjustment accomplishes sound wave penetration through the uterus. (b) Supine position is critical to accurate results. (c) Center the urine pool image over the cross-hatch on the ultrasonic grid.

> ***Red Flag***
>
> **Potential Problems Associated with Renal Ultrasounds**
>
> Renal ultrasounds cannot be done over open wounds or dressings. A kidney scan must be performed before radiographic studies involving barium; if not possible, at least 24 hours must elapse between barium procedure and the kidney scan. (Note: renal biopsy may be done with ultrasound guidance.)

Radiographic Studies

There are a variety of radiographic studies that are used in diagnostic testing of the renal system. Each test has specific nursing implications that the nurse should know to meet the educational needs of the patient. The descriptions of the tests and the nursing care involved is provided in Table 52-5.

Renal Ultrasound (Kidney Scan)

A renal ultrasound visualizes the parenchyma and associated structures including the renal blood vessels. Doppler ultrasonography is a noninvasive test that uses ultrasound waves over the flank areas to identify occlusions of the veins or arteries. Ultrasound waves are transmitted and received from the transducer while it is placed over the circulatory system locations. The returning echoes are amplified and images are recorded on a video and strip recorder. The kidney is visualized by using the liver or the spleen as comparative structures. The renal ultrasound may be performed with an intravenous pyelogram (IVP) to define or characterize masses or lesions and can be used in people with iodine allergy (Noble & Brown, 2004).

TABLE 52-1 Urine Studies

STUDY	PURPOSE	NURSING MANAGEMENT
Urine Dipstick	Screening urine study used primarily to identify gross abnormalities and determine need for further study	Follow instructions on the package. Store according to manufacturers guidelines to ensure test strip reliability. Collection is appropriate at any time of day; the first void of the day provides the optimal specimen. It is usually important to collect expediently. Send to the laboratory within one hour of the void. Avoid contamination by menses or feces.
Urine culture	Determine bacterial count and identify infecting bacteria for best choice of antibiotic. A bacterial count greater than 100,000 indicates treatable infection.	Males: Cleanse the glans penis with the appropriate cleansing solution following institutional procedure and attending any patient allergies. Retract foreskin, if present. Have the patient start to void; then collect a midstream urine sample. Keep inside of cover and container free of contamination from the hands or surroundings. Females: Separate the labia and cleanse the vulva as above. A catheter specimen is warranted during menses or conditions that will not allow a reliable midstream collection into a sterile container.
Timed urine collection	The most common is the 24-hour creatinine clearance to determine renal filtering efficiency. Normal clearance range is 70–140 mL/minute.	Have the patient void and discard the specimen or drain the collecting system and discard urine to start the collection. Place the collection receptacle on ice and carefully add each void to the collection. If the patient has an indwelling catheter, place the catheter bag on ice and empty regularly into the collection bottle. End the collection by having the patient void or by emptying the drainage system and adding the specimen to the collection receptacle. Label and keep on ice for delivery to the laboratory.
Voiding cystometrogram	A graphic recording of bladder filling pressure and abdominal pressure during the filling and voiding cycle. A urinary catheter is inserted into the urinary bladder for filling and emptying during the procedure. In addition, a catheter may be inserted into the vagina or rectum to measure abdominal pressures. Each has an attached manometer for measurement purposes. The patient will be asked about sensations while the catheter fills the bladder. A Valsalva maneuver is required at some point during the test. Alert the health care provider or technician of any patient prone to vasovagal reactions. Postprocedure, the patient may experience an increase in urinary symptoms from the use of the urethral catheter. Inform him or her to alert the health care provider of fever, chills, low back pain, or hematuria.	
Cystography	Bladder injury and suspicion of **vesicoureteral reflux** (backward propulsion of urine through the valve the normally closes the bladder and ureteral junction to backward flow of urine) are indications for this study. Radiopaque dye is instilled via a catheter directly into the bladder. As with the voiding cystometrogram, pressure recordings can be obtained. Check for allergies to contrast media. Postprocedural hydration, unless contraindicated, is important for nephrotoxic dye excretion.	

TABLE 52-2 Blood Studies

STUDY (NORMAL VALUE)	NURSING MANAGEMENT (EVALUATION AND PATIENT EDUCATION)
Blood urea nitrogen (BUN) (10–20 mg/dL)	Nonrenal causes of variance include high-protein diet, gastrointestinal (GI) bleed, rapid cell destruction as in chemotherapy or severe burns, and hydration status.
Serum creatinine normal (0.6–1.4 mg/dL)	Endogenous in source, creatinine is a by-product of muscle metabolism. It is a much more reliable indicator of renal dysfunction than is the BUN. The normal BUN/creatinine ratio is 10:1.
Sodium (135–145 mEq/L)	Abnormal levels of blood sodium are reliable indicators of intravascular hydration. Dilute or concentrated sodium indicates intravascular fluid overload (dilute) or dehydration (concentrated).
Potassium (3.5–5 mEq/L)	Serious cardiac arrhythmias or asystole are potential consequences of the high fluctuations in potassium levels associated with renal dysfunction.
Carbon dioxide content (CO_2) (22–30 mEq/L)	Indicator of metabolic acid-base balance. Variance is most commonly due to renal dysfunction. Most patients in chronic renal failure demonstrate significant metabolic acidosis.
Calcium (8.5–10.5 mg/dL)	Decreased renal secretion of phosphorus is the primary cause of hypocalcemia in renal failure. Correction is accomplished by correcting high phosphorus levels.
Phosphorus (2.5–4.5 mg/dL)	Phosphorus control is critical to prevention of renal osteodystrophy. Increased phosphorus levels result in low calcium levels and secondary hyperparathyroidism when inadequately treated.
Hematocrit (Males: 42–52 percent; Females: 35–47 percent)	Renal secretion of **erythropoietin** (**[EPO]** a hormone produced by the kidney in response to low oxygen states or a low hematocrit, which stimulates red blood cell production in the bone marrow) is compromised in renal failure and is reflected in chronically low red blood cell counts. The hematocrit is followed to adjust the dose of recombinantly produced EPO or determine need for red blood cell transfusion. Most chronic renal failure patients have hematocrit maintained in the high 20th to mid-30th percentile.

TABLE 52-3 BUN and Creatinine Levels

BUN (blood urea nitrogen)	Normal in adult 5–20 mg/dL; older adult 8–21 mg/dL; child 5–18 mg/dL	BUN measures the nitrogen fraction of urea, which is the chief end-product of protein metabolism. It is formed by the liver from ammonia and excreted by the kidney. BUN reflects protein intake, the liver's ability to metabolize, and the renal excretory ability. BUN exists in a normal ratio with serum creatinine, and they often arise together in pathological conditions of the renal system.
Creatinine	Normal in adult 0.4–1.5 mg/dL (blood) Range depends on age and gender: from as low as 52 in older females to as high as 146 in young men.	Creatinine clearance (mL/min/1.73 m^2) Creatinine is a catabolic by-product of muscle energy metabolism and is excreted by the kidneys. It is dependent on muscle mass. Kidney disorders hinder creatinine excretion; creatinine clearance is the rate at which the kidneys are able to clear creatinine from the blood.

Adapted from Daniels, R. (2004). Nursing fundamentals: Caring and clinical decision making. *New York: Thomson Delmar Learning.*

BOX 52-6

PATIENT EDUCATION FOR A RENAL ULTRASOUND

The nurse can assist and educate the patient with a renal ultrasound by providing the following information:

- You will be positioned in a supine position. Your flank will be exposed and appropriately draped.
- Your abdomen will be lubricated with an acoustic gel.
- You will be asked to take a deep breath and hold it. This is done so that various parts of the kidney can be visualized.
- The technician will use a transducer to visualize various regions of the kidney and surrounding areas.

Source: Daniels, R. (2003). Delmar's manual of laboratory and diagnostic tests. *New York: Thomson Delmar Learning.*

TABLE 52-4 Common Causes of Urinary Retention

Bladder outlet obstruction	Prostatic enlargement
	Benign prostatic hyperplasia (BPH)
	Prostate cancer
	Prostatitis
	Bladder neck dyssynergia (dyssynergia of the smooth muscle of the sphincter mechanism)
	Detrusor sphincter dyssynergia (dyssynergia between detrusor and striated muscle of sphincter)
	Urethral stricture
	Urethral tumor (rare)
	Constipation
	Pelvic organ prolapse
	Cystocele
	Uterine prolapse
Deficient detrusor contraction strength	Transient conditions
	Fecal impaction
	Acute immobility
	Side effect of drugs, including anticholinergics and tricyclic antidepressants
	Side effect of recreational drugs, including hallucinogens
	Herpes zoster of sacral dermatomes
	Vitamin B_{12} deficiency
	Established conditions
	Lesions of the sacral spine
	Cauda equina syndrome
	Diabetes mellitus (late stages)
	Tabes dorsalis
	Poliomyelitis
	Chronic alcoholism

Adapted from Daniels, R. (2004). Nursing fundamentals: Caring and clinical decision making. *New York: Thomson Delmar Learning.*

Nursing Management

The correct procedures for the nurse to follow for administration of a renal ultrasound are described in Box 52-6.

Renal Biopsy

A needle biopsy via ultrasonic guided imagery offers the least intrusive method to obtain samples of the renal cortex for microscopic examination. Surgical biopsy (open biopsy) may be required. Indications for renal biopsy include unexplained renal failure, glomerular dysfunction, and transplant rejection (Mittal, Rennke, & Singh, 2005).

Nursing Management

Preprocedure, the patient will be instructed not to eat or drink for four to six hours. Forewarn of the approximate two-hour period of bedrest required for transplant graft biopsy and the four to six hours of bedrest for **native kidney**

TABLE 52-5 Radiographic Diagnostic Tests for the Renal System

STUDY	NURSING MANAGEMENT
KUB—abdominal X-ray study of the kidneys, ureters, and bladder	Constipation can interfere with the viewing field. The KUB show kidney size, shape, and position and presence of calculi. Hydronephrosis, cysts, and tumors may be visualized.
Computed-assisted tomography (CAT or CT) scan	Contrast media must be ingested in a brief period of time prior to going to the radiology department. Inform the patient that he or she must lie still while strapped onto a gently moving table for a considerable period of time. The table will move through a large cylindrical opening. Though alone in the room, the patient will be in voice contact with the technician. Sedation should be considered for patients with anxiety issues.
Magnetic resonance imaging (MRI)	Similar to the CAT scan, though MRI does not require contrast media. A metal screening is mandatory prior to the MRI. If the patient has had significant exposure to metal, facial X-rays will be ordered to deem the patient safe to proceed with the MRI. The patient will need an IV access and all jewelry and metal removed. Metal implants will likely exclude the patient as an MRI candidate.
	Claustrophobia is a real concern because of the confined space and continual loud noises while images are taken. Sedation is often needed. Noninvasive, the MRI and CT scans offer detailed images of soft tissue.
Nuclear scans	**Radioisotopes** (a compound that contains radioactive materials, which are used in nuclear scans; the activity of these tagged materials allows the study of substances as they course through the body), such as technetium or iodine, are injected prior to the study. A scintillation camera follows passage through the renal vascular system. Nuclear scans evaluate renal blood flow and renal masses. Allergies to technetium are rare; iodine allergies must be considered.
	Alert the patient that he or she will go to radiology for the injection and return to radiology about two hours later for the actual study. He or she will be required to lie still for about 30–45 minutes in a quiet environment.
	Postprocedure care: Unless the patient is fluid restricted, encourage the patient to drink liberal amounts of fluid to promote isotope excretion.
Intravenous pyelogram (IVP)	A radiopaque contrast agent is injected intravenously. This renders the urine radiopaque as the contract agent is excreted in the urine. Abnormalities of the lumen, calculi, and masses can be detected. It is imperative to check for dye allergies and to hydrate the patient for posttest dye excretion to avoid nephrotoxic damage.
Renal angiography	An invasive procedure, renal angiography evaluates renal artery stenosis, tumors, and trauma. A catheter is threaded through the femoral artery allowing direct injection of a radiopaque substance. Preprocedure, shave the groin and mark the pedal pulses. Inform the patient that he or she may feel a temporary surge of warmth when the dye is injected. Iodine allergy must be considered.
	Postprocedure care includes approximately four hours of bedrest, frequent vital signs, groin check for hematoma, peripheral circulation status check distal to the injection site (color, warmth, and pulses), and hydration to clear the potentially nephrotoxic contrast agent.

Source: Daniels, R. (2003). Delmar's manual of laboratory and diagnostic tests. *New York: Thomson Delmar Learning.*

(one's own kidney as opposed to a transplant graft) biopsy. Less bed rest is required for transplant biopsy due to less strain on the renal capsule with the graft located in a lower abdominal quadrant.

Postprocedure care focuses on the potential for bleeding. Nursing interventions are shown in Box 52-7.

Cystoscopy

The surgical procedure of a cystoscopy allows direct visualization via a self-contained visual lens system. An illustration of a cystoscopy is presented in Figure 52-8, while an illustration of a flexible cystoscope is presented in Figure 52-9. Although the procedure could be done under local anesthesia, gen-

BOX 52-7

NURSING CARE OF PATIENTS HAVING A RENAL BIOPSY

- Frequent vital signs and inspection of the biopsy site for hematoma. Typical frequency is every 15 minutes during the first hour then gradually increasing the interval if no bleeding occurs. Follow provider protocol.
- Monitor for any evidence of bleeding. Signs and symptoms include significant change in blood pressure, tachycardia, nausea or vomiting (often associated with hypotension), or a reduction in the hematocrit.
- Anything more than minimal pain. Ureteral colic could signal a clot occluding the ureter. Back pain may indicate a retroperitoneal or intrarenal bleed.
- Monitoring the urine for hematuria or clots. Serial samples of urine are saved in urinalysis tubes, dated, timed, and placed in a rack for color comparison.
- Educate the patient to avoid heavy lifting for an average of two weeks and notify the health care provider of flank pain, light-headedness or dizziness, rapid pulse, dysuria, or hematuria.

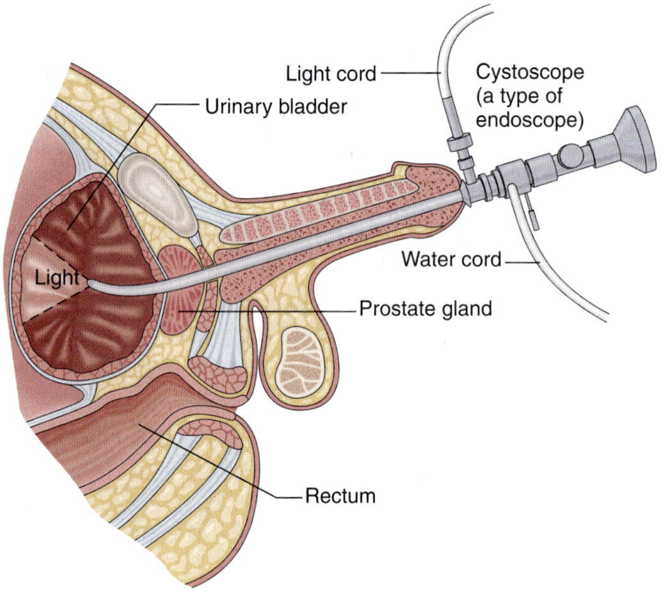

Figure 52-8 Cystoscopy.

eral anesthesia is most often chosen to prevent ureteral spasm when probing with the ureteral catheter. Complete visualization of the entire macroscopic urinary system as catheters ascend into the renal pelvis. Calculi removal, biopsy, and urine sampling from each kidney are possible with this procedure.

Nursing Management

The patient must avoid food and fluids for four to eight hours prior to the procedure if receiving general anesthesia. Postprocedural care includes monitoring the patient for urinary obstruction secondary to swelling and hematuria related to biopsy or inadvertent injury to urinary structures. Light hematuria and pain during first void(s) may not be abnormal depending on the extensiveness of the procedure (Forsyth, Shaikh, & Gunn, 2005).

The patient should be educated to notify the health care provider for problems voiding, gross hematuria, excessive pain, fever or chills, and continued **dysuria** (painful urination).

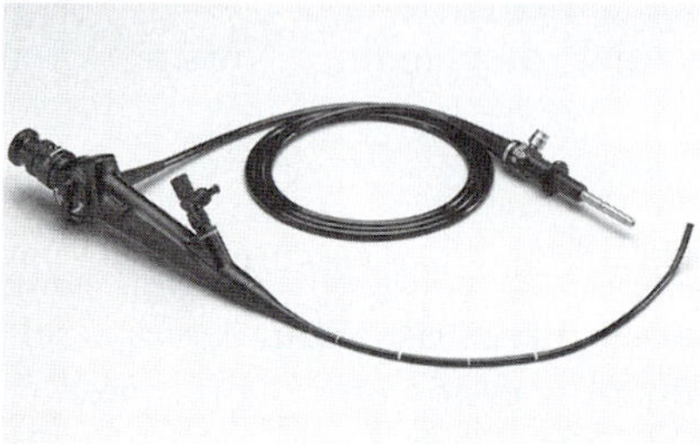

Figure 52-9 Flexible cystoscope.

KEY CONCEPTS

- The renal system controls the fluid balance of the body, controls many of the metabolic processes within the body and provides stabilization for the human body circulation.
- Composed of smooth muscle, the ureter propels urine toward the bladder by peristalsis.
- The bladder neck plays a critical role in continence and in dysfunctions of bladder emptying.
- The cumulative action seen in the renin-angiotensin cycle causes vasoconstriction and yields an increase in blood pressure.
- Hypertension, extensive cardiovascular disease, diabetes, gout, and autoimmune disease are among the more common causes of renal problems.
- Daily weight is a critical assessment components for a patient with renal failure.
- Adherence to specimen collection and test prep protocols is critically important to accurately diagnose and treat urinary system disorders.
- Serum creatinine is a by-product of muscle metabolism and is a much more reliable indicator of renal dysfunction than BUN.
- An abdominal X-ray study of the kidneys, ureters, and bladder is a KUB.
- A needle biopsy via ultrasonic guided imagery offers the least intrusive method to obtain samples of the renal cortex for microscopic examination.
- The surgical procedure of a cystoscopy allows direct visualization vial a self-contained visual lens system.

REVIEW QUESTIONS

1. Which of the following is a definitive method to monitor for bleeding into the urinary system post renal biopsy?
   1. Ask the patient if he or she has noticed blood in his or her urine
   2. Check the urine with a dipstick before discarding it
   3. Collect a small sample of each voiding and place in a rack for comparison over time
   4. Use a Foley catheter to collect a urine specimen

2. You must collect a 24-hour creatinine clearance on Mr. Jones. What will you do to begin the urine collection?
   1. Have the patient void and place the sample in the collection container
   2. Have the patient void and discard urine, noting this as the beginning of the 24-hour urine collection
   3. Wait until the patient voids to start the 24-hour urine collection
   4. All of the above are appropriate options

3. Which of the following is most appropriate intervention to protect the kidney in the presence of nephrotoxic contrast media?
   1. Hydration, administration of acetylcysteine, or administration of IV sodium bicarbonate
   2. Radiologist adjustment of nephrotoxic contrast media dosage
   3. Withhold contrast media in all cases of renal concern
   4. None of the above

4. You must send a patient for a magnetic resonance imaging (MRI) study of his kidneys. Identify two primary nursing considerations in preparation for the MRI.
   1. Coordinating the MRI with other patient care activities and informing the patient about the test
   2. Giving all scheduled medications and completing the bath before the test
   3. Report metal screening findings to the MRI department and sedate for claustrophobia before sending him or her to the MRI department
   4. Make sure the patient is NPO and hold all medications until the test is completed

5. Your patient reports, "I'm just clumsy. I dropped the cap of specimen cup on the bathroom floor, but I don't think it got dirty." What do you do now?
   1. Hope that he or she is right and send the specimen to the laboratory
   2. Discard the specimen and collect another specimen with review of instructions
   3. Clean the cover, cap the specimen, and send it to the laboratory
   4. Find a new cover to put on the specimen container and then send it to the laboratory

Continued

REVIEW QUESTIONS—cont'd

6. What position must your patient assume to obtain an accurate postvoid residual with the bladder scan?
   1. Semi-Fowler
   2. Supine
   3. Head slightly elevated
   4. Prone
7. What is the primary significance of constipation to an X-ray of the kidneys, ureters, and bladder (KUB) or other abdominal study?
   1. Resolving constipation may prevent the patient from needing the KUB.
   2. Constipation can interfere with the viewing field.
   3. The patient may have the urge to defecate during the study.
   4. There is no relationship between constipation and KUB results.
8. Identify the evidence that the kidney is an organ with high oxygen demand and the primary homeostatic organ of the body.
   1. The kidney has 2 million functioning units.
   2. The kidney filters nearly approximately 180 L water a day.
   3. The kidney receives 20 percent of the cardiac output.
   4. None of these are evidence of a high oxygen demand.
9. Nursing care of the patient who has had a cystoscopy include all of the following *except:*
   1. Warm sitz baths
   2. Monitor intake and output
   3. Mild analgesics for pain
   4. Restrict fluids
10. A patient is suspected to have a urinary tract infection. Which of the following laboratory tests would be appropriate to determine if an infection is present?
    1. Creatinine clearance
    2. Blood culture
    3. Residual urine
    4. Urine culture and sensitivity

REVIEW ACTIVITIES

1. State and describe the organs of the renal system.
2. Perform a concise health history related to the renal system on an adult patient.
3. Describe age-related changes seen in the renal system.
4. Describe any two of the diagnostic tests used for the renal system.
5. In the clinical setting, identify the location of (a) test strips for urinalysis; (b) specimen cups for collecting urine samples; and (c) Foley catheter kits.

Urinary Dysfunction: Nursing Management

CHAPTER 53

Paul Chamberland, MSN, APRN, BC, CMSRN

Leslie H. Nicoll, PhD, MBA, RN, BC

CHAPTER TOPICS

- Urinary Tract Infections
- Interstitial Cystitis
- Pyelonephritis
- Glomerulonephritis
- Nephrotic Syndrome
- Renal Tuberculosis
- Urinary Tract Calculi (Urolithiasis)
- Renal Trauma
- Renal Vascular Disorders
- Renal Cancer
- Bladder Cancer
- Urinary Diversion
- Urinary Retention
- Urinary Incontinence

Urinary tract dysfunctions cover a wide spectrum. Dysfunction in any segment of the system easily creates disorder in other areas. For example, a simple bladder infection may ascend upward along the urinary tract and evolve into nephritis with significant threat to renal function. Similarly, obstruction distal to the kidney can create pressure damage to the renal parenchyma from unrelieved or repetitive episodes of **hydronephrosis** (stretching of the renal pelvis as a result of obstruction to urinary outflow). This chapter explores nursing management of infectious, noninfectious, obstructive, calculus, and vascular disorders of the entire urinary system. Surgical diversion of urinary flow into continent or incontinent systems will also be discussed. Acute and chronic renal failure will be discussed at length in chapter 54. Although these are urinary tract disorders, discussion is lengthy because of homeostatic disturbance and the extensive treatments that are involved.

KEY TERMS

Anasarca
Cystectomy
Dysuria
Hematuria
Hydronephrosis
Hypercholesterolemia
Hypoalbuminemia
Malaise
Nephrectomy
Nephrolithiasis
Nocturia
Nosocomial
Oliguria
Proteinuria
Pyelonephritis
Ureteral strictures
Urethral strictures
Urinary tract infection (UTI)
Urolithiasis (calculi)

URINARY TRACT INFECTION

Urinary tract infection (UTI) is an infection involving the kidneys, ureters, bladder, or urethra. Synonyms for UTI include bacteriuritis, asymptomatic bacteriuritis, bacterial cystitis, urethritis, pyelonephritis, and prostatitis. A UTI can cover a wide variety of conditions, ranging from asymptomatic infections with low bacterial counts not requiring intervention to severe infection of the kidney and sepsis with threat to survival. Early intervention has the potential to save costs, prevent significant incapacity, and save lives.

A UTI is labeled according to the region of infection. In general terms, reference is made to lower urinary tract (e.g., urethra, bladder, or prostate) and upper urinary tract infections (e.g., ureters or kidney). In addition, a UTI may be classified by events such as initial or recurrent, acute or chronic. A UTI may be identified as drug-resistant. Combinations of these labels offer critical information to the provider for assessment, care planning, and patient education purposes. For example, an initial, lower tract UTI most likely prompts a lower level of concern than does a diagnosis of a chronic, recurrent, upper tract UTI.

Further, a UTI may be classified as uncomplicated in patients without structural abnormalities or altered urodynamics or complicated in patients with a structural abnormality or altered urodynamics, or any urinary infection in males.

Epidemiology

UTIs prompt over five million office visits annually in the United States. Uncomplicated infections incur annual health care costs in excess of $350 million. UTIs are more common in females because of a shorter urethra and the proximity of the urethra to the vagina and anus (Table 53-1). Sexual intercourse and forward cleansing following defecation offer primary sources of contamination. Incidence increases in the aging female because of bladder prolapse. Recurrent infection is common.

In the male, the incidence of bladder infection is higher in the uncircumcised than in the circumcised. Incidence in all males increases with age because of problems of prostatic hypertrophy.

TABLE 53-1 Epidemiological Factors Associated with UTI

Incidence	Females: 12 cases per 1,000 women per year in the United States.
	Males: 0.3 cases per 1,000 men per year.
Prevalence	Females: 10–40 per 1,000 women per year.
	Males: Less than 1 per 1,000 males per year.
	Note: Asymptomatic bacteriuria occurs in up to 40 percent of elderly men and women.
Gender	Most prevalent in sexually active adult females.
	After 65 years of age, equal numbers of men and women are affected.
Age	In infants up to six months of age; UTI is more common in boys, who have a higher incidence of abnormalities of the urinary tract than girls.
	Between 1 and 65 years of age, UTI is predominantly a disease of females, presumably because of the anatomy of the female urethra, which allows bacteria to access the urinary tract relatively easily.
	Over 65 years of age, bacteriuria affects men and women roughly equally (approximately 40 percent), with the majority of infections being asymptomatic. Routine screening and treatment has not been found to decrease morbidity or mortality in this population.

Etiology

Bacteria causing a UTI usually originates from the bowel as normal flora of the host. *Escherichia coli (E. coli)* are the most common infective bacterial organism in acute cystitis and represent 80 present of all cases requiring treatment. *E. coli* bacteria are present in feces, adhere easily to the epithelium of the urinary tract, and have the capability to resist destruction by the white blood cells.

Hospital-acquired (nosocomial) infection adds a significant health care dollar burden to the public and to the institution. UTIs are of particular significance. Physical and psychological stress response to hospitalization predisposes patients to acquired infection. Hospitalized patients frequently require procedure-associated bladder catheterization. Catheter intrusion into the urinary system predisposes the patient to inoculation with bacteria-contaminated equipment or bacterial entry along the in-place catheter. In addition to *E. coli* exposure from episodes of fecal incontinence or compromised hygiene, the environment offers exposure to more virulent organisms such as *Pseudomonas* and *Staphylococcus.* More recently, interdisciplinary health faces the challenge of limiting the spread of drug-resistant organisms, such as vancomycin-resistant enterococcus (VRE). See Table 53-2 for a summary of the common causes of UTI sorted according to their frequency of occurrence.

Pathophysiology

The epithelium of the kidneys, ureter, and bladder is sterile in the healthy individual. An infection occurs when bacteria enter the urine and begin to grow. The infection usually starts at the opening of the urethra where the urine leaves the body and moves upward into the urinary tract.

Usually, the act of emptying the bladder (urinating) flushes the bacteria out of the urethra. If there are too many bacteria, this will not stop them. The bacteria can travel up the urethra to the bladder, where they can grow and cause an infection. The infection can spread further as the bacteria move up from the bladder via the ureters. If they reach the kidney, they can cause a kidney infection (pyelonephritis), which can become a serious condition if not treated promptly.

Complications of a simple lower tract infection are rare and typically involve resistant microorganisms or indicate undiagnosed structural abnormalities or abnormal urodynamics. Primary complications of complicated and resistant UTI are ascending infection and spread to the blood stream. Nephritis and sepsis place the patient at high risk have potential for chronic illness or death.

Assessment with Clinical Manifestations

In lower urinary tract infection (e.g., cystitis), the lining of the urethra and bladder becomes inflamed and irritated. The symptoms that can be seen with lower urinary tract infection include:

- **Dysuria**—Pain or burning during urination
- Frequency—More frequent urination (or waking up at night to urinate)
- Urgency—The sensation of not being able to hold urine
- Hesitancy—The sensation of not being able to urinate easily or completely (or feeling a need to urinate but only a few drops of urine come out)
- Cloudy, bad smelling, or bloody urine
- Lower abdominal pain
- Mild fever (less than 101° F [38.3° C]), chills, and not feeling well (malaise)

In upper UTI (e.g., pyelonephritis), symptoms develop rapidly and may or may not include the symptoms for a lower urinary tract infection (see Red Flag).

Red Flag

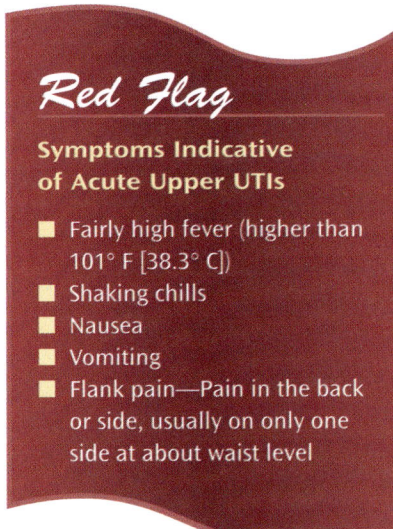

Symptoms Indicative of Acute Upper UTIs

- Fairly high fever (higher than 101° F [38.3° C])
- Shaking chills
- Nausea
- Vomiting
- Flank pain—Pain in the back or side, usually on only one side at about waist level

TABLE 53-2 Causes of UTIs and Their Frequency

Common	Gram-positive organisms:
	Staphylococcus saprophyticus (5–15 percent)
	Enterococcus faecalis
	Gram-negative organisms:
	Escherichia coli (80–85 percent)
	Klebsiella pneumoniae
	Proteus species
	Pseudomonas aeruginosa
	Enterobacter species
Rare	*Salmonella* species
	Mycobacterium tuberculosis
	Chlamydia trachomatis
	Candida species
	Multiple microbial organisms causing infection may be found in patients with renal calculi, chronic renal abscesses, or indwelling urinary catheters
Serious	*S. aureus*—commonly a result of bacteremia producing renal or perinephric abscesses
	Candida species—found in critically ill, immunosuppressed, and chronically catheterized patients
Contributory or predisposing factors	Female gender is an independent frisk factor for UTI
	Recent sexual intercourse
	Use of spermicides or diaphragm
	Pregnancy
	Antecedent antibiotic use—antimicrobials used 15–28 days before a UTI may alter urogenital normal flora in favor of pathogen-dominated flora
	Obstruction of urinary tract (e.g., benign prostatic hyperplasia, tumors, or cholinergic drugs)
	Residual urine in bladder caused by prostatic hypertrophy, urethral strictures, cystocele, hypotonic bladder, renal calculi, urolithiasis, tumors, bladder diverticula, or anticholinergic drugs
	Incomplete bladder emptying caused by neurological pathology (e.g., stroke or spinal cord injuries)
	Retrograde urinary reflux gives an increased risk of acute and chronic pyelonephritis
	Urinary catheterization
	Mechanical instrumentation

In newborns, infants, children, and the elderly, the classic symptoms of a UTI may not be present. Other symptoms may indicate a UTI:

- Newborns—Fever or hypothermia (low temperature), poor feeding, or jaundice
- Infants—Vomiting, diarrhea, fever, poor feeding, or not thriving
- Children—Irritability, eating poorly, unexplained fever that does not go away, loss of bowel control, loose bowels, or change in urination pattern
- Elderly people—Fever or hypothermia, poor appetite, lethargy, or change in mental status

Typically pregnant women do not have unusual or unique symptoms. A urine sample should be checked during prenatal visits, because an unrecognized infection can cause pregnancy complications.

Although most people have symptoms with a UTI, some do not. The symptoms of UTI can resemble those of sexually transmitted diseases. The complete assessment of a UTI is based on information given relating to one's symptoms, medical and surgical history, medications, habits, and lifestyle (Table 53-3). A physical examination and lab tests complete the evaluation.

Diagnostic Tests

Performing a dipstick of the urine offers a quick, easy, and readily available prediction of UTI. A result that is positive for nitrates and leukocyte esterase indicate treatable infection, but it does not identify the exact location within the urinary system. To perform a dipstick test, follow instructions on the package. Verify that the dipsticks have been stored according to manufacturer's guidelines to ensure test strip reliability.

Urinalysis screens that are positive for heme, protein, leukocytes, or nitrites need further study. Collection is appropriate at any time of day; the first void of the day provides the optimal specimen. It is usually important to collect expediently. Send it to the laboratory within one hour of the void. Avoid contamination by menses or feces.

Urine culture determines bacterial count and identifies infecting bacteria for best choice of antibiotic. A bacterial count of more than 100,000 indicates treatable infection. Sensitivity may be added to the culture to determine antibacterial sensitivity or resistance. This is especially important in recurrent or complicated infections.

Collection technique for males include cleansing the glans penis with the appropriate cleansing solution following institutional procedure and attending any patient allergies. Retract foreskin, if present. Have the patient start to

TABLE 53-3 Clinical Assessment for UTIs: Subjective and Objective Data

Subjective Data	
Focused past health history	Previous UTIs and how treated, urinary calculi, ureteral or urethral strictures, bladder cancer or prostate problems, recent hospitalization or surgery, sexually transmitted disease, vaginal infection, diabetes, or pregnancy.
Current history	Burning on urination, urine color and odor, fever, chills, nausea or vomiting, voiding pattern and any changes. Pain character and location. Query especially for flank or low back pain, suprapubic discomfort or feeling unrelieved with voiding, bladder spasm or burning on urination, vaginal or penile discharge, and menses.
Medications	History of taking anticholinergic or antispasmodic medications. Complete listing of current medications including over-the-counter (OTC) and herbal preparations.
Personal data	Fluid and nutritional intake, hygiene habits, adherence to prescribed medications, smoking, and caffeine and alcohol intake.
Objective Data	
Systemic	Fever, chills, nausea, diarrhea, and skin turgor.
Urinary	Cloudy urine, hematuria, foul smelling urine, distension, or suprapubic or costovertebral tenderness.
Laboratory findings	Elevated white blood cell count. Urine positive for nitrites, leukocytes, red blood cells, or bacteria.

Adapted from Estes, M. (2006). Health assessment and physical examination *(3rd ed.). New York: Thomson Delmar Learning.*

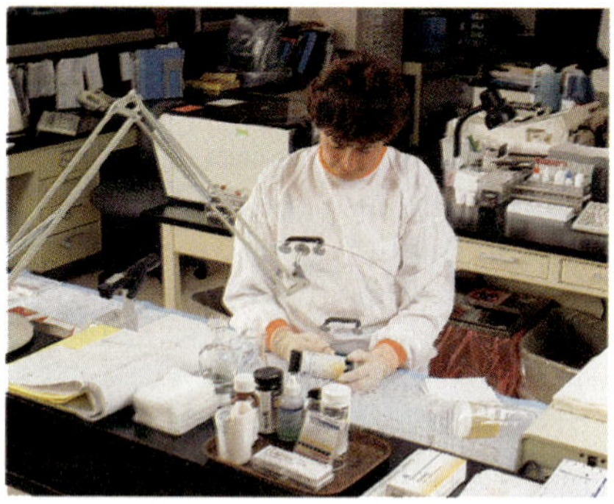

Figure 53-1 Laboratory technician examining urinalysis sample for physical, chemical, or microbiological properties from a patient with glomerulonephritis.

void then collect a midstream urine sample. Keep inside of cover and container free of contamination from the hands or surroundings. Collection technique for females include: separating the labia and cleansing the vulva. A catheter specimen is warranted during menses or conditions that will not allow a reliable midstream collection into a sterile container (Estes, 2006).

The culture is usually sent for special populations, including men, because they are less likely to get UTIs. It is not necessary to send a culture for everyone because the majority of UTIs are caused by the same bacteria. For example, a urine culture may not be required for uncomplicated cystitis in women (Figure 53-1).

Some species (e.g., *Chlamydia* and *Mycoplasma*) require special cultures to be detected. Special tests should be ordered if a patient has signs and symptoms of a UTI, but a laboratory culture fails to grow bacteria.

Imaging studies are not needed in the vast majority of patients with UTI. However, appropriate imaging studies should be done if structural abnormality or altered urodynamics are suspected. Pelvic ultrasound may be indicated in young women with pelvic tenderness, cervical discharge, and unilateral adnexal tenderness or elderly patients with abdominal pain and pyuria with no classic symptoms for UTI.

When a patient has a persistent infection that does not resolve after appropriate antibiotic therapy or suffers from recurrent infections, referral may be necessary for further tests to identify structural or functional abnormalities (Box 53-1).

BOX 53-1

SUMMARY OF DIAGNOSTIC TESTS FOR UTI

Initial Tests

- Macroscopic urinalysis: A simple, noninvasive test that should be performed on all patients suspected of having a UTI
- Dipstick nitrite tests: Detection of nitrite in urine indicates presence of nitrate-reducing bacteria. Sensitivity 0.35; specificity 0.95
- Leukocyte esterase dipstick tests: Sensitive and highly specific test for detecting greater than 10 white blood cells/mm^3 of urine (pyuria). Sensitivity 0.75-0.90; specificity 0.70
- Microscopic urinalysis: Can reveal bacteruria and pyuria
- Quantitative urine culture: Differentiates between contamination of urine and infection by quantification of bacteria; allows identification and susceptibility testing of microorganisms

Additional tests to consider if structural or functional abnormalities of the urinary tract are suspected, or with history of recurrent infections; may be performed by a specialist if warranted:

- Renal and bladder ultrasound: May demonstrate structural abnormalities
- Voiding cystourethrogram (VCUG): May demonstrate abnormalities of the collecting system, particularly vesicoureteral reflux
- Intravenous pyelogram (IVP): May demonstrate abnormal renal function, abnormalities of the collecting system, or obstruction
- Postvoid residual volume: May demonstrate significant urinary retention (greater than 100 mL is abnormal)
- Radionuclide scan: May demonstrate abnormal renal function and structure
- Cystoscopy: Allows direct visualization of bladder and distal collecting system and the collection of urine from various areas of the renal system

Adapted from Daniels, R. (2003). Delmar's manual of laboratory and diagnostic tests. *New York: Thomson Delmar Learning.*

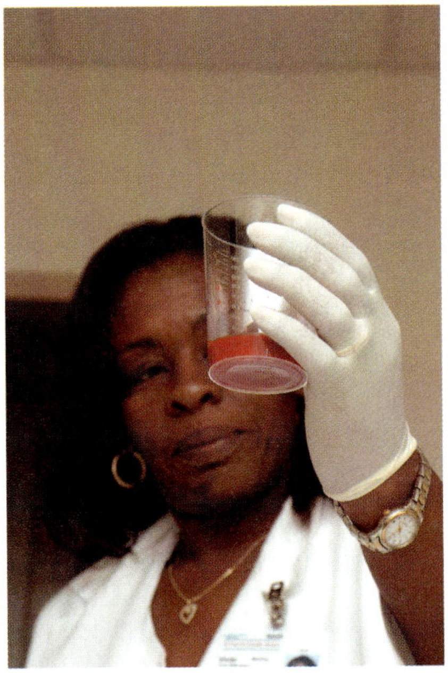

Figure 53-2 Nurse examining and measuring hematuria sample from a patient with a UTI.

Nursing Diagnoses

Based on the information gathered, examples of nursing diagnoses in the person with a UTI may include the following:

- Infection related to frequency or burning on urination, fever, elevated white blood cell count, foul-smelling urine, and suprapubic tenderness
- Impaired urinary elimination related to excessive urgency and pain with bladder filling
- Acute pain related to inflammation of urinary mucosa as evidenced by suprapubic discomfort and dysuria

Planning and Implementation

There are focused interventions to use for patients who have UTIs. The primary considerations are prevention of the UTI in the first place. Then, if a person contracts the UTI, prompt identification of the presence of the UTI is essential, followed with quick responsive antibiotic therapy (Figure 53-2). The American Urological Association (2006) is one source of referral for patients with UTIs (www.auanet.org).

Goals

The overall goals for treating a person with a UTI include: to prevent (or treat) the systemic consequences of the infection; to eradicate pathogenic organisms in the person's urine; and to prevent the recurrence of infection.

Pharmacology

It is not uncommon to have a clinically insignificant bacterial infection of this system. In such case, the patient is asymptomatic with a urinary bacterial count significantly less than 100,000 colony forming units (CFU) per milliliter. UTI are considered clinically significant and warrant treatment when presenting symptoms of UTI (irrespective of a low bacterial count) or with a bacterial count is greater than 100,000 CFU/mL. However, a health care provider should not wait to obtain the culture report before treating. Empiric antibiotic therapy should be initiated on the basis of the patient's symptoms and urinalysis results before urine culture results are obtained (Box 53-2).

Evaluation of Outcomes

Potential patient outcomes for each of the example nursing diagnoses for the patient with the UTI are shown in Table 53-4.

INTERSTITIAL CYSTITIS

The common clinical picture of interstitial cystitis (IC) presents with urgency, frequency, **nocturia** (urination at night), and dysuria in the presence of noninfected urine. **Hematuria** (blood in the urine) may be present. Pain associated with the bladder is a major complaint. IC is often confused with recurrent UTI as presenting symptoms are markedly similar. Because of its uncertain etiology, IC is regarded by many as more of a clinical syndrome than a disease entity.

Epidemiology

In general, IC affects both men and women. Although 90 percent of these people are middle-aged women, it can occur in children or older adults (Table 53-5).

PATIENT PLAYBOOK

Considerations for Patient Teaching

Health care providers should instruct all patients to completely empty the bladder when voiding; and to not put off the urge to urinate, particularly after intercourse.

It is also important to validate (or instruct, as needed) that women cleanse and dry from front-to-back when completing perineal care.

Diet

- Drinking six to eight glasses of water daily helps to prevent UTI.
- Cranberry juice may help to prevent UTI.

Sexual behavior

- Urinating before and after sexual intercourse may help to prevent UTI.
- Limiting the number of sexual partners may help to prevent UTI.

Medication history

- Always instruct the patient to finish taking the medications as the health care provider prescribed.
- Use of anticholinergic medications cautiously, as they may leave residual urine in bladder, predisposing to UTI.

Other

- If there is a family history of UTI, a genetic predisposition for bacterial adherence to bladder may be present. Awareness of and adherence to lifestyle and wellness issues, sexual behavioral practices, and dietary considerations may offer protection from UTI.
- Self-catheterization or mechanical instrumentation may introduce bacteria into urinary tract. Assist or instruct the patient on the proper and appropriate self-catheterization technique.

BOX 53-2

COMMON MEDICATIONS USED WITH PATIENTS WITH UTI

Antifolates

- Effective against common UTI pathogens except *Pseudomonas aeruginosa*. Inexpensive. Appropriate as a short course, first choice in uncomplicated UTI. Inexpensive.
- Trimethoprim-sulfamethoxazole D.S. (TMP/SMZ, Bactrim). Drink large amounts of fluids to prevent sediment in urine and calculus formation.
- Trimethoprim (Primsol, Proloprim, and Trimpex) may be prescribed alone in an attempt to limit TMP/SMZ side effects.

Fluoroquinolones

- Indicated for *Pseudomonas aeruginosa* and multidrug-resistant gram-negative infections. Expensive. Also indicated for patients with sulfa allergies.
- Ciprofloxacin (Cipro or Ciloxan) should not be administered within two hours of taking antacids.

Cephalosporins: First Generation

- Cephalexin (Biocef, Keflex, and Keftab). Typical pathogens are frequently resistant to cephalexin (20 to 30 percent nationally). Probably less effective than other alternatives for short-course (three-day) treatment, owing to its rapid clearance from urine. Is not effective in elimination of *Escherichia coli* from vaginal flora.

Penicillins

- Amoxicillin and clavulanic acid (Augmentin) is effective against beta-lactam-resistant organisms. Probably less effective than other alternatives for short-course (three-day) treatment, owing to its rapid clearance from urine. Typical pathogens are frequently resistant to amoxicillin or clavulanic acid (20 to 30 percent nationally).

Nitrofurantoin (Macrobid, Furalan, Macrodantin) attains a high concentration in the bladder because it is excreted unchanged into urine. Documented lower cure rate in short-course (three-day) treatment than other alternatives. Fifteen to 20 percent of typical organisms are resistant to nitrofurantoin. Take with food or milk to increase absorption; urine may appear dark yellow or brown.

Adapted from Broyles, B. E., Reiss, B. S., & Evans, M. E. (2007). Pharmacological aspects of nursing care *(7th ed.). New York: Thomson Delmar Learning.*

Etiology

The cause of this debilitating condition is not clearly known. Theories include obstruction to lymphatic flow, thrombophlebitis secondary to acute infections, prolonged arteriolar spasm, and neuropathic or endocrine dysfunction. Clearly this is a confusing anomaly. More recently, researchers are focusing on the activity of mucosal mast cells capable of releasing histamine and other irritants to the bladder mucosa.

Pathophysiology

The pathophysiology of IC is poorly understood. Various causes have been proposed, none of which sufficiently explain the differing clinical presentations, clinical courses, or responses to therapies. The most frequently cited cause of the presenting symptoms is that the bladder mucosa becomes thinned or

TABLE 53-4 UTIs: Nursing Diagnosis, Patient Outcomes, and Interventions

Patient with a UTI

Nursing Diagnosis: Acute pain related to inflammation of urinary mucosa as evidenced by suprapubic discomfort and dysuria

OUTCOMES (NOC)	INTERVENTIONS (NIC) AND RATIONALE
Pain Control (1605)	Pain Management (1400)
Uses resources appropriately.	Teach principles of pain management.
Reports changes in pain symptoms or sites to the health care professional.	Ensure that patient receives attentive analgesic care.
Outcome Scale	Explore with patient factors that relieve or worsen pain.
1 = Never demonstrated	Teach use of nonpharmacological techniques (heat to lower back or pubis)
2 = Rarely demonstrated	Perform a comprehensive assessment of pain to include location, characteristics, onset and duration, frequency, quality, intensity or severity of pain, and precipitating factors
3 = Sometimes demonstrated	
4 = Often demonstrated	
5 = Consistently demonstrated	

Nursing Diagnosis: Impaired urinary elimination related to UTI.

OUTCOMES (NOC)	INTERVENTIONS (NIC) AND RATIONALE
Urinary Elimination (0503)	Urinary Elimination Management (0590)
Achieves established fluid intake.	Teach patient to drink an additional eight ounces of liquid with meals, between meals, and in early evening.
Urine regains clarity and dysuria is relieved.	Consult with dietary to include additional liquids, such as soups and juices with meals.
1 = Never demonstrated	Instruct patient to respond immediately to urge to void.
2 = Rarely demonstrated	Teach patient the signs and symptoms of UTI and inform of potential for recurrence.
3 = Sometimes demonstrated	Monitor urinary elimination including frequency, consistency, odor, volume, and color.
4 = Often demonstrated	
5 = Consistently demonstrated	

Adapted from NANDA International. (2005a). Nursing diagnoses: Definitions & classifications 2005–2006. *Philadelphia: NANDA International.*

TABLE 53-5 Epidemiological Factors Associated with IC

Incidence	The incidence rate of IC is 2.6 cases per 100,000 women per year in the United States.
Prevalence	Estimated at up to 60–70 per 100,000
Frequency	1 in 4.5 women are affected; rare in men.
Race	Of patients with IC, 94 percent are white. IC appears to be slightly more common in Jewish women.
Gender	Approximately 90 percent of patients with IC are female.
Age	Median age at presentation is 40 years. IC may occur in children.
Associated medical conditions	Patients with IC are more likely to have prior gynecological surgery or a history of UTIs and are 10–12 times more likely to report childhood bladder problems. Associations exist with chronic illnesses, including inflammatory bowel disease, systemic lupus erythematosus, irritable bowel syndrome, fibromyalgia, and atopic allergy

Adapted from Rosenberg, M. T., & Hazzard, M. (2005). Prevalence of interstitial cystitis symptoms in women: A population based study in the primary care office. Journal of Urology, 174*(6), 2231–2234.*

denuded. The exposed detrusor muscle is progressively damaged and develops fibrosis. Losing its stretch capacity, bladder pain is elicited as the bladder fills. The irritating effect of urine constituents further elicits pain in the presence of an intact mucosa. The disease has rapid progression at onset and tends to plateau though in a debilitated state. Bladder capacity is reduced, voiding dysfunction or vesico-ureteral valvular incompetence develops. For clinical purposes, IC is often divided into two groups, ulcerative (i.e., classic) and nonulcerative (i.e., Messing-Stamey) types.

During a cystoscopic examination, a diffusely reddened appearance to the bladder surface epithelium can be seen in association with one or more ulcerative patches. These patches can also be surrounded by local areas of inflammation and mucosal ulceration (Hunner's ulcer), this being a hallmark of classic IC, and increased capillary formation resembling glomeruli (hence the term glomerulations), submucosal petechiae, and hemorrhage. These bladders demonstrate more fibrosis and scarring with progressive reduction in bladder capacity. The ulcers may become apparent only after the bladder is overdistended because areas of mucosal scarring rupture during the procedure (Ottem & Teichman, 2005). In the United States, this type of interstitial cystitis is rarely seen (less than 10 percent of cases), and some authors consider this type to be more resistant to therapy (Moldwin & Sant, 2002). The nonulcerative type of IC is characterized by similar clinical symptoms (i.e., frequency, urgency, or pelvic pain) but without the cystoscopic findings noted previously.

Genetics

Although traditionally IC has not been considered a hereditable condition, a recent study from the University of Maryland reports a higher occurrence of IC in monozygotic versus dizygotic twins, suggesting the disease has at least a partial genetic predisposition.

Assessment with Clinical Manifestations

A complete history as described for lower UTI is essential. Most importantly, it is critical to believe the patient about persistent reports of pain. People with IC have pain that ranges from mild to severe. Pain is most prominent as the bladder fills between voiding. Suprapubic pain is a common finding, but a person may also feel pain in the bladder, the urethra, the area below the umbilicus, the lower back, or the area around the vagina. Men may also feel pain in the scrotum, testes, or penis. Pain can come and go or it can be constant. It can increase during sex, and some women find that it is worse when they are having their period.

Absence of negative laboratory findings may tempt the health care provider to view the patient as a complainer and to minimize reports of pain. On the contrary, pain characteristics, frequency, duration, precipitating factors, and relieving factors are among the more important findings prompting cystoscopic examination and diagnosis. Empathetic listening and questioning are the nurse's greatest tools in treating a patient with IC. People with IC also feel the need to urinate often. Some people urinate up to 16 times a day and need to get up during the night to urinate. Whereas an urgent and frequent need to urinate combined with pain are common symptoms, not everyone has both symptoms. A person may have one but not the other. Symptoms can become worse or better over time.

Diagnostic Tests

IC is difficult to diagnose, and health care providers do not agree on the best way to identify it. No other laboratory test is definitive of or specific for IC: No urine cytology findings specifically suggest a diagnosis of IC; no serological or hematological abnormalities are known to be specific for IC; no known radiographic, ultrasonographic, or other imaging findings are specific for IC; and urodynamic studies are not helpful as part of the routine IC evaluation.

Most health care providers will begin by examining the person and asking about his or her symptoms. The first step in diagnosing IC is to rule out other diseases that cause similar symptoms. The differential diagnosis of urinary frequency, urgency, or pain is summarized in Box 53-3.

If the health care provider cannot find any other disease that is causing the person's symptoms, the provider may order or perform one of two tests commonly used to help diagnose IC. The first test often used to check for IC is cystoscopy. For this test, the procedural provider will insert a hollow tube that contains lenses and a light into the urethra and bladder. This tube, or cystoscope, allows the health care provider to directly examine the patient's bladder. In addition, most procedural providers will fill the patient's bladder with gas or liquid to test how well it can stretch.

Another common test for IC is the potassium sensitivity test. For this test, liquid that contains potassium is put into the bladder. After a few minutes, the patient will be asked to urinate. Plain water is then put into the patient's bladder. If the potassium causes more pain or a greater need to urinate than the water does, the person may have IC.

A number of other tests may be performed, depending on the patient's symptoms and medical history.

Nursing Diagnoses

Based on the information gathered, examples of nursing diagnoses in the person with IC may include the following:

- Impaired urinary elimination related to excessive urgency and pain with bladder filling
- Impaired comfort related to pain with bladder filling
- Potential for alteration in coping related to person's perception of possible chronic nature of this disease

BOX 53-3

DIFFERENTIAL DIAGNOSIS OF URINARY FREQUENCY, URGENCY, OR PAIN

Infectious or Inflammatory Conditions

Recurrent UTI, urethral diverticulum, infected Bartholin gland or Skene gland, vulvovestibulitis, tuberculous or eosinophilic cystitis, vaginitis (e.g., bacterial, viral [e.g., herpes]), or schistosomiasis

Gynecological Causes

Pelvic malignancy or mass (e.g., fibroid or endometrioma), endometriosis, mittelschmerz, pelvic inflammatory disease, or genital atrophy

Urological Causes

Bladder cancer or carcinoma in situ (CIS), radiation cystitis, overflow incontinence, acontractile detrusor, prostatodynia, chronic pelvic pain syndrome, bladder outlet obstruction (e.g., urinary retention with overflow incontinence), or open bladder neck (e.g., intrinsic sphincteric deficiency, urolithiasis, or urethritis)

Neurological Causes

Detrusor hyperreflexia, Parkinson disease, lumbosacral disk disease, spinal stenosis, spinal tumor, multiple sclerosis, or cerebrovascular accident

Other Possible Diagnoses

Dysfunctional voiding, vulvodynia, pelvic floor myalgia, degenerative joint disease, hernia, inflammatory bowel disease, GI neoplasm, diverticulitis, or adhesions from prior surgery

Planning and Implementation

Because no discrete pathological criteria exist for assessing and monitoring disease severity, indications and goals for treatment are based on the degree of patient symptoms. Despite considerable research, universally effective treatments do not exist, and therapy usually consists of various supportive, behavioral, and pharmacological measures. Surgical intervention is rarely indicated.

Nutrition

Some people find that changing their diet helps. Possible items to avoid include alcohol, tomatoes, spices, chocolate, caffeinated drinks, acidic foods, and artificial sweeteners.

Pharmacology

There is no general agreement about the best treatment for IC because no one knows with certainty what causes it. Many believe that each person must find a treatment that works best for him or her. There are two treatments for IC that are used by many health care providers. One is an oral agent called pentosan polysulfate sodium (Elmiron) that is taken three times a day to help the bladder heal. The other medicine for IC is a liquid solvent called dimethyl sulfoxide (abbreviated as DMSO) that is put into the bladder via a urinary catheter. It is given once or twice a week for six to eight weeks. Other drugs are sometimes given to patients with IC (Van Ophoven, Polupic, Heinecke, & Hertle, 2004). A summary of these medications is provided in Box 53-4.

BOX 53-4

COMMON MEDICATIONS USED WITH PATIENTS WITH IC

Specific for IC

Pentosan polysulfate sodium (Elmiron) is the specific for IC. Oral tablet dosage is 100 mg three times daily. The mode of action is not precisely known. It appears that Elmiron structurally and chemically resembles the lining of the bladder and offers similar protection against irritating substances. Pain reduction has been noted as soon as four weeks after the onset of treatment.

Anti-Inflammatory Agents

Cortisone acetate (Cortone, Cortone or Acetate): 100 mg daily for anti-inflammatory effect

Predinisone: 10–20 mg in divided doses daily for 21 days then in decreasing doses for another 21 days for anti-inflammatory effect

Antihistamine

Tripelennamine (Pyribenzamine): 50 mg four times a day for antihistamine effect. [Note that the side effect of this medication is bladder discomfort.]

Catheter Installation

Instillation of 50 mL of 50 percent dimethyl sulfoxide (DMSO) and letting it dwell for 15 minutes. This is repeated every two weeks and offers only symptomatic relief.

Catheter Bladder Lavage

Bladder lavage with increasing strengths of silver nitrate (1:500–1:100) for symptom relief

Adapted from Broyles, B. E., Reiss, B. S., & Evans, M. E. (2007). Pharmacological aspects of nursing care (7th ed.). New York: Thomson Delmar Learning.

PATIENT PLAYBOOK

Patient and Family Teaching for Patients with IC

The nurse should perform the following patient teaching interventions:

- Instruct the patient and family regarding signs and symptoms of upper and lower UTI.
- Instruct the patient diagnosed with IC and his or her family to distinguish between the defining characteristics of this disease and those for a UTI.
- Instruct the patient and family regarding the factors that could possibly relieve and worsen the painful episodes. Explore with the patient what was experienced with each new episode.
- Instruct the patient and family regarding the needed comfort measures.
- Review with the patient and family and explain all potentially threatening and unfamiliar procedures.
- Encourage the patient and family to identify the needed support and assist them, as appropriate, to seek and obtain it.

Health Care Resources

The International Interstitial Cystitis Patient Network Foundations offers support to patients, patient support groups, and health professionals. The latest literature, research and news are available on the World Wide Web at http://www.iicpn-foundation.org.

The Interstitial Cystitis Association (ICA) plays a vital role in research funding, disability, promoting development of new treatments, advocacy, information sharing, public awareness, and education for patients and health professionals. The association is available on the World Wide Web at http://www.ichelp.org/.

Surgery

Electrocoagulation of any splits in the bladder mucosa to relieve the painful irritation of submucosal structures may be indicated. To do this procedure, cystoscopy is required. Cystectomy with urinary diversion may be considered but only in the most severe cases. Urinary diversion is discussed later in this chapter.

Alternative Therapy

Overdistension of the bladder with water to gradually improve the capacity has been found to be successful in some cases. To do this, the person may require anesthesia. Other treatments, such as electrical stimulation or exercises to train the bladder muscles, may be prescribed. People with severe pain or major problems with urination may need surgery.

People with IC need to work with their clinical providers to find the therapy that helps them the most. Therapy can stop working over time, and most people with IC need to continue trying new therapies.

Evaluation of Outcomes

Potential patient outcomes for each of the example nursing diagnoses for the person with IC are:

- Impaired urinary elimination related to excessive urgency and pain with bladder filling. The patient is continent of urine or verbalizes satisfactory management.
- Impaired comfort related to pain with bladder filling. The patient should verbalize an adequate relief of pain along with the ability to realistically cope with the pain if it is not completely relieved.
- Potential for alteration in coping related to person's perception of possible chronic nature of this disease. The patient identifies own maladaptive coping behaviors, available resources, and support systems, describes and initiates alternative coping strategies, and describes positive results from new behaviors.

PYELONEPHRITIS

Pyelonephritis is an infection of the upper urinary tract. It may involve the ureters, renal pelvis, and the papillary tips of the collecting ducts. Unchecked, it can extend into the tubules of the nephron creating a potential for renal failure.

Etiology

Commonly, pyelonephritis is caused by urinary retention or an ascending and unresponsive lower UTI. Retained urine provides a breeding ground for bacteria. Repetitive antibacterial treatment may lead to drug resistance and extension of infection. In addition, drugs may cause necrosis of the renal papillae and sloughed papillae tissue may then cause ureteral blockage thus extension the pyelonephritis.

PATIENT PLAYBOOK

Renal Assessment

Subjective

The nurse can ask the following questions when obtaining a renal assessment from the patient:

- What is the general state of health?
- Is there a history of neurological deficit, diabetes, or other debilitating disease that could lead to urinary stasis, damage to the nephron, or impaired healing?
- Have there been recent hospitalizations and drug therapy?
- Is there a history of urinary calculi or prostate gland hypertrophy?
- Is there a recent history of catheterization?
- Has he or she experienced burning on urination, cloudy urine, suprapubic pain, colicky abdominal pain, or flank or back pain?
- How long have the symptoms persisted and how were they treated in the past?

Objective

The physical examination must include:

- Palpation of the abdomen for masses and tenderness.
- Palpation of CVA with a gentle tap of the fist over the kidney to elicit diagnostic discomfort in the presence of an inflammatory process.
- Urine inspection for clarity with sample collection for laboratory analysis. Key point: Catheter specimen will be necessary for females during menses or for those patients who lack the capacity to produce a reliable, noncontaminated specimen.

Pathophysiology

Prostate gland hypertrophy, masses, urinary calculi, or ureteral obstruction from sloughed papillae are common causes of urinary retention. Pooled urine promotes bacterial growth and the continuous urine pathways offer easy access for bacterial ascension to the renal pelvis. In addition, the presence of catheters or fecal incontinence increases the potential for UTI by providing an entry point for *E. coli,* one of the more common infecting organisms. Unchecked, bacteria in the urethra or bladder have easy access to the kidney via the ureters and renal pelvis.

Assessment with Clinical Manifestations

Acute pyelonephritis is described as a clinical syndrome presenting with bacteriuria accompanied by flank pain at the costovertebral angle (CVA), fever, and chills. In addition, the patient may experience painful urination, frequency, nocturia, nausea, vomiting, and colicky abdominal pain (Tolkoff-Rubin, Cotran, & Rubin, 2004). Conversely, chronic pyelonephritis may have a deceptively quiet presentation of frequency, dysuria, and nocturia. Mild, intermittent fever or intermittent back or flank pain may accompany the urinary symptoms (Kelly & Nielson, 2004).

Diagnostic Tests

There are a variety of diagnostic tests for detection of pyelonephritis. Urinalysis and urine culture may be sufficient in mild, initial cases of pyelonephritis in an uncomplicated presentation. Correct urine sample collection technique is critical to proper treatment. Catheterization may be necessary to collect a reliable specimen for the patient who is unable to stand, cleanse, and collect a midstream specimen.

Computed tomography (CT) is the standard diagnostic tool for pyelonephritis unresponsive to 72 hours of antibiotic therapy. CT is valuable in diagnosing obstructive etiology as well as identifying complications, such as perinephric abscess (Daniels, 2003).

Ultrasound is used when CT scanning is contraindicated, such as in pregnancy or in preexisting renal compromise. Renal ultrasound is used to place nephrostomy tubes for direct drainage of the renal pelvis in cases of complicated urinary obstruction.

Nursing Diagnoses

Based on the information gathered, examples of nursing diagnoses in the patient with pyelonephritis may include the following:

- Risk for imbalanced body temperature
- Pain related to ureteral colic
- Fear in response to the diagnosis of pyelonephritis
- Deficient knowledge related to completion of drug therapy, optimal fluid intake, or need to empty bladder every four hours to reduce bacterial count
- Ineffective coping related to anxiety, **malaise** (body discomfort and fatigue), and lowered activity level

Planning and Implementation

There are several strategies to providing care for patients with pyelonephritis. The implementation of these strategies may provide quick recovery and positive outcomes for the patient with this disorder.

Goals

The primary goal for providing care for pyelonephritis is to eradicate the UTI and to prevent damage to the renal parenchyma. Additionally and of equal importance, the secondary goal of preventing further infection must be promoted through patient education.

Evidence-Based Care

The nurse is positioned to play a significant role in preventing UTI. Evidence points to avoiding catheterization and early removal of catheters as critical to preventing UTI. The nurse must resist viewing catheters as nursing convenience or an easy answer to incontinence.

The nurse must always employ effective hand washing between patients to prevent patient-to-patient contamination and **nosocomial** (hospital acquired) infection. In addition, the practice of strict aseptic technique in catheter insertions and thorough, regular perineal and catheter site cleansing in the presence of a urinary catheter should be used. The nurse must practice preventive measures with prevention of an ascending UTI in mind.

Collaborative Management Including NIC

The collaborative management for pyelonephritis includes:

- Monitor vital signs and fluid balance.
- Ensure adequate hydration via an accurate intake and output record, encourage and provide at least 2 liters per day fluid intake or maintain a patent intravenous (IV) access.
- Monitor electrolytes, white blood count (WBC), blood urea nitrogen (BUN), and creatinine.
- Provide adequate pain management via usual analgesics and urinary antiseptics, such as phenazopyridine (Pyridium) or a combination urinary antiseptic or antispasmodic agent such as Urised (Urisedon or Urisedamine) or Urisept (Uriseptic).
- NIC: Assist with hygiene.

Population-Based Care

The elderly may have must be carefully assessed as they may have reduced sensation and therefore are not aware of a UTI prior to an advanced stage. The elderly may present with only minor complaints and may not have an elevation in temperature even with advanced infection.

The nurse must determine if the elderly patient uses fasting as a health practice and educate about the need for adequate fluid intake to prevent infection hypovolemia of the kidneys and bladder (Eliopoulos, 2005).

Patient and Family Teaching

The primary aspects of patient and family teaching are to educate about the importance of completing the full course of antibiotic therapy and maintaining the prescribed schedule to ensure continuous therapeutic blood levels. In addition, there needs to be information regarding the value of these above activities in preventing drug resistance. The NIC for the patient with pyelonephritis is to appraise the patient's current level of knowledge related to the disease process.

Evaluation of Outcomes

Potential patient outcomes for each of the example nursing diagnoses for the patient with pyelonephritis are:

- Risk for imbalanced body temperature. The patient maintains body temperature within a normal range.

- Fear in response to the diagnosis of pyelonephritis. The patient will manifest positive coping behaviors and verbalize how to effectively treat the disease and prevent its recurrence.
- Ineffective coping related to anxiety, malaise, and lowered activity level. The patient identifies own maladaptive coping behaviors, available resources, and support systems, describes or initiates alternative coping strategies, and describes positive results from new behaviors. The patient regains energy and participates in self-care.
- Acute pain related to ureteral colic or bladder spasm. Patient will verbalize maintenance of identified comfort level.
- Deficient knowledge related to completion of drug therapy, optimal fluid intake, or need to empty bladder every two hours to reduce bacterial count. The patient will verbalize the drug therapy regimen, the need to complete full dose on schedule to prevent drug resistance or continued infection. The patient will verbalize need to flush urinary system via adequate fluid intake and fully empty bladder every two hours to reduce the amount of bacteria available for growth.

GLOMERULONEPHRITIS

Glomerulonephritis is an inflammation of the glomerular capillaries. In patients with glomerulonephritis, the glomeruli become inflamed and impair the kidney's ability to filter urine. Eventually, the glomeruli become inflamed and scarred, and slowly lose their ability to remove waste and excess water from the blood to make urine. Glomerulonephritis can be acute, occurring as a sudden attack of inflammation, or chronic, which develops gradually. Glomerulonephritis can be part of a systemic disease, such as lupus or diabetes, or it can be a disease by itself, which is known as primary glomerulonephritis. Treatment varies depending on the type of glomerulonephritis that has been diagnosed.

Epidemiology

Glomerulonephritis represents 10 to 15 percent of glomerular diseases. Variable incidence has been reported in part because of the subclinical nature of the disease in more than half the affected population (Kazzi & Tehranazdeh, 2005). Incidence of poststreptococcal glomerulonephritis has fallen over the last few decades in western countries. This is believed to be a result of more rapid and effective treatment of a streptococcal infection with antibiotics, better health care delivery, and improved socioeconomic conditions. The disease remains much more common in regions such as Africa, the Caribbean, India, Pakistan, Malaysia, Papua New Guinea, and South America.

Etiology

There are many causes of glomerulonephritis. They include those related to infections, immune diseases, inflammation of the blood vessels (vasculitis), and conditions that scar the glomeruli. Often, however, the exact cause is initially unknown. Glomerulonephritis after infection includes poststreptococcal glomerulonephritis, bacterial endocarditis, and viral infections.

Poststreptococcal glomerulonephritis may develop after an infection of group A beta hemolytic streptococcus, usually in the pharynx (strep throat) or skin (impetigo). Postinfectious glomerulonephritis is becoming more uncommon because of rapid and complete antibiotic treatment of most streptococcal infections. Bacterial endocarditis is known as a cause of glomerulonephritis. Those at greatest risk are patients with a heart defect, such as a damaged or artificial heart valve. Among the viral infections that may trigger glomerulonephritis are the human immunodeficiency virus (HIV), which causes acquired immune deficiency syndrome (AIDS), and the hepatitis B and hepatitis C viruses, which affect the liver and can become chronic infections.

Systemic lupus erythematosus (SLE) is a chronic inflammatory disease and has been shown to cause glomerulonephritis. Goodpasture's syndrome is a rare immune lung disorder that may mimic pneumonia. It causes hemorrhage in the lungs as well as glomerulonephritis. Immunoglobulin A (IgA) nephropathy is characterized by recurrent episodes of blood in the urine. This condition results from deposits of the protein IgA in the glomeruli. IgA nephropathy can progress for years with no noticeable symptoms. Men seem more likely to develop this disorder than women.

Polyarteritis is a form of vasculitis that affects small and medium blood vessels in many parts of the body, including heart, kidneys, and intestines. Wegener's granulomatosis is a form of vasculitis that affects small and medium blood vessels in the lungs, upper airways, and kidneys. In both cases, the damage to the kidneys results in glomerulonephritis.

Pathophysiology

Immune complexes form in situ and deposit on the glomeruli, forming lesions. Except for poststreptococcal glomerulonephritis, the exact triggers for the formation of the immune complexes are unclear. Histopathologically, the glomerular tufts will appear swollen and infiltrated with polymorphonucleocytes. On gross examination, the kidneys may be enlarged by 50 percent.

There are a number of conditions that cause scarring of the glomeruli, including hypertension, diabetic nephropathy, and glomerulosclerosis. Hypertension damages the kidneys and impairs their ability to perform their normal functions. Glomerulonephritis can also cause high blood pressure because of its impact on kidney function. Diabetic nephropathy, also known as diabetic kidney disease, is one of the leading causes of end-stage kidney disease in the United States. It usually takes years to develop diabetic nephropathy. Damage may be slowed or prevented by in patients who maintain good control of their blood sugar. Glomerulosclerosis is characterized by scattered scarring of some of the glomeruli. This condition may result from another disease or occur for no known reason.

Chronic glomerulonephritis sometimes develops after a bout of acute glomerulonephritis, but in many patients there is no history of kidney disease. Often, the first indication of chronic glomerulonephritis is chronic kidney failure. Infrequently, chronic glomerulonephritis runs in families. In many cases, the cause is unknown.

In poststreptococcal glomerulonephritis, long-term prognosis is generally good. More than 98 percent of individuals are asymptomatic after five years. Chronic renal failure is a possibility, however, and has been reported 1 to 3 percent of the time.

For patients with other forms of glomerulonephritis, long-term outcomes generally depends on the underlying agent, which must be identified and treated and can range from complete recovery to total renal failure. In the latter case, treatment with dialysis and possibly a kidney transplant may be required. The prognosis for patients with cardiopulmonary or neurological complications is generally poorer.

Some patients become critically ill during the acute phase. Patients with anuria, nephrotic syndrome, massive proteinuria, significant hypertension, encephalopathy, or pulmonary symptoms will require hospitalization. Complications can lead to end-organ damage in the central nervous and cardiopulmonary systems. Other complications include hypertensive retinopathy, hypertensive encephalopathy, nephrotic syndrome, and chronic renal failure.

Assessment with Clinical Manifestation

In patients with poststreptococcal glomerulonephritis, there is a latent period between the streptococcal infection and the onset of signs and symptoms of acute glomerulonephritis. In general, the latent period is one to two weeks after a strep throat infection and three to six weeks after an impetigo infection (Geetha, 2004). If glomerulonephritis occurs within one to four days of a streptococcal infection, that is suggestive of preexisting renal disease.

The first clinical symptom is often dark urine, which is described as brown or tea- or cola-colored. It is caused by the hemolysis of red blood cells that have penetrated the glomerular basement membrane and have passed into the tubular system. Periorbital edema occurs suddenly. It is usually most noticeable on waking. Edema is a result of the defect in renal excretion of salt and water. The severity of the edema is not necessarily related to the degree of renal impairment. Hypertension is present in approximately 80 percent of patients. This cluster of symptoms: hematuria, edema, and hypertension, is known as nephritic syndrome. Approximately 95 percent of patients have at least two of these symptoms; 40 percent have all three.

Patients may complain of flank pain, due to stretching of the renal capsule. Approximately 10 to 50 percent of patients often have a low urine output **(oliguria)**. In this group, 15 percent have a urine output of less than 200 mL/day. Other symptoms include general malaise, weakness, and anorexia, which are present in about 50 percent of patients. Approximately 15 percent of patients complain of nausea and vomiting.

Patients with underlying systemic diseases that have caused the glomerulonephritis may present with symptoms of those diseases. For example, patients with SLE often have arthralgias or skin rashes. Patients with Wegener's granulomatosis often present with a triad of sinusitis, pulmonary infiltrates, and nephritis.

Diagnostic Tests

Laboratory tests include a complete blood count (CBC), electrolytes, including BUN and creatinine, urinalysis, and cultures of throat and skin to rule out *Streptococcus.* The BUN and creatinine will be elevated, reflecting the decrease in glomerular filtration rate. This elevation is usually transient. The urinalysis is always abnormal. Hematuria and proteinuria are present in 100 percent of cases. The specific gravity is greater than 1020 osm. Red blood cells and red blood cell casts are present in the urine. Blood cultures should be obtained in patients with fever, immunosuppression, a history of IV drug use, or those with indwelling shunts or catheters. Chest X-ray (CXR) may be necessary in patients with a cough, with or without hemoptysis.

Nursing Diagnoses

Based on the information gathered during the assessment, the following nursing diagnoses may be appropriate for the patient with glomerulonephritis:

- Excess fluid volume
- Risk for infection
- Deficient knowledge

Planning and Implementation

The management for glomerulonephritis is ideally implemented early in the disorder to prevent complications. Renal system involvement and more serious systemic problems can occur as the disorder exacerbates.

Goals

The major goals of care are to control edema and blood pressure. Therapy is symptomatic and depends on the clinical severity of the illness.

Nutrition

To control edema, the patient should be prescribed a low sodium diet (2 g per day) and placed on a fluid restriction (1 L per day). In the hospitalized patient, it is important to maintain a careful record of intake and output.

Pharmacology

In patients with positive cultures for *Streptococcus,* the infection must be treated. Penicillin is indicated in nonallergic patients. Oral penicillin G is usually prescribed as 250 mg four times a day for 7 to 10 days. Patients who are allergic to penicillin can be prescribed erythromycin, 250 mg four times a day for 7 to 10 days. Obtain throat cultures from family members and close personal contacts, and treat those who are infected.

In patients with severe edema, loop diuretics, such as furosemide (Lasix), may be prescribed. This is to increase urinary output, which will consequently improve cardiovascular congestion and hypertension. In adults, the usual dose is 20 to 40 mg orally or intravenously, given every six to eight hours. Potassium-sparing diuretics are contraindicated because of an increased risk of hyperkalemia.

Hypertension may be severe and may not be controlled by the diuretic. In this case, calcium channel blockers or angiotensin-converting enzyme (ACE) inhibitors may be prescribed. Amlodipine (Norvasc) is an example of the former and usually prescribed in a dose of 5 to 20 mg orally, twice a day. Captopril (Capoten) is an ACE inhibitor and is prescribed as 25 mg orally, two or three times per day. Total daily dose should not exceed 150 mg.

Steroids, immunosuppressive agents, and plasmapheresis are generally not indicated.

Population-Based Care

As noted above, family members and close personal contacts should have throat cultures and be treated if a streptococcal infection is present. In some areas of the world, streptococcal infection, leading to epidemics, may occur. In this case, it is recommended that close contacts and family members receive prophylactic antibiotic therapy.

Surgery

Renal biopsy may be required, especially in the following cases: (a) absence of a latent period between the streptococcal infection and acute disease; (b) anuria; (c) rapidly deteriorating renal function; (d) no improvement or continued decrease in the glomerular filtration rate at two weeks; and (e) persistent hypertension beyond two weeks. During the recovery phase, renal biopsy may be warranted if the glomerular filtration rate is not normal by four weeks or proteinuria lasts beyond six months.

Patient and Family Teaching

The patient must be taught the basics of a low-sodium diet and fluid restriction. Advise the patient to continue the diet until edema, hypertension, and urine abnormalities have resolved. If the patient is taking a diuretic, high-potassium foods, such as bananas and avocados, should be avoided.

The patient should be taught to have moderate activity until the symptoms subside; strenuous exercise can exacerbate proteinuria and hematuria. Bed rest may be required during the acute phase of the illness.

Stress to the patient the importance of follow-up care. Blood pressure should be monitored at every visit, or every month for six months, and then every six months after that. Blood work to monitor BUN and creatinine needs to be done at 2, 6, and 12 weeks, then every three months for one year. Urinalysis for hematuria and proteinuria needs to be done every two, four, and six weeks and then again at 4, 6, and 12 months. Lab values should be normal within six weeks, although it can take much longer for microhematuria in the urine to resolve.

Teach patients about their medications and side effects. Most patients will not require any medications after the acute phase of their illness, although antihypertensive medications may be required if the blood pressure remains high.

If the patient has a skin infection, stress the importance of meticulous personal hygiene.

Evaluation of Outcomes

Potential patient outcomes for each of the example nursing diagnoses for the patient with glomerulonephritis:

- Excess fluid volume. The patient with glomerulonephritis will:
  - Remain free of edema and effusion; weight will be appropriate for the patient.
  - Maintain urine output within 500 mL of intake with normal urine osmolality and specific gravity.
  - Explain measures that can be taken to treat or prevent excess fluid volume, especially diet, fluid restriction, and medications.
- Risk for infection. The patient with glomerulonephritis will:
  - Remain free from signs and symptoms of infection.
  - State symptoms of infection of which to be aware.
  - Maintain good personal hygiene.
  - State the importance of having family members tested and treated for streptococcal infection.
- Deficient knowledge. The patient with glomerulonephritis will:
  - Explain dietary and drug therapy.
  - Explain the schedule for follow-up visits and the need for long-term follow-up.
  - Discuss the need to balance activities with rest if fatigue is present.

NEPHROTIC SYNDROME

Nephrotic syndrome (nephrosis) is not a single disease but a group of symptoms. Symptoms include heavy **proteinuria** (increase in protein in the urine), **hypoalbuminemia** (decrease in albumin in the blood), edema, **hypercholesterolemia** (high serum cholesterol), and normal renal function. Nephrotic syndrome can be primary or secondary. Primary nephrotic syndrome occurs as part of a recognized systemic disease.

Epidemiology

Nephrotic syndrome is often described a disease of children and is relatively rare. It is 15 times more common in children than in adults. The reported annual incidence rate is 2 to 5 per 100,000 children younger than 16 years. The cumulative prevalence rate is approximately 15.5 per 100,000 individuals (Travis, 2005). Nephrotic syndrome prevalence is difficult to establish in adults, because the condition is usually a result of an underlying disease. In adults, diabetes mellitus is emerging as a major cause of nephrotic syndrome, thus American Indians, Hispanic (Americans), and African Americans have a higher incidence of nephrotic syndrome compared to Caucasians (Agraharkar, 2004).

BOX 53-5

PRIMARY CAUSES OF NEPHROSIS

- Collagen vascular disease, such as systemic lupus erythematosus or rheumatoid arthritis
- Sickle cell disease
- Diabetes mellitus
- Amyloidosis
- Malignancy, such as leukemia, lymphoma, Wilms tumor, or pheochromocytoma
- Toxins, such as bee sting, poison ivy or oak, or snake venom
- Medications, including probenecid, fenoprofen, captopril, lithium, or warfarin
- Heroin use

Etiology

There are both primary and secondary causes of nephrotic syndrome. Examples of primary causes are listed in Box 53-5. Secondary nephrotic syndrome occurs after an infectious disease, such as infection with group A beta-hemolytic streptococci, syphilis, malaria, tuberculosis, or viral infections, including varicella, hepatitis B, HIV, and infectious mononucleosis.

Pathophysiology

Nephrotic syndrome results from damage to the kidneys' glomeruli, the tiny blood vessels that filter waste and excess water from the blood and send them to the bladder as urine. They consist of capillaries that are fenestrated, that is, have small openings, which allow fluid, salts, and other small solutes to flow through but normally not proteins. Damage to the glomeruli from diabetes, glomerulonephritis, or even prolonged hypertension, causes the membrane to become more porous, so that small proteins, such as albumin, pass through the kidneys into urine. As protein continues to be excreted, serum albumin is decreased, which in turn decreases the serum osmotic pressure. Capillary hydrostatic fluid pressure becomes greater than capillary osmotic pressure, which results in generalized edema. As fluid is lost into the tissues, the plasma volume decreases, stimulating secretion of aldosterone to retain sodium and water, which decreases the glomerular filtration rate to retain water. This additional water also passes out of the capillaries into the tissue, leading to even greater edema.

Assessment with Clinical Manifestations

The major clinical manifestation is edema, which is the presenting symptom in about 95 percent of cases. In adults, the edema is usually present in dependent parts, such as ankles or legs, and is pitting in nature. In children, periorbital edema is common. Patients may have fluid in the pleural cavity, causing pleural effusion, or in the abdominal area, causing ascites. The edema may progress rapidly or quite slowly. Eventually, the edema is present throughout the body, which is known as **anasarca.** Some patients may notice foamy urine, due to a lowering of the specific gravity by the high amount of proteinuria. Actual urinary complaints, such as hematuria or oliguria, are uncommon. Other symptoms may include anorexia, irritability, fatigue, abdominal discomfort, and diarrhea (Travis, 2005).

When taking a history, many patients report a viral upper respiratory tract infection immediately preceding the first clinical signs of the disease but its relevance to the nephrotic syndrome is unknown. A history of prior allergic events is common. Children should be questioned about insect stings, immunizations, or poison ivy. In adults, it is important to ask about underlying diseases that may be the cause of nephrotic syndrome.

Diagnostic Tests

Laboratory tests include a urinalysis for protein and cellular elements and serum tests for protein and lipid analysis. Protein in the urine usually exceeds 100 mg/dL and values as high as 1000 mg/L are common. Protein can also be tested with a dipstick and may be as high as +3 to +4. The protein-to-creatinine ratio may vary from 1 to 20 (normal is less than 0.2). Hematuria may or may not be present. Hypoalbuminemia is common, with serum albumin levels following below 2 g/dL. Values as low as 0.5 g/dL are not uncommon. Hyperlipidemia is common and typically correlates inversely with the concentration of serum albumin. Values for lipids may remain moderately elevated for one to three months after remission of proteinuria (Daniels, 2003).

No routine imaging studies are indicated. CXR may reveal pleural effusion. The presence of pleural effusion correlates directly with the degree of edema and indirectly with the serum albumin concentration.

Nursing Diagnoses

Based on the information gathered during the assessment, the following nursing diagnoses may be appropriate for the patient with nephrotic syndrome:

- Imbalanced nutrition, less than body requirements
- Risk for infection
- Deficient knowledge

Planning and Implementation

The nurse plans a variety of strategies for caring for patients with nephritic syndrome. Nutrition and pharmacology are part of the areas of focus for the management of these patients.

Goals

The major goal of care is to preserve renal function. Secondary goals include the prevention of infection and receiving an adequate diet. In many patients, nephrotic syndrome is chronic and relapsing; they need to be taught to monitor their urine for protein and to be awareness of signs and symptoms of a recurrence of the disease.

Nutrition

In patients with nephrotic syndrome, the tubular function of the kidney to conserve sodium is not affected, thus, total body sodium is uniformly increased. Patients are often treated with glucocorticoids, which further curtails renal sodium excretion. Patients with nephrotic syndrome will usually be prescribed a sodium-restricted diet. Alterations in protein are not indicated, and fluid restriction is unnecessary unless the patient's thirst is so excessive that fluid intake is extreme.

Pharmacology

Glucocorticoid therapy has become the primary agent of choice in the treatment of patients with nephrotic syndrome. In most cases, oral prednisone or prednisolone is started in a dosage of 2 mg/kg/day. The total daily dose is usually split into two doses and given daily for four to eight weeks. Maintenance therapy should be tailored to the individual patient, with gradual weaning from the glucocorticoid.

Patients with nephrotic syndrome are at high risk for infection and immunosuppression as a result of steroid therapy, which increases this risk. If the patient becomes febrile, blood and urine cultures should be obtained. If an infection is present, it should be promptly treated with an appropriate antibiotic.

Diuretic therapy may be beneficial, especially in patients with symptomatic edema. A loop diuretic, such as furosemide, may be given orally (1–2 mg/kg/day). Patients should be carefully observed for hypovolemic shock. If the edema is severe enough to warrant IV diuretic therapy, then salt-poor albumin should be infused concurrently. The usual dose is 1 g/kg given intravenously over two to four hours.

Pneumococcal vaccine is indicated in all patients after remission is obtained.

Population-Based Care

It has been found that viral respiratory illness can initiate an exacerbation of nephrotic syndrome, therefore, the patient should avoid exposure to others with obvious respiratory tract infections.

Patient and Family Teaching

Because nephrotic syndrome can be a chronic and relapsing problem, patient education about awareness of symptoms and self-management is essential. Patients should be taught to keep a log of treatment and progress. Clinical notes, including presence, absence, or degree of edema; blood pressure; other illnesses; urine protein results; and administration of medications should all be recorded in the log on a daily basis.

Home monitoring of urine protein and albumin is an important aspect of patient education. Patients should be taught how to monitor urine protein by means of a dipstick; this should be recorded in the log. It is recommended that urine be tested daily, usually the first urine of the day. Monitoring should continue after the urine has become free of protein, during the maintenance period, and beyond. If a patient should experience a relapse, the log can give clues to the progression of the disease before edema recurs.

Evaluation of Outcomes

Potential patient outcomes for each of the example nursing diagnoses for the person with nephrotic syndrome:

- Imbalanced nutrition, less than body requirements. The patient with nephrotic syndrome will:
  - Eat a diet high low in sodium with adequate calories to meet nutritional requirements.
  - Will maintain a stable weight.
- Risk for infection. The patient with nephrotic syndrome will:
  - Remain free from signs and symptoms of infection.
  - State symptoms of infection of which to be aware.
  - State the importance of avoiding people with upper respiratory infection.
- Deficient knowledge. The patient with nephrotic syndrome will:
  - Explain dietary and drug therapy.
  - Demonstrate how to test urine for protein and maintain a clinical log.
  - Discuss the importance of monitoring ongoing health status and the need to obtain health care promptly if there is any change in status.

RENAL TUBERCULOSIS

Renal tuberculosis is the most common site of extrapulmonary tuberculosis. This infection can result in cessation and destruction of renal mass and healing can lead to strictures, obstruction, and infection, causing renal functional loss and failure. If identified early it is a completely curable condition (Casaccia, et al., 2003).

Etiology

Usually, renal tuberculosis results from silent bacillemia accompanying pulmonary tuberculosis. However, active lesions in the kidney may not manifest clinically for many years. Also, many cases remain clinically silent for years while irreversible renal destruction takes place.

Pathophysiology

The pathophysiology is that of tuberculosis and renal tuberculosis is usually secondary to tuberculosis (TB) of the lung. In a small percentage, the tubercle bacilli reaches the kidney via the bloodstream. The healing process can lead to stricture, obstruction, secondary calculi, and infection causing renal functional loss and failure.

Assessment with Clinical Manifestations

The most frequent clinical features reported have been frequency, dysuria, urgency, hematuria, and flank pain. In addition, unexplained sterile pyuria or hematuria can exist and should prompt the health care provider to undertake an evaluation for renal tuberculosis. Sometimes, patients can have a late presentation with advanced disease including renal insufficiency. Most renal tuberculosis patients are asymptomatic, and slow but continuous infection causes destruction of renal mass and the healing process leads to renal functional loss (Matsumura, Yamamoto, Hirohashi, & Kitano, 2005).

Diagnostic Tests

A detailed history including past and family history of pulmonary tuberculosis and thorough clinical examination is important. Laboratory investigations will include a urine examination with pH, acid-fast bacillus (AFB) smear, routine and AFB cultures, hemogram, serum chemistry specific to renal function (e.g., BUN and creatinine), CXR, plain abdominal X-ray, intravenous pyelogram (IVP), and tuberculin test. A CT scan is usually performed on selected patients to confirm findings on IVP and cystoscopy may be performed to get histological diagnosis (Daniels, 2003). The definitive diagnosis of tuberculosis is by culturing tubercle bacilli from urine.

Nursing Diagnoses

Based on the information gathered, examples of nursing diagnoses in the patient with renal tuberculosis may include the following:

- Acute pain as related to burning on urination
- Risk for imbalanced body temperature related to infectious process of tuberculosis

Planning and Implementation

The earlier the detection and treatment is initiated, the less the damage to the renal system. If prolonged disease, there may be renal scarring, the development of ureteral strictures, and even renal failure. The patient may require specific follow-up on the renal system to prevent complications. Specific drug therapy and nursing management are discussed in chapter 32.

Evaluation of Outcomes

Potential patient outcomes for each of the example nursing diagnoses for the patient with renal tuberculosis are:

- Acute pain as related to burning on urination. The patient should verbalize an adequate relief of pain along with the ability to realistically cope with the pain if it is not completely relieved.
- Risk for imbalanced body temperature related to infectious process of tuberculosis. The patient maintains body temperature within a normal range.

URINARY TRACT CALCULI (UROLITHIASIS)

Urolithiasis (calculi) refers to stones in the urinary tract. The formation of urinary calculi formation remains somewhat of a perplexity. The often unilateral formation of urinary stones challenges questions of environment and diet. One would assume both kidneys to be creating the same environment for stone formation. Their ability to resist the velocity urinary stream long enough to grow in size is further perplexing. Many of the people that develop renal calculi require hospitalization, and the pain associated with renal stones is often unmistakably acute.

Epidemiology

Urinary calculi afflict males more often than females at approximately a 3:1 ratio. Incidence in the United States averages 20 cases per 10,000 persons. Incidence is higher in warmer regions and is most likely related to dehydration. The incidence is primarily between 20 and 55 years of age. Whites have a greater occurrence than African Americans. Untreated, stones recur 10 percent in 1 year and up to 50 percent in 10 years. The lifetime prevalence of symptomatic **nephrolithiasis** (kidney stone disease) is approximately 10 percent in men and 5 percent in women, and more than $2 billion is spent on treatment each year.

Etiology

The etiology of renal calculi is unclear. Factors directly contributing to stone formation include an acid urine and concentration of precipitating elements in the urine. Increased rate of calcium absorption from the gut may be a more important contributory factor than is dietary intake. The likelihood of stone formation is influenced by urinary, dietary, and genetic factors as well as the presence of other medical conditions. A number of dietary factors have been associated with a reduced risk of stone formation, including higher intakes of dietary calcium, potassium, and phytate and lower intakes of animal protein, sodium, and sucrose. Systemic factors also influence risk independent of dietary intake, including higher body mass index (particularly in women), gout, and primary hyperparathyroidism (Curhan, 2005).

Pathophysiology

There are a variety of stones, each with potential to form in a different environment. Calcium composes the majority of renal stones. Struvite stones are composed of magnesium, phosphate, and ammonium and frequently present as staghorn calculi lodged in the pelvis of the kidney. Uric acid stones claim less than 5 percent of all urinary calculi. Cystine and xanthine stones are associated with hereditary factors. Indinavir, triamterene, and silicate stones are associated with medications.

Approximately 85 percent of stones in men and 70 percent in women contain calcium, most commonly as calcium oxalate. Overall, UTI or systemic disorders, such as primary hyperparathyroidism, are responsible for less than 10 percent of stones in men and 25 percent in women. The other stone types, such as cystine, uric acid, and struvite, are much less common. However, these types of stone also deserve careful attention, because recurrences are common.

A kidney stone may form when the concentrations of urinary constituents exceed their solubility. The causes of stone formation differ for different stone types. Cystine stones form only in individuals with the autosomal recessive disorder of cystinuria. Uric acid stones form only in individuals with persistently acid urine, with or without hyperuricosuria. Struvite stones form only in the setting of an upper UTI with a urease-producing bacterium. Stones may occasionally result from precipitation in the urinary tract of medications, such as acyclovir and indinavir (Curhan, 2005).

Assessment with Clinical Manifestations

The typical presentation of renal stones is sudden-onset unilateral flank pain of sufficient severity that the individual usually seeks medical attention, often at an emergency department. Although the term colic is used, this is a mis-

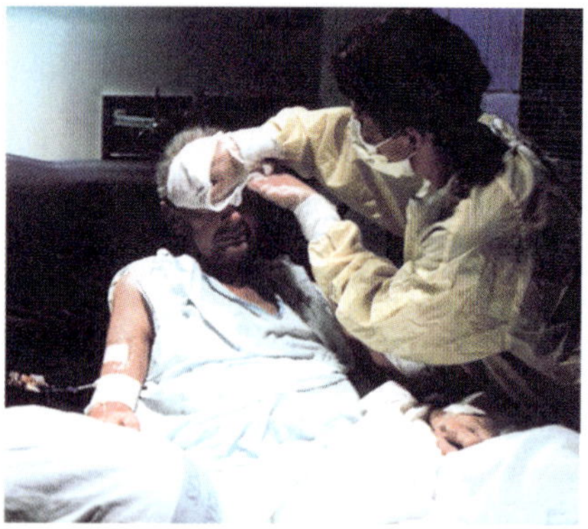

Figure 53-3 Nurse is applying cool wash cloth to man experiencing severe acute pain from renal calculi.

nomer, because the pain does not completely remit but rather waxes and wanes. The pain is often accompanied by nausea and occasionally vomiting. The pain can radiate to a variety of locations depending on the location of the stone: when the stone is in the upper ureter, pain may radiate anteriorly to the abdomen; when the stone is in the lower ureter, pain can radiate to the ipsilateral testicle in men or ipsilateral labium in women; or if the stone is lodged at the ureterovesical junction, the major symptoms may be urinary frequency and urgency. A less common acute presentation is gross hematuria without pain (Curhan, 2005). The patient may also experience the first stage of shock with cool, diaphoretic skin. In addition, the patient may develop a UTI and have the symptoms of fever, nausea, and vomiting (Figure 53-3).

Diagnostic Tests

Although the physical examination alone will not completely make the diagnosis, there are clues to help guide the evaluation. The patient will typically be in obvious pain and cannot find a comfortable position. There may be ipsilateral CVA tenderness, or in cases of obstruction with infection, signs and symptoms of sepsis may be present. In addition, the familial history may lend information to confirm renal calculi.

The serum chemistries are typically normal, but leukocytosis may be present because of stress or infection. The urinalysis classically reveals red and white blood cells and occasionally may have crystals. If the ureter is completely obstructed due to the stone, there may be no red blood cells, as no urine will be flowing from that ureter into the bladder. Clinically, patients with an asymptomatic renal stone often have microscopic hematuria.

Helical CT scan is the imaging modality of choice because of its sensitivity, ability to visualize uric acid stones (traditionally considered radiolucent), and lack of need for radiocontrast. Helical CT can detect small stones that may be missed by IV urography, which requires IV radiocontrast. Typically, CT will show a ureteral stone or evidence of recent passage whereas plain abdominal X-ray (kidney-ureters-bladder [KUB]) can miss a stone in the ureter or kidney, even if radiopaque, and provides no information on obstruction (Curhan, 2005).

Ultrasound has the advantage of avoiding radiation but can only image the kidney and possibly the proximal ureter; thus, ureteral stones are typically not seen by ultrasound.

The differential diagnosis of someone with suspected renal colic includes muscular or skeletal pain, herpes zoster, acute cholecystitis, duodenal ulcer, appendicitis, diverticulitis, pyelonephritis, abdominal aortic aneurysm, gynecological causes, ureteral obstruction due to other intraluminal factors, such as a blood clot or sloughed papilla, and ureteral stricture.

Nursing Diagnoses

Based on the information gathered, examples of nursing diagnoses in the patient with renal calculi may include the following:

- Acute pain as related to renal calculi
- Ineffective coping related to anxiety, lower activity level and the inability to perform normal activities of daily living
- Impaired urinary elimination related to renal calculi
- Risk for infection

Planning and Implementation

Renal colic is one of the most excruciating types of pain that a patient will experience; therefore, the first and foremost treatment is pain control. IV fluids are routinely given for volume repletion, and some experts believe this will increase the likelihood of stone passage, but no prospective data are available (Curhan, 2005). Overall, the management for urinary calculi focuses on relieving the pain, destroying or removing the renal stones, and preventing continued formation of calculi.

Nutrition

In general, dietary management for prevention of renal calculi focuses on changing the urine composition. Increasing fluid intake to 2.5 to 3 liters per day is advised with an intake that is spread throughout the day, as well as even drinking fluids at night.

Calcium intake is limited in regard to dietary calcium and vitamin D enriched foods. Decreasing vitamin D limits the absorption of calcium from the gastrointestinal (GI) tract. In addition, both phosphate and oxalate can also be limited from the diet.

Animal proteins are limited to prevent uric acid stones, as indicated in the Patient Playbook. Also, maintaining urine pH at higher levels (alkaline) decreases the potential development of uric acid and cystine stones. Examples of foods that alkalinize are: fruits, green vegetables, legumes, milk, and milk products.

PATIENT PLAYBOOK

Self-Care Nutrition Advice

Self-care for kidney stones can be approached in a number of ways, but starting with these simple steps first may help prevent further renal stone development:

- Drink plenty of fluids
- Water, lemonade, and most fruit juices can help dilute the substances in the urine that form kidney stones; avoid grapefruit juice and soft drinks
- Do not eat too much animal protein
- Diets high in animal protein are linked to increased calcium in the urine, which contributes to oxalate stones
- Avoid foods with organic acids (oxalates) that can help stones form
- Limit intake of spinach, rhubarb, beet greens, nuts, chocolate, tea, bran, almonds, peanuts, and strawberries, which appear to significantly increase urinary oxalate levels
- Supplement with vitamin B_6 and magnesium
- Taking 50 mg a day of the supplement vitamin B_6 with 200 to 400 mg a day of the mineral magnesium (preferably in the form of magnesium citrate) can inhibit oxalate stone formation
- Monitor calcium intake
- If the health care provider has determined that a patient does not overabsorb calcium, take 800 mg a day of calcium (in the form of calcium citrate or calcium citrate-malate) with meals

Pharmacology

Acute pain from renal calculi is typically treated with analgesia and hydration. Evidence from many randomized controlled trials suggests that parenteral nonsteroidal anti-inflammatory drugs (NSAIDs) are as effective as narcotics in relieving the pain of renal colic. There are no clinically important differences in terms of rapidity of action or magnitude of relief. A variety of types of medications, dosages, and routes of administration have been compared, but there is no one clearly superior approach. Local active warming may also be an adjunctive treatment. Newer medications that may be effective include antispasmodics, alpha-blockers, trigger point injection with lidocaine, desmopressin, and NSAIDs combined with nitrates (Curhan, 2005).

Thiazide diuretics are often administered for calcium calculi to reduce urinary calcium excretion, which prevents further stones. Potassium citrate causes the pH of urine to move in an alkaline direction, which prevents stones from form in acidic urine (e.g., uric acid and cystine).

Surgery

Surgical options for stone removal are driven by stone size, location, and composition; urinary tract anatomy; and availability of technology. Extracorporeal shock wave lithotripsy (ESWL) is the least invasive; it is most effective for stones that are smaller than 2 cm, located in the renal pelvis, and composed of calcium oxalate dihydrate, apatite, uric acid, or struvite. If available, ESWL for acute ureteral colic may be successful and reduce the morbidity associated with stone passage (Figure 53-4).

Cystoscopic stone removal, by either basket extraction or fragmentation, is invasive but effective and can now be used to remove stones even in the kidney. Percutaneous nephrostolithotomy is more invasive but is necessary for large stone burdens or stones that cannot be removed cystoscopically and is the standard for making a patient stone free (Curhan, 2005).

The treatment of existing stones in morbidly obese individuals is challenging. The ability to image the urinary tract may be limited if the patient's size prohibits access to scanning by CT. ESWL may not be an option, as morbid obesity may impede stone localization and the ability of the shock waves to reach the calculus. Percutaneous approaches can be used but may be more difficult in the morbidly obese patient; thus, the preferred approach is ureteroscopy (Casaccia, et al., 2003).

Evaluation of Outcomes

Potential patient outcomes for each of the example nursing diagnoses for the patient with renal calculi are:

- Acute pain as related to renal calculi. The patient should verbalize an adequate relief of pain along with the ability to realistically cope with the pain if it is not completely relieved.
- Ineffective coping related to anxiety, lower activity level, and the inability to perform normal activities of daily living. The patient identifies own maladaptive coping behaviors, available resources, and support systems, describes and initiates alternative coping strategies, and describes positive results from new behaviors.
- Impaired urinary elimination related to renal calculi. The patient is continent of urine or verbalizes satisfactory management.
- Risk for infection. The patient remains free of infection, as evidenced by normal vital signs and absence of purulent drainage from wounds, incisions, and tubes. Infection is recognized early to allow for prompt treatment.

RENAL SYSTEM TRAUMA

The kidney is the most common organ in the urinary tract to be injured by severe trauma. Trauma is injury caused by an external force that may be either blunt; such as a car accident, or penetrating, such as a gunshot wound. Blunt trauma injuries to the kidney may show no evidence of external injury, or bruises may appear over the back or abdomen where the kidney is located. Penetrating kidney injury may also be difficult to detect. For example, the external point of entry of the bullet may be small and at a distance far enough away from the location of the kidney for it not to be a consideration.

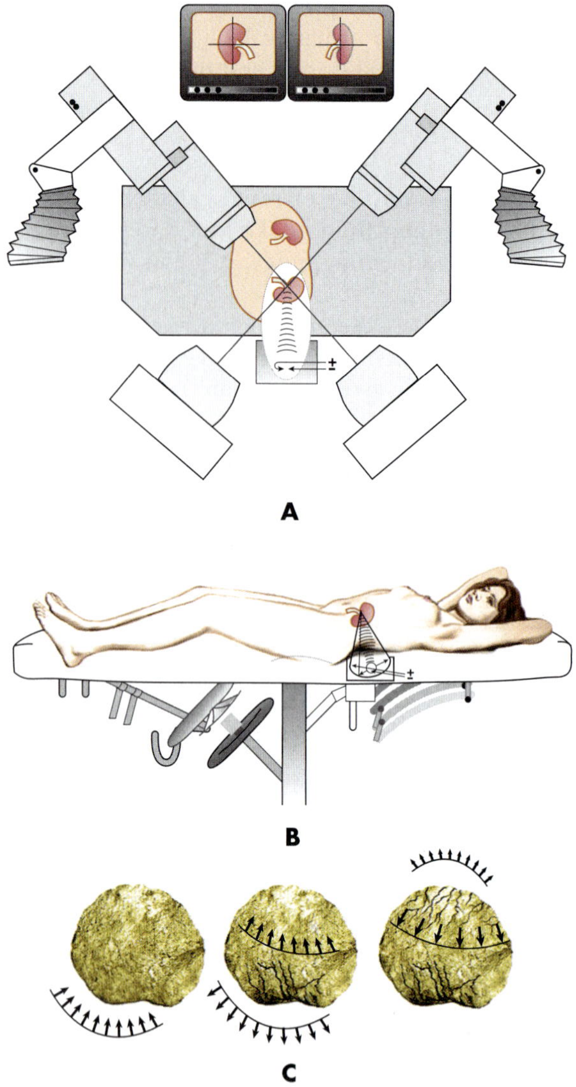

Figure 53-4 ESWL: A. Two X-ray beams crossing at focal point for proper positioning on stone, B. Focal point, C. Reflection of shock waves at first and second acoustical interfaces of the stone and surrounding fluid with fracture of the stone.

Etiology

Renal contusions, superficial cortical lacerations, and small perirenal hematomas account for 90 percent of all renal injuries. Renal injuries occur in 15 to 40 percent of patients with abdominal trauma. Blunt renal trauma can be classified according to the severity of injury and the most common is the renal contusion. The kidney can be damaged from a blow in the abdomen anteriorly, just below the rib cage, particularly in road traffic accidents, such as when the victim is thrown onto the steering column or some other projecting object. Abdominal injuries due to seat belts include 11 percent that involve the urinary tract, and half of those are renal.

Penetrating injuries (usually from gunshot or stab wounds) account for 20 percent of renal traumas in an urban setting. The damage from a bullet will depend not only on direction but also on the velocity of the missile. Also, a knife or stiletto stab can readily cut the cortex of the kidney if the weapon is driven more than three inches into the victim. Although a perirenal hematoma usually develops, the patient may not show hematuria unless the weapon has reached the calyces or renal pelvis.

There is also the possibility of iatrogenic injuries, which can occur in the passage of a catheter up the ureter (damage of renal pelvis), when a renal biopsy is done or when there is an infection carried indirectly into the renal pelvis.

Red Flag

Ureteral and Urethral Strictures

Ureteral strictures (a narrowing of the lumen of the ureter) can be caused by surgical interventions as a result of scarring. These strictures can decrease the actual function of the kidney. The nurse can assess for strictures when renal pain increases if the patient drinks large amounts of fluids in a short period of time. Correction is made with stent placement.

Urethral strictures (a narrowing of the lumen of the urethra) occur as a result of inflammation of the urethra from causes such as trauma, urethritis, congenital defects, and surgery. The nurse can assess for strictures of the urethra by noticing a diminished force of the urine stream, a split urine stream, and spraying of urine. In addition, the patient may develop urethritis and potentially a UTI. Correction is made by a urethral dilation and potentially stent placement.

Pathophysiology

The classification of renal injuries is based on the extent and depth of parenchymal lacerations, the integrity of the renal collecting system, and the status of the renal pedicle. Major renal injuries include deep cortical lacerations with or without disruption of the collecting system, comminuted renal fractures, and vascular pedicle injuries with either avulsion, intimal dissection, or traumatic occlusion. These injuries often require surgical intervention.

The most common complications in renal trauma are urinary leakage or delayed bleeding from the damage (Box 53-6). Other complications, such as the development of an abscess surrounding the kidney, can also occur. Finally, some patients develop hypertension after significant kidney trauma. This may be treated by medications, angiographically, or surgically (including removal of the kidney), if conservative treatment fails.

Assessment with Clinical Manifestations

The cardinal sign of a renal trauma is hematuria, which can be massive or microscopic, but the extent of the injury cannot be measured by the volume of hematuria or appearance of the wound. Other signs that can be present in renal trauma are lumbar and abdominal pain, sometimes with rigidity of the anterior abdominal wall and local tenderness. The health care provider should assess for such injuries as rib fractures, pelvic fractures, or vertebral injury, which can elicit renal trauma. In addition, nausea and vomiting can be present. Extensive blood loss and shock may result from retroperitoneal bleeding (Figure 53-5).

If the patient presents with a small flattening of the normal contour of the loin, a perinephric hematoma should be suspected. In the case of retroperitoneal hematoma or effusion, the renal injury may be associated with paralytic ileus, which produces a danger confusing diagnosis of intra peritoneal trauma.

Diagnostic Tests

Once injury is suspected, it is important to perform imaging studies of both kidneys to confirm clinical suspicion and determine injury severity. In past years, an X-ray in the form of an IVP was used. Currently, a CT scan with contrast is the investigation of choice to obtain a reliable and quick way of assessing kidney injury. Ultrasonography is another effective tool that may be utilized in the diag-

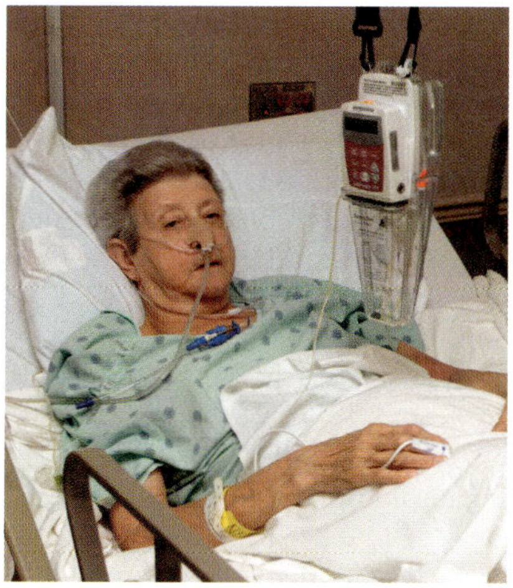

Figure 53-5 Patient with nausea while experiencing recent renal trauma.

BOX 53-6

POSSIBLE COMPLICATIONS OF RENAL TRAUMA

The most common and possible complications of renal injuries are:

- Secondary hemorrhage, usually due to infection (10 to 14 days after trauma)
- Paralytic ileus (4 to 5 days) as a result of retroperitoneal hematoma
- Hypertension as a result of the constricting effect of reorganizing perirenal hematoma
- Arterio-venous fistula
- Renal failure
- Renal atrophy
- Hydronephrosis
- Chronic pyelonephritis
- Renal calculi
- Renal artery stenosis

nosis of kidney trauma. However, it may not provide the best details of the degree of injury and may need to be supplemented by either an IVP or a CT scan.

In patients with multivisceral trauma requiring emergent laparotomy, imaging evaluation is usually limited to emergency excretory urography prior to surgery. In more stable patients, CT allows accurate diagnosis and staging of major renal injuries. CT can determine the depth of cortical laceration, the amount of infarcted renal parenchyma, the extent of perirenal hemorrhage, the status of the renal collecting system, and the vascular pedicle. Although excretory urography (ultrasonography) is the most cost-effective screening modality in the evaluation of stable patients with isolated flank trauma, its accuracy falls significantly with more severe renal injuries. The majority of patients with extensive renal injuries are not adequately staged by excretory urography alone. Therefore, contrast-enhanced CT should be performed in patients with suspected major renal trauma, multivisceral injuries, or inadequate staging with excretory urography.

Nursing Diagnoses

Based on the information gathered, examples of nursing diagnoses in the patient with renal trauma may include the following:

- Deficient fluid volume related to hematuria
- Acute pain in the lumbar and abdominal areas related to renal trauma
- Nutrition imbalance, less than body requirements, related to nausea from renal trauma

Planning and Implementation

Treatment of kidney trauma depends on the condition of the patient, the severity of kidney injury, and the presence of other injuries. If the patient's condition is stable and injury to other organ systems has been ruled out, conservative, nonsurgical treatment is an option. In the cases of parenchymal lacerations, that are restricted to the cortex, the patient should be hospitalized, kept on bed rest, and given broad-spectrum antibiotics until the blood in the urine clears. When there is deep parenchymal laceration, the patient should be treated conservatively and assessed for clinical manifestations of abscess, infection, hypertension, and secondary hemorrhage. Even after discharge from the hospital, the patient needs to be monitored for the possibility of late bleeding from the injured kidney or development of high blood pressure as the result of the kidney injury.

Surgery

Patients with the more significant parenchymal lacerations (major injuries), extensive extravasation, vascular injuries, or pulsatile hematoma, will likely undergo exploratory surgery. Penetrating injuries from gunshot or stab wounds could require surgical exploration, but it is not necessary if the CT scan or arteriography show a minor injury, without extravasation of contrast medium, which confirms preservation of vascular vessels. When surgery is necessary, the aim is to try to repair and preserve the injured kidney. However, if it is not possible to save the kidney, because it is too severely injured, surgical removal of the kidney (**nephrectomy**) may be required.

Evaluation of Outcomes

Potential patient outcomes for each of the example nursing diagnoses for the patient with renal trauma are:

- Deficient fluid volume related to hematuria. The patient experiences adequate fluid volume and electrolyte balance as evidenced by urine output greater than 30 mL/hour, normotensive blood pressure, heart rate 100 beats/minute, consistency of weight, and normal skin turgor.

- Acute pain in the lumbar and abdominal areas related to renal trauma. The patient should verbalize an adequate relief of pain along with the ability to realistically cope with the pain if it is not completely relieved.
- Nutrition imbalance, less than body requirements, related to nausea from renal trauma. The patient verbalizes and demonstrates selection of foods or meals that will achieve a cessation of weight loss and weighs within 10 percent of ideal body weight.

RENAL VASCULAR DISORDERS

There are primarily three conditions of renal vascular disorders: (a) renal artery stenosis, (b) renal vein thrombosis, and (c) nephrosclerosis. Table 53-6 depicts the primary differences for each of these conditions:

RENAL CANCER

Several different types of cancer can affect the kidneys. Although it is not a common cancer overall, renal cell carcinoma is the most common kidney cancer, affecting approximately 40,000 people in the United States each year.

Epidemiology

Renal cell carcinoma accounts for approximately 3 percent of adult malignancies and 90–95 percent of neoplasms arising from the kidney. The age-adjusted incidence of renal cell carcinoma has been rising by 3 percent per year. Approximately 31,200 new cases of renal cell carcinoma were diagnosed in the year 2000, and more than 11,900 affected individuals died.

Renal cell carcinoma is more common in people of Northern European ancestry (Scandinavians) and North Americans than in those of Asian or African descent. In the United States, its incidence has been equivalent among Caucasian

TABLE 53-6 Renal Vascular Disorders

RENAL VASCULAR DISORDER	DESCRIPTION AND PATHOPHYSIOLOGY	CLINICAL MANIFESTATIONS	MGMT CONSIDERATIONS
Renal artery stenosis	Partial blockage of renal arteries caused by such disorders as atherosclerosis and fibromuscular hyperplasia	Hypertension (1 to 2 percent of all hypertension cases is caused by renal artery stenosis)	Renal angioplasty Surgical revascularization Nephrectomy as most critical care technique
Renal vein thrombosis	Caused by such disorders as: renal cancer, trauma, nephritic syndrome, pregnancy	Hematuria Flank pain Fever Pulmonary emboli	Corticosteroids Anticoagulants Surgical therapy (removal of thrombi)
Nephrosclerosis	Sclerosis of small vessels of kidney	Intermittent areas of ischemia from lack of blood flow Hypertension Loss of renal function, even to the extent of renal failure	Antihypertensive medication treatment Supportive mgmt if patient develops renal failure

BOX 53-7

CAUSES FOR RENAL CANCER

- Cigarette smoking doubles the risk of renal cell carcinoma and contributes to as many as one third of all cases. The risk appears to increase with the amount of cigarette smoking in a dose-dependent fashion.
- Obesity is another risk factor, particularly in women; increasing body weight has a linear relationship with increasing risk.
- Additional factors associated with development of the disease include the following: hypertension, treatment for hypertension, unopposed estrogen therapy, and occupational exposure to petroleum products, heavy metals, solvents, coke-oven emissions, or asbestos.

and African Americans, but incidence among African Americans is increasing rapidly. Renal cell carcinoma is twice as common in men as in women. This condition occurs most commonly in the fourth to sixth decades of life, but the disease has been reported in younger people who belong to family clusters.

Etiology

A number of cellular, environmental, genetic, and hormonal factors have been studied as possible causal factors for renal cell carcinoma. These are shown in Box 53-7.

Pathophysiology

Renal cell carcinoma (e.g., renal adenocarcinoma and hypernephroma) is the development of cancerous changes in the cells of the renal tubules. The tissue of origin for renal cell carcinoma is the proximal renal tubular epithelium. Renal cancer occurs in both a sporadic (nonhereditary) and a hereditary form. In the past these tumors were believed to derive from the adrenal gland; therefore, the term hypernephroma often was used.

Renal cancer is staged with two different systems. The first, the Robson modification of the Flocks and Kadesky system, is uncomplicated and is used commonly in clinical practice. The Robson staging system has stages I to IV. The second system is the tumor, nodes, and metastases (TNM) classification which is endorsed by the American Joint Committee on Cancer (AJCC). The major advantage of the TNM system is that it clearly differentiates individuals with tumor thrombi from those with local nodal disease.

Genetics

Genetic studies of the families at high risk for developing renal cancer led to the cloning of genes whose alteration results in tumor formation. These genes are either tumor suppressors or oncogenes. At least four hereditary syndromes associated with renal cell carcinoma are recognized: (a) von Hippel-Lindau (VHL) syndrome, (b) hereditary papillary renal carcinoma (HPRC), (c) familial renal oncocytoma (FRO) associated with Birt-Hogg-Dube syndrome (BHDS), and (d) hereditary renal carcinoma (HRC). VHL disease is transmitted in an autosomal dominant familial multiple-cancer syndrome, which confers predisposition to a variety of neoplasms,

Assessment with Clinical Manifestations

Renal cell carcinoma symptoms include blood in the urine, abnormal urine color, flank or back pain, a lump or mass in the kidney area, abdominal pain or swelling, weight loss, testicle enlargement, fatigue, fever, and anemia. However, several less serious conditions can cause similar symptoms, including UTIs (from simple cystitis to more complex infections, such as pyelonephritis), kidney stones, or a cyst. These alternatives must be considered before establishing a diagnosis.

As renal cell carcinoma grows, it may invade organs near the kidney such as the liver, colon, or pancreas. Kidney cancer cells may also spread (metastasize) to other areas, such as the lymph nodes, brain, lungs, or bone. These advances in renal cancer lead to a wide variety of other clinical manifestations.

Diagnostic Tests

Laboratory studies in the evaluation of renal cell carcinoma should include a workup such as: urine analysis, CBC count with differential, electrolytes, renal profile, liver function tests, calcium, erythrocyte sedimentation rate (ESR), prothrombin time (PT), and activated partial thromboplastin time (APTT).

A large proportion of patients diagnosed with renal cancer have small tumors discovered incidentally on imaging studies. A number of diagnostic modalities are used to evaluate and stage renal tumors, such as, excretory urography, CT scan, ultrasonography, arteriography, venography, and magnetic resonance imaging (MRI). In addition, radiologic studies can be tailored to enable further characterization of renal masses, so that nonmalignant tumors can be differentiated from malignant ones. A bone scan is recommended for bony symptoms with elevated alkaline phosphatase level. Percutaneous cyst puncture and fluid analysis is used in the evaluation of potentially malignant cystic renal lesions detected by ultrasonography or CT imaging (Lake & Hafez, 2005).

Nursing Diagnoses

Based on the information gathered, examples of nursing diagnoses in the patient with renal cancer may include the following:

- Fear in response to the diagnosis of renal cancer
- Knowledge deficit related to the diagnosis of renal cancer
- Ineffective coping related to anxiety, lower activity level and the inability to perform normal activities of daily living

Planning and Implementation

Usually the management of renal cancer uses a combination of treatments, although surgery, including full or partial kidney removal, is the mainstay of renal cell carcinoma treatment. Other treatments, depending on individual cases, include biological therapy to trigger the body's immune system, hormone therapy, radiotherapy, chemotherapy, or arterial embolization, which blocks the blood supply to the tumor. Other treatments are under study including molecular markers and additional chemotherapy agents (Fromer, 2005). The nursing care of patients with renal cancer is illustrated in detail in chapter 15.

Pharmacology

A variety of chemotherapy agents are used in the treatment of renal cancer. Floxuridine (FUDR), 5-fluorouracil (5-FU), vinblastine, paclitaxel (Taxol), carboplatin, ifosfamide, gemcitabine, and anthracycline (doxorubicin) all have been used (Anderson, Woltman, Kovach, & Konety, 2004).

Immunotherapy stimulates the immune system to attack cancer. The most commonly used immunotherapy agents are Proleukin and interferon. The interferons (biological therapy) are natural glycoproteins with antiviral, antiproliferative, and immunomodulatory properties. The interferons have a direct antiproliferative effect on renal tumor cells (Coppin, et al., 2005).

Surgery

Surgery is always utilized for the treatment of patients with renal cell cancer unless the patient is too ill to tolerate the procedure. Currently, most health care providers think that the primary cancer should be removed even when there is widespread cancer present at diagnosis. In many patients with renal cancer, surgery alone can be curative and when the cancer is more extensive the surgery can be palliative. There also is the general concept that immunotherapy will work better if as much cancer as possible is removed before treatment. There are several surgical approaches that are utilized, depending on the extent of disease and the condition of the patient.

The most commonly performed surgery to treat renal cell cancer is radical nephrectomy. During a radical nephrectomy, the entire cancerous kidney, the attached adrenal gland, and the fatty tissue immediately around the kidney are removed. The lymph nodes around the kidney are often removed and examined under the microscope to determine if they contain cancer. Radical nephrectomy is associated with a greater than 90 percent five-year survival in patients with stage I and II cancer (Galli, Munver, Sawczuk, & Kochis, 2005).

Partial nephrectomy is performed to preserve as much normal kidney tissue as possible; however its complication rate may be slightly higher than radical nephrectomy. Open partial nephrectomy is usually the treatment of choice when radical nephrectomy may result in either immediate dialysis or a high risk for subsequent dialysis.

Laparoscopic radical nephrectomy is a surgical technique that is less extensive and invasive than a typical radical nephrectomy. Compared to open radical nephrectomy, laparoscopic radical nephrectomy involves longer operative time, less postoperative pain, shorter hospital stay, and shorter recovery time.

Tumor ablation is a process that destroys the tumor without excising it. Examples of ablative technologies include cryotherapy, interstitial radiofrequency, high-intensity focused ultrasound, microwave therapy, and laser coagulation.

Patient and Family Teaching

A vital need for nursing management of patients with renal cancer is patient teaching. Patients in the high-risk group should be made aware of the early signs and symptoms, and the need for early intervention for possible cure should be stressed. Patients in early stages who have undergone treatment should be educated about possible relapse. In addition, the consequences of the treatment strategies (e.g., chemotherapy, surgery, or radiation) are described in a thorough manner in chapter 15.

Evaluation of Outcomes

Potential patient outcomes for each of the example nursing diagnoses for the patient with renal cancer are:

- Fear in response to the diagnosis of renal cancer. The patient should manifest positive coping behaviors and verbalize a reduction in the amount of fear of having this disease.
- Knowledge deficit related to the diagnosis of renal cancer. The patient should demonstrate motivation to learn, identify perceived learning needs, and verbalize an understanding of desired content.
- Ineffective coping related to anxiety, lower activity level, and the inability to perform normal activities of daily living. The patient identifies own maladaptive coping behaviors, available resources, and support systems, describes or initiates alternative coping strategies, and describes positive results from new behaviors.

BLADDER CANCER

Bladder cancer is a common urological cancer. The most common type of bladder cancer in the United States is urothelial carcinoma, formerly known as transitional cell carcinoma (TCC). The urothelium in the entire urinary tract may be involved, including the renal pelvis, ureter, bladder, and urethra. The clinical course of bladder cancer carries a broad spectrum of aggressiveness and risk. Low-grade, superficial bladder cancers have minimal risk of progression to death; however, high-grade muscle-invasive cancers are often lethal. Smoking is the greatest single risk factor for bladder cancer and exposure to certain toxic chemicals and drugs also predispose the patient to bladder cancer.

Epidemiology

Bladder cancer is the 4th most frequently diagnosed cancer in men and the 10th most frequently diagnosed cancer in women. Most people who develop the disease are older adults with less than 1 percent of cases occurring in people younger than 40. People over the age of 70 develop the disease two to three times more often than those aged 55 and 15 to 20 times more often than those aged 30. According to the National Cancer Institute, the highest incidence of bladder cancer occurs in industrialized countries, such as the United States, Canada, and France. Incidence is lowest in Asia and South America, where it is about 70 percent lower than in the United States. An annual cohort of 300,000 to 400,000 patients with bladder cancer is reported in the United States. Bladder cancer is more prevalent in Caucasians than in African Americans and Hispanic (Americans); however, African Americans have a poorer prognosis than Caucasians (Schrag, et al., 2005).

Etiology

Cancer-causing agents (carcinogens) in the urine may lead to the development of bladder cancer. Cigarette smoking contributes to more than 50 percent of cases, and smoking cigars or pipes also increases the risk. Other risk factors include the following: age, chronic bladder inflammation, diet high in saturated fat, external beam radiation, family history of bladder cancer, infection with *Schistosoma haematobium* (parasite found in many developing countries), and treatment with certain drugs (e.g., cyclophosphamide). Exposure to carcinogens in the workplace also increases the risk for bladder cancer (Bosetti, Pira, & La Vecchia, 2005).

Pathophysiology

A review of chapter 15 addresses the pathophysiology of cancer. Almost all bladder cancers are epithelial in origin (Steinberg & Kim, 2005). The urothelium consists of a three- to seven-cell mucosal layer within the muscular bladder. Of these urothelial tumors, more than 90 percent are transitional cell carcinomas. However, up to 5 percent of bladder cancers are squamous cell in origin, and 2 percent are adenocarcinomas. The World Health Organization classifies bladder cancers as low grade (grade 1 and 2) or high grade (grade 3). Carcinoma in situ (CIS) is a flat, noninvasive, high-grade urothelial carcinoma. The most significant prognostic factors for bladder cancer are grade, depth of invasion, and the presence of CIS.

Assessment with Clinical Manifestations

Approximately 80 to 90 percent of patients with bladder cancer present with painless gross hematuria, which is the classic presentation. Consider the likelihood that patients with gross hematuria to have bladder cancer until proven otherwise. More common conditions (e.g., UTI, kidney disease, or renal calculi) also cause hematuria. Twenty to 30 percent of patients with bladder cancer experience irritative bladder symptoms (e.g., dysuria, urgency, or frequency of urination). Patients with advanced disease can present with pelvic or bony pain, lower-extremity edema from iliac vessel compression, or flank pain from ureteral obstruction.

Diagnostic Tests

Diagnosis of bladder cancer includes urological tests and imaging tests. A complete medical history is used to identify potential risk factors (e.g., smoking or exposure to dyes). Laboratory tests may include the following: BladderChek (a urine test used to detect elevated levels of a nuclear matrix protein called NMP22 to detect elevated levels of tumor markers in the urine), urinalysis with microscopy, urine cytology, and urine culture.

Various imaging tests may also be performed; IVP is the standard imaging test for bladder cancer. Other imaging tests include CT scan, MRI, bone scan, and ultrasound. If bladder cancer is suspected, cystoscopy and biopsy are performed. If the sample is positive, the cancer is staged using the TNM system. In addition, the primary procedure used for diagnosis is a cystoscopy with biopsy. Staging for bladder cancer uses the International Union Against Cancer and the American Joint Committee on Cancer Staging developed the TNM staging system, which is used to stage bladder cancer (Bassi, et al., 2005).

Nursing Diagnoses

Based on the information gathered, examples of nursing diagnoses in the patient with bladder cancer may include the following:

- Fear in response to the diagnosis of bladder cancer
- Knowledge deficit related to the diagnosis of bladder cancer
- Ineffective coping related to anxiety, lower activity level and the inability to perform normal activities of daily living

In addition, refer to the section on renal cancer.

Planning and Implementation

Management for bladder cancer depends on the stage of the disease, the type of cancer, and the patient's age and overall health. Options include surgery, chemotherapy, radiation, and immunotherapy. In some cases, treatments are combined (e.g., surgery or radiation and chemotherapy, preoperative radiation). Further descriptions of these broad forms of management are available in chapter 15, along with specific information regarding the nursing care for patients with cancer.

Pharmacology

Chemotherapeutic drugs commonly used to treat bladder cancer include valrubicin, thiotepa, mitomycin, and doxorubicin. Side effects can be severe and include such things as: abdominal pain, anemia, bladder irritation, excessive bleeding or bruising, malaise, infection and anorexia (Manoharan, et al., 2005).

Radiation therapy is also used to relieve symptoms (called palliative treatment) of advanced bladder cancer. The typical side effects include inflammation of the rectum (proctitis), incontinence, skin irritation, hematuria, fibrosis, and impotence (Logue & McBain, 2005).

Immunotherapy (biological therapy) may be used in some cases of superficial bladder cancer. This treatment is used to enhance the immune system's ability to fight disease. A vaccine derived from the bacteria (BCG) that causes tuberculosis is infused through the urethra into the bladder, once a week for six weeks to stimulate the immune system to destroy cancer cells. Sometimes BCG is used with interferon. The side effects include inflammation of the bladder (cystitis), inflammation of the prostate (prostatitis), and flu-like symptoms.

Photodynamic therapy is a new treatment for early bladder cancer. It involves administering drugs to make cancer cells more sensitive to light and then shining a special light onto the bladder. This treatment is being studied in clinical trials.

Surgery

The type of surgery depends on the stage of the disease. In early bladder cancer, the tumor may be removed through the urethra (transurethral resection; see section on urinary diversion for more specifics of surgical intervention). Bladder cancer that has spread to surrounding tissue usually requires partial or radical removal of the bladder (cystectomy). Radical cystectomy also involves the removal of nearby lymph nodes and may require a urostomy (opening in the abdomen created for the discharge of urine). Complications include infection, urinary stones, and urine blockages. Bladder cancer has a high rate of recurrence. Urine cytology and cystoscopy are performed every three months for two years, every six months for the next two years, and then yearly (Martis, D'Elia, Diana, Ombres, & Mastrangeli, 2005).

In men, the standard surgical procedure is a cystoprostatectomy (removal of the bladder and prostate) with pelvic lymphadenectomy (removal of the lymph nodes within the hip cavity). In women, the standard surgical procedure is radical cystectomy (removal of the bladder and surrounding organs) with pelvic lymphadenectomy. Radical cystectomy in women also involves removal of the uterus (womb), ovaries, fallopian tubes, anterior vaginal wall, and urethra.

Evaluation of Outcomes

Potential patient outcomes for each of the example nursing diagnoses for the patient with bladder cancer are:

- Fear in response to the diagnosis of bladder cancer. The patient should manifest positive coping behaviors and verbalize a reduction in the amount of fear of having this disease.
- Knowledge deficit related to the diagnosis of bladder cancer. The patient should demonstrate motivation to learn, identify perceived learning needs, and verbalize an understanding of desired content.
- Ineffective coping related to anxiety, lower activity level, and the inability to perform normal activities of daily living. The patient identifies own maladaptive coping behaviors, available resources, and support systems, describes or initiates alternative coping strategies, and describes positive results from new behaviors.

In addition, refer to the section on renal cancer.

URINARY DIVERSION

Urinary diversion is a term used when the bladder is removed or diseased, or the normal structures are being bypassed and an opening is made in the urinary system to divert urine. The flow of urine is diverted through an opening in the abdominal wall. Individuals who might require urinary diversion would be those whose bladders were nonfunctional or needed to be removed either because of cancer or injury. For almost 150 years, surgeons have been performing urinary tract diversions. In 1852, Simon performed the first ureteroproctostomy on a patient with exstrophy. The procedures have since become more refined and patient outcomes have improved. Today, patients may be divided into two standard categories, those with continent diversions and those with noncontinent diversions, who require external ostomy collecting devices.

Etiology

The most common indications for urinary system diversion are as follows: bladder cancer requiring cystectomy, neurogenic bladder conditions that threaten renal function, intractable incontinence in females, chronic pelvic pain syndromes, and severe radiation injury to the bladder. The condition of the bladder, the age of the patient, the status of renal function, the pathology of ureteral dilation, and the general health of the patient are all risk factors for urinary diversion.

Assessment with Clinical Manifestations

Most often, patients who are candidates for urinary diversions present with an appearance indicating obvious illness. The typical presentation of these patients consists of easy fatigability, weakness, anorexia, weight loss, polydipsia, nausea, vomiting, and diarrhea.

> **Red Flag**
>
> **Anaphylaxis to Contrast Medium**
>
> The nurse needs to assess the patient having an IVP for allergies to iodine. Clinical manifestations are those of anaphylaxis and should immediately be reported and epinephrine administered per order. For prevention purposes, the patient should be asked if they have allergies to iodine, eggs, and shellfish and if they are allergic to any of these, the test is contraindicated.

The major contraindications to urinary diversion are anomalies of the bowel. For example, bowel injured by radiation should not be used for diversion. Patients with poor renal function, severe metabolic abnormalities, and significant proteinuria should not undergo diversion with continent reservoirs. Additionally, patients who lack motivation or are unable to catheterize a continent reservoir should not undergo diversion in this manner.

Diagnostic Tests

The laboratory studies assessed prior to urinary diversion are focused on assessing the patient's renal function. A minimum creatinine clearance of 60 mL/min is necessary prior to performing continent diversion. In addition, the laboratory studies for patients with urinary diversion should be primarily directed toward excluding infection and assessing metabolic status. Therefore, arterial blood gases (ABGs), complete blood count, urinalysis and urine culture, electrolytes, BUN, and creatinine are assessed.

A variety of imaging studies may be performed prior to a urinary diversion. An ultrasound is a desirable method for imaging the upper urinary tracts, because it requires no nephrotoxic agents. A nuclear scan can be used, with the main drawback being the lack of information obtained regarding the precise location of obstruction or integrity of the urinary tract. A CT scan is valuable for demonstrating the presence of urinary calculi and for assessing a ruptured continent urinary reservoir or for determining the presence of fistulous communication of the urinary tract with the GI or genital tracts. An MRI may be performed to rule out recurrent cancer in a patient who has equivocal findings on CT scan images and for imaging the drainage of a tract in a patient who is azotemic or allergic to intravenous contrast.

Planning and Implementation

Patients requiring urinary diversion often are monitored for a time by their urologist, and the decision for surgical intervention is made after conservative management fails. The topic of urinary diversion is essentially a surgical set of interventions and is discussed in the following section.

Surgery

Urinary diversions may be divided into two categories: (a) noncontinent diversions, and (b) continent diversions. Noncontinent urinary diversion into a noncontinent conduit is considered less technically demanding and is associated with the fewest postoperative complications; therefore, this technique is the criterion standard. Noncontinent urinary diversion is performed by either directly anastomosing the ureters to the anterior body wall (i.e., cutaneous ureterostomy) or using a segment of bowel to anastomose in a similar manner to the anterior wall for ostomy bag drainage. The bowels most commonly used for noncontinent conduit diversion are 15 to 25 cm of ileum, colon, and, least often, jejunum bowel segments (Deliveliotis, et al., 2005).

The second form of urinary diversion, continent urinary diversion, is subdivided into two basic types: (a) those with a surgical opening brought out of the abdomen, and (b) those in which a replacement bladder is made out of part of the intestine. Those with a new bladder are able to urinate spontaneously, whereas those patients with a surgical opening need to place a tube into the opening periodically to drain the accumulated urine. The advantage of the two types of continent urinary diversion is that no permanent ostomy bag needs to be worn. Continent urinary diversion describes all forms of urinary diversion that enable the patient to urinate at his or her own discretion without the use of any form of appliance or collecting device. All patients undergoing anticipated continent urinary diversion should be prepared for the possibility that a traditional ileal conduit might be performed (Figure 53-6). Therefore, prior to

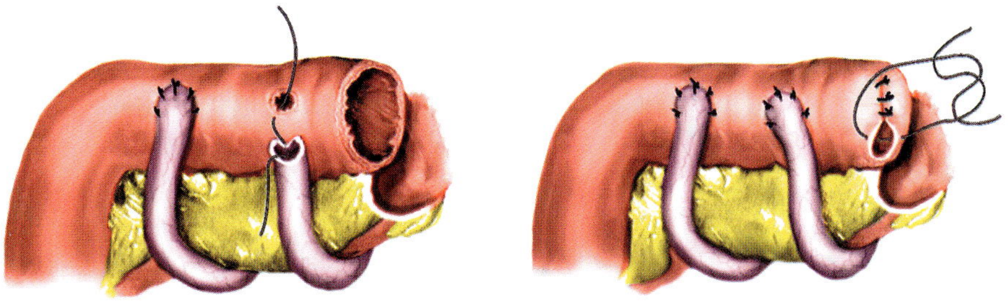

Figure 53-6 Ileal conduit: A. Ureters implanted into ileal segment, B. Closure of proximal end of ileal conduit.

the operation, the site for an external stoma should be selected in conjunction with an enterostomal therapist (Gronau & Pannek, 2005).

The removal of the bladder **(cystectomy)** will always be preceded by complete bowel preparation. A Go-Lytely one-gallon bowel preparation is administered, following a liquid dinner on the night prior to surgery. Oral antibiotics are also given to help sterilize the intestinal tract and reduce the chance of infection. All forms of urinary diversion require the placement of drainage tubes in the new bladder and the kidneys, and these will be present when the patient wakes from surgery. Certain drainage tubes will remain in place for two to three weeks postoperatively. Before removal of the drainage tubes, X-ray studies may be performed to ensure that the new bladder has healed and has no leakage. Postoperatively, patients are taught to wash out the urethral catheter at home every four to six hours. In the early postoperative period, the new bladder may hold only a small volume of urine and patients are required to empty frequently (Ludwig, et al., 2005).

Some metabolic complications that can result from use of the intestinal tract in urinary diversion are UTI, urinary stone formation, vitamin B_{12} deficiency, changes in bowel habits, and changes in pH balance. Early complications of urinary diversions include postoperative ileus or bowel obstruction, which, as a group, is more common in continent diversions. Other early complications may include ureter-bowel anastomotic leak and acute pyelonephritis. Late complications are metabolic disturbances that may result from the interaction of urine with the absorptive surface of the bowel used for the procedure. In addition, a vitamin B_{12} deficiency may develop as the terminal ileum is the exclusive site of vitamin B_{12} absorption. Patients with urinary retention usually present with abdominal pain and distension; and this condition is an emergency, and drainage of the reservoir is indicated. In addition, patients with continent reservoirs are at risk for secretory and osmotic diarrhea, depending on the length of ileum used and whether or not the ileocecal valve was resected for construction of the urinary pouch (Tolhurst, et al., 2005).

Patient and Family Teaching

The lifelong care of a stoma created with noncontinent urinary diversions may be psychologically stressful, and the nurse must provide referral services for the patient (see chapter 50 for stoma care and implications seen in lower GI managements). The patient wears an ostomy bag into which the urine continuously drains and is educated that it is still possible to participate in strenuous physical activity in addition to daily routines. Also, patients undergoing continent diversion should also be aware of the functional complications and results of this form of urinary tract reconstruction (e.g., nocturnal enuresis). Nocturnal incontinence can be expected following neobladder diversion particularly in the first six to nine months following surgery. This problem can usually be managed by external collecting devices in the male (condom catheter) or fluid restriction before bed.

Fast Forward ▶▶▶

Robotic Forms of Surgery for Urinary Diversions

The use of robotics is currently purported for a variety of surgical interventions (e.g., prostatectomy). Robotic surgery is the latest minimally invasive treatment option available for patients with localized muscle-invasive bladder cancer. The robotic laparoscopic procedure offers advantages over open radical cystectomy (removal of the bladder using a relatively large abdominal incision) in that there is a quicker recovery time and only a few small adhesive strip-sized incisions.

URINARY RETENTION

Urinary retention, or bladder-emptying problems, is a common urological problem with many possible causes. Normally, urination can be initiated voluntarily and the bladder empties completely. Urinary retention is the abnormal holding of urine in the bladder. Acute urinary retention is the sudden inability to urinate, causing pain and discomfort. Causes can include an obstruction in the urinary system, stress, or neurological problems. Chronic urinary retention refers to the persistent presence of urine left in the bladder after incomplete emptying. Urinary retention always requires medical attention, sometimes hospitalization, for treatment, symptom relief, and detection of the underlying cause. Failure to treat the condition can lead to infections or damage to the urinary tract and kidneys.

Epidemiology

Urinary retention is not an unusual condition and is more common in men than in women. The average age of patients is over 60, and hospitalization may be required for treatment.

Etiology

Urinary retention develops when the duct that drains the bladder (the urethra) becomes blocked (e.g., an enlarged prostate gland). Acute urinary retention may be caused by stones lodged in the urethra or urethral strictures (often from gonorrhea); fecal impaction, prostatitis, prostatic carcinoma, or benign prostatic hypertrophy; retroverted gravid uterus, after an operation, urethral rupture, and tumor or clots in the bladder (Lau & Lam, 2004). Any drug with anticholinergic effects or alpha adrenergic effects; such as, antihistamines, ephedrine sulfate, and phenylpropanolamine, can precipitate urinary retention. Neurological etiologies include cord lesions, spinal anesthesia, and multiple sclerosis. Patients with genital herpes may develop urinary retention from nerve involvement. Acute urinary retention has also been reported following vigorous anal intercourse.

Chronic urinary retention has a much more protracted course. It is usually relatively painless and may be reflective of renal impairment, late-onset enuresis, hypertension, and present with symptoms of bladder outflow obstruction.

Pathophysiology

As the bladder enlarges, the tension in the walls required to empty it rises in keeping with LaPlace's law so that if the bladder becomes overdistended, it is difficult or impossible to empty it naturally. The risk is greatest when production of urine is high at a time when sensation is impaired. Even if the patient is passing urine, if there is a large, palpable bladder, there is retention of urine. If the bladder is large, palpable, and tender whilst the patient complains of pain with an urge to void that cannot be fulfilled, the diagnosis is clear. If there is a mass that is not painful, it may be a bladder in chronic retention, but other considerations include a large uterus from fibroids, pregnancy, ovarian cysts, or ovarian carcinoma. It is also imperative to ascertain that failure to pass urine is not because of failure to produce urine as in acute renal failure.

Assessment with Clinical Manifestations

Acute urinary retention always presents with acute onset pain of intolerable severity, while chronic retention of urine is associated with almost no pain, and a history of gradually developing symptoms, which have suffered neglect by the patient. In acute urinary retention, the patient may complain of increasing dull low abdominal discomfort and the urge to urinate, without having been able to urinate for many hours. A firm, distended bladder can be palpated between the symphysis pubis and umbilicus (note: palpation can be difficult in the obese or in pregnancy). Rectal examination may reveal an enlarged or tender prostate or suspected tumor. Sometimes hematuria develops midway through bladder decompression, probably representing loss of tamponade of vessels injured as the bladder distended. This should be watched until the bleeding stops (usually spontaneously) to be sure there is no great blood loss, no other urological pathology responsible, and no clot obstruction (Elkhodair, Parmar, & Vanwaeyenbergh, 2005).

In chronic retention, the patient with chronic retention may be passing some urine. There is often retention with overflow so that the complaint is one of urinary frequency rather than inability to void. Small volumes are passed often. Painful bladder is not a complaint.

BOX 53-8

DIAGNOSTIC TESTS FOR URINARY RETENTION

- Urinalysis may give a clue to underlying UTI
- BUN and serum creatinine may reflect acute renal failure
- WBC: raised in prostatitis and UTI
- Urinalysis and electrolytes are essential as renal failure often follows chronic retention. If urinary calculus, check urate, calcium, and phosphate
- Check PSA in prostatic enlargement for carcinoma
- Renal ultrasound, IVP, urethrography

Diagnostic Tests

Typical diagnostic tests for urinary retention are shown in Box 53-8.

Nursing Diagnoses

Based on the information gathered, examples of nursing diagnoses in the patient with urinary retention may include the following:

- Urinary retention
- Acute pain as related to acute urinary retention

Planning and Implementation

Acute urinary retention may be an indication of surgical intervention. Initial management should be urethral catheterization followed by at least one voiding trial, because acute urinary retention is reversible in some patients. In the elderly, especially the male population, routine enquiry into problems of micturition that may be regarded as a normal feature of aging can permit treatment of the underlying cause before retention of urine occurs. At high risk times (e.g., postoperative or trauma), encouragement of the patient to pass urine may prevent overdistension and retention. Urine charts and awareness of failure to pass urine are essential. In addition, avoid drugs, like tricyclic antidepressants, in elderly men. The patient can be instructed to drink small volumes of water or tea or to sit in a warm bath or take a warm shower. In addition, the patient can be asked to void every three to four hours, regardless of his or her urgency (Griffiths, Fernandez, & Murie, 2004).

Red Flag

Catheterizing a Patient with Urinary Retention

- If the catheterization fails to drain a significant volume of urine, the diagnosis will be reconsidered.
- If there is difficulty in passing the catheter, do not use force, do not inflate catheter balloon until urine has been seen in the catheter, and do not use a catheter introducer unless adequately trained in its use.
- Note: If unable to pass a urethral catheter, the use a suprapubic puncture may be indicated.

Evaluation of Outcomes

Potential patient outcomes for each of the example nursing diagnoses for the patient with urinary retention are:

- Urinary retention. The patient empties the bladder completely and has a residual of less than 30 mL.
- Acute pain as related to acute urinary retention. The patient should verbalize an adequate relief of pain along with the ability to realistically cope with the pain if it is not completely relieved.

URINARY INCONTINENCE

Urinary incontinence (UI), loss of bladder control, is the involuntary passage of urine. This can range from an occasional leakage of urine to a complete inability to hold any urine. There are many causes and types of incontinence and many treatment options. Treatments range from simple exercises to surgery. Women are affected by urinary incontinence more often than men. Approximately $12 to $15 billion is spent annually on UI.

Epidemiology

UI has a prevalence of 15 to 30 percent in community-residing elderly patients, 50 to 84 percent among older adults in long-term care institutions, and 33 percent in older people in acute care settings. UI affects more than 10 million Americans, 85 percent of whom are women. UI affects at least 13 million American women, with an estimated cost to society of $16 to $26 billion. UI affects up to 7 percent of children older than 5 years. Incidence is 1.4 percent of adults aged 15 to 24 years and 2.9 percent of those aged 55 to 64 years. There is no clear evidence of racial differences in prevalence of UI. Age itself is not a cause of UI; however, age-related changes may predispose or contribute to UI (e.g., diabetes, medications, sleep disturbances, restricted mobility, hormonal changes, and mentation) (American College of Obstetricians and Gynecologists, 2005).

Etiology

Incontinence may be sudden and temporary or ongoing and long term. Causes of sudden or temporary incontinence include such things as UTI, prostate infection, stool impaction from severe constipation, side effects of medications (e.g., diuretics, tranquilizers, antihistamines, and antidepressants), poorly controlled diabetes, pregnancy, or weight gain). Causes for long-term UI includes spinal injuries, urinary tract anatomical abnormalities, CVA, benign prostatic hypertrophy, pelvic prolapse in women, and bladder cancer (Madersbacher & Madersbacher, 2005).

Pathophysiology

Usually development of incontinence involves the bladder, the outlet (sphincter), or both. In bladder hyperactivity, the bladder's compliance is decreased, as seen in the decrease in the volume-pressure curve during filling or bladder contractions. Patients may have a painful bladder sensation on filling. Incontinence also can be because intermittent decreases in urethral pressure below that of bladder pressure, which occurs during abdominal straining and is unrelated to bladder hyperactivity. Episodic decrease in sphincter pressure (urethral instability) and loss of closure potential at the bladder outlet (intrinsic sphincter deficiency) are other causes of incontinence. Incontinence may be chronic and progressive, a manifestation of an underlying disease, or transient, such as that seen with a bladder infection or after childbirth. There are several different types of UI, which are shown in Box 53-9.

Assessment with Clinical Manifestations

The nurse must carry out a thorough examination, including a brief psychiatric and neurological evaluation. A goal is to eliminate any serious disease that may be the underlying cause of incontinence and any transient cause or functional impairment. The nurse can assess the abdomen, looking at the flanks and checking for masses, distended bladder after voiding, and signs of fluid overload. In addition, neurologic concerns can be fecal impaction and changes in sphincter tone. A pelvic examination is necessary for women, and the examination should be made with the patient's bladder empty to check organs and with the bladder full to check for prolapse, cystocele, rectocele, or incontinence. A stress test can assess for stress-induced leakage when the bladder is full. A stress test is performed by having the patient relax and asking the

BOX 53-9

TYPES OF INCONTINENCE

1. Stress incontinence is loss of urine with increased intra-abdominal pressure without detrusor contraction. Anatomy of the sphincter is normal, but it has lost some of its efficacy due to excessive mobility and loss of support. Stress incontinence happens when urine leaks during exercise, coughing, sneezing, laughing, lifting heavy objects, or other body movements that put pressure on the bladder. It is the most common type of bladder control problem in younger and middle-age women (Kielb, 2005).
2. Urge incontinence (true, detrusor overactivity, or reflex) is precipitous loss of urine, preceded by a strong urge to void, with increased intravesical pressure and detrusor contraction. Urge incontinence can occur in healthy persons, but it is often found in people who have chronic disorders (e.g., diabetes, stroke, or Alzheimer's disease). It is also sometimes an early sign of bladder cancer.
3. Overflow incontinence is loss of urine because of chronic urinary retention or secondary to a flaccid bladder. It usually is due to an obstructive or neuropathic lesion and occurs when small amounts of urine leak from a bladder that is always full (BPH or spinal cord injury).
4. Functional incontinence happens in many older people who have normal bladder control. They just have a hard time getting to the toilet in time because of arthritis or other disorders that make moving quickly difficult.

PATIENT PLAYBOOK

Bladder Training Techniques

The nurse instructs the patient to:

- Start by trying to not urinate for 10 minutes every time you feel an urge to urinate.
- Then try upping the waiting period to 20 minutes, with the goal to lengthen the time between trips to the toilet until you are urinating every two to four hours.
- Bladder training may also involve double voiding (urinating, then waiting a few minutes and trying to urinate again).
- When you feel the urge to urinate, relax, breathe slowly and deeply, or distract yourself with an activity.
- Nighttime bladder training may be reinforced with devices, such as moisture alarms, which wake you up when you begin to urinate. They are particularly helpful for children who wet the bed at night.
- Schedule toilet trips (timed urination) by going to the toilet according to the clock rather than waiting for the need to go (usually every two to four hours).

patient to cough or strain once vigorously; instantaneous leakage is typical of stress UI, delayed leakage is typical of stress-induced detrusor overactivity.

Diagnostic Tests

The history of the patient is the first assessment tool used for diagnosing UI. Then, the diagnostic tests that may be performed for UI include urinalysis, urine culture, cystoscopy, urodynamic studies (tests to measure pressure and urine flow), uroflow, and post void residual (PVR) to measure amount of urine left after urination. Other tests may be performed to rule out pelvic weakness as the cause of the incontinence. One such test is called the Q-tip test. This test involves measurement of the change in the angle of the urethra when it is at rest and when it is straining. An angle change of greater than 30 degrees often indicates significant weakness of the muscles and tendons that support the bladder.

Nursing Diagnoses

Based on the information gathered, examples of nursing diagnoses in the patient with UI may include the following:

- Impaired urinary elimination
- Deficient knowledge related to self-care and risk prevention

Planning and Implementation

The management of UI falls into four broad categories: behavioral techniques, devices, medications, and surgery. The behavioral techniques include strengthening the muscles of the pelvic floor with: bladder retraining (urinating on a schedule); Kegel exercises (voluntary contraction of the pelvic floor muscles); regulating bowels to avoid constipation; quit smoking to reduce coughing and bladder irritation; avoid alcohol and caffeinated beverages, par-

> **PATIENT PLAYBOOK**
>
> **Performing Kegel Exercises**
>
> The nurse can instruct the patient to do the following when learning Kegel exercises:
>
> - To find the pelvic muscles when you first start Kegel exercises, stop your urine flow midstream. The muscles needed to do this are your pelvic floor muscles.
> - Perform the exercises for 10 seconds, then relax them for 10 seconds and repeating this action three times per day.
> - Do not contract your abdominal, thigh, or buttocks muscles.
> - Do not overdo the exercises. This may tire the muscles out and actually worsen incontinence.

ticularly coffee, which can overstimulate the bladder; avoid foods and drinks that may irritate the bladder, like spicy foods, carbonated beverages, and citrus fruits and juices; and keep blood sugars under good control if a diabetic.

There are devices in the forms of catheters, if the behavioral methods fail or are found unacceptable. Catheters must be managed with great care to avoid infection and stone formation. The patient can use clean intermittent catheterization for problems with emptying the bladder. The catheterization techniques may be taught to the patient or family members. In addition, a condom catheter may be used when men prefer a drainage system that fits over the penis like a condom. The patient must be taught to take the same care to avoid infection as with other catheters. Condom catheters can also carry a risk of skin breakdown.

Pharmacology

Drugs commonly used to treat incontinence include anticholinergics, antidepressants, hormone replacements, and antibiotics. The anticholinergic drugs calm an overactive bladder, so they may be helpful for urge incontinence. Examples include tolterodine (Detrol), oxybutynin (Ditropan), and hyoscyamine (Levsin). These drugs can be effective at controlling incontinence, but a side effect is dry mouth. To combat dry mouth, the patient may be tempted to drink more water, which is contraindicated with the incontinence.

Antidepressants may be used to treat incontinence (e.g., imipramine). It causes the bladder muscle to relax, while causing the smooth muscles at the bladder neck to contract.

Hormone replacements are effective after menopause; a drop in estrogen can contribute to changes in the skin lining the urethra and vagina, which can contribute to the development of incontinence. Applying estrogen in the form of a vaginal cream, ring, or patch may help relieve some of the symptoms of incontinence in these women. Also, in children, nighttime incontinence may be because of a shortage of the nighttime production of a hormone called antidiuretic hormone (ADH). This hormone slows the making of urine. Therefore, a synthetic version of ADH (desmopressin [DDAVP]) is available as a nasal spray or pill for children to use before bedtime.

Antibiotics can be used if the incontinence is because of a UTI or an inflamed prostate gland (prostatitis).

Surgery

Surgery may be required to relieve an obstruction or deformity of the bladder neck and urethra. Uterine or pelvic suspension operations are sometimes needed in women. Men may require prostatectomy (removal of the prostate gland). Incontinence can sometimes be managed by artificial sphincters. These are synthetic cuffs that are surgically placed around the urethra to help retain urine. Urethral injections are another method to help keep the urethra closed. A fat-like substance (e.g., collagen) is injected into the area that surrounds the opening of the bladder into the urethra. A variety of bulking agents are available for injection.

Evaluation of Outcomes

Potential patient outcomes for each of the example nursing diagnoses for the patient with urinary incontinence are:

- Impaired urinary elimination. The patient is continent of urine or verbalizes satisfactory management.
- Knowledge deficit related to self-care and risk prevention. The patient should demonstrate motivation to learn, identify perceived learning needs, and verbalize an understanding of desired content.

Case Study

Nursing Care Plan

Mrs. Lockwell, 51 years of age and an active and energetic female, arrived at her gynecologist's office for her scheduled annual appointment. Mrs. Lockwell has had an annual gynecological evaluation for the past 7 years. She is married and has two adult children. She does not drink alcohol or smoke. She exercises three times per week at the local health club. She works as an elementary educator and has been teaching third grade for 26 years. She is active in her local church group and has an active social life. Mrs. Lockwell reports that for the past two weeks she has had to "go to the bathroom a lot and it burns when I urinate" and that her urine "smells strong and is a dark orange." When asked how much fluid she consumes daily, Mrs. Lockwell responded, "I drink one big cup of coffee in the morning, one can of diet soda at lunch, one glass of skim milk at dinner, and maybe one glass of water at bedtime." She also stated that, "My skin feels very dry and my lower back hurts."

Vital signs revealed a temperature of 37.8° C (100° F), pulse 96 beats per minute, lying blood pressure of 136/74, and a standing blood pressure of 128/70. Height is 5 feet 5 inches, and weight is 125 pounds. A urine specimen for urinalysis and for culture and sensitivity were ordered by the health care provider. The nurse observed that Mrs. Lockwell's urine was foul smelling, dark amber, cloudy, and thick. Her skin turgor revealed tenting with the shape remaining for 15 seconds. Her fluid intake for the past 24 hours was 930 mL. The urinalysis revealed a specific gravity greater than 1.030, and the culture and sensitivity report disclosed the presence of *Escherichia coli* with a sensitivity to all penicillins. Her hemoglobin was 14, hematocrit was 45 percent; and WBC count was 12,000. In addition, Mrs. Lockwell guards her lower back on movement.

Assessment

Patient is a 51-year-old female with a UTI that has existed for the past two weeks. She is febrile and has subjective complaints of pain from the infection, and her urine is concentrated, dark colored, and foul smelling.

Nursing Diagnosis 1: Impaired urinary elimination related to irritation of bladder secondary to infection as evidenced by foul smelling, dark amber, cloudy, thick urine; oral temperature 37.8° C (100° F); urine culture reveals *Escherichia coli.*

NOC: Urinary elimination; Urinary continence

NIC: Urinary elimination management

Expected Outcomes

The patient will:

1. Experience no urinary urgency as evidenced by voiding every 240 to 400 mL every 6 to 8 hours within three days of initiating treatment.
2. Report no pain or burning on urination within 24 hours of initiating treatment.
3. Be free of infection as evidenced by clear, urine that is not foul smelling, pain-free urination, WBCs between 5,000 and 10,000 within three days of initiating treatment.

Planning, Interventions, Rationales

1. Evaluate previous patterns of voiding. *Voiding patterns are unique to each patient and can vary. UTIs can cause retention, but it is more likely to cause frequency.*

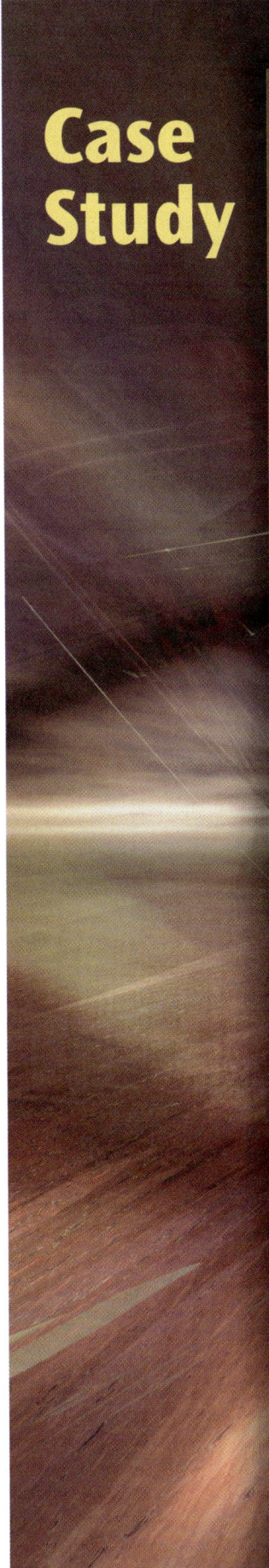

Case Study

2. Assess the balance between intake and output. *Intake greater than output may indicate retention.*
3. Monitor results of urinalysis, urine culture, and sensitivity. *Retention of urine can predispose the patient to UTIs.*
4. Every 4 hours assess patient description of pain: quality, nature, and severity using a pain rating scale. *UTIs are described as burning on urination; if renal involvement, may experience back or flank pain.*
5. Encourage fluids by offering fluids of choice every 2 hours. *Fluid intake should be 1,500 mL per 24 hours to promote renal blood flow and flush bacteria from urinary tract.*

Evaluation

Patient's urine is clear and does not smell foul, and WBC count is between 5,000 and 10,000 within three days of initiating treatment. The patient is free of urinary urgency, voids 240 to 400 mL every 6 to 8 hours within three days of initiating treatment. In addition, within 24 hours of initiating treatment, the patient rates the severity of burning on urination as a 0 on a severity rating scale of 0 to 5, with 0 being no burning and 5 severe burning on urination.

Nursing Diagnosis 2: Deficient knowledge related to lack of information about causes for UTIs and not seeking health care treatment.

NOC: Knowledge of disease process, health behaviors, health resources, infection control, treatment procedures, and treatment regimen.

NIC: Teaching: Disease process; Teaching: Individual

Expected Outcomes

The patient will:

1. Accurately verbalize measures to prevent or reduce risk of reinfection by eliminating beverages with caffeine, by consuming liquids or products that acidify urine, and by drinking at least 1,500 mL of fluids every 24 hours within 7 days of initiation of treatment and at the follow-up appointment visit.
2. Implement measures that will reduce the risk for introduction of pathogens into the urethra.

Planning, Interventions, Rationales

1. Assess knowledge of nature of UTIs. *To identify patient's knowledge and understanding of the risk factors for UTIs.*
2. Teach patient the importance of adequate fluid intake. *Keeps tissues hydrated and decrease bladder irritation.*
3. Teach patient to consume products or liquids that acidify urine (e.g., cranberry juice). *Bacteria grow poorly in acidic environment.*
4. Teach patient to avoid or reduce caffeine intake. *Caffeine is a diuretic, which may lead to dehydration.*

Evaluation

1. Patient verbalizes measures to prevent or reduce risk of reinfection by eliminating beverages with caffeine, by drinking fluids that acidify urine, and by drinking at least 1,500 mL of fluids every 24 hours within 7 days of initiation of treatment and at the follow-up appointment visit. In addition, the patient verbalizes that showering, wiping from front to back after voiding, and voiding immediately after sexual intercourse decrease the concentration of pathogens that may enter the urethra.

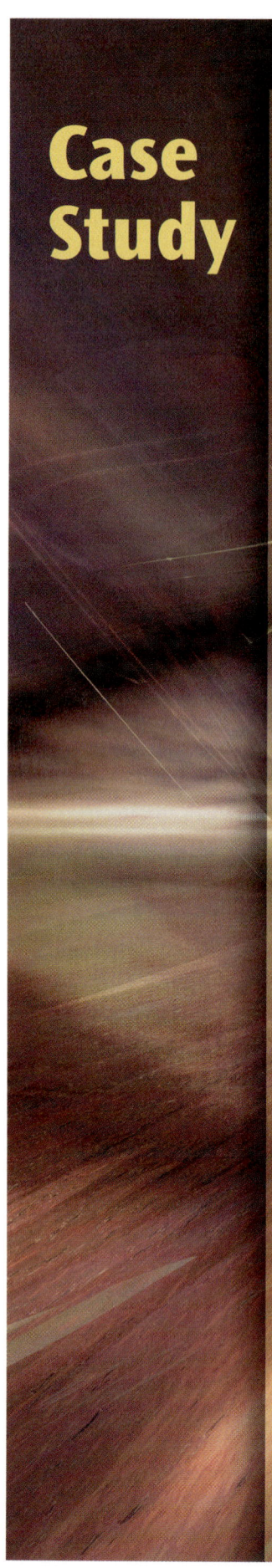

KEY CONCEPTS

- UTIs can cover a wide variety of conditions ranging from asymptomatic infections with low bacterial counts to severe infection of the kidney and sepsis.
- IC presents with urgency, frequency, nocturia, and dysuria in the presence of noninfected urine.
- Pyelonephritis is an infection of the upper urinary tract and may involve the ureters, renal pelvis, and the papillary tips of the collecting ducts.
- Glomerulonephritis is categorized into acute and chronic conditions.
- Nephrotic syndrome (nephrosis) is not a single disease but a group of symptoms.
- Renal tuberculosis is the most common site of extrapulmonary tuberculosis
- Many of the people that develop renal calculi require hospitalization, and the pain associated with renal stones is acute.
- The kidney is the most common organ in the urinary tract to be injured by severe trauma
- There are three conditions of renal vascular disorders: (a) renal artery stenosis, (b) renal vein thrombosis, and (c) nephrosclerosis.
- Renal cell carcinoma accounts for approximately 3 percent of adult malignancies and 90 to 95 percent of neoplasms arising from the kidney.
- Bladder cancer is the 4th most frequently diagnosed cancer in men and the 10th most frequently diagnosed cancer in women.
- Urinary diversion is a term used when the bladder is removed or diseased, and an opening is made in the urinary system to divert urine.
- Urinary retention is the abnormal holding of urine in the bladder.
- UI is the involuntary passage of urine and can range from an occasional leakage of urine, to a complete inability to hold any urine.

REVIEW QUESTIONS

1. Which of the following is true concerning the patient teaching for UTIs?
  1. Drinking 10 to 12 glasses of water daily helps to prevent UTI.
  2. Completely empty the bladder when voiding and do not put off the urge to urinate.
  3. Advise patients to use anticholinergics for their UTIs without restriction.
  4. Self-catheterization should be discouraged because of contamination problems.

2. IC is often confused with which of the following disorders, as their presenting symptoms are markedly similar?
  1. Recurrent UTI
  2. Renal cancer
  3. Renal tuberculosis
  4. Urinary retention

3. What is the most common cause of pyelonephritis?
  1. Urinary retention and ascending infection of the urinary tract
  2. Renal calculi
  3. Delayed voiding
  4. Previous UTI

4. Which of the following disorders is more common in children than in adults?
  1. Bladder cancer
  2. Pyelonephritis
  3. Nephrotic syndrome
  4. UTI

5. The nurse is performing discharge teaching for a patient who was admitted with pyelonephritis. The patient asks the nurse, "What is pyelonephritis?" Based on the nurse's knowledge, the best response would be:
  1. Pyelonephritis is an inflammation of the bladder.
  2. Pyelonephritis is a rupture of the bladder.
  3 Pyelonephritis is an infection of the kidney.
  4. Pyelonephritis is an infection of the lower urinary tract.

6. Which of the following tests are most appropriate after experiencing renal trauma?
  1. A CT scan with contrast and ultrasonography
  2. An IVP and a paracentesis
  3. A cystoscopy and histological examination
  4. Staging using the TNM system

Continued

REVIEW QUESTIONS—cont'd

7. Which of the following statements is true concerning renal cancer?
   1. BladderChek is the best lab study to confirm the presence of cancer in the bladder.
   2. The most commonly performed surgery to treat renal cell cancer is radical nephrectomy.
   3. Partial blockage of renal arteries and hypertension are the most common clinical manifestations.
   4. Renal cancer is usually secondary to tuberculosis of the lung.
8. Which of the following disorders presents with painless gross hematuria as the classic presentation?
   1. Pyelonephritis
   2. Nephrotic syndrome
   3. Bladder cancer
   4. Urinary retention
9. Which of the following uses a traditional ileal conduit for management?
   1. Continent urinary diversion
   2. Noncontinent urinary diversion
   3. Urinary retention
   4. Renal calculi
10. A patient with multiple sclerosis is unable to move about easily. Which of the following types of incontinence is the patient most likely to experience?
    1. Urge incontinence
    2. Stress incontinence
    3. Overflow incontinence
    4. Functional incontinence

REVIEW ACTIVITIES

1. Evaluate the urinalysis results of a patient in the clinical setting.
2. Describe the clinical manifestations seen in acute pyelonephritis.
3. Describe the clinical manifestations seen in patients with renal calculi.
4. Identify possible complications of renal injuries.
5. Describe the most common surgical interventions for patients with renal cancer.

Renal Dysfunction: Nursing Management

CHAPTER 54

Irene Eaton-Bancroft, RN, MSN, CS

CHAPTER TOPICS

- Pyelonephritis
- Polycystic Kidney Disease
- Goodpasture Syndrome
- Rhabdomyolysis
- Acute Renal Failure
- Chronic Renal Failure

The kidneys are one of the most efficient organs in the human body. Complex in function, the kidneys maintain homeostasis of elements important to critical body functions. Sensing altered states, the kidneys are able to adjust fluid and electrolyte retention or excretion and increase excretion of protein waste products. The kidney's endocrine function allows secretion of hormones for blood pressure control in low volume output states or increased production of red blood cells in low oxygen states. In addition, the kidneys facilitate calcium absorption and metabolism through conversion of vitamin D to its enzyme form. Changes in kidney function can go relatively undetected until one has lost nearly 65 percent of total function. Signs and symptoms of renal failure are common regardless of the cause. This chapter explores the many causes of renal failure and the stages of failure. Thorough assessment and prompt, focused nursing response are critical to promote optimal recovery.

KEY TERMS

Allogeneic
Allograft
Amyloid
Anuria
Azotemia
Casts
Disequilibrium
Effluent
Fasciotomy
Hematuria
Hypervolemia
Hypovolemia
Intrarenal
Malaise
Myoclonus
Nephropathy
Normovolemia
Nosocomial
Oliguria
Parenchyma
Perinephric
Phenotypes
Postrenal
Prerenal
Proteinuria
Pyelonephritis
Xenogeneic

PYELONEPHRITIS

Pyelonephritis is an infection of the upper urinary tract. It may involve the ureters, renal pelvis, and the papillary tips of the collecting ducts. Unchecked, it can extend into the tubules of the nephron creating a potential for renal failure.

Etiology

Commonly, pyelonephritis is caused by urinary retention or an ascending and unresponsive lower urinary tract infection (UTI). Retained urine provides a breeding ground for bacteria. Repetitive antibacterial treatment may lead to drug resistance and extension of infection. In addition, drugs may cause necrosis of the renal papillae, and sloughed papillae tissue may then cause ureteral blockage and thus extension of the pyelonephritis.

Pathophysiology

Prostate gland hypertrophy, masses, urinary calculi, or ureteral obstruction from sloughed papillae are common causes of urinary retention. Pooled urine promotes bacterial growth, and the continuous urine pathways offer easy access for bacterial ascension to the renal pelvis. In addition, the presence of catheters or fecal incontinence increases the potential for UTI by providing an entry point for *Escherichia coli,* one of the more common infecting organisms. Unchecked, bacteria in the urethra or bladder have easy access to the kidney via the ureters and renal pelvis.

Assessment with Clinical Manifestations

Acute pyelonephritis is described as a clinical syndrome presenting with bacteriuria accompanied by flank pain at the costovertebral angle, fever, and chills. In addition, the patient may experience painful urination, frequency, nocturia, nausea, vomiting, and colicky abdominal pain (Tolkoff-Rubin, Cotran, & Rubin, 2004). Conversely, chronic pyelonephritis may have a deceptively quiet presentation of frequency, dysuria, and nocturia. Mild, intermittent fever, or intermittent back or flank pain may accompany the urinary symptoms (Kelly & Nielson, 2004).

Diagnostic Tests

There are a variety of diagnostic tests for detection of pyelonephritis. Urinalysis and urine culture may be sufficient in mild, initial cases of pyelonephritis in an uncomplicated presentation. Correct urine sample collection technique is critical to proper treatment. Catheterization may be necessary to collect a reliable specimen for the patient who is unable to stand, cleanse, and collect a midstream specimen.

Computed tomography (CT) is the standard diagnostic tool for pyelonephritis unresponsive to 72 hours of antibiotic therapy. CT is valuable in diagnosing obstructive etiology, as well as identifying complications, such as perinephric abscess (Daniels, 2003).

Ultrasound is used when CT scanning is contraindicated, such as in pregnancy or in preexisting renal compromise. Renal ultrasound is used to place nephrostomy tubes for direct drainage of the renal pelvis in cases of complicated urinary obstruction.

Nursing Diagnoses

Based on the information gathered, examples of nursing diagnoses in the patient with pyelonephritis may include the following:

- Risk for imbalanced body temperature

PATIENT PLAYBOOK

Renal Assessment

Subjective

The nurse can ask the following questions when obtaining a renal assessment from the patient:

- What is the general state of health?
- Is there a history of neurological deficit, diabetes, or other debilitating disease that could lead to urinary stasis, damage to the nephron, or impaired healing?
- Have there been recent hospitalizations and drug therapies?
- Is there a history of urinary calculi or prostate gland hypertrophy?
- Is there a recent history of catheterization?
- Have they experienced burning on urination, cloudy urine, suprapubic pain, colicky abdominal pain, or flank or back pain?
- How long have the symptoms persisted, and how were they treated in the past?

Objective

The physical examination must include:

- Palpation of the abdomen for masses and tenderness.
- Palpation of costovertebral angle with a gentle tap of the fist over the kidney to elicit diagnostic discomfort in the presence of an inflammatory process.
- Urine inspection for clarity with sample collection for laboratory analysis. Vital point: Catheter specimen will be necessary for females during menses or for those patients who lack the capacity to produce a reliable, noncontaminated specimen.

- Pain related to ureteral colic or bladder spasm
- Fear in response to the diagnosis of pyelonephritis
- Deficient knowledge related to completion of drug therapy, optimal fluid intake, or need to empty bladder every two hours to reduce bacterial count
- Ineffective coping related to anxiety, **malaise** (body discomfort and fatigue), and lowered activity level

Planning and Implementation

There are several strategies to providing care for patients with pyelonephritis. The implementation of these strategies may provide quick recovery and positive outcomes for the patient with this disorder.

Goals

The primary goal for providing care for pyelonephritis is to eradicate the UTI and to prevent damage to the renal parenchyma. Additionally and of equal importance, the secondary goal of preventing further infection must be promoted through patient education.

Evidence-Based Care

The nurse is positioned to play a significant role in preventing UTI. Evidence points to avoiding catheterization and early removal of catheters as critical to preventing UTI. The nurse must resist viewing catheters as nursing convenience or an easy answer to incontinence.

The nurse must always employ effective hand washing between patients to prevent patient-to-patient contamination and **nosocomial** (hospital acquired) infection. In addition, the nurse should practice strict aseptic technique in catheter insertions and thorough, regular perineal and catheter site cleansing in the presence of a urinary catheter. The nurse must practice preventive measures with prevention of an ascending UTI in mind.

Collaborative Management including Nursing Intervention Classifications (NIC)

The collaborative management for pyelonephritis includes:

- Monitor vital signs and fluid balance.
- Ensure adequate hydration via an accurate intake and output record, encourage and provide at least 2 liter a day fluid intake or maintain a patent intravenous (IV) access.
- Monitor electrolytes, white blood count (WBC), blood urea nitrogen (BUN) and creatinine.
- Provide adequate pain management via usual analgesics and urinary antiseptics, such as phenazopyridine (Pyridium) or a combination urinary antiseptic or antispasmodic agent, such as Urised (Urisedon or Urisedamine) or Urisept (Uriseptic).
- NIC: Assist with hygiene.

Population-Based Care

The elderly must be carefully assessed as they may have reduced sensation and therefore are not aware of a UTI prior to an advanced stage. The elderly may present with only minor complaints and may not have an elevation in temperature even with advanced infection.

The nurse must determine if the elderly patient uses fasting as a health practice and educate about the need for adequate fluid intake to prevent infection hypovolemia of the kidneys and bladder (Eliopoulos, 2005).

Patient and Family Teaching

The primary aspects of patient and family teaching are to educate about the importance of completing the full course of antibiotic therapy and maintaining the prescribed schedule to ensure continuous therapeutic blood levels. In addition, there needs to be information regarding the value of these above activities in preventing drug resistance. The NIC for the patient with pyelonephritis is to appraise the patient's current level of knowledge related to the disease process.

Evaluation of Outcomes

Potential patient outcomes for each of the example nursing diagnoses for the patient with pyelonephritis are:

- Risk for imbalanced body temperature. The patient maintains body temperature within a normal range.
- Acute pain related to ureteral colic or bladder spasm. Patient will verbalize maintenance of identified comfort level.
- Fear in response to the diagnosis of pyelonephritis. The patient should will manifest positive coping behaviors and verbalize how to effectively treat the disease and prevent its recurrence.
- Deficient knowledge related to completion of drug therapy, optimal fluid intake, or need to empty bladder every two hours to reduce bacterial count. Patient will verbalize the drug therapy regimen, the need to complete full dose on schedule to prevent drug resistance or continued infection. Patient will verbalize need to flush urinary system via adequate fluid intake and fully empty bladder every two hours to reduce the amount of bacteria available for growth.
- Ineffective coping related to anxiety, malaise, and lowered activity level. The patient identifies own maladaptive coping behaviors, available resources, and support systems, describes or initiates alternative coping strategies, and describes positive results from new behaviors. The patient regains energy and participates in self-care.

POLYCYSTIC KIDNEY DISEASE

Polycystic kidney disease is a genetically inherited kidney disease and may be autosomal dominant (ADPKD) or autosomal recessive (ARPKD). Genetic mutation causes cysts to form in the renal tubules. As the cysts enlarge, the kidney's functioning units are destroyed.

Epidemiology

Prevalence in the United States is approximately 400,000 with about 1,800 developing dialysis dependent end-stage renal disease (ESRD) each year. Polycystic kidney disease is found throughout the world and shows no preference for race or ethnicity (O'Sullivan & Torres, 2003). As polycystic kidney disease is explored regarding the nature, assessment, and treatment of this disorder, the focus will be on the autosomal dominant form as this is the form most seen in the adult population. ADPKD is commonly referred to as polycystic kidney disease.

Genetics

ADPKD is caused by genetic mutations on chromosomes 4 and 16; it is a multisystem disorder (O'Sullivan & Torres, 2003). ADPKD occurs in 1 of every 500 to 1,000 individuals. Eighty-five percent of the gene carriers will evidence the disease by their seventh decade, and 50 to 75 percent will advance to ESRD (Grantham & Winklhofer, 2004).

ARPKD, on the other hand, occurs in only 1 in every 6,000 to 55,000 individuals, is more aggressive, and usually causes patient death by age 15 (Grantham & Winklhofer, 2004).

There are two genetic types of ADPKD. ADPKD-2 is the milder of the two **phenotypes** (the expression of the genes present in an individual) of ADPKD. Patients with PKD-2 will have an onset of hypertension and develop renal failure at an older age then does the patient with PKD-1.

Pathophysiology

Cysts form in the renal tubules. As the cysts advance in number and size, the kidney becomes grossly enlarged. Enlarged cysts create pressure against the normal renal parenchyma interfering with both renal filtration and renal circulation. Stretching and occlusion of the renal tubular vasculature causes decreased filtration and renin release that leads to hypertension (Grantham & Winklhofer, 2004). The developing hypertension causes renal parenchyma fibrosis and accelerates the trajectory toward renal failure. Aggressive hypertensive control is needed to slow progression toward failure.

Polycystic kidneys have been found to be many times normal size and can weigh as much as 7 to 8 kg. Many cysts are able to actively secrete chloride and water, thus the normal fluid output seen in most cases of polycystic kidney disease. Solute clearance is compromised and will require medical management as renal function declines.

Pain, the most common presenting symptom in ADPKD, may be unilateral or bilateral and range from dull and achy to knife-like, stabbing pain. Pain is caused by blood vessel rupture with bleeding into the cyst or perinephric tissues. As the hemorrhagic cyst empties, the patient may present a sudden onset of **hematuria** (blood in the urine) ranging from mild to severe and obstructive (Grantham & Winklhofer, 2004). Gross hematuria is another source of pain.

Polycystic liver disease is the most common expression of the disease outside the kidney. Nearly 75 percent of those with ADPKD will develop cystic livers by their seventh decade. Nearly 8 percent will develop cranial aneurysms. Cysts may develop in other organs systems, such as the pancreas, arachnoid membrane, spleen, ovaries, testicles, or seminal vessels (O'Sullivan, & Torres, 2003). One can appreciate that pain and related symptoms may not follow a regular pattern.

The patient with ADPKD is susceptible to urinary obstruction from hemorrhage into large cysts, particularly those located near the renal pelvis. Advanced disease may impose renal failure and need for dialysis or transplantation.

Assessment with Clinical Manifestations

There is tremendous value to the assessment of patients with polycystic kidney disease. First, the nurse must assess the subjective components of the patient by beginning with obtaining a complete medical and family history focusing on renal disease, family history of polycystic kidney disease, pain, hematuria, increase in abdominal girth, and symptoms of UTI. Next, the nurse assesses the objective aspects of the patient with a complete physical examination, which must include careful palpation of the abdomen and costovertebral angle. Possible findings include enlarged, irregular shaped kidneys and enlarged liver with palpable cysts. The urine may be positive for blood. Proteinuria indicates an advanced stage of the disease (Grantham & Winklhofer, 2004). Any of these findings should raise one's suspicions, yet not lead to a conclusive diagnosis. Imaging studies are the most common positive identifier of PKD.

Diagnostic Tests

Ultrasound is the most useful diagnostic tool in combination with a family history or gene linkage to ADPKD. Renal ultrasound is the most reliable and least expensive test for identifying ADPKD. Advantages include avoidance of contrast media in the patient with renal disease or pregnancy.

Nursing Diagnoses

Based on the information gathered, examples of nursing diagnoses in the patient with polycystic kidney disease may include the following:
- Anxiety related to potential for renal failure and to the possibility for genetic transfer of disease to offspring
- Acute pain related to blood vessel rupture with bleeding into the cyst or perinephric tissue
- Injury, potential for related to fluid, electrolyte, and metabolic acid-base balance
- Knowledge deficit related to related genetics, disease process, and treatment regimen

Planning and Implementation

There are several strategies to providing care for patients with polycystic kidney disease. The implementation of these strategies may provide quick recovery and positive outcomes for the patient with this disorder.

Goals

Primary goals of treatment for patients with polycystic kidney disease include:
- Maintaining homeostasis in each state of renal function decline and prevent or minimize cardiovascular complications.
- The patient will feel free to express the dynamic of guilt associated with genetic disease transmission and be given appropriate resources to meet any family planning goals.
- The patient will receive support with the coping mechanism of denial in dealing with the disease.
- The patient will receive adequate pain control with consideration to need for increased doses related to drug tolerance.
- The patient will acquire full knowledge of the disease process and measures to minimize complications.

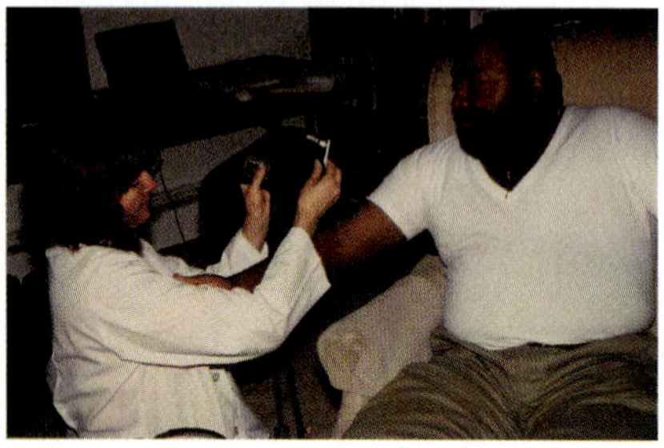

Figure 54-1 Nurse taking blood pressure of a hypertensive patient with ADPKD.

Evidence-Based Based Care

Cardiovascular complications are the primary cause of death in patients with ADPKD. Blood pressure control has proven clinically important in preventing death from left ventricular hypertrophy in the patient with ADPKD (Schrier, et al., 2002). The nurse is assigned a major therapeutic role in dispensing antihypertensive medications according to as needed within parameters medication orders (Figure 54-1).

Collaborative Management with NIC

The collaborative management for polycystic kidney disease includes:
- Pain management to prevent disability from chronic pain or analgesics.
  - NIC: Notify health care provider if measures are unsuccessful or if current complaint is a significant change from patient's past experience of pain.
  - Teach patients that nonsteroidal anti-inflammatory drugs (NSAIDs) pose a hazard to remaining kidney function via further compromise to intrarenal blood flow.
  - Prepare the patient for guided ultrasound drainage of troublesome cysts or for surgical intervention, as appropriate.
- Blood pressure control to prevent complications.
  - NIC: Monitor blood pressure after patient has taken medication, if possible.
  - Early diagnosis and management of infected cysts or parenchymal infection as evidenced by fever, deep tenderness over kidney, diaphoresis, bacteremia, leukocytosis, and bacteriuria (Grantham & Winklhofer, 2004).
  - NIC: Notify health care provider if measures are unsuccessful or if current complaint is a significant change from patient's past experience of pain.
  - NIC: Monitor WBC, hemoglobin, and hematocrit levels.

- Antibiotic therapy for infected cysts. See Box 54-1 for pharmacological agents.
  - NIC: Promote adequate fluid and nutritional intake; administer antipyretic medications, as appropriate.
- Provide counseling to consider both the benefits and consequences of genetic testing in asymptomatic adult patients.
- Facilitate social work referral, as appropriate.

Health Care Resources

Emotional support and education for patients and their families are available through the Polycystic Kidney Foundation (www.PKDcure.org).

Surgery

Hemorrhagic cyst and cyst dome removal may be necessary for those individuals with frequent or obstructive episodes of bleeding. Nephrectomy may be necessary following repeated resistant infections, cysts creating uncontrollable pain, or uncontrollable hypertension with significant loss of renal function (Figure 54-2).

Patient and Family Teaching

The nurse can promote showers rather than tub baths for female patients, frequent voiding, good perineal hygiene, and voiding immediately after intercourse. The rationale is to minimize opportunity for an ascending UTI. In addition, the nurse can promote and teach to adhere to a low-sodium diet, weight control, and exercise for those patients presenting with hypertension. And, the nurse can make dietary referral, as appropriate. The nurse must be aware that a positive finding of ADPKD genes may compromise employment opportunities and prohibit health and life insurance.

BOX 54-1

ANTIBIOTIC THERAPY FOR INFECTED CYSTS IN PATIENTS WITH POLYCYSTIC KIDNEY DISEASE

First line antibiotics for management of cysts in polycystic kidney disease:

Cephalosporins

Penicillin derivatives

Aminoglycosides

Resistant infection following use of the above may call for a lipid-soluble antibiotic to penetrate the less permeable cysts:

Clindamycin and newer derivatives

Gentamicin

Evaluation of Outcomes

Potential patient outcomes for each of the example nursing diagnoses for the patient with polycystic kidney disease are:

- Anxiety related to potential for renal failure and to the possibility for genetic transfer of disease to offspring. The patient maintains activity level within capabilities, as evidenced by normal heart rate and blood pressure during activity, as well as absence of shortness of breath, weakness, and fatigue.

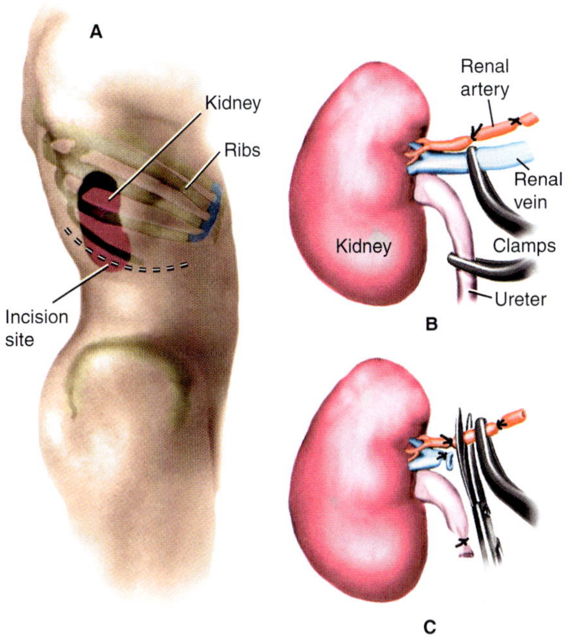

Figure 54-2 Simple nephrectomy: A. Subcostal incision, B. Renal artery ligated first, C. Renal artery transected.

- Acute pain related to blood vessel rupture with bleeding into the cyst or perinephric tissue. The patient should verbalize an adequate relief of pain along with the ability to realistically cope with the pain if it is not completely relieved.
- Injury, potential for related to fluid, electrolyte, and metabolic acid-base balance. The patient maintains adequate fluid volume, electrolyte balance, and acid-base balance as evidenced by vital signs within normal limits, clear lung sounds, pulmonary congestion absent on X-ray, resolution of edema, and arterial blood gases (ABGs) within normal limits.
- Knowledge deficit related to related genetics, disease process, and treatment regimen. The patient should demonstrate motivation to learn, identify perceived learning needs, and verbalize an understanding of desired content.

IMMUNOLOGICAL AND VASCULAR DISEASES OF THE KIDNEY

There is a group of somewhat mysterious disease phenomena that affect the renal vasculature via immune complex deposit or necrosis. Each has a potential to destroy kidney function through the common mechanism of vascular damage. Renal failure may present acutely during periods of exacerbation. With adequate treatment and response, the acute renal failure may resolve or progress with varying intensity to ESRD and chronic renal failure. The more common disorders in the group will be presented with a focus on the renal component of the disease. Note: systemic lupus erythematosus (SLE) is also a dysfunction that affects renal function and is considered in this group of disorders, but SLE is covered in detail in chapter 42. Assessment will be discussed in the sections covering acute renal failure and chronic renal failure.

Alport Syndrome

Alport syndrome is a complex genetic disorder. The genetic anomaly varies; thus patients have differing presenting syndromes. Renal dysfunction, deafness, or visual disturbance may occur dependent on genetic mutation.

Epidemiology

The genetic frequency for Alport syndrome is estimated to be one case in a population of 5,000. According to the 2005 annual data report of the United States renal data system, Alport syndrome accounts for approximately 2.5 percent of pediatric patients with ESRD In Europe, Alport syndrome may be responsible for as many as 2.3 percent of cases of ESRD.

Etiology

Alport syndrome encompasses a group of heterogeneous inherited disorders involving the basement membranes of the kidney and frequently involving the cochlea and the eye. These disorders are the result of mutations in type IV collagen genes. The mode of inheritance is X-linked in 80 percent, autosomal recessive in 15 percent, and autosomal dominant is reported in about 5 percent of individuals with Alport syndrome.

Pathophysiology

Alport syndrome may vary even within a family group. The form most affecting the renal system is X-linked Alport syndrome. Collagen anomaly in the glomerular and tubular basement membranes results in a characteristic thickening and thinning of the membrane. Focal ruptures develop in the basement membrane allowing spillage of red blood cells and protein leakage. Hematuria is a common finding. Males presenting with hematuria before age 10 commonly develop the greatest degree of renal failure (Kashtan, 2003).

Red Flag

Respiratory Occlusion

Patients with subglottal lesions or stenosis may present with a sense of breathlessness and stridor. This signals need for emergent attention to avoid complete respiratory occlusion.

Genetics

There are three genetic forms of Alport syndrome. X-linked dominant form, autosomal recessive form, and autosomal dominant form each have differing molecular genetics. X-linked Alport syndrome accounts for approximately 80 percent of the cases (Kashtan, 2003).

Diagnostic Tests

The primary methods for diagnosing Alport syndrome are by renal biopsy and a complete family history.

Small Vessel Vasculitis: Wegener Granulomatosis

Wegener granulomatosis, Churg-Strauss' syndrome, microscopic polyangiitis, and Schönlein-Henoch purpura are a group of diseases that characteristically cause small vessel pathology. Small vessel vasculitis with inflammatory or necrotizing lesions in the vasculature is common to all of these diseases, but there may be variance in presentation. All manifest multisystem involvement in varying degrees. Renal involvement is significant in 45 to 90 percent of all cases. Wegener granulomatosis is the only one of these disorders that will discussed in this section.

Wegener granulomatosis is a multisystem disease. It presents with respiratory disease in 75 percent of the cases with classic necrotizing and cavitating lesions of the pulmonary **parenchyma** (functional elements of an organ), trachea, and subglottal region (Appel, Radhakrishnan, & D'Agati, 2004). Shortness of breath and hemoptysis may be the presenting symptoms.

Wegener granulomatosis may cause nasal crusting or septal defect, hearing loss, chronic sinusitis, or ophthalmological disorders. Fever, weakness, malaise, and cough with hemoptysis are common presenting symptoms. Renal involvement develops in up to 95 percent of all cases and is varied in the clinical presentation (Appel, et al., 2004). Evidence of renal involvement includes microscopic hematuria, **proteinuria** (protein in the urine), decreased glomerular filtration, and hypertension.

Epidemiology

The literature evidences discrepancy in incidence and demographics of this vasculitis disease set. Advances in diagnostics and knowledge of disease characteristics prompt dynamic change in available data. The collective incidence of small vessel vasculitis is 19.8 cases per million. There appears to be seasonal variance with more cases presenting in the late fall and early spring.

Incidence of Wegener granulomatosis is only slightly higher in males than in females. Peak incidence is in the fourth and fifth decades. Though more than one family member has been found to have Wegener granulomatosis, there is no conclusive evidence of genetic transmission (Appel, et al., 2004).

Etiology

There is no clear etiology of this disease group. Autoimmune humoral and cell-mediated immune responses are implicated.

Pathophysiology

Wegener granulomatosis produces granulomatous necrotizing lesions in small- and medium-sized blood vessels. A multisystem disease, Wegener granulomatosis is associated with necrosis and granulomatous inflammation of the small vessels of the respiratory tract and glomeruli (Appel, et al., 2004). Associated renal pathology includes obstruction from associated ureteral lesions with sclerotic narrowing and immunosuppression treatment-associated malignancies.

Relapse has become the major challenge in treating Wegener granulomatosis. It is postulated that the resulting granulomatous areas in the connective

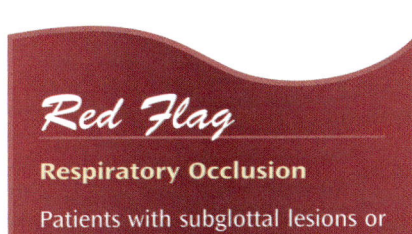

> **Skills 360°**
>
> **Assessment of Wegener Granulomatosis**
>
> The following are assessment findings that may be present in Wegener granulomatosis:
>
> - Upper and lower respiratory symptoms, including hoarseness, shortness of breath, cough, hemoptysis, or nasal drainage; inspect for nasal crusting or septal defect
> - Recent hearing deficit, tinnitus, pain; inspect ear for drainage or perforation of the tympanic membrane
> - Sinus infection; pain or tenderness over the sinuses
> - Visual disturbances or conjunctivitis
> - Joint and muscle aches
> - Changes in urine quantity and quality

tissue may be the source of remission (Bacon, 2005). Intensive study is ongoing. Nurses must stay alert to changes in early diagnostics and treatment.

Assessment with Clinical Manifestations

The clinical presentation of Wegener granulomatosis varies, which affects the assessment processes. Wegener granulomatosis may be mild and obscure or present with fulminant respiratory and renal involvement. The nurse must first obtain a complete health history and perform a complete physical examination. In addition, the nurse must keep the focus broad to include those physical responses shown in the Soft Skills feature.

Diagnostic Tests

The diagnostic tests for Wegener granulomatosis are CT of the lungs, bronchoscopy with lung biopsy, and renal biopsy. In addition, the laboratory tests are antineutrophil cytoplasmic antibodies (ANCA), electrolytes, CBC, and urine studies.

Planning and Implementation

Wegener granulomatosis was formerly a lethal disease. Advances in diagnosis and treatment have decreased mortality rates but have not yet affected a cure. The primary treatment for Wegener granulomatosis is the pharmacological treatment, which uses glucocorticoids and cyclophosphamide (Appel, et al., 2004). Repeated exacerbations and related chronic health changes have resulted in considerable work disability and diminished quality of life (Reinhold-Keller, et al., 2005). Social work referral to address insurance and disability challenges is critical. Referral to or consult with the mental health nurse specialist, when available, may be of real value to this patient population.

GOODPASTURE'S SYNDROME

Goodpasture's syndrome is a glomerular basement membrane disease (GBM). Primary sites of vascular membrane destruction occur in the capillary beds of the lungs and the kidneys. Goodpasture's syndrome, by definition, must include the three characteristics of proliferative glomerulonephritis, pulmonary hemorrhage, and the presence of anti-GBM antibodies.

Epidemiology

Goodpasture's syndrome has an incidence of one in one million, occurs slightly more in males than in females, and is more prominent in Caucasians. Most diagnoses are made in the third and fifth decades (Bergs, 2005). ESRD develops in 40 to 70 percent of those with renal involvement.

Etiology

The exact cause of Goodpasture's syndrome is unknown. It is believed that the disease process may be triggered when genetically predisposed individuals are exposed to upper respiratory infection, irritants, or toxins (Bergs, 2005). Inhalation of hydrocarbon fumes, cigarette smoke, or cocaine and exposure to hair dye, metallic dust, and D-penicillamine have all been associated with syndrome exacerbations (Appel, et al., 2004).

Pathophysiology

Circulating antibodies react with antigens against type IV collagen specific to the basement membranes of glomerular and pulmonary capillaries (Appel, et al., 2004). Immune globulins deposited in the basement membranes, causing an inflammatory response, glomerulonephritis, and breakdown in the basement membrane with crescent formation. The complications of Goodpasture's syndrome include pulmonary hemorrhage, respiratory failure and dialysis dependent ESRD. Goodpasture's Syndrome carries a 50 percent mortality rate without early recognition and intervention.

Genetics

Autoimmune response has been linked to genes in q35 to q37 region of chromosome 2 (Appel, et al., 2004). It is suggested that one may have a genetic predisposition to Goodpasture's syndrome (Bergs, 2005).

Assessment with Clinical Manifestations

The primary clinical focus must be pulmonary function. The patient may first present with mild shortness of breath or severe, exsanguinating pulmonary hemorrhage (Appel, et al., 2004; Bergs, 2005). Presenting flulike symptoms of weakness, malaise, and pallor may be related to anemia secondary to chronic blood loss. Renal involvement may be evidenced by hematuria, decreased urine output, edema, and hypertension.

Diagnostic Tests

The principal indicator of Goodpasture's syndrome is laboratory finding of circulating anti-GBM antibodies, proteinuria, and iron deficiency anemia. Chest X-ray (CXR) may show hemorrhagic infiltrates, atelectasis, and pulmonary edema (Appel, et al., 2004).

Planning and Implementation

Early diagnosis and intervention have drastically decreased mortality related to Goodpasture's syndrome. Current treatment includes high dose oral or IV corticosteroid therapy to control the inflammatory process in conjunction with plasmapheresis to reduce the circulating immune complexes.

RHABDOMYOLYSIS

Rhabdomyolysis is a condition of muscle tissue destruction with release of myoglobin in the urine. It is a major cause of acute renal failure.

Etiology

A myriad of conditions contribute to rhabdomyolysis. Direct muscle injuries, drugs and toxins, infection, excessive muscular activity, ischemia, electrolyte imbalances, endocrine or metabolic disturbances, and immunological disorders are major categories of etiology. Among these categories are severe burns, crush injuries, tetanus, gas gangrene, excessive exercise, diabetic ketoacidosis, hypothermia, and polymyositis.

Pathophysiology

Lethal levels of intracellular ionized calcium occur with disruption in normal muscle structure or metabolism. Degrading enzymes are activated, causing cell death. Lysis of the cell membrane releases cell content, inclusive of myoglobin, into the system. The exact pathophysiology is unclear and believed to be a combination effect of hypovolemia, tubular toxicity, and tubular obstruction.

Safety First 1

Safety Considerations for Rhabdomyolysis

Health care and medical advances enable the elderly to live independently longer. Potential for falls with a period of prolonged immobility before assistance arrives expose them to the risk of rhabdomyolysis. Education and persuasion to the advantages of a personal medical alert system has the potential to minimize complications of fractures, electrolyte imbalances, or dehydration in this population. A myriad of service providers are available. Many community emergency services and or community hospitals offer these services.

PATIENT PLAYBOOK

Assessment of Rhabdomyolysis

The nurse must examine carefully for:

- Redness, swelling, and induration over tender or painful muscles
- Muscle stiffness or weakness varying from mild at onset to severe with the development of muscular necrosis
- Muscle paralysis that may develop with severe muscular necrosis
- Hypotension or hypertension
- Signs of hypovolemia and reduced urine output
- Dark urine from the characteristic brown debris and sediment

Genetics

Hereditary enzyme deficiencies predispose to rhabdomyolysis. They include deficiency of myophosphorylase (McArdle's syndrome), phosphofructokinase, or carnitine palmityl transferase with resultant decreased intracellular energy production.

Assessment with Clinical Manifestations

The initial data collection must include learning what the patient was doing and what the environmental conditions were prior to the onset of symptoms (Russell, 2005). An example is running an unusually long distance in hot, humid conditions with adequate hydration before, during, or after the exercise.

Diagnostic Tests

The diagnostic tests for rhabdomyolysis are primarily blood and urine. Blood studies that are used for diagnostics are elevated creatinine kinase (CK-MM) which confirm muscle injury; CK-MM which is the specific diagnostic serum marker for rhabdomyolysis; hyperkalemia is the most life-threatening consequence of muscle necrosis; hyperphosphatemia and hypocalcemia; elevated BUN and the creatinine ratio; and elevated uric acid levels. In addition, urine studies will show myoglobin, and have an acid pH and be positive for red blood cells.

Safety First 1

Safety Considerations with Rhabdomyolysis

It has been demonstrated that many patients presenting with rhabdomyolysis do not admit to muscle pain or tenderness and do not present with swelling. This emphasizes the need for repeated patient questioning and thorough examination for early intervention and optimal recovery.

Planning and Implementation

Rhabdomyolysis can cause acute renal failure, which is covered extensively later in this chapter. In addition, the primary goal for the management of rhabdomyolysis is to minimize complications and to intervene effectively as complications of muscle necrosis occur. For example, in the development of compartment syndrome requiring fasciotomy occur, the wounds must be kept infection free and the muscle tissue moist for successful closure.

ACUTE RENAL FAILURE

Acute renal failure (ARF) presents as a rapid decline in renal function. This decline may occur within a few hours or over a period of several weeks. Relatively asymptomatic, ARF is most often detected by laboratory studies. ARF is evidenced by oliguria elevated blood levels of BUN and creatinine (Brady, Clarkson, & Lieberthal, 2004).

Epidemiology

ARF occurs in approximately 5 percent of all hospital admissions and 30 percent of all intensive care unit admissions (Brady, et al., 2004). ARF contributes to an increase in morbidity and mortality in the hospitalized patient. Most patients recover from ARF. Optimal recovery is dependent on early recognition, identifying the cause, and instituting appropriate clinical management (Figure 54-3) (Toto, 2004).

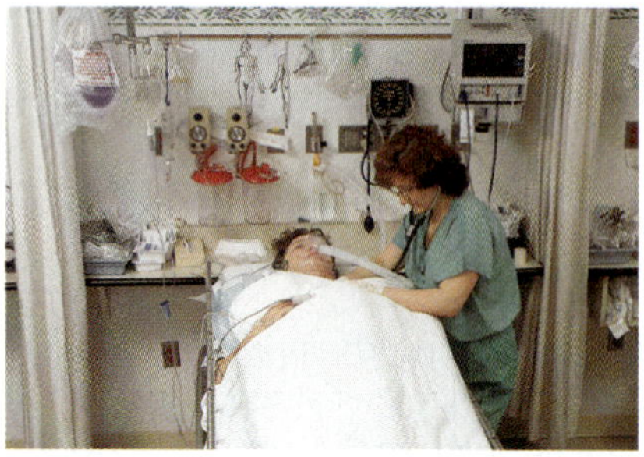

Figure 54-3 Patient in critical condition with ARF.

Etiology

There are many causes for ARF, which are presented in the following pathophysiology section and in Table 54-1.

TABLE 54-1 Etiology of ARF

INTRARENAL CAUSES OF ACUTE OR PROGRESSIVE RENAL FAILURE	PATHOPHYSIOLOGY AND ETIOLOGY
Ischemic acute tubular necrosis (ATN)	ATN infers damage to the renal parenchyma. Multiple sources of tubular injury resulting in ATN include major and prolonged surgery, burns, overwhelming sepsis, myoglobin release, and nephrotoxic drugs. Though often associated with **hypovolemia** (insufficient intravascular fluid), ATN has occurred in states of **normovolemia** (state of normal blood volume). It is not to be confused with perfusion-deficit related ATN. Recovery potential is directly correlated to the extent of intrarenal damage (Brady, et al., 2004).
Drug toxicity	NSAIDs inhibit renal prostaglandin production thereby contribute to intrarenal vascular constriction and potential acute tubular necrosis. The potential for renal function impairment secondary to NSAIDs increases in the presence of hypovolemia, decreased arterial blood volume, or chronic renal insufficiency.
Renal artery stenosis or thrombosis	Loin pain and hematuria are the classic signs of acute renal artery occlusion. Chronic renal artery occlusion is generally asymptomatic until a precipitous event occurs. Collateral circulation from the adrenal glands will often allow chronic stenosis go undetected for some time. Causes include emboli, thrombi, hypercoagulable states, and aortic dissection or occlusion. The transplant patient may be predisposed secondary to immunosuppression or vascular rejection or constriction at the site of vascular anastomosis.
Hemolytic uremic syndrome (HUS)	Occlusion of glomerular capillaries by capillary wall thickening and thrombus formation. HUS may be associated with pregnancy as a complication of preeclampsia and may occur in the first three months postpartum. It is also seen after receiving the chemotherapeutic agent mitomycin or the antirejection medication cyclosporine.
Multiple myeloma	Protein-like **casts** (materials in a space that fills the contours of the space) in distal nephron segments, interstitial calcification, and **amyloid** (extracellular protein-like substance) deposits in nephron glomeruli and blood vessels.
Radiation nephritis	Endothelial cell swelling causes decreased intrarenal blood flow and results in tubular atrophy within the nephron.
Contrast-induced nephropathy	Ischemia resulting from dye-induced vasoconstriction is the probable cause of decreased kidney function following IV contrast media. Acute decline in renal function is seen within 24 to 48 hours of dye administration with a peak creatinine in three to five days and resolution in uncomplicated cases in about one week. At-risk populations are associated with existing renal impairment, diabetes mellitus, repeated use of contrast media, and concurrent use of nephrotoxic drugs including NSAIDs and the elderly. Preventive measures include: Infusion of 0.45% normal saline 1 mL/kg for 12 hours prior to and following contrast media Administration of oral acetylcysteine in combination with hydration (600 mg twice daily 24 hours before and after contrast media) Infusion of 154 mEq/L sodium bicarbonate as a bolus of 3 mL/kg/hour for 1 hour before the procedure and 1 mL/kg/hour for 6 hours following the procedure.

Adapted from Brady, H., Clarkson, M., & Lieberthal, W. (2004). Acute renal failure. In B. Brenner (Ed.), Brenner and Rector's the kidney *(7th ed., vol. 1, pp. 1215–1292). Philadelphia: W. B. Saunders Co.; Karnib, H., & Badr, K. (2004). Microvascular diseases of the kidney. In B. Brenner (Ed.),* Brenner and Rector's the kidney *(7th ed., vol. 2, pp. 1601–1623). Philadelphia: W. B. Saunders Co.; Kelly, C., & Nielson, E. (2004). Tubulointerstitial diseases. In B. Brenner (Ed.),* Brenner and Rector's the kidney *(7th ed., vol. 2, pp. 1483–1511). Philadelphia: W. B. Saunders Co.*

Red Flag

Compartment Syndrome in Rhabdomyolysis

Compartment syndrome may develop with extensive muscle damage. The mechanism of injury is acute swelling in a muscular compartment. Rigid, nonexpanding fascia surrounds each muscle group forming a compartment for the muscle. Fascia is rigid and unable to accommodate swelling. Increased pressure within the constrictive compartment causes further muscle necrosis, vascular constriction, and nerve damage. This can occur immediately or may be delayed for up to three days. The health care team must monitor for development of or increase in neurovascular deficit. This presents a surgical emergency to relieve the compartment pressure before permanent damage occurs. The treatment of choice is **fasciotomy** (incision through a fibrous layer that separates muscles) with closure following resolution of swelling.

Pathophysiology

ARF is a sudden and near complete cessation of kidney function and may occur suddenly and last for days in certain situations. ARF is seen in acute care patients and may occur in other arenas of health care as well (e.g., convalescent care, home care, or out-patient care). ARF begins with oliguria, anuria, or even normal urine output. **Oliguria** (less than 400 mL per 24 hours of urine) is the most common clinical manifestation, with **anuria** (less than 50 mL per 24 hours of urine), and normal urine output being less common in occurrence. ARF can be a critical condition, and there is an associated mortality percentage even with management in the acute care settings.

The etiology of ARF is varied. Classification follows the source of failure in relation to the kidney. **Prerenal** causes of ARF are those that result in decreased blood flow to the kidney. This may be something as simple as dehydration from fluid loss or as complex as the vascular expansion of sepsis or the deficient pumping of cardiac failure. Prerenal ARF is the most common cause of ARF (Kieran & Brady, 2003). **Intrarenal** causes of ARF are intrinsic to the kidney. These include inflammation of the renal parenchyma, intrarenal vascular thrombosis, or tubular necrosis from nephrotoxic agents. **Postrenal** failure is caused by obstruction to urine flow. More commonly the obstruction is caused by an enlarged prostate gland or a calculus. There simply is no route for the urine to exit the system.

There are myriad causes of ARF. Many are presented in Table 54-1. It is important to note that any ARF event is a potential precursor to chronic renal insufficiency (CRI)) or chronic renal failure (CRF). Factors influencing resolution or progression of failure episode are early diagnosis, adequacy of treatment, and the presence of preexisting kidney disease. Major complications of ARF include hyperkalemia, hyponatremia, hypocalcemia, hyperphosphatemia, and hyperuricemia (Kieran & Brady, 2003) (Figure 54-4).

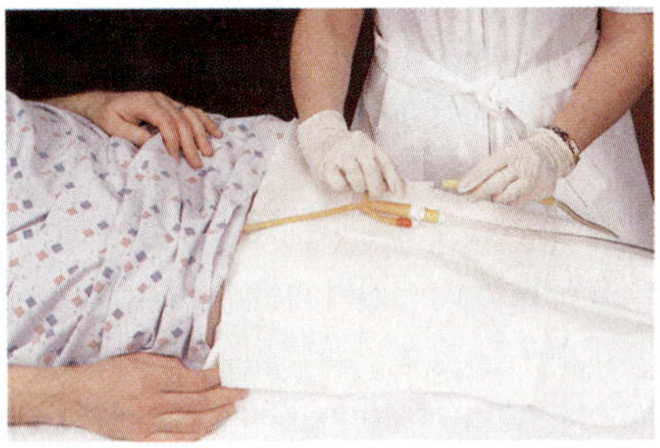

Figure 54-4 Nurse connecting irrigation tubing to irrigation port of a catheter for a postrenal cause of ARF.

Assessment with Clinical Manifestations

The assessment for the patient with ARF needs to be comprehensive and includes the entire body system. Specific assessment components are shown in the Patient Playbook.

Diagnostic Tests

In addition to the cessation or change of urine output, there are many diagnostic tests to determine the presence of acute renal failure. The following are the diagnostic tests for ARF: plain abdominal X-ray of the kidneys, ureters and bladder (KUB) to determine calculi or renal vascular calcification; a renal ultrasound to identify renal vascular blood flow and to rule out obstruction, and a bladder scan to detect urinary retention. In addition, laboratory studies are several blood chemistry tests (e.g., BUN, serum creatinine), a basic metabolic panel (BMP), and a CBC.

Nursing Diagnoses

Based on the information gathered, examples of nursing diagnoses in the patient with ARF may include the following:

- Risk for imbalance in fluid volume
- Impaired tissue integrity related to alterations in internal regulatory function
- Risk for infection related to invasive lines and altered immune response secondary to ARF and uremic toxins
- Anxiety related to sudden change in health status
- Knowledge deficit related to disease process and related diagnostic studies

PATIENT PLAYBOOK

Assessment of Patients with ARF

Subjective

The nurse will gather a history with focus on hydration and medications. Questions for the nurse to ask may include:

- Have you had any nausea, vomiting, diarrhea, fever, or profuse sweating recently? Quantify the amount and duration.
- Have you felt light-headed or dizzy?
- Have you been able to drink fluids in good amounts?
- Have you experienced any change in the amount of urine or the number of times you have urinated?
- Have you noticed shortness of breath, weakness, or fatigue?
- Have you had any recent injuries?
- Have you taken any antibiotics recently?
- How much do you use NSAIDs? Name the NSAIDs: Advil, Aleve, Excedrin, ibuprofen, Indocin, Motrin, Naprosyn, Pamprin, and Voltaren.

Objective

The nurse will complete a physical examination with diagnostic studies. System alterations in acute renal failure reflect the kidneys inability to maintain homeostasis. Table 54-2 lists homeostatic losses and evidence of alteration. Table 54-3 identifies questions to ask when suspecting urinary dysfunction.

Planning and Implementation

There are many interventions and strategies for the nurse to be aware of in the management of ARF. Often patients are transferred to the critical care settings as they experience ARF, and the mortality percentages are relatively high for patients with the diagnosis of ARF.

Goals

The primary goal is to reverse the causative process with full recovery of renal function. When this is impossible, the goal is always to minimize renal compromise.

Collaborative Management including NIC

ARF presents a dynamic management challenge. The clinical presentation can rapidly change and requires intricate teamwork among health care providers. The patient can go from a state of intravascular hypovolemia to fluid overload and pulmonary edema in just a few hours and require skilled, dynamic assessment and alertness to management change. Among the considerations are:

- Treat the underlying cause of acute renal failure.
- Keep the patient informed of the disease process and the treatment plan.
- NIC: Determine patient's understanding of common medical terminology, such as *azotemia, creatinine,* and *acute renal failure.*
- Fluid replacement in primary hypovolemia and high output failure in the recovery phase.
- NIC: Offer fluids regularly throughout the day, as appropriate.
- Fluid restriction in low output failure and hypervolemia.
- Intermittent hemodialysis or continuous renal replacement therapy (Box 54-2).
- Diuretics, as appropriate and with evidence of tubular response.
- Maintain accurate intake and output records and obtain a daily weight. Day-to-day weight gain in the hospital reflects fluid gain. One liter of fluid is equivalent to 1 kilogram of weight.

BOX 54-2

CONTINUOUS RENAL REPLACEMENT THERAPY (CRRT)

Continuous renal replacement therapy (CRRT) offers lower fluid removal and solute clearance rates than intermittent HD. Hemodynamic stability is more easily attained in the hypotensive critically ill patient.

The procedure is performed in the critical care setting utilizing an inline hemofilter. Arteriovenous hemofiltration relies on the driving force of the systemic blood pressure for blood flow through the extracorporeal circuit. Venovenous hemofiltration requires a blood pump for blood flow through the extracorporeal circuit.

Vascular access is achieved by percutaneous insertion of a single-lumen catheter into a central artery and vein for arteriovenous hemofiltration. A dual-lumen catheter inserted into a central vein is sufficient for venovenous hemofiltration.

Complications include hemofilter clogging and clotting, emboli distal to arterial puncture, vascular damage, and hemorrhage.

Source: Marshall, M., & Golper, T. (2003). Other dialysis modalities. In R. Johnson & J. Feehally (Eds.), Comprehensive clinical nephrology *(2nd ed., pp. 1025–1034). St. Louis, MO: Mosby.*

TABLE 54-2 Alterations in ARF and the Mechanisms of the Alterations

ALTERATIONS IN ACUTE RENAL FAILURE	MECHANISM OF ALTERATION
Alterations in fluid volume	Intravascular fluid overload in oliguric states: edema, hypertension, shortness of breath, abnormal lung sounds, and acute weight gain Intravascular dehydration in high output failure: thirst, reduction in skin turgor, dry mucous membranes, hypotension, tachycardia, decreased urine output, and acute weight loss
Alterations in intravascular sodium (Na^+) Normal range: 135 to 145 mEq/L	Hyponatremia due to dilution in **hypervolemia** (excess intravascular fluid): disorientation, apathy, depression, depressed deep tendon reflexes, and agitation. The elderly are especially susceptible. Hypernatremia due to concentration in hypovolemia: thirst. Note: be alert to the development of muscle weakness, restlessness or lethargy, and coma.
Alterations in intravascular potassium (K^+) Normal range: 3.5 to 5 mmol/L	Hypokalemia in hypervolemic state because of dilution or diuretic phase of recovery because of loss. Anticipate need for potassium replacement. Watch for broad flat T waves, ST depression, or prolonged QT. The elderly and patients on digoxin or antiarrhythmic drugs are most prone to arrhythmia secondary to low potassium levels. Hyperkalemia in hypovolemic state because of concentration and retention. Respiratory acidosis promotes potassium movement out of the intracellular space into the extracellular space compounding hyperkalemia in any form of renal insufficiency. Hyperkalemia signals a medical emergency. Peaked T-waves characteristic of hyperkalemia. Severe and prolonged hyperkalemia will increasingly prolong the PR and QRS intervals with a potential for cardiac arrest.
Alterations in intravascular magnesium (Mg^{2+}) Normal range: 1.8 to 2.3 mg/dL	Mg^{2+} blood levels may be low because of high output kidney failure, through GI loss or dietary deficiency. All three conditions often exist in the patient with ARF. There may be no clinical signs of low magnesium levels. Retention of Mg^{2+} in the oliguric state can cause high blood levels of magnesium. Anticipate muscle weakness or twitching and cardiac arrhythmias when accompanied by low levels of K^+ and Ca^{2+}.
Alterations in bicarbonate	Metabolic acidosis occurs with retention of sulfuric acid and phosphoric acid from protein metabolism. As failure progresses, acidosis is compounded by retention of hydrogen ions and decreased production of bicarbonate.
Elevations in BUN and creatinine levels (azotemia)	Urea nitrogen is excreted exclusively by the kidney. Elevations may be caused by renal dysfunction, higher levels of protein catabolism, GI bleed, or severe burn or even excessive protein intake. Creatinine, on the other hand, is exogenous in source. A muscle enzyme, it is excreted exclusively by the kidney. Creatinine provides an easy, first look at kidney function.
Alteration in urine studies	Decreased sodium output as indicated by a fractional excretion of sodium of less than 1 is indicative of prerenal failure and useful in determining need for fluid challenge. Cells, casts and crystals are indicative of intrarenal damage.

Adapted from Kieran, N., & Brady, H. (2003). Clinical evaluation, management, and outcome of acute renal failure. In R. Johnson & J. Feehally (Eds.), Comprehensive clinical nephrology *(2nd ed., pp. 183–206). St. Louis, MO: Mosby; Mount, D., & Zandi-Nejad, K. (2004). Disorders of potassium balance. In B. Brenner (Ed.),* Brenner and Rector's the kidney *(7th ed., vol. 1, pp. 997–1040). Philadelphia: W. B. Saunders Co.; Pollak, M., & Yu, A. (2004). Clinical disturbances of calcium, magnesium, and phosphate metabolism. In B. Brenner (Ed.),* Brenner and Rector's the kidney *(7th ed., vol. 1, pp. 1040–1076). Philadelphia: W. B. Saunders Co.*

Red Flag

Hypokalemia in Renal Failure

Hypokalemia can occur in renal failure patients. The nurse must remember that hypokalemia can cause a cardiac arrest when: (a) the potassium level is less than 2.5 mEq/L, and (b) the patient is taking digitalis (an inotropic medication that strengthens the contraction of the myocardium and slows down the rate of the heart). Hypokalemia enhances the action of digitalis and therefore causes toxicity.

TABLE 54-3 Questions the Nurse Can Ask Patients Who Have Altered Patterns of Urinary Elimination Caused by Renal Dysfunction

Diurnal Voiding Habits
How long can you postpone urination?
Can you postpone urination for two hours?
Nocturia (awakening from sleep to urinate)
How many times do you wake up at night and urinate?
Does the urge to urinate interrupt your sleep?
Urinary Incontinence
Do you leak urine or lose bladder control?
Does this leakage cause any problems for you?
Urinary Retention
Do you feel you completely empty your bladder?
Have you ever been unable to urinate at all?
Do you strain to start your stream?
Does your stream start and stop?

Red Flag

Geriatric Differences regarding Urinary Output

Older patients may have a larger amount of debris in their urine. Their urine or irrigant output must be monitoring closely for potential blockages or retention.

- Monitor respiratory status; anticipate acute changes, particularly with fluid challenges or with acutely diminished urine output.
- Monitor blood chemistries and respond appropriately.
- Manage serum potassium: replacement in high output failure and restriction in low output failure. Hyperkalemia is considered a medical emergency when greater than 6.5 mmol/L (Kieran & Brady, 2003). Treatment of hyperkalemia is outlined in Box 54-3.
- Maintain blood pressure control. Hypertension: During periods of reduced tubular filtration, renin is likely secreted and the angiotensin system activated with resulting increase in blood pressure. Nursing plays an important role in maximizing recovery from ARF. Timely administration of as needed antihypertensive medications has the potential to prevent tubular necrosis or its advance.
- Maintain blood pressure control. Hypotension. In the acute setting, it is important to maintain renal perfusion. Low dose (1 to 3 mcg/kg/min) dopamine has been utilized in oliguric ARF.

Evidence-Based Care

Dopamine is the immediate precursor of norepinephrine. Low-dose dopamine has been used to increase renal perfusion by stimulating dopamine receptors by infusing a dose intended to prevent stimulation of related alpha and beta receptors (Pierce, Morris, & Clancy, 2002). Commonly referred to as renal dose dopamine, research has challenged its use in the critically patient. Tachycardia, increase in cardiac index, respiratory drive suppression, and pulmonary arteriovenous shunting have been observed in the critically ill patient (Kieran & Brady, 2003). In addition, renal dose dopamine has not been shown effective in preventing ischemic acute tubular necrosis.

The challenge to nursing is significant. Dopamine at renal doses continues in use. Many institutions have approved its use outside of the critical care units. Nurse-patient ratios in noncritical care settings range four to six or more

BOX 54-3

MANAGEMENT OF HYPERKALEMIA

Emergent: Regular insulin 10 units and 50 mL of 50% Dextrose intravenously; Insulin provides active transport to shift potassium from the bloodstream into the intracellular compartment. Glucose is required to prevent hypoglycemia. Frequent monitoring of blood sugar is required. Insulin and glucose are given consecutively and in the same time frame. This is a stabilizing measure only. It will usually be followed by dialysis or an exchange resin, removal of potassium from IV fluids and dietary restriction.

Sodium bicarbonate 50 mmol is given over five minutes in cases of acidosis. The addition of bicarbonate to the insulin-glucose regimen prevents continued potassium efflux from the cell in acidosis. This is a temporary measure. The acidosis must be corrected and is often accomplished by diuretic or dialysis correction of hypervolemia.

Cardiac protective: Calcium gluconate or calcium chloride (10 mL of 10% solution intravenously over five minutes) to antagonize the cardiac effect of hyperkalemia.

Intermediate: Exchange resin such as sodium polystyrene sulfonate (Kayexalate). 15 to 30 grams in 50 to 100 mL of 20% sorbitol. The exchange resin exchanges sodium ions for potassium ions in the gut. Sorbitol provides catharsis to remove the potassium complex from the gut. This is appropriate in non–life-threatening hyperkalemia. Loose bowel movements following administration and lowered serum potassium levels are indicative of successful treatment.

Maintenance: Potassium dietary restriction of 2 g/day.

Adapted from Kieran, N., & Brady, H. (2003). Clinical evaluation, management, and outcome of acute renal failure. In R. Johnson & J. Feehally (Eds.), Comprehensive clinical nephrology *(2nd ed., pp. 183–206). St. Louis, MO: Mosby.*

patients per nurse. Close observation of the respiratory, cardiovascular, and urinary systems of these ill patients need be taken seriously. Patient advocacy is critical at the sign of toxicity.

Nutrition

Dietary management in ARF requires the nurse, dietitian, and health care provider to put forth a concerted effort. Nutritional goals include preventing exacerbation of azotemia and maintaining mineral and electrolyte balance. The nutritional care for ARF involve caloric intake adequate to prevent protein catabolism and starvation ketoacidosis; protein intake restriction, except in highly catabolic patients of 0.8 to 1 g/kg/day, and phosphate restriction, as appropriate. This may require limiting dairy foods though a reduced protein diet provides phosphate restriction. In addition, there should be potassium restriction in patients at risk for hyperkalemia at 2 g/day.

Patients should be taught to avoid the following foods that are high in potassium: fresh fruits and vegetables, particularly citrus, tomatoes, and potatoes; reduce the potassium content of potatoes by boiling and replacing water during the cooking process; dried fruits and vegetables, legumes and nuts; chocolate; and protein-rich foods.

Uncovering the Evidence

ARF in Varying Regions of the World

Discussion: Although ARF is believed to be common in the setting of critical illness and is associated with a high risk of death, little is known about its epidemiology and outcome or how these vary in different regions of the world. This study's objective was to determine the prevalence, differences in etiology, illness severity, and clinical practices associated with ARF in intensive care unit (ICU) patients in multiple countries.

A prospective observational study of ICU patients who either were treated with renal replacement therapy (RRT) or fulfilled at least one of the predefined criteria for ARF from September 2000 to December 2001 at 54 hospitals in 23 countries. The main outcome measures were the occurrence of ARF, factors contributing to etiology, illness severity, treatment, need for renal support after hospital discharge, and hospital mortality.

Implications for Practice: Of 29,269 critically ill patients admitted during the study period, 1,738 had ARF during their ICU stay, including 1,260 who were treated with RRT. The most common contributing factor to ARF was septic shock (47.5 percent). Approximately 30 percent of patients had preadmission renal dysfunction. The overall hospital mortality was 60.3 percent, and dialysis dependence at hospital discharge was 13.8 percent for survivors. In conclusion, in this multinational study, the period prevalence of ARF requiring RRT in the ICU was between 5 and 6 percent and was associated with a high hospital mortality rate.

Source: Shigehiko, U., Kellum, J., Bellomo, R., Doig, G., Morimatsu, H., Morgera, S., et al. (2005). Acute renal failure in critically ill patients. JAMA, *294(7), 813–818.*

Population-Based Care

The elderly are a particularly vulnerable population. Reduced glomerular capacity along with preexisting cardiac and respiratory illness makes them an easy target for ARF. Incontinence and altered mental states make early detection a challenge.

Surgery

Surgery or other invasive procedure may be implicated for the patient in ARF. Procedures include:

- Angioplasty or renal artery bypass surgery for renal artery stenosis or renal vein thrombosis.
- Ureteral stents placed by cystoscopy for obstructive conditions involving the ureters.
- Percutaneous nephrostomy tubes for obstructive conditions that will not allow ureteral stent passage. Nephrostomy tube is the treatment of choice in the obstructed patient who has hyperkalemia or sepsis (Mellon, 2003).

Patient and Family Teaching

The patient and family will have a totally new and frightening illness experience when they develop any level of renal failure. Language and tests compounded by the effects of the illness will present a confusing situation. They may need ongoing education relative to the disease process, medications inclusive of over-the-counter medication use, and nutrition.

Evaluation of Outcomes

Potential patient outcomes for each of the example nursing diagnoses for the patient with ARF are:

- Risk for imbalance in fluid volume. The patient's fluid balance is evidenced by 24-hour intake and output are balanced, orthostatic hypotension not present, normal skin turgor with moist mucous membranes, and urine-specific gravity is normal.
- Impaired tissue integrity related to alterations in internal regulatory function. The patient will improve the condition of their impaired tissue integrity as evidenced by decreased redness, swelling, and pain.
- Risk for infection related to invasive lines and altered immune response secondary to ARF and uremic toxins. The patient remains free of infection, as evidenced by normal vital signs and absence of purulent drainage from wounds, incisions, and tubes. Infection is recognized early to allow for prompt treatment.
- Anxiety related to sudden change in health status. The patient should be able to recognize the signs of anxiety, demonstrate positive coping mechanisms, and describe a reduction in the level of anxiety experienced.
- Knowledge deficit related to disease process and related diagnostic studies. The patient explains disease state, recognized need for medications, and understands treatments.

CHRONIC RENAL FAILURE

Chronic renal failure (CRF) is a progressive and irreversible decline in renal function ranging from mild with nearly normal function to ESRD requiring renal replacement therapy. The kidney disease quality initiative have classified chronic kidney disease into five stages based on glomerular filtration rate (GFR) (Table 54-4) (Nahas, 2003).

Epidemiology

CRF is a worldwide health problem. The incidence in the United States in 2000 was 252 new patients per million with a prevalence of 1,624 patients per million (Nahas, 2003). The incidence of CRF is higher in African Caribbeans, Native Americans, and Asian (Americans) and increases with aging in all populations (Winearls, 2003).

TABLE 54-4 Stages of Chronic Kidney Disease

STAGE	DESCRIPTION	GFR (ML/MIN/1.73M^2)
1	Kidney damage with normal or increased GFR	Greater than or equal to 90
2	Kidney damage with mildly decreased GFR	60–89
3	Moderately decreased GFR	30–59
4	Severely decreased GFR	15–29
5	Kidney failure	Less than 15 (or dialysis)

Etiology

Diabetes mellitus and hypertension are the two most common causes of CRF in the United States. All conditions causing ARF discussed in this chapter may cause progression to CRF.

Modifiable risk factors deserve discussion. Proteinuria has been shown to exacerbate progression to CRF. Dietary modification and angiotensin-converting enzyme (ACE) inhibitors have been shown to reduce the level of proteinuria. Hypertension is less damaging to patients with proteinuria when kept at or below 125/75. Hyperglycemia is a major cause of CRF, and hyperlipidemia has been shown to hasten the progression to ESRD (Nahas, 2003). All modifiable risk factors can be better controlled by the patient and health care providers alike (Box 54-4).

BOX 54-4

THREE CATEGORIES OF FACTORS AFFECTING PROGRESSION OF CRF

Nonmodifiable:

Age
Gender
Genetics
Race

Factors Necessary to Initiate CRF in Susceptible Individuals:

Immune pathology
Hemodynamic changes
Metabolic disorders
Infections

Modifiable Risk Factors:

Systemic hypertension
Hyperglycemia
Dyslipidemia
Proteinuria

Pathophysiology

The common underlying cause of progression to CRF is glomerulosclerosis (Nahas, 2003). Regardless of the initial insult, glomerulosclerosis is the end result. As the level of glomerular function declines, need for intervention increases. Failure of the kidney to maintain homeostasis has significant health implications. Cardiovascular disease is the major cause of death in the patient with ESRD.

Assessment with Clinical Manifestations

Clinical manifestations are many and varied as shown in Table 54-5.

Diagnostic Tests

There are many diagnostic tests used to determine the presence and severity of chronic kidney failure. The blood chemistries performed are: a complete blood count for general CRF, a urinalysis for cellular debris, sediment, casts, and elevated white blood cell count; and a twenty-four-hour urine collection for creatinine clearance to determine GFR. A CXR can be performed to view pulmonary status relative to fluid overload or to confirm dialysis catheter placement; and an electrocardiograph can determine the presence of severe hyperkalemia. In addition, studies relative to underlying pathologies or complications of CRF can be done.

Nursing Diagnoses

Based on the information gathered, examples of nursing diagnoses in the patient with CRF may include the following:

- Anxiety related to major health, lifestyle, role, and financial income changes
- Injury, potential for, related to alteration in homeostatic mechanism
- Imbalanced nutrition, less than body requirements, related to anorexia, nausea, vomiting, altered taste sensation, and dietary intake
- Excess fluid volume related to inability of the kidneys to excrete excess fluid, excessive daily intake, or inadequate dialysis
- Potential for injury related to phosphate clearance by pharmacological binding in the gut and highly dependent on dispensing promptly at mealtime
- Disturbed body image related to visible dialysis access, edema, and skin changes
- Readiness for enhanced family coping related to managing chronic illness and potential role changes

Skills 360°

Bathing the Patient Who Has a Renal System Disorder

The nurse may have the opportunity to be involved in bathing a patient with an acute care admission because a renal disturbance. The nurse should recognize that baths are an excellent time to perform a complete skin assessment. For example, during the bath, ischemic frost conditions due to **azotemia** (a buildup of nitrogenous waste products) may be assessed. In addition, the bathing process provides time for the nurse to meet the patient's psychosocial needs through assessment and counseling. Last, bathing provides time to educate the patient on basic and special hygienic needs, which often accompany renal disturbances.

TABLE 54-5 Clinical Manifestations of Chronic Kidney Failure

SYSTEM	MANIFESTATION
Cardiovascular	Volume overload, hypertension, anemia-related increased cardiac output with left ventricular dysfunction, and dyslipidemia
Endocrine	Anemia secondary to decreased secretion of erythropoietin in low oxygen states. Decreased production of 1,25-dihydroxyvitamin D (calcitriol).
Skeletal	Renal bone disease related to high levels of phosphorus competing with calcium and to the kidney's decreased production of 1,25-dihydroxyvitamin D (calcitriol) and increased levels of parathyroid hormone (PTH).
Dermatological	Dry scaly skin with brown pigmentation with brownish discoloration of the nails. Pruritus is a consequence of hyperphosphatemia and thought also to be caused by histamine release.
GI	Occult blood loss, anorexia, nausea, and vomiting. Constipation is common and secondary to dietary restrictions, fluid restrictions, decreased mobility, and phosphate binders.
Hematological disturbances	Metabolic acidosis, hyperkalemia, hyponatremia secondary to dilution, hypermagnesemia, hypocalcemia, and hyperphosphatemia
Genitourinary	Hormonal changes lead to sexual dysfunction in males and infertility in females
	Menses range from severe and erratic to amenorrhea
Neurological	Uremic encephalopathy manifested as cognitive impairment in its mildest form and ranging to uremic coma
	Myoclonus (restless legs) ranging to uncontrollable twitching
	Mixed sensorimotor polyneuropathy in ESRD manifested primarily as a prickly, burning sensation
	Autonomic neuropathy causing diminished cardiovascular reflexes causing dialysis fluid removal-related hypotension
Immunological	Immunosuppression with increased risk of infection, the second cause of death in ESRD
Psychological	Anxiety and depression related to disease process, lack of knowledge, changes in lifestyle, sexual dysfunction, rising health care costs, or loss of income

Adapted from Gonzales, E., & Martin, K. (2003). Bone and mineral metabolism in chronic renal failure. In R. Johnson & J. Feehally (Eds.), Comprehensive clinical nephrology *(2nd ed., pp. 873–885). St. Louis, MO: Mosby; Winearls, C. (2003). Clinical evaluation and manifestations of chronic renal failure. In R. Johnson & J. Feehally (Eds.),* Comprehensive clinical nephrology *(2nd ed., pp. 857–871). St. Louis, MO: Mosby.*

Planning and Implementation

There are many varieties of nursing strategies for the care of patients with CRF. Providing care often involves a tremendous level of complexity for these patients. In addition, many of the problems associated with CRF are similar to ARF and have been previously discussed.

In general, the patient with CRF has three options: (a) dialysis, (b) renal transplantation, and (c) do nothing. If the patient chooses either dialysis or renal transplant, they will have implications associated with chronic care for the rest of their life. If the patient chooses to do nothing, then he or she will die from renal failure (see Ethics in Practice). The nurse must be aware that death from uremia is peaceful and should be painless. Priority is to ensure that the patient and family or significant others are comfortable with the decision (Winearls, 2003). Remember that the whole family is involved in this process. Offer consideration of their needs. Encourage breaks from the bedside vigilance while respecting the needs to be present.

ETHICS IN PRACTICE

Patient Refuses Treatment for CRF

Probably one of the most challenging times will be allowing the patient to refuse life-dependent dialysis treatments or to cease dialysis treatments with the certain outcome of death. Refusing treatment may leave the care provider with the uncertain feeling that the patient had not really tried the therapy or that it had not been well enough explained.

The patient is told that he or she can try therapy, and it will be stopped if not acceptable. This is stressful for the patient and the care provider. If the decision is made in a depressed state, the health care provider will most likely ask for a mental health consult to establish decision reliability.

As the patient progresses into uremic coma, any stressful symptoms can be controlled. Management issues and treatment of choice include:

- Nausea and decreased appetite. Antiemetic and allow the patient to eat small, frequent meals in preference to large, regular meals. Offer snacks as visiting family members change shifts.
- Dry, crusty mouth with uremic fetor. Cleanse frequently with refreshing, mild mouth rinse.
- Twitching or clonic jerks. Benzodiazepines, such as clonazepam (Winearls, 2003).
- Breathing difficulties from pulmonary edema and acidosis. Morphine sulfate infusion.
- Supportive care to the family.

Goals

The overall goals of therapy for CRF are to halt progression to a higher level of dysfunction and to prevent or minimize complications.

Evidence-Based Care

Evidence-based care demonstrates that early intervention is critical to arresting progression in renal failure and in minimizing complications. Cardiovascular and skeletal diseases are particularly vulnerable to pathology with late intervention (Winearls, 2003). Late referral to the nephrology team places the patient at greater health risk.

Collaborative Management

CRF demands the highest level of collaborative management (Box 54-5). Competent patient self-management is pivotal in optimizing health at all stages of CRF. This is best accomplished by promoting self-efficacy (Thomas-Hawkins & Zazworsky, 2005). A concerted team effort to promote skill building and peer group modeling and support while practicing positive attitude interpreting symptoms and demonstrating a can-do attitude is essential to building patient self-efficacy.

Pharmacology

There are many medications used in the management of CRF. Examples of these medications are provided in Box 54-6.

Fast Forward ▶▶▶

ABG Monitoring

There are monitoring system for ABGs that can give a continuous ABG recording. As these machines become less expensive and more available, the many acid-base imbalances associated with kidney failure (e.g., metabolic acidosis) may be more specifically monitored. The continuous digital readout of ABGs allows the nurse in the patient with CRF to more accurately note the current status of the patient with these conditions.

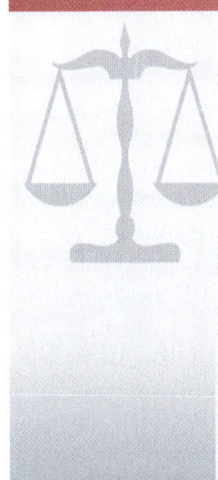

BOX 54-5

NIC CARE AND CRF

NIC: Facilitate communication of concerns or feelings between patient and family or between family members.
NIC: Maintain fluid balance utilizing fluid restriction, diuretics, or dialysis.
NIC: Weight will remain within 2 to 3 kg of dry weight. Dry weight is evidenced by:

- No evidence of elevated venous jugular pressure, edema, or other signs of fluid overload.
- A predialysis blood pressure of less than 140/90.
- Low susceptibility to hypotension and cramping during the dialysis treatment.

NIC: Maintain electrolyte and mineral balance utilizing dietary restriction, phosphate binders, pharmacological therapy or dialysis.
NIC: Provide adequate nutrition. Consult with dietitian, and together provide dietary education.
NIC: Manage anemia with recombinant erythropoietin and blood transfusions, as appropriate.
NIC: Manage hyperglycemia, as necessary to maintain optimal glycemic control.
NIC: Maintain patent and infection-free dialysis access and prevent infection; maintain integrity of dialysis access.

Adapted from Farrington, K., Greenwood, R., & Ahmad, S. (2003). Hemodialysis: Mechanisms, outcome, and adequacy. In R. Johnson & J. Feehally (Eds.), Comprehensive clinical nephrology *(2nd ed., pp. 975–990). St. Louis, MO: Mosby.*

BOX 54-6

PHARMACOLOGICAL THERAPY IN CRF

- Phosphate binders (to be taken with each meal) (e.g., calcium carbonate (TUMS), calcium acetate (PhosLo), sevelamer HCl (Renagel)
- Recombinant erythropoietin (Epogen or Procrit) for CRF-related anemia. Dose adjusted for target hematocrit
- 1,25 Dihydroxyvitamin D_3 (e.g., Calcitriol, Rocaltrol)
- Water-soluble replacement because of dialysis loss: includes folate, vitamins C and B (e.g., Berocca and Nephrocap)
- Avoid magnesium-containing antacids and cathartics
- Opioids: Monitor closely for respiratory depression and adjust dose and interval, as appropriate
- Drug dose or interval adjustment is necessary for most drugs dependent on renal clearance
- Schedule daily drugs for after dialysis to prevent dialysis loss. Alternatively, check with a pharmacist for information on drugs used during dialysis.

Hemodialysis

Hemodialysis (HD) is the mainstay of RRT. The patient's blood is pumped through semipermeable capillaries in a hemodialyzer. Dialysate fluid containing a premixed concentrate of electrolytes flows countercurrent to blood flow through the intercapillary spaces of the dialyzer. Solute clearance is directly related to concentration gradient and flow rate. Prescribed fluid removal is facilitated by transmembrane pressure and the ultrafiltration capacity of the hemodialyzer. Typical HD treatment duration is three to four hours on a three times weekly schedule. Outpatients are assigned a regular time for their HD procedure at an outpatient facility (usually three times a week) or taught to do HD in their home with a dedicated partner (Figures 54-5 and 54-6).

Disequilibrium syndrome is a preventable complication of initial dialysis on a uremic patient. **Disequilibrium** refers to an imbalance in solute concentration across the blood-brain barrier. Rapid reduction in intravascular solutes can precipitate rapid fluid osmosis across the blood-brain barrier with net flow of water into the cerebrospinal space in a homeostatic attempt to equalize solute concentration. The resulting increased intracranial pressure may be evidenced by headache, nausea, vomiting, muscle twitching, and seizure. Daily initial treatments for the disequilibrium syndrome utilizing reduced dialysis blood flow rates and shorter treatment time with gradual increase of flow rate and treatment time over a few days maintains equilibrium safety.

Dialysis Vascular Access

To perform HD, there is a need to access both the arterial and venous circulation of the patient. Therefore, a temporary dialysis vascular access is achieved by insertion of a dual lumen dialysis catheter. Dialysis catheters are placed in a femoral, subclavian, or jugular vein. Insertion of a noncuffed catheter is the first choice for acute dialysis as it is easily accomplished at the bedside. Complications include subclavian stenosis, pneumothorax, venous rupture with hemorrhage, and infection. Imposed bedrest and higher infection rates are the primary disadvantage of femoral catheters (Conlon & Giblin, 2003).

Dual lumen, cuffed dialysis catheters are placed surgically for longer term use. Primary use is providing vascular access for short-term dialysis in recovering ARF or in CRF when vascular access for arteriovenous fistula (AVF) has been exhausted by complications. The dialysis catheter should be reserved for

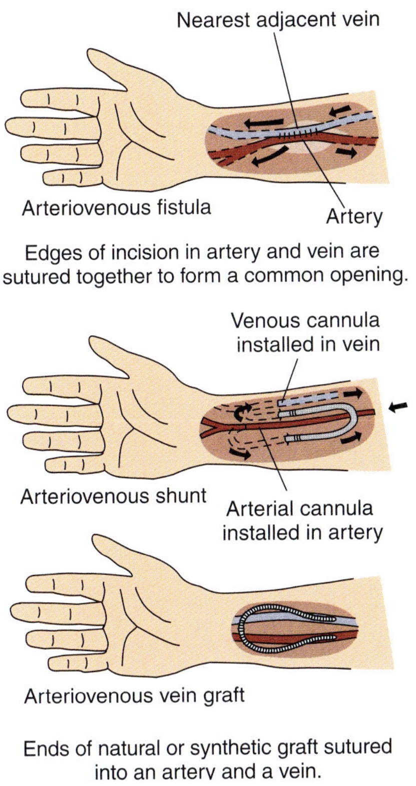

Figure 54-5 HD access sites.

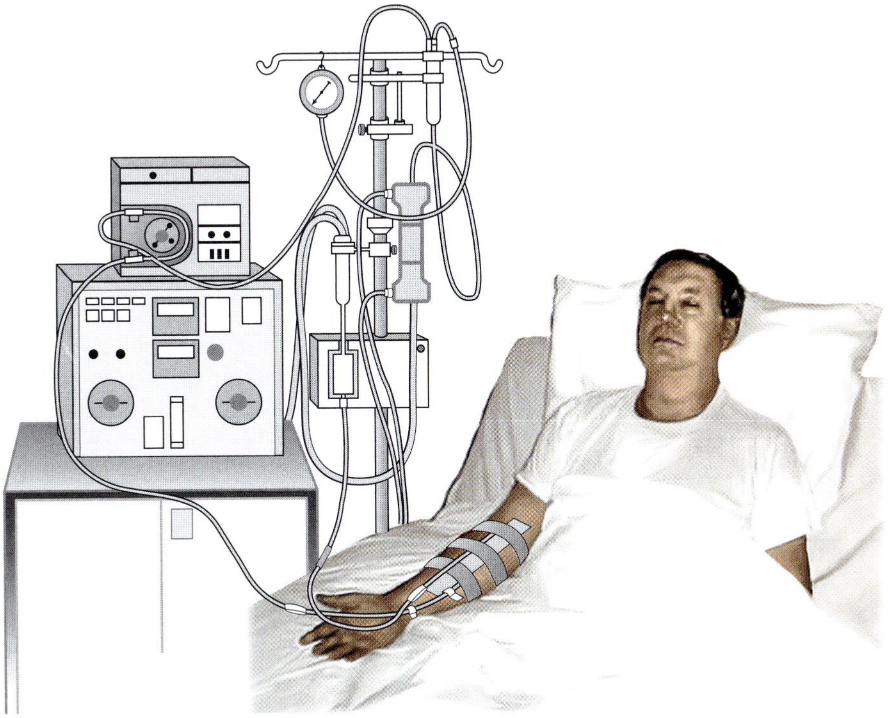

Figure 54-6 HD.

> *Red Flag*
>
> **Medication Safety and Renal Dysfunction**
>
> The nurse must evaluate the medications that are ordered for patients with renal disturbances. If a specific medication is excreted in the urine and the patient has a renal problem, the patient may experience symptoms of toxicity.

dialysis use only as it is the patient's lifeline. Meticulous care aimed at preventing dislodgement or infection is imperative (Box 54-7).

AVF is preferable for permanent dialysis vascular access. The AVF may be created by direct anastomosis of an artery to a vein (natural or native fistula). More commonly, a polytetrafluoroethylene (PTFE) graft is employed to create a fistula between an artery and a vein. Comprising 80 percent of the AVF in use in the United States, PTFE grafts are advantageous in patients with poor-quality blood vessels (Conlon & Giblin, 2003). An AVF is preferably placed in the nondominant lower arm. Other sites include the dominant lower arm, upper arms, and upper anterior thighs.

Complications from AVF include graft thrombosis, failure to mature enough to allow adequate blood flow (native), infection, and arterial steal syndrome. Steal syndrome occurs with disruption of adequate blood flow to the distal region of the extremity. Early intervention is imperative to prevent loss of hand function. Steal syndrome is evidenced by pain, coolness, and paresthesias. Symptoms may exacerbate during the dialysis treatment. Banding to diminish volume of blood flow diverted from the hand or ligation may be required to preserve hand function (Conlon & Giblin, 2003).

Peritoneal Dialysis and Chronic Ambulatory Peritoneal Dialysis

Peritoneal dialysis (PD) is being used by more than 120,000 patients worldwide (Davies & Williams, 2003). The capillaries of the peritoneal membrane allow solute clearance down a concentration gradient between the instilled dialysate and the plasma. Fluid removal is by osmotic gradient with dialysate dextrose concentration providing the higher osmotic pressure. Capillary pore size will allow some protein loss but is not large enough to allow phosphate clearance. Phosphate binding is required.

Insertion of a Dacron cuffed, tunneled Silastic PD catheter affords easy access. The catheter is allowed to rest for tunnel healing for approximately one month prior to use. Meticulous exit site care according to local practice protocols is imperative. Tunnel integrity is maintained by taping the catheter

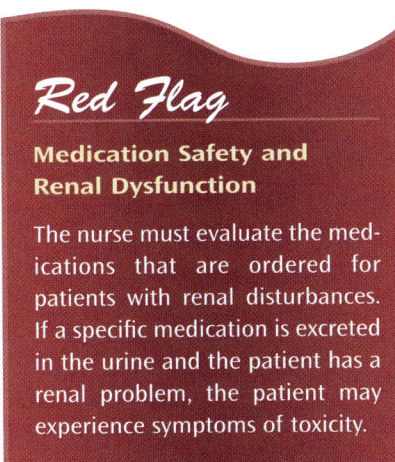

BOX 54-7

MANAGEMENT OF VASCULAR ACCESS DEVICES IN DIALYSIS

The nurse should do the following when caring for patients with vascular assessment care:

Dialysis Catheter

- Maintain sterile dressing according to institution protocol.
- Confirm that caps are secure and clamps are closed.
- Prevent tugging or pulling on the catheter.
- Provide or promote meticulous patient hygiene.
- Teach patient to handle unexpected catheter dislodgement. Apply direct pressure over catheter site to control bleeding. When bleeding has ceased, cover with dry dressing and notify health care provider.

AVF

- Confirm patency; presence of thrill (palpated pulsation) and bruit (whooshing sound heard with a stethoscope) along course of the AVF.
- Nephrology precautions to prevent thrombosis and infection. This includes no blood pressure measurement, IV accesses, or laboratory blood draws on affected extremity.
- Teach patient to avoid constrictive clothing and to check fistula patency daily. Report absence of thrill or bruit promptly.
- Teach patient to handle posttreatment bleeding at cannula site: apply direct pressure for several minutes to control bleeding, apply dry dressing, and call health care provider as appropriate.

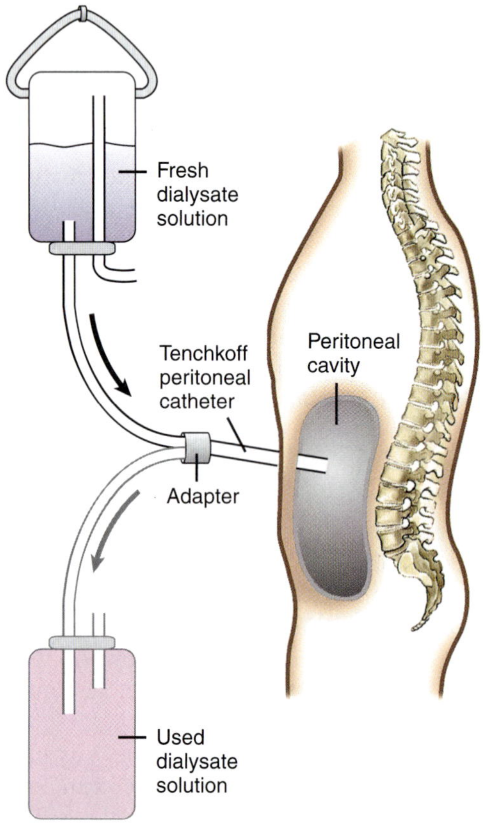

Figure 54-7 PD.

securely to the abdomen to prevent pull at the exit site. Tunnel integrity is vital to prevention of tunnel site infection and PD catheter loss. It is imperative that strict sterile technique and environmental control of circulating contaminants be practiced on every occasion when the catheter is uncapped or any related equipment is exposed to the air.

PD requires filling the peritoneal cavity with a prescribed volume of peritoneal dialysate, allowing it to dwell for a prescribed period of time then draining and discarding the **effluent** (waste materials). Continuous ambulatory peritoneal dialysis (CAPD) requires manual dialysate instillation and removal on a predetermined schedule. Continuous cyclic peritoneal dialysis is delivered by a computerized cycler. The dialysis cycler is programmed for length of therapy and desired fill volumes. The computer tracks volumes filled and drained for accurate ultrafiltration information. CAPD is usually a nighttime procedure allowing the patient to sleep through the process. CAPD requires manual fills and drains. Determining ultrafiltration volume requires weighing effluent bags.

Advantages to PD include portability (patient can perform the PD relatively easily at home or when traveling), higher level of self-efficacy and independence, daily maintenance dialysis with constant lower levels of azotemia, and moderation in dietary and fluid restrictions (Figure 54-7). Disadvantages include protein loss and potential for life-threatening peritoneal infection

Complications include changes in peritoneal vascular and interstitial structure and function, peritonitis, tunnel and exit site infection, fluid leaks, catheter malfunction, and ultrafiltration failure. While any has

BOX 54-8

ANTIBIOTIC THERAPY FOR PD

Antibiotic treatment of peritonitis for the patient on PD according to the Advisory Committee on Peritonitis Management of the International Society of Peritoneal Dialysis:

- Initial empirical therapy with first generation cephalosporin (cefazolin, or cephalothin). Loading dose in first bag and maintenance dose in each following bag of PD dialysate.
- Negative culture: continue cephalosporin for two weeks.

Once an organism is identified, the regimen is altered accordingly.

Adapted from Davies, S., & Williams, J. (2003). Peritoneal dialysis: Principles, techniques, and adequacy. In R. Johnson & J. Feehally (Eds.), Comprehensive clinical nephrology *(2nd ed., pp. 1003–1011). St. Louis, MO: Mosby.*

the potential for major disruption in health practices, peritonitis is probably the most important complication and cause of treatment failure (Davies & Williams, 2003). Cloudy effluent and abdominal pain are the sentinel signs of developing peritonitis and require immediate intervention. Immediate effluent sample collection for WBC count and microbiology is imperative. Empirical, intraperitoneal antibiotic treatment is usually initiated prior to culture return (Box 54-8).

Nutrition

Dietary management is crucial to minimizing disease progression and azotemia, preventing malnutrition, and preventing complications of hyperkalemia and hyperphosphatemia. The National Kidney Foundation's Kidney Disease Outcomes Quality Initiative (K/DOQI) guidelines herald nutrition as a primary determinant in ESRD patient outcomes.

Nurses have a major role in preventing malnutrition in this patient population (Wells, 2003). Assessment must include appetite, weight change, decreased muscle mass, and decreased strength and endurance are all markers of malnutrition. Positive findings coupled with a serum albumin less than 4 should prompt intervention from the health care team.

PD patients require greater amounts of protein related to protein and amino acid loss in the dialysis exchange process. In addition, daily dialysis with PD results in less electrolyte and mineral restrictions. HD patients experience some amino acid loss and may have increased catabolism. Daily dietary management includes:

- Protein intake: HD, 1.2 g/kg/day with 50 percent of high biological value; PD, 1.2 to 1.3 g/kg/day with 50 percent biological value and increases to 1.5 g/kg/day with malnutrition or peritonitis (Wells, 2003).
- Sodium is restricted in ESRD to minimize thirst. Daily recommendations are: HD, 1,000 to 3,000 mg/day; PD 2,000 to 4,000 mg/day.
- Potassium: HD, 40 to 70 mEq/day; PD 75 to 100 mEq/day.
- Phosphate: HD and PD, less than 17 mg/kg/day.
- Fluid intake: HD, 1,000 mL/day plus volume to replace any urinary output. The goal is to limit weight gain between dialysis treatments to 2 to 5 percent of the established dry weight (Wells, 2003).

Renal Transplantation

Transplantation can be both a blessing and a challenge. The health care professional experiences the excitement of successful graft function and is subjected to the trauma of graft loss or immunosuppressive complications. The recipient hopes for release from the constraints of chronic illness and resumption of a fuller life. They hope for the best and brace themselves to accept all the adverse potentials for which they have been informed.

Transplantation is not an automatic choice. Though 70 has been considered maximal age for eligibility, a good state of health will make the patient a reasonable candidate to consider (Hostima & Hilbrands, 2003). Recurrent and persistent noncompliance, acute or chronic infection, malignancy, substance abuse, unstable psychosis that would impair consent and compliance, ABO incompatibility, and a positive cross-match will render the patient ineligible for transplantation (Hostima & Hilbrands, 2003).

Patients with diabetic nephropathy and in reasonable health are prime candidates for a kidney transplant and may be considered for a pancreas or kidney transplant. It has been shown that patients with diabetic **nephropathy** (disease of the kidneys) have a better quality of life and longer term survival following transplantation (Hostima & Hilbrands, 2003).

Pretransplantation counseling and testing are completed before the patient is placed on the transplant list as eligible for a cadaver kidney (graft) or a living donor graft. The recipient undergoes extensive testing to deem them a safe immunosuppression candidate.

Transplant immunology has made successful allogeneic transplantation possible. A basic understanding of terminology and immune response facilitates appreciation and more active participation in the care of the transplant patient. **Allogeneic** signifies a genetic relationship between two individuals of the same species. An allogeneic organ is referred to as an **allograft. Xenogeneic** signifies a genetic relationship between individuals of differing species. Of interest, organ shortage is prompting research in xenogeneic transplantation.

Cell surface molecules vary in structure from individual to individual. It is this polymorphic (antigenic) phenomenon that lies at the root of the immune response to the allograft. Major histocompatibility complex (MHC), so named for the chromosomal region where encoded, evokes the most powerful rejection response. MHC in combination with the antigen presenting cell (APC) of the graft attracts cytotoxic T cells. Without intervention, this would result in graft cell death. Interestingly, graft MHC together with the presenting antigen mimics the intended receptor for the T cell and sets up a cascade of events resulting in full-scale T cell activation.

T cells are lymphocytes that mature in the thymus, thus the name T cell. T cells are divided into two classes according to their activity. CD4 T cells are classified as cytolytic. Their primary action is to kill the target cell. CD4 T cells are classified as helper cells with two primary helper activities. They stimulate B cell growth and differentiation for antibody production (humoral immunity) and secrete cytokines for phagocyte activation (Abbas & Lichtman, 2004). Cytokine release is inclusive of interleukins and tissue necrosis factor (TNF). Normally, CD4 T cells account for 50 to 60 percent, and CD8 T cells account for 20 to 25 percent of the total lymphocyte count. Significantly, each has CD3, CD4, and CD8 coreceptors on the cell surface. The CD3 coreceptor activates multiple enzymes, including calcineurin, when stimulated by the cytoplasmic tail of the other two receptors. Calcineurin is a significant target of immunosuppression.

Adhesion molecules provide another mechanism of rejection. Cells from lymphoid organs infiltrate the graft. These cells adhere to vascular endothelium and cause cytokine release (Abbas & Lichtman, 2004). Interference with this activity is another target of transplant immunosuppression.

Agents of immunosuppression and their targets are:

- Glucocorticoids: Block cytokines and migration of phagocytes indirectly block T cell activation.
- Azathioprine: Blocks DNA to prevent lymphocyte proliferation following antigenic stimulation.

> **BOX 54-9**
>
> **LIVE DONOR EXCLUSION CRITERIA**
>
> Live donor exclusion criteria include:
>
> - Age younger than 18 years
> - Severe hypertension (HTN) or end-organ damage secondary to HTN
> - Diabetes mellitus or a strong family history of diabetes mellitus
> - Impaired renal function including proteinuria and hematuria
> - Family history of polycystic kidney disease or hereditary nephritis
> - History of nephrolithiasis or hypercoagulability
> - Morbid obesity
> - Uncontrolled psychiatric disorder
> - Infection, HIV, hepatitis B, or hepatitis C

- Mycophenolate: Selective inhibition of T and B lymphocyte proliferation.
- Cyclosporine: Inhibits calcineurin, blocks interleukins and TNF.
- Tacrolimus (FK506): Inhibits calcineurin and T cell activation.
- Rapamycin (Sirolimus): Inhibits T cell activation.

Cross-match and tissue typing by blood sample are utilized to align recipient with a histocompatible organ. Two primary considerations are ABO blood group antigens and human leukocyte antigens (HLA) molecules. Of the blood group type, antigen findings infer the following compatibility profile. Group A and B develop antigens to each other and to Group O; incompatible. Group O does not develop antigens against A or B, compatible donor. The rhesus Rh factor is not a concern in cross-match for organ transplantation. There is hesitation in using Group O organs for Group A or B recipients as this would diminish the organ pool for Group O recipients in this time of organ shortage.

HLA, also called MCH antigens, are found on the short arm of chromosome 6. Each set of alleles on the chromosome is called a haplotype and given a numerical designation (Abbas & Lichtman, 2004). HLA-A, HLA-B, and HLA-DR are primary concerns in organ transplantation.

Living donors include living related (biological and nonbiological), living nonrelated, paired kidney exchange, and nondirected live donation (McKay & King, 2004). The paired kidney exchange program allows willing and incompatible living donors assist the intended recipient to obtain a kidney. When two recipients have willing unmatched donors matching the opposite recipient, they may swap donors (Fisher, Kropp, & Fleming, 2005). Because of advances in immunology and continued organ shortage, live donation has increased significantly (Box 54-9).

Most often, donor nephrectomy can be accomplished by laparoscopic surgery. An approximate 2 to 3 inch incision in the lower quadrant suffices for delivering the kidney. Postoperative care follows routine postoperative guidelines. Hospital stay is minimal.

Cadaver acquired kidneys must evidence no damage by clinical testing and by history. Complete donor screening includes viral screening for all groups of hepatitis virus herpes viruses, human T cell lymphotropic virus type 1, and human immunodeficiency virus (HIV). In addition, Centers for Disease Control and Prevention (CDC) guidelines are followed to screen the donor for history of high-risk HIV behavior. Blood, urine, and sputum cultures are obtained as well as a screen for malignancy (McKay & King, 2004).

The transplanted kidney is placed in either the left or right lower abdominal quadrant anterior to the peritoneal space. The transplanted ureter is secured to the bladder wall by a technique designed to prevent urinary reflux. A urinary catheter is left in place for up to five days to allow ureteral implant healing without bladder filling. A ureteral stent may be in place if there is concern for swelling or stricture at the site of ureteral implant.

The graft may have immediate and excellent urinary output beginning in the operating room at the time of vascular anastomosis or function may be delayed for an extensive period (Figure 54-8). Ischemic acute tubular necrosis is the most common cause of delayed graft function (Magee & Milford, 2004). Managing fluid and electrolyte balance is a priority. The nurse must anticipate renal ultrasound for graft blood flow studies, graft biopsy for rejection studies, and supportive dialysis as a form of treatment (Box 54-10).

Complications include rejection, vascular thrombosis, and ureteral anastomosis failure. Renal artery thrombosis presents as an acute cessation of urine output and rapid increase in creatinine. Renal vein thrombosis may have the additional sign of sudden acute abdominal pain. The usual consequence is graft loss (Magee & Milford, 2004). Rejection presents with continuous rise in creatinine and biopsy finding of cellular or vascular changes consistent with rejection. Ureteral anastomosis failure will present

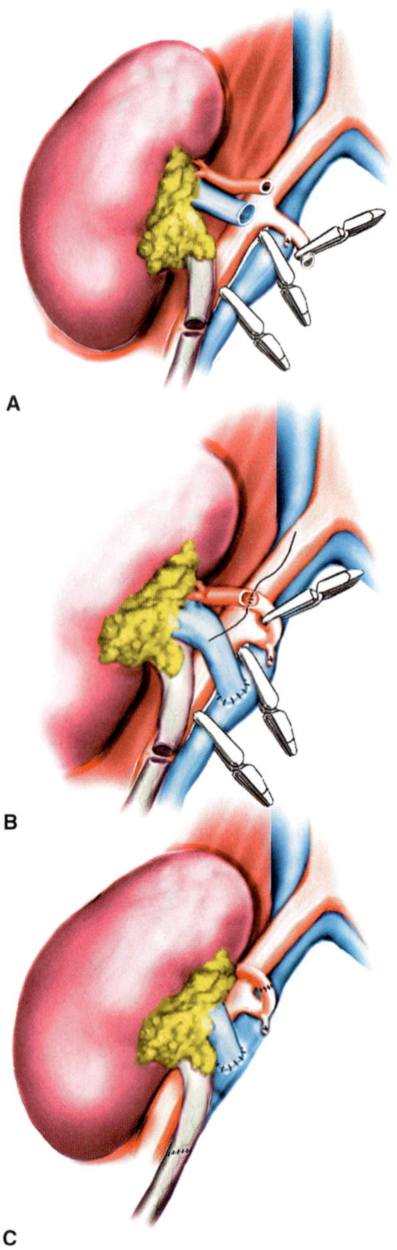

Figure 54-8 Renal transplantation (adult recipient): A. Iliac vessels exposed, B. Renal artery and vein anastomosis, C. Donor kidney in place.

BOX 54-10

NURSING MANAGEMENT FOR A RENAL TRANSPLANT

The nurse must perform the following as part of the nursing management of a patient experiencing a renal transplant:

- Maintain fluid balance by closely monitoring urinary output and providing expedient replacement.
- Monitor laboratory studies for graft function and electrolyte balance.
- Monitor for abrupt decrease in urine output or abruptly increased pain or swelling at graft site as this may be indicative of renal vascular thrombosis or acute rejection.
- Monitor wound drainage for any signs of ureteral anastomosis failure.
- Adhere to immunosuppression schedule and facilitate accurate timing of phlebotomy blood drawing of samples for related drug levels.
- Monitor blood glucose and anticipate changes related to high-dose glucocorticoids.
- Arrange for supply of medications prior to discharge to prevent any disruption in immunosuppression.
- Teach patient medication management, follow-up protocols, signs of transplant rejection or infection and appropriate response, importance of adequate hydration, and infection prevention.
- Offer patient support during periods of delayed graft function or graft failure.
- Arrange postdischarge follow-up appointments.

with **perinephric** (surrounding the kidney) graft fluid collection, increased wound drainage, or rise in creatinine. Wound sample creatinine level compared to serum creatinine is the primary diagnostic tool for ureteral anastomosis failure.

There are many medications necessary for the patient following a renal transplant. In addition, there are important considerations for the patient as he or she receives his or her medications. And, there are a wide variety of side effects to consider when the patient is given these medications. Table 54-6 enumerates a number of the typical medications given to patients as they live after having a renal transplant.

Health Care Resources

There are three valuable resources for patients, families, and health care professionals. They provide up-to-date and reliable information on the latest research, understanding diseases process, and progression and state-of-the-art patient self-management.

The National Kidney Disease Education Program (NKDEP) is an initiative of the National Institute of Diabetes and Digestive and Kidney Diseases (NIDDK), National Institutes of Health (NIH), U.S. Department of Health and Human Services (DHHS). Life options is designed to help people live long and live well with kidney disease. A multidisciplinary national health care team reviews all materials presented through Life options.

Evaluation of Outcomes

Potential patient outcomes for each of the example nursing diagnoses for the patient with CRF are:

- Anxiety related to major health, lifestyle, role, and financial income changes. The patient should be able to recognize the signs of anxiety,

TABLE 54-6 Drug Therapy for Patients after a Renal Transplant

IMMUNOSUPPRESSIVE AGENTS	IMPORTANT CONSIDERATIONS	SIDE EFFECTS
Corticosteroids: IV: Methylprednisolone Oral: Prednisolone or prednisone	Be alert to tapering doses	Cataracts, infection, osteoporosis, and avascular necrosis of the head of the femur
Calcineurin inhibitors Cyclosporin (Neoral) Tacrolimus (FK506, Prograf)	Schedule phlebotomy to facilitate accurate serum level samples	Diabetes mellitus, hypertension, hyperlipidemia, nephrotoxicity, seizures and thrombocytopenia, hemolytic uremic syndrome, and gingival hyperplasia
Sirolimus (Rapamune)	Adhere strictly to 12-hour dosing	Lymphoma, malignancy, lymphocele, thrombocytopenia, and leukopenia
Azathioprine (Imuran and AZA San)	Adhere strictly to 12-hour dosing Encourage use of sun block	Bone marrow suppression, leukopenia, thrombocytopenia, and anemia; increased risk of malignancy, hepatotoxicity, and hair loss
Mycophenolate mofetil (CellCept)	Adhere strictly to 12-hour dosing	Diarrhea, increased cytomegalovirus (CMV) infection, leukopenia, and mild anemia
Thymoglobulin	Premedicate with acetaminophen, Benadryl, and corticosteroids to minimize or prevent flulike response	Thrombocytopenia, neutropenia, secondary infection, secondary malignancy, lymphoproliferative disorders, and sepsis
OKT3	Premedicate as per thymoglobulin	Pulmonary edema and acute renal failure

demonstrate positive coping mechanisms, and describe a reduction in the level of anxiety experienced.

- Injury, potential for, related to alteration in homeostatic mechanism. The patient does not experience any skin breakdown from uremia or falls from fatigue.
- Imbalanced nutrition, less than body requirements, related to anorexia, nausea, vomiting, altered taste sensation, and dietary intake. The patient verbalizes and demonstrates selection of foods or meals that will achieve a cessation of weight loss and weighs within 10 percent of ideal body weight.
- Excess fluid volume related to inability of the kidneys to excrete excess fluid, excessive daily intake, or inadequate dialysis. The patient maintains fluid balance as evidenced by skin turgor, blood pressure and weight within designated limits.
- Disturbed body image related to visible dialysis access, edema, and skin changes. The patient demonstrates enhanced body image and self-esteem as evidenced by ability to look at, touch, talk about, and care for actual or perceived altered body part or function.
- Readiness for enhanced family coping related to managing chronic illness and potential role changes. The patient and family identify own maladaptive coping behaviors, available resources, and support systems, describes or initiates alternative coping strategies, and describes positive results from new behaviors.

Financial Outcomes

CRF can be financially devastating. Many people are unable to continue employment because of work time lost to dialysis, reduced energy levels, and depression. Social work involvement is crucial. Assistance with travel arrangements to dialysis facilities, disability assistance applications, and interpretation of insurance coverage are critical at this time. Counseling is primary to facilitate adjustment to the overwhelming demands and limitations of chronic illness and family adjustment to role change.

KEY CONCEPTS

- Pyelonephritis is an infection of the upper urinary tract and may involve the ureters, renal pelvis, and the papillary tips of the collecting ducts.
- Polycystic kidney disease is a genetically inherited kidney disease and may be autosomal dominant (ADPKD) or autosomal recessive (ARPKD).
- ARF presents as a rapid decline in renal function, and this decline may occur within a few hours or over a period of several weeks.
- CRF is a progressive and irreversible decline in renal function ranging from mild with nearly normal function to ESRD requiring RRT.
- Diabetes mellitus and hypertension are the two most common causes of CRF. in the United States.
- It has been shown that patients with diabetic nephropathy (disease of the kidneys) have a better quality of life and longer term survival following transplantation.

REVIEW QUESTIONS

1. A 21-year-old woman is admitted to the hospital with a diagnosis of acute renal failure. She is oliguric and has proteinuria. She asks the nurse, "How long will it be before I start to make urine again?" Which of the following would be the correct response?
   1. This phase of renal failure will last for one to two days.
   2. This phase of renal failure will last for three to seven days.
   3. This phase of renal failure will last for one to two weeks.
   4. This phase of renal failure will last for three to four weeks.

2. You are caring for a patient who is admitted to the hospital in acute renal failure. The appearance of a U wave on the electrocardiogram (ECG) should alert you to check for which of the following laboratory values?
   1. Hyperkalemia
   2. Hypokalemia
   3. Hypernatremia
   4. Hyponatremia

3. You are caring for a man who is on hemodialysis. He has an AVF. Which of the following is expected when assessing the fistula?
   1. Ecchymotic area
   2. Enlarged veins
   3. Pulselessness
   4. Redness

4. A male patient with end-stage renal disease receives HD three times a week. You conclude that dialysis is effective when:
   1. The patient does not have a large weight gain.
   2. The patient has no signs and symptoms of infection.
   3. The patient says that he can catch up on his rest while on dialysis.
   4. The patient is able to return to work.

Continued

REVIEW QUESTIONS—cont'd

5. You are performing discharge teaching for a patient who was admitted with pyelonephritis. The patient asks the nurse, "What is pyelonephritis?" Based on your knowledge of pyelonephritis, your best response would be:
   1. Pyelonephritis is an inflammation of the bladder.
   2. Pyelonephritis is a rupture of the bladder.
   3. Pyelonephritis is an infection of the kidney.
   4. Pyelonephritis is an infection of the lower urinary tract.
6. A patient is admitted to your care with ARF. Which of the following must you continually assess for?
   1. Hyponatremia and hyperkalemia
   2. Decreased BUN and creatinine
   3. Alkalosis
   4. Hypercalcemia
7. A patient with CRF complains of irritating white crystals on his skin. You recognize this finding as uremic frost. Which of the following nursing actions do you take?
   1. Administer an antihistamine, because the physician would prescribe one to relieve itching
   2. Increase fluids to prevent crystal formation and decrease itching
   3. Provide skin care with tepid water and apply lotion to the skin to relieve itching
   4. Permit the patient to soak in a bathtub to remove crystals
8. Immediately following a kidney transplant, you should assess your patient for which of the following?
   1. Fluid and electrolyte imbalance
   2. Infection
   3. Hepatotoxicity
   4. Respiratory complications
9. You are caring for a patient receiving PD. You are completing the exchange by draining the dialysate. You notice it is cloudy. How do you interpret this finding?
   1. It is the normal appearance of draining dialysate.
   2. It is a sign of infection.
   3. It is an indication of an impending lower back problem.
   4. It is a sign of a vascular access occlusion.
10. You are providing patient education to a patient on CAPD. You determine that he understands is treatment when he states:
    1. I must increase my carbohydrate intake daily.
    2. I must maintain a positive nitrogen balance by decreasing protein.
    3. I must take prophylactic antibiotics to prevent infection.
    4. I must be aware of the signs and symptoms of peritonitis.

REVIEW ACTIVITIES

1. Describe the clinical manifestations seen in acute pyelonephritis?
2. Compare and contrast autosomal dominant (ADPKD) and autosomal recessive polycystic kidney disease (ARPKD)?

Continued

REVIEW ACTIVITIES—cont'd

3. Describe the assessment findings that may be present in Wegener granulomatosis.

4. What are reasons that patients with rhabdomyolysis have safety issues?

5. Compare and contrast HD and CAPD.

6. What would you teach a donor regarding his or her giving up a kidney in a renal transplantation?

Visit the Contemporary Medical-Surgical Nursing online companion resource at www.delmarhealthcare.com for additional content and study aids. Click on Online Companions then select the Nursing discipline.

UNIT

XIII

Alterations in Endocrine Function

Chapter 55 Assessment of Endocrine Function

Chapter 56 Endocrine Dysfunction: Nursing Management

Chapter 57 Diabetes Mellitus: Nursing Management

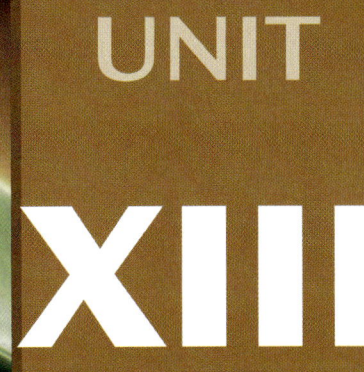

CHAPTER 55

Assessment of Endocrine Function

Martha K. Carlson, MSN

KEY TERMS

Adrenocorticotropic hormone (ACTH)
Aldosterone
Antidiuretic hormone (ADH)
Calcitonin
Corticosteroids
Cortisol
Endocrine glands
Exocrine glands
Glucagon
Growth hormone (GH)
Hormones
Insulin
Negative feedback
Parathyroid hormone (PTH)
Prolactin
Target tissues
Thyroid-releasing hormone (TRH)
Thyroid-stimulating hormone (TSH)
Thyroxine (T_4)
Triiodothyronine (T_3)

CHAPTER TOPICS

- Anatomy and Physiology of the Endocrine system
- Hormones
- Assessment of the Endocrine System
- Diagnostic Tests for the Endocrine System

The endocrine system, in conjunction with the nervous system, is responsible for the control of multiple body systems. It can be thought of as a communication system that uses hormones to help maintain homeostasis. **Hormones** are chemical messengers produced and secreted by specialized endocrine cells and released into the bloodstream to act on target cells at another location in the body. Hormones help to maintain homeostasis by regulation of metabolism and energy, cardiac output and blood pressure, reproduction, and growth and development. The hormones of the endocrine system are affected by the central nervous system (CNS); more specifically, the hypothalamus, and in turn, these hormones affect the nervous system. The hypothalamus coordinates the activity of the endocrine system through the pituitary gland using releasing hormones. Simply stated, the hypothalamus translates messages from the nervous system into chemical messengers, hormones. Hormones affect the nervous system in a variety of complex mechanisms. For example, a deficiency of thyroid hormone may result in emotional depression, and adrenaline causes increased mental activity. Hormones affect the nervous system by enhancing the rapid transmission of signals between neurons from localized synapses. The hormones cause fast outcomes and occur quickly. In contrast the endocrine system uses more generalized signals that require less energy than the synapses of the nervous system. The signals from the hormones travel by the blood stream to the specific target organs. These effects of the hormones are slower and of a longer duration than the nervous system's transmission of signals. Another system that interacts closely with the endocrine system is the immune system. Hormones secreted from the adrenal cortex regulate the immune system responses. Hormones are vital in regulating the body's internal environment.

Hormones exert their effects on target organs or tissues. A feedback system is commonly found in the endocrine system. The feedback can be direct or indirect. The most common type of feedback is negative or inhibitory, preventing excessive hormone secretion. A thermostat on a furnace controls the heat in the house by negative feedback. When the internal temperature of the house drops below a set point, the thermostat signals the furnace to turn on and produce heat. As the temperature of the house rises to a preset level, the thermostat signals the furnace to shut off. An example of negative feedback in the body is the secretion of insulin in response to rising blood glucose levels. When blood glucose levels in the body rise, **insulin,** the hormone produced by the beta cells of the pancreas to lower blood glucose, is secreted. Insulin acts on the cells, causing them to take up the excess glucose in the bloodstream. The blood glucose level then falls and insulin secretion stops. Some of the negative feedback occurring in the endocrine system is much more complex than this example, involving stimulation of more than one gland (Griffin & Ojeda, 2004).

ANATOMY AND PHYSIOLOGY

The endocrine system is comprised of the pituitary, hypothalamus, thyroid, parathyroids, pancreas, adrenals, thymus, ovaries, and testes. The endocrine system is not easily assessed as compared with other body systems. When discussing endocrine system imbalances, there are often increased or decreased variations (e.g., hyperthyroidism versus hypothyroidism).

Glands

Glands in the body are classified as endocrine or exocrine. **Exocrine glands** are those glands that secrete substances into ducts that empty into a body cavity or onto a body surface. Sweat glands and lacrimal glands (tear ducts) are examples of exocrine glands. **Endocrine glands** are those glands that produce hormones, which are secreted into the blood stream and travel to their target organs or tissues (Figure 55-1). **Target tissues** are tissues or organs in the body that are affected by specific hormones. The thyroid, parathyroid, pituitary, and adrenals are examples of endocrine glands. The pancreas is both an endocrine and an exocrine gland. Insulin and glucagon production is an endocrine function while digestive enzymes from the pancreas make up its exocrine function (Tierney, Mc Phee, & Papakakais, 2004).

Hormones

Hormones are chemicals that are produced and secreted by specific tissues or organs in the body. They travel via the bloodstream to the target organ, where they bind to specific receptors on the cell membrane or in the cell. Hormones change the metabolism of the target cells by either altering the cell membrane permeability to nutrients or by alteration of the synthesis or activation of hormones. Hormones may be either water or lipid soluble based on their chemical structure. They may stimulate an organ to release a hormone, to act, or both. Additionally, hormones can inhibit the release of other hormones and do so in a variety of locations throughout the body (Table 55-1). The pituitary produces the stimulating hormones called follicle-stimulating hormone (FSH). The hypothalamus stimulates the releasing hormones. These hormones then can change the behavior of other organs or tissues. Lipid soluble hormones (steroid and thyroid) are able to pass through cell membranes of the target organs. Hormones that are protein based are not able to pass through the cell membranes. They bind to receptors on specific cells and trigger actions with in the cell (Tierney, et al., 2004).

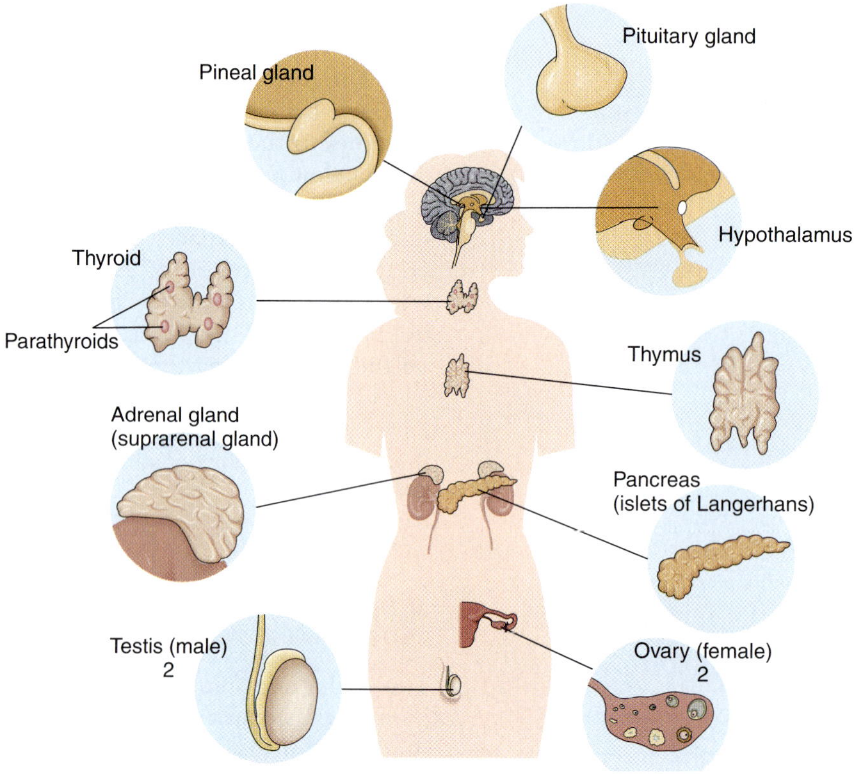

Figure 55-1 Structures of the endocrine system.

Regulation of Hormones

There are several complex mechanisms for controlling hormone levels. These body system controls are interrelated and actually are occurring simultaneously as homeostatic balances to the body system.

Negative Feedback Mechanisms

The pituitary gland and feedback mechanisms are responsible for controlling hormone levels. The majority of the feedback mechanisms are **negative feedback** (the response of a gland by increasing or decreasing the secretion of a hormone) or inhibitory, similar to a thermostat in the house. The endocrine system contains sensors that detect and alter hormone secretion to maintain balance in the body's internal environment. When the sensors detect low hormone levels, they stimulate actions that will result in an increase in hormones. Conversely, when the sensors detect elevated hormone levels, they cause a decrease in the production and release of hormones. Insulin secretion by the pancreas related to the blood glucose level is an example of negative feedback. The pancreas produces insulin when the blood glucose level rises. As the blood glucose level decreases from the insulin, the pancreas decreases the production of insulin (Greenspan & Gardner, 2004).

Positive Feedback Mechanisms

Positive feedback mechanisms occur when increasing the level of one hormone produces an increase in the level of another hormone. For example, during the follicular stage in the female menstrual cycle there is an increase in the production of estradiol. This increase in estradiol causes an increase in the production of FSH by the anterior pituitary.

Nervous System Controls

The nervous system also controls endocrine function through the CNS and the sympathetic nervous system (SNS). When stress is experienced by the body, it is detected by the CNS. The SNS then releases catecholamines that cause the

TABLE 55-1 Endocrine Gland Hormones

HORMONE	FUNCTION
Pancreas	
Glucagon	Raises blood glucose
Insulin	Lowers blood glucose
Somatostatin	Inhibits secretion of insulin, glucagon, and growth hormone from the anterior pituitary and gastrin from the stomach
Anterior Pituitary	
Thyroid-stimulating hormone (TSH)	Stimulates thyroid growth and secretion of the thyroid hormone
Adrenocorticotropic hormone (ACTH)	Stimulates adrenal cortex growth and secretion of glucocorticoids
Follicle-stimulating hormone (FSH)	Stimulates ovarian follicle to mature and produce estrogen; in the male, stimulates sperm production
Luteinizing hormone (LH)	Acts with FSH to stimulate estrogen production; causes ovulation; stimulates progesterone production by corpus luteum; in male, stimulates testes to produce testosterone
Melanocyte-stimulating hormone (MSH)	Causes increase in synthesis and spread of melanin (pigment) in skin
Growth hormone (GH)	Stimulates growth
Prolacting or lactogenic hormone	Stimulates breast development during pregnancy and milk secretion after delivery of baby
Posterior Pituitary	
Antidiuretic hormone (ADH)	Stimulates water retention by kidneys to decrease urine secretion
Oxytocin	Stimulates uterine contractions; causes breast to release milk into ducts
Thyroid Gland	
Thyroid hormone (thyroxine T_4 and triiodothyronine T_3)	Increases metabolic rate
Calcitonin	Decreases blood calcium concentration
Parathyroid Gland	
Parathyroid hormone	Increases blood calcium concentration
Adrenal Cortex	
Glucocorticoids (cortisol, hydrocortisone)	Stimulates gluconeogenesis and increases blood glucose; antiinflammatory; antiimmunity; antiallergy
Mineralocorticoids	Regulates electrolyte and fluid homeostasis
Sex hormones (androgen)	Stimulate sexual drive in females; in males, negligible effect
Adrenal Medulla	
Epinephrine (adrenalin)	Prolongs and intensifies sympathetic nervous response to stress
Norepinephrine	Prolongs and intensifies sympathetic nervous response to stress

blood pressure and heart rate to increase in an attempt to assist the body to deal with the stress more effectively. In addition, various rhythms from the brain affect the release of hormones. The circadian rhythm is an example of a 24-hour rhythm while the menstrual cycle is an example of the ultradiam rhythm, which is of longer duration.

Hypothalamus Gland

The hypothalamus can be considered the major regulating organ of the body, as it is the connection between the nervous system and the endocrine system. Input from the circulatory system and the nervous system give information to the hypothalamus about the homeostasis of the body. The hypothalamus, located centrally in the brain, secretes hormones that release or inhibit secretion of hormones from the anterior pituitary gland. The hormones from the hypothalamus are secreted in a circadian rhythmic pattern, and do not directly affect the peripheral endocrine tissues. The amount of hormones secreted by the hypothalamus is small. The hypothalamus contains neurons that produce hormones called antidiuretic hormone and oxytocin that are stored in the posterior pituitary. These neurons in the hypothalamus also interact with the brainstem, spinal cord, and limbic system.

Pituitary Gland

The pituitary gland, or hypophysis, is a small gland located under the hypothalamus in the sella turcica at the base of the brain (Figure 55-2). The pituitary gland is often labeled the master gland, because it directly or indirectly stimulates the release of a variety of hormones. It is connected to the hypothalamus by the hypophyseal stalk and is made up of two parts, the anterior stalk, the adenohypophysis, and the posterior stalk, the neurohypophysis. Hormones from the pituitary do act on the peripheral endocrine tissues. Patients with tumors of the pituitary often present with visual disturbances because of the location of the gland within the cranial vault. The pituitary response to the stimulus of the hypothalamus remains relatively constant throughout the life span with the exceptions of puberty, ovulation, and aging.

Anterior Pituitary Gland

The anterior pituitary gland is controlled by the hypothalamus and is the largest lobe of the gland (Figure 55-3). It produces more hormones than the posterior pituitary, several of which are called tropic hormones. Tropic hormones regulate the secretion of hormones by other glands. **Adrenocorticotropic hormone (ACTH)** from the anterior pituitary stimulates the secretion of corticosteroids by the adrenal cortex. Other tropic hormones secreted by the anterior pituitary include **thyroid-stimulating hormone (TSH),** FSH, and luteinizing hormone (LH). **Growth hormone (GH)** is a hormone that affects all tissues of the body, is secreted from the anterior pituitary, and is one of the counter regulatory hormones. GH is also secreted by the anterior pituitary and affects the growth of the long bones and skeletal muscles. It also plays a role in the metabolism of fat, protein, and carbohydrates. **Prolactin** is a hormone from the anterior pituitary that stimulates the breast to cause lactation.

Posterior Pituitary Gland

The posterior pituitary gland can be thought of as an extension of the hypothalamus. It is made up of nerve tissue and communicates with the hypothalamus through the median eminence. **Antidiuretic hormone (ADH)** and oxytocin are produced in the posterior pituitary. ADH regulates the reabsorption of water in the kidneys thereby regulates fluid volume. ADH secretion is controlled by the osmolality of the circulating plasma. When the osmolality of the plasma increases, sensors located in the hypothalamus are activated and ADH is released. A drop in blood pressure, orthostatic hypotension, decreased circulating blood volume, nausea, vomiting, and pain, can also trigger ADH release. When fluid volume is increased, secretion of ADH decreases, the kidneys do not reabsorb water and more dilute urine is excreted.

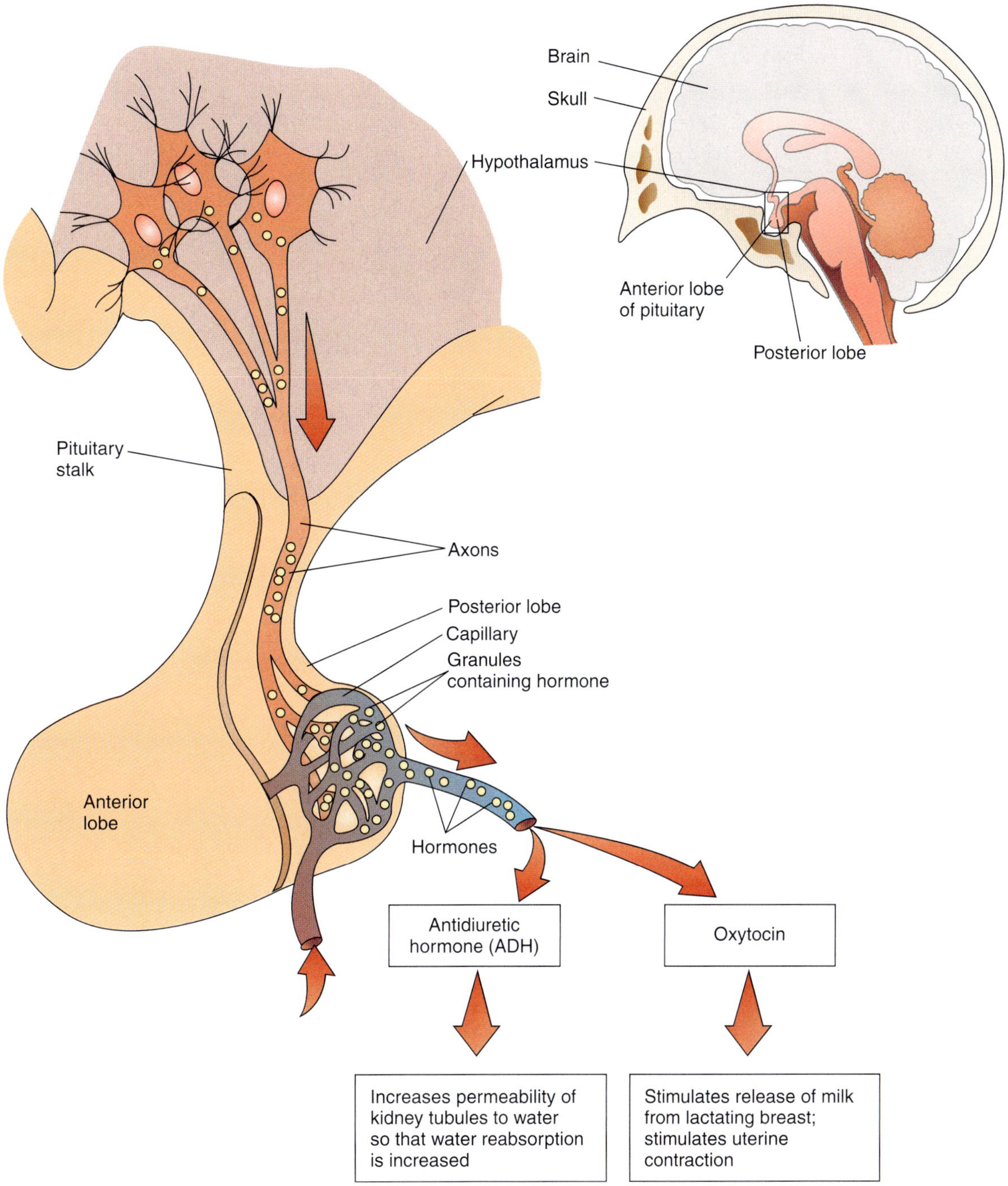

Figure 55-2 Pituitary gland.

Thyroid Gland

The thyroid gland is a vascular organ, consisting of two lobes connected by an isthmus (Figure 55-4). It is located in the anterior portion of the neck, anterior to the trachea. TSH from the anterior pituitary regulates the function of the thyroid. Hormones produced and secreted by the thyroid gland include thyroxine, triiodothyronine, and calcitonin. **Thyroxine (T_4)** is the most abundant thyroid hormone, and makes up approximately 90 percent of the thyroid hormone secretion. **Triiodothyronine (T_3)** is the most powerful thyroid hormone with 10 percent secreted by the thyroid and the remainder converted from T_4 by peripheral tissues. T_4 and T_3 are produced, stored, and released in the thyroid. A lesser amount of T_3 is produced, but it is a more potent hor-

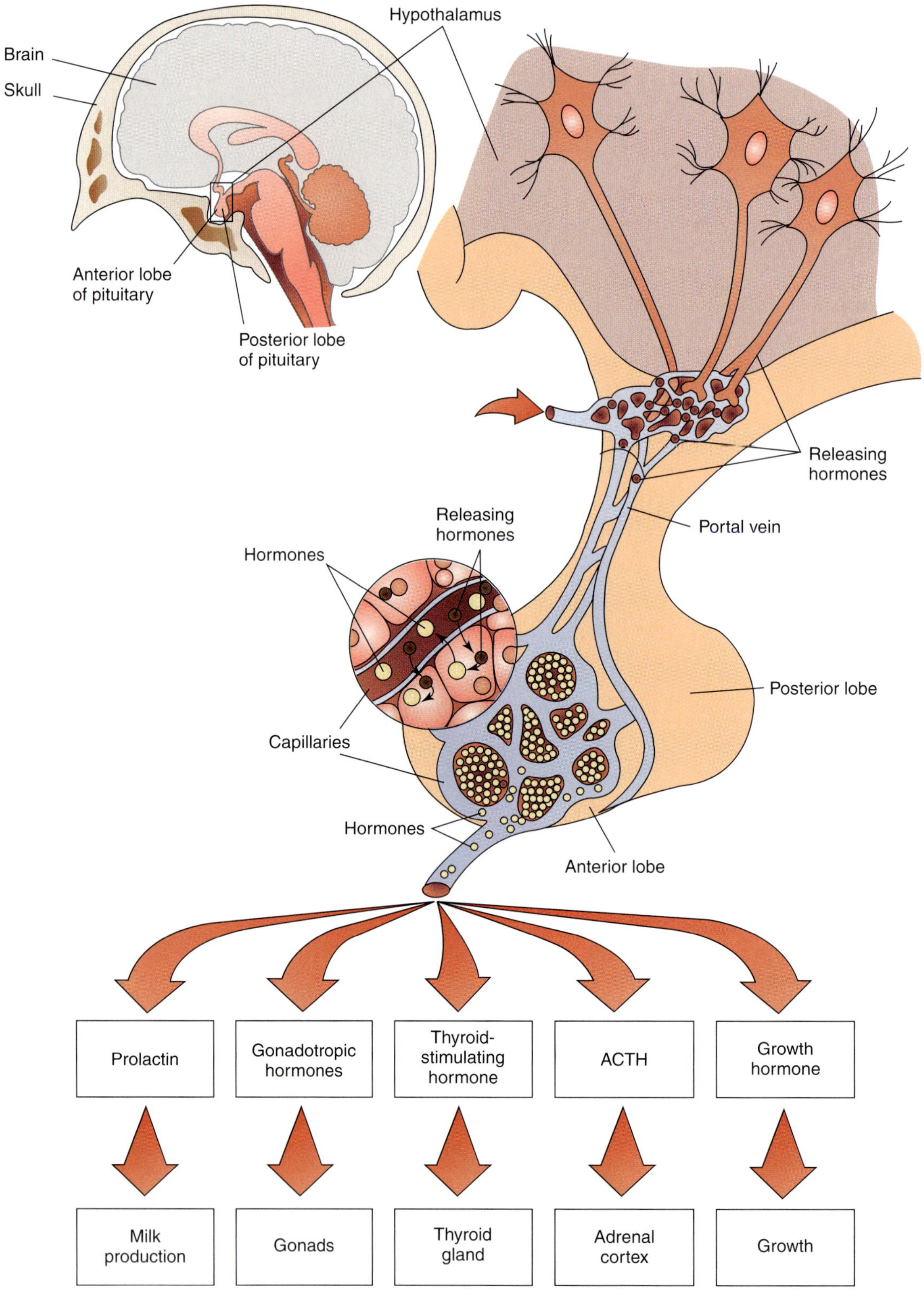

Figure 55-3 Anterior and posterior pituitary glands.

mone than T_4, having a greater effect on metabolism. Only about 10 percent of circulating T_3 is secreted by the thyroid gland. The remainder is converted from T_4. Synthesis of thyroid hormones requires the presence of iodine. T_3 and T_4 are lipid soluble and directly enter the cell. They affect the metabolism of lipids, metabolic rate, oxygen consumption, caloric requirements, nervous system activity, growth and development, and functions of the brain. Approximately 99 percent of the thyroid hormones are bound to plasma pro-

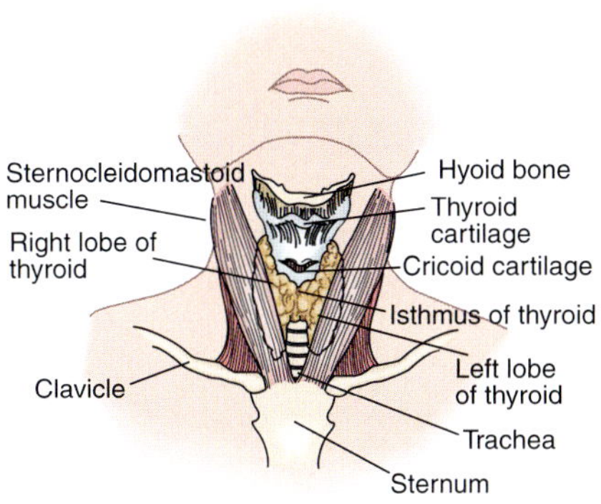

Figure 55-4 Structures of the thyroid gland.

teins. It is only the unbound or free hormones that are active and circulate within the body system (Liebert, 2003a).

Production and secretion of thyroid hormones is controlled by TSH from the anterior pituitary. The hypothalamus releases **thyroid-releasing hormone (TRH)** when circulating levels of thyroid hormones are low. TRH is the hormone that stimulates the anterior pituitary to release TSH. If the levels of circulating thyroid hormone are high, the secretion of TRH and TSH will be inhibited (Liebert, 2003b). The rate of thyroxin exchange, or turnover, changes with age, being highest in infants and children. The turnover rate of T_4 will decline to adult levels at puberty and stabilize until age 60. After age 60 the rate declines again (Greenspan & Gardner, 2004).

Calcitonin is a hormone produced by the thyroid gland when the circulating levels of calcium are elevated. Calcitonin has an inhibitory affect on the reabsorption of calcium from the bone and increases the storage of calcium in the bone. Calcitonin lowers circulating levels of calcium by promoting the excretion of calcium and phosphate by the kidneys.

Parathyroid Glands

The parathyroid glands are small glands located behind the thyroid gland and usual occur in pairs. Commonly there are four parathyroid glands. Like the thyroid, the parathyroid glands are vascular. **Parathyroid hormone (PTH)** is secreted by the parathyroids, and its main function is the regulation of the blood level of calcium in the body. The secretion of PTH is controlled by a negative feedback mechanism. PTH is secreted when serum calcium levels are low, and it is inhibited when serum calcium levels increase. PTH acts on the bone to inhibit bone formation and stimulate bone resorption, releasing phosphate and calcium in the blood. PTH stimulates the excretion of phosphate and reabsorption of calcium by the kidneys (Griffin & Ojeda, 2004).

Adrenal Glands

The two adrenal glands are located on the upper portion of each kidney. They are small vascular glands made up of a medulla and cortex. The medulla and cortex of each adrenal gland have separate and distinct functions and play a major role in the body's ability to adapt to internal and external stress.

Adrenal Medulla

The catecholamines, epinephrine, norepinephrine, and dopamine are secreted by the adrenal medulla, with epinephrine being secreted in the largest amount. Epinephrine and norepinephrine are considered hormones when they are secreted by the adrenal medulla, but they are often classified as neurotransmitters. As hormones, they are secreted and released into the circulation and act on a target organ. They play a primary role in the body's response to stress.

Adrenal Cortex

The adrenal cortex is the largest part of the gland and makes up the outer portion. It secretes steroid hormones that are classified as glucocorticoid, mineralocorticoid, and androgens. In addition, **corticosteroids** are any of the hormones, except androgen, synthesized by the adrenal cortex. Glucocorticoids (cortisol) affect the metabolism of glucose, mineralocorticoids (e.g., **aldosterone,** which is a mineralocorticoid synthesized in the adrenal cortex that functions to maintain extracellular fluid volume) maintain fluid and electrolyte balance.

Cortisol is a major glucocorticoid that functions in the regulation of blood glucose levels. By facilitating hepatic gluconeogenesis, cortisol increases blood glucose levels.

Glucocorticoids are also anti-inflammatory and play a role in the body's response to stress. Cortisol secretion is controlled by a negative feedback mechanism and the secretion of cortisol-releasing hormone (CRH) from the hypothalamus. Hypoglycemia, surgery, burns, stress, and fever stimulate the secretion of cortisol.

Pancreas Gland

The pancreas is both an endocrine and exocrine gland. The pancreas is located behind the stomach. The islets of Langerhans are the portions of the pancreas that secrete hormones. These islets are made up of four types of cells: alpha, beta, delta, and F cells. Glucagon is produced and secreted by the alpha cells, and insulin is produced and secreted by the beta cells of the pancreas. The delta cells are responsible for the production and secretion of somatostatin and the F cells secrete pancreatic polypeptide.

Glucagon

Glucagon is a hormone released from the pancreas in response to low levels of blood glucose and is a counter-regulatory hormone. Glucagon stimulates glycogenolysis, gluconeogenesis, and ketogenesis to raise the blood sugar levels.

Insulin

Insulin is a hormone produced by the beta cells of the pancreas to lower blood glucose levels. Insulin regulates the metabolism and storage of carbohydrates, fats, and proteins. Without insulin, glucose is unable to enter the cells in most tissues. The exceptions are the brain, lens of the eye, nerves, kidney tubules, and intestinal mucosa. Insulin is secreted in response to elevated blood glucose and is inhibited by hypoglycemia, glucagon, hypokalemia, and catecholamines.

At the peripheral level, insulin acts to transport glucose into the cells and triglycerides into the adipose tissue. For this reason, insulin is often referred to as a storage hormone. Insulin acts on the liver to inhibit gluconeogenesis.

Effects of Aging on the Endocrine System

Aging affects several functions of the endocrine system. The thyroid gland becomes smaller with age, decreasing the basal metabolic rate. There is an increased production of ADH resulting in more dilute urine and polyuria. The pancreas secretes less insulin, and the cells become more resistant to insulin, leading to the development of diabetes and decreased glucose tolerance. Estrogen function decreases in women leading to osteoporosis (Greenspan & Gardner, 2004).

It can be a challenge for the nurse to assess for abnormal endocrine functioning because of the presence of chronic illnesses, changes in sleep patterns that occur with normal aging, or the use of multiple medications that may affect hormone functions. Regular screenings for glucose tolerance, thyroid functioning, and calcium levels should be encouraged in the aging population.

ASSESSMENT

Effects of the endocrine system can be found in nearly every body system. The nurse uses his or her understanding of pathophysiology as a guide for assessment of this system. Following are suggestions for areas to be covered in an assessment of the endocrine system.

Subjective Data

Inquire about the energy level of the patient as the endocrine system regulates metabolism and energy production. Questions about lethargy, fatigue, increased need for sleep, and performance of activities of daily living should be assessed. The nurse should assess sleep patterns and should inquire about sleep disturbances, such as frequent awakenings. Heat and cold intolerance should also be assessed. Childhood exposure to ionizing radiation is associated with an increased risk of thyroid diseases and thyroid cancer. Use of iodine in cough medications or contrast media may increase the occurrence of hypothyroidism, hyperthyroidism, or goiter (Tierney, et al., 2004). Family history should include information about presence of thyroid disease and goiter, thyroid cancer, and diabetes. In addition, exploring whether or not the patient has ever had a crisis condition associated with their endocrine disorder is important information to obtain. An example is seen in a patient with hyperthyroidism and the condition labeled thyroid crisis (see Red Flag feature). The nurse should gather specific information regarding when the thyroid crisis occurred, what the clinical manifestations were, and what types of treatment measures were employed.

> *Red Flag*
>
> **Thyroid Crisis**
>
> A patient with hyperthyroidism is susceptible to experiencing a thyroid crisis. Often caused by increased medications, a thyroid crisis (also known as thyroid storm) is a rare but often life-threatening emergency. The clinical manifestations are marked by fever, sweating, restlessness, tachycardia, congestive heart failure, shock, and cardiac arrhythmias. Early detection and identification of the thyroid crisis is essential.

Integumentary

Questions should include assessment of hair loss (alopecia), dry skin, coarse hair, brittle nails, or changes in pigmentation. The nurse should ask patients for their history of the conditions of each of these integumentary components.

Head and Face

Inquire about puffiness of the face or eyelids, changes in the appearance of the eyes, or increased redness of the eyes. The nurse should assess for changes in the voice or enlargement of the neck. In addition, the patient needs to be assessed for alterations in self-esteem from the abnormalities often associated with endocrine disorders.

> **Skills 360°**
>
> **Professional and Caring Communication**
>
> Patients with endocrine disorders may have disfigurement related to their physical appearance (e.g., acromegaly, dwarfism, Grave's disease, or goiter). The nurse must remember to focus on maintaining an objective assessment and still provide a caring and supportive style of communication with the patient.

Cardiovascular

Palpitations are common with alterations in endocrine functioning. The patient should be asked if they ever "feel" his or her heart beat and if there seems to be an increase in the strength of the heartbeat. Ask if the patient feels if he or she has enough energy to complete their tasks of daily living. Inquire about exercise habits, including frequency, duration, and types of exercise.

Gastrointestinal

Common alterations include changes in weight, either loss or gain. Polydipsia, polyphagia, and polyuria occur with diabetes. Patients may also experience dysphagia with alterations in the endocrine system so assess for changes in swallowing or chewing. Assess the patient's typical daily food intake, including meals, snack, and use of supplements or vitamins. Ask about daily fluid intake including types and amounts ingested. Inquire about changes in appetite or weight.

Changes in bowel habits, constipation, and diarrhea should be assessed. Determine the patient's usual bowel habits, character of stool, use of laxatives or aids, and discomfort.

Neurological

The nervous system is closely associated with the functioning of the endocrine system, and alterations in neurological functioning are common. Common findings include tremors, memory loss, jitteriness or nervousness, and decreased sensation in the hands and feet. Depression is a common finding in the elderly patient.

Assess the patient's sleep patterns. Ask about difficulty falling asleep, number of hours per night spent sleeping, and use of sleep aids. Inquire about number of times the patient awakens at night and difficulty getting back to sleep. Is the patient bothered by nightmares? Do they feel rested when they awaken in the morning?

Genitourinary

Changes in the menstrual pattern are common in alterations of the endocrine system. Amenorrhea (absence of menses), menorrhagia (prolonged or excessive menses), and oligomenorrhea (decrease in the frequency of menses) may occur. There may also be an increase in urination (polyuria). Inquire about urinary frequency, amount, color, clarity, and odor of urine.

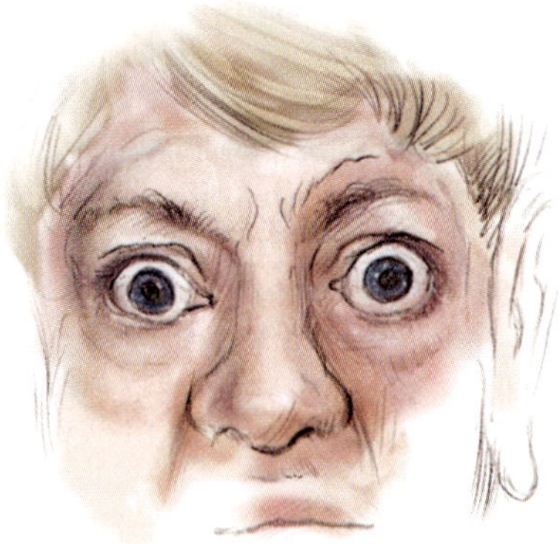

Figure 55-5 Exophthalmos of Graves' disease.

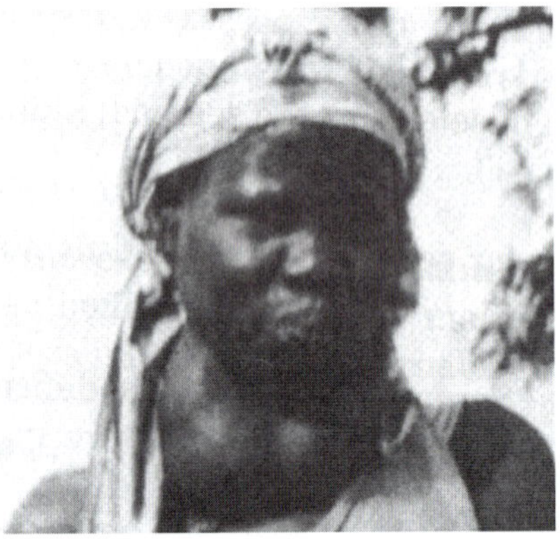

Figure 55-6 Goiter from iodine deficiency Courtesy of the Food and Agriculture Organization of the United Nations.

TABLE 55-2 Assessing the Endocrine System

SYSTEM	ASSESSMENTS
Integumentary	Skin is assessed for integrity, lesions, warmth, hair growth, pigmentation, color, and turgor. Hair is assessed for distribution, texture, quantity, and quality. Nails are assessed for color, thickness, growth, curvature, and clubbing.
Head and face	Assess the head and face for symmetry, exophthalmus, presence or absence of lid lag, periorbital, or facial edema.
Neck	Observe the neck for symmetry and position of the trachea (midline or deviated). Palpate the thyroid gland for size, symmetry, shape, consistency, and tenderness.
Heart	Inspect the anterior chest for heaves. Palpate the anterior chest for thrills and the apical impulse. Auscultate the heart sounds, noting rate, rhythm and presence of extra heart sounds.
Neurological	Assess for changes in mental status, especially in the elderly patient. Deep tendon reflexes should be assessed at the biceps, triceps, brachioradialis, patella, and Achilles tendons. Assess for presence or absence of ankle clonus. Vibratory sensation should be evaluated with a percussion hammer.

Adapted from Estes, M. (2006). Health assessment and physical examination *(3rd ed.). New York: Thomson Delmar Learning.*

Respecting Our Differences

Assessment of Integument with Regard to Ethnic Differences

When assessing the integument of non-Caucasian patients who have endocrine disturbances, the nurse must remember the obvious differences. For example, the patient with Addison's disease (hypofunction of the Adrenal gland) in a Caucasian patient will have a bronze-colored skin. However, in an African American patient, the skin coloration related to pigmentation hormonal influences will not be as pronounced.

Assess female patient's menstrual history, including age of menarche, menstrual pattern, pregnancy history, and use of contraceptives. Males and females should be assessed for interest in sexual activity or any noted changes.

Musculoskeletal

Muscle weakness and aching frequently occur and can have an impact on the patient's activities of daily living. Inquire about the patient's ability to perform the tasks of feeding, bathing, dressing, toileting, general mobility, shopping, cooking, and home maintenance tasks.

Objective Data

Vital signs, weight, nutritional status, apparent age as compared to chronological age, facial expression, and general appearance are important in the assessment of the endocrine system (Table 55-2). There are a wide variety of endocrine disturbances that exhibit themselves in identifiable appearances. For example, in hyperthyroidism, exophthalmos associated with Graves' disease causes the eyes to protrude in an obviously pathological manner (Figure 55-5). Another example is a goiter caused by hyperthyroidism as illustrated in Figure 55-6. In addition, inspection and palpation of the thyroid gland and the gonads are the two objective methods for assessing specific endocrine glands.

DIAGNOSTIC TESTS

Alterations in endocrine function are diagnosed by the use of blood and urine tests as well as radiological tests that may include computed tomography (CT) (Figure 55-7) and magnetic resonance imaging (MRI) (Table 55-3). Nursing interventions with diagnostic testing includes explanation of the procedure to the patient and significant others.

TABLE 55-3 Common Diagnostic Tests for Endocrine System Disorders

Pancreas Diagnostic Tests	***Thyroid Gland Diagnostic Tests—cont'd***
Blood glucose, fasting blood sugar (FBS)	Thyroxine, T_4, Thyroxine screen
2-Hour postprandial glucose (2hPPG) or 2-hour post-prandial blood sugar (2hPPBS)	Triiodothyronine, T_3 radioimmunoassay, T_3 by RIA
Glucose tolerance test (GTT)	Radioactive iodine uptake, (RAIU), iodine uptake test uptake
Pituitary Gland Diagnostic Tests	Thyroid scan, thyroid scintiscan
Adrenocorticotropic hormone (ACTH), corticotropin	Thyroid ultrasound, thyroid echogram, thyroid sonogram
Antidiuretic hormone (ADH), vasopressin	Thyroid biopsy
Follicle-stimulating hormone (FSH)	***Parathyroid Gland Diagnostic Tests***
Growth hormone (GH), human GH (HGH), somatotropin hormone (SH)	Parathyroid hormone (PTH), Parathormone
Growth hormone (GH) stimulation test, GH provocation test, insulin tolerance test (ITT), Arginine test	Calcium, total/ionized Ca^{++}
Luteinizing hormone (LH) assay	Phosphorus
Prolactin levels (PRL)	***Adrenal Glands Diagnostic Tests***
Thyrotropin-releasing hormone (TRH) test, thyrotropin-releasing factor (TRF) test	Adrenocorticotropic hormone (ACTH) stimulation test, Cortisol stimulation test, Cosyntropin test
Urine specific gravity	Corisol, Hydrocortisone
Long bone x-rays	Dexamethasone suppression test (DST), Cortisol suppression test, ACTH suppression test
Sella turcica x-ray	Plasma renin assay, Plasma renin activity (PRA)
Computed tomography of head (CT scan of head), Computerized axial transverse tomography (CATT)	Progesterone assay
Thyroid Gland Diagnostic Tests	Aldosterone assay
Antithyroid microsomal antibody, Antimicrosomal antibody, Microsomal antibody, Thyroid autoantibody, Thyroid antimicrosomal antibody	17-Hydroxycorticosteroids (17-OHCS)
Calcitonin, HCT, Thyrocalcitonin	17-Ketosteroids (17-KS)
Serum free triiodothyronine (T_3)	Urine cortisol, Hydrocortisone
Thyroid-stimulating hormone (TSH), Thyrotropin	Vanillylmandelic acid (VMA) & catecholamines, VMA & epinephrine, Norepinephrine, Metanephrine, Normetanephrine, Dopamine
Thyroid-stimulating hormone (TSH) stimulation test	Adrenal angiography, Adrenal arteriogram
Thyroxine index free, FTI, FT_4 Index	Adrenal venography
	Computed tomography of adrenals (CAT scan of adrenal CT scan of adrenals)

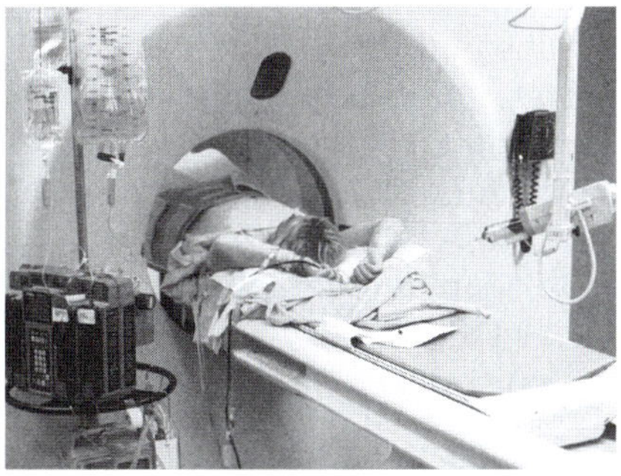

Figure 55-7 CT testing.

Thyroid Scan

A thyroid scan utilizes a scintillation camera or scintiscanner to evaluate the thyroid gland following administration of a radioactive isotope or technetium. Hyperactive areas in the thyroid will appear as black or gray regions (hot spots) while areas of hypoactivity will appear as white (cold spots). Hot spots are generally indicative of benign nodules while malignancies will appear as cold spots (Daniels, 2003).

Nursing Management

Instruct the patient that this test evaluates the structure and function of the thyroid gland. The patient is ensured that the amount of radioactive material used is not harmful to the patient or others. Ask if the patient has received any radiographic contrasts from other diagnostic tests in the past three months as these may interfere with the scan. Patients who are taking medications with iodine (e.g., Lugol's solution, cough syrups, or multivitamins) may be instructed by the practitioner to discontinue their use for two weeks prior to the scan. Thyroid medications may be discontinued for four to six weeks prior to the scan. If I 123 or I 131 is used, the patient will be required not to eat anything (NPO) after midnight. The patient will remain NPO for 45 minutes after ingesting the isotope, and the scan is performed 24 hours later. If technetium is used, it is administered 30 minutes before the scan. IV administration eliminates the need for fasting.

Thyroid Ultrasound

Thyroid ultrasound is useful in differentiation of fluid filled cysts or tumors. It involves the use of ultrasonic pulses that are directed at the thyroid gland. The sound waves bounce back and are displayed on an oscilloscope. Fine needle aspiration or biopsy may be performed if a tumor is suspected.

Nursing Management

The procedure takes about 30 minutes and requires no special preparation. The patient just needs to be educated as to the expectations of the results of the ultrasound. In addition, young children will likely need to be restrained or potentially mildly sedated during this procedure.

Thyroid Biopsy

A biopsy may be performed as a surgical procedure, requiring general anesthesia or with the use of fine needle aspiration and local anesthesia (Liebert, 2003c). A 21-gauge needle is inserted into the thyroid nodule; tissue from the thyroid is withdrawn and placed on a slide for examination. The possibility of hematoma formation and edema postprocedure are the major complications, which may present as respiratory difficulty. If the test is to be completed using general anesthesia, the patient will be required to fast. It is common for the patient to experience a sore throat after a thyroid biopsy.

Nursing Management

Explain the test procedure and the purpose of the test. Assess for the patient's knowledge of the test. Provide preprocedure sedation and analgesia as prescribed. The older patient may find it difficult to maintain positions when required to do so for lengthy periods of time during the biopsy. Obtain a signed consent form.

KEY CONCEPTS

- The endocrine system is made up of a variety of organs that secrete hormones.
- Hormones are the chemicals produced and stored by the endocrine system that help regulate metabolism and energy.
- The hypothalamus can be considered the major regulating organ of the body.
- The pituitary gland is often labeled the master gland, because it directly or indirectly stimulates the release of a variety hormones.
- PTH is secreted by the parathyroids, and its main function is the regulation of the blood level of calcium in the body.
- The medulla and cortex of each adrenal gland have separate and distinct functions and play a major role in the body's ability to adapt to internal and external stress.
- The catecholamines, epinephrine, norepinephrine, and dopamine are secreted by the adrenal medulla.

Continued

KEY CONCEPTS—cont'd

- The adrenal cortex secretes steroid hormones that are classified as glucocorticoid, mineralocorticoid, and androgens.
- The pancreas is both an endocrine and exocrine gland.
- Glucagon is a hormone released from the pancreas in response to low levels of blood glucose and is a counter-regulatory hormone.
- Insulin is a hormone produced by the beta cells of the pancreas to lower blood glucose levels.
- Common alterations of the endocrine system include changes in weight, either loss or gain.
- Vital signs, weight, nutritional status, apparent age as compared to chronological age, facial expression, and general appearance are important in the assessment of the endocrine system.
- Alterations in endocrine function are diagnosed by the use of blood and urine tests as well as radiological tests (e.g., CT, MRI).

REVIEW QUESTIONS

1. Which of the following is *not* produced by the thyroid gland?
   1. Calcitonin
   2. T_4
   3. T_3
   4. TSH

2. What is the correct label for the body parts that secrete substances into the ducts that empty into a body cavity or onto a body surface?
   1. Endocrine glands
   2. Target tissues
   3. Exocrine glands
   4. Hormones

3. Which of the following is true of the hypothalamus gland?
   1. It is often called the master gland.
   2. It stimulates the secretion of corticosteroids.
   3. It is located in the anterior portion of the neck.
   4. It secretes hormones that release or inhibit hormones from the anterior pituitary gland.

4. Which of the following are the two major hormones secreted by the adrenal medulla?
   1. Epinephrine and norepinephrine
   2. Insulin and glucagon
   3. Cortisol and aldosterone
   4. Calcitonin and PTH

5. When blood glucose levels are elevated, the pancreas secretes insulin. When the blood glucose declines, the stimulus for the secretion of insulin decreases. This is an example of:
   1. Circadian rhythm
   2. Negative feedback
   3. Complex feedback
   4. Neural or hormonal interaction

6. All of the following statements about parathyroid hormone are correct *except:*
   1. PTH is regulated by the pituitary and hypothalamus.
   2. PTH regulates the blood level of calcium.
   3. PTH stimulates bone reabsorption.
   4. PTH stimulates the kidneys to convert vitamin D to its most active form.

7. Which organ in the endocrine system consists of two lobes, connected by an isthmus, and secretes T_4, calcitonin, and T_3?
   1. Thyroid gland
   2. Hypothalamus gland
   3. Parathyroid gland
   4. Adrenal cortex

8. Which of the following are clinical manifestations of a patient having a thyroid crisis?
   1. Chilling, coma, and dyspnea
   2. Nausea, seizures, and apprehension
   3. Fever, tachycardia, and restlessness
   4. Double vision, mental deterioration, and diarrhea

9. Which organ controls serum calcium?
   1. Adrenal gland
   2. Thyroid gland
   3. Hypothalamus gland
   4. Parathyroid gland

10. A negative feedback mechanism refers to:
   1. The response of the cardiovascular system to hormone regulation
   2. The response of a gland by increasing or decreasing the secretion of a hormone
   3. The response seen when increasing one hormone causes another hormone to increase
   4. The response of the autonomic nervous system when stimulated by the adrenal cortex

REVIEW ACTIVITIES

1. Compare and contrast the endocrine and the exocrine glands.

2. Describe a negative feedback system related to hormone control.

3. Select two of the glands in the endocrine system and describe their location and function.

4. Develop three to five questions to ask a patient regarding his or her endocrine system.

5. Perform an assessment of the thyroid gland and document your results.

Visit the Contemporary Medical-Surgical Nursing online companion resource at www.delmarhealthcare.com for additional content and study aids. Click on Online Companions then select the Nursing discipline.

CHAPTER

56

Endocrine Dysfunction: Nursing Management

Joyce Campbell, RN, MSN, CCRN, FNP-C

KEY TERMS

Adenoma
Amenorrhea
Anovulation
Euthyroid
Galactorrhea
Gynecomastia
Hirsutism
Oligomenorrhea
Osteopenia
Panhypopituitarism
Proptosis

CHAPTER TOPICS

- Hypersecretion and Hyposecretion of the Anterior Pituitary Gland
- Diabetes Insipidus
- Syndrome of Inappropriate Antidiuretic Hormone
- Hyposecretion and Hypersecretion of the Adrenal Gland
- Thyroid Disorders
- Parathyroid Disorders

The endocrine system along with the nervous system influences all body functions including metabolism, maturation, growth, reproduction, and adaptation to changes within the internal environment. The endocrine system regulates body function through the secretion of chemical substances called hormones, which exert action on specific target tissue by binding to a receptor site. Disease occurs when there is hyposecretion or hypersecretion of these hormones, or when target cells become nonresponsive to the hormone (Asp, 2005).

Beginning with general pituitary dysfunction, this chapter will address each target organ and the disease entities that occur when there is hyper or hypo functioning related to hormone secretion or tissue nonresponsiveness.

HYPERSECRETION OF THE ANTERIOR PITUITARY GLAND

Pituitary dysfunction may present with a variety of clinical signs and symptoms including those related to hyposecretion or hypersecretion of the pituitary hormones and sellar turcica enlargement. The importance of the pituitary gland to system function contributes to the variety of illnesses when the gland is diseased. Ten to 15 percent of all intracranial neoplasms are pituitary adenomas (Ferri, 2005).

Hyperfunction of the pituitary gland occurs when there is excess hormonal activity. Most commonly, secretory tumors cause hypersecretion of one or more of the pituitary hormones. Autoimmune stimulation is another reason for hyperfunction of the pituitary gland.

Etiology

The most common cause of pituitary hyperfunction is a pituitary **adenoma** (a benign tumor made of epithelial cells, usually arranged like a gland), which can cause hypersecretion of prolactin, growth hormone (GH) or adrenocorticotrophin (ACTH) hormone (Jameson, 2005).

Pathophysiology

Patients who have hyperfunction of the pituitary gland may present with hormonal or neurological symptoms. Located in the sella turcica, the pituitary gland is positioned in close proximity to the cavernous sinuses, cranial nerves, and optic chiasm. Therefore, in addition to the hormonal symptoms, enlargement of the gland may cause localized symptoms, such as visual changes, cranial nerve impingement, and headache.

> **Red Flag**
>
> **Visual Changes**
>
> Patients presenting with an unexplained visual field defect or bitemporal hemianopsia, or visual loss should be considered to have a pituitary or hypothalamic disorder until proven otherwise (Aron, Finding, & Tyrrell, 2004a).

Hyperprolactinemia

Hyperprolactinemia is a prolactin secreting pituitary tumor. This condition is the most common pituitary tumor, accounting for 60 percent of primary pituitary tumors.

Epidemiology

Prolactin secreting tumors are more common in women. In women the tumors are usually microadenomas, which do not grow even with oral contraceptives or with pregnancy. Men more commonly have macroadenomas (Ferri, 2005).

Etiology

Etiology of hyperprolactinemia includes pituitary adenoma, primary hypothyroidism, traumatic injury, or surgery to the pituitary stalk, breast disease, estrogen therapy, pregnancy, and drugs. Renal and liver disease and hypothyroidism should also be considered a potential cause. Hyperprolactinemia is also seen in multiple sclerosis, spinal cord lesions, systemic lupus erythematosus, and other diseases. The most common cause of hyperprolactinemia is ingestion of drugs, including dopamine antagonist, haloperidol, risperidone, metoclopramide, opioids, cimetidine, verapamil (Aron, et al., 2004a).

Pathophysiology

Most commonly, prolactinomas arise from the lateral wings of the anterior pituitary. As growth of the tumor continues, the sella turcica is filled, and the normal anterior and posterior lobes are compressed. The size of the tumor varies from the more common microadenomas to large tumors, which invade the extracellular area.

Assessment with Clinical Manifestations

Clinical manifestations of hyperprolactinemia in women include **galactorrhea** (excessive secretion of milk), **amenorrhea** (absence of menstruation), **oligomenorrhea** (scanty or infrequent menstrual flow) with **anovulation** (failure to ovulate), and infertility. In men, hyperprolactinemia causes a decrease in testosterone secondary to an inhibition of gonadotropin secretion leading to decreased facial and body hair, erectile dysfunction, decrease in libido, small testicles and infertility; **gynecomastia** (enlargement of breast tissue) in the male occurs less frequency in men. Since hyperprolactinemia is associated with a decrease in estrogen, women with prolactinomas often have an estrogen deficiency with resulting symptoms of vaginal dryness, hot flashes, and more seriously **osteopenia** (a significant amount of decrease in bone mineral density), and osteoporosis. The patient may also experience weight gain, irritability, **hirsutism** (condition characterized by the excessive growth of hair or the presence of hair in abnormal places), anxiety, and depression. In some incidences, pituitary prolactinomas secrete GH simultaneously and cause acromegaly (Jameson, 2005).

Diagnostic Tests

Patients who present with symptoms of hyperprolactinemia should have a basal prolactin level, thyroid panel, and gonadal function test done. Tests to rule out renal and liver disease are advised. In addition, women with amenorrhea should have a pregnancy test. In most incidences, a PRL level of greater than 200 ng/mL is diagnostic of a prolactinoma. A prolactin level of less than 200 ng/mL does not rule out a pituitary tumor (Aron, et al., 2004a). Other causes for hyperprolactinemia should be excluded.

Computed tomography (CT) scan or magnetic resonance imaging (MRI) is recommended when prolactin levels are elevated for the purpose of identifying a microadenoma or macroadenoma. Macroadenomas are greater than 1 cm in size. Microadenomas are less than 1 cm. Tumor size usually correlates with the prolactin level (Jameson, 2005) (Box 56-1).

> **BOX 56-1**
>
> **PROLACTIN LEVELS**
>
> Normal prolactin levels in nonpregnant women: 0–23 ng/mL or 0–23 mcg/L. Normal prolactin levels in men: 0–20 ng/mL or 0–10 mcg/L.
>
> After fasting for 12 hours, blood for the prolactin test should be drawn between 8:00 and 10:00 a.m. It is also recommended that all prescribed medications be discontinued if possible two weeks prior to prolactin test (Daniels, 2003).

Nursing Diagnoses

Based on the information gathered, examples of nursing diagnoses in the patient with hyperprolactinemia may include the following:

- Disturbed body image related to gynecomastia and galactorrhea.
- Sexual dysfunction or ineffective sexuality patterns related to altered gonadal function.

Planning and Implementation

The patient will require psychosocial support to deal with altered body image and issues related to sexual function. Reversal of signs and symptoms is promising with medical or surgical treatment. Special attention must be given to instruction and preparation regarding treatment plan, (e.g., medications, surgery).

Goals

Goals of treatment include normalization of prolactin level, alleviation of the suppressive effect of gonadal function, halting of galactorrhea, and preservation of bone density (Jameson, 2005). Long-term remission is possible when the adenoma is small in size, and the prolactin levels are less than 200 ng/mL. If asymptomatic, microadenomas are usually not treated; however, close monitoring is required. For tumors larger than 2 cm, surgical treatment (see transsphenoidal resection) will usually provide an initial remission. Because there is often remaining tumor, medical interventions may be required at some time postoperatively.

Pharmacology

There are specific medications that are used to treat hyperprolactinemia. Dopaminergic medications, which stimulate dopamine receptors, are used to medically manage prolactinomas. They are capable of controlling hyperprolactinemia, shrinking tumor, and restoring menses and fertility. These drugs include bromocriptine (Parlodel) and cabergoline (Dostinex). Bromocriptine, the first available dopamine agonist, has effects at both the hypothalamic and pituitary levels. Dosage is 2.5 to 10 mg a day orally in divided dosages. Side effects include postural hypotension and gastrointestinal (GI) problems. Cabergoline, (Dostinex), a newer dopaminergic agonist, is administered once or twice weekly and has fewer side effects. Ninety percent of patients have success in treatment with cabergoline (Aron, et al., 2004a).

Surgery

Conventional radiation therapy is reserved for patients who do not respond to medications or who have persistent hyperprolactinemia after surgery or medical treatment. Fifty to 60 percent of the patients experience impairment of anterior pituitary function with the radiation therapy. A newer modality for treating pituitary tumors is stereotactic radiosurgery (gamma knife). Multiple ports allow high dose ionizing radiation to be delivered with minimal irradiation to surrounding tissues (Ferri, 2005). See the National Institutes of Health Web site (www.cancer.gov) for elaboration of the gamma knife treatment procedure used for brain tumors.

Evaluation of Outcomes

Potential patient outcomes for each of the example nursing diagnoses for the patient with hyperprolactinemia are:

- Disturbed body image related to gynecomastia and galactorrhea. Patient will have resolution of gynecomastia and amenorrhea.
- Sexual dysfunction or ineffective sexuality patterns related to altered gonadal function. The patient will verbalize satisfaction with the way he or she expresses physical intimacy.

Acromegaly (Gigantism)

Acromegaly, a Greek word, *akro* (extremity) and *megas* (large) is a condition occurring in adults, that is caused by hypersecretion of the pituitary GH over a long period of time. Hypersecretion of GH in childhood causes gigantism.

Etiology

In most incidences gigantism and acromegaly are secondary to a benign tumor of the pituitary gland. Other rare causes include hypothalamus tumors producing excess GH releasing hormone (GHRH), bronchial tumors (carcinoid), and pancreatic islet cell tumors.

Epidemiology

Acromegaly occurs equally between men and women and is a rare disease with only three cases occurring per 1 million people per year. The average age for diagnosis of acromegaly is 42 years, though the duration of symptoms is usually 5 to 10 years prior to diagnosis. Diagnosis is often missed or delayed. When undiagnosed, untreated, or undertreated, there is increase morbidity and mortality due to the chronic effect of GH on body organs resulting in increase incidence of cardiovascular, cerebrovascular, respiratory disease, malignancies, and diabetes (Asp, 2005).

Pathophysiology

Most pituitary tumors, which secrete GH and cause acromegaly, are usually over 1 cm in diameter when the diagnosis is made. The tumors evolve from the outer wings of the anterior pituitary gland. In about 15 percent of the tumors, lactotrophs are present, and therefore both GH and prolactin are secreted.

Clinical manifestations of acromegaly occur due to an excess of GH, which once released into circulation stimulates production of insulin growth factor

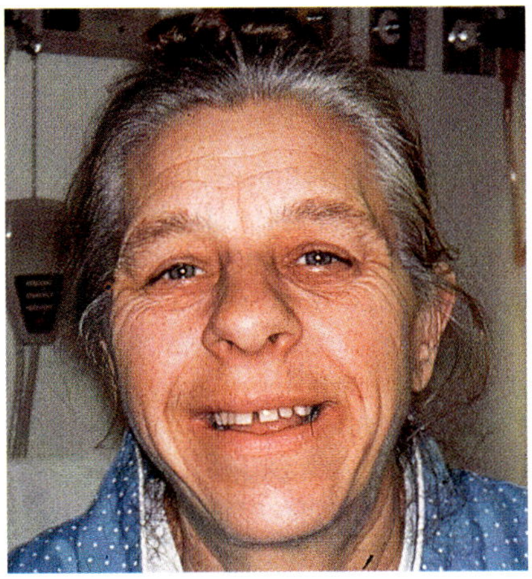

Figure 56-1 Acromegaly (note wide nose, spaced teeth, and large lips).

(IGF-1) or somatomedin C. IGF-1 is produced mainly by the liver and is the primary mediator of the growth-promoting effects of GH. In children and adolescence, gigantism occurs because GH stimulates growth in all body tissues prior to fusion of the growth plate. A child may grow to seven feet or taller. In adults, acromegaly occurs because GH causes continued growth of soft tissues and small bones of the hands and feet and the membranous bones of the skull and face (Figure 56-1). Excess GH also causes an alteration in fat and carbohydrate metabolism. The multiple effects of GH on carbohydrate metabolism include hyperglycemia, which occurs due to a decreased glucose uptake by peripheral tissues and an increased production of glucose by the liver. Rather than normal use of carbohydrates for energy, GH boosts the creation of ketones and the utilization of free fatty acids for energy. These events lead to glucose intolerance, hyperinsulinemia, and the probability of developing diabetes. Thirty percent of the patients will have some form of cardiac disease, including coronary artery disease, cardiac dysrhythmias, left ventricular hypertrophy (LVH), or cardiomyopathy (Jameson, 2005). Acromegaly has also been associated with colon polyps.

Assessment with Clinical Manifestations

There are several identifying characteristics seen in patients with acromegaly. Table 56-1 clearly represents both the history and physical findings of this disorder.

Diagnostic Tests

Diagnostic tests to determine the presence of excess GH include serum growth hormone (hGH), IGF-1, and GH suppression test. Normally growth hormone (hGH) is less than 5 ng/mL or is less than 226 pmol/L in men and is less than 10 ng/mL or is less than 452 pmol/L in women. Increased values of hGH may be associated with certain medications (e.g., glucagon, levodopa, insulin, estrogens, or oral contraceptives). In acromegaly, the hGH level is greater than 10 ng/mL (Aron, et al., 2004b). Prior to the hGH test the patient should be fasting and the test should be drawn at eight in the morning because of the circadian cycle.

TABLE 56-1 Assessment of the Patient with Acromegaly

HISTORY	PHYSICAL FINDINGS
Skin: Changes in facial features; excessive sweating	Oily skin, thickening of heal pads, acanthosis nigricans, macroglossia, hirsutism.
Neuro/HEENT: Headaches, lethargy, photophobia, headache	Prognathism (Underbite)
	Visual changes, paresthesia, carpal tunnel syndrome. Enlargement of tongue
Respiratory: Sleep apnea, hypersomnolence	Obesity
CV: History of: hypertension, atherosclerotic disease Hypercholesterolemia	LVH, cardiomyopathy
Reproductive: Decreased libido, impotence, infertility	Galactorrhea, gynecomastia
Oligomenorrhea	
GU: renal colic	
MS: arthralgias, muscle weakness	Proximal myopathy, soft tissue overgrowth
	Glucose intolerance
General: Fatigue, weight gain, and heat intolerance	

Adapted from Asp, A. (2005) Mechanisms of endocrine control. In K. Copstead & J. L. Banasik, Pathophysiology *(pp. 639–645). St. Louis, MO: Elsevier Saunders.*

Glucose suppression test involves measuring GH following the administration of 100 g of glucose. Normally, GH secretion is lowered to less than 2 ng/mL. A result greater than 2 ng/mL is considered conclusive of a diagnosis of acromegaly (Ferri, 2005).

Somatomedin C (SM-C): Insulin-like growth factor (IGF-1) results are interpreted according to patient's age and sex. Elevated GH levels increase IGF-1 levels and are usually diagnostic of acromegaly (Daniels, 2003). IGF-1 levels are two to three times higher in pregnancy. Additional tests include postprandial plasma glucose, serum phosphorous, and urine calcium levels, which are often elevated in the patient who has hypersecretion of GH.

Plain films will often show sellar turcica enlargement due to a pituitary tumor. Thickening of the calvarium, enlargement of the sinuses and jaw can also be seen on X-ray. An MRI will usually show tumor location and size.

Nursing Diagnoses

Based on the information gathered, examples of nursing diagnoses in the patient with acromegaly may include the following:

- Disturbed body image related to changes in skin, facial features, hair, and musculoskeletal system.
- Chronic pain related to arthralgia and myalgia from cartilage overgrowth.
- Deficient knowledge related to the disease, complications, and management.
- Sleep deprivation related to sleep apnea.

Planning and Implementation

The nurse should work with the endocrinologist or health care provider experienced in managing acromegaly. Treatment of choice is surgical removal of tumor. For patients who are not candidates for surgery treatment, elect not to have surgery, or have residual tumor following surgery, treatment may be radiotherapy or medical therapy. Conventional supervoltage irradiation successfully treats patients in 60 to 80 percent of the cases. Often there is a prolonged delay in achieving reduction of GH levels with radiotherapy. Hypopituitarism with resulting hypoadrenalism, hypogonadism, and hypothyroidism may occur with irradiation. Other complications of radiotherapy include cranial nerve dysfunction, radionecrosis, and cognitive abnormalities (Ferri, 2005). Another approach that has been used to treat tumors of the sella turcica is stereotactic technique with gamma knife.

A comprehensive plan for instruction and follow-up of the patient regarding proposed surgery or radiotherapy and prescribed medications should be implemented. Patients who are hyperglycemic due to hypersecretion of GH will need to have diabetic management involving glucose monitoring, diet, exercise, and medications to normalize glucose. Measures to prevent complications of diabetes must be implemented. Cardiovascular problems, such as hypercholesterolemia and hypertension, must be monitored closely and treated expeditiously. The nurse plays a major role in the management of the patient with acromegaly. Teaching involved in prevention and treatment of complications of the disease is of paramount importance.

Fast Forward ▶▶▶

A Gamma Knife

A gamma knife is a new treatment modality used in the treatment of pituitary tumors. It is referred to as a stereotaxic approach for treating pituitary tumors. The stereotaxic approach is a viable alternative to radiation therapy and may continue in use in the near future. An interesting source is the National Institute of Health Web site (www.cancer.gov) for current treatment of brain tumors including gamma knife stereotaxic approach.

Pharmacology

Octreotide is a drug that can be used to treat patients who have residual GH hypersecretion following surgery. Octreotide (Sandostatin) may be administered subcutaneously three times daily by the patient or administered intramuscularly in a long-acting form that lasts up to four weeks. Side effects may occur due to the inhibition of gastric and pancreatic function and include alteration in gastric motility, nausea, flatus, fat malabsorption, and gallstones. An alternative medication is bromocriptine (Parlodel). Though less effective than octreotide, it is less expensive and can be taken in oral form. (Ferri, 2005).

Surgery

Patients who undergo successful treatment for GH hypersecretion may expect a marked improvement and reversal of most signs and symptoms with successful therapy. Bone overgrowth will cease, and soft tissue bulk in extremities and facial puffiness will decrease (Aron, et al., 2004a).

Evaluation of Outcomes

Potential patient outcomes for each of the example nursing diagnoses for the patient with acromegaly are:

- Disturbed body image related to changes in skin, facial features, hair, and musculoskeletal system. Patient will relate an understanding of the cause for change in physical appearance.
- Chronic pain related to arthralgia and myalgia from cartilage overgrowth. Patient will report a decrease in skeletal muscular pain.
- Deficient knowledge related to the disease, complications, and management. Patient will verbalize understanding of disease, complications, and management.
- Sleep deprivation related to sleep apnea. Patient will report relief from symptoms of sleep deprivation.

Cushing's Disease (Hypercortisolism)

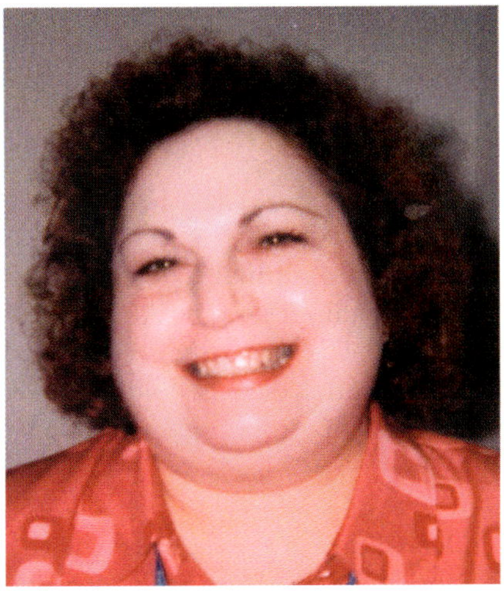

Figure 56-2 Cushing's syndrome.

Hypercortisolism is most often caused by excessive production and release of ACTH by a pituitary secreting adenoma. This form of hypercortisolism is called Cushing's disease (Figure 56-2).

Epidemiology

Most commonly Cushing's disease occurs in women between 20 and 40 years of age. ACTH secreting adenomas (Cushing's disease) make up approximately 20 percent of pituitary tumors. The most common cause of Cushing's syndrome is the use of corticosteroids, which are prescribed for multiple inflammatory, immune, and numerous other conditions. Consequently, the condition of increased ACTH, which causes Cushing's disease or Cushing's syndrome (discussed later), could be included under: (a) the pituitary section from the etiology of a tumor of the pituitary gland or (b) excessive stimulation from the adrenal cortex. The clinical manifestations and management strategies are similar for either causation.

Etiology

When Cushing's disease is primary in its etiology the condition is due to a pituitary adenoma. Less often Cushing's disease may occur because of excessive corticotropic releasing hormone (CRH), which stimulates an increase in ACTH secretion. Because excess production of ACTH results in bilateral hyperplasia of the adrenal glands and hypercortisolism, the disease is often referred to as ACTH dependent. Mass effect or localized symptoms occur less frequently than other types of pituitary tumors because the adenoma is generally small, 5 to 10 mm in diameter (Aron, et al, 2004b).

Another cause for hypercortisolism is an ACTH secreting neoplasm (ectopic ACTH). The most common ACTH ectopic secreting tumor is small cell carcinoma of the lung. A nonpituitary or non-ACTH dependent hypercortisolism called Cushing's syndrome (non-ACTH dependent) is often due to the iatrogenic effects of chronic glucocorticoid therapy. Less frequent causes for Cushing's syndrome are adrenal disease, neoplasm, or hyperplasia (Aron, et al., 2004a).

Pathophysiology

Ninety percent of the patients with Cushing's disease have a pituitary adenoma. Up to 90 percent of these tumors are microadenoma (less than 10 mm). The tumors are usually basophilic or chromophobe adenomas and can appear anywhere within the anterior pituitary gland. The tumor is rarely greater than 10 mm and invasive, causing a mass effect. Malignant ACTH secreting tumors are seldom reported. Under the influence of ACTH secretion, the adrenal glands are enlarged, with thickened cortex due to hyperplasia (Aron, et al., 2004a).

Assessment with Clinical Manifestations

Clinical manifestations of hypercortisolism occurring from pituitary disease, ectopic tumor, primary disease of the adrenal gland, or iatrogenic effects of glucocorticoid are similar. Symptoms from excess cortisol and androgen are usually present. If an iatrogenic cause or other disease that causes hypercortisolism is not identified, a thorough diagnostic workup must be implemented to determine the etiology to develop a treatment plan. Many of the clinical manifestations of hypercortisolism can be interpreted as exaggeration action of cortisol, which affects glucose, protein, and fat metabolism. Some of the symptoms are easy bruising, poor wound healing, excess hair growth in females, hypertension, edema of extremities, accumulation of fat in the face (moon face), voice changes, hyperlipidemia, dysrhythmias, emotional liability, irritability, depression, poor memory, euphoria, psychosis, suicidal tendencies, protein breakdown and muscle wasting, osteopenia, osteoporosis, renal calculi, polyuria, amenorrhea in females, decrease in libido, impotence, decrease in body hair (males), protruding abdomen, subclavicular fat pads (buffalo hump), hyperinsulinemia, and abnormal glucose tolerance test. Additional clinical manifestations that may be present due to fluid and electrolyte imbalance are hypokalemia and sodium imbalances.

Diagnostic Tests

There are a number of diagnostic tests for hypersecretion of the adrenal glands: serum ACTH (elevated in hyperfunction of the pituitary; decreased in hypofunction of the pituitary), plasma cortisol, dexamethasone, ACTH suppression test, urine free cortisol (UFC) (requires 24 hour urine collection), salivary cortisol, CT and MRI of pituitary and adrenal glands, and inferior petrosal sinus sampling (IPSS). More information is provided in Box 56-2.

> **BOX 56-2**
>
> **ADVANCES IN DIAGNOSING PITUITARY SECRETING TUMOR**
>
> Inferior petrosal sinus sampling (IPSS), a diagnostic test that is yielding close to 100 percent accuracy is currently being done in some hospitals. The test requires the skills of an interventional radiologist (Aron, et al., 2004a). Blood leaves the pituitary gland and drains into the cavernous sinus and then on to the inferior petrosal sinuses and then into the jugular bulb and vein. Simultaneous ACTH measurement of samples of blood taken from the posterior petrosal sinus and peripheral circulation before and after CRH stimulation has high sensitivity for identifying a pituitary secreting adenoma.

Nursing Diagnoses

Based on the information gathered, examples of nursing diagnoses in the patient with hypersecretion of the adrenal glands may include the following:

- Activity intolerance related to congestive heart failure, and weakness due to hypercortisolism, which causes proximal muscle weakness, decreased muscle mass, and hypokalemia.
- Disturbed body image related to appearance changes.
- Risk for infection related to altered resistance to infection due to compromised immune system, altered production of cytokines, hyperglycemia, and negative nitrogen balance.
- Risk for injury related to fractures from osteoporosis.
- Impaired skin integrity related to loss of tissue strength with increase capillary fragility.
- Ineffective sexuality patterns related to loss of libido in females secondary to elevated androgens; impotence and decreased libido in males secondary excess cortisol.

Planning and Implementation

The patient with hypercortisolism due to Cushing's disease or Cushing's syndrome presents with a complex number of problems. Priorities of care include fluid and electrolyte imbalances, which require careful monitoring for fluid excess and symptoms of electrolyte imbalance. The nurse must be prepared to monitor the patient for symptoms of heart failure and implement the medical plan of care, which may include diuretic, antihypertensive, and cardiotonic drug therapy. Providing assistance with activities of daily living is paramount,

Safety First 1

Preventing Falls in Patients with Cushing's Disease

Safety measures to prevent falls must be implemented, because the patient is prone to fractures related to osteoporosis. Assistance with ambulation and getting in and out of bed should be included in the plan of care. Discharge planning needs to include measures to maintain a safe environment at home, including adequate lighting, clutter-free environment, and use of nonskid slippers. It is important to ensure that the patient's vision is normal or corrective lenses are available. The patient should have ongoing monitoring for fatigue, weakness, and other factors that may predispose to a fall.

because the patient may be short of breath and have activity intolerance. Weakness may also be due to hypokalemia, which requires cardiac monitoring and potassium replacement.

Special attention must be given to prevent the patient from acquiring an infection. The compromised immune system makes the patient with hypercortisolism susceptible to opportunistic or bacterial infections. Even minor wounds and infections heal slowly. The patient may not respond normally to an infection with increased body temperature and pulse rate. Even a low-grade temperature may be a red flag for the patient with hypercortisolism. The patient and significant others should be instructed to assess and report any symptoms of infection. Principles of medical and surgical asepsis must be implemented as indicated when caring for the patient.

An altered body image is of great concern for these patients. It is not uncommon for the patient's physical appearance to change to the point at which they are not recognizable. Weight gain between 25 and 100 pounds, acne, excess body hair redistribution of fat, and striae on abdomen and breast completely changes the physical appearance. Encourage the patient to explore his or her feelings. Thorough explanations about the disease and its prognosis can help the patient deal with his or her feelings.

Helping the patient to understand the cause for weight gain is important. The appetite is described as excessive by most patients. Instruction in healthy eating and measures to decrease portion size and replacement of excess eating with lower calorie snacks is important. Exercise to tolerance should be encouraged. The patient should be told that it is likely that body changes will be reversible with treatment. In addition, the patient may have to deal with cortisol induced diabetes (see chapter 57).

Pharmacology

No drugs are available to successfully suppress pituitary ACTH secretion. Ketoconazole, metyrapone, and aminoglutethimide are expensive drugs, which have been shown to have limited success in treating Cushing's disease (Aron et. al., 2004a). The initial treatment of choice is selective transsphenoidal resection with tumor removal to correct the hypercortisolism. Radiotherapy may be prescribed. In extreme cases, bilateral adrenalectomy has been done when all other therapies have failed. Lifelong hormone replacement therapy is required following the surgery.

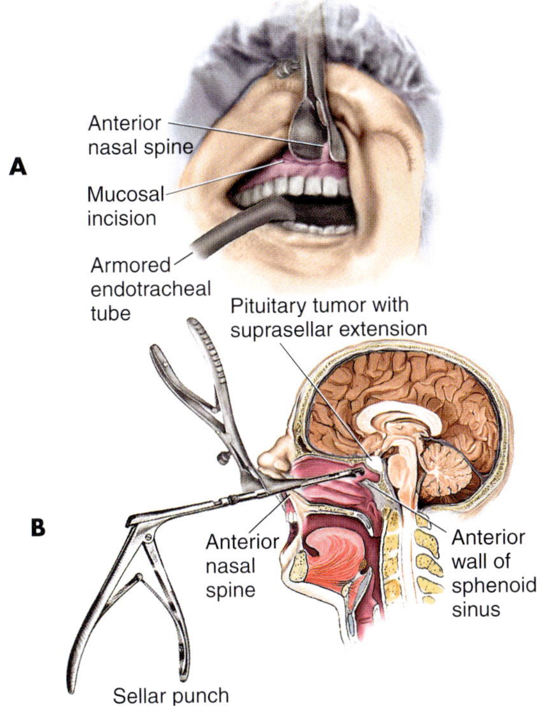

Figure 56-3 Transsphenoidal approach to hypophysectomy: A. A bivalved speculum is inserted, B. The floor of the sphenoid is removed with a sellar punch.

Surgery

Transsphenoidal hypophysectomy is the treatment of choice for most pituitary adenomas (Figure 56-3). It entails a horizontal incision at the intersection of the inner part of the upper lip and the gingival extending bilaterally from the center of the upper lip and gum. From this incision, instrumentation is made underneath the nasal cartilage and splenoid sinus up to the floor of the sella turcica, where excision of the adenoma can be made (Ghorayeh, 2005). Following removal of the tumor, the incision is closed and fascia or muscle obtained from the abdomen or a muscle is implanted at the surgical site to prevent leakage of cerebrospinal fluid (CSF) and assist in healing of the wound. The nasal passage is usually packed for 24 to 48 hours, and a gauze dressing is secured under the nose to absorb drainage.

A newer approach for removal of a pituitary tumor is the endonasal approach, which is considered to be less invasive, requiring no incision. A small endoscope is inserted through the nostril and into the skull base, through the splenoid sinus and into the sella turcica, where visualization of the tumor takes place. Overall recovery time is reported to be reduced.

The initial preoperative workup will usually be done on an outpatient basis. The patient should have a well-documented head-to-toe assessment to use as a baseline. Preoperative teaching includes informing the patient about incision sites, including both the oral incision and the donor site for removing the fascia or muscle. Discomfort regarding the packing should be explained. The necessity of receiving a liquid diet initially and use of toothettes for cleaning the teeth should be included in the teaching plan. Instructions related to deep-breathing exercises should be emphasized, along with information regarding the need for breathing through the mouth because the nostrils will be temporarily blocked. Leg exercise to prevent clot formation should be demonstrated. Diagrams and information regarding the actual procedure should be provided by the surgeon.

Following surgery the patient is positioned supine with the head of the bed elevated 30°. In addition to monitoring and ensuring that the patient has respiratory and circulatory stability postoperatively, the following potential problems should be addressed. Symptoms of meningitis or encephalitis should be addressed immediately. The patient should be monitored for signs and symptoms of infection. Clear drainage from the nasal passages or frequent swallowing (postnasally) is suggestive of a CSF leak. The patient is supplied a drip pad under the nose, which is changed as needed. Drainage amounts will vary among patients. Usually the drainage decreases within 24 hours. A CSF leak is suspected if there is an appearance of a halo ring on the dressing or if the clear drainage is positive for glucose. Lab analysis to verify that the drainage is CSF should be carried out. If it is determined that the patient has a CSF leak, bed rest with head of bed elevated should be implemented. Although, normally the leak will cease spontaneously, the patient will be at a higher risk for infection, therefore antibiotics are usually ordered. Ongoing assessment for clinical manifestations of infection is warranted. In rare situations, the patient will need additional surgery to repair the leakage site in the sella turcica. If fascia has been removed for packing, the donor site should be assessed for signs and symptoms of infection. Because the nasal passage is packed, the patient will breathe though the mouth. Frequent mouth and lip care is necessary. Liquids help to decrease the discomfort from dry mouth.

An anterior transsphenoidal hypophysectomy may cause edema or trauma to the posterior pituitary. Clinical manifestations of diabetes insipidus should be assessed. The patient's fluid status should be carefully monitored. Intake and output and daily weight are important. Neurological assessment, including cranial nerves, should be assessed initially and every hour as indicated by unit policy. Changes in neurological status may indicate an increase in intracranial pressure or other complications related to surgery.

The patient is usually discharged 48 to 72 hours after surgery. The patient should be instructed to avoid lifting, straining, stooping, blowing nose, swimming, aerobic exercise, all of which could cause pressure in the sella turcica and disrupt the healing process The nurse should stress the importance of follow-up with the endocrinologist as prescribed. Due to surgical trauma (Aron, et al., 2004b), a small percentage of patients may develop syndrome of inappropriate antidiuretic hormone (SIADH) 5 to 10 days after surgery (Prather, Forsyth, Russell, & Wagner, 2003). The patient and family should be instructed to report symptoms of SIADH including confusion, headache unrelieved by typical analgesics, and lethargy. A serum sodium and urine osmolality are used to diagnose SIADH. Serum sodium will be elevated and urine osmolality decreased. The patient should also be alerted to report symptoms of diabetes insipidus, including increased urine output, light yellow urine, and thirst. Symptoms of infection should also be reported. An antibiotic is usually prescribed for several days postsurgery.

At the follow-up appointment, pituitary hormone levels will be determined. Often patients will have transient secondary adrenocortical insufficiency requiring glucocorticoid support until the hypothalamic-pituitary-adrenal (HPA) axis recovers. If there has been total removal of the anterior pituitary, the patient will require lifelong replacement of thyroid hormone and glucocorticoids. Males will also need testosterone replacement (Aron, et al., 2004a). Follow-up MRIs will be used to monitor patient's progress.

When hypercortisolism is caused by an adrenal secreting tumor, a partial or complete removal of the adrenal gland (adrenalectomy) is usually the treatment of choice. An adrenalectomy may be done by laparoscope procedure or general surgery. General postoperative nursing care is required in addition to careful monitoring for and treatment for hypoadrenalism. If bilateral adrenalectomy is performed, the patient will require immediate and lifetime replacement of glucocorticoids and mineralocorticoids. When unilateral adrenalectomy is performed, glucocorticoid and mineralocorticoid replacement will be needed until the remaining adrenal gland regains full function.

Evaluation of Outcomes

Potential patient outcomes for each of the example nursing diagnoses for the patient with Cushing's disease (or Cushing's syndrome) are:

- Activity intolerance related to congestive heart failure, and weakness due to hypercortisolism, which causes proximal muscle weakness, decreased muscle mass, and hypokalemia. Patient will report increase in strength and will demonstrate increased participation in activities of daily living.
- Disturbed body image related to appearance changes. Patient will discuss the cause for change in body image.
- Risk for infection related to altered resistance to infection due to compromised immune system, altered production of cytokines, hyperglycemia, and negative nitrogen balance. Patient will identify ways to avoid contacting an infection.
- Risk for injury related to fractures from osteoporosis. Patient will demonstrate safety measures to help prevent a fracture.
- Impaired skin integrity related to loss of tissue strength with increased capillary fragility. Patient will maintain intact skin and not experience skin breakdown.
- Ineffective sexuality patterns related to loss of libido in females secondary to elevated androgens; impotence and decreased libido in males secondary to excess cortisol. Patient will share feelings related to altered sexuality.

HYPOSECRETION OF THE ANTERIOR PITUITARY GLAND

Hypofunction of the pituitary gland occurs with decreased hormonal activity of one or more of the pituitary hormones. When all cell types in the pituitary gland fail to synthesize and secrete hormones it is called **panhypopituitarism.**

Etiology

There are a broad number of causes for hypopituitarism, including idiopathic conditions. In the event of tumors, there are space-occupying lesions that can cause the hypopituitarism. In addition, there can be ischemic damage to the pituitary from infarctions, traumatic head injuries, and infections. There are also infiltrative diseases (e.g., sarcoidosis, hemochromatosis, and histiocytosis X) and immunological causes for the hypofunction of the pituitary gland. There can be iatrogenic causes, as well, such as surgical and radiation therapy (Aron, et al., 2004b).

Pathophysiology

Dysfunction may be caused by destruction of the anterior pituitary gland or a secondary event resulting in a shortage of hypothalamic stimulatory factors. The deficiency of stimulation to the anterior pituitary gland causes clinical manifestations congruent with an alteration in the normal function of the pituitary gland.

Assessment with Clinical Manifestations

Clinical manifestations of hypopituitarism occur in relation to the hyposecretion of the pituitary hormones, which in addition to secreting GH, controls the secretion of hormones by the ovaries, gonads, adrenal, thyroid, and parathyroid glands. Hyposecretion of GH causes decreased growth in children. In children and adults, it is associated with a diminished sense of well-being and altered level of health-related life. Hypogonadism causes amenorrhea in women and impotence in men Thyroid-stimulating hormone (TSH) deficiency causes hypothyroid symptoms similar to those of primary hypothyroidism. ACTH deficiency causes symptoms similar to those in primary adrenal failure. Often the signs of hypopituitarism are subtle and require careful attention. The patient may be mildly overweight. The face may have fine wrinkles, and the skin is fine, smooth, and pale. Pubic and body hair may be sparse, and atrophy of the genitalia may be noted. In more severe cases, the patient may have orthostatic hypotension, bradycardia, and a decreased in muscle strength (Aron, et al., 2004a).

Planning and Implementation

The nursing care plan should be focused on assessment of the patient for signs and symptoms of pituitary dysfunction. Initially the plan of care involves preparation of the patient for the test to determine the cause of the hypofunction of the pituitary gland. After the cause is identified, the patient is prepared for treatment. This may involve pituitary surgery or treatment of underlying disease. In most all incidences, hormone replacement therapy will be a priority of care. A plan of care should evolve that assists the patient to know about the importance of compliance with hormone replacement therapy.

POSTERIOR PITUITARY DISORDERS

The posterior pituitary gland secretes antidiuretic hormone (ADH). Problems can arise either because of hyposecretion of the antidiuretic hormone, which causes diabetes insipidus, or hypersecretion of ADH, which is known as SIADH. Both disorders have a pronounced effect on fluid balance.

Diabetes Insipidus

Diabetes insipidus is a disorder that occurs due either to an insufficiency of ADH, which is referred to as central diabetes insipidus, or loss of sensitivity of the nephrons of the kidney to the circulating ADH.

Etiology

Central diabetes insipidus is common following surgery for tumors of the hypothalamus or pituitary gland. Other causes are hypopituitarism, tumors, aneurysms, thrombosis, infections, and immunological disorders of the hypothalamus and pituitary gland.

Pathophysiology

When ADH is insufficient, the kidney is not adequately able to concentrate urine and there is immediate excretion of large amount of urine. When the person is conscious, thirst will be experienced because the osmoreceptors in the hypothalamus are stimulated. In turn, the patient will have induced polydipsia. Output can be more than 20 liters per day.

Assessment with Clinical Manifestations

Polyuria with daily urine ranging from 2.5 to 20, and thirst with strong preference for ice water are the two primary symptoms of diabetes insipidus. The conscious patient will experience extreme thirst, thereby drinking and helping to prevent dehydration. In an unconscious patient or patient who cannot drink, severe dehydration and hypovolemia may occur.

Diagnostic Tests

Urine osmolarity decreases to 50 to 100 mOsm/kg; serum osmolality is elevated greater than 300 mOsm/kg. Urine specific gravity will range between 1.001 and 1.005. Hypernatremia, hypercalcemia, and hypokalemia may be present (Daniels, 2003).

Nursing Diagnoses

Based on the information gathered, examples of nursing diagnoses in the patient with diabetes insipidus may include the following:

- Deficient fluid volume related to excess diuresis due to decreased ADH.
- Fatigue related to weakness secondary to hypokalemia.

Planning and Implementation

Because patients may have up to 20 liters of urinary output daily, volume replacement is a priority. Dehydration is treated by administering a hypotonic solution, such as NaCl O.45%. The flow rate is usually ordered to match the urinary output. Additional fluids may be needed to treat dehydration and hypovolemia. ADH replacement is a necessity to help resolve the fluid imbalance and to maintain fluid balance (Ferri, 2005).

Pharmacology

Aqueous pitressin (Vasopressin) may be administered subcutaneously in relation to the amount of urinary output in hospitalized patients. Desmopressin acetate a synthetic analogue of vasopressin is administered intranasally as a metered dose nasal spray or be taken orally. These agents usually control the polydipsia and polyuria in patients with central diabetes insipidus (Broyles, Reiss, & Evans, 2007). Desmopressin may be ordered for discharge maintenance if diabetes insipidus does not resolve.

Evaluation of Outcomes

Potential patient outcomes for each of the example nursing diagnoses for the patient with diabetes insipidus are:

- Deficient fluid volume related to excess diuresis due to decreased ADH. Patient will have restoration of fluid volume and electrolyte balance.
- Fatigue related to hypokalemia. Patient will demonstrate improved energy and will maintain a normal serum potassium.

Syndrome of Inappropriate Antidiuretic Hormone

Another abnormality of the posterior pituitary gland is hypersecretion of ADH, known as SIADH.

Etiology

Conditions that cause SIADH include malignant lung disease and tumors such as lymphoma and sarcoma in different organs of the body. Many central nervous system (CNS) disorders, such as infections, and trauma cause the disease. Other causes are medications that stimulate ADH release, such as thiazides, phenothiazines, vincristine, opioids, severe pain, and emotional stress. Certain endocrine diseases, such as adrenal insufficiency and hypopituitarism, are associated with SIADH.

Pathophysiology

In SIADH, the posterior pituitary gland continues to release ADH even though the normal stimulants (an increase in osmolality and hypovolemia) are not present. When plasma levels of ADH are high, hyponatremia and hypoosmolality occur. The hyponatremia, which occurs with SIADH, can lead to cerebral edema, which is the primary cause for the clinical manifestations of the illness. The urine is usually inappropriately concentrated.

Assessment with Clinical Manifestations

The patient with SIADH must be assessed for neurological symptoms that occur as a result of cerebral edema, which is related to the hypoosmolality of hyponatremia. Symptoms occurring early include headache, weakness, muscle changes, and some weight gain. Later the patient will be observed to have personality changes, hostility, and sluggish reflexes. Nausea, vomiting, and diarrhea may also be present. An impending crisis may be predicted if the patient develops confusion, lethargy, and change in respirations. When serum sodium reaches 110 mmol/L, the nurse should anticipate that seizures may occur. Additional symptoms that may occur include headache, confusion, irritability, somnolence, seizures, and coma.

Diagnostic Tests

The primary forms of diagnostic tests for SIADH are serum and urine studies. Hyponatremia and low serum osmolality (less than 280 mosm/kg) confirm the condition. And, the urine is inappropriately concentrated (greater than 100 mOsm/kg; urinary sodium is greater than 20 mmoL/d) (Daniels, 2003).

Nursing Diagnoses

Based on the information gathered, examples of nursing diagnoses in the patient with SIADH may include the following:

- Excess fluid volume related to SIADH.
- Disturbed sensory perception related to cerebral edema.

Planning and Implementation

Identifying and eliminating the underlying cause are the initial steps of treatment. Fluid restriction of 600 to 1,200 mL per day is the simplest form of treatment. Special attention must be given to nonliquid fluid intake. In the event that the patient is unable to adhere to fluid restriction, demeclocycline, an antibiotic that decreases the availability of ADH, may be prescribed. When demeclocycline is administered, water restriction is not advocated. In other situations, sodium supplements are administered along with a loop diuretic to increase urinary solute excretion (Gardner & Greenspan, 2004). Intravenous NaCl 0.9% may also be prescribed.

When the patient has acute symptomatic hyponatremia, intravenous NaCl 3% may be the treatment of choice. NaCl 3% must be administered cautiously. Rate of administration should not exceed 50 mL/hour. Rapid administration may cause fluid over load and congestive heart failure. Too rapid correction of hyponatremia may lead to central pontine myelinolysis. (Gardner & Greenspan, 2004).

Evaluation of Outcomes

Potential patient outcomes for each of the example nursing diagnoses for the patient with SIADH are:

- Excess fluid volume related to SIADH. Patient's serum sodium level will be within normal levels.
- Disturbed sensory perception related to cerebral edema. Patient will have a normal neurological assessment.

HYPOSECRETION OF THE ADRENAL GLAND

Adrenal insufficiency occurs because of one of two major reasons. Primary adrenal insufficiency results from destruction or dysfunction of the cortex of the adrenal gland. Secondary adrenal insufficiency results from deficient

ACTH secretion due to dysfunction of the pituitary-hypothalamic axis or a disorder of pituitary gland.

Epidemiology

There are five cases of Addison's disease per 100,000 population. In addition, there is a 2:1 ratio of women to men (Ferri, 2005).

Etiology

Primary adrenal insufficiency, also known as Addison's disease, is rare. The leading cause is autoimmune disease. Other causes include adrenal hemorrhage, infections, metastatic cancer or lymphoma, amyloidosis, hemochromatosis, congenital adrenal hyperplasia, familial glucocorticoid deficiency, and hypoplasia. Certain drugs, such as ketoconazole, metyrapone, aminoglutethimide, and etomidate, have been associated with the disease. Though *Mycobacterium tuberculosis* was the leading infection in the past to cause adrenal insufficiency, in the United States today histoplasmosis is the leading infectious cause (Aron, et al., 2004a). Tuberculosis continues to be the leading cause of adrenal insufficiency worldwide. Thirty percent of patients with AIDS develop adrenal insufficiency (Ferri, 2005).

Pathophysiology

Addison's disease occurs insidiously over weeks and even months. By the time of diagnosis there is often a loss of 90 percent of the cortices of both adrenal glands. The gradual loss of adrenal function may go unnoticed because both mineralcorticoids and glucocorticoids continue to be secreted from a reserve. When the basal reserve is depleted chronic manifestations of adrenal insufficiency will manifest. An acute crisis can occur if the patient is predisposed to stressful situations, such as trauma, surgery, and the like. When the adrenals are affected by hemorrhage, both glucocorticoid and mineralocorticoid secretion is loss causing an acute adrenal crisis (Aron, et al., 2004a).

Assessment with Clinical Manifestations

Clinical manifestations of chronic adrenal insufficiency include weakness, fatigue, anorexia, GI symptoms, orthostatic hypotension, hypotension, salt craving, and hyperpigmentation. Hyperpigmentation and hyperkalemia occur only in primary hypoadrenalism. Weight loss and malnutrition can occur due to diminished appetite and nausea. The patient with secondary adrenal insufficiency may also have deficiencies in testosterone, GH, thyroxine, and ADH.

Secondary adrenal insufficiency can occur due to tumors of the hypothalamus or pituitary gland resulting in deficiency of ACTH (Table 56-2). Removal of a tumor from the pituitary gland may result in permanent deficiency in ACTH, causing cortisol and adrenal androgen deficiency. Usually in secondary adrenal insufficiency, aldosterone function is not affected. Another common cause of secondary adrenal insufficiency is the rapid withdrawal of glucocorticoid therapy. Twenty milligrams of hydrocortisone, or its equivalent, taken for longer than 7 to 10 days, has the potential for suppressing the HPA axis. If the glucocorticoid is stopped abruptly, the patient may experience an adrenal crisis (Hudak, Morton, Galle, & Fontaine, 2005).

> **Red Flag**
>
> **Acute Adrenal Crisis**
>
> Acute adrenal crisis is a serious life-threatening complication. Minor illness, stress, trauma, or pregnancy may be the precipitating event.

Diagnostic Tests

In addition to the tests in Table 56-2, suppression and stimulation tests may be done to differentiate between primary and secondary insufficiency. The management of both of these types of insufficiency is linked closely to the outcomes of the diagnostic tests.

TABLE 56-2 Comparison of Clinical Manifestations of Primary and Secondary Adrenal Insufficiency

CLINICAL MANIFESTATION	PRIMARY	SECONDARY
Skin	Skin	Absent because there is a deficiency in ACTH
Hyperpigmentation due to an increase in ACTH secretion and melanocyte stimulation	Present	
Loss of axillary and pubic hair due to decrease in androgens	May occur	
Cardiovascular Hypotension with orthostatic symptoms (lower peripheral resistance)	Present	Usually not present because aldosterone secretion is usually not deficiency
Occasionally syncope due to loss of mineralocorticoid activity		Hypotension may occur in acute situations
Neurological: Anxiety and mental irritability		
GI	Present	Present
Anorexia, nausea, vomiting		
Musculoskeletal myalgias, arthralgias	Present	May occur
Reproductive amenorrhea	Often present	
Hyponatremia	Present	May occur due to water retention
Hyperkalemia	Present	Not present
Hypoglycemia	May be provoked by fasting, infection, fever, and so on	Usually not present
Deficiencies in thyroxin, testosterone, and GH	Not present because pituitary deficiency is not the problem	Possible if pituitary or hypothalamus dysfunction is present
Plasma cortisol less than 5 mg/dL at 8 a.m.	Yes	Yes
ACTH Level	Greater than 200 pg/mL	Low or normal
Antibodies	Antiadrenal antibodies present in autoimmune Addison's disease	

Adapted from Aron., D., Finding, J. Tyrell, B. (2004). Hypothalamus and pituitary. In F.S. Greenspan & D. G. Gardner (Eds.), Basic and clinical endocrinology *(pp. 537–542). St. Louis, MO: Lange Medical Books.*

Nursing Diagnoses

Based on the information gathered, examples of nursing diagnoses in the patient with adrenal insufficiency may include the following:

- Activity intolerance related to weakness and fatigue.
- Deficient knowledge related to disease and treatment.
- Risk for injury related to syncope from hypotension.
- Deficient fluid volume related to sodium depletion.

Planning and Implementation

The patient who presents in an adrenal crisis must be provided with aggressive care. Major goals include restoration of extracellular fluid volume, reversal of shock, and replacement of corticosteroids and mineralcorticoids. Monitor cardiovascular and respiratory status, urinary output, and neurological status every hour. Provide fluids and electrolytes to restore fluid balance and correct hypoglycemia. Electrocardiogram (ECG) monitoring should be instituted to assess the cardiac effects of hyperkalemia and hypercalcemia. Hyperkalemia and acidosis are usually corrected with replacement of fluid volume and cortisol levels. The electrolytes and creatinine should be monitor daily and as needed. Environmental stress should be minimized. Dietary assessment should be completed and caloric nutrients provided as tolerated. Nausea and anorexia should resolve with the normalizing of cortisol levels.

Goals

The following are goals for the patient with adrenal insufficiency:

- The patient will state the rationale for lifelong therapy.
- The patient will state the rationale for increasing corticosteroid dosage in the event of illness or stress.
- The patient will give the rationale for seeking medical assistance in the event that oral medication cannot be taken during time of illness.
- The patient will be normotensive.
- The patient will have a normal electrolyte profile.
- The patient will have access to a medical alert identification.

Pharmacology

Patients who have adrenal insufficiency need to be taught to adhere carefully to medication plan for hydrocortisone and fludrocortisone replacement. They will need an increase in dosage during stress or illness. With minor illness, the cortisol dose should be increased to 60 to 80 mg/day. The patient should avoid fasting and may need to increase his or her salt intake. It is recommended that the patient with adrenal insufficiency keep a kit with hydrocortisone for self-injection in an emergency and in the event that oral intake is not possible. The patient should wear a medical alert bracelet at all times. Family members need to be taught emergency care (Broyles, et al., 2007).

The patient who has adrenal insufficiency due to an ACTH insufficiency will require only glucocorticoid replacement. Mineralocorticoid replacement is not necessary. Patients who are receiving exogenous corticosteroids should be instructed to taper the dosage gradually, decreasing the dosage daily to allow the adrenal gland to return to normal function. This will help to prevent a secondary adrenal insufficiency. Patients treated with corticosteroids should be monitored for osteoporosis. A minimum maintenance dose is recommended because research shows there is a correlation between high corticosteroid dose and bone loss.

Evaluation of Outcomes

Potential patient outcomes for each of the example nursing diagnoses for the patient with adrenal insufficiency are:

- Activity intolerance related to weakness and fatigue. Patient will identify measures to conserve energy.
- Deficient knowledge related to disease and treatment. Patient will discuss pertinent information concerning the disease and treatment.
- Risk for injury related to syncope from hypotension. Patient will identify and implement measures to prevent syncope episodes.
- Deficient fluid volume related to sodium depletion. Patient will have normal fluid and electrolyte balance.

HYPERSECRETION OF THE ADRENAL GLAND (HYPERALDOSTERONISM)

An increased stimulation of the adrenal glands may lead to hyperaldosteronism. There are a variety of causes for this disorder and there are serious implications for patients with hyperaldosteronism.

Epidemiology

One to two percent of the patients who have hypertension have primary aldosteronism. It occurs more often in females (Ferri, 2005).

Etiology

Primary aldosteronism may be due to a unilateral adrenal adenoma or bilateral hyperplasia of the adrenal glands. Sixty percent of the cases are caused by an aldosterone producing adenoma. Other causes are aldosterone-producing carcinoma, glucocorticoid-suppressible hyperaldosteronism, and idiopathic hyperaldosteronism, which cause more than 30 percent of the cases (Ferri, 2005).

Pathophysiology

Involvement of the zona glomerulosa causes an increase production of aldosterone, which initiates a cascade of events that includes retention of sodium and fluid and potassium depletion. With the expansion of extracellular fluid, there is an increase in cardiac output and subsequent hypertension. As mineralocorticoid excess continues, there is an increase in total peripheral vascular resistance that contributes to the problem of hypertension (Huether, 2004).

Assessment with Clinical Manifestations

There are no characteristic physical manifestations that occur with excessive mineralocorticoids. Patients usually are diagnosed with mild to severe hypertension. Some patients may have only an elevation in diastolic pressure. Their primary complaint may be that of nonspecific loss of energy, weakness, and lassitude. In situations in which potassium depletion is more severe, dysrhythmias, decrease in gastric motility, polyuria, polydipsia, and paresthesia may be reported. Because the most common cause of hypokalemia in patients with hypertension is diuretic therapy, diuretic therapy would need to be discontinued for up to three weeks to accurately evaluate the serum potassium. Other causes of hypertension and hypokalemia must be eliminated when diagnosing hyperaldosteronism. Excessive ingestion of real licorice, oral contraceptives, Cushing's syndrome, and renal vascular disease can cause hypertension and hypokalemia (Burl, Schambelan, & Lo, 2004).

Diagnostic Tests

Urinary aldosterone excretion over a 24-hour period best measures aldosterone production. Plasma aldosterone levels should be drawn around 8:00 a.m. while the patient is supine after overnight recumbency. A plasma renin test must be done at the same time. For both urinary and serum testing for aldosterone, it is important that the patient receive normal salt intake with NaCl supplementation, because with any decrease in salt intake aldosterone production will increase causing a high serum aldosterone level and increase urinary excretion. A low plasma renin (less than 5 mcg/dL) with a 24-hour urinary test for aldosterone greater than 20 mcg/dL indicates hyperaldosteronism A plasma aldosterone greater than 20 mcg/dL supports a diagnosis of adrenal adenoma (Burl, et al., 2004).

Following a positive serum and urine test for hyperaldosteronism, a CT scan of the adrenals can identify the presence of an adenoma with 80 percent success. In the event that the CT scan is negative, adrenal vein catheterization for aldosterone or radioisotope test can be utilized for confirming diagnosis.

Nursing Diagnoses

Based on the information gathered, examples of nursing diagnoses in the patient with hyperaldosteronism may include the following:

- Fatigue related to weakness secondary to hypokalemia.
- Activity intolerance related to weakness secondary to hypokalemia.
- Decreased cardiac output related to alteration in cardiac contraction and dysrhythmias secondary to hypokalemia.
- Excess fluid volume related to sodium retention due to excess aldosterone.

Planning and Implementation

Because hypokalemia can cause cardiac conduction abnormalities, the patient with hyperaldosteronism needs to have continuous cardiac monitoring. Serum potassium levels are monitored sometimes as often as every four to six hours. Because the body cannot conserve potassium, it has to be replaced daily. Cardiac and respiratory assessment should be completed every four hours or more often as needed. Monitor vital signs in relation to activity. Daily weights and intake and output are important interventions for assessing fluid balance. Provide assistance with activities of daily living since the patient may have increasing muscle weakness related to the hypokalemia. Assess for signs and symptoms of hypertension as indicated. Lying, sitting, and standing blood pressure monitoring may be necessary if the patient has symptoms of orthostatic hypotension, which may occur with some antihypertensive medications. Discharge instructions for the patient are shown in the Patient Playbook feature.

> **PATIENT PLAYBOOK**
>
> **Discharge Plan for Postoperative Unilateral Adrenalectomy**
>
> The nurse should discuss the following as discharge criteria for the patient:
>
> - Discuss specific symptoms of infection (fever, fatigue, or diaphoresis) for the patient to report to their health care provider.
> - Instruct the patient to monitor their blood pressure on a regular basis (at least weekly) and to document the date and time.
> - Educate the patient regarding the symptoms of hypertension (e.g., headache, ringing of the ears).
> - Describe the clinical manifestations of electrolyte imbalances, particularly hypokalemia (e.g., muscle weakness, fatigue).

Pharmacology

Patients with aldosterone-producing adenomas are treated with spironolactone until the blood pressure and serum K^+ are normal. Spironolactone blocks the mineralocorticoid receptor, reducing extracellular fluid volume, and promotes potassium retention. Patients diagnosed with aldosterone-producing adenoma are recommended to have a unilateral adrenalectomy if there are no contraindications. Following a unilateral adrenalectomy, blood pressure and electrolytes must be monitored frequently. Several months may elapse before blood pressure and electrolytes, particularly potassium becomes normal.

Evaluation of Outcomes

Potential patient outcomes for each of the example nursing diagnoses for the patient with hyperaldosteronism are:

- Fatigue related to weakness secondary to hypokalemia. Patient will demonstrate improved energy; potassium level will be normal.
- Activity intolerance related to weakness secondary to hypokalemia. Patient will daily increase participation in activities of daily.
- Decreased cardiac output, related to alteration in cardiac contraction and dysrhythmias secondary to hypokalemia. Patient will have normal cardiac output as indicated with normal vital signs and sinus rhythm.
- Excess fluid volume related to sodium retention due to excess aldosterone. Patient will have absence of signs and symptoms of fluid volume excess.

Pheochromocytoma

A pheochromocytoma is a tumor of the adrenal gland that secretes catecholamines. It is affecting and causes severe hypertension with those patients that are afflicted with this disorder.

Red Flag

Diagnosing Pheochromocytomas

Consider the possibility of pheochromocytomas when the patient has severe hypertension and suspicious symptoms, such as, palpitations, diaphoresis, headache lasting minutes to hours, and chest or abdominal pain that is not explainable. More than one third of patients who have pheochromocytomas die from a stroke or cardiac arrhythmia prior to diagnosis.

Epidemiology

Though considered a rare disorder, pheochromocytomas are found in less than 0.1 percent of hypertensive individuals; autopsy suggests a higher incidence. A rare endocrine disorder, pheochromocytomas occur in two patients per million people annually. Pheochromocytomas occur most often in the fourth or fifth decade; males are more frequently affected.

Patients who should be screened for pheochromocytoma include young hypertensives, patients with symptoms of catecholamine excess, marked lability of blood pressure, family history, shock or severe hypotensive episodes with surgery, anesthesia, or antihypertensive drugs. The signs and symptoms result from persistent hypersecretion of catecholamines (epinephrine or norepinephrine) by the tumor.

Assessment with Clinical Manifestations

Most adult patients have paroxysmal symptoms that may last minutes or hours. Symptoms begin abruptly and slowly subside. Severe headache, palpitations, and profuse sweating are the most common symptoms. In addition, patients can have palpitations, chest discomfort, anxiety, visual disturbances, constipation, weight loss, and cold hands or feet. Greater than 30 percent of pheochromocytomas cause a fatal cardiac arrhythmia or stroke prior to diagnosis.

Diagnostic Tests

A single 24-hour urine specimen to measure catecholamines, specifically metanephrines, is the most common and sensitive test for diagnosing pheochromocytoma. Typically, patients with pheochromocytomas have elevations of catecholamines or metanephrines that are more than twice normal, particularly after a paroxysmal episode.

CT scan is used to detect adrenal pheochromocytomas. If not found on the adrenal gland, CT scanning is used to scan the whole pelvis, abdomen, and chest. MRI is not as sensitive but is considered a safer test because it can be done without contrast.

Nursing Diagnoses

Based on the information gathered, examples of nursing diagnoses in the patient with pheochromocytoma may include the following:

- Risk for injury related to hypertension leading to stroke and cardiovascular events.
- Anxiety related to excess catecholamines.

Planning and Implementation

Monitoring the patient's vital signs along with neurovascular, cardiac, and respiratory assessment is a priority in caring for the patient with a pheochromocytoma. Because patients may experience orthostatic hypotension, they must be instructed to rise slowly and recognize symptoms to avoid falls.

Preparing the patient psychologically and physically for upcoming surgery should be included in the plan of care. Patients need to be instructed in the rationale and side effects of medications used to control symptoms prior to surgery. The patient should have blood pressure readings in lying, sitting, and standing positions as the blood pressure medications are increased.

Postoperative complications include shock and cardiovascular collapse. Large volumes of saline or colloids may be needed to regain extracellular volume. In some incidences intravenous norepinephrine may be required. Blood glucose should be monitored. Hypoglycemia may be prevented by administering dextrose solutions.

Goals

Goals for patients with pheochromocytoma are:

- The patient will demonstrate blood pressure monitoring.
- The patient will state plan to monitor blood pressure daily and report abnormal findings.
- The patient will convey an understanding for follow-up within designated times following surgery for a 24-hour urine collection to determine fractionated catecholamines, metaphrines, and creatinine.
- Abnormal levels of catecholamines and elevation of blood pressure may indicate that the tumor has recurred and indicates a need for more thorough work-up.

Pharmacology

The risks involved with pheochromocytoma surgery are decreased by the administration of alpha-adrenergic blocking drugs. Calcium channel blockers and alpha-adrenergic blockers, such as phenoxybenzamine and angiotensin-converting enzyme (ACE) inhibitors, each may play a role in treating the hypertension occurring with a pheochromocytoma. A beta-adrenergic blocker, such as propranolol, is used for treating the symptoms, such as tachycardia, palpitations, and flushing.

Surgery

The treatment of choice is laparoscopic removal of the tumor(s) under 6 cm in diameter. With laparoscopic surgery, the patient generally has a shorter time for eating to resume, reduced postoperative pain, and fewer hospitalization days. A laparotomy may be necessary if the tumor is large and invasive.

The major postoperative complication from pheochromocytoma surgery is shock and hypoglycemia. To treat shock, large volumes of intravenous normal saline or colloids may be used. Some incidences require intravenous norepinephrine. Hypoglycemia is prevented by postoperative infusion of dextrose 5% in water at 100 mL/hour.

Evaluation of Outcomes

Potential patient outcomes for each of the example nursing diagnoses for the patient with pheochromocytoma are:

- Risk for injury related to hypertension leading to stroke and cardiovascular events. Patient's blood pressure will be within safe parameters.
- Anxiety related to excess catecholamines. Patient will report a decrease in symptoms of anxiety.

THYROID DISORDERS

Thyroid hormones influence all major body systems, thus alteration in function can have a widespread effect on the body. Patients may present with symptoms of thyroid deficiency or excess, which affect cardiac and neurological function as well as overall energy. Other patients may have thyroid enlargement. Complications of thyroid disease may be the first symptom to be identified, such as exophthalmos that occurs with Graves' disease or cardiac problems, which occur with hypothyroidism. It is not uncommon for the patient to have cardiac or mental changes because of an excess or deficit in thyroid hormone. The diagnosis may be difficult because symptoms are often insipidus and ill-defined (Greenspan, 2004).

Hypersecretion of the Thyroid Gland

Frequently seen in primary care, 0.5 percent of Americans have hyperthyroidism. Though not the same, hyperthyroidism and thyrotoxicosis are often used interchangeably. Hyperthyroidism refers to the continuous secretion of thyroid hormones by the thyroid gland with resultant abnormal elevation of triiodothyronine (T_3) and thyroxine (T_4) hormones and an abnormally low TSH level. Thyrotoxicosis is a term used for the acceleration of metabolism with toxic manifestations that occur when thyroid hormones are extremely elevated. Subclinical hyperthyroidism is a term used to define a situation in which the patient has a low TSH, normal free T_4, and free T_3 levels with few or no clinical manifestations (White, 2004).

Epidemiology

Graves' disease (diffuse toxic goiter) is the most common cause of thyrotoxicosis. This disorder occurs most often in women between and during the second through fourth decade.

Etiology

Diseases that cause overproduction of thyroid hormones include Graves' disease (diffuse toxic goiter), toxic multinodular goiter, follicular adenoma, and pituitary adenoma. Destruction of the thyroid gland with subsequent release of stored hormones occurs in lymphocytic thyroiditis and Hashimoto's thyroiditis. Administration of exogenous thyroid medications or excessive exposure of iodine in drugs, such as amiodarone or radiopaque dyes, are other causes for hyperthyroidism.

Pathophysiology

Hyperthyroid disease may occur due to overproduction of thyroid hormone or because of destruction of the thyroid gland. In Graves' disease, a TSH receptor autoantibody stimulates the thyroid gland to produce high concentrations of T_3 and T_4. The thyroid gland is enlarged and there is a marked increase in vascularity. Considered a familial disease, 50 percent of patients have close relatives who have circulating thyroid autoantibodies and 15 percent of patients have a close relative with the same diseases (Greenspan, 2004). Other autoimmune diseases that may be associated with Graves' disease are diabetes mellitus, pernicious anemia, vitiligo, and myasthenia gravis (Lingappa, 2003).

Assessment with Clinical Manifestations

The clinical manifestations of Graves' disease occur because of the excessive activity of T_3 and T_4 hormones, which cause a hypermetabolic state with an increase in oxygen consumption. There is also an increase in sympathetic nervous system activity, which suggests that the body is hyperreactive to catecholamines. All body tissues are affected, as demonstrated by the clinical manifestations described in Table 56-3. Common clinical manifestations include enlarged thyroid gland, cardiac palpitations, fatigue, excessive perspiration, heat intolerance, and weight loss without a loss of appetite, and eye changes. Eye disease (ophthalmopathy) may range from lid lag and soft tissue and extraocular muscle problems to involvement of the cornea and some vision loss.

Diagnostic Tests

There are several tests (refer to Table 56-4) used to detect thyroid disease. The most sensitive and cost-effective test is serum TSH. Combined use of the third-generation assay TSH test and T_4 provide the highest sensitivity and specificity for diagnosing thyroid disorders. An elevation of FT_4 and a suppressed TSH supports a diagnosis of hyperthyroidism. Eye signs plus an elevation of FT_4 and a suppressed TSH support a diagnosis of Graves' disease. Additional tests for Graves' disease include thyroid autoantibodies. Both Graves' disease and Hashimoto's thyroiditis will be positive for TgAb and TPO Ab, but TSH-R Ab is specific for Grave's disease (Greenspan, 2004).

TABLE 56-3 Assessment of the Patient with Thyrotoxicosis or Graves' Disease

HISTORY	PHYSICAL FINDINGS
History of other autoimmune diseases	
Medications:	Nails—ridges; discolored, splitting.
Skin: Heat intolerance. Change in temperature preference. Change in nails and hair. Pruritus	Moist warm skin. Hair loss, fine consistency. Hyperpigmentation of lower extremities. Oily skin
HEENT: Prior neck radiation, thyroid surgery, family history of thyroid disease. Presence of neck lumps, fullness, tenderness, or swelling: onset, location, size texture. Increased prominence of the eyes, difficulty swallowing. Puffiness in periorbital area. Blurred or double vision. Increase in lacrimination	Enlarged thyroid gland or goiter. Eyes: Ophthalmopathy: **Proptosis** (forward placement of the eye) (unilaterally or bilaterally), lid retraction. Diplopia, redness, congestion, conjunctival and periorbital edema.
Gritty sensation in eyes	Hyperactive reflex response
Neuromuscular: insomnia, irritability, nervousness, lethargy, or muscular weakness	Fine motor tremor
Skeletal:	Low bone mineral density
CV: palpitations, tachycardia,	Supraventricular dysrhythmias, atrial fibrillation, increase systolic blood, tachycardia at rest, "high output" congestive heart failure, murmur; decrease in vital capacity
Resp: shortness of breathe, exertional dyspnea	
GI: Increased frequency of bowel movements. Excessive appetite with high caloric intake	Documented high caloric intake with weight loss.
Reproductive: Diminished or scant menses	
Psychosocial: Emotional lability, mania and psychosis	
General: Fatigue, weight loss	

Adapted from Estes, M. (2006). Health assessment and physical examination *(3rd ed.). New York: Thomson Delmar Learning.*

Nursing Diagnoses

Based on the information gathered, examples of nursing diagnoses in the patient with hyperthyroidism may include the following:

- Anxiety related to fear of the unknown.
- Deficient knowledge related to disease and treatment (radioactive iodine therapy or surgery).

Planning and Implementation

Following assessment and diagnosis of the patient with Graves' disease, nursing management includes planning and implementation of a plan of care, which will decrease the patient's body metabolism, prevent tissue and organ damage, and restore normal body function. A collaborative approach between

TABLE 56-4 Diagnostic Tests for Thyroid Function

TESTS	RATIONALE
Serum T_4 Normal value: 5–12 mcg/dL	Measures by direct assay the biologically active thyroxine capable of binding with a T_3 or T_4 receptor Increased in hyperthyroidism
Serum Total T_3 Normal value: 80–200 ng/dL	Measures total amount of circulating T_3
TSH Normal 0.31–5 mLU/L	Third-generation assay is best indicator of endogenous thyroid function Undetectable or less than 10 in hyperthyroid patients is high; greater than 7 in hypothyroid patients is high. Exogenous corticosteroids and dopamine may suppress TSH
Thyroid scan	Tests the capacity of thyroid cells to trap and store iodine. Differentiates between the thyroid glands ability to trap iodine throughout the gland or whether a hypofunctioning cold nodule or hyperfunctioning hot nodule is present. Can differentiate between functioning metastasis and thyroid carcinoma
Thyroid antibodies	Antibodies against thyroid peroxidase enzyme or against thyroglobulin are frequently found in patients with Graves' disease and Hashimoto's thyroiditis
Radioactive iodine uptake (RIU)	Measures quantitatively the ability of the thyroid gland to confine radioactive iodine. The patient is administered a dosage of iodine; 24 hours later, the absorption is measured. RIU is elevated in patients with Graves' disease, multinodular goiter, or autonomous nodule
Thyroid sonogram	Distinguishes cystic from solid lesions Identify and define the size or number of thyroid nodule(s). Use for follow-up evaluation of nodules
Fine needle biopsy	Rule out cancer when nodule is present
CT scan or MRI	Diagnose substernal extension of nodule or identify deep thyroid nodules

Adapted from Daniels, R. (2003). Delmar's manual of laboratory and diagnostic tests. *New York: Thomson Delmar Learning.*

the nurse, health care providers, and dietitian is of paramount importance. The patient with thyrotoxicosis has several major nursing problems.

A nutrition imbalance that is often less than body requirements related to high metabolic needs is a major concern. Weight loss is often pronounced. The outcome for the patient is that the patient will have cessation of weight loss and will continue to gain until normal weight has been acquired. The patient with hyperthyroidism needs to have a thorough nutritional assessment. In collaboration with a dietitian, calorie count should be carried out and a plan be formulated for caloric intake that will meet nutritional demands.

Consultation with the dietitian to determine ways of increasing intake of high-energy foods will be beneficial. A prealbumin test helps to determine the body's protein reserve or deficit. The patient may need 4,000 to 6,000 calories a day or more to meet metabolic needs. Provision for six meals daily should be implemented. Daily weights are an essential part of the care. Interventions for nutritional needs include nutrition management.

Because of the increased energy requirements, the patient is fatigued and may be to the point of exhaustion. The patient's physical limitations should be assessed, and a plan should be developed to ensure adequate time for rest. Inform the patient that as the hypermetabolic state decreases, rest and relaxation will be easier. Interventions recommended for fatigue include energy management and sleep enhancement.

Anxiety is a common problem with the patient who has Graves' disease because to CNS irritability. Promotion of optimum rest and relaxation will assist in decreasing the patient's anxiety. Knowledge of the disease process and proposed treatment outcomes will help to decrease fears related to the symptoms that the patient is experiencing. Treatment with beta-adrenergic blockers will decrease the sympathetic response and reduce some of the symptoms of anxiety. Other interventions for anxiety include simple massage, relaxation therapy, and guided imagery.

Two major complications associated with Graves' disease are ophthalmopathy and toxic storm. Ocular manifestations including proptosis may occur as the extraocular muscles and tissue within the orbit enlarge due to infiltrative changes and edema. Paralysis of the extraocular muscles, damage to the retina and optic nerve may also occur. (Huether, 2004). The patient may experience a gritty sensation in the eye, diplopia, photophobia, lacrimation, inflammation, and edema. Catecholamine excess is thought to contribute to lid lag and stare that is associated with Graves' disease. With some patients, the eye symptoms regress as the hyperthyroidism is brought under control. Time and reassurance may be all that are needed. More severe ophthalmopathy will require aggressive therapy. Removal or destruction of the thyroid gland is recommended to prevent recurrence of thyrotoxicosis, which can reactivate residual ophthalmopathy (Greenspan, 2004). Other treatments include glucocorticoids to modify the immune response and treat the inflammation, orbital radiation therapy, plasmapheresis to remove circulating pathogenic antibodies, and decompression surgery to allow orbital tissue to expand into adjacent areas. Extraocular and or cosmetic surgery may be required to correct eyelid malposition. Minor degrees of diplopia may require special lenses.

A nursing priority in caring for the patient with ophthalmopathy is to protect the eye from injury. Nursing interventions include instructing the patient to protect the cornea against wind-borne particles, suggesting tinted or dark glasses to relieve light sensitivity, and providing artificial tears or ointment to decrease the sensation of having a foreign body in the eye. A protective shield and light taping of the lid at night with nonallergic tape may help to protect the cornea. Elevation of the head at night may help to alleviate periorbital edema.

Thyroid Crisis (Thyroid Storm)

Thyroid crisis or thyroid storm is a serious form of thyrotoxicosis, which is life-threatening. It is most likely to occur in people who have been inadequately treated or undiagnosed. Infection, stress or emotional trauma, pregnancy, comorbidity, or medications may precipitate this event. Clinical manifestations include: extremely high fever, severe neurological signs and symptoms (e.g., restlessness, delirium, agitation, psychosis, and coma) and cardiovascular problems (e.g., atrial fibrillation, heart failure, and angina). Most patients will have a high systolic blood pressure with a wide pulse pressure. One of the earliest clues to the onset of a thyroid storm is high fever and diaphoresis, which is out of proportion to an infection.

Patients with thyroid storm should be treated in the intensive care unit. It is important that expedient treatment be provided. Respiratory support should be provided immediately. Hemodynamic instability is a major priority. Intravenous access is a priority to correct volume and electrolyte depletion and administer nutrition as indicated. Vasopressors may be ordered to restore or maintain blood pressure. The nurse must be prepared to implement measures to treat congestive heart failure. Measures to reduce fever must be immediately implemented. A cooling blanket and the administration of acetaminophen as ordered is standard care.

Treatment includes adrenergic blocking drugs to interrupt the sympathetic nervous system effects. Drugs to inhibit synthesis of thyroid hormones and block production and secretion are utilized for treating thyroid storm. Because the patient may experience adrenal insufficiency with the stress related to the thyroid storm, glucocorticoids, such as hydrocortisone may be prescribed. Effort is made to identify any underlying disease that may have precipitated the storm, and antiallergy, antibiotics, and special postoperative care may be indicated. Aspirin should be avoided, because it displaces free thyroxin from protein carriers and releases more thyroxin into circulation. Heart failure may be treated with digoxin and diuretics. Plasmapheresis, or peritoneal dialysis, is emergency measures that may be implemented to remove circulating antibodies (Greenspan, 2004)

In elders the most frequent complications that present with hyperthyroidism are cardiovascular, including atrial fibrillation, congestive heart failure, angina, and acute myocardial infarction or CNS symptoms, such as apathy, depression, and confusion. A hypermetabolic state may be present with muscle wasting. Bone loss and fractures are other problems. Readjustments of medications may be necessary because an increase in metabolism may alter dose requirements (Greenspan & Resnick, 2004).

Pharmacology

Treatment of Graves' disease includes radioiodine therapy, surgery, and antithyroid medications. Newly diagnosed patients are placed on thiamazole (antithyroid drugs) medications to correct their hypermetabolic state. Examples of the thiamazole are propylthiouracil (PTU) and methimazole. These drugs are used to assist the patient to reach a euthyroid state. Young patients with small glands and mild symptoms respond most readily to medication. Outcome of therapy with the antithyroid drugs is variable. Though in many incidences the treatment is effective, there can be serious side effects to the antithyroid medications. The thioamides can cause agranulocytosis; therefore, the patients have to be monitored carefully for leukopenia. PTU can cause liver injury. Prior to the treatment, the patient should have a baseline complete blood count, comprehensive metabolic profile, including liver function test and a thyroid panel (TSH; free T_4; total T_3). PTU is the drug of choice for treating hyperthyroidism in a pregnant or breastfeeding patient, because it has limited transfer across the placenta or into breast milk. Methimazole promotes compliance because of once a day dosing. Nursing interventions for the patient receiving thioamides involve the following assessing for thrombocytopenia and hepatotoxicity; teaching the patient to report symptoms of adverse reactions: skin rash, yellowing of eyes, sore throat, chills, fever, or painful joints; reporting bruising or unexplained bleeding; and instructing patient about the importance of frequent laboratory tests to detect adverse effects and response to treatment.

In addition to the thioamides, patients can receive beta blockers (e.g., propranolol, atenolol) to decrease the beta-adrenergic activity of a stimulated thyroid gland. The beta blockers may be contraindicated for patients with congestive heart failure, asthma, or diabetes. The nurse must monitor the heart rate and blood pressure. In addition, the nurse must assist the patient alleviate symptoms of anxiety, palpitations, tremor, and heat intolerance. Side effects of beta blockers include nausea, headache, fatigue, insomnia, hypotension, bradycardia, and dysrhythmias.

A last type of medication to treat thyroid conditions is potassium iodide (SSKI). This medication blocks thyroid hormone release by decreasing vascularity preoperatively before thyroid surgery. The nursing implication for this medication is to assess for allergies to iodine and shellfish. In addition, the nurse can disguise the iodine taste by diluting in water or juice. Lithium carbonate may be given if prescribed as an alternative to iodine (Broyles, et. al., 2007).

> **PATIENT PLAYBOOK**
>
> **Nursing Strategies for Radioiodine Tests**
>
> The nurse should instruct the patient:
>
> Before the test: verify that the patient is not pregnant and advise the patient to avoid pregnancy for six months and be aware that allergies to iodine do not contraindicate use.
>
> After the test: instruct the patient to avoid sharing food and eating utensils, avoid having close contact with children and kissing for several days, flush toilet twice after use, and avoid breastfeeding.
>
> *Adapted from Grigsby, P. W. (2004). Thyroid. In C. Perez, E. Halperm, L. Brady, R. Schmidt-Ullrich (Eds.),* Principles and practices of radiation oncology *(pp. 211–215). New York: Lippincott, Williams & Williams.*

Radioiodine Therapy

Radioiodine therapy is the treatment of choice in the United States for hyperthyroidism in patients over 21 years and for patients who have not responded to antithyroid therapy. Pregnant patients are absolutely contraindicated from having radioiodine therapy. Prior to 131I therapy, patients may require antithyroid agents for the purpose of obtaining a **euthyroid** state (having a normal functioning thyroid gland). To reach a euthyroid state, methimazole rather than propylthiouracil is the preferred drug, because the inhibitory effect of methimazole on radioiodine uptake dissipates in 24 hours. The antithyroid drug is stopped for five to seven days prior to the treatment with radioactive iodine. Iodine therapy may also be prescribed prior to the radioiodine therapy (see prethyroidectomy care). Prior to the therapy, a radioactive iodine uptake measurement is performed to determine the appropriate dose of 131I. Following the therapy, 80 percent of patients who are adequately treated with radioiodine therapy will develop hypothyroidism This complication of therapy actually may be considered beneficial because the patient will no longer be susceptible to Grave's disease. The patient will need to be monitored for hypothyroidism and when diagnosed be treated promptly with replacement thyroid medication (Greenspan, 2004). A variety of nursing strategies are shown in the Patient Playbook feature.

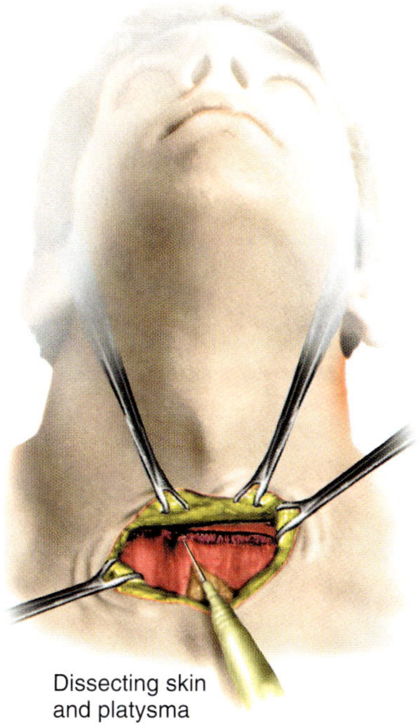

Figure 56-4 Thyroidectomy.

Surgery

Though surgery is rarely required for patients with thyroid disorders, a subtotal thyroidectomy may be the treatment of choice for patients with large glands or multinodular goiters or for patients who fail other treatments (Figure 56-4). Prior to surgery, the patient will be prescribed antithyroid medications to promote a euthyroid state; this usually takes around six weeks. Saturated solution of potassium iodide may be administered to reduce the vascularity of the gland (Greenspan, 2004).

Prior to thyroid surgery, the patient needs thorough preoperative teaching. An explanation regarding the medications prescribed, their action, side effects, and such should be provided. The importance of compliance to the treatment should be stressed. Ample time should be provided to answer questions. The patient will have concerns and fears about the site of the incision and the scar that may be present afterward. The patient can be reassured that minimal scarring should be present; a scarf or necklace will most likely cover the site. Complications of thyroid surgery include hypoparathyroidism, bleeding, and injury to the recurrent laryngeal nerve.

Priority in care postoperatively is prevention and detection of complications. Assess for respiratory distress, which may occur due to hemorrhage and edema, or laryngeal spasms, which may occur if there is injury to the parathyroid glands during surgery resulting in hypocalcemia and tetany. The unit code cart should be available in the event that intubation or tracheostomy is warranted.

The patient should be assessed for early symptoms of hypocalcemia. Symptoms and signs include paresthesia of the mouth, toes, fingers; generalized muscle twitching; and positive Chvostek's and Trousseau's signs. Intravenous calcium gluconate or calcium chloride should be on hand for treatment of hypocalcemia. Ionized calcium levels should be drawn to monitor calcium. Though hoarseness may be the result of irritation due to intubation during surgery, there is potential for injury to the laryngeal nerve, which can cause permanent hoarseness.

Evaluation of Outcomes

Potential patient outcomes for each of the example nursing diagnoses for the patient with hyperthyroidism are:

- Anxiety related to fear of the unknown. Patient will report signs of anxiety and relate a decrease in symptoms of anxiety.
- Deficient knowledge related to disease and treatment (radioactive iodine therapy or surgery). Patient will verbalize an understanding of disease and treatment.

Nontoxic Goiter

Nontoxic goiter is the enlargement of the thyroid gland from TSH stimulation, which occurs due to inadequate thyroid hormone synthesis. At one time it was prevalent in the United States because of iodine deficiency. Though the problem is no longer common in the United States, because of the wide availability of iodine in food sources, there are still large areas of the world where iodine intake is deficient. Daily iodine requirements for adults range from 150 to 300 mcg a day. Other causes for nontoxic goiter include Goitrogen diet, Hashimoto's thyroiditis, neoplasm (benign and malignant), and inherited defect in thyroid hormone synthesis (Greenspan, 2004).

Thyroiditis

Thyroiditis may be classified as chronic lymphocytic (Hashimoto's) thyroiditis due to autoimmunity, subacute thyroiditis, suppurative thyroiditis, and Riedel's thyroiditis. The most common form of thyroiditis in the United States is Hashimoto's thyroiditis. A familial disease, it is six times more common in women.

Clinical manifestations of Hashimoto's thyroiditis include a diffuse, enlarged firm and nodular thyroid gland. The patient often complains of painless neck tightness. Thyroid function tests are variable. Antithyroid antibody tests are usually positive. Rarely, the patient may present with thyrotoxicosis due to destruction of thyroid tissue and sudden release of thyroid hormones. Most often the patient progresses to hypothyroidism, which is 95 percent of the time permanent.

Thyroid Nodules and Neoplasms

Other disorders of the thyroid gland are nodules and neoplasms. Either of these anomalies requires treatment and have varying levels of affects on the patients with these conditions.

Epidemiology

It is estimated that 4 percent of the adult population has a thyroid nodule, and there is a gender relationship for incidence of thyroid cancer (Greenspan, 2004). Women are more prone to thyroid nodules than men.

Etiology

Causes of thyroid nodules include: adenomas, cysts, carcinomas, multinodular goiters, Hashimoto's thyroiditis, and subacute thyroiditis (Braimon, Naaznin, Lokhandwala, & Walczak, 2003). Follicular adenoma, a solitary firm nodule, up to 5 cm, is the most common nodule occurring in the thyroid gland. It accounts for 30 percent of all nodules. In less than 10 percent of follicular adenomas, malignant change will occur. Cancer of the thyroid occurs more often in women and is rare (0.0004 percent). Cancers are classified as either papillary or follicular; these types are often mixed. Other types are Hürthle cell, anaplastic, and medulla (Table 56-5).

Predisposing factors to thyroid cancer include childhood exposure to radiation in the head or neck and genetic predisposition. Children exposed to high degrees of radiation during the Chernobyl accident have had a high incidence of thyroid cancer. Papillary and follicular cancers usually pursue a long clinical course of 15 to 20 years. Papillary cancer tends to metastasize to regional lymph nodes in the neck, and follicular thyroid cancer follows a pattern of distant metastasizes to the lung or bone (Greenspan, 2004; Lingappa, 2003).

Planning and Implementation

Patients with papillary and follicular carcinoma can be classified into high- and low-risk groups. For patients under 45 who have primary lesions that are 1 cm or less in size and no evidence of metastasis, a lobectomy is standard of care. All other patients should be considered at high risk, and a total thyroidectomy is the recommended treatment. A modified neck resection may be recommended if there is any evidence of lymphatic spread. Following surgery it is usually recommended that the patient receive radioiodine ablation therapy for any remaining thyroid tissue. See Box 56-3 for management strategies for the patient receiving high dose radioactive therapy.

Thyroid suppression therapy has been shown to reduce growth of papillary or follicular thyroid cancer. Suppression therapy involves the prescribing of levothyroxine daily. With an increase in circulating thyroid hormone, the feedback to the pituitary gland will decrease the release of TSH, thereby depressing the function of the thyroid gland and hopefully the growth of the tumor, if it is TSH dependent. Radiation therapy may also be useful in situations in which the patient does not respond to other treatments (Greenspan, 2004). The National Cancer Institute outlines the staging and treatment of thyroid cancers.

Hypothyroidism

Hypothyroidism is a clinical state in which there is a deficient production of thyroid hormone by the thyroid gland. This disorder may be primary or secondary. All body functions are affected by a thyroid deficiency, which causes an

TABLE 56-5 Comparison of Benign and Malignant Thyroid Lesions

	BENIGN	MALIGNANT
History	Lives in area where goiter is endemic Family history of benign goiter	Family history of thyroid medullary cancer History of irradiation of neck or head Recently diagnosed with thyroid nodule Symptoms: hoarseness or dysphagia
Sex/Age	Female sex, older women	Male; child, young adults
Clinical manifestations	Soft nodule; multinodular goiter	Firm, usually single nodule different from other thyroid tissue; vocal cord paralysis, suspected metastases, and enlarged firm nodes
Thyroid scan	Hot nodule	Cold nodule
Echo	Cyst (pure)	Solid or semicystic
Fine needle biopsy	Cytologic exam—benign	Cytologic exam malignant
Levothyroxine therapy (TSH suppression therapy)	Decrease in size	No change

Adapted from Greenspan, F. S. (2004). The thyroid gland. In F.S. Greenspan & D. G. Gardner (Eds.), Basic and clinical endocrinology *(pp. 215–294). St. Louis, MO: Lange Medical Books.*

BOX 56-3

CARING FOR THE PATIENT RECEIVING HIGH-DOSE RADIOACTIVE IODINE THERAPY

1. Isolation principles are employed.
2. Patient wears foot coverings when ambulating.
3. The outer door is kept closed, and the bathroom door is kept open. (Flush twice after each use.)
4. Shower and wash hands frequently.
5. Personnel and visitors must wear gloves, gown, and mask, and the patient must wear hospital gown with a "chuck" wrapped around neck (visitors are discouraged, and no children or pregnant women are allowed entry).
6. If specimen is needed, urine should be collected in a lead container.
7. At 24 hours and 48 hours the patient's radiation level is measured. The radiation level must be less than 30 mC131 prior to discharge.
8. Patients should drink copious amounts of water to promote release of radioactive iodine.
9. Male patients are instructed to sit to void.
10. Because traces of radioactive iodine remains in the urine and blood up to a week, the patient is instructed to not have close contact with children; sleep alone; avoid prolonged intimate contact; practice good personal hygiene; launder linens, towel, and clothes daily; and avoid preparing food with bare hands.

Adapted from Grigsby, P. W. (2004). Thyroid. In C. Perez, E. Halperm, L. Brady, R. Schmidt-Ullrich (Eds.), Principles and practices of radiation oncology *(pp. 211–215). New York: Lippincott, Williams & Williams.*

overall decline in metabolic processes. The disease may present in a range from a mild form with vague symptoms to severe symptoms, which occur with myxedema. Early in the disease the most common symptoms are fatigue, weakness, lethargy, cold intolerance, constipation, and dry skin. As the disease progresses more physical manifestations occur, including puffy face and hands, hoarseness, slow mentation, and slow reflexes.

Epidemiology

Hypothyroidism is a common disease. One and one-half percent to 2 percent of women have the disease. It occurs in 0.2 percent of the male population. More commonly it is found in the elderly patients (over 60 years); 6 percent of women and 2.5 percent of men have laboratory evidence of hypothyroidism (Ferri, 2005).

Etiology

The most common cause of hypothyroidism is Hashimoto's thyroiditis. Other primary causes are due to thyroid failure and include thyroidectomy (surgical removal of thyroid gland), radioiodine therapy resulting in destruction of the gland, or congenital defects resulting in a deficiency of thyroid hormone during infancy. Certain medications, such as lithium (a drug used to treat mania) and antithyroid drugs used in treating hyperthyroid disease, can block synthesis of thyroid hormones. Ingestion of large amounts of iodine will also result in blockage of thyroid hormone production. Products that contain iodine in abnormal amounts include kelp tablets, iodide containing cough medicines, radiographic contrast media, and the antiarrhythmic drug amiodarone, which has 75 mg of iodine per 200 mg. Rarely, hypothyroidism occurs in the United States because of iodide. Secondary causes include diseases of the pituitary gland, such as a pituitary tumor, which results in deficiency or absence of TSH. Tertiary causes include an alteration in hypothalamus function resulting in a deficiency of thyrotropin and consequential decrease in TSH (Greenspan, 2004; Huether, 2004).

Assessment with Clinical Manifestations

A careful history should be taken from the patient and family. Information is obtained regarding the patient and their history of thyroid surgery, radioiodine therapy, or previous thyroid disease. Other common symptoms, which should be checked out for thyroid disease, are fatigue and unexplained weight gain (Table 56-6).

Diagnostic Tests

A diagnosis of primary hypothyroidism is supported by a low serum FT_4 and an elevated TSH (greater than 1). T_3 results may be in the normal range. If the hypothyroidism is due to a pituitary problem, the TSH will not be elevated and the FT_4 will be low.

TABLE 56-6 System Assessment of Patient with Hypothyroidism

CLINICAL MANIFESTATIONS OF HYPOTHYROIDISM	RATIONALE
General	Thyroid deficiency results in general metabolic depression and alters the function of almost all body system.
Skin	An increase in the deposition of protein polysaccharide complexes lead to retention of sodium and water causing puffiness.
Dry skin, puffy skin, and thin hair. Skin may have yellow tint. Cold intolerance and sometimes decrease in body temperature.	Loss of sweat and sebaceous gland secretion causes dryness. Reduction of carotene to vitamin A may give skin a yellowish tint. Decrease in metabolic rate, oxygen consumption, and heat production with a decrease circulation to the skin contributes to cold intolerance.
HEENT: Hoarseness, large tongue	Hoarseness may occur because of accumulation of mucopolysaccharides in the larynx.
Cardiac: Bradycardia or decreased cardiac output, cardiac enlargement	Interstitial edema, nonspecific myofibrillar swelling may lead to cardiac enlargement. Insufficient thyroid hormones results in interruption of normal cardiac contraction.
Respiratory: Shallow slow respirations	Decrease in thyroid hormone alters normal ventilatory responses to carbon dioxide and hypoxia. Respiratory muscle changes occur as thyroid deficiency continues. Pleural effusions may occur with the myxedematous changes.
GI: Chronic constipation	Altered GI motility and tone with decrease in secretion of digestive juices occurs with insufficient thyroid hormones.
Renal: Impaired ability to excrete fluid	Blood flow to the kidney is reduced with resultant decrease in filtration rate.
Neuromuscular: Paresthesia, muscle weakness, diminished DTR CNS: Confusion, fatigue, slow cognition	Decrease in muscular contraction and relaxation results in slow movement. Reduction in cerebral blood flow leads to cerebral hypoxia.
Genitourinary: Severe menorrhagia anovulatory cycles, impotence, and infertility in men	Alteration in the metabolism of estrogens and androgens.
Hematological: Normocytic, normochromic, and macrocytic anemia.	Decrease in RBC production; vitamin B_{12} deficiency; inadequate iron and folate absorption related to the deficiency in thyroid hormone with resultant decrease metabolic rate and decrease in oxygen requirements.

Adapted from Greenspan, F. S. (2004). The thyroid gland. In F.S. Greenspan & D. G. Gardner (Eds.), Basic and clinical endocrinology *(pp. 215–294). St. Louis, MO: Lange Medical Books; Huether, S. E. (2004). Alterations of hormonal regulation. In S. E. Huether & K. L. McCance (Eds.),* Understanding pathophysiology *(pp. 356–362). St. Louis, MO: Mosby.*

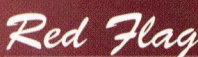

> **Red Flag**
>
> **Subclinical Hypothyroidism**
>
> Subclinical hypothyroidism is defined as normal serum free T_3 and T_4 levels with TSH suppressed below the normal range. A detailed clinical history should be completed because patients do not generally present with overt symptoms of hypothyroidism. Patients, particularly the elderly, who have subclinical hypothyroidism are at risk for developing cardiac abnormalities, such as atrial fibrillation and osteoporosis.

Nursing Diagnoses

Based on the information gathered, examples of nursing diagnoses in the patient with hypothyroidism may include the following:

- Activity intolerance related to decrease in metabolism.
- Constipation related to decreased activity and decreased metabolic rate.
- Risk for injury related to hypersensitivity to sedatives, narcotics, and anesthetics.
- Disturbed sensory perception (numbness of the hands or feet) related to mucin deposits and nerve compression.

Planning and Implementation

When first diagnosed the patient may need assistance with activities of daily living. Fatigue and activity intolerance may be major problems. Cardiorespiratory response to activities should be monitored. Nutritional intake and sleep patterns should be also monitored and appropriate interventions taken to ensure sufficient calories and rest. Patient and family should be informed that as the medication takes effect tiredness should resolve. Constipation may have been a chronic problem if the patient has had undiagnosed hypothyroidism. Dietary assessment will help to identify nutritional needs. Discuss methods to increase dietary fiber. Encourage intake of a minimum of eight glasses of fluid daily unless contraindicated.

Cardiovascular disease is more common in patients who have hypothyroidism. Signs include bradycardia, impaired muscular contraction, and diminished cardiac output. Some patients have heart enlargement; this may be due to left ventricular dilation or pericardial effusion.

Pharmacology

The treatment of choice for hypothyroidism is levothyroxine (T_4), which is available in pure form and is inexpensive and stable. Even though only T_4 is administered, levothyroxine is converted to T_3 so that both hormones available in the tissues. Because of variable hormone content, desiccated thyroid is not satisfactory for use. Instruct patient to take oral medication one hour before a meal or two hours afterward to ensure proper absorption. Dosage will vary according to age and weight. Thyroid medications potentiate medications, such as digoxin and Coumadin. The patient should be monitored for digoxin toxicity and bleeding problems. In addition, the patient should be monitored for cardiovascular insufficiency (e.g., chest pain, shortness of breath, palpitations, tachycardia, or peripheral edema).

Evaluation of Outcomes

Potential patient outcomes for each of the example nursing diagnoses for the patient with hypothyroidism are:

- Activity intolerance related to decrease in metabolism. Patient will perform activities of daily living independently or with assistive devices as needed; patient will be free of complications of immobility, as evidenced by intact skin, absence of thrombophlebitis, and normal bowel patterns.
- Constipation related to decreased activity and decreased metabolic rate. Patient will report normal bowel elimination pattern.
- Imbalanced nutrition, more than body requirements, related to intake greater than metabolic needs. Patient will verbalize and demonstrate selection of foods or meals that will achieve and maintain weight within 10 percent of recommended body mass index.
- Impaired skin integrity related to dryness and edema secondary to movement of fluid into the interstitial tissues. Patient skin condition will show improvement as demonstrated by decreased redness, swelling, and pain.

> **Red Flag**
>
> **Hypothyroidism in the Elderly**
>
> Hypothyroidism may be overlooked in the elderly because euthyroid patients have similar symptoms. Elderly are more likely to present with complications of the disease, (e.g., congestive heart failure, angina, neurological problems, confusion, or depression) (Greenspan & Resnick, 2004). In addition, subclinical hypothyroidism occurs in 5 to 10 percent of elderly people. The patient should be carefully assessed for symptoms of hypothyroidism. Each person must be carefully evaluated for risk before the decision to treat is made (Huether, 2004).

Myxedema Coma

Myxedema is a medical emergency. The patient will present with a diminished level of consciousness due to severe hypothyroidism. Symptoms include hypothermia, hypoventilation, hypotension, and bradycardia. Preceding the coma, the patient may be depressed, confused, paranoid, and sometimes even manic.

Nursing Diagnoses

Based on the information gathered, examples of nursing diagnoses in the patient with myxedema coma may include the following:

- Impaired gas exchange related to hypercapnia or hypoxia due to hypoventilation.
- Hypothermia related to hypometabolism.
- Decreased cardiac output related to heart failure, or fluid volume deficit.

Planning and Implementation

Priorities of care for the patient with myxedema coma include respiratory and hemodynamic support. The patient will be admitted to an intensive care unit, and ventilator support is usually necessary. Respiratory and cardiovascular assessment must be provided continuously. The patient will require continuous cardiac and respiratory monitoring. Arterial blood gases should be done at intervals. Associated illnesses that may have precipitated the coma should be looked for and treated. Intravenous fluids should be given slowly because the patient may easily become overloaded with fluids. Gastric absorption of medication is poor in the myxedema patient; therefore, thyroid replacement should be administered intravenously. For patients who have had hypothyroidism for long periods and for diagnosed cardiac patients, thyroid replacement is started slowly. In the event that angina or dysrhythmias occur, the dosage is usually reduced. Therapeutic response to treatment will be indicated by increase in temperature and an improved respiratory and cerebral functioning. Patients with myxedema often have adrenal insufficiency also; therefore, glucocorticoids may be prescribed (Greenspan, 2004).

Evaluation of Outcomes

Potential patient outcomes for each of the example nursing diagnoses for the patient with myxedema coma are:

- Impaired gas exchange related to factors of hypercapnia or hypoxia due to hypoventilation. Patient's arterial blood gases will be within normal limits.
- Hypothermia related to factors of hypometabolism. Patient will have normal body temperature.
- Decreased cardiac output related to factors of heart failure and fluid volume deficit. Patient will have normal cardiac rhythm and vital signs.

HYPERPARATHYROIDISM

The parathyroid glands (normally four) are located in the neck in the posterior aspect of the thyroid gland. These small glands are easily overlooked and can be removed accidentally during thyroid surgery (Lal & Clark, 2004). When the parathyroid glands are stimulated to excess, the condition of hyperparathyroidism exists.

Epidemiology

Primary hyperparathyroidism is found in approximately 0.1 percent of adult patients examined. It occurs three times more frequently in women. Primary hyperparathyroidism accounts for about 90 percent of the cases of hypercalcemia. Over half of cases of hyperparathyroidism occur in patients over 60 years of age.

Etiology

Hyperparathyroidism is usually sporadic and most often due to a single enlarged gland or adenoma. Other causes of hyperparathyroidism include parathyroid carcinoma and hyperplasia. Studies show that there has been a decline in cases of hyperthyroidism since 1970. Earlier detection of primary hyperparathyroidism occurs today because of incidental hypercalcemia, which is found when patients have comprehensive metabolic blood profiles. Those patients who have early detection of the disease are less likely to be symptomatic.

Pathophysiology

Hyperparathyroidism leads to excessive excretion of calcium and phosphate by the kidney. Even though parathyroid hormone stimulates the renal tubules to reabsorb calcium causing hypercalcemia, the excessive calcium in the glomerular filtrate overwhelms tubular reabsorption and results in hypercalciuria. Polyuria and polydipsia may occur as a result of the nephrogenic diabetes insipidus, which hypercalcemia can induce. Kidney stones occur in 18 percent of patients with newly diagnosed primary hyperparathyroidism. Excessive PTH can cause excessive bone reabsorption, which leads to diffuse demineralization, cystic bone lesions, and pathological fractures.

Assessment with Clinical Manifestations

Patients with hyperparathyroidism have clinical manifestations that affect many of the body's systems. Neurological symptoms can occur from mild (e.g., lethargy, fatigue, personality change, paresthesia, or depression) to severe stupor and coma. GI symptoms, such as, dyspepsia, nausea, and constipation, are also common.

Diagnostic Tests

In hyperparathyroidism, serum calcium and ionized calcium levels are elevated. A serum calcium greater than 10.9 mg/dL is the hallmark of primary hyperparathyroidism when corrected for serum albumin. When serum albumin is low, the serum calcium results may also be low, therefore ionized calcium is more accurate, because it is not bound to protein and provides a more accurate measurement of calcium. Urine calcium is also high to normal, and urine phosphorus is high. To distinguish the parathyroid from nonparathyroid causes of hypercalcemia, a parathyroid hormone assay test is warranted. A diagnosis of primary hyperparathyroidism is confirmed by a parathyroid assay test, which is high normal to elevated (Daniels, 2003).

Imaging techniques for localizing parathyroid adenomas include ultrasonography, CT, MRI, and Tc-99m MIBI studies. The expertise of the technical personnel and available equipment influence the sensitivity and specificity of the procedure. A bone survey by shoe evidence of bone resorption indicates excess of PTH. Osteitis fibrosa cystica is the classic bone disease of primary parathyroidism (Ferri, 2005).

Nursing Diagnoses

Based on the information gathered, examples of nursing diagnoses in the patient with hyperparathyroidism may include the following:

- Acute or chronic pain related to renal stone or bone discomfort.
- Risk for injury related to pathological fracture.

Planning and Implementation

Management of fluid and electrolytes is the priority problem when a patient presents with hypercalcemia. Severe hypercalcemia requires hospitalization. Intensive hydration with intravenous normal saline (fluid resuscitation with normal saline: 500 to 1,000 mL over the first hour followed by 250 to 500 mL hourly) is the treatment of choice unless contraindicated. The patient may need three to five liters of fluid each a day. Ensuring that the patient receives sodium chloride greater than 400 mEq every day is important to facilitate calcium excretion.

Patients who have mild, asymptomatic hyperparathyroidism should be followed closely by their health care provider. The patient should be encouraged to exercise and drink adequate fluids. Vitamin D and A supplements, calcium containing medications, such as antacids and laxatives, and thiazide diuretics should be avoided. Recommendations for follow-up includes serum calcium and albumin twice yearly, renal function and urine calcium once each year, and bone density every two years. There is caution in use of digitalis preparations because patients with hypercalcemia are more sensitive to toxic effects. A calcium channel blocker may be prescribed to help in preventing adverse cardiac effects from the hypercalcemia.

Surgery

Parathyroidectomy is the definitive treatment of choice leading to 95 percent cure rate of parathyroid adenoma. With parathyroid hyperplasia the cure rate is somewhat lower, because there is a 20 percent incidence of recurrent hypercalcemia. Preoperative and postoperative care is similar to the care of the patient having a thyroidectomy.

Because the parathyroid glands lie within 1 cm of the point of intersection of the recurrent laryngeal nerve, there is danger of injury with resultant hoarseness. Hypocalcemia with resulting tetany will occur if there is inadvertent removal of all parathyroid tissue. The patient needs to be observed closely the evening after surgery or on the following day. Frequent monitoring of ionized calcium is advisable. Calcium carbonate is provided orally to prevent hypocalcemia after the hypercalcemia has resolved. Intravenous calcium gluconate and calcium chloride should be available if hypocalcemia occurs. Because adequate magnesium is required for functional recovery of the remaining suppressed parathyroid glands, magnesium may be required. The patient should be monitored for hyperthyroidism immediately after parathyroid surgery because stored thyroid hormone may be released during surgery.

Evaluation of Outcomes

Potential patient outcomes for each of the example nursing diagnoses for the patient with hyperparathyroidism are:

- Acute or chronic pain related to renal stone or bone discomfort. Patient should relate that pain has been decreased and discuss measures to cope with the pain if it is not completely relieved.
- Risk for injury related to pathological fracture. Patient will not experience of fractures.

HYPOPARATHYROIDISM

By secreting PTH, the parathyroid gland and vitamin D function to maintain a normal serum calcium. Either the failure to secrete PTH or respond to PTH or vitamin D results in hypocalcemia, which is the major problem occurring with hypoparathyroidism.

Epidemiology

Hypoparathyroidism is a rare disorder, occurring equally between males and females. It is speculated that the United States has similar rates of hypoparathyroidism as does Japan, which reports 7.2 cases of idiopathic hypoparathyroid cases per one million and 3.4 cases per one million of pseudohypoparathyroidism.

Etiology

Hypoparathyroid may be familial, idiopathic, caused by infection, autoimmune disease, or surgical removal of the parathyroid glands. Hypoparathyroidism most commonly occurs following a thyroidectomy; it is usually transient, rarely, it may be permanent. Other causes of hypoparathyroidism include autoimmune syndrome, functional due to poor absorption of magnesium sulfate, and pseudohypoparathyroidism, which occurs as a result of renal resistance to parathyroid hormone.

Pathophysiology

When there is inadequate parathyroid hormone, calcium levels decrease and phosphorus levels increase. Calcium reabsorption from the bone ceases and regulation of calcium reabsorption from the renal tubules are impaired. A decrease in calcium reduces the threshold for nerve and muscle excitation so that a nerve impulse may occur by a slight stimulus along the nerve fiber. This leads to alteration in nerve transmission and in more severe incidences tetany. Serum calcium levels may be further reduced by high phosphorus levels, which impede conversion of vitamin D to its active form by inhibiting the renal enzyme that is necessary for the vitamin D to become active.

Assessment with Clinical Manifestations

Symptoms of hypoparathyroidism mirror those of hypocalcemia, and therefore are mainly due to increased neuromuscular excitability and deposition of calcium in soft tissues. Acute symptoms of hypocalcemia include numbness and tingling of lips and hands, tetany, carpopedal spasms (Trousseau's sign), Chvostek's sign, muscle and abdominal cramps, and psychological changes. Chronic clinical manifestations include lethargy, personality changes, anxiety, and blurring of vision due to cataracts. ECG may show prolonged QT intervals and T wave abnormalities.

Diagnostic Tests

Refer to the diagnostic tests section for parathyroid dysfunction.

Nursing Diagnoses

Based on the information gathered, examples of nursing diagnosis in the patient with hypoparathyroidism may include the following:

- Risk for injury related to hypocalcemia with resultant tetany

Planning and Implementation

The goal of treatment for hypoparathyroidism is to normalize calcium levels. The nurse must be prepared to recognize early symptoms of hypocalcemia. If tetany occurs, laryngospasm can result in inadequate airway calling for emergency tracheostomy. To prevent and or treat symptoms (e.g., tetany) intravenous calcium gluconate is administered. The patient will be prescribed oral calcium supplements and vitamin D for maintenance therapy. Dietary instruction for foods high in calcium should be provided. The nurse should provide a thorough explanation for the importance of compliance to the therapeutic plan.

Evaluation of Outcomes

Potential patient outcomes for each of the example nursing diagnoses for the patient with hypoparathyroidism are:

- Risk for injury related to hypocalcemia with resultant tetany. Patient will be not experience tetany and ionized calcium level will return to normal.

KEY CONCEPTS

- Hyperfunction of the pituitary gland occurs when there is excess hormonal activity.
- Hyperprolactinemia causes mainly problems with the fertility and sexual function.
- Acromegaly, though causing changes in body appearance with increase growth of body tissues, has effect on all body systems, leading to many comorbidities.
- Hypercortisolism (Cushing's disease and Cushing's syndrome) alters the function of practically all tissues and organs of the body.
- Transsphenoidal hypophysectomy is the recommended treatment for most pituitary tumors.
- Hypofunction of the pituitary gland occurs with decrease hormonal activity of one or more of the pituitary hormones.
- Both diabetes insipidus and SIADH alter fluid and electrolytes.
- Adrenal insufficiency can be life-threatening.
- An increased stimulation of the adrenal glands may lead to hyperaldosteronism.
- Pheochromocytomas are rare but have a high mortality rate because of predisposing the patient to stroke and myocardial infarction.
- An excess or decrease in available thyroid hormone alters function of all body organs.
- Hyperthyroidism refers to the continuous secretion of thyroid hormones by the thyroid gland.
- Primary hypothyroidism is usually treatable with replacement thyroid therapy.
- The treatment of choice for hyperthyroidism is radioiodine therapy.
- The major problems related to hyperparathyroidism are kidney stones and fractures.
- Hypoparathyroidism can cause hypocalcemia, which may cause tetany, a life-threatening event.

REVIEW QUESTIONS

1. When assessing a patient who is diagnosed as having acromegaly, what signs and symptoms will the nurse most likely assess? Select all that apply.
   1. Decrease in peripheral vision
   2. Hypotension
   3. Muscle weakness
   4. Large tongue

2. Which statement by a 28-year-old female patient would support a diagnosis of hyperprolactinemia?
   1. "I have progressively become hoarse over the past six months."
   2. "I am experiencing deep bone pain."
   3. "I have not had a menstrual period in 12 months."
   4. "I have had a problem with weight loss."

3. When instructing a patient who is to have a transsphenoidal hypophysectomy. What information should the nurse include?
   1. Nasal passage will be packed with gauze for 24 to 48 hours.
   2. A soft bulky head dressing will be present.
   3. A pureed diet will be provided immediately after surgery.
   4. Teeth will need brushing four to six times daily after surgery.

4. Which nursing intervention should the nurse anticipate providing for a patient with hypercortisolism?
   1. Monitoring for hypotension
   2. Fall prevention measures
   3. Assessing for symptoms of hyperkalemia
   4. Dietary instruction to promote weight gain

Continued

REVIEW QUESTIONS—cont'd

5. What statement by a patient with Addison's disease indicates that discharge teaching has been effective?
   1. "I will taper off of my glucocorticoid medications after I start feeling better."
   2. "The dietary supplements will help decrease my need for medications."
   3. "My glucocorticoid medications will need to be increased when I am ill or experiencing stress."
   4. "I will recognize that my symptoms are worsening when I experience extreme thirst."
6. When presenting an inservice on endocrine diseases, which statement by the nurse would be correct?
   1. Patients who have acromegaly have primary involvement of the soft tissues and joint. Major organs are spared.
   2. Patients who have diabetes insipidus should be monitored for fluid overload.
   3. Patients with hyperprolactinemia may experience breast engorgement.
   4. Patients with Cushing's syndrome often have episodes of hypotension.
7. Which outcome would be most appropriate to include in the plan of care for a patient who has been diagnosed with a pheochromocytoma?
   1. Fasting glucose will be less than 100 mg/dL
   2. Blood pressure will be within normal limits
   3. Serum sodium will be greater than 135 mg/dL
   4. ECG will demonstrate no ectopy
8. Which clinical manifestation should the nurse assess for when caring for a patient with a diagnosis of hyperthyroidism?
   1. Fine hand tremor
   2. Slow, irregular pulse
   3. Cool, pale extremities
   4. Diminished bowel sound
9. What discharge teaching would be most important for the nurse to include for the patient who is prescribed methimazole (Tapazole)?
   1. Report sore throat and fever to health care provider
   2. Take medication with full glass of water before breakfast
   3. Weight daily and record
   4. Mild headaches should be expected
10. Which statement by a patient who has received instruction about radioiodine therapy for hyperthyroidism would require further explanation by the nurse?
    1. "My infant son breastfeeds every 4 hours."
    2. "I am allergic to iodine."
    3. "I will need to flush the toilet 3 times after each use."
    4. "I will use disposable eating utensils for several days after the treatment."
11. Following a parathyroidectomy, a patient complains of numbness and tingling in the tips of the fingers and around the mouth. The nurse should anticipate the physician writing which order?
    1. Serum albumin
    2. Serum thyroxin
    3. Ionized calcium
    4. Parathyroid hormone level
12. Which therapeutic response should the nurse anticipate when vasopressin is administered?
    1. The patient relates that thirst has resolved.
    2. The patient reports that he is urinating more often.
    3. The patient states his headache has subsided.
    4. The patient demonstrates improvement in appetite.

REVIEW ACTIVITIES

1. A 21-year-old female is admitted to the floor complaining of severe abdominal pain. Routine lab work including an electrolyte panel is ordered. The lab results are as follows: Na = 115 mmol/L; K = 3.6 mmol/L; BUN = 10 mg/dL; Glucose = 126 mg/dL; Hgb = 10 g/dL; and Hct = 30%.
   a. Which lab result should require the nurse's most immediate attention?
   b. Which system assessment is a priority when the sodium is at this level?
   c. What are the priority nursing interventions when caring for a patient with SIADH?
2. A 28-year-old male patient comes to the emergency department complaining of his heart racing. After the history and physical is done, the physician plans to workup the patient for having hyperthyroidism.
   a. State one clinical manifestation that relates to the following body systems, which the nurse should assess the patient.
      Skin:
      Eyes:
      Neuromuscular:
      Respiratory:
      GI:
      Cardiovascular:
   b. Which lab test is most cost-effective and sensitive for diagnosing hyperthyroidism?
   c. What medication should the nurse anticipate the patient being prescribed to control his tachycardia.
3. A 21-year-old female patient is diagnosed as having a prolactinoma.
   a. What clinical manifestations should the nurse anticipate finding during the interview?
   b. The nurse should be aware that a patient who has an untreated prolactinoma is likely to develop what bone disease?
4. a. When caring for a patient with Cushing's syndrome, which electrolyte problem should the nurse monitor most carefully? Why?
   b. What clinical manifestations of hypokalemia should the nurse assess for?
5. Compare an alert patient who has diabetes insipidus with an unconscious patient who has diabetes insipidus. What is more likely to occur in the unconscious patient? Why? What is the priority nursing diagnosis? How is this problem corrected?

Visit the Contemporary Medical-Surgical Nursing online companion resource at www.delmarhealthcare.com for additional content and study aids. Click on Online Companions then select the Nursing discipline.

Diabetes Mellitus: Nursing Management

CHAPTER 57

Martha K. Carlson, MSN

CHAPTER TOPICS

- Type 1 Diabetes
- Type 2 Diabetes
- Management of Diabetes
- Acute Complications of Diabetes
- Chronic Complications of Diabetes

Nurses will potentially encounter patients with diabetes in a wide variety of settings. Therefore it is necessary to have a fundamental knowledge of diabetes and the nursing care involved. The patient's ability to manage diabetes is an important focus for the nurse. This chapter includes information on the pathophysiology of diabetes, diagnosis and management of the disease, and acute and chronic complications. Nursing diagnoses and interventions are included along with expected outcomes.

KEY TERMS

Diabetes mellitus
Endogenous
Euglycemia
Exogenous
Glucagon
Gluconeogenesis
Glycogenolysis
Hyperesthesia
Hyperglycemia
Insulin
Lipodystrophy
Self-monitoring of blood glucose (SMBG)
Syndrome X (insulin resistance syndrome)

DIABETES MELLITUS

Diabetes mellitus refers to a group of chronic disorders of metabolism characterized by elevated blood glucose levels and disturbances in metabolism of carbohydrate, fats, and protein. Diabetes affects approximately 16 million people in the United States, and this number is expected to rise in the future. The majority of patients, approximately 1.4 million have type 1 diabetes, and the remaining 14.5 million have type 2 diabetes.

Annually nearly 18 percent of deaths in people age 25 and older is attributed to diabetes. The American Diabetes Association (ADA) places the remainder of the 16 million patients in a category of diabetes referred to as other specific types (e.g., gestational diabetes). Additionally, numerous people have impaired glucose tolerance, prediabetes, or insulin resistance. The incidence of diabetes increases with age, and there is no variation in gender. African Americans, Hispanic (Americans), Native Americans, Asian (Americans), and Pacific Islanders are at increased risk for development of diabetes. Obesity and advancing age are major contributors to the increased incidence of diabetes regardless of ethnicity or race (Cleator & Wilding, 2003).

Patients with diabetes are twice as likely to experience heart disease as the general population. The mortality rate of heart disease in patients with diabetes is six times greater in males and four times greater in females then in the general population. Type 1 diabetes results from insufficient insulin, and type 2 is a disease of insulin resistance. There has been a dramatic increase in the incidence of diabetes in the past 20 years, particularly type 2 diabetes. In the past, type 2 diabetes was thought to be a disease of adult onset. It is now common to find type 2 diabetes in children and adolescents as well. As a chronic disease, diabetes requires long-term management and is associated with subsequent development of heart disease, hypertension, stroke, kidney disease, and lower limb amputation. Patients with either type 1 or type 2 diabetes can and frequently do develop complications. Patients with diabetes are major consumers of health care, and the nurse can expect to care for them in hospitals, homes, nursing homes, schools, and communities.

It is not uncommon for patients and families to believe that diabetes treated with oral medications is less severe than diabetes treated with insulin. The nurse can play a major role in helping them understand that they do have diabetes and are not just borderline with their blood sugars.

Pathophysiology

ADA has categorized diabetes into four categories as shown in Box 57-1. Of these four types of diabetes, type 1 and type 2 are the most common. Gestational diabetes occurs with pregnancy, with the blood glucose levels typically returning to normal after delivery. These women do, however, have an increased risk of developing diabetes later in life. Impaired glucose tolerance or prediabetes exists when patients have a blood sugar that is higher than normal but not high enough to meet the criteria for diabetes. Studies indicate that many people with prediabetes can delay or even prevent the occurrence of diabetes with regular exercise and weight reduction (Fong, Aiello, Ferris, & Klein, 2004).

BOX 57-1

FOUR TYPES OF DIABETES MELLITUS

Type 1 diabetes mellitus
Type 2 diabetes mellitus
Gestational diabetes
Impaired glucose tolerance (prediabetes)

Type 1 Diabetes

Type 1 diabetes results from a defect or failure of the beta cells of the pancreas' islet cells. The islet cells are destroyed by an interaction of genetics and environmental factors or autoimmunity. This loss of beta cells causes an absolute lack of insulin. Historically, type 1 diabetes was called juvenile onset and thought to have an acute onset. Recent studies now suggest a genetic predisposition with a preclinical period followed by destruction of the beta cells from autoimmune mechanisms, which results in a deficiency of insulin and hyperglycemia. Some authors suggest specific environmental factors are linked to diabetes (Mundy, 2004; Robinson, 2004). Diabetes can also result from pancreatitis or other diseases of the pancreas.

Insulin is one of the hormones produced by the pancreas (beta cells) with a function of lowering blood sugar. **Glucagon** is another hormone released by the alpha cells of the pancreas and it functions to raise blood sugar levels. Beta cell destruction is present long before the patient develops **hyperglycemia** (an elevated blood sugar level). Approximately 90 percent of the beta cells must be destroyed before hyperglycemia occurs, causing a lack of insulin. There is also an increase in glucagon production by the alpha cells of the pancreas. The hyperglycemia from lack of insulin fails to inhibit the production of glucagons. Virtually every form of diabetes is associated with elevated glucagon levels (Griffin & Ojeda., 2004).

Insulin is a storage hormone that moves glucose from the bloodstream into the cells of the liver, muscles, and fat cells. Insulin facilitates the storage of glucose as glycogen in the liver and muscle. It also helps to store fat from the diet in adipose tissue. Insulin stops the body from breaking down stores of protein, glucose, and fat.

The pancreas secretes a basal amount of insulin during times when a food is not being ingested, as during sleep or fasting. Glucagon is also secreted from the pancreas when the blood glucose levels decrease, and the liver is then stimulated to release glucose. The counter-regulatory hormones, insulin and glucagon, keep a homeostatic condition of glucose in the bloodstream.

In type 1 diabetes, there is a destruction of the beta cells of the pancreas and therefore a lack of insulin. As previously stated, the cause of type 1 diabetes is thought to be a combination of genetic, environmental, and immunological factors. Type 1 diabetes is not hereditary; however, there is a genetic predisposition for type 1 to develop in patients with certain human leukocyte antigens (HLA) types. Type 1 diabetes is consequently more common in children and adolescents but can develop at any time. Regardless of the cause, in type 1 diabetes, fasting hyperglycemia occurs as the liver continues to produce glucose. Glucose ingested in the diet is also not able to be utilized and remains in the bloodstream. As the blood glucose elevates, the kidneys are no longer able to filter it effectively, and glucose is spilled into the urine. Fluid and electrolytes are lost in the urine as well. This is referred to as an osmotic diuresis.

Insulin is required by the body for the synthesis of glucose from amino acids **(gluconeogenesis)**. It also stops the physiological process of the breakdown of stored glucose **(glycogenolysis).** With an insulin deficiency, there is no regulatory effect, and the blood sugar elevates as the cells starve. As the body breaks down fats, ketones are produced, which disrupt the acid-base balance in the body.

Type 2 Diabetes

Type 2 diabetes was previously classified as adult onset. A comparison between type 1 and type 2 diabetes is shown in Table 57-1. While patients with type 2 diabetes are generally older, there is a dramatic increase in type 2 diabetes in children and adolescents. Commonly, patients with type 2 diabetes will have insulin resistance syndrome with hypertension, central obesity, and hyperlipidemia for years before diagnosis. The major abnormalities of pathophysiology that occur in patients with type 2 diabetes are: (a) defective beta cell secretion with early loss of first phase insulin production; (b) insulin resistance in the peripheral tissues, especially muscle and liver; and (c) increased production of glucose from the liver as the disease progresses.

First phase insulin secretion inhibits the production and output of glucose by the liver. When there are defects in the beta cells, this inhibitory effect is lost, resulting in fasting hyperglycemia. The body compensates by increasing second phase insulin secretion, which results in hyperinsulinemia. The beta cells may

TABLE 57-1 Comparison of Type 1 and Type 2 Diabetes

TYPE	CHARACTERISTICS	CLINICAL MANIFESTATIONS	MANAGEMENT
Type 1	Destruction of beta cells with absolute lack of insulin. Genetic predispositions and markers determine immune response. Strong hereditary link. Peak onset age 11–13. Onset may be acute, often following long preclinical period Prone to ketoacidosis	Hyperglycemia, polydipsia, polyuria, polyphagia, weight loss, and fatigue	Medications—insulin, diet, exercise, and SMBG
Type 2	Insulin resistance with insulin deficiency. Decrease in number and size of beta cells. Insidious onset. Strong genetic predisposition. Usually occurs over 40 years of age but increasing in frequency in children	Hyperglycemia, obesity, polydipsia, polyuria, skin infections, blurred vision, or fatigue. Not prone to ketosis but can develop with stress	Medications—oral agents or insulin, diet, exercise or SMBG

Adapted from DeLaune, S., & Ladner, P. (2006). Fundamentals of nursing *(3rd ed.). New York: Thomson Delmar Learning.*

continue to secrete high levels of insulin for years to regulate the blood glucose levels. Eventually the beta cells fail, and insulin secretion diminishes. The production of glucose from the liver increases, and then hyperglycemia results. The beta cells are not able to produce sufficient insulin for the demand but are able to produce enough to prevent the breakdown of fat and protein (ketosis).

The tissues develop a decreased sensitivity to insulin and as a result, the body produces more insulin. Hyperinsulinemia does not prevent gluconeogenesis so hyperglycemia occurs. The cells' sensitivity to insulin can decrease as much as 70 percent before fasting plasma glucose levels elevate to an abnormal level. This type 2 diabetes has a slower, more insidious onset, as long as 20 years in some cases. Although there is some uncertainty about the mechanisms of insulin resistance in the tissues, the role of obesity, especially central obesity is clear. Patients will exhibit an impaired glucose tolerance, as the beta cells are able to continue to produce enough insulin to keep the blood sugar elevated but below the level required for a diagnosis of diabetes. This slow progression of glucose tolerance manifests itself with vague symptoms of fatigue, weight gain, irritability, frequent urinary tract infections, and poor skin healing. Often, the diagnosis of type 2 diabetes is made when the patient presents for health care with a complication of the disease. Obesity is associated with type 2 diabetes because of the insulin resistance. Type 2 diabetes has a familial tendency and probably a genetic link.

Syndrome X, also known as **insulin resistance syndrome,** is a group of abnormalities of metabolism that act together to increase the risk of cardiovascular disease. Patients with syndrome X will exhibit high levels of triglycerides, insulin, hypertension, and low-density lipoproteins (LDLs), and decreased levels of high-density lipoproteins (HDLs). The risk factors for syndrome X include abdominal obesity, family history, sedentary lifestyle, gestational diabetes, polycystic ovary disease, and increased age. Programs of weight loss and exercise can prevent or delay the onset of type 2 diabetes in patients at risk for the disease.

Assessment with Clinical Manifestations

Patients with both type 1 and type 2 diabetes will present with the three Ps of diabetes (i.e., polydipsia, polyphagia, and polyuria). Type 1 diabetes is a disorder of metabolism of fat, protein, and carbohydrates. Without the presence of insulin, glucose is unable to enter the cells and remains in the bloodstream. As a result, the cells are starving, and the patient experiences hunger (polyphagia) with weight loss. The increased concentration of glucose in the circulation causes an osmotic diuresis, causing large amounts of urine to be produced (polyuria). Increased blood sugar levels will cause water to be drawn from the cells by osmosis, resulting in cellular dehydration. This triggers the thirst center in the hypothalamus, and the patient drinks large volumes of water (polydipsia). The patient will experience weight loss as the body uses proteins and fats for energy and loses fluids from the osmotic diuresis.

Type 1 diabetes typically has a rapid onset, and the patient presents with the three Ps, fatigue, and weight loss. There may be ketoacidosis present as well. Type 2 diabetes has a more insidious onset, and the patient may already have complications when presenting for health care. Symptoms that induce the patient with type 2 diabetes to seek treatment include frequent infections, delayed wound healing, or fatigue. Patients with type 2 diabetes may also experience polydipsia, polyphagia, and polyuria. Diabetics who are obese will commonly display thin muscular extremities with increased deposits of fat in the abdomen, chest, neck, and face. A waist hip/ratio of greater than 0.9 in men and greater than 0.8 in women is associated with diabetes (Tierney, McPhee, & Papakakais, 2004).

Past health history should include childhood illnesses (rubella, mumps, or other viral illnesses) recent surgery, trauma, stress or infection, pregnancy history, birth weight of infants, and history of pancreatitis. The nurse should inquire about medications used, especially diuretics, corticosteroids, and use of insulin and oral agents. A continued assessment is shown in Box 57-2.

BOX 57-2

ASSESSMENT OF PATIENTS WITH DIABETES

Nutritional—Metabolic

Assess for obesity, changes in weight, increased thirst and hunger, nausea, vomiting, delayed wound healing especially involving the feet, and daily food intake pattern.

Elimination

Inquire about constipation, diarrhea, frequency of urination, nocturia, urinary tract infections, and incontinence.

Activity—Exercise

Assess for the presence of fatigue and muscle weakness.

Cognitive—Perceptual

Assess for the presence of headache, abdominal pain, pruritus, numbness, and tingling in extremities or blurred vision.

Eyes

Inspect for vitreal hemorrhages and cataracts.

Skin

Inspect for pigmentation on legs, ulcers on feet, and loss of hair on legs and feet.

Respiratory

Assess for Kussmaul breathing (rapid, deep respirations).

Cardiovascular

Assess for weak rapid pulse and hypotension.

GI

Assess for fruity breath, vomiting, and dry oral mucous membranes.

Neurological

Assess for restlessness, confusion, stupor, coma, and altered deep tendon reflexes.

BOX 57-3

DIAGNOSTIC CRITERIA FOR DIABETES

Fasting plasma glucose level greater than 126 mg/dL

Random plasma glucose level greater than 200 mg/dL with clinical signs of diabetes

Two-hour oral glucose tolerance test greater than 200 mg/dL with a 75 g glucose load

Diagnostic Tests

There are three standard tests used to determine the presence of diabetes, no matter what type. Diagnosis is not made on a single lab finding but is confirmed with a subsequent test (Box 57-3). If the fasting plasma glucose is elevated on one occasion, it will be confirmed by repeating the test a second day. Fasting plasma glucose is the preferred method of diagnosis. Generally a true elevation of plasma glucose is indicative of diabetes mellitus. There are factors that can elevate the blood glucose level, such as stress (surgery, trauma, general anesthesia, infections, or age), caffeine, and medications (tricyclic antidepressants, corticosteroids, or diuretics).

A patient with a random plasma glucose greater than 200 mg/dL should have a fasting plasma glucose the next day. If the fasting plasma glucose is greater than 126 mg/dL, the diagnosis of diabetes can be made, because it meets the criteria of two occasions of hyperglycemia. If the fasting plasma glucose is less than 126 mg/dL, the patient will likely be given a 75 g glucose challenge for the oral glucose tolerance test (OGTT) and a two-hour plasma glucose level drawn. If this two-hour plasma glucose is greater than 200 mg/dL, the diagnosis of diabetes can be made.

A fasting plasma glucose level is a snap shot in time, giving information about the current state of blood glucose. Another useful test is the glycosylated hemoglobin (hemoglobin A_{1C}). This test measures the amount of glucose attached to hemoglobin molecules and red blood cells over their life span of approximately 120 days. Information from this test provides assessment information about the patient's metabolic control.

The diagnosis of prediabetes is made if the fasting plasma glucose is between 110 to 125 mg/dL. Impaired fasting glucose is currently defined by the ADA as a fasting plasma glucose of 100 to 125 mg/dL. This criterion will effectively increase the number of people with prediabetes. This group may benefit from lifestyle changes of weight reduction and exercise to prevent the onset of diabetes. Screening recommendations for diabetes and prediabetes includes patients with risk factors for the disease (e.g., obesity, family history, older than age 45, or a history of gestational diabetes). Retesting is recommended in three years if the test is normal. Patients diagnosed with prediabetes or impaired glucose tolerance have a greater risk of developing diabetes in 10 years. Lifestyle modifications are recommended for this group (Burden, 2003).

Fast Forward ▶▶▶

Complications for People with Diabetes while Traveling

Patients with diabetes will need extra planning when they travel. Their supplies for their disease management should be readily available in carry-on luggage, including blood glucose monitoring meters, insulin, and syringes. With the increase in homeland security, the patient should bring a letter from his or her health care provider explaining the medical necessity of the syringes. The patient should bring along fast-acting carbohydrate sources to reverse hypoglycemia. Extra medications and food should be included in the event of long delays, canceled flights, and closed restaurants. Patients with diabetes should wear identification stating that they are diabetic. It is also recommended that the patient carry identification with the names of their medications and health care providers.

Nursing Diagnoses

Patients with diabetes may have a large variety of nursing diagnoses. These diagnoses will likely change as the patient learns to manage his or her chronic illness or as other associated problems or complications arise. Based on the information gathered, examples of nursing diagnoses in the patient with diabetes may include the following:

- Deficient knowledge regarding disease process or treatment and individual care needs.
- Imbalanced nutrition less than body requirements.
- Risk for impaired adjustment.
- Risk for infection.
- Risk for disturbed sensory perception.
- Interrupted family processes.

Planning and Implementation

Nursing care for diabetes involves a combination of diet, glucose monitoring, medications, and exercise. As with any chronic disease, the patient is responsible for day-to-day management of his or her disease. Nurses play a major role in education, screening, and follow-up of patients with diabetes. The goals of

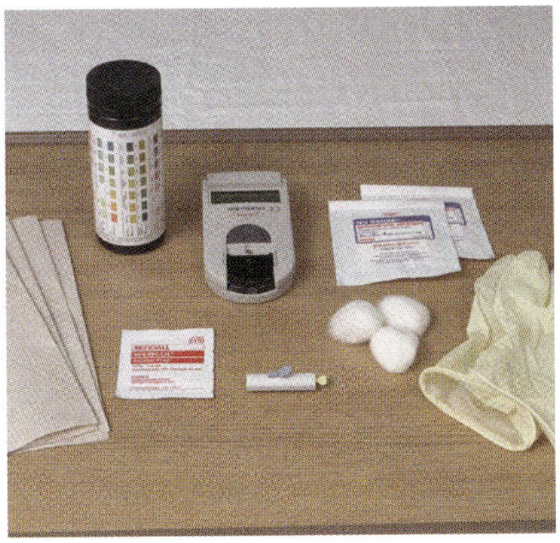

Figure 57-1 Self-monitoring blood glucose equipment.

PATIENT PLAYBOOK

Management of Diabetic People in the Home Environment

Much of the management and care of the patient with diabetes is done by the patient and family at home. The goal is to allow the patient to reach or maintain the optimal level of self-care. The diabetic patient often has difficulty reaching this goal, because patients with diabetes have an increased risk for the development of other chronic illnesses. Often the patient's visual acuity is impaired or his or her functional mobility is limited. Nursing care for diabetic patients in the home involves assessing the patient and caregiver's knowledge and technique with SMBG, insulin preparation and administration, adjustment of insulin dosage, side effects of insulin, exercise pattern, and nutritional therapy. As with any patient teaching, the nurse must first assess the patient's readiness to learn, identify barriers, and determine the meaning of the illness to the patient. It is important to identify the patient's support system and involve the family in the patient's plan of care. The family must understand the plan of care while allowing the patient to manage the disease as long as he or she are able.

nursing management are to reduce hyperglycemia and prevent or delay the onset of acute and long-term complications. Glycemic control is the most likely way to meet these goals, and it is imperative that the patient understand the management of the disease. Patients with type 1 diabetes will require insulin therapy in addition to diet and exercise. Some patients with type 2 diabetes will be successful with weight control, diet modifications, and exercise; however, the majority of patients with type 2 diabetes will require medication to control their blood sugar.

Patients just beginning to use insulin are assessed by the nurse to determine their ability to understand the relationship between insulin, food intake, and exercise. The patient must know the signs and symptoms of hypoglycemia, hyperglycemia, and the actions needed to correct them. If the patient is unable to understand or manage the care, the nurse works with the caregiver to ensure compliance. Regular evaluations of the patient's techniques with insulin therapy, including management of hypoglycemia and self-monitoring of blood glucose, are conducted. The nurse will review the patient's blood glucose log to assess patterns and glycemic control. If the patient is managing the disease with oral agents, the nursing care is similar. The nurse assesses the administration and response to the medications. The nurse must remember to advise the patient with diabetes as they live out their lives and go about their daily routines (see Fast Forward).

Blood glucose monitoring by patients has dramatically increased care in diabetes. Frequent monitoring of blood glucose levels allows the patient to adjust and manage their regimen for optimal glycemic control. Normalization of blood glucose levels helps to prevent the long-term complications of diabetes. **Self-monitoring of blood glucose (SMBG)** is a method whereby a patient tests his or her own blood glucose levels (Figure 57-1). SMBG also allows patients who take insulin the ability to detect and treat asymptomatic hypoglycemia. The Diabetes Control and Complications Trial (DCCT) determined that there are significant health benefits for patients treated with insulin that achieve normal or near normal blood glucose levels (Gordon, 2004). Based on the results of the DCCT, the recommendation from the ADA encourages the use of SMBG for daily routine monitoring, especially patients treated with insulin to maintain and prevent asymptomatic hypoglycemia. For most patients SMBG is required three times a day but the frequency may vary by individual. There are no data to suggest the optimal number of times type 2 diabetics should monitor their blood sugar, but the frequency should be enough to facilitate reaching the glycemic goals. The frequency of hyperglycemic and hypoglycemic events will be decreased with frequent SMBG. Whenever diet, exercise, or medications are modified, both type 1 and type 2 patients should increase the frequency of monitoring. Home management for diabetics is complicated and requires a great deal of instruction by nurses. This is illustrated in the patient playbook feature.

The accuracy of SMBG is dependent on the instrument and the operator. Health care providers should periodically and regularly evaluate the patient's monitoring technique. The patient should regularly use calibration and control solutions with their testing equipment to ensure accuracy of readings. The patient also needs to be taught to interpret and use the data from SMBG to achieve and maintain optimal glycemic control.

There are a variety of SMBG methods on the market. Most require application of a drop of blood from the fingertip to a reagent strip (Figure 57-2). The blood remains on the strip for a specified period of time, and the meter gives a reading of the blood glucose level. The nurse has a major role in the initial patient teaching about SMBG. Patients are instructed to keep a logbook of their blood glucose readings so patterns can be assessed. Patients should be given guidelines when to contact their health care provider. Those on intensive insulin regimens may be given algorithms to follow for changing their insulin dose based on blood glucose levels. Electronic diaries or PDAs can also

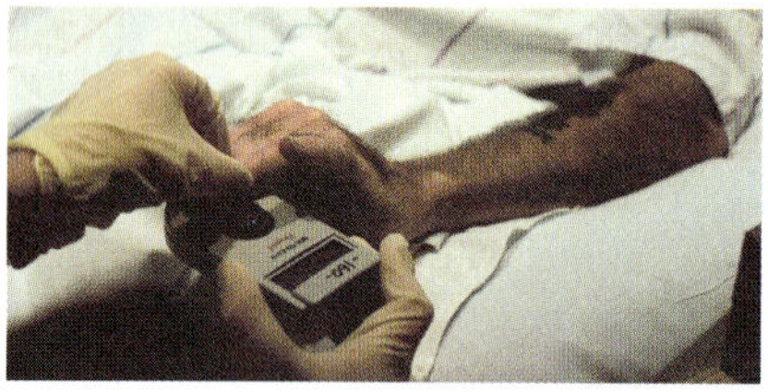

Figure 57-2 A nurse obtaining a sample of blood for glucose testing.

be used to track blood glucose results and activity levels. Data collected in this manner can be shared among patient and primary and other health care providers (Kerkenbusch, 2003).

Nutrition

Nutritional therapy is based on a well-balanced diet and is one of the mainstays in the treatment of diabetes. Because of the social and psychological issues associated with eating, this aspect of therapy can likely be one that the patient has the most difficulty controlling. A multidisciplinary health care team approach may be the most effective. There are many misconceptions about diet and diabetes, and in fact the plan of eating for diabetics is based on healthy eating, which would benefit anyone. Patients with diabetes can eat the same types of foods as people who do not have diabetes. The goals of nutritional therapy are shown Box 57-4.

Patients with type 1 diabetes will have a food plan based on activity, food intake, and insulin requirements. Patients with type 2 diabetes will have a food plan with an emphasis on maintaining blood glucose levels, lowering blood pressure, and weight reduction, as there is a high incidence of obesity. The meal plan will be formulated by the dietitian, reinforced by the nurse, and will include decreased fat intake, particularly saturated fats, and a decrease in simple sugars. Even a small weight loss of 5 to 7 percent can improve glycemic control. Weight loss can be accomplished with a program of exercise.

General dietary guidelines for patients with diabetes include the identification of the percentage of calories to come from carbohydrates, protein, and fats. Carbohydrates have the greatest effect on blood sugar, because of their rapid absorption and conversion to glucose. The ADA (2006) now recommends 60 to 70 percent of the caloric intake came from carbohydrates and monosaturated fats. This amount may vary for obese type 2 diabetics as their goals include weight loss, glucose, and lipid controls. This group of patients is taught to limit carbohydrate intake and substitute monosaturated lower cholesterol oils, such as olive oil, canola oil, or the oils in avocados and nuts. Patients with type 1 diabetes using intensive insulin therapy with near normal blood glucose levels can also use this approach. Patients are taught carbohydrate counting to administer one unit of regular or lispro insulin for 10 to 15 g of carbohydrate at a meal. Carbohydrates play a major role in the regulation of blood glucose levels. Managing carbohydrate intake can be accomplished by use of an exchange list or counting grams of carbohydrates consumed. Low-carbohydrate diets are not recommended as they are a major source for energy, water-soluble vitamins and minerals, and fiber. The current recommendation for carbohydrate intake is 45 to 65 percent of the total caloric intake.

> **BOX 57-4**
>
> **NUTRITIONAL THERAPY FOR PATIENTS WITH DIABETES**
>
> The following are goals for nutritional therapy for diabetes:
>
> - Maintenance of blood glucose levels to near normal to prevent complications.
> - Lifestyle modifications for the treatment of obesity and prevention of cardiovascular disease and dyslipidemia.
> - Reduction in blood pressure.
> - Selection of healthy food choices.
>
> *Adapted from Roth, R. (2007).* Nutrition and diet therapy *(9th ed.). New York: Thomson Delmar Learning.*

Current recommendations for both type 1 and type 2 diabetes includes a protein intake of 15 to 20 percent of total calories and limitation of cholesterol to 300 mcg daily (Bartels, 2004). There are still no conclusions about the long-term effects of diets high in protein and low in carbohydrates (e.g., Atkins diet). While these diets produce a short-term weight loss and improve glycemia, there is no proof of long-term weight loss, and there is a concern about the effects of the diet on LDL cholesterol.

The goal for dietary fat intake for patients with diabetes is to limit saturated fats and cholesterol. Use of lower fat or fat-free foods and beverages will reduce the amount of high fat intake in the diet, and these substances are approved by the Food and Drug Administration. Regular use of these products may not reduce weight however. Polyunsaturated fats should make up approximately 10 percent of the caloric intake.

Dietary fiber has been shown to improve blood glucose levels and decrease endogenous insulin requirements. Fiber is classified as soluble or insoluble. Soluble fiber is found in legumes, some fruits, and oats. This type of fiber seems to play a larger role in reduction of blood glucose and lipid levels than insoluble fibers, but the clinical significance is probably small. Soluble fiber

Fast Forward ▶▶▶

The Use of Personal Digital Assistants (PDAs) in Blood Glucose Monitoring

Traditionally, patients recorded their blood glucose measurements using paper and pencil. The technology of PDAs offers some advantages over this traditional method of recordkeeping. Findings in a study demonstrated a significant lowering of hemoglobin A_{1C} when electronic diaries were used. The blood glucose level was tracked over a three-month period. The PDAs were able to give feedback on the amount of carbohydrate, fat, and protein in the patient's meals. This was accomplished by downloading the data via the phone lines. PDAs have also been used also in patients with migraine headaches. The technology offers promise for improving outcomes for patients with diabetes (Kerkenbush, 2003).

Respecting Our Differences

Age and the Relationship to Complications of Diabetes

Approximately 20 percent of patient's age 65 and older will have diabetes, and this number is expected to increase. Currently there are no available long-term studies of people 65 and older that examines the effects of glycemic, lipid, and blood pressure control (Fong, et al., 2004). Patients in this age-group often present with other chronic illnesses and different levels of cognitive ability that must be factored into their plan of care. Evidence suggests that greater benefits in reduction of morbidity and mortality may be possible by reduction and control of all cardiovascular risk functions instead of aiming for tight glycemic control alone. Less stringent glycemic target goals may be reasonable for older patients with advanced complications of diabetes, cognitive impairment, or other comorbidities affecting life span.

slows emptying of the stomach by forming a gel in the gastrointestinal (GI) tract. The slower rate of absorption caused by the fiber gel may contribute to lowering of the blood glucose levels. Insoluble fiber, found in whole grains, cereals, and some vegetables, increases bulk in the stools and prevents constipation in diabetes. Both types of fiber are beneficial in weight loss and produce a feeling of satiety.

Alcohol is permitted for patients with diabetes, but the patient should be aware of the affects of alcohol on diabetes. Alcohol decreases gluconeogenesis and will contribute to hypoglycemia. Additionally, alcohol has no nutritional benefits, is high in calories, and is damaging to the liver. Abuse of alcohol can make control of blood sugar more difficult, and the patient should carefully and honestly discuss this with their health care provider. Moderate use of alcohol can be incorporated into the dietary plan, if the patient has good blood sugar control. To reduce the risk of hypoglycemia from alcohol, the patient can eat carbohydrates while drinking. Alcoholic drinks provide empty calories, approximately 135 calories per drink. In addition to eating food while drinking alcohol, the patient with diabetes should drink dry, light wines, and use sugar-free mixes.

The ADA (2006) states that the clinical dietician is the team member to provide medical nutritional therapy. Often it is the nurse who is responsible for teaching dietary management to the patient and family. A useful tool is the Food Pyramid Guide, which provides visual cues to the patient about recommended amounts of foods to be eaten from each food group daily. The Food Pyramid Guide was reshaped with a new emphasis on the type of calories eaten with an emphasis on fruits, vegetables, whole grains, lower fat milk products, and exercise. Patients may also be given exchange lists, which divide foods into three main groups: carbohydrate, meat and meat substitutes, and fats. The carbohydrate group includes starches, fruit, milk, other carbohydrates, such as grains, and vegetables. The meat group is further divided into very lean, lean, medium-fat, and high-fat groups. The fat group has small serving sizes and is divided into monounsaturated, polyunsaturated, and saturated fats.

It is important for the diabetic patient and family members to learn to read food labels. Caution is advised about portion size as the serving sizes on food labels may not be the same size as those recommended in the patient's nutritional plan. The patient can compare the serving size on the food label to the serving sizes in the exchange list. They will need to check the number of grams of carbohydrate, protein, and fat in the serving size as well as the number of calories. If the food contains less than 20 calories per serving it is considered a free food.

Another way for the nurse to teach the basics of nutrition is to use the plate method. This allows the patient to visualize the portions of vegetables, meat, and carbohydrates that should fill up a 9-inch plate. At lunch and dinner, nonstarchy vegetables and meat will fill up half the plate, one fourth is 2 to 3 ounces of lean meat, and the remaining one fourth is filled with a carbohydrate. The patient should have a fruit and glass of low-fat milk to complete the meal. Breakfast is made up of one half of the plate filled with carbohydrates, one fourth filled with an optional protein, and the remaining fourth is made up of a fresh fruit and low fat milk.

It is essential to include the patient's family and significant others in the dietary teaching and planning. Identify the person who will be cooking and make sure they understand the diet. The responsibility for maintaining the diet is the patient.

Pharmacology

The storage and metabolism of carbohydrates, proteins, and fats are controlled by insulin, particularly in the liver, muscle, and adipose tissue. It is the key that unlocks the door to the cell allowing transport of nutrients inside. Because of the insulin deficiency of beta cells, patients with type 1 diabetes will require administration of **exogenous** (originating outside an organ) insulin to maintain blood glucose control. Patients with type 2 diabetes produce insulin and have functioning beta cells. Patients with type 2 diabetes may require insulin if diet, exercise, weight reduction, and oral hypoglycemics do not maintain adequate blood sugar control.

Insulin

Insulin preparations in the past were from pork or beef pancreas. Currently the majority of insulin used is human insulin. Human insulin is produced using strands of *Escherichia coli* and DNA technology. Human insulin has fewer incidences of allergic reactions than animal insulins. There are a wide variety of insulin preparations available to facilitate control of blood glucose levels and to adjust to the lifestyles of patients with diabetes. Each patient's dose of insulin is individualized to maintain **euglycemia** (a normal concentration of glucose in the blood) and avoid hyperglycemia and hypoglycemia. The measurement of insulin is units and injections are standardized with each milliliter containing 100 USP units of insulin (U100) (Broyles, Reiss, & Evans, 2007). Insulins are classified according to onset, peak action, and duration. Human insulins have a shorter duration of action than insulin from animal sources. Regular insulin is the base for all insulin preparations. Additives of protamine, zinc, and acetate buffers alter the onset, peak, and duration of insulin action. Lente insulin contains zinc; NPH insulin contains zinc and protamine. The additives in the insulin may cause allergic reactions at the injection site. The additives alter the appearance of the insulin, making it cloudy, rather than the clear appearance of regular insulin.

Lispro insulin (Humalog) is classified as an ultra short-acing insulin that peaks in one hour after subcutaneous injection, and it has a duration of action of four hours regardless of the dose. Food intake must be with in 15 minutes of injection to avoid hypoglycemia. Regular insulin is short-acting insulin with an onset of action in 30 minutes and duration of five to seven hours. Regular insulin is also administered intravenously in hyperglycemic emergencies.

Lente insulin is an intermediate-acting insulin with an onset of action in 2 hours, peak in 8 to 12 hours, and a duration of action of 18 to 24 hours. It is commonly given in two daily injections. NPH insulin is also an intermediate-acting insulin with onset and duration comparable to those of Lente. It is usually given twice daily and mixed with regular insulin to mimic the body's own insulin pattern. Premixed insulins (70% NPH, 30% Regular) are also available for patients who may have difficulty mixing insulins.

Insulin glargine (Lantus, Aventis) has a long duration of action, up to 24 hours after one subcutaneous injection. Insulin gargline is indicated for adults and children (age 6 and up) with type 1 diabetes and adults with type 2 diabetes requiring a basal (long-acting) insulin. Insulin gargline provides a constant insulin concentration similar to an insulin infusion. It requires a once daily injection at bedtime. If a patient becomes hypoglycemic with insulin gargline, the prolonged effects may delay the recovery.

Insulin is administered to mimic the body's normal insulin release and control blood glucose levels. With normal pancreatic functioning there is a continuous secretion of insulin throughout the day and night with increased secretion of insulin after eating. There are several insulin regimens used, ranging from a single dose of insulin to multiple doses requiring frequent monitoring of blood glucose. Commonly patients use a combination of short-acting and longer-acting insulin to achieve glycemic control (Table 57-2).

Insulin is administered with plastic disposable syringes that are available in 1 mL, 0.3 mL, and 0.5 mL sizes. The 0.3 mL syringe is referred to as the low-dose syringe and is popular among diabetics. Except in cases of severe insulin resistance, patients should not take more than 30 units of insulin in one injection. The syringes are available in short (8 mm) and long (12.7 mm) needle lengths, with the longer length preferable for obese patients. Patients at home may reuse the disposable syringes three to five times until the needle begins to blunt. Recapping the syringes at home after use provides sufficient sterility. It is not necessary to clean the needle with alcohol, and this practice may in fact alter the silicone coating on the needle and increase the pain with subsequent injections. Before recommending the recapping of syringes, consideration must be given to the patient's vision and manual dexterity. The patient should be taught to hold the syringe firmly in one hand and recap the needle using a straight motion of the forefinger and thumb (Figure 57-3). It is important that the syringe be stabilized to avoid needle-stick injury. Several pen-like devices are available for insulin delivery as well. These pens contain insulin cartridges and are useful for patients who are neurologically impaired.

Insulin may be given using a single type of insulin (Regular) or in a mixed dose (Regular and NPH). Longer acting insulins will have a cloudy appearance and should be rotated gently in the palms to resuspend the insulin. Insulin requires special storage considerations. As a protein, insulin is affected by heat and freezing. Extremes of temperature will alter the molecule of insulin. An insulin vial that is currently in use can be stored at room temperature as long as four weeks if the temperature of the room remains between 37 and 86 degrees.

TABLE 57-2 Types of Insulins

TYPE	ONSET	PEAK	DURATION
Humalog (Lispro)	Less than 15 minutes	30–90 minutes	4 hours
Regular	30–60 minutes	2–4 hours	5–7 hours
NPH	3–4 hours	6–12 hours	18–28 hours
Lente	1–3 hours	8–12 hours	18–28 hours
Ultra Lente	4–6 hours	18–24 hours	36 hours
70/30	15–30 minutes	2–3 hours and 8–12 hours	18–24 hours
Insulin glargine	1.1 hour	5 hours	24 hours

Adapted from Broyles, B. E., Reiss, B. S., & Evans, M. E. (2007). Pharmacological aspects of nursing care *(7th ed.). New York: Thomson Delmar Learning.*

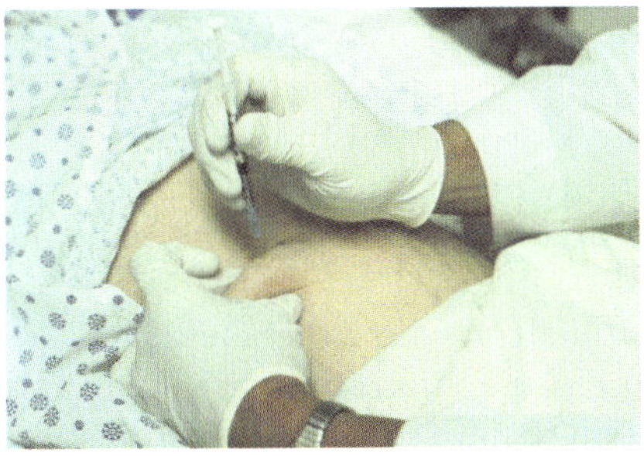

Figure 57-3 Performing a subcutaneous injection of insulin.

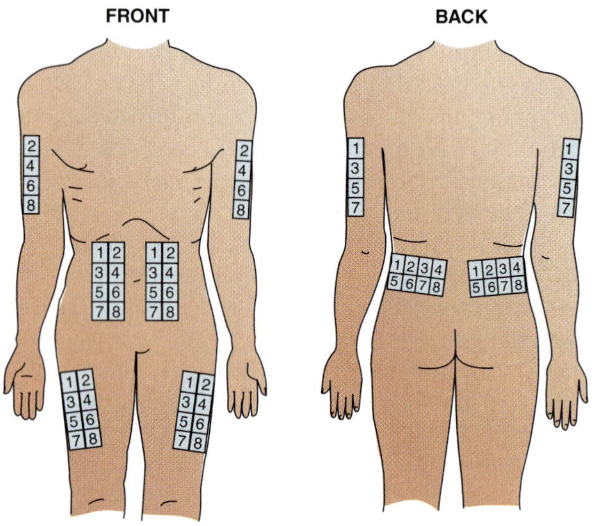

Figure 57-4 Possible sites and rotation for insulin administration.

The vials should be protected from direct sunlight. Insulin not in use should be stored in the refrigerator. Insulin that is kept at room temperature is less likely to irritate the injection site than insulin that is cold.

Newly diagnosed patients requiring insulin therapy will need education on preparing and administering an insulin injection. The nurse should review insulin injection procedures with patients to ensure a correct technique as diabetes is a lifelong disease. The rate of absorption of insulin varies with the anatomic location of the injection site. Insulin is absorbed fastest from the abdomen, followed by the arm, thighs, and buttocks. Exercise of the thigh or arm will increase the absorption time and rate of onset of action. The abdomen remains the preferred site of injection because of the convenience and its good absorption rates.

Prior to the use of purified human insulins, rotation of insulin sites was a part of patient education. The rotation of sites was used to prevent **lipodystrophy,** a localized complication of insulin administration characterized by changes in the subcutaneous fat at the site of the injection. This is not a problem with human insulin, and it is no longer necessary to recommend rotation of insulin sites. Patients are instructed to inject into the abdomen and rotate the injection sites in that area (Figure 57-4).

Insulin is injected subcutaneously at a 90° angle. It is not necessary to aspirate with the injection. The needle should remain in the skin for five seconds after the injection to ensure that a complete dose of insulin has been administered. This is particularly true if an insulin pen is used. If blood or clear fluid is visible at the injection site after withdrawing the needle, pressure should be applied to the injection site for 5 to 10 seconds without rubbing. If this occurs, the patient should monitor their blood glucose more often that day. Suggestions for minimizing pain with insulin injections are shown in the Skills 360° feature.

Skills 360°

Injection of Insulin

Pain with the insulin injection can be minimized by:

- Injecting insulin at room temperature.
- Ensuring no air bubbles are in the syringe prior to injection.
- Allowing topical alcohol to evaporate prior to injection.
- Using a quick wrist motion to puncture the skin quickly.
- Avoiding reuse of needles.

Insulin pumps provide a continuous administration of short-acting insulin subcutaneously. These pumps are small battery operated devices that can be worn on a belt. The pump is connected to a catheter inserted in the subcutaneous tissue in the patient's abdomen. The patient will change the insertion site every 48 to 72 hours and refill the pump with insulin. The pump delivers a basal rate of insulin 24 hours a day. The user programs the pump to deliver boluses at mealtime based on the amount of carbohydrates ingested. Because the insulin pump closely mimics normal insulin secretion and uses only rapid-acting insulin, which has the least variable absorption rate, tighter glycemic control is possible. Because the insulin is absorbed more efficiently, patients often require 25 percent less insulin with a pump than with multiple daily injections. Patients who use the pump must be knowledgeable about carbohydrate counting, because the pump delivers boluses based on carbohydrates eaten at a meal. Use of a pump offers the advantage of more flexibility with mealtimes and a more normal lifestyle (Figure 57-5).

Intensive insulin therapy is another option with a goal of near normal blood glucose levels between 80 and 120 mg/dL. Multiple daily insulin injections and frequent SMBG make up this regimen. The outcomes of this type of insulin administration compares favorably with administration by insulin pump. It has the disadvantage of three or more insulin injections daily. Long-acting or intermediate-acting insulins are used for to stabilize the patient's blood glucose levels.

Oral agents are commonly used for treatment of type 2 diabetes. They are not insulin but affect the manner in which glucose and insulin are made and used by the body. It is necessary for the patient to have some **endogenous** (produced or originating from within a cell or organism) insulin for the oral hypoglycemics to take effect.

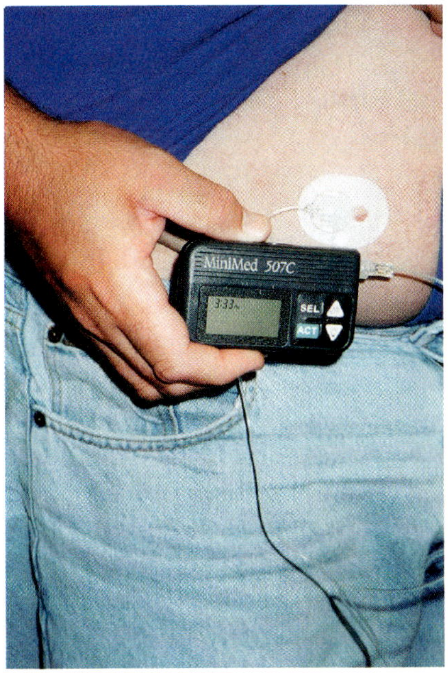

Figure 57-5 The Insulin Pump.

Sulfonylureas were introduced in the 1950s for treatment of diabetes. This classification includes Tolinase (tolazamide), Dymelor (acetohexamide), and Orinase (Tolbutamide). These drugs are referred to as first generation, because they have been used the longest. There are several second-generation sulfonylureas available today including Glucotrol and Glucotrol XL (glipizide), Micronase, DiaBeta, and Glynase (glyburide), and Amaryl (glimepiride). The second-generation drugs have a longer duration of action and fewer side effects.

Sulfonylureas act to increase the production of insulin by the pancreas, and therefore a functioning pancreas is necessary. They also improve the action of insulin at the cellular level and are thought to decrease glucose production in the liver. They tend to have better effectiveness early in the course of the disease.

Alpha glucosidase inhibitors (e.g., Precose) delay the absorption and digestion of carbohydrates in the small intestine, resulting in a smaller increase in blood glucose after eating. This classification of drugs does not alter insulin production and does not produce hypoglycemia. Because they are not absorbed systemically, they are safe to use. They can be used as monotherapy or in combination with sulfonylureas, thiazolidinediones, or meglitinide. The patient may experience hypoglycemia when used in combination with sulfonylureas and thiazolidinediones.

Biguanides (e.g., Glucophage) are another type of oral hypoglycemic agent that acts by decreasing absorption from the intestines and glucose production in the liver. Additionally, peripheral insulin sensitivity is increased. Because it does not act on the beta cells in the pancreas, there is no change in the secretion of insulin and no hypoglycemia. Lactic acidosis is a potentially serious side effect with this medication.

Meglitinide (e.g., Prandin) is another agent to lower blood glucose by stimulation of the beta cells of the pancreas. It is shorter acting than the sulfonylureas. There must be some functioning of the pancreas for this drug to be effective. It is to be taken before meals to stimulate the body to secrete insulin in response to the meal. Hypoglycemia is a side effect of meglitinide.

Thiazolidinediones (e.g., Actos, Avandia) lower insulin resistance by resensitization of the body to its own insulin and are most effective in patients with insulin resistance. They will not cause hypoglycemia when used as monotherapy, because they do not increase the production of insulin.

Patients who are using these oral hypoglycemic agents need to understand that the drugs are in addition to other types of therapy, namely diet and exercise. The patients may not always respond to the oral agents and may need to be started on insulin if the oral agents are no longer effective. Combination therapy with the oral agents is commonly used, and patients need to know the signs and symptoms of hypoglycemia (Table 57-3).

Exercise

Regular exercise is an essential part of the treatment of diabetes because of its ability to lower blood sugar and decrease cardiovascular risk factors (Blair & Church, 2003). Exercise increases the body's uptake of glucose by the muscles and therefore lowers blood sugar levels. Strength or resistance training will increase lean muscle mass and increase the metabolic rate. This is helpful in weight reduction. Exercise will aid in the reduction of cardiovascular risks by increasing HDLs and lowering cholesterol and triglyceride levels. There are additional exercise benefits resulting in decreased stress, decreased depression, and increased self-esteem.

Patients should work toward a goal of 30 minutes of exercise daily. The intensity of exercise should allow both breathing and talking with ease during the exercise. Patients can be taught to gauge the intensity of exercise by determining their desired heart range and checking the pulse to see if their heart rate falls in the target range. Target range is estimated by subtracting the patient's age from 220. This value is multiplied by 60 percent to determine the lower

TABLE 57-3 Oral Hypoglycemics

GENERIC (BRAND)	USUAL DOSE	ONSET TIME (HOURS)	DURATION (HOURS)
First-Generation Sulfonylureas			
tobutamide (Orinase)	500–2,000 mg divided dose	1	6–12
acetohexamide (Dymelor)	250–1,500 mg single or divided dose	1	12–24
tolazamide (Tolinase)	100–1,000 mg single or divided dose	4–6	12–24
chlorpropamide (Diabanese)	100–750 mg single dose	1	60
Second-Generation Sulfonylureas			
glipizide (Glucatrol)	2.5–40 mg single or divided dose	1–1½	10–16
glimepride (Amaryl)	1–4 mg single dose	1	24
glyburide (Diabeta, Micronase)	1.25–20 mg single or divided dose	2–4	24
Biguanides			
metformin hydrochloride (Glucophage)	500–2,500 mg two or three divided doses	24–48	6–12
Alpha-Glucosidase Inhibitors			
acarbose (Precose)	25–100 mg with meals (tid)	1	No data
miglitol (Glyset)	25–100 mg with meals (tid)	2–3	4–6
Thiazolidenediones			
troglitazone (Rezulin)	200–600 mg with a meal (qd)	2–3	No data

Adapted from Broyles, B. E., Reiss, B. S., & Evans, M. E. (2007). Pharmacological aspects of nursing care *(7th ed.). New York: Thomson Delmar Learning.*

limit and by 80 percent to obtain the upper limit. Patients just beginning an exercise program should use the lower limit as their target heart rate initially.

Those patients who have pacemakers, or take beta blockers, have arrhythmias, or autonomic neuropathies should use this heart rate formula with caution. The lower limit of 60 percent may overtax the heart. Patients should be taught to stop exercising and get immediate help if they experience shortness of breath, chest tightness or pain, dizziness, palpitations, or weakness.

Exercise can cause fluctuations in blood sugar levels, and the patient should be taught how to prevent these. Patients using insulin or oral medications that promote insulin secretion should be familiar with the symptoms of hypoglycemia because physical exercise lowers insulin resistance and can cause hypoglycemia for up to 48 hours after. Commonly blood glucose levels will drop between 6 and 15 hours after exercise as insulin resistance is decreased, and the muscles and liver replace the glycogen stores. The patient can reduce the risk of hypoglycemia during exercise by checking the blood sugar level before exercise and eating a carbohydrate snack for a blood sugar reading less than 100 mg/dL. It is safe to start exercise if the blood sugar level is between 100 and 200mg/dL. The patient should be taught to monitor blood glucose levels before, during, and after exercise and to eat a carbohydrate snack if the exercise session lasts longer than 60 minutes.

If the patient becomes hypoglycemic during exercise, they should immediately stop and monitor their blood sugar every 15 minutes until the level is higher than 89 mg/dL. The patient should always have a ready supply of glucose sugars and carbohydrates on hand. Exercise-induced hypoglycemia should be treated with such substances as 15 grams of carbohydrate, one half cup of fruit juice, 8 ounces of low fat milk, 6 ounces of sweetened carbonated beverage, or 4 glucose tablets.

Exercise can also cause hyperglycemia in diabetics. This typically happens when the circulating level of insulin is low and occurs more commonly in type 1 diabetes. The patient should check the blood sugar level prior to exercise. If the blood sugar level is greater than 250 mg/dL, the urine should be checked for ketones. If the ketone level in the urine is moderate to high, the patient should not exercise until the blood sugar and ketone levels are lower. Patients with type 1 diabetes can exercise with an elevated blood glucose level (250 to 300 mg/dL) as long as there are no ketones present. The blood sugar level should decrease within 15 minutes of exercise. Type 2 diabetics should not exercise if the blood sugar level is greater than 400 mg/dL. It is important to remember that type 1 diabetes is associated with ketoacidosis. Patients who participate in high-intensity physical activity may experience a transient blood glucose elevation that should fall within several hours. This elevation is a result of hormonal factors and should not be treated with insulin but should be carefully monitored.

Evaluation of Outcomes

Nutritional therapy is a mainstay in the patient's management of diabetes. The patient with diabetes should be able to maintain glycemic control utilizing their prescribed therapeutic nutritional plan. If the patient is overweight, it is expected that a slow steady weight loss will be attained using the prescribed nutritional therapy. A reduction in blood pressure may be expected with weight reduction. The patient should be able to demonstrate the selection of healthy food choices in the amounts outlined in their therapeutic nutritional plan.

There may be a localized allergic reaction at the site of the insulin injection. This is manifested as redness, tenderness, swelling, and induration or appearance of a 2- to 4-mm wheal within one to two hours after the injection. These rare reactions will occur early in the course of insulin therapy and will decrease as insulin therapy continues. Local allergic reactions are rare now with the increased use of human insulins.

Systemic allergic reactions to insulin rarely occur but may be associated with anaphylaxis. Immediately the patient will experience a localized skin reaction that increases to generalized urticaria (hives). Lipodystrophy, as previously described, can occur at the site of the injection. This reaction occurs less commonly with the use of human insulin. Fibrous, fatty changes occur at the site of repeated injections, leaving a lumpy area on the skin. Insulin injected into these scarred areas will be absorbed more slowly. In the past, lipoatrophy also occurred with repeated injections at the same site. With lipoatrophy, there is a loss of the subcutaneous fat resulting in a dimpling or pitting of the skin. Again, the occurrence of this is now rare because of the increased use of human insulins.

Respecting Our Differences

Aging and Diabetes

Geriatric patients with diabetes should be given a comprehensive geriatric history and physical in addition to a preexercise screening. Issues to be considered include an assessment of balance and gait, nutritional status, visual changes, cognitive level, and functional capacity. Elderly patients should avoid high-intensity exercise that can increase the risk of myocardial ischemia, which may be asymptomatic in diabetes. Strength training with low resistance for the legs, trunk, arms, and stomach will help to prevent functional decline and loss of muscle mass.

ACUTE COMPLICATIONS OF DIABETES

Acute complications of diabetes include hyperglycemia from too little insulin and hypoglycemia from too much insulin. In both diabetic ketoacidosis (DKA) and hyperosmolar hyperglycemic nonketotic syndrome (HHNS), there is an imbalance among circulating insulin levels and the counter regulatory hormones. The hormones stimulate increase glucose production in the liver and cause decreased utilization of glucose in the peripheral tissues. Infection is one of the most common causes for the development of DKA or HHNS. Medications affecting the metabolism of carbohydrates, such as corticosteroids or thiazides, may also contribute to the development of DKA and HHNS.

The management of both DKA and HHNS is aimed at monitoring and correcting the frequent dehydration, hyperglycemia, and electrolyte imbalances of the patient. Nurses must be able to clinically differentiate the two events. Hypoglycemia can rapidly develop causing serious threat to the patient's well-being.

Diabetic Ketoacidosis

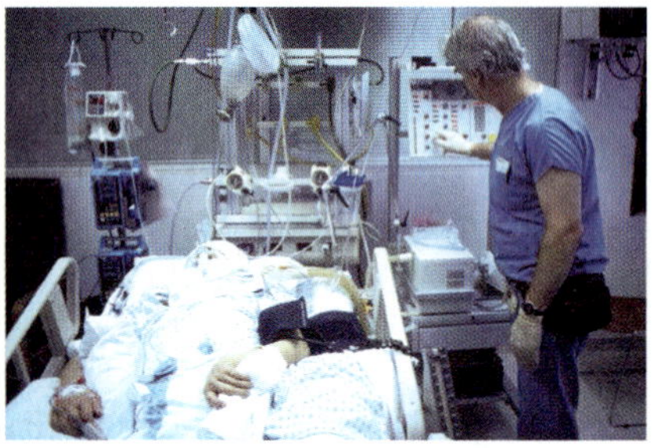

Figure 57-6 Patient on a ventilator in a critical care unit for the complication of DKA.

DKA results from a marked insulin deficiency and is manifested by hyperglycemia, ketosis, acidosis, and dehydration. DKA is associated with type 1 diabetes but may also occur in type 2. It is a life-threatening medical emergency associated with a mortality rate of approximately 5 percent (Figure 57-6). Factors contributing to the development of DKA include illness, infection, inadequate management of the disease, insufficient insulin, and undiagnosed type 1 diabetes. Noncompliance with the therapeutic regimen is the most common causes of recurrent ketoacidosis (Tierney, et al., 2004).

In DKA, there is insufficient insulin to metabolize glucose, and the body begins to break down protein stores for energy. Ketones are by-products of protein breakdown and are acidic in nature. As the ketone level in the blood increases, the pH is altered, and metabolic acidosis develops.

Assessment with Clinical Manifestations

The patient often will experience fatigue, polydipsia, and polyuria prior to the development of ketoacidosis. Nausea, vomiting, and change in the level of consciousness (LOC) can occur as well. Physical examination reveals dehydration from the hyperglycemia and the characteristic acetone or fruity odor of the breath. There is fluid and electrolyte depletion with the dehydration, and the patient will have hypotension and tachycardia. Abdominal pain is accompanied by nausea and vomiting. Kussmaul breathing is associated with DKA. The respiratory rate increases in rate and depth in an attempt to blow off the carbon dioxide accumulating with the acidosis state. Laboratory findings include hyperglycemia greater than 250 mg/dL, acidic pH in the arterial blood (less than 7.35), and low serum bicarbonate levels (less than 15 mEq/L). Ketones and glucose are present in the urine in large amounts. Serum potassium may be elevated as potassium shifts with the acidosis. Potassium levels may also be near normal or low. This represents a severe total body depletion of potassium and requires careful monitoring as the treatment of DKA will further lower the potassium levels. The patient is typically slightly hypothermic, and an infection should be suspected if an elevation in temperature is present. Hypothermia occurs because of peripheral vasodilatation and is considered a poor prognostic sign (Hurlock-Chorostecki, 2004).

Nursing Diagnoses

Based on the information gathered, examples of nursing diagnoses in the patient with diabetes may include the following:

- Deficient fluid volume related to active losses.
- Disturbed thought processes related to physiological causes.
- Risk for imbalanced body temperature related to decreased sensitivity of thermoreceptors.

Planning and Implementation

Patients with DKA can now be managed at home if the dehydration is not severe. The decision to manage the patient at home takes into consideration other accompanying symptoms, such as change in LOC, presence of fever, increased fluid losses through nausea, vomiting and diarrhea, and the ability for frequent communication with the health care practitioner.

The patient's fluid volume deficit is life-threatening and must be treated immediately. Fluid replacement of the intravascular and extravascular space is the goal of treatment. Intravenous (IV) fluids of 0.9% normal saline (NS) or 0.45% NS are used to reestablish an adequate urine output of 30 to 60 mL/hour and reverse the hypotension. When the blood glucose level is down to 250 mg/dL, 5% dextrose is added to the IV fluids to prevent hypoglycemia. Particular attention is given to correction of potassium imbalances. At the onset, the potassium levels may be high or normal, but these levels will fall with the administration of IV insulin. Insulin will move the potassium from the circulation into the cells and hypokalemia develops. This is a lethal complication of DKA. Potassium replacement will be administered to prevent hypokalemia. The potassium replacement will be started when the serum potassium level falls below 5.5 mEq/L.

Regular insulin is administered intravenously after fluid therapy has begun. Insulin will move water, potassium, and glucose into the cells. The movement of fluids into the cells acts to deplete the vascular volume. IV insulin therapy begins with a bolus of insulin, after determining that there is no hypokalemia present, followed by a continuous infusion.

Evaluation of Outcomes

Overall, DKA is resolved when the plasma glucose is less than 200 mg/dL. In addition, blood glucose levels are monitored, as are vital signs, LOC, cardiac monitoring, urine output, and O_2 saturation. The patient must be assessed for fluid volume overload with the fluid resuscitation. Potassium will be given to correct hypokalemia, and potassium levels will be closely monitored.

Hyperosmolar Hyperglycemic Nonketotic Syndrome

Patients with diabetes who produce sufficient insulin to prevent protein breakdown and ketoacidosis may not produce sufficient insulin to prevent or reverse severe hyperglycemia. HHNS is a life-threatening emergency associated with severe hyperglycemia, an osmotic diuresis, and a profound fluid volume deficit. The absence of ketosis is the distinguishing feature between DKA and HHNS.

Assessment with Clinical Manifestations

HHNS has a slower onset, days to weeks, with polydipsia, polyuria, and weakness. Blood glucose levels can rise extremely high (e.g., above 400 mg/dL), which increases the osmolality of the blood. This leads to neurological changes that include seizures, aphasia, somnolence, and coma. HHNS occurs more often in the older adult. Often these patients will have congestive heart failure and renal insufficiency. The presence of either of these will make the prognosis for the patient worse. Common precipitating factors include infection or recent surgery. The onset is frequently attributed to a decreased fluid intake. The patient will present with blood glucose levels greater than 400 mg/dL and the absence of ketones. The serum osmolality will be greater than 310 mOsm/kg, and no evidence of acidosis. The serum sodium level may be greater than 140 mEq/L.

Nursing Diagnoses

Nursing diagnoses for the patient experiencing HHNS include but are not limited to the following:

- Deficient fluid volume related to active losses.

- Risk for ineffective therapeutic regimen management.
- Disturbed sensory perception related to biochemical imbalance.

Planning and Implementation

As with DKA, fluid resuscitation is of utmost importance in treating a patient with HHNS. IV therapy is initiated with 0.9% NS if oliguria and hypotension are present. If hypotension and oliguria are not present, fluid therapy is initiated with 0.45% NS, because the patient is hyperosmolar. It is common to deliver large volumes of fluid, as much as 6 to 8 liters in the first 8 to 10 hours of therapy. When the blood glucose level reaches 250 mg/dL 5% dextrose will be added to the IV solution. A goal of therapy is maintenance of the blood glucose levels between 250 and 300 mg/dL to decrease the risk of cerebral edema. Urine output of 50 mL/hour is a goal of fluid therapy. The patient will be given IV regular insulin, but HHNS may require less insulin than DKA. If the fluid volume deficit is corrected the hyperglycemia lessens. Correction of the hypovolemia will increase the functioning of the kidneys and the excretion of glucose in the urine (Tierney, et al., 2004). Potassium imbalances occur with HHNS as insulin drives the glucose and potassium in to the cells. The patient with HHNS will have fewer problems with potassium than the patient with DKA because of the absence of acidosis. As with any administration of potassium, adequate renal function must be established.

Evaluation of Outcomes

HHNS has a higher rate of mortality than DKA because of the increased incidence in elderly patients. The elderly are at increased risk because of decreased cardiovascular functioning and the slower recognition of the onset of dehydration. The nurse will monitor the vital signs, lung sounds, cardiac rhythm, LOC, urine output, and potassium levels while caring for the patient with HHNS. Patients should be taught to care for themselves, because infection is a leading cause of DKA and HHNS.

Hypoglycemia

Another acute complication of diabetes is hypoglycemia (blood glucose levels less than 70 mg/dL). Hypoglycemia must be recognized and treated quickly, because the brain requires constant sufficient supplies of glucose to function. Hypoglycemia results from too much insulin.

Assessment with Clinical Manifestations

The patient with hypoglycemia presents with irritability, increasing confusion, tremors, hunger, sweating, weakness, and visual disturbances. The patient presentation is similar to alcohol intoxication and if not treated rapidly, coma and death may occur. Causes of hypoglycemia are too little food, too much insulin, increased exercise, or delay in eating. It is more common with insulin therapy but can occur in patients treated with oral agents as well.

Patients may not be able to recognize the symptoms of hypoglycemia (hypoglycemia unawareness). This can occur because of neuropathy in the autonomic nervous system of the diabetic. This neuropathy interferes with the release of counter-regulatory hormones by the body to compensate for the low blood sugar levels. Hypoglycemia can occur in both type 1 and type 2 diabetes (Table 57-4). Hypoglycemia unawareness is common in the elderly patients and also in patients who take beta blockers (see Red Flag feature). Patients with hypoglycemic unawareness will usually be allowed to have higher blood glucose levels to prevent undetected episodes of hypoglycemia.

A patient may exhibit symptoms of hypoglycemia in the presence of blood glucose levels that are above normal. This can occur when the blood glucose level has been extremely high and decreases rapidly. Patients may experience the symptoms of hypoglycemia when the hyperglycemia was treated aggressively.

Red Flag

Hypoglycemia in the Frail Elderly

Patients who live at home by themselves and have inadequate support systems are at increased risk if they are using an oral agent that causes hypoglycemia. This is especially true in the frail elderly who often do not detect the onset of severe hypoglycemia and often live alone. These patients need monitoring by their health care providers and safety alert mechanisms to contact emergency health care givers. The crisis of severe hypoglycemia can be life-threatening and ultimately fatal in this population.

TABLE 57-4 Hypoglycemia in Type 1 and Type 2 Diabetes

ONSET/CAUSE	Occurs with both type 1 and type 2 diabetes
	Rapid onset
	Too much insulin or dose error
	Insufficient food intake
RISK FACTORS	Trauma
	Illness
	Exercise
	Renal failure
	Alcohol intake
	Surgery
CLINICAL MANIFESTATIONS	Cool, moist skin
	Pallor
	Headache
	Nausea
	Sweating
	Tremors
	Hunger
	Lethargy
	Confusion
	Slurred speech
	Anxiety
TREATMENT	15 grams of fast acting carbohydrate, i.e., 3–4 glucose tablets, 4–6 ounces of fruit juice or regular soda
	Glucagon 1 mg subcutaneously or intramuscularly followed by concentrated source of carbohydrate when patient fully alert

Adapted from DeLaune, S., & Ladner, P. (2006). Fundamentals of nursing *(3rd ed.). New York: Thomson Delmar Learning; Greenspan, F. S., & Gardner, D. G. (2004).* Basic and clinical endocrinology *(7th ed.). New York: Lange Medical Books.*

Nursing Diagnoses

Nursing diagnoses for patients experiencing hypoglycemia may include but are not limited to the following:

- Imbalanced nutrition related to imbalance of food, insulin, and activity.
- Knowledge deficit regarding diabetes self-care.
- Disturbed sensory perception related to biochemical imbalance.

Planning and Implementation

Recognition of hypoglycemia is important. The blood glucose level should be assessed quickly with the onset of the first symptom. In the absence of blood glucose monitoring equipment, the patient should be treated for the hypoglycemia. If the blood glucose level is assessed at less than 70 mg/dL, treatment is begun. The patient should be given 10 to 15 g of a simple carbohydrate (fast acting), i.e., 8 ounces of low-fat milk or 4 ounces of fruit juice or a carbonated soft drink. The treatment should be moderate but quick, with the blood glucose levels monitored every 15 minutes. If the blood glucose is low (less than 70 mg/dL) after the initial treatment, the treatment is repeated. The nurse can teach the patient that 15 g of carbohydrate are given every 15 minutes until the blood glucose level is above 70 mg/dL. Once that level is reached the patient should eat a regular meal or snack and recheck the blood glucose in 45 minutes. If the hypoglycemia does not reverse after two or three doses of carbohydrates or if the swallowing is impaired, an injection of 1 mg of glucagon may be given intramuscularly or subcutaneously. Glucagon will make glucose more available by stimulating the liver to convert some glycogen stores to glucose. Foods that are sweet and contain fat should not be given, such as candy bars or cookies. The presence of fat in the food slows the absorption of the sugar. The patient may use glucose tablets or gel to treat hypoglycemia.

The patient should be assessed for reasons for the occurrence of the hypoglycemic episodes. Patient and family education may be indicated. The patient and family must recognize the danger of hypoglycemia and the potential for cognitive impairment if not treated.

Dawn Phenomenon and Somogyi Effect

The dawn phenomenon manifests itself as morning hyperglycemia present on awakening. This hyperglycemia results from predawn release of counter-regulatory hormones. It is likely that cortisol and growth hormones are factors in the occurrence of the dawn phenomenon. It is most common in adolescence and young adults.

The Somogyi effect presents as wide variations in early morning or fasting blood glucose levels. The Somogyi effect is a result of too much insulin and occurs during sleep. Too much insulin activates the counter-regulatory hormones, and gluconeogenesis and glycogenolysis occurs, resulting in hyperglycemia and ketosis. When the blood sugar is measured in the morning and hyperglycemia is present, the patient or the health care worker may increase the dose of insulin. This action is incorrect because the Somogyi effect is a result of too much insulin. The Somogyi effect causes headaches on awakening, nightmares, and night sweats. When the Somogyi effect is suspected the patient's blood sugar should be monitored between 2 and 4 a.m. to check for the presence of hypoglycemia at that time. If the patient is hypoglycemic then, the insulin dose affecting the morning blood sugar level should be reduced.

Treatment for the dawn phenomenon is an increase in insulin or an adjustment in the administration. Treatment for the Somogyi effect is less insulin. The patient and the nurse should be aware that careful assessment is necessary to determine the cause of the early morning rise in blood sugars as the treatment for Somogyi effect is different than the treatment for the dawn phenomenon.

CHRONIC COMPLICATIONS OF DIABETES

Chronic complications include macrovascular and microvascular problems. These complications include angiopathy or vessel disease, retinopathy, neuropathy, and nephropathy. These conditions are caused by damage to the large and small vessels from chronically elevated blood glucose. The risk of development of microvascular complications (e.g., integumentary problems or infections) can be dramatically decreased with optimal control of blood sugar levels. These results were achieved with an intensive insulin therapy regimen. Additionally the study indicated that intensive insulin therapy reduces the risk of retinopathy and nephropathy. Patients with diabetes require regularly scheduled follow-up treatment to prevent and monitor the occurrence of long-term complications.

Angiopathy or Vessel Disease

Macrovascular complications cause changes in the large vessels. These changes may occur in patients who do not have diabetes but are more frequent and earlier in patients who do have diabetes. As a disease of metabolism, diabetes affects the metabolism of lipids. Plaque formation from atherosclerosis is associated with diabetes. The incidence of vessel disease can be decreased with optimal glycemic control. The diseases of the larger vessels include cardiovascular, cerebral, and peripheral vascular diseases. Patients should understand the risk factors associated with macrovascular disease, because many of the risk factors are modifiable with lifestyle changes. These risk factors include obesity, smoking, sedentary lifestyle, high blood pressure, and increased fat intake. Patient education efforts should be aimed at reduction of these modifiable risk factors (refer to chapter 23 for assessment considerations).

Microvascular Complications

Microvascular complications are specific to diabetes and result from the chronic presence of hyperglycemia. The elevated blood glucose levels lead to a thickening in the capillaries and arterioles. Most common sites of occurrence include the eyes with diabetic retinopathy, the kidneys with nephropathy, and skin. These do not usually appear until the first or second decade after the onset of diabetes.

Diabetic Retinopathy

Chronic hyperglycemia causes damage to the small vessels of the retina in patients with diabetes. It is a common complication, present in approximately 60 percent of patients with type 2 diabetes and nearly every patient with type 1 diabetes for longer than 20 years. Diabetic retinopathy is the most frequent cause of new blindness among adults ages 20 to 74. During the first two decades of the disease, nearly all patients with type 1 diabetes and more than 60 percent of patients with type 2 diabetes have retinopathy.

Assessment with Clinical Manifestations

The most common form of retinopathy is nonproliferative. This manifests itself as microaneurysms in the retinal capillaries. Capillary fluid leaks from the weakened aneurysms and retinal edema occurs. If the macular area of the eye is involved, the vision will be affected.

Proliferative retinopathy is more severe, involving the vitreous humor and the retina. New blood vessels are formed in the retina as the smaller capillaries become occluded. This is called neovascularization. The new blood vessels are extremely friable (broken) and subject to hemorrhage. As the vessels tear and bleed in the vitreous, the patient's vision is changed. The patient will report the appearance of red or black lines or spots. There may be retinal detachment or involvement of the macula.

Diagnostic Tests

Examination with an ophthalmoscope allows direct visualization of the retina. A fluorescein angiograph may be performed as well to provide information about the presence and type of retinopathy. This procedure involves a venous injection of a dye that is carried throughout the body but accumulates in the vessels of the retina. The ophthalmologist is then able to visualize the retinal vessels in greater detail than with an ophthalmoscope alone. This procedure is associated with minor side effects of nausea with the injection of the dye, a yellow fluorescent color of the urine and skin for 12 to 24 hours and occasionally an allergic reaction with hives and itching. Patient instructions are shown in the patient playbook feature.

> **PATIENT PLAYBOOK**
>
> **Instructions for a Fluorescein Angiogram**
>
> The nurse should inform the patient that is going to have a fluorescein angiogram of the following information:
>
> - This is a painless procedure.
> - The steps involved in the diagnostic test.
> - The potential side effects of the procedure.
> - There could be brief discomfort associated with the camera flash.

Planning and Implementation

Prevention of retinopathy is first and foremost. The importance of near normal glycemic control is stressed. The main medical treatment of diabetic retinopathy is laser photocoagulation to destroy the areas of revascularization and leaking vessels. This procedure may have a profound impact on slowing the progression of vision loss. These treatments are done on an outpatient basis, with most patients returning to usual activities of daily living the next day.

Evaluation of Outcomes

The procedure may cause some discomfort, but intense pain is rare. The patient will be pretreated with an analgesic eye drop. Occasionally patients may develop permanent visual changes from the treatment, including loss of peripheral vision or decreased ability to adapt to the dark. These changes are much less than those that result from progressive retinopathy.

If a large hemorrhage occurs in the vitreous, the blood combines with the vitreous fluid and hampers the ability of light to pass through the eye, resulting in blindness. This fluid can be removed with a drill-like instrument in a procedure called a vitrectomy. The space is then filled with saline. Patients are candidates for this surgery if the hemorrhage has persisted for six months, and they are experiencing visual loss. Vision should improve after the procedure, but a return to near normal vision is not to be expected.

Nursing care is focused on patient education regarding the importance of regular eye exams and glycemic control. The nurse emphasizes to the patient the importance of early diagnosis and treatment. If vision loss occurs, the nurse will need to incorporate the use of assistive devices to aid the patient in self-care. The patient should be reminded that retinopathy occurs after having diabetes for several years and does not indicate that the diabetes is getting worse. If the patient maintains optimal blood sugar control and optimal blood pressure, the chances for loss of vision are lessened. The patient must understand and comply with regular eye examinations.

Nephropathy

Renal disease, secondary to microvascular changes associated with diabetes, is common, accounting for approximately one half of the cases of newly diagnosed end-stage renal disease (ESRD) annually. About one quarter to one third of patients with type 1 and type 2 diabetes will exhibit nephropathy. A lesser number of type 2 diabetics progress to ESRD. Symptoms of renal disease will manifest within 10 to 15 years for type 1 diabetics and within 10 years for type 2 diabetics. Because of the slow development of type 2 diabetes, frequently patients will also develop evidence of renal disease at the time of diagnosis of type 2 diabetes. The DCCT study concluded that intensive treatment of diabetes with maintenance of hemoglobin A_{1C} levels as close to normal as possible decreased the occurrence of early signs of renal disease. Microalbuminuria was reduced by 39 percent, and albuminuria was reduced by 54 percent in that study. A similar study in the United Kingdom showed a decreased incidence of nephropathy in type 2 diabetics with good glycemic control.

When glycemic control is not adequate allowing elevated levels of blood glucose, the kidneys filtration will decrease, and protein from the blood is excreted in the urine. Protein has fluid attracting properties, and the pressure in the blood vessels of the kidneys increases. This increased blood pressure is thought to be the mechanism for nephropathy.

Assessment with Clinical Manifestations

Signs and symptoms of kidney disease are not specific to the diabetic. The diabetic patient may have an increase in the occurrence of hypoglycemia as the breakdown of insulin (exogenous and endogenous) decreases. Insulin requirements will change as a result of the kidney disease and the treatments. It is not uncommon for multiple body systems to fail as the kidney disease progresses, including visual impairment, foot ulcerations, nocturnal diarrhea, and heart failure. Patients in the early stages of renal disease will frequently develop hypertension.

Diagnostic Tests

Albumin in the urine is a hallmark of renal disease. Clinical nephropathy will develop in approximately 85 percent of patients with microalbuminuria. Albumin in the urine may be detected with a urine dipstick or 24-hour urine collection. If significant amounts of albumin are present, a blood urea nitrogen (BUN) and creatinine are obtained.

Nursing Diagnoses

Please refer to chapter 55 for specific nursing diagnoses on nephropathy conditions.

Planning and Implementation

Nursing management includes maintenance of glycemic control. Additionally, the nurse must stress prevention of urinary tract infections and management of hypertension. The nurse should adjust the patient's medications in an attempt to meet the challenging demands of decreased renal functioning. In addition, nursing care must involve nutritional changes, which will include a low-protein, low-sodium diet. Patients with microalbuminuria in excess of 30 mg in 24 hours on two consecutive tests will be started on an angiotensin-converting enzyme (ACE) inhibitor to lower the blood pressure and reduce the microalbuminuria. Another option is the use of angiotensin-receptor blocking agents and a low-protein diet.

Patients in ESRD are often placed on hemodialysis. There is a trend toward use of continuous ambulatory peritoneal dialysis for patients with diabetes. This type of dialysis allows the patient more freedom in their lifestyle. Insulin can be added to the dialysate to achieve better glycemic control. Some patients may need to increase their insulin requirements because of the glucose in the dialysate. Infection is a complication of peritoneal dialysis.

Evaluation of Outcomes

Please refer to chapter 55 for explanation of specific evaluation of outcomes for patients with nephropathy conditions.

Peripheral Neuropathy (Sensory Neuropathy)

Diabetic neuropathies involve the peripheral, autonomic, and spinal nerves. The diabetic neuropathies are a group of disorders that increase in occurrence as the diabetic patient ages and with the increasing duration of diabetes. The cause of the neuropathies is chronic elevation of blood glucose levels. The two most commonly occurring types are autonomic and sensorimotor (peripheral) neuropathy. Peripheral neuropathy most often involves the nerves of the lower extremities, affecting the body symmetrically, and proceeding proximally (Mchugh, 2004).

The peripheral neuropathies are sensory disorders that are associated with diabetes. The most common type seen in diabetes is the polyneuropathies, or bilateral sensory disorders, that begin in the toes and feet and progress upward. These conditions can become serious and lead to complete tissue destruction, gangrene, and may even require limb amputations or the development of septic shock (Figure 57-7). The presentation of symptoms will be based on the nerve fibers that are involved. In addition, infections are increased with diabetes, which also prolongs wound healing (Aragon, 2003).

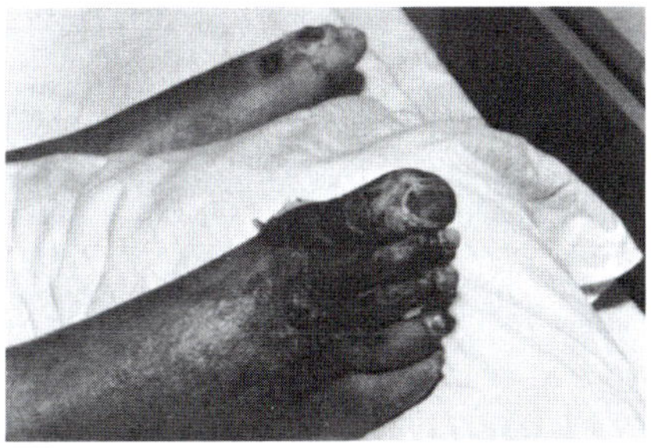

Figure 57-7 Gangrene of the toes and foot as a result of peripheral neuropathy.

Assessment with Clinical Manifestations

Assessment will reveal symptoms of generalized tingling or a prickly sensation (paresthesia) and burning sensations, particularly at night. The patient may experience **hyperesthesia** (increased sensitivity of the skin) and may report that even light pressure from bedcovers is intolerable. As the neuropathy advances, sensation in the feet decreases markedly, leaving the feet numb. This decreased sensation makes the patient susceptible to injury, as he or she is unaware of pain or pressure sensations. Peripheral neuropathy is also associated with deformities of the feet, such as Charcot's joints. Peripheral neuropathy causes atrophy of the muscles in the foot. With peripheral neuropathy, the foot assumes a rocker bottom with an abnormal weight distribution on the joints. The patient may have decreased deep tendon reflexes on exam.

Nursing Diagnoses

Nursing diagnoses for patients with diabetic neuropathies may include but are not limited to the following:

- Disturbed sensory perception, tactile, related to biochemical imbalance.
- Impaired skin integrity related to altered metabolic state.

Planning and Implementation

The best management for diabetic neuropathy is optimal glycemic control. It will be effective in some but not all cases. Symptoms are managed with medications that include topical anesthetics (e.g., capsaicin), tricyclic antidepressants (e.g., amitriptyline), and antiseizure drugs (e.g., gabapentin).

Capsaicin is produced from chili peppers. As a topical medication, it acts locally to decrease the chemicals that mediate pain. It is used with a fair amount of success when applied three to four times daily. The patient may initially experience an increase in symptoms. Within two weeks of therapy, the patients will begin to have pain relief. Tricyclic antidepressants decrease the pain sensation by inhibiting the reuptake of serotonin and norepinephrine and decrease the transmission of pain sensation at the spinal level. The exact mechanism of action of gabapentin is not understood, but it has been shown to relieve the pain of peripheral neuropathy.

Evaluation of Outcomes

Potential patient outcomes for each of the example nursing diagnoses for the patient with peripheral neuropathies are:

- Disturbed sensory perception, tactile, related to biochemical imbalance: The patient will experience not problems with peripheral neurovascular function by a specified date.
- Impaired skin integrity related to altered metabolic state: The patient will not experience any alteration in skin integrity by a specified date.

Autonomic Neuropathies

Autonomic neuropathies are widespread, and they affect nearly every body system. Essentially, the pathology of this diabetic complication is the breakdown of the autonomic nervous system.

Assessment with Clinical Manifestations

Autonomic neuropathy leads to bowel and bladder incontinence, hypoglycemic unawareness, and delayed gastric emptying (gastroparesis). Gastroparesis presents as anorexia, nausea and vomiting, feelings of fullness, and gastroesophageal reflux. The delay of absorption of food that occurs with gastroparesis can lead to the development of hypoglycemia. The effects of autonomic neuropathy on the cardiovascular system lead to postural hypotension, asymptomatic myocardial infarction, and a resting tachycardia.

Sexual functioning can be affected in males or females. Males may experience erectile dysfunction, and females may experience decreased libido. The patient may develop a neurogenic bladder with urinary retention.

Nursing Diagnoses

Potential complications or collaborative problems for the patient with autonomic neuropathies may include:

- Diarrhea.
- Constipation.
- Urinary retention.
- Decreased sexual functioning.

Planning and Implementation

Nursing management is aimed at the symptoms. No treatment is available for the painless myocardial ischemia within the cardiovascular system. Patient education should include the avoidance of strenuous exercise. Patients are cautioned about changing positions slowly in the presence of postural hypotension. Antiembolic stockings may alleviate some of the postural hypotension by decreasing the pooling of blood in the lower extremities. Gastroparesis is treated with glycemic control, a low-fat diet in small frequent feedings, and medications to increase gastric emptying (metoclopramide). If the patient experiences diarrhea from diabetes, bulk-forming agents can be used. Constipation is treated with increased fluids and fiber. Neurogenic bladder is treated by emptying the bladder every three hours and use of the Credé's method (downward pressure on the abdomen over the bladder area) Patients may need to learn self-catheterization.

Evaluation of Outcomes

Nursing care is aimed at alleviation of the symptoms. The patient may be expected to exhibit no diarrhea or constipation and increased bladder emptying.

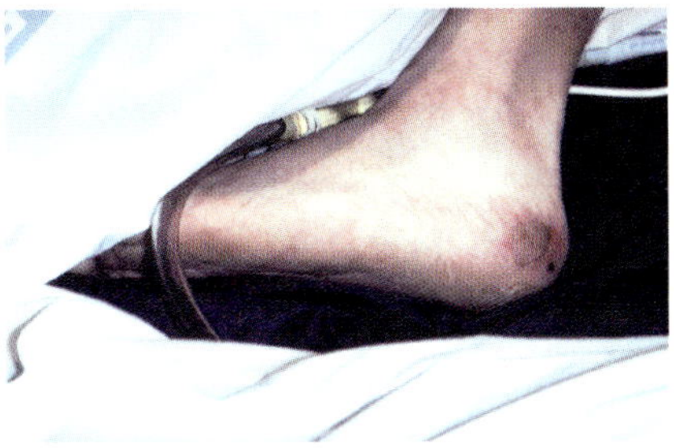

Figure 57-8 The beginnings of a pressure ulcer on the foot for the patient with diabetes can become a serious problem.

Peripheral Vascular Complications of the Lower Extremities

The most common cause of hospitalization for the diabetic patient is the complication of the lower extremities and specifically, the foot. These complications are a result of the peripheral vascular changes that occur with diabetes, both microvascular and macrovascular (Figure 57-8). An alteration in the shape and mechanics of the foot from neuropathy contributes as well. Other risk factors include the presence of peripheral vascular disease and smoking. Patients who are male, have had diabetes for more than 10 years, have poor glycemic control, or microvascular or macrovascular complications are at increased risk of ulcerations or amputations. Peripheral vascular disease decreases the blood flow, and therefore the supply of nutrients and oxygen to the tissues. This increases the risk for infection and delays wound healing.

Assessment with Clinical Manifestations

Assessment for peripheral vascular dysfunction (PVD) include diminished or absent pedal pulses, cool feet, pain at rest, intermittent claudication, hair loss on the extremity, rubor of the skin (e.g., redness) when the extremity is dependent, and slower capillary filling. Doppler studies or angiography will confirm the diagnosis. The loss of sensation from peripheral neuropathy is another major risk factor for the development of foot ulcers in patients with diabetes. Loss of sensation removes the protective function of pain, and the patient is unable to sense pressure or discomfort or even injury. Pain sensation is assessed by use of a monofilament on the plantar aspect (sole) of the patient's foot.

Nursing Diagnoses

Nursing diagnoses for patients with PVD may include but are not limited to the following:

- Disturbed sensory perception, tactile, related to biochemical imbalance.
- Impaired skin integrity related to altered metabolic state.

Planning and Implementation

Early identification and prevention of risk factors is the optimal patient management. The feet of the diabetic should be assessed at every visit to a health care practitioner and inspected daily at home by the patient or family member. Sensation should be checked annually using the Semmes-Weinstein monofilament. The exam should also include an assessment of the foot structure and mechanics, the vascular status, and integrity of the skin.

Patients with neuropathy will require well-fitted shoes. If the patient has signs of increased pressure on the plantar aspect of the foot, such as calluses, redness, or warmth, cushioning with shoe inserts can be used to redistribute the pressure on the foot. Foot deformities are common in the diabetic and may require extra wide or deep shoes.

Management of PVD includes reduction or control of risk factors, especially smoking, hypertension, and elevated cholesterol levels. Patients may require surgery, including a bypass graft or amputation.

Patient and family member's knowledge and practice of foot care should be assessed regularly. Patients should be instructed to wash their feet daily with warm water and mild soap. Decreased sensation increases the risk of burn injuries; therefore the patient should first test the water temperature with his or her hands. The feet should be patted dry, particularly between the toes. Feet should be examined daily for cuts, blisters, and reddened areas. Patients are advised not to use over-the-counter (OTC) preparations to treat calluses and corns. Toe nails should be cut with the corners rounded; they are easier to trim following a bath or shower. The nails should be cut straight across to avoid ingrown toe nails. Shoes should fit properly and not be open-toed styles or high heels. Socks are to be clean cotton and colorfast. Cotton socks are more absorbent and are therefore preferable. Cuts are to be cleansed with warm water and mild soap. The use of alcohol or iodine is to be avoided. Injuries to the skin or infections are to be reported immediately to the health care provider.

Evaluation of Outcomes

Potential patient outcomes for each of the example nursing diagnoses for the patient with PVD are:

- Disturbed sensory perception, tactile, related to biochemical imbalance: The patient will not experience problems with peripheral neurovascular function by a specified date.
- Impaired skin integrity related to altered metabolic state: The patient will not experience any alteration in skin integrity by a specified date.

Skin Complications

The microangiopathy associated with diabetes increases the chances of skin changes and infections. It is common for patients with diabetes to have infections of the skin, especially *Candida albicans.* Localized skin infections, such as boils and furuncles, are common and recurrent in patients with diabetes. Often it is the history of recurrent skin infections that leads the health care provider to suspect diabetes.

Assessment with Clinical Manifestations

Assessing the skin in the diabetic patient is extremely important to his or her well-being. The appearance of the skin may change on the lower extremities. Red-yellow lesions, called necrobiosis lipoidica diabeticorum, present along the anterior aspect of the lower extremities, commonly along the shin. These spots are caused by the breakdown of collagen. Skin around the area atrophies and thins, making it susceptible to injury and ulceration. These are not common but often are present before other clinical signs of diabetes and occur more often in young women. It is common to find small brown spots along the shin. These brown spots are usually less than 1 cm in diameter and are harmless.

Case Study

Nursing Care Plan

Mrs. Ballenger, age 78, is hospitalized in the intensive care unit (ICU) with complications of type 1 diabetes mellitus. Most recently, she is experiencing diabetic ketoacidosis with a blood glucose of 320 mg/dL. In addition, she has coronary heart disease (CHD) from the microvascular complications of her diabetes; she has a pulmonary artery catheter to monitor his hemodynamic status. Her primary clinical manifestations from the CHD are hypertension, tachycardia, and occasional arrhythmias. At present her level of consciousness (LOC) is impaired, she is breathing with Kussmaul respirations, her breath is acetone in nature, and she is extremely fatigued.

Assessment

A 78-year-old female with complications associated with type 1 diabetes mellitus. Specifically, she has a primary diagnosis of diabetic ketoacidosis ([DKA] blood glucose = 320 mg/dL. In addition she has hypertension, atrial cardiac arrhythmias, and a decreased LOC. She is being monitored in an intensive care unit.

Nursing Diagnosis #1: Deficient fluid volume related to osmotic diuresis associated with hyperglycemia.

NOC: Electrolyte and Acid-Base Imbalance; Fluid balance; Hydration; Nutritional status; Food and fluid intake.

NIC: Fluid management; Hypovolemia management; Shock management: Volume

Expected Outcomes

The patient will:

1. Maintain a blood glucose level in the 150–180 mg/dL range within 72 hours.
2. Demonstrate no signs or symptoms of dehydration during her admission in the ICU.
3. Maintain a cardiac output in the normal range of 4–6 L/min during her admission to the ICU.

Planning/Interventions/Rationale

1. Measure blood glucose levels every hour and administer insulin per sliding scale orders. *Blood glucose levels are at a crisis level, and close monitoring prevents further complications of DKA.*
2. Evaluate cardiac output by assessing cardiac system with vital signs, hemodynamic monitor (pulmonary artery catheter), and electrophysiology. *Allows for close cardiac monitoring, which is necessary for the patient's critical condition.*
3. Assess hydration status every hour by monitoring: urine specific gravity, intake and output (hourly urine output), skin turgor, and vital signs. *Frequent assessment detects subtle changes in hydration status during the critical complication of DKA.*

Evaluation

The patient has a blood glucose within a controlled range, stable hemodynamic readings of the pulmonary artery catheter, and no clinical manifestations of dehydration during her admission to the ICU.

Nursing Diagnosis #2: Ineffective breathing pattern of Kussmaul respirations related to metabolic acidosis associated with DKA.

NOC: Respiratory status: Ventilation; Vital signs status; Respiratory status; Airway patency

NIC: Airway management; Respiratory monitoring

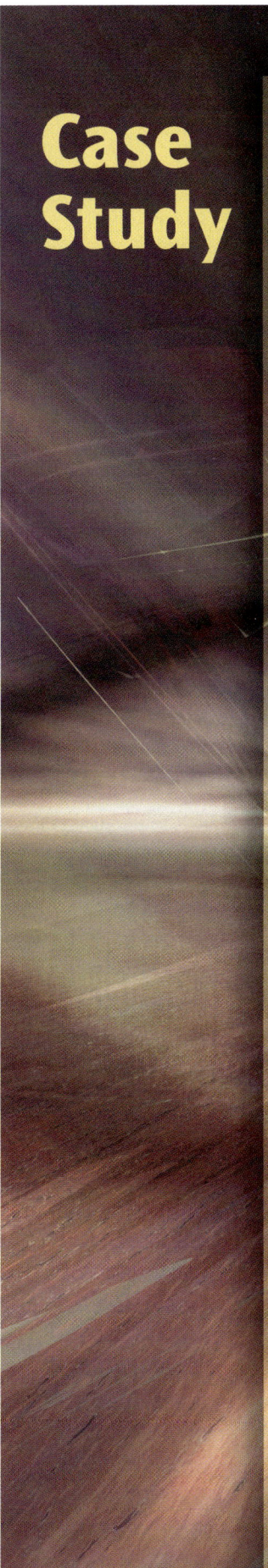

Case Study

Expected Outcomes

The patient will:

1. Demonstrate an effective respiratory rate of 12–16 breaths per minute with an oxygen saturation level of at least 94 percent within 24 hours.
2. Progressively regain level of consciousness within 24–48 hours.
3. Decrease sense of energy and experience less generalized fatigue within 24–48 hours.

Planning/Interventions/Rationale

1. Monitor oxygen saturation levels and assess depth or rhythm of respirations every hour. *Detects respiratory compensation during a time of the respiratory crisis of Kussmaul breathing (caused by the DKA).*
2. Assess LOC by evaluating neurological responses and patient's ability to effectively answer questions every hour. *Provides constant monitoring of neurological status.*
3. Ask patient questions regarding her level of energy and ask patient to quantify from 1–10 the level of her fatigue every hour. *Evaluates fatigue levels on constant basis.*

Evaluation

The patient has a progressive decrease in the Kussmaul breathing pattern, an increasing LOC, and an increasing level of energy.

KEY CONCEPTS

- Diabetes mellitus refers to a group of chronic disorders of metabolism characterized by elevated blood glucose levels as well as disturbances in metabolism of carbohydrate, fat, and protein.
- There are four types of diabetes mellitus: type 1 diabetes mellitus, type 2 diabetes mellitus, gestational diabetes, and impaired glucose tolerance (prediabetes).
- Insulin is one of the hormones produced by the pancreas (beta cells) with a function of lowering blood sugar.
- Glucagon is a hormone released by the alpha cells of the pancreas, and it functions to raise blood sugar levels.
- Patients with both type 1 and type 2 diabetes will present with the three Ps of diabetes (i.e., polydipsia, polyphagia, and polyuria).
- Nutritional therapy is based on a well-balanced diet and is one of the mainstays in the treatment of diabetes.
- Regular exercise is an essential part of the treatment of diabetes because of its ability to lower blood sugar and decrease cardiovascular risk factors.
- Diabetic ketoacidosis results from a marked insulin deficiency and is manifested by hyperglycemia, ketosis, acidosis, and dehydration.
- HHNS is a life-threatening emergency associated with severe hyperglycemia, an osmotic diuresis, and a profound fluid volume deficit.
- Hypoglycemia is an acute complication of diabetes where the blood glucose levels are less than 70 mg/dL.
- Chronic complications include macrovascular and microvascular problems. These complications include angiopathy or vessel disease, retinopathy, neuropathy, and nephropathy.
- Macrovascular complications in diabetes cause changes in the large vessels.
- Diabetic neuropathies involve the peripheral, autonomic, and spinal nerves.
- The most common cause of hospitalization for the diabetic patient is the complication of the lower extremities; specifically, the foot.

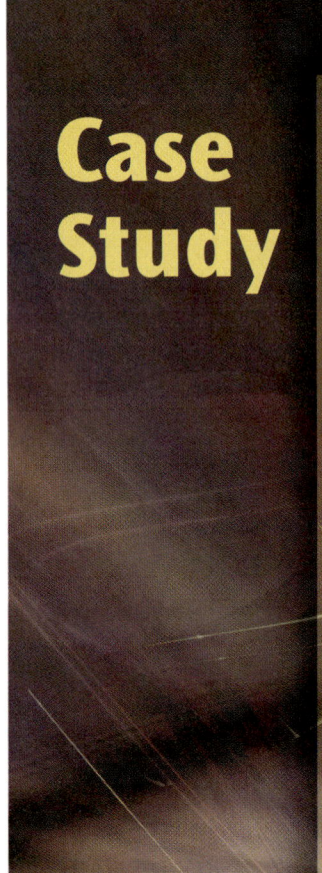

REVIEW QUESTIONS

1. A patient has just been admitted to the emergency department after being found disoriented at the grocery store. His medical alert bracelet indicates that he has type 1 diabetes. Which of the following clinical signs do you anticipate finding upon assessment? Check all that apply.
   1. Hyperglycemia
   2. Fruity odor of breath
   3. Tachycardia
   4. Hypertension
2. A patient with diabetes has just finished the teaching session on mixing insulins. The nurse knows that more teaching is needed when the patient:
   1. Injects air into the NPH insulin first followed by injecting air into the regular insulin vial
   2. Withdraws too much NPH insulin and injects the extra back into the Lente vial
   3. Withdraws too much regular insulin and injects the extra back into the regular insulin vial
   4. Uses separate syringes to draw up 5 units of regular insulin and 4 units of NPH
3. Which of the following lab tests offers the best information about glycemic control?
   1. $HgbA_{1C}$
   2. Fasting plasma glucose
   3. Glucose tolerance test
   4. Capillary glucose measurement
4. A patient is admitted to the hospital with DKA. The nurse can anticipate which of the following solutions will be administered initially intravenously?
   1. 5% dextrose in water
   2. Ringer's lactate
   3. 0.9% NS
   4. 5% dextrose in 0.45% NS
5. Which of the following types of insulin can be administered intravenously?
   1. Regular
   2. Lente
   3. Semi-Lente
   4. NPH
6. Diabetes is a chronic condition that requires effective long-term management. This management includes:
   1. Initial treatment of all types of diabetes with dietary modifications for a three-month time period
   2. Initial treatment of all diabetics with insulin administration to prevent complications
   3. Initial treatment of all diabetics with an oral glucose lowering agent and an exercise program
   4. Use of a glucose lowering agent, diet, and activity
7. What is the primary difference between DKA and HHNS?
   1. The absence of ketosis is the distinguishing feature.
   2. HHNS has much higher blood glucose levels.
   3. DKA has associated hyperkalemic levels.
   4. HHNS is usually caused as a reaction to previous conditions of hypoglycemia.
8. What are clinical manifestations of hypoglycemia?
   1. Severe abdominal pain, accompanied with nausea
   2. Cardiac arrhythmias
   3. Neurological responses of the parasympathetic nervous system
   4. Irritability, increasing confusion, tremors, hunger, sweating, weakness and visual disturbances
9. Which of the following is true of the dawn phenomena?
   1. It manifests itself as morning hypoglycemia.
   2. The corresponding hyperglycemia results from predawn release of counter-regulatory hormones.
   3. It is best managed by decreasing the administration amounts of insulin.
   4. The patient is not allowed to take insulin in any form when diagnosed with the dawn phenomena.
10. Which of the following is true regarding the autonomic neuropathy conditions associated with diabetic complications?
    1. They result in bradycardia and profuse diaphoresis.
    2. They are seldom seen in adult-onset diabetic conditions.
    3. They lead to bowel and bladder incontinence and delayed gastric emptying.
    4. They result in foot ulcers due to a lack of adequate circulation.

REVIEW ACTIVITIES

1. Describe what information is to be included in teaching a patient with newly diagnosed diabetes about sick day management.

2. List information to be included in teaching a patient newly diagnosed with diabetes about foot care.

3. A patient with diabetes is admitted to the emergency department with a blood sugar level of 52. The patient is still conscious. Describe the treatment that you will administer.

4. A patient with type 2 diabetes is admitted to the hospital with a diagnosis of pneumonia and is started on insulin injections. The patient questions the use of insulin, stating that he has been able to control his diabetes with pills and diet. What information should the nurse give to the patient?

5. Explain the following symptoms and their cause: polydipsia, polyphagia, and polyuria.

6. Locate a diabetes educator in your area. What are the educational requirements for the position of diabetes educator? Observe some teaching sessions with the diabetic educator and patients. What are some of the teaching strategies utilized, and how do they vary based on the age and education level of the patient? How frequently are patients seen by the diabetic educator, and how is this determined? Is a referral from a health care provider required or can the patients self refer for services? Is there an interdisciplinary team for patients with diabetes? Who makes up that team?

Visit the Contemporary Medical-Surgical Nursing online companion resource at www.delmarhealthcare.com for additional content and study aids. Click on Online Companions then select the Nursing discipline.

UNIT

XIV

Alterations in Musculoskeletal Function

Chapter 58 Assessment of Musculoskeletal Function

Chapter 59 Musculoskeletal Dysfunction: Nursing Management

Chapter 60 Musculoskeletal Trauma: Nursing Management

CHAPTER

58

Assessment of Musculoskeletal Function

Anita M. Zehala, RN, MS, ONC, CNS

KEY TERMS

Acetylcholine
Actin filaments
Arthroscopy
Articulation
Bone scan
Bone marrow aspiration and biopsy
Bursae
Cancellous
Clonus
Cortical or compact (bone)
Deep vein thrombosis (DVT)
Displaced fracture
Dual energy X-ray absorptiometry (DEXA) scans
Epiphyses
Homans' sign
Hyaline
Isokinetic
Joint aspiration
Lacunae
Lamellar bone
Ligaments
Myelogram
Myosin
Osteogenesis
Osteopenia
Periosteum
Remodeling
Resorption
Sarcomere
Synovium
Tendons
Trabecular

CHAPTER TOPICS

- Anatomy and Physiology of the Bony Skeleton
- Anatomy and Physiology of Skeletal Muscles
- Musculoskeletal Assessment
- Diagnostic Studies Related to the Musculoskeletal System

The years 2000 to 2010 have been declared the Bone and Joint Decade with a goal of improving the health-related quality of life for people with musculoskeletal disorders throughout the world (Bone and Joint Decade Organization, 2004). Sanctioned by the United Nations and the president of the United States, as well as others, participants include the National Association of Orthopaedic Nurses (NAON) and the American Academy of Orthopaedic Surgeons (AAOS). Because musculoskeletal diseases affect so many lives throughout the world, one of the major efforts of the participating organizations is to increase awareness of musculoskeletal diseases. By becoming familiar with the basic anatomy and physiology and assessment of the musculoskeletal system (as well as learning about musculoskeletal dysfunction and trauma in the following two chapters) providers will be able to assist in keeping musculoskeletal diseases in the forefront. Nurses will also be able to speak with confidence regarding issues that may arise during discussions with patients and family members.

ANATOMY AND PHYSIOLOGY OF THE BONY SKELETON

The anatomy and physiology of the bone are complex and consist of multiple layers of collagen, noncollagen, protein, and mineral components. These components continually renew themselves, giving bones the strength, integrity, and structure necessary to support the human form. Bone formation is triggered by multiple sources including physical force, hormones, and genetics.

During the 19th century, surgeon Julius Wolff made an impressive discovery, known as Wolff's law, involving the formation of bone. This dynamic remodeling process called **osteogenesis** (the process of bone formation and remodeling) is thought to be a direct response to physical stresses caused by the amount and direction of physical forces placed on bones (Childs, 2002).

TABLE 58-1

Types of Bone

BONE TYPE	BONE NAMES
Flat (mostly composed of cancellous bone)	Scapula, iliac crest, and sternum
Short (length equals width)	Tarsal and metatarsal bones and carpal and metacarpal bones
Long (length less than width and thickness)	Femur, tibia, fibula, humerus, ulna, and radius
Irregular (unable to be place in a category listed above)	Vertebrae

Macroscopic Structure of Bone

Embryonic development influences the distribution of bone cells (Schneider, Miclau, & Helms, 2002). Bones are woven in structure from infancy until 4 years of age. Woven bone is considered immature bone with collagen arranged randomly rather than in the uniform structure of lamellar bone. **Lamellar bone** (thin layer of mature bone tissue) is considered mature bone.

Four types of bones can be distinguished in the body. These types are flat, short (cuboidal), long, and irregular bones. Table 58-1 categorizes some of the bones of the body into type. Lamellar bone can be separated into two types: **cortical or compact** (dense, hard, and forms the protective exterior portion of all bones) and **cancellous, trabecular,** or spongy (inside the compact bone and porous). Cortical bone forms the hard outer layer of bone surfaces. Cancellous bone is found in the ends of the long bones (e.g., tibia) and in smaller amounts in some of the flat bones (e.g., iliac crest) (Scott & Fong, 2004).

Long bones are differentiated into three sections (Figure 58-1). The diaphysis is the shaft of a long bone, between the two ends (epiphysis), and consists of compact bone enclosing the medullary cavity or canal (the hollow tube located within the diaphysis). Within the medullary cavity is the bone marrow, in which hematopoietic activity takes place. The **epiphyses,** the widened ends of the long bone, contain mostly cancellous bone and are covered by a thin layer of cortical bone. The bone marrow system continues into the epiphyseal cavity. The metaphysis is the area of transition between the diaphysis and the epiphysis. The amount of cortical bone becomes gradually thinner as the metaphysis moves from diaphysis to epiphysis but the amount of cancellous bone increases from diaphysis to epiphysis. In the maturing child, the epiphyseal plate, or growth plate, is where active longitudinal growth occurs. The epiphyseal plate is located between the epiphysis and the metaphysis. If a fracture occurs in or through the epiphyseal plate, growth in that extremity may be delayed or stopped. When maturity is reached, the epiphyseal plate disappears when the epiphysis and the metaphysis merge (Childs, 2002).

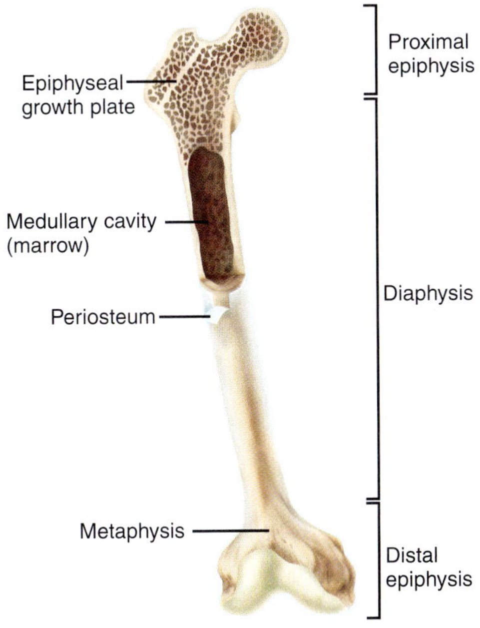

Figure 58-1 Structure of a long bone.

Surrounding most bone surfaces is a layer of connective tissue containing blood vessels and osteoblasts known as the **periosteum** (Childs, 2002). The periosteum supplies nutrients to the outer portion of the cortical bone and provides a blood supply to the bone. This outer layer is essential for the repair and remodeling of bone after fractures. Within the medullary canal and cancellous bone is a layer of tissue involved in **resorption** (the removal of bone tissue by normal physiological process or as part of a pathological process such as an infection) of bone cells. This layer of tissue is known as the endosteum (the thin layer of cells lining the medullary cavity of a bone).

Microscopic Structure of Bone

Full understanding of the minute structure and physiology of the bone would take a great deal of time and effort for the nurse. Therefore, only the basic anatomy and physiology necessary for nurses to understand how a bone matures and repairs will be discussed. For a more in depth review of the anatomic makeup and physiologic processes of the bone and bone repair, refer to the references to this chapter.

Osteon (Haversian System)

Cortical bone is made up of Haversian canals or osteons (channels running through a bone in which blood vessels and nerves are located), which allow the flow of fluid throughout the bone. This fluid supplies water and nutrients to the bone. Also within the cortical bone are canaliculi, which extend from the Haversian canals to the **lacunae.** Lacunae are "the little 'lakes'" in which the mature bone cells are embedded" (Childs, 2002). The osteons are surrounded by rings of lamellae, which characterize mature bone or lamellar bone (Figure 58-2).

Cell Types

There are three characteristic cell types found in bone. Osteoblasts (bone building cells) originate from stem cells and produce bone marrow. Osteoblasts reside within the periosteum and mature into calcified bone cells (osteocytes) or remain as bone lining cells (Sims & Baron, 2002). Osteocytes are calcified mature bone cells that are transported to the lacunae to reside. Osteocytes give bone its hard structure. These cells are thought to activate bone turnover and have a part in the regulation of extracellular calcium, but the exact function is unknown. Osteoclasts demineralize bone and are responsible for resorption of osteocytes and other bony debris. Similar to osteocytes, they originate from stem cells. These cells line bones and behave in a manner similar to phagocytes. The activity of osteoclasts is regulated by both locally acting cytokines and systemic hormones (Sims & Baron, 2002).

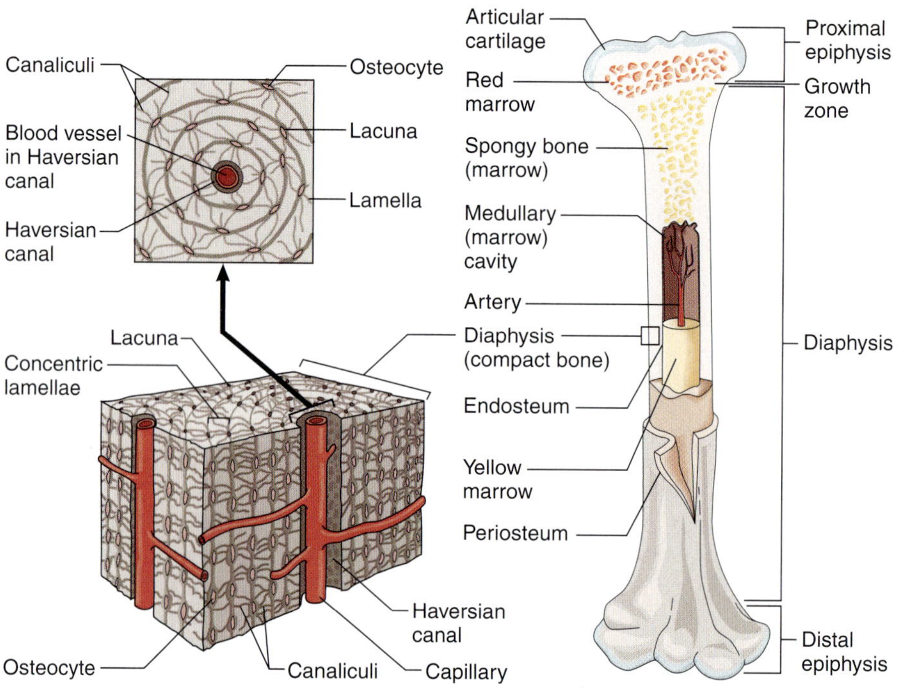

Figure 58-2 The Haversian system.

Physiological Processes

There are five physiological processes of the bone: (a) growth; (b) modeling; (c) remodeling; (d) repair; and (e) blood-bone exchange. Growth starts approximately two months after conception and continues to maturity. Lengthening and thickening of the bones occur during the growth process. The periosteum, as it becomes vascularized in utero, becomes the center of osteogenesis and continues this function throughout the life span. Modeling can be altered when genetic or nutritional circumstances affect the supply of nutrients to the bone (e.g., osteogenesis imperfecta, Paget's disease, or vitamin-deficiency rickets). Modeling also occurs in cartilage and fibrous tissue as well (Childs, 2002).

Turnover of the bone at the microscopic level is known as **remodeling.** Remodeling is a series of events continuously occurring in the bone. To maintain the structure and integrity of the bone, the bony tissue must be continually replaced. Bone cells fully replace themselves on average every 87 days. Roughly 30 percent of the total skeletal mass is renewed every year in a normal adult. There appears to be a balance of osteoclastic and osteoblastic activity that maintains and equalizes the overall skeletal mass. The exact trigger for remodeling is not known, but it is thought to occur after osteoclastic activity has occurred on the endosteal surface of the bone (Sims & Baron, 2002).

Blood-bone exchange is the physiological process in which electrolytes and acid-base substances move between the blood and bone tissue via the interstitial fluids. Bone tissue contributes to the modulation of hypercalcemia or hypocalcemia. Hydrogen ions (in acid-base balance), as well as other electrolytes, may also be influenced by tissue response within the bone. The osteocytes probably play a role in this influence (Childs, 2002).

Bone Repair/Fracture Healing

Bone repair or fracture healing occurs in much the same way as remodeling, however the trigger, such as trauma or surgery, is usually well defined. With any injury in the body, inflammation is the first stage, which occurs with an injury. Inflammation results from the ruptured blood vessels within the bone, the torn periosteum, and any damage to the surrounding soft tissue. A hematoma forms around the fracture within 24 hours. The hematoma releases hormones and inflammatory agents that stimulate the healing process. Within the hematoma, a fibrin network forms that serves as a framework for the formation of new blood vessels and cartilage. The inflammatory stage lasts several days.

In the first 24 to 48 hours after the injury, red blood cells continue to disintegrate and provide a stimulus for repair. Vascular congestion occurs and leukocytes, mainly neutrophils, invade the area causing significant edema. Approximately 48 hours after the injury, the area is flooded with macrophages to clean up remaining debris. At this time fibroblasts and chondroblasts invade the area to assist in forming a cartilage callus (new blood vessels and cartilage over the fracture site). This is stage is called the cellular proliferation stage. Chondrocytes (cartilage cells that make the structural components of cartilage), which are present in the cartilage callus, regulate the calcification of the cartilage. This usually occurs by the end of the first week. The calcified cartilage is then invaded by blood vessels and becomes resorbed by chondroblasts (a cell that arises from the mesenchyma and forms cartilage) and osteoclasts. The cartilage callus is then replaced by woven bone similar in structure to the growth plate. The callus is the beginning of bony formation but is weak.

With simple fractures the callus will reach its maximal size in two to three weeks after the injury. The callus continues to increase in strength from the precipitation of bone salts. During this time, osteoblastic and osteoclastic activity at the fracture site or injury, in response to external stresses, such as weight bearing activity, reform the bone. The ossification stage can take three to four months to complete. Remodeling also includes the growth of fine bone and the maturation of osteoblasts into osteocytes. Complete remodeling of a fracture can take months to years depending on the extent of the injury. Should the fracture be comminuted (a fracture in which the bone is splintered or crushed) or other complications be present, such as a patient with diabetes, the healing time may be increased.

Functions of Bone

The main functions of bones are to support the structure of the body, provide form, and enable movement. The skeleton is the ridged framework for the body and serves to protect the vital organs. It serves as the lever to which muscles attach. Bones store mineral, calcium and phosphate ions, lipids, and much of the hematopoietic system (the bodily system of organs and tissues, primarily the bone marrow, spleen, tonsils, and lymph nodes, involved in the production of blood), which forms new red blood cells and other blood components.

Aging and the Skeletal System

As a person ages, the physiology of the bone normally becomes thinner and weaker. This process is called **osteopenia** (the presence of less than normal amount of bone). If osteopenia is not treated it may result in osteoporosis. Osteoblastic activity slows between the ages of 30 and 40. After age 40, women lose approximately 8 percent of their bone mass every decade. In men the loss is 3 percent per decade.

ANATOMY AND PHYSIOLOGY OF SKELETAL MUSCLES

Skeletal muscle makes up the largest mass of tissue in the body and is responsible for approximately 50 percent of a person's body weight. The main functions of skeletal muscle are to produce movement, maintain posture and position, support soft tissues, guard entrances and exits to the digestive and urinary tracts, and to assist in maintaining body temperature (Scott & Fong, 2004).

Unlike cardiac and smooth muscle, skeletal muscle is voluntary. The voluntary nature of the skeletal muscle makes it unique in composition and action. Muscles are encapsulated epimysium (the external sheath of connective tissue surrounding a muscle). The long and cylindrical muscle cells contain subcellular units called myofibrils, which are surrounded by sarcoplasm (the cytoplasm of a striated muscle fiber). The myofibrils run lengthwise in the muscle and are made up of two types of subunits: myosin and actin filaments. The **myosin** (the protein that makes up the thick filaments of a myofibril) and **actin filaments** (the contractile part of a myofilament) slide together and compose the **sarcomere** (the contractile unit of the muscle). Tropomyosin and troponin are also contained within the myofibril. These components act as inhibitors to muscle contraction by preventing the interaction of myosin with actin (Childs, 2002).

The sarcoplasm reticulum releases large amounts of calcium into the vicinity of the myofibrils during contraction of the muscle. Through removal of the

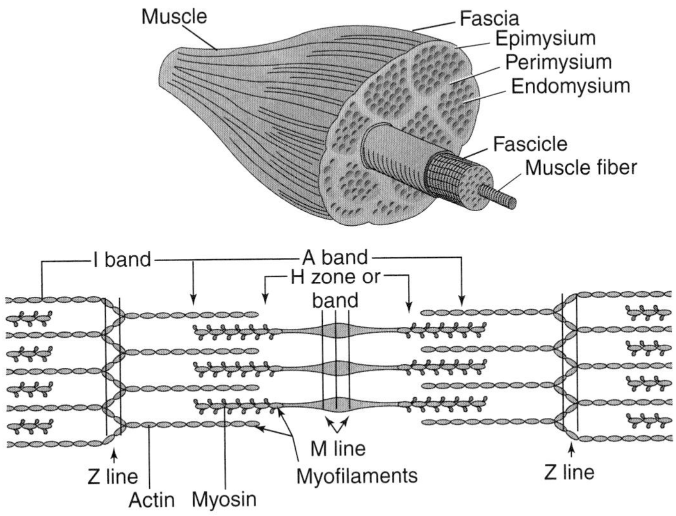

Figure 58-3 Illustration of muscle fibers.

tropomyosin-troponin block, the rise in calcium concentration initiates muscle contraction. As a result, the myosin and actin filaments slide past each other and enable myofibrillar contraction or the shortening of the sarcomere (Figure 58-3) (Childs, 2002).

Nerve and Blood Supply

There are generally one or two nerves that innervate each muscle. The nerve is necessary for the muscle to contract. When a nerve root ends within a muscle it is referred to as the neuromuscular junction. When the nerve root receives the signal from the brain to contract, **acetylcholine** (a neurotransmitter in both the central and peripheral nervous system) is released. The release of acetylcholine stimulates the sarcoplasm reticulum to release calcium and the muscle contraction begins (Childs, 2002).

Tendons, Ligaments, and Bursae

Tendons connect muscle to bone. This attachment allows the bone to move once the muscle has contracted. Tendons offer strength, extensibility, and flexibility to the muscle insertion sites.

Ligaments are strong bands of connective tissue that attach bone to bone or bone to cartilage. Ligaments help to give joints stability, guide the joint movement, and prevent excess motion within the joint (Childs, 2002).

Bursae are synovial fluid-filled sacs near joints. They are seen where tendons rub against bone, ligaments, or other tendons, as well as skin over bony prominences. Bursa provide cushion and minimize friction.

Aging and the Muscular System

In general, lean muscle mass decreases with age. Atrophy from disuse can lead to muscle wasting. Muscle contraction time is decreased in response to a reduction in acetylcholine and increased resorption of calcium. After disuse as a result of calcium resorption, fatigue is often increased and endurance decreased. Ligaments and tendons lose elasticity and resiliency. With trauma or repetitive stress, ligaments and tendons shorten, resulting in stiffness and loss of flexibility and range of motion (ROM). Furthermore, during the reparative phase, calcium can be deposited in muscle, tendon, and ligamentous structures, creating pain and further decreasing function. In light of the above information, it is essential that early rehabilitation be initiated when an injury occurs to return the patient to preinjury status and prevent further deterioration (Childs, 2002).

JOINTS

A joint or **articulation** is formed when a bone meets another bone. Joints function to provide stability and mobility. The amount of stability and mobility depend largely on the location of the joint as well as the muscular and structural (ligaments and tendons) support surrounding the joint.

Classifications

Three classes of joints can be identified according to the amount of movement allowed: synarthrosis (immovable), amphiarthrosis (slightly movable), and diarthrosis (freely movable) (Crowther, 2004). Another method of classification is based on the connective structure of the joints. Fibrin, cartilage, and **synovium** (a fibrous envelope that produces a fluid to help to reduce friction and wear in a joint) are the connective structures seen in joints. Fibrous tissue is generally found in synarthrosis joints. In amphiarthrosis joints, cartilage is the predominant connective tissue. Within the joint capsule of the diarthrosis joints is the synovium. The diarthrosis joints are the most movable and most commonly injured joints in the body.

Structural Aspects of the Diarthrosis Joint

Hyaline (articular) cartilage covers the end of each bone to reduce friction and distribute weight-bearing forces. This cartilage is either thick or thin depending on the size of the joint, the fit of the bones, and the amount of weight bearing and shearing forces to which the joint is subjected (Crowther, 2004). For example, the knee joint cartilage is thicker than the shoulder joint cartilage due to the amount of weight bearing the knee withstands.

The synovial cavity is the space between the two bones that allows movement. This cavity is surrounded by the synovial membrane and filled with synovial fluid. The synovial membrane is the smooth fragile lining of the joint capsule, which is found in the nonarticulating portions of the joint. The synovial membrane is vascular and contains phagocytic cells as well as cells that secrete hyaluronate. Hyaluronate gives the synovial fluid its viscous quality. Synovial fluid also contains an ultrafiltrated solution that lubricates the joint surfaces, provides nourishment for the articular cartilage, and covers the ends of bones. The synovial fluid contains synovial cells and leukocytes that phagocytose joint debris and microorganisms (Crowther, 2004).

Motions

Diarthrosis joints, in conjunction with muscles, tendons, ligaments, and nerves allow body movement, which enables people to perform activities of daily living.

MUSCULOSKELETAL ASSESSMENT

Limitation in movement or pain is the chief reason patients seek musculoskeletal treatment. A thorough examination of the complaint is necessary to assist the patient in the relief or abatement of the symptoms. A complete health history is important to collect when interviewing a patient. Tools needed for a musculoskeletal assessment include a goniometer, tape measure, and flashlight.

Guidelines for Assessment

The NAON publishes the *Core Curriculum for Orthopaedic Nursing*. The core curriculum lists some general guidelines to use when performing a focused orthopedic assessment (Box 58-1).

Focused Health History

When completing an adult orthopedic musculoskeletal health history, the nurse should focus on four key areas: (a) pain, (b) onset of symptoms, (c) deformity, and (d) paralysis. It is also important to consider the special circumstances of trauma and chronic conditions that may affect the musculoskeletal system.

Pain

Pain is the most common symptom associated with a musculoskeletal complaint. When assessing the patient's level of pain the nurse should ask questions that clarify the type, location, severity, duration, and precipitating or alleviating factors related to the patient's pain.

Onset of Symptoms

Knowledge of when and how the symptoms of the chief complaint first occurred helps the nurse assess the mechanism of injury. Questions to ask include: (a) What are the symptoms? (b) What occurred to cause the symptoms? (c) When did they occur? (d) Did the symptoms come on gradually or was it a sudden onset? (e) Have the symptoms gotten worse or better? (f) What have you done to treat the symptoms? (g) Where these treatments effective? (h) Has anything increased the intensity of the symptoms?

Deformity

Physical deformities can be associated with edema, pain, and stiffness. While examining the deformity the nurse may discover when the changes first appeared. The nurse may also ask questions related to heredity. Deformities occur with dislocations, fractures, sprains, and strains. The nature of inflammatory diseases can lead to multiple deformities in the joints. For example, rheumatoid arthritis may cause lateral deviations in the joints of the fingers

BOX 58-1

ORTHOPAEDIC ASSESSMENT GUIDELINES

1. The examination should be performed after providing privacy to the patient.
2. The patient should be dressed in a way that allows full visualization of the body and facilitates examination without needless exposure.
3. Wash your hands before beginning the examination.
4. The examination should proceed in an orderly fashion from head to toe, proximal to distal.
5. Compare one side of the body to the other, frequently alternating the assessment of one part of the body to the other side.
6. Examination should reflect the influence on activities of daily living, including impact on school and work.
7. Questions should be worded in a way that helps ascertain information. For example:
   a. Are you able to get into and out of the bathtub?
   b. Can you stand at work?
   c. Can you comb your hair?
   d. Can you lift your backpack?

Safety First 1

A Case Study

The victim involved in a motor vehicle accident explains to you that he was a restrained passenger in the front seat of a minivan when the accident occurred. He twisted around to the left to check on his son in the back seat at the time the van slammed into the back of the car in front of them. The air bag went off. He suffered a fractured left distal femur. On further investigation you find that the distal portion of his knee (the proximal portion of the tibia) hit a portion of the console between the front two seats. This caused the distal portion of the left femur to be pushed back while the patient's body was moving forward (even with the airbag). As a result, a tremendous amount of force was applied to the distal end of the femur going in the opposite direction of his body and resulted in a distal femur fracture. Under these circumstances, it is also important to look for complaints of hip pain as the femoral head may have been forced into the acetabulum, causing major or minor fractures in the hip joint.

and hands. Congenital anomalies can also cause deformities. The nurse should ask questions about the usual shape and position of the affected area and compare these against expected findings.

Paralysis

When examining any paralysis, the nurse needs to explore the time of onset, what limbs or areas are affected, the extent of the paralysis, and the progression or regression of the paralysis. It is also important to note the presence or absence of sensory disturbances, such as numbness or tingling.

Trauma

Trauma can be highly emotional for patients and their families. Focusing on the exact cause of the injury will help make assessment and treatment of the entire patient more effective. Some causes of trauma may include motor vehicle accidents, sports-related injuries, and physical abuse. If the trauma was emotionally disturbing, the nurse should be sensitive to the patient's physical and psychological needs. Care also needs to be taken so that the more obvious injuries do not overshadow less apparent but potentially life-threatening injuries.

When investigating a motor vehicle accident it is important to note the force and direction of the impact. These details may reveal the cause and severity of the injury. The nurse should ascertain the object(s) involved in the trauma. This information is necessary to determine the mechanism of injury.

Chronic Conditions

When completing a health history, it is important to remember that patients with chronic conditions have a unique set of needs. Health care professionals should focus questions on those directed specifically at the chronic condition (Box 58-2).

Physical Examination of the Musculoskeletal System

There are three basic maneuvers used in assessing the musculoskeletal system: (a) inspection; (b) palpation; and (c) evaluation of passive and active ROM.

BOX 58-2

HEALTH HISTORY: CHRONIC CONDITIONS

The following questions be asked when assessing a chronic problem:

- When did the symptoms begin?
- How long have the symptoms been present?
- Are the symptoms continuous or intermittent?
- How did the symptoms begin?
- What caused the symptoms?
- What helps or irritates the condition?
- What interventions have been used (both traditional and nontraditional)? What was their effect?
- What is your response to heat and cold?
- What position causes pain?
- What medications, herbs, or over-the-counter products have been used?
- What was their effect?
- What complementary or alternative therapy have been used, such as therapeutic massage, acupuncture, or aromatherapy? What was their effect?

Inspection

When performing a focused assessment involving the musculoskeletal system, the nurse needs to consider the entire body. If the patient is able to ambulate, the nurse should observe the patient's gait and ROM while entering the examination room and sitting in a chair. The nurse's assessment should focus on the patient's ROM and observed ease or discomfort associated with position changes.

Palpation

When palpating an affected area the nurse should note the firmness of the skin and muscle, any report of tenderness, warmth, texture, presence of masses under the skin (measure for accuracy, if appropriate), and crepitus (a sign of fracture). It is important to note the presence of any deformity in shape of the bone or marked changes in muscle shapes, tone, or resistance to pressure.

Neurovascular Assessment

Considered a hallmark of musculoskeletal assessment, the neurovascular assessment is a simple, yet telling method of investigating musculoskeletal complaints or assessing for complications resulting from treatment of musculoskeletal injuries. The neurovascular assessment combines a focused neurological assessment with the assessment of the vascular system.

Skills 360°

Inspection

Performing the focused assessment starts with inspecting the area where the chief complaint occurs. When inspecting look for obvious deviations, observe the contour of the musculature, the color of the skin, the presence of any scars, bruises or open areas, edema, or atrophy. You may need to use a flashlight to illuminate subtleties in contour, which can indicate edema. Always compare the area in question to the opposite side of the body. Should there be an amputation (surgical removal of a limb of the body) on the side to which you are trying to compare, ask the patient if what you observe is normal. The patient should be able to tell you if what you are observing is normal or not. For example, a male patient with a right above-the-knee amputation is complaining of left knee pain. You observe edema in the knee area. The patient should be able to tell you if this is the normal size of his knee. Remember that it is normal for the dominant upper extremity, or a limb that is used frequently in a repetitive manner, to be slightly larger than the opposite extremity.

Skills 360°

Neurovascular Assessment

Focused on the extremities, the neurovascular assessment uses the techniques of inspection and palpation. You can begin by observing the color of the skin on the toes or fingers as well as the rest of the extremity, comparing the color to that of the opposite extremity. Observe for normality of color for the patient. Palpate the most distal pulse in the affected extremity. You then need to compare that pulse to the opposite extremity, looking for a similar pulse quality in both extremities. If you are unable to compare the most distal pulses, assess the next most distal comparable pulses. For example, if the patient has a below-the-knee amputation on one extremity, use the popliteal pulses for comparison. While palpating the pulses, make note of the temperature of the skin in the foot or hand and compare this to another portion of the extremity or body to assess for consistency. If you find it difficult to feel the pulses, it is often useful to use the middle finger of your non-dominant hand to attempt the palpation. This finger tends to be more sensitive then the others. Pulses which you will assess in the upper extremity include the radial, ulnar, and brachial. In the lower extremity you will assess the dorsalis pedis, posterior tibialis, popliteal, and femoral. The dorsalis pedis (often documented as the pedal pulse) is on the dorsum or top of the foot. The posterior tibialis is located behind the medial malleolus on the inside of the ankle. These two pulse points are often confusing to the beginning practitioner; therefore special care should be taken in assessment and documentation to obtain the correct assessment.

The neurological component of the neurovascular assessment evaluates both sensory and motor function. To test the sensory nerves simply ask if the patient can feel you touch his or her toes or fingers without the patient looking. In assessing motor function, ask the patient to dorsiflex and plantar flex in the lower extremity and then to make a fist, open the hand, and spread their fingers. Compare these assessments with the opposite extremity (Figure 58-4). During the assessment be sure to note differences between the extremities. In a postoperative patient, report these differences to the health care provider if it is the first time the difference has been noted, as this may be a sign of an impending complication.

Range of Motion

A unique aspect of the musculoskeletal assessment is the assessment of ROM at each joint. Joint function is essential to perform activities of daily living. There are essentially seven types of motions made by the joints: (a) flexion and extension; (b) circumduction; (c) abduction and adduction; (d) internal rotation and external rotation; (e) pronation and supination; (f) plantar flexion and dorsiflexion; and (g) inversion and eversion (Figures 58-5 through 58-9).

Measuring ROM requires the use of a goniometer to measure joint angles (Figure 58-10). For example, the knee joint when straight is at 0° of flexion. Angles can range from minus 15° in extension to as far as 130° of flexion. Table 58-2 describes the normal range of motion for joints.

Muscle Tone and Muscle Strength Grading

Muscle tone and muscle strength grading can be integrated with the assessment of ROM To assess the muscle's tone, while putting the muscle through passive ROM, the nurse should be aware of any spasticity or fasciculations (quivering) (Maher, 2002). To assess muscle strength, the nurse should ask the patient to flex the muscle and then flex the muscle again while applying resistance. It is important to also test the opposing muscle (e.g., tricep to bicep) (Figure 58-11). To assess the appropriateness of muscle strength a graded numerical scale is commonly used. See Table 58-3 for this graded scale.

Analysis of Gait

The way in which a person walks can reveal much about the musculoskeletal system. A person's gait provides evidence of pain, muscle atrophy, leg length discrepancy, as well as hip, knee, and ankle complications.

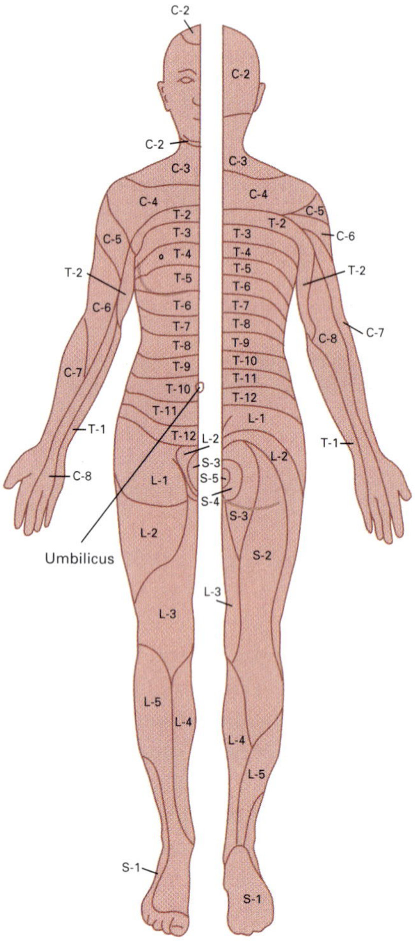

Figure 58-4 Illustration of sensory innervation of the body.

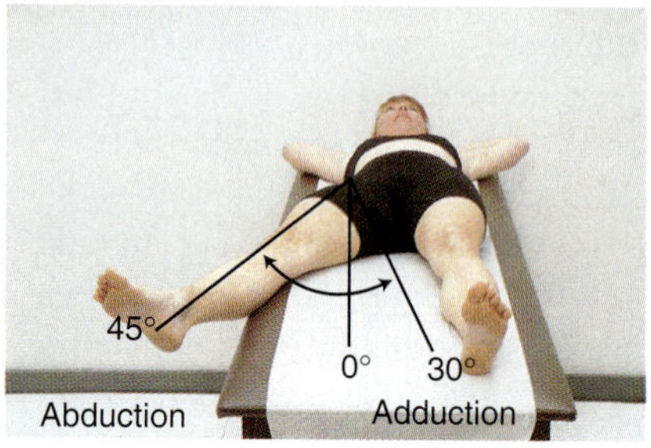

Figure 58-5 Abduction and adduction.

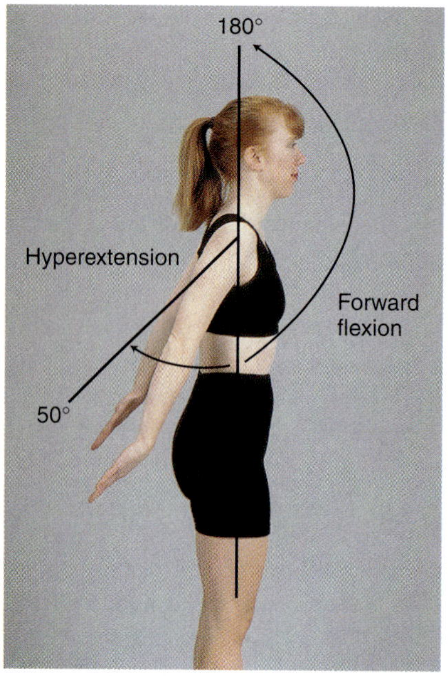

Figure 58-6 Forward flexion, hyperextension/circumduction.

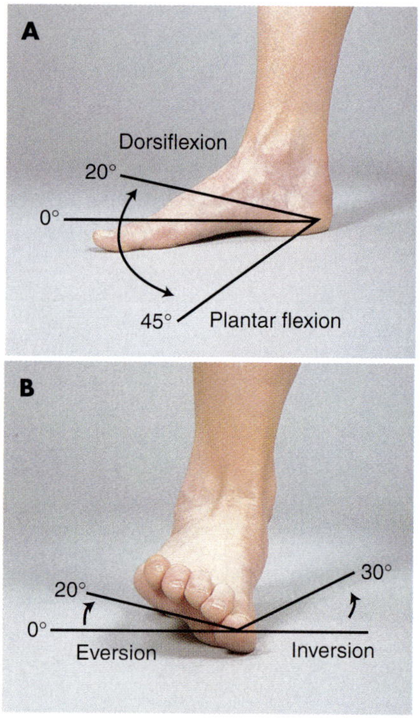

Figure 58-7 A. Plantar flexion and dorsiflexion, B. Eversion and inversion.

The gait has two phases: the stance or weight-bearing phase and the swing or non–bearing-weight phase. While the patient is walking a straight line, the nurse should note the stance phase. Particular attention should be paid to the patient's heel, how flat the foot is at midstance, and how the patient pushes off the ball of the foot. During the swing phase the nurse should assess the rate and rhythm of acceleration, midswing, and deceleration. It is important to compare the left and the right sides, looking for similarities and discrepancies during both phases of the gait.

The nurse needs to observe the alignment of the head, shoulders, spine, pelvis, knees, and feet; the rhythm of the pelvis (normal rotation during arm swing is 40° forward); the width of gap between legs (ankle to ankle should be 2 to 4 inches); the length of the step (approximately 15 inches); and the center of gravity should be midline. Any lack of coordination, use of assistive devices, such as cane or crutch, or use of equipment, such as splints or special shoes, should be noted. To observe the areas of greatest wear, the clinician should ask to see the soles of the patient's shoes. Listening to the patient walk, paying particular attention to the noises made while walking, such as the foot slapping or scraping the floor, can also reveal areas of concern in the musculoskeletal system.

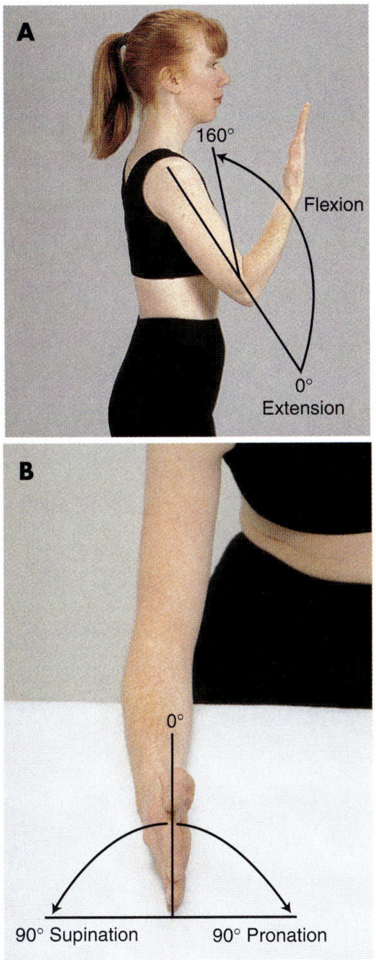

Figure 58-8 A. Elbow joint flexion and extension, B. Supination and pronation.

Assessment of Injuries to the Musculoskeletal System

When assessing for muscle injuries or strains (occurs when a muscle or the tendon that attaches it to the bone is overstretched or torn), it is best to palpate gently from the origin (the more proximal and fixed end) to the insertion site (the end close to the center of the body). Injuries can occur throughout the muscle, but 40 percent of the injuries occur in the muscle body.

Sprains or ligamentous injuries occur because the ligament is stretched beyond its capability. The ligament is pliable but not elastic, and consequently, it is easy to sustain a ligament injury when the joint is unduly stretched.

Both muscle and ligament injuries can be classified into three different grade levels. Table 58-4 lists the grading for muscles and ligaments.

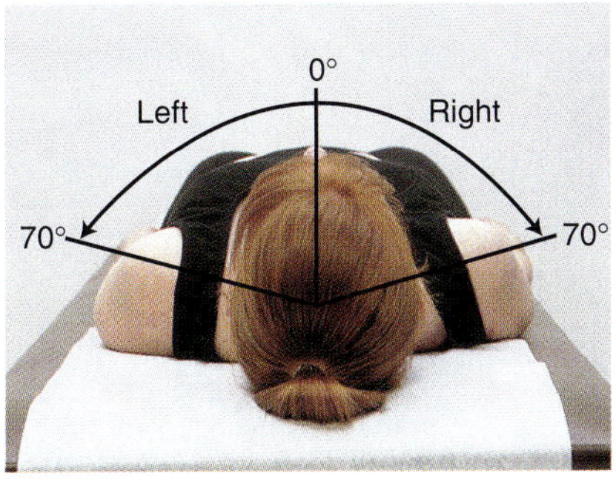

Figure 58-9 Cervical spine rotation.

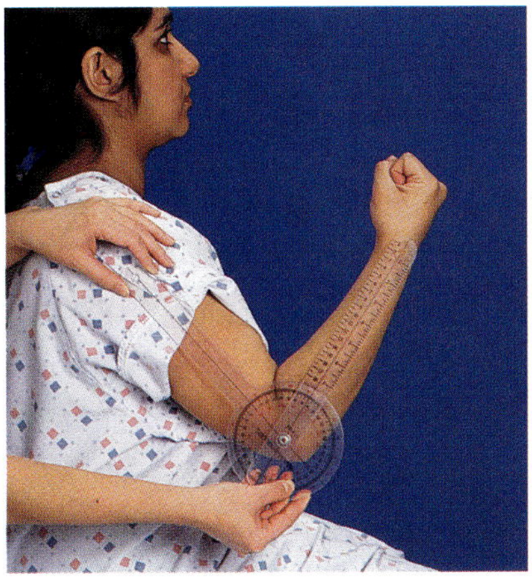

Figure 58-10 A Goniometer in use.

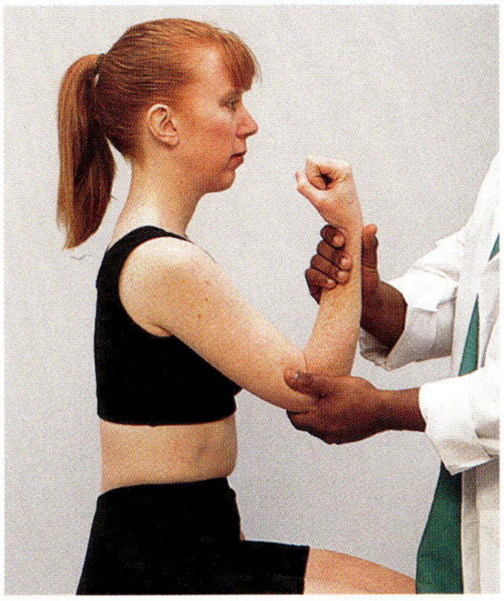

Figure 58-11 Assessment of strength in upper extremity.

Red Flag

Homans' Sign

A test that can be easily integrated into the neurovascular assessment is the **Homans' sign.** This test is used to assess for the presence of a **deep vein thrombosis** ([**DVT**] a blood clot in a deep vein that accompanies an artery). DVT affects mainly the veins in the lower leg. To perform this test, passively dorsiflex the patient's foot feeling for **clonus** (a slight involuntary pushing against your foot) and ask if the patient has any pain in his or her calf. A positive Homans' sign is the presence of extreme pain with or without clonus. Homans' sign is not a reliable predictor of the presence of DVT, but it is frequently used as a cursory assessment when a problem is suspected.

TABLE 58-2 Range of Motion

JOINT	RANGE OF MOTION	JOINT	RANGE OF MOTION
Cervical Spine			
Flexion	80–90 degrees	Radial deviation	15 degrees
Extension	70 degrees	Pronation	85–90 degrees
Lateral flexion	20–45 degrees	Supination	85–90 degrees
Rotation	70–90 degrees	***Hip***	
Lumbar Spine		Flexion	110–120 degrees
Flexion	40–60 degrees	Extension	10–15 degrees
Extension	20–35 degrees	Abduction	30–50 degrees
Lateral flexion	15–20 degrees	Adduction	30 degrees
Rotation	3–18 degrees	External rotation	40–60 degrees
Shoulder		Internal rotation	30–40 degrees
Flexion	160–180 degrees	***Knee***	
Extension	50–60 degrees	Flexion	0–130 degrees
Abduction	170–180 degrees	Extension	0–15 degrees
Adduction	50–75 degrees	Medial rotation	20–30 degrees
External rotation	80–90 degrees	Lateral rotation	30–40 degrees
Internal rotation	60–100 degrees	***Ankle***	
Circumduction	200 degrees	Plantar flexion	50 degrees
Elbow		Dorsiflexion	20 degrees
Flexion	140–160 degrees	Inversion	30 degrees
Extension	0–10 degrees	Eversion	20 degrees
Supination	90 degrees	Subtalar inversion	5 degrees
Pronation	80–90 degrees	Subtalar eversion	5 degrees
Wrist		Forefoot adduction	20 degrees
Flexion	80–90 degrees	Forefoot abduction	10 degrees
Extension	70–90 degrees	Great toe flexion	45 degrees
Ulnar deviation	35–45 degrees	Great toe extension	70 degrees

TABLE 58-3 Graded Muscle Strength

GRADING	DESCRIPTION	LOVETT SCALE
0	No palpable contraction of muscle	Zero (0)
1	Palpable contraction of muscle; no joint motion	Trace (T)
2	Complete range of motion (ROM) with gravity eliminated	Poor (P)
3	Complete ROM against gravity; no added resistance	Fair (F)
4	Complete ROM against gravity: some added resistance	Good (G)
5	Complete ROM against gravity with full resistance	Normal (N)

Adapted from Maher, A. B. (2002). Assessment of the musculoskeletal system. In A. B. Maher, S. W. Salmond, & T. A. Pellino (Eds.), Orthopaedic nursing *(3rd ed., pp. 189–210). Philadelphia, PA: W. B. Saunders Company.*

TABLE 58-4 Muscle and Ligament Injury Classification

GRADE	MUSCLE	LIGAMENT
One	Strain–stretch on muscle fibers. Less than 10 percent muscle fibers involved.	Stretched. No tear to up to 20 percent torn.
Two	Partial tear in muscle. Palpation reveals defect. Ten to 50 percent of muscle fiber involved.	Twenty to 75 percent torn.
Three	Extensive tear or complete rupture. Fifty to 100 percent muscle fibers torn to complete rupture of the muscle.	Seventy-five percent to complete rupture of the ligament.

Adapted from Crowther, C. L. (2004). Structure and function of the musculoskeletal system. In S. E. Huether & K. L. McCance (Eds.), Understanding pathophysiology *(3rd ed., pp. 1047–1070). St. Louis, MO: Mosby.*

Assessment of Fractures

Although most accurately diagnosed with X-ray, if a fracture is suspected, assessment can be performed on the area by keeping the following principles in mind. A stress fracture (fracture caused by nontraumatic, cumulative overload on bone) is the most difficult to diagnose on X-ray despite the patient's ability to point to the area that hurts. There may be soft tissue swelling with painless active ROM as well as painless resisted active movement of the joint. A callous may form over the stress fracture site and may confirm the presence of a fracture. The gait may also be affected if the fracture is in the lower extremity due to pain at the fracture site with weight-bearing.

A **displaced fracture** is a fracture in which the bones have gone out of natural alignment. Immediate edema will occur with a displaced fracture. Pain may occur with movement and deformity may be seen. A fracture is considered a stable fracture if the edges of the fracture do not move. An unstable fracture is when motion is present at the fracture site causing a potential for trauma to the surrounding tissue, such as an unstable rib fracture that may puncture the lung.

Sports Injury Considerations

Whether a person is a weekend warrior or a professional athlete, sports injuries can occur at any time. Fortunately, many sports-related injuries heal without professional intervention. Guidelines to follow when deciding to see medical assistance include:

- Prolonged or nonsubsiding pain continuing two weeks after the episode.
- Any injury that occurs in or near a joint.
- Any loss of function.
- Any injury that does not heal in three weeks or in which the structure is apparently abnormal *or* any sign of infection on or under the skin, presence of pus, red streaks, swollen lymph nodes or fever.
- Any alteration in sensation, such as numbness or tingling.

The key to assessing sports injuries is to determine the severity and extent of the injury before permanent damage takes place. The following points will assist the nurse while assessing a sports-related injury: (a) because different areas of the body are developed depending on the sport, other areas may not be as developed; (b) unbalanced opposing muscle groups leave the athlete at risk to injury; and (c) it may be necessary to refer the athlete to a physician that specializes in sports-related injuries.

One of the best methods to evaluate muscle balance is to test the strength of opposing muscle groups with isometric measuring devices (muscle contraction without movement at the joint). These devices may be used for **isokinetic** exercise as well (exercise involving resistance through full range of movement).

DIAGNOSTIC STUDIES RELATED TO THE MUSCULOSKELETAL SYSTEM

Musculoskeletal assessment can be completed by physical examination. However, modern tools are available to pinpoint exact causes of musculoskeletal dysfunction and allow the diagnostician to develop thorough and complete plans of care.

Laboratory Studies

From a musculoskeletal assessment perspective, blood and urine study results show indications of disease and extent of disease progression. These studies also can be assistive in monitoring a patient's recovery from a surgical procedure or trauma. Although there are many studies that can be performed on the blood and urine, only those studies that can be used specifically in the assessment of the musculoskeletal system will be addressed here.

To monitor a patient's recovery from a surgical procedure or trauma, it is helpful to know the baseline hematology, chemistry, and coagulation studies. Blood loss is often a factor that deters a patient's ability to participate in recovery efforts postsurgery or posttrauma. Being able to compare the patient's current hemoglobin and hematocrit to preoperative levels allows the nurse to anticipate the health care provider's orders for iron supplements or administration of blood products. Basic chemistry levels allow comparisons to be made to monitor fluid balance, kidney function, and if the patient is diabetic, the reaction to the physiological stressors that the patient has endured. Elevated blood glucose levels in response to stress may necessitate a change in the patient's normal insulin or oral medication routine.

Warfarin (Coumadin) and heparin are often used as prophylactic therapy in the prevention of DVT and pulmonary embolism. Partial thromboplastin time (PTT), prothrombin time (PT), and the international normalized ratio (INR) are the laboratory values that monitor the effectiveness of aforementioned medications.

Radiographic Studies

Radiology technology has developed rapidly in recent years and has been instrumental in the diagnosis and treatment of musculoskeletal conditions. The radiographic studies described in this section are a combination of gold standard studies and new technologies to assist in making accurate diagnoses. As with the laboratory studies discussed previously, only musculoskeletal implications will be discussed for the radiologic tests presented.

Angiogram

For patients with musculoskeletal disorders, angiogram is most often used after trauma or surgery to confirm a diagnosis of a DVT or a pulmonary embolism. An angiogram is an invasive procedure that can have serious complications. A catheter is inserted in the femoral, brachial, subclavian, or carotid artery and a contrast dye is injected to visualize the vessels. The most serious complication is an embolus forming due to catheter clot formation. Another precaution to take is to assess for a potential allergy to the contrast dye. Questions about allergies to seafood, iodine, or contrast dye may prevent any allergic reactions (Kee, 2002).

Arthrography

Arthrography is a radiological examination used to diagnose complaints in the joints. Knees and shoulders are the most commonly assessed using this method. Air, contrast dye, or both are injected into the joint space to visualize the structures of the joints. Arthrography is an outpatient procedure usually done with a local anesthetic (Kee, 2002).

Preprocedure nursing interventions include reviewing the patient's medical history to obtain allergy information, obtaining signed consent, and patient teaching related to the procedure. Postprocedure interventions may include instructing the patient about the importance of limiting movement of the affected joint and maintaining compression dressings for 12 hours. Analgesia and ice may be used to reduce pain.

Bone Scan

A **bone scan** is a nuclear scan used to detect early bone disease, bone metastasis, and bone response to therapeutic regimens (Kee, 2002). Bone scans assist in detecting fractures, abnormal healing of fractures, and degenerative bone diseases (Kee, 2002). The patient is injected with the isotope because radioisotopes are used in the bone scan. Depending on the type of isotope used, the scan may take two to four hours to complete. Once the isotope is injected and has been distributed in the body, the body is scanned for hot spots. Dark spots on the scan indicate an area where the radioisotope uptake is greater, usually indicating an abnormality in that region.

Preprocedure nursing interventions include obtaining a health history, a signed consent form, and patient teaching related to the procedure. Patients are required to drink four to six glasses of water during the waiting period, remove all jewelry or metal objects, and void before the procedure. Postprocedure nursing interventions include encouraging the patient to continue increased fluid intake, observation for allergic reactions to the radioisotopes, and avoiding any other radionuclide tests for 24 to 48 hours.

Computed Tomography Scan

Also known as computed axial tomography (CAT or CT), the CT scan is a radiographic study that is 100 times more sensitive than normal X-rays (Kee, 2002). The CT scan can be done with or without contrast dye. For long bones and joints, CT scans can give a detailed examination of cross-sections of the areas examined. Defects that can be seen include tumors and fractures. Contrast may be used in joint examination. CT scans are generally tolerated well. Timing for the scan ranges from 30 to 90 minutes.

Preprocedure nursing interventions include obtaining a health history regarding possible pregnancy or allergies, a signed consent form, and patient teaching related to the procedure. The procedure requires the patient to remain still and may cause some patients to feel claustrophobic. Antianxiety medications are often helpful to alleviate these reactions. Patients are required to remove all jewelry or metal objects and void before the procedure. Postprocedure there are no physical restrictions.

Dual Energy X-ray Absorptiometry Scan

Dual energy X-ray absorptiometry (DEXA) scans measure bone density. These scans assist in the early diagnosis of osteoporosis. Using a computer analysis, the scans can determine size, thickness, and mineral content of the bone (Kee, 2002).

Preprocedure nursing interventions include obtaining a health history, a signed consent form, and patient teaching related to the procedure. Patients are required to remove all jewelry or metal objects. Postprocedure there are no physical restrictions.

Indium (White Blood Cell) Scan

The indium (white blood cell [WBC]) scan is used to detect osteomyelitis. A blood sample is obtained from the patient. An indium-111 radioisotope is then mixed with the blood to tag the WBCs. Once the blood has been mixed, it is reinfused in the patient. At 6 and 24 hours the patient's body is scanned. The scan takes 1 to 2 hours. The tagged WBCs will migrate to areas where tissue destruction from inflammation or infections is occurring (*WBC nuclear scan*, 2003)

Magnetic Resonance Imaging

Although costing approximately 30 percent more than a CT, magnetic resonance imaging (MRI) is being extensively used to confirm the diagnosis of musculoskeletal dysfunction by orthopaedic surgeons. This technique uses a magnet field and radio frequency waves that create images to be analyzed by computer technology. The computer can produce cross-sectional images, similar in detail to CT images. Kee (2002) states that MRIs are "now the most sensitive technique for defining the structure of internal organs and for detecting edema, infarction, hemorrhage, blood flow, tumors, infections, and plaques on the myelin sheath that cause Multiple Sclerosis" (p. 560). Kee also states that bone, joint, and soft tissue injuries can be seen without bone artifact and can distinguish whether a tumor is within or adjacent to a bone.

Most areas of the body can be visualized with a MRI. Because the magnets of the MRI are housed in a tubular machine that allows the magnetic field to be formed, claustrophobia can be an issue. Open MRIs are available but may not give as clear of an image as the closed system.

Preprocedure nursing interventions include obtaining a health history to determine possible pregnancy and the presence of metal implants, a signed consent form, and patient teaching related to the procedure. The procedure requires the patient to remain still and may cause some patients to feel claustrophobic. Antianxiety medications are often helpful to alleviate these reactions. Patients are required to remove all jewelry or metal objects, and void before the procedure. Postprocedure there are no physical restrictions.

Myelogram

A **myelogram** is used to diagnose defects in and around the spinal column. Using fluoroscopy and radiography, a contrast dye is injected into the subarachnoid space of the spinal canal. Defects are revealed when a smooth flow of contrast is not seen. Herniated discs, tumors, and spinal nerve root injury are examples of defects that may be seen (Kee, 2002).

Preprocedure nursing implications include obtaining a health history to determine allergies to contrast dye. Metrizamide is sometimes used as the contrast dye (water based). If it is used it is necessary to find out if the patient is taking any medications that lower the seizure threshold (phenothiazines, tricyclic antidepressants, central nervous system stimulants, or amphetamines) as metrizamide can cause seizures. Patients are often required to force fluids the night before the procedure and then have nothing by mouth (NPO) four to eight hours prior to the procedure. Other nursing interventions include obtaining a signed consent form and patient teaching related to the procedure. Patients are required to void before the procedure.

Postprocedure nursing interventions include prevention of lumbar puncture headaches and other complications. For the water-based test, the patient's head should be elevated 15 to 40° for 8 hours and then progress to supine bed rest with bathroom privileges for 16 hours. It is important to avoid phenothiazines or drugs that lower the seizure threshold. For the oil-based test the patient will be required to lie supine in bed for 12 to 24 hours. The patient may turn from side-to-side. For all patients, the nurse should encourage them to increase their fluid intake, monitor for bladder distension, perform neurological vital signs and assessments, and administer pain medications for headaches or discomfort. Possible complications include bleeding or leakage at the injection site, nausea and vomiting, headache, fever, seizure (most likely to occur 4 to 8 hours after the procedure), paralysis, arachnoiditis (inflammation of coverings of spinal cord, neck stiffness, sterile meningitis reaction, severe headache, and slow electroencephalogram [EEG] patterns), brainstem compression, and brainstem herniation.

X-rays

X-rays are the gold standard of diagnosis in the assessment of skeletal complaints. X-rays assist in the diagnosis of fractures, abnormal fracture healing, tumors, arthritic conditions, and osteomyelitis (Kee, 2002). Although brief exposure to radiation is necessary, X-rays are well tolerated by most patients.

Preprocedure nursing interventions include obtaining a health history to determine the possibility of pregnancy, a signed consent form, and patient teaching related to the procedure. Postprocedure there are no physical restrictions, but the patient may require analgesia if the procedure was prolonged.

Special Tests

Arthrometry

Arthrometry is a method used to measure and document cruciate ligament laxity of the knee both passively and actively. The arthrometer measures the distraction forces on the knee. These measurements are taken passively, actively, and manually. Measurements are taken on both the noninjured and injured knee. Surgeons use this method to diagnose anterior cruciate ligament (ACL) or posterior cruciate ligament (PCL) tears. The surgeon will evaluate and confirm ACL or PCL stability intraoperatively and postoperatively with this method of assessment.

Preprocedure nursing interventions include obtaining a health history, a signed consent form, and patient teaching related to the procedure. Postprocedure there are no physical restrictions.

Arthroscopy

Most often performed in the knee joint, an **arthroscopy** is an endoscopic procedure used to diagnose and repair meniscal, patellar, extrasynovial, and synovial diseases. Biopsies can also be performed. As with arthrography, this procedure is done on an outpatient basis. Local, spinal, or general anesthesia can be used (Kee, 2002).

Preprocedure nursing interventions include obtaining a health history to determine the possibility of pregnancy, a signed consent form, and patient teaching related to the procedure. Preprocedure medications should be administered and vital signs recorded. Patients should be instructed to remove all jewelry, contact lenses, glasses, dentures, or plates. Postprocedure, the patient will return to the recovery room for routine postoperative monitoring and assessment. Depending on type of anesthesia, activity, rehabilitation, diet, and medications may be resumed as soon as tolerated.

Bone Marrow Aspiration and Biopsy

Bone marrow aspiration and biopsy is used to examine the bone marrow for abnormal tissue growth or to monitor the progress of bone marrow disease. This procedure is performed under local anesthesia. The aspiration can be performed at the iliac crest or the sternum. Bone marrow is aspirated using a needle that is inserted into the cancellous bone (Kee, 2002).

Preprocedure nursing interventions include obtaining a health history to determine the possibility of pregnancy, a signed consent form, and patient teaching related to the procedure. Postprocedure the biopsy site should be assessed frequently for bleeding or hemorrhage and vital signs should be monitored closely. Diet, medications, and activity may be resumed as tolerated. The patient and family should be instructed to assess the site for signs of infection.

Joint Aspiration

Joint aspiration is performed to examine the synovial fluid in the joint cavity. It is also used to relieve pain in the joint resulting from edema and effusion. The procedure involves inserting a needle into the joint space and withdrawing fluid using a syringe. The fluid is then sent to the laboratory to be analyzed for infection or abnormal cells. The procedure is generally done under local anesthetic in the health care provider's office.

Preprocedure nursing interventions include patient teaching related to the procedure. Postprocedure the site will need pressure applied for 5 to 10 minutes. There are no physical restrictions.

Nerve Conduction Studies

Electromyography (EMG) measures electrical activity of skeletal muscle at rest and during voluntary muscle contraction (Kee, 2002). EMG is used to diagnose neuromuscular diseases and nerve damage. Kee states that the EMG can be used to differentiate between muscle and nerve damage. Needles are inserted into the muscle to detect electrical activity and printed as a graph. This procedure may be uncomfortable for the patient.

Preprocedure nursing interventions include obtaining a signed consent form and patient teaching related to the procedure. Patients are required to refrain from nicotine and caffeine two to three hours before the procedure. Postprocedure there are no physical restrictions.

Somatosensory Evoked Potentials (Evoked Potentials)

Somatosensory evoked potentials (SEP) are used to measure time in meters per second from the stimulation of a peripheral nerve through the response. It is used when EMG is not appropriate. This measurement documents axonal continuity when sensory potential cannot be measured due to nerve trauma. It is useful in the evaluation of radiculopathies and peripheral nerve function and the diagnosis of Charcot-Marie-Tooth disease. Electrodes are placed on the skin, stimulus is applied, and time intervals are calculated based on the time it takes from the stimulus to be given at one electrode and reach the next electrode along the peripheral nerve pathway. This procedure can be uncomfortable because of the electric nature of the stimulus.

Preprocedure nursing interventions may include patient teaching related to the procedure.

KEY CONCEPTS

- Anatomy and physiology of the bone consist of collagen, noncollagen, protein, and mineral components, which continually renew themselves.
- Bone formation is triggered by physical force, hormones, and genetics.
- There are four types of bones in the body: flat, short, long, and irregular.
- Long bones have three sections: the diaphysis, the medullary cavity, and the epiphyses.
- In the maturing child, the epiphyseal plate is the growth plate.
- Haversian canals, or osteons, allow the flow of fluid and nutrients to the bones.

Continued

KEY CONCEPTS—cont'd

- The five physiological processes of the bone are: (a) growth; (b) modeling; (c) remodeling; (d) repair; and (e) blood-bone exchange.
- Growth begins at two months after conception and continues until maturity.
- Remodeling of the bone occurs at the microscopic level through a balance of osteoclastic and osteoblastic activity.
- The main functions of the bones are to support the structure of the body, provide form, and enable movement.
- As a person ages, bones often become thinner and weaker and lean muscle mass decreases.
- A joint is formed when a bone meets another bone. It provides stability and mobility.
- The three classes of joints are synarthrosis (immobile), amphiarthrosis (slightly moveable), and diarthrosis (freely moveable).
- To reduce friction and distribute weight-bearing faces, hyaline cartilage covers the end of each bone.
- Synovial fluid lubricates joint surfaces.
- The nurse should focus on pain, onset of symptoms, deformity, and paralysis when completing an adult orthopedic musculoskeletal health history.
- The three maneuvers used in assessing the musculoskeletal system are: (a) inspection; (b) palpation; and (c) evaluation of passive and active ROM.
- Analysis of muscle tone, muscle strength, and gait are important aspects of identifying problems in the musculoskeletal system.
- Fractures can be classified as stress, displaced, stable, or unstable.
- The key to assessing sports-related injuries is to determine the severity and extent of the injury before permanent damage takes place.
- Radiographic studies are instrumental in the diagnosis and treatment of musculoskeletal conditions.
- Preprocedure nursing interventions for any testing include obtaining a health history, a signed consent form, and patient teaching related to the procedure.

REVIEW QUESTIONS

1. Wolff's law states what?
   1. The direction of growth is in opposite proportion to the amount of physical force placed on the bone.
   2. Bone forms and remodels itself in direct proportion to the amount and the direction of physical forces placed on it.
   3. Muscle tone and muscle strength increase with use.
   4. Myofibrils will contract with the release of actin and myosin.

2. A 7-year-old boy has fallen while roller-skating and fractured his radius along the epiphyseal plate. What is a likely consequence of the fracture?
   1. Fracture healing will proceed as normal and be fully remodeled in four weeks.
   2. The arm will always have a noticeable deformity, even after the fracture is healed.
   3. The fracture site has a 95 percent chance of developing an infection.
   4. Growth in the arm may be delayed or stopped.

3. All of the following statements are true regarding bone growth and remodeling *except*:
   1. Osteoblastic activity increases after the age of 30.
   2. Remodeling of a fracture can take several months to several years.
   3. Bones in children resemble cartilage more so than mature bone.
   4. The inflammation stage of fracture healing is the initial phase.

4. A few of the main functions of skeletal muscle are to (circle all that apply):
   1. Store minerals
   2. Maintain posture and body position
   3. Produce enzymes responsible for movement
   4. Guard entrances and exits to the digestive and urinary tracts

5. The mineral necessary to trigger a muscular contraction is:
   1. Potassium
   2. Calcium
   3. Magnesium
   4. None of the above

Continued

REVIEW QUESTIONS—cont'd

6. Ligaments have all the following characteristics *except*:
   1. Strong bands of connective tissue
   2. Give joints stability
   3. Elasticity
   4. Guide the joint movement
7. The three classes of joints are:
   1. Synarthrosis, amphiarthrosis, and diarthrosis
   2. Synarthrosis, biarthrosis, and amphiarthrosis
   3. Amphiarthrosis, biarthrosis, and lunarthrosis
   4. Synarthrosis, acetylarthrosis, and diarthrosis
8. Most patients come to a health care provider seeking assistance with musculoskeletal complaints because of:
   1. Obvious defects
   2. Limitation of movement
   3. Increase in the flexibility
   4. Decrease in pain
9. Physical assessment techniques used during the musculoskeletal system assessment include:
   1. Palpation and auscultation
   2. Inspection and range of motion
   3. Observation and auscultation
   4. Interview and palpation
10. Mrs. Dibble fell when getting off the bus and fractured her right ankle. The nurse is performing a neurovascular assessment (NVA). Important aspects to remember when performing a NVA are:
    1. Palpating the most distal pulse on the right lower extremity only using the nondominant hand
    2. Assessing for the patient's ability to feel the nurse touching her feet
    3. Asking the patient to dorsiflex and plantar flex her left foot only
    4. Compare the temperature of the left foot and toes to the left thigh

REVIEW ACTIVITIES

1. The patient has been diagnosed with a fractured radius and is placed in a cast. Explain to the patient why the health care provider stated the fracture would take about six weeks to heal. What would you tell the patient to look for when teaching about signs of circulatory and neurological impairment?
2. Search for a nursing article about osteoporosis, care of a patient with a joint replacement, or care of a patient with a congenital musculoskeletal problem, such as hip dysplasia, clubfoot, or muscular dystrophy. What does the article say about nursing assessment of the patient? What nursing interventions are done to minimize mobility problems? Does the article describe the collaborative nature of the relationship between the nurse and the health care provider or advanced practice nurse?
3. A neighbor tells you he has been diagnosed with bursitis in his elbow. He asks why he experiences pain when he flexes or extends his elbow. What explanation will you give?
4. Identify the orthopaedic nursing unit in your facility. Observe a nurse assessing his postoperative patient. What assessments does he perform? When performing the neurovascular assessment does he assess both extremities?
5. After being examined by the health care provider for complaints of hip and leg pain, your patient tells you that he is being scheduled for an MRI. He asks why an MRI and not a simple X-ray or CT scan. What explanation will you give him? What preparatory information can you tell him about the MRI testing procedure?

CHAPTER 59

Musculoskeletal Dysfunction: Nursing Management

Anita M. Zehala, RN, MS, ONC, CNS

Debra Davis, BSN, RN

Rebecca Sears, RN

CHAPTER TOPICS

- Osteoarthritis
- Gout
- Lyme Disease
- Spondyloarthropathies Polymyositis/Dermatomyositis
- Fibromyalgia
- Metabolic Bone Disease
- Osteomyelitis
- Tumors of the Musculoskeletal System
- Spinal Disorders

KEY TERMS

Adams Bending Forward Test
Bouchard's nodes
Chondrosarcoma
Crepitus
Dactylitis
Enthesitis
Ewing's sarcoma
Fibromyalgia
Heberden's nodes
Hyperuricemia
Hypokyphosis
Keratitis
Kyphosis
Onycholysis
Osteoarthritis (OA)
Osteomalacia
Osteomyelitis
Osteoporosis
Osteosarcoma
Papilledema
Sacroilitis
Sarcoma
Scoliometer
Tendosynovial
Tophus

Musculoskeletal disorders (MSDs) affect nearly everyone. Whether a problem occurs because of overuse, sports, or an accident, there is some alteration, temporary or permanent, in a person's activities of daily living. MSDs occur in one in seven people in the United States. In a review of gender differences in upper extremity musculoskeletal disorders (UEMDs), the current literature supported the hypothesis that UEMDs did indeed occur more commonly in women than in men. Many nonfatal occupational injuries involving days away from work were MSDs. However, work-related musculoskeletal injuries occurred more often in men than women.

Because so many people are affected by MSDs, this chapter will cover the most common nontraumatic disorders in adults and children. Chapter 60 covers MSDs that are related to trauma.

OSTEOARTHRITIS

Osteoarthritis (OA) is noninflammatory degenerative joint disease characterized by degeneration of the articular cartilage, hypertrophy of bone at the margins, and changes in the synovial membrane. It is also accompanied by pain and stiffness, particularly after prolonged activity. More common than rheumatoid arthritis (RA), OA also affects the joint cavity. Unlike RA, OA is a noninflammatory arthritis. OA slowly progresses from deterioration of the articular cartilage to new bone formation in the joint margins and synovial hyperplasia and capsular thickening in diarthrodial (movable) joints. OA does not have systemic involvement.

Epidemiology

OA is the most common form of joint disease. OA, also known as degenerative joint disease (DJD), shows no favoritism with regard to race, age, or geographical area. At least 20 million adults in the United States suffer from the effects of OA. The incidence of OA increases with age, weight, and incidence of injury within a joint. The incidence of OA is twice as great in women over age 55.

Patients with OA find that physical limitations pose the greatest challenge. Seventy-eight percent of the elderly and one third of all patients report a limitation that affects performance of activities of daily living. Gait disturbance is also a common. Falls are, therefore, risks. Coping with a chronic illness, pain, and physical limitations can be challenging. Assessment of emotional and social coping is imperative.

Etiology

There are two types of OA, idiopathic (primary) and secondary. Idiopathic refers to the development of OA without any known or obvious trigger. A decrease in the quality and quantity of proteoglycans with aging is seen as an important factor that may influence the development of OA. There is evidence that idiopathic OA may be inherited as an autosomal recessive trait with gene defects causing premature cartilage destruction.

Secondary OA is the result of a known cause. Generally, the development is related to a known trauma in the area (e.g., fracture or sprain), prolonged mechanical stressors (e.g., obesity or athletics), inflammation in joint structures (not associated with RA), joint instability (e.g., damage to ligaments or tendons), neurological disorders (e.g., lost of proprioceptive reflexes leading to a tendency for abnormal movement, positioning, or weight-bearing), congenital or acquired skeletal deformities (e.g., dislocated hip or Legg-Calvé-Perthes disease), hematological or endocrine disorders (e.g., hemophilia with chronic bleeding into the joints or hyperparathyroidism with calcium loss from the bone) or selected drug use (collagen-digesting enzymes are stimulated in the synovial membrane by the drugs, such as colchicines, indomethacin, and steroids).

Sex hormones and other hormones seem to play a role in disease development and progression. For example, excessive growth hormone produces progressive overgrowth of bone and excessive parathyroid hormone results in hypercalcemia, which can produce skeletal changes. Unlike RA, OA is usually presents in only one joint (asymmetrical development).

Pathophysiology

OA occurs because of damage to articular cartilage and the metabolic response that results at the chondrocyte level. As a result of articular cartilage damage occurs, enzymes are released that breakdown the cartilage. This leads to a softening of the cartilage matrix (made up of type II collagen and pro-

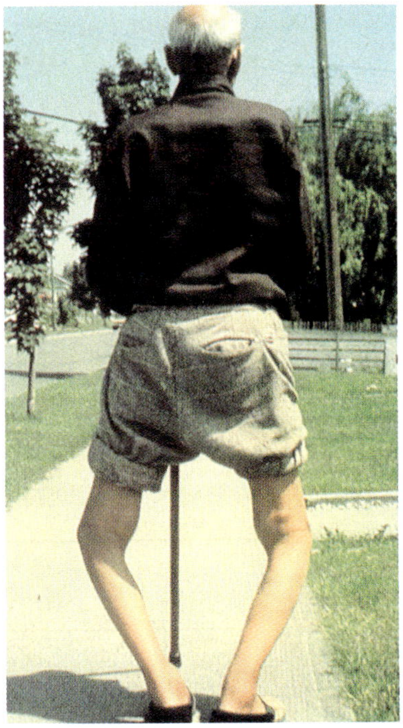

Figure 59-1 A patient with osteoarthritis of both knee joints.

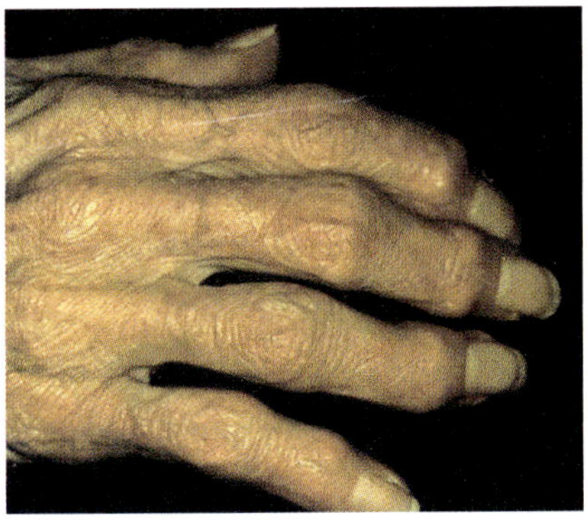

Figure 59-2 Bouchard's nodes and Heberden's nodes.

teoglycans) as well as a loss of elasticity, and the cartilage becomes more fibrous. The resulting compensatory response is not enough to keep up with the destruction of the cartilage. This makes the articular surface more susceptible to joint friction.

With decreased cushioning, increased friction and tendency to become more fibrous, cartilage loses its ability to resist wear and utilize nutrients from the synovial fluid. The normally white, glistening, and smooth surface of the articular cartilage becomes yellowish, dull, and granular. The cartilage is gradually worn down to subchondral bone in the center of the joint surface. This bony friction triggers fibroblast production in the periphery of the joints, leading to the development of bone spurs in these areas.

With spurs present, the articular cartilage left in the periphery of the joint may shear off. The debris formed attracts phagocytes in to the areas, initiating an inflammatory response. This results in synovitis and an enlarged joint capsule. The inflammatory response also leads to an increase in synovial fluid production that further increases the edema in the joint. The early pain and stiffness of OA are results of the inflammatory response (Figure 59-1).

Assessment with Clinical Manifestations

Joint pain is the first and most common symptom reported by patients with OA. The joint pain is often described as aching. This symptom is what distinguishes it from other disease processes.

Physical examination will be focused on the joint(s) in which the main complaint is noted. The nurse should always compare the affected joint to the same joint in the opposite extremity. It is helpful to assess the joints most distal and proximal to the affected joint to assess if the chief complaint is actually a referred pain. For example, knee and thigh pain may be related to OA of the hip.

Patients with OA will complain of tenderness in the affected joint. Joint warmth and soft tissue swelling will indicate local inflammation—usually seen in early disease. While assessing for range-of-motion (ROM) the health care worker will note a limitation in the movement as well as **crepitus** (a crinkly, crackling, or grating feeling or sound in the joints, skin, or lungs), which is present in more than 90 percent of patients. **Heberden's nodes** (hard nodules or enlargements of the tubercles of the last phalanges of the fingers) and **Bouchard's nodes** (bony enlargements of the proximal interphalangeal joints) may develop as a result of osteophyte formation and loss of joint space (Figure 59-2). OA in the knee may lead to a varus deformity because of medial cartilage damage. Effusion around the knee can be because of synovitis. The effusion is usually only slight to moderate. Large effusions are uncommon in OA. Advanced OA in the hip can result in leg length discrepancy. This can be seen easily on a person wearing a belt—one hip is obviously higher than the other. Muscle atrophy may develop secondary to guarding of the hip.

Diagnostic Testing

There is no specific laboratory test for the diagnosis of OA. Synovial aspiration may be used to rule out an infectious process if the joint is tender and swollen.

Radiographic images can confirm diagnosis. X-rays can reveal joint space narrowing, however, magnetic resonance imaging (MRI) is much more sensitive in identifying the progression of joint destruction.

Nursing Diagnoses

Based on the information gathered, examples of nursing diagnoses in the patient with OA may include:

- Acute pain.
- Chronic pain.
- Impaired physical mobility.

- Activity intolerance.
- Bathing/hygiene self-care deficit.
- Dressing/grooming self-care deficit.

Planning and Implementation

The management goals for patients with OA are to maintain joint mobility and minimize pain and inflammation. These can be accomplished by many methods, from rest to surgical joint replacement. The various options for treatment will be discussed below.

Collaborative Management

A variety of management therapies are a mainstay of recommendations by the ACR. These therapies include general aerobic type exercise as well as formal physical and occupational therapy assistance. Aerobic exercise will maintain joint mobility and muscle strength as well as assist with weight reduction, should the patient be overweight. These exercises can be done at home with a walking program at virtually no cost or in a structured environment in a gym or spa at varying costs.

Formal physical therapy does require a physician's prescription for insurance to cover some or all of the costs. Physical therapists will assess the patient's muscle strength, joint stability, and mobility; recommend heat or cold therapy; provide instruction for strength training, maintenance of joint mobility; and suggest the use of devices, such as canes or walkers (Estes, 2006). Occupational therapists can assist with joint protection and energy conservation as well as provide assistive devices and techniques for activities for daily living.

A review of literature found that home-based exercise programs were more likely to be adhered to than center-based exercise programs (gyms or with physical therapists) in the long-term (Ashworth, Chad, Harrison, Reeder, & Marshall, 2005). The literature also states that exercise of most types and intensities will assist in reducing pain and improving function in patients with osteoarthritis of the knee.

Nutrition

Many nutritional supplements have been studied examining their effect on OA. The *Alternative Medicine Review* published a review of multiple studies that looked at the effectiveness and safety of different nutritional supplements (Wang, Prentice, Vitetta, Wluka, & Cicuttini, 2004). With regard to prevention of OA, the review found that vitamin deficiencies, such as vitamin D, when treated with a vitamin supplement might play a role in preventing or treating OA (Wang, et al., 2004). The article also found that some supplements, such as avocado-soybean unsaponifiables, glucosamine, and chondroitin, may assist in providing symptom relief (pain and stiffness) and may have "structural effects" (p. 291). The theory is that these supplements may increase the lubrication in the joint.

Pharmacology

Because of the nature and cause of OA pharmacological therapy is aimed at pain control versus repair of joint damage. Traditionally, first line medication is acetaminophen for pain control. The belief is that there are fewer side effects associated with this medication (Broyles, Reiss, & Evans, 2007). Acetaminophen is available over the counter (OTC) and is inexpensive.

The next line of medication for pain management is the class of nonsteroidal anti-inflammatory drugs (NSAIDs). Nonsteroidal anti-inflammatory drugs include ibuprofen (Motrin or Advil) and naproxen sodium (Naprosyn or Aleve), diclofenac (Voltaren), and COX-2 inhibitors, such as rofecoxib (Vioxx), celecoxib (Celebrex), and valdecoxib (Bextra). Like acetaminophen, ibuprofen, and naproxen are readily available OTC and are relatively inexpensive.

Uncovering the Evidence

Treatment of OA

Discussion: The authors performed a meta-analysis comparing efficacy and safety of recommended dosages of nonsteroidal anti-inflammatory drugs with acetaminophen in the treatment of symptomatic hip and knee OA. Using a standardized form to abstract all data, Medline and EMBASE searches were performed on original clinical trials directly comparing NSAIDs with acetaminophen. Seven articles met the inclusion criteria.

NSAIDs were found to be statistically superior in reducing rest and walking pain compared with acetaminophen. They also found that safety was not statistically different between NSAID and acetaminophen groups.

Implications for Nursing Practice: There is an emphasis that includes the ability to safely recommend the use of OTC NSAIDs to patients with osteoarthritis who may find acetaminophen in ineffective for pain control.

Citation: Lee, C., Straus, W., Balshaw, R., Barla, S., Vogel, S., & Schnitzer, T. J. (2004). A comparison of the efficacy and safety of nonsteroidal antiinflammatory agents versus acetaminophen in the treatment of osteoarthritis: A meta-analysis. Arthritis and Rheumatism, 51*(5), 746–754.*

Diclofenac and higher doses of ibuprofen and naproxen sodium are available with a physician prescription.

Ibuprofen, naproxen and diclofenac all have been known to produce the side effect of gastrointestinal (GI) bleeding. The ACR recommends that NSAIDs be given with medications to treat or prevent GI symptoms should the patients be in a high-risk category for GI side effects.

Because of the potential side effects, a different type of NSAID was developed. Cyclooxygenase-2 (COX-2) inhibitors have fewer GI complications yet still produce the desired effects of pain relief and decreased inflammation that the NSAIDs deliver.

In cases where pain cannot be controlled with other medications, opioid analgesics (tramadol, oxycontin, hydrocodone, morphine, or diluadid) can be used to decrease pain. However, opioids do nothing to combat inflammation in the joint or surrounding musculature.

Intra-articular injections (viscosupplementation) with hyaluronic acid and glucocorticoids have been used to replace the lost synovial fluid and decrease local inflammation, respectively. ACR recommendations suggest intra-articular therapy for those patients who have been unresponsive to a program of nonpharmacological therapy and simple analgesics—especially for those who are at risk when taking NSAIDs or COX-2 inhibitors (Broyles, Reiss, & Evans, 2007). Payment from insurance companies varies for intra-articular injections.

In addition, steroid injections can be used to manage musculoskeletal disorders. They provide 2 to 6 weeks of pain relief and begin to have affects within the first 24 hours. Also, topical medication (e.g., capsacin, methylsalicylate, lidocaine patches) are recommended by the ACR.

Health Care Resources

In addition to home health nurses, physical therapists, and occupational therapists, a vocational guidance counselor can be consulted to assist with adaptations that may need to be used for those employed and have arthritis. Indeed, the changes needed for someone who is employed and has OA (or RA) can have an impact on productivity or days lost from work. A vocational guidance counselor would be able to assist the employee and the employer with the types of changes that need to be made. Most human resource departments should be able to assist in making contact with a vocational guidance counselor.

Surgery

Because the numbers of joints that can be affected by OA are numerous, only a few will be addressed below. Today, most joints can be replaced or modified in structure to return joint mobility and reduce pain.

When pain and limitations in mobility become too great for the patient, the assistance of an orthopedic surgeon is often sought. The patient's primary professional caregiver, a medical specialist (such as an internist, a pain specialist, or rheumatologist), or a concerned family member or friend often recommends the surgeon. The surgeon will need X-rays of the affected joint and sometimes an MRI to view thoroughly the source of the problem. The surgeon will interview the patient to determine if the patient has the necessary qualifications to be a candidate for surgery.

The types of surgeries that can be performed are arthroscopy, tibial osteotomy, and arthroplasty (joint replacement). Arthroscopy is used for the removal of loose bodies and resection of torn tissue when the joint space is sufficiently wide yet causing pain and mobility issues. Tibial osteotomy is employed when the patient has knee OA with a relatively small varus (inward) angle and stable ligament support (Figure 59-3). Arthroplasty is used with the patient has severe varus or valgus deformity (knock knees or bow legged), advanced OA of the hip and knee or other joint, and ineffective pain relief with other modalities. Boxes 59-1 through 59-3 provide guidance on patient care throughout the perioperative experience.

Evaluation of Outcomes

Generally OA has a good prognosis, if recommended treatment is followed. Potential outcomes for each of the example nursing diagnoses for the patient with OA are:

- Acute pain: The patient's pain should be adequately controlled, as assessed by the patient on scale of 1 to 10.

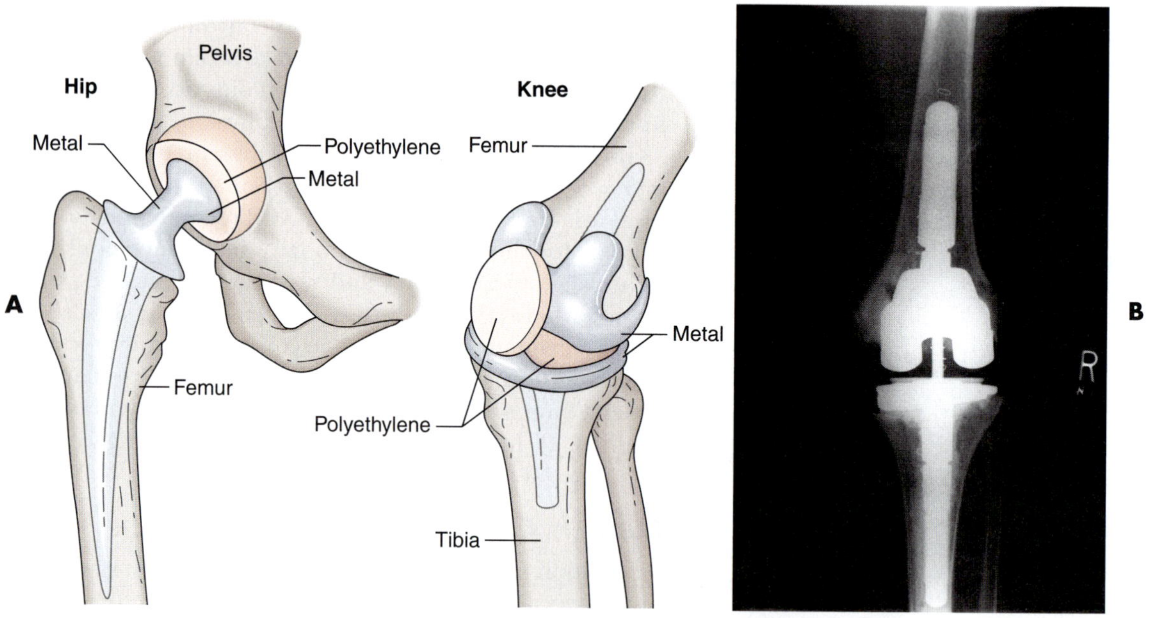

Figure 59-3 A. Total hip and knee replacement, B. Radiograph of a total knee replacement (anterior-posterior view).

BOX 59-1

CARE OF THE PATIENT WITH A TOTAL JOINT ARTHROPLASTY (PREOPERATIVE)

Assessment

- History and Physical: Gather information on past medical and surgical history. Is there any medical condition(s) that may cause postoperative concerns (e.g. hypertension, chronic obstructive pulmonary disease, or bleeding disorders)? What are the current medications taken (prescribed, OTC, and herbal or natural medications)? If the patient has had surgery in the past, was there any reaction to anesthesia? Assess patient's gait and use of any mobility devices used. What is the patient's preoperative range of motion in the affected extremity?
- Social History: Gather information regarding who the patient lives with. If the patient is alone will the person have a support individual to assist him or her in the home after surgery, will he or she go to a family member's residence after surgery, or does the patient anticipate needing to go to an extended care facility (ECF) for a short while to recover? Does the home have a first floor restroom? How many steps will the patient need to negotiate to get into the home? Does the patient have access to the necessary equipment for assistance with activities of daily living (e.g., walker, elevated toilet seat, reachers)?
- Financial Information: Are there any referrals that are needed by the insurance company? Is a social work consult necessary to assist with payment for the surgery?

Planning and Implementation

- History and Physical: Ensure patients that any medical conditions that they currently have will be addressed by the surgeon, anesthetist, and nursing staff that their other conditions will not adversely affect his recovery from surgery. Patient teaching should include what medications that patient should stop taking before surgery and when they should stop taking them. Explain the operative procedure (preoperative room, what happens during surgery and postanesthesia care unit). If available, provide written or video material that explains the surgical experience and postoperative recovery requirements that the patient can take home with him and will reinforce teaching you have already done.
- Social History: Help the patient to explore options about posthospital recovery regarding where he or she will be staying and equipment needed. Usually the hospital can provide resources for equipment for the patient. However, the patient may have relatives or friends who have had to use this type of equipment and might be able to loan or give it to the patient. Also, some churches keep such equipment that can be borrowed. If the patient anticipates going to an extended care facility after being discharged from the hospital, does he know which facility he or she would like to use? Also, consider involving social workers now or early on during the hospital stay.
- Financial Information: Make the appropriate referrals and contact the insurance company if preauthorization is necessary.

Evaluation

- History and Physical: Patient verbalizes an understanding of the basics of what will happen on the day of surgery and the general course during the hospital stay. He or she will verbalize what medications to stop taking before surgery.
- Social History: Patient verbalizes where he or she will be staying after discharge from the hospital and who will be available to assist him or her. The patient will verbalize where equipment can be obtained.
- Financial Information: Patient verbalizes any financial concerns.

BOX 59-2

IN HOSPITAL POSTOPERATIVE RECOVERY

Assessment

- Routine physical assessment consists of neurological, pulmonary, cardiac, GI, psychological, and neurovascular assessments as well as assessing the operative site. (See chapter 58 for method to perform neurovascular assessment.) Pain will also be an assessment you need to make. Arthroplasties tend to be painful (a different pain than experienced preoperatively). Adequate pain assessment and control will enhance the patient's recovery.
- Potential complications (most common): Deep vein thrombosis (DVT), wound infection, hematoma at the surgical site, neurovascular compromise, dislocation (hip).
- Also assess any patient or family concerns regarding the patient's progress.
- Assess the patient's learning of correct mobility techniques and precautions related to the specific surgery (e.g., patient verbalizes that he should not cross his legs after a total hip arthroplasty).

Planning and Implementation

- Administering pain medications, antibiotics, and anticoagulants as ordered. Emphasize to the patient that keeping pain under control will assist in the recovery process by making it easier to ambulate and rest more comfortably.
- Report any questionable assessments to the health care provider immediately to minimize adverse effects from complications.
- Generally physical therapy (PT) is the first to instruct a patient in how to get out of bed and to ambulate. Nursing is capable of doing the initial teaching but most generally reinforces the teaching of PT. Encourage the patient to gradually increase mobility, without pushing himself too far.
- Encourage patient and family to verbalize concerns and questions to you and any member of the nursing or medical staff.

Evaluation of Outcomes: Potential outcomes for the patient following surgery include:

- Patient verbalizes adequate pain control and willingly participates in therapy.
- Patient does not suffer from any postoperative complications.
- Patient's mobility steadily increases.
- Patient and family are freely able to express concerns and have concerns and questions addressed promptly.

- Chronic pain: The patient's pain should be adequately controlled, so that the patient is able to minimize disruptive effects for day-to-day living.
- Impaired physical mobility: The patient should demonstrate coordinated movement with active joint mobility. The patient should be able to perform self-care and manage activities of daily living. The patient should be able to demonstrate the proper way to transfer from bed to chair, chair to standing. The patient should be able to verbalize knowledge of prescribed activity level.
- Activity intolerance: The patient should be able to tolerate activity within normal limits and verbalize knowledge of endurance.
- Bathing/hygiene self-care deficit: The patient should demonstrate the ability to perform activities of daily living, bathing, toileting, and personal hygiene, using mobility aids if needed.
- Dressing/grooming self-care deficit: The patient should demonstrate the ability to dress.

BOX 59-3

AFTER DISCHARGE FROM THE HOSPITAL

Assessment

- Medications: Assess patient's understanding of prescribed postoperative medications and what preoperative medications the patient should continue taking after discharge.
- Mobility and exercise: Assess patient's need to obtain or maintain prescribed postoperative mobility and therapy. Does the person have a walker, crutches, or cane to for home use.
- Wound care: Assess patient's knowledge of appropriate wound care postoperatively.
- Home environment: If being discharged to a private residence, assess physical layout of the unit by asking questions. How many steps? Are there throw rugs? Are there chairs high enough to sit on (for hip patients)?
- Follow-up Care: Does the patient or caregiver understand when to see the surgeon for a follow-up appointment?

Planning and Implementation

- Medications: Teach patient which medications should be taken at home and continued. Often, antibiotics and anticoagulants are sent home with the patient. If the patient is sent home on warfarin (Coumadin), arrangements will need to be made to draw weekly or biweekly INR levels with a home health agency or a local clinic or health care provider's office. Encourage the patient to take all the prescribed antibiotics and to take the warfarin as prescribed. Caution the patient that the health care provider may change the warfarin prescription after blood tests are drawn to prevent excess bleeding. Pain medication prescriptions are most always sent home with the patient. Encourage the patient to take the pain medication about 30 minutes before exercising to keep pain to a minimum. Teach the patient about not driving when on this medication as it can cause drowsiness. Also caution the patient not to share his medications with others. Tell the patient to flush any unused pain medication down the toilet.
- Mobility and exercise: If formal therapy is prescribed, contact a home health agency to arrange this. Reinforce the necessity to increase amount of mobility each day to strengthen the muscles in the affected extremity.
- Wound care: Teach the patient appropriate wound care at home.
- Home environment: Encourage the caregiver to remove any throw rugs in the home. The health care provider will recommend how many times a patient can go up and down stairs. The rule of thumb is up and down stairs once a day for the first two weeks, then increase as the patient tolerates after that.
- Follow-up Care: Tell the patient when the surgeon wants schedule a follow-up appointment. You may make the appointment or allow the patient to do so.

Evaluation

- The patient recovers and returns to normal activities of daily living without complications.

GOUT

Gout is a metabolic disorder that primarily affects men and stems from elevated urate levels in the body. Gout has a hereditary tendency.

Epidemiology

Primary gout is more commonly found in Pacific Islanders (e.g., Filipinos or Samoans). Ninety percent of patients with secondary gout are men, generally over 30 years old. Women who develop gout are usually postmenopausal.

Etiology

As with osteoarthritis, there are two types of gout: (a) primary and (b) secondary. Primary gout is a result of excessive purine synthesis, accelerated nucleotide breakdown, or increase nucleic acid turnover. Secondary gout is a result of a known cause. The cause can be from acquired diseases (e.g., **hyperuricemia,** which is an abnormal amount of uric acid in the urine, hemolytic anemia, psoriasis, and renal insufficiency); obesity or starvation; lead toxicity; use of certain drugs (e.g., salicylates, diuretics, nicotinic acid, alcohol); or organ transplant recipients (especially renal or cardiac allografts) who take cyclosporine and diuretics. Primary gout is seen in about 90 percent of all diagnosed cases. Secondary gout only accounts for 10 percent of occurrences.

Pathophysiology

Hyperuricemia is the primary cause of the pathology of gout. Hyperuricemia is caused by an overproduction or underexcretion of uric acid. Unlike RA and OA, gout usually develops in only one joint, frequently the great toe, which accounts for 50 percent of all acute attacks. The characteristic nodule that develops is known as the **tophus.** The tophus consists of uric acid crystals. The presence of the crystals, which are not normally found in joints, causes a foreign body reaction. This leads to an acute arthritis attack.

Because of the chronic hyperuricemia, systemic problems can occur. In addition to joints, tophi can be found in cartilage, subcutaneous and periarticular tissues, tendon, bone, kidneys, as well as other areas. Kidney stones develop as a result of the elevated uric acid levels. These stones develop in 5 to 10 percent of patients with gouty arthritis. Patients with chronically elevated uric acids, especially those who are already predisposed to renal failure, can progress into chronic renal failure.

Complications

The major complications from chronic gout are soft tissue damage and deformity; joint destruction resulting in a crippling deformity; nerve compression syndrome; and nephrolithiasis and gouty nephropathy.

Assessment with Clinical Manifestations

The patient will report a rapid development (within hours) of pain and edema in the one affected joint. Pain that develops over weeks or months is more likely to be some other condition. When gathering history, the nurse should keep in mind the factors that may contribute to the development of gout (e.g., trauma, alcohol use, medications, acute illness, or family history). Physical examination will reveal swelling, pain, and decreased range of motion in the affected joint. Fever, complaints of headache, and hypertension may also be present. Tophi may be seen on external ears, hands, feet, the olecranon process and prepatellar bursas.

Diagnostic Tests

Laboratory findings will reveal the following: Uric acid levels will be elevated (7 to 10 mg/dL); urine albumin will be greater than100 mg/24 hours; urinary uric acid will be elevated; leukocytosis will be present, and there will be an elevated sedimentation rate. Radiographic studies can be useful in identifying tophi that are not visible in early disease. In chronic disease, bony abnormalities will be shown, such as the punched out erosion of bone with sclerotic borders. An overhanging rim of cortical bone may also be seen (Daniels, 2003). An MRI may be needed to differentiate tophi from infection or tumor.

Performing synovial fluid aspiration is controversial in diagnosing gout, as 80 percent of patients can be diagnosed using physical examination only. However, aspiration may have a therapeutic effect from the decompression that accompanies fluid withdraw. If differential diagnosis between septic arthritis, pseudogout, and gout is needed, the only way to confirm a diagnosis is with a synovial fluid aspiration. The fluid aspirated from a joint with gout will reveal distinctive needle-like intracellular crystals of sodium urate.

Renal and cardiovascular system evaluation is necessary because of the systemic complications from chronic hyperuricemia. This workup would include a complete blood count (CBC), serum creatinine, serum uric acid, blood urea nitrogen (BUN), and urinalysis.

Nursing Diagnoses

Based on the information gathered, examples of nursing diagnoses in the patient with gout may include:

- Acute pain.
- Chronic pain.
- Impaired physical mobility.
- Activity intolerance.
- Bathing/hygiene self-care deficit.
- Dressing/grooming self-care deficit.

Planning and Implementation

Although medication is a vital in the management and prevention of gouty arthritis, the role the nurse plays in teaching about lifestyle and nutritional changes is integral in overall management. The management goals in treating gout are to treat the arthritis symptoms first (pain and edema) and secondarily treat the hyperuricemia (Hellman & Stone, 2004).

During an acute attack, bed rest is the exercise of choice. This assists in allowing the inflammation to recede and promotes pain relief. Bed rest should be continued for approximately 24 hours. Heat, ice, and elevation will assist in relief of pain and edema during an acute attack.

Nutrition

A diet low in purines is helpful to reduce serum uric acid. Low-purine foods are refined cereals, white bread, pasta, and flour, milk and milk products, sugar, sweets, and gelatin, all fats, fruits, nuts and peanut butter, vegetables (except those listed), and cream soups. Moderate-purine foods are beef, chicken, duck, pork, and ham, shellfish (except mussels) and oysters, asparagus, mushrooms, and spinach, and kidney beans, lentils, and lima beans. High-purine foods are alcoholic beverages, anchovies, sardines, herring, mussels, codfish, scallops, trout, haddock, bacon, turkey, veal, venison, and organ meats.

Pharmacology

The medications used to treat gouty arthritis and hyperuricemia fall into four categories: (a) nonsteroidal anti-inflammatory drugs (NSAIDs); (b) gout medications; (c) corticosteroids; and (d) analgesics. Nonsteroidal anti-inflammatory medications are the drugs of choice in treating acute gout. They assist with inflammation and pain reduction. Indomethacin (Indocin) has been the traditional drug of choice. However, Hellman and Stone (2004) point out that any of the newer NSAIDs are equally effective. COX-2 inhibitors (e.g., celecoxib) work well when there is a risk of ulcer or renal problems exist.

Medications used to specifically treat the hyperuricemia have two purposes: to treat the acute attack and to assist in the prevention of further attacks. Colchicine is used for the acute attack phase. Effective within the first few hours of the attack, it is thought to work by interfering with the inflammatory response to the uric acid crystals in the joint. Unfortunately, patients poorly tolerate colchicine. Up to 80 percent of patients treated develop abdominal cramping, diarrhea, nausea, or vomiting (Hellman & Stone, 2004). Colchicine is generally used in the first 24 hours. Allopurinol, probenecid, or sulfinpyrazone (Anturane) is used to lower serum uric acid levels. Because acute attacks can happen when uric acid levels are lowered quickly, colchicine may be added to the treatment to prevent an acute attack.

Corticosteroids are used to provide symptomatic relief during acute attacks. Corticosteroids are best used when a patient is unable to take NSAIDs (Hellman & Stone, 2004). Analgesics, such as acetaminophen, may be needed to control the acute pain of gout (Broyles, Reiss, & Evans, 2007).

Patient and Family Teaching

Teaching should include proper use of medications and instruction on side effects. Dietary teaching and reinforcement are necessary. It is important to remind the patient to maintain a urinary output of 2,000 mL or more per day to minimize the precipitation of uric acid in the urinary tract (Hellman & Stone, 2004).

Evaluation of Outcomes

Generally gout has a good prognosis, if recommended treatment is followed. Potential outcomes for each of the example nursing diagnoses for the patient with gout are:

- Acute pain: The patient's pain should be adequately controlled, as assessed by the patient on scale of 1 to 10.
- Chronic pain: The patient's pain should be adequately controlled, so that the patient is able to minimize disruptive effects for day-to-day living.
- Impaired physical mobility: The patient should demonstrate coordinated movement with active joint mobility. The patient should be able to perform self-care and manage activities of daily living. The patient should be able to demonstrate the proper way to transfer from bed to chair, chair to standing. The patient should be able to verbalize knowledge of prescribed activity level.
- Activity intolerance: The patient should be able to tolerate activity within normal limits and verbalize knowledge of endurance.
- Bathing/hygiene self-care deficit: The patient should demonstrate the ability to perform activities of daily living, bathing, toileting, and personal hygiene, using mobility aids if needed.
- Dressing/grooming self-care deficit: The patient should demonstrate the ability to dress.

Red Flag

Preventing Recurrent Gout Attacks

- Proper use of NSAIDs or corticosteroids as prescribed.
- Adequate bed rest.
- Adequate support both physically and emotionally during the attack.
- Knowledge of when to notify the health care provider if the attack is not controlled within a specified time period to prevent complications.

LYME DISEASE

Lyme disease (LD) is a multisystem inflammatory process with devastating long-term effects if not treated early or effectively (American College of Physicians, 2004). Lyme disease is a bacterial infection that occurs after the bite of an infected tick.

Epidemiology

LD symptoms have been described since the early twentieth century (Knisley & Johnson, 2004). Until a group of children in Lyme, Connecticut developed juvenile rheumatoid arthritis, the disease was not recognized in the United States. This occurred in 1977.

The CDC reports that 23,763 cases of LD were reported in 2002, which is a 40 percent increase from 2001. It is speculated that the increase occurred because of increased deer population, increased residential development in wooded areas, tick dispersal to new areas, improved disease recognition, and enhanced reporting (Edlow, 2002). In reviewing the 2002 data, the majority of cases fell into two age-group ranges: (a) 5 to 14 years old and (b) 50 to 59 years old. The northeastern and north central states in the United States are where 95 percent of all cases were reported (CDC, 2004d).

Etiology

Lyme disease is caused by the spirochete *Borrelia burgdorferi*. It is transmitted to humans by the bite of the deer tick (Figure 59-4). The deer tick in the nymphal stage is the size of a pinhead (3.5 mm to 5.5 mm in length) (CDC, 2004d). Therefore the bite often goes unnoticed. Once the tick is attached it must remain in place 36 to 48 hours for the spirochete to be transmitted. The symptoms can develop in 7 to 14 days, but Knisley and Johnson (2004) report symptoms can begin as soon as three days or as late as 30 days after the bite.

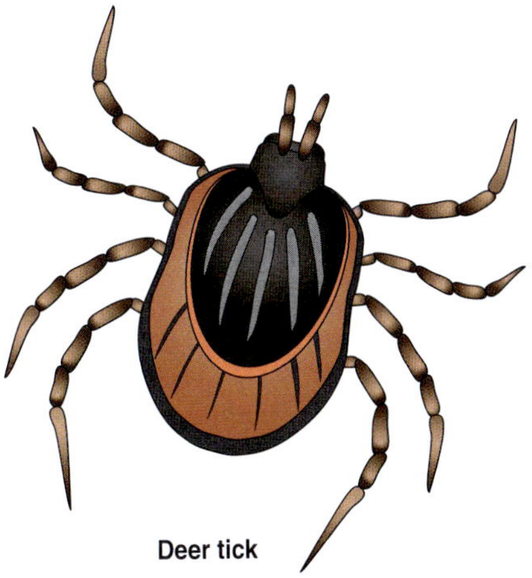

Figure 59-4 Lyme disease is transmitted with the help of a vector, such as the deer tick.

Assessment with Clinical Manifestations

Patients will generally present with flu-like symptoms. Knisley and Johnson (2004) point out that the symptoms include but are not limited to low-grade fevers, fatigue, muscle, bone aches, chills, and malaise. Patients may or may not report a history of tick bite. They may report being physically active out of doors in the previous two to four weeks before symptoms occurred when questioned. Fifty percent to 75 percent of patients present with the classic symptom erythema migrans (EM), which is definitive of the disease (Edlow, 2002). EM presents as a circular rash that continues to grow and often resembles a bullseye.

The American College of Physicians (ACP, 2005) reports that symptoms of LD occur in three indistinct stages. Flu-like symptoms, as described above, represent the early LD stage. The second stage's symptoms reflect the spread of the bacterium throughout the body. If a patient does not get EM, then he or she may first appear to the health care provider with second-stage symptoms (early disseminated LD). These symptoms include numbness and pain in the arms and legs, paralysis of facial muscles (usually unilaterally, as in Bell's palsy), meningitis, and rarely, an abnormal heart rhythm. The third stage can occur weeks, months, or even years after infection in patients who either never received antibiotic treatment for early LD or where treatment did not kill all of the bacteria. Late LD symptoms include chronic Lyme arthritis, central nervous system (CNS) symptoms, and chronic pain in muscles or restless sleep. The arthritis symptoms revolve around bouts of pain and edema in one or more of the larger joints, but these symptoms tend to present more frequently in the knees (Edlow, 2002). Memory loss and difficulty concentrating are CNS symptoms. Arthritic symptoms may be the only clinical symptoms seen in children (Knisley & Johnson, 2004).

More serious, but rare, is ocular involvement. Symptoms range from conjunctival erythema and retinal hemorrhages to **keratitis** (inflammation of the cornea) and **papilledema** (edema of the optic disk) (Edlow, 2002).

The physical examination should include a head to toe skin assessment looking for EM. The nurse should be especially diligent when examining areas of the body with creases (e.g., groin and axilla). Erythema migrans is sometimes best seen when the skin is warm, such as in a bath (Knisley & Johnson, 2004). Therefore, the patient should be questioned about such occurrences when performing the examination.

Other assessments include neurological examination, assessment of range of motion, complaints of muscular pain, and a thorough cardiac examination including an electrocardiogram (ECG). Although rare, LD can cause atrioventricular block and lead to complete heart block (Knisley & Johnson, 2004).

Diagnostic Tests

Although blood tests cannot diagnose LD alone, they can be used to confirm diagnosis. LD antibody can be assessed for, but it can be positive in patients with a high rheumatoid factor. An enzyme-linked immunosorbent assay (ELISA), which tests for antibody rise, is more often used to confirm an LD diagnosis. Because the anti–*Borrelia burgdorferi* antibodies do not appear for two to six weeks after transmission, the ELISA is not performed until this time. The ELISA can show antibodies in the presence of other bacterial infections and other disease processes. A Western blot test, which is more specific to LD is performed to confirm positive ELISA tests (Daniels, 2003).

Nursing Diagnoses

Nursing diagnoses with LD will revolve around the stage of the disease in which the patient presents. Based on the information gathered, examples of nursing diagnoses for the patient with all stages of LD include activity intolerance related to fatigue or weakness; risk for infection related to longer term antibiotic use; and anxiety related to unknown progression of the disease.

Nursing diagnoses for early disseminated LD may include those similar to OA as well as disturbed body image related to facial paralysis and decreased cardiac output related to atrioventricular (AV) block. Impaired role performance and self-care deficit related to memory and concentration difficulties or chronic pain may be encountered in the late LD stage.

Planning and Implementation

LD is a curable disease, therefore the ultimate management goal is to recognize the symptoms early and start antibiotic therapy as soon as possible. If treated early, LD can be prevented from progressing to a more serious and chronic condition.

Pharmacology

Much research has been done exploring the subject of LD. In a query on the subject over 110,000 global articles were found. The articles researched and discussed identification of the responsible organism, transmission of the disease, clinical manifestations, and treatment of LD. Eppes (2003) reviewed and summarized relevant literature and found that the most effective treatment of LD was with oral antibiotics. The drug of choice is doxycycline. When doxycycline cannot be tolerated or for children less than 8 years old, amoxicillin or cefuroxime can be used orally in both the early LD stage as well as the early disseminated stage. If neurological symptoms are present, intravenous (IV) ceftriaxone is the treatment of choice in both the early disseminated stage and the late LD stage. When arthritis is present in the late LD stage, oral doxycycline is utilized. The duration of treatment is generally two to four weeks, depending on symptoms and stage.

A vaccination against LD was introduced in 1998 but was pulled from market in 2001. Controversy exists over the reason for discontinuation. Other adjuvant therapies may be helpful in controlling symptoms. Eppes (2003) suggests nonsteroidal anti-inflammatory medications can be used to assist with complaints from myalgias and arthralgias.

Surgery

When synovitis accompanies arthritic symptoms, a synovectomy may be used to reduce edema and pain in the joint.

Patient and Family Teaching

As oral antibiotic is the treatment of choice for LD, it is essential that all antibiotics be taken as prescribed, because the bacterium can live in the body for years if not completely eradicated early on (ACP, 2005).

As with any infectious disease, a prevention focus is important when providing information about LD. The CDC (2004d) recommends using personal protection measures, such as tucking pants into socks and wearing long sleeves when in areas where tick exposure is likely. The use of insect repellents on exposed skin and clothing that contains diethyl toluamide (DEET) can reduce the risk of tick attachment (CDC, 2004d). Tick checks should be done when returning from outdoor activities.

Evaluation of Outcomes

Generally LD has a good prognosis, if recommended treatment is followed. Potential outcomes for each of the example nursing diagnoses for the patient with LD are:

- Acute pain: The patient's pain should be adequately controlled, as assessed by the patient on scale of 1 to 10.
- Chronic pain: The patient's pain should be adequately controlled, so that the patient is able to minimize disruptive effects for day-to-day living.
- Impaired physical mobility: The patient should demonstrate coordinated movement with active joint mobility. The patient should be able to perform self-care and manage activities of daily living. The patient should be able to demonstrate the proper way to transfer from bed to chair, chair to standing. The patient should be able to verbalize knowledge of prescribed activity level.
- Activity intolerance: The patient should be able to tolerate activity within normal limits and verbalize knowledge of endurance.
- Bathing/hygiene self-care deficit: The patient should demonstrate the ability to perform activities of daily living, bathing, toileting, and personal hygiene, using mobility aids if needed.
- Dressing/grooming self-care deficit: The patient should demonstrate the ability to dress.

In addition, response to antibiotic and adjuvant therapy is seen in abatement of the symptoms. For those who present in the later stages of disease progression, antibiotic therapy may need to be extended to allow time to kill the bacterium and for symptoms to disappear.

DOLLARS AND SENSE

Keeping the Cost of Treatment for LD Reasonable

Eppes' (2002) review of the LD literature found that traditional treatment with doxycycline and the minimal use of diagnostic tests for confirmation of diagnosis appeared to be the most cost-effective course when dealing with LD. Prolonged IV antibiotic therapy will add to the cost of treatment. IV therapy is utilized in the early and late disseminated stages when CNS symptoms are present and as alternatives to oral therapy.

SPONDYLOARTHROPATHIES

Spondyloarthropathies are a group of systemic, inflammatory, rheumatic-type syndromes. These syndromes all have common symptoms. The symptoms can make initial diagnosis challenging. The nurse's responsibility is to assess accurately the patient's complaints or lack thereof to assist in making a specific diagnosis and to provide education and support to the patient and family.

These syndromes include ankylosing spondylitis (AS), reactive arthritis (Reiter's syndrome), arthritides associated with psoriasis, Crohn's disease, and ulcerative colitis, and a form of juvenile chronic arthritis. There are also several forms of undifferentiated spondyloarthropathies that are often underdiagnosed or undiagnosed (Khan, 2002). Khan (2002) described the common features of the spondyloarthropathies: **sacroilitis** with or without spondylitis; variable inflammatory peripheral arthritis (single or multiple joints); **enthesitis** (inflammation at the bony insertion sites of ligaments and tendons); **dactylitis;** tendency for ocular inflammation; familial tendency; no rheumatoid factor; strong association with the HLA-B27 gene.

Etiology

The etiology for these syndromes is generally unknown. The majority of patients with spondyloarthropathies can identify a hereditary link or have the HLA-B27 antigen.

Pathophysiology

The mechanisms that cause inflammation in the joints and elsewhere in spondyloarthropathies are not fully understood. Similar to RA, elevated levels of T cells, macrophages and an increase in cytokine release is seen in the inflamed joints. With continued inflammation, bony erosions and new bone formation can occur. Unlike RA, there is no synovial membrane involvement. Explanation for the extra-articular symptoms may occur by the transport of triggers (T cells and others) via the lymphatic system or macrophages (Khan, 2002).

AS, reactive arthritis, and psoriatic arthritis will be described later in the chapter. General considerations for the spondyloarthropathies as a group will then be discussed.

Assessment with Clinical Manifestations

Resembling RA, arthritic symptoms will be seen worse in the morning, with complaints of pain and stiffness in the affected joint(s). The symptoms and pain will lessen within an hour and become less intense during the day. Timing of the onset of symptoms helps to identify the correct diagnosis. Symptoms of AS tends to be a gradual onset. Reactive arthritis tends to occur within four weeks after the onset of an aforementioned infection. Psoriatic arthritis is always associated with psoriasis and usually appears months to years after initial diagnosis of psoriasis. However, psoriatic arthritis can precede or occur simultaneously with the onset of skin lesions (Hellman & Stone, 2004).

Physical examination will focus on the areas of complaint. AS often shows limited motion in the back; lateral flexion and extension and forward flexion will be limited.

Reactive arthritis shows symptoms of asymmetric polyarticular complaints, with or without effusions. Again, with Reiter's syndrome the provider will see the "sausage" toes and complaints of arthritis symptoms in the knees and ankles (Khan, 2002). There will also be symptoms associated with the infectious process that precedes the arthritic symptoms. Urethritis symptoms, such as edema, redness at, and purulent drainage from, the urethral meatus may be present. Conjunctivitis or uveitis may also be seen. Psoriasis-like lesions on the soles of the feet and other body surfaces may be visible. With psoriatic arthritis sausage digits and erythema may be present in small peripheral joints. Other symptoms are psoriasis lesions and pitted and discolored nails.

When enthesitis is present in any of these syndromes, palpation along the spine will elicit tenderness. The enthesitis can also be seen with complaints of heel pain because of inflammation of the Achilles tendon and plantar fascia (Kataria & Brent, 2004). There may also be tenderness when the sacroiliac joints are palpated while the patient is flexed at the hips.

Diagnostic Testing

Diagnosis is made mainly by physical examination. X-rays in AS will show bilateral symmetrical sacroilitis and squaring of the vertebrae. As the disease progresses, total fusion of the sacroiliac joint and the involved vertebrae will occur. Eventually, spine X-rays will show a classic "bamboo spine," which is indicative of the vertebral fusion. For psoriatic arthritis, erosions may be seen in the distal interphalangeal (DIP) joints of the hands and feet.

Blood drawn to detect the presence of HLA-B27 gene is not necessary to diagnose, but it is often done to confirm the diagnosis. Rheumatoid factor may be drawn to make a differential diagnosis. Evidence of infection is frequently seen in the blood work of a patient with reactive arthritis.

Nursing Diagnoses

Based on the information gathered, examples of nursing diagnoses in the patient with spondyloarthropathies may include:

- Acute pain.
- Chronic pain.
- Impaired physical mobility.
- Activity intolerance.
- Bathing/hygiene self-care deficit.
- Dressing/grooming self-care deficit.

Planning and Implementation

The goals of care for the spondyloarthropathies involve minimizing the inflammation, maintaining functional ability, controlling pain, and minimizing the effects of systemic complications. Research on the spondyloarthropathies focuses on a wide range of subjects from causative factors to successful treatments to patients' reactions to the syndromes. Evidence will be discussed that supports multidisciplinary therapeutic interventions used with patients who have spondyloarthropathy.

As noted earlier, arthritic symptoms associated with the spondyloarthropathies are generally worse in the early morning and get better with use. Therefore, activity is a mainstay of treatment. Many studies have been done looking at the effect of exercise on the progression of symptoms, maintenance of functional ability, and patient coping.

Falkenbach (2003) found that the greater the disability in patients with AS, the greater the motivation to exercise. Ward (2002) found that functional disabilities increased as the patient's age increased and if the patient smoked. He found that the disability decreases if the patient exercised and had better social support. Intense physical therapy also increases mobility in patients for the short term.

Analay, Ozcan, Karan, Diracoglu, and Aydin (2003) studied patients to determine whether an at home exercise program would be more effective in promoting exercise than a structured program. They found that the participants in the structured program faired better and were more likely to participate.

A review of organizations with information on spondyloarthropathies (National Institute of Health, Spondylitis Association of America, The Arthritis Foundation, American College of Rheumatologists and American College of Physicians-American Society of Internal Medicine) showed unanimous agreement on the use of exercise in promoting musculoskeletal function and decreasing pain.

The use of splints, braces, and other joint support devices are not encouraged. These devices immobilize the joint, leading to further stiffness and decreased mobility as well as the potential for the development of permanent contractures. With spondyloarthropathies, rest does not decrease the symptoms.

Pharmacology

A mainstay to any treatment plan is the administration of medication. Because spondyloarthropathies share symptoms similar to RA, it is logical to believe that the medications used with RA would be effective in the treatment of the spondyloarthropathies. To some extent this is true. First-line treatment tends to be with NSAIDs. This is followed up by the use of sulfasalazine (Alzulfidine) when the NSAIDs are no longer effective in relief of the inflammatory symptoms. Kataria & Brent, (2004) reviewed five separate studies noting the positive effects of tumor necrosis factor-alpha (TNF-alpha) inhibitors (etanercept [Enbrel] and infliximab [Remicade or Centocor]) in treating the inflammation.

Disease-modifying antirheumatic drugs (methotrexate and cyclosporine) have shown some effectiveness against inflammation. Corticosteroid injections can decrease local inflammation.

Surgery

Joint replacement and stabilization may be appropriate for patients with severe arthritic symptoms. Spinal fusion can be performed when AS gets to the point of causing major functional disability.

Patient and Family Teaching

Teaching involves the proper use of medications; encouragement, and instruction in appropriate exercise therapy (with or without a therapist) and pain relief measures. Heat and cold as well as mild analgesics can be used to assist with pain relief.

Evaluation of Outcomes

Generally spondyloarthropathies have a good prognosis, if recommended treatment is followed. Potential outcomes for each of the example nursing diagnoses for the patient with spondyloarthropathies are:

- Acute pain: The patient's pain should be adequately controlled, as assessed by the patient on scale of 1 to 10.
- Chronic pain: The patient's pain should be adequately controlled, so that the patient is able to minimize disruptive effects for day-to-day living.
- Impaired physical mobility: The patient should demonstrate coordinated movement with active joint mobility. The patient should be able to perform self-care and manage activities of daily living. The patient should be able to demonstrate the proper way to transfer from bed to chair, chair to standing. The patient should be able to verbalize knowledge of prescribed activity level.
- Activity intolerance: The patient should be able to tolerate activity within normal limits and verbalize knowledge of endurance.
- Bathing/hygiene self-care deficit: The patient should demonstrate the ability to perform activities of daily living, bathing, toileting, and personal hygiene, using mobility aids if needed.
- Dressing/grooming self-care deficit: The patient should demonstrate the ability to dress.

Ankylosing Spondylitis

Ankylosing spondylitis (AS) is a chronic, progressive, inflammatory arthritis that primarily affects the synovial joints of the spine and soft tissue surrounding the spine (Chou, Lo, Kao, Jim & Cho, 2002). AS refers to fusion (ankylosis) of inflamed vertebrae (spondylitis).

Epidemiology

Ankylosing spondylitis appears more frequently in men, ages of 16 and 35. AS is seen in less than 1 percent of the U.S. population. It is three times more likely to occur in men than in women. African Americans are 25 percent more likely to develop AS than Caucasians. Five percent of AS begins in childhood. Boys develop it at a greater rate than girls. In children symptoms usually begin in the hips, knees, bottoms of heels, or big toes and may later progress to involve the spine.

Assessment with Clinical Manifestations

The typical patient has a gradual onset of symptoms of low back pain. There is often no incident that can be linked to the onset of the back pain. The pain is worse in the morning and lessens with activity. The pain may radiate to the gluteal region. A decrease in spine mobility (range of motion) will be seen as the syndrome progresses. Typically the decrease in mobility affects the lumbar spine, then moves to the sacroiliac joints, and then gradually up the spine to include the cervical spine. As the disease progresses, thoracic kyphosis is exaggerated, and the cervical spine becomes hyperextended (Kataria & Brent, 2004).

Other problems that occur with AS include: (a) uveitis (edema of the upper eyelid, excessive lacrimation, small irregular pupil, and swollen iris); (b) aortic and mitral valve dilation leading to regurgitation; and (c) fibrosis of the upper lobes of the lungs (Kataria & Brent, 2004).

Reactive Arthritis

Also known as Reiter's syndrome, reactive arthritis is associated with an infectious process, often chlamydia or enteritis secondary to gram-negative enterobacteria (Khan, 2002). Of those affected greater than two thirds have the HLA-B27 antigen. The symptoms usually appear in a series of three: nongonococcal urethritis, conjunctivitis, and arthritis. The arthritis symptoms seen usually involve the lower extremities and are asymmetrical. A classic symptom for patients with reactive arthritis is the sausage toe. The toe becomes uniformly edematous and reddened and resembles a sausage. In addition, the condition of enthesitis leads to inflammation with a tendency toward fibrosis and calcification can develop. This condition causes heel pain as a distinguishing characteristic of reactive arthritis. Low back pain is a common symptom secondary to sacroilitis. Conjunctivitis occurs in approximately 50 percent of patients (Kataria & Brent, 2004). Onset of symptoms occurs within one to four weeks after the initial infection.

Reactive arthritis is usually an acute episode. The symptoms are generally present for five days to five months. A small percentage of patients will have mild symptoms for up to a year. Fifteen to 30 percent of patients will develop chronic musculoskeletal symptoms (Khan, 2002).

Etiology

Because of wide variation in recognition and clinical severity the true incidence of reactive arthritis is difficult to assess. In Sweden the incidence was 28 reported cases in 100,000 adults (Söderlin, Börjesson, Kautiainen, Skogh, & Leirisalo-Repo, 2002). The incidences occurred equally in men and women.

Psoriatic Arthritis

Psoriatic arthritis (PsA) develops in association with the diagnosis of psoriasis. PsA is a progressive, chronic, inflammatory form of arthritis accompanied by fatigue, severe joint pain, and swelling. Psoriatic arthritis exhibits in five different patterns: arthritis in the DIP; arthritis mutans; symmetrical polyarthritis similar to RA; asymmetrical oligoarthritis; and spondyloarthropathy (Tam & Geier, 2004). Up to 60 percent of patients will often present with one typical pattern of arthritis and then transition into another pattern.

With PsA, nail lesions occur in about 80 percent of patients. These nail lesions are pitting and include **onycholysis** (the loosening of the nails starting at the border). Uveitis also tends to be present and chronic (Kataria & Brent, 2004).

Etiology

It is estimated that one million people have PsA. This is roughly 0.5 percent of the U.S. adult population. An estimated 4.5 million people have psoriasis. Psoriatic arthritis generally appears between the ages of 30 and 55 equally in men and women.

POLYMYOSITIS AND DERMATOMYOSITIS

Polymyositis (PM) and dermatomyositis (DM) are another set of autoimmune disorders that affect the musculoskeletal system. These syndromes produce muscle weakness secondary to muscle inflammation which, if left unchecked, can lead to respiratory failure and death.

Epidemiology

PM is mostly seen in adults. DM can be seen in both adults and children. The incidence of occurrence for both is 8.4 per million people in the general U.S. population. African Americans tend to develop the disorder more often than Caucasians. Women are twice as likely to develop the syndromes (Hellman & Stone, 2004).

Pathophysiology

The causes of PM and DM are not known. It is known that the autoimmune disorder causes extensive necrosis and destruction of muscle fibers. As with most autoimmune disorders, autoantibodies develop and start destroying target areas. In the case of PM, the autoantibodies (CD-8 positive cells) invade the target muscle fibers. With DM, complement C3 forms a membranolytic attack complex that is deposited in the capillaries of the muscle tissue. This complex leads to the development of edematous endothelial cells, capillary necrosis, perivascular inflammation, ischemia, and destruction of muscle fibers.

Another inflammatory myopathy can be seen that does not fit all of the diagnostic criteria of PM. Inclusion-body myositis can be sporadic, but it is less responsive to treatment (Hellman & Stone, 2004).

DM is also associated with an increased risk of cancer, especially in older adults (Hellman & Stone, 2004). The cancers seen are ovarian, in the GI tract, lung, breast, and non-Hodgkin's lymphomas.

PM and DM are sometimes seen in association with other autoimmune and connective tissue disorders (e.g., lupus). Often the symptoms overlap, making the diagnosis of new onset PM or DM challenging.

Assessment with Clinical Manifestations

The patient will present with a gradual and insidious onset of bilateral, generalized muscle weakness. Rarely is the onset acute with PM. Patients with DM often present with the characteristic rash that precedes the muscle weakness. The rash can be seen on the upper eyelids with a blue-purple discoloration (heliotrope rash), often with edema. There can also be a reddish rash on the face and anterior chest in a V shape or over the back and shoulders (which is labeled the shawl sign), knees, elbows, or malleoli. Another characteristic rash is known as Gottron rash or sign. This red rash appears on the knuckles of the hands and fingers.

Muscle weakness usually develops in a pattern. The muscle weakness starts in the proximal muscles of the arms and legs and then moves distally. Eventually, without treatment, the muscles of the fingers are affected, making fine motor movements difficult. Holding a pencil or feeding oneself is a challenging task.

Because cancer is associated with DM, cancer screening may be indicated. This is especially true if the patient is greater than 60 years of age or is in a high-risk category for cancer development.

Diagnostic Tests

There are three hallmark tests which confirm the diagnosis of PM or DM: elevated muscle enzymes, an abnormal electromyogram, and positive results in a muscle biopsy.

The muscle enzymes which specifically indicate either PM or DM are creatinine kinase (CK) and aldolase. The CK can be increased as much as 50 times the normal value for CK. These enzymes can also be monitored to indicate response to treatment.

The muscle biopsy is the definitive diagnostic test for PM and DM. In PM, the biopsy will show muscle fiber inflammation and necrosis. With DM, the inflammation is seen primarily in the perivascular areas of the muscle.

Other cancer screening diagnostic tests may need to be completed at the same time, especially for high-risk patients with DM.

Nursing Diagnoses

Based on the information gathered, examples of nursing diagnosis in the patient with PM and DM may include the following:

- Bathing/hygiene self-care deficit.
- Impaired physical mobility.
- Fear.
- Anxiety.
- Deficient knowledge.
- Risk for injury.

Planning and Implementation

The goals of therapy are to improve the ability to carry out activities of daily living by increasing muscle strength and to ameliorate extramuscular manifestations.

Pharmacology

The first-line of treatment is pharmacological care. Prednisone, in doses of 40 to 100 mg per day are prescribed for several weeks to decrease the inflammation that is causing the muscle weakness (Hellman & Stone, 2004). Prednisone is eventually tapered to a dose that effectively treats the symptoms and lowers the serum enzyme levels and is often administered on an every-other-day regimen.

Should the patient be intolerant to prednisone or the disease does not respond to the prednisone, immunosuppressive drugs are the next line of therapy. Azathioprine (Imuran or Azasan) is the most commonly used immunosuppressive agent. Other immunosuppressive therapies include methotrexate (Rheumatrex), cyclosporine (Neoral or Sandimmune), and mycophenolate mofetil (CellCept).

Collaborative Management

Therapies can be initiated to assist in regaining strength, once pharmacological therapy has been initiated. Occupational therapist may be especially helpful in the early stages to assist in providing activities of daily living equipment.

Health Care Resources

Health care providers and nurses can lend a good deal of support and information to the patient about the disease processes. There are many organizations that can lend support and encouragement for patients and their families who suffer with PM or DM. A Google search on the Internet found over 100,000 hits on PM alone. Just three organizations that were listed that had support information and access to support groups were the National Institute of Neurological Disorders and Stroke (NINDS), the Muscular Dystrophy Foundation, and the Arthritis Foundation.

Patient and Family Teaching

The focus of teaching will be disease information, medication and symptom management, safety, and for patients with DM, cancer screening. Including all applicable health care providers during the teaching phase of care ensures that all necessary aspects are covered. As the nurse, you can be a consistent contact person for questions, which is also assistive. A special contact person for the patient can coordinate care and information and clarify any questions the patient may have.

Evaluation of Outcomes

Positive patient outcomes focus on improvement of the rash and muscle weakness. Trends of decrease muscle enzymes will also show that the medication is effective. Assessing for patient reaction to the medication in the form of side effects is an important nursing responsibility.

FIBROMYALGIA

Fibromyalgia is most frequently defined as a clinical syndrome or condition involving chronic widespread diffuse musculoskeletal pain, stiffness, and tenderness. A lack of restorative or deep sleep is a prominent feature of fibromyalgia and has been described as both a contributing factor to and a symptom of the disorder (Henriksson, 2003). Fatigue and insomnia are frequently cited as accompanying features of fibromyalgia.

Fibromyalgia is a common disorder and represents the second most common disorder seen by rheumatologists in North America. The majority of sufferers are women. Although it is seen in all age-groups, prevalence appears to increase with age, reaching a peak among individuals 60 to 80 years of age (Inanici & Yunus, 2002).

Epidemiology

The incidence of fibromyalgia varies with the specifics of patient samples studied as well as the geographical location. Incidence has been described from 7 percent within the general population to 2.1 to 5.7 percent in general medical clinics or primary care practices to 10 to 20 percent in rheumatology clinics. Prevalence in Europe has been reported as between 1 to 2 percent, whereas North America reports a prevalence of 2 percent. The prevalence of fibromyalgia among women is 3.4 percent as compared to men at 0.5 percent (Inanici & Yunus, 2002).

Etiology

The etiology of fibromyalgia is unclear, although it has been suggested that the condition is not the result of a single etiological factor. The role of infectious agents as causative factors has been the subject of investigation, with Epstein-Barr virus, cytomegalovirus, human herpes virus 6, human immunodeficiency virus (HIV), and *Borrelia Burgdorferi* representing the most frequently cited organisms. The basis for an infectious origin is supported by the presence of a viral syndrome at the time of diagnosis by a reported 55 percent of patients. A genetic predisposition has been suspected but not confirmed (Inanici & Yunus, 2002).

Pathophysiology

Although some muscle abnormalities have been reported, fibromyalgia differs from other musculoskeletal disorders in its absence of clear inflammatory or structural musculoskeletal pathology. Instead, current research suggests pathology related to dysfunction within the neuroendocrine system. It is this dysfunction within the neuroendocrine system that is thought to provoke the abnormalities in pain sensitivity characteristic of fibromyalgia. Central sensitization of neurons, deficits in the functioning of the descending inhibitory system, and ongoing activity within the afferent nerves result in functional changes within the nociceptive system. A number of associated pathophysiological mechanisms responsible for the regulation of mood, sleep, and pain perception have been considered as contributory including a low serotonin level and increased substance P in the cerebrospinal fluid (Henriksson, 2003).

Abnormalities in the hypothalamic pituitary-adrenal axis are also seen. A decreased level of insulin-like growth factor 1 is common and may be a pathogenic marker in fibromyalgia. The characteristics of growth hormone deficiency, such as, diminished energy, dysphoria, impaired cognition, poor general health, reduced exercise capacity, muscle weakness, and cold intolerance parallel symptoms seen in fibromyalgia.

Fibromyalgia shares clinical features with a number of other conditions, including irritable bowel syndrome (IBS), chronic fatigue syndrome (CFS), and temporomandibular pain syndrome. Common attributes among these disorders include the increased prevalence among women, pain without tissue damage, fatigue, poor sleep, and responsiveness to similar groups of medications. Similarities are particularly striking with CFS. An estimated 70 percent of fibromyalgia patients meet the criteria for CFS. The difference appears to be largely related to the degree of pain versus the degree of fatigue experienced by the patient. Similarities between the two entities suggest the possibility of commonalities in the pathology of fibromyalgia and CFS. The evidence of central sensitization seen in fibromyalgia, CFS, IBS, and temporomandibular pain syndrome suggests central sensitization as the common physiological feature that binds these entities together and may provide clues to an underlying pathology (Inanici & Yunnus, 2002).

Assessment with Clinical Manifestations

As a clinical entity, fibromyalgia has been the subject of much debate. Historically, the subjective parameters used in the diagnosis of fibromyalgia have resulted in challenges to the existence of fibromyalgia as a distinct clinical entity. Concerns have included the subjective nature of the tender point examination, the subjective nature of chronic pain, the lack of a standardized definitive laboratory test, and the absence of clear objective pathology. Although both rheumatologists and the World Health Organization (WHO) now recognize fibromyalgia, the subjective nature of fibromyalgia continues to plague effective diagnosis and management. It is not unusual for patients to have fibromyalgia for five to seven years before a diagnosis is confirmed (Inanici & Yunus, 2002).

Diagnosis of fibromyalgia is based entirely on signs and symptoms characteristic of the syndrome. The American College of Rheumatology (ACR) established criteria in 1990 for the diagnosis of fibromyalgia based on the occurrence of both subjective and objective findings (Table 59-1). Musculoskeletal pain is typically characterized as widespread aching, in addition to tenderness on palpation with multiple tender points. Eighteen locations have been identified as common tender points in the diagnosis of fibromyalgia. The presence of at least 11 out of the 18 tender points is considered diagnostic according to ACR criteria.

A number of other clinical features and syndromes have been associated with fibromyalgia. These include restless leg syndrome, IBS, irritable bladder

TABLE 59-1 Criteria for the Classification of Fibromyalgia

History of Widespread Pain

Definition: Pain is considered widespread when all of following are present: pain in the left side of the body, pain in the right side of the body, pain above the waist, and pain below the waist. In addition, axial skeletal pain (cervical spine or anterior chest or thoracic spine or low back) must be present. In this definition, shoulder and buttock pain is considered as pain for each involved side. Low back pain is considered lower segment pain.

Pain in 11 of 18 tender point sites on digital palpation.

Definition: Pain, on digital palpitation, must be present in at least 11 of the following 18 sites:

Occiput: Bilateral at the suboccipital muscle insertions.

Low cervical: Bilateral at the anterior aspects of the intertransverse spaces at C5 to C7.

Trapezius: Bilateral at the midpoint of the upper border.

Supraspinatus: Bilateral at origins above the scapula spine near the medial border.

Second rib: Bilateral at the second costochondral junctions, just lateral to the junctions on upper surfaces.

Lateral epicondyle: Bilateral 2 cm distal to the epicondyles.

Gluteal: Bilateral in upper outer quadrants of buttocks in anterior fold of muscle.

Greater trochanter: Bilateral posterior to the trochanteric prominence.

Knee: Bilateral at the medial fat pad proximal to the joint line.

Digital palpation should be performed with an approximate force of 4 kg.

For tender point to be considered positive the subject must state that the palpation was painful.

"Tender" is not considered "painful."

For classification purposes, patients will be said to have fibromyalgia if both criteria are satisfied. Widespread pain must have been present for at least three months. The presence of a second clinical disorder does not exclude the diagnosis of fibromyalgia.

syndrome, interstitial colitis, headaches (particularly migraine), ocular and vestibular complaints, cognitive dysfunction, cold intolerance, multiple sensitivities, and dizziness. The coexistence of associated features supports the diagnosis of fibromyalgia in situations where only 8 to 10 tender points are noted on physical examination.

Diagnostic Tests

Although there are no definitive standardized diagnostic tests specific to the diagnosis of fibromyalgia, various laboratory tests and radiography should be performed to evaluate for any possible coexisting conditions noted by history and physical examination and to eliminate other conditions that may be responsible for the patient's symptomatology. These might include a CBC, measurement of ESR, C-reactive protein, serum electrolyte level, blood glucose level, liver enzyme tests, renal function tests, thyroid function tests, urinalysis, and various radiological exams. In some cases, a moth-eaten appearance in type 1 fibers and atrophy in type 2 fibers may be seen on muscle biopsy. An ANA, serum complement, and rheumatoid factor tests are generally not performed unless the patient shows indication of rheumatic disease (Inanici & Yunnus, 2002).

Nursing Diagnoses

Based on the information gathered, examples of nursing diagnoses in the patient with fibromyalgia may include:

- Acute pain.
- Chronic pain.
- Impaired physical mobility.
- Activity intolerance.
- Bathing/hygiene self-care deficit.
- Dressing/grooming self-care deficit.

Planning and Implementation

Central to the goal of therapy in the treatment of fibromyalgia is the alleviation of pain and the management of any associated symptoms, conditions, and contributing factors. Common approaches include both pharmaceutical and nonpharmaceutical therapy. Pharmaceutical therapy is inclusive of pain management and the medical management of coexisting conditions and symptoms. Primary to effective nonpharmaceutical management is the restoration of sleep hygiene, increasing physical fitness, and elimination of psychological distress.

Pharmacology

Analgesia, antidepressants, and muscle relaxants represent pharmaceutical therapies common in the treatment of fibromyalgia. Antidepressant therapy has been shown to improve sleep, fatigue, and pain severity in patients regardless of the presence of clinical depression. The effectiveness of NSAIDs in the treatment of pain has been debatable, although some patients have reported benefit. The most effective pharmaceutical approaches appear to employ combination therapies, such as combinations of analgesics and antidepressants or antidepressants and muscle relaxants. Amitriptyline, cyclobenzaprine, a fluoxetine and amitriptyline combination, citalopram, and tramadol have been shown to be efficacious in the treatment of fibromyalgia as reported in various research studies. Lidocaine injections into tender points can be administered to ease pain at particularly bothersome sites. A graduated and individualized approach to pharmacological therapy may be employed with doses or medications chosen to manage varying degrees of pain and other symptomatology (Inanici & Yunnus, 2002).

Nutrition

Although a specific dietary regimen has not been established in the literature, a number of concerns exist that may warrant assistance from a dietitian. Some evidence exists that implicates the role of certain foods in the exacerbation of fibromyalgia symptoms similar to what has been found with migraine and IBS. In particular the limitation of caffeine and alcohol is recommended because of their ability to act as muscle irritants. Vitamin and mineral supplements may be warranted to assist with stress, immune support, and the correction of any deficiencies. While other specific recommendations were inconclusive, agreement in the need for a healthy meal plan, avoidance of foods that patients have identified as contributory to flares, and nutritional management of coexisting conditions, such as migraine and IBS were consistently seen.

Collaborative Management

Physical deconditioning is a common feature of fibromyalgia and likely the result of physical inactivity related to patient attempts to minimize pain. The impact of physical fitness on pain has been inconsistent in studies examining the outcomes of aerobic exercise in patients with fibromyalgia. However, studies suggest that aerobic activity does contribute to improvements in physical functioning, psychological well-being, and improvements in overall quality of life. The type, duration, and intensity of the exercise program should be individualized to the needs and abilities of each patient focusing on the goal of preventing physical inactivity and improving the level of physical fitness. The added benefit of combating the muscle weakness and fatigue associated with fibromyalgia is seen with the involvement of physical therapy and cardiovascular fitness training.

The benefits of gentle low-impact aerobic exercise must be balanced with individual patient abilities to prevent the exacerbations of fibromyalgia symptoms. One suggested approach involves 3 to 5 minutes of aerobic activity per day gradually increasing to 20 to 30 minutes per day for patients who are deconditioned. A variety of methods has been suggested, including walking, bicycling, and the use of various types of home equipment. Aerobic water exercise may be best tolerated in patients who are unable to tolerate other forms of exercise. Care should be taken to avoid extremes in water temperature that may prevent patients from doing well.

Health Care Resources

The complexity of fibromyalgia demands the expertise of a comprehensive health care team including the physician, nurse, dietitian, and social worker or counselor working in collaboration with the patient and his or her family. In addition, a number of resources are available to assist patients with fibromyalgia. The Arthritis Foundation and The National Fibromyalgia Association both offer information and connecting resources.

Alternative Therapy

In addition to traditional therapy, roughly two thirds of patients with fibromyalgia seek assistance from alternative therapy. However, mind-body techniques, acupuncture, and manipulative therapies represent the only therapies supported by research as potentially beneficial in the treatment of fibromyalgia.

Patient and Family Teaching

The role of patient self-management in fibromyalgia underlines the critical importance of patient and family education. A thorough understanding related to the nature of the disease, its symptoms, variability, and the likelihood of periods of exacerbation versus remission is essential to the ongoing participation and well-being of the patient. Education should be ongoing and address the main areas of pain management, physical fitness, sleep, and psychological well-being. Pain management includes adherence to medication regimens, monitoring of pain characteristics, participation in physical activity, and prompt follow-up with health care team members regarding changes in and exacerbations of pain. Physical activity should be stressed but balanced with rest needs during periods of exacerbation. Patients should be cautioned to avoid overuse of physical activity during flares and use of the most painful muscles. Patients should be instructed to start exercise at a low level and to increase gradually on a regular basis. The keeping of an exercise diary or graph that includes exercise time, intensity, and pulse rate achievements are useful in evaluating exercise programs. Sleep can be enhanced through the avoidance of caffeine; alcohol; or heavy meals before bedtime; the elimination of disturbing factors, such as noise and light; and the establishment of a regular sleep schedule. Interventions to maintain psychological well-being may include relaxation training, coping skills training, reduction of negative pain behaviors, and the fostering of a positive attitude. A referral to counseling would be appropriate for patients struggling with anxiety and depression (Inanici & Yunus, 2002).

Evaluation of Outcomes

Fibromyalgia is a condition characterized by remissions and exacerbations. Therefore, the importance of ongoing care and follow-up can not be underestimated. Acute flares can frequently be managed with support, physical therapy, rest, and medication management. Systemic disease and other conditions may develop over time warranting a thorough evaluation of new or changes in present symptoms. Cognitive dysfunction may present as impairments in recall, concentration, and memory (Inanici & Yunus, 2002).

The impact of fibromyalgia on quality of life can be tremendous. Fibromyalgia represents a major cause of disability in the United States. As many as 25 percent of patients with fibromyalgia receive some form of disability payment or injury compensation suggesting the existence of issues with the ability to obtain and maintain suitable work environments. Self-assessments of disability parallel that of RA and OA. Pain, fatigue, and weakness are the most frequently cited causes. While most patients are able to continue working, modifications in the work environment inclusive of changes in the ergonomic structure and reductions in work hours may be required (Inanici & Yunus, 2002).

> *Red Flag*
>
> **Risk Factors for Developing Osteoporosis and Related Fractures**
>
> The major risk factors include:
> - Personal history of fracture as an adult
> - History of fragility fracture in a first-degree relative
> - Low body weight (less than about 127 pounds)
> - Current smoking
> - Use of oral corticosteroid therapy for more than three months
>
> The minor risk factors are:
> - Impaired vision
> - Estrogen deficiency at an early age (younger than 45)
> - Dementia
> - Poor health or frailty
> - Recent falls
> - Low calcium intake (lifelong)
> - Low physical activity
> - Alcohol in amounts greater than two drinks per day

OSTEOPOROSIS

Osteoporosis is defined as being characterized by low bone mass, microarchitectural deterioration, compromised bone strength, and an increase in the risk of fracture.

Epidemiology

Based on the 2000 census data, NOF estimates that 20 percent (7.8 million) of postmenopausal Caucasian women in the United States will have osteoporosis, and 52 percent of (21.8 million) other women will have low density at the hip in 2002. Given these numbers, it is not surprising that osteoporosis is the most frequently diagnosed bone disease in humans.

Etiology

Although the exact cause of primary osteoporosis is not known, it is known that the rate of bone loss is strongly correlated with genetics, estrogen, and other risk factors, which will be discussed in further detail (Sedlak & Doheny, 2002). Secondary osteoporosis can be linked to nutritional deficiencies, endocrine function abnormalities, and disuse. Table 59-2 summarizes the known links leading to secondary osteoporosis.

Pathophysiology

As discussed in chapter 58, bone remodeling is never static. Bone formation and remodeling take place because of the balance of osteoblastic and osteoclastic activity. With osteoporosis, this activity slowly becomes less balanced, with osteopenia developing first. At about the age of 30 osteoclastic activity starts to over take osteoblastic activity. This process is more rapid during the first years after menopause and then slows down but continues throughout the rest of a female's life. Men do suffer from the effects from the imbalance, but because men generally start with a larger bone mass, the process takes longer (Crowther & McCance, 2004).

> "In normal bone, the frequency of [multicellular] unit activation, the rate of resorption and the rate of new bone formation are relatively constant, so that replacement follows resorption immediately and the amount of bone replaced equals the amount of bone resorbed. In bone affected by osteoporosis, this equilibrium can be disrupted by (1) an increase in the number of basic [multicellular] unit activated, (2) an increase in the frequency of basic [multicellular] unit activation, (3) an increase in the rate of resorption, (4) a delay in the rate of bone formation, or (5) a deficiency of cells in the [multicellular] unit. Any one of these changes will cause a net decrease in total bone mass" (Crowther & McCance, 2004, p. 1083).

TABLE 59-2 Contributing Factors to Secondary Osteoporosis

Nutritional deficiencies
Vitamin C deficiency (scurvy)
Mild malabsorption syndrome (lactose intolerance)
GI and hepatic diseases (those that impair absorption of calcium, phosphate, and vitamin D)
Acid diets
Calcium-deficient diets
Chronic alcohol abuse (alcohol is a direct inhibitor of osteoblasts and may directly inhibit calcium absorption)
Endocrine function abnormalities
Hyperthyroidism
Hyperparathyroidism
Cushing's syndrome
Acromegaly
Hypogonadism
Corticosteroids
Disuse—reduces stressors on bones (Wolff's law)
Bed rest
Inactivity common in elderly

PATIENT PLAYBOOK

Risk Assessment Tool for Osteoporosis

1. Have either of your parents broken a hip after a minor bump or fall?
   Yes No
2. Have you broken a bone after a minor bump or fall?
   Yes No
3. Have you taken corticosteroid tablets (cortisone, prednisone, etc.) for more than three months?
   Yes No
4. Have you lost more than 3 cm (just over 1 inch) in height? Yes No
5. Do you regularly drink heavily (in excess of safe drinking habits)? Yes No
6. Do you smoke more than 20 cigarettes a day?
   Yes No
7. Do you suffer frequently from diarrhea (caused by problems such as celiac disease or Crohn's disease)?
   Yes No

For women:

1. Did you undergo menopause before the age of 45?
   Yes No
2. Have your periods stopped for 12 months or more (other than because of pregnancy)?
   Yes No

For men:

1. Have you ever suffered from impotence, lack of libido, or other symptoms related to low testosterone level?
   Yes No

Answering yes to any of these questions does not mean that you have osteoporosis. You should show this test to a health care provider or nurse practitioner and discuss the questions you have with him or her.

The presence of the above factors leads to an increased risk of fractures (Figure 59-5).

Assessment with Clinical Manifestations

Osteoporosis is often considered a silent disease with the first indication of a problem often being when the patient suffers a fracture. Unfortunately, this can be indicative of advanced disease. Another presenting condition most often because of osteoporosis is a decrease in height, sometimes accompanied by **kyphosis** (hunchback). Kyphosis is the result of the vertebral column becoming brittle, weak, and misshapen as the bone loses volume (Crowther & McCance, 2004).

A risk assessment is in order when osteoporosis is suspected or a familial history of osteoporosis in known. This can be done during a routine physical examination, accompanying a more focused examination or after a fracture has occurred. Knowing the amount and types of risk factors the patient has will assist the nurse in planning your teaching and anticipating health care provider orders.

Sedlak and Doheny (2002) note that an annual loss of height (approximately 0.09 percent of total height) is normal after the age of 45 They state that a loss greater than this will need investigation as height loss is often a first sign of osteoporosis. Kyphosis will be obvious on physical examination. Back pain is a common complaint.

The most common fracture sites seen with osteoporosis are the forearm, femur (hip), ribs, and spine (Crowther & McCance, 2004). Care should be taken to assess these areas assessing for pain, edema, deformity, and crepitus. Should a fracture be suspected, referral to the physician will be necessary for follow-up diagnostic studies.

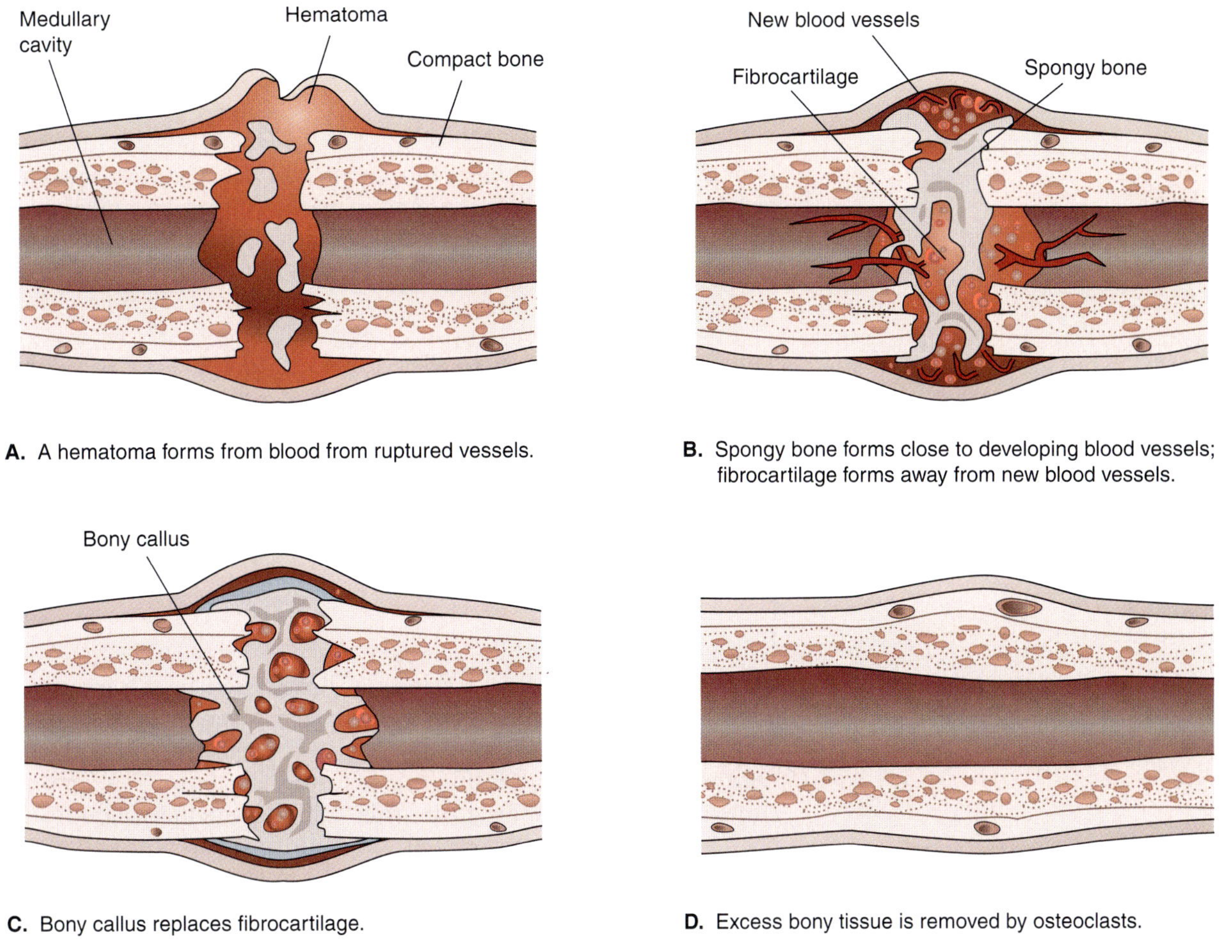
Medullary cavity
Hematoma
Compact bone
New blood vessels
Fibrocartilage
Spongy bone
A. A hematoma forms from blood from ruptured vessels.
B. Spongy bone forms close to developing blood vessels; fibrocartilage forms away from new blood vessels.
Bony callus
C. Bony callus replaces fibrocartilage.
D. Excess bony tissue is removed by osteoclasts.

Figure 59-5 Steps of bone repair.

Diagnostic Tests

When a fracture is suspected, the most common test is a simple X-ray. When osteoporosis is suspected or the patient has several risk factors, measurement of bone mineral density is in order. The gold standard in determining bone mineral density and diagnosing osteoporosis is with a dual X-ray absorptiometry (DEXA) scan. Refer to chapter 58 for information on this scan.

Laboratory studies that may be conducted to assess the patient are calcium, magnesium, phosphate, vitamin D, alkaline phosphatase, and protein electrophoresis. In looking for secondary causes parathyroid hormone levels may be drawn. Further testing for thyrotoxicosis and hypogonadism may be required once a definitive diagnosis is made (Fitzgerald, 2004).

Nursing Diagnoses

A multitude of nursing diagnoses are appropriate the diagnosis of osteoporosis. For those who have just been diagnosed, deficient knowledge related to the new diagnosis of osteoporosis should be the major focus of nursing care. Anxiety related to fear of fracture may be another that may apply early on. Potential nursing diagnoses for patients with osteoporosis are:

- Impaired physical mobility (actual or high risk for) related to effects of osteoporosis
- Potential for injury related to impaired physical mobility
- Pain related to injury or effects of osteoporosis
- Alteration in nutrition: less than body requirements related to poor appetite, change in taste or smell, nutritional intake imbalance or lack of funds

Constipation and ineffective breathing patterns may be an issue when kyphosis is present (Crowther & McCance, 2004).

Planning and Implementation

With diagnosis and treatment of osteoporosis management outcomes will focus on preventing further bone loss and injuries. A multipronged approach to osteoporosis care is essential to treat the disorder and manage the sequelae of the disease process. Pharmacological, physical, and nutritional therapy will be reviewed.

Nutrition

The NIH recommends a total of 1,000 mg to 1,500 mg of calcium a day to maintain good bone health. That is equivalent to five 8-ounce glasses of milk. Most American diets do not allow for this level of calcium consumption. Therefore, calcium supplementation is necessary. It has been shown that the addition of a vitamin D supplement to the calcium can reduce the incidence of hip fractures in patients with a current diagnosis of osteoporosis (Gillespie, Avenell, Henry, O'Connell, & Robertson, 2004; Homik, Suarez-Almazor, Shea, Cranney, Wells, & Tugwell, 2004).

Pharmacology

There are several different classes of drugs used in the treatment of osteoporosis: bisphosphonates; selective estrogen receptor modulators; hormones; prescribed supplements; and skeletal anabolics. Bisphosphonates have been utilized since 1995 as inhibitors of osteoclast bone resorption (Sedlak & Doheny, 2002). The drugs in this category include alendronate sodium (Fosamax), risedronate (Actonel), and etidronate (Didronel).

Homik, et al. (2004) performed a meta-analysis of the usefulness of bisphosphonates for steroid induced osteoporosis. The findings from this review showed that bisphosphonates were effective in preventing and treating the steroid-induced bone loss at the lumbar spine and femoral neck. Other such reviews that risedronate was effective in the reduction of both vertebral and nonvertebral fractures and etidronate increased bone density in the lumbar spine and femoral neck.

Selective estrogen receptor modulators (SERM) are used for both the prevention and treatment of osteoporosis. Raloxifene (Evista) is a SERM used to "maximize the effect of estrogen on bone and minimize the negative effects on the breast and endometrium" (Sedlak & Doheny, 2002, p. 436).

Hormone replacement therapy (HRT) has become controversial because of the increased risk of breast and uterine cancer. More research is needed to look at the long-term effects and efficacy of HRT with regard to reducing bone loss versus cancer risk.

Calcitonin (Miacalcin) is a hormone that has been used in the treatment of postmenopausal and corticosteroid-induced osteoporosis. It is available both orally and as a nasal spray. Calcitonin shows a preservation of bone mass in the lumbar spine after the first year of steroid therapy when compared to placebo, but no effect was made at the femoral neck. It is suggested that more research is needed to conclude that calcitonin is effective in preventing fractures in steroid-induced osteoporosis.

A prescribed supplement that has been utilized in osteoporosis treatment is fluoride. Fluoride is known to stimulate bone formation. Fluoride should be taken with calcium. A review of the literature revealed no evidence to support that the use of fluoride prevented vertebral fractures but did show an ability to increase bone mass density at the lumbar spine.

A relatively new class of drugs used to combat osteoporosis and bone loss are skeletal anabolics. Skeletal anabolics stimulate bone formulation, produce large increases in bone mineral density, improve bone quality, and reduce bone fractures (Broyles, Reiss, & Evans, 2007).

Exercise, Physical, and Occupational Therapy

Long established as a preventive and therapeutic measure, weight-bearing exercise is a simple and low-cost treatment in the fight against osteoporosis.

Walking is the easiest therapy. Prescribed, formal exercise with the supervision of a physical therapist can be beneficial and prove to be a motivator for some. Should assistive devices be needed, an occupational therapist can be consulted. Exercises of all types (aerobics, weight-bearing, and resistance training) are effective in increasing bone mineral density (BMD) of the spine in postmenopausal women. Walking is also shown to be effective in increasing BMD in the hip.

Health Care Resources

Many local resources are available to assist patients and their families in learning about osteoporosis and its treatment. Most primary care providers (physicians and nurse practitioners) can provide good basic information. A useful source of information is a registered dietitian. As calcium supplementation is often the key in prevention of bone loss, dietitians can offer a myriad of alternatives to assist in providing the supplementation. In addition, there are also many resources available on the World Wide Web.

Surgery

See osteoarthritis for applicable surgical procedures related to fractures associated with osteoporosis.

Patient and Family Teaching

Prevention is the focus of much of the teaching associated with osteoporosis. Teaching prevention needs to start early in life to promote good nutrition habits. Family members will benefit from education and can assist the patient in applying their new found knowledge. Focuses of teaching will be on dietary needs and changes and physical activity. Handouts that a patient and family member can take home with them are useful to reinforce the messages the nurse is delivering.

When the diagnosis is confirmed, teaching should be given about the disease process, dietary needs and changes, physical activity, and any medication information that is necessary. Sedlak and Donheny (2002) add that instructions on fracture and falls prevention and pain management are needed. It is often helpful to give this abundance of information a little at a time. Information overload is always a concern. The health care worker should schedule time with the patient more than once to provide all information needed. Collaborative instruction from the physician, nurse, physical therapist, and a dietitian often assists in helping the patient get a well-rounded perspective of the disease process.

Evaluation of Outcomes

Management of osteoporosis is a lifelong process. Prevention of further bone loss is vital to prevent the sequela of fractures. Disease progression or regression can be monitored through BMD scans and biochemical markers of bone turnover found in the urine.

Fractures are the most frequent and serious complication of osteoporosis. Other problems can include weakness and fatigue from pain, kyphosis, and a risk for falls.

OSTEOMALACIA

Osteomalacia is a metabolic disease that causes poor and delayed mineralization of the bone cells in mature bones (Crowther & McCance, 2004).

Epidemiology

Fortunately, osteomalacia is rare in the United States and Western Europe. Osteomalacia is a significant problem in Great Britain, Ethiopia, Pakistan, Iran, and India. In the United States, osteomalacia secondary to vitamin D deficiency can be seen in the elderly, in premature infants with low birth weights, and in vegetarians on a strict macrobiotic diet (Crowther & McCance, 2004).

Etiology

The main cause of osteomalacia is a vitamin D deficiency. Risk factors for this deficiency include a diet deficient in vitamin D; low endogenous production of vitamin D (lack of sunlight exposure); malabsorption; renal tubule disease; and anticonvulsant therapy. Liver disease interferes with metabolism of vitamin D to its more active form, and diseases of the pancreas and biliary system cause a deficiency of bile salts needed for normal absorption of vitamin D (Crowther & McCance, 2004).

Pathophysiology

Bone cell mineralization requires adequate levels of calcium and phosphate. Vitamin D regulates the absorption of calcium ions from the intestine. Lack of vitamin D interrupts the absorption of calcium. The low calcium levels lead to the stimulation of parathyroid secretion. Although calcium levels increase, it also stimulates an increase in renal clearance of phosphate. With the ever-decreasing phosphate levels, bone cell mineralization cannot occur (Crowther & McCance, 2004).

Assessment with Clinical Manifestations

The patient generally presents with a history of generalized skeletal pain and tenderness without a history of injury. The site in which the most frequent complaint of pain is experienced is in the hips. The patient may report a reluctance to ambulate. Other complaints include low back pain, pain in the ribs, feet, and other areas. The patient will present with a waddling gait. When obtaining all history information, the provider should be sure to obtain a diet history, a medical history, and obtain a list of medications.

Diagnostic Tests

Blood tests that are obtained to assist in diagnosis are as follows: Serum calcium, phosphate, alkaline phosphatase, parathyroid hormone, 25-hydroxy vitamin D, as well as BUN and creatinine (Daniels, 2003).

Bone densitometry and X-rays will be performed to examine the extent of the disease. In adults with sporadic onset hypophosphatemia, hyperphosphatemia, or low serum 1, 25 hydroxy D levels, a tumor may be suspected, and an MRI of the whole body is recommended (Daniels, 2003).

Nursing Diagnoses

Based on the information gathered, examples of nursing diagnoses for the patient with osteomalacia may include the following:

- Impaired physical mobility related to osteomalacia.
- Risk for impaired skin integrity related to compromised tissue perfusion.
- Acute pain as related to osteomalacia.

Planning and Implementation

The goals of therapy are to prevent osteomalacia and to prevent further bone loss in already established disease.

Nutrition

Milk fortified with vitamin D is readily available in the United States. An 8-ounce glass of milk provides 25 percent of the recommended daily allowance (RDA) of vitamin D and 50 percent of the RDA for calcium.

Pharmacology

To prevent a vitamin D deficiency, sunlight exposure and vitamin D supplementation are recommended. The RDA of vitamin D is 10 g (400 international units) per day. Patients with low sunlight exposure, the RDA is 1,000 international units per day. Patients taking phenytoin (Dilantin), the RDA for prophylactic treatment is 50,000 international units orally every two to four weeks (Fitzgerald, 2004). Vitamin D is available OTC or by prescription.

For established osteomalacia, the deficiency is treated with ergocalciferol (D_2) 50,000 international units orally one or two times per week for 6 to 12 months, then 1,000 international units per day. For malabsorption problems the dose is 25,000 to 100,000 international units per day. In addition, the patients will receive calcium citrate (0.4 to 0.6 g of elemental calcium) or calcium carbonate (1 to 1.5 g of elemental calcium) per day (Fitzgerald, 2004).

For osteomalacia secondary to hypophosphatemia, aluminum-containing antacids are discontinued. Patients with renal tubule acidosis are given bicarbonate therapy. For idiopathic hypophosphatemia or hyperphosphatemia, oral phosphate supplements are used on an ongoing basis with calcitriol (Rocaltrol) given to combat decreased calcium absorption caused by the oral phosphate (Fitzgerald, 2004).

Patient and Family Teaching

Teaching about the disease itself will need to be initiated. Medication and nutrition education will focus on prevention with vitamin D and sunlight exposure or correction of deficiencies or other causes of the osteomalacia. Proper dosage and schedule will be the focal points for the medication teaching. For sunlight exposure, encourage the use of sunblock, explaining that the sunblock will not stop the necessary exposure to stimulate vitamin D production.

Evaluation of Outcomes

Fortunately, osteomalacia is treatable, and therefore the prognosis for patients who suffer from osteomalacia is good. Complications can include fractures and bone growth deformities.

Financial Outcomes

Fortunately the prevention and treatment of osteomalacia is relatively inexpensive, especially if caused by a dietary deficiency. Expenses can be high if the deficiency is secondary to other disease processes (e.g., renal tubule disease with dialysis required).

PAGET'S DISEASE

Paget's disease is the second most common bone disease after osteoporosis in the United States. It often goes undiagnosed until the disease is in the advanced stages. It is difficult to diagnosis, because the pain associated with Paget's disease is similar to arthritis. Paget's disease is a chronic bone disorder with no definitive cure. However, an early diagnosis along with effective treatment can lessen the impact of the disease and decrease the complications associated with Paget's disease (The Paget Foundation, 2005).

Epidemiology

Paget's disease is rare before the age of 40 and increases with age with an incidence of 1.5 to 8 percent of the population over the age of 50. It affects men slightly more than women. It is more commonly seen in people of Anglo-Saxon ancestry, and it is rarely seen in people of Asian, Indian, and Scandinavian descent (The Paget Foundation, 2005). Overall, the incidence of Paget's disease has been declining. The reason for this is unknown.

Etiology

The cause of Paget's disease remains unknown. However, Paget's disease tends to run in families and several genes have been linked to the disorder, but no specific abnormality can explain Paget's disease. Paramyxovirus has also been linked to the etiology of Paget's disease, but once again there is a lack of conclusive evidence (Binder, 2003).

Pathophysiology

Paget's disease begins with an increase in bone absorption. To compensate for this, bone formation increases along with bone remodeling. This newly formed bone is highly vascular and weak, which leads to deformity and fractures. The areas most often affected are the long bones, pelvis, lumbar vertebrae, and skull (Maher, Salmond, & Pellino, 2002).

Assessment with Clinical Manifestations

Assessment should begin with a thorough history including family incidence of Paget's disease and previous fractures. Patients with Paget's disease are often asymptomatic. For patients who experience symptoms, the most common symptom is pain in the hip and pelvis. The pain is often described as a deep aching that worsens with weight bearing. The patient may also have deficits in hearing, vision, swallowing, speech, movement of eye and facial muscles, and balance (Maher, Salmond, & Pellino, 2002).

Physical examination begins with inspection of the skeleton for deformities. Bowing of the long bones of the arms and legs is a common finding. Bowing of the tibia can cause increased pain to the knee and ankle and an increased risk of fracture. The skull is often enlarged with the bone becoming soft and thick. In more advanced cases, the spine may also show kyphosis or scoliosis. Palpation of the skin over areas of Pagetic bone may reveal areas that are warm to touch because of the increased blood flow to the newly formed bone (Maher, Salmond, & Pellino, 2002).

Diagnostic Tests

An increase in serum alkaline phosphatase (ALP) is often the first indicator that the patient's symptoms are associated with Paget's disease and not arthritis. Normal serum ALP is 30 to 115 international units/L. A slightly higher level is often found in a patient with a healing fracture. However, values two to three times the normal amount indicates Paget's disease. ALP is an enzyme produced by bone, liver, and the intestines. It can further be broken down into isoenzymes to pinpoint the origin of the enzyme. An increase in the bone-specific ALP (bAP) indicates an increase in bone formation. There are also several markers for bone formation, turnover, and reabsorption that can be detected in the urine. These include calcium, hydroxyproline, N-telopeptide, and deoxypyridinolines (The Paget Foundation, 2005). However, these are less sensitive than serum bAP.

X-rays and a bone scan are the two diagnostic studies used in the diagnosis on Paget's disease. Bones affected by Paget's disease have characteristic features that show well on X-ray. Early in the disease osteolytic lesions are observed in the long bones and the skull. As the disease progresses, the bones become enlarged with coarse and irregular borders (Maher, Salmond, & Pellino, 2002). A radioactive bone scan is a more sensitive diagnostic tool. A radioactive bisphosphonate is injected intravenously. This substance collects in areas of bone where there is an increase in blood flow and bone formation. This test is used to determine the full extent of the disease.

Nursing Diagnoses

Based on the information gathered, examples of nursing diagnoses in the patient with Paget's disease may include:

- Acute pain.
- Chronic pain.
- Impaired physical mobility.
- Activity intolerance.
- Bathing/hygiene self-care deficit.
- Dressing/grooming self-care deficit.

In addition, based on information gathered, examples of nursing diagnoses for the patient with Paget's disease may include the following shown in Table 59-3. This table shows additional nursing diagnoses, NIC, and NOC classifications that may be applicable for patients with Paget's disease.

Planning and Implementation

The three major areas of focus for a patient diagnosed with Paget's disease are symptom management, limiting disability, and complication prevention. In the past only patients with symptoms were treated. Now, the standard is to treat all patients with active disease including asymptomatic patients. Active disease is defined as ALP level twice the upper limit of normal (Rakel & Bope, 2003). Treatment of Paget's disease may not correct existing damage to hearing, deformities to bone, or osteoarthritis caused by the disease. The goal is to prevent any further complications by restoring the normal pattern of new bone formation. Treatment of Paget's disease is comprised of four main options that are used in conjunction with each other. These options are physical therapy, pharmacological therapy, analgesics, and surgery.

Also, although Paget's disease is an incurable disease, there are few life-threatening complications. The prescribed treatment is usually effective in decreasing pain and slowing the progression of the disease. Fractures usually develop in the weight-bearing portion of long bones and may start out as stress fractures. Neurological complications are also seen because of the pagetic bone pressing on nerves and include hearing loss, changes in vision, impairment of the eye and facial muscles, and problems with swallowing, speech, and

TABLE 59-3 Nursing Diagnoses, NIC, and NOC Classifications for Paget's Disease

NURSING DIAGNOSIS	NURSING INTERVENTION CLASSIFICATIONS (NIC)	NURSING OUTCOMES CLASSIFICATIONS (NOC)
Potential injury	Fall prevention Environment management	Fall prevention behavior
Fear related to potential injury	Anxiety reduction Coping enhancement Security enhancement	Fear self-control

balance (Maher, et al., 2002). Other neurological complications may include hydrocephalus, radicular neuropathies, and spinal stenosis.

The pagetic bone is highly vascularized and prone to bleeding. Because of this there is a potential complication of hemorrhage and an increase in blood loss during bone surgery. Bisphosphonates may be given prior to surgery to reduce the bleeding from the operative bone during the surgery (Rakel & Bope, 2003).

Another potential complication of Paget's disease is hypercalcemia. It is imperative that the patient continues with weight-bearing exercises to keep the bones strong. Any amount of prolonged bed rest, especially after surgery, will increase bone demineralization and hypercalcemia. Hypercalcemia can contribute to hypertension, weakness, urinary lithiasis, or mild bowel disturbances (Rakel & Bope, 2003).

Pharmacology

Pharmacological therapy is a major component of the treatment plan. Antiresorptive agents inhibit osteoclastic activity therefore suppressing bone turnover. Calcitonin was the first osteoclastic inhibitor to be used in the treatment of Paget's disease. It is a hormone that binds to the osteoclast receptor site and inhibits bone resorption and turnover. It is given as a subcutaneous injection, and it is expensive. Because of these two disadvantages, this treatment is not widely used any more unless the patient is unable to tolerate other medications. Bisphosphonates are other types of antiresorptive agents used to slow the progression of Paget's disease and to treat the bone pain associated with the disease. They can also be used prior to surgery to reduce the bleeding from the bone that is being repaired (Rakel & Bope, 2003). The disadvantage of these medications is that they must be taken orally on waking with a full glass of water on an empty stomach, and the patient must stay upright for 30 minutes after taking the medication. These instructions must be followed to reduce the risk of reflux that may cause esophagitis. Food, milk, and other dairy products prevent the absorption of this drug; therefore, the patient must take the medication on an empty stomach. Hypocalcemia is a potential side effect; therefore the patient should be taking oral calcium and vitamin D. Refer to Table 59-4 for a list of bisphosphonates.

Exercise, Physical, and Occupational Therapy

Physical therapy is another vital component in the treatment of Paget's disease. The focus of physical therapy is to improve muscle strength and to promote mobility by encouraging weight-bearing exercises, which may improve bone strength. Occupational therapy along with physical therapy may help the patient become more functional and independent by providing advice on assistive devices used for activities of daily living and for walking aids, heels lifts, and corsets (Maher, Salmond, & Pellino, 2002). Physical therapy may also help control chronic pain.

Surgery

Surgery may be a necessary treatment option for some patients. Surgery may include repair of a pathological fracture, realignment of the knee to decrease pain, total joint arthroplasty for arthritic changes from the disease process. It is important to mobilize the patient as soon as possible and to avoid bed rest. Periods of immobilization can lead to bone demineralization and hypercalcemia, which can further increase the patient's risk of pathological fractures (Rakel & Bope, 2003).

Patient and Family Teaching

Patient and family teaching begins with education regarding the disease process and support for the patient and family as they cope with the impact the disease may have on the patient's quality of life. Another important component

TABLE 59-4 Bisphosphonates used with Paget's Disease

DRUG	DOSE	SPECIAL INSTRUCTIONS
Etidronate (Didronel)	200–400 mg once daily for six months; 400 mg dose is preferred	Available in oral form Must be taken with six to eight ounces of water on an empty stomach No food, beverages, or other medication two hours before or after dose Treatment should not exceed six months Repeat courses can be given after a three to six month rest period
Pamidronate (Aredia)	30 mg intravenously over four hours for three consecutive days	Available in IV form only May be readministered as needed
Alendronate (Fosamax)	40 mg once daily for six months	Available in oral form Must be taken on an empty stomach, with six to eight ounces of water, in the morning. No food, beverages, or other medication for 30 minutes after dose. Do not lie down for at least 30 minutes after taking dose.
Tiludronate (Skelid)	400 mg once daily for three months	Available in oral form Must be taken on an empty stomach with six to eight ounces of water. It may be taken any time during the day, as long as there is no food, beverage, or other medication taken two hours before or after the dose.
Risedronate (Actonel)	30 mg once daily for two months	Available in oral form Must be taken on an empty stomach, with six to eight ounces of water. No food, beverages, or other medication for 30 minutes after dose. Do not lie down for at least 30 minutes after taking dose.

Adapted from Broyles, B. E., Reiss, B. S., & Evans, M. E. (2007). Pharmacological aspects of nursing care *(7th ed.). New York: Thomson Delmar Learning.*

of teaching is medication administration. The patient needs to know the potential side effects of the prescribed medications and the correct way to take these medications to decrease the risk of these side effects. Another area of needed information is in regard to pain management. Simple strategies like anti-inflammatory drugs and nonnarcotic analgesics may be all that are needed to reduce the patient's bone pain (Rakel, & Bope, 2003). Positioning and following the treatment modalities may also decreased the patient's pain.

Evaluation of Outcomes

Generally Paget's disease has a good prognosis, if recommended treatment is followed. Potential outcomes for each of the example nursing diagnoses for the patient with Piaget's disease are:

- Acute pain: The patient's pain should be adequately controlled, as assessed by the patient on scale of 1 to 10.

- Chronic pain: The patient's pain should be adequately controlled, so that the patient is able to minimize disruptive effects for day-to-day living.
- Impaired physical mobility: The patient should demonstrate coordinated movement with active joint mobility. The patient should be able to perform self-care and manage activities of daily living. The patient should be able to demonstrate the proper way to transfer from bed to chair, chair to standing. The patient should be able to verbalize knowledge of prescribed activity level.
- Activity intolerance: The patient should be able to tolerate activity within normal limits and verbalize knowledge of endurance.
- Bathing/hygiene self-care deficit: The patient should demonstrate the ability to perform activities of daily living, bathing, toileting, and personal hygiene, using mobility aids if needed.
- Dressing/grooming self-care deficit: The patient should demonstrate the ability to dress.

OSTEOMYELITIS

Osteomyelitis is a serious infection of the bone that is often difficult to treat. Osteomyelitis can be categorized as acute or chronic, which occurs when the symptoms are present for longer than three months.

Epidemiology

Acute osteomyelitis occurs commonly in children under 13 (1 in 5,000) (Zorn, 2001). Forty percent of all cases occur in children under age 20, with 35 percent of cases occurring in adults over age 50. Chronic osteomyelitis is responsible for one to three percent of all hospital admissions and occurs after orthopaedic surgery from 0.5 to 1.5 percent of the time (Zorn, 2001). The most common site is the tibia, following an open fracture.

Etiology

Osteomyelitis can stem from an infection that has spread through the blood to the site of infection (site varies with the individual). It can also be caused by a soft tissue infection that spreads to the bone. It is also associated with patients who have diabetes or vascular problems. With these patients the site of infection is often the foot or ankle (Hellman & Stone, 2004).

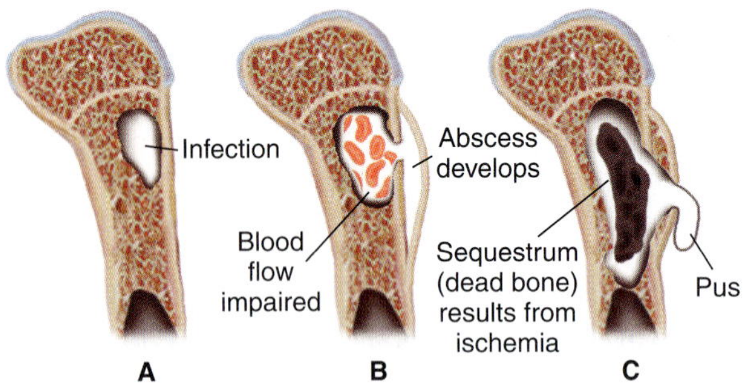

Figure 59-6 Pathology and progression of osteomyelitis: A. Osteomyelitis, B. Without early treatment, an abscess forms, C. Bone dies (sequestrum) and pus forms.

Pathophysiology

The infection is spread through the bloodstream to the medullary canal. Cellulitis develops in the bone marrow. As the infection develops, bacteria and white blood cells cause exudate to form and pressure increases within the medullary canal. The infection continues to invade the inner layers of the bone until it spreads to the periosteum leading to necrosis and devascularization of the cortex of the bone (Zorn, 2001) (Figure 59-6).

Assessment with Clinical Manifestations

In acute osteomyelitis the patient will have manifestations of acute infection. There may be a report of recent acute infection, puncture wound, mild trauma, or obvious fracture. Adults may present with history of diabetes, vascular insufficiency, or other process that leads to a compromised immune system.

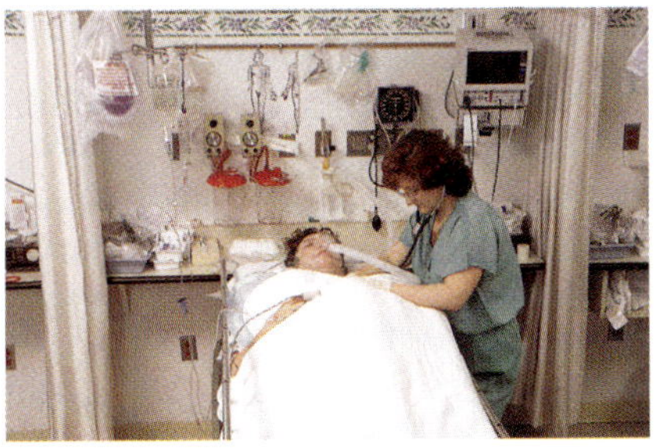

Figure 59-7 Acute osteomyelitis has caused an uncontrolled infectious process in this patient is in an ICU.

Children present with a variety of symptoms. Infants will present with symptoms that range from irritability to pseudoparalysis or signs of sepsis. Most children will complain of localized pain. Younger children may refuse to use the affected extremity.

Chronic osteomyelitis patients will present with mild systemic symptoms, have periods of remissions and exacerbations, pain (from mild to severe), and soft tissue abscesses and draining wounds may occur. There will generally be a history of surgery or trauma to the affected extremity or site. There may be a previous history of acute osteomyelitis, and the patient may have continued or intermittent symptoms. These patients may also have histories of immune system compromise. Fever is common with acute osteomyelitis but not with the chronic form of the infection.

Complications of osteomyelitis include loss of function of the joint above or below the infection, leg-length discrepancies or deformities, and renal insufficiency or hearing loss related to nephrotoxic or ototoxic antibiotics (Figure 59-7).

Diagnostic Tests

There are a variety of diagnostic tests for both acute and chronic osteomyelitis. These diagnostics are shown in Box 59-4.

Nursing Diagnoses

Based on the informative gathered, examples of nursing diagnoses for the patient with osteomyelitis may include the following:

- Acute or chronic pain due to the osteomyelitis.
- Fear due to the diagnosis of osteomyelitis.
- Impaired physical mobility due to the osteomyelitis.
- Risk for impaired skin integrity related to compromised tissue perfusion.
- Deficient knowledge related to self-care and risk prevention.

Planning and Implementation

Management goals are to eliminate the infection and prevent complications.

BOX 59-4

DIAGNOSTIC TESTING FOR OSTEOMYELITIS

Acute Osteomyelitis

- X-rays will not show changes until 10 to 14 days after the infection occurs
- Sedimentation rate and white blood cells will be elevated
- Blood cultures are positive in about half of the samples
- Bone scans will be positive in the area of the infection
- Bone wound cultures will need to be taken to identify the microorganism present

Chronic Osteomyelitis

- X-rays will show bone and soft tissue changes
- Sedimentation rate will be mildly to moderately elevated
- May see a minimal elevation of white blood count and mild anemia
- C-reactive protein will be elevated
- CT scans will show changes in the bone and can show pockets of exudates
- Wound cultures will need to be take

Pharmacology

Traditional pharmacological therapy is for four to six weeks of IV antibiotic therapy based on the results of wound cultures for acute osteomyelitis. Chronic osteomyelitis is treated with six to eight weeks of oral antibiotic therapy, based on the wound culture results (Hellman & Stone, 2004).

Surgery

Localized wound debridement will be necessary to rid the site of the necrotic bone.

Patient and Family Teaching

Teaching will be focused on the disease process and management.

Evaluation of Outcomes

Potential patient outcomes for each of the example nursing diagnoses for the patient with osteomyelitis are:

- Acute or chronic pain due to the osteomyelitis. The patient should verbalize an adequate relief of pain along with the ability to realistically cope with the pain if it is not completely relieved.
- Fear due to the diagnosis of osteomyelitis. The patient should manifest positive coping behaviors and verbalize a reduction in the amount of fear of the having this disease.
- Impaired physical mobility due to the osteomyelitis. The patient should perform physical activity independently or with assistive devices as needed. In addition, the patient should be free of complications of immobility, as evidenced by intact skin, absence of thrombophlebitis, and normal bowel patterns.
- Risk for impaired skin integrity related to compromised tissue perfusion. The condition of the skin should be improved as evidenced by decreased redness, swelling, and pain.
- Deficient knowledge related to self-care and risk prevention. The patient should demonstrate motivation to learn, identify perceived learning needs, and verbalize an understanding of desired content.

TUMORS OF THE MUSCULOSKELETAL SYSTEM

Tumors of the musculoskeletal system can arise in any of the structures that make up this system. They are classified as either benign or malignant and are found in children and adults. A malignant neoplasm of the musculoskeletal system is called a **sarcoma.** According to the American Cancer Society, in 2005 there will be an estimated 11,990 newly diagnosed cases of cancer of the bones, joints, and soft tissues. The estimated number of deaths for musculoskeletal cancers in 2005 is 4,700.

Primary Bony and Soft Tissue Tumors

Primary bone cancers are rare. There are an estimated 2,500 new case of primary bone cancer each year. Primary bone cancers are generally considered pediatric cancers. Most cases are diagnosed between the ages of 10 and 25. **Osteosarcoma** is the most common type of primary bone cancer. Other primary bony tumors include **Ewing's sarcoma** (a diffuse endothelioma or endothelial myeloma forming a fusiform swelling on a long bone) and **chondrosarcoma** (cartilaginous sarcoma). These tumors are aggressive and tend to recur if not completely excised. They also tend to metastasize to the lungs early in the disease process especially if they are high-grade tumors.

Malignant soft tissue tumors arise from or resemble connective tissues of the body. These tissues include muscle, fat, cartilage, fibrous tissue, **tendosynovial** tissue, vessels, and peripheral nerves. Most soft tissue malignancies are considered intermediate in nature, meaning that they tend to be locally aggressive but have a low-to-moderate tendency to metastasize to distant areas. These primary soft tissue tumors occur twice as often as primary bone sarcomas and are seen more often in men than in women. They are seen in the lower extremity 45 percent of the time and the upper extremity 15 percent of the time. They are seen less often in the head and neck, retroperitoneum, abdomen, chest wall, and in the connective tissue of organs. Soft tissue sarcomas are typically seen in the older adult with the exception of rhabdomyosarcoma, which is typically seen in children and young adults.

Epidemiology

Bony sarcomas are considered pediatric cancers. They are usually diagnosed in people ages 10 to 25 years. Soft tissue sarcomas usually occur in adults over the age of 55 (Maher, et al., 2001). Sarcomas appear in males slightly more often than females. There is a second peak of osteosarcoma in the seventh decade, which is most likely due with osteosarcomas association with Paget's disease. Secondary chondrosarcomas can also appear later in life from benign cartilage lesions.

Etiology

The exact cause of primary sarcomas is not known, and there are no definitive risk factors. Factors that may play a role in the development of sarcomas are previous high-dose irradiation, exposure to chemicals, prior treatment with chemotherapy drugs, immunosuppression, preexisting bone conditions (Paget's disease), and skeletal maldevelopment. Environmental factors, such as trauma or a past injury, have also been associated with the development of primary sarcomas (Maher, et al., 2002).

Pathophysiology

As the sarcoma grows, it forms a ball-like mass that penetrates the bony cortex (Wittig, et al., 2002). High-grade tumors are aggressive and quickly metastasize to the lung. Once this occurs, the prognosis worsens.

Assessment with Clinical Manifestations

Clinical symptoms of a bony sarcoma include a dull, aching pain that worsens at night. Often, the pain may be associated with a prior injury. Other symptoms may include swelling, localized enlargement of the extremity, fever, night sweats, and occasionally, pathological fracture. In early stages of soft tissue sarcomas there are often no symptoms. Symptoms start to appear once the tumor has grown enough to put pressure on surrounding structures, such as nerves and muscles causing pain.

During the physical examination a mass may be visible. It may be firm and warm to the touch. It can be painless, or the patient may have some localized tenderness around the mass. Range of motion of the adjacent joints may be compromised. The patient may also have a limp or a decrease in muscle strength if the tumor is located in the lower extremity. It is important to note the size of the mass and to compare it to the bilateral extremity or side.

Diagnostic Tests

The definitive diagnostic test for a sarcoma is a biopsy. In most cases a percutaneous needle biopsy is recommended. It is minimally invasive, associated with lower risk of infection, contamination, and postbiopsy fractures (Wittig, et al., 2002). In osteosarcoma a plain film X-ray will show a destructive lesion with a mixture of osteolytic and osteoblastic areas. Staging of the tumor is important in planning course of treatment. MRI and computed tomography (CT) scans are used to determine the local extent of the disease. Plain film X-rays, CT scans of the chest, and a bone scan are used to check for metastases to the lungs and other bone. A bone marrow aspirate is also used to check for metastasis in the bone marrow.

Blood tests may reveal an elevation in serum lactate dehydrogenase and ALP levels due to the increase in bone formation and cell turnover. This elevation is seen in about 50 percent of patients, so it is not useful in the diagnosis of sarcoma. However, it has been linked to a poorer prognosis.

Nursing Diagnoses

Based on the informative gathered, examples of nursing diagnoses for the patient with sarcomas may include the following:

- Acute or chronic pain due to the sarcoma.
- Fear due to the diagnosis of sarcoma.
- Impaired physical mobility due to the sarcoma.
- Risk for impaired skin integrity related to compromised tissue perfusion.
- Deficient knowledge related to self-care and risk prevention.

Planning and Implementation

The overall goal of treatment of sarcoma is to destroy or remove the tumor from the primary site and to treat any metastatic lesions. Prior to 1970, treatment of choice for sarcoma was amputation. For Ewing's sarcoma the treatment varied from other sarcomas because of the tumor's response to radiation therapy. However, sarcomas still had an overall mortality rate of 70 to 80 percent because of metastases to the lung. With the improvement in chemotherapy, radiotherapy, and surgical techniques, amputation is only seen in advanced stages of the disease, and the survival rate is 70 percent. Limb-sparing surgery is the standard of care with chemotherapy and radiation if tumor is radiation sensitive, before and after surgery to shrink the tumor and to decrease the risk of the tumor returning or metastasis occurring. Amputations are only necessary in about 5 percent of cases. Some of the contraindications for limb-sparing surgery include inability to achieve wide surgical margins, invasion of major neurovascular structures, patients with extensive skin involvement, pathological fractures, and sepsis (Hosalkar & Dormans, 2004).

The current treatment of osteosarcoma involves a course of chemotherapy before surgery. This shrinks the size of the tumor and kills the microscopic metastases before they have a chance to multiply. A second round of chemotherapy is administered to the patient after surgery to ensure that any cells left behind are destroyed. Surgery may not always be a viable option if the location of the tumor is axial (involving spine or pelvis) or if the surgery will result in an amputation. In these cases, radiotherapy for local control may be another option for some patients who respond to chemotherapy.

Complications of bony sarcoma include weakened bone and pathological fractures. Other complications are related to reconstructive surgery and can include prosthetic loosening, infection, and mechanical failure (Wittig, et al., 2002). Infection can be a serious complication if it delays chemotherapy or radiation treatment. Delaying adjuvant therapy could increase the patient's risk of metastasis and local recurrence. Another complication for some patients who have undergone a resection involving the lymph system is lymphedema. Lymphedema may also be a complication of radiation therapy.

Pharmacology

Table 59-5 lists common chemotherapy drugs used to treat sarcoma.

Exercise, Physical, and Occupational Therapy

Therapy following a limb-sparing surgery or an amputation is crucial in allowing the patient to obtain the highest level of function possible and independence in daily activities. The rehabilitation program is initiated by the physical and occupational therapist. However, the nurse plays an important role by reinforcing the program and ensuring the patient is adequately

TABLE 59-5 Common Chemotherapy Drugs Used in Treatment of Sarcoma

CLASSIFICATION AND DRUG NAME	ACTION	NURSING IMPLICATIONS
Methotrexate	A folate antimetabolite that inhibits enzyme production for DNA synthesis, leading to strand breaks or premature chain termination	Follow with leucovorin and calcium rescue Mucositis is common, mouth care is needed Photosensitivity precautions needed Patient to avoid multivitamins that contain folic acid
Cisplatin	Causes cross-linkage and breaks in the DNA helix strand, thereby inhibiting DNA replication	Hold drug if serum creatinine is greater than 1.5 mg/dL to prevent renal damage.
Dacarbazine	Causes cross-linkage and breaks in the DNA helix strand, thereby inhibiting DNA replication	Flu-like syndrome may occur up to seven days after drug administration Dacarbazine can cause severe pain and burning at injection site.
Ifosfamide	Causes cross-linkage and breaks in the DNA helix strand, thereby inhibiting DNA replication	Always administer Ifosfamide with Mesna to prevent hemorrhagic cystitis.
Dactinomycin	Binds with DNA inhibiting DNA and RNA	Dactinomycin is a vesicant.
Doxorubicin	Binds with DNA inhibiting DNA and RNA	Doxorubicin is a vesicant.
Vincristine	Prevents formation of mitotic spindles, preventing cell division	Cardiotoxicity, check baseline ejection fraction. May cause flare reaction. Vincristine is a vesicant. Assess for peripheral neuropathy Constipation is a common side effect

Adapted from Broyles, B. E., Reiss, B. S., & Evans, M. E. (2007). Pharmacological aspects of nursing care *(7th ed.). New York: Thomson Delmar Learning.*

medicated for pain prior to therapy to maximize the patient's participation during the therapy session.

Alternative Therapy

Alternative and complementary therapy are becoming more popular in the treatment of cancer. Some therapies have shown to increase quality of life, but others have been shown to do harm or interfere with the traditional medical regimen. Nutrition and dietary supplements are becoming more commonplace. The goal of these therapies may be to strengthen the immune system, increase energy, promote cell health, or ease the side effects associated with chemotherapy or radiation therapy. Other complementary or alternative therapy may be used to treat pain, such as massage or acupuncture. It is important for the nurse to encourage the patient to discuss openly other therapy the patient is using and to document these on the medical record.

Patient and Family Teaching

Patient and family teaching starts with the initial diagnosis of the sarcoma. The patient and family may be overwhelmed with all of the new information related to the diagnosis and treatment options. After the physician initially speaks with the family and patient regarding the diagnosis, the nurse should be available to explain things with simpler terms, answer questions, or just to offer support. This education with the patient and family is ongoing and continuous. The patient and family may need to hear the information more than once and may need to have it presented in different ways using printed material, pictures, or audiovisual modalities.

Evaluation of Outcomes

After the initial treatment phase the patient will need to continue follow-up with the orthopedic or medical oncologist. Radiographic tests will be ordered on a routine basis to monitor for local recurrence and metastatic disease.

Metastatic Tumors

Metastatic tumors of the bone are detrimental consequences of cancer. Metastatic tumors greatly affect the patient's quality of life and increase morbidity (Wilfred & Muttarak, 2002). They are more commonly seen than primary bone sarcomas.

Epidemiology

The three most common sites of metastases in order of occurrence are the lung, liver, and bone (Reich, 2003). The primary cancers that most frequently metastasize to the bone are breast, prostate, kidney, thyroid, and lung. Ninety percent of metastatic bone lesions are found on the vertebrae, pelvis, proximal parts of the femur, ribs, proximal part of the humerus, and skull.

Pathophysiology

Malignant tumor cells tend to break off from the primary site and travel through the bloodstream or through the lymphatic system to other areas. The tumor can also invade nearby tissues as the tumor grows beyond the normal limits of the primary site. Metastatic bone lesions can be categorized into three different categories: osteolytic, osteoblastic, and mixed. Osteolytic lesions occur in patients with multiple myeloma due to the osteoclastic activity caused by excessive proteins. Osteoblastic lesions are areas where new bone has grown over existing bone and are seen in patients with prostate cancer. The last type of lesion is called mixed osteoblastic and osteolytic and are seen most often in patients with breast cancer.

Assessment with Clinical Manifestations

The number one symptom of bone metastases is pain. The pain is usually described as a dull, aching pain that increases at night and with weight bearing. Other complications that can be caused by metastatic bone disease include hypercalcemia, myelosuppression, pathological fractures, and spinal cord compression (Reich, 2003).

Diagnostic Tests

Diagnostic testing begins with X-rays; however, X-rays can only detect large lesions. Therefore, skeletal scintigraphy (bone scan) is the standard in staging and monitoring bone metastases. The disadvantage of a bone scan is that while it is sensitive in detecting bone metastases, it is unable to provide information regarding the type of lesion (Wilfred & Muttarak, 2002). Plain film radiography is the standard in characterizing the type of lesion seen on bone scan and in determining the response of the bone. Positron emission tomography (PET) scan is another option in detecting and staging bone metastases.

However, it is unclear if the sensitivity of PET scan is comparable to the bone scan (Folgelman, Cook, Israel, & Van der Wall, 2005).

Nursing Diagnoses

Based on the informative gathered, examples of nursing diagnoses for the patient with bone metastases may include the following:

- Acute or chronic pain due to the bone metastases.
- Fear due to the diagnosis of bone metastases.
- Impaired physical mobility due to the bone metastases.
- Risk for impaired skin integrity related to compromised tissue perfusion.
- Deficient knowledge related to self-care and risk prevention.

Planning and Implementation

The management goals of treatment for metastatic bone disease are pain control, prevention of complications, and remission through a multimodal approach. Therapy, much like those for primary bone tumors, includes pain medication, hormone therapy, chemotherapy, surgery, radiation therapy, and the use of bisphosphonates.

Radiotherapy is the first treatment used for a bone lesion. An external beam of radiation is used to kill the tumor cells directly at the site of the lesion. In a review of 43 studies, radiotherapy has been shown to be clearly effective in providing pain relief in patients with metastatic bone disease (Licata, 2005).

Bisphosphonates, however, have not been proven as effective in reducing pain associated with bone metastases. In a review of over 50 randomized controlled studies, the results show modest pain relief at best. Therefore, bisphosphonates are not used as first-line therapy for pain relief. Bisphosphonates may be used in the treatment of bone metastases to prevent complications, such as pathological fractures, and to prevent new osteolytic lesions (Licata, 2005).

Evaluation of Outcomes

Potential patient outcomes for each of the example nursing diagnoses for the patient with bone metastases are:

- Acute or chronic pain due to the bone metastases. The patient should verbalize an adequate relief of pain along with the ability to realistically cope with the pain if it is not completely relieved.
- Fear due to the diagnosis of bone metastases. The patient should manifest positive coping behaviors and verbalize a reduction in the amount of fear of the having this disease.
- Impaired physical mobility due to the bone metastases. The patient should perform physical activity independently or with assistive devices as needed. In addition, the patient should be free of complications of immobility, as evidenced by intact skin, absence of thrombophlebitis, and normal bowel patterns.
- Risk for impaired skin integrity related to compromised tissue perfusion. The condition of the skin should be improved as evidenced by decreased redness, swelling, and pain.
- Deficient knowledge related to self-care and risk prevention. The patient should demonstrate motivation to learn, identify perceived learning needs, and verbalize an understanding of desired content.

SPINAL DISORDERS

Spinal disorders are relatively common and require assistance from the health care team. The more common ones are scoliosis, kyphosis, lordosis, and spinal stenosis (Figure 59-8).

A
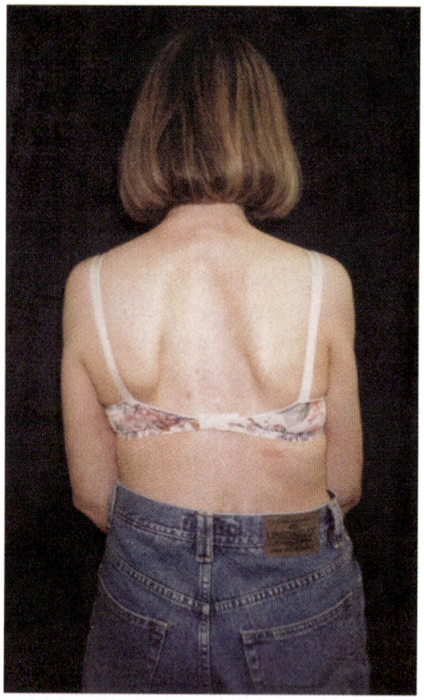

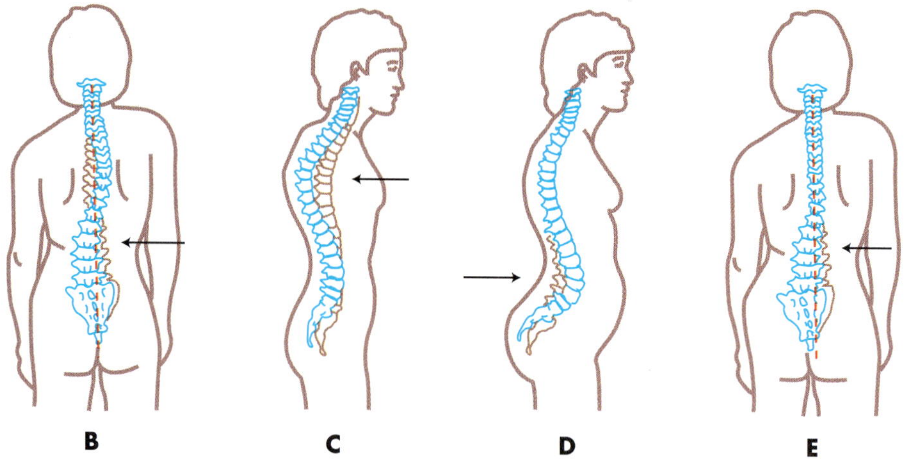

Figure 59-8 Abnormalities of the spine: A. Scoliosis, B. Scoliosis, C. Kyphosis, D. Lordosis, and E. List.

Scoliosis

Scoliosis is defined as a spinal deformity that is characterized by a lateral curve, spinal rotation causing rib asymmetry, and thoracic **hypokyphosis** (less than normal curvature in the thoracic spine) (Hockenberry &Brown, 2003).

Epidemiology

An estimated 2 to 3 percent of 10 to 16 year-olds are affected by curvatures of 10 degrees or more.

Etiology

Scoliosis can be congenital or developmental during infancy or childhood. Most often it is detected early in adolescence. The cause of scoliosis is most often unknown but can be associated with a number of neuromuscular disorders.

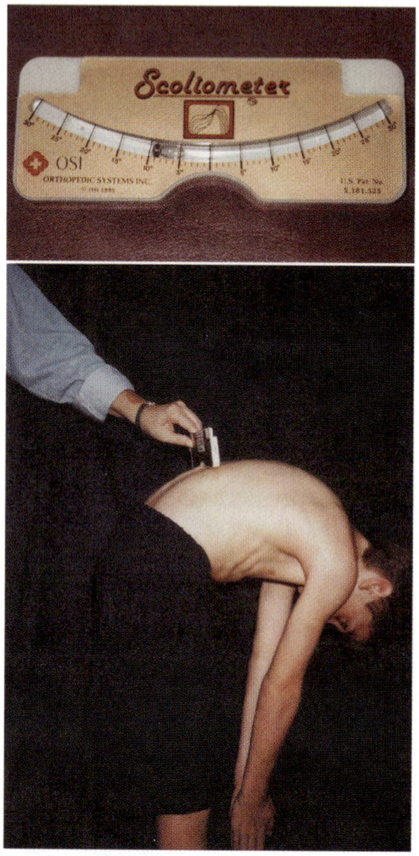

Figure 59-9 Use of scoliometer.

Assessment with Clinical Manifestations

Scoliosis is seldom seen before the age of 10 and parents will be referred to a health care provider after a school screening; or they may notice uneven pant lengths or skirt hems (Hockenberry & Brown, 2003). Pain is usually not an issue until the deformity has progressed.

The physical assessment technique used in school screenings is known as the **Adams Bending Forward Test** (a test to assess for scoliosis). The patient, wearing only underwear, bends forward at the waist with both arms hanging toward the floor, palms together. Viewing the patient from behind, the health care worker observes the back for curvature by observing the symmetry of the shoulders, scapulae, flank shapes, hip heights, and pelvis. A **scoliometer** (an instrument for measuring curves, especially those in lateral curvature of the spine) can be used to measure the trunk rotation during the Adams Test (Figure 59-9). Authors do note that the reliability of these tests are questionable but do not make recommendations for other screening tools (Hockenberry & Brown, 2003; Slote, 2002).

Diagnostic Tests

Standing spinal X-rays are performed, and curvature is measured. The amount of curvature noted determines actual diagnosis and the degree of deformity. It will also help to determine the type of treatments recommended (Hockenberry & Brown, 2003).

Nursing Diagnoses

Based on the informative gathered, examples of nursing diagnoses for the patient with scoliosis may include the following:

- Acute or chronic pain due to the scoliosis.
- Fear due to the diagnosis of scoliosis.

- Impaired physical mobility due to the scoliosis.
- Risk for impaired skin integrity related to compromised tissue perfusion.
- Deficient knowledge related to self-care and risk prevention.

Planning and Implementation

The goal of treatment, whether surgical or nonsurgical, is to correct the deformity and prevent complications. For mild curvature, exercise and bracing are the treatments of choice. Exercise is used in conjunction with bracing. Bracing allows the scoliosis progression to be stopped or slowed because of the limitation in truncal mobility. Usually utilized in growing children, braces are used until the child reaches maturity (Hockenberry & Brown, 2003). Two types of braces are used: the Boston brace and the thoracolumbar sacral orthotic (TLSO).

Left untreated, scoliosis can lead to back pain, compromised cardiopulmonary function, GI tract disturbances, and gait abnormalities. Surgical complications include postoperative paralysis, paralytic ileus, and urinary retention (Hockenberry & Brown, 2003). A long-term complication may be a failure in the hardware used in the surgery. This failure can be include broken hardware or failure of the hardware to stay in place, sometimes due to poor bone quality, although this is more frequent in older people after a spinal fusion.

Surgery

Spinal fusion is used to fuse the vertebrae to correct the curvature as well as the rotation of the spine. Surgery is recommended for curves greater than 40 degrees with continued development of the curve over time (Slote, 2002). Fusion of the vertebrae is performed two vertebrae above the curve and two vertebrae below the curve. Bracing is continued after the surgery to provide additional support while recovery takes place.

Patient and Family Teaching

Patient and family teaching include defining the disorder, discussion of treatment for the level of severity (may include bracing and exercise or surgery options), and understanding of the developmental support (both social and emotional) for the child.

Evaluation of Outcomes

Potential patient outcomes for each of the example nursing diagnoses for the patient with scoliosis are:

- Acute or chronic pain due to the scoliosis. The patient should verbalize an adequate relief of pain along with the ability to realistically cope with the pain if it is not completely relieved.
- Fear due to the diagnosis of scoliosis. The patient should manifest positive coping behaviors and verbalize a reduction in the amount of fear of the having this disease.
- Impaired physical mobility due to the scoliosis. The patient should perform physical activity independently or with assistive devices as needed. In addition, the patient should be free of complications of immobility, as evidenced by intact skin, absence of thrombophlebitis, and normal bowel patterns.
- Risk for impaired skin integrity related to compromised tissue perfusion. The condition of the skin should be improved as evidenced by decreased redness, swelling, and pain.
- Deficient knowledge related to self-care and risk prevention. The patient should demonstrate motivation to learn, identify perceived learning needs, and verbalize an understanding of desired content.

In addition, successful interventions provide the successful outcomes of halting the progress of the spinal curvature and supporting the growing body into an anatomically correct position. Other successful outcomes include adequate coping by the patient and family with the treatment of the disorder. Slote (2002) emphasizes psychological support and empowering the patient.

Family and peer support groups can take a proactive role in the patient's emotional and physical healing by providing the support and empowerment the patient needs. The involvement of these support groups can and will make the relatively long treatment and recovery period a positive experience, especially after surgery.

Kyphosis

Kyphosis (posterior curvature of the thoracic spine) is abnormal when the curvature of the thoracic spine is greater than 45 degrees. Kyphosis often results from osteoporosis (hunchback) or AS. Treatment can be accomplished with bracing or spinal fusion should the defect cause cardiopulmonary problems or pain.

Spinal Stenosis

Spinal stenosis is a degeneration of the spine that causes narrowing of the spinal canal secondary to bony overgrowth (osteophytes) at the facet joints, hypertrophy of the ligaments supporting the spine, or protrusion of intervertebral disks (Hellman & Stone, 2004). The most common site of stenosis is the lumbar region of the spine. The result of the narrowing of the canal is impingement on the nerves and subsequent low back pain and/or leg pain as well as leg fatigue and reduced physical activity tolerance.

The incidence of spinal stenosis increases with age. Spinal stenosis can be a complication of many processes traumatic back injury, arthritis, or Paget's disease.

Assessment with Clinical Manifestations

The patient will usually present with a gradual onset of difficulty walking or low back pain. Pain may also radiate down one leg. The patient may complain of the inability to stand or sit in one position for long because of the pain or fatigue (Hellman & Stone, 2004). A neurological assessment may be unremarkable. Gait assessment may reveal unsteadiness or a limp.

Diagnostic Tests

An MRI is the most useful diagnostic tool when spinal stenosis is suspected.

Nursing Diagnoses

Based on the information gathered, examples of nursing diagnoses in the patient with spinal stenosis (and other spinal disorders) may include the following:

- Chronic and acute pain related to spinal stenosis.
- Activity intolerance.
- Ineffective coping.
- Ineffective role performance.

Planning and Implementation

The goals of treatment are to reduce pain and return the patient to normal physical activity. Exercises to strengthen back muscles and flexibility are often prescribed. These exercises can be done in conjunction with a therapist's or nurse's instruction or by simple written instructions.

Nutrition

Weight loss is recommended to reduce the lumbar lordosis that causes strain on the back. A consult with a dietitian may be in order.

Surgery

To treat continuing pain, a decompression laminectomy may be performed. The laminectomy relieves the pressure within the spinal canal and reduces the pain. Some patients may need to have a spinal fusion in order to stabilize the spine. Refer to the section on scoliosis for more on spinal fusions. Risks of surgical complications increase with age and comorbid conditions. The potential postoperative complications are: hematoma, dural tears, spinal cord injury, nonunion of the fusion, infection, and delayed wound healing.

Patient and Family Teaching

Teaching will revolve around the disease process, the prescribed exercises and pain medications as well as the importance of weight control. Teaching may also need to be done regarding potential surgical options.

Evaluation of Outcomes

A review of the literature found that patients with mild symptoms of spinal stenosis did better with conservative treatment whereas patients with moderate to severe symptoms did better with surgical treatment (Snyder, Doggett, & Turkelson, 2004). However, a study performed on long-term effects of spinal fusions in lumbar spinal stenosis showed that although the surgical group had initially better results than the nonsurgical group, the benefit of surgery decreased with time (Chang, Singer, Wu, Keller, & Atlas, 2005).

Concept Map Case Study

Mr. Juan Rodriguez

Juan Rodriguez, age 76, is a retired schoolteacher. He is widowed and lives alone in the home that he and his wife shared for 37 years. His two adult sons and their wives live in the city, and they visit him at least once each week. His two grandchildren attend college in another state. A cleaning woman comes to his home every two weeks. Mr. Rodriguez enjoys his independence, still drives his car, attends his church regularly, and likes to garden. He manages the routine cooking and household tasks rather well. He also belongs to a group of retired teachers that has breakfast meetings once a month.

Mr. Rodriguez has hypertension and is taking daily doses of lisinopril, an angiotensin-converting enzyme (ACE) inhibitor medication, of 40 mg and pravastatin, an antilipemic medication, of 10 mg, and low-dose aspirin of 81 mg. He takes Tylenol (over-the-counter) for arthritis pain. He is scheduled for cataract surgery next month.

Yesterday, he tripped and fell when he was retrieving his mail from the post box by his driveway. He felt a sharp pain in his right hip and leg and was unable to get up. His next door neighbor heard his shouts for help and ran out to assist him. She notified Mr. Rodriguez's son and called 911. After being examined in the emergency department, he was diagnosed with a femoral neck fracture. He was transferred to the orthopedic unit and was scheduled for a total hip replacement (arthroplasty).

Postoperative orders include: thigh high support hose, an indwelling catheter (for two to three days), legs must remain abducted, and Mr. Rodriguez cannot be turned. The wound dressing and Hemovac drainage must be assessed. He has an intravenous (IV) fluid running. Intake and output are to be measured. Narcotic analgesics will be administered via a patient controlled analgesia device (PCA) for the first two days with transition to oral analgesics the third day, if needed. Heparin is to be administered via IV as a prophylactic measure against thrombophlebitis. Vital signs and neurovascular status of the lower extremities are to be evaluated on a routine basis.

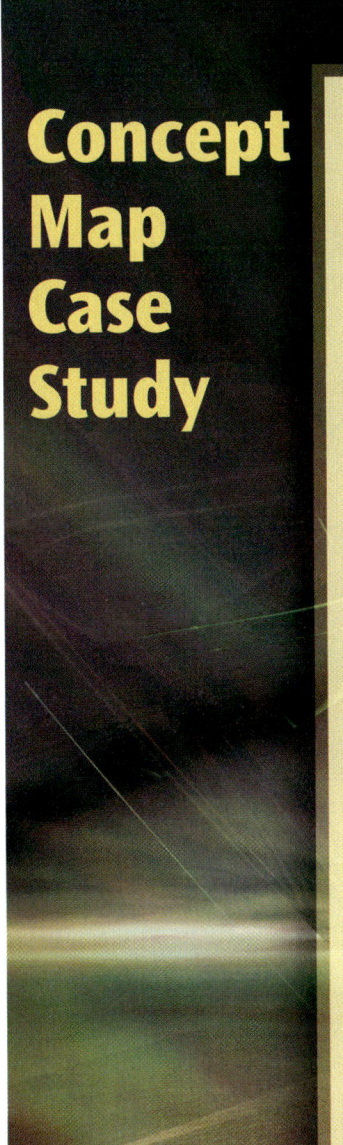

Concept Map Case Study

Note: There is a current trend for using clinical pathways for managing the interdisciplinary care for total hip replacement. Patients can usually return to their regular presurgical diet on the second postoperative day. Hospitalization for this type of surgery is four to five days. The patient is usually discharged to a rehabilitation facility for a period of time. Physical and occupational therapies and education related to transferring techniques, weight bearing, exercises, modifications in the home, and so on begins early in the postoperative treatment time. The nurse is also involved in education and monitoring the patient's progress. The recovery period is approximately four to six weeks. As you respond to the discussion questions for this case study, consider the special needs of the geriatric patient as they relate to the holistic mental, physical, spiritual, environmental, and safety needs. Refer to the sample concept map for assistance in designing a map for Mr. Rodriguez. Add concepts where you believe they belong. (Note: some concepts may belong in more than one area.)

Suggested References

Current Nurses Drug Guide or Pharmacology Text
Current Medical/Surgical Nursing Text
Nanda International. (2005). *NANDA nursing diagnoses: Definitions and classification 2005–2006.* Philadelphia: Author.

1. Describe the potential complications due to immobility. What are the nursing actions to prevent these complications?
2. What precautions should be taken when transferring Mr. Rodriguez from the bed to a chair?
3. What clinical manifestations (respiratory, gastrointestinal, mental, and so on) would alert you to the adverse side effects of the narcotic medications?
4. Describe discharge instructions that you would provide for Mr. Rodriguez.
5. If you were assigned to evaluate Mr. Rodriguez's home what safety precautions or adaptations would you suggest to minimize falls and to promote his progress toward independent living?

KEY CONCEPTS

- OA occurs because of damage to articular cartilage and the metabolic response that results at the chondrocyte level.
- Patients with gout will report a rapid development (within hours) of pain and edema in the one affected joint.
- LD is preventable by taking simple precautions.
- The common features of the spondyloarthropathies are sacroilitis variable inflammatory peripheral arthritis, enthesitis, dactylitis, tendency for ocular inflammation, familial tendency, no rheumatoid factor, and strong association with the HLA-B27 gene.
- There are three hallmark tests which confirm the diagnosis of polymyositis or dermatomyositis: elevated muscle enzymes; an abnormal electromyogram; and positive results in a muscle biopsy.
- Fibromyalgia is most frequently defined as a clinical syndrome or condition involving chronic widespread diffuse musculoskeletal pain, stiffness, and tenderness.
- Osteoporosis is the most frequently diagnosed bone disease in humans.
- The main cause of osteomalacia is a vitamin D deficiency and is rare in the United States.

Continued

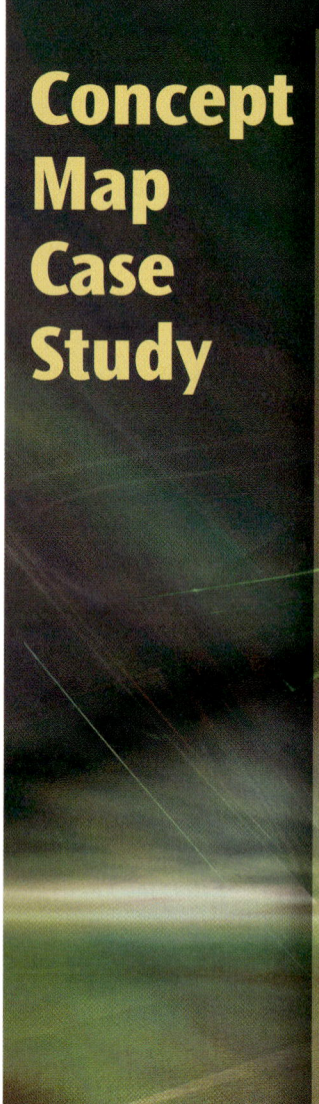

KEY CONCEPTS—cont'd

- Paget's disease is a chronic bone disorder characterized by weakened bone structure with no definitive cause or cure.
- Musculoskeletal infections can have devastating results if not treated promptly or completely.
- Primary bone cancers are rare. Metastatic tumors of the bone are detrimental consequences of cancer and are more common than primary bone cancers.
- For mild scoliosis curvature, exercise and bracing are the treatments of choice. For greater curves, spinal fusion is used.
- Spinal stenosis causes impingement on the nerves and subsequent low back pain or leg pain, as well as leg fatigue and reduced physical activity tolerance.

REVIEW QUESTIONS

1. Mrs. Jones is newly diagnosed with osteoarthritis of her knees. She told you the health care provider prescribed acetaminophen or ibuprofen for pain. She asks you how she can afford this medication. Your best response would be:
   1. "Dr. Cho thinks your pain is only minimal, and the cheap drugs are a good way to keep you out of the office."
   2. "Dr. Cho knows that these medications will help your pain and are relatively inexpensive and available over-the-counter at your local grocery or pharmacy."
   3. "I'll call the social worker."
   4. "Dr. Cho knows that these medications are covered by insurance and you shouldn't worry."

2. Mr. Cooper, a 65 year-old white male, has just been diagnosed with gout. Your teaching would include instructions to:
   1. Check his feet everyday for ulcers
   2. Avoid alcohol and turkey
   3. Avoid fats and milk products
   4. Take his antigout medications only when his toe hurts

3. Your patient is admitted for an appendectomy and states he has been suffering with Reiter's syndrome. You remember that patient's with Reiter's syndrome can present with all of the following symptoms *except:*
   1. The patient's eyes may be red and irritated.
   2. One of your patient's toes may be swollen and red.
   3. Your patient will complain of headaches.
   4. Your patient will complain of low back pain.

4. Your 55-year-old female patient with ankylosing spondylitis has been taking NSAIDs for years and finds these are no longer effective. A disease-modifying antirheumatic drug (DMARD) is now being prescribed. You tell you patient the following about DMARDs:
   1. They will help to increase the lubrication in the joint.
   2. They are analgesics.
   3. They assist with reducing inflammation.
   4. They should be taken with milk.

5. A 10-year-old boy is brought into your clinic. The parents state he has been complaining of pain in his knees and elbows for the past couple of days. On physical examination you find a bullseye-shaped rash on his upper back. Which of the following do you suspect?
   1. LD
   2. Reactive arthritis
   3. Fibromyalgia
   4. Extra pulmonary tuberculosis

6. A 59-year-old female is presenting to the clinic for a workup for suspected fibromyalgia. You know the following about fibromyalgia:
   1. The patient will have pulmonary function tests performed.
   2. The patient will be tested for rheumatoid factor and serum complement.
   3. The patient will be tested for electrolyte panel and ESR.
   4. The patient will have a liver biopsy.

7. A 67-year-old female presents with progressively worsening pain in the lower back with numbness and pain down the right leg. She reports she has lost about an inch in height over the last 10 years. You suspect spinal stenosis because:
   1. Spinal stenosis causes impingement of the nerve roots and can lead to back and leg pain.
   2. Disc space in the spinal column shrinks with spinal stenosis causing height loss.
   3. She was a long distance runner in her earlier years and the constant jarring from running causes spinal stenosis.
   4. Her X-rays show hypokyphosis.

Continued

REVIEW QUESTIONS—cont'd

8. A woman who has had rheumatoid arthritis for several years is admitted to the hospital. On physical examination of this patient, you should expect to find:
   1. Asymmetrical joint involvement
   2. Heberden's nodes
   3. Obesity
   4. Small joint involvement
9. A 50-year-old man has suffered from low back pain and sciatica for over two years. He is admitted to the hospital for evaluation and treatment of this problem. A thorough assessment of his level of discomfort from low back pain is important primarily because:
   1. This will provide a baseline for later comparison.
   2. This is a method for identifying patients with low back neurosis.
   3. Patients who have pain localized to the back and radiating to one extremity are probably not candidates for surgery.
   4. Surgery is contraindicated for patients who have had pain for less than two years.
10. A 52-year-old woman has RA and is taking prednisone. In creating a teaching plan, you will be certain to tell the patient which of the following?
    1. The patient should expect to be on corticosteroids for the rest of her life.
    2. It may take three to six months for the patient to notice any effect from the medication.
    3. The patient should notify the health care provider of any stomach upset.
    4. The patient should avoid bananas and spinach while she is taking this drug.

REVIEW ACTIVITIES

1. During a rotation in the operating room, ask to see an orthopedic surgery (preferably a joint replacement). What were there surgical instruments like? Did they look familiar? If you were present for a joint replacement how was the surgical team dressed? How was the patient placed during surgery? Was there any type of traction put on the patient during this surgery?
2. Visit the orthopedic nursing unit in your hospital. Does your hospital have a designated orthopedic nursing unit? What types of patient's do you see admitted? Why are these types of patient's admitted and others not? How long is the typical stay for an orthopedic patient after joint replacement?

Continued

REVIEW ACTIVITIES—cont'd

3. Your patient with osteoarthritis is concerned about the long-term effects of the disease. What can you tell the patient about the prognosis to allay any fears? What support programs are available to the patient or her family? How can you assess the patient's acceptance of this information?

4. Perform a search on the World Wide Web for information about Lyme disease. Look at both sites directed toward laypersons and medical personnel. What sort of information do you see? Is the information factual on the layperson sites? Who sponsors these sites? How can you tell if they are reliable sources? What information can you give to your patients about searching for medical information on the web?

Visit the Contemporary Medical-Surgical Nursing online companion resource at www.delmarhealthcare.com for additional content and study aids. Click on Online Companions then select the Nursing discipline.

Musculoskeletal Trauma: Nursing Management

CHAPTER 60

Rebecca Sears, RN

Anita M. Zehala, RN, MS, ONC, CNS

CHAPTER TOPICS

- Sports Injuries
- Overuse Syndrome/Repetitive Motion Injuries
- Shoulder Dislocations
- Rotator Cuff Tears
- Lateral Epicondylitis
- Carpal Tunnel Syndrome
- Patellar Tendonitis
- Knee Ligament Injuries
- Meniscal Injuries
- Ankle Sprain
- Achilles Tendon Injuries
- Plantar Fasciitis
- Stress Fractures
- Fractures
- Hip Fractures
- Complications
- Amputation

KEY TERMS

Ankle sprain
Arthroscopy
Closed reduction
Compartment syndrome
Cryotherapy
Drawer test
Fascia
Fasciotomy
Fracture
Inversion stress test
Lateral epicondylitis
Mechanism of injury
Microtrauma
Occult fracture
Overuse syndrome
Phalen's maneuver
Phantom limb sensation
Prosthesis
Radiculopathy
RICE
Rotator cuff tears
Sports medicine
Thenar
Tinel's sign
Valgus
Varus

Unintentional trauma is the leading cause of death for Americans between the ages of 1 and 44. Overall, unintentional injuries are the fifth leading cause of death for all age-groups. Males are injured two to three times more often than females, however, after the age of 65 this trend reverses, and females sustain more injuries than males (National Center for Health Statistics, 2004). Motor vehicle accidents are the leading cause of unintentional injuries for all age groups, followed by poisonings and falls. Sports injuries and occupational injuries are also a musculoskeletal concern. In 2002, 2.5 million workplace injuries and illnesses resulted in either days away from work, job transfer, or job restrictions (National Center for Health Statistics, 2004). Injuries place a heavy burden on our health care system and it resources. According to a 2000 report from the Center for Disease Control and Prevention (CDC), the United States spent $117 billion on medical expenditures related to injuries. This is equal to 10 percent of the total amount of medical expenditures for 2000. On an annual basis, injuries accounted for 9 million inpatient hospital days, 36 percent of total visits to the emergency department, and 1.8 million discharges, with fractures being the most common type of injury (National Center for Health Statistics, 2004).

SPORTS INJURIES

Sports medicine can be defined as the application of professional knowledge to the understanding, prevention, treatment, and rehabilitation of sports-related and exercise-related problems. It entails a multidisciplinary team approach, including the health care providers, nurses, physical therapists, athletic trainer, coaches, and exercise physiologists. The initial treatment of sports-related injuries consists of protection, rest, ice, compression, and elevation **(RICE),** and pain control. The rehabilitation phase begins when the pain is gone, and the injury is healed. The overall goal of rehabilitation is to return the patient back to preinjury status, and in the case of the competitive athlete, back to full participation in the sport activity. Rehabilitation consists of four areas of focus: full range of motion of the joint, optimal flexibility, strength, and endurance.

BOX 60-1

FACTORS ASSOCIATED WITH OVERUSE SYNDROME

- Repetitive tasks
- Forceful exertions
- Exposure to vibration
- Exposure to cold temperatures
- Awkward positioning
- Poor ergonomics and work place design
- Lack of job satisfaction
- Physiological makeup
- Boredom at work

OVERUSE SYNDROME/REPETITIVE MOTION INJURIES

Overuse syndrome (also called repetitive motion injuries or cumulative trauma disorders) is caused by a repetitive motion or sustained exertion, causing **microtrauma** to the involved tissue (usually a muscle or tendon). The injured tissue is not given sufficient time to rest and heal before being subjected to more stress, which leads to pain, swelling, fatigue, and numbness. Overuse syndrome is an umbrella term and is used to describe many work-related injuries and injuries seen in athletes. The injury can take weeks or years to develop, and the symptoms may start to appear gradually. Many factors play a role in development of these injuries (Box 60-1).

Many occupations and sports have also been associated with a high level of overuse syndromes. These are listed in Box 60-2.

BOX 60-2

OCCUPATIONS AND SPORTS WITH HIGH INCIDENCE OF OVERUSE SYNDROME

- Grocery store clerks
- Computer keyboard operators
- Dental hygienists
- Frozen food workers
- Assembly line workers
- Health care workers
- Meat packers and butchers
- Professional dancers
- Musicians

DISLOCATION OF THE SHOULDER

The shoulder is an important joint and is used in most activities of daily living. Therefore when it is injured it can cause disability and great inconvenience to the patient and family.

Epidemiology

In 2002, 12.3 million people in the United States visited a health care provider for a shoulder-related problem. Shoulder dislocations account for almost 50 percent of all joint dislocations. About 90 percent are anterior dislocations and 2 to 10 percent are posterior dislocations. In younger patients the dislocation is caused by direct trauma and sports injuries. In the elderly the number one cause is a fall and a fracture is also commonly sustained (Quillen, Wuchner, & Hatch, 2004).

Etiology

The **mechanism of injury** for an anterior dislocation is a fall on an outstretched hand and arm that is abducted and externally rotated. It can also be caused by a direct blow to the posterior humerus. In a posterior dislocation, the force is applied while the arm is adducted and internally rotated.

Pathophysiology

The shoulder joint is a ball-and-socket joint, which allows a great amount of range and movement, but because of this, it is more vulnerable to dislocation. The shoulder is supported by the joint capsule, cartilage, and the muscles of the rotator cuff. In most adults the cause of a shoulder injury is a traumatic force. In the older adult, collagen fibers have fewer cross-links, which makes the shoulder joint weaker and more likely to dislocate (Price & Wilson, 2005).

Complications

After conservative treatment, recurrent dislocation can occur in 67 to 97 percent of cases with a higher incidence occurring in patients younger than 30 years. Athletes also have a higher incidence of recurring dislocation (82 percent) when compared to nonathletes (30 percent) (Welsh & Veenstra, 2004). Many studies have shown that early surgical treatment may prevent recurring dislocation (Davy & Drew, 2002).

Assessment with Clinical Manifestations

Assessment begins with a history of the traumatic event, including the position of the arm before and after the event. History of a prior dislocation is a risk factor for future dislocations. During the physical assessment any movement of the affected arm will cause severe pain because of muscle spasms. The affected arm is often guarded and cradled with the contralateral arm. The affected shoulder will appear lower, and the humeral head can be palpated in the front of the shoulder (Welsh & Veenstra, 2004). A neurovascular assessment is extremely important. Any changes in pulses, color, temperature, or sensation to the limb may be because of the impingement of the axillary nerves and radial artery. See chapter 58 for instructions on how to perform a neurovascular assessment.

Diagnostic Tests

Radiographic films are often used to confirm diagnosis and to assess for any accompanying fractures. However, relocation of the shoulder should not be delayed because of diagnostic testing. The longer the time between injury and relocation, the more difficult the relocation can become.

Nursing Diagnoses

Based on the information gathered, examples of nursing diagnoses, interventions, and outcomes in the patient with upper extremity trauma include:

- Acute pain.
- Risk for peripheral neurovascular dysfunction.
- Impaired physical mobility.
- Anxiety.
- Bathing/hygiene self-care deficit.
- Dressing/grooming self-care deficit.

Planning and Implementation

Closed reduction should be accomplished as soon as possible after the injury. As time passes, the muscles in the shoulder will become more spastic, and the joint itself will become more inflamed and swollen making reduction more difficult. Sedation and analgesics are often used in addition to a muscle relaxant to make reduction easier. Traditionally, treatment after reduction follows a conservative approach. The affected shoulder is immobilized in a sling for four to six weeks. External rotation and abduction is avoided (Welsh & Veenstra, 2004). After the initial rest period, rehabilitation is started, which includes strengthening of the shoulder girdle, flexibility, and regaining full range of motion.

ROTATOR CUFF TEARS

Rotator cuff tears are a common cause of shoulder pain in the adult population. They are most commonly seen in adults over the age of 40 years. In younger patients they are seen following a traumatic event or a sports-related injury (Fischer, 2005). The rotator cuff is made up of four muscles: the supraspinatus, infraspinatus, teres minor, and subscapularis (Figure 60-1).

The primary function of the rotator cuff is providing stability to the shoulder joint. It also provides some movement to the shoulder.

Epidemiology

The incidence of full thickness tears range from 5 to 40 percent and increases with age (Malanga, Andrus, & Bowen, 2004).

Etiology

Injury to the rotator cuff can occur by direct trauma, such as a fall, motor vehicle accident, or shoulder dislocation, or it can be caused by an overuse syndrome as seen in sports and activities that require extensive overhead movements

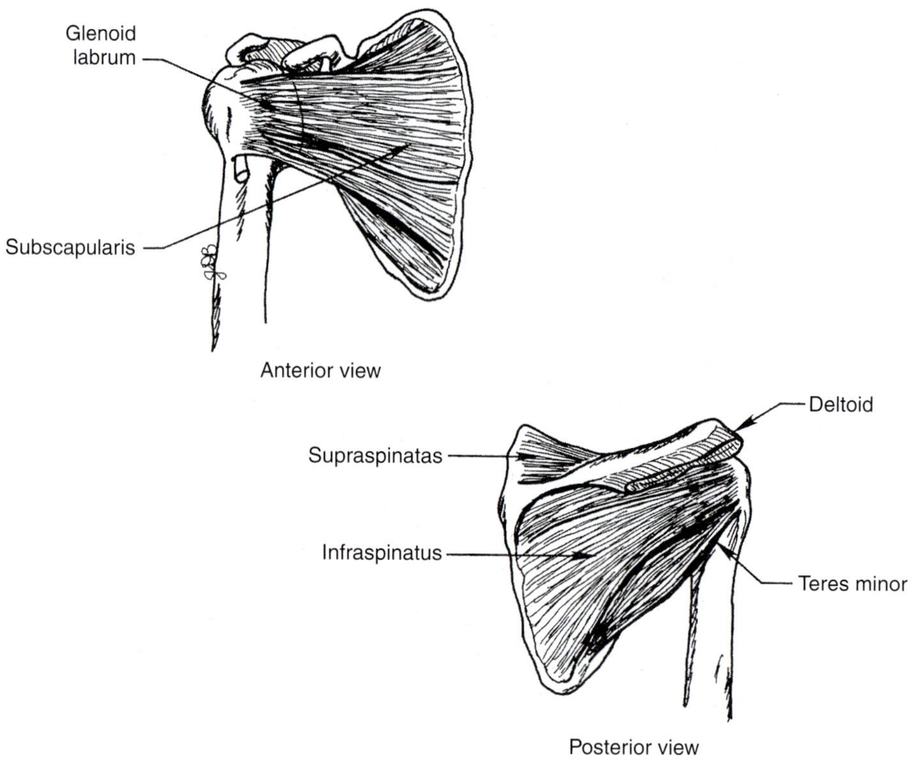

Figure 60-1 Rotator cuff tear.

(Quillen, et al., 2004). In overuse syndromes, poor posture, improper technique, and direct injury cause swelling and microtears to the muscles. If the microtrauma continues, eventual rupture of the rotator cuff can result. Rotator cuff tears are most commonly seen in sports that requires extensive use of the upper extremities, such as baseball, softball, tennis, swimming, and volleyball.

Assessment with Clinical Manifestations

A detailed history of the injury is needed to help rule out other causes of the symptoms, such as **radiculopathy** of the cervical nerves and pain that is of cardiac origin (Malanga, et al., 2004). History should include onset of pain, description of symptoms, and aggravating factors.

The physical assessment begins with inspection and comparison of the shoulder with the contralateral shoulder, noting any swelling, muscle atrophy, or asymmetry. Palpation will reveal localized tenderness. Assessment of the strength and range of motion (both passive and active) is important in determining the existence of a rotator cuff injury. With a rotator cuff tear, pain and reduced range of motion are experienced when the arm is abducted and externally rotated.

Diagnostic Tests

Diagnostic testing includes plain radiographs to view the bony structures of the shoulder and magnetic resonance imaging (MRI) to detect the size, location, and severity of the tear (Malanga, et al., 2004).

Nursing Diagnoses

Based on the information gathered, examples of nursing diagnoses, interventions, and outcomes in the patient with a rotator cuff tear include:

- Acute pain.
- Potential for impaired neurovascular status.
- Impaired physical mobility.

Planning and Implementation

The goals of treatment during the initial phase of the injury are rest and immobilization. Overhead activity is restricted, and a sling is usually worn. Pendulum exercises are started to reduce loss of range of motion (Quillen, et al., 2004). Ice, nonsteroidal anti-inflammatory drugs (NSAIDs), and acetaminophen are also used during this time to relieve inflammation and pain. During the recovery phase, physical therapy focuses on restoration of the range of motion, strengthening, proprioception, and joint stability (Malanga, et al., 2004).

Surgical Procedures

Surgical treatment is usually indicated for partial-thickness and full-thickness tears in active patients when three to six months of conservative treatment have failed to improve pain and function (Malanga, et al., 2004). Competitive athletes usually have better outcomes with surgical treatment (Quillen, et al, 2004). For smaller tears, the surgical procedure is usually performed by **arthroscopy.** The rotator cuff is derided, and measures may be taken to increase the subacromial space to prevent recurrence. For larger tears the procedure is performed using an open surgical technique.

Patient and Family Teaching

Patient teaching should focus on the rehabilitation plan of care. It is extremely important to stress to the patient the reasoning behind the program and why certain exercises may not be preformed until healing has occurred to protect the surgical site and to prevent fibrosis and reinjury to the rotator cuff.

Evaluation of Outcomes

Potential patient outcomes for each of the example nursing diagnoses for the patient with a rotator cuff tear are:

- Acute pain. The patient should verbalize an adequate relief of pain along with the ability to realistically cope with the pain if it is not completely relieved.
- Potential for impaired neurovascular status. The patient will have intact nervous system as evidenced by normal movement and sensation.
- Impaired physical mobility. The patient should perform physical activity independently or with assistive devices as needed. In addition, the patient should be free of complications of immobility, as evidenced by intact skin, absence of thrombophlebitis, and normal bowel patterns.

LATERAL EPICONDYLITIS

Lateral epicondylitis, or tennis elbow, is a common injury seen in athletes and in the general population. It is an overuse injury that involves the extensor/supinator muscles that attach to the distal humerus.

Epidemiology

Lateral epicondylitis has been seen in up to 50 percent of tennis players. The risk of injury increases with the hours of play and with the age of the athlete. Prevalence in relation to occupation varies widely from 1.6 to 23.1 percent (Hong, et al., 2003). There are no differences between men and women (Owens, et al., 2004).

Etiology

Although tennis is most commonly associated with lateral epicondylitis, any activity involving an extensive amount wrist extension or supination can cause lateral epicondylitis, such as many different manufacturing workplace activities. In younger patients, lateral epicondylitis tends to be associated with tennis and other sport activities, and in older patients, it is associated with occupational causes. In regard to tennis players, risk factors include improper technique, size of racquet handle, and racquet weight (Owens, Murphy, & Kuklo, 2004).

Pathophysiology

Although named lateral epicondylitis, many studies have failed to find evidence of an inflammatory process (Hong, Durand, & Loisel, 2003). The cause has been attributed to microinjuries with an inadequate repair response leading to macroscopic tearing and structural failure of the tendon (Owens, et al., 2004).

Assessment with Clinical Manifestations

The most common presenting symptom is pain at the lateral aspect of the elbow and in the forearm that is exacerbated with use (Owens, et al., 2004). The ability to grip is also impaired, thus everyday activities become difficult (Hong, et al., 2003).

Tenderness slightly distal to epicondyle is found with palpation of the elbow. Wrist extension and supination against resistance will cause an increase in pain; however, wrist flexion and pronation will not. The chair raise test examines the patient's ability to grip and lift. The patient stands behind a chair and places their hands on the chair back. The patient then attempts to raise the chair. If pain is experienced over the lateral elbow, lateral epicondylitis may be present (Owens, et al., 2004).

Diagnostic Tests

As with many overuse and sport injuries, the diagnosis is based on clinical findings during the examination of the patient. X-rays may be useful in ruling out other causes of elbow pain, such as osteochondral loose bodies and osteophytes (bone spurs). If the condition is chronic, calcification of the tendon may also be seen on X-ray. MRI can also be useful in the diagnosis, but usually it is not needed.

Nursing Diagnoses

Based on the information gathered, examples of nursing diagnoses, interventions, and outcomes in the patient with lateral epicondylitis include:
- Acute pain.
- Potential for impaired neurovascular status.
- Impaired physical mobility.

Planning and Implementation

The goal of treatment is to return the patient to preinjury status. Most patients respond to conservative treatment, which includes avoiding the activity that causes the pain, bracing and splinting of the elbow and wrist, and use of NSAIDs for short-term pain relief.

Once the patient is no longer experiencing pain, rehabilitation therapy can begin with strengthening exercises (Owens, et al., 2004). The first phase is stretching of the wrist with the elbow extended. This includes flexion, extension, and rotation of the wrist. The next phase is strengthening of the wrist using light weights in both extension and flexion. Forearm pronation and supination is then added along with having the patient squeeze a tennis ball.

If the patient is still experiencing symptoms after six months of conservative treatment, surgery is needed. The procedure is usually performed on an outpatient basis. Debridement of the muscle, removal of the portion of diseased epicondyle, and release of the tendon is performed.

Once the patient's strength is back to baseline, the focus of therapy turns to prevention of further injury to the elbow. Education on correct technique, equipment in relation to sports, and modification of occupational activities is important in preventing further irritation to the lateral elbow.

Evaluation of Outcomes

Potential patient outcomes for each of the example nursing diagnoses for the patient with a lateral epicondylitis are:
- Acute pain. The patient should verbalize an adequate relief of pain along with the ability to realistically cope with the pain if it is not completely relieved.
- Potential for impaired neurovascular status. The patient will have intact nervous system as evidenced by normal movement and sensation.
- Impaired physical mobility. The patient should perform physical activity independently or with assistive devices as needed. In addition, the patient should be free of complications of immobility, as evidenced by intact skin, absence of thrombophlebitis, and normal bowel patterns.

CARPAL TUNNEL SYNDROME

Carpal tunnel syndrome (CTS) is a median nerve entrapment neuropathy. It is the most common compression neuropathy of the upper extremity.

Epidemiology

CTS is most often seen between the ages of 30 and 60. Women are five times as likely to experience CTS as men (Wright, 2003).

Etiology

CTS is seen in conjunction with many other conditions. It is often seen during pregnancy, premenstrual period, and menopause; suggesting a hormonal link. It is also seen in patients with a history of arthritis, lipomas, ganglion, and after a fracture or trauma to the hand or wrist (Figure 60-2). Diabetes mellitus impairs peripheral nerve conduction and repair, therefore CTS is commonly seen in these patients as well (Kennedy & Zochodne, 2005). Anything that may cause the tendons of the wrist to become inflamed or swollen can also place pressure on the median nerve. Besides these above conditions, CTS is also associated with repetitive motion of the hand and wrist. Any activity where hand use is vigorous and routine can lead to CTS. The activities that have been associated with CTS are computer keyboarding or typing, playing a musical instrument, driving a motor vehicle or motorcycle, and flying a plane. There is also an increase in incidence in occupations that subject workers to a cold environment, such as meat packers, butchers, and frozen food workers (Falkiner & Myers, 2002).

Pathophysiology

The carpal tunnel is a canal in the wrist made up of the carpal bones and the transverse carpal ligament through which the flexor tendons and median nerve pass through to the hand. It is located at the base of the palm. CTS is the result of increased pressure inside the canal, which causes ischemia to the medial nerve. The damaged nerve is unable to function properly resulting in impaired nerve conduction, paresthesia, muscle weakness, and pain to the wrist and hand.

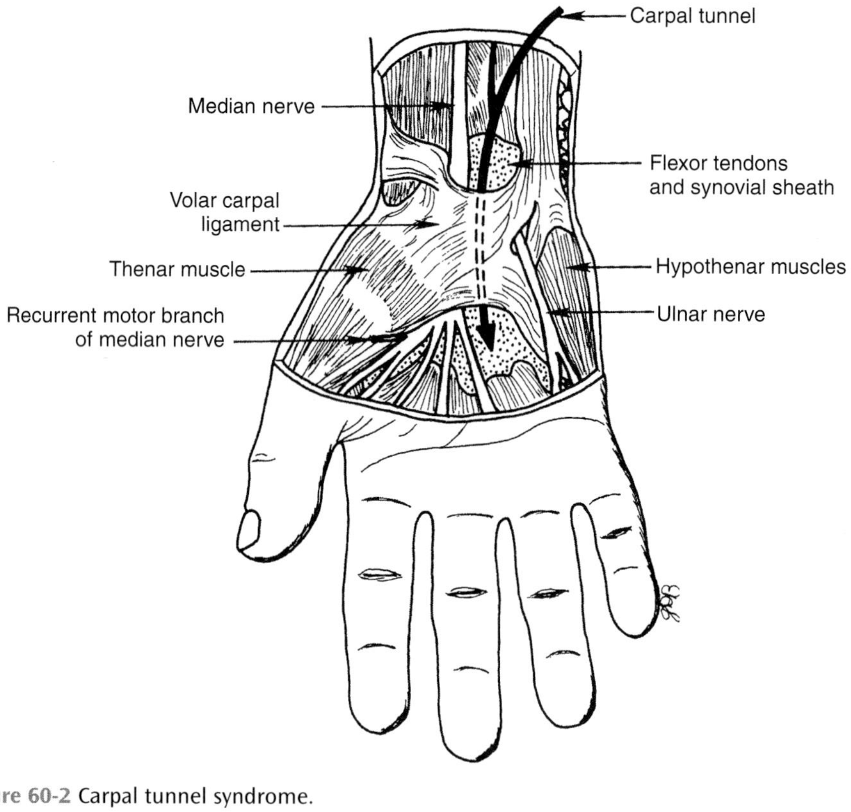

Figure 60-2 Carpal tunnel syndrome.

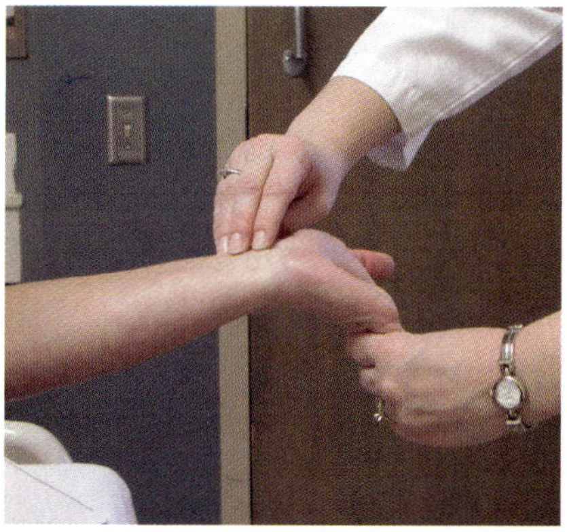

Figure 60-3 Tinel's sign.

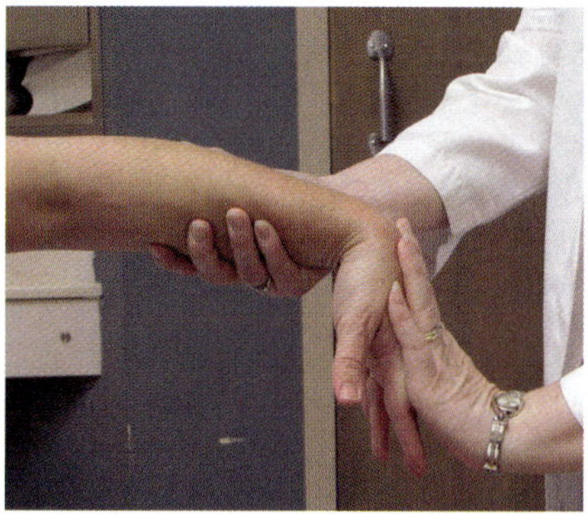

Figure 60-4 Phalen's maneuver.

Assessment with Clinical Manifestations

The diagnosis of CTS begins with a thorough history of symptoms. The patient may present with a combination of paraesthesia, numbness, and pain. The pain is usually described as a deep aching, or throbbing that is diffuse in nature and radiates up the forearm (Wright, 2003). The pain typically worsens at night. To attribute these symptoms to CTS, they must occur in the areas of the hand supplied by the median nerve, which includes the palmar aspect of the thumb, index finger, middle finger, and radial half of the ring finger. The patient may also report that the symptoms improve when the affected hand is placed in a dependent position and is shaken. This is known as the "flick test" (Katz & Simmons, 2002).

The physical examination consists of two classic tests to determine if the medial nerve has been compromised. The **Tinel's sign** (Figure 60-3) is a way to determine if the nerve is irritated. The area over the median nerve is lightly tapped. If the patient experiences a sensation of tingling or "pins and needles" the test is positive. The **Phalen's maneuver** (Figure 60-4) is more sensitive in the diagnosis of CTS. In this test the patient's wrist is put into flexion for 30 seconds. If the patient experiences a burning, tingling, or numbness the test it considered positive. Loss of two point discrimination along the area of the hand supplied by the median nerve and **thenar** (the palm of the hand or the sole of the foot) atrophy are late signs of CTS (Katz & Simmons, 2002).

Diagnostic Tests

Diagnostic testing is only used to confirm the diagnosis of CTS. Electromyography is used to test the function of the nerve. A mild electric current is used to stimulate the median nerve to see if there is a delay in motor response, which could indicate CTS.

Planning and Implementation

Conservative treatment starts with splinting of the affected wrist. The splint is used to maintain the wrist in the neutral position. This is important especially during sleep. Activity modifications along with exercises of the wrist may help to alleviate symptoms as well. If after four to six weeks of conservative treatment, symptoms remain or worsen, or the patient has thenar muscle atrophy or weakness, corticosteroid injection is recommended (Wright, 2003).

Pharmacology

If the symptoms are mild, NSAIDs are used to decrease the inflammation of the tendon and to help with pain control.

Health Care Resources

Annually, estimated 3 of every 10,000 workers lost time from work and half of these workers missed more than 10 days of work because of CTS. The average lifetime cost of carpal tunnel syndrome, including medical bills and lost time from work, is estimated to be about $30,000 for each injured worker (National Institute of Neurological Disorders and Stroke, 2002).

Surgery

If conservative treatment, including corticosteroid injection, does not improve symptoms after three months, surgery is considered. Surgical options include an open release of the ligament either by a mini or standard incision or by endoscopic surgery. It is performed on an outpatient basis using a regional block. After surgery, the patient is placed in a splint with instructions on range of motion exercises of the fingers. After, a few days, the splint is removed and more active physical therapy may begin. Most patients return to work within

2 to 14 days depending on the type of occupation and surgery. There is some debate over the use of surgery versus corticosteroid injection. In a study comparing the two treatments local steroid injections showed a slightly better outcome in the short term, but at 12 months, the outcomes for both groups were comparable (Ly-Pen, Andreu, de Blas, Sanchex-Olaso, & Millan, 2005).

Alternative Therapy

In a study by O'Connor, Marshall, & Massey-Westropp (2005), 21 trials comparing nonsurgical treatments for CTS other than steroid injection were reviewed. The results showed that there is significant short-term benefit from oral steroids, splinting, ultrasound, yoga, and carpal tunnel mobilization. However, magnet therapy, laser acupuncture, exercise, or chiropractic care did not show a significant benefit in symptom relief when compared to placebo or control.

Patient and Family Teaching

Patient teaching focuses on changes in ergonomics when completing daily activities. Teaching the patient proper hand and wrist alignment and stretching exercises can improve the symptoms and prevent further problems. Relaxing the force of grip on pens and other objects and taking frequent short breaks can also dramatically reduce the symptoms.

PATELLAR TENDINOPATHY

Patellar tendinopathy, also known as jumper's knee, is seen in athletes who participate in activities that require a lot of jumping, such as basketball and volleyball. It can be a challenge to treat the athlete, whether professional or recreational, and in some cases, he or she will no long be able to participate in those activities that cause the pain.

Epidemiology

Patellar tendinopathy occurs in 20 percent of jumping athletes and affects men twice as often as females (Hyman, et al., 2005).

Etiology

Patellar tendinopathy is caused by functional stress overload that is applied to the patellar tendon with jumping (Hyman, Malanga, & Alladin, 2005). Risk factors include overtraining, jumping on hard surfaces, poor quadriceps and hamstring flexibility, and poor jumping or landing technique (Hyman, et al., 2005).

Pathophysiology

In the past, patellar tendinopathy was thought to be an inflammatory process, but now it is thought to be a degenerative process from overuse (Peers & Lysens, 2005). When strain is applied to the tendon, microinjuries occur. If the amount of injuries outnumbers the ability of the tendon to repair itself, the tendon will start to degenerate (Hyman, et al., 2005).

Assessment with Clinical Manifestations

Patients usually describe anterior knee pain with an aching quality to it. It usually has an insidious onset, and most athletes will not be able to remember a specific precipitating event but may remember noticing the pain during an increase in activity or training. The extent of functional impairment is also important to assess. If the athlete is unable to participate in activities that require jumping, or if the pain continues long after the activity has ended, the tendinopathy may be more severe (Peers & Lysens, 2005).

During palpation of the knee joint, point tenderness may occur at the inferior patella pole and hamstring and quadriceps tightness may also be present (Hyman, et al., 2005). Range of motion should still be within normal limits.

Diagnostic Tests

Radiographic imaging is rarely needed to make a diagnosis, but it may be used to exclude other bony abnormalities (Hyman, et al., 2005). Ultrasound and MRI can also be used to visualize a degenerative process in the patella tendon (Peers & Lysens, 2005).

Nursing Diagnoses

Based on the information gathered, examples of nursing diagnoses, interventions and outcomes in the patient with inflammatory and connective tissue disorders include:

- Acute pain
- Impaired physical mobility
- Anxiety

Planning and Implementation

The goal of treatment is getting the patient back to preinjury state. Most patients respond to conservative management, which includes avoiding jumping and squatting. The patient should be encouraged to do other exercises that do not cause pain to the knee. Total immobilization of the knee joint is contraindicated because of risk of muscle or joint contracture (Hyman, et al., 2005). Physical therapy consists of strengthening and stretching programs for the quadriceps and hamstring muscles to help prevent the injury from returning. Surgical repair is only recommended if pain and functional disability remains after six months of conservative treatment (Hyman, et al., 2005).

Pharmacology

NSAIDs are used more for acute pain relief than for their anti-inflammatory properties, because inflammation is not part of the disease process. Corticosteroids are used only when conservative treatment has failed, and the pain is disrupting performance in a sport activity because of the risk of further damaging the tendon (Hyman, et al., 2005).

Evaluation of Outcomes

Potential patient outcomes for each of the example nursing diagnoses for the patient with patellar tendinopathy are:

- Acute pain: The patient should verbalize an adequate relief of pain along with the ability to realistically cope with the pain if it is not completely relieved.
- Impaired physical mobility: The patient should perform physical activity independently or with assistive devices as needed. In addition, the patient should be free of complications of immobility, as evidenced by intact skin, absence of thrombophlebitis, and normal bowel patterns.
- Anxiety: The patient should be able to recognize the signs of anxiety, demonstrate positive coping mechanisms, and describe a reduction in the level of anxiety experienced.

LIGAMENT INJURIES

Two set of ligaments in the knee provide a four-plane stability force to the knee. The collateral ligaments and are located on each side of the knee. The medial collateral ligament (MCL) connects the femur to the tibia and protects the knee from **valgus** (lateral) stress and external rotation. The lateral collateral ligament (LCL) connects the femur to the fibula and provides protection from **varus** (medial) forces. The other set of ligaments are called the cruciate ligaments and are located inside the knee joint and crisscross as they connect the femur to the tibia. The anterior cruciate ligament (ACL) is located in the front of the knee and prevents the tibia from excessive anterior movement. The posterior cruciate ligament (PCL) is located in the back of the knee (Figure 60-5).

Etiology and Pathophysiology

The MCL is the most commonly injured ligament (Gundel, 2004). The injury occurs when the foot is firmly planted and a direct valgus force is applied to the knee or the leg sustains an external rotational force. This injury is commonly seen in athletes who participate in football or basketball. The LCL is rarely injured, but if exposed to a contact varus force while the foot is planted, an injury can occur.

An ACL tear can result from several different mechanisms of injury. A sudden change in direction with the foot planted, sudden deceleration with some or no knee flexion, landing from a jump or by a direct valgus stress applied to an externally rotated leg. Any sport or activity that requires pivoting, twisting, rapid deceleration, or contact are associated with ACL injury, including basketball, football, skiing, soccer, and volleyball. ACL and meniscal injuries often coexist. The PCL is rarely injured, and the usual mechanism of injury involves an anterior force to the tibia with the knee flexed. This type of injury is commonly referred to as a dashboard injury.

Epidemiology

According to the American Academy of Orthopaedic Surgeons, more than eight million people visit an orthopaedic surgeon each year because of pain and other problems associated with the knee. Souryal and Adams (2005) reviewed several epidemiological studies and estimated that about 1 in 3,000 people sustain an ACL injury every year in the United States. Female athletes sustain injury to the ACL 3 to 10 times more frequently than male counterparts.

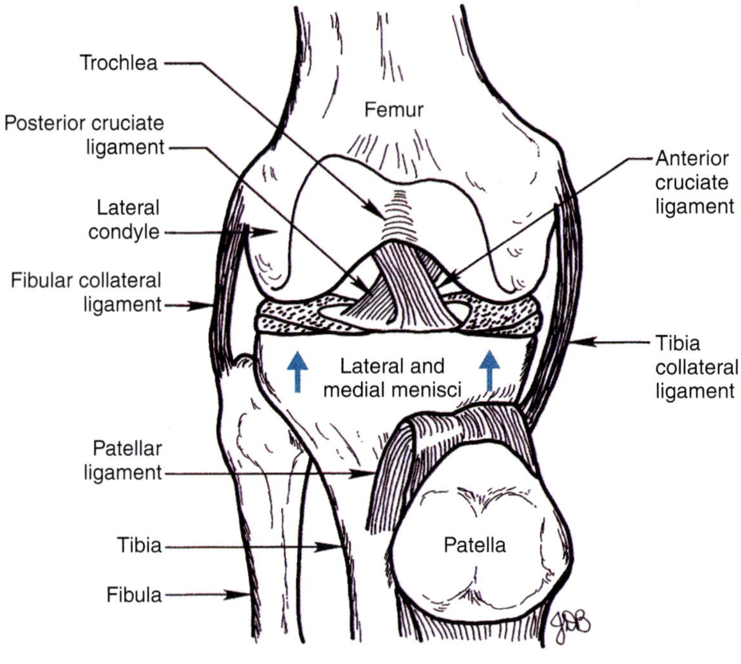

Figure 60-5 Normal anatomy of the knee with ligaments.

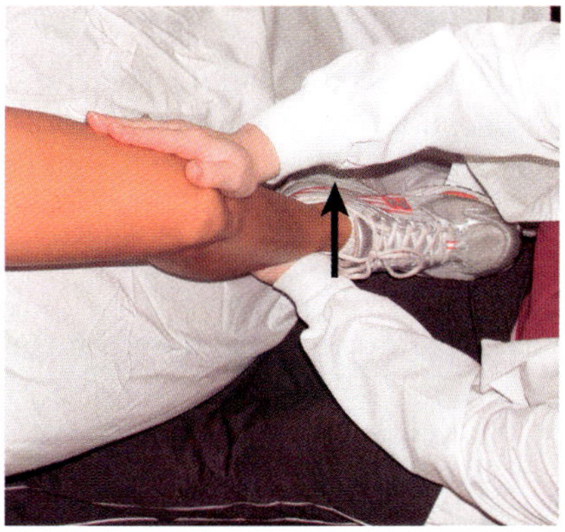

Figure 60-6 Varus stress test.

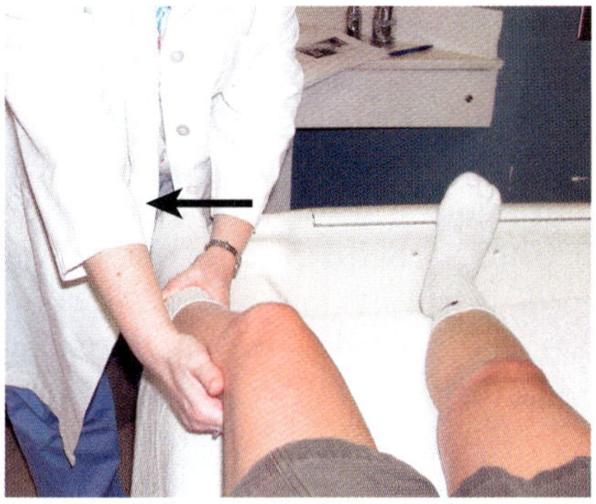

Figure 60-7 Valgus stress test.

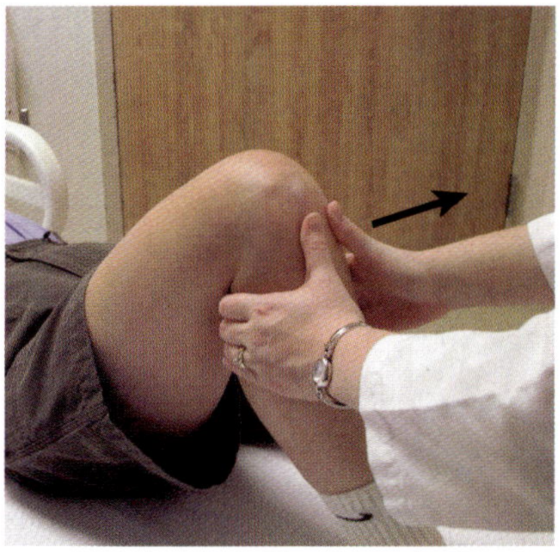

Figure 60-8 Drawer test.

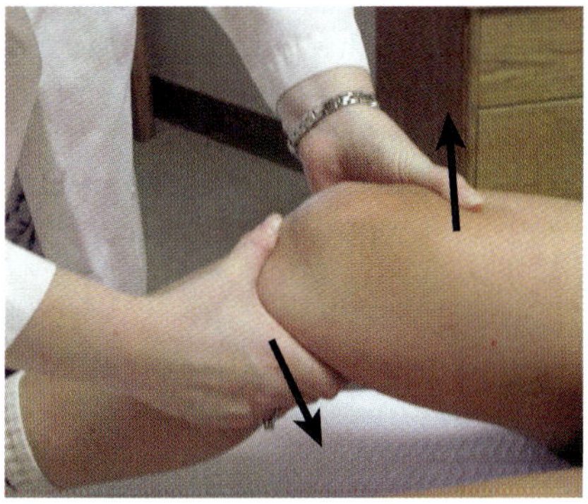

Figure 60-9 Lachman's test.

The reasons for the gender difference are not known, but many studies have linked possible factors, such as size and strength of the athlete and anatomical and hormonal differences.

Assessment

A history of the traumatic event is helpful in the diagnosis of a ligament injury. Details of how the injury occurred, position of the knee and foot, and any sounds of popping or tearing should be explored. Physical assessment begins with inspecting and comparing both knees while the patient sits, walks, stands, and is supine. Assess for the presence of pain, swelling, and any difficulty walking. Localized tenderness at the site of injury and joint effusion are often present during palpation of the knee joint. Stability of the knee is also an important area of assessment. The valgus stress test and varus stress tests are used to assess the stability of the LCL and MCL and the Drawer and Lachman stress tests are used to assess the stability of the ACL and PCL (Figures 60-6 through 60-9).

Diagnostic Tests

Plain radiographs are used when a clinically significant fracture is suspected. MRI is used to view both the soft tissue and the bone to further confirm the diagnosis of a ligament injury.

Nursing Diagnoses

Based on the information gathered, examples of nursing diagnoses, interventions, and outcomes in the patient with ligament injury include:

- Acute pain
- Impaired physical mobility
- Anxiety

Planning and Implementation

The goal of treatment is obtaining the best functional level possible. Return to preinjury status and ability to participate in high level sport activity is an indicator of successful treatment (Kvist, 2004). Immediately following the injury, ice and elevation are recommended until the patient can be seen by a health care professional. The decision to treat the ligament tear by conservative measures versus surgical repair involves consideration of many factors, such as severity of the tear, patient's age, level of athletic activity, occupation, and lifestyle expectations. Conservative treatment includes RICE and rehabilitation. Severe ACL tears are usually treated with surgical repair.

Early rehabilitation is the key to success whether or not the treatment plan includes surgical repair or conservative treatment with the rehab program being similar to both groups (Souryal & Adams, 2005). Early range-of-motion, strengthening, and flexibility exercises are the cornerstone of the rehab program. The patient must be committed to the program to achieve a successful outcome and return to preinjury status.

Surgery

Surgical repair of the ACL can be performed either by arthroscopy or by open incision. Repair may include reconstruction of the ACL by using a piece of the patellar tendon or a portion of the hamstring muscle. In some cases a synthetic material is used. Recommending that the patient wear a brace when involved in strenuous sport activity remains controversial. The theory behind this practice is that the brace will protect the knee from recurrence of a ligament injury, However, McDevitt, et al. (2004) showed that there was no difference in the rate of recurrence of injury with or without functional bracing.

Patient and Family Teaching

Successful rehabilitation requires a commitment from the patient. Teaching the patient and family on why it is important to follow the program and not to participate in activities until cleared by the health care provider is needed to gain the full benefit of the therapy program.

Evaluation of Outcomes

Potential patient outcomes for each of the example nursing diagnoses for the patient with knee ligament injury are:

- Acute pain: The patient should verbalize an adequate relief of pain along with the ability to realistically cope with the pain if it is not completely relieved.
- Impaired physical mobility: The patient should perform physical activity independently or with assistive devices as needed. In addition, the patient should be free of complications of immobility, as evidenced by intact skin, absence of thrombophlebitis, and normal bowel patterns.
- Anxiety: The patient should be able to recognize the signs of anxiety, demonstrate positive coping mechanisms, and describe a reduction in the level of anxiety experienced.

The main complication of a knee ligament injury is symptomatic instability of the knee, which may inhibit the patient from participating in competitive sports at the same level prior to injury. Chronic instability may also cause damage to the other structures of the knee, such as the menisci and the articular surfaces of the joint, which may lead to osteoarthritis.

MENISCAL INJURIES

The menisci are crescent-shaped pieces of fibrocartilage found inside of the knee joint. The function of the menisci are to absorb the loading forces the knee joint experiences during movement and weight bearing and aid in maintaining the stability of the joint.

Epidemiology

The incidence of acute meniscal tears is 60 per 100,000, with a 60 percent incidence of degenerative meniscal tears after age 60 years.

Etiology

Meniscal injuries are caused by a rotational force as the flexed knee is moving toward extension. When the foot is planted, the femur is internally rotated and a valgus force is applied to the flexed knee, the medial meniscus is at risk for injury. If the femur is externally rotated and a varus force is applied, the lateral meniscus is at risk. The medial meniscus is injured more often than the lateral. The reason for this has to do with the way the menisci are attached inside the joint capsule. The medial meniscus is more tightly tethered to the tibial plateau and therefore is less able to move when a force is applied. Because of this, it is torn more easily than the lateral meniscus. The peripheral third of the meniscus has minimal blood supply, which limits its ability to heal when torn or injured. The most common location of injury is in the posterior section, with longitudinal tears being the most common type. A history of a previous meniscal injury predisposes the menisci to additional injury from a lesser force than in a healthy knee. Also with aging the menisci start to degenerate, placing them at higher risk for tears and injury (Miller, 2003).

Assessment with Clinical Manifestations

If a specific traumatic event caused the symptoms, a detailed history of the trauma, with positioning of the leg, foot, and knee is helpful in determining a diagnosis. The patient may remember hearing a popping or tearing sound at the time of the injury. If the tear is degenerative, the onset of pain may be more gradual, or it may have been caused by minimal movement such as rising from a squatting position (Miller, 2003). Symptoms can include pain over the area of the injury, swelling, stiffness, locking, catching or popping of the knee, and buckling of the knee.

During the physical assessment, the most common finding is tenderness along the joint line. Inspect the knee for joint effusion, comparing it with the contralateral knee. Meniscal injuries usually accompany ligament injuries, so stability of the knee should also be assessed (refer to section on ligament injuries).

Diagnostic Tests

Plain radiographs are used to rule out fractures and other possible causes of symptoms, but they are of little value in diagnosing torn menisci. MRI is highly specific and sensitive in the diagnosing of a tear.

Nursing Diagnoses

Based on the information gathered, examples of nursing diagnoses, interventions and outcomes in the patient with meniscal injuries include:
- Acute pain
- Impaired physical mobility
- Anxiety

Planning and Implementation

The goals of treatment are to return the patient back to preinjury status and restoring full strength and range of motion to the knee. Traumatic meniscal tears are usually treated with surgical repair. If the tear is small and of degenerative origin, conservative treatment is tried first. Conservative treatment includes the use of RICE, with strict activity restriction. A knee immobilizer is used for four to six weeks or until the pain and swelling has subsided. Once this occurs rehabilitation can begin. If the pain and swelling continue and locking of the knee is present surgery is considered.

During conservative treatment isometric exercises are used to maintain strength of the leg and to help in the rehabilitation process once the brace is removed (Miller, 2003). During the rehabilitation phase, the focus is on quadriceps strengthening and range of motion. Full return to participation in sports is usually three to six months (Miller, 2003).

For small tears, surgery usually entails suturing of the tear or partial removable when suturing is not an option. It is performed by arthroscopy and on an outpatient basis. Removal of the entire meniscus is avoided when possible due to the risk of developing osteoarthritis later in life (Englund, Roos, & Lohmander, 2003; Miller, 2003).

The patient teaching focuses on the rehabilitation program and ways to protect the knee from future injury. Following the therapy and exercise regimen is stressed to get the patient back to preinjury state. Explaining to the patient theory behind the rehabilitation will help in compliance. Strategies for future injury prevention includes having strong thigh and hamstring muscles, stretching before and after exercise, wearing shoes that fit properly and that are appropriate for the activity the patient is doing, and when skiing, ensuring that ski bindings are set correctly by a trained professional so that skis release with a fall.

Evaluation of Outcomes

Potential patient outcomes for each of the example nursing diagnoses for the patient with meniscal injuries are:

- Acute pain: The patient should verbalize an adequate relief of pain along with the ability to realistically cope with the pain if it is not completely relieved.
- Impaired physical mobility: The patient should perform physical activity independently or with assistive devices as needed. In addition, the patient should be free of complications of immobility, as evidenced by intact skin, absence of thrombophlebitis, and normal bowel patterns.
- Anxiety: The patient should be able to recognize the signs of anxiety, demonstrate positive coping mechanisms, and describe a reduction in the level of anxiety experienced.

ANKLE SPRAIN

Ankle sprain is extremely common, occurring at a rate of one injury per 10,000 people per day (Struijs & Kerkhoffs, 2005). They occur in both athletes and nonathletes and in people of all ages.

Etiology

The ligaments of the ankle act as stabilizers by preventing the ankle from movements, such as twisting, turning, or rolling of the foot. When the ankle is displaced or a sudden force is applied the ligaments are stretched beyond their normal stretching capacity and a sprain of the ligament occurs. The most common type of ankle sprain is a lateral sprain. The mechanism of injury is a combination of plantar flexion and inversion. Medial ankle sprains are less common but can occur with excessive eversion and dorsiflexion of the foot.

Ankle sprains are categorized according to severity (Table 60-1.)

TABLE 60-1 Ankle Sprain

GRADE OF SPRAIN	TYPE OF TEAR	SYMPTOMS
Grade I (mild)	Partial tear	No instability Mild tenderness, minimal swelling Able to bear weight and walk
Grade II (moderate)	Partial disruption of one or more ligaments	Mild instability Tenderness and swelling more diffuse May or may not be able to bear weight
Grade III (severe)	Complete disruption of at least one ligament	Moderate to severe instability Severe swelling inability to bear weight

Source: Gehrig, L. (2005). Sprained ankle. *Retrieved on September 26, 2005, from http://orthoinfo.aaos.org/.*

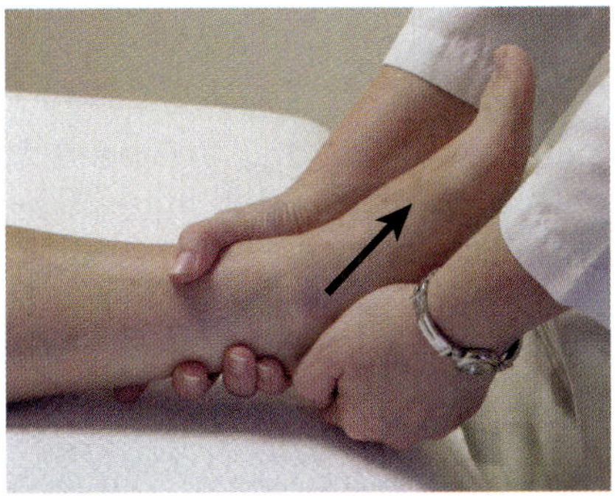

Figure 60-10 Anterior drawer test.

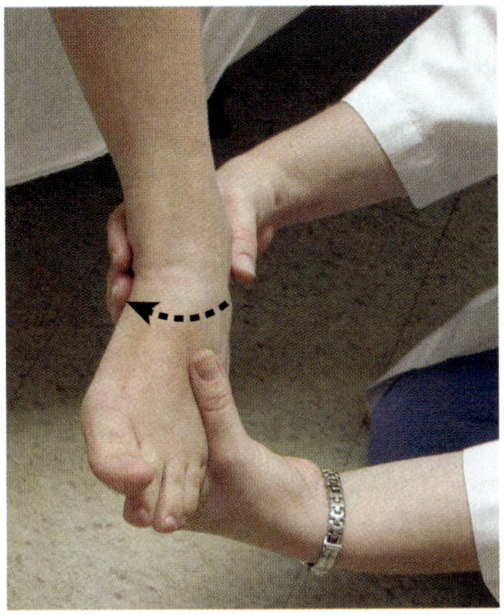

Figure 60-11 Inversion stress test.

Assessment with Clinical Manifestations

Assessment begins with a history of how the injury occurred. The patient may remember hearing a pop or a snap at the time of injury. Have the patient describe the exact motion of the foot and ankle and the position of the foot before and after the traumatic event. It is also important to ask about previous injuries to the ankle. In chronic ankle problems little force is needed to reinjure the ligaments.

The physical examination begins with observation of the joint for any gross deformities that may indicate a fracture. The amount of swelling is best determined 24 hours after the initial injury. Minimal swelling immediately after the injury may not be a reliable indication of the severity of the injury. Physical assessment should also include neurovascular status, range of motion, and presence of crepitus. Palpation of the ankle will reveal tenderness. The anterior **drawer test** and the **inversion stress test** are used in determining the stability of the ankle joint (Figures 60-10 and 60-11).

Diagnostic Tests

Plain radiographic films are useful in ruling out fractures in the ankle and foot, but are only indicated when a fracture is suspected by the presence of tenderness in the posterior half of the lower fibula and tibia or in the fifth metatarsal and if the patient is unable to bear weight. For symptoms that persist for more than six weeks, a computed tomography (CT) or a MRI is indicated to further rule out other complications.

Nursing Diagnoses

Representative nursing diagnoses for the patient with an ankle sprain include:
- Acute pain
- Impaired mobility

Planning and Implementation

The immediate goals of treatment are to prevent swelling and to maintain range of motion to the ankle joint. Immediate interventions include RICE. The amount of weight bearing to the ankle will be determined by the amount of pain. Crutches may be needed for two to three days to allow for rest of the ankle joint and to relieve pain. For more sever sprains cast boots or air splints may be used. Ice should be immediately applied. Apply for 20 to 30 minutes three to four times a day. An elastic bandage should be used to further reduce the amount of swelling and to provide support to the joint. Finally, the ankle is elevated above the level of the heart for the first 48 hours after injury to facilitate venous and lymph drainage.

Rehabilitation starts at one or two weeks after the injury. The focus is on restoring the range of motion and strengthening the ankle joint to prevent complications of chronic instability. Proprioception and flexibility training is also important improve balance and to prevent recurring injury to the joint.

Complications usually result from returning to activities too soon and not allowing the ankle to fully heal. Complications may include abnormal proprioception, imbalance, weakness, and instability of the ankle joint. A chronic ankle sprain is defined as frequently respraining of the ligaments and having symptoms for more than four to six weeks. Surgery may be indicated if the joint remains unstable after several months of conservative treatment.

Pharmacology

Anti-inflammatory drugs, such as NSAIDS, may be used to control pain and inflammation.

ACHILLES TENDON INJURIES

The Achilles tendon is the strongest tendon in the body (McGuigan & Aierstok, 2005). It absorbs large stresses during running and jumping. The tendon itself moves in two directions, lengthening and concentric contracting. This puts it at a higher risk for injury and degenerative changes.

Epidemiology

Tendon ruptures occur in men three times as often as in women. The peak incidence of rupture is in middle age.

Etiology

Injury to the Achilles tendon is seen in athletes that participate in activities that require a lot of running, jumping, and stop and go movements, such as tennis and basketball. Tendonitis is seen more commonly seen in runners from overuse and repetitive loading of the tendon. Rupture of the tendon is more commonly seen in tennis and basketball players. Many ruptures are also seen in middle age adults who lead sedentary lives who participate in physical activity (Koike, et al., 2004). There has also been a link between the use of fluoroquinolone antibiotics and Achilles tendonitis.

Pathophysiology

The Achilles tendon is located in the posterior distal third of the lower extremity. It attaches the calf muscles to the calcaneus. The blood supply to the distal portion of the tendon is poor, which predisposes this area to a higher incidence of injury. Tendonitis is seen more often in the proximal portion of the tendon and is two to three times more common than rupture (McGuigan & Aierstok, 2005). Tendonitis can result from a sudden and persistent change in the tightness of the tendon. This change causes pain and inflammation. An example of this is a woman who routinely wears high-heeled shoes and begins to wear athletic shoes while doing physical activity

Rupture of the tendon is thought to be caused by a combination of earlier injury and degenerative and regenerative changes (Koike, et al., 2004).

Assessment with Clinical Manifestations

A detailed history of the pain is necessary to make a accurate diagnosis. Tendonitis initially causes pain after physical activity. If the patient continues with activity the tendonitis will progress and cause pain during physical activity (Koike, et al., 2004). Patient with a rupture may describe a sharp severe pain and hearing a popping sound at the time of injury followed by difficulty walking.

The ankle, foot, and tendon should be inspected for deformity and swelling. On palpation, tenderness, local heat, crepitation, and a possible nodule may be present. With a rupture a gap between the tendon and the heel may also be palpated. The Thompson test is used to help in diagnosis of a rupture. The foot will normally plantar flex when the calf is squeezed just distal to the maximum girth. In a patient with a ruptured tendon the foot does not plantar flex (Koike, et al., 2004).

Diagnostic Tests

A plain radiographic film will not pick up a tendon injury. If the tendonitis is chronic, calcium deposits may be seen (McGuigan & Aierstok, 2005). MRI is often used and will show inflammation, tearing, and degenerative changes.

However, ultrasound may be the best method of visualizing the tendon because of the availability and low cost (Koike, et al., 2004).

Nursing Diagnoses

Nursing diagnoses for a patient with an injury to the Achilles tendon include:
- Acute pain
- Impaired mobility

Planning and Implementation

Treatment of tendonitis begins with resting the tendon. A heel lift or fracture boot is often used to decrease the stress on the tendon (McGuigan & Aierstok, 2005). **Cryotherapy** (cold therapy) is also used to decrease inflammation and swelling. Early treatment is crucial in preventing chronic tendonitis, which may predispose the patient to a rupture.

Tendon rupture is also treated nonoperatively. The patient is placed in a cast or brace with the foot in plantar flexion for up to six weeks. Surgical repair is indicated when the tendon ends have receded and in athletes who want to retain strength and power with plantar flexion (Koike, et al., 2004). Surgical treatment also requires cast immobilization. Physical therapy is a crucial part of the treatment plan if the patient is to return to preinjury state. The exercise regimen focuses on strengthening of the lower leg and ankle (McGuigan & Aierstok, 2005). Rehabilitation usually takes five to six months.

It is important to teach the patient the importance of following the treatment course. It may be difficult for athletes to abstain from activity to rest the tendon. However, it is important for the athlete to understand the consequences of too much activity, which may include chronic tendonitis and rupture. Once the rehabilitation phase is over, it is important to teach the patient the importance of proper warm up and conditioning before participation in high-impact sports and running to prevent another injury.

There is no hard evidence in the literature to support a consensus in the treatment of acute and chronic tendonitis (McLauchlan & Handoll, 2005). However, the goal of treatment is to return the patient back to preinjury status. This goal may be more important for an athlete than for the average individual.

Pharmacology

NSAIDs are usually helpful in the treatment of tendonitis. Steroid injections are not recommended (McGuigan & Aierstok, 2005).

Evaluation of Outcomes

Potential patient outcomes for each of the example nursing diagnoses for the patient with tendonitis are:
- Acute pain: The patient should verbalize an adequate relief of pain along with the ability to realistically cope with the pain if it is not completely relieved.
- Impaired mobility: The patient should perform physical activity independently or with assistive devices as needed. In addition, the patient should be free of complications of immobility, as evidenced by intact skin, absence of thrombophlebitis, and normal bowel patterns.

PLANTAR FASCIITIS

Plantar fasciitis is a common cause of heel pain and mobility problems from young athletes to the elderly.

Etiology

The exact cause of plantar fasciitis is unknown, but many factors may be involved. Risk factors include obesity, low arches (pes planus), reduced dorsiflexion of the ankle, and occupations that require prolonged standing (Roxas, 2005). In athletes, risk factors can include running on hard surfaces, changing the intensity or duration of an exercise or training program, and improper footwear. In the elderly, poor muscle strength of the foot and ankle and a decrease in the body's ability to heal may also play a role.

Pathophysiology

The plantar fascia extends from the heel to the toes. When the arch of the foot is flattened during walking or running the fascia is stretched. Plantar fasciitis is thought to be a degenerative process from repeated trauma that has caused microinjuries or microtears to the fascia. Inflammation of the fascia may or may not be present.

Assessment with Clinical Manifestations

The diagnosis of plantar fasciitis relies on a detailed history of symptoms. Most patients will report heel pain that is usually worse in the morning or after a prolonged period of inactivity. The pain tends to improve through out the day but may increase again at night, especially if the patient is on his or her feet all day. Recent changes in a training or exercise program, foot wear, and weight should also be explored.

The patient may experience pain and tenderness with palpation of the heel and foot. The pain may be exacerbated by passive dorsiflexion of the toes or by having the patient stand on their tip toes. Signs of inflammation, such as swelling, redness, and warmth in the area, may or may not be present.

Diagnostic Tests

Plain radiographs and bone scan may be useful in ruling out other causes of heel pain, such as a stress fracture of the heel. However, the diagnosis of plantar fasciitis is usually based on clinical assessment alone.

Nursing Diagnoses

Representative nursing diagnoses for the patient with plantar fasciitis include:
- Acute pain
- Impaired mobility

Planning and Implementation

Plantar fasciitis is considered a self-limiting condition, which means that even without treatment the symptoms will subside. However, it can take 6 to 18 months before plantar fasciitis is resolved. Because of this, treatment is focused on relieving the symptoms and returning the patient back to original baseline. Treatment begins with rest, avoidance of intense weight-bearing activity, avoidance of walking barefoot on hard surfaces, and replacing old footwear with better fitting footwear. Ice may also be use to reduce pain and inflammation after activity.

Physical and occupational therapy play a major role in the treatment of plantar fasciitis. Stretching and strengthening programs can help to correct functional risk factors, such as muscle weakness and inflexibility of the foot and ankle. Night splinting and orthotics may also be useful in more severe cases.

Vitamin C and zinc are essential components in connective tissue repair; therefore, a deficiency may contribute to changes seen in plantar fasciitis.

More research is needed to discover the full impact of vitamin C and zinc in plantar fasciitis (Roxas, 2005).

The surgical intervention of a plantar fascia release is performed only when all other therapies have failed. Complications that can occur with surgical intervention include nerve damage, which may cause a small amount of numbness to the heel area, wound infection, and osteomyelitis. An acquired flatfoot deformity may also develop requiring the patient to wear supportive footwear with good heel support.

Pharmacology

Oral NSAIDs may be useful in temporarily relieving the pain and inflammation, however, they are not curative (Roxas, 2005). Corticosteroid injections are usually given for chronic heel pain that has not responded to conservative treatment. There are many risk factors and potential complications with the use of locally injected corticosteroids, such as weakening and rupture of the fascia and atrophy of the fat pad that cushions the heel (Tallia & Cardone, 2003).

Teaching begins with the treatment course. It is important for the patient to truly rest the foot and avoid intense weight-bearing activity, to be successful in resolving plantar fasciitis. Teaching proper stretching before and after intense weight-bearing activity may be useful in preventing plantar fasciitis from recurring. Also, selecting proper footwear, which offers good arch support and cushioning may also prevent a recurrence of plantar fasciitis.

Evaluation of Outcomes

Potential patient outcomes for each of the example nursing diagnoses for the patient with plantar fasciitis are:

- Acute pain: The patient should verbalize an adequate relief of pain along with the ability to realistically cope with the pain if it is not completely relieved.
- Impaired mobility: The patient should perform physical activity independently or with assistive devices as needed. In addition, the patient should be free of complications of immobility, as evidenced by intact skin, absence of thrombophlebitis, and normal bowel patterns.

STRESS FRACTURES

Stress fractures are a common sports-related injury. They are most commonly seen in the metatarsals and tibia, and less commonly in the fibula, calcaneus, femur, and pelvis. Stress fractures in the upper extremities and in the ribs are not as common as in the lower extremity. Stress fractures of the tibia occur in the distal third of the bone and are more common in activities that involve running and jumping. Stress fractures in the metatarsals occur most frequently in the distal second or third metatarsals. These fractures are commonly seen in military recruits and in runners. Stress fractures of the calcaneus are often misdiagnosed as plantar fasciitis. They can occur at any age and are a common cause of chronic heel pain. Stress fractures of the femur are often seen in endurance athletes and are difficult to diagnosis. They also have a high incidence of complications, such as nonunion, complete fracture, and avascular necrosis (Sanderlin & Raspa, 2003). Stress fractures that occur with normal activity are called insufficiency fractures and are caused by an underlying bone disease, such as osteoporosis.

Epidemiology

Stress fractures are more commonly seen in track and field sports. In one study, 20 percent of track and field athletes developed a stress fracture, and these stress fractures made up 20 percent of the total injuries experienced by

BOX 60-3

RISK FACTORS FOR STRESS FRACTURES

- Participation in sports requiring running and jumping
- Rapid increase in amount or speed of an activity
- Rapid increase in distance with running
- Hormonal or menstrual disturbances
- Female
- Nutritional deficiencies (including dieting)
- Running on irregular or angled surfaces
- Changing surface that activity is performed on
- Inappropriate footwear
- Inadequate muscle strength
- Poor flexibility

these athletes. Many studies have also shown that stress fractures occur more often in women, especially in those who diet or exercise to the point of amenorrhea. Stress fractures tend to recur. In one study 60 percent of those with a stress fracture had a history of a previous stress fracture.

Etiology

Stress fractures frequently occur in preseason training or when there is a rapid increase in the amount or speed of activity or training or a significant increase in distance with running. They are seen in athletes who participate in tennis, track and field, gymnastics, and basketball. For risk factors, see Box 60-3.

Pathophysiology

Stress fractures occur as a result of repetitive use injury. There are two theories that may explain the development of stress fractures. The first theory is when there is an increase in activity there is a delay in the remodeling of the bone cells. The osteoclasts eats away the old bone, but the osteoblasts take a few weeks to lay down new bone cells. During this period the bone may be more at risk for microfractures, which can go on to form stress fractures. The second theory focuses on the repetitive stress on the bone at the insertion point of the muscles which can stress the bone to the point of fracture (Sanderlin & Raspa, 2003).

Assessment with Clinical Manifestations

The assessment begins with a detailed history of the pain. The patient may report an insidious onset of pain that is dull with activity. The pain usually subsides with rest and returns with the causative activity. The patient usually cannot remember a specific incidence of trauma to the injured area. Exploring recent changes in exercise and training programs can also offer clues that the injury is a stress fracture.

Palpation will reveal local tenderness at the fracture site. Redness and swelling may also be observed. The pain may be reproducible with weight bearing or with stress to the injured bone.

Diagnostic Tests

Plain radiographs may not reveal a fracture until two to four weeks after injury (Martinez & Tsai, 2004). Bone scans and MRI are more sensitive in detecting stress fractures (Martinez & Tsai, 2004; Sanderlin & Raspa, 2001).

Nursing Diagnoses

Nursing diagnoses for the patient with a stress fracture include:

- Acute pain
- Impaired mobility

Planning and Implementation

The goals of treatment focus on conservative therapies to returning the patient back to preinjury state or in the case of an athlete, back to participating in sport activity. The first step is resting the involved bone for six to six weeks. This includes complete avoidance of the activity that causes pain or a significant reduction of that activity followed by a gradual return (Martinez & Tsai, 2004). Substitution of a non–weight-bearing exercise or activity may be used to allow the athlete from becoming deconditioned, such as swimming. Patients who experience pain with walking may be placed in a walking cast or a short leg brace to achieve rest.

> **BOX 60-4**
>
> **PREVENTION OF STRESS FRACTURES**
>
> Avoidance of overtraining
> Gradual increase of intensity of 10 percent per week
> Use of proper footwear
> Attention to proper technique
> Adequate warm-up exercises
> Use of shock absorbing insoles

Rehabilitation consists of a stretching and flexibility program, cross training, and a gradual return to the offending activity. The use of air casting may be beneficial in returning the athlete to preinjury state sooner (Rome, Handoll, & Ashford, 2005).

Surgery is indicated for stress fractures that are displaced or that fail conservative treatment as indicated by nonunion or delayed union. The best cure for stress fractures is prevention (Box 60-4).

Pharmacology

There is some controversy on whether anti-inflammatory drugs should be used in the treatment of stress fractures. There is thought that to heal properly the bone needs to go through an inflammatory process. The use of NSAIDs may in fact lead to a higher incidence of nonunion. More research is needed in this area before a definitive decision can be made (Wheeler & Batt, 2005).

Evaluation of Outcomes

Potential patient outcomes for each of the example nursing diagnoses for the patient with stress fractures are:

- Acute pain: The patient should verbalize an adequate relief of pain along with the ability to realistically cope with the pain if it is not completely relieved.
- Impaired mobility: The patient should perform physical activity independently or with assistive devices as needed. In addition, the patient should be free of complications of immobility, as evidenced by intact skin, absence of thrombophlebitis, and normal bowel patterns.

FRACTURES

A **fracture** is defined as any disruption in the continuity of a bone. The fracture can result from a direct blow or from an indirect force. A fracture occurs when the bone is exposed to more stress than it can absorb. The amount of force or stress needed to cause a fracture depends on several factors including size and density of bone, the type and mount of force, and individual biological factors, such as age and underlying disease. As an individual gets older, bone becomes more brittle, and less force is needed to cause a fracture. A pathological fracture occurs when bone is weakened by an underlying disease process, and the force needed to cause a fracture is less than what is needed for normal, healthy bone. Refer to Box 60-5 for causes of pathological fractures.

> **BOX 60-5**
>
> **CAUSES OF PATHOLOGICAL FRACTURES**
>
> Osteogenesis imperfecta
> Rickets
> Osteomalacia
> Osteoporosis
> Hyperparathyroidism
> Cushing's syndrome
> Paget's disease
> Neoplasms
> Cystic bone disease
> Primary benign bone tumor
> Primary malignant bone tumor
> Infection
> Irradiation fracture

Epidemiology

According to the National Center for Health Statistics, 17,789 deaths in 2002 were attributed to fractures (2004). Between the years 2000 and 2002 the average annual number of emergency department visits for nonfatal fractures was 3,894,000 with 992,000 of these patients requiring hospitalization.

Pathophysiology

Fractures are classified by how they look on a plain radiograph and by clinical assessment. Anatomy is used to describe the bones involved, the location within the bone and if any articular surface was involved. Description also includes any displacement, angulations, or rotations that may have occurred as seen on the radiograph. Shortening, fragmentation, and soft tissue involvement are also included in the description of a fracture (see Figure 60-12 for types of fractures).

Fractures can be classified as complete or incomplete. A complete fracture is a break across the entire section of bone producing two bone fragments. An incomplete fracture occurs through only one cortex of the bone. Fractures are also described as closed or open. A closed fracture has intact skin over the site of injury while an open fracture has a break in the skin over the injury, which may have been caused by the mechanism of injury or the bone fragments themselves. An open fracture places the patient at a higher risk for infection because of contamination of the wound. See Table 60-2 for classification of types of open fractures.

Complications of fractures can be divided into immediate and delayed complications. Immediate complications include shock, fat, embolism, compartment syndrome, deep vein thrombosis, pulmonary embolism, and infection.

Delayed complications include joint stiffness, malunion, delayed union, nonunion, and refracture. Joint stiffness can result from edema, joint contractures, and immobilization. It is most common in fractures that involve the upper extremities. Malunion occurs when the fracture has healed in an abnormal position or alignment. It is caused by improper reduction or inadequate immobilization. A malunion can impair how the bone functions in several ways. It can cause irregular weight bearing in a joint, which can lead to arthritis. If the malunion occurs in the lower extremities it can interfere with the patient's gait, balance, and coordination (Whittle, 2003). Many malunions do not impede function and therefore are not surgically repaired even if a visual deformity is present. Surgical repair is considered when a deficit in function is present.

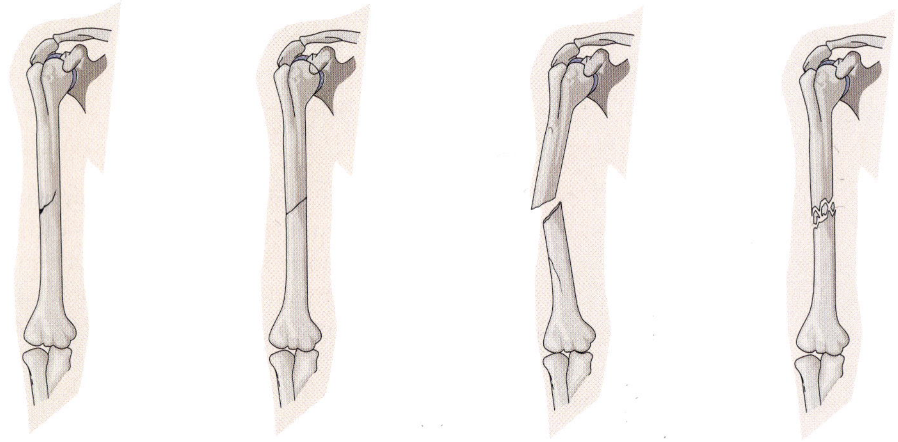

Figure 60-12 Types of fractures.

TABLE 60-2 Classification of Open Fractures

Type I	Length of wound less than 1 cm, low-energy injury, clean
Type II	Length of wound longer than 1 cm, low-energy injury, clean
Type III	Length of wound longer than 1 cm with significant soft tissue damage, fracture is comminuted, high-energy trauma
Type III A	Sufficient soft tissue to cover bone, no reconstruction surgery is needed for closure
Type III B	Damage to soft tissue is extensive requires reconstruction surgery for wound closure
Type III C	Any open fracture associated with arterial damage. Requires involvement of vascular surgeon.

Delayed union is diagnosed when healing has not advanced for three months to one year after the fracture has occurred. It is usually treated with a cast that allows as much function of the limb as possible. In the lower extremities a snug walking cast is often used that will promote healing (Lavelle, 2003). Delayed union can be a sign of infection or in the case of internal fixation a fracture at the site of the fixation. Once the cause is identified and solved, conservative treatment is usually successful (Lavelle, 2003). If conservative treatment fails, then the delayed union is treated as a nonunion.

A nonunion is when healing at the site of the fracture has ceased and union is highly unlikely. Factors that may lead to nonunion are a poor metabolic or nutritional state, overall poor health, low activity level, tobacco or alcohol intake, and having an open fracture. Surgery is required for healing to take place. The fragments are realigned and a bone graft is inserted. Another option for treatment of certain types of nonunion and malunion is the use of external fixation to achieve solid union and to correct any deformities and limb-length discrepancies caused by the nonunion or malunion (Katsenis, Bhave, Paley, & Herzenberg, 2005).

Assessment with Clinical Manifestations

Assessment begins with emergency management and the basic principles of trauma care. The initial primary assessment focuses on the general condition of the patient, which includes airway maintenance, bleeding or shock management, and stabilization of any life-threatening injuries. In multiple traumas, most fractures are not life-threatening so their management is a second priority. Once the patient is stabilized, assessment of the fracture can begin with focus on neurovascular status and pain (Keany, 2005). The mechanism of injury and a detailed description of the accident can help determine the nature and extent of the fracture and can also lead to injuries that otherwise might be missed.

Physical assessment starts with observing for any ecchymosis, edema, deformity, or other soft tissue injury, which may point to a possible fracture site. Other abnormal findings may include muscle spasms, tenderness, pain, numbness, loss of function, abnormal movement, or crepitus. If a femur or hip fracture is suspected the lower extremity may appear shortened and externally rotated (Keany, 2005). Assessment for hypovolemic shock should be completed when a femoral, tibial, or pelvic fracture is suspected because of the possibility of high-volume blood loss and the risk for exsanguinations. Signs and symptoms of hypovolemic shock include hypotension, tachycardia, tachypnea, and dyspnea.

A peripheral neurovascular assessment should be performed and documented on a frequent basis. This comprehensive examination should include a vascular assessment, comparing color, temperature, capillary refill, peripheral pulses, and edema of the involved extremity to the contralateral extremity whenever possible. The peripheral neurological examination includes assessing sensation and function. Assessment of pain is also important in determining the location of injury and the severity. Pain will increase in severity until the fracture is mobilized.

Diagnostic Tests

Radiographs should include the joint above and below the suspected fracture in order to see the extent of the injury. The patient who has sustained multiple trauma should also have a CT scan of the chest and pelvis to rule out the possibility of further injury.

Nursing Diagnoses

Nursing diagnoses for the patient with a stress fracture include:
- Acute pain
- Impaired mobility

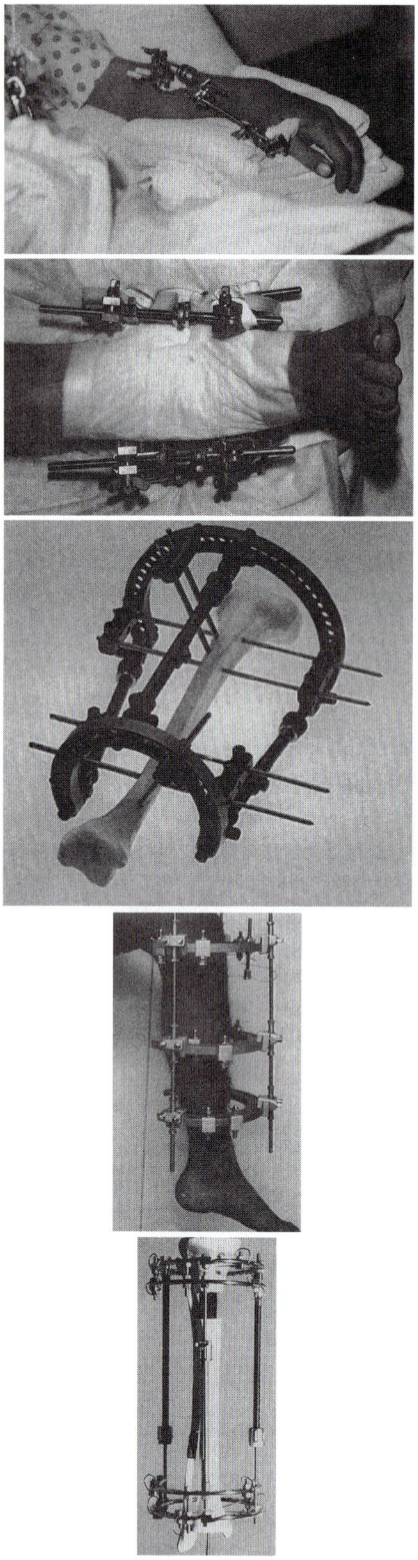

Figure 60-13 Examples of external fixation devices: A. Hoffman external fixation to the forearm, B. To the tibia and fibula, C. Ace-Fischer external fixator, D. Monticelli-Spinelli external fixator, E. Ilizarov external fixator.

Planning and Implementation

The primary goals for fracture management are the prevention of complications and the return to preinjury state. In emergency treatment, the first step is covering any open wounds or fractures with a sterile normal saline dressing to control bleeding and prevent further contamination. The next step for a closed or open fracture is splinting. Whenever possible, this should be accomplished before moving the patient. The purpose of splinting is to minimize bleeding, edema, and pain. Splinting can also prevent further injury to the tissues and structures surrounding the fracture, such as nerves, vessels, muscles, and tendons. Complications from improper handling or splinting can include increase bleeding, a significant increase in pain, and a decrease in sensation and function, which may be temporary or permanent. The incidence of fat embolism and shock are also increased.

Depending on the type of fracture, location, and other associated injuries, treatment may include closed or open reduction, internal or external fixation, amputation, or a combination of the above. If the fracture is stable and the bone fragments are properly aligned, the patient is placed in a splint or cast to maintain alignment as healing occurs.

Management of a displaced fracture starts with reduction. Reduction is the manipulation of bone segments to obtain proper natural alignment of the bone involved. It can be a painful procedure; therefore, local anesthesia or sedation may be required. Reduction can be accomplished by several different methods. Closed reduction is when manual traction is applied to move the bone segments back into alignment. Realignment is confirmed with a radiograph and then a splint or cast is applied to keep the bone segments in place. When a cast or splint is applied it usually immobilizes the joint below and above the fracture site to maintain immobilization of the fracture segments.

Open reduction is the realignment of bone segments under direct visualization through an incision. Open reduction is indicated for fractures with multiple bone segments, for widely separated bone segments, or when there is soft tissue in between the bone segments. For unstable fractures casts may not be adequate in maintaining bone alignment. Complications of not maintaining proper alignment include nonunion, delayed union, or displacement of the fracture segments. Casts also immobilize the muscles and joints next to the fracture site causing weakness, wasting, stiffness, and contractures (Gugenheim, 2004). Because of these disadvantages, internal fixation is often used for unstable fractures. Internal fixation is a surgical procedure where the surgeon implants metal wires, plates, rods, pins, screws, or nails to support the bone directly. Open reduction and internal fixation is contraindicated when there is an active infection, fractures that have multiple bone fragments, or severe osteoporosis. There are several disadvantages to internal fixation as well. It is an invasive procedure and introduces a foreign body into the patient. It is also difficult to eliminate contamination in open fractures and places the patient at higher risk for infection. It also can cause osteoporosis of the bone directly surrounding the hardware because of stress shielding (Gugenheim, 2004).

Another option in the treatment of fractures is external fixation (Figure 60-13). External fixation is the use of percutaneous pins or wires that is connected to a rigid external frame. The advantages of external fixation are listed in Box 60-6.

Patient and Family Teaching

Patient and family education begins with the type of injury and treatment options. Once a treatment option is chosen, education focuses on the treatment plan, normal bone healing, care of immobilization devices (e.g., splints, casts, external fixators), use of assistive devices, and signs and symptoms of complications.

It is important to assess the patient's and family's readiness to learn. Look for teachable moments, when the patient and family are most ready to learn. This is

BOX 60-6

ADVANTAGES OF EXTERNAL FIXATION

Minimally invasive procedure

Allows for acute and gradual fracture reduction

Immediate motion of the joints above and below the fracture

Direct visualization of soft tissue

Allows for treatment of soft tissue injuries surrounding fracture

Can be used to treat chronic infections, contractures, limb length discrepancy, acute nonunion fractures, or fractures with extensive soft tissue injury

Once healing has been accomplished, the pins or wires and external frame are removed leaving no foreign material in the extremity

Adapted from Gugenheim, J. J. (2004). External fixation in orthopedics. Journal of the American Medical Association, *291, 2122–2124.*

Uncovering the Evidence

Discussion: The National Association of Orthopaedic Nurses (NAON) has developed this guideline to present evidence-based recommendations for the care of the skin around the skeletal pin site using current knowledge gleamed from critical reviews of research literature and from expert opinion. CINAHL and MEDLINE databases were searched from 1995 through mid-2004. Only seven studies were found that linked a method of pin site care to infection rates. These studies were diverse in populations studied and definitions of infection. Therefore, the authors concluded through a meta-analysis of these studies that there is insufficient evidence on which to recommend a particular pin site care method. The evidence did provide a basis for recommendations on several actions over others until more specific answers are offered through additional research. The use of the expert panel also provided a basis for these recommendations as well. These recommendations are:

- Pins located in areas with considerable soft tissue should be considered at greater risk for infection.
- After the first 48 to 72 hours (when drainage may be heavy), pin sites care should be done daily or weekly for sites with mechanically stable bone-pin interfaces.
- Chlorhexidine 2 mg/mL solution may be the most effective cleansing solution for pin site care.
- Patients or their families should be taught pin site care before discharge from the hospital. They should be required to demonstrate whatever care needs to be done and should be provided with written instructions that include signs and symptoms of infection.

Implications for Practice: Nursing implications from this study is to be more diligent in pin site care in areas where there is more soft tissue, perform pin site care on a routine basis either daily or weekly, use of chlorhexidine 2 mg/mL as the preferred solution and to make sure the patient and family is knowledgeable in pin site care and in knowing what signs and symptoms to report to the orthopedic surgeon.

Source: Holmes, S. B., & Brown, S. J. (2005). Skeletal pin site care: National Association of Orthopaedic Nurses guideline for orthopaedic nursing. Orthopaedic Nursing, *24(2), 99–107.*

usually when the patient's pain is best controlled and the level of distraction is low (Hohler, 2004). Start with assessing what the patient already knows and build on it, giving information in small amounts so the patient and family have time to absorb the information and think of questions. Teaching is a team effort, passing on to the next nurse where the patient and family is in their educational needs will help to provide continuity. It is also important to evaluate what the patient and family has learned. This is best achieved by asking open-ended questions.

Physical therapy and occupational therapy play pivotal roles in the rehabilitation and in the prevention of complications. The physical therapist will teach the patient the proper technique for using assistive devices, such as walkers or crutches. Exercises are also important to build and maintain muscle strength and endurance. The occupational therapist's role is important in making sure the patient is as independent as possible with activities of daily living. There are many aids that may help the patient maintain his or her independence with dressing, such as dressing sticks, shoe horns, sock aids, and reachers.

PATIENT PLAYBOOK

Casts

The nurse can instruct the patient to care for their cast by the following:

Plaster casts

- The type of cast hardens within 5 to 10 minutes, but may take two to three days to completely dry.
- To move or reposition the cast, use the palms of your hands to prevent denting the cast.
- Place the cast on a soft, flexible surface to prevent the cast from flattening until fully dry.
- Reposition the cast every 2 hours to help the cast dry.
- If weight bearing is allowed, do not do so until the cast is completely dry, usually about 48 hours.
- Keep the cast dry.

Synthetic casts (Fiberglass)

- The type of cast will harden rapidly, so you can bear weight (if allowed) within 30 minutes after application.
- If the surface of the cast is rough, a sock or stockinette can be applied to protect the skin on the opposite limb, and to prevent it from snagging on clothes or blankets.
- It can be immersed in water but check with your health care provider first. To dry the cast, use a hair dryer on a low heat setting.

Helpful hints for both types of casts

- If you are not allowed to get the cast wet, protect it well with a waterproof covering, such as plastic bag. Place a cloth at the top of the cast and tape the plastic bag into place.
- If the cast does become wet or damp, dry it using a towel and a hair dryer on a low heat setting.
- Elevate the limb above the level of the heart whenever possible to decrease swelling.
- Do not scratch under your cast or poke anything down into the cast to scratch. The skin under the cast can become irritated and an infection can develop. Instead, if itching occurs, try knocking on the cast or use a hair dryer on a low heat setting.
- Inspect the cast daily, looking for cracks, soft spots, excessive flaking, or flattening.

When to call the physician

- Numbness or tingling to the fingers or toes or any part of the limb.
- Extreme pain not relieved by prescribed medication.
- Extreme tightness of the cast.
- Swollen or discolored fingers or toes.
- Cracks, soft spots, or any other problems with the integrity of the cast.
- Foul odor from the cast.
- Hot spots which may point to an infection.

Source: Altizer, L. (2004). Casting for immobilization. Orthopedic Nursing, *23(2), 136–141.*

Evaluation of Outcomes

Potential patient outcomes for each of the example nursing diagnoses for the patient with fractures are:

- Acute pain: The patient should verbalize an adequate relief of pain along with the ability to realistically cope with the pain if it is not completely relieved.
- Impaired mobility: The patient should perform physical activity independently or with assistive devices as needed. In addition, the patient should be free of complications of immobility, as evidenced by intact skin, absence of thrombophlebitis, and normal bowel patterns.

HIP FRACTURES

Hip fractures are one of the most serious health consequences of falls and are the most frequently seen injury requiring hospitalization. The problem is on the rise and is only expected to become a larger health concern for several reasons. First of all the general life expectancy of the general population is increasing along with the escalation of the total number of people over the age of 65. Secondly, the number of people age 65 or older living in nursing homes is also rising. In 1997, 1.5 million people lived in nursing homes, and by 2030 that number is expected to increase to 3 million. In 2002, nearly 13,000 people over the age of 65 and older died of fall-related injuries. Many, if not most, of these falls, and the injuries caused by the fall, are preventable. When a hip fracture occurs in people younger than 50 years of age it is usually the result of contact sports, industrial accidents, or motor vehicle accidents. This type of trauma is classified as high energy as compared to a fall, which is a low-energy trauma. Osteoporosis is a major contributing factor to the cause of hip fractures from falls. Low bone mineral density is one of the most consistent risk factors in predicting hip fractures in older women. In one study women with a low bone mineral density were three times more likely to sustain a hip fracture than women who had a higher bone mineral density. See chapter 59 for more information on osteoporosis. However, the normal aging process may also have a component in the cause of hip fractures as well. As a person ages and is less active, there is not as much mechanical load to the femur. This causes the bone to thin and weaken making a hip fracture more likely (Mayhew, et al., 2005). Other factors that increases fracture risk include lack of physical activity or exercise in the last year, reduced vision, and a fall within the last year.

Epidemiology

Based on the 2000 census, there are 360,000 to 480,000 fractures a year that are fall-related. This equals to about one in three people over the age of 64 falling each year. Women are more likely to sustain a hip fracture from a fall at a rate of 4:1. Caucasian men have the highest death rate because of a fall, followed by Caucasian women, African American men, and African American women.

Pathophysiology

The hip is classified as a ball-and-socket joint. The classification of hip fractures is based on the anatomical location of the fracture within the hip. The fracture may occur in the femoral head, neck, intertrochanter, subtrochanter, or acetabular area. Treatment depends on the location of the fracture. With a femoral neck fracture, blood supply to the femoral head may be disrupted placing the patient at risk for avascular necrosis (AVN) and degenerative changes to the femoral head especially if the fracture is displaced. Therefore this type of fracture is treated with a hemiarthroplasty. With a hemiarthroplasty, the entire head and neck of the femur is replaced with an implant. If the fracture is not displaced internal fixation with a cannulated screw is the treatment of choice (Altizer, 2005). Intertrochanteric fractures are usually repaired with a nail fixation. Subtrochanteric fractures are usually treated with an intramedullary nailing.

Complications

Infection can severely disrupt the patient's rehabilitation. Function and range of motion to the affected joint or bone can be compromised. The fracture healing process slows or stops completely, because the cells normally involved in fracture repair are now focused on fighting the infection. Patient characteristics that may increase the risk of infection include diabetes mellitus, nicotine use, steroid use, malnutrition, prolonged preoperative hospital stay, and a perioperative blood transfusion.

Inspection and observation of the incision area includes looking for erythema, edema, drainage, and tenderness. Another clue that an infection may be present is the presence of persistent pain in the joint area especially with movement (Altizer, 2005). Other signs and symptoms may include elevated sedimentation rate (ESR), progressive narrowing of the joint space on X-ray, loss of bone density, or loosening of the internal fixation devices (Altizer, 2005).

Assessment with Clinical Manifestations

Assessment begins with a history of the fall and a general medical history, including past fractures and presence of osteoporosis.

The physical assessment starts with the basics of trauma care. Refer to the section on fractures for detailed information. The fractured extremity is usually shortened and externally rotated. There may also be bruising and swelling in the groin area and inner thigh. A neurovascular assessment is critical in making sure that there is no compromise of the nerves or blood vessels in that extremity.

Diagnostic Tests

Radiographs should include a two-dimensional view of the hip including a right-angle view of the site to diagnosis the anatomical location of the fracture. An oblique view may also be helpful in determining any rotation and the extent of displacement (Altizer, 2005). The views should also include the joint above and below the site of injury to rule out any further fractures. Not all hip fractures are easily diagnosed with an X-ray. An **occult fracture** is defined as a fracture that does not show up on plain radiographic films until the healing process begins and calcification is seen. If the patient is experiencing hip pain, difficulty bearing weight, and difficulty ambulating, a nuclear bone scan or a MRI may be useful in determining the presence of a fracture (Lubovsky, Liebergall, Mattan, Weil, & Mosheiff, 2005). CT has not been proven to be effective in the diagnosis of occult hip fractures (Lubovsky, et al., 2005). Failure to diagnose the fracture can lead to serious consequences, including displacing of a stable fracture and a longer, more complicated surgery and rehabilitation.

Nursing Diagnoses

Nursing diagnoses for the patient with a hip fracture include:

- Acute pain
- Impaired mobility

Planning and Implementation

The goal of treatment is to return the patient back to his or her preinjury level of functioning. This is completed by surgical intervention and an intensive rehabilitation program.

Physical therapy and occupational therapy play important roles in helping the patient achieve preinjury state. The patient will need an exercise program to strengthen the muscles of the injured extremity as well and to increase endurance. Teaching the patient the correct use of assistive devices and providing dressing tools will help the patient regain independence.

Patient and family teaching should focus on fall and fracture prevention. If the patient is returning to the community, either to his or her own home or to a family member's home, interventions can include gait training and a long-term exercise program, review of current medications focusing on the use of psychotropic medications, and use of proper assistive devices. For patients going to a long-term or assisted living, interventions also include staff education programs. To further reduce the risk of falls, the environment should be assessed and hazards removed. Things that can be done to decrease the risk of falling include removing throw rugs and clutter in the hallway, placing nonslip mats on the shower floor, installing grab bars next to the toilet and shower, installing handrails on both sides of stairs, and improving the lighting throughout the house and outside in the garage and porch. The patient should also see his or her health care provider yearly for a routine assessment of risk factors and should have his or her vision tested yearly as well. A bone mineral density test should be completed and measures taken to raise levels if they are low.

Evaluation of Outcomes

Unfortunately the prognosis for recovery from a hip fracture is not always positive. Patients who are age 75 and older are four to fives times more likely to be admitted into a nursing home for a year or longer. Many patients never get back to their preinjury level and sustain complications because of immobility, such as pneumonia, pulmonary embolism, and future fall-related injuries. Half of older adults who suffer a hip fracture never regain their previous level of functioning and an estimated 13,000 people die each year from complication of a hip fracture.

Potential patient outcomes for each of the example nursing diagnoses for the patient with a hip fracture are:

- Acute pain: The patient should verbalize an adequate relief of pain along with the ability to realistically cope with the pain if it is not completely relieved.
- Impaired mobility: The patient should perform physical activity independently or with assistive devices as needed. In addition, the patient should be free of complications of immobility, as evidenced by intact skin, absence of thrombophlebitis, and normal bowel patterns.

COMPARTMENT SYNDROME

A compartment is an area in the body where muscles, nerves, and blood vessels are enclosed within tissue, such as bone or fascia. **Fascia** is a nonelastic connective tissue that covers and separates muscles, tendons, and ligaments.

A total of 46 compartments are found through out the body with a total of 36 found in the limbs. The most common compartments affected are the anterior compartment of the leg and the volar compartment of the forearm. Acute **compartment syndrome** can be caused by either an increase in the amount of contents inside the compartment or a decrease in the size of the compartment itself. Pressure inside the compartment can be caused by trauma especially fractures of the tibia and other long bones, severe crush syndrome, and hypotension. Peripheral vascular disease also increases the risk of compartment syndrome. See Box 60-7 for a list of causes of acute compartment syndrome.

Chronic or exertional compartment syndrome is seen with exercise and overuse that cause inflammation and edema. It is seen in long distance runners, new military recruits, or patients who have made a major change in activity. The result is an increase in pressure, which causes an aching pain and tightness. It is usually relieved by rest and rarely causes permanent damage.

The rest of this section discusses acute compartment syndrome only.

BOX 60-7

CAUSES OF ACUTE COMPARTMENT SYNDROME

Trauma

Fractures
Crush injuries
Hypothermia
Snake or spider bites
Burns

External pressure

Positioning
Tourniquets
Tight dressings
Casts
Splints
Excessive traction

Bleeding

Vascular injury
Coagulopathies

Venous obstruction

IV infiltration

Pathophysiology

When there is an increase in pressure inside the compartment no matter the cause, the result is ischemia, which causes damage to the nerves, muscles, and blood vessels. This causes a secondary elevation in the venous pressure, which obstructs blood outflow. This viscous cycle will evidentially increase pressure inside the compartment to the point that it supersedes arterial pressure, and the compartment is left without a blood supply. If the blood flow is not returned within a period of time usually four to eight hours, the structures inside the compartment will die. The result is a Volkman's contracture (Figure 60-14).

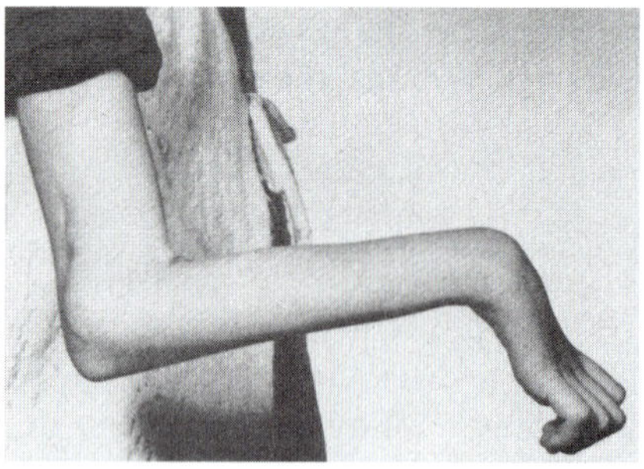

Figure 60-14 Volkman's contracture.

Assessment with Clinical Manifestations

Signs and symptoms may occur as soon as 30 minutes after the ischemia begins. Early recognition of the signs and symptoms are critical in preserving the limb. The classical symptoms include the 6 P's: pain, paresthesia, paresis, pressure, pallor, and pulselessness. The two earliest symptoms are pain disproportionate to the injury especially on passive stretching on the long muscle inside the affected compartment and a change in sensation distal to the ischemic compartment. Late symptoms include pallor, paralysis, tight or rigid compartment, and pulselessness. Neurovascular and pain assessments should be performed at least every four to eight hours for all orthopedic patients and more often, such as every one to two hours in the immediate postoperative phase. The health care provider should be notified right away if the patient develops any of the signs or symptoms of compartment syndrome.

Diagnostic Tests

Direct measurement of the pressure inside the compartment can confirm diagnosis. The measurement can be preformed by a wick, continuous infusion, or by an injection method.

A normal compartment pressure is 0 to 10 mm Hg. Compartment syndrome is diagnosed when the diastolic pressure minus the intracompartment pressure is less than or equal to 30 mm Hg.

Goals

The primary goal is prevention. This includes making sure that edema and bleeding within the compartment is minimized by preventing motion at the fracture site and minimizing soft tissue damage. This can be accomplished by splinting, traction, early closed reduction with casting, and when needed, early internal fixation. Elevating the limb to the level of the heart will also help to decrease edema in the affected limb. Elevation above the level of the heart is contraindicated, because this makes it more difficult for arterial blood flow to enter into the compartment.

Once compartment syndrome is suspected the goals of treatment include relieving the pressure in the compartment, restoring blood flow back to the structures inside the compartment and preserving the function of the limb. If the patient has a constrictive cast, splint, or dressing, the first step in relieving pressure and restoring blood flow is to bivalve the cast and loosen the underlying dressings or splints. Ice should be avoided once compartment syndrome is suspected, because it will further decrease blood flow and mask symptoms of pain. Fluid balance should also be monitored carefully, and fluids replaced as needed to ensure an adequate blood volume and arterial pressure. If the above interventions do not relieve the pressure in the compartment, a **fasciotomy** is the next step. A fasciotomy is the surgical opening of the fascia that surrounds the affected compartment. The incision is usually done length wise and the wound is left open to allow the contents of the compartment to decompress. Wet dressings are applied, and once the swelling subsides closure is accomplished. Complications of a fasciotomy include loss of fracture stabilization, necrosis of the bone, delayed union or nonunion, and infection.

FAT EMBOLISM SYNDROME

Fat embolism syndrome (FES) is seen following trauma in the presence of long bone fractures, pelvic fractures, multiple fractures, and intramedullary manipulation during internal fixation procedure. The most common causes are fractures of the pelvis, femur, tibia, or ribs (Fort, 2003). FES occurs when fat globules are released into the bloodstream and travel to the lungs and brain where they produce ischemia and inflammation. It is a serious complication of trauma and can lead to acute respiratory insufficiency, thrombocytopenia, deteriorating mental status, and death. The incidence of FES is 1 to 2 percent with tibia or femoral shaft fractures. The incidence rises to 5 to 10 percent when there are fractures of both the tibia and femoral shaft or multiple fractures as seen in pelvic fractures. The mortality rate ranges from 10 to 20 percent (Kirkland, 2005).

Pathophysiology

There are two different theories on the cause of FES. The first theory is that fat globules are released from the marrow of injured bone or injured soft tissues and enter the venous circulation through torn veins at the site of injury. The fat droplets deposit in other parts of the body including the lungs, brain, kidney, retina, or skin and cause damage to these areas. The second theory is a biochemical theory, and it proposes that hormonal changes due to trauma trigger the release of free fatty acids into the circulation, such as chylomicrons, a type of lipoprotein. The chylomicrons join together to form fat globules that deposit through out the body. This theory helps to describe how nontraumatic FES can occur (Goer & Lacey, 2005; Kirkland, 2005).

The severity of FES depends on the amount of fat released into the circulation and the overall health of the patient. The patient is at high risk for hypovolemia, shock, hypoxia, and right-sided heart failure.

Assessment with Clinical Manifestations

The most critical period for the occurrence of FES is 24 to 72 hours after the injury. The classical symptoms are hypoxemia, changes in mental status, and petechiae on the upper body. Seizures may also occur. Rales or rhonchi may be auscultated throughout the lung fields. Other signs and symptoms may include use of accessory muscles, tachypnea, dyspnea, restlessness, apprehension, anxiety, agitation, or confusion (Fort, 2003). Gurd's criteria are used to diagnosis the presence of FES. It is named after a health care provider who established the system for diagnosing FES (Box 60-8).

BOX 60-8

GURD'S CRITERIA FOR DIAGNOSIS OF FES

The diagnosis is made in the presence of one major and three minor criteria or in the presence of two major and two minor criteria.

Major Criteria

Nonpalpable reddish brown petechial rash over upper body in a vest distribution

Respiratory symptoms: hypoxia with a PaO_2 less than 60 mm Hg, pulmonary edema, bilateral CXR changes, tachypnea, and dyspnea

Cerebral changes: agitation, seizures, or coma

Minor Criteria

Tachycardia

Temperature greater than 101.3° F (38.5° C)

Retinal hemorrhages

Fat globules in the urine or sputum

Sudden decrease in hemoglobin and hematocrit levels and platelet count

Increase in sedimentation rate

Diagnostic Tests

Arterial blood gases will show an initial drop of the $PaCO_2$ due to hyperventilation, but as the compensatory mechanisms fail, $PaCO_2$ will rise and metabolic acidosis will occur.

Chest x-ray (CXR) films will show diffuse bilateral infiltrates. CT scan of the brain may show diffuse fatty infiltrates as well.

Planning and Implementation

The first priority is to prevent FES from occurring. This includes proper splinting of the fractured long bone, avoiding unnecessary handling of the fracture, and early reduction. Other ways to protect the lungs is to have the patient cough and breathe deeply and regularly to minimize atelectasis and improve pulmonary function, provide adequate oxygenation, maintain adequate hydration to prevent shock, protect kidneys, and prevent mobilization of fat, and record baseline assessments and frequently assess patient for changes in condition (Goer & Lacey, 2005).

Once FES develops, treatment is supportive and focused on preserving oxygenation. Supplemental oxygen is provided and intubation and mechanical ventilation may be necessary. Prevention of shock is another focus. Maintaining adequate circulatory volume is a must. Adequate blood pressure is also critical to ensure that the body is receiving the necessary oxygen. Hypotension is treated immediately and aggressively.

BOX 60-9

RISK FACTORS FOR DEVELOPING A DVT

- Immobility
- Surgical procedure longer than two hours
- Long bone, pelvic, or multiple fractures
- Pregnancy
- Hormone therapy
- Cancer
- History of prior DVT or PE
- Congestive heart failure
- Extensive soft tissue damage
- Venous injury
- Femoral central venous catheter
- Obesity
- Hypotension
- Chronic obstructive pulmonary disease

VENOUS THROMBOEMBOLISM

Deep vein thrombosis (DVT) and pulmonary embolism (PE) together are known as venous thromboembolism (VTE). They are major causes of morbidity and mortality in the orthopedic patient. A thrombosis is a blood clot in a vessel, when this clot breaks off and travels through the circulatory system to the lungs it is called a PE. The rate of fatal PE in orthopedic patients who do not receive any antiembolism prevention is 40 percent in total joint replacements or multiple trauma patients. Risk factors are based on Virchow's triad: trauma to the vessel, venous stasis, and hypercoagulability (Box 60-9).

Pathophysiology

Virchow's triad, which is damage to vessels, venous stasis, and hypercoagulability, contributes to the formation of the thrombosis. Injury to the vessel initiates the clotting cascade and platelet aggregation. Venous stasis develops from immobility caused by the injury itself or by the treatment. This causes the clotting factors to accumulate. Finally, the injury itself or the surgical treatment can cause hemorrhage, shock, or hypothermia, which modifies the coagulability of the blood (Fort, 2003).

Assessment with Clinical Manifestations

The diagnosis of a DVT can be difficult. The signs and symptoms are often nonspecific, and some patients have no signs or symptoms at all. The most common symptoms are pain and tenderness at or below the site of the thrombosis. The patient may describe the pain as aching, cramping, sharp, dull, severe, or mild. During the physical assessment, swelling at or below the site of the thrombosis may be present. If tenderness or pain is associated with the presence of swelling, a DVT may be present. The site may also be red and warm to touch. Homans' sign is not a reliable predictor of the presence of a thrombosis.

The signs and symptoms of a PE include unexplained dyspnea and chest pain. Other signs and symptoms may include hypoxia, apprehension, confusion, and anxiety. Breath sounds are often diminished, but rales and wheezes may also be heard. Cough, fever, diaphoresis, and hemoptysis are other less common symptoms.

Diagnostic Tests

Venous ultrasound is a sensitive and accurate diagnostic test in diagnosing the presence of a DVT. It is noninvasive and can be preformed at the bedside. Venous Doppler is also done at the bedside and is noninvasive, but it is not as sensitive and may provide false readings. Other available diagnostic tests include venography and impedance plethysmography. Both have disadvantages and are not used as often as the ultrasound and Doppler methods.

A ventilation/perfusion (V/Q) scan is often the first test ordered when a PE is suspected. The gold standard is a pulmonary angiogram, but the V/Q scan is less invasive and readily available. The V/Q test measures two areas. The first is ventilation. During this part, the patient inhales a radiolabeled gas and then X-rays are taken looking at the distribution of the gas throughout the lung fields. The second part looks at the perfusion to the lung fields. This involves injection of radiolabeled albumin into the circulatory system and X-rays are taken to show the distribution of blood flow to the lungs. A normal V/Q scan can effectively rule out a PE. Large perfusion defects that do not show up on the ventilation scan are associated with a high probability for a PE.

Planning and Implementation

The primary goal is the prevention of the DVT. This is achieved by using a mechanical form and an anticoagulant method of prophylaxis (Geerts, et al., 2004). The mechanical methods include early ambulation, elevation of the foot of the bed with the knees in extension, ankle exercises, graded compression elastic stockings, and intermittent external pneumatic compression devices. Anticoagulation choices include warfarin, unfractionated heparin, low molecular weight heparin, and aspirin. Aspirin alone is not recommended without a mechanical method (Geerts, et al., 2004).

One a DVT is suspected, the treatment goals turn to preventing additional clots, and to prevent the movement of the clot to the lungs (PE). The traditional therapy for a DVT is intravenous (IV) unfractionated heparin (Fort, 2005). This requires frequent monitoring and blood tests to monitor the level of the activated partial thromboplastin time (APTT). Platelet counts are also monitored for the presence of thrombocytopenia. Low molecular weight heparins are now being used as well in the treatment of a DVT. They do not require the IV access or the high level of monitoring as unfractionated heparin does, so often the patient does not need to be in an acute hospital setting. Oral warfarin is started within 24 hours after heparin therapy is initiated. The therapeutic international normalized ratio (INR) is 2 to 3, with a goal of 2.5. Patients receiving anticoagulants need to be monitored carefully for signs and symptoms of bleeding. This includes changes in mental status and monitoring stool, urine, and emesis for the presence of blood. The patient is usually on bedrest until a therapeutic APTT is achieved. Elevation of the leg is recommended, but the use of other mechanical devices, such as compression stockings and pneumatic devices, should be stopped to prevent a PE.

Treatment of a PE includes anticoagulation with unfractionated heparin. Even though it does not have the ability to dissolve clots, it prevents new clots and emboli. Oral warfarin is started within three days of initiation of heparin therapy. Thrombolytic therapy may also be indicated in the presence of a large PE. Thrombolytic therapy hastens clot lysis, promotes pulmonary tissue reperfusion, and can reverse right-sided heart failure. Other treatments include insertion of a vena cava filter and a pulmonary embolectomy.

AMPUTATION

Amputation is the oldest of surgical procedures. Advancements in surgical technique and prosthetic design have been motivated by the consequences of war. There have also been major advances in microvascular surgery, antibiotic therapy, treatment for musculoskeletal tumors, and orthopedic reconstructive surgery that have allowed for limb salvage in many cases where amputation would have been performed in the past. The only absolute indication for amputation is irreversible ischemia either caused by disease or trauma.

Epidemiology

According to the latest information from the National Limb Loss Information Center ([NLLIC]2002), there are approximately 1.2 million people living in the United States without at least one limb and about 185,000 hospital discharges related to an amputation every year. The number of new cases of amputation is highest in the diabetic patient population with 1 in every 185 diabetic patients undergoing an amputation of a digit or limb (NLLIC, 2002). Congenital limb deficiency rate is 2.6 per 10,000 live births (NLLIC, 2002).

Etiology

The most frequent indication for elective lower extremity amputation is peripheral vascular disease, with over half of the amputations attributed to diabetes mellitus (National Limb Loss Information Center, 2002). Trauma is the leading cause of amputation in the younger population and is more common in men because of higher exposure to vocational and recreational hazards. Amputation may also be indicated in thermal or electrical burns, severe frostbite, and gangrene. Malignant tumors may also warrant amputation, but this is less common because advances in limb salvage. Refer to chapter 60.

Pathophysiology

In peripheral vascular disease the muscle group involved (usually the calf muscle) does not receive adequate arterial blood supply either caused by obstruction or occlusion. In diabetes mellitus, this is caused by arteriosclerosis. This will evidentially lead to irreversible ischemia. In trauma, every effort is made to salvage the limb, with the only absolute indication for amputation being irreparable vascular injury.

A hematoma may form at the incision site and can delay wound healing and can also predispose the patient to infection. A hematoma can be prevented by using a drain for the first 24 to 48 hours after surgery and by using a dressing with good compression to the stump. If a hematoma does develop, it is treated conservatively with a compression dressing. If this fails the patient may be taken back to surgery to evacuate the hematoma.

Infection is also another risk associated with amputation. It is more commonly seen in patients with peripheral vascular disease, especially those with diabetes mellitus. Antibiotics can be used, but a debridement may be necessary to manage the infection.

Assessment with Clinical Manifestations

If the amputation is from chronic disease, the patient's history should include past medical history to find the cause of the amputation or impending amputation. If the cause is because of peripheral vascular disease, assess the patient for a history of intermittent claudication which includes pain (usually in the calf muscles) with activity that is relieved by rest. Also ask the patient about the presence of pain in the toes and feet at rest that improves with placing the extremity in a dependent position. If the cause is from trauma or burns, the mechanism of injury is obtained.

Physical examination starts with a thorough neurovascular assessment of the affected extremity and also of the opposite extremity. Refer to chapter 59 for instructions on how to perform a neurovascular assessment. Further assessment should include observing for discoloration of the ankles, edema, skin integrity, presence of ulcerations, presence or absence of hair on the legs, and presence of any necrosis or gangrene. Another assessment technique is the elevation-dependency test, which assesses collateral arterial blood supply. If there is a sudden blanching with elevation and significant redness when the leg is placed in a dependent position, poor collateral circulation is present (Chojnowski, 2005).

After the amputation, the postoperative assessment should include pain level, limb color, temperature, and presence of drainage and edema. Inspect the stump, making sure the stitches or staples are intact and the incision is well approximated. Mild serosanguineous drainage, edema, and inflammation may be expected, but if there is excessive edema or drainage, heat, or odor, an infection may be suspected and the health care provider should be contacted.

Diagnostic Tests

A noninvasive diagnostic test commonly used is the ankle-brachial index. This test compares the blood pressure of the arm with the leg using a Doppler ultrasound device (Rice, 2005). The most common invasive test is the angiogram. During an angiogram, radiopaque dye is injected into a blood vessel and then radiographs are taken in rapid succession to determine the size and shape of the vessel.

Nursing Diagnoses

Based on the information gathered, examples of nursing diagnoses in the patient with an amputation may include the following:
- Acute pain
- Impaired physical mobility

Planning and Implementation

With vascular disease the goals of treatment is to restore the circulation to the limb (femoropopliteal bypass) if this fails and additional bypass surgery is not possible, or the patient's pain cannot be controlled then amputation is the next step. The goal of treatment then becomes providing the patient with the highest level of functioning. To achieve this, the amputation is preformed at the most distal level that has sufficient blood supply to allow for healing.

In the traumatic amputation, the primary goal is to salvage and reattach the limb. Many guidelines and scoring systems have been established to aid in determining, which limbs are salvageable. One of the most widely used scoring system is the mangled extremity severity score (MESS) (Table 60-3).

When the amputation is performed due to trauma, the contaminated tissue must be derided and irrigated to reduce the risk of infection. Often this type of amputation will be left open to allow further debridement, and skin flaps are closed at a later time. If there is not enough tissue to create flaps to close the wound, bone revision and skin grafting may be necessary.

No matter if the amputation was caused by chronic disease, trauma, or other causes, the patient will need to adapt and accept the changes in physical appearance and functionality. Common reactions that patients may experience include postamputation depression, anxiety, feelings of vulnerability, and changes in body image, social support changes, and grief (Rybarczyk, Edwards, & Behel, 2004). Nurses are in a vital position to offer emotional support to the patient and family and to assess for depression and inadequate coping (Norris & Spelic, 2002). The patient should be encouraged to express his or her emotions and be allowed to convey grief. This will promote a full recovery by helping the patient reach his or her maximum functional level. Several factors may influence the progress and quality of coping. These include individual values and interpretations, access to health care technologies, social support, life experiences, and self-esteem (Norris & Spelic, 2002). Referrals for further treatment should be offered if the patient is struggling or exhibiting inadequate coping mechanisms. Information on local support groups and other resources should also be made available to the patient with the help of the social services department.

Patient and family teaching is crucial in the achievement of the treatment goals. The first decision the patient may need to make in a traumatic amputation is whether to attempt limb salvage (if this is an option) or to have an immediate amputation with a prosthetic fitting. With limb salvage the patient may need multiple surgical procedures to obtain soft tissue coverage. External fixation may also be necessary. Other possible complications with limb salvage are infection, nonunion, or loss of a muscle flap. The patient may also be at

TABLE 60-3 Mangled Extremity Severity Score

TYPE	CHARACTERISTICS	INJURIES	POINTS
A. Skeletal and Soft Tissue Injury			
1	Low energy	Stab wounds	1
		Simple closed fractures	
		Small caliber gunshot wounds	
2	Medium energy	Open or multiple fractures	2
		Dislocations	
		Moderate crush injuries	
3	High injury	Close range shotgun	3
		High-velocity gunshot wounds	
4	Massive crush	Logging, railroad, or oil rig accidents	4
		Gross contamination	
		Tissue avulsion	
B. Shock			
1	Normotensive	Blood pressure stable in field and in operating room	0
2	Transient hypotensive	Blood pressure unstable in field but responsive to intravenous fluids	1
3	Prolonged hypotensive	Systolic blood pressure less than 90 mm Hg in field and responsive to IV fluids only in operating room	2
C. Limb Ischemia			
1	None	Pulse present, perfusion normal	0[a]
2	Mild	Diminished pulses without signs of ischemia	1[a]
3	Moderate	No pulse by Doppler, sluggish capillary refill, paresthesia, diminished motor activity	2[a]
4	Advanced	Pulseless, paralyzed, and numb without capillary refill	3[a]
D. Age			
1	0–30 years		0
2	30–50 years		1
3	50+ years		2

[a]Points are doubled for ischemia greater than 6 hours.
Score less than 7 means that the patient has a salvageable extremity.
Score 7 or greater means that the patient has a nonsalvageable extremity.

higher risk for chronic pain, drug addiction, and greater financial difficulties. Even with all the advances in limb salvage, the patient also needs to realize that the procedure may fail and may require an amputation or the patient may end up with a limb that is not functional.

Care of the stump is important in preventing skin breakdown and to provide a good fit for the **prosthesis.** A daily skin care routine of cleansing and inspecting for redness, abrasions, and any skin breakdown is essential. Until the incision has healed the patient will need an analgesic about 30 minutes prior to stump care and dressing change. Instruct the patient to wash the stump with a mild soap and warm water. The stump must be dried thoroughly before applying a dressing, compressive bandage, or shrinking device. Often the patient can leave the stump open to air for about 10 minutes to allow the stump to dry completely. This time also allows the patient the opportunity to look at the stump and aid in acceptance. The next step in stump care is massage. This is performed on a routine basis as well to desensitize the residual limb. It also prevents adherence of the underlying tissue to the skin, which can cause complications once the prosthesis is worn. The patient should be encouraged to perform stump care and massage to increase the patient's independence and to help the patient accept the amputation. Immediately after surgery a sterile dressing is kept in place along with a compressive bandage. The compressive bandage should be applied using a figure eight method (Figure 60-15) with the greatest compression applied to the distal end of the stump to prevent edema. Instruct the patient to be cautious in using clips or pins in securing the compression dressing because of the risk of causing cuts or abrasions on the residual limb.

Before the patient is fitted for the prosthesis, a stump shrinker is used to decrease edema and to shape the residual limb for the prosthesis. To prevent other complications, such as hemorrhage, neurovascular damage, infection, abduction, external rotation, and flexion contractures, guidelines for positioning the stump must be followed. In the first 24 hours after surgery the limb

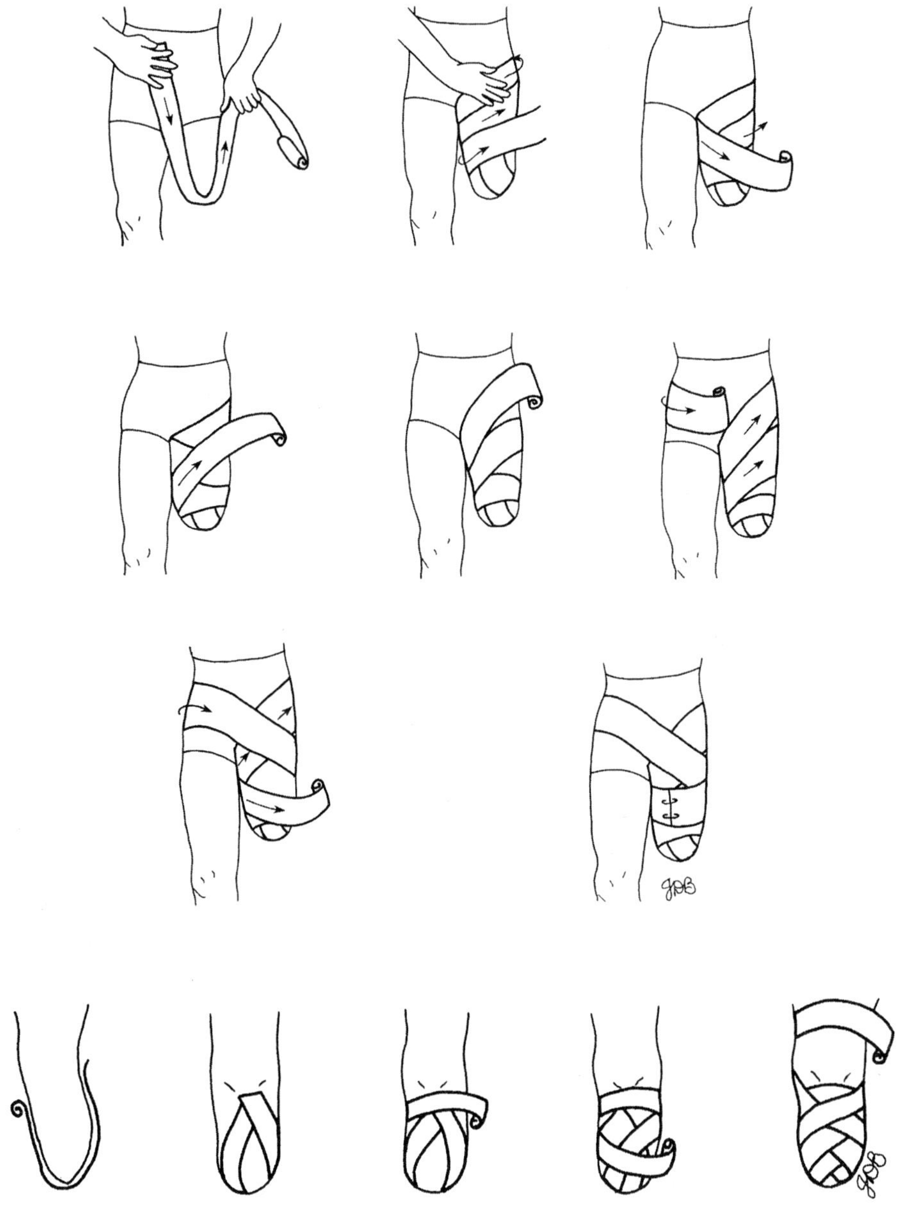

Figure 60-15 Illustration of a figure eight method of wrapping a stump.

BOX 60-10

GUIDELINES FOR POSITIONING A STUMP.

Keep residual limb elevated on a padded surface at the level of chair or toilet

Do not place pillows under the stump or bend the knee of the bed

Position legs close together

Change position every hour in a chair and every two hours in bed

Encourage use of trapeze

Lie flat on back several times a day for 10 to 20 minutes

Avoid use of pillow under stump, do not elevate past level of chair cushion

Avoid excessive hip abduction, flexion, or external rotation

can be elevated to reduce edema. After this initial period of time the stump should not be elevated or propped up with pillows because of the risk of causing contractures. A dependent position should be also avoided to help with circulation and prevention of increasing edema. While the patient is sitting in the chair or on the toilet the stump should be maintained on a padded surface at the same level as the chair or toilet. Instruct the patient to keep legs positioned together to prevent hip abduction. The patient should be encouraged to change position every hour while in the chair and every two hours while in bed. The patient can achieve this through using a trapeze. The patient should also be instructed to lie prone several times a day for 10 to 20 minutes to promote hip extension and prevent hip flexion contractures. A summary of guidelines is listed in Box 60-10.

Contractures can be prevented by good positioning. Refer to Box 60-10 for instructions on properly positioning the stump. If a contracture does occur, the prosthesis can be modified to adapt. In severe cases surgical release may be necessary.

There are several types of pain that the patient may experience after the postoperative pain has subsided. Residual limb pain or chronic stump pain may be because of several factors. The first step in assessing the cause of the pain is to inspect the prosthesis and stump. Look for any areas of abnormal pressure or edema that may indicate a poor-fitting prosthesis. Modification of the prosthesis will usually solve the problem.

A neuroma formation too close to the end of the stump can cause irritation to the nerve. The patient will experience a neuropathic type of pain, which may include burning, or a sharp shooting pain. Treatment starts with modification of the prosthesis and the use of pain medication, but if this is unsuccessful, the neuroma may need to be removed.

Phantom limb sensations are when the patient has the perception that the limb is there. They are not painful and should be expected. Over time the sensations will diminish. If these sensations are painful, then they are referred to as phantom limb pain. Most patients describe these pains as tingling, burning, throbbing, itching, cramping, stabbing, or shocking, and the pains are localized to the distal area of the limb (Talu & Erdine, 2005). The pain can be continuous or intermittent. Phantom limb pain is experienced by 50 to 80 percent of patients who have had an amputation. In many patients the pain will eventually dissipate, but for some it is ongoing. Various medications have been used in the treatment of phantom limb pain. Most narcotics are not useful because this type of pain is neuropathic in nature. The most commonly used drugs are antidepressants and anticonvulsants. Other medications that have been found effective are beta blockers, calcitonin, and ketamine. Other therapies that have been used in the treatment of phantom limb pain include nerve blocks, transcutaneous electrical nerve stimulation (TENS), acupuncture, neurostimulation, and neuroablation (Talu & Erdine, 2005). Other techniques include guided imagery, music therapy, biofeedback, and distraction. Although there is no psychological component in the cause of phantom pain, anxiety may increase the pain sensation because of the release of noradrenalin and adrenalin. Therefore, anxiolytic medications may be useful along with other stress reducing techniques to decrease this reaction.

Exercise, Physical, and Occupational Therapy

Rehabilitation is a true team effort and includes the patient, nurse, health care provider, prosthetist, physical therapist, occupational therapist, psychologist, and vocational counselor. A comprehensive approach is needed to address all aspects of the patient's life. Exercises are used to increase muscle strength and flexibility in the residual limb and the other extremities. The goal is to obtain maximum function of the residual limb as well as allowing for maximum use of the prosthesis. A pool program may help the patient achieve these goals and increase endurance, strength, balance, coordination, and mobility. The type of prosthesis chosen depends on the level of amputation, the patient's lifestyle and occupation, and patient preference. Age, agility, weight, endurance, general medical condition, and mobility are also considered. Gait training is initiated with the use of parallel bars and is progressed to crutches and then to a cane. Other important aspects of therapy are walking on uneven surfaces, mastering stairs, and learning how to fall and how to get up.

Evaluation of Outcomes

Potential patient outcomes for each of the example nursing diagnoses for the patient with an amputation are:

- Acute pain: The patient should verbalize an adequate relief of pain along with the ability to realistically cope with the pain if it is not completely relieved.
- Impaired physical mobility: The patient should perform physical activity independently or with assistive devices as needed. In addition, the patient should be free of complications of immobility, as evidenced by intact skin, absence of thrombophlebitis, and normal bowel patterns.

KEY CONCEPTS

- Unintentional trauma is the leading cause of death for Americans between the ages of 1 and 44.
- The initial treatment of sports related injuries consists of protection, RICE, and pain control.
- Patient teaching should focus on the importance of adherence to the rehabilitation schedule to achieve the best functional outcome.
- Treatment for a shoulder dislocation includes immediate closed reduction and immobilization for four to six weeks followed by rehabilitation.
- Surgical repair for a rotator cuff repair is indicated for partial-thickness and full-thickness tears in active patients once a six-month trial of conservative treatment as failed.
- The common signs and symptoms of carpal tunnel syndrome are paraesthesia, numbness, and a deep aching or throbbing pain that worsens at night to the area innervated by the median nerve (palmar aspect of the thumb, index finger, middle finger, and radial half of the ring finger).
- The most common complication after a knee ligament injury is instability of the knee.
- Meniscal injuries of the knee are caused by rotational forces as the flexed knee is moving toward extension.
- Achilles tendon injuries are most often seen in athletes whose sport or activity involves a great deal of running, jumping, and stop-and-go movements. The prognosis for an Achilles tendon rupture is good.
- Plantar fasciitis is a self-limiting condition; however, it may take 6 to 18 months before the symptoms resolve.
- Stress fractures can result from repetitive use or may be a result of an underlying pathological condition, such as osteoporosis.
- The primary goals in the management of a fracture are the prevention of complications and a return to preinjury states of function.
- The advantages of external fixation over internal fixation and immobilization with a cast include acute and gradual reduction, immediate mobility of adjacent joints, and direct visualization of soft tissues.
- Injuries from falls are a major health concern for the elderly population.
- In the elderly population the prognosis for a full recovery from a hip fracture is poor with many never returning to preinjury status.
- The first signs and symptoms of compartment syndrome are extreme pain with passive stretching and change in sensation distal to the affected compartment.
- The signs and symptoms of a PE are unexplained dyspnea, chest pain, and a feeling of apprehension or anxiety.
- Common reactions that a patient may experience after an amputation include depression, anxiety, feelings of vulnerability, changes in body image, and grief.
- It is important for the nurse to encourage the amputee to express his or her feelings and to provide the patient with additional resources, such as support groups.
- The majority of patients who have had an amputation will experience phantom limb pain; however, chronic phantom limb pain is rare.

REVIEW QUESTIONS

1. The home health nurse is teaching a patient with osteoporosis about reducing the risk for falls. Which of the following recommendations is not necessary to include in the teaching plan?
   1. Installing grab bars in the bathroom
   2. Use of nightlights
   3. Installing railings to both sides of stairs
   4. Removing wall-to-wall carpeting
2. A patient enters the emergency department for a lower leg injury. There is a visible deformity to the lower aspect of the leg, and it appears shorter than the other leg. The area is painful, swollen, and beginning to show signs of bruising. The nurse understands that the patient has experienced a:
   1. Contusion
   2. Sprain
   3. Fracture
   4. Strain
3. The nurse witnesses a patient fall in the bathroom, and the patient is now lying on the floor. The nurse suspects that the hip may be fractured. Which of the following interventions is of the highest priority of the nurse?
   1. Immobilize the leg before moving the patient
   2. Notify the patient's family of the fall
   3. Call the radiology department for an X-ray
   4. Reassure the patient that everything will be alright
4. Which of the following is *not* true concerning a plaster cast?
   1. The patient will need to keep the cast dry
   2. The patient will be able to bear weight on the cast in 30 minutes
   3. The cast can be elevated to the level of the heart
   4. The cast will give off heat as it dries
5. The patient has a fiberglass cast and asks the nurse when the patient will be able to walk on the cast. The nurse tells the patient:
   1. In 30 minutes
   2. In 8 hours
   3. In 24 hours
   4. In 48 hours
6. The nurse is assessing a patient with a fiberglass cast to the lower leg. Which of the following signs and symptoms is indicative of an infection?
   1. Coolness and pallor of the extremity
   2. Diminished pedal pulse
   3. Pain with passive stretching of toes
   4. Presence of a hot spot on the cast
7. Which of the following patients is at most risk for FES?
   1. A patient with a hip fracture
   2. A patient with a sprained ankle
   3. A patient with a mid shaft femur fracture
   4. A patient with a shoulder dislocation
8. Which of the following symptoms is not indicative of FES?
   1. Restlessness
   2. Decrease in pedal pulses
   3. Dyspnea
   4. Petechial rash over chest
9. Which of the following symptoms are early indicators of compartment syndrome?
   1. Pulselessness and pallor
   2. Swelling at the site and inability to move joints
   3. Fever and erythema
   4. Pain with passive motion and loss of sensation
10. Which of the following diagnostic tests is used for the diagnosis of a pulmonary embolism?
    1. Ventilation/perfusion scan (V/Q scan)
    2. CXR
    3. Nuclear bone scan
    4. MRI
11. Which of the following interventions is not appropriate for caring for a stump postoperatively?
    1. Allow patient to lay prone every day for 20 to 30 minutes
    2. Elevate the stump on two to three pillows
    3. Encourage patient to look at stump
    4. Remove and rewrap ACE bandage or elastic stump shrinker three to four times a day

REVIEW ACTIVITIES

1. Complete a rotation visit an outpatient rehabilitation facility. What type of injuries do the patients have? What treatments have they had? What type of exercises are they doing with the therapist? What activity restrictions do they have?

2. Complete a rotation visit to an emergency department that receives a high number of trauma patients. What kinds of trauma patients are seen? What treatments did the paramedics give the patients in the field? How did they immobilize any fractures that are seen?

3. Visit an inpatient orthopaedic unit. How many hip fracture patients are admitted? What is the ratio of hip fracture patients to other types of orthopaedic patients? Describe the type of hip fractures seen and the surgical treatment used to fixate the fractures. Does the surgeon give a rationale for the surgical treatment chosen? If not, list why you think that particular surgical treatment was chosen? Which surgical procedures require that the patient follow hip precautions?

4. Develop a teaching plan for an elderly patient who is at risk for falls. How do you personalize the plan for the individual patient? List some of the important questions you would ask the patient. What are the main elements of the teaching plan?

5. Perform a search of the local resources available for a patient who has recently undergone an amputation. How would you find these resources? What vital people would you ask? What Web sources are available? Who sponsors these sites? How can you tell if these sites are reliable sources?

Visit the Contemporary Medical-Surgical Nursing online companion resource at www.delmarhealthcare.com for additional content and study aids. Click on Online Companions then select the Nursing discipline.

UNIT

XV

Alterations in Reproductive Function

Chapter 61 Assessment of Reproductive Function

Chapter 62 Female Reproductive Dysfunction: Nursing Management

Chapter 63 Breast Alterations: Nursing Management

Chapter 64 Male Reproductive Dysfunction: Nursing Management

CHAPTER

61

Assessment of Reproductive Function

Mary Fry, PhD, RN

KEY TERMS

Androgens
Azoospermia
Climacteric
Detumescence
Gametes
Menarche
Menopause
Menstrual cycle
Myotonia
Oligospermic
Oocytes
Ovulation
Parity
Sexual dysfunction
Spermatogenesis

CHAPTER TOPICS

- Anatomy and Physiology of the Male and Female Reproductive Systems
- Sexual Response Cycle
- Assessment of Reproductive and Sexual Function
- Diagnostic Studies of Reproductive Function

Reproductive health assessment should be a part of every complete physical assessment. Reproductive health issues are relevant to lifestyle, healthy intimate relationships, and reproductive choices to bear children or prevent unintended pregnancies. Reproductive system dysfunction and disease take a high and costly toll in loss of life, infertility, and epidemic numbers of sexually transmitted infections, as well as the emotional stresses of **sexual dysfunction** and intimate relationship problems. Because of the sensitive nature of sexual concerns, health care providers must first become comfortable with their own sexuality and develop a professional manner in addressing sexual concerns with patients so that patients are able to initiate discussion of any reproductive health concerns they are experiencing.

ANATOMY AND PHYSIOLOGY

When comparing males and females, many of the structures and functions of the reproductive systems are more similar than different, with the exception of women's unique role of pregnancy and birth and the associated menstrual cycling. Healthy sexuality, sexual function, and reproductive function are integral with, and dependent on, overall health and emotional well-being.

Male Reproductive System

The primary functions of the male reproductive system are (a) production of sperm, (b) transport and deposit of sperm in the female reproductive tract, and (c) secretion of testosterone. The testes are the primary reproductive organs. Testosterone is necessary for the development of reproductive functions of **spermatogenesis** (formation of mature functional spermatozoa from the testes, usually beginning during puberty and continuing throughout the life of the adult male), sexual libido, and secondary sex characteristics of the male. The secondary reproductive organs are the ducts (epididymis, vas deferens, ejaculatory ducts, and the urethra), sex glands (prostate gland, bulbourethral gland, and seminal vesiclcs), and the external genitalia (scrotum and penis) (Figure 61-1).

Testes

The testes are two oval, firm, smooth organs that produce spermatozoa and testosterone. They are 4 to 5 cm long and 2 to 3 cm wide. The testes are suspended from the body by the spermatic cord, which contains the vas deferens and testicular blood and lymph vessels and nerves. Each testicle is covered by a sac derived from the peritoneum acquired during its descent from the abdomen during fetal development. Under the sac each testis is surrounded by a thick capsule of collagenous connective tissue. The posterior surface of

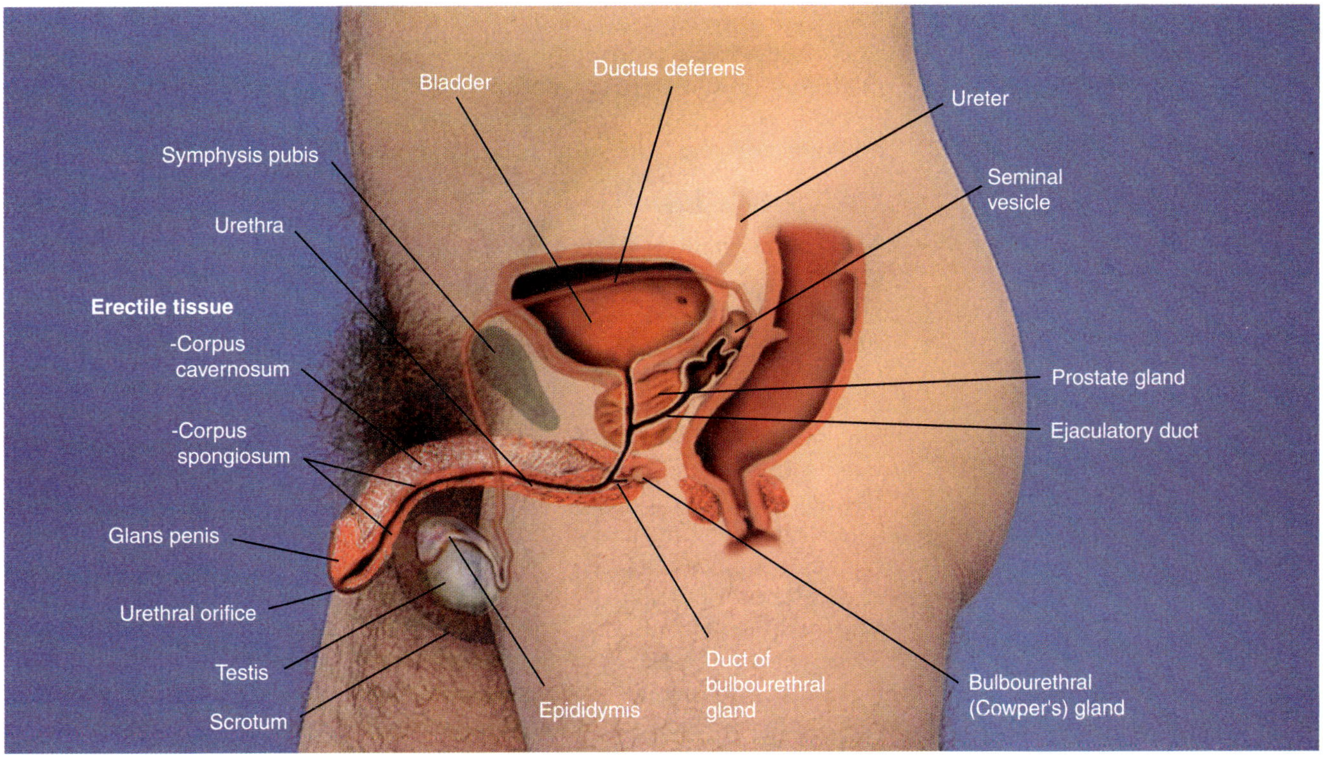

Figure 61-1 Male genitalia.

the sac is thickened to form the mediastinum from which septa extend into the gland to separate it into about 250 lobules. Each lobule is filled with 1 to 4 seminiferous tubules, connective tissue, vascular supply, lymphatic vessels nerves, and interstitial cells.

Spermatozoa are produced within the seminiferous tubules. The interstitial cells produce testosterone. Within each testis there are about 200 meters of seminiferous tubules accounting for 80 to 90 percent of the testicular mass. Seminiferous tubules contain a lining of germ cells and specialized Sertoli cells that partially envelop and nurture the developing **gametes** (a mature male or female reproductive cell). The Sertoli cells are joined to one another by tight junctions so that substances cannot freely flow from the blood to the tubular lumen. This testis-blood barrier is important in protecting the sperm from antibodies in the blood. Follicle-stimulating hormone (FSH) from the pituitary gland stimulates Sertoli cells to produce androgen-binding protein, which is excreted into the lumen of the tubule. This provides for a high concentration of testosterone within the lumen necessary for spermatogenesis. The rete testes, a meshwork of ducts, collect sperm from the seminiferous tubules. The sperm are transported to the epididymis by testicular fluid pressure, ciliary action, and contraction of the efferent ductules.

Epididymis and Vas Deferens

The epididymis is a hood-like structure lying on the top and back side of each testis. It consists of about 6 meters of tightly coiled tubule. As they travel through the epididymis over 12 days, spermatozoa are functionally and morphologically readied for fertilization. The sperm leave the epididymis during sexual arousal and travel through the vas deferens that propels sperm forward by muscular peristaltic contractions into the ejaculatory duct. Supported within the spermatic cords, the vas deferens is continuous with the tail of the epididymis, passing through the superficial inguinal ring, inguinal canal, and deep inguinal ring to reach the posterior surface of the bladder, where it joins with the duct of the seminal vesicle to form the ejaculatory duct.

Seminal Vesicles

The seminal vesicles are glandular sacs that reside behind the bladder. The thick alkaline fluid secreted by the glandular epithelium of the seminal vesicle contributes about 60 percent of the seminal fluid volume. This fluid is rich in fructose, citric acid, amino acids, proteins, and prostaglandins for the health and nutrition of the sperm.

Prostate Gland

The prostate gland is located in front of the rectum just under the bladder and surrounds a portion of the urethra. The prostate is comprised of 30 to 50 branched glands, weighing about 20 g and measuring 4 by 2 by 3 cm. It is surrounded by a fibroelastic capsule that penetrates the gland to divide it into lobes. The capsule and the stroma within the gland contain smooth muscle cells capable of contracting to expel the prostatic fluid. The ejaculatory ducts join the urethra within the prostate gland. The prostate gland produces a milky alkaline fluid rich in citric acid, spermine, cholesterol, phospholipids, fibrinogenase, fibrinolysin, zinc, and acid phosphatase, and other proteins. The alkalinity helps to neutralize the acidity of the male urethra and female vagina. It contributes about 30 to 35 percent of the total seminal fluid volume.

The central portion of the prostate contains pseudostratified epithelium. The peripheral zone is composed of stratified epithelium, occupies some 70 percent of the gland's volume, and is the most prevalent site of prostatic cancer. The prostate cells, as well as prostate cancer cells, produce a protein called prostate specific antigen (PSA), which is used as a biomarker for metastatic cancer of the prostate. The transitional zone between these types of tissue is the most common site of benign prostatic hyperplasia. Benign prostatic hypertrophy (BPH) occurs in about 50 percent of men over the age of 50 years. The prostate remains normal size until the age of 40 or 50 when, in some men, in association with decreasing testosterone, it degenerates without any symptoms.

Bulbourethral Glands

The bulbourethral glands (Cowper's) are two pea-sized glands located just below the prostate gland. They are connected to the urethra by small ducts. During sexual arousal the glands secrete alkaline mucus into the penile urethra. The alkalinity of the mucus protects sperm by neutralizing any residual acidic urine in the urethra.

Penis

The penis functions as the external male sex organ and also a passageway for urine. Its structure consists of two dorsally paired corpus cavernosa, and one ventrally located corpus spongiosum that surrounds the urethra. These three cylindrical masses are wrapped in thick membranous sheaths and are surrounded by a loose layer of skin. The corpus spongiosum expands at the terminal end to form the glans penis. The erectile tissues are composed of venous spaces lined with epithelial cells separated by connective tissue and smooth muscle cells. The arterial supply to the penis originates at the internal pudendal arteries. Nutritive arteries supply oxygen and nutrients to the vascular tissues. Other arteries empty directly into the erectile tissues, and when activated by sexual arousal greatly increase the flow into the penis. The glans is highly innervated with sensory neurons that are sensitive to contact and friction during sexual stimulation, which may result in pleasure sensations, erection, orgasm, and ejaculation of semen. The glans is naturally covered by a retractable foreskin. As newborns many men had the foreskin removed in a procedure called circumcision for religious or sociocultural reasons.

Spermatogenesis

Male contribution to reproduction is through spermatogenesis, a process that requires endocrine regulation from the hypothalamus and pituitary interacting with interstitial cells within the testes to produce, mature, and eject sperm in sufficient numbers to effectively fertilize the ovum in the female. The process of mating requires that the penis becomes erect through sexual stimulation and that erection is maintained for penetration and ejaculation into the female vagina. These complex functions require functional endocrine, neurological, and vascular interactions within the male genitalia. Psychological, relational, and sociocultural factors can also play important roles in creating healthy sexual responses for many men.

Spermatogenesis is the process of sperm generation in the seminiferous tubules in the testes. When the male enters puberty, the gonadotropin-releasing hormone (GnRH) produced by the hypothalamus is received by the anterior pituitary gland, which in turn releases FSH and luteinizing hormone (LH). FSH establishes the function of the Sertoli cells in the interstitial tissue of the testes and stimulates mitotic division of spermatogonia. Sertoli cells also regulate sperm production by producing inhibin, which provides negative feedback to reduce pituitary FSH. LH increases testosterone production by the interstitial cells in the interstitial tissue of the testes. Testosterone in turn promotes Sertoli cell function and maintains spermatogenesis.

The process of spermatogenesis takes 70 days for cells to mature in an orderly process along the length of the seminiferous tubules. It occurs in three phases: (a) proliferation of the stem cell spermatogonia by mitotic division, (b) production of the haploid gamete by meiotic division, and (c) morphological maturation of spermatids into spermatozoa. Mature males continue to produce spermatozoa throughout their lives, with several hundred million sperm produced each day.

Spermatogonia are labile and can be affected by seasonal hormonal and temperature cycles, disease, trauma, or heat. As external structures, the testes are able to maintain a lower than core body temperature necessary for healthy sperm production. Spermatozoa that are not ejaculated die and are reabsorbed within the body.

Semen Production

Semen is composed of secretions produced by the testes, seminal vesicles, prostate gland, and bulbourethral glands. Normal ejaculate volume is between 2 and 6 mL, 60 percent of the volume from the seminal vesicles, 30 to 35 percent from the prostate gland, and a small amount of the volume from sperm and bulbourethral secretions. Normal semen pH is 7.2 to 8.0. Prostatic secretion is more acidic, and seminal vesicle fluid is alkaline due to the presence of fructose. Infections can increase the alkalinity of semen.

Androgen Hormone Production

The male sex hormones are called **androgens.** Most androgens are produced by the testes, although the adrenal cortex also produces a small amount. Testosterone, the primary androgen, is responsible for the growth and development of the masculine characteristics. It directly influences the maturation of the male sex organs. After puberty, sperm development and sexual drive, as well as erectile function are maintained by testosterone. The secondary male sex characteristics (facial hair patterns, thickened vocal chords, and increased muscle mass) are also under the influence of testosterone. Testosterone secretion appears to decline slowly and continuously throughout adult life in men, with plasma levels decreasing about 35 percent between 20 and 85 years of age.

Because testosterone is the main hormonal mediator of libido, when testosterone levels decline, sexual desire decreases. Testosterone also has a critical role in stabilizing the levels of intracavernosal nitric oxide synthase, the enzyme responsible for triggering the nitric oxide cascade required to have an erection.

Erection and Ejaculation

Healthy erectile response requires functional neurological and vascular systems. The neural pathways involved in erection are located in the sacral segments of the spinal cord between the S3 and T12 vertebrae. Input from sensory endings in the genitalia and descending tracts carrying impulses generated from erotic stimuli are integrated in the spinal cord. Sensory signals from physical stimulation of the penis are sent via the pudendal nerve to the erection center. Incoming signals activate connector nerve cells, which in turn stimulate nearby parasympathetic neurons. These neurons then transmit erection-inducing signals from the sacral spine to the endothelial linings of penile arterioles. Endothelial linings of the arterioles in the corpus cavernosa release nitric oxide, which activates the enzyme guanylate cyclase, which in turn increases cyclic guanosine monophosphate (American Association of Clinical Endocrinologists Male Sexual Dysfunction Task Force, 2003). The smooth muscles in the arterioles relax and allow increased inflow of blood. This reflex arc needs to remain intact for an erection to be possible. When these systems are functioning, the male has the ability to achieve and maintain an erection of sufficient duration and firmness to complete satisfactory intercourse through vaginal penetration as desired.

Pharmacological treatments of erectile dysfunction, such as sildenafil (Viagra), target the enzymatic processes in the epithelium of the erectile tissues. Erectile functions may be affected by injury and disease factors, such as lumbar neurological injuries; vascular disease affecting large or small vessels, neurological conditions, such as multiple sclerosis, Parkinson's disease, peripheral neuropathies, and endocrine disorders.

Ejaculation is the reflexive phenomenon that ejects the seminal fluid through the penis. Ejaculation is usually preceded by erection of the penis and can occur during copulation, masturbation, or as a nocturnal emission. Effective sexual stimulation of the penis results in buildup of neural excitation to a critical level. When the threshold is reached, several internal events are triggered. Ejaculation occurs in two stages. In the emission phase, the prostate, seminal vesicles, and upper portions of the vas deferens undergo contractions bringing the seminal fluids into the ejaculatory ducts and prostatic urethra. The urethral sphincters (to the bladder and below the prostate) trap the seminal fluid in the urethral bulb. The male experiences this as a sense that orgasm is imminent.

The second stage of ejaculation, called the expulsion phase, occurs when strong, rhythmic contractions of pelvic muscles that surround the urethral bulb and root of the penis expel the collected semen through the urethra. The external sphincter below the prostate relaxes while the internal sphincter remains contracted to prevent the escape of urine.

Although male orgasm is associated with ejaculation, these processes are not one and the same, nor do they necessarily occur together. Prior to puberty, orgasms may not involve ejaculation. If several orgasms occur within a sexual encounter, some orgasms may be nonejaculatory. Some men may experience retrograde ejaculation into the bladder with little or no ejaculation from the penis, particularly after prostate surgery if internal sphincter damage has occurred.

Female Reproductive System

The primary functions of the female reproductive system are (a) production of ova, (b) secretion of hormones, (c) pregnancy and birth of a fetus, and (d) breastfeeding the infant. The main reproductive organs of the female are the ovaries, oviducts, uterus, vagina, external genitalia, and breasts.

The female reproductive functions of **ovulation,** pregnancy, birth, and lactation are regulated by a complex neuroendocrine process referred to as the reproductive axis. The hypothalamus, pituitary gland, and ovaries function to produce hormones that interact to regulate the **menstrual cycle;** facilitate the maturation and release of ova; maintain an enriched endometrial lining in the uterus, which is shed and replenished monthly; maintain the endometrium in response to embryonic hormones in pregnancy; and interact with placental-fetal hormones that sustain the pregnancy, prepare for lactation, and produce milk to meet infant nutritional needs after birth. Because of the complex and multiple levels of function, when menstrual disorders and or fertility issues arise it is sometimes difficult to determine the cause because dysfunctions in the system may occur at any of the functional levels.

Ovaries

The ovaries are solid, paired, oval bodies about 3 cm long by 1.5 cm wide. Each ovary is divided into a medulla and a cortex. The medulla is composed of loose connective tissue, blood vessels, lymphatics, and nerves. The cortex is composed of Graafian vesicles, which contain the ovum. At birth the ovaries contain between 2 to 4 million ova. Most of these ova will degenerate across time until there are only 300,000 to 400,000 ova present at puberty. These begin maturing one or more at a time during monthly menstrual cycling after the age of puberty through to menopause. The woman may release fewer than 500 mature ova during monthly ovulation across her reproductive years.

Fallopian Tubes

The fallopian tubes are 8 to 14 cm long, extending from a fimbriated end over the ovary to a narrowed insertion point in the upper uterine wall. The lumina are internally continuous with the uterine cavity. The fimbriae create a small current that pulls ova released from the ovaries into the tube. The tubes are lined with longitudinal ciliated and secretory columnar epithelial cells. Along with the cilia, the fallopian tubes produce contractions that can move the ovum toward the uterus, a 2- to 3-day journey. Secretory cells provide nutrients for the ovum during transport. Fertilization of the ovum usually occurs within the fallopian tube.

Uterus

The uterus is a hollow, pear-shaped, muscular organ, approximately 7.5 cm long by 5 cm wide by 2.5 cm thick. The walls of the uterus are composed of three layers: the external peritoneum, the middle muscular myometrium, and the internal endometrium. Its size varies slightly according to **parity** (the number of viable births) a woman has experienced.

The fundus or body of the uterus is covered by the peritoneal layer, which separates the uterus from the abdominal cavity. The lining flows from the uterus on the anterior side to form a pouch with the bladder wall called the vesicouterine pouch. On the posterior side, the peritoneal lining forms the rectouterine pouch (Douglas' cul-de-sac) between the uterus and the vaginal-rectal wall. The uterus is held into position by several ligaments. The round ligaments extend laterally from the uterine wall and down to the internal inguinal ring, through the inguinal canal where they blend with the labia majora. The broad ligaments are folds of peritoneum that envelope the fallopian tubes and extend to the lateral pelvic wall. The uterosacral ligaments extend posteriorly from the uterus to the sacrum. The body of the uterus is usually flexed anteriorly but may also be retroflexed.

The myometrium of the uterus is formed by three overlapping layers of smooth muscles that are interlaced with blood vessels. These muscles stretch and grow in size to accommodate a growing fetus, contract at intervals during labor to expel the fetus, and then contract tightly to minimize bleeding after childbirth. The smooth muscle cells shrink in size after childbirth, allowing the uterus to return to normal size within a few weeks.

The inner endometrial layer of the uterus is composed of tubular glands and arteries that can be divided into two functional segments. The outer layer is built up each month under the influence of estrogen and progesterone to form a rich nutrient bed prepared to receive a fertilized ovum. This portion is shed during the menstrual period when fertilization of an ovum did not occur. The base of epithelial and glandular cells remains in tact, supplying the replicative cells to regenerate the lining after menstruation.

Cervix

The cervix is the portion of the uterus that extends into the vagina. The cervix is composed of fibrous, muscular, and elastic tissue and is lined by simple columnar and stratified squamous epithelium. The fibrous connective tissue is the predominant component. Smooth muscle, making up about 15 percent of the cervix, is mainly located in the upper portion. The vaginal portion has rare smooth muscle fibers.

The cervical canal is approximately 2.5 cm long and provides the passageway for sperm to enter the uterus and menstrual flow to exit the uterus. The internal os of the cervical canal is located at the junction with the uterine corpus. The endocervical surface and the infolding that create glands are lined by a simple columnar mucin-producing epithelium. The cervical mucus is subject to profound cyclic changes. Under estrogen stimulation, the endocervical secretions are profuse, watery, and alkaline, facilitating sperm penetration. During the postovulatory phase, secretions are scant, thick, and acid, contain numerous leukocytes, and act as a barrier for sperm penetration. The external os is located centrally on the vaginal portion of the cervix. The os is circular in women who have not borne children and is slit-like in women who have borne children.

The outer cervix is covered with squamous epithelium. Where the endocervical glandular epithelium joins the squamous epithelium is the transformational zone known as the squamocolumnar junction. The clinical identification of the transformation zone is important, because almost all cervical squamous neoplasia and their precursors begin in this area. During the reproductive period, the transformation zone is located on the exposed portion of the cervix and can be visualized.

Vagina

The vagina is a 7.5- to 10-cm canal that extends upward and backward from the vulva to the uterus. It is situated behind the bladder and in front of the rectum and its axis forms an angle of over 90 degrees with that of the uterus. Its walls are ordinarily in contact, and the usual shape of its lower part on transverse section is that of a collapsed H. It is constricted at its commencement, dilated in the middle, and narrowed near its uterine extremity. It surrounds the vaginal portion of the cervix, its attachment extending higher up on the posterior than on the anterior wall of the uterus. The recess behind the cervix is called the posterior fornix, while the smaller recesses in front and at the sides are called the anterior fornix and lateral fornix.

The vagina consists of an internal mucous lining and a muscular coat separated by a layer of erectile tissue. The mucosal lining is stratified squamous epithelium. The epithelium contains elastic fibers and a rich venous and lymphatic network. Although the vaginal mucosa contains no glands, its surface is lubricated by cervical mucus and by direct transudate through the mucosa during sexual stimulation. Secretions from the vaginal epithelial cells contain glycogen and liquid. The amounts of glycogen and transudates secreted by the vaginal mucosa are influenced by ovarian hormones. Normal vaginal flora, particularly *Lactobacillus acidophilus,* interact with the glycogen to produce lactic acid, maintaining an acidic pH of 4 to 5 in the vagina. This acidity reduces susceptibility to vaginal infections.

The vaginal mucous membrane is continuous above with that lining the uterus. The presence of longitudinal ridges along with numerous transverse ridges, or rugae, on the vaginal wall allows the vagina to be highly distensible during intercourse and the birth process. The submucosa is loose erectile tissue, containing numerous large veins, which by their anastomoses form a plexus, together with smooth muscular fibers derived from the muscular coat. The muscular coat consists of two layers: an external longitudinal layer and an internal circular layer. The longitudinal fibers are continuous with the superficial muscular fibers of the uterus.

Vaginal tissues receive their blood supply from uterine arteries and sometimes branches of the internal iliac artery. Blood returns to the venous system through veins that empty into the internal iliac veins. Lymphatic drainage is via the external and internal iliac lymph nodes and superficial inguinal lymph nodes. The muscles of the pelvic floor provide important support to the vagina and uterus.

External Genitalia

The external genitalia, also known as the vulva, extend from the mons pubis anteriorly to the anus posteriorly and laterally to the inguinal-gluteal folds. The vulva include the mons pubis, the clitoris, the labia majora and minora, the hymen, Bartholin's and Skene's glands and ducts, and the vaginal introitus (Figure 61-2).

Mons Pubis

The mons pubis is a fatty layer covered with coarse pubic hair, lying over the pubic bone. It provides some protective padding during intercourse. Touch and pressure on the mons can be sexually pleasurable because of the presence of numerous nerve endings.

Labia Majora and Labia Minora

The labia majora are tissue folds covered by hair-bearing skin and contain both smooth muscle and fat. The labia majora fuse anteriorly with the mons pubis and posteriorly with the perineum. The skin of the labia majora is usually darker that the skin of the thighs. The nerve endings and underlying fatty

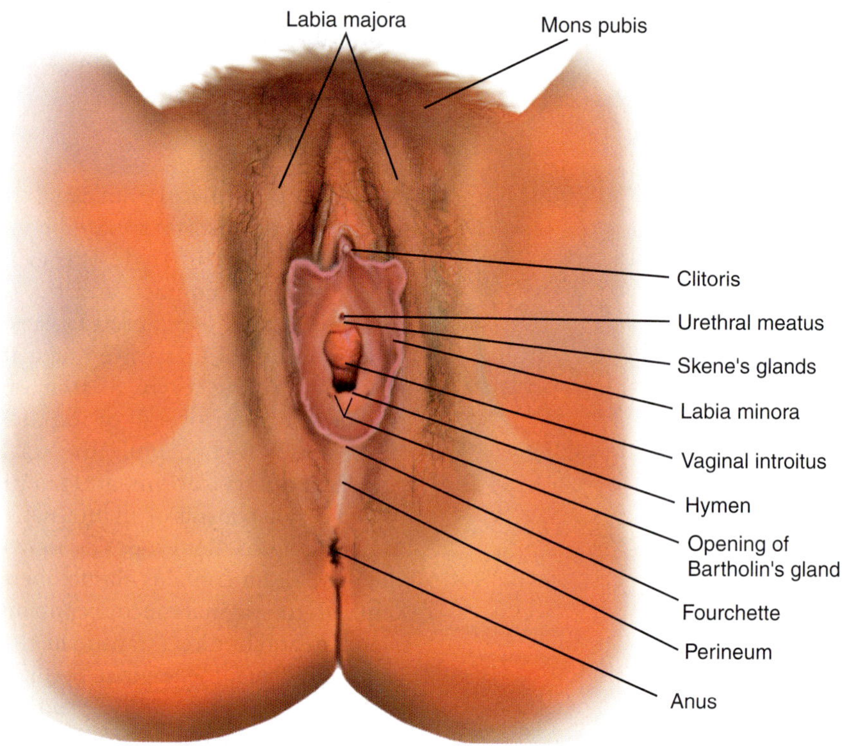

Figure 61-2 External female genitalia.

tissue are similar to those in the mons. Vestibular bulbs analogous to the corpus spongiosum in the male lie behind the folds of the labia majora.

The labia minora are smaller thin folds covered by skin that bears no hair laterally and by vaginal mucosa medially. The folds fuse anteriorly to form the hood or prepuce of the glans of the clitoris. Posteriorly along the lower edge of the vaginal opening, the labia minora form a thin, flat tissue called the fourchette. The labia minora are devoid of fat but are rich in elastic fibers and blood vessels forming erectile tissue. Sebaceous glands are present on both surfaces of minora and produce thick cheesy secretions called smegma.

Clitoris

The clitoris is analogous to the male phallus. It is comprised of a glans, a shaft, and crura. The glans is the portion externally visible just under the hood formed by the labia minora. The glans is highly sensitive to touch, resulting in sexual arousal and pleasure. The clitoral shaft is composed of vascular erectile tissue that engorges with blood during sexual arousal. The crura divide in two conjoined cavernous bodies, which branch near the base of the clitoris and lie along the pubic bone behind the labia majora. The corpora cavernosa are composed of endothelial lined lacunar spaces, cavernosal arteries, smooth muscle, and connective tissue similar to these structures in the male penis. Although other sexual organs, both male and female, have combined functions of reproduction and waste elimination, the only known function of the clitoris is arousal and sexual pleasure. This exclusive purpose of the clitoris for sexual pleasure confounds notions in some cultures that women are less sexual than men.

Hymen

The hymen is a fold of mucous membrane that partially marks the introitus or entrance to the vagina. It may appear smooth in nonparous women. In parous women, it may have irregular tags because of stretching and small lacerations during birth. Occasionally the hymen may completely or partially occlude the vaginal opening. If the occlusion interferes with menstrual flow or sexual activity, a surgical incision may be necessary to open it. Contrary to assumptions in some cultures, the degree of intactness of the hymen cannot be used to prove or disprove virginity or history of sexual intercourse.

Perineum

The perineum is the area of smooth skin between the vaginal introitus and the anus, composed of vascular tissue and nerve tissue. A transverse fold of mucous membrane called the posterior fourchette is formed by connecting the ends of the labia minora. It may disappear after initiation of sexual intercourse and childbearing, leaving the vulva more open.

Paraurethral (Skene's) Glands

The paraurethral glands (Skene's), equivalent to the prostate in the male, are composed of mucus-secreting columnar epithelium. The openings are located just inside of, and on the posterior area of, the urethra. The glands can become infected by bacteria present in the vulvar area.

Bulbourethral (Bartholin's) Glands

The vestibular glands (Bartholin's), equivalent to the bulbourethral (Cowper's) glands in the male, are located on each side of the vestibule of the vagina inside the labia minora. These glands are composed of alveoli lined with columnar cells that produce mucus that is excreted through small ducts near the vaginal opening. Mucus produced by these glands may contribute somewhat to vaginal lubrication during sexual activity. The glands are usually not palpable unless infection occludes the ducts creating an abscess or cyst.

Breasts

The breasts are mammary glands that produce milk to nourish an infant after birth. As such, they function as accessories to the reproductive process and are considered part of the secondary female sex characteristics. Their growth, development, and functions are regulated by hormonal influences from the hypothalamus, pituitary gland, and the ovaries. Breasts also function as organs for sexual arousal in some cultures and can be responsive to sexual stimuli.

Extending from the second to the sixth ribs, the breasts are dome-shaped and are composed of alveolar glands clustered in 15 to 20 lobes separated from each other by interlobular septa. Each lobe is drained by a lactiferous duct that opens at the tip of the nipple. The nipple, located centrally on the dome of the breast, contains nerve endings and erectile tissue. The nipple is surrounded by the areola, a pigmented area that contains sebaceous glands (Montgomery's). Usually the nipple protrudes from the areola, though in some women one or both nipples may be flat or inverted. Inverted nipples may cause some problems with initiation of breastfeeding.

Fibrous and fatty tissue surrounding the glandular tissue provides support and accounts for the varying sizes and shapes in the breasts of different women. Part of the mammary gland may extend along the inferolateral edge of the pectoralis major toward the axilla (armpit), forming an axillary tail (of Spence). Approximately 50 percent of breast cancer tumors are located in this portion of breast tissue.

Under the influence of increasing estrogen production during puberty, the glandular and ductal tissues undergo growth and development. With menstrual cycling, some women experience tenderness and fullness in the breast tissue related to increased production of ovarian hormones. Over half of women 30 to 50 years of age may experience benign fibrocystic changes in their breasts. These usually recede after menopause.

Changes in the breast occur during pregnancy. Increasing amounts of estrogen and progesterone are secreted first by the corpus luteum of the ovary and later by the placenta. Progesterone works along with the estrogen to complete the development of the alveoli. After birth, prolactin hormone from the pituitary gland initiates milk production. In response to nerve stimulation of the nipple, oxytocin is released from the posterior pituitary gland and induces smooth muscles surrounding the alveoli and within the ductal system to contract and bring the milk down from the glands during suckling by the infant.

Menarche

Menarche refers most specifically to the initiation of the first menstrual period. Menarche results from a rapid maturation of the reproductive axis. The average age of menarche is around 12 years of age, though it can range from 9 to 16 years of age. Age of onset is mediated by genetics, race, and possibly nutritional and socioeconomic status.

The functions of the menstrual cycle are mediated by the hypothalamus, which begins to secrete GnRH directly to the pituitary gland. The pituitary is stimulated to produce FSH, which is picked up by the ovaries where a number of primary **oocytes** (the early or primitive ovum before it has developed completely) begin the maturational process. Granulosa and thecal cells surrounding these oocytes increase in number and form the follicles. Usually one follicle exceeds the others in size and activity. The follicles that have lagged behind in their development atrophy, and those oocytes die and are absorbed. The maturing follicle continues to expand, pushing through to the exterior wall of the ovary. The granulosa cells surrounding the ovum produce estrogen in increasing amounts along with lower levels of progesterone.

Under the influence of a second pituitary hormone, LH, and along with peak levels of FSH, the follicle ruptures releasing the ovum coated with follicular fluid into the peritoneal cavity. The fimbriated ends of the fallopian tube create currents that pull the ovum into the tube. The follicular cells at the site of ovulation, now called the corpus luteum, continue to produce estrogen and even higher levels of progesterone. These hormones are picked up by endometrial tissue that continues to grow in vascularity and glandular activity. The follicular cells also produce inhibin, a glycoprotein, which provides negative feedback to the pituitary gland to decrease the production of FSH.

If fertilization of the ovum has not occurred, approximately 10 to 12 days after ovulation the corpus luteum decreases its production of estrogen and progesterone. The dropping levels of these ovarian hormones cause the vessels of the endometrial lining to constrict resulting in cellular death and the sloughing of the endometrial lining in menses. The drop in estrogen now creates a negative feedback to the hypothalamus to increase production of GnRH, which again stimulates release of FSH from the pituitary gland and the menstrual cycle begins again.

If the ovum has been fertilized, the developing zygote produces human chorionic gonadotropin (hCG). The hCG is picked up by the ovary, causing the corpus luteum to continue production of estrogen and progesterone for several more weeks until the placenta can produce levels of estrogen and progesterone sufficient to maintain the pregnancy.

Estrogen and progesterone produced by the ovaries are also responsible for the development of female secondary sex characteristics, such as the development of the mammary glands, feminine patterns of fat distribution, and pubic and body hair patterns. During pregnancy these hormones also contribute to the growth of the uterus and increased vascularization of the breasts, pelvic, and perineal tissues.

Menopause

Menopause specifically refers to the last menses, which marks the end of the menstrual cycling. This event occurs between the ages of 40 and 58 and occurs within the perimenopausal period, or **climacteric,** which occurs two to eight years prior to menopause and up to one year after the final menses. The quality and quantity of follicular development undergoes decline about 20 to

25 years after menarche. Variation in the menstrual cycle length may be related to anovulation or irregular maturation of follicles. A shorter menstrual cycle is the most common change that occurs during the perimenopausal period.

Because there is a decrease in the number of functional follicles that respond to FSH, the follicular phase of the menstrual cycle shortens and may become anovulatory. The luteal phase remains fairly constant at 14 days. Although fertility declines, women may still conceive during the perimenopausal period. As the follicular tissue becomes more resistant to gonadotropin stimulation along with a decreased production of inhibin, which regulates, particularly, LH, there are increases in production of FHS and LH.

Hypothalamic-pituitary insensitivity to estrogen feedback may also play a significant role in perimenstrual symptoms (Weiss, Skurnick, Goldsmith, Santoro, & Park, 2004). Symptoms such as hot flashes and sleep disturbances occur more commonly in perimenopausal women and are related to decreasing levels of estrogen and increasing levels of LH. However, early in the perimenopausal phase, levels of LH are higher in perimenopausal women even in the presence of estrogen levels similar to younger women. Elevated FSH and LH levels lead to stromal stimulation of the ovary, which increases the production of estrone levels and decreases estradiol levels. With fewer functioning follicles, inhibin levels also drop during this time causing further rises in FSH levels.

Systems affected by the perimenopausal phase include neuroendocrine, cardiovascular, genitourinary, skeletal, and skin and hair. Hot flashes are defined as transient periods of intense heat in the upper body, arms, and face, which are followed by flushing of the skin and sweating. Core body temperature may drop a degree or two after the hot flash because of heat lost through increased blood flow to the skin and evaporation. From 40 to 70 percent of women experience hot flashes and of these 10 to 20 percent may seek attention from their health care professional. Hot flashes may be experienced for months or years but average around three years for most women. Hot flashes may disturb sleep patterns and result in fatigue, irritability, and negative impact on life activities. It remains unclear whether hot flashes are caused by the high levels of FSH and LH or low levels of estrogen and inhibin. It is possible that both of these factors may be required to increase the incidence of hot flashes (Whiteman, Staropoli, Benedict, Borgeest, & Flaws, 2003).

The risk of atherosclerotic disease, including coronary heart disease increases with age. Women demonstrate lower incidences of cardiovascular diseases than men before age 50. However, after the age of 50 the incidence of disease increases until women's rates are similar to the rate in men. Total cholesterol, low-density lipoprotein (LDL) cholesterol, and triglyceride levels increase after menopause, whereas high-density lipoprotein (HDL) cholesterol levels decline, promoting atherosclerosis.

Vaginal mucosal thinness and dryness progresses later in the perimenopausal period and is related to estrogen withdrawal. Skin and hair changes may also be noted. The incidence of osteoporosis increases substantially after menopause. The cause is not fully understood but may be related to loss of estrogen influence on parathyroid activity and production of the active form of vitamin D, resulting in bone reabsorption.

SEXUAL RESPONSE CYCLE

The sexual response is a complex interplay between psychological and physiological factors. Humans usually move from sexual neutrality to interactive sexual behavior for reasons related to enhancement of emotional closeness, desire to increase a sense of attractiveness and attraction to a partner, and a desire to share sexual pleasure. Masturbation or self-stimulation is more commonly related to sexual tension or hunger. Sexual desires, or at least willingness to be receptive to sexual stimuli, are important cognitive components to sexual arousal, which may also require adequate levels of gonadal hormones to maintain libido.

Physiologically, sexual function is dependent on functional endocrine, neurological, and vascular systems. During puberty, male testosterone levels increase approximately 10 to 20 times, triggering the maturation of male genitalia, secondary sex characteristics, and behavioral changes, particularly a fourfold increase in sexual activity. Clinical literature shows that testosterone levels directly and indirectly influence the fundamental components of male sexual function including sex drive, erectile function, and ejaculation. Although testosterone levels are much lower in women, the presence of testosterone in women seems important in maintaining libido. Changes in testosterone levels through puberty in the female have not been documented. A woman's testosterone level begins to decline in the perimenopause (5 to 10 years before menopause) and tends to stabilize at lower levels several years after menopause.

The two fundamental physiological responses to effective sexual stimulation that occur in both males and females are vasocongestion and **myotonia** (tonic spasm of a muscle or temporary rigidity). Vasocongestion is the engorgement of blood in the genital and breast tissue in response to sexual stimuli. Myotonia refers to building muscle tension in the muscles of the pelvic floor and throughout the body. Myotonia is evident in the facial grimaces, spasmodic contractions of the hands and feet, and the muscular spasms that occur during orgasm. These responses follow the same general pattern regardless of the method of sexual stimulation. Masters and Johnson (1966) first distinguished four phases in the physiological sexual response pattern in both males and females: excitement, plateau, orgasm, and resolution. These phases, as well as some variations in male and female expression of the phases are described in Table 61-1. Kaplan (1985) adds the psychological phase of desire to the response cycle.

Healthy and safe sexuality involves intentional decisions to live a lifestyle that maintains maximum health for reproduction if and when one might desire to become a parent. This includes establishing a healthy intimate relationship, preventing unintentional impregnation, and planning pregnancy when the decision is mutual and the couple is prepared for the role of parenting, as well as avoidance of contracting or spreading sexually transmitted infections.

Male Sexual Response Cycle

The physiological components of male sexual response include erection, orgasm, and ejaculation. These components are discussed here as a basis for understanding both sexual function and dysfunction as these are related to selected treatment protocols. An erection is a process coordinated by neural input generated from sensory erotic and fantasy experiences and stimulation of sensory endings in the genitalia. The penis is maintained in a flaccid state by sympathetic nervous system stimulation of the penile blood vessels and smooth muscle contractions within the vessel walls of the lacunar spaces of the cavernosa of the penile shaft. When the penis is flaccid the intralacunar smooth muscle is in a contracted state, and the tone is maintained by norepinephrine. When a male becomes sexually aroused vasodilator impulses are delivered by the parasympathetic nervous system. Dilation of the arterioles of the penis and relaxation of the smooth muscles of the lacunar spaces cause the erectile tissue of the penis to fill with blood. The veins are compressed by this engorgement so that outflow is blocked. The effect of these vascular changes is to increase penile distension. The testes also experience increased blood flow and increase 50 percent in size during sexual arousal.

When fully distended, the penis is rigid and capable of penetrating the vagina, facilitating sperm deposits into the vaginal vault with ejaculation. The

TABLE 61-1 Physiological Phases of the Sexual Response Cycle

MALE RESPONSES	FEMALE RESPONSES	SHARED RESPONSES
Excitement		
Penis becomes erect. Erection may be partially lost and regained during a prolonged phase. Testes enlarge and elevate. Scrotum tightens, flattens, and skin thickens. When fully distended, the penis is rigid and capable of penetration.	Clitoris swells, glans becomes tumescent, and shaft increases in diameter and length. Vagina lubricates and expands. Uterus elevates and breasts enlarge.	Myotonia spreads; some evidence of involuntary muscle activity. Heart rate increases in direct proportion to rising sexual tension. Sex flush may be visible in some women. Nipples become erect.
Plateau		
Erection is stabilized. Increase in penile circumference at coronal ridge. Full testicular elevation; enlargement of testes reaches 50 percent over unstimulated size. Secretions from Cowper's appear at urethral opening.	Continued vaginal expansion; uterine and cervical elevation. Development of orgasmic platform. Retraction of clitoris under labial hood. Secretions of Bartholin's gland. Further enlargement of breasts.	Increased muscle tension; superficial and deep vasocongestion. Rapid respiration and increase in heart rate and blood pressure; hyperventilation may be present. Sex flush appears in some men, becomes more pronounced in women.
Orgasm		
Contractions of vas deferens, seminal vesicles, prostate gland moves sperm and semen to penile bulb; emission phase of orgasm. Contractions of pelvic floor muscles around urethral bulb causes ejaculation of semen and creates sensations of orgasm	Contractions of muscles of pelvic floor and uterus create sensations of orgasm	Same pelvic floor muscles are contracting in men and women. Length and strength of orgasmic responses are similar in men and women. Hyperventilation and increased heart rate and blood pressure and sex flush continue.
Resolution		
Loss of most of penile erection within 30 seconds. Testes descend into relaxed scrotum. Refractory period limits the return of an erection and orgasm.	Loss of vaginal and clitoral vasocongestion. Clitoris returns to prestimulated position. With continued stimulation vasocongestion and myotonia may recur for multiple orgasms.	Loss of muscle tension and nipple erection. Sex flush disappears. Heart rate, breathing, and blood pressure return to normal.

Adapted from Kaplan, H. S. (1985). Comprehensive evaluation of disorders of sexual desire. *Washington, DC: American Psychiatric Press.*

firmness in the erection may come and go within a sexual encounter as the male's focus on his own sensations vary, such as when his attention is given to his partner. As he nears orgasm the erection stabilizes. Following orgasm arterial blood flow into the penis decreases to nonaroused levels, vasocongestion is relieved, and the penis becomes flaccid.

Although an erection is basically a physiological response, it also involves psychological components. In healthy sexual relationships, sexual interactions with a desired partner can involve intense emotional feelings of intimacy and attachment along with the personal pleasure from the experience. When other psychological issues are involved within the relationship or within the individual, altered sexual responsiveness can inhibit erectile functions.

Ejaculation is a neurophysiological reflexive process by which semen is expelled through the penis to the outside of the body. When effective sexual stimulation of the penis results in a buildup of neural excitation to a critical level, several internal physiological events are triggered in the ejaculatory process. During the emission phase of the process, the ampulla of the vas deferens, the seminal vesicles, and the prostate gland undergo contractions. The contractions eject the glandular secretions into the urethral bulb. Two sphincters, one located where the urethra exits the bladder and the other below the prostate, enclose the semen in the urethral bulb. Next, in the expulsion phase, the collected semen is expelled out of the urethra by strong, rhythmic contractions of the pelvic floor muscles that surround the urethral bulb and the root of the penis. The external sphincter relaxes, allowing the semen to pass through, while the internal sphincter remains contracted to prevent the loss of urine.

Orgasm is the series of contractions of the levator ani and pubococcygeus muscles of the pelvic floor and is associated with pleasure and the release of the sexual tension. The first few muscular contractions are quite strong and occur at close intervals. Most of the seminal fluid is expelled in spurts with each contraction. Several more muscular contractions occur in decreasing intensity and frequency. The entire expulsion stage may last from 3 to 10 seconds.

Following orgasm the blood flow decreases and the vasocongestion is relieved, a process known as **detumescence.** Detumescence begins within seconds of the orgasm, but may take 10 to 30 minutes to return the penis to a flaccid nonaroused state. If orgasm is not experienced, the release of vasocongestion may take longer. The male may also experience aching in the testes until the testicular vasocongestion is relieved.

Female Sexual Response Cycle

Although the anatomical appearance of female genitalia differs from male genitalia, the physiological sexual response is the same within analogous tissues and includes sexual arousal, lubrication, and orgasm. In the nonaroused state, the clitoral body and vaginal smooth muscles are under contractile tone. Following sexual stimulation, the neurogenic and endothelial release of nitric oxide relaxes the smooth muscles in the clitoral cavernosum and coiled arteriolar smooth muscles. Increased arterial inflow creates increased intracavernosal pressure and clitoral engorgement resulting in the extrusion of the glans clitoris and enhanced sensitivity.

Within the vaginal wall, neurotransmitters including nitric oxide and vasoactive intestinal peptide (VIP) are released modulating vaginal vascular and nonvascular smooth muscle relaxation. Dramatic increase in capillary flow in the submucosa leads to production of 3 to 5 mL of vaginal transudate that provides vaginal lubrication. Vaginal smooth muscle relaxation results in increased vaginal length and diameter, especially in the distal two thirds of the vagina.

Because the cavernous bodies in the female lie out along the pelvic floor, rather than being contained within a shaft of skin as in males, engorgement of these spongy tissues is less visible. Vasocongestion can be visualized through magnetic resonance imaging (MRI) during sexual arousal in the female, demonstrating that clitoral and cavernous tissues doubles in size (Maravilla, et al., 2005). The female can experience a more diffuse vasocongestion than males.

During orgasm, the female experiences a series of rhythmic, rapidly occurring contractions of the orgasmic platform, the outer third of the vagina and the engorged tissues surrounding it. Females experience a variety of orgasmic responses from intense contractions of the pelvic floor muscles to mild contractions that are perceived as pleasurable and relieve sexual tension, though release of vasocongestion may take longer. A mild orgasm may be accompanied by 3 to 5 contractions; intense orgasms may continue for 12 or more contractions. The intervals between contractions lengthen in duration after the first few and intensity diminishes progressively.

Following orgasm, the vasocongestion is relieved and both the outer third and inner two thirds of the vagina return to their unstimulated state. The vagina loses its deep coloration and regains its normal appearance about 10 to 15 minutes after an orgasm. If the female does not experience orgasm, relief of vasocongestion may take longer and may result in dull aching heaviness similar to premenstrual abdominal heaviness.

Interactive Sexual Intimacy

Adequate functioning of the neurological and vascular systems is important in physiological sexual responsiveness. Establishing and maintaining a positive interpersonal relationship with one's sexual partner also contributes to sexual interest, desire, and willingness to participate in sexual intimacy. Cognitive components, such as negative past experiences, anxiety, emotional distress, and depression, may influence the ability to respond to sexual situations with sexual arousal and to experience sexual satisfaction as desired or expected. When a patient or a couple expresses concerns about sexual functioning, contributing factors within the individual or within the couple relationship should be explored. If serious personal or relationship issues are present the patient or couple should be referred to counseling.

Sexual Dysfunction

Sexual dysfunction is a disturbance or disorder in desire, excitement, or orgasm of the sexual response cycle. Sensory arousal combines with emotional arousal and conscious thoughts to trigger and interdependently direct the hormonal, neurological, and circulatory systems that develop and maintain the sexual response cycle. Thus, levels of performance and satisfaction may vary situationally, relationally, and across the life span related to aging or disease. Sexual dysfunction may be caused by factors such as the patient's perception and beliefs about gender role or aging. Sexual functioning must always be examined in the context of the whole person and the intimate partner relationship not just physical or psychological status.

Physical, Medical, or Surgical Causes of Sexual Dysfunction

Patients who have chronic illness, physical disability, or episodic acute illness often have difficulties with sexual functioning. Although physical demands of sexual activity are high, there are rarely significant restrictions on sexual activities. However, couples may need to alter their usual sexual patterns and activities to accommodate any limitations they may experience. Psychological effects on sexual functioning may result from disinterest, anxiety, fatigue, pain, or misconceptions about their ability to experience sexual activities (Nusbaum, Hamilton, & Lenahan, 2003).

Chronic medical illnesses tend to disrupt the desire and arousal phases of sexual response. Negative body image and perception of self as a sexual being may result from medical diagnoses and required lifestyle changes. Neurological disorders can potentially affect desire, arousal, and orgasm. Treatments of chronic illnesses can also interfere with sexual functioning. Many drugs contribute to changes in sexual response. Antihypertensive and psychotropic drugs particularly affect arousal and possibly disrupt orgasm. Sometimes alternative drugs can be prescribed that have less effect on sexual functioning. But when selected drugs are essential, the patient may require information on alternative ways to experience intimacy. Surgery may disrupt sympathetic and parasympathetic neural pathway.

Substance-Induced Sexual Dysfunction

Substance-induced sexual dysfunction can affect any stage of the sexual response cycle. For diagnosis, a link needs to be established between a clinically diagnosed sexual dysfunction and a specific substance, legal or illegal. Diagnostic criteria include the following: (a) the sexual dysfunction must cause

Respecting Our Differences

Reproductive Issues Accompanying Aging

Fecundity and fertility are reduced as both males and females grow older. A woman's fertility starts to decline in her late 20s, and for men, fertility begins to drop after age 35. A woman is born with her lifetime supply of ova, which diminishes to about 300,000 by the time she reaches puberty. By the time she reaches her late 30s, the risks of abnormal haploid cell division and other chromosomal abnormalities increase. As men and women approach middle age, chronic disorders, such as diabetes mellitus and hypertension, may reduce fertility in both men and women and increase the risks associated with childbearing in women. In association with chronic conditions, the incidence of miscarriage increases with age as does preterm birth and low-birth-weight babies. Medications used to treat some health conditions may also interfere with sexual function and fertility, and some pose risks of congenital anomalies.

marked distress or interpersonal difficulty; (b) the condition may involve impaired desire, arousal, or orgasm, or sexual pain and is fully explained by the direct effects of the substance; and (c) the recurring or persistent dysfunction is not better accounted for by a dysfunction that is not substance induced. Both psychotropic drugs and somatotropic drugs may have side effects that can produce sexual dysfunction.

A significant number of prescribed drugs, combinations of prescribed drugs, or over-the-counter (OTC) drugs are known to affect sexual functioning (e.g., antiandrogens, antiarrhythmics, anticholinergics, antihistamines, corticosteroids, decongestants, and diuretics). Sexual side effects of some drugs may be present in some patients and not in others. Health care practitioners must review the known side effects of drugs taken by patients, providing information as indicated. If patients are unaware of potential side effects, the cause of the sexual dysfunction may be assumed to be unrelated to medication and not be reported to the practitioner. Patients with chronic diseases who must take more that one medication regularly are particularly susceptible. The effects can range from a simple additive effect (the effect on one medication added to the effect of the other) to a synergistic effect (the effects of two or more drugs creating a third, enhanced, and often unpredictable effect). Patients should be informed to not mix some medically prescribed drugs or OTC medications with alcohol or illegal substances.

As with all psychoactive drugs, the patient's psychological well-being and environment can affect the outcome of the drug activity. Antidepressants, tranquilizers, barbiturates, and alcohol are all central nervous system depressants, reducing or slowing down neurological functioning. Mild tranquilizers and alcohol are sometimes used to reduce anxiety and improve mood in an attempt to enhance sexual desire and induce a relaxed, less inhibited state of mind. In higher doses, these drugs may impair the patient's judgment, impacting sexual decisions, or the drugs may decrease the ability to function sexually. Narcotic medications usually create a loss of sexual desire, arousal, and orgasm.

Psychological Issues

Childhood learning shapes many fundamental attitudes, values, and beliefs about sexuality. The need for close bonding with other humans and the need for sensual touch are present from birth to death. When life experiences fail to meet these needs in healthy ways, psychological issues can result that impact psychosexual development and negatively influence intimate relationships. Psychological issues affecting sexual functioning may be related to sexual ignorance, fear of failure, or communication or relationship issues with a partner. Life issues such as restrictive upbringing, rigid gender roles, traumatic sexual experiences, or conflict with sexual orientation also can contribute to sexual dysfunction. Sometimes psychological factors can be resolved with information and education; other times professional psychiatric counseling may be required.

ASSESSMENT

Sexuality is an integral component of physical and emotional health for all people, incorporating gender identity, self-worth, the ability to establish healthy intimate relationships, and expressions of sexual behaviors. Thus, all patients should be provided opportunity to discuss sexual concerns that are related to health issues. All women of reproductive age should be assessed for the need for contraception, assistance with pregnancy planning, and sexual practices that may place them at risk for sexually transmitted diseases (STDs). Adolescent males and females are particularly vulnerable to STDs because of greater likelihood of inadequate education and self comfort, and the social skills necessary to practice safer sexual behaviors. Because STDs can have serious impacts on reproductive function, as well as be life-threatening, sexual practices must be assessed for all patients. Patients deemed at risk must be screened for STDs and be provided education regarding safer sex behaviors.

Populations known to be at higher risk for STDs are adolescent women age 15 to 19 years and young adults (male and female) aged 20 to 24 years. Rates of human immunodeficiency virus (HIV) infection remain high, especially among minority populations. Of newly diagnosed HIV infections in the United States during 2005, the Centers for Disease Control and Prevention (CDC) estimated that approximately 62 percent were men who were infected through sexual contact with other men, 51 percent were African Americans, 31 percent were Caucasians, and 17 percent were Hispanic (Americans). Studies of HIV infection among young men who have sex with men (MSM) in the mid- to late-1990s revealed high rates of HIV prevalence, incidence, and unrecognized infection, particularly among young African American MSM. Although some populations, such as lesbian women and older adults, are sometimes assumed to be at lower risks for STDs and unsafe sexual practices, there is sufficient incidence to mandate that all patients need to be assessed.

General Health and Medical History

Sexual health concerns should be included in a matter-of-fact manner in the general review of body systems. If health care professionals do not inquire about sexual concerns, patients may believe them to be unimportant, insignificant, or not amenable to treatment. These concerns are often not addressed because of discomfort or anxiety on the part of the health care provider, which can leave the patient unable to bring up issues of a sexual nature. Health care providers must learn to be comfortable and nonjudgmental in asking questions about sexuality and responding to issues that arise from questioning the patient or from the patient's efforts to address concerns. The health care provider should initiate the discussion to let the patient know that sexuality is an important aspect of health.

When basic questions about sexuality are included in preconsultation questionnaires that are given to patients, the patients may feel more comfortable about discussing concerns. Questions should be sensitive but direct enough to clarify issues. Emphasizing the commonality of concerns about sexual functioning may ease patient discomfort. In a patient who has arthritis, for example, the health care practitioner may begin by saying "It is common for people who have arthritis to notice changes in their sexual lives. Has your pain affected your sexual activity?" Often patients become more comfortable when the practitioner begins with open questions, such as "How can I help you?" and "What do you think is the cause of the difficulty?"

Sexual Health History

Depending on the complexity and severity of a sexual concern, a brief sexual history may be adequate (Box 61-1). With more severe concerns, a comprehensive history may be indicated. The patient may need to be referred to a psychiatrist, psychologist, or sexual counselor.

Intimate Partner Violence

The rate of family violence is approximately 2 victims per 1,000 U.S. residents age 12 or older. Family violence accounts for about 1 in 10 violent victimizations. intimate partner violence (IPV) occurs in some degree across all social, economic, religious, and cultural groups (Heise & Garcia-Moreno, 2002). Women and those in families living below the poverty line are more likely to be affected. In the study 30 percent of the women who had married or had lived with a man as part of a couple reported violence by a husband or male

PATIENT PLAYBOOK

Promoting Optimal Health of the Reproductive System

The nurse can suggest the following to instruct the female patient how to promote optimum reproductive health:

- Become comfortable with your own body. Examine your genitals to become familiar with normal appearance and to note any changes, such as inflammation, lesions, or masses.
- Become familiar with the amount, color, consistency, and odor of your normal daily discharge. If the discharge changes, consult a health care provider
- Maintain a record of your menstrual cycle.
- Be actively involved in your own health care. Wash the vulva daily with warm soapy water and avoid douching, scented hygiene sprays, and perfumed soaps.
- Never force vaginal penetration. Make sure your vagina is well-lubricated before inserting anything into it and be careful about what you insert into your vagina.
- Be sure that a condom is used during sexual intimacy when there may be any risk of exposure to STDs or unintended pregnancy if permitted by religious beliefs.

The nurse can suggest the following to instruct the male patient how to promote optimum health:

- Become comfortable with your own body. Examine your genitals to become familiar with normal appearance and to note any changes.
- Be actively involved in your own health care. Seek out information. Ask questions. If you are at risk, seek regular checkups.
- Retracting the foreskin when intact, wash your genitals daily with warm soapy water.
- Urination before and after intercourse can help to reduce urinary tract infections (UTIs).
- Be sure that a condom is used during sexual intimacy when there may be any risk of exposure to STDs or unintended pregnancy. You are fully responsible to protect yourself and to protect your partner.
- Do not progress from anal intercourse to vaginal intercourse without first washing your penis. If a condom is used, the condom should be changed.
- Strive to be in a mutually satisfying, infection-free relationship with one person.
- If you desire or intend to become a parent, select behaviors and a lifestyle that maintains fertility.

Adapted from Stewart, E. G., & Spencer, P. (2002). The V book: A doctor's guide to complete vulvovaginal health. *New York: Bantam.*

BOX 61-1

SHORT FORM OF SEXUAL HISTORY

- Are you currently sexually active: with one, or more than one, partner? Male, female, or both?
- Is sex satisfying to you? For your partner?
- How has your present illness (concern) affected your sexual functioning?
- Do you experience any pain during vaginal penetration? Under what circumstances? Is vaginal dryness a problem?
- Do you have difficulty achieving an orgasm when you want to? If so, in what situations?

Pertinent Questions for Postmenopausal Women

- Has your interest in sexual activity changed?
- Do you have discomfort with intercourse?
- Do you lubricate adequately with sexual stimulation?
- Is your partner able to have an erection? Maintain an erection?
- Are you taking hormone replacement therapy? Other medications?

Adapted from Estes, M. (2006). Health assessment and physical examination *(3rd ed.). New York: Thomson Delmar Learning.*

cohabitant. All adult and teenage women should be routinely screened for IPV. The possibility of abuse should also be considered in elder adults, same sex relationships, and men. Of note is that 11 percent of women living with another woman reported IPV. Approximately 15 percent of males living with a male intimate partner report IPV compared with 7.7 percent of males who were married or living with a woman as a couple. American Indian/Alaska Native women and men report more violence than do other cultural groups. Hispanic (American) women are more likely to report instances of intimate partner rape. Barriers to screening for domestic violence include the assumption of time constraints, care provider discomfort with the topic, discomfort about offending the patient, and perceptions of powerlessness to change the situation. Prevention and early intervention can occur by routinely asking simple and direct nonjudgmental questions regarding abuse and sexual assault (Box 61-2).

BOX 61-2

A SHORT ABUSE ASSESSMENT SCREEN

- In the last year (since I saw you last), have you been hit, slapped, kicked, or otherwise physically hurt by someone? (If yes, by who? Number of times? Nature of injury?)
- Within the last year has anyone made you do something sexual that you did not want to do? (If yes, who?)
- Are you afraid of your partner or anyone else?

Adapted from Norton, L. B., Peipert, J. F., Zierler, S., Lima, B., & Hume, L. (1995). Battering in pregnancy: An assessment of two screening methods. Obstetrics and Gynecology, 85*(3), 321–325.*

Screening for violence must be based on more than observed injuries. Psychological abuse or unseen injuries may also be occurring. Previous health care visits should be monitored for a pattern of injuries, history of abuse or assault, chronic pelvic pain, headaches, irritable bowel syndrome, depression, substance use, suicide attempts, and anxiety. Such symptoms may be warning signs of IPV. However, violence can exist in the absence of warning signs in the patient's medical history or behavior. Patients may not present with symptoms, especially those who experience psychological or emotional abuse. They may conceal what they are experiencing out of shame or fear. Thus, it is essential to screen every patient routinely. Partner control is often an important factor in violence and abuse. Thus, it is essential to ask questions in private, apart from the partner and apart from children, family, or friends. Behaviors of the partner during a health care visit that may be indicative of abuse include never leaving the patient's side, being over solicitous, being hostile and demanding, or answering questions for the patient. The patient must be assessed for safety and ensured that they are not in immediate danger.

When IPV is occurring, the patient may present with a flat affect or as frightened, depressed, or anxious. Symptoms of posttraumatic stress disorder (PTSD), such as dissociation, psychic numbing, or negative responses to touch, may be present in severe cases. Abused women may appear overly compliant and may have learned not to question authority. Conversely, because of the fear and shame associated with the abuse and the possibility of its detection, an abused woman may exhibit distrust of health care providers.

In cases where violence is identified, findings must be documented in the patient's chart. Explanations about issues of confidentiality must be given, but awareness of any state mandatory reporting laws is important. Most states have mandatory reporting laws that require health care providers to contact local domestic violence and child protection agencies. Patients must be informed of any such requirement when abuse is documented. The patient's options should be reviewed with him or her and referrals provided.

Sexual Abuse and Assault

According to the National Violence Against Women Survey, 1 in 6 women and 1 in 33 men in the United States have experienced an attempted or completed rape at some time in their lives. Immediate physical and psychological trauma must be addressed. Pregnancy and sexually transmitted diseases can result from sexual assault. Long-lasting physical symptoms and illnesses have been associated with sexual abuse and assault. Symptoms may include chronic pelvic pain, gastrointestinal (GI) disorders, and a variety of chronic pain disorders, including headaches and back pain.

Sexual violence victims exhibit immediate reactions that can include shock, disbelief, fear, confusion, and anxiety; symptoms associated with PTSD. Longer term effects of PTSD, which may continue for months or become chronic, include anxiety, nervousness, phobias, sleep disturbances, substance abuse, depression, alienation, flashbacks, emotional detachment, and sexual dysfunction. Recognition of the uniqueness of each individual's expression of outcomes is important in understanding their trauma and facilitating their healing.

People who have experienced sexual assault are more likely than those who are not victims to express risky behavior patterns that make them vulnerable to further victimization. Such behaviors include having unprotected sex, having sex at a younger age, and having multiple sexual partners. Other victims may use alcohol, drugs, or overeating to cope with their stress. Women, particularly those under age 18 or minority women are significantly more likely to experience sexual assault.

Physical Examination of Male Genitalia

Unless the male patient seeks health care for a reproductive or genital tract problem, physical examination of the genitalia may not be performed, depending on the health care setting and age of the patient. Some male patients may be embarrassed or anxious about assessment of their genitalia. Before beginning the examination the health care practitioner should consider the patient's cultural background and what beliefs or attitudes he may have about the examination. His culture may prohibit female practitioners from examining him. The patient's level of apprehension should be addressed, ensuring him as necessary that this is normal. The assessment techniques should be explained. If an erection occurs in response to touch during the examination, this should be explained in a professional and matter-of-fact manner as a common response. The examination should take place in a comfortable room that ensures privacy and freedom from interruptions. After undressing, the patient may be asked to lie supine on an examination table or stand in front of the seated examiner. Clean gloves should be worn to prevent spread of infection.

The examiner notes the secondary sex characteristics and assesses appropriateness for developmental stage, including distribution of pubic hair, size of penis, size of scrotum, and size and descent of testes. Presence of pubic lice, scabies, or lesions is noted. The foreskin, glans, and shaft of the penis are inspected for lesions, swelling, and inflammation. If the patient is uncircumcised, he is asked to retract the foreskin. The foreskin should retract easily and completely over the glans. The glans should appear smooth, with the urinary meatus located centrally at the distal tip. The glans is compressed between the thumb and forefinger to determine whether any discharge is present. Any discharge should be considered abnormal and a specimen for culture should be obtained. The shaft of the penis is palpated noting tenderness, hard areas under the skin, or signs of inflammation.

The examiner can ask the patient to hold the penis to one side for inspection of the size and shape of the scrotum. Using the thumb and two fingers, the examiner should gently palpate the scrotum, testes, epididymis, and spermatic cord for size, shape, consistency, tenderness, and presence of masses. The testes should have smooth borders, with the epididymis extending from the posterior surface. This portion of the examination can be used to teach the patient about monthly testicular self-examination (TSE), encouraging him to palpate his own testes while the shape and contours are explained to him. The spermatic cord is palpated on each side along its length from the epididymis to the inguinal ring noting nodules or swelling.

The final assessment of the male reproductive system is inspection of the rectum and prostate. The patient may be positioned in a knee-chest position, lying in a lateral position with knees flexed, or standing and leaning over the examining table. The anal area is visually examined for lesions, ulcerations, or fissures. Then the examiner gently inserts a lubricated index finger through the anus in direction of the umbilicus. The prostate gland is palpated through the anterior rectal wall, noting the size, shape, and consistency of the lateral posterior lobes. The contour is symmetrical and bilobed, with a palpable vertical groove in the center. The prostate should feel firm, smooth, slightly mobile and tender.

Commonly, some patients may experience the urge to urinate when the gland is being palpated. All male patients over 50 years of age should have the prostate gland examined annually by digital rectal examination (DRE). Because only the posterior lobes are palpable, when prostatic tumors or hypertrophy is suspected, additional diagnostic tests may be necessary.

Abnormal findings of the male reproductive system are most often related to benign or malignant growths or inflammations and lesions associated with infections. Penile growths or masses related to malignancy may be nodular or ulcerated. Chancre lesions are indurated, smooth, and disk-like in appearance. Chancroids are more papular to irregular-shaped ulcerations that drain pus. Condyloma may be flat, wart-like nodules or elevated, fleshy, elongated projections. Painful vesicles, erosions, or ulcers may be indicative of herpes, chancroid, or other inflammatory infections. Painless, singular, small erosions with eventual lymphadenopathy may be related to lymphogranuloma venereum or cancer.

Scrotal masses with localized swelling and tenderness unilaterally or bilaterally can be indicative of epididymitis, orchiditis, or testicular torsion. Incarcerated intestinal hernia is evidenced by a tender or painful swelling up through the groin. Hydroceles present as unilateral or bilateral translucent scrotal swelling without much pain. Spermatoceles are firm and within the epididymal tissue, varicoceles, dilations of the veins that drain the testes, palpate as cordlike or wormlike in texture. Testicular cancer tends to be a firm and nodular unilateral mass.

Penile discharge indicative of infections, such as chlamydia or gonorrhea, can be clear to purulent and minimal to copious. Urination may or may not be painful. The presence of macules or papules on the penis or scrotum may indicate scabies or pubic lice. Cultures must be taken whenever infections are suspected.

Gynecological Examination of the Female

Assessment of the female reproductive system consists of breast examination, inspection and palpation of the external genitalia, speculum assessment of the internal genitalia, collection of specimens for laboratory analysis, bimanual examination, and rectovaginal assessment. The patient may be apprehensive about the examination. If the patient is anxious, explanations of each step of the process, along with relaxation and breathing techniques, can be provided as the examination proceeds. Women experiencing their first pelvic examination and women who have a history of sexual abuse or assault may benefit from the presence of a support person during the examination. The examination should take place in a comfortable room that ensures privacy and freedom from interruptions.

Breasts are first examined by visual inspection for size, shape, contour, and symmetry (see chapter 63). The skin of the breasts, areolae, and nipples are inspected for color, pigmentation, vascularity, surface characteristics, discharge, and lesions. The breasts are inspected in various postures for bilateral pull, symmetry, and contour. The breast tissue and axillary nodes are palpated for lesions or masses. Instruction in breast self-examination (BSE) should be provided to women who have not yet been instructed. The examination provides the opportunity to have the patient feel her own breast tissue and recognize the usual textures of her own breast tissue. Review of the procedure and the regularity of practice should be included in all subsequent health visits.

During the gynecological examination, with the patient in recumbent position, the abdomen is palpated for symptomatic or asymptomatic abdominal or pelvic masses. The masses may originate from reproductive, GI, or renal organs. Gynecological masses, such as ovarian, adnexal, or uterine masses, may be differentiated through the bimanual pelvic portion of the examination.

The mons pubis and vulva are observed for hair distribution, age-appropriate development, skin coloration, and condition. The labia majora and minora are inspected and palpated for pigmentation and surface characteristics. The skin pigmentation of the labia majora is slightly darker than the patient's general skin. The labia minora should be dark pink and moist, with no evidence of nodules, tenderness, drainage, or lesions. The clitoris is noted and should be smooth, pink, and moist, about the size of a pea.

The urethral meatus should be centrally located and close to, or slightly within, the vaginal introitus. The vaginal introitus may be a thin vertical slit or a larger orifice with irregular edges from hymenal remnants related to vaginal birth. The skin surface of the perineum between the vaginal introitus and the anus should appear smooth and free from lesions. An episiotomy scar may be present in some women who have given birth vaginally. The anus is inspected for color and lesions, including hemorrhoids.

The Skene's glands are located in the periurethral area and are not visible. The glands are palpated by placing the index finger into the vagina, exerting pressure on the anterior vaginal wall and milking the glands toward the vaginal opening. The glands should be tender and without discharge. If discharge is present, a specimen should be obtained for culture.

Next the Bartholin's glands are palpated. These glands are not visible but are located in the posterolateral portion of the labia majora. Using the thumb and index finger, the examiner can palpate the perineal tissue between the vaginal wall and the lower portion of the labia majora. The surface should appear smooth and pink, and it should be tender, without discharge.

If there is a history of incontinence or discomfort in a woman who has had children, then the examiner can assess vaginal wall tone. While holding the labia apart, the patient is asked to bear down and to cough. The vaginal wall is observed for bulging indicative of a cystocele, rectocele, or uterine prolapse, which may be the result of injury, childbirth, or age.

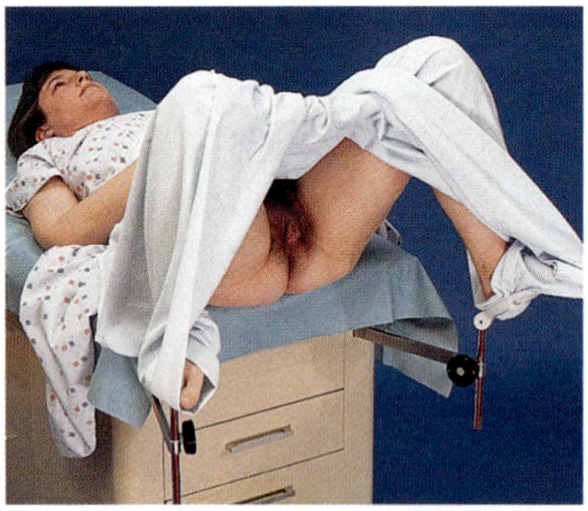

Figure 61-3 Patient positioning and draping for gynecological examination.

Speculum Examination

Every woman should have a Papanicolaou (Pap) smear as part of a complete pelvic examination beginning when she becomes sexually active or reaches 18 years of age but no later than 21 years. These examinations should continue throughout her reproductive years. Current guidelines from the National Cancer Institute recommend that Pap tests need not be repeated within two years of a prior negative test (Sawaya, et al., 2003). Women ages 65 to 70 who have had at least three normal Pap tests and no abnormal Pap tests in the last 10 years may decide, after talking with their health care practitioner, to stop having Pap tests (National Cancer Institute, 2003).

The internal organs of the pelvis are examined bimanually. The patient is placed in a lithotomy position with Trendelenburg and draped (Figure 61-3). With clean gloves, the middle and index fingers are gently placed in the vagina. The vaginal wall is palpated for surface characteristics and discomfort. The wall should be smooth and nontender. The cervix is located with the fingers of the internal hand. The hand on the abdominal should gently hold the uterus downward against the internal hand so that the cervix and vaginal fornices can be palpated. The cervix should feel smooth, slightly round, and firm. It is located in the midline position and slightly mobile in either direction without causing discomfort. The examiner moves the fingers in the vagina into the anterior fornix while positioning the other hand on the abdomen "trapping" the uterus between the two hands to assess its position, size, shape, and mobility. The ovaries may not always be palpable, but if felt, they should feel smooth, firm and ovoid. Oviducts are soft and normally not palpable. The rectovaginal portion of the examination involves palpating the rectal wall for surface characteristics, such as masses, fistulas, fissures, or tenderness. The posterior wall

Red Flag

Abdominal pain

Because ruptured ectopic pregnancy can be life-threatening if hemorrhage and shock ensue, alternative diagnoses of abdominal pain must be pursued. Ultrasound and pregnancy testing are carried out when ectopic pregnancy must be ruled out. When infection is suspected, cultures are obtained.

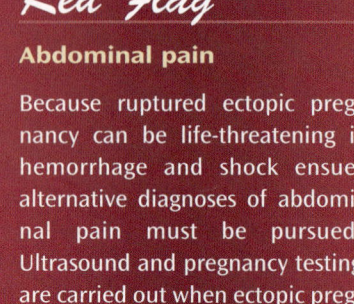

of the uterus is palpated by stabilizing the cervix with the internal hand and palpating with the abdominal hand. As the internal fingers are withdrawn, the anal sphincter is evaluated for tone.

Abnormal Findings

Common abnormalities of the female reproductive system notable on assessment include vulvar or vaginal discharges, erythema, masses or lesions, and abdominal masses, pain, or tenderness. Candidiasis may present as vulvovaginal discharge that is odorless and plaque-like in consistency, accompanied by itching and inflammation. Bacterial vaginosis also creates vulvar irritation but with a grayish, copious, "fishy," malodorous discharge. Bloody discharge not directly associated with menstruation may be caused by trauma or vaginal, cervical, or uterine infections. With the use of some lower dosage oral contraceptives, or during the first few cycles of oral contraceptive use until the hormonal cycle adapts, breakthrough bleeding may occur. Vulvar erythema may often be related to vulvovaginal sexually transmitted infections. Vulvovaginal lesions associated with genital herpes may present with a reddened base, painful vesicles, or ulcerations. Herpes lesions may be on the labial folds, surrounding or inside the vestibule, on the vaginal walls, or on the cervix. Genital warts are nontender, soft, flat or fleshy growths that may be warty in appearance. Chancres are indurated, firm ulcers that tend to be nonpainful. Abdominal pain or tenderness may result from ectopic pregnancy, salpingitis, endometritis, pelvic inflammatory disease (PID), cystitis, ovarian cysts, or abscesses that may or may not have ruptured.

> **PATIENT PLAYBOOK**
>
> **Pap Test**
>
> The nurse can instruct the patient in the following prior to her Pap test:
>
> - Schedule your examination when you are not menstruating (ideally 10 to 20 days after the first day of the last menstrual period).
> - For 2 days before the test, avoid douching, vaginal creams, or jellies.
> - You will be asked to empty your bladder before the examination, and you will put on a patient gown.
> - The examiner will wear gloves during the examination.
> - The speculum should be warmed and lubricated using warm water, and you will be asked to bear down, while breathing slowly.
> - The cervix is examined for color, shape, modules, masses, erosions, discharge, or bleeding.
> - Specimens are obtained cytological studies, if indicated, and a specimen for culture obtained from any suspicious discharge.
>
> *Adapted from Estes, M. (2006).* Health assessment and physical examination *(3rd ed.). New York: Thomson Delmar Learning.*

DIAGNOSTIC TESTS

The reproductive system has many disorders that require extensive diagnostic tests to determine the nature of the dysfunction. In general, there are specific tests for the male and specific tests for the female. Males have unique serum tests of such areas as the prostate gland and semen. Females have diagnostic tests of specific areas that are unique to their gender; such as the cervix and breast. This section of the chapter will examine the diagnostic tests for each gender separately.

Male Diagnostic Tests

Studies for assessment of health and disease in the male reproductive system include diagnosing infection, fertility issues, sexual dysfunction, structural abnormalities, and tissue masses. When indications of genitourinary infection are present, discharge or lesions may be swabbed or aspirated to obtain potential microorganisms for microscopic examination. To obtain a urethral smear, the male patient should not urinate prior to specimen collection. A small swab is inserted into the urethra. An anoscope is used to collect a rectal smear specimen and sample areas containing pus.

The smear of a specimen to which a gram stain is applied can distinguish gram-positive from gram-negative bacteria. A gram stain can provide important diagnostic information concerning the type of organisms present and the appropriate therapy to initiate while waiting for other test results. The gram stain is used to aid in the diagnosis of gonorrhea and candidal infections and in the assessment of urethritis, proctitis, and other infections characterized by a discharge.

Infections within the urethra, prostate, and bladder can contribute to urogenital dysfunction. Urinalysis detects bacteria, white blood cells, and red blood cells. Patient complaints, such as pain related to tissue inflammation, pain or irritation during voiding, bladder spasms, or alterations in urinary elimination, should be assessed by urinalysis. A clean-catch specimen may also be collected for examination.

Analysis of the semen for quality and presence of sperm is a primary diagnostic tool in infertility assessment. Semen specimens are obtained by masturbation into a sterile wide-mouthed container after two to five days of abstinence. The specimen must be analyzed within two hours of collection. Usually, two to three specimens, each separated by at least a month, are analyzed to ensure a meaningful evaluation. An obstruction of the ejaculatory duct is usually implied when **azoospermia** (absence of spermatozoa in the semen) is coupled with low ejaculate volume of nonclotting watery fluids that are fructose-negative. If the vasa are palpable, a transrectal ultrasonography (TRUS) can be diagnostic. Patients who are not azoospermic but are **oligospermic,** or have low sperm motility with a low semen volume, may have partial ejaculatory duct obstruction or retrograde ejaculation. Retrograde ejaculation is commonly seen in diabetics, as well as in men who have had transurethral surgery at, or near, the bladder neck. To assess for retrograde ejaculation a postejaculatory urine specimen is obtained. The specimen is obtained by first having the patient empty his bladder, then ejaculate. Following ejaculation the patient voids again into a separate container. Computer-assisted semen analysis (CASA) is available but is primarily used as a research tool and does not provide information that alters therapy at this time.

Prostate fluid is assessed when bacterial infection is suspected to be localized in the prostate gland. To obtain a specimen from the lower urinary tract for culture, the patient is asked to urinate a few drops into a sterile container. Then a midstream urine sample is collected in a second container. A prostate examination and massage are performed, and the prostate fluid is collected for culture and microscopic examination. The patient is then asked to urinate into a third container. A diagnosis of chronic bacterial prostatitis is made if the bacterial count of the postmassage urine sample is ten-fold higher than in the first urine samples.

DRE is performed by the practitioner to detect abnormalities of the prostate gland. Abnormalities such as induration, marked asymmetry, and frank nodularity are associated with clinically significant intracapsular prostate tumors. The examination can be performed in any of three positions: the patient can stand with flexed hips and lean over an examination table, lie on his side and curl inward, or kneel, face-down on top of the examination table. The examiner inserts the index finger into the rectum and palpates the prostate, which is situated between the examining finger and the symphysis pubis. While the DRE may detect abnormalities present in the posterior and lateral aspects of the glands, masses located on the anterior surface cannot be directly palpated. Used alone, DRE has been shown to miss approximately 40 percent of cancers detected during an initial screening (Daniels, 2003).

Basic endocrine evaluation includes measurement of serum testosterone and FSH, LH, and prolactin. LH abnormalities are rare and thus, LH levels need be obtained only in men with abnormal testosterone levels. Elevated serum FSH can result from impaired secretion of inhibin, which is produced by the Sertoli cell and provides feedback at the pituitary and hypothalamus to turn off FSH secretion. Elevated serum FSH can imply abnormalities in the seminiferous epithelium and subsequently spermatogenesis. Prolactin, another pituitary hormone, may affect fertility by decreasing LH production, resulting in a decrease in testosterone and subsequently, decreased libido. Low levels of FSH, LH, and testosterone are also diagnostic of hypogonadotropic hypogonadism resulting in a delay or failure in the onset of puberty and therefore poorly developed secondary sexual characteristics and small, firm testes. Serum estrogens, prolactin, and adrenal steroids are only measured if clinically indicated due to low serum testosterone, decreased libido, gynecomastia, or a history of precocious puberty.

PSA testing is used to evaluate men at risk for prostate cancer, to assist in pretreatment staging of prostate cancer, to monitor the posttreatment, and manage treatment of this disease. Produced exclusively by the epithelial cells of the prostate, periurethral, and perirectal glands, PSA is excreted by normal, hyperplastic, and malignant cells of the prostate. PSA increases yearly after age 40, but especially after age 50, by approximately 3 percent per year in healthy 60-year-olds without cancer. In conjunction with the DRE, PSA is used to investigate or evaluate an enlarged prostate gland or masses palpable on the prostate gland when cancer is suspected. PSA levels are determined in a 5-mL blood specimen, and a PSA reading of 4 nanograms and below is considered normal. A reading of up to 10 nanograms may be an indication of cancer. Men with PSA levels of 4.1 to 9.9 nanograms should undergo prostate biopsy. PSA levels may be repeated three or more times over a period of one to three years to determine PSA velocity. This can indicate the potential presence of prostate cancer and the need for a prostate biopsy before the total PSA becomes abnormally elevated. If the PSA increase is greater than 0.75 ng/mL over the last year, prostate cancer is likely present.

Prostate biopsy is the primary screening test for prostate cancer, though less than 25 percent of all biopsies contain cancer. Prostatic biopsy is performed by inserting a needle through the perineum (external) or via the rectum through the rectal wall to penetrate areas of nodularity or induration of the prostate. Multiple random needle biopsies may be performed to determine if a tumor is multifocal.

Ultrasonography measures and records high-frequency sound waves as they pass through tissues of variable density. Ultrasonography helps to identify masses greater than 3 cm, such as tumors within the prostate or nodal enlargement associated with metastasis or infections. Ultrasonography can also determine the adequacy of arterial circulation in the genital organs. TRUS is performed to view prostate tissue and is usually carried out in conjunction with prostatic biopsy.

After pathological confirmation of prostate cancer, MRI is used to determine the staging of the cancer. MRI can determine the extent of malignant involvement by exhibiting capsular penetration, seminal vesicle and neurovascular invasion, regional lymph node metastasis, or diffuse body metastasis.

In patients with PSA levels of 20 nanograms and higher, a radionuclide bone scan is done to rule out metastasis. Radionuclide can also localize in soft tissue areas, demonstrating calcification as well as infarction, inflammation, trauma, and tumor. Computed tomography (CT) scan detects grossly enlarged lymph nodes but does not provide clear pictures of intraprostatic features.

Testicular biopsy is used to determine if men with either azoospermia or severe oligospermia have an absence or deficiency of sperm production or whether obstruction is present at some point along the pathway from seminiferous tubule to ejaculatory duct. The procedure may also be performed to confirm presence of neoplastic tissue. Under local anesthesia, a 3- to 4-mm incision is made through the scrotum into the testis exposing about a pea-sized sample of seminiferous tubule. The procedure is often carried out in an operative setting where the patient may undergo immediate exploration and microsurgical reconstruction or sperm retrieval for immediate use in an in vitro fertilization (IVF) or intracytoplasmic sperm injection (ICSI) cycle or cryopreservation.

Cavernosometry and cavernosography are procedures that evaluate the flow of blood and pressure functions of the penis. These tests assess the integrity of the arterial and venous circulatory systems of the penis during an erection. Local anesthesia and an intracavernosal injection of a vasoactive drug are given prior to initiation.

Duplex ultrasonography is used to diagnose marked arterial insufficiency as the major cause of erectile dysfunction. Duplex ultrasonography entails high-resolution sonography with pulsed Doppler blood flow analysis to evaluate the penile arterial status. An injected vasodilator drug (e.g., papaverine hydrochloride, phentolamine mesylate, and prostaglandin E_1) is given prior to the test to enhance assessment of arterial or venous insufficiency.

The penile brachial index (PBI) is calculated by comparing the penile systolic blood pressure, determined by a Doppler, with the brachial systolic blood pressure at rest and after exercise. An intracavernosal injection of a vasoactive drug may be administered prior to the test. The normal range for PBI is equal to or more than 0.75, while abnormal range for PBI is equal to or less than 0.6. A PBI that is not within the normal range may indicate a vascular cause of erectile dysfunction.

Female Diagnostic Tests

This section will examine the diagnostic tests that are specific to disorders of the reproductive system of the female. Studies for assessment of health and disease in the female reproductive system include diagnosing infection, fertility issues, sexual dysfunction, structural abnormalities, and tissue masses. To begin, mammography is a radiographic image of the breast to screen for cancerous lesions in the breast tissue. The U.S. Preventive Services Task Force (USPSTF) recommends screening mammography, with or without clinical breast examination (CBE), every one to two years for women age 40 and older (U. S. Department of Health and Human Services, Agency for Health Care Research and Quality, 2002). Mammography, in combination with breast self-examination (BSE) and breast examinations during routine physical assessment, detects about 85 to 90 percent of existing breast cancers. The health history of women at increased risk for breast cancer (family history, genetic tendency, and past breast cancer) should be evaluated to determine the benefits and limitations of starting mammography screening earlier, having additional tests (breast ultrasound or MRI), or having more frequent examinations. Abnormalities of the breast determined by mammography or palpation should be further evaluated by fine needle biopsy or core needle biopsy that provides a larger sample, to determine the histology of the tissue mass or lesion. These procedures may be performed under local anesthesia in a clinic setting. Ultrasound may be used to guide the placement of the needle to targeted areas. If cancer is diagnosed, further treatment, such as surgery, chemotherapy, hormone therapy, or radiation, is also initiated.

Screening, particularly for STDs, can be performed by culture of blood samples, lesions, or any discharge from the reproductive tract. Chlamydia and gonorrhea are the two most common STD infections of the female reproductive tract. Both produce similar symptoms and may occur simultaneously. Because symptoms may be asymptomatic or mild, periodic screening is recommended among sexually active women.

Cervical cytological screening (Pap smear) is used to detect cancer and precursors of cancer in the uterine cervix. A sampling of exfoliated cells from the cervix is examined microscopically using a technique developed by Papanicolaou in 1942, thus, the current abbreviated name of Pap smear. Widespread use of Pap smears in routine gynecological screening in the United States has reduced deaths from cervical cancer by 75 percent. A description of the Pap test (e.g., speculum exam) and instructions to patients were described previously in the chapter. Women with atypical Pap smear results and evidence of high-risk type HPV should receive further evaluation with colposcopy.

Colposcopy involves examination of the cervix, the vagina, and at times, the vulva with magnification using a colposcope, a special binocular microscope and light system that magnifies the mucosal surfaces. A 3 percent solution of acetic acid is applied to improve the contrast between tissue types. Photographs for future reference and biopsy samples may be taken of any lesions that appear to be abnormal or suggestive of dysplasia or invasive cancer.

A culdoscopy is the examination of the viscera of the female pelvic cavity after introducing a flexible endoscope via the posterior vaginal fornix. It is use as a diagnostic procedure for infertility and for pelvic pain. Surgical procedures, such as tubal ligation, excision of an ovarian cyst, lysis of adhesions, and biopsy of endometriosis, may also be performed using culdoscopy. These procedures can be done using local, regional, or general anesthesia.

When cervical cytological studies reveal atypical squamous cells, a diagnostic excisional procedure should be carried out by the health care practitioner to obtain a specimen from the cervical transformation zone and endocervical canal for histological evaluation and to remove the area of cervical dysplasia. The specimen may be collected by several methods, including laser conization, cold-knife conization (CKC), loop electrosurgical excision (LEEP), and loop electrosurgical excision of transformational zone (LEETZ). All these procedures create a raw wound on the cervix and bleeding may require cauterization. Laser conization is performed with a carbon dioxide laser. The procedure may be performed with the use of colposcopy, which allows precise determination of the margins of the cervical lesion. Cold knife cone biopsy is the surgical excision of a wedge-shaped portion of the ectocervix and endocervix, including the removal of the entire squamocolumnar junction of the cervix. LEEP uses high-frequency electromagnetic currents to obtain a specimen by passing a thin wire loop through the transformation zone of the cervix approximately 1 cm in depth (Figure 61-4).

When abnormal uterine bleeding occurs an endometrial biopsy is performed to differentially diagnose hormonal imbalances or an anatomical cause for bleeding (e.g., polyps, hyperplasia, or cancer). The procedure involves taking a small sample of endometrial tissue from the inside of the uterus by inserting an endometrial suction catheter through the cervix and into the fundus of the uterus, where suction is applied to the catheter as it is gently rotated within the uterus. Endometrial tissue is collected by this process and sent for microscopic examination. In infertility treatment, endometrial biopsy is performed to evaluate the endometrial changes indicative of normal

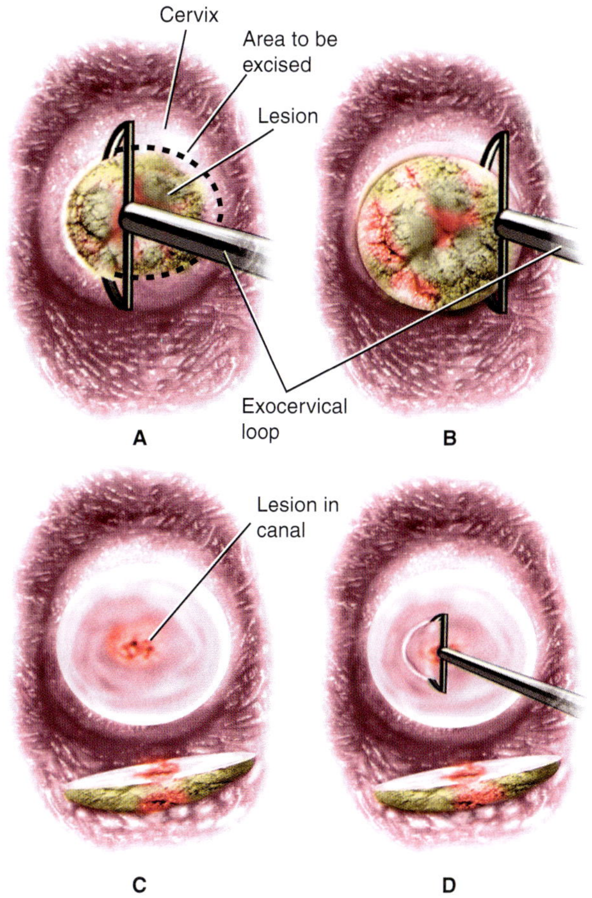

Figure 61-4 Cervical conization—LEEP technique: A. Path of electrosurgical loop through distal cervix, B. Loop near completion of excision, C. Lesion identified in cervix, D. Loop excision of lesion.

endometrial growth and cycling to determine endometrial readiness to accept embryo transplants.

Dilation and curettage (D & C) is a surgical procedure in which the cervical canal is dilated using dilators of graduated size and the endometrial tissue of the uterus is scraped out using a sharp curette. This procedure may be performed to evaluate infertility, to treat endometrial hyperplasia and other abnormal uterine bleeding, and as an abortion procedure.

Menstrual cycling, sexual responses, fertility, pregnancy, and menopause are all regulated by complex interactive endocrine activities involving the pituitary, ovaries, uterus, and other endocrine systems. When there are indications of abnormal functioning in any of these processes, there are a range of diagnostic endocrine studies that may be performed. FSH and LH studies are performed using a serum specimen and immunoassay. These studies are indicated in a range of reproductive disorders and assessments of abnormal functional patterns (gonadal failure, menstrual disturbances, and infertility). Estrogen and progesterone levels may be measured to determine the presence of dysfunction (e.g., gonadal dysfunction, menstrual abnormalities, or responses to hormone replacement therapy). Testosterone levels in women are normally 10 percent of the levels found in men. Levels in perimenopausal women may fall slightly more in relationship to age than to menopausal status.

Pregnancy tests are designed to detect hCG, a hormone produced by the placenta, using immunochromatographic assay. In normal pregnancy, hCG can be detected in serum as early as seven days following conception, doubling every 1.3 to 2 days and reading 100 mIU/mL at the first missed menstrual period. Serum levels less that 5 mIU/mL indicate that the woman is not pregnant. When using hCG-based urine tests, including those available OTC, the highest possible screening sensitivity conducted on the first day of a missed period is 90 percent. Pregnancy tests also assist in the diagnoses of suspected ectopic pregnancy, threatened abortion, incomplete abortion, and hCG-producing tumors.

Pelvic organs and tissues can be visualized by a range of endoscopic examinations. These procedures are usually performed on an outpatient basis even when performed under general anesthesia. Instructions for endoscopy may include bowel preparation and clear liquids or fasting on the day of the procedure. Postoperative instructions include the expectation of abdominal or referred pain and vaginal bleeding or discharge. Normal activities often are resumed within two to three days. Because these procedures are invasive, abdominal pain, fever, significant bleeding, or nausea and vomiting may indicate complications and need to be reported to the care provider immediately.

For reproductive assessments, laparoscopy using a fiberoptic scope may be performed to inspect the uterus, oviducts, ovaries, and lower pelvic region. Common indications for laparoscopy are unexplained pelvic pain, infertility procedures, suspected endometriosis, or ovarian masses. Procedures that can be performed under laparoscopic visualization include tubal sterilization, lysis of adhesions caused by endometriosis, and uterine fibroidectomy.

Hysteroscopy is a procedure in which direct visual examination of the uterus is used to investigate reproductive system problems, such as dysfunctional uterine bleeding, uterine fibroids, or suspected uterine cancer. The patient is given a local anesthetic and placed in the lithotomy position. Either carbon dioxide or fluid is inserted into the uterine cavity, and the hysteroscope is inserted through the vagina into the uterus. The uterine cavity is inspected for abnormalities and biopsies may be taken. Problems diagnosed with hysteroscopy include the cause of abnormal bleeding; fibroid tumors that arise within the uterine cavity; intrauterine polyps; location of a lost intrauterine device, uterine abnormalities, such as a uterine septum, bicornate uterus and, in some cases, endometrial cancer.

Basal body temperature (BBT) is a noninvasive method of determining the probable time of ovulation as well as determining ovulatory versus anovulatory cycles. The patient should use a digital basal thermometer and chart her oral temperatures taken after at least five hours of sleep and before arising from bed. A slight drop in temperature often occurs just before ovulation. After ovulation the temperature raises 0.2° to 0.4° C (0.4° to 0.8° F) and remains up through the remainder of the menstrual cycle. Records should be kept for at least three months to ascertain ovulation patterns.

The patient is taught to collect vaginal mucus using toilet tissue or her fingers and to document changes throughout her menstrual cycle. Before ovulation and after ovulation the cervical mucus is normally scant, thick, sticky, and opaque. When this ovulatory phase mucus is present, it indicates that ovulation has likely occurred. Postcoital examination of cervical mucus is used to evaluate the characteristics of cervical mucus and sperm function. Assessments include characteristics of the cervical mucus, correlated with the phase of the woman's menstrual cycle and with the number, morphology, motility, and ability of the sperm to cross the cervical mucus. The test should be scheduled one to two days before ovulation is anticipated and within two to three hours after intercourse.

When the female patient is experiencing infertility or recurrent pregnancy loss, the uterine cavity is evaluated through hysteroscopy, hysterosalpingogram, or sonohysterography. Hysterosalpingography involves instillation of contrast media through the cervix into the uterine cavity and out into the oviducts to determine abnormalities. The recent development of the falloposcope has increased the use of falloposcopy in evaluation of the oviducts in the infertile patient (American Infertility Association, 2005). Saline infusion sonohysterography (SHG) creates an image of the uterus and uterine cavity using ultrasonography after sterile saline is instilled into the uterine cavity. The purpose of SHG is to detect abnormalities of the uterus and endometrial cavity (e.g., abnormal uterine bleeding, infertility, or recurrent spontaneous miscarriage). The procedure begins with a transvaginal ultrasound examination. The uterine cavity is filled with sterile saline to improve the detail of the images of the uterine cavity. Pelvic ultrasound may be performed transabdominally, transvaginally, or endovaginally in women and transrectally in men. In reproductive system assessment in women pelvic ultrasound is most often used to examine the uterus and ovaries and, during pregnancy, to monitor the health and development of the embryo or fetus. Sonography can assist in determining the causes of pelvic pain, abnormal bleeding, or other menstrual problems and identifying palpable masses, such as ovarian cysts, uterine fibroids, and ovarian or uterine cancers.

A CT scan is an X-ray procedure that combines many X-ray images with the aid of a computer to generate cross-sectional views and three-dimensional images of the internal organs and structures of the body. A CT scan is used to define normal and abnormal structures in the body, as well as to accurately guide the placement of instruments or treatments during procedures. For reproductive assessment, CT scans are used to verify the presence or absence of tumors, infection, or abnormal anatomy, as well as to assist in certain procedures, such as biopsies of suspicious masses, draining of abscesses, or removal of fluids for diagnostic tests.

MRI uses radiofrequency waves and a strong magnetic field to provide clear and detailed images without exposing pelvic organs and tissues to radiation. MRIs can contrast uterine myometrium and endometrium; identify evidence of endometriosis; differentiate cervical, epithelial, and mucous tissue; and differentiate ovarian cysts and masses.

Prevention and control of STDs is based on education and counseling of persons at risk, identification of infected people, effective diagnosis and treatment of infected persons, evaluation and treatment of sex partners, and preexposure vaccinations of people at risk for vaccine-preventable STDs. As part of the clinical interview, health care providers can obtain a sexual history from their patients. If risk factors are identified, providers should encourage patients to adopt safer sexual behaviors. Patients seeking treatment or screening for STDs

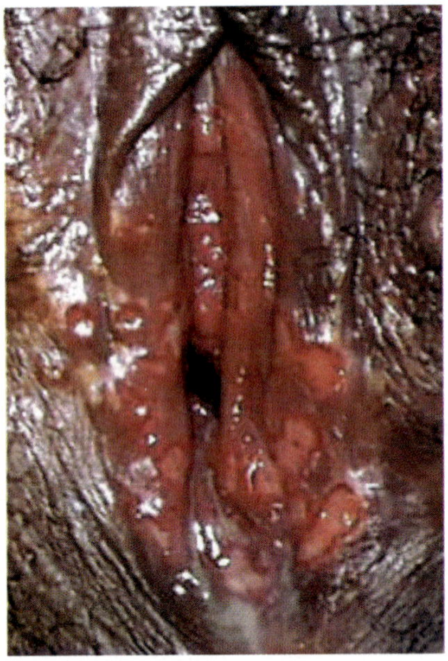

Figure 61-5 Primary HSV, first episode. Serology tests are negative for HSV. Copyright GlaxoSmithKline. Used with permission.

may expect evaluation for all common STDs (e.g., *Chlamydia trachomatis, Neisseria gonorrhoeae,* syphilis, herpes simplex virus [HSV], human papillomavirus, HIV).

A number of STDs can be diagnosed by point of care testing (POCT), which is defined as testing performed outside of clinical laboratories. This may be particularly relevant in clinical settings that provide care to transient populations, patients who may not be motivated to return for care after confirmation of an STD, or with patients who do not have access to regular health care. However, most STD POCT should be verified by additional standard testing within a clinical laboratory. In addition, physical examination can detect STD abnormalities (Figure 61-5). Most patients whose STDs are treatable with antibiotics should return for a test of cure, ensuring that the treatment regimen was effective.

Laboratory-based tests are available for many of the STD disorders. POCT has long included the gram-stained smear for *N. gonorrhoeae* and *C. trachomatis.* In addition, cultures are also performed on endocervical swab specimens in the female, or for male patients, on an intraurethral swab specimen. Specimens may also be obtained from rectal or pharyngeal swab specimens. The screening tests for syphilis are the Venereal Disease Research Laboratory (VDRL) and rapid plasma reagin (RPR) tests that detect a rise in antibody titers following infection (U.S. Department of Health and Human Services, Centers for Disease Control and Prevention, 2003).

KEY CONCEPTS

- The primary functions of the male reproductive system are production, transport, and deposit of sperm and secretion of testosterone.
- The primary functions of the female reproductive system are production of ova, secretion of hormones, pregnancy and birth of a fetus, and breastfeeding an infant.
- The physiological components of male sexual response include erection, orgasm, and ejaculation.
- Adequate functioning of the neurological and vascular systems is important in physiological sexual responsiveness.
- Sexual dysfunction is a disturbance or disorder in desire, excitement, or orgasm of the sexual response cycle.
- Sexuality is an integral component of physical and emotional health for all people, incorporating gender identity, self-worth, the ability to establish healthy intimate relationships, and expressions of sexual behaviors.
- Sexual violence victims exhibit immediate reactions that can include shock, disbelief, fear, confusion, and anxiety, symptoms associated with PTSD.
- Assessment of the female reproductive system consists of breast examination, palpation of the external genitalia, speculum assessment, laboratory analysis, bimanual examination, and rectovaginal assessment.
- Women with specific concerns about premenstrual symptoms, irregular menstrual cycles, or dysmenorrhea should be assessed for further diagnostic work.
- Assessment of the male reproductive system includes self testicular examination, laboratory analysis, prostate examination, and palpation of external genitalia.

REVIEW QUESTIONS

1. Sperm generation in the male is dependent on testosterone production, which is mediated by which pituitary gland hormones?
   1. Gonadotropin-releasing hormone and FSH
   2. FSH and LH
   3. Gonadotropin-releasing hormone and Sertoli hormone
   4. LH and Sertoli hormone
2. Menstruation is the result of:
   1. Withdrawal of human chorionic gonadotropin
   2. Decreasing production of LH and progesterone
   3. Decreasing production of estrogen and progesterone by the corpus luteum
   4. Withdrawal of FSH and LH
3. In both the male and female body, the fundamental physiological responses to effective sexual stimulation are:
   1. Vasocongestion and muscle tension (myotonia)
   2. Erections and increased blood pressure and heart rate
   3. Lubrication from the Cowper's gland and the Bartholin's glands
   4. Excitement and plateau
4. Why is it essential for the health care practitioner to address sexual health concerns in routine health assessment?
   1. To ensure the patient that sexual health concerns are an important aspect of health
   2. To ensure the patient that sexual concerns can be discussed in the health care setting
   3. To provide opportunity to discuss preventive sexual health lifestyles with the patient
   4. All of the above
5. Which of the following questions is not part of a sexual history?
   1. Are you currently sexually active?
   2. Is sex satisfying to you?
   3. How has your present illness (concern) affected your sexual functioning?
   4. Which sexual positions do you prefer?
6. Which of the following symptoms is commonly associated with sexually transmitted infections in the male?
   1. Penile discharge with pain on urination
   2. Difficulty initiating a steady urine stream
   3. Heavy tenderness in the scrotum
7. A 22-year-old woman returns to the health clinic with her concerns about pelvic pain. Although her pelvic examination revealed no apparent abnormalities beyond the general tenderness, the nurse notes bruises on her upper arms and chest. An important question to ask would be:
   1. Are your injuries work-related?
   2. Do you bruise easily? Does your family have a history of a clotting disorder?
   3. Violence is a problem for many women. Has someone been hurting you?
   4. Have you been raped?
8. Which of the following descriptions of vaginal discharge is indicative of possible bacterial vaginosis?
   1. Odorless, white, opaque mucus that is sticky
   2. Copious, green, frothy, somewhat malodorous discharge
   3. Odorless, plaque-like patches accompanied by vulvar redness
   4. Copious, gray, malodorous, or "fishy" odor discharge
9. A 3-cm nodule was palpated during the digital rectal examination of the prostate gland? What diagnostic tests would be recommended to evaluate the nodule?
   1. Prostate ultrasonography, biopsy of nodule, and PSA
   2. PSA, serum testosterone level, and MRI
   3. MRI, serum testosterone level, and PSA
   4. Prostate ultrasonography and serum testosterone level
10. The Pap smear as part of routine pelvic assessment of the female patient examines what specific tissue for potential precancerous or cancerous changes?
    1. The transformation zone between columnar epithelial cells of the cervical canal and the squamous cells covering the outer cervix
    2. The squamous cells of the cervix on the posterior surface and along the posterior fornix of the vagina
    3. The cervical mucus, which contains sloughed cells from the uterine lining as well as the cervical canal
    4. Any cervical lesions showing evidence of HPV

Continued

REVIEW QUESTIONS—cont'd

11. What is the rationale for teaching an 18-year-old male how to perform self-examination of his genitals?
1. Self-examination can prevent him from acquiring an STD.
2. Testicular torsion is a surgical emergency that requires prompt identification and treatment.
3. Self-examination can help determine when he has achieved fully developed genitalia.
4. Testicular cancer is the most common type of cancer in young men.

12. A female patient indicated that she has sex with multiple partners and she does not use condoms because she is on oral contraceptives. Which of the following responses is most appropriate?
1. How long have you been on oral contraceptives?
2. You should avoid sex until you are married.
3. Even though you are on oral contraceptives, you should use condoms to protect yourself from sexually transmitted disease.
4. How well do you know your partners?

REVIEW ACTIVITIES

1. Role-play taking a sexual health history with a peer to increase your comfort in asking appropriate questions.
2. Provide nursing care for a person of the opposite gender who is close to your age. Describe the potential difficulties of patient education regarding self-examinations that are characteristic of reproductive function (e.g., TSE, BSE).
3. Describe the sexual response cycle to a peer and afterward discuss together the areas that you believe will be somewhat uncomfortable for you to verbalize with a patient.
4. Compare four diagnostic tests in the reproductive system, which are performed with a male.
5. Compare four diagnostic tests in the reproductive system, which are performed with a female.

Visit the Contemporary Medical-Surgical Nursing online companion resource at www.delmarhealthcare.com for additional content and study aids. Click on Online Companions then select the Nursing discipline.

Female Reproductive Dysfunction: Nursing Management

Mary Franklin, MSN, CNM

CHAPTER 62

CHAPTER TOPICS

- Menstrual Disorders
- Reproductive Tract Infections
- Benign Reproductive Tract Conditions
- Female Genital Mutilation
- Reproductive Tract Malignancies
- Infertility
- Sexual Dysfunction

The female reproductive system is complicated both in terms of anatomical structures and of hormonal regulation. A result of that complexity, reproductive dysfunctions are common. Nurses play a crucial role in the care of women with reproductive dysfunctions, and there is strong nursing collaboration with other disciplines that also provide care for women. Nurses with basic clinical preparation, advanced practice nurses, and certified nurse midwives work in the area of women's reproductive health care. The social and psychological consequences of female reproductive dysfunctions require skilled and sensitive nursing care. The topics discussed in this chapter are menstrual disorders, reproductive tract infections, benign reproductive tract conditions, female genital mutilation, reproductive tract malignancies, infertility, and sexual dysfunction.

KEY TERMS

Anovulation
Condyloma
Didelphic
Dysfunctional uterine bleeding (DUB)
Dysmenorrhea
Dyspareunia
Endometriosis
Imperforate hymen
Leiomyomata
Menopause
Menorrhagia
Metrorrhagia
Müllerian dysgenesis
Myomectomy
Oligomenorrhea
Perimenopause
Primary amenorrhea
Primary anorgasmia
Secondary amenorrhea
Secondary anorgasmia
Vaginitis

MENSTRUAL DISORDERS

Menstrual disorders are varied and have many different consequences in females. The menstrual disorders included in this section are: dysmenorrhea, amenorrhea, menopause, and premenstrual disorders.

Dysmenorrhea

Dysmenorrhea or pain during the menstrual cycle, affects 75 percent of menstruating women, and 90 percent of adolescents experience it with the onset of ovulatory cycles. Menstrual pain is commonly described by women as a cramping pain but may also include backache and leg pain. The release of prostaglandin hormone with the onset of menses is a main factor in dysmenorrhea. Increased prostaglandin release also accounts for the nausea, sweating, and bowel emptying experienced by some women at the start of their cycles.

Dysmenorrhea is not as common in the first 12 to 24 months after menarche, before cycles become ovulatory. Dysmenorrhea occurring with the first few menstrual cycles can be caused by an outflow obstruction and should be evaluated. **Leiomyomata** (benign smooth muscle tumors of the uterus commonly called fibroids), infection, ovarian cysts (globular sacs on the ovaries that are filled with fluid or semisolid material), or **endometriosis** (growth of the functioning endometrial tissue that lines the uterus somewhere outside of the uterus) may cause a significant worsening or new onset of dysmenorrheal (Figure 62-1). Therefore, dysmenorrhea not responsive to nonsteroidal anti-inflammatory drugs (NSAIDs) or combined oral contraceptives must be evaluated.

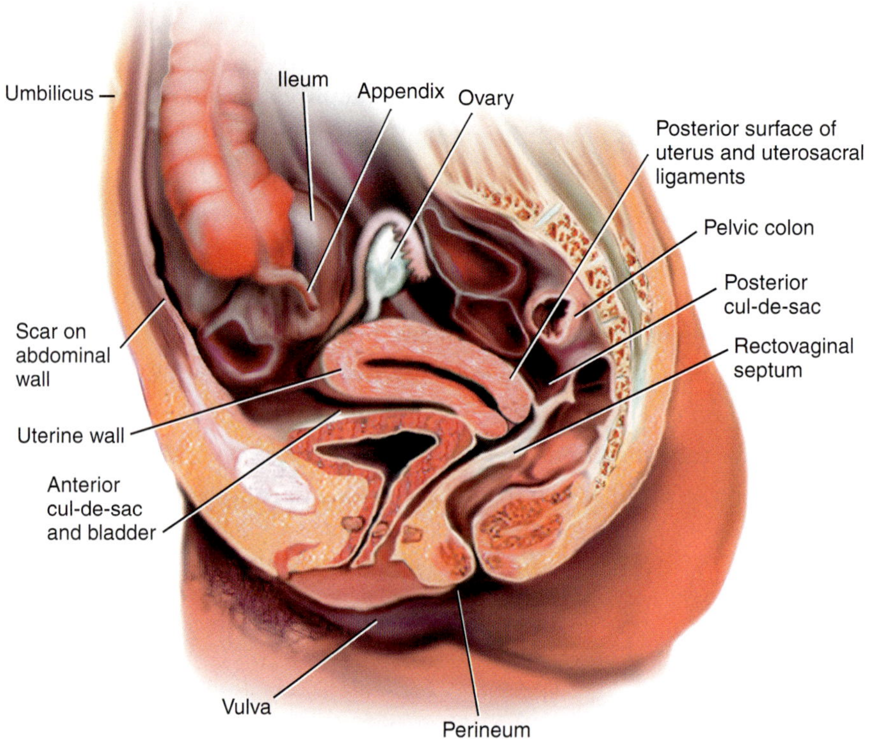

Figure 62-1 Common areas of endometriosis.

Amenorrhea

The average age of menarche in the United States is 12.8 years. In **primary amenorrhea** menstrual cycles have not started by age 16. In **secondary amenorrhea** menstrual cycles start normally but then stop. Of prime importance in evaluating any woman with amenorrhea is ruling out pregnancy.

Distinguishing primary from secondary amenorrhea is done to rule out the structural abnormalities that only need to be considered in primary amenorrhea. Primary amenorrhea can be caused by a congenital absence of a part of the reproductive tract, such as the ovaries, uterus, or vagina. Another cause is when the hymenal opening at the exit of the vagina does not form **(imperforate hymen),** and there is no exit from the vagina. Imperforate hymen occurs in 1 in 1,000 women. When imperforate hymen is the only abnormality menstrual cycles occur normally, but menstrual flow cannot be released to the outside and considerable pain and pelvic distension occurs. Treatment of imperforate hymen is excision of the hymen. This is usually a simple office procedure, performed under local anesthesia, which provides immediate resolution of the problem without sequelae.

Amenorrhea, either primary or secondary, can also occur because of disruptions in the hypothalamic system, elevated prolactin levels, thyroid disorders, premature ovarian failure, lack of sufficient body fat, or as a side effect of medication, stress, surgery, or local trauma. Unexplained secondary amenorrhea that lasts three months or longer or **oligomenorrhea** (menstrual cycles that occur farther apart than usual) of nine cycles or less per year needs evaluation (Practice Committee of the American Society for Reproductive Medicine, 2004). Amenorrhea is sometimes an expected event not requiring evaluation. Breastfeeding women will commonly be amenorrheic for up to 10 months postpartum. Amenorrhea is an expected and sometimes desired side effect of medications such as long-acting progesterone contraceptives and gonadotropin-releasing hormone (GnRH) agonists.

Athletes and women with anorexia nervosa can be amenorrheic if fat comprises less than 10 percent of their body. The female athlete triad includes the following three components: a menstrual disorder (amenorrhea or oligomenorrhea), an eating disorder, and decreased bone mineral density (Sherman & Thompson, 2004). Obese women also have a higher incidence of amenorrhea. Excessive scraping of the uterine lining with curettage, usually after childbirth or abortion, can cause permanent damage to the uterine lining and an absence of further menstruation. This is called Asherman's syndrome.

Women with amenorrhea always have **anovulation** (failure of the ovaries to grow or failure to release ova) except when amenorrhea is caused by a structural problem (American College of Obstetricians and Gynecologists [ACOG], 2002). Treatment of amenorrhea depends on its cause. Correcting pituitary disorders, thyroid disorders, or gaining sufficient body fat usually results in a resumption of menses.

For women with a hypothalamic disorder, progesterone therapy can be used to initiate a cycle. For example, a course of 10 mg of Provera for 10 days may be prescribed. Most amenorrheic women without other disorders will have a cycle within two weeks of taking Provera. If Provera alone does not initiate a cycle, particularly if amenorrhea is long-standing, estrogen therapy to prime the endometrium prior to taking Provera may prove effective. If there is no menses with estrogen followed by progesterone therapy, then expert consultation is required. Continued therapy for amenorrhea includes repeated courses of Provera, or hormonal contraceptives, to induce a cycle at least once every three months. Provera therapy will not protect against a pregnancy. If conception is desired, ovulation induction may be required.

Menopause

The average age of natural **menopause** (cessation of menses) in the United States is 51.4 years, with an age range of 42 to 58 years. By the time women are in their early 50s, 90 percent will have experienced menopause. Smoking accelerates the age of menopause by 1.5 to 2 years. That means that about 50 million women are currently in the menopausal transition or in menopause. Women are considered to be menopausal if they have not had a menstrual cycle for 12 months. Cessation of menstrual cycles is caused by cessation of ovarian function and estrogen depletion. When life expectancy was age 50, few women experienced menopause. With an average life expectancy of 70 to 80 years, women now spend up to one third of their life in menopause.

The **perimenopause** transition includes the 5 to 10 years before menses cease. As the ovaries begin to decline in function, hormonal fluctuations are common. Women may have irregular cycles and some inconsistent menopausal symptoms. Anovulatory menses is common.

The depletion of estrogen with onset of menopause can lead to vasomotor symptoms including hot flashes and night sweats, difficulty with memory and concentration, sleep disturbances, skin changes, vaginal dryness, and an increased risk of osteoporosis and cardiovascular disease. The incidence and severity of hot flashes is variable, although most hot flashes are mild to moderate and decrease in intensity and frequency over time. Women typically report that hot flashes last six months to 2 years, although some women report hot flashes for as long as 10 years. Increased environmental temperatures, higher body mass index (BMI), cigarette smoking, sedentary lifestyle, and lower socioeconomic status (SES) have all been related to an increased incidence of hot flashes (North American Menopause Society [NAMS], 2004).

In the past, replacement of estrogen was considered beneficial for women's health, not only in terms of symptom relief, but also for prevention of cardiovascular disease and osteoporosis. It was routine to offer and encourage women to take estrogen therapy as they became postmenopausal. In July, 2002, a large study of postmenopausal estrogen and progesterone therapy was ended early when investigators found an increased risk of coronary heart events, stroke, breast cancer, and pulmonary embolism (Writing Group for the Women's Health Initiative Investigators, 2002). In 2004 the Food and Drug Administration (FDA) evaluated the research evidence and decided to require a boxed warning of harm for estrogen/progesterone formulations. They strongly recommend that estrogen preparations not be used to prevent

Uncovering the Evidence

Perimenopausal Symptoms and Age

Discussion: In this study of 418 women ages 30 to 50, the authors found that the following perimenopausal symptoms increased with age: sleeplessness, moodiness, depression, and poor concentration. Headache ranked first among symptoms for severity. The study subjects did not often recognize the symptoms of perimenopause.

Implications for Practice: Education and anticipatory guidance for women entering perimenopause should be included in women's health care.

Source: Lyndaker, C., & Hulton, L. (2004). The influence of age on symptoms of perimenopause. Journal of Obstetric, Gynecologic, and Neonatal Nursing, *33(3), 340–347.*

Fast Forward ▶▶▶

Tibolone for Menopause Symptoms

Tibolone is used to treat postmenopausal symptoms in more than 70 countries and approval by the FDA is pending in the United States. Tibolone is related to the progestins in oral contraceptive agents, but it acts differently on selected tissues. Tibolone has been demonstrated to give relief for the vasomotor symptoms of menopause, vaginal dryness, and for osteoporosis prevention. It does not seem to increase the risk for endometrial proliferation, cardiovascular events, or breast cancer. Tibolone may be the next news in hormone therapy for postmenopausal women (Speroff & Clarkson, 2003).

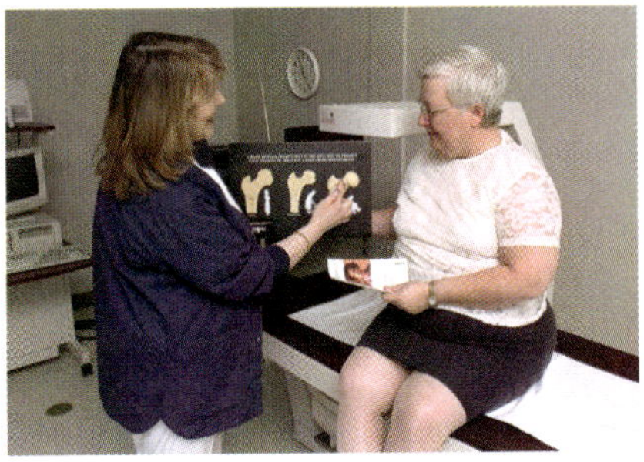

Figure 62-2 As women approach menopause, osteoporosis prevention education is critical in promoting optimal health.

coronary disease or osteoporosis. In addition, the following recommendations are made for using estrogen therapy:

- Estrogen and progesterone should not be used to prevent coronary events, strokes, or osteoporosis.
- There are risks with the use of postmenopausal estrogen, and each woman must have an individual assessment of whether the benefits outweigh the risks.
- Estrogen therapy is the most effective relief for vasomotor symptoms and vaginal dryness, but estrogen should be used for the shortest amount of time and in the lowest doses and with full knowledge of risks and benefits.

Estrogen therapy should be done on an individual basis, taking into consideration a woman's complete health and family history, particularly her risk for cardiovascular disease and breast cancer. When estrogen therapy is prescribed for a woman who still has her uterus, progesterone therapy must also be prescribed to reduce the risk of endometrial cancer.

Topical vaginal therapy is an effective treatment for vaginal atrophy and dryness. Vaginal rings, cream, and tablets are available. Vaginal lubricants, moisturizers, and maintaining regular sexual activity can help relieve and prevent vaginal dryness. Progesterone therapy to protect the endometrium is not necessary when only vaginal therapy is used. Ultra-low-dose estradiol therapy in a transdermal patch (Meno star) has been developed to prevent osteoporosis. This therapy is not indicated to relieve the vasomotor symptoms.

Risk reduction for heart disease and osteoporosis must be part of the health care of menopausal women (Figure 62-2). This includes education on diet, exercise, calcium and vitamin D intake, and screening for cholesterol and bone density. Other therapies for osteoporosis prevention and treatment should be considered for women not taking hormone therapy.

In addition to natural menopause, women of all ages can experience surgical menopause induced by oophorectomy, the surgical removal of one or both ovaries. Women with removal of the uterus without removal of the ovaries will experience amenorrhea without other accompanying menopausal symptoms until the ovaries stop functioning at the usual age of menopause, because the ovaries continue to produce estrogen. When the ovaries are removed, either with or without the uterus, amenorrhea and menopausal symptoms begin immediately. The therapies for treating vasomotor symptoms in women experiencing surgical menopause are the same as for women experiencing natural menopause except that progesterone therapy is not required if estrogen is prescribed. The decision to use estrogen therapy for women experiencing surgical menopause must be made on an individual basis, taking into account the woman's age, significance of symptoms, and health status.

Premenstrual Syndrome and Premenstrual Dysphoric Disorder

Premenstrual syndrome (PMS) is a collection of symptoms associated with the last half of the menstrual cycle and usually relieved shortly after the onset of menstruation. Symptoms can be physical, such as bloating, headache, and breast tenderness or mental and emotional, such as irritability, depression, anxiety, food cravings, and mood swings. Social withdrawal and difficulty concentrating may also be present. The symptoms are severe enough to prompt 30 to 40 percent of women with PMS to seek treatment (Reid & Bruce, 2003). To diagnose PMS, charting of symptoms is helpful to establish a pattern of symptoms clustered in the last half of the cycle and relieved shortly after the onset of menses.

Premenstrual dysphoric disorder (PMDD) is a form of PMS with more severe emotional symptoms. Only 3 to 8 percent of women have PMDD. PMDD has not been officially adopted as a diagnosis by the American Psychiatric Association but has been identified as a proposed diagnosis requiring further study. The main symptoms of PMDD are markedly depressed mood, marked anxiety, marked affective lability, and decreased interest in activities. To establish a diagnosis these symptoms should have occurred during the last week of the luteal phase of the menstrual cycle during most cycles in the previous 12 months. The symptoms begin to resolve during the week of menses and are always absent in the week after the menses. PMS and PMDD resolve once menopause occurs.

To diagnose PMDD, five or more of the following symptoms must have been present most of the time during the last week of the luteal phase:

- Feeling sad, hopeless, or self-deprecating
- Feeling anxious
- Mood swings or tearfulness
- Persistent irritability
- Anger and increased conflicts in relationships
- Feeling fatigued, lethargic, or lacking in energy
- Marked changes in appetite with binges or food cravings
- Increased sleep or insomnia
- Feeling overwhelmed
- Physical symptoms
- Suicidal thoughts

When these symptoms are severe enough to impair the ability to function in everyday life, evaluation by a health care provider is needed. It is important to distinguish PMDD from clinical depression, anxiety, or panic disorders or the premenstrual exacerbation of an underlying psychiatric disorder. The hallmark of PMDD is that there is always a symptom-free period every month. Diagnosis of PMS and PMDD is done with charting of symptoms each month for at least three months and exclusion of other diseases.

Polycystic Ovary Syndrome

Polycystic ovary syndrome (PCOS) is an endocrine disorder usually characterized by multiple ovarian cysts, oligomenorrhea or amenorrhea, hirsutism, acne, obesity, and infertility. Alopecia and hypertension may also be present. The incidence of PCOS is approximately 5 to 10 percent, making it the most common endocrine disorder in women of childbearing age. A recent study conducted in Alabama of 400 premenopausal women found an incidence of 6.6 percent (Azziz, et al., 2004). PCOS is considered to be an endocrine disorder involving insulin resistance and higher than usual testosterone levels.

The exact cause of PCOS is not known, but genetic mutations are being studied, because there is a strong genetic tendency for PCOS. Women with PCOS may have male or female relatives with adult-onset diabetes, elevated triglyceride levels, and hypertension and female relatives with infertility, hirsutism, and menstrual disorders (McKittrick, 2002). Women with PCOS should also have testing for diabetes and hyperlipidemia, because they are at risk for diabetes and coronary artery disease due to insulin resistance.

Lifestyle recommendations for PCOS include weight loss as a first priority, exercise including aerobic and weight resistance training, identifying and correcting behavioral impediments to healthy eating and exercising, adding 1,000 to 1,500 mg of calcium and a multivitamin supplement to their diet, and avoiding smoking. Correcting insulin resistance with metformin can result in resumption of regular menstrual cycles and fertility. Metformin plus clomiphene citrate to induce ovulation is also used to induce ovulation to achieve pregnancy. Combined oral contraceptives regulate menstruation, reduce androgen levels, and help clear acne.

Hair removal products help with hirsutism. Topical eflornithine HCL (Vaniqa) reduces unwanted facial hair in women (Cowan & Graham, 2003). Studies have shown that a significant problem with PCOS is body image and self-esteem. Depression or emotional lability are common and may be related to insulin resistance, physical symptoms of androgen excess, such as hirsutism and acne, or infertility. A small qualitative study in the United Kingdom found that women with PCOS felt abnormal as women because of hirsutism, disordered menstruation, and infertility (Varcoe, 2002).

Dysfunctional Uterine Bleeding

Dysfunctional uterine bleeding (DUB) is defined as abnormal uterine bleeding in the absence of pathology and includes **menorrhagia** (prolonged or excessive, but regular, menses), **metrorrhagia** (bleeding between menstrual cycles), and postmenopausal bleeding. DUB is often related to anovulation and is therefore common at both ends of the age spectrum. Adolescents often have irregular cycles in the first year or two of initiating cycles, and women in the perimenopause often have irregular or disordered bleeding. Anovulation results in continued endometrial growth without progesterone-induced bleeding and results in unpredictable bleeding in terms of both timing and volume. Assessment of DUB includes a careful history. Menstrual cycles that are shorter than 21 days in length or longer than 7 days in duration are usually considered abnormal. Menorrhagia affects 15 to 20 percent of women who have DUB.

One defining characteristic of DUB is the absence of reproductive pathology. DUB may be caused by thyroid disorders, hormonal imbalances, clotting disorders, or as a side effect of medications, among other etiologies. Abnormal uterine bleeding that can be associated with pathology is distinct from DUB and can be caused by polyps (small tumor like growths that project from mucous membrane), leiomyomata, infection, carcinomas, local trauma, ovarian cysts (globular sacs on the ovaries filled with fluid or semisolid material), and pregnancy complications.

When DUB occurs in adolescents, inherited clotting disorders, such as platelet disorders, prothrombin deficiencies, idiopathic thrombocytopenia, and von Willebrand's disease should be considered. The incidence of von Willebrand's disease is approximately 1 percent of the population. There is a clear genetic component for von Willebrand's disease, so a family history should be obtained. Leukemia should be ruled out in adolescents with menstrual hemorrhages. Perimenopausal and postmenopausal bleeding should be a cause to suspect reproductive tract carcinomas until these are excluded.

The incidence of endometrial cancer increases with age, therefore all women over age 40 need evaluation of anovulatory bleeding with endometrial biopsy. Endometrial biopsy, typically done in the outpatient setting, involves removing a sample of the uterine lining. Usually, no anesthesia is required for the procedure. A thin catheter is placed through the cervical canal into the endometrium, and a small amount of endometrial lining is removed and sent to the pathology lab for examination. If dilation of the cervix is necessary to allow for passage of the catheter, then a local anesthetic, either a topical spray or injectable anesthesia is used. The patient commonly experiences menstrual-like cramping during and for a short time following the procedure. Endometrial biopsy may be performed by a physician, an advanced practice nurse, or a physician's assistant.

Therapy for DUB depends on the cause of the disordered bleeding. Initial treatment is often antiprostaglandin therapy with NSAIDs or cyclooxygenase inhibitors. An antiprostaglandin is started with the first day of the cycle and continued throughout the menses. Treatment may include hormonal therapies, such as combined or progesterone-only oral contraceptives, injectable progesterone or GnRH agonists, the levonorgestrel-containing intrauterine system, destruction of the uterine lining using heat or laser, or treatment of fibroids. Tranexamic acid, a fibrinolytic agent, has been studied in the United Kingdom, Pakistan, and Australia and has shown to be an effective treatment for DUB.

Endometrial ablation, or destruction of the uterine lining with heat, results in amenorrhea for 50 percent of women. Endometrial ablation is done under

Dollars and Sense

DUB

Hysterectomy is one of the most common surgical procedures performed on women. According to the Centers for Disease Control and Prevention (CDC, 2002a). After cesarean section, hysterectomy is the second most frequently performed major surgical procedure for women of reproductive age in the United States. Approximately 600,000 hysterectomies are performed annually in the United States, and an estimated 20 million women have had a hysterectomy. Hysterectomy accounts for a significant proportion of health care costs for reproductive women, including the cost in terms of lost wages during recovery. This has led to an abundance of research into the cost effectiveness of alternatives to hysterectomy in the treatment of DUB. In one study of the levonorgestrel-releasing intrauterine system (IUS) to treat DUB, patient satisfaction for the IUS and hysterectomy were comparable. The cost for treatment with the IUS was approximately half the cost of treatment with hysterectomy (Hurskainen, et al., 2004). Expect the scrutiny of various alternative treatments for improvement in quality of life and cost-effectiveness to continue, with perhaps a future debate on which patients are appropriate hysterectomy candidates.

general anesthesia, and patient satisfaction with the procedure is 90 to 95 percent. Hysterectomy, surgical removal of the uterus, also has high patient satisfaction ratings for relief of dysfunctional bleeding (Kuppermann, et al., 2004).

Acute uterine hemorrhage commonly occurs during a spontaneous abortion or in prolonged perimenopausal bleeding but may also occur secondary to uterine fibroids or other uterine conditions. Hemorrhage that occurs in the postpartum or postoperative period is classified as a complication rather than as a reproductive dysfunction. Most commonly, a woman presents at the emergency department with a complaint of uncontrolled vaginal bleeding. The treatment for acute vaginal hemorrhage involves stabilizing the patient and making a rapid decision whether to implement medical therapy or operative therapy. The unstable patient usually requires an immediate dilatation of the cervix and removal of the uterine lining by scraping (dilatation and curettage [D & C]), to stop the hemorrhage. Hysterectomy is always a consideration, especially if childbearing is not an issue and there is a failure of medical therapy.

If the patient is stable, fluids, blood, and high-dose intravenous (IV) conjugated estrogens, 25 mg, are administered every four hours until the hemorrhage stops. High-dose estrogens have three actions that stop uterine hemorrhage: initiation of endometrial proliferation, increase in clotting factors, and promotion of platelet clumping and clotting at the capillary level.

Nursing management of the woman experiencing acute uterine hemorrhage includes a rapid assessment of status including vital signs, amount of visible hemorrhage, skin turgor, presence and location of pain, level of consciousness and orientation, and the possibility of pregnancy. The physician is immediately notified and IV fluid therapy is initiated. Lab work for complete blood count, clotting indices, pregnancy hormone level, and type and crossmatch is obtained. Administration of blood products and medications is done according to the physician's orders. Urinary catheterization may be required to most accurately monitor intake and output. Continuous monitoring of vital signs, intake and output, and level of consciousness is done until the patient has either stopped hemorrhaging and is stable, or is transferred to surgery. Support of the patient and family includes explanation of procedures and treatment, relieving anxiety, and helping the patient and family be prepared for surgery, if necessary.

Endometriosis

Endometriosis is a condition involving implantation of segments of endometrium outside of the uterus in the pelvis or abdomen. These implants behave as though they were located within the uterus. They bleed during the menstrual cycle and cause internal bleeding, pain, inflammation, and scarring. There are theories about how the endometrium becomes implanted outside the uterus, but there is no one explanation of how this happens. Implants can be on the ovaries, on the pelvic wall, on the fallopian tubes, on the colon, or elsewhere in the peritoneal cavity. Occasionally the implants occur in remote areas of the body.

Typically endometriosis is diagnosed between the ages of 25 and 35 and affects between 5 and 15 percent of women of reproductive age (Denny, 2004). Endometriosis among family members is common, and patients with an affected first-degree relative have 10 times the risk of developing endometriosis. Infertility affects 30 to 40 percent of women with endometriosis and is more common as the disease progresses. Symptoms are quite varied, depend on the location of the endometrial implants, and can include pelvic pain, severe dysmenorrhea, **dyspareunia** (painful intercourse), abnormal uterine bleeding, and infertility. Intestinal symptoms of abdominal cramping and diarrhea or constipation can also occur.

Diagnosis of endometriosis can be quite difficult, because there are no specific tests short of surgery to confirm the diagnosis. This means that there is often a delay in diagnosis, and a delay of several years between onset of symptoms and diagnosis is common. Once other causes for pain have been excluded, laparoscopic surgery is considered for diagnosis and removal of the implants.

If pregnancy is desired, conception is advised as soon as possible after surgery, because endometrial implants tend to recur and the best chance for successful conception is immediately after surgery. Hormonal therapy, such as Provera, norethindrone, depo-medroxyprogesterone acetate (DMPA), danazol, or leuprolide, can also be used. A limiting factor in leuprolide therapy is the cost—each three-month injection can cost $1,400 or more. Surgical treatments include excising implants or ablating them with laser. Hysterectomy is also a treatment option.

> **Skills 360°**
>
> **Reproductive Health History**
>
> Nurses, as well as patients, may feel uncomfortable about discussing reproductive health history. Here are some suggestions for helping to desensitize the history process. Nurses often use open-ended history questions, but in assessing menstrual cycles more directed questioning may be helpful. Helping women remember when their last menstrual cycle started may include use of a calendar, or questions such as "Your birthday was last month; was your period before or after your birthday?" When obtaining a reproductive history it is important to use language that is inclusive and nonjudgmental. Use phrases such as "your sexual partner" rather than "your husband." Avoid assumptions. If you ask "How many children do you have?" you may get an answer that is not the same as the answer to the question "How many pregnancies have you had?" Using a brief preface to the section of reproductive history questions paves the way for the history section and can make the patient more receptive to the questions. Here is an example of an introduction: "I'm going to ask you a series of questions about female health issues. The answers to these questions help give us an idea of your complete health status. If you don't understand the question I am asking or feel uncomfortable giving me an answer, please let me know."

Assessment with Clinical Manifestations

When assessing patients with actual or potential menstrual disorders, a careful history is most important. Women should be asked about their age at menarche, the date of the first day of last menstrual period (LMP), length of cycles and any recent changes, number of days of bleeding, amount of bleeding during cycles (light, moderate, or heavy), presence of clots, and any intermenstrual bleeding. Every woman should be encouraged to write down the days she has bleeding each month. Reviewing a history of bleeding days may reveal that a bleeding pattern that a woman thought was abnormal is just a variation of normal. Women can be assisted to determine cycle length by calculating the number of days between the first day of bleeding and the day before menses starts again.

Asking direct and concrete questions about the number of tampons or sanitary pads used, the amount of bleeding on each tampon or pad, and the presence or absence of clots gives a good indication of the amount of blood loss. Pain should be evaluated as to location, type, severity, relieving and aggravating factors, any changes in pain over time, and other symptoms associated with the pain. Women with painful cycles need to be asked questions about the impact of pain on their functioning and activities of daily living, as well as about the therapies that they use to treat the pain.

A history should be obtained about the type of contraception being used, recent surgeries or traumas, medications, chronic illness, family history—particularly of bleeding disorders, endometriosis and PCOS—usual type of physical activity, and eating disorders. Women should be asked about any constitutional symptoms, such as weight loss or gain, hot flashes, night sweats, heat or cold intolerance, fatigue, or insomnia. Queries regarding medications should include over-the-counter (OTC) medicines and herbal therapies, as well as prescription medications.

The treatment of menstrual disorders often changes depending on a woman's age and desires for childbearing, so women should be asked if they are currently planning a pregnancy, have a need for contraception, or have completed their families. It is important not to assume that all younger women want to become pregnant and that women over 35 with multiple children have completed their families. Women should be asked about the effect of their menstrual disorder on work and activities, relationships, sleep patterns, eating patterns, elimination patterns, and sexual interest and function. Pregnancy must be ruled out in cases of amenorrhea or irregular bleeding, and all women should be asked about the possibility of pregnancy. The history is not usually relied on to determine pregnancy status, however, and a routine pregnancy test is often ordered even if women deny sexual activity.

Diagnostic Tests

Diagnostic testing for dysmenorrhea includes a pelvic exam, cultures for gonorrhea (a sexually transmitted infection of the cervix caused by *Neisseria gonorrhoeae*), and chlamydia (a sexually transmitted infection of the cervix caused by *Chlamydia trachomatis*), and ultrasound, if structural abnormalities are a concern. Diagnostic tests for amenorrhea include the physical and pelvic examination and lab studies, such as a pregnancy test, prolactin level (to rule out prolactin-stimulating tumor), thyroid-stimulating hormone (TSH) level (to rule out thyroid disease), and follicle-stimulating hormone (FSH) level (to rule out premature ovarian failure). Ultrasound may be indicated if absence of reproductive organs is suspected as a cause of primary amenorrhea.

Menopause is diagnosed by a physical with a pelvic examination. FSH and estradiol levels can be drawn if the diagnosis of menopause is uncertain. Screening for osteoporosis risk (bone density scan), hyperlipidemia risk (cholesterol level), and breast cancer (mammogram) may be indicated.

No specific diagnostic tests exist for endometriosis short of laparoscopy. The diagnosis of endometriosis is made by eliminating other causes of pelvic pain, so cultures for infection, ultrasound, physical, and pelvic examination are often performed. A physical examination and pelvic exam are performed to diagnose PCOS. Lab testing may include testosterone level, insulin level, glucose testing, and serum dehydroepiandrosterone sulfate (DHEAS). Ultrasound can be done to verify polycystic ovaries but is not required for diagnosis.

PMS and PMDD are diagnosed by reviewing symptom diaries and excluding other causes of physical or emotional symptoms. Evaluation of DUB includes physical and pelvic examinations. Lab studies include a complete blood count and TSH. Diagnostic tests may include pregnancy testing, pelvic exam and Pap smear, ultrasound examination, saline-infusion sonogram, hysteroscopy, endometrial biopsy, D & C, and laparoscopy. Saline-infusion sonogram is an ultrasound study performed in the outpatient ultrasound area. A thin catheter is inserted through the cervix into the uterus, and saline is injected into the uterine cavity. The saline expands the endometrial cavity and helps with visualization of any anomalies. No anesthesia is typically needed unless dilation of the cervix is required.

Hysteroscopy is a procedure done in the operating room. It may be performed under local, regional, or general anesthesia and may be done in conjunction with D & C or laparoscopy. The cervix is dilated and the hysteroscope is inserted through the cervix into the uterus. Liquid or gas is used to improve visualization. Using light through the hysteroscope, the health care provider can directly view the uterine cavity and the opening of the fallopian tubes into the uterus.

D & C is done under regional or general anesthesia in the operating room. The cervix is dilated and the health care provider uses one or more instruments to scrape out the lining of the uterus. Samples of the uterine lining are often sent to the pathology lab for examination. D & C may provide both diagnosis and treatment of DUB. Lab work for DUB may include prolactin level, TSH, FSH, complete blood count, and screening for von Willebrand's disease.

Nursing Diagnoses

Based on the information gathered, examples of nursing diagnoses in the patient with menstrual disorders may include the following:

- Anxiety related to the impact of menstrual dysfunction on relationships, daily functioning, plans for childbearing, or implications of the disease.
- Deficient knowledge related to relief measures available for dysmenorrhea, range of normal menstrual patterns, or changes in health status associated with menopause.
- Acute or chronic pain related to dysmenorrhea or pain of endometriosis.
- Disturbed body image related to negatively viewing physical changes associated with PCOS.

Planning and Implementation

Care of the patient with menstrual disorders includes education, support, therapeutic interventions, and prevention measures. Collaborative management of the patient with dysmenorrhea requires evaluation by a physician, advanced practice nurse, or physician's assistant. Once other disorders are eliminated, relief of dysmenorrhea with prescription and nonprescription pain relief can be ordered by the evaluating provider. The nurse provides patient education about relief measures for dysmenorrhea, side effects and instructions for medications ordered, and symptoms that should prompt contact with the health care provider.

The patient with amenorrhea also needs a full evaluation. If the athletic triad is present, physical therapists can be an important part of the health care team in terms of making the assessment and its treatment and prevention (Papanek, 2003). Psychological counseling can be helpful for women with eating disorders. Nutritionists can assist with diet counseling for women with anorexia-related amenorrhea. Women with primary amenorrhea caused by imperforate hymen will need a hymenectomy performed in the physician's office by a gynecologist. Women with primary amenorrhea caused by congenital absence of reproductive organs will need consultation with a gynecologist and reproductive endocrinologist. A management plan for amenorrhea is outlined by the evaluating provider. The nurse provides the patient with education about the plan, when menses may be expected, the contraceptive effect (if any) of the medication provided, and what symptoms should prompt contact with the health care provider.

The patient in menopause needs an evaluation by a health care provider. A management plan for menopause is outlined by the evaluating provider. A nutritionist may assist the woman in modifying her diet to reduce vasomotor symptoms. The nurse plays an important role in education for women in menopause, because many of the health care interventions for women in menopause include strategies to maintain health and prevent symptoms and disease.

The patient with PMS/PMDD symptoms requires evaluation by a physician, advanced practice nurse, or physician's assistant. Psychological counseling may help with relationship issues and communication difficulties. A management plan for PMS/PMDD is outlined by the evaluating provider. The nurse provides the woman with PMS/PMDD education about monitoring her cycles, adjunctive therapies to relieve symptoms, and symptoms that should prompt contact with their health care provider.

The patient with PCOS needs an evaluation by a physician, advanced practice nurse, or physician's assistant. Consultation with an endocrinologist may be required. A nutritionist can assist the woman with PCOS in planning meals and snacks to reduce cravings and promote weight loss, and provide education and support. Psychological counseling may be helpful for women experiencing anxiety or self-esteem issues as well as those women with eating disorders. Spiritual counseling may be helpful for those with PCOS that has an effect on fertility. The nurse provides education, especially about the long-term implications of PCOS for the woman's overall health. The nurse also helps the patient problem-solve to maximize compliance to the treatment regimen and achieve the patient's goals such as fertility.

The patient with DUB requires an evaluation by a physician, advanced practice nurse, or physician's assistant. Gynecologists will perform hysteroscopy, laparoscopy, or other indicated surgery, such as hysterectomy. Hematologists may be consulted for women with von Willebrand's disease or other hematological disorders. If surgery is indicated, the nurse provides preoperative and postoperative care and education. The nurse also gives prescribed medications and monitors the patient for resolution of DUB. Nursing care includes educating women about monitoring cycles, adjunctive therapies to relieve symptoms, and symptoms that should prompt contact with the health care provider.

Women on antipsychotic medications may have prolactin abnormalities causing amenorrhea and may need hormonal therapy to have regular cycles (Miller, 2004). Women with cystic fibrosis can have amenorrhea related to poor weight gain and delayed puberty. Women with cystic fibrosis also may have congenital absence of pelvic organs (Jarzabek, et al., 2004). Chronic debilitating diseases, such as uncontrolled diabetes, end-stage renal disease, cancers, acquired immune deficiency syndrome (AIDS), or malabsorption, can result in amenorrhea from anovulation, probably caused by stress-induced hormonal changes (Practice Committee of the American Society for Reproductive Medicine, 2004).

Women with endocrine disease, cancer, systemic lupus erythematosus (SLE), anemia, or infection may have cyclical aggravation of their symptoms. Women with trauma or who have surgery can have short-term menstrual disturbances in their recovery phase. Inherited clotting disorders, such as idiopathic thrombocytopenia and von Willebrand's disease, can be the cause of DUB in adolescents. Migraines, asthma, allergies, and seizure disorders may be exacerbated during the premenstrual phase of the cycle, and it is important to distinguish between one of these aggravated conditions and PMDD.

Nutrition

Calcium-intake and a healthy diet should be addressed for postmenopausal women. Adequate intake of vitamin B_6, vitamin B_{12}, folic acid, and magnesium during the menopause are necessary to prevent cardiovascular disease and prevent osteoporosis. It is prudent for postmenopausal women to take a multivitamin supplement. For women with PMS/PMDD and physical symptoms, nutritional counseling on a diet low in salt, refined carbohydrates, caffeine, and alcohol, and increased calcium intake as well as small frequent meals may be beneficial. Supplementation with calcium, magnesium, vitamin B_6, and vitamin E may be helpful.

It is important to assess the learning needs of postmenopausal patients before giving advice or teaching about lifestyle recommendations. Although calcium intake is typically low in women older than 50, some women have a diet high in dairy products and do not need calcium supplementation. Women with adequate dietary calcium instead need messages of positive reinforcement about their calcium intake. In addition, some women have medical conditions in which calcium supplementation is not advised or a particular calcium supplement is not advised. Women with hypercalcemia or a history of calcium kidney stones may be advised not to take a calcium supplement. Women with diabetes need to consider their calcium supplement carefully, because some calcium supplements contain sugars. Tailoring the basic message of adequate calcium intake to the particular patient improves the effectiveness of teaching and enhances patient compliance (Roth, 2007).

Weight loss and regular exercise are recommended as part of the treatment regimen for PCOS. If obesity is present, weight loss is the first priority in treating PCOS. Nutrition counseling should include correcting behavioral impediments to healthy eating and advise adding 1,000 to 1,500 mg of calcium and a multivitamin supplement.

Pharmacology

There are five classes of medications used in the pharmacological management of menstrual disorders. The first class of medications used in treatment of menstrual disorders is the hormones. The second class of medications includes the pain relievers used to treat dysmenorrhea and menorrhagia. The third class of medications includes the selective serotonin reuptake inhibitors (SSRIs) used to treat PMS/PMDD and the mood disorders of menopause. The fourth class of medications includes the antihyperglycemic drug used to treat insulin resistance in PCOS. The final class of drugs includes the topical cream used to prevent unwanted facial hair in PCOS. Table 62-1 summarizes the medications used to treat menstrual disorders.

Surgery

DUB may be treated with endometrial ablation or hysterectomy. Endometriosis may be diagnosed and treated laparoscopically or with hysterectomy. Hysterectomy may include removal of only the body of the uterus without the cervix (partial hysterectomy) or the total uterus (complete hysterectomy).

TABLE 62-1 Medications Used to Treat Menstrual Disorders

DRUG	INDICATION	SIDE EFFECTS
Hormones		
Estrogen (Alora, Climara, FemPatch; Ogen; Premarin; Estrace; Estratab, etc.)	Suppression of vasomotor symptoms Prevention of urogenital atrophy	Breast tenderness; nausea; depression; headache; bleeding or spotting
Progestin (Provera; Hylutin; Aygestin; Megace; Depo Provera; Mirena; etc.)	DUB Amenorrhea Endometriosis	Breast tenderness; irregular bleeding
Combo oral contraceptives (Ortho Novum; Norinyl; Ovcon; Levlen; Modicon; Necon; Nelova; Estrostep; etc.)	Suppression of vasomotor symptoms Prevention of urogenital atrophy DUB Amenorrhea	Breast tenderness; nausea; depression; headache; bleeding or spotting
GnRH agonists (Lupron)	DUB Endometriosis	Amenorrhea; hot flashes; headache; vaginal dryness; reversible bone loss
Danazol (Danocrine)	Endometriosis	Weight gain; acne; hirsutism; deepening of voice
Nonsteroidal Anti-inflammatory Agents		
Motrin; Advil; Orudis; Mylan; Anaprox; Aleve; Ponstel; etc.	Relief of dysmenorrhea and menorrhagia	Gastric upset; heartburn; nausea; bleeding; renal impairment
Selective Serotonin Reuptake Inhibitors		
Celexa; Prozac; Luvox; Zoloft; Lexapro; Paxil	Relief of PMS/PMDD Relief of menopausal mood disorders	Irregular heartbeat; blood pressure changes
Hypoglycemic Drugs		
Glucophage	Reduce insulin resistance in PCOS	Nausea; vomiting; diarrhea; abdominal pain; decreased appetite
Topical Cream		
Vaniqa	Prevention/treatment of hirsutism in PCOS	Skin irritation; folliculitis

Adapted from Broyles, B., Reiss, B., & Evans, M. (2007). Pharmacological aspects of nursing care *(7th ed.). New York: Thomson Delmar Learning.*

Removal of the ovaries and fallopian tubes is called a salpingo-oophorectomy. The hysterectomy may be performed abdominally. Removal of the uterus, ovaries, and fallopian tubes through the abdominal incision is called total abdominal hysterectomy and bilateral salpingo-oophorectomy (TAH and BSO). Hysterectomy may also be performed vaginally. During a vaginal hysterectomy, the laparoscope can be used to help with visualization and removal of organs. This is called laparoscopically assisted vaginal hysterectomy (LAVH).

Nursing care for patients undergoing hysterectomy includes preoperative and postoperative care. Preoperative care includes patient education about the surgical procedure, anticipatory guidance about expected recovery and monitoring for complications, and assessing the patient's feelings about the loss of the uterus and childbearing ability. Nursing interventions to reduce anxiety and improve knowledge are most important. Postoperative nursing care is discussed in detail in chapter 22.

Alternative Therapy

Dysmenorrhea can often be relieved by drugs that have antiprostaglandin activity, such as NSAIDs. Other relief measures include heat and exercise. Studies have found fish oil to be of some benefit in dysmenorrhea relief, and preliminary studies from Germany found that magnesium supplementation reduced prostaglandin levels and relieved pain (Health Gate Data Corp, 2003). Supplementation with thiamine (vitamin B_1) or calcium has shown some effect on dysmenorrhea and herbal therapies, such as black cohosh, have been proposed as relief measures. Acupuncture and biofeedback have been shown to be of some benefit (Sidani & Campbell, 2002).

The dramatic shift away from traditional hormone therapy has led to a proliferation of alternative therapy to treat the vasomotor symptoms of menopause including black cohosh, evening primrose oil, soy supplements, vitamin E, antidepressants, such as venlafaxine, paroxetine, or fluoxetine, the anticonvulsant gabapentin, antihypertensives clonidine, methyldopa, or Bellergal (Fitzpatrick, 2003; NAMS, 2004). Acupuncture and yoga have been used to treat the vasomotor symptoms of menopause. Lifestyle modifications recommended to relieve hot flashes include reducing the environmental temperature and dressing in layers, increasing physical activity, weight reduction, smoking cessation, and relaxation techniques.

Botanical therapy with chasteberry, black cohosh, gingko biloba, or St. John's wort has been used to relieve PMS and PMDD symptoms (Girman, Lee, & Kligler, 2003; Sidani & Campbell, 2002). Evening primrose oil has been used to treat PMS. For emotional symptoms, psychological therapy, education and counseling about communication strategies may help with relationship issues. Relaxation therapy, biofeedback, guided imagery, cognitive behavior therapy, light therapy, massage, and yoga have all been used to treat PMS. Lifestyle changes, such as increased exercise, quitting smoking and stress management, may also help relieve symptoms. Acupuncture may be of some benefit for women with PCOS and anovulation. Complementary treatment options for endometriosis may include traditional Chinese medicine, nutritional approaches, homeopathy, allergy management, and immune therapy.

Patient and Family Teaching

Patients and their family need to be taught to recognize normal and abnormal menstrual patterns. When dysmenorrhea occurs, teaching of the most effective pain management strategies is needed. Information on procedures to evaluate and treat menstrual disorders may become necessary. Once diagnosed, the implications for altered health status with PCOS or menopause should be taught to both patients and their family.

All women need to know that any postmenopausal bleeding is an abnormal finding that must be reported to their health care provider. When surgery is required, the nurse should teach postoperative care. Patients and their family need to anticipate the possibility of disrupted menstrual cycles following trauma, surgery, or selected treatment regimens.

Evaluation of Outcomes

Potential patient outcomes for each of the example nursing diagnoses for the patient with menstrual disorders are:

- Anxiety related to the impact of menstrual dysfunction on relationships, daily functioning, plans for childbearing, or implications of the disease. The patient should be able to recognize the signs of anxiety, demonstrate positive coping mechanisms, and describe a reduction in the level of anxiety experienced.
- Deficient knowledge related to relief measures available for dysmenorrhea, range of normal menstrual patterns, or changes in health status associated with menopause. The patient should demonstrate motivation to learn, identify perceived learning needs, and verbalize an understanding of desired content.
- Acute or chronic pain related to dysmenorrhea or pain of endometriosis. The patient should verbalize an adequate relief of pain along with the ability to realistically cope with the pain if it is not completely relieved.

- Disturbed body image related to negatively viewing physical changes associated with PCOS. The patient demonstrates enhanced body image and self-esteem as evidenced by ability to look at, touch, talk about, and care for actual or perceived altered body part or function.

INFECTIONS

Vaginitis and Bartholin's (Skene's) gland infections are the most common vaginal infections. These infections are sometimes considered sexually transmitted diseases ([STDs] contagious diseases usually contracted through sexual contact), because the causative organisms may be passed to sexual partners. Many infections develop without sexual contact and sexual partners do not always become infected.

Vaginitis

Strictly defined, **vaginitis** is inflammation of the vagina, and the term is commonly used for any vaginal inflammation, regardless of the underlying etiology. Vaginal infections are one of the most common reasons that women seek gynecological care. The three most common types of vaginitis are candida, bacterial vaginosis (BV), and trichomoniasis. Candidal vaginal infections are commonly known as yeast infections. Ninety percent of vaginal yeast is caused by *Candida albicans.* Candida infections can be caused by a shift in vaginal flora (such as with antibiotic administration) or a change in vaginal pH, or an environment conducive to yeast growth (a high blood sugar or suppressed immune system). Glucose tolerance testing for diabetes and human immunodeficiency virus (HIV) screening are recommended for women with chronic candida infections. Routine douching for hygiene purposes has been shown to double the risk of contracting vaginitis and to increase the risk of pelvic inflammatory disease (PID) and endometritis and should be discouraged. Itching is a hallmark presenting symptom. Typically there is thick, white discharge that is adherent to the vaginal walls. Treatment is with either oral or vaginal antifungal preparations. Exogenous lactobacillus either orally or vaginally can be used to prevent and treat chronic candida infections (Jeavons 2003; Reid & Bruce, 2003).

BV is a condition of an overgrowth of the bacteria normally present in the vagina. BV is the most common vaginal infection in women of reproductive age. The cause of BV is not clearly understood, although it rarely occurs in women who are not sexually active. It is often associated with douching, having a new sex partner, or having multiple partners. BV can be spread through contact with a female sex partner. Presenting symptoms are discharge that is white or gray, thin, watery and with an odor. Treatment is with oral or vaginal metronidazole (Flagyl) or clindamycin (Cleocin). Male sex partners generally do not need treatment, because men do not seem to get BV; so treating partners is not generally helpful in preventing recurrences. Female partners may need treatment. BV has been associated with premature rupture of membranes and preterm labor, and pregnant women with BV should be treated. Women with a history of preterm labor, particularly with preterm rupture of membranes, should have a wet mount to check for BV.

Trichomoniasis is infection with a small parasite, *Trichomonas vaginalis.* Trichomonas can be transmitted through sex with either men or women, although men rarely have symptoms. An estimated 7.4 million cases occur each year in men and women (CDC, 2004g). Trichomonads reside in the female vagina, urethra, bladder, and Skene's glands. Presenting symptoms is discharge that is frothy and may be green or white. Irritation or itching is common. Treatment is with metronidazole (Flagyl). Male and female partners must be treated to prevent reinfection.

Although trichomoniasis can be transmitted through sexual contact, candida and BV are not usually classified as infections that can be transmitted by sexual contact. However, this depends on women's sexual practices. Women can transfer candida and BV to female sexual partners. Histories should be taken in a nonjudgmental way that allows women the opportunity to share all their pertinent sexual information and get their questions answered.

Vaginal infections and cystitis share many of the same symptoms, and the organisms that cause vaginitis may also infect the urethra and Skene's glands. Infections with the herpes virus, a virus that produces small, transient fluid-filled blisters on skin and mucous membrane, can have dysuria as the presenting symptom. A careful history can help reveal those women with dysuria who need more than an evaluation for cystitis. Women with dysuria must have an evaluation for vaginitis if their urinalysis or culture is negative or inconclusive for cystitis or if their history and symptoms suggest an underlying or coexisting vaginitis or vulvitis.

Bartholin's or Skene's Gland Infection

The Bartholin's and Skene's glands may become obstructed, inflamed, or infected. In women without a cervix, the urethra and Skene's glands may be the primary site of infection for gonorrhea, caused by the bacterium *N. gonorrhoeae* or chlamydia, caused by the bacterium *C. trachomatis.* A Bartholin's cyst is an obstruction of the duct causing an enlargement of the Bartholin's gland. The enlargement may be significant, but it is typically soft and painless or mildly uncomfortable. Treatment of Bartholin's cysts primarily involves hot soaks with water and observation. Some women have minor enlargements of the Bartholin's glands that persist but are without symptoms and do not in any way obstruct the vaginal entrance, and these do not need treatment.

When the Bartholin's glands become infected the symptoms include pain, progressive enlargement of the gland, redness of the skin around the gland, exquisite tenderness to the touch and, often, induration. If there is an opening in the gland to the skin, there may be purulent or bloody discharge around the gland. The pain and gland enlargement are usually progressive until the contents are released through the skin, either naturally or through surgical draining. Gonorrhea and chlamydia are common causes of Bartholin's gland abscesses, so culture of the gland contents and antibiotic treatment are indicated. If the infection is more than superficial long-term or multiple antibiotic treatments may be indicated.

The Skene's glands can be a site for STDs, particularly gonorrhea, chlamydia, and trichomoniasis. The Skene's glands are assessed during a pelvic examination. With one finger in the vagina, the Skene's gland is milked between the examining finger and the vagina. If there is an infection, purulent discharge will be noted coming out of the glands. Culture of this discharge may be helpful and antibiotics are indicated. If trichomoniasis is suspected because there is a concomitant vaginal infection, then metronidazole should resolve the Skene's infection as well as the vaginal infection.

Sexually Transmitted Disease

Sexually transmitted diseases (STD) are infections that include gonorrhea, chlamydia, syphilis (caused by the spirochete *Treponema pallidum*), human papillomavirus ([HPV] the cause of genital warts), herpes virus infections, hepatitis B (a form of viral hepatitis), and human immunodeficiency virus (HIV). Gonorrhea and chlamydia typically infect the cervix in women. These infections are most common in young women under the age of 24. Having multiple partners increases the risk of contracting an STD. The location of the transformation zone of the cervix in adolescents and young women makes their cervices more susceptible to STD infections. The CDC estimates that 700,000 people in the United States have gonorrhea each year.

Gonorrhea is a bacterial infection that infects the cervix, anus, or throat. Many women are asymptomatic, but if women have symptoms they can include a purulent vaginal or cervical discharge, dysuria, and abdominal pain. Gonorrhea is treated with antibiotics. Antibiotic-resistant strains of gonorrhea are a recurrent problem. Treatment for gonorrhea shifted away from penicillin when penicillin-resistant strains of gonorrhea became prevalent. Gonococcal strains may also be resistant to spectinomycin (Trobicin) and fluoroquinolones. Changes in antibiotic treatments have so far kept pace with the resistant strains.

Chlamydia is caused by the bacteria *C. trachomatis*. It infects the cervix, urethra, anus, or pharynx. Chlamydia is the most frequently reported bacterial STD in the United States. An estimated 2.8 million Americans are infected each year. For both gonorrhea and chlamydia, partner notification and treatment are important. The CDC recommends that all sexually active women under age 25 have annual screening cultures for chlamydia.

Blood-borne infections include hepatitis B, syphilis, and HIV. HIV is discussed in chapter 42. Hepatitis B can be spread by sexual contact and contact with infected blood. Symptoms of hepatitis B include jaundice, fatigue, nausea, anorexia, and weight loss. Hepatitis B can resolve or can become a chronic infection, and treatment with antiviral drugs is sometimes needed.

Syphilis is caused by the bacteria *Treponema pallidum*. Syphilis is contracted by direct contact with a syphilis sore or by contact with syphilis-infected blood. Primary syphilis is characterized by a painless genital ulcer. This will resolve without treatment. If syphilis progresses to the secondary stage, symptoms usually include a rash on the palms of the hands and soles of the feet. Tertiary syphilis is characterized by brain and nervous system involvement.

Herpes Simplex Virus

The CDC estimates that one out of every five people over age 12 in the United States has had a genital herpes infection caused by the *Herpes simplex* virus (HSV). The number of Americans diagnosed with a genital herpes infection increased by 30 percent between the late 1970s and the early 1990s. Herpes virus type 1 and type 2 both cause identical genital herpes viral infections. Of all the HSV genital infections, 75 to 85 percent are caused by type 2 herpes virus and 15 to 25 percent are caused by type 1. One-third of women ages 20 to 45 have been exposed to the type 2 herpes virus. Of all women with antibodies to the type 2 herpes virus, 60 to 85 percent never have a recognized genital infection.

Symptoms of HSV can be significant or mild and subtle and usually include blisters that break open and form a sore or an ulcer. This ulcer is painful and often causes dysuria. It usually occurs three to seven days after exposure. Initial outbreaks often include flu-like symptoms of malaise, fever, swollen inguinal lymph nodes, and muscle aches. Subsequent outbreaks are usually not as painful, they do not last as long, the symptoms are usually more localized, and women do not have as many accompanying symptoms. Transmission of type 2 herpes virus usually occurs from sexual contact with someone who has type 2 genital herpes. More women than men are likely to have infection with type 2 herpes virus, possibly because transmission of the type 2 virus is more common from men to women than it is from women to men (CDC, 2004c).

Transmission of type 1 herpes virus can occur from sexual contact with someone who has type 1 genital herpes but can also happen from genital-to-oral contact, because type 1 herpes virus also causes oral lesions or cold sores. Type 1 lesions tend to recur less frequently, but the diagnosis and treatment is the same. Diagnosis is obtained by culturing the lesion. The herpes virus resides in the nerve ganglia between outbreaks, and it is not possible to eradicate the virus. Transmission of the virus is possible even if lesions are not present, and condoms are not as effective at preventing the transmission of the herpes virus as they are at preventing the transmission of infections that affect mucous membranes.

Human Papillomavirus

The human papillomavirus (HPV) is associated with genital warts and cervical cancer (a neoplasm of the uterine cervix). The CDC (2004) estimates that 20 million people currently have HPV. HPV is present in 30 to 45 percent of women. The link between HPV and cervical cancer is clear. Regular Papanicolaou test, or Pap smears, help detect precancerous lesions and allow for treatment. The increase in the performance of routine screening Pap smears accounts for the 74 percent decline in the incidence of cervical cancer between 1955 and 1992 (American Cancer Society [ACS], 2004b).

There are more than 100 different strains of HPV virus, and types 16, 18, 31, 33, and 35 are considered high risk and are associated with high-grade cervical dysplasia (atypical or abnormal cervical cells) and cervical cancer. The prevalence of HPV decreases with increasing age. HPV viral infection is usually asymptomatic. Women may have genital warts **(condyloma)** present. All types of HPV virus can cause abnormalities in Pap smears, but the presence of a high-risk type of HPV indicates that those Pap smear abnormalities need close follow-up. Along with traditional Pap smear testing, HPV genetic typing (HPV digene) is done for mildly abnormal Pap smears, using either the original sample or by obtaining a sample just for HPV typing.

Each year approximately 3.5 million women in the U.S. (7 percent of all women obtaining Pap smears) have an abnormal result requiring follow-up or evaluation. Postmenopausal women are less likely to have significant cervical abnormalities with Pap smears that only show atypical cells. Pap smear test results are reported as one of the following: negative for intraepithelial lesions (normal), atypical squamous cells of undetermined significance (ASCUS), low-grade squamous intraepithelial lesion (LGSIL), high-grade squamous intraepithelial lesion (HGSIL), carcinoma-in-situ, and invasive cervical cancer.

A more unusual finding is atypical glandular cells of undetermined significance (AGUS). Premenopausal women with AGUS are more at risk for cervical

Safety First 1

Pap Smear Follow-up

Having a plan to manage Pap smears is not sufficient to ensure that patients get appropriate treatment and follow-up. If a system is not in place to ensure that Pap smear results are received from the pathology lab, women can have progression of cervical lesions and more extensive disease at time of treatment. An example of a problem with Pap smear follow-up is as follows. A patient went to her gynecologist's office for a yearly Pap smear. All her Pap smears up to this point had been normal. In this gynecology office, nurses were responsible for keeping a log book, recording all Pap smears that went to the lab, and logging in all results as they returned. The log book was not checked in a timely fashion, and it was not noticed that this patient's Pap smear results were never logged in. The patient returned the following year for her annual examination, and the results of that Pap smear showed HGSIL. When the previous year's Pap smear result was obtained from the lab, it showed LGSIL that could have been treated before progression to a high-grade lesion. The nurses in the office instituted the following procedures to fix this problem:

- The pathology lab was contacted and asked to send out a follow-up letter to the office asking for confirmation that patients with results of LGSIL or worse had been notified.
- The nurses established a schedule to check the Pap log book on a daily basis.
- Patient postcards indicating normal test results were sent out as the normal Pap smear results came into the office. Patients were instructed to call the office in four weeks to find out their results if they had not received a postcard.
- Charts of patients with abnormal Pap smears were covered with a green folder to remind the health care providers that the patients with green charts had an abnormal Pap smear.

BOX 62-1

CRITERIA FOR INPATIENT TREATMENT OF PID

- Pregnancy
- Inability to comply with outpatient therapy
- Failure of outpatient therapy
- Severe infection with temperature hotter than 39° C (102.2° F)
- Suspected tubo-ovarian abscess

Red Flag

Emergency Treatment of TSS

Immediate treatment for TSS includes hospital admission, removal of tampon or diaphragm, IV fluids to maintain blood pressure, and antibiotics. Intubation, vasopressors, and dialysis may all be indicated. There is a 3 percent incidence of fatality with supportive therapy. Antibiotics reduce the recurrence rate from 30 to 50 percent. Nursing management of the patient with TSS includes removal of the tampon or diaphragm, rapid assessment of vital signs and level of consciousness and orientation, and immediate notification of the physician. Lab work is drawn for complete blood count, clotting functions, sedimentation rate, and chemistries as indicated. IV fluids, blood products, and antibiotics are administered as ordered by the health care provider. Insertion of a urinary catheter may be required to monitor intake and output. Close monitoring of vital signs and level of consciousness continues until the patient is stable or transferred.

abnormalities, and postmenopausal women with AGUS are more at risk for endometrial hyperplasia and cervical cancer. Treatment is often required for cervical lesions associated with high risk HPV. However, in adolescent or postmenopausal women with LGSIL on Pap smear testing, it is possible to avoid aggressive treatment and expectantly follow Pap smears.

Pelvic Inflammatory Disease

The CDC estimates that one million women each year have pelvic inflammatory disease (PID), an inflammatory condition of the female pelvic organs. PID can lead to abscess formation, scarring and occlusion of the fallopian tubes, reinfection, and chronic pelvic pain. Scarring of the fallopian tubes can lead to infertility and risk of ectopic pregnancy. Fallopian tube occlusion associated with untreated chlamydia infections is a major cause of infertility.

PID is a common cause of hospitalization for young women. It is an expensive illness in terms of costs for hospitalization, medications, follow-up, and risks for infertility. The symptoms of PID include abdominal pain, fever, elevated white count, purulent cervical discharge, acute cervical pain on palpation, and adnexal tenderness or enlargement.

Treatment of PID includes antibiotic therapy. Outpatient antibiotic therapy can be considered for a compliant patient with the ability to return for close follow-up, but hospitalization is considered if these conditions cannot be met because the risk for tubo-ovarian abscess and significant morbidity associated with untreated or inadequately treated PID is great. The criteria for inpatient treatment of PID can be seen in Box 62-1.

Management of PID includes treatment of the infection, close follow-up, partner evaluation and treatment, and education to maximize compliance with therapy and followup to prevent reinfection. Possible intravenous treatment regimens for PID are cefotetan, cefoxitin plus doxycycline, clindamycin plus gentamicin, ofloxacin, levofloxacin with or without metronidazole, ampicillin/sulbactam plus doxycycline.

Toxic Shock Syndrome

Toxic shock syndrome (TSS) is an acute illness caused by toxin-producing *Staphylococcus aureus* bacteria. Six percent of women carry *S. aureus* in their vagina, but only 2 percent of women have the type capable of producing the toxin. TSS is highly associated with menstruation and tampon use but has also occurred in the postpartum and postoperative periods. It has also been described with contraceptive diaphragm use. All women should avoid prolonged and overnight use of tampons, although this is of uncertain effectiveness.

Symptoms include a high fever greater than 102° F (38.9° C), a diffuse rash, falling blood pressure, systemic symptoms of nausea, vomiting, diarrhea, myalgia, hyperemia of mucous membranes, possibly disorientation, and coma. Blood urea nitrogen (BUN), creatinine, and liver enzymes are elevated and thrombocytopenia is present.

Complications

PID is the most common serious complication of chlamydia. Up to 40 percent of untreated women with chlamydia will develop PID. Chlamydia-associated PID is a common cause of infertility. Reiter's syndrome, which is a combination of arthritis, skin lesions, inflammation of the eye, and urethra, is a rare complication. Women with chlamydia are up to five times more likely to be infected with HIV, if exposed (CDC, 2004a). If left untreated, complications of gonorrhea can include PID, perihepatic inflammation, or gonococcal arthritis. Neonatal eye infections with gonorrhea and chlamydia are also possible if the mother has an untreated infection at the time of delivery. Untreated chlamydia can also cause neonatal pneumonia.

Chronic hepatitis is a complication of hepatitis B infections. Irreversible brain and nervous system impairment is a consequence of untreated syphilis that progresses to tertiary syphilis. Infants can also contract hepatitis B and congenital syphilis during birth if the mother is infected and untreated. An infant that comes in contact with an active herpes outbreak during delivery may contract systemic neonatal herpes infection. A woman with an active genital herpes virus infection at the time of labor is recommended to deliver by cesarean section to reduce this risk. Cervical cancer is a complication of HPV infection.

Assessment with Clinical Manifestations

In evaluating women for infections a nonjudgmental history needs to be taken. Information is obtained about the specific symptoms and their timing, any symptoms the sexual partner may have, an assessment of the possibility of pregnancy, and any history of infections. Pain must be evaluated as to location, type, severity, and relieving and aggravating factors, any changes in pain over time, and other symptoms associated with pain. The history for patients with infections should include the number of sexual partners and whether those partners are male, female, or both, and the types of sexual contact. Information on contraceptive method, LMP, any chronic illness, and routine medications should be obtained. Information on the timing and results of the last Pap smear is important to obtain.

Diagnostic Tests

The diagnosis of vaginitis involves taking a small sample of the vaginal discharge during a speculum examination, checking the pH, and examining the discharge under the microscope. The discharge is mixed with normal saline to prevent drying of the sample and placed on a microscope slide. This is called a wet mount and is examined under the microscope for the presence of trichomonads, bacteria-studded epithelial cells indicative of bacterial vaginosis called clue cells, and budding forms of yeast called hyphae. After this examination, a drop of potassium hydroxide is added to the discharge and the "whiff test" is performed to check for the presence of a fishy odor indicative of BV. The sample with potassium hydroxide can then be examined under the microscope for hyphae, as these are easier to identify in the potassium hydroxide sample.

Diagnosis of gonorrhea or chlamydia is made by taking a swab from the area of sexual contact and sending the specimen to be cultured. Visual inspection is necessary to diagnose external infections and genital warts. Other diagnostic tests include Pap smears, colposcopy with biopsies, and the pelvic exam. Cultures for HSV are obtained as indicated. The HPV digene test is done as indicated. Blood testing is done to detect syphilis, hepatitis B, and HIV infections. When one STD is diagnosed, it is important to test for the other sexually transmitted infections as the presence of one makes a woman more susceptible to others. TSS is diagnosed by site-specific cultures for *S. aureus* and exclusion of other illnesses such as Rocky Mountain spotted fever, leptospirosis, and measles (Daniels, 2003).

Women with AGUS Pap smears are usually evaluated with colposcopy and endometrial biopsy. Diagnosis of cervical pathology with HPV infection usually includes colposcopy, cervical biopsy, and endocervical curettage. Colposcopy is the use of a microscope to evaluate the cervix. The cervix is usually washed with an acetic acid solution, because this aids in the detection of lesions. Cervical biopsies are usually taken through the colposcope from the site of abnormalities. Colposcopy and Pap smears are ideally done at least 24 hours after any douching, use of tampons, intercourse, or use of vaginal medications. An endocervical scraping or curettage is generally also done during colposcopy, except if the patient is pregnant. A small amount of bleeding or discharge is normal after colposcopy, but continued bleeding, fever, chills, severe lower abdominal pain, or malodorous discharge should be reported.

Nursing Diagnoses

Based on the information gathered, examples of nursing diagnoses in the patient with infections of the reproductive system may include the following:

- Acute pain related to HSV, PID, or other painful infection.
- Risk for infection, reinfection, or infecting others related to sexually transmitted infections.
- Deficient knowledge related to knowledge of disease transmission and prevention.

Planning and Implementation

Care of the patient with gynecological infections include education, support, therapeutic interventions, and prevention measures. An advanced practice nurse, physician's assistant, or physician performs a pelvic examination, obtains cultures, wet mount, or other diagnostic tests, and orders antibiotics or antifungal therapy. For women who are hospitalized with acute infections, infectious disease specialists may be consulted. Advanced practice nurses or physician's assistants may perform colposcopy, but physicians are usually responsible for treatment of abnormal cervical pathology. An oncologist may be consulted for significant cervical pathology. The nurse administers therapies as ordered and assists with diagnostic tests. The nurse is responsible for monitoring women who are hospitalized with infections, including response to therapy and readiness for discharge. A crucial role for nurses is patient education.

Women with diabetes and altered immune systems from diseases, such as HIV, are more prone to yeast vaginitis. Women with chlamydia infections are more susceptible to HIV. Immunosuppressed women are more likely to have significant cervical abnormalities with Pap smears that only show atypical cells, and immunosuppressed women are more likely to be infected with high risk types of HPV.

Nutrition

Lactobacillus has been proposed as a preventive for candidal yeast infections. Lactobacillus can be obtained by eating yogurt, as a supplement, or in applications directly to the vagina. Lysine supplementation has been shown to reduce the frequency and intensity of herpes virus infections.

Pharmacology

The medications used to treat gynecological infections can be found in Table 62-2.

Population-Based Care

Control of sexually transmitted infections depends on partner identification, notification, and treatment. Measures to make notification and treatment of partners easier include preprinted cards that can be given to sexual contacts with information from health care providers on the specific infection and treatment needed. Screening programs for STDs and other infections, such as HIV, should be concentrated in the populations where these infections are most prevalent. Screening all women under age 25 for gonorrhea and chlamydia may help reduce the incidence of PID and infertility. With a few exceptions, all adolescents in the United States can consent to STD screening and treatment without parental notification or consent (Workowski & Levine, 2002).

TABLE 62-2 Medications for Gynecological Infections

DRUG	INDICATION	SIDE EFFECTS
Antifungal		
Monistat; Terazol; Mycelex; Femstat; Nystatin; Diflucan	Treatment of candida vaginitis and candida vulvitis	Nausea; abdominal pain; headache; local irritation
Antibacterial		
Flagyl; Cleocin	Treatment of trichomoniasis and bacterial vaginosis	Nausea; vomiting; GI upset; metallic taste
Penicillin G; Doxycycline; Tetracycline	Treatment of syphilis	Nausea; vomiting; GI upset; discoloration of teeth
Azithromycin, Erythromycin, Doxycycline	Treatment of chlamydia	Nausea; vomiting; GI upset; hepatic injury
Cefixime; Ciprofloxacin; Spectinomycin	Treatment of gonorrhea	Nausea; vomiting; skin rash; dizziness; headache
Antiviral		
Zovirax; Famvir; Valtrex	Treatment of HSV lesions	Nausea; vomiting; GI upset
Wart Removal Agents		
Podocon; Tri-chlor; Condylox; Aldara	Treatment of condyloma caused by HPV	Skin irritation

Adapted from Broyles, B., Reiss, B., & Evans, M. (2007). Pharmacological aspects of nursing care *(7th ed.). New York: Thomson Delmar Learning.*

Health Care Resources

Syphilis, gonorrhea, chlamydia, and HIV are infections reportable to local health departments in every state. Health departments have the responsibility to prioritize the infections to track and to carry out personal notification and treatment of partners. Since the early 1980s, most health departments have concentrated their resources on partner notification and treatment for HIV and AIDS.

Surgery

Surgery is not commonly needed to treat infections. When surgical draining is performed on Bartholin's gland infections, the skin is cleansed with Betadine, local anesthetic is usually injected, and an incision is made with a scalpel to allow for draining. A syringe may be used to release as much of the gland's contents as possible and to collect a sample for culture. It is important that the skin not close before all the contents of the gland have released or the infection may not resolve, so packing is sometimes done. Whether or not packing is done, close follow-up must be done to ensure that the Bartholin's gland infection resolves. Surgery may be required to remove a tubo-ovarian abscess associated with PID. Treatment for cervical abnormalities caused by HPV includes cryotherapy, loop electrosurgical excision procedure (LEEP), cone biopsy, electrocautery, laser and, rarely, hysterectomy.

Cryotherapy involves freezing the cervical lesion using the colposcope for visualization. Typically, no anesthesia is needed for cryotherapy, and it is done as an outpatient procedure. The LEEP procedure involves the use of a thin wire loop with an electric current that removes a thin layer of surface cells. LEEP is done as an outpatient procedure. A speculum is inserted, the colposcope is used, and the cervix is cleaned with an acetic acid solution. The cervix is anesthetized. The LEEP is used to remove a thin layer of surface cells, and Monsel's solution is used to ensure hemostasis, if necessary. Vaginal bleeding, mild cramping, and a brownish-black discharge from the Monsel's solution are expected side effects. Patients should consult their health care provider if heavy bleeding, severe abdominal pain, fever, chills, or malodorous discharge is experienced. If pregnancy occurs after a LEEP procedure is done, cervical competency may need to be assessed by ultrasound during the pregnancy.

A cone biopsy is done under general anesthesia. A cone-shaped piece of tissue is removed from the cervix with a small knife or a laser. Cervical tissue regenerates in four to six weeks. One concern after conization is the ability of the cervix to be competent with a subsequent pregnancy. If more than one cone biopsy has been done, the risk of incompetent cervix increases.

Alternative Therapy

Lactobacilli recolonization to treat and prevent yeast vaginitis and BV with yogurt and lactobacillus capsules is done by oral and intravaginal administration. Betadine vaginal suppositories or douches have been used to treat BV. Vaginal boric acid capsules, 600 mg/day at bedtime for two weeks, have been successfully used as treatment for recurrent or chronic yeast infections. Boric acid is not recommended for use during pregnancy.

Tea tree oil has been used as an antifungal and antibacterial. Garlic, one clove wrapped in unbleached gauze, and crushed before vaginal insertion nightly for six nights has been used to treat yeast vaginitis. Supplementation with L-lysine, vitamin C, and zinc has been used to prevent recurrent HSV infections. Herbal therapy with an herb from the rain forest of Peru, cat's claw, has been used to prevent recurrent HSV infections.

Patient and Family Teaching

Along with treatment of the woman, partner identification, notification, treatment, and ways to prevent reinfection must be discussed. Prevention of reinfection includes avoiding contact with untreated partners, use of condoms, and avoiding sexual contact if symptoms (e.g., HSV) are present. Patient education to avoid reinfection is an integral part of therapy. Male condoms are an effective prevention for the spread of HIV, if they are used consistently and correctly, and they can reduce the risk of spreading other infections, such as gonorrhea, chlamydia, and trichomoniasis. Condoms are most effective in preventing infections transmitted by contact with mucosal surfaces, such as HIV, gonorrhea, chlamydia, and trichomoniasis. They are less effective in preventing those infections transmitted by skin contact, such as HSV, HPV, and syphilis. Incorrect use, not breakage, is usually the cause of condom failure (CDC, 2002a).

Patient teaching includes education on disease transmission and prevention, avoidance of douching, use of condoms for STD prevention, completing the course of antibiotic therapy even if symptoms have resolved, symptoms that indicate medical evaluation is necessary, and importance of regular Pap screening. Patients may need explicit instructions on the use of vaginal medications. The use of a demonstration applicator for vaginal medications may be helpful. Patients should be made aware of the limitations on the use of condoms and the correct application of condoms. If one sexually transmitted infection is diagnosed, patients must be advised to obtain testing for the other infections.

Evaluation of Outcomes

Evaluation of outcomes allows the nurse to determine the effectiveness of interventions and change or refocus care as needed.

- Acute pain related to HSV, PID, or other painful infection. The patient should verbalize an adequate relief of pain along with the ability to realistically cope with the pain if it is not completely relieved.
- Risk for infection, reinfection, or infecting others related to sexually transmitted infections. The patient remains free of infection, as evidenced by normal vital signs and absence of purulent drainage from wounds, incisions, and tubes. Infection is recognized early to allow for prompt treatment.
- Deficient knowledge related to knowledge of disease transmission and prevention. The patient should demonstrate motivation to learn, identify perceived learning needs, and verbalize an understanding of desired content.

STRUCTURAL ABNORMALITIES AND BENIGN CONDITIONS

There are many structural abnormalities and benign conditions of the female reproductive system. Women have a variety of clinical manifestations and complications related to these disorders. The conditions included in this section are: polyps, pelvic relaxation, anatomic deviation, leiomyomata, and ovarian cysts.

Polyps

Polyps are fleshy growths on the cervix or in the endometrial cavity. Cervical polyps can be found in approximately 4 percent of all gynecology patients. Polyps may be located on the exterior or exocervix, in the cervical canal, or in the endometrial cavity. Polyps are usually asymptomatic. If symptoms do occur, they include bleeding and unusual vaginal discharge. Carcinoma with polyps is rare. Polyps are treated by removal. This is accomplished by grasping the polyp with a ring forceps and twisting it off, usually a painless procedure. In pregnancy, stable and benign polyps are followed conservatively by observation only, so that minimal disruption of the cervix occurs prior to delivery. In postmenopausal women, cervical polyps can be associated with endometrial polyps that can cause postmenopausal bleeding, so a diagnosis of cervical polyps may warrant further evaluation, such as uterine ultrasound or endometrial biopsy.

Pelvic Relaxation

Urethrocele is defined as relaxation of the anterior vaginal wall causing prolapse of the urethra into the vagina. Cystocele is relaxation of the anterior vaginal wall causing prolapse of the bladder neck or bladder into the vagina. Urethrocele and cystocele are associated with parity or childbearing. The greater number of pregnancies with a high percentage resulting in vaginal births increases the likelihood that some degree of pelvic relaxation will have occurred. The symptoms of urethrocele and cystocele are a sensation of suprapubic fullness or pressure, stress incontinence, urgency to void, and a feeling of incomplete emptying after voiding.

Management of urethrocele and cystocele includes teaching of Kegel's exercises (a regimen of isometric exercises to increase contractility of the vaginal introitus), pessary insertion, estrogen cream to correct vaginal atrophy if there are no contraindications, and operative repair. Pessaries are devices of different shapes that are inserted into the vagina to provide support to relaxed pelvic structures. Pessaries are typically left in and removed on a regular basis for cleaning and reinsertion. This is done either by the patient or by a health care provider. The use of vaginal therapy to minimize irritation is helpful when a pessary is used. Either estrogen vaginal cream or Trimo-San cream can be used. Trimo-San cream modulates the pH of the vagina and helps prevent bacterial infection and irritation.

Rectocele is defined as relaxation of the posterior vaginal wall causing prolapse of the rectum into the vagina. Symptoms of rectocele include a feeling of pressure in the vagina, constipation, and a sensation of incomplete rectal emptying. Rectoceles are also associated with parity. Therapy for rectocele includes instruction in Kegel's exercises, estrogen vaginal cream to correct vaginal atrophy if there are no contraindications, and operative management.

Enterocele is defined as the herniation of the intestines into the space between the vagina and the rectum. Enteroceles are difficult to diagnosis and are usually found during operative repairs for other conditions of pelvic relaxation. The treatment for an enterocele is operative repair.

Uterine prolapse is caused by relaxation of the support structures holding up the uterus. The result is the descent of the uterus into the vagina. The symptoms of uterine prolapse are a feeling of something falling out of the vagina, and the cervix may eventually be seen protruding from the vagina. Temporary descent of the cervix may occur immediately following a vaginal delivery, but it usually corrects itself within a few weeks after delivery. Urination and defecation changes are also common.

Uterine prolapse often occurs in conjunction with cystocele or rectocele. If the cervix appears low in the vagina but is not visible from the outside, no therapy is needed unless symptoms are present. Therapy is often indicated for the cervix that is visible external to the vagina, because irritation and ulcerations of the cervix can occur. Therapy includes insertion of pessaries to hold the uterus up and surgical repair, usually including hysterectomy. These conditions of pelvic relaxation can be present singly or in any combination. Risk factors for pelvic relaxation include obesity, family history of pelvic relaxation, and parity.

Leiomyomata

Commonly called uterine fibroids, leiomyomata are benign growths originating from the smooth muscle cells of the uterus. Fibroids may be single or multiple, small or large, and are located within the uterine cavity, in the muscle wall of the uterus itself, or external to the uterus. Leiomyomata are the most common solid pelvic tumors in women, and 20 to 40 percent of women have fibroids during their childbearing years. Fibroids are the most common reason for hysterectomy in the United States. Leiomyomata are estrogen-dependent tumors, and they predictably shrink during menopause (Wallach & Vlahos, 2004).

Most women with fibroids do not have symptoms. If women do have symptoms, the most common ones are excessive menstrual bleeding and pelvic pressure. Increased dysmenorrhea may be associated with fibroids. Depending on the location of the fibroid, gastrointestinal (GI)or urinary symptoms may be present. Constipation, increased abdominal girth, urinary retention, and dyspareunia may all be present. Uterine leiomyomata located in the uterine cavity may be associated with infertility and pregnancy loss. Asymptomatic fibroids need no therapy.

Symptomatic fibroids can be evaluated with ultrasound or hysterosalpingography. The choice of therapy depends on factors, such as age, desires for childbearing, severity of symptoms, size, number, and location of fibroids, and associated medical conditions. Fibroids can be followed expectantly, managed with medical therapy, removed with preservation of the uterus **(myomectomy),** reduced or destroyed by eliminating the blood supply to the fibroid through interventional radiology (uterine artery embolization), or treated by hysterectomy. Medical therapy with hormones can include progestins (either oral or injectable), combined estrogen-progesterone oral contraceptives, or GnRH analogues, such as leuprolide. Medical management should be adjusted individually for each woman. Costs and side effects of medical management may limit their use long-term.

Unless infertility or recurrent losses are an issue, women do not need to have fibroids removed to prevent possible pregnancy complications. Additional surveillance of pregnancy may be indicated if the placenta is implanted over the fibroid (Lefebvre, et al., 2003). When acute hemorrhage happens in women with fibroids, medical management, D & C, or hysteroscopy may be considered, but hysterectomy may be needed to control the hemorrhage.

Ovarian Cysts

Ovarian cysts are a common finding. There are follicular cysts, corpus luteum cysts, dermoid cysts, and endometriomas. Follicular cysts form in the first half of the menstrual cycle. The dominant follicle fails to ovulate, becomes fluid-filled, and does not regress right away. Follicular cysts are typically fluid-filled cysts within the ovaries that last up to two months and spontaneously resolve. Most follicular ovarian cysts are asymptomatic, have no known specific cause, and do not require treatment.

Follicular ovarian cysts usually occur during the childbearing years. If symptoms occur, they include pelvic pain, dyspareunia, abnormal menstruation or amenorrhea, and abdominal bloating, and distension. Follicular ovarian cysts can present with signs of rupture and intraperitoneal bleeding. Treatment includes combined oral contraceptives, which help resolve and prevent the reoccurrence of ovarian cysts. However, use of estrogen and progesterone oral contraceptives may not be an acceptable alternative for women with chronic illnesses, such as migraines, diabetes, and cardiovascular disease. If cysts do not resolve spontaneously, surgical removal may be indicated.

Corpus luteum cysts form in the last half of the menstrual cycle. They are less common but are often filled with blood and fluid. Rupture is possible, but most regress spontaneously. Persistent corpus luteum cysts are associated with menstrual irregularities and often amenorrhea. There may be cramping abdominal pain on the same side of the abdomen as the cyst, or if rupture has occurred, sharp, generalized abdominal pain is present. The pain may radiate to the back, shoulders, or legs, and bladder or rectal discomfort is possible.

Dermoid cysts are benign complex cystic growths that commonly contain different kinds of tissue such as fat, hair, and teeth. They are ovarian germ cell tumors and are the most frequent ovarian tumor in women under age 20. The peak incidence is ages 20 to 40. Dermoids are often asymptomatic, but pressure, achiness, or abdominal pain may be present.

Endometriomas (or chocolate cysts) are formed when endometrial tissue attaches to the outside of the ovary. They are usually associated with endometrial implants elsewhere in the pelvis. Endometriomas contain old blood. They are typically painful and cause dysmenorrhea and dyspareunia. Endometriomas may need to be removed through a laparoscopic procedure or during laparotomy.

Genetics

Any defect in the development of the müllerian system, typically before the eighth week of embryonic development, can result in structural or functional defects in the reproductive system. There may be congenital absence of the ovaries, fallopian tubes, uterus, or vagina. **Müllerian dysgenesis** is defined as abnormally developed or absent uterus, cervix, or upper part of the vagina. Ovaries, however, are present and develop normally.

Congenital absence of the ovaries is called ovarian agenesis or Turner's syndrome. Women with Turner's syndrome have an absence of one of the X chromosomes in all body cells caused by a lack of disjunction of the sex chromosomes. The typical woman with Turner's syndrome is short in stature and has neck webbing, lateral placement of the nipples on the chest, and an absence of breast development. Axillary and pubic hair is also lacking. Turner's syndrome is associated with coarctation of the aorta and absence of one kidney, but these typical features may not be present.

There are other chromosomal abnormalities that cause abnormal reproductive function. People with 46XY karyotypes have feminine or ambiguous genitalia with intra-abdominal testes. Breast development takes place, but the vagina is a blind pouch and there is no uterus or ovaries and no axillary or pubic hair. When an XY karyotype is detected the reproductive tissue is usually removed, because of the high risk of malignant changes, and hormone therapy is started. Sex-hormone insensitivity is associated with the 46XY karyotype.

Absent or anomalous fallopian tube formation results from failure of müllerian duct fusion. Tubal absence usually occurs with absence of the uterus. Any complete absence of ovaries, tubes, or uterus results in infertility. The absence of the uterus is usually diagnosed when primary amenorrhea exists and is identifiable during a pelvic examination. Absence of a vagina is rarc, with an incidence of 1 in 4,000 to 1 in 10,000. The absence of a vagina is usually accompanied by absence of a uterus, caused by failure of müllerian duct fusion during embryonic development (ACOG, 2002).

Patients with absence of the vagina and uterus have a normal 46XX karyotype, normal ovarian formation and function, and normal secondary sex characteristics. Agenesis of the vagina is usually diagnosed as a consequence of primary amenorrhea and must be distinguished from sex-hormone insensitivity, a low-lying transverse vaginal septum, and imperforate hymen. Patients with vaginal agenesis may also have other congenital anomalies of the urinary tract and skeleton. Psychological support is necessary, and the adolescent with vaginal agenesis needs to be aware of the implications of the disorder. A normal sex life is possible with construction of a neovagina, but infertility is a consequence of the disorder. Harvesting of the woman's eggs and pregnancy achieved through surrogacy is a possibility for these patients.

Imperforate hymen is the most common müllerian duct defect and is a disorder of descent of the müllerian ducts. The hymenal membrane does not regress and obstructs the lower vagina, causing accumulation of menstrual blood behind the hymen.

Duplication of the müllerian system also exists. Deviations in the normal fusion of the müllerian duct buds result in duplication of all or part of the uterus, cervix, or upper vagina. Estimates are that müllerian duct defects occur in 1 in 700 women. Most of these defects are asymptomatic.

If a **didelphic,** or duplicated, uterus and cervix are present, fertility and childbirth are usually not affected, as long as both uteri and cervices communicate with a vagina and have a normal intrauterine cavity. The unicornuate uterus usually also has no affect on pregnancy, except that it may take longer to conceive if there is only one tubal connection with the uterus. Bicornuate uterus or uterus with septum may complicate fertility and pregnancy outcome if there is not sufficient space in the endometrial cavity to allow the pregnancy to implant, grow, and develop. Uterine septi are disorders of müllerian duct descent and are frequently associated with recurrent spontaneous pregnancy losses. Therefore, septi may need to be removed to allow for sufficient uterine function.

Assessment with Clinical Manifestations

Assessment includes a complete history and physical assessment with questions about menstrual cycles, pain symptoms, pregnancy history, and family history. Information about plans for future childbearing is crucial in developing plans for treatment of fibroids, pelvic relaxation, and other disorders where hysterectomy may be indicated for definitive treatment. Physical assessment includes observation of external genital features and in the case of suspected genital developmental abnormalities, assessment of secondary sex characteristics.

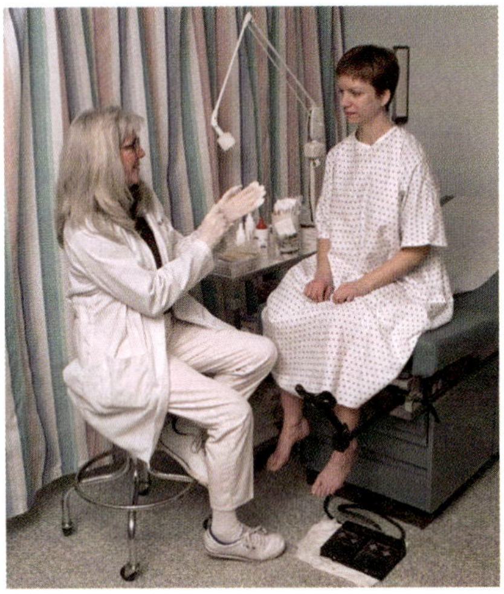

Figure 62-3 The nurse and patient prepare for a pelvic examination.

A comprehensive pelvic examination is the most helpful assessment for structural abnormalities and benign conditions.

Diagnostic Tests

The diagnosis of urethrocele and cystocele is made by observing a soft bulging mass of the anterior vaginal wall during a speculum or pelvic examination (Figure 62-3). Straining or coughing makes the bulging mass more apparent. If a urethrocele or cystocele is suspected, it is helpful to use only the posterior half of the speculum, insert it into the vagina and place downward pressure. This allows for unobstructed observation of the anterior vaginal wall.

Diagnosis of rectocele is made by observing a soft, bulging mass of the posterior vaginal wall during a speculum examination. To evaluate the rectocele, the posterior half of the speculum is inserted along the anterior vaginal wall and upward traction is applied, allowing for unobstructed observation of the posterior vaginal wall. Having the patient cough or strain will make the bulge in the posterior vaginal wall more apparent. Uterine prolapse may be diagnosed by observing the cervix protruding from the vaginal opening, but it is usually diagnosed by observing descent of the cervix into the vagina during a speculum examination.

Diagnostic tests for fibroids and structural abnormalities may include ultrasound, saline infusion sonogram, and hysterosalpingogram (HSG). An HSG is an X-ray study of the interior of the fallopian tubes and uterus. It is typically done to evaluate tubal patency and the structure of the uterine cavity. With the patient lying on an X-ray table, a speculum is inserted into the vagina, the cervix is numbed with an anesthetic, a thin tube is inserted through the cervix into the uterus, and then dye is inserted through the uterus into the fallopian tubes. X-rays are then taken, and the progress of the dye through the tubes is monitored. An HSG typically takes 10 to 20 minutes to perform. Rare complications of an HSG include infection or a recurrence of a chronic infection, allergic reaction to the dye, bleeding, and damage to the uterine wall or fallopian tubes. If fibroids are symptomatic, a complete blood count may be needed to assess the severity of anemia and the urgency for treatment. Chromosomal studies may be indicated if congenital structural abnormalities are suspected (Daniels, 2003).

Diagnostic tests for ovarian cysts include a pelvic exam, ultrasound examination, and serum hCG levels to rule out pregnancy. Lab tests may also include tumor markers, such as cancer antigen 125 (CA125) and alpha fetoprotein (AFP) to rule out ovarian cancer, a malignant neoplasm of the ovaries. Endometriomas are usually evaluated with ultrasound and possibly other imaging such as magnetic resonance imaging (MRI) or computerized tomography (CT) scan, or direct visualization with laparoscopy. Hysteroscopy can be used for diagnosis or treatment of disorders, such as abnormal uterine bleeding, infertility due to a structural uterine defect, repeated miscarriages due to structural defect, adhesions, polyps, fibroids, or displaced intrauterine devices.

Nursing Diagnoses

Based on the information gathered, examples of nursing diagnoses in the female patients with structural abnormalities may include the following:

- Situational low self-esteem or risk for situational low self-esteem related to physical changes and infertility associated with structural abnormalities.
- Disturbed body image related to negatively viewing physical changes associated with structural abnormalities.
- Acute or chronic pain associated with ovarian cysts.
- Impaired urinary elimination related to relaxed pelvic support.

Planning and Implementation

Care of the patient with structural abnormalities includes education, support, therapeutic interventions, and prevention measures. The initial physical and pelvic examination may be performed by an advanced practice nurse, physician's assistant, or physician. Any of these providers can order initial ultrasound or imaging studies and can remove cervical polyps. Gynecologists generally perform surgery to correct structural abnormalities, ovarian cysts, fibroids, and pelvic relaxation, although a urogynecological specialist may be consulted for reconstruction involving the urinary system. Physical therapists may be involved in bladder training and pelvic therapy to treat pelvic relaxation. Psychological or spiritual counseling may be helpful for women with congenital anatomical deviations, particularly those affecting fertility and body image. Patient education and patient preparation for any testing may be ordered. The nurse provides preoperative and postoperative care and discharge instructions, and plays a crucial role in teaching Kegel's exercises.

Uterine prolapse is associated with intra-abdominal pressure. This can come from ascites, pelvic, or intra-abdominal tumors, sacral nerve disorders (particularly injuries to S1 through S4), or diabetic neuropathy. Increased abdominal pressure and uterine prolapse can also be associated with coughing, such as occurs in chronic bronchitis, asthma, or bronchiectasis.

In a New York study of elderly women with chronic medical conditions undergoing pelvic reconstructive surgery, the women had no mortality and no significant morbidity. The women did find that the corrective surgery provided an immediate, substantial, and long-lasting improvement to the quality of life. The conclusion of the investigators was that pelvic reconstructive surgery should be an option even for women with chronic medical conditions (Vetere, Putterman & Kesselman, 2003). Conditions of pelvic relaxation are associated with parity and multiple vaginal births.

Nutrition

Women with fibroids may need nutritional counseling regarding foods that are a high source of iron to correct iron-deficiency anemia. Women with symptomatic pelvic relaxation who are obese may benefit from nutritional counseling for weight loss.

Pharmacology

Estrogen vaginal cream is indicated to relieve vaginal atrophy and improve symptoms associated with cystocele, rectocele, and uterine prolapse. The GnRH agonist leuprolide is used in treating fibroids to correct anemia and shrink fibroids, particularly prior to surgical intervention. Combined estrogen and progesterone oral contraceptive are used in the treatment of fibroids and the prevention and treatment of follicular ovarian cysts. Progesterone therapy, both oral progesterone and long-acting intramuscular progesterone are used in the treatment of fibroids. The hormonal therapies that may be used are listed previously in Table 62-1.

Surgery

Cervical polyps that cannot be removed in the outpatient setting and endometrial polyps may require surgical removal (Box 62-2). Anatomical structural defects may need to be corrected or removed surgically. The absence of a vagina can be corrected with surgical reconstruction or dilation of the blind pouch with dilators. Creating the vagina with dilators takes several months of progressive dilation (ACOG, 2002). Surgery to create a vagina is an option if dilation is unsuccessful or not a preferred option. Symptomatic pelvic relaxation is often treated with anterior or posterior repair, usually with hysterectomy. Fibroids may be treated with

BOX 62-2

INDICATIONS FOR SURGICAL MANAGEMENT OF FIBROIDS

- Abnormal bleeding not responsive to medical therapy
- High level of suspicion of malignancy
- Growth of fibroids after menopause
- Infertility from distortion of the uterine cavity, particularly if there are recurrent pregnancy losses
- Symptoms that interfere with quality of life
- Urinary tract symptoms from obstruction
- Iron deficiency anemia from chronic blood loss

removal of only the fibroids in the uterus-sparing myomectomy or with removal of fibroids along with the entire uterus in hysterectomy. Uterine artery embolization is not a surgical procedure but is an intervention performed by a radiologist.

If surgery is contemplated, a course of leuprolide may be prescribed to shrink the fibroids and correct anemia before surgery is performed. Hysterectomy is a definitive treatment, for a woman who has completed their childbearing and is associated with a high level of patient satisfaction (Lefebvre, et al., 2003). Women choosing uterine artery embolization must be carefully counseled that they preserve their uterus, but long-term data on effectiveness, potential fertility, pregnancy outcomes, and patient satisfaction are not complete. Ovarian cysts may be removed with minimal disruption to the ovary or may be accomplished by complete removal of the ovary or associated hysterectomy.

Alternative Therapy

Pessaries are a nonsurgical alternative used to treat all the pelvic relaxation disorders. Each pessary has a specific function and specific directions for fitting and removal. The choice of the appropriate type of pessary is made by the care provider who fits the pessary. The pessary can be inserted and then removed and cleaned at intervals by the patient or by a health care provider. Vaginal therapeutic creams can be used to prevent vaginal irritation from the pessary. Trimo-San cream can be used to adjust the vaginal pH and prevent bacterial infection, and estrogen cream can be used to prevent atrophy. If pessary removal and cleaning is done in the gynecology office, the vagina and cervix should be inspected for unusual discharge, bleeding, or areas of irritation.

Patient and Family Teaching

Teaching includes information about the patient's specific diagnosis, particularly if there are implications for fertility. Teaching should also include information on treatment options, instruction in the use of pessaries, and medication instruction. If surgery is indicated, preoperative and postoperative teaching is indicated. Ways to cope with pain and pain relief measures should be reviewed. Teaching Kegel exercises is an important part of the treatment plan for problems of pelvic relaxation. Recognition of symptoms indicating the need for medical attention should be reviewed with women who have asymptomatic cervical polyps, fibroids, and ovarian cysts.

Evaluation of Outcomes

Potential patient outcomes for each of the example nursing diagnoses for the patient with structural abnormalities and benign conditions are:

- Situational low self-esteem or risk for situational low self-esteem related to physical changes and infertility associated with structural abnormalities. The patient demonstrates acceptance of self and condition of infertility.
- Disturbed body image related to negatively viewing physical changes associated with structural abnormalities. The patient demonstrates enhanced body image and self-esteem as evidenced by ability to look at, touch, talk about, and care for actual or perceived altered body part or function.
- Acute or chronic pain associated with ovarian cysts. The patient should verbalize an adequate relief of pain along with the ability to realistically cope with the pain if it is not completely relieved.
- Impaired urinary elimination related to relaxed pelvic support. The patient is continent of urine or verbalizes satisfactory management.

FEMALE GENITAL MUTILATION

Female circumcision (FC) or female genital mutilation (FGM) involves removal of part or all of the external genital structures. Removal of the clitoris and labia minora is the most common type of procedure. FC and FGM comprise all

> **PATIENT PLAYBOOK**
>
> **Kegel Exercises**
>
> The nurse should instruct the patient in the following to perform Kegel exercises:
>
> - Locate the pubococcygeus muscle by placing your finger inside your vagina and tightening the muscle around your finger.
> - If you are unwilling, or unable, to place your finger in your vagina, an alternative approach is to contract the muscles around your anus, without contracting the buttocks or abdominal muscles, as if you were attempting to stop the passage of gas.
> - Hold the contraction to a count of 10 and then release.
> - Contract the muscle using both slow muscle squeezes and fast muscle squeezes.
> - Repeat the muscle contraction-relaxation cycle 10 to 20 times in a row.
> - The exercise should be repeated three times a day.
> - After six weeks, symptom improvement should be noted.
> - These exercises can be done while performing everyday tasks, such as standing in line, doing dishes, and driving.

procedures involving partial or total removal of the external female genitalia or other injury to the female genital organs whether for cultural, religious, or other nontherapeutic reasons. The World Health Organization (WHO) estimates that between 100 and 140 million women, particularly in African countries, are affected. FGM also occurs in Asia and the Middle East. Female emigrants from these countries who have undergone the procedure can also be found in Europe, Australia, Canada, and the United States.

Immediate health consequences associated with FGM include pain, difficulty with urination, infection, and hemorrhage. Hemorrhage and infection can cause subsequent shock and death. Later health consequences include pain, infection, sexual dysfunction, urinary incontinence, scarring, and childbirth complications (Nour, 2004). Dyspareunia and psychosexual dysfunctions are common. The United Nations Children's Fund, the United Nations Population Fund, and the WHO have jointly issued a statement that FC and FGM cause unacceptable harm and issued a call for the elimination of this practice worldwide.

Nursing care for women who have had FGM must include an understanding of the physical and psychological effects of the procedure. Vaginal exams and gynecological procedures may be painful and produce anxiety, and women require sensitive, empathetic care. Women may suffer anxiety, depression, and impairment to psychosexual and psychological health. The FGM procedure itself may cause a direct or indirect barrier to childbirth because of scarring or infectious complications, resulting in a long or obstructed labor. Episiotomy often relieves soft tissue obstruction, and episiotomy and lacerations are the most common complication of labor and birth with FGM. Increased postpartum pain and postpartum hemorrhage may be present. Fear of labor and birth may be evident. Urinary retention may happen during labor.

Assessment with Clinical Manifestations

Culturally competent providers should care for women with FGM to the extent possible. Assessment must be tactful and respectful of the cultural and religious roots of FGM practices. Assumptions about the effect of FGM on a woman's self-esteem or body image must not be made. The nurse needs to explore the woman's view of FGM and any implications for her emotional, psychological, and sexual health. The type of mutilation must be ascertained to understand what physical effects can be expected as a result of it. Any symptoms relating to FGM, such as urinary problems, pain, or infection, should be elicited. The nurse must assess for the immediate complications of FMG including pain, difficulty with urination, infection, as well as hemorrhage, shock, and death. Later complications include pain, infection, sexual dysfunction, urinary incontinence, scarring, and childbirth complications (Nour, 2004).

Diagnostic Tests

Diagnosis of female mutilation involves inspection of the external genitalia. The care provider confirms which parts have been excised and determines any scarring or restriction of function that is evident. In addition, related laboratory tests, radiologic tests, or CT scans can also confirm the presence of injury.

Nursing Diagnoses

Based on the information gathered, examples of nursing diagnoses in the patient with female mutilation may include the following:

- Chronic pain related to the FGM procedure or its sequelae.
- Impaired urinary elimination related to FGM.
- Disturbed body image related to changes in external genitalia.
- Sexual dysfunction related to alterations in external genitalia.

BOX 62-3

EMPATHY FOR OTHERS

Nurses have a crucial role in the care of women with genital mutilation including support and reassurance, providing nonjudgmental care, and helping the woman maintain her modesty during examinations and procedures. Nurses can assist women in avoiding complications such as urinary retention. It is most important that the nurse not react to the sight of altered external female genitalia with visible shock, because this can be psychologically devastating to the woman who has experienced genital mutilation.

Planning and Implementation

Care of the patient with female genital mutilation includes education, support, therapeutic interventions, and prevention of complications. Psychological counseling, particularly with a counselor who is culturally competent, can be invaluable in helping patients who have experienced FGM (Box 62-3). Mutilating procedures can be associated with religious practices, and a spiritual advisor may be helpful to the woman experiencing complications. A physician or nurse-midwife may need to surgically revise the FGM outcome to assist in childbirth and relieve symptoms. FGM is closely associated to the woman's culture of origin and may have religious significance. Childbirth may be associated with complications of FGM, if there is perineal trauma and repair. Patient teaching should include hygiene measures that will minimize urinary tract infections (UTIs) and knowledge of symptoms requiring medical evaluation. There is no special nutritional therapy for FGM, although a diet that is generally well-balanced will help make tissues as strong as possible for any healing that must occur as a result of childbirth and make urinary infection less likely. Surgery may be necessary to revise FGM to relieve symptoms, particularly during and after childbirth.

Pharmacology

There is typically no medical therapy indicated for FGM. If recurrent urinary infections are a concern, prophylactic antibiotics can be used to prevent UTIs. If disruption and repair of FGM was performed during childbirth, a short-term course of topical estrogen cream may assist with healing and prevent atrophy and scarring.

Population-Based Care

The prevalence of FGM will vary in areas of the country. Areas with large numbers of emigrants from Africa will likely have more women with FGM. Women with FGM are reluctant to seek care, particularly from care providers unfamiliar with FGM, as they are afraid they will be subject to embarrassing questions and painful examinations.

Evaluation of Outcomes

Potential patient outcomes for each of the example nursing diagnoses for the patient with FGM are:

- Chronic pain related to the FGM procedure or its sequelae. The patient should verbalize an adequate relief of pain along with the ability to realistically cope with the pain if it is not completely relieved.
- Impaired urinary elimination. The patient is continent of urine or verbalizes satisfactory management.
- Disturbed body image related to changes in external genitalia. The patient demonstrates enhanced body image and self-esteem as evidenced by ability to look at, touch, talk about, and care for actual or perceived altered body part or function.
- Sexual dysfunction related to alterations in external genitalia. The patient will verbalize satisfaction with the way they express physical intimacy.

MALIGNANCIES

There are several gynecological malignancies with different prognoses, clinical manifestations, and consequences for the patient. This section will examine the following malignancies: vulvar, vaginal, cervical, endometrial, and ovarian cancers. In general, refer to chapter 15 for more information regarding the various types of management strategies for patients that have cancer.

Vulvar Cancer

Vulvar cancer is a malignant neoplasm of the vulvar tissue that accounts for 4 percent of all cancers of the female reproductive tract. Over 90 percent of vulvar cancers are squamous cell cancers. These cancers begin with precancerous changes confined to the epithelial layer called vulvar intraepithelial neoplasia (VIN). VIN can be further divided into VIN1, VIN2, and VIN3. VIN1 is the earliest stage of precancerous changes, and VIN3 is the latest stage toward cancerous changes. Not all women with VIN will progress to vulvar cancer, but it is difficult to determine which lesions will progress and which will not, so all women with VIN are treated.

Melanomas account for 2 to 4 percent of vulvar cancers. A small percentage of vulvar cancers develop from the glands, particularly the Bartholin's glands, and these are called adenocarcinomas. When vulvar cancer is detected early the prognosis is good. If lymph nodes are not affected the five-year survival rate is 90 percent. When lymph node involvement is present, the five-year survival rate drops to 50 to 70 percent. Risk factors for vulvar cancer include HPV infection, smoking, HIV infection, VIN, lichen sclerosis, other genital cancers, and a personal or family history of melanoma. Lichen sclerosis is a skin condition which makes the skin thin and atrophic, and therefore susceptible to cancerous changes. Women with vulvar cancer usually are symptomatic. When symptoms are present they include persistent vulvar itching, vulvar skin color changes, a white warty bump or sore that does not heal, new darkly pigmented mole, or an atypical mole.

Vaginal Cancer

Primary vaginal cancers are much rarer than other cancers of the genital tract. Only about 3 percent of genital tract cancers are vaginal. Squamous cell carcinomas account for 85 to 90 percent of vaginal cancers, most occurring in the upper area of the vagina near the cervix. Adenocarcinomas account for 5 to 10 percent of vaginal cancers.

Adenocarcinomas are usually found in women over 50 years of age. Clear cell carcinoma is a specific type of adenocarcinoma typically found in younger women with diethylstilbestrol (DES) exposure. The risk for vaginal cancer increases with age. More than half the women diagnosed with vaginal cancer are over age 60. Other risk factors include vaginal adenosis (replacement of the usual squamous lining of the vagina with glandular cells) caused by DES exposure, HPV infection, cervical cancer, and smoking.

Vaginal intraepithelial neoplasia (VAIN) is an indicator of precancerous changes. VAIN is diagnosed with colposcopy and treated with laser surgery or topical chemotherapy. VAIN is usually asymptomatic, but lesions may be noted during a routine examination or on colposcopy. Vaginal cancers are usually symptomatic, and if symptoms are present, they include abnormal vaginal discharge, abnormal vaginal bleeding, a vaginal mass, or dyspareunia. Dysuria, constipation, or pelvic pain may occur with advanced disease.

Cervical Cancer

Most cervical cancer originates in the transformation zone between the endocervical canal and the ectocervix. Squamous cell carcinomas account for 80 to 90 percent of cervical cancers, with the rest being adenocarcinomas. Most cervical cancer is diagnosed in women in their postreproductive years, and half of all cancers are diagnosed in women between 35 and 55 years of age. The five-year survival rate for the earliest stage of cancer is 92 percent, and the overall five-year survival rate is 71 percent.

The most important risk factor for cervical cancer is infection with high-risk type HPV. The likelihood of contracting an HPV infection increases with the

Fast Forward ▶▶▶

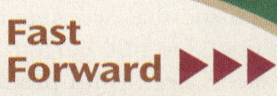

HPV Vaccination

In the future, vaccines may be available to immunize young women against HPV. A clinical trial for a vaccine against HPV type 16 showed 100 percent effectiveness over an 18-month study. One cost-benefit analysis estimated that vaccinating 12-year-old girls and doing Pap screening every three years would result in a 92 percent reduction of cervical cancer (Goldie, et al., 2004).

first sexual contact occurring at an early age, having multiple partners, and having sexual contact with uncircumcised men. Although HPV infection must be present, other risk factors for cervical cancer include smoking, HIV infection, past or current chlamydia infection, obesity, low SES, multiple pregnancies, DES exposure, and family history of cervical cancer (ACS, 2004c). Most cervical cancer is asymptomatic. If symptoms are present, they can include abnormal vaginal discharge or vaginal bleeding, particularly after intercourse, and dyspareunia.

The ACS (2004b) has identified four factors that influence the quality of life that people with cancer have: physical, social, psychological, and spiritual. Women with cervical cancer are often concerned about: the opportunity for pregnancy, fear of recurrence, the presence of pain, sexual problems, fatigue, guilt for behaviors that caused the cancer or delayed screening or treatment, changes in physical appearance, depression, sleep disorders, changes in activities of daily living, the impact on finances, and the effect on their relationships with loved ones.

Endometrial Cancer

Most endometrial cancers are adenocarcinomas. Cancer of the endometrium is the most common cancer of the female reproductive system. Women over age 40 account for 95 percent of all women with endometrial cancer. The five-year survival rate for all types of endometrial cancer is 84 percent. The lifetime probability for a woman to develop endometrial cancer is 1 in 38 (ACS, 2004d).

Risk factors for endometrial cancer include early age at menarche, late menopause, infertility or nulliparity, obesity, use of tamoxifen, estrogen therapy unopposed by progesterone, ovarian tumors, a diet high in animal fat, diabetes, age greater than 40, family history of hereditary nonpolyposis colon cancer, breast or ovarian cancer, and prior pelvic radiation therapy. Tamoxifen is a selective estrogen receptor modulator (SERM) used as adjunctive therapy for breast cancer and to prevent breast cancer in women at high risk. Tamoxifen therapy is associated with endometrial proliferation, hyperplasia, polyp formation, and endometrial cancer. The risk is two to three times that of women the same age not taking tamoxifen. Women taking tamoxifen should be closely monitored for endometrial hyperplasia and should have a gynecological examination once a year. In addition, women taking tamoxifen should be educated about the risks of endometrial proliferation and cancer and be educated about warning signs, such as unusual vaginal discharge and unusual spotting or bleeding.

Oral contraceptives protect against the risk of developing endometrial cancer, as does taking progesterone therapy along with estrogen replacement therapy. If hyperplasia develops, treatment with progesterone and D & C can prevent development of endometrial cancer. The main symptom of endometrial cancer is irregular vaginal bleeding, primarily postmenopausal bleeding. Weight loss, the presence of pelvic pain, and a pelvic or an abdominal mass may also be present in the late stages.

Ovarian Cancer

Excluding nonmelanoma skin cancers, ovarian cancer is the fifth most common cancer in women and the second most common female reproductive cancer. Epithelial ovarian carcinomas account for 85 percent of ovarian cancers (ACS, 2004c). The lifetime probability for women to develop ovarian cancer is 1 in 59.

Most ovarian cancers occur in women after menopause. Half of all ovarian cancers are in women over the age of 63. More women die from ovarian cancer than from cervical and uterine cancer combined. Risk factors for ovarian cancer include increased age; early menstruation; late menopause; no children or first child after age 30; prolonged use of clomiphene citrate to induce ovulation; family history of breast, ovarian, or colorectal cancer; personal history of breast cancer; possibly postmenopausal estrogen therapy; and possibly the use of talcum powder.

Ovarian cancers are often asymptomatic. If symptoms occur, they include abdominal pain and swelling, bloating, nausea, vomiting, indigestion, change in bowel or bladder habits, unexplained weight loss, leg and back pain, and pelvic pain (ACOG, 2002, ACS, 2004c). The breast cancer genes BRCA1 and BRCA2 are associated with a high risk of breast and ovarian cancer. These two genes are responsible for about 9 percent of all cases of ovarian cancer. If there is a family history of breast and ovarian cancer, consideration should be given to offering genetic counseling and testing for the BRCA1 and BRCA2 genes, because prophylactic treatments can be offered for women carrying these genes. Hereditary ovarian cancer accounts for 5 to 10 percent of all ovarian cancers. The lifetime risk of developing ovarian cancer for a woman with the BRCA1 or BRCA2 gene is 15 to 45 percent. If prophylactic treatments are not done, regular screening with pelvic examinations, ultrasound, and CA125 is indicated. Oral contraceptives, hysterectomy, tubal ligation, having a child before age 30, and prolonged breastfeeding all offer a protective effect against ovarian cancer (ACS, 2004c).

Assessment with Clinical Manifestations

The nursing assessment of a patient with a genital cancer should include a complete health history, including the presence of any chronic illness, the possibility of pregnancy, any lifestyle issues that may need to be addressed, such as smoking, the woman's age and plans for childbearing, and relationship support. Family history should also be obtained, particularly the history of breast or ovarian cancer. Refer to chapter 15 for further development of the assessment of patients with cancer.

Diagnostic Tests

Diagnostic tests include colposcopy with cervical biopsy, endocervical curettage, and possibly cone biopsy for evaluation of cervical cancer. Diagnosis of endometrial cancer is usually done by endometrial biopsy or D & C. Ultrasound evaluation may also be helpful. Ultrasonography, other imaging such as MRI or CT scan, and tumor markers such as hCG, CA125, and AFP are used to evaluate ovarian cancer.

Ultrasound and CA125 tests are not recommended as routine screening for women without risk factors because CA125 may be falsely positive, and as many as half of all women with ovarian cancer have a falsely reassuring CA125 result. CA125 is not recommended for premenopausal women, because an elevated level of CA125 may be associated with benign conditions, such as leiomyomata, PID, endometriosis, adenomyosis, pregnancy, and even menstruation (ACOG, 2002). Vulvar and vaginal cancer are evaluated with direct inspection, colposcopy, and tissue biopsy. Other imaging or lymph node biopsy may be necessary. Staging of cancers may include imaging studies such as CT or MRI, chest X-ray, and intravenous pyelogram (IVP).

Nursing Diagnoses

Based on the information gathered, examples of nursing diagnoses in the patient with malignancies may include the following:

- Anxiety related to loss of reproductive function and fear of cancer.
- Altered body image related to surgical changes in genital organs.
- Acute pain related to treatment for genital cancer.
- Deficient knowledge for self-care related to diagnosis or treatment of cancer.
- Sexual dysfunction related to anxiety, altered body image, or treatments for cancer.

Planning and Implementation

Care of the patient with a gynecological malignancy includes education, support, therapeutic interventions, and prevention measures. Treatment of reproductive cancers requires a team approach including nurses, gynecological surgeons, oncologists, physical therapists, nutritionists, sex therapists, and psychological counselors. A diet low in animal fat has been proposed to reduce the risk of certain types of cancer. Women with reproductive tract cancers should be encouraged to regularly eat green, leafy vegetables. Cervical cancer is more prevalent in women who are obese, who smoke, who have HIV or chlamydia, have low SES, and in women with DES exposure, or a family history of cervical cancer. When a diagnosis of cervical cancer is made in a woman who is pregnant, the woman may choose early termination or may choose to continue the pregnancy and obtain treatment after delivery. Endometrial cancer is more common in women with infertility, diabetes, a family history of hereditary nonpolyposis colon cancer, or prior pelvic irradiation. Women with breast cancer are at risk and are at an additional risk if they have used tamoxifen to treat the breast cancer. Ovarian cancer also contributes to the risk of endometrial cancer. Ovarian cancer is more common in women with a family history of ovarian or breast cancer and in women with infertility, particularly with prolonged use of clomiphene citrate to stimulate ovulation. Most reproductive cancers are treated surgically or with radiation. Chemotherapeutic agents also may be used, which are discussed in chapter 15.

Population-Based Care

Minority women are more likely to develop cervical and endometrial cancer, and Caucasian women are more likely to develop ovarian cancer. Vietnamese women have the highest rates of incidence of cervical cancer. The cervical cancer death rate for African Americans is twice that of the national average. Hispanic (American) women and American Indian women also have higher death rates than Caucasian women. Caucasian women have a higher risk of developing and dying from ovarian cancer than do African American women. African American women are twice as likely to die from endometrial cancer as are white women (ACS, 2004c).

Health Care Resources

In August 1990, Congress enacted the Breast and Cervical Cancer Mortality Prevention Act. This act authorized the CDC to establish programs to increase breast and cervical cancer screening among low-income women who are uninsured. The current priority of the cervical cancer screening project is to target women who have never had a Pap smear or have not had a Pap smear for five years or longer.

Surgery

Treatment for reproductive cancers may include surgery, chemotherapy, and radiation therapy. Treatment for cervical cancer often involves surgery, which may include local laser excision, cryosurgery, or cone biopsy if the cancer is in the earliest stages and the woman wants to preserve her fertility. Typically, early cervical cancer is treated with hysterectomy, although pelvic exenteration (removal of the uterus and pelvic structures, lymph nodes, bladder, vagina, rectum, and part of the colon) may be necessary for recurrent cervical cancer. Radiation or chemotherapy may be used for more extensive cervical cancer.

Surgery for endometrial cancer involves hysterectomy and potentially, removal of the ovaries. Surgery for ovarian cancer usually involves removal of the ovaries and uterus. Treatment for vulvar cancer may include laser or surgical excision, vulvectomy, pelvic exenteration, radiation, or chemotherapy. Treatment of vaginal cancer may involve radiation, chemotherapy, or surgery. Local excision may be done for small lesions. If the vagina needs to be removed, a replacement vagina is reconstructed from a graft.

Patient and Family Teaching

Patient and family teaching is extremely important for patients with malignancies of the female reproductive system. For example, an important part of the teaching for women with ovarian cancer is the information that a strong family history of breast and ovarian cancer may indicate the presence of the BRCA1 or BRCA2 gene, and the possibility for other family members to be offered genetic counseling, testing, and prophylactic treatment. Teaching includes information on the specific diagnosis. Lifestyle modifications that can reduce the risk of recurrence, such as smoking cessation, should be discussed. Patients may need information on treatment options. Preoperative and postoperative teaching will also need to be done.

Women undergoing vulvectomy have specific educational needs. Such women may experience discomfort from tight clothing after a vulvectomy. The vaginal opening looks different and scarring may be present; this may cause sexual difficulties for women if they fear their partner's reaction. This may be particularly true for women who enjoy oral stimulation as part of sex. Women who have a vulvectomy have difficulty reaching orgasm and may have numbness in their genital area. Light touching and lubrication may help irritation.

Scar tissue may narrow the entrance to the vagina, causing painful penetration. Vaginal dilators can assist with stretching the vaginal opening. If lymph nodes have been removed, women may have swelling of their genital areas or legs. This can result in pain, fatigue, and difficulty with intercourse. Nurses need to assist women to anticipate problems and help them with communication skills and solving difficulties. Partner education and support is, of course, essential. Sexual issues need to be explored with women who have had vaginal reconstruction. The replacement vagina has no natural lubrication, and sensation during intercourse is varied and different.

Evaluation of Outcomes

Evaluation of outcomes allows the nurse to determine the effectiveness of interventions and change or refocus care as needed.

- Anxiety related to loss of reproductive function and fear of cancer. The patient should be able to recognize the signs of anxiety, demonstrate positive coping mechanisms, and describe a reduction in the level of anxiety experienced.
- Altered body image related to surgical changes in genital organs. The patient demonstrates enhanced body image and self-esteem as evidenced by ability to look at, touch, talk about, and care for actual or perceived altered body part or function.
- Acute pain related to treatment for genital cancer. The patient should verbalize an adequate relief of pain along with the ability to realistically cope with the pain if it is not completely relieved.
- Deficient knowledge for self-care related to diagnosis or treatment of cancer. The patient should demonstrate motivation to learn, identify perceived learning needs, and verbalize an understanding of desired content.
- Sexual dysfunction related to anxiety, altered body image, or treatments for cancer. The patient will verbalize satisfaction with the way they express physical intimacy.

INFERTILITY

Infertility must be considered as the problem of the couple, not an individual, and must be evaluated as such (Figure 62-4). Approximately 14 percent of couples will have difficulty conceiving. Infertility is a concern for 2.7 million U.S. women. The definition of infertility is one year of unprotected intercourse without conception.

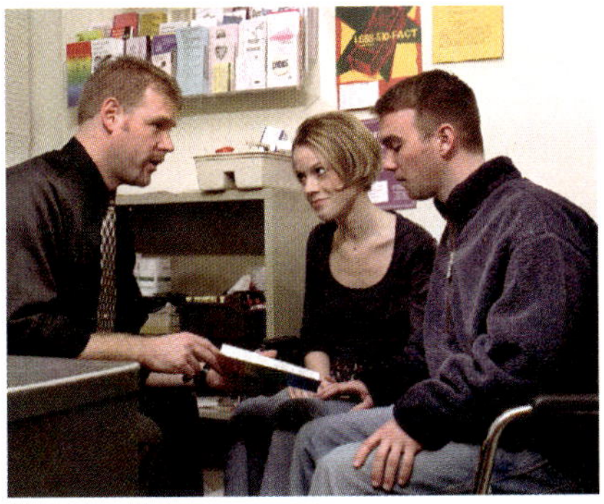

Figure 62-4 An important element in fertility counseling is sharing information with both members of the concerned couple.

The male factor in infertility accounts for 30 percent of infertility, anovulation for 25 percent, tubal damage for 20 percent, and unexplained factors for 25 percent. Among women with anovulation, 70 percent have PCOS. Regular menstrual cycles of 22 to 35 days with premenstrual symptoms and dysmenorrhea suggest that ovulation is occurring. Infertility is associated with a higher (above 27) BMI.

Anovulation may be caused by PCOS, disorders of the hypothalamic system, hyperprolactinemia, and premature ovarian failure. If hypothalamic disruption is caused by a low BMI of less than 20, weight gain may result in the resumption of normal menses and ovulation (ACOG, 2002). Much of infertility treatment includes support and counseling.

Assessment with Clinical Manifestations

The nursing assessment includes questions about pregnancy history, menstrual cycle characteristics, timing of intercourse, and length of time patient and partner have been attempting pregnancy. A complete medical history should be obtained including medication use (prescription, OTC, and herbal), chronic illness, and any surgeries. A social history should be obtained including the use of cigarettes, marijuana, other recreational drugs, and alcohol. A history should be obtained to screen for tubal patency. If there is a history of STDs, PID, ruptured appendix, exposure to DES, or previous pelvic surgery, hysterosalpingography should be considered (ACOG, 2002). DES is a form of estrogen that was given to women from 1940 to 1971 to prevent spontaneous abortion. The daughters of mothers who took DES are at increased risk to develop clear cell adenocarcinoma of the vagina and other reproductive problems.

The partner's history should be obtained including any pregnancies with a prior partner, chronic illness and medication use, surgical history, history of any trauma to the testes or radiation therapy, any use of recreational substances, alcohol, smoking, and type of underwear worn. A family history including questions about endometriosis, PCOS, and infertility should be obtained. Occasionally, the process of obtaining the nursing assessment will uncover an underlying explanation for failure of conception. Sometimes this explanation will be as simple as couples not having an opportunity to have sex at midcycle because of work schedules and not understanding that conception only occurs when ovulation happens.

Diagnostic Tests

A semen analysis for the male partner should be conducted at the beginning of the evaluation of the woman for infertility. The first goal in assessing a woman for infertility is diagnosis of ovulation or anovulation. Laboratory methods to determine ovulation include basal body temperature (BBT) charting; measurement of urine luteinizing hormone (LH), the test used in OTC ovulation predictor kits; measurement of luteal phase serum progesterone; and endometrial biopsy. Serial ultrasounds can be used to identify the growth and rupture of ovarian follicles. The BBT record is reviewed after three months and used in conjunction with ovulation prediction kits to determine the ovarian cycle. If ovulation is occurring, and the semen analysis is normal, the next step is usually to ensure tubal patency with HSG. HSG is discussed in the section on structural abnormalities.

Nursing Diagnoses

Based on the information gathered, examples of nursing diagnoses in the patient with infertility may include the following:

- Anxiety related to inability to conceive.
- Altered body image related to inability to fulfill role as woman.
- Deficient knowledge related to infertility.

Planning and Implementation

Care of the patient with infertility includes education, support, therapeutic interventions, and prevention measures. The nurse caring for a woman experiencing infertility generally collaborates with a primary care practitioner who evaluates and manages the overall care plan and process. This might be a physician, advanced practice nurse, or physician's assistant. If surgery is necessary, this is performed by the general gynecologist or reproductive specialist. Referral to reproductive endocrinologists or fertility specialists may be necessary. Psychological and spiritual counseling is often helpful to support the couple through the process. It is important to verify with the couple at each step that continuing with the plan is what they wish to do. Each couple will have their own financial and emotional threshold for continuing with the infertility process and it is important not to assume what each couple will decide.

Women with PCOS or endometriosis have a higher risk of infertility. For these women, it is not generally advisable to wait an entire year before seeking consultation about infertility. Patients with a diagnosis of PCOS or endometriosis will benefit from anticipatory guidance about trying for pregnancy and the interventions that can maximize their success. Women with other chronic illnesses may find conceiving difficult because of anovulation, fatigue, lack of sexual desire, or use of medications that are contraindicated in pregnancy.

Women with chronic illnesses who are contemplating pregnancy should consult the health care provider managing their chronic illness about taking medication that is effective yet the safest for pregnancy. Women sometimes seek evaluation of infertility because their partners have a chronic illness with a related decrease in sexual functioning. If the patient has a BMI over 30, or diabetes is suspected, testing for diabetes is indicated before attempting to

ETHICS IN PRACTICE

Multifetal Pregnancy Reduction

If the result of infertility treatment is a multiple gestation of more than two fetuses, the couple may need to make difficult choices about carrying a multiple pregnancy or selectively terminating one or more fetuses. Selectively terminating one or more fetuses from a multiple pregnancy is called multifetal pregnancy reduction. The ethical decisions to be made regarding selective reduction of fetuses are difficult for the parents and for their health care providers.

Patients who have gone through extensive time, testing, and procedures to become pregnant may be faced with the following choices: terminate the entire pregnancy, continue the pregnancy and take the risk of delivering severely preterm infants with a high likelihood of neonatal mortality and morbidity, or have selective reduction performed in an effort to decrease the risks of delivering extremely preterm babies. The decision is especially difficult if the parents do not agree on a plan. The plan that parents make in the hypothetical case of what if there is a multiple pregnancy may not be a plan they can live with once a multiple gestation pregnancy is a reality. Spiritual advice from religious advisers may help some couples, as well as talking with couples who have had to make similar choices.

induce ovulation. Diabetes mellitus should be controlled prior to trying for pregnancy to reduce the risks of congenital defects (ACOG, 2002).

Pharmacology

Clomiphene citrate is used to induce ovulation. When clomiphene citrate is used, most successful pregnancies occur within the first three cycles of using the clomiphene, and almost all occur within six months of initiating its use. Gonadotropins (LH and FSH or only FSH) can be used to treat anovulation in women with PCOS, and combined LH and FSH treatment can be used to treat anovulation in women with hypothalamic disorders. Metformin can be used in PCOS, along with clomiphene citrate to induce ovulation if indicated. Dopamine-agonist drugs, such as bromocriptine, pergolide, and cabergoline, are used to induce ovulation in women with hyperprolactinemia. The drugs in Table 62-3 are used in the treatment of infertility.

Health Care Resources

Some health insurance plans cover infertility services, usually to a set end point or to a dollar amount. The most expensive types of infertility evaluation and treatment are not usually covered by health care insurance. This limits infertility treatment to those who can pay for the procedures.

Surgery

Surgery may be used to correct blocked fallopian tubes, for artificial insemination, for egg retrieval, and for in vitro fertilization (IVF). If ovulation is not occurring, then treatment is ovulation induction. If ovulation induction does not work, then options include artificial insemination, or directly introducing sperm into the cervix, uterus, or fallopian tubes. The sperm used may be the woman's partner's sperm, referred to as artificial insemination husband (AIH) or donor sperm, referred to as artificial insemination donor (AID).

IVF involves inducing ovulation, removing the eggs, fertilizing them and then implanting the fertilized eggs inside the uterus. Zygote intrafallopian transfer (ZIFT) involves the same steps as IVF, but the fertilized eggs are transferred into

TABLE 62-3 Medications Used in the Treatment of Infertility

DRUG	INDICATION	SIDE EFFECTS
Ovulation Inducer		
Clomid; Milophene; Serophene	Induction of ovulation in conditions of anovulation	Vasomotor symptoms; lower abdominal tenderness; nausea; headache; ovarian cysts
Gonadotropins		
Gonal-F; Bravelle Follistim; Profasi; Pergonal; Choron; Ovidrel; etc.	Induction of ovulation in PCOS or hypothalamic dysfunction	Ovarian hyperstimulation; increased risk of multiple gestation
Dopamine Agonists		
Parlodel; Permax; Dostinex	Ovulation induction in women with hyperprolactinemia	Hypotension; nausea

Note: Metformin is also used in infertility treatment associated with PCOS.
Adapted from Broyles, B., Reiss, B., & Evans, M. (2007). Pharmacological aspects of nursing care *(7th ed.). New York: Thomson Delmar Learning.*

the fallopian tube instead of into the uterus. Gamete intrafallopian transfer (GIFT) involves induction of ovulation, harvesting the eggs, mixing the eggs with sperm, and implanting the egg-sperm combination in the fallopian tube for fertilization to occur within the tube.

Women may have complications from surgical procedures, such as infection or hemorrhage. The process of evaluation and treatment for infertility can be a significant stressor for the couple and can lead to relationship difficulties and psychological trauma.

Alternative Therapy

Yoga has been described as an adjunctive therapy to help with relaxation, making decisions, and feeling positive about treatment choices. Multivitamin supplements and acupuncture have been suggested to increase fertility.

Patient and Family Teaching

There is much helpful teaching that can maximize couples' chances of conceiving. Women should be taught how to predict their ovulation and time intercourse for maximum success. Women and their partners should be counseled to stop smoking cigarettes and marijuana, drinking alcohol, and using other illicit substances. The partner should be encouraged to wear boxer shorts because tighter, restrictive underwear reduces sperm counts. Women should be given clear guidance on when to present for an evaluation, based on their age, history, and likelihood of conceiving.

Evaluation of Outcome

Potential patient outcomes for each of the example nursing diagnoses for the patient with infertility are:

- Anxiety related to inability to conceive. The patient should be able to recognize the signs of anxiety, demonstrate positive coping mechanisms, and describe a reduction in the level of anxiety experienced.
- Altered body image related to inability to fulfill role as woman. The patient demonstrates enhanced body image and self-esteem as evidenced by ability to look at, touch, talk about, and care for actual or perceived altered body part or function.
- Deficient knowledge related to infertility. The patient should demonstrate motivation to learn, identify perceived learning needs, and verbalize an understanding of desired content.

SEXUAL DYSFUNCTION

Sexual dysfunction is any disorder of the female sexual system, including dysfunctions of desire, arousal, orgasm, or pain. By definition, sexual dysfunction results in personal distress and has an effect on interpersonal relationships. Risk factors associated with sexual dysfunction are emotional problems or difficulties coping with stress, deterioration in economic standing, history of sexual trauma, and lower educational levels. Fatigue and emotional exhaustion can contribute to sexual dysfunction.

Sexual dysfunction may occur in up to 35 percent of U.S. women (Walton & Thorton, 2003). Lack of libido is the most common reported symptom. In postmenopausal women, decreased lubrication, decreased arousal, difficulty achieving orgasm, and pain with intercourse are commonly reported. Frequency of sexual activity and desire for sexual activity both decrease in the menopausal years and may relate to the increase in dyspareunia.

A lack of sexual desire (sexual arousal disorder) is the persistent or recurrent deficiency of sexual desire sufficient to maintain sexual excitement that causes personal distress. Depression is often associated with lack of libido. The lack of sexual desire should first be treated by correcting psychological, relationship, and situational issues, such as mental or physical exhaustion. A healthy lifestyle with exercise and rest may help correct a lack of desire, but the woman may need to be referred for professional counseling.

Disorders of sexual arousal can result from a lack of vaginal lubrication, poor genital vascularity, or neurological conditions. Sexual arousal disorders may be caused by physical factors, such as insufficient foreplay, lack of vaginal lubrication, lack of vaginal muscle relaxation, decreased sensitivity of external genitalia, pelvic trauma, medication use, or postsurgical changes. Sexual arousal disorders may also be caused by psychological factors, such as emotional distraction or inability to relax.

An orgasmic disorder is the persistent or recurrent difficulty in obtaining orgasm. Orgasmic disorders are associated with communication difficulties with the partner, negative attitudes toward masturbation, and greater sexual guilt. Women who have never achieved orgasm **(primary anorgasmia)** may need referral to a sex therapist. **Secondary anorgasmia** (loss of the ability to achieve orgasm in a woman who was previously orgasmic) may result from depression or medications used to treat depression. Changing from SSRIs to bupropion may provide relief. Pelvic floor rehabilitation can be used to correct secondary anorgasmia caused by surgery or menopause.

Pain disorders include dyspareunia, vaginismus, vulvar vestibulitis syndrome, and nonsexual pain. Dyspareunia is recurrent or persistent genital pain associated with sex. Dyspareunia can be caused by endometriosis, vulvar vestibulitis syndrome, interstitial cystitis, atrophy of genital tissues, infection, or adhesions. Smoking may decrease blood flow to the vagina and make atherosclerotic changes in the pelvic blood vessels worse and should be discouraged. Women with pain disorders may have suffered sexual trauma in the past.

Vaginismus is the recurrent or persistent involuntary spasm of the muscles at the entrance of the vagina, interfering with penetration and causing pain and personal distress. Vulvar vestibulitis syndrome (VVS) is characterized by pain on insertion of the penis into the vagina, redness at the vaginal entrance, and tenderness when pressure is exerted within the vaginal vestibule. VVS is one of the most common causes of dyspareunia for women of childbearing age. There is no specific etiology for VVS. A careful history and physical must be done if VVS is suspected. Any vaginal infection must be diagnosed and treated, particularly if chronic candida infection is present (Graxiottin & Brotto, 2004).

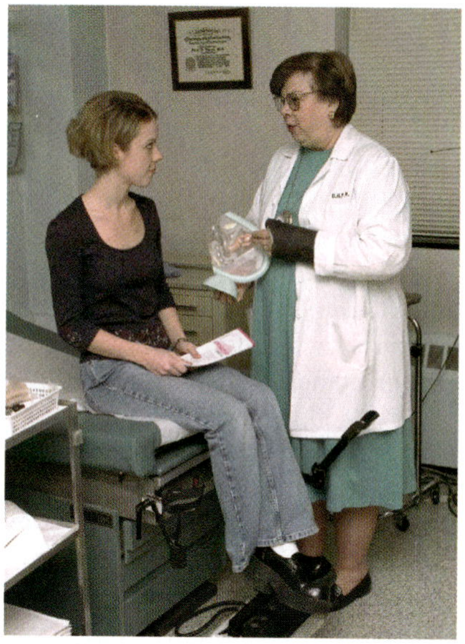

Figure 62-5 Nurses play an important role in helping patients understand their sexual health and development.

Assessment with Clinical Manifestations

History taking from a woman with sexual dysfunction should use gender inclusive terminology so that heterosexuality is not assumed. The interview should be private—this may be an issue in the hospital setting—and confidentiality must be ensured (Figure 62-5). Assessment includes a complete history to include the timing of the symptoms and their history; the presence of any chronic illness; injuries; surgical and psychiatric history; the relationship dynamics and the level of partner support; as well as any medications, alcohol use, recreational drug use or therapies that may interfere with sexual activity. A complete history and a physical need to be done for women with pain disorders. Pain may be associated with endometriosis, pelvic adhesions, interstitial cystitis, or postmenopausal atrophic vaginitis. A medication history is important. The partner's sexual functioning must also be assessed.

Diagnostic Tests

Inspection of external genitalia is performed, and areas of tenderness are assessed. Vaginal atrophy is assessed with a speculum exam. The presence of vaginismus is evaluated by examination with a finger. The presence of pain should be evaluated. If possible, the pain should be reproduced. Muscle tone and strength are evaluated during the pelvic examination. If vaginal atrophy or thyroid disorders are suspected, lab work for estrogen levels and thyroid hormone profiles need to be drawn. Testosterone levels are often drawn before testosterone supplementation is considered.

Nursing Diagnoses

Based on the information gathered, examples of nursing diagnoses in the patient with sexual dysfunction may include the following:

- Sexual dysfunction related to a specific etiology.
- Risk for situational low self-esteem related to sexual difficulties.
- Chronic pain related to vulvar vestibulitis.

Planning and Implementation

Care of the patient with sexual dysfunction includes education, support, therapeutic interventions, and prevention measures. The woman with sexual dysfunction should have a gynecological examination by a health care provider with experience in sexual dysfunction. Psychological counselors and sex therapists are often involved in developing the management plan. Physical therapists may be involved in pelvic physical therapy including biofeedback and strength, relaxation, and exercise training. Gynecologists may evaluate and treat some aspects of sexual dysfunction, and urologists may need to be consulted to correct interstitial cystitis or urethral disorders. The nursing role in sexual dysfunction includes patient support, education, and referral, as indicated.

Women with chronic illnesses or surgery may have sexual dysfunction. Postoperative pain from surgery to correct incontinence or prolapse may be associated with dyspareunia. Women with endometriosis commonly have dyspareunia. Lack of sexual desire can be a consequence of medical conditions or psychological or emotional disorders. Neurological conditions can cause a disorder of sexual arousal or the inability to achieve orgasm. Lack of sexual arousal can be the result of medical or surgical treatment, pelvic floor disorders, or a lack of ability to relax the pelvic floor muscles.

The inability to achieve orgasm may be caused by nerve injury from pelvic surgery or spinal cord injury. The use of beta-adrenergic blockers, central nervous system (CNS) depressants, anticholinergics, or antidepressants can have sexual side effects. Depression is often associated with decreased libido. Vascular effects related to sexual arousal are noted in women with hypertension, smoking, high cholesterol levels, and cardiac disease. Women with arthrosclerosis may have decreased pelvic blood flow and decreased lubrication and clitoral engorgement. Cardiovascular disease may indirectly interfere with sexual activity due to dyspnea. Impaired pelvic floor muscles from episiotomy or significant lacerations with poor healing may contribute to muscular dysfunction leading to vaginismus and sexual pain disorder.

If sexual dysfunctions are not treated, disorders may become progressive, multifaceted, and difficult to treat. Relationships and self-esteem may suffer. Sexual pain syndromes can become chronic pain syndromes that are difficult to treat.

Pharmacology

Postmenopausal women may have relief of atrophic changes with estrogen therapy. Estrogen can be administered with creams, tablets, or a vaginal ring. Women with bilateral oophorectomy and postmenopausal women may benefit from testosterone therapy. Tricyclic antidepressants, such as amitriptyline, and the anticonvulsant gabapentin have also been used to treat VVS (Graxiottin & Brotto, 2004). A common dosage schedule for amitriptyline is 10 to 25 mg orally, with the dose increased, up to three times a day if necessary. Table 62-4 displays the drugs used to treat sexual dysfunction.

TABLE 62-4 Medications Used to Treat Sexual Dysfunction

DRUG	INDICATION	SIDE EFFECTS
Androgens		
Delatestryl; Depo-Testosterone; Testopel; Testim; AndroGel; Danazol	Increase sexual desire, arousal, activity, and orgasm frequency	Acne; hirsutism; voice deepening; clitoromegaly; lipoprotein alterations
Impotence Agents		
Viagra	Treatment of orgasmic disorders or sexual dysfunction	Potentiates nitrates; headache

Note: Oral and topical estrogen therapy is used to treat atrophy of vaginal tissues.
Adapted from Broyles, B., Reiss, B., & Evans, M. (2007). Pharmacological aspects of nursing care *(7th ed.). New York: Thomson Delmar Learning.*

Population-Based Care

Hispanic (American) women have less incidence of sexual dysfunction. Caucasian women have a slightly higher incidence of pain disorders, and almost twice as many African American women have a lack of sexual desire when compared to Caucasian women.

Alternative Therapy

The clitoral therapy device is an FDA approved therapy to treat sexual arousal disorder. It is a battery-powered vacuum device that enhances clitoral blood flow and clitoral enlargement, improving sexual arousal. Several herbal formulations are marketed to promote libido and sexual arousal. Sentia contains epimedium, damiana leaf, dodder seed, black cohosh, isoflavones, valeriana root, ginger root, gingko biloba, bayberry fruit, licorice root, capsicum pepper, and red raspberry leaf. Avlimil contains sage leaf, red raspberry leaf, kudzu root extract, red clover, capsicum pepper, licorice root, bayberry fruit, damiana leaf, valeriana root, ginger root, and black cohosh.

Treatment of sexual disorders may include behavior modification. Exercise improves body image, decreases depression, increases libido, and increases testosterone levels. Strength training exercise may benefit postmenopausal women who have decreased desire. Pelvic floor rehabilitation includes Kegel's exercises, vaginal weights, biofeedback, or pelvic floor physical therapy. Cognitive behavioral therapy, Kegel's exercises, relaxation, and biofeedback have been used for VVS.

Women with vaginismus may benefit from pelvic-floor physical therapy and psychological counseling. Muscle relaxation and progressive vaginal dilation may be used to treat vaginismus. Muscle relaxation, is taught by having the patient isolate and concentrate on the musculature during an examination, and practice contracting and relaxing the vaginal muscles. Dilators are available commercially or tampons of increasing diameter can be used. The dilators or tampons are placed in the vagina for 15 minutes twice a day by the patient to facilitate muscle relaxation and dilation. Reactive muscle tension of the pelvic floor may be treated by teaching relaxation, use of lubricants, self-stretching with dilators, Kegel's exercises, and massage. Physical therapy with relaxation and biofeedback may also be effective. Pain may be treated with surface electroanalgesia, local injection of interferon, topical anesthetics, SSRIs, or oral analgesia. Couples' sex therapy and cognitive behavioral therapy has also been used to treat VVS.

Patient and Family Teaching

Patients should be taught to recognize signs of sexual dysfunction and be made aware that treatment is available. It is important to assist patients to recognize the goals of therapy. Explanations of how treatments such as physical therapy may help correct sexual dysfunction are also important.

Evaluation of Outcomes

Potential patient outcomes for each of the example nursing diagnoses for the patient with sexual dysfunction are:

- Sexual dysfunction related to a specific etiology. The patient will verbalize satisfaction with the way they express physical intimacy.
- Risk for situational low self-esteem related to sexual difficulties. The patient demonstrates enhanced body image and self-esteem as evidenced by ability to look at, touch, talk about, and care for actual or perceived altered body part or function.
- Chronic pain related to vulvar vestibulitis. The patient should verbalize an adequate relief of pain along with the ability to realistically cope with the pain if it is not completely relieved.

Case Study

Nursing Care Plan

Tim and Karen, both 61 years old, have been married for 32 years. For the past several years Karen has suffered from increasingly painful osteoarthritis. She is in the hospital after receiving a right knee replacement. As you are reviewing her discharge plans, Tim comments that now he hopes they can be intimate again. When you ask for clarification, Karen blushes and states that she avoids sex, because it is so painful for her.

Assessment

A married couple who are having difficulty in their sexual activities for a variety of reasons. They do not communicate well and are not open in their expressions regarding their sexual activities. In addition, the wife has osteoarthritis that causes her to have pain and consequently this interrupts her outlook on sexual behaviors.

Nursing Diagnosis 1: Ineffective sexual patterns related to painful and swollen joints

NOC: Risk of Ineffective role performance; Situational low self-esteem; Sexual dysfunction

NIC: Sexual counseling

Expected Outcomes

The patient will:

1. Verbalize a sexually satisfying relationship with spouse by second counseling appointment.
2. Acknowledge strategies to decrease pain by end of first counseling appointment.

Case Study

Planning, Interventions, Rationales

1. Explore with patient current methods used to enhance sexual function, including open communication. *Increases knowledge level.*
2. Encourage patient to take a hot bath or shower prior to sexual activity. *Potentially increases libido.*
3. Apply anti-inflammatory creams over joints prior to sexual activity. *Decreases pain during sexual activities and increases satisfaction during sexual intercourse.*
4. Explores alternative positions for sexual activity. *Decreases the amount of strain on arthritic joints.*
5. Explore the best time of day for sexual activity. *Pain may be lowest in the morning or after gentle physical activity.*

Evaluation

After two months, Tim and Karen both verbalize satisfaction with sexual function. Morning is the best time for Karen to participate in sexual intercourse, after taking ibuprofen followed by a hot shower and gentle range of motion exercises. The couple is most satisfied with a side-lying position for sex. They have also incorporated more massage and touch in sexual activity, lengthening the amount of foreplay and leading to more satisfactory sexual activity for both Tim and Karen. Both also acknowledge that improved communication has lead to less misunderstandings and frustrations.

KEY CONCEPTS

- The female reproductive system is complicated both in terms of anatomical structures and hormonal regulation.
- Pregnancy must always be the first consideration in women with the complaint of amenorrhea or dysfunctional bleeding.
- Women with endometriosis commonly experience a delay in diagnosis and this increases the emotional distress associated with the disease.
- The hallmark of PMS/PMDD is a symptom-free period with every cycle shortly after the menstrual cycle begins.
- Routine douching for hygiene purposes increases the risk for vaginal infection and should be discouraged.
- Antiviral therapy can be used to both treat HSV outbreaks and to help prevent outbreaks.
- Uterine fibroids are the most common solid pelvic tumor in women and the most common reason for hysterectomy.
- Some structural abnormalities of the reproductive tract have implications for childbearing.
- Pessaries are a nonsurgical option used in treating pelvic relaxation disorders.
- FGM is commonly associated with urinary complications.
- Cervical cancer rates have dramatically decreased because of routine Pap smear screening.
- The breast cancer genes (BRCA1 and BRCA2) are associated with the development of ovarian cancer.
- Most reproductive cancers in the early stages are treated surgically.
- Surgeries for reproductive tract cancers are associated with significant psychological, sexual, and body image issues.
- The top three reasons for infertility are male factors, anovulation, and tubal damage or obstruction.
- Anovulation caused by PCOS can often be corrected with the use of metformin and clomiphene citrate.
- Loss of libido is the most common sexual dysfunction.
- Diagnosis and treatment of sexual dysfunction is important to prevent complications and progression of the disorders.
- Amitriptyline is a useful treatment for VVS.
- Physical therapy can be a useful treatment for some sexual dysfunctions.

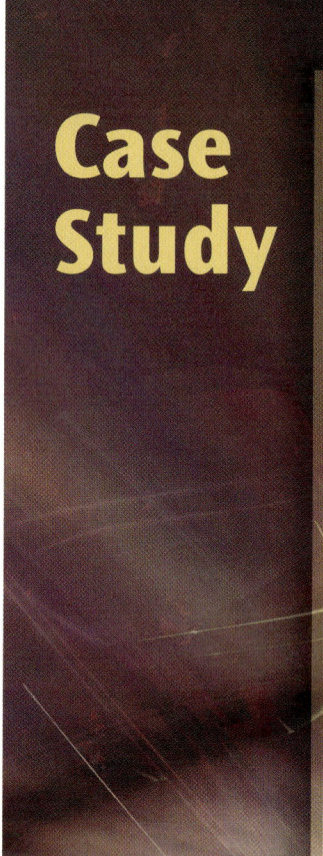

REVIEW QUESTIONS

1. A patient complains of dysmenorrhea. Which of the following are nonprescription relief measures you can suggest that she try?
1. Heat, exercise, NSAIDs, and oral contraceptives
2. Oral contraceptives, vitamin E, and COX-2 inhibitor
3. Aspirin, soy supplements, and NSAIDs
4. Heat, exercise, and NSAIDs

2. A 30-year-old patient has severe dysmenorrhea that suddenly started two cycles ago. Which of the following might be an explanation for this?
1. Ovarian cancer
2. Imperforate hymen
3. Fibroids
4. Late-onset menarche

3. What of the following is not a long-term health implication for a woman diagnosed with PCOS?
1. Cervical cancer
2. Hyperlipidemia
3. Insulin resistance and diabetes
4. Infertility

4. What is the first priority for managing PCOS?
1. Inducing ovulation with clomiphene citrate
2. Weight loss
3. Checking cholesterol level
4. Tracking menstrual cycles with a calendar

5. If a woman is experiencing menopausal symptoms and does not want to take hormone therapy, which intervention can you recommend that she try to reduce hot flashes?
1. Dress in layers
2. Reduce the environmental temperature
3. Exercise
4. Black cohosh supplements
5. All of the above

6. What is the most common serious consequence of untreated chlamydia?
1. Neonatal eye infection
2. Arthritis
3. Infertility related to tubal damage of PID
4. Cervical cancer

7. Which of the following messages should be included in the patient teaching session for women who have been diagnosed with an STD?
1. Condoms are not a perfect protection against STDs.
2. Take all medication until it is gone.
3. Sexual partners should be contacted and treated.
4. Keep all follow-up appointments.
5. All of the above

8. Most hysterectomies in the United States are performed for what indication?
1. Cervical cancer
2. Vaginal infections
3. PCOS
4. Fibroids

9. You are providing nursing care for a teenager who has just been diagnosed with a didelphic reproductive system. She asks you about the implications for pregnancy. Which of the following is the correct answer?
1. Pregnancy is not possible, but adoption or surrogate pregnancy is an option.
2. Pregnancy is possible, but there is a high risk of complications and the pregnancy will have to be closely monitored.
3. Pregnancy is possible, but conception may take longer than usual.
4. Pregnancy is not usually affected as long as there are two separate uteri, cervices, and vaginas that open to the outside.

10. A woman comes into the family practice office where you work. She has been trying to conceive for eleven months without success. What diagnostic testing might be included in the initial evaluation for this patient?
1. BBT and semen analysis
2. HSG and BBT
3. Semen analysis and D & C
4. Ultrasound and HSG

11. Cervical cancer is associated with what virus?
1. HSV
2. Coxsackie virus
3. Rubella
4. HPV

12. What accounts for the large decrease in cervical cancer seen in the last half of the 20th century?
1. Increased hysterectomy rate
2. Improved antibiotics
3. Increased incidence of regular Pap smear screening
4. Improved nutrition

13. Women with strong family histories of ovarian and breast cancer may need to be referred for genetics counseling. What role does genetics play in the development of ovarian cancer?
1. The ovarian cancer gene has been isolated and is responsible for developing ovarian cancer.
2. The breast cancer genes are associated with the development of ovarian cancer.

Continued

REVIEW QUESTIONS—cont'd

3. The gene that makes women susceptible to HPV infection increases the risk for developing ovarian cancer.
4. Ovarian cancer is inherited through the paternal cell line.

14. What is the most common reproductive cancer in women?
1. Vaginal
2. Vulvar
3. Endometrial
4. Ovarian

15. Which of the following is the most common complication of FGM?
1. Urinary complications
2. Infertility
3. Delayed menopause
4. Vulvar cancer

16. Which of the following is the most common sexual dysfunction?
1. Vaginismus
2. Anorgasmia
3. Dyspareunia
4. Decreased libido

REVIEW ACTIVITIES

1. Write a sample patient education sheet on PCOS.

2. Interview a patient who is going to have or has had a hysterectomy. About what issues is she most concerned?

3. Write sample nursing diagnoses and expected outcomes for a patient who has been diagnosed with PCOS.

4. Find out the incidence of cervical cancer for your local community or state. Can you suggest any improvements that could be made in local cervical cancer screening programs?

5. Interview five postmenopausal women. What are their attitudes about hormone therapy for menopausal symptoms?

Visit the Contemporary Medical-Surgical Nursing online companion resource at www.delmarhealthcare.com for additional content and study aids. Click on Online Companions then select the Nursing discipline.

CHAPTER

63

Breast Alterations: Nursing Management

Ruth Grendell, MSN, RN

Marilyn Moorhouse, RN, MSN

CHAPTER TOPICS

- Anatomy and Physiology of the Breast
- Assessment and Diagnosis of Breast Problems of the Breast
- Breast Disorders
- Mammoplasty
- Breast Cancer

KEY TERMS

Atypia
Breast augmentation
Fibroadenomas
Galactorrhea
Gynecomastia
Intraductal papilloma
Lumpectomy
Mammary duct ectasia
Mammoplasty
Mastalgia
Mastitis
Mastodynia
Paget's mammary disease
Periductal mastitis
Supernumerary nipples

Although breast disease can occur in the male, such disease is primarily viewed as a female issue. Both the male and the female breast is commonly associated with physical beauty and perceived as a symbol of sexuality and sexual desire. The female breast is also viewed as a symbol of motherhood and nurturing. Most societies place considerable significance on the cosmetic appearance of the breast, making it difficult to separate the social aspects from the physical aspects of breast disorders. Alterations of the breast can generate negative perceptions of body image, which in turn, can negatively impact the individual's feelings about self-worth. Therefore, addressing the social and psychological implications of breast alterations is essential. This chapter addresses the pathology, collaborative treatment, and nursing care of diseases and conditions that affect the breast.

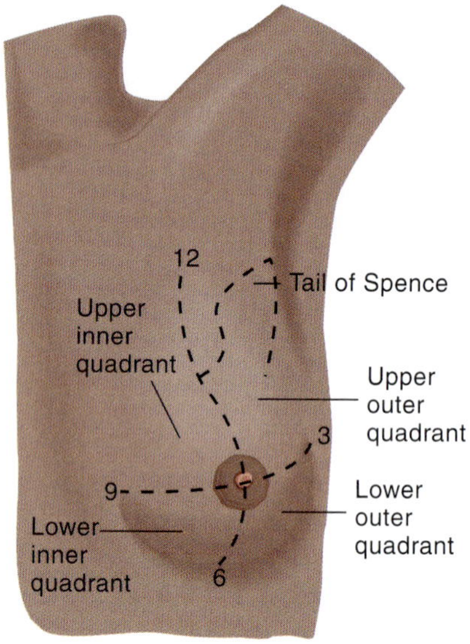

Figure 63-1 Quadrants of the left breast.

ANATOMY AND PHYSIOLOGY OF THE BREAST

The sole physiological function of the female breast, or mammary gland, is to secrete milk for nourishment of an infant. This function is directed and mediated by the same hormones that regulate the reproductive system, and the breast is considered an accessory organ of that system. Each breast is composed of a mound of glandular, adipose, and fibrous tissue located between the third and seventh ribs of the anterior chest wall. For ease in locating structures or areas of the breast, it is conceptually divided into four quadrants. Figure 63-1 shows the quadrants of the left breast. The quadrants of the right breast are a mirror image of those of the left breast.

The breasts are supported by the pectoralis major muscles shown in Figure 63-2 and by fibrous bands called Cooper's ligaments. The ligaments are suspensory ligaments that extend in a radial fashion from the outer boundaries of the breast to the nipple area, similar in configuration to the spokes of a wheel. The ligaments divide the breast into 15 to 20 breast lobes of lactiferous (milk-carrying) ducts and help to shape the breast. The ligaments are attached to the deep layer of the subcutaneous fascia of the dermis. The skin of the breast is attached to the superficial connective and glandular tissues. This is an important contributing factor to visualizing the movement of the skin over the breast during self-examination.

Each woman's breasts are shaped differently. Individual breast appearance is influenced by the volume of a woman's breast tissue and fat, her age, her history of pregnancies and lactation, her heredity, the quality and elasticity of her breast skin, and the influence of hormones. Normal anatomy on a mammogram will image differently depending on a woman's weight, age, and the presence of surgical scars or implants, as well as the amount of fatty tissue in her breasts. The Cooper's ligaments also affect the image of the glandular tissue seen on the mammogram (Daniels, 2003). Because the breast is made up

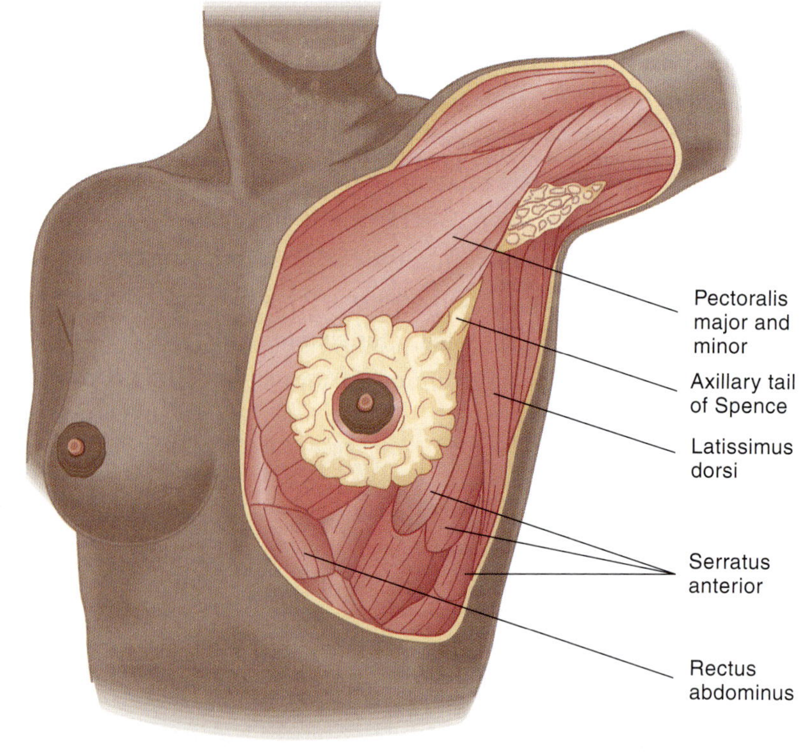

Figure 63-2 Muscles supporting the breast.

of tissues with different textures, it may not have a smooth surface and often feels lumpy. This irregularity is especially noticeable when a woman is thin and has little breast fat to soften the contours; it becomes less obvious after menopause when the cyclic changes and endocrine stimulation of the breast have ceased and the glandular tissue.

Breast Alterations during Maturational Phases

Breasts undergo significant changes during specific maturational phases of a person's life. Initially, there are changes in the breast that correlate with the onset of hormonal influences. Later, various changes in the way breast tissue develops may occur related to pregnancy, lactation, and during menopause. The growth and development stages of the human body and the changes in breast tissue are detailed in the following section.

Effects of Hormones on Breast Tissue

The breast is responsive to a complex interplay of hormones that cause the breast tissue to develop, enlarge, and produce milk. The three major hormones affecting the breast are estrogen, progesterone, and prolactin. These hormones cause glandular tissue in both the breast and the uterus to change during a woman's menstrual cycle. Because of reduced hormonal levels, the breasts are less full for one to two weeks after menstrual flow. Therefore, it may be easier to detect breast lumps during this time. Reduction of hormonal levels is also responsible for the breast's return to its prepregnant state after breastfeeding is concluded.

Changes at Birth

Both female and male infants are born with rudimentary breast tissue that has ducts lined with epithelium. An inspection should reveal a symmetrical location of the nipples in the mid-clavicular line at the fourth to sixth ribs of the anterior chest. Infrequently, small dark spots on the chest may indicate undeveloped nipples and areola called **supernumerary nipples** that can be mistaken for moles. The presence of the extra nipples may be associated with congenital renal or cardiac anomalies (Littleton & Engebretson, 2002).

Changes at Puberty and Adolescence

The release of follicle-stimulating hormone (FSH), luteinizing hormone (LH), and prolactin from the pituitary gland in females at puberty stimulates the release of estrogen from the ovaries. The estrogen stimulates the growth of the ductile system in the breasts. At the onset of the ovulation cycles progesterone is released stimulating the growth of the ductile system and the secretory epithelium of the alveoli. Breast development is the first pubertal change for females. The female breast assumes the characteristic contour by the time of adolescence. Feelings of fullness and discomfort in the breasts are common during the menstrual cycle.

Changes during Pregnancy

Changes in the breast during pregnancy are significant because of the increased levels of estrogen and progesterone. The alveolar epithelium and the ductile system are being prepared for the lactation process. The cellular changes that occur are considered to be beneficial in altering the susceptibility to estrogen-influenced changes in later life.

Prolactin, a hormone secreted by the anterior pituitary gland stimulates the secretion of milk by the alveolar cells. The release of oxytocin from the posterior pituitary gland influences the ejection of the milk from the alveolar cells to the ductile system. Suckling by the infant further stimulates ejection of the milk by providing feedback to the hypothalamus and on to the posterior pituitary.

Leakage of milk often occurs during the later stages of pregnancy. Following the termination of breastfeeding, a woman may have milk leakage for a period of three months to a year until the hormones return to the nonlactating level. Leakage can also occur from overzealous stimulation of the breast even when the woman is not pregnant.

Changes with Menopause

The levels of estrogen and progesterone are gradually reduced at the onset of menopause. The breasts lose glandular tissue; the lobular-alveolar structures atrophy; adipose tissue, connective tissue, and the ducts remain. The breasts decrease in mass and become pendulous. Estrogen supplements after menopause can cause continued lumpiness. As discussed previously, the breast glands drain into a collecting system of ducts that go to the base of the nipple. The ducts then extend through the nipple and open on its outer surface. In addition to serving as a channel for milk, these ducts are often the source of breast problems. Experts now believe that most breast cancer begins in the lining of the ducts and sometimes the milk glands. Benign fibrocystic changes also originate from these ducts.

Gynecomastia in Males

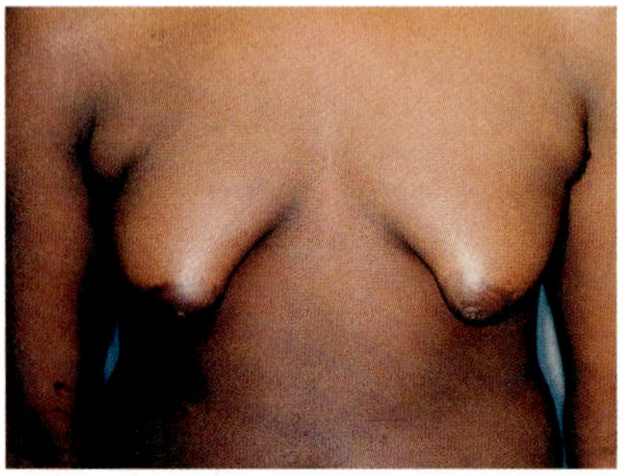

Figure 63-3 Gynecomastia. *Courtesy of Steven M. Lynch, M.D.*

Gynecomastia, a Greek word meaning woman-like breasts, is used to describe the enlargement of male breast tissue shown in Figure 63-3. Although gynecomastia in men is not often talked about, it can occur in 40 to 60 percent of all males. Gynecomastia may be transitory at birth, arise at puberty, and then gradually subside, or it may occur later in life. There may be multiple causes. For instance, digoxin is weakly estrogenic and can cause gynecomastia in some men. Spironolactone, a diuretic, can also cause gynecomastia. Breast development in the male is frequently caused by a shift in the estrogen/androgen ratio because of increased circulating estrogens or decreased circulating androgens. Pseudo-gynecomastia is the enlargement of the male breast because of an increase in fatty tissue. Gynecomastia can result in feelings of embarrassment or feelings of increased self-consciousness in individuals who are affected. Plastic surgery to reduce the glandular tissue or breast fat is an option.

ASSESSMENT AND DIAGNOSIS OF BREAST PROBLEMS

Nurses are instrumental in the education and assessment of women and men with breast disorders. Nurses are also pivotal sources of education and assessment of all individuals for prevention of cancer. Understanding the normal physiology of the breast and the steps in the examination process is essential to providing care for this population.

Examination of the Breast

Examination of the breast is performed in both the upright and supine positions. The examination involves bilateral inspection and palpation of the breasts, areola, axillary, and supraclavicular areas. Adequate lighting is needed for optimal examination, with the woman standing or sitting with hands on hips and disrobed to the waist. Visual inspection focuses on the contour and symmetry of the breasts; skin changes, such as scaling, puckering, dimpling, or scars; the position of nipples; nipple discharge or retraction; and presence or absence of masses.

Variations between breasts are not uncommon, but the breasts should be fairly symmetrical. Findings should include the surface contours of both breasts being round and the skin being smooth, with uniform and matching skin tone. The areola can range from pink to dark brown depending on hormonal factors and normal skin tone. Vascular patterns should be diffuse and symmetrical. Pregnant, obese, or fair-skinned individuals may have hypervascular patterns on examination. Unilateral or focal patterns are considered abnormal and are generally produced by dilated superficial veins that may occur in malignant conditions because of increased blood flow to the area (Estes, 2006).

The areola and nipples are inspected for shape and size. Both areolae and nipples are generally equal in size. Montgomery tubercles may be irregularly spaced around the areola. Nipples should be soft and smooth and usually point in the same direction. If the nipples have been inverted since puberty, it is considered normal. If, however, nipple inversion is a new change, investigation must take place.

Dimpling, a sign of possible underlying tumor, can be detected by asking the woman to slowly raise both arms over her head. The tension created in the breast by contracting the pectoral muscle makes any dimpling evident. Retraction can be assessed with the woman sitting with both hands at waist level with her palms pressed together. For large breasts, have the woman lean forward while standing. This allows the nurse to watch the movement of the breasts to assess that there is no fixation of the breasts to the chest wall.

Palpation of the breasts begins with the lymph nodes. The axillary, subclavicular, and supraclavicular lymph nodes are palpated for firmness and for lumps. While the patient is encouraged to relax the muscles in the arm, the provider palpates the axilla for enlarged nodes. The palpation then progresses down along the chest wall, the anterior border of the axilla, along the posterior border of the axilla, and along the inner aspect of the upper arm.

The supraclavicular nodes are palpated with the woman sitting with the neck flexed slightly forward and turned slightly to the side. The primary purpose of palpation is to discover masses. The examination needs to be completed in a systematic manner. Developing a specific system used for each patient is necessary to ensure all areas of the breast are palpated. The upper outer quadrant of the breast to the axilla (tail of Spence) is an area that needs to be evaluated well. The greatest proportion of malignancies is found in this area of the breast. The breast examination should be completed with the woman in the sitting and supine positions with the provider using the pads of the fingers to palpate. This is done first with the patient sitting with arms down at the sides and then with the patient in the supine position with the arm of the side being examined raised over the head. If a mass is felt, the mass should be identified by the location, size, shape, consistency, distance from the nipple, and quadrant. Nipple discharge is best assessed in the upright position. Collection of the liquid can be done by bringing a slide in contact with the fluid.

The last portion of the breast examination is the patient demonstrating breast self-examination (BSE) as shown in Figure 63-4. This provides an opportunity for teaching, answering questions, and enforcing the importance of monthly self-examinations.

PATIENT PLAYBOOK

BSE

The nurse needs to teach BSE using clear and understandable methods and terminology. The following is one example:

1. First the patient must be advised that BSE should be performed once a month, eight days following menses or on any given fixed date. Advise the patient to avoid the time when her breasts might be tender because menstruation or ovulation. Encourage her to put the BSE on her calendar and include her significant other in the process.
2. Think "B" (bed): Show the patient how to palpate her breast while supine in bed using the palmar surfaces of her fingers. She should start by placing her right arm over her head and palpating the right breast with the left hand, moving in concentric circles from the periphery inward and including the periphery, tail of Spence, and areola. Finally, instruct the patient to squeeze the nipple to examine for discharge. Using the reverse procedure, the woman should examine the other breast.
3. Think "S" (standing): Instruct the patient to repeat the above palpation method while standing.
4. Think "E" (examination before a mirror): The patient should stand in front of a mirror and examine her breasts for symmetry, retractions, dimpling, inverted nipples, or nipple deviation with her arms at her sides, then with her arms raised over head, and finally, with her hands pressed into her hips.

BREAST DISORDERS

The majority of breast disorders are benign. However, it is imperative that breast disorders are diagnosed accurately and treated early to have the most optimal outcome. The emotional distress that a potential breast disorder creates in the patient with breast alteration symptoms is significant. Even when the final diagnosis is of a benign nature, the period of waiting for confirmation can be a time of intense fear and anxiety. Unfortunately, some women delay seeking health care attention because of their fear of a dreaded diagnosis. The following discussion is related to several of the benign breast problems.

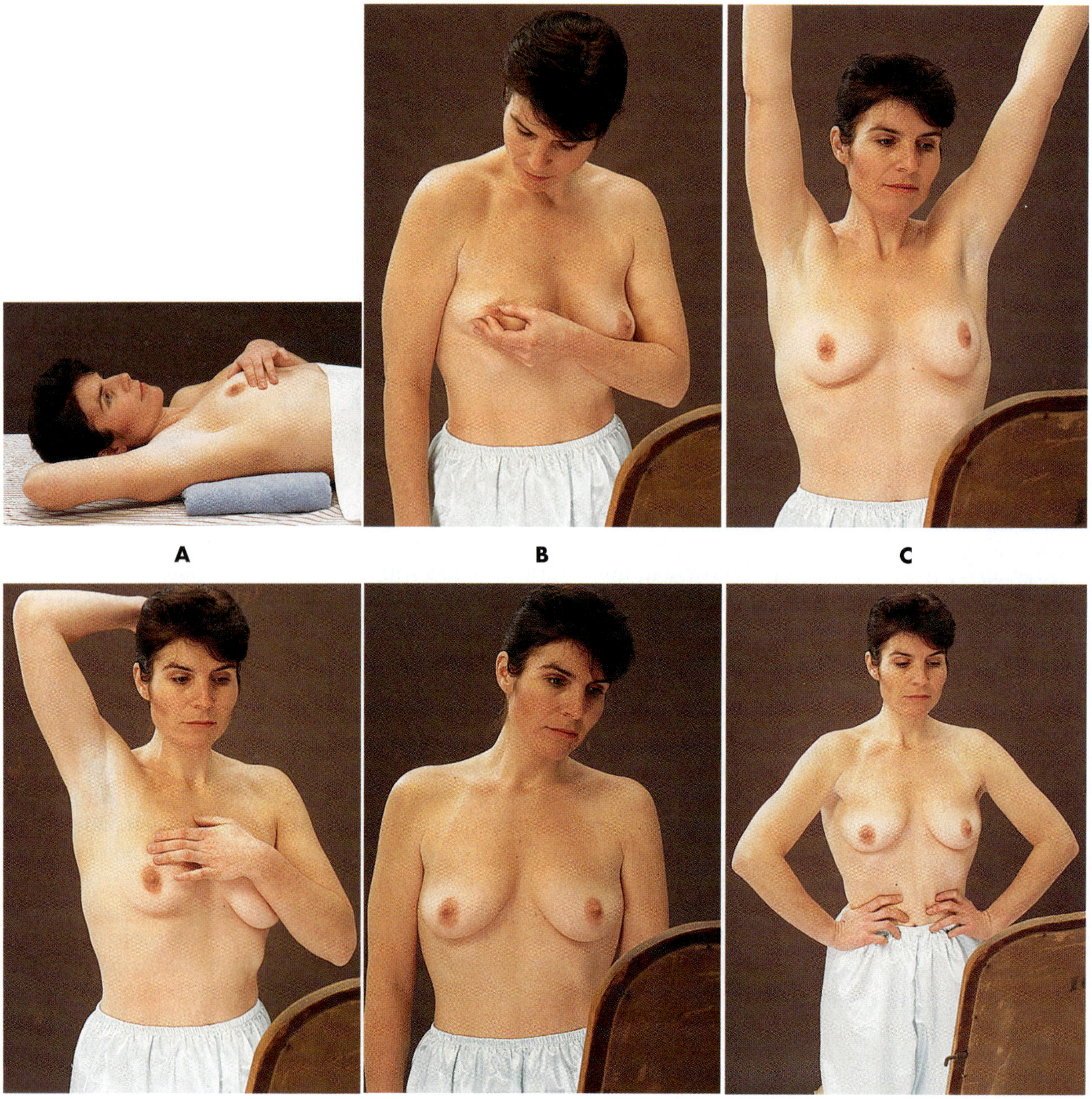

A B C D E F

Figure 63-4 Breast Self-Examination (BSE).

Mastodynia and Mastalgia

Mastodynia and **mastalgia** are used synonymously to refer to breast pain, the most common breast complaint. However, pain is not generally associated with breast cancer. Women with cyclic premenstrual mastodynia also may have lumpy breasts about one week prior to the menses. Examination is performed to rule out any problems. A well-fitting supportive brassiere worn particularly during jogging and other vigorous exercise may be helpful. Decreasing the intake of coffee may also be beneficial.

Nipple Disorders

There are three primary pathological conditions of the nipple: (a) bleeding, (b) discharge, and (c) fissures. A bloody discharge is generally produced when there is an increase of pressure in the areola. Usually, bleeding in this manner

Skills 360°

Cultural Influences on Breast Examination

The women's health nurse practitioner is to conduct a well-woman examination on a 31-year-old new patient. The woman made this appointment at the insistence of her husband, who wants to begin a family. The woman has been in the United States four years and has never had a well-woman checkup. She comes from a culture that highly respects women's privacy and modesty. The female nurse practitioner spends 12 minutes explaining the examination and what the woman will experience. In addition, the equipment that will be used is shown to the patient. The patient has no questions, so the nurse leaves the room to let the patient undress in privacy. The nurse returns a few minutes later to find the woman wearing the paper gown. The nurse tells the patient that the breast examination will be performed first. The nurse inspects the woman's breasts. As soon as the nurse begins to palpate the breasts, the patient grabs the gown around herself, stands up, and states that she has had enough for the day.

The nurse practitioner suspects that the woman may be feeling offended, because the nurse practitioner touched her breasts. The nurse practitioner asks the woman whether she is feeling upset about having her breasts manually examined. In addition, the nurse practitioner expresses respect for the woman's cultural beliefs and empathy for the woman's feelings. The nurse practitioner encourages the woman to talk about her beliefs to better understand how the examination might be modified to be acceptable, drawing the woman out about whether doing the examination through a fabric or with another person from her own culture present might be an option. Through using a soft, caring tone of voice the nurse practitioner attempts to elicit suggestions for alternative approaches from the woman herself, without frightening her with admonitions about what she is risking if she refuses the breast examination.

Red Flag

Examining Nipple Discharge

If a woman is found to have abnormal nipple discharge:

1. Don gloves before proceeding with the assessment.
2. Note the following: color, odor, consistency, amount, whether it is unilateral or bilateral, whether it is spontaneous or provoked.
3. With a sterile, cotton-tipped swab, obtain a sample of the discharge so that a culture and sensitivity, as well as a gram stain can be obtained.
4. Consider checking the sample for occult blood.
5. Follow your institution's guidelines for sample preparation.

is because of a benign condition, but it may accompany malignancy. Bleeding can also occur from trauma to the breast that causes blood to be released through the nipple. Generally, if bleeding is noticed, women should be encouraged to seek their health care professional's consultation immediately to pursue diagnostics.

Discharge from the nipples, other than lactation, can be related to several possible causes. For example, cancer, pituitary adenoma, cystitis, and a variety of medications can cause fluid discharge from the nipples. Some discharge may be normal in many women, but following up on any discharge is the responsibility of the health care provider. The discharge will be examined to see if it is lactation products, sanguine discharge, or infectious products.

Fissures of the nipple are ulcers that most commonly develop in lactating women. In the presence of fissures, the patient should wash the breast and nipple area carefully with water, massage with lanolin, and expose to air to dry. If the fissure is too painful or bleeding occurs, the lactating woman may be advised to stop breastfeeding. Referral to a lactation specialist should be suggested.

Fibrocystic Changes

Fibrocystic change is the most frequently occurring pathological breast problem. The etiology of fibrocystic conditions is unknown, but there is some evidence that it is related to hormonal regulation. Typical changes include fluid-filled cysts that are round, soft or hard, and movable. The cysts may increase in size premenstrually. These changes are most common during the childbearing years but can also occur after menopause. Breast tenderness and pain may be present, but there should not be any nipple discharge. If nipple discharge is noted a health care provider should be contacted. For women with fibrocystic changes it is critically important to do monthly BSEs to be familiar with the breast tissue so that any change is noticed as soon as possible. Although this is often called a disease, it is classified as a condition. There is no specific treatment for fibrocystic breast changes. Aspiration of a cyst may be necessary depending on the symptoms it causes. A biopsy is performed if the cyst recurs after an aspiration procedure. Fibrocystic disease is considered to be a risk factor for breast cancer when there it is accompanied by cellular proliferation and **atypia** (deviation from the standard cell form). Regular examinations by a health care professional and regular mammograms are recommended in addition to BSEs (Estes, 2006).

Fibroadenoma

Fibroadenomas are benign, fibrous growths, or tumors, of the glandular epithelium in breast tissue. They usually occur in women between the ages of 15 and 30 years. These growths are generally solid, painless, rubbery masses that do not attach to any structures in the breast. The movability of the tumor is its most distinctive characteristic, and it can be diagnosed by cytology. The tumor may form a dense stroma (a collection of serosanguineous fluid). A fibroadenoma is usually removed surgically using a local anesthetic.

Galactorrhea

Galactorrhea is the secretion of a white, milk-like fluid in a nonlactating breast. This may be because of vigorous nipple stimulation; medications, such as exogenous hormones, blood pressure medications, or antidepressants; herbal preparations, including nettle, fennel, anise, fenugreek seed, and blessed thistle; street drugs, such as opiates and marijuana; internal hormonal imbalance; or local chest infection or trauma. Large amounts of prolactin hormone from a pituitary tumor may also be the cause. Galactorrhea is usually benign. A health care provider should be contacted for further assessment if the breast liquid is reddish or blood-tinged (serosanguineous).

Cyst

Cysts are fluid-filled sacs. The cause of a cyst is unknown, and the majority of cysts are not harmful. Cysts may cause pain and may disappear spontaneously. Surgical removal may be necessary if the cysts continue to be problematic and painful.

Abscess

An abscess of the breast is a collection of pus resulting from infection. Antibiotics are given and local comfort measures are used to relieve pain. In some cases, draining the cyst may be necessary.

Intraductal Papilloma

Intraductal papilloma is a small, benign tumor that grows within the terminal portion of a solitary milk duct of the breast. Papillomas occur in women mainly between the ages of 25 and 55, and the cause is unknown. Solitary intraductal papillomas are usually not precancerous. They are usually too small to palpate but often cause serosanguineous nipple discharge. In the presence of serosanguineous discharge, it is required that malignancy be ruled out. Surgical excision is the primary treatment.

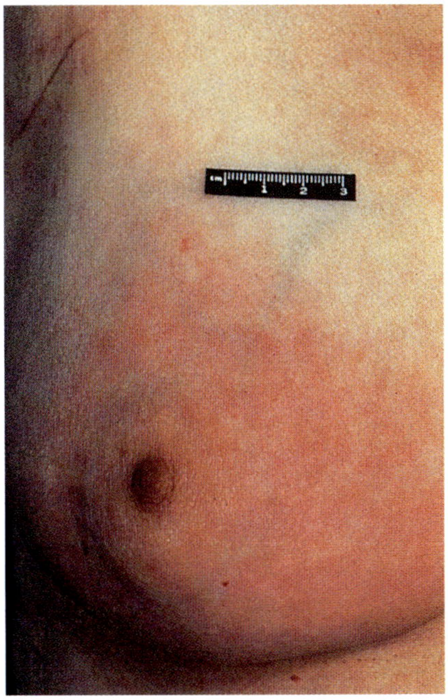

Figure 63-5 Inflamed breast with erythema.

Mastitis

Mastitis is inflammation of the breast. It can be caused from irritation, injury, or infection, and while it most commonly occurs within the first three months after childbirth, it can occur at any age. Mastitis can develop at any time so long as a woman is breastfeeding. Causes of mastitis during breastfeeding include bacterial or, occasionally, fungal infections, poorly fitting bras, and breastfeeding in only one position. The sentinel symptoms of mastitis include erythema (usually wedge-shaped redness with swelling), pain, and breast tissue that feels warm to touch accompanied by general malaise and fever. An inflamed breast with erythema is shown in Figure 63-5. Cracked nipples also commonly accompany mastitis. The treatment includes warm compresses, continued breastfeeding to completely empty the affected breast, antibiotics, pain medications, bed rest, increased fluid intake, and improved support. If an abscess forms, it may be necessary to drain the breast. Nursing care and education of the woman with mastitis is essential. Reassurance that the baby will not be affected by continued breastfeeding from the inflamed breast or from the medications being given can ease the concerns of the mother.

Periductal Mastitis

Periductal mastitis is an inflammation of the breast that can occur in nonlactating older women. Milk ducts near the nipple become inflamed and breast pain results. There may be other changes noted including a mass, dimpling, and nipple retraction. There is a great need to be followed by a health care provider. Treatment includes antibiotics and, in some cases, surgery. Thorough examination is recommended as breast cancers can present in this manner.

Inflammatory breast cancer can be confused with mastitis. This is a rapidly growing, aggressive, deadly cancer, and treatment needs to be initiated quickly. One differentiating symptom between mastitis and inflammatory breast cancer is fever. The woman with mastitis generally complains of a fever.

Mammary Duct Ectasia

Mammary duct ectasia is a noncancerous condition of the breast in which the milk ducts beneath the nipple become dilated and sometimes inflamed. It occurs most often in women during or after menopause. Causes may include smoking, hormonal changes, vitamin A deficiency, or inverted nipples. Symptoms include breast and nipple tenderness, dirty white or greenish nipple discharge, breast redness, and a lump. This condition may improve without treatment, but more often, antibiotics, warm compresses and excision of the affected ducts are needed.

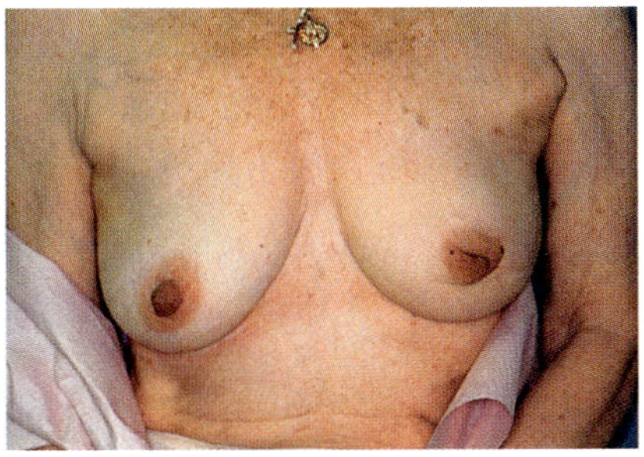

Figure 63-6 Nipple retraction of left breast.
Courtesy of Steven M. Lynch, M.D.

Breast Tumor

A breast tumor that is precancerous or cancerous usually is evident as a white area on a mammogram even before it can be palpated. In cases where the tumor is cancerous, it may appear as a white area with radiating arms. A cancerous tumor may have no symptoms, or it may cause swelling, tenderness, and discharge from the nipple or indentation of the nipple called retraction. Nipple retraction is shown in Figure 63-6. There may be a dimpled appearance to the skin over the tumor. A breast biopsy is the choice to determine whether a lesion is cancerous.

Paget's Mammary Disease

Paget's mammary disease is an uncommon skin cancer characterized by a chronic eczema-like rash of the nipple and adjacent areolar skin. It most commonly occurs between 50 and 60 years of age and is much more common in women than in men. Paget's mammary disease is associated with an underlying cancer, either in situ carcinoma of the breast or a more widespread infiltrating cancer, although this is sometimes difficult to detect on clinical examination or by mammogram.

Most patients go to their health care provider with the chief complaint of an itchy rash in the breast area. Additional symptoms may include nipple discharge that is often bloody, redness, scaling, inversion or ulceration, and swelling around the nipple. The diagnostic workup includes a skin biopsy to determine the presence or absence of Paget's cells. Mammography may also be helpful in assessing the patient for underlying breast cancer. Because Paget's disease is associated with underlying cancer the diagnostic workup must be extensive.

MAMMOPLASTY

Mammoplasty is a surgical procedure to increase or decrease the size or shape of the breast. It is usually considered an elective procedure. Generally speaking, there are two categories of mammoplasty: (a) breast augmentation and (b) breast reduction. Both of these interventions are discussed in the following section.

Breast Augmentation

Many women who seek **breast augmentation** (surgical enlargement of the breasts) are young individuals who are dissatisfied with the appearance of their breasts. However, mature women also choose to have breast revisions for various reasons. Health care providers need to be nonjudgmental toward the woman's desire to alter the appearance of her breasts as she strives to alter her body image. It is also important to be aware of the cultural values placed on the woman's breasts. The number of women seeking breast augmentation has increased steadily over the past 10 years. Breast augmentation is the most popular cosmetic procedure performed by plastic surgeons in the United States (American Cancer Society, 2004a). From a historical perspective, the American Society of Plastic Surgeons (2002) reported that 206,354 breast augmentation surgeries had been performed in 2001. This represents a 56 percent increase from 1998 and a 533 percent increase since 1992.

Many factors influence a woman's decision to seek breast augmentation. Included in the decision-making process is consideration of at least five factors: (a) intrapsychic or internal motivation that is affected by body image, feelings about physical appearance, female identity, focused dissatisfaction with breast appearance, and quality of life; (b) interpersonal reasons related to the importance of breasts in social or romantic situations; (c) available information about breast augmentation; (d) medical risks, including pain and complications; and (e) the out-of-pocket cost of cosmetic surgery.

Over the centuries women have attempted to create the look of a full bosom. This look was initially attempted through the modification of clothing as early as 3,000 B.C. Minoan women used primitive corsets and bras to enhance breast contour. With the exception of brief periods of time in the 15th and 20th centuries when the fashion was to attempt to deemphasize the size of the female breast, large breasts have been one of the standards that define beauty in society.

In the 18th century women underwent disfiguring and painful surgeries to enhance the breasts. These procedures were invasive and used materials such as rubber, glass, ivory, and metal as implants. Not only were these procedures unsuccessful in enhancing breast size, the procedures caused many medical problems for the women who underwent these surgeries. Interest in breast enlargement continued and other materials were used for injection in to the breasts. These included olive oil, paraffin, and petroleum jelly. Again, the outcomes were extremely negative, resulting in complications and terrible cosmetic results.

In 1992 silicone breast implants were banned because of concerns with potential leaking, physical symptoms, and nonspecific illnesses in women with such implants. Saline implants soon replaced the banned silicone implants. There has been an increasing number of women who have undergone breast augmentation surgery with saline implants. In 1999 the Institute of Medicine released the investigational results of silicone breast implants and concluded that there is no association between autoimmune disease or other health problems and silicone breast implants.

Investigators have become increasingly concerned regarding the ability to accurately screen and diagnosis women for breast cancer after they have undergone breast augmentation surgery. It has been suggested that women who have undergone breast augmentation are at higher risk for presenting with advanced disease. The studies have been limited by small sample sizes and have reported conflicting findings. A multicentered study found that the sensitivity level for screening women with breast augmentation was significantly lower than for those without augmentation. Another study found that sensitivity was significantly higher in women with augmentation than without and that there was no significant difference for asymptomatic women diagnosed with breast cancer with or without breast augmentation on the basis of tumor characteristics, i.e., stage, invasiveness of the disease, nodal status tumor size, or estrogen receptor status (Miglioretti, et. al., 2004). This study identified that breast augmentation does present difficulties with accurately diagnosing women with breast cancer on mammography. However, the study also suggests that women with breast augmentation are no more likely to be diagnosed with advanced disease than women without augmentation.

Breast augmentation techniques have improved over the past decade. The size of the incision has decreased and the materials used are less toxic to the patient. The use of saline-filled implants has decreased the potential for connective tissue or autoimmune diseases. However, saline implants still carry a risk for potential complications including infection, hematoma, and hypertrophic scarring. Such complications are estimated to occur in 1 to 3 percent of all surgeries. More frequent complications include mammographic interference; breastfeeding problems; decrease in, or loss of, nipple sensation; and capsular contracture. The occurrence rate for these issues is 10 to 35 percent of surgical cases. The latter complications may occur immediately after surgery or may take years to surface.

The current prostheses are safe, durable, and seamless silicone rubber casings filled with saline, dextran, or silicone. Soybean oil implants are sometimes used. This implant has an outer shell of silicone filled with highly refined soybean oil. (X-rays can easily penetrate the implant to allow for better visualization of the underlying breast tissues.) The prosthesis is placed beneath existing breast tissue or beneath the pectoralis muscle. The incision may be made under the breast or around the nipple. Mammography is performed prior to the surgery to rule out breast cancer in women older than 35 years of age or in younger women with a family history of cancer or with a suspicious lump. The surgery is usually performed under general anesthesia as an outpatient procedure, but the patient may stay overnight in the hospital. Drains are usually placed in the surgical wound to prevent hematoma formation. The drains are removed two to three days postoperatively if the drainage is normal.

Postoperative complications can occur including changes in sensation or the development of a hematoma, infection, or leakage from the prosthesis, but the complication that occurs in as many as 70 percent of cases is formation of fibrous sacs of collagen, or scar tissue, around the implant that contract and compress the breast into the shape of a hard, round ball. The breast becomes hard, immobile, painful, and distorted. This generally happens within the first six months after surgery and is beginning to be considered a natural outcome by researchers, rather than a complication. Breast massage may be prescribed to deter such scar tissue formation. The woman's temperature should be monitored, and sterile dressings changed as needed. The health care provider may instruct the woman to wear a supportive brassiere continuously for a few days.

Breast Reduction

Surgical breast reduction is performed to relieve the neck and shoulder pain that can lead to degenerative nerve changes because of overly large breasts. Large breasts can also interfere with daily activities, such as writing, typing, or driving a car, and it may be difficult to find appropriate clothing. Overly large breasts may be a source of embarrassment and affect the woman's self-esteem and self-image. Breast reduction can have psychological as well as physiological benefits. The reduction consists of removing wedges of tissue from the upper and lower quadrants of the breast. Excess skin is removed, and the nipple and areola are repositioned on the breast. The woman may be able to breastfeed if a large amount of tissue is not removed and the nipples remain connected during the surgery.

Nursing Diagnoses

Nursing diagnoses that may be appropriate for a woman with mammoplasty may include the following:

- Disturbed body image related to mammoplasty.
- Fear in response to diagnosis of breast cancer.
- Ineffective coping related to uncertainty and anxiety regarding surgical outcome and compromised ability to perform normal activities of daily living postoperatively.

Planning and Implementation

During the nursing assessment of the patient undergoing a breast-related diagnostic workup, problems that require management by other health care disciplines, such as medicine, physical therapy, nutrition, or pharmacy, may be discovered. The nurse is responsible for recognizing the need for collaboration across the health care team and for initiating team action. Nurses are able to bridge the issues and coordinate care, as well as monitor the response of the patient and inform the specific disciplines involved. The opportunity to case manage a patient, minimize complications, and promote the patient's safe passage along the health care continuum are important aspects of the collaborative process. The nursing care required for patients with breast diagnoses includes significant emphasis on social and psychological support. In addition to the need for emotional support, the opportunity for teaching and enhancing health management in relationship to breast health is paramount.

Evaluation of Outcomes

Potential patient outcomes for each of the example nursing diagnoses for the patient with mammoplasty are:

- Disturbed body image related to mammoplasty. The patient demonstrates enhanced body image and self-esteem as evidenced by ability to look at, touch, talk about, and care for actual or perceived altered body part or function.
- Fear in response to diagnosis of breast cancer. The patient should manifest positive coping behaviors and verbalize a reduction in the amount of fear of the having this disease.
- Ineffective coping related to uncertainty and anxiety regarding surgical outcome and compromised ability to perform normal activities of daily living postoperatively. The patient identifies her own maladaptive coping behaviors, available resources and support systems, describes and initiates alternative coping strategies, and describes positive results from new behaviors.

BREAST CANCER

It has only been within the last 20 years that breast cancer and treatment have been openly discussed. Well-known women have been sharing their personal experiences with breast cancer, treatment and the importance of early detection by discussing their stories with the media. This disease is no longer kept a secret as it was previously.

Epidemiology

Breast cancer is the most common type of cancer in women and is a major public health problem in the United States, with one in eight women expected to be diagnosed sometime during their lives. In 2004 the number of reported cases of invasive breast cancer in the United States was 217,440. This number includes only 1,450 men. In women, breast cancer is the most frequently diagnosed nonskin cancer. In addition to invasive breast cancer 59,390 cases of cancer in situ were documented in 2004. The increase in reporting and detection is directly related to the use of screening mammography and the ability to detect breast lesions before they can be palpated.

Breast cancer rates have continued to increase since the 1980s with some slowing in the 1990s. The increased incidence of breast cancer in women 50 years of age and older has persisted. Most breast abnormalities are benign, do not grow uncontrollably, and are not life-threatening. Careful evaluation must take place to ensure an accurate diagnosis.

Etiology

Although men are diagnosed with breast cancer, it remains a predominately female disease. Besides being female, age is the most important risk factor for breast cancer. Currently, a woman in the United States has a 13.2 percent, or one in eight, chance of developing breast cancer in her lifetime. The rate of breast cancer has gradually increased over the past 30 years, in part because of longer life expectancies and also that more women are diagnosed with breast cancer because of improved screening techniques.

A personal history of cancer has been shown to increase the risk of breast cancer. Women with a family history of breast cancer of a first-degree relative have an increased risk. The risk increases if more than one relative has a positive family history, and the risk also increases inversely to the age of that relative at the time of diagnosis. It is estimated that 5 to 10 percent of breast cancer cases result from inherited mutations or alterations in the breast cancer susceptibility genes, BRAC1 and BRAC2. These mutations are found in less than 1 percent of the population. Some women who know they carry one of the genes use the information to decide whether to use medication (e.g., tamoxifen) prophylactically. It is impossible to predict if or when these women may be diagnosed with breast cancer, and it is uncertain as to whether genetic predisposition and other factors combine to increase an individual's risk.

Risk factors related to diet, exercise, alcohol consumption, or immune system issues are thought to make a difference in the risk of contracting breast cancer. Environment is also being studied as a source of risk for the development of breast cancer. Some pesticides have chemical similarities to estrogen and may actually attach to receptor sites in the same manner as estrogen.

Caucasian women continue to have the highest breast cancer rates. However, African American women have later diagnostic testing and poorer responses to treatment. This population often enters treatment at later stages of the disease, thus negatively influencing the outcomes and life expectancy of those diagnosed and treated.

Hormones are thought to increase breast cancer risk by affecting cell proliferation, damaging deoxyribonucleic acid (DNA) and promoting cancer cell growth. Early menarche (younger than 12 years of age) and later menopause (older than 50 years of age), older age at first full-term pregnancy (older than 30 years of age), and fewer number of pregnancies are thought to impact a woman's risk by affecting the endogenous reproductive hormones (Kumle, et al., 2003). Recent use of oral contraceptives may increase the risk of breast cancer, but women who have not used oral contraceptives for 10 years have the same risk as those who have never used hormones. Use of hormone replacement therapy (HRT) has been shown to increase breast cancer risk with a higher risk associated with the duration of use (Li, Malone, & Porter, 2003). When given to women without a uterus, estrogen alone does not increase the risk of developing breast cancer as much as HRT does (Beral, 2003). Breastfeeding has consistently been shown to decrease a woman's risk of breast cancer slightly, with greater benefit for those who breastfeed for a longer duration.

Increased weight or obesity increases the risk of postmenopausal women for breast cancer. Some studies suggest that weight gain during adulthood increases the risk. The rationale for this association is that in postmenopausal women fat produces circulating estrogen, and an increase in fatty tissue can therefore increase estrogen levels and the potential for developing breast cancer. A study by the American Cancer Society showed that overweight women are 1.3 to 2.1 times more likely to die from breast cancer compared to women of normal weight (Calle, Rodriguez, Walker-Thurmond, & Thun, 2003).

Alcohol intake is consistently associated with an increased risk of breast cancer. Studies have suggested that the equivalent of two drinks, or 24 ounces, of alcohol per day may increase breast cancer risk by 21 percent. This risk is dose dependent, and it does not matter what type of alcohol beverage is consumed. It is thought that the increase is attributed to an increase in androgen and estrogen levels.

Smoking has continued to be controversial. In a recent report from Reuters regarding a study from Canada, the investigator calculates that women who smoke have a 46 percent increased risk of breast cancer and that women exposed to passive smoke have an overall increased risk of 27 percent. Physical activity has been suggested to provide a small amount of protection against breast cancer. A recent study suggests that regular exercise, regardless of intensity, may reduce the risk of breast cancer in postmenopausal women (McTiernan, Kooperberg, & White, 2003).

Red Flag

Risk Factors for Benign Breast Disease

The following risk factors enhance a woman's potential for benign breast disease:

1. Caffeine use
2. Imbalance between estrogen and progesterone
3. Estrogen excess
4. Hyperprolactemia
5. Age 20 to 50 years

Pathophysiology

Some cancers are classified as in situ, which means they have not spread beyond the area where they began. In situ breast cancer is confined within the ducts (ductal carcinoma in situ or DCIS) or lobules (lobular carcinoma in situ or LCIS). Nearly all cancers at this stage can be cured. Many oncologists believe that lobular carcinoma is not a true cancer, but that it is an indicator of increased risk for developing invasive cancer at a later date.

The remaining breast cancers are invasive or infiltrating. This type of cancer begins in the lobules or ducts of the breast and then spreads through the duct or gland wall to invade the surrounding fatty breast tissue. The degree of seriousness of invasive carcinoma depends on the stage of the disease and the extent to which it has spread when it is diagnosed. Two different staging or classifications of tumors are used. The American Joint Committee on Cancer (AJCC) uses stages I, II, III, or IV with stage I being an early stage, and stage IV being an advanced stage based on information about the tumor size, lymph node involvement, and the presence or absence of distant metastases (American Cancer Society, 2004a). A broader system used for staging of most cancers is known as the SEER summary stage system. The SEER classifications are local stage (confined to the breasts, regional stage (tumors that have spread to surrounding tissue or nearby nodes), and distant stage (cancers that have metastasized to distant organs.

Red Flag

Breast Mass

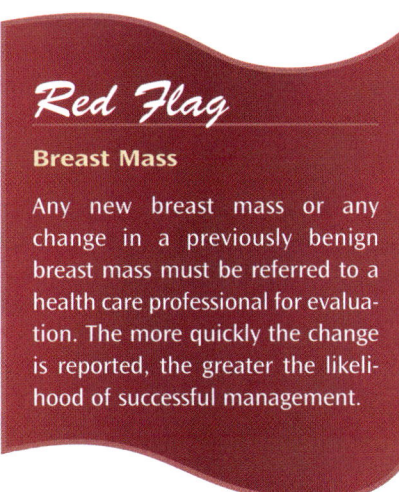

Any new breast mass or any change in a previously benign breast mass must be referred to a health care professional for evaluation. The more quickly the change is reported, the greater the likelihood of successful management.

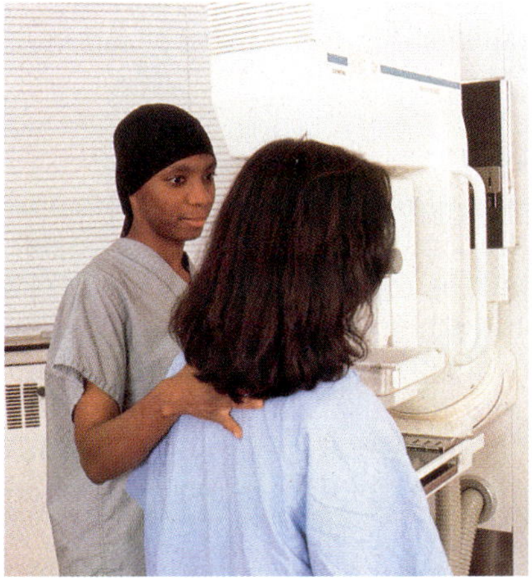

Figure 63-7 The patient is being positioned for a mammogram by a radiology technologist.

Diagnostic Tests

There are several primary tests used to diagnose alterations of the breast in addition to physical examination. The most common are mammography, ultrasonography, and biopsy. This section will discuss the specifics of these tests.

Mammography

Mammography is low dose X-ray visualization of the internal structures of the breast. It is highly accurate. Mammography has been shown to significantly increase the early detection of breast cancers and thus the ability to initiate treatment at an earlier stage of the disease. Mammography is the single most effective method for early detection of breast cancer. On average, mammography will detect about 80 to 85 percent of breast cancers in asymptomatic women. Testing is a little more accurate in postmenopausal than in premenopausal women. There is a 5 to 10 percent false-positive reporting requiring further testing. Figure 63-7 shows a woman being positioned for a mammography examination.

Recommended screening intervals are based on the duration of time a breast cancer is detectable by mammography before symptoms develop. Many breast cancers are not diagnosed until they become large, more advanced cancers because too much time lapses between mammography examinations. In an effort to detect breast cancer while it is optimally treatable, women are having mammograms at earlier ages. There are some studies that question the use of mammography and that suggest that mammograms have the potential to increase a woman's risk of developing breast cancer. Some researchers are questioning whether radiation exposure at earlier ages might be related to earlier development of the disease.

Recent reports from the behavioral risk factor surveillance system found that 61.5 percent of U.S. women age 40 and older have had a mammogram within the past year. A woman with less than a high school education, who has no health insurance, or who is a recent emigrant to this country is much less likely to have had a recent mammogram. While utilization of mammograms in general has been increasing, women below the poverty level are less likely to have had a mammogram within the last two years (Miglioretti, et al., 2004).

Breast Ultrasound

The increased use of breast ultrasonography has paralleled the augmented use of screening mammography. Unlike mammography, however, ultrasonography is not an effective screening tool; it is mainly used in the office setting for further characterization and biopsy of breast masses and suspicious axillary nodes. However, ultrasonography is particularly useful for differentiating cystic from solid breast lesions. Sonographically, simple cysts tend to be oval or lobulated and anechoic (echo free) with well-defined borders. Solid masses are characterized sonographically with respect to shape, compressibility, height-width ratio, margins, internal echo pattern, and presence of shadowing versus posterior enhancement. Carcinomas are typically hypoechoic (echoes are weaker than normal) with masses that are taller than they are wide, irregular borders, and broad acoustic shadowing. As with mammography, some malignancies cannot be visualized with ultrasonography. Therefore all clinically suspicious breast masses should undergo biopsy. In the operating room, ultrasonography can help the surgeon locate and excise nonpalpable breast lesions and achieve clean lumpectomy margins. It is also being used to guide various investigational tumor-ablating procedures.

Biopsy

Cytological, or tissue, diagnosis of a palpable breast mass may be obtained by means of fine needle aspiration (FNA) biopsy, core needle biopsy, and open incisional or excisional biopsy. Needle biopsy techniques are less invasive, less costly, and more expeditious than open biopsy, but they are significantly more

PATIENT PLAYBOOK

Breast Sonogram

The nurse needs to explain the following to the patient prior to the ultrasound of the breast:

1. Explain the test procedure and the purpose of the test.
2. Assess the patient's knowledge about the test.
3. Instruct the patient that there will be no discomfort during this diagnostic test.
4. Ask the patient to remove clothing from the waist up and provide privacy.
5. Instruct the patient to not apply any deodorant, powder, or lotions to the breast or axillary area prior to the test.
6. Obtain a history of breast implants, surgeries, and previous or existing abnormalities of the breast.
7. After the test, encourage the patient to verbalize their feelings about the test results and teach, or review, how to perform monthly BSEs.

likely to yield false-negative results. The choice of a biopsy technique should be individualized on the basis of the clinical and radiographic features of the lesion, the experience of the health care provider, and the patient's condition and preference.

Fine Needle Aspiration Biopsy

FNA biopsy permits the sampling of cells from breast lesions for cytological analysis. It is an appropriate first step in the evaluation of dominant breast masses, but it requires substantial experience on the part of both the operator and the cytopathologist. FNA biopsy is usually the diagnostic procedure of choice for T3 and T4 primary lesions, as well as chest wall and axillary recurrences for which systemic chemotherapy or irradiation is indicated as the first treatment modality. Because of sampling error, the procedure is less useful in evaluating small masses and areas of vague thickening or nodularity. In addition, it often cannot reliably distinguish invasive from noninvasive cancer.

Discrete masses discovered on physical examination may be either cystic or solid. Unless previous ultrasonographic examination has shown the mass to be solid, the needle used should be large enough (20 or 21 gauge) to permit aspiration of potentially viscous fluid if the lesion proves to be cystic. If the mass is known to be solid, a smaller needle (22 to 25 gauge) is sufficient for obtaining diagnostic tissue and will cause the patient less discomfort. For sufficient suction to be generated, a syringe with a capacity no smaller than 10 mL should be used. A variety of syringe holders are available that facilitate application of suction with a single hand.

Image-Guided Core Needle Biopsy

Needle biopsy techniques are increasingly being used to diagnose nonpalpable breast lesions. In general, FNA biopsy of nonpalpable lesions is inadvisable because of its high false negative rate. Little is lost by attempting an FNA biopsy of a palpable lesion in the office setting, but performing a stereotactic or ultrasound-guided FNA biopsy of a nonpalpable mass carries a significant cost in terms of time, patient discomfort, and expense. The diagnostic accuracy currently achievable with FNA biopsy in this setting does not justify this cost. Consequently, image guided core needle biopsy is the preferred approach for needle biopsy of nonpalpable lesions.

In choosing core needle biopsy, both patient and health care provider must be comfortable with the fact that the lesion will only be sampled rather than excised, recognize that the possibility of a sampling error that will cause the examiner to miss the lesion is higher with core needle biopsy than with open biopsy, and realize that equivocal findings will necessitate follow-up with open biopsy. The trade-off for these limitations is that core needle biopsy generally costs less than open biopsy, takes less time, and leaves only a tiny scar. After a core needle diagnosis of malignancy, the surgeon may proceed directly to wide local excision and will often be able to obtain clean margins with a single open procedure.

Open Biopsy

The vast majority of open breast biopsies are now performed with either local anesthesia alone or local anesthesia with intravenous sedation (monitored anesthesia care). General anesthesia is reserved for situations in which multiple lesions must be excised and the amount of local anesthetic required would exceed the maximum safe dose.

Open biopsy incisions should generally be curvilinear and should be placed directly over the lesion to minimize tunneling through breast tissue. Resection of a portion of overlying skin is not necessary unless the lesion is extremely superficial. In case the lesion proves to be malignant, all open biopsy incisions should also be oriented so that they can be excised with any subsequent lumpectomy or mastectomy incision. Accordingly, if an open biopsy is to be done at an extremely lateral or medial site, it may be best approached via a radial incision placed over the lesion rather than via a more vertical curvilinear incision.

Stereotactic Versus Ultrasound Guided Core Needle Biopsy

Whenever feasible, core needle biopsy is performed with ultrasonographic guidance that permits real-time documentation of needle position within the lesion. Stereotactic mammography guided core needle biopsy is performed if the lesion is not visualized ultrasonographically. Stereotactic biopsy is appropriate for lesions that are favorably located within the breast for achieving stable positioning in the biopsy window of the machine. Lesions close to the chest wall or the areola may not be accessible to stereotactic biopsy and are best approached via open biopsy with needle localization.

Clustered microcalcifications may also be approached by stereotactic core needle biopsy. If the cluster is not large enough for calcifications to remain to guide subsequent wide excision if a malignancy is found, a clip should be placed to mark the biopsy site. Alternatively, if the surgeon has experience with breast ultrasonography, this imaging modality may be used intraoperatively to identify the hematoma that results from stereotactic core needle biopsy.

As is the case for open biopsy of palpable lesions, the vast majority of needle-localized breast biopsies are now performed with local anesthesia or local anesthesia with intravenous sedation. General anesthesia is reserved for excision of multiple lesions or other special circumstances. The lesion to be excised is localized by inserting a thin needle and a fine wire under mammographic or ultrasonographic guidance immediately before surgery. To facilitate incision placement, images should be sent to the operating room with the wire entry site indicated on them. With superficial lesions, the wire entry site is usually close to the lesion and thus may be included in the incision. With some deeper lesions, the wire entry site is on the shortest path to the lesion and so may still be included in the incision. The incision is placed as directly as possible over the mass to minimize tunneling through breast tissue. Once the incision is made, a core of tissue is excised around and along the wire in such a way as to include the lesion. This process is easier and involves less excision of tissue if the localizing wire has a thickened segment several centimeters in length that is placed adjacent to, or within, the lesion. The surgeon then follows the wire itself into the breast tissue until the thick segment is reached. Only then is the excision extended away from the wire to include the lesion in a fairly small tissue fragment.

Nursing Diagnoses

Based on the information gathered, examples of nursing diagnoses in the patient with breast cancer may include the following:

- Acute pain as related to breast surgery.
- Fear in response to the diagnosis of breast cancer.
- Ineffective coping related to anxiety, lower activity level and the inability to perform normal activities of daily living.
- Activity intolerance related to fatigue after breast surgery.

Planning and Implementation

There are a variety of treatment modalities for cancer of the breast. These treatment choices are divided into those that do not require surgery and those requiring surgical intervention.

Nonsurgical Treatment

Systemic therapy includes hormonal and biological therapy and chemotherapy. This is called neoadjuvant treatment, and it has been found to be as effective as adjuvant therapy given after surgery to kill any undetected cancer cells that may

Fast Forward ▶▶▶

Diagnostic Tests That Are Definitive for Breast Cancers

There are several forms of diagnostic tests that are currently being used for the refinement of diagnoses related to breast cancers. These tests are continuing to be studied for their effectiveness and likely will progress to more specific value in the near future.

Ductal Lavage

The majority of breast cancers originate from the epithelium of the mammary ducts. Ductal lavage is a method of recovering breast duct epithelial cells for cytological analysis via a microcatheter that is inserted into the duct. It has several promising potential applications, such as identifying high-risk women, predicting risk with the help of molecular markers, monitoring the effectiveness of chemopreventive agents as evidenced by regression of cellular atypia, and delivering drugs directly into the ducts. At present, however, ductal lavage remains investigational and its predictive value and clinical utility await further definition.

Ductoscopy

Advances in endoscopic technology have made visualization and biopsy of the mammary ducts possible. Mammary ductoscopy is a procedure in which a microendoscope is employed to directly visualize the ductal lining of the breast and to provide access for retrieval of epithelial cells by means of lavage. At present, this technology is only available at a few centers, and as with all new technological developments, there is a learning curve associated with its application.

Ductoscopy is currently being evaluated for use in three main areas: (a) evaluation of patients with pathological nipple discharge; (b) evaluation of high-risk patients; and (c) evaluation of breast cancer patients to determine the extent of intraductal disease and, perhaps, define the extent of resection more precisely. Further study will be required to determine the precise role of this investigational technique in the evaluation and management of breast disease (Lind, Smith, & Souba, 2005).

have migrated to other parts of the body. This therapy often shrinks the tumor enough to make surgical removal possible. In some cases this neoadjuvant therapy has decreased tumor size enough to allow women whose larger tumors would require mastectomy to have breast conserving surgery instead.

Herceptin biological therapy is a monoclonal antibody that directly targets the HER2 protein of breast tumors and offers significant survival benefit for some women with metastatic disease. It is currently being used to treat women with late stage, recurring cancer. It has been suggested that women with early cancers may also benefit from this therapy.

Radiation therapy may be used to destroy cancer cells remaining in the breast, chest wall, or axilla after surgery. The ability to more accurately target radiation therapy has increased dramatically over the past decade, thus decreasing radiation therapy side effects. When used in conjunction with surgery and chemotherapy, long-term survival has been improved in women with lymph node positive disease.

Surgery

There are several surgical options for primary treatment of breast cancer. It should be emphasized that for most patients, wide local excision (lumpectomy) to microscopically clean margins coupled with axillary dissection and radiation therapy yields long-term survival equivalent to that associated with modified radical mastectomy. Currently, indications for mastectomy include patient preference, inability on the part of the surgeon to achieve clean margins without unacceptable deformation of the remaining breast tissue, the presence of multiple primary tumors, previous chest wall irradiation, pregnancy, and the presence of severe collagen vascular disease (e.g., scleroderma). Nonmedical indications for mastectomy include the lack of access to a radiation therapy facility and any other patient factors that would prevent completion of a full course of radiation therapy.

Lumpectomy

Lumpectomy, also referred to more precisely as wide local excision or partial mastectomy, involves excision of all cancerous tissue to microscopically clean margins. Reexcision or lumpectomy without axillary dissection may be performed with the patient under local anesthesia, but sedation or general anesthesia is usually advisable if a significant amount of tissue is to be excised or if there is tenderness from a previous biopsy. Lumpectomy with axillary dissection usually calls for general anesthesia, but it may be performed with thoracic epidural anesthesia supplemented by local anesthesia as needed.

Like open breast biopsy incisions, lumpectomy incisions should generally be curvilinear, should be placed directly over the lesion, and should also be oriented so as to be included within a subsequent mastectomy incision if margins prove positive. Extremely lateral or medial incisions may be better approached via a radial incision placed over the lesion. Because accurate assessment of margins is of central importance in a lumpectomy, it is critical that the incision be long enough to allow removal of the specimen in a single piece rather than in several pieces (Lind, et al., 2005).

Along with the mass itself, it is generally necessary to remove a 1- to 1.5-cm margin of tissue that appears normal beyond the edge of the palpable tumor or, if excisional biopsy has already been performed, around the biopsy cavity. In the case of nonpalpable lesions diagnosed via needle biopsy, the position of the lesion must be determined by means of wire localization, and 2 to 3 cm of tissue should be excised around the wire to obtain an adequate margin. The specimen should be oriented by the surgeon and the margins inked by the pathologist; this orientation is useful if reexcision is required to achieve clean margins. Reexcision of any close margins may be performed during the same surgical procedure if the specimen margins are assessed immediately by the pathologist. Surgical clips may be left in the lumpectomy site before closure to assist the radiation oncologist in planning the radiation boost to the tumor bed.

Minimally Invasive Ablative Techniques

The next step in the evolving application of less invasive techniques to breast cancer is to determine whether ablative local therapies can be effective substitutes for extirpative local therapies. Cryotherapy, laser ablation, radiofrequency ablation (RFA), and focused ultrasound ablation have all been studied as means of eradicating small breast cancers (Simmons, 2003). In most of these techniques a probe is placed percutaneously into the breast lesion under the guidance of an imaging modality, and tumor cell destruction is achieved by means of either heat or cold.

Cryotherapy has been successfully used for some time in the treatment of nonresectable liver tumors. It kills tumor cells by disrupting the cellular membrane during the freeze/thaw cycle. Unfortunately, early results of studies evaluating cryotherapy in breast cancer patients indicate that it does not always achieve complete tumor destruction. In addition, ultrasonographic monitoring of cell death may not be precise enough to allow accurate determination of the adequacy of treatment.

Laser ablation causes hyperthermic cell death by delivering energy through a fiberoptic probe inserted into the tumor. Because of the precise targeting required, ensuring complete tumor destruction has proved difficult with this technique.

RFA is a minimally invasive thermal ablation technique in which frictional heat is generated by intracellular ions moving in response to alternating current. Currently, RFA appears to be the most promising ablative method for small breast cancers. Like cryotherapy, RFA has also been extensively used to treat liver tumors. The RFA probe is percutaneously placed in the tumor under imaging guidance, and a star-shaped set of electrodes is extruded from the tip of the probe. Postprocedural MRI may help confirm complete tumor destruction, not only after RFA, but also after other ablative techniques as well.

Experience with ablative breast therapies is still relatively scant, and these techniques remain investigational. To date, most of the studies examining ablative breast cancer techniques have been single institution pilot studies involving highly selected patients with small, well-defined lesions who do not have extensive intraductal cancer or multifocal disease. In addition, these techniques have been restricted to lesions that are neither superficial nor deep, so as to avoid injury to the skin or the chest wall. Most of the initial ablative series involved subsequent surgical excision to obtain histological evidence of cell death. Unfortunately, when ablative therapies are used alone, the benefits of pathological assessment of the specimen, including evaluation of margin status, are lost; and positive surgical margins are associated with increased local recurrence rates. Preliminary data from the initial studies demonstrate acceptable short-term results, but the long-term results must be evaluated against those of standard breast conservation techniques (Simmons, 2003). The minimally invasive ablative techniques clearly are technically feasible, and they appear to offer some potential advantages, but it remains to be determined to what extent they are oncologically appropriate.

Lymphatic Mapping and SLN Biopsy

The histological status of the axillary nodes is the single most important predictor of outcome for breast cancer patients. Traditionally, axillary dissection has been a routine part of the management of breast cancer, but it has become clear that axillary dissection can be associated with sensory morbidities and lymphedema. The growing recognition of the morbidity of axillary dissection, together with the increasing ability of mammography to detect smaller and smaller node-negative tumors, gave rise to the need for a less morbid axillary procedure. Lymphatic mapping and SLN biopsy is a minimally invasive method of determining occult lymph node metastasis that is less morbid and more accurate than axillary dissection. SLN biopsy is based on the principle that the SLN is the first node to which tumor spreads; thus, if the SLN is tumor free, patients can be spared the morbidity associated with axillary dissection (Lind, et al., 2005).

The technique of SLN biopsy continues to evolve, but at present, the most common method of identifying the SLN employs both a vital dye and a radionuclide. Lymphatic mapping is a critical part of the procedure. A radionuclide is injected before surgery and dynamic gamma camera imaging is subsequently employed to delineate sites of drainage. Several imaging series examining various sites of injection (peritumoral, intradermal, and subareolar) concluded that the breast and its overlying skin may drain to the same few SLNs. In the operating room, a vital blue dye is injected (usually peritumorally), and the breast is massaged to stimulate lymphatic flow. The surgeon then makes a small incision in the axilla and uses a handheld gamma probe to remove lymph nodes that are "hot" (i.e., radioactive), blue, or both. At the time of breast surgery, the SLN can be examined by means of frozen section analysis or touch-print cytology. If metastases are present in the SLN, axillary dissection may then be performed.

Because SLN biopsy involves analysis of only one or two nodes, the pathologist can carry out a more intensive pathological examination than would be possible with a standard axillary lymphadenectomy specimen containing multiple nodes. Newer techniques (e.g., immunohistochemical and molecular assays) can also be used to identify micrometastases that light microscopy would fail to detect, but the therapeutic and prognostic significance of tumor cells identified by such means remains unclear.

Because there is a learning curve for SLN biopsy, the success rate varies with the surgeon's experience. Accordingly, it is recommended that surgeons first learning the technique use axillary dissection as a backup for the first 20 procedures to gain experience in identifying the SLN. Surgeons competent in SLN biopsy should be able to identify the SLN with better than 85 percent accuracy and a false-negative rate lower than 5 percent. (Classe, Curtet, & Campion, 2003). Currently, axillary dissection is recommended for patients who have a positive SLN; however, prospective, randomized trials are required to determine to what extent this step is necessary in SLN-positive patients. A number of studies have confirmed that the absence of metastases in the SLN reliably predicts the absence of metastases in the remaining axillary nodes.

SLN biopsy has also been employed in DCIS patients. Women with DCIS have high survival rates without undergoing any axillary procedure, and there is concern that indiscriminate application of SLN biopsy to these patients may result in unnecessary axillary dissection and subsequent systemic chemotherapy. Therefore, SLN biopsy should be limited to (a) patients with extensive DCIS in whom percutaneous biopsy may have missed areas of invasion and (b) patients with extensive DCIS who are undergoing mastectomy that would preclude SLN biopsy if occult invasive disease were found on pathological examination. The SLN identification rates and false-negative rates reported when SLN biopsy is performed after neoadjuvant chemotherapy are similar to those seen when the procedure is performed after diagnosis, but before systemic chemotherapy. Contraindications to SLN biopsy include the presence of palpable axillary nodes suggestive of metastatic disease, the presence of large or locally advanced breast cancers, prior axillary surgery, and pregnancy or lactation.

Axillary Dissection

Before the advent of SLN biopsy, axillary dissection was routinely performed in breast cancer patients; it provided prognostic information that guided subsequent adjuvant therapy, it afforded excellent local control, and it may have contributed a small overall survival benefit. Axillary dissection for clinically node-negative breast cancer includes resection of level I and level II lymph nodes and the fibrofatty tissue within which these nodes lie. The superior border of the dissection is formed by the axillary vein laterally and the upper extent of level II nodes medially; the lateral border of the dissection is formed by the latissimus dorsi from the tail of the breast to the crossing point of the axillary vein; the medial border is formed by the pectoral muscles and the anterior serratus muscle; and the inferior border is formed by the tail of the breast. Level II nodes are easily removed by retracting the greater and smaller pectoral muscles medially; it is not necessary to divide or remove the smaller pectoral muscle. In general, level III nodes are not removed unless palpable disease is present.

Mastectomy

The goal of a mastectomy is to remove all breast tissue, including the nipple and the areola, while leaving well-perfused, viable skin flaps for primary closure or reconstruction. This is the case whether the mastectomy is performed for treatment of breast cancer or for prophylaxis in high-risk patients. Proper skin incisions and good exposure throughout the procedure are the important components of a well-performed mastectomy. The borders of dissection extend superiorly to the clavicle, medially to the sternum, inferiorly to where breast tissue ends on the costal margin below the inframammary fold, and laterally to the border of the latissimus dorsi. The fascia of the greater pectoral muscle forms the deep margin of the dissection and should be removed with the specimen.

A

B

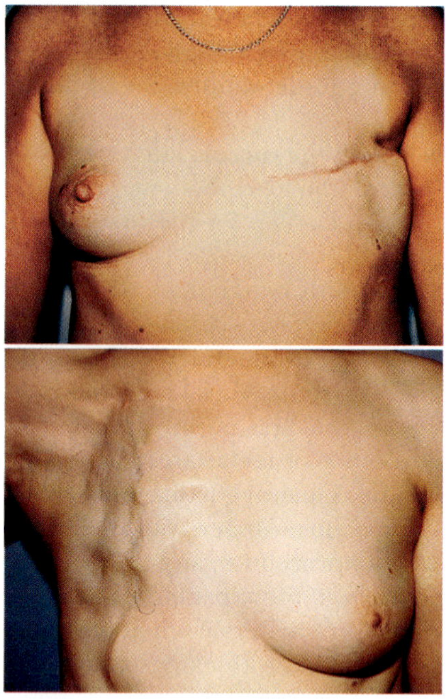

Figure 63-8 Mastectomy patients. *Courtesy of Steven M. Lynch, M.D.*

Mastectomy usually calls for general anesthesia, but it may be performed with thoracic epidural anesthesia supplemented by local anesthesia as needed. When a simple mastectomy is to be performed in a frail patient for whom general anesthesia poses unacceptable risks (particularly if the patient is elderly and has a narrow-based, pendulous breast), local anesthesia with sedation is appropriate.

Simple mastectomy is performed: (a) to treat DCIS; (b) as a prophylactic measure; (c) as a follow-up to lumpectomy and axillary dissection if lumpectomy margins are positive for malignancy; (d) to treat local recurrence of breast cancer after lumpectomy, node dissection, and irradiation; and (e) in elderly patients in whom coexisting medical conditions or other factors constitute contraindications to axillary dissection. Simple mastectomy is also indicated for treatment of sarcomas of the breast, because lymphatic spread to axillary nodes is not part of the natural history of this disease (Lind, et al., 2005).

Modified radical mastectomy is performed to treat invasive breast cancer when (a) there are contraindications to breast preservation or (b) the patient or the health care provider prefers mastectomy. Simple mastectomy in conjunction with SLN biopsy is an increasingly common alternative to modified radical mastectomy for patients with clinically negative axillary nodes. If the nodes are positive for tumor on pathological examination, the surgeon may then elect to perform a completion axillary dissection. Postoperative views of two patients who underwent mastectomy are shown in Figure 63-8.

An increasingly popular approach for women requiring mastectomy is skin-sparing mastectomy (SSM) (Hultman & Daiza, 2003). This procedure consists of resection of the nipple-areola complex, any existing biopsy scar, and the breast parenchyma, followed immediately by breast reconstruction. It is somewhat demanding technically in that the effort expended in preserving the skin makes it difficult for the oncologist to ensure removal of as much breast tissue as possible. Because the inframammary fold is preserved and a generous skin envelope remains after SSM, cosmetic results after reconstruction are optimized. SSM is oncologically safe and is not associated with an increased incidence of local recurrence. The recurrences that do occur typically develop below the skin flaps and thus are easily detectable. Deep recurrences beneath the reconstruction are comparatively uncommon. Patients with locally advanced breast cancer are not appropriate candidates for SSM with immediate reconstruction. In general, immediate reconstruction should be reserved for patients at low risk for postoperative adjuvant therapies.

Breast Reconstruction

Advances in reconstructive techniques have made breast reconstruction increasingly popular. Reconstruction may be done either at the time of the mastectomy (immediate reconstruction) or later (delayed reconstruction). It is well recognized that immediate breast reconstruction after mastectomy is safe, does not significantly delay subsequent administration of chemotherapy or radiation therapy, and does not prevent detection of recurrent disease. Either implants or autologous tissue may be used in reconstruction.

The option of breast reconstruction is presented to the mastectomy patient by her breast surgeon during preoperative discussion of mastectomy or in the case of delayed reconstruction, during follow-up after an earlier mastectomy. The patient, the plastic surgeon, and the oncologist or general surgeon will decide among the several reconstruction options available: implants with tissue expansion, the transverse rectus abdominis myocutaneous (TRAM) flap, the latissimus dorsi myocutaneous flap, and various free flaps on the basis of patient preference and lifestyle, the availability of suitable autologous tissue, and the demands imposed by any additional cancer therapies required. Familiarity with the strengths and drawbacks of these reconstruction options facilitates this decision.

Perhaps the simplest method of reconstruction is to place a saline-filled implant beneath the greater pectoral muscle and the anterior serratus muscle to recreate a breast mound as shown in Figure 63-9. Even after SSM, the greater pectoral muscle is usually so tight that unless the patient is small-breasted, expansion of this muscle and the skin is necessary before an implant that matches the opposite breast can be inserted. Serial expansions are performed on an outpatient basis: saline is injected into the expander every 10 to 14 days until an appropriate size has been attained. A second operative procedure is then required to exchange the expander for a permanent implant. A nipple and an areola are constructed at a later date (Lind, et al., 2005).

The major advantage of implant reconstruction is that there is no need to harvest autologous tissue, and the patient is spared the discomfort, scarring, and loss of muscle function that would occur at the donor site. Accordingly, implant reconstructions are commonly performed in patients who require bilateral mastectomies and reconstructions. The initial operating time is significantly shorter for implant reconstruction than for autologous tissue reconstruction, and there is no need for autologous blood donation or transfusion. Hospital stay and recuperation time are also significantly shorter. The main drawbacks are the prolonged time and the multiple office visits required to achieve a symmetrical reconstruction if tissue expansion is required and the necessity of a second surgical procedure to place the permanent implant. In addition, the final cosmetic result often is not as good as what can be achieved with autologous tissue reconstruction, and it may deteriorate over time as a consequence of capsule formation or implant migration (Lind, et al., 2005). The implant-reconstructed breast is significantly firmer than the contralateral breast. The life expectancy of currently available saline implants has not been established, but it may be less than a decade, which means that many patients who have received or are receiving implants may need replacements at some point. Patients who have previously undergone irradiation of the breast or the chest wall may have tissue that cannot be adequately expanded and thus is unsuitable for implant reconstruction.

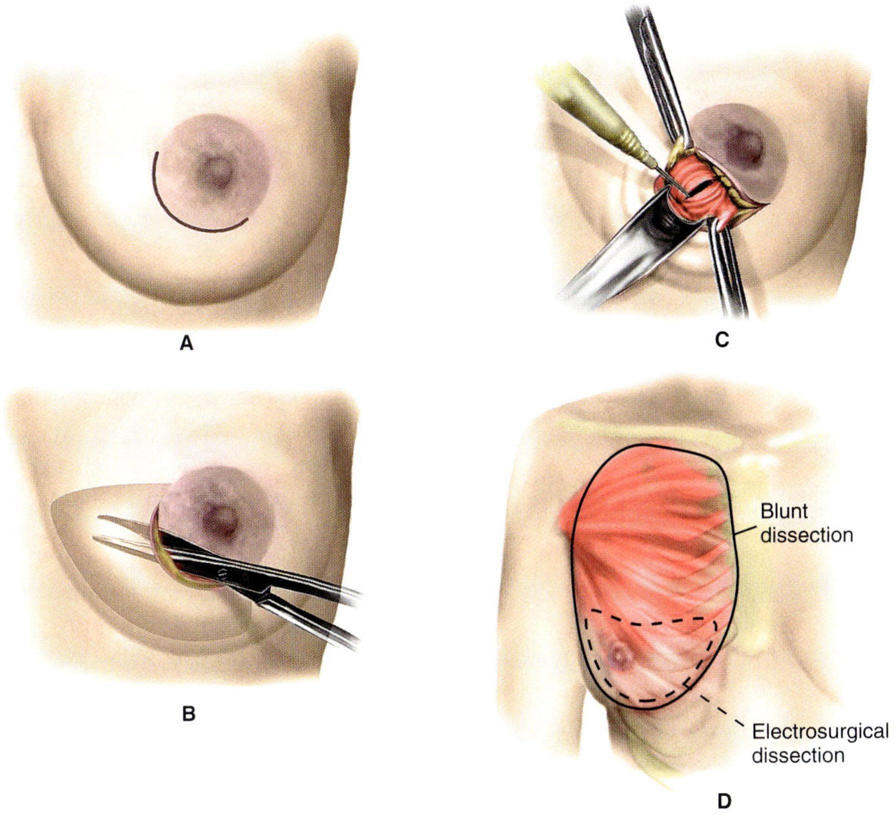

Figure 63-9 Augmentation mammoplasty: A. Areolar incision, B. Creation of pocket, C. Pectoral muscle incision, D. Implant position.

A second approach to reconstruction is to transfer vascularized muscle, skin, and fat from a donor site to the mastectomy defect. The most commonly used myocutaneous flaps are the TRAM flap and the latissimus dorsi flap. Use of the free TRAM flap is advocated by certain centers. Other free-flap options, including the free gluteus flap, are used in special circumstances, such as when other donor sites are unsuitable.

The major advantage of autologous tissue reconstruction is that it generally yields a superior cosmetic result. Often the size and shape of the opposite breast can be matched immediately with no need for subsequent office or operative procedures. The reconstructed breast has a soft texture that is similar to that of the contralateral breast. In addition, the cosmetic result is stable over time. The main drawbacks are the magnitude of the surgical procedure required for the reconstruction (involving both a prolonged operating time and longer inpatient hospitalization); the potential need for autologous blood donation or transfusion; and the pain, scarring, and loss of muscle function that arise at the donor site. Smokers and patients with significant vascular disease may not be ideal candidates for autologous tissue reconstruction. Partial necrosis of the transferred flap may create firm areas, while on rare occasions complete necrosis and consequent loss of the flap can occur (Lind, et al., 2005).

A number of factors are considered in choosing between the TRAM flap and the latissimus dorsi flap. In a TRAM flap reconstruction, the contralateral rectus abdominis is transferred along with overlying skin and fat to create a breast mound. This procedure yields a flatter abdominal contour, but it calls for a long transverse abdominal incision and necessitates repositioning of the umbilicus (Lind, et al., 2005). A major advantage of the TRAM flap is that it can provide enough tissue to match all but the largest contralateral breasts. Some patients, however, such as those who have undergone an abdominal procedure that compromises the TRAM flap's vascular supply, are not ideal candidates for TRAM flap reconstruction. Postoperative discomfort is greater with TRAM flap reconstruction than with other flap reconstructions because of the extent of the abdominal portion of the procedure. In young, healthy, and motivated patients who require bilateral reconstructions it is often possible to perform two TRAM flap procedures in the same operation (Hultman & Daiza, 2003).

In a latissimus dorsi myocutaneous flap reconstruction, the ipsilateral latissimus dorsi is transferred along with overlying skin and fat to create a breast mound. Either a horizontal or a vertical donor site incision may be made on the back. The operative technique for the latissimus dorsi flap reconstruction is complex. Patients who have undergone irradiation of the breast, chest wall, or axilla (including irradiation of the thoracodorsal vessels) may not be eligible for this procedure.

A major advantage of the latissimus dorsi flap is that its donor site is associated with less postoperative discomfort than the abdominal donor site of the TRAM flap. In addition, transfer of the latissimus dorsi results in substantially less functional impairment than transfer of the rectus abdominis. A drawback of the latissimus dorsi flap is that in many women, the latissimus dorsi is not bulky enough to provide symmetry with the contralateral breast. In such cases, an implant must be added to the flap to match the size and shape of the opposite breast, which means that the drawback of the implant's limited life span is added to the drawbacks already associated with autologous tissue reconstruction.

Free flap reconstruction options are utilized primarily when other autologous and implant reconstruction options are not available, do not provide sufficient tissue volume, or have failed. They are more complex procedures, requiring microvascular anastomoses and carrying a higher risk of total flap loss. The two most commonly employed free flap options are the free TRAM flap and the free gluteus flap. TRAM flap reconstruction is shown in Figure 63-10.

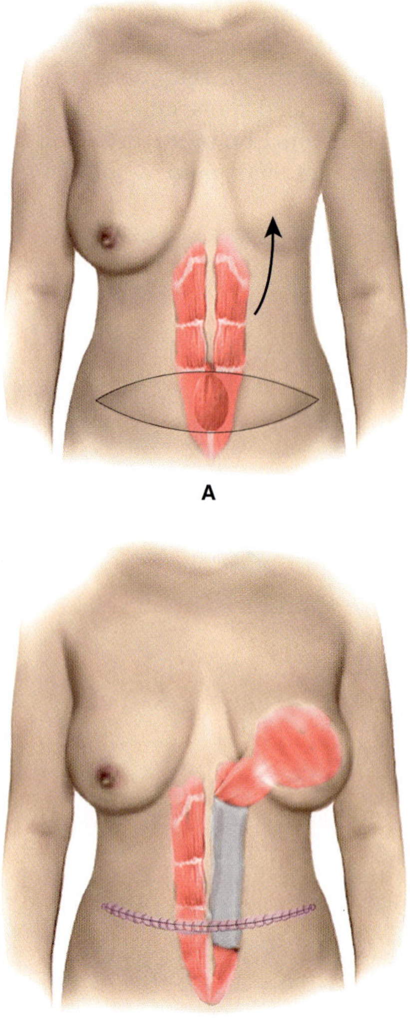

A

B

Figure 63-10 TRAM flap reconstruction: A. Abdominal incision, B. TRAM flap rotated into position.

Donor site morbidity, including postoperative pain, wound healing complications, decreased abdominal muscle strength, and hernia formation, is a prime disadvantage of pedicled or free TRAM flap reconstruction. As a result, muscle-sparing alternatives to autogenous breast reconstruction have been developed, such as the deep inferior epigastric perforator (DIEP) flap (Craigie, Allen, DellaCroce, & Sullivan, 2003). In this approach, free flaps are used that comprise skin and fat alone, without the rectus abdominis. Avoidance of muscle sacrifice in the abdomen ultimately translates into greater patient satisfaction, but careful patient selection is essential to optimize outcomes. The disadvantages of the DIEP flap include the considerable technical expertise and long operating time required, as well as the greater potential for flap loss, because this flap has a more tenuous blood supply than the standard TRAM (Lind, et al., 2005).

Evaluation of Outcomes

Potential patient outcomes for each of the example nursing diagnoses for the patient with breast cancer are:

- Acute pain as related to breast surgery. The patient should verbalize an adequate relief of pain along with the ability to realistically cope with the pain if it is not completely relieved.
- Fear in response to the diagnosis of breast cancer. The patient should manifest positive coping behaviors and verbalize a reduction in the amount of fear of the having this disease.
- Ineffective coping related to anxiety, lower activity level, and the inability to perform normal activities of daily living. The patient identifies own maladaptive coping behaviors, identifies available resources and support systems, describes or initiates alternative coping strategies, and describes positive results from new behaviors.
- Activity intolerance related to fatigue after breast surgery. The patient maintains activity level within capabilities, as evidenced by normal heart rate and blood pressure during activity, as well as absence of shortness of breath, weakness, and fatigue.

KEY CONCEPTS

- The sole physiological function of the breast, or mammary gland, is to secrete milk for nourishment of the infant.
- There are varying ways that the breast tissue develops during pregnancy, lactation, and during menopause.
- Gynecomastia is frequently caused by a shift in the estrogen/androgen ratio because of increased circulating estrogens or to decreased circulating androgens.
- The breast exam involves bilateral inspection and palpation of the breasts, areola, axillary, and supraclavicular areas.
- The majority of breast disorders are benign, but it is imperative that breast disorders are diagnosed accurately and treated early to have the most optimal outcome.
- There are three primary pathological conditions of the nipple: (a) bleeding, (b) discharge, and (c) fissures.
- Fibrocystic breast changes are the most frequently occurring pathological breast problem.
- Mastitis (inflammation or infection) of the breast may be caused from irritation, injury, or infection and most commonly occurs within the first three months after childbirth; however it can occur at any age.
- Mammoplasty is a surgical procedure to increase or decrease the size or shape of the breast and is usually considered an elective procedure.
- Surgical breast reduction is performed to relieve the neck and shoulder pain that can lead to degenerative nerve changes due to overly large breasts.
- Breast cancer is the most common type of cancer in women and is a major public health problem in the United States, with one in eight women expected to be diagnosed sometime during their lifetime.
- In situ breast cancer is confined within the ducts (ductal carcinoma in situ, DCIS) or lobules (lobular carcinoma in situ).
- Cytological (tissue) diagnosis of a palpable breast mass may be obtained by means of FNA biopsy, core needle biopsy, or open incisional or excisional biopsy.

Continued

KEY CONCEPTS—cont'd

- Lumpectomy is a wide local excision or partial mastectomy that involves excision of all cancerous tissue to microscopically clean margins.
- The goal of a mastectomy is to remove all breast tissue, including the nipple and the areola, while leaving well-perfused, viable skin flaps for primary closure or reconstruction.
- Breast reconstruction may be done either at the time of the mastectomy (immediate reconstruction) or later (delayed reconstruction).

REVIEW QUESTIONS

1. The three major hormones that cause the breast tissue to develop, enlarge, and produce milk are:
   1. Estrogen, progesterone, and LDH
   2. Progesterone, FSH, and estrogen
   3. Estrogen, progesterone, and prolactin
   4. LDH, FSH, and MSH

2. Which of the following is true concerning an examination of the breast?
   1. Only examine the patient in the supine position
   2. Variations between breast size is not uncommon, but breasts should be fairly symmetrical.
   3. Dimpling of the nipples on large-breasted women is best detected by having the woman lean backward.
   4. Palpation of the breasts begins with the nipples.

3. Which of the following is true concerning pathological conditions of the nipples?
   1. Bleeding in the discharge generally suggests malignancy.
   2. A variety of medications can cause fluid discharge from the nipples.
   3. Fissures in the nipples are most often caused by puberty.
   4. It is not necessary for health care providers to follow-up on discharge from the nipples.

4. Which of the following is correct regarding changes and disorders of the breast?
   1. Fibrocystic breast changes involve the secretion of a white, milk-like fluid in a nonlactating breast.
   2. Fibroadenomas are benign, fibrous growths of the glandular epithelium in breast tissue.
   3. Intraductal papillomas usually occur in women over the age of 60.
   4. Mastitis occurs in all ages of women, but primarily at puberty in adolescence.

5. Which of the following is true concerning the risk factors for breast cancer?
   1. Other types of cancer history have no correlation with breast cancer.
   2. Environment is not a risk factor for breast cancer.
   3. Ethnicity is a risk factor for breast cancer.
   4. Hormones are not a risk factor for breast cancer.

6. Which of the following is true of a breast biopsy?
   1. A fine needle aspiration biopsy permits the sampling of cells from breast lesions.
   2. FNA biopsy of nonpalpable lesions has the highest level of accuracy for diagnostics.
   3. Open biopsies usually are performed under a general anesthetic.
   4. Stereotactic mammography-guided biopsy is performed only if the lesion is easily visualized.

7. Ms. Jones has a ductoscopy. Which of the following is true of this test?
   1. It involves recovering breast duct epithelial cells for cytological analysis.
   2. It is particularly useful in evaluating patients with nipple discharge.
   3. It is not diagnostic in patients who are in the high-risk category for cancer.
   4. It is predictive of whether or not the patient may not be a good risk for breast augmentation.

8. Which of the following is the least invasive form of surgery?
   1. Modified radical mastectomy
   2. Simple mastectomy
   3. Lumpectomy
   4. Skin-sparing mastectomy

Continued

REVIEW QUESTIONS—cont'd

9. Which of the following is the single most important predictor of outcome for breast cancer patients?
    1. The age of the patient
    2. The presence of nipple discharge at the time of diagnosis
    3. The histological status of the axillary nodes
    4. The presence of mastitis and an infection process upon diagnosis

10. What is the major advantage of implant reconstruction of the breast using a prosthetic saline-filled implant?
    1. It is less expensive.
    2. It does not require harvesting of autologous tissue and a loss of muscle function.
    3. It allows for fewer office visits and additional surgical interventions.
    4. It lasts virtually forever and therefore does not require surgical revision.

REVIEW ACTIVITIES

1. Describe the changes in the breast tissue during the maturational phases of a woman.

2. Teach a patient how to perform a BSE.

3. Evaluate the differences in cultures as related to breast examinations.

4. Describe the history of breast augmentation surgery.

5. Describe one of the common diagnostic methods for determining alterations of the breast.

6. Compare and contrast minimally ablative techniques to breast cancer.

Visit the Contemporary Medical-Surgical Nursing online companion resource at www.delmarhealthcare.com for additional content and study aids. Click on Online Companions then select the Nursing discipline.

CHAPTER 64

Male Reproductive Dysfunction: Nursing Management

Pam Hamre, RN, MS, CNM

CHAPTER TOPICS

- Prostatitis
- Benign Prostatic Hyperplasia
- Prostate Cancer
- Testicular Disorders
- Disorders of the Penis and Urethra

KEY TERMS

Balanitis
Balanoposthitis
Embolization
Epididymitis
Epispadias
Hypospadias
Infertility
Orchitis
Paraphimosis
Phimosis
Posthitis
Priapism
Prostatitis
Spermatocelectomy
Testicular self-examination (TSE)
Urethritis
Urethroplasty
Urethrotomy
Varicocele
Varicocelectomy
Vasectomy

Disorders of the male reproductive system can impact the urinary system, as well as the emotional stability and social lifestyle of the patient and his family across the life span. Regardless of whether such disorders involve minor inconveniences or major lifestyle and self-concept issues, assessing problems of the reproductive system requires gentle and thoughtful therapeutic communication that is open, frank, and educational with close attention to detail. The nurse must constantly be alert to verbal and nonverbal indicators of patients' sensitivity or embarrassment about their genitals, their sexual behaviors, and conditions that could be interpreted as assaults on their masculinity.

PROSTATITIS

Prostatitis is inflammation of the prostate gland. The inflammation is classified as either acute or chronic, by the causative agent (bacterial or nonbacterial), and by whether the patient is aware or unaware of symptoms. If there is an acute infectious process present, the condition is termed acute bacterial prostatitis. If the infection is recurrent, it is termed chronic bacterial prostatitis. In the absence of demonstrable infection, prostatitis is classified as chronic nonbacterial prostatitis or chronic pelvic pain syndrome (CPPS). In the absence of symptoms, prostatitis is classified as asymptomatic inflammatory prostatitis (AIP) (Theodorescu & Krupski, 2005).

Epidemiology

Approximately 50 percent of men experience symptoms of prostatitis at some time in their life, with the highest incidence occurring between ages 35 and 65. However, only about 10 percent of prostatitis is bacterial in origin. When the prostate gland becomes inflamed and enlarges, creating pressure on the bladder, urinary symptoms result.

Etiology

The most common causes for prostatitis are bacteria, mycoplasma, and fungi. In addition, other causes are urethral strictures and prostatic hyperplasia. The most common bacterial cause is *Escherichia coli* and is usually carried from the urethra to the prostate. In cases of bacterial prostatitis, common bowel bacteria (*E. coli, Enterobacter,* or *Enterococcus*) or sexually transmitted organisms (*Chlamydia trachomatis* or *Gonococcus*) invade the prostate by ascending the urethra.

Pathophysiology

Chronic prostatitis can create hard nodules of scarring on the prostate gland, that can be mistaken for prostate cancer on digital rectal examination (DRE) and that can cause chronic pelvic pain. Nonbacterial prostatitis is thought to be either an autoimmune disorder or the result of neurological damage to tissues surrounding the prostate during bacterial prostatitis.

Assessment with Clinical Manifestations

Prostatitis is usually characterized by acute onset of urinary burning, frequency, urgency, and dysuria. Patients with bacterial prostatitis often experience fever and malaise. Pain experienced in the testes, rectum, low back, or perineum may also be present. The assessment for prostatitis includes questions that are shown in the Patient Playbook.

PATIENT PLAYBOOK

Assessment of Prostatitis

The nurse can ask the patient the following questions in assessing for the presence of prostatitis:

- When did the dysuria begin?
- Were there precipitating factors for the urinary frequency and urgency?
- Is urethral discharge present, and if so, what color is it?
- When were malaise and fever noticed?
- What is your sexual history, including episodes of unprotected intercourse or sexual contact with partners with sexually transmitted infections?

Diagnostic Tests

A variety of diagnostic tests can be used to verify prostatitis. Urethral and prostatic secretions may be tested for the presence of white blood cells and cultured for organisms. Diagnosis of bacterial prostatitis is made by culturing spontaneous or expressed urethral discharge, or prostate fluid (Daniels, 2003). Urine can also be cultured to detect which bacteria is the causative organism. Prostate fluid is obtained by collecting a clean, divided specimen. The patient voids about 20 mL, the amount of urine lying in the urethra, and then prostatic massage is performed until the prostate secretions are collected. The patient then voids again to provide a specimen containing a combination of bladder urine and prostate secretions. The presence of cytotoxic T-cells in the expressed prostate fluid may indicate an autoimmune inflammatory response, indicative of nonbacterial prostatitis.

Nursing Diagnoses

Based on the information gathered, examples of nursing diagnoses in the patient with prostatitis may include the following:
- Pain related to prostatic enlargement and inflammation.
- Risk for imbalanced body temperature secondary to acute bacterial prostatitis.
- Risk for infection related to prostatitis.

Planning and Implementation

If the prostatitis is bacterial in nature, elimination of the bacteria causing the infection is the primary goal. The secondary goal is to eliminate the pain and urinary symptoms. Prevention of chronic pain is a third goal. In addition to the primary health care provider and nurse, the team of health care providers may need to include several other professionals. A pharmacist and an infection control provider may help manage the infection. Mental health professionals may be needed to assist the patient to cope with emotional distress. A public health nurse or social worker may need to carry out case finding if the infection was sexually transmitted.

Pharmacology

Medications prescribed for prostatitis are dependent on the cause of the inflammation. In the case of bacterial prostatitis, ciprofloxacin (Cipro) and doxycycline are commonly utilized. A severe infection may require intravenous (IV) antibiotics and hospitalization. Acetaminophen or ibuprofen may be used to control fever and pain. Nonsteroidal anti-inflammatory drugs (NSAIDs) are optimally effective because of their anti-inflammatory properties and thus are more commonly recommended for those patients who can tolerate them (Broyles, Reiss, & Evans, 2007).

Patient and Family Teaching

Teaching focuses on eradication of the infection and helping the patient feel more comfortable. The nurse needs to ensure that the patient understands and accepts the importance of careful adherence to the treatment plan and the importance of completing the antibiotic regimen, because prostatitis is prone to recur. Patients should be given written and verbal information on the cause of their prostatitis. If a sexually transmitted infectious organism is found to be the bacteria involved, state mandates regarding notification of sexual partners must be implemented.

Comfort may be enhanced by sitz baths and avoiding long periods in a sitting position. Foods and beverages that have diuretic action or that increase prostatic secretions, such as alcohol, coffee, tea, chocolate, cola, and spices, should be avoided. The patient also needs to be cautioned to avoid sexual arousal and intercourse while the acute infection persists.

Evaluation of Outcomes

Potential patient outcomes for each of the example nursing diagnoses for the patient with prostatitis are:
- Pain related to prostatic enlargement and inflammation. The patient should verbalize an adequate relief of pain along with the ability to realistically cope with the pain if it is not completely relieved.
- Risk for imbalanced body temperature secondary to acute bacterial prostatitis. The patient maintains body temperature within a normal range.
- Risk for infection related to prostatitis. The patient remains free of infection, as evidenced by normal vital signs and absence of purulent drainage from wounds, incisions, and tubes. Infection is recognized early to allow for prompt treatment.

Respecting Our Differences

Prostate Enlargement and Elderly Males

BPH is obviously common among elderly males. Nurses must make certain that they do not assume that the patient with BPH is accepting his disorder without reservations. The nurse must remember to communicate well with the patient and ask open-ended questions regarding how the patient feels about the new diagnosis. In addition, the nurse must remember that issues of sexuality and incontinence may be of great importance to the patient, even though the patient is elderly.

BENIGN PROSTATIC HYPERPLASIA

Benign prostatic hyperplasia (BPH) is enlargement of the prostate gland because of an overgrowth in the number of cells. The enlargement of the prostate creates pressure on the neck of the bladder, requiring intrabladder pressures to be higher than normal to overcome the prostate pressure so that urine can be released. The increased pressure exerted on the neck of the bladder is responsible for the symptoms of BPH that together are referred to as prostatism: weak and dribbling urine stream, difficulty in starting the stream of urine, nocturia, and voiding small amounts frequently.

Epidemiology

BPH is a common condition affecting middle-aged and elderly men and the greatest risk factor for BPH is age. According to the National Cancer Institute virtually all men over age 50 have some degree of prostatic hyperplasia resulting in enlargement of the prostate gland. In addition, 50 percent of men over age 60 and 90 percent of men over age 70 have symptomatic BPH (National Cancer Institute, 2005d). Family history may also have a contributory effect. Men of southern European descent have the highest risk, while men of Asian and Scandinavian descent have a slightly lower risk. When men do not recognize that prostatic hyperplasia is a normal aging process for which effective treatment is available they may not seek treatment.

Pathophysiology

The prostate gland normally undergoes two periods of active growth. At puberty the prostate doubles in size, and at about age 25 additional growth of the prostate begins to occur. This latter growth is ongoing and over time, develops into BPH. As the cells continue to replicate they crowd against the urethra, causing the urinary stream difficulties. The additional prostatic tissue results in an abnormally high total amount of dihydrotestosterone (DHT), causing the smooth muscle cells of the urethra and prostate tissue to spasm slightly. The spasms further increase the difficulty in voiding.

The hyperplastic prostate cells are not precancerous. Hyperplasia creates an enlargement of the prostate that is soft in consistency in an inward expansion of the transitional portion of the prostate tissue that wraps around the urethra. In contrast, prostate cancer is usually firm and nodular to palpation and is located in the periphery of the prostate gland.

Assessment with Clinical Manifestations

Assessment for BPH involves taking a careful history about urinary function. The ease with which the stream of urine is started, the strength of the stream, the perceived amount of urine eliminated each voiding, along with the patient's sense about whether his bladder is completely emptying and the presence of nocturia or dribbling are important indicators of urethral compression. A DRE is performed to assess the size and consistency of the prostate.

Diagnostic Tests

The primary concern when evaluating BPH is the potential for having a malignancy of the prostate. To assist in differentiating BPH from prostate cancer a prostate specific antigen (PSA) blood test is also obtained to rule out prostate cancer. Rectal ultrasonography of the prostate may be undertaken if prostate cancer is suspected. A postvoiding bladder scan may be done to assess how effectively the bladder is emptying, and a cystoscopy may be performed to assess the degree of urethral compression and bladder wall integrity. Renal function tests, such as creatinine, may be done to ascertain any renal impairment secondary to elevated retrograde pressure.

Nursing Diagnoses

Based on the information gathered, examples of nursing diagnoses in the patient with BPH may include the following:

- Risk for infection from frequent urinary tract infections.
- Impaired urinary elimination related to BPH.
- Risk for disturbed sleep pattern secondary to nocturia.

Planning and Implementation

The goal of treatment for BPH is a reduction in prostate size that improves bladder outflow and decreases urinary system issues. The primary methods of correcting this disorder are surgery and management with medications. In general, the health care provider is also concerned that the condition does not become malignant, and the patient will be evaluated based on preventing cancer from developing.

Surgery

BPH is often treated through surgical removal of the hypertrophied prostate tissue. Transurethral resection of the prostate (TURP) is the most common procedure used. The surgery is usually performed under regional anesthesia and involves laser ablation of prostatic tissue during cystoscopy. Resection of the prostate can also be accomplished using a laser to vaporize or necrotize prostate tissue with less bleeding than occurs with the traditional TURP.

Following the surgery a double lumen indwelling catheter is placed into the urinary bladder. Normal saline is instilled through one lumen of the catheter

Uncovering the Evidence

Quality of Life While Living with Prostate Cancer

Discussion: The aim of the study was to investigate men with prostate cancer and BPH in comparison with men from the general population. In addition, the study investigated the impact of micturition problems on quality of life.

The samples consisted of 155 men with prostate cancer, 131 with BPH, and 129 from the general population. Micturition problems were assessed with four different instruments. Parametric and nonparametric statistics were applied. The findings revealed that the most troublesome urinary problems were leakage, feelings of discomfort, and disrupted urinary function, and frequency. Men with urological diagnosis had more micturition problems, fatigue, and sleeping difficulties than men from the general population, but the cancer diagnosis did not add to the problems. Role and social functioning (prostate cancer), emotional functioning (BPH), and grade of fatigue (general population) showed itself vital for overall quality of life.

Implications for Practice: The results of this study show that assistance in solving issues of micturition problems, fatigue, and sleeping disturbances may contribute to maintenance of role, social, and emotional aspects of life.

Source: Jakobsson, L., Loven, L., Hallberg, I. R. (2004). Micturition problems in relation to quality of life in men with prostate cancer or benign prostatic hyperplasia: Comparison with men from the general population. Cancer Nursing, *27(3), 218–229.*

and flows into the bladder, where it flushes or washes out the blood that oozes from the operative site. The second lumen of the catheter drains the saline, blood, and urine out of the bladder. Immediately postoperatively, the urine is bright red, and the saline must be run in fast enough to prevent clotting of the blood within the bladder that could plug the outflow holes of the catheter. Large 5 liter bags of 0.9% saline are used for this continuous bladder irrigation. The presence of the catheter often creates bladder spasms that are treated with antispasmodic medications.

An alternative to a TURP is transurethral microwave procedure (TUMP). In this hour-long outpatient procedure the enlarged prostatic tissue that impinges into the urethra is heated to 111° F (43.8° C) through a transurethral catheter, while a water cooling system protects the urethra from damage. This microwave therapy does not achieve a cure of the BPH and does not correct incomplete emptying of the bladder. TUMP merely reduces the urinary flow symptoms. A third surgical procedure is the transurethral needle ablation (TUNA). In this procedure low-level radiofrequency energy is emitted through twin needles to burn away the enlarged prostate tissue impinging the urethra. TUNA improves urine flow and relieves urinary symptoms with fewer side effects than TURP.

Pharmacology

Medications can be used instead of surgery in the treatment of mild to moderate BPH. Commonly used medications include nonselective alpha blockers, such as terazosin (Hytrin), alfuzosin (Uroxatral), and doxazosin (Cardura). These medications do not decrease the size of the hypertrophic cells but instead create smooth muscle relaxation of the bladder neck and prostate (Broyles, et al., 2007). Such muscle relaxation leads to an almost immediate improvement in urinary flow. The nonselective alpha blockers can cause orthostatic hypotension. Tamsulosin (Flomax) is a highly selective alpha blocker that maximizes urinary flow with fewer side effects. Finasteride is an antiandrogen agent that prevents conversion of testosterone to DHT helping to shrink the hyperplastic cells. However, finasteride may cause erectile dysfunction and gynecomastia (breast enlargement).

Alternative Therapy

The herb saw palmetto (*Serenoa repens*) has been shown to improve urinary tract symptoms. Saw palmetto has fewer side effects (e.g., orthostatic hypotension, and erectile dysfunction) than the traditional medications. In addition, using the herbal therapy is much less expensive and may have reliable results.

Patient and Family Teaching

Patient teaching for BPH initially focuses on conservative measures to control the primary symptoms associated with impaired urinary flow. Establishment of a consistent medication routine, avoidance of large quantities of late evening fluid intake, and emptying the bladder immediately before going to bed can help to control nocturia that interrupts restful sleep. In social situations, emptying the bladder regularly can help avoid sudden onset of urgency. If surgery becomes the treatment plan, teaching the patient and family what will happen on the day of surgery, how he will feel postoperatively, what treatments will be used postoperatively, and how long he can expect to be hospitalized become paramount.

> **Red Flag**
>
> **Urine Evaluation**
>
> It is especially important to alert the patient and family that the urine will normally appear bloody for several hours postoperatively. The patient and family should be taught to assess for clinical manifestations of low blood volume (e.g., fatigue, skin pallor, or tachycardia), in which case the health care provider should be notified.

Evaluation of Outcomes

Potential patient outcomes for each of the example nursing diagnoses for the patient with BPH are:

- Risk for infection from frequent urinary tract infections. The patient remains free of infection, as evidenced by normal vital signs and absence of purulent drainage from wounds, incisions, and tubes. Infection is recognized early to allow for prompt treatment.

- Impaired urinary elimination related to BPH. The patient is continent of urine or verbalizes satisfactory management.
- Risk for disturbed sleep pattern secondary to nocturia. The patient is able to sleep without wakefulness and awakens rested in the morning.

PROSTATE CANCER

Prostate cancer is a condition in which the cells of the prostate gland become abnormal in their morphology. Prostate cancer is the second most commonly diagnosed cancer in men. Only skin cancer is more common. About 70 percent of men diagnosed with this disease are over the age of 65. It has been estimated that 80 percent of the men over age 80 have prostate cancer. A total of 232,090 new cases of prostate cancer and 30,350 deaths from the disease occurred in 2005 (National Cancer Institute, 2005d).

Epidemiology

African American men die from prostate cancer twice as often as Caucasian men. Asian (American) men generally have low rates of prostate cancer. Men of northern European descent have the highest incidence of this disease. There is a 2 to 11 percent increase in risk of developing the disease if a first-degree relative has also had it. However, this risk factor only accounts for 5 to 10 percent of prostate cancer cases. As for other correlates for causation of cancer itself, refer to chapter 15.

Pathophysiology

As in most cancers, prostate cancer develops when the rate of cell division is greater than the rate of cell death. Prostate cancer begins most commonly in the outer portion of the prostate gland. It is accepted that most prostatic cancers are preceded by the development of prostatic intraepithelial neoplasia, characterized by rapid proliferation of both glandular and ductal tissues. These epithelial abnormalities are thought to progress in terms of degree of abnormality and tissues involved until cellular changes are extensive and widespread. Most of the prostate cancer cases are multifocal with multiple areas of simultaneous cancer development. Therefore multiple biopsies (6 to 12) are required for optimal diagnostic detection. Bone is the most common site of metastases (The Prostate Cancer Foundation, 2004).

Assessment with Clinical Manifestations

Incontinence is a common first symptom in men, but it is not unusual for younger men to experience no symptoms. Men over the age of 50 are recommended to have an annual screening digital rectal examination (DRE) (Figure 64-1). Prostate cancer is suspected when the DRE reveals an enlarged, nodular, and hard prostate gland.

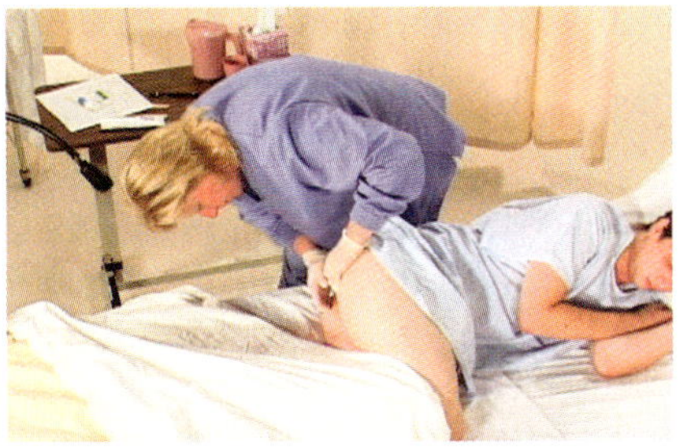

Figure 64-1 Nurse performing a DRE.

Another screening tool used for men over age 50 is the serum PSA. The normal PSA level gradually increases with age so the level at which the PSA is considered abnormal is dependent on the patient's age (Table 64-1).

It must be remembered that conditions, such as BPH, and even recent sexual activity will cause an elevated PSA. Most health care provider will progress to biopsy when the PSA is greater than 4.0 (Dreicer, 2004).

Diagnostic Tests

Transrectal ultrasonography is useful for differentiating between BPH and prostate cancer. A definitive diagnosis is accomplished through biopsy, which is usually a needle biopsy of multiple sites obtained transrectally under ultrasound guidance. Based on the analysis of the biopsy results, the

TABLE 64-1 PSA Levels

Normal PSA Levels Across Age Ranges

Age younger than 40	40–50	51–60	61–70	Older than 70
Less than 2 ng/mL	Less than 2.5 ng/mL	Less than 3.5 ng/mL	Less than 4.5 ng/mL	Less than 6.5 ng/mL

Elevated PSA Levels

0.25 ng/mL	2.6–10 ng/mL	10.1–19.9 ng/mL	More than 20 ng/mL
Low	Mildly elevated	Moderately elevated	Significantly elevated

Adapted from Daniels, R. (2003). Delmar's manual of laboratory and diagnostic tests. *New York: Thomson Delmar Learning; Dreicer, R. (2005).* Prostate cancer. *Retrieved July 19, 2006, from http://www.clevelandclinicmeded.com.*

TABLE 64-2 Gleason Grading System

GLEASON GRADE	1	2	3	4	5
Prostate tissue	Closely packed, well-defined glands	Less uniformly shaped glands	Irregular glands of varying shape	Mass of fused glands	Few if any glands, little difference

Adapted from National Cancer Institute. (2004d). National Cancer Institute cancer facts radiation therapy for cancer: Questions and answers. *Retrieved June 16, 2006, from http://cis.nci.nih.gov.*

TABLE 64-3 Cancer Staging System

STAGE A OR T1	STAGE B OR T2	STAGE C OR T3	STAGE D OR T4
Not palpable during DRE, confined to prostate	Palpable during DRE, confined to prostate	Palpable, spread beyond prostate but not to other organs	Palpable, spread to organs and often distant sites such as bones or lymph nodes

Adapted from American Joint Committee on Cancer. (2002). Staging systems. *Retrieved June 16, 2005, from http://training.seer.cancer.gov.*

cancer is then graded and staged. Grading refers to the aggressiveness of the cancer, while staging refers to the localization or spread of the disease. The Gleason Grading System is a commonly used scale for grading prostate cancer (Table 64-2).

At least two separate biopsy specimens are graded based on their differentiation from normal prostate cells. The scores of the two specimens are then added to obtain a score of 2 to 10. A tumor score less then 4 is considered a low-grade cancer that is well differentiated. A score of 5 to 7 is considered an intermediate-grade cancer with moderate differentiation. A score of 8 or greater indicates a high-grade cancer with poor differentiation that tends to be growing rapidly (Theodorescu & Krupski, 2005).

Staging of prostate cancer designates how far beyond the prostate the cancer has spread (Table 64-3). The stage of a cancer often dictates what type of treatment is recommended. Staging is usually reported with either an A to D system or a numeric system. Ultimately, the size of the tumor, how rapidly it is growing, the age of the patient, and the treatment combine to determine life expectancy.

Nursing Diagnoses

Based on the information gathered, examples of nursing diagnoses in the patient with cancer of the prostate may include the following:

- Risk for impaired urinary elimination.
- Fear secondary to the diagnosis of cancer.
- Deficient knowledge related to self-care and risk prevention.

Planning and Implementation

The management strategies for cancer of the prostate are varied with the staging of the cancer and its virility. Treatment options for prostate cancer usually take an interdisciplinary approach and are based on the grade and stage of the disease, as well as the age of the patient. The typical therapies are surgery, medications, and radiation. In general, surgery has good success with treating prostate cancer when surgery is indicated. And, often the growth of the cancer of the prostate is slow enough, that when the cancer is less advanced, and diagnosed early, the patient has a good survival rate with treatment. The primary goal in the treatment of prostate cancer is to prevent the spread of the disease. Nursing care must also focus on assisting the patient to manage the physical and emotional implications of incontinence and impotence.

Radiation Therapy

Radiation therapy is commonly used to treat prostate cancer. Traditional external beam radiation is used, as is intensity modulated radiation therapy (IMRT). IMRT applies computer technology to plan and administer three-dimensional radiation treatment that is both powerful and more specific to the tumor tissue, sparing surrounding tissue. Brachytherapy is the implantation of radioactive seeds directly into the tumor. Brachytherapy is indicated when the tumor is confined to the prostate. About 25 percent of patients experience impotence following definitive radiation therapy (National Cancer Institute, 2005d).

Surgery

The standard surgical procedure for treating early stage, potentially curable prostate cancer in a patient with greater than 10 years' life expectancy is the radical prostatectomy. In this procedure the entire prostate gland and seminal vesicles are removed along with several lymph nodes. Radical prostatectomy can be done via a transabdominal, laparoscopic, transperitoneal or extraperitoneal route (Figure 64-2). Postoperative urinary incontinence occurs in 5 to 10 percent of patients, and sexual impotence can be anticipated because of the risk for nerve damage during manipulation of tissues while accessing the posterior prostate. Currently, there is a newer form of robotic surgery for a prostatectomy. This method is more expensive and has qualifying criteria for those that could have this form of surgery. The robotic method has fewer postoperative complications, and the patient returns to normal activities of daily living more quickly than the suprapubic or other surgical approaches.

Pharmacology

In cases of metastatic or recurrent prostate cancer, androgen deprivation therapy through the use of orchiectomy or medications that suppress the release of luteinizing hormone, such as leuprolide, goserelin, and triptorelin, is sought to decrease or eliminate the availability of testosterone. Approximately 90 percent of cases are tumors dependent on testosterone. Chemotherapy, most often with taxane-based medications, is also commonly used in treating prostate cancer. For general information on chemotherapy, refer to chapter 15.

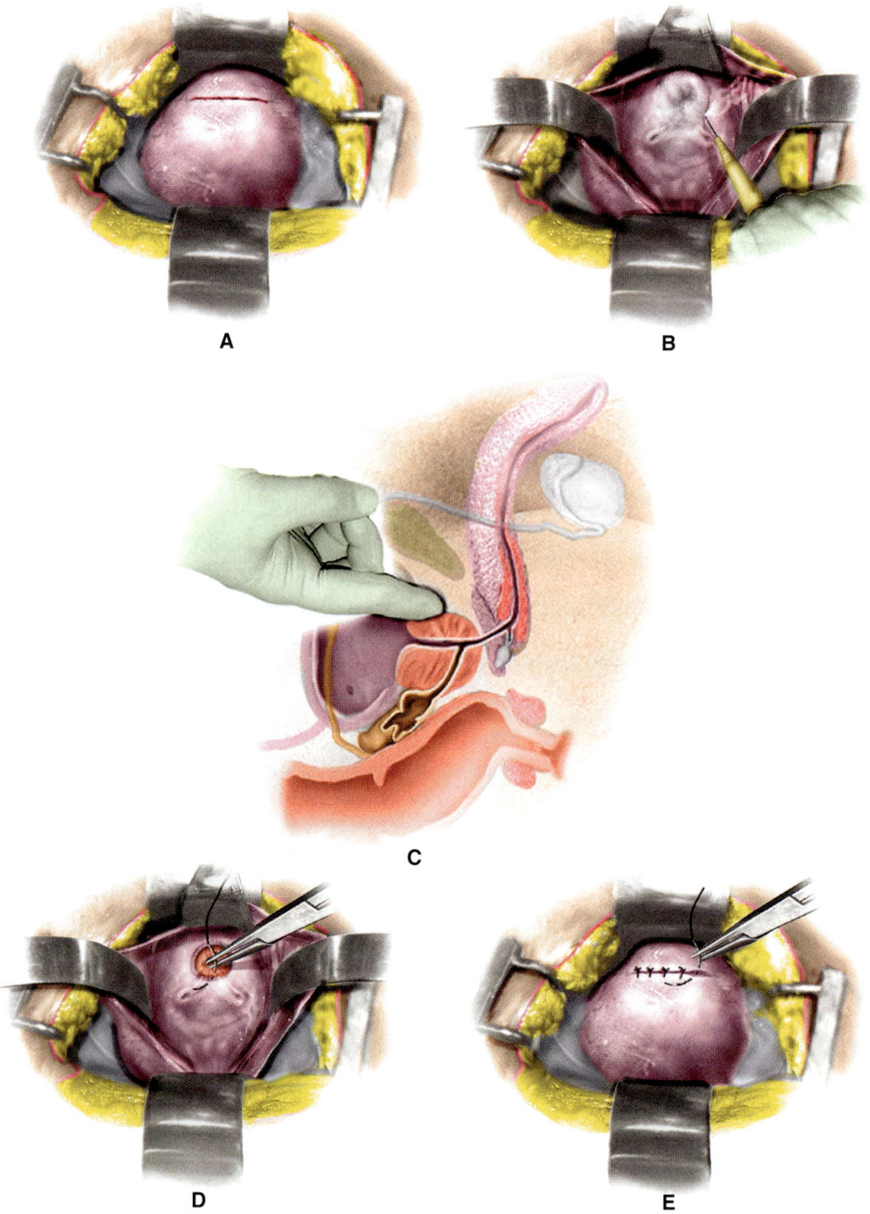

Figure 64-2 Suprapubic prostatectomy: A. Bladder exposed through low transverse incision, B. Bladder entered, C. Blunt dissection of prostate, D. Prostate fossa sutured to bladder mucosa.

Alternative Therapy

Alternative therapy for treatment of prostate cancer includes the herb saw palmetto and oral ingestion of shark or bovine cartilage. The use of these substances results in a decrease in the size of the prostate. Human studies using cartilage administration trials reveal improved outcomes with use of cartilage, but none of the studies was done exclusively on patients with prostate cancer. The study can be reviewed at http://www.cancer.gov.

Patient and Family Teaching

As with any patient with a diagnosis of malignancy teaching must be sensitive, as well as thorough and accurate. Information may need to be provided repeatedly over several sessions when the patient's (or family's) anxiety, fear, and pain are barriers to his being able to focus on the teaching. Facilitating open discussion about an uncertain future, as well as about the important private functions and behaviors associated with urination and sexuality can be challenging. The nurse may need to open such discussions by suggesting some ways the patient must be feeling or some issues that must be concerning to the patient (Mayo Clinic, 2003). Pain management, fluid intake, nourishment, catheter care, perineal muscle exercises to help manage incontinence, wound care, symptoms to report to the health care provider (e.g., infection, bleeding, urinary bladder pain, or leg pain), recommended activity level, fatigue management, and feelings of hopelessness or embarrassment could all be fertile areas for teaching both the patient and those who support him.

Evaluation of Outcomes

Potential patient outcomes for each of the example nursing diagnoses for the patient with cancer of the prostate are:

- Risk for impaired urinary elimination. The patient is continent of urine or verbalizes satisfactory management.
- Fear and anxiety secondary to the diagnosis of cancer. The patient should be able to recognize the signs of anxiety, demonstrate positive coping mechanisms, and describe a reduction in the level of anxiety experienced.
- Deficient knowledge related to self care and risk prevention. The patient should demonstrate motivation to learn, identify perceived learning needs, and verbalize an understanding of desired content.

TESTICULAR CANCER

Cancer of the testes is the most common form of cancer in men ages 15 to 35. It is estimated that 8,010 new cases will be diagnosed in the United States in 2005, resulting in 390 deaths (National Cancer Institute, 2005d). Rates of testicular cancer have more than doubled in the past 40 years, but mortality rates have decreased 60 percent. Testicular cancer is highly treatable and usually a form of curable cancer.

Epidemiology

Scandinavian and Swiss men have the highest incidence, while African and Asian men have the lowest; the United States is in the midrange. Men with untreated congenital cryptorchidism (undescended testis) have a 10 to 40 times increased risk of testicular cancer. Males who have an XXY genotype also have an increased risk of developing testicular cancer and men who were exposed to diethylstilbestrol (DES) in utero may also face a higher risk. At the time of diagnosis, 60 percent of testicular cancers are localized, 24 percent regionalized, and 14 percent have spread to lymph nodes or other organs.

Pathophysiology

The two types of testicular cancer are germinal and nongerminal. Germinal tumors grow from the germinal cells of the testes and may be seminomas or nonseminomas. Seminomas are the most common, are susceptible to treatment by radiation, and have upward of a 90 percent treatment success rate, because they tend to remain localized. The nonseminomas are also referred to as germ cell tumors, are cancers of remaining embryonic tissue, and include choriocarcinoma, yolk sac carcinoma, and teratoma. These are rapid-growing tumors. Nongerminal tumors originate in epithelium. Approximately 95 percent of testicular cancers are germinal and of those, approximately 40 percent are seminomas.

Assessment with Clinical Manifestations

The most common presentation is an otherwise healthy male with a painless lump in the testicle. Testicular self-examination (TSE) is one of the best methods of detecting testicular cancer in its beginning stages (reviewed more specifically later in this section). The appropriate diagnosis and treatment can be delayed if the practitioner merely suspects testicular trauma and prescribes watchful waiting to allow a suspected trauma to resolve spontaneously.

Diagnostic Tests

Painless enlargement of a testis is generally diagnostic of testicular cancer. Transillumination of the scrotum can detect thickened areas or lumps that are potential areas of cancer. However, this is a nonspecific approach and generally regarded as a screening tool. Scrotal ultrasonography more definitively evaluates testicular lumps. An initial needle biopsy of the lump is usually undertaken, although some surgeons will proceed directly to lumpectomy in young patients with negative computerized tomography (CT) scans. The CT scan is performed to detect metastases to other organs, especially to the pelvis and lungs (Daniels, 2003). Lymphangiography can identify lymph node involvement.

Nonseminoma tumors produce alpha fetoprotein (AFP), beta human chorionic gonadotropin (hCG), and lactate dehydrogenase (LDH.) Immunocytochemical analyses are used to identify the malignant cells that produce them. These serum markers are measured at the time of diagnosis and after treatment; if the levels rise after treatment, cancer remains or has recurred and additional treatment is required. Staging of the cancer is based on a variety of factors, including location and spread of the primary tumor, involvement in regional lymph nodes, presence or absence of distant metastases, and the levels of serum tumor markers.

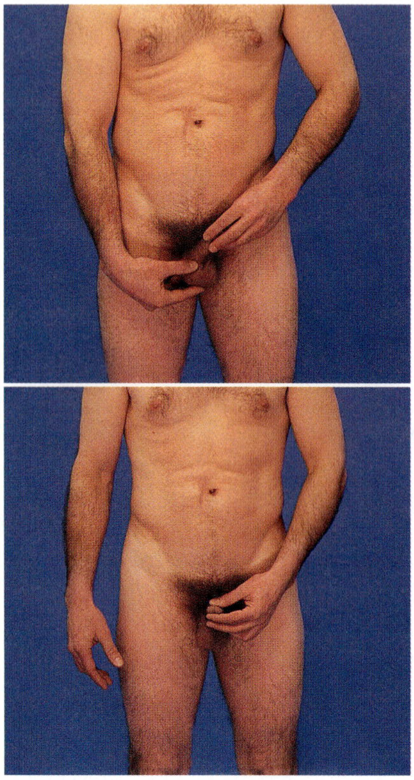

Figure 64-3 Performing a TSE.

Nursing Diagnoses

Based on the information gathered, examples of nursing diagnoses in the patient with testicular cancer may include the following:

- Fear in response to the diagnosis of testicular cancer.
- Ineffective coping related to anxiety, lower activity level, and the inability to perform normal activities of daily living.
- Disturbed body image related to testicular cancer.

Planning and Implementation

The first nursing goal related to testicular cancer is early detection, which is best accomplished through regular **testicular self-examination (TSE)** (a method of a male assessing their testicles for any changes as a preventive measure against testicular cancer) (Estes, 2006). This technique should be taught to young men, and should be performed on a monthly basis (Figure 64-3). The goal of medical treatment is to eradicate the existing disease and prevent metastases. It is important to note that testicular cancer with multiple metastases is still curable. The well publicized case of bicyclist Lance Armstrong illustrates the value of early management.

Most commonly treatment involves surgery, either lumpectomy or orchiectomy (surgical removal of at least the affected testicle) (Figure 64-4). Nonseminoma tumors are more difficult to stage via CT scanning, and surgical lymph node dissection is frequently required. Patients who have been treated for cancer in one testicle have a 2 to 5 percent rate of recurrent disease in the remaining testicle within 25 years of treatment (National Cancer Institute, 2005d). External beam radiation is also commonly utilized, especially for less invasive cases. Chemotherapy is utilized prior to surgery in patients with symptomatic metastases and after surgery in many cases. All treatment options will at least temporarily decrease sperm production, which may lead to subfertility or infertility after treatment. Prior to the onset of treatment many men will choose to donate and store sperm in a commercial sperm banking facility for use when fertility is desired.

Pharmacology

Testicular cancers are quite successfully treated with chemotherapy. Cisplatin (Platinol) is the most successful chemotherapeutic agent for testicular cancer (National Cancer Institute, 2005d). Bleomycin (Blenoxane) vinblastine (Velban), and ifosfamide (Ifex) are other chemotherapy medications that usually achieve remission. Combined chemotherapy, radiation therapy, and surgery are notable for success even after metastasis is evident.

Patient and Family Teaching

In addition to teaching the patient and family about the positive prognosis for eradication of testicular cancer, the nurse needs to teach them about comfort measures. After the surgical intervention, ice and a scrotal support may help relieve discomfort during recovery.

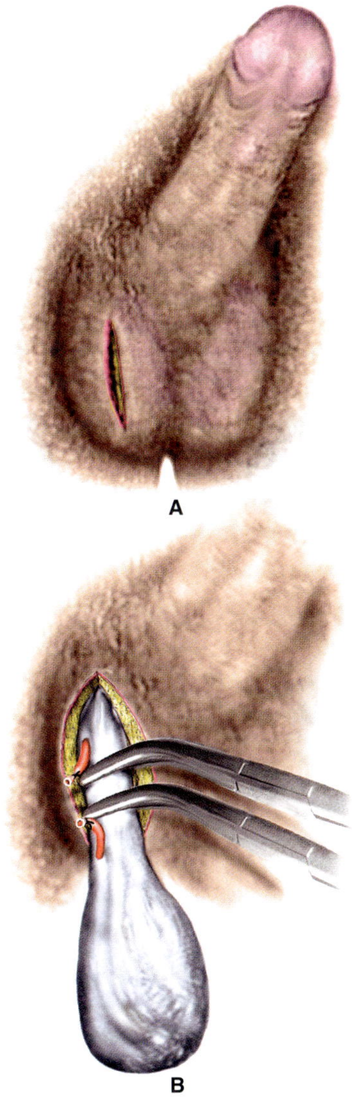

Figure 64-4 Simple orchiectomy: A. Scrotal incision, B. Removal of testicle.

Evaluation of Outcomes

Potential patient outcomes for each of the example nursing diagnoses for the patient with testicular cancer are:

- Fear in response to the diagnosis of testicular cancer. The patient should manifest positive coping behaviors and verbalize a reduction in the amount of fear of the having this disease.
- Ineffective coping related to anxiety, lower activity level and the inability to perform normal activities of daily living. The patient identifies own maladaptive coping behaviors, available resources and support systems, describes or initiates alternative coping strategies, and describes positive results from new behaviors.
- Disturbed body image related to testicular cancer. The patient demonstrates enhanced body image and self-esteem as evidenced by ability to look at, touch, talk about, and care for actual or perceived altered body part or function.

TESTICULAR TORSION

Testicular torsion is a condition where the testis twists on the spermatic cord within the scrotum, creating venous, lymphatic, and arterial obstruction leading to occlusion with resultant hypoxia of the testicle. The development of testicular torsion may be related to sexual activity or exercise but can also occur during sleep. Testicular torsion is a urological emergency. Incidence in the United States is approximately 1 in 4,000, with the left testicle more commonly involved.

Epidemiology

Testicular torsion occurs most commonly in adolescents and almost always prior to the age of 30. Patients describe a rapid onset of acute pain with scrotal edema developing rapidly after the onset of pain.

Pathophysiology

Testicular torsion is more common in men who have bell clapper deformity, a condition where the tunica vaginalis does not anchor normally to the posterior scrotum. This deformity, which occurs in approximately 12 percent of males, allows the testicle to swing like a bell clapper inside the scrotum. The freedom of movement can lead to torsion. Most torsions occur inward toward the midline of the body.

Assessment with Clinical Manifestations

The primary symptomatology with testicular torsion is the acute pain experienced in the testicular region. The nurse must assess the patient for his subjective response to the pain and have the patient verbalize the level of their pain on the 1 to 10 pain scale (see chapter 16). In addition, the nurse can assess for other clinical manifestations of pain (e.g., hypertension, facial grimacing, or diaphoresis). And, the nurse can assess the patient for their restriction of movement and whether their activities of daily living are affected by the testicular torsion.

Diagnostic Tests

Men with testicular torsion present with an exquisitely tender and enlarged testicle. The affected testicle is usually in a horizontal position and often is higher in the scrotum than the nonaffected testicle. Urinalysis is performed to rule out urinary tract involvement. C-reactive protein levels may be elevated as a result of the inflammatory response to hypoxia. The diagnosis is largely clinical, based on the symptoms. Although diagnostic imaging studies can be performed to assess testicular blood flow, many believe ordering such examinations delays treatment and subsequently decreases the possibility for testicular salvage.

Nursing Diagnoses

Based on the information gathered, examples of nursing diagnoses in the patient with testicular torsion may include the following:

- Acute pain related to testicular torsion.
- Impaired physical mobility secondary to pain.
- Potential for disturbed body image related to orchiectomy secondary to testicular torsion.

Planning and Implementation

The goal of testicular torsion treatment is to untwist the spermatic cord and thus reestablish normal blood flow to the testicle quickly so that the testicle can be salvaged. In the emergency department, the testicle may be manually untwisted to promote blood flow to the testicle; two or three twists may be required to replace the testicle to anatomic position. This procedure is successful in 30 to 70 percent of cases. Orchiopexy is a surgical procedure where the testicle is untwisted on the spermatic cord, and the testicle is then sutured to the scrotum on two sides to prevent recurrence. If surgical treatment occurs within 6 hours of the onset of pain, the testicle is salvaged at least 80 percent of the time; if treatment is delayed 12 hours or more, the hypoxia of the testicle progresses to necrosis and thus the testicle must be removed. Analgesics are the medications used to treat the pain of testicular torsion and to treat postoperative pain. No medications will cure the torsion. Patient teaching is focused on providing comfort. Application of ice and use of a scrotal support can be recommended.

Evaluation of Outcomes

Potential patient outcomes for each of the example nursing diagnoses for the patient with testicular torsion are:

- Acute pain related to testicular torsion. The patient should verbalize an adequate relief of pain along with the ability to realistically cope with the pain if it is not completely relieved.

- Impaired physical mobility secondary to pain. The patient should perform physical activity independently or with assistive devices as needed. In addition, the patient should be free of complications of immobility, as evidenced by intact skin, absence of thrombophlebitis, and normal bowel patterns.
- Potential for disturbed body image related to orchiectomy secondary to testicular torsion. The patient demonstrates enhanced body image and self-esteem as evidenced by ability to look at, touch, talk about, and care for actual or perceived altered body part or function.

ORCHITIS

Orchitis is acute inflammation of the testes, usually as a result of infection and most commonly during concurrent **epididymitis,** infection of the epididymis. Orchitis can be caused by viral, spirochetal, parasitic, or bacterial infections. In the United States, orchitis is most often a result of having contracted a sexually transmitted infection, such as chlamydia (responsible for about 30 percent of orchitis cases) or gonorrhea. Mumps is the most common viral cause of orchitis, with the orchitis occurring four to seven days after the onset of mumps in about 30 percent of males who experience puberty and then contract mumps. Mumps is particularly devastating to men because approximately 30 percent of men who suffer orchitis will develop testicular atrophy and subsequent sterility (Gilbert, 2004). Orchitis can also develop secondary to urinary tract instrumentation, such as an indwelling urinary catheter or cystoscopy.

Pathophysiology

Infection of the genitourinary tract can progress to infection of the testis. The infection causes inflammation, which in turn creates edema. The causative organism in men under age 35 is most often gonorrhea or chlamydia. In men over age 35 and in sexually active gay men the causative organism is more likely to be gram-negative bacteria (Mycyk & Moyer, 2004).

Assessment with Clinical Manifestations

Symptoms of orchitis include fever with painful erythema and edema of the groin, testicles, and scrotum. Pain is often exacerbated by movement or straining for a bowel movement. Dysuria, urethral discharge, and blood in the semen may also be present. Although dysuria can be severe with chlamydia or gonorrhea, there usually is no mechanical blockage of the bladder from orchitis, thus urinary retention is rarely a problem (American Urologic Association, 2004).

Diagnostic Tests

There are several diagnostic tests used to confirm orchitis. There is not a single laboratory study or test that is positive for orchitis. Rather, a compilation of the following tests confirms the presence of orchitis. A complete blood count (CBC) is performed to assess for an elevated white count indicative of infection. When a bacterial cause is suspected, urine and urethral discharge cultures are done to identify the bacteria. Doppler ultrasonography is used to verify increased blood flow to the testis, a sign of inflammation, and rule out testicular torsion.

Nursing Diagnoses

Based on the information gathered, examples of nursing diagnoses in the patient with orchitis may include the following:

- Pain secondary to orchitis.
- Risk for imbalanced body temperature secondary to orchitis.

Planning and Implementation

The goal of management for orchitis is first to identify the organism involved and then treat the underlying cause of the infection. The secondary goal is alleviation of symptoms. While awaiting the lab results to verify the organism involved, broad-spectrum antibiotics may be initiated based on the suspected causative organism as determined from the patient's history. Viral causes have no direct treatment. Common antibiotics for treatment of chlamydia are oral doxycycline or azithromycin (Zithromax). Common antibiotics for gonorrhea treatment include intramuscular (IM) ceftriaxone (Rocephin) or oral (PO) ciprofloxacin (Cipro) or ofloxacin (Floxin). Trimethoprim (Bactrim DS) and sulfamethoxazole (Septra DS) are commonly used for urinary tract infections (Broyles, et al., 2007). NSAIDs may be used to decrease inflammation and pain. Patient teaching is directed toward rapid and effective relief of the symptoms. Bed rest is advised and elevation of the scrotum may decrease pain. Cold packs applied to the area may also decrease pain.

Evaluation of Outcomes

Potential patient outcomes for each of the example nursing diagnoses for the patient with orchitis are:

- Pain secondary to orchitis. The patient should verbalize an adequate relief of pain along with the ability to realistically cope with the pain if it is not completely relieved.
- Risk for imbalanced body temperature secondary to orchitis. The patient maintains body temperature within a normal range.

EPIDIDYMITIS

Epididymitis is inflammation of the epididymis and vas deferens. Inflammation of the epididymis and vas deferens usually develops secondary to bacterial infection in the urinary tract or prostatitis, most commonly chlamydia or gonorrhea. Rarely, noninfectious chemical epididymitis can occur from backflow of urine into the vas deferens during heavy lifting or straining. The epididymis is located like a hood on the top of the testis, extending down the posteriolateral side to the juncture of the vas deferens. That location causes epididymitis to present much like orchitis.

Most cases occur in adults and can be either unilateral or bilateral, but most cases are unilateral. Acute epididymitis presents with a rapid onset of severe symptoms. Chronic epididymitis tends to have a longer, more gradual onset and may never be completely eradicated. As in orchitis, inflammation creates fever along with pain and edema in the scrotum and groin. Chronic epididymitis usually presents only with pain in the scrotum; edema is not usually present (American Urologic Association, 2004).

As in orchitis, bacteria from sexually transmitted infections or urinary tract infections ascend into the epididymis and into the vas deferens. Because of their proximal location, infections of the epididymis and testis often occur simultaneously. For that reason the assessment, diagnostic tests, nursing diagnoses, planning and implementation, and patient and family teaching for epididymitis are identical to those for orchitis (see preceding section).

HYDROCELE, HEMATOCELE, AND SPERMATOCELE

Hydrocele is a fluid-filled sac located along the spermatic cord and within the scrotum. It is a fairly common finding in newborns. This condition may accompany an inguinal hernia, develop from an adjacent infection, or develop secondary to a systemic infection, such as mumps. Trauma to the scrotum may cause hydrocele, especially in older men. Hematocele is similar to hydrocele, but is a blood-filled sac. Spermatocele is a cyst-like structure within the scrotum that contains fluid and dead sperm cells.

Pathophysiology

During fetal development the testes form in the low abdomen and descend along the inguinal canals. If a canal fails to close properly, peritoneal fluid can flow into the scrotum, creating a hydrocele. If hydrocele occurs later in life, the cause is thought to be either overproduction of fluid associated with inflammation, or from reabsorption problems because of lymphatic or venous obstruction (Gilbert, 2003). Hematocele usually results from direct scrotal trauma and is painful. The etiology of spermatocele development is unknown. It has been hypothesized that the condition develops as a result of epididymal duct obstruction that results in a bulging cyst of fluid and sperm.

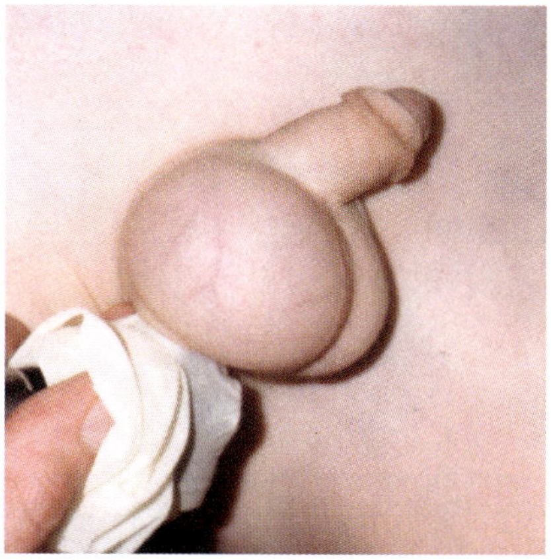

Figure 64-5 Transillumination of a hydrocele.

Assessment with Clinical Manifestations

Hydrocele, hematocele, and spermatocele all present with painless swelling or bulging in the scrotum. Hydroceles transilluminate clearly (Figure 64-5), whereas an inguinal hernia, hematocele, and spermatocele do not. The condition is usually unilateral, and the affected side feels much like a water-filled balloon to palpation. If a large amount of fluid is present, the testis can be difficult to palpate. Spermatocele often palpates as a discrete firm mass in the scrotum, located at the epididymis.

Diagnostic Tests

Scrotal ultrasonography accurately detects these conditions and is used to differentiate among the three conditions. A history of scrotal trauma, systemic illness, or orchitis and epididymitis can help identify the underlying etiology.

Nursing Diagnoses

Based on the information gathered, examples of nursing diagnoses in the patient with any of these cysts may include the following:

- Risk for pain secondary to treatment of hydrocele or hematocele.
- Risk for body image disturbance related to diagnosis.

Planning and Implementation

Most often no treatment is undertaken for these cysts. In the newborn most cases of hydrocele resolve spontaneously within a few months after birth. When treatment is undertaken, it is usually surgery with the goal is to improve comfort or to promote spermatogenesis.

Surgery

In older men, if a hydrocele or hematocele becomes uncomfortably large or disrupts blood flow, surgical repair may be undertaken. Spermatocele may also become significantly uncomfortable and require treatment. Surgical correction may be undertaken if infertility is associated with the spermatocele. Surgical removal of the spermatocele **(spermatocelectomy)** is performed under local anesthesia.

Sclerotherapy is an alternative to surgical treatment. Sclerotherapy is done by inserting a large-bore needle into the spermatocele, aspirating the contents thoroughly, and then injecting a substance that causes inflammation. The inflammatory response causes scarring of the spermatocele to prevent reformation. Approximately 32 percent of patients undergoing sclerotherapy for treatment of spermatocele require a second treatment for complete resolution of the condition (Alsakafi & Kuznetsov, 2004). Analgesics are usually the medications used to manage any of these conditions.

Evaluation of Outcomes

Potential patient outcomes for each of the example nursing diagnoses for the patient with any of these cysts are:

- Risk for pain secondary to treatment of hydrocele or hematocele. The patient should verbalize an adequate relief of pain along with the ability to realistically cope with the pain if it is not completely relieved.
- Risk for body image disturbance related to diagnosis. The patient demonstrates enhanced body image and self-esteem as evidenced by ability to look at, touch, talk about, and care for actual or perceived altered body part or function.

VARICOCELE

Varicocele is a group of varicose veins within the scrotum. A varicocele can enlarge during increased intra-abdominal pressure during a Valsalva maneuver, such as a sneeze or bowel movement.

Pathophysiology

It has been hypothesized that the varicocele has a torturous system of enlarged blood vessels within the scrotum that develops along the spermatic cord as a result of incompetent valves in the left internal spermatic vein. This group of vessels often increases in size with age. **Infertility** or subfertility often occurs in conjunction with varicocele because the increased blood flow in the varicocele raises the scrotal temperature beyond 93.2° F (34° C), the ideal temperature for spermatogenesis.

Assessment with Clinical Manifestations

Pain and tenderness in the scrotum and inguinal discomfort may be evident. About 10 percent of the male population, however, has an asymptomatic varicocele of which they are unaware. When palpated, a varicocele often feels like a bag of worms that is apparent when the patient is upright and greatly diminishes or disappears when the patient is supine.

Diagnostic Tests

The patient with a varicocele disorder is identified primarily by confirmation with the patient history. In addition, scrotal ultrasonography can assist in diagnosis, as can Doppler ultrasonography.

Nursing Diagnoses

Based on the information gathered, examples of nursing diagnoses in the patient with varicocele dysfunction may include the following:

- Acute pain related to the varicocele.
- Deficient knowledge related to self-care and risk prevention.
- Disturbed body image related to infertility.

Planning and Implementation

The goal of therapy is primarily to improve comfort. A secondary goal may be to improve or preserve fertility. The treatment undertaken varies with the age of the patient, the size of the varicocele, the amount of discomfort present, and whether infertility is an issue. If the patient is experiencing discomfort, surgical removal of the varicocele (**varicocelectomy**) may be undertaken. Varicocelectomy is done under local anesthesia and involves ligating the internal spermatic vein. **Embolization** can also be undertaken. Embolization involves introduction of an angiocatheter into the internal spermatic vein, fluoroscopic visualization of the vein, and insertion of steel or platinum springs or detachable silicone balloons into the beginning of the venous defect to correct the dysfunction. Medications used in the treatment of varicocele are primarily analgesics.

Patient and Family Teaching

Teaching for varicocele is focused on postoperative comfort measures. Cold packs to control edema and bleeding from the operative site and elevating the scrotum usually contribute to improved comfort. The nurse needs to ensure that the patient recognizes signs of bleeding or infection that must be reported to the care provider.

Evaluation of Outcomes

Potential patient outcomes for each of the example nursing diagnoses for the patient with varicocele dysfunction are:

- Acute pain related to the varicocele. The patient should verbalize an adequate relief of pain along with the ability to realistically cope with the pain if it is not completely relieved.
- Deficient knowledge related to self-care and risk prevention. The patient should demonstrate motivation to learn, identify perceived learning needs, and verbalize an understanding of desired content.
- Disturbed body image related to infertility. The patient demonstrates enhanced body image and self-esteem as evidenced by ability to talk about and care for actual or perceived altered body part or function and express feelings regarding potential infertility.

VASECTOMY

Vasectomy is surgical sterilization of men through removal, ligation, or destruction of a small portion of the vas deferens to prevent passage of sperm to the urethra. Approximately 500,000 men in the United States choose vasectomy as permanent birth control each year (Johnsen & Davis, 2005.) There is mixed and indefinite evidence linking vasectomy to prostate and testicular cancer.

Assessment with Clinical Manifestations

The most important aspect of assessing a patient prior to vasectomy is to be certain that he understands the permanent nature of the procedure and under no circumstances wants additional children. Men who are uncertain about their decision, considering having children in the future, making the decision during times of great life change, or are undergoing the procedure because of coercion by their partners should be counseled to reconsider their decision. Sperm banking prior to undergoing the procedure may be a consideration.

Nursing Diagnoses

Based on the information gathered, examples of nursing diagnoses in the patient having a vasectomy may include the following:

- Acute pain related to the vasectomy.
- Fear and anxiety related to actual or potential lifestyle changes from the vasectomy.

Planning and Implementation

The goal of a vasectomy is permanent sterilization with minimum side effects. The surgery is performed on an outpatient basis under local anesthesia. A small one-fourth inch incision is made on each side of the scrotum, a portion of the vas deferens is lifted up through the incision and a small section of the vas deferens is removed. The ends of the vas deferens are then cauterized, ligated, or crushed. The vas deferens is then replaced into the scrotum. One small suture is placed to close the incision. In the no-incision method, a puncture is made in the scrotum, the vas deferens is pulled through the puncture wound, and the rest of the surgery proceeds as in the incisional method, except that no suture is needed. Recanalization of the vas deferens can occur if there is leakage into the scrotum from the severed end of the proximal vas deferens. The medications used for vasectomy are primarily analgesics. If necessary, antibiotics are used to treat infection.

Patient and Family Teaching

The nurse's teaching for a vasectomy focuses on comfort measures that promote both physical and psychological health. Initial use of ice packs to control postoperative bleeding and edema and cotton jockey type briefs to provide scrotal support followed by warm sitz baths has been demonstrated to be useful. The patient needs to feel confident that any postoperative edema and discoloration are normal and temporary. The nurse needs to provide the signs and symptoms of infection and of bleeding in writing for the patient's reference, along with instructions about how to notify the health care provider if such symptoms become evident. It is important that the nurse validates that the patient and the partner understand the difference between sterility and impotence and that there will be no effect on sexual capability (erection or ejaculation); that there will be no noticeable change in the amount or consistency of ejaculate, but that it will contain no sperm; that the patient's body will simply reabsorb the sperm; and that vasectomy does not protect against sexually transmitted diseases. The patient will need to be instructed to use contraceptives until all sperm are cleared from the distal vas deferens. The health care provider may order an examination of ejaculate for the presence of sperm approximately one month postoperatively.

Evaluation of Outcomes

Potential patient outcomes for each of the example nursing diagnoses for the patient having a vasectomy are:

- Acute pain related to the vasectomy. The patient should verbalize an adequate relief of pain along with the ability to realistically cope with the pain if it is not completely relieved.
- Fear and anxiety related to actual or potential lifestyle changes from the vasectomy. The patient should be able to recognize the signs of anxiety, demonstrate positive coping mechanisms, and describe a reduction in the level of anxiety experienced.

CRYPTORCHIDISM

Cryptorchidism is also referred to as undescended testes when it is present at birth. In about 70 percent of cases, one testicle has not descended fully and either remains in the inguinal canal or the abdomen. Cryptorchidism occurs in about 3 percent of males and is the most common pediatric genital abnormality. The condition affects about 30 percent of preterm males, because the testis normally descends into the scrotum toward the end of 28 to 40 weeks gestation (Kolon, 2005).

Pathophysiology

Mechanical or hormonal obstruction to the descent of the testes occurs in utero. During the first trimester the testes are formed and migrate into the inguinal canal under the influence of testosterone. If there is inadequate production of testosterone the testes may not descend. If the epididymis does not develop normally the testes will not descend. Occasionally the testes are located ectopically or not within the inguinal canal. Cryptorchidism may occur concurrently with other conditions including Wilms' tumor, cerebral palsy, hypospadias, abnormal epididymis, and abdominal wall defects, such as gastroschisis or omphalocele (hernia of the navel).

Assessment with Clinical Manifestations

The testes may be palpable or nonpalpable. If they are palpable, they are located in the inguinal canal and will usually descend by one year of age. Nonpalpable testes are associated with higher degrees of epididymal abnormalities. Approximately 9 percent of male infants with nonpalpable testes actually have absent testes. Such absence is thought to be caused by a late prenatal vascular occlusion that resulted in hypoxia and necrosis of the testes.

Diagnostic Tests

Cryptorchidism is identified with a thorough assessment of the testes of the patient. In addition, ultrasonography of the groin, pelvis, and lower abdomen usually reveal the location of the testes.

Nursing Diagnoses

Based on the information gathered, examples of nursing diagnoses in the patient with cryptorchidism may include the following:

- Acute pain related to the vasectomy.
- Fear and anxiety related to actual or potential lifestyle changes from the vasectomy.

Planning and Implementation

The goal of care is permanent appropriate location of the testes with surgical intervention. Orchiopexy is the surgical procedure to relocate the testis down through the inguinal canal into the scrotum, where it is anchored. If spontaneous resolution of cryptorchidism does not occur by around one year of age, orchiopexy is usually performed. This procedure is undertaken to prevent progressive failure of spermatogenesis that occurs in undescended testes because of the increased core temperature in the abdomen as compared to the scrotum and to allow earlier detection of testicular cancer if it occurs.

In addition, human chorionic gonadotropin may be given IM to promote bilateral testicular descent. From 250 to 1,000 international units is administered IM (dosage varies by age of the patient) two to three times per week for up to six weeks (Broyles, et al., 2007).

Patient and Family Teaching

The nurse is responsible for providing the parents of a child with an orchiopexy with a written list of the signs and symptoms of bleeding and of infection, as well as information about how to contact a care provider in the event that those symptoms become evident. Comfort measures such as the appropriate application of ice to the scrotal area and use of a soft support are important. It is also critical that the nurse provide information and reassurance to the parents adequate to ensure that parent/child attachment is completed.

Evaluation of Outcomes

Potential patient outcomes for each of the example nursing diagnoses for the patient with cryptorchidism are:

- Acute pain related to the vasectomy. The patient should verbalize an adequate relief of pain along with the ability to realistically cope with the pain if it is not completely relieved.
- Fear and anxiety related to actual or potential lifestyle changes from the vasectomy. The patient should be able to recognize the signs of anxiety, demonstrate positive coping mechanisms, and describe a reduction in the level of anxiety experienced.

PHIMOSIS AND PARAPHIMOSIS

Phimosis is the inability of the foreskin to be stretched and retracted over the glans of the penis. Phimosis can occur congenitally or be acquired as a result of infection or edema. It is important to note that the foreskin is not retractable at birth but becomes retractable usually between two and four years of age. Nearly all infant males have enough movement in the foreskin prepuce that the urethral meatus is visible and urine can flow out. By age 16 less than 1 percent of uncircumcised males continue to experience phimosis (Cantus, 2004).

Congenital phimosis is present at birth and can cause urinary retention when the urethral opening is covered by unretractable foreskin. Acquired phimosis usually develops in situations where penile hygiene to cleanse normal secretions is inadequate and balanitis (inflammation) and adhesions develop. Thickened secretions become encrusted with urinary salts and calcify, forming calculi in the prepuce. Eventually, uncorrected phimosis may predispose the patient to the development of cancer of the penis. Acquired phimosis can result if the foreskin is forcibly retracted and inflammation results. Foreskin piercing can lead to acquired phimosis if infection accompanies the piercing. Phimosis only becomes a surgical emergency when the urethral opening is covered and urine is unable to escape. Surgical correction of phimosis is circumcision.

Paraphimosis is the entrapment of the retracted foreskin behind the glans penis of an uncircumcised male. Paraphimosis is characterized by edema of the foreskin, pain, and erythema. Foreskin piercing can lead to development of paraphimosis if pain from the piercing prevents replacement of a retracted foreskin.

Pathophysiology

The foreskin of an infant is not retractable until the progression of keratinization of the epithelial tissues located between the foreskin and the glans is complete. In acquired phimosis, long-term poor hygiene resulting in chronic balanitis causes fibrotic tissue to form near the prepuce, which adheres the foreskin to the glans. Paraphimosis develops when the foreskin has been retracted for an extended period of time. As edema of the foreskin develops, edema and venous engorgement of the glans quickly follow.

Assessment with Clinical Manifestations

Phimosis, whether congenital or acquired, is diagnosed when the foreskin is not able to be retracted behind the glans penis. Paraphimosis is diagnosed when the foreskin is not able to be replaced over the glans after being retracted.

Diagnostic Tests

Phimosis and paraphimosis are identified by clinical history and assessment. In addition, there are no specific diagnostic tests available to determine the presence of phimosis or paraphimosis.

Nursing Diagnoses

Based on the information gathered, examples of nursing diagnoses in the patient with phimosis and paraphimosis may include the following:

- Impaired urinary elimination.
- Pain related to paraphimosis.

Planning and Implementation

In the case of congenital phimosis the primary goal is to explain to parents and caretakers of the male infant that an unretractable foreskin is a normal finding. This is especially important if the father of the child is circumcised and has no personal experience with care of an uncircumcised penis. In the case of acquired phimosis and paraphimosis, the main goal is that the patient will learn and consistently practice good hygiene.

Surgery

If urinary obstruction exists, either circumcision or dorsal slit surgery is performed to free the urethral opening and allow for urine to flow. If paraphimosis is not resolvable through lubrication of the glans and manual replacement of the foreskin because of inflammation or extensive edema, dorsal slit surgery may be required to restore foreskin mobility.

Patient and Family Teaching

In the case of congenital phimosis without urinary obstruction, adequate education of parents of newborn males must include information on foreskin care including: the foreskin will not be retractable yet; complete retractability of the foreskin can take several years to develop; no parental manipulation of the foreskin is required; forcible retraction of the foreskin can cause paraphimosis; hygiene of the retractable foreskin and glans involves retraction, cleaning, and replacement of the foreskin. In acquired phimosis the patient must be instructed in appropriate hygiene and antibiotic treatment, if balanitis is present. With paraphimosis, appropriate penile and foreskin hygiene must be taught, including the need to both retract and replace the foreskin.

Evaluation of Outcomes

Potential patient outcomes for each of the example nursing diagnoses for the patient with phimosis and paraphimosis are:

- Impaired urinary elimination. The patient is continent of urine or verbalizes satisfactory management.
- Pain related to paraphimosis. The patient should verbalize an adequate relief of pain along with the ability to realistically cope with the pain if it is not completely relieved.

BALANITIS AND POSTHITIS

Balanitis is inflammation of the glans penis. Balanitis usually occurs in uncircumcised or partially circumcised males. **Posthitis** is inflammation of the foreskin and thus only occurs in uncircumcised or partially circumcised males. If posthitis occurs concurrently with balanitis, the condition is termed **balanoposthitis.**

Etiology

Usually a bacterial infection is the causative agent for balanitis and posthitis. In extreme cases urinary obstruction can occur as a result of balanitis. Phimosis can also occur. Balanitis accounts for 11 percent of adult visits to urology clinics (Leber, 2005). Diabetes is the most common cause of balanitis, but chemical irritation from soaps or other products applied to the penis can also be to blame. Right-sided congestive heart failure (CHF) can also contribute to balanitis because of the edema that develops as a result of the CHF. In cases of morbid obesity, hygiene may be extremely difficult or impossible to perform, resulting in balanitis. In addition, if the foreskin is not retracted, the glans then cleaned, and the foreskin replaced, balanitis can occur. Bacterial, viral, or fungal infections can create balanitis.

Pathophysiology

The pathology of these infection-induced conditions is primarily the result of the inflammatory processes. Thus, the initiation of the typical infection increases in swelling of fluids to the areas of infection, warmth and redness in the areas of the infection, and other cellular responses to the inflammation of these conditions.

Assessment with Clinical Manifestations

The typical clinical manifestations for balanitis and posthitis include penile discharge, pain, erythema, and edema. In addition, it is important that the history includes hygienic practices along with the onset and severity of symptoms.

Diagnostic Tests

Diagnostic tests include culture of any discharge present to identify the causative organism involved. A wet mount to detect fungi is performed and serology for syphilis may also be obtained. If the patient is known, or suspected, to be diabetic, serum glucose or hemoglobin A_{1C} may be ordered as part of a comprehensive diabetes workup.

Nursing Diagnoses

Based on the information gathered, examples of nursing diagnoses in the patient with balanitis and posthitis may include the following:

- Impaired urinary elimination related to phimosis secondary to balanitis.
- Pain related to balanitis.

Planning and Implementation

In order that appropriate treatment can be quickly undertaken, identification of the causative organisms is the first goal. Prevention of recurrence is another goal and must be directed at the appropriate cause. Medications that treat the causative organism are utilized. If bacterial infection is suspected, topical antibiotic ointments, such as Neosporin, are used. If fungal infection is detected, topical clotrimazole (Lotrimin) is applied twice daily. Patients are instructed to retract the foreskin and soak in warm water daily to thoroughly clean the glans. Appropriate treatment of causative organisms should be undertaken. If phimosis leading to urinary obstruction is present, dorsal slit surgery may be required.

Evaluation of Outcomes

Potential patient outcomes for each of the example nursing diagnoses for the patient with balanitis and posthitis are:

- Impaired urinary elimination related to phimosis secondary to balanitis. The patient is continent of urine or verbalizes satisfactory management.
- Pain related to balanitis. The patient should verbalize an adequate relief of pain along with the ability to realistically cope with the pain if it is not completely relieved.

URETHRITIS

Urethritis is inflammation of the urethra, which most commonly occurs with a genitourinary tract infection but can also be due to trauma. Posttraumatic urethritis occurs in up to 20 percent of men who must self-catheterize for urinary elimination and is 10 times more common with latex catheters than with silicone catheters. Urethritis can accompany other infectious processes, such as orchitis or prostatitis or even otitis media. Symptoms include dysuria, penile discharge, and erythema.

Pathophysiology

Urethritis inflammation secondary to cystitis is frequently caused by gram-negative bacteria, but sexually transmitted infections, such as gonorrhea and chlamydia, comprise at least 80 percent of urethritis cases. Both gonorrhea and chlamydia will often present initially as urethritis, because the urethra is the portal of entry for the infectious organisms. Sudden onset of dysuria with penile discharge is suggestive of either gonococcal or chlamydial infection. Traumatic urethritis can lead to urethral stricture.

Assessment with Clinical Manifestations

Urethritis is assessed by evaluating the onset of symptoms, sexual history, and medical history including self-catheterization. Temperature and white blood cell count should be assessed for elevations that suggest the presence of urethritis. Urinary frequency or urgency are rarely present in males with urethritis, and suggest, instead, prostatitis. The penis must be palpated for painful localized fluctuant areas that may indicate abscess formation.

Diagnostic Tests

Diagnostic tests for urethritis include urine culture if cystitis or prostatitis is also suspected, and urethral discharge culture or polymerase chain reaction testing for suspected gonorrhea and chlamydia infections. A retrograde urethrogram may be ordered if a foreign body is suspected.

Nursing Diagnoses

Based on the information gathered, examples of nursing diagnoses in the patient with urethritis may include the following:

- Impaired urinary elimination related to urethritis.
- Pain related to urethritis.

Planning and Implementation

The goals of care for urethritis are to prevent recurrence and complications and to encourage compliance with the treatment regimen to ensure a complete cure of the infection. In addition, appropriate antibiotic therapy is administered. Common antibiotics for treatment of chlamydia are oral doxycycline or azithromycin (Zithromax). Common antibiotics for gonorrhea treatment include IM ceftriaxone (Rocephin) or PO ciprofloxacin (Cipro) or ofloxacin (Floxin). Trimethoprim and sulfamethoxazole (Bactrim DS or Septra DS) are commonly used for urinary tract infections. NSAIDs may be used to decrease inflammation and pain (Broyles, et al., 2007).

Traumatic urethritis cases should be managed by an urologist to help prevent complications such as urethral stricture. Patient education on safer sex practices, including monogamy and consistent use of condoms, should be provided for patients with suspected or documented cases of sexually transmitted infections. Patients should also be educated about the need to complete the entire course of antibiotics to achieve complete eradication of the infection.

Evaluation of Outcomes

Potential patient outcomes for each of the example nursing diagnoses for the patient with urethritis are:

- Impaired urinary elimination related to urethritis. The patient is continent of urine or verbalizes satisfactory management.
- Pain related to urethritis. The patient should verbalize an adequate relief of pain along with the ability to realistically cope with the pain if it is not completely relieved.

URETHRAL STRICTURE

Urethral stricture is a narrowing or stenosis of the urethra. The main symptom is difficulty voiding and a noticeably decreased urine stream that can develop either gradually or suddenly. Dysuria, pelvic pain, and increased urinary frequency or urgency are also often present. The risk factors for development of urethral stricture are men who have experienced multiple episodes of urethritis, prostatitis, sexually transmitted infections, BPH, or trauma to the urethra (including instrumentation). Rarely, complete urinary obstruction develops.

Pathophysiology

Urethral stricture is caused by inflammation. Severe or repeated episodes of inflammation can lead to the development of fibrotic scar tissue, which in turn, narrows the urethral diameter as the scarring builds up. Recurrence is high after treatment (Gilbert, 2004).

Assessment with Clinical Manifestations

The description of the onset of symptoms and presence of risk factors (e.g., self-catheterization or recent instrumentation) must be assessed. In addition, the patient history is important to evaluate the clinical manifestations for suspected urethral stricture.

Diagnostic Tests

Diagnostic tests for suspected urethral stricture include urinary flow rate, ultrasound postvoiding residue measurement, urinalysis with culture, tests for gonorrhea and chlamydia. Also if indicated either a retrograde urethrogram or cystoscopy is performed for confirmation of urethral stricture.

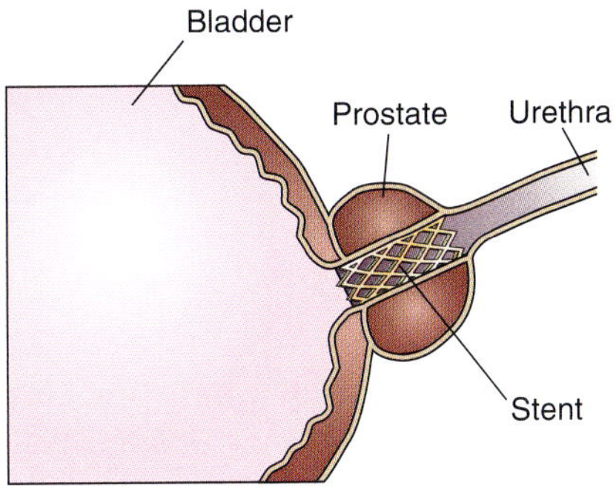

Figure 64-6 Urethral stent.

Nursing Diagnoses

Based on the information gathered, examples of nursing diagnoses in the patient with urethral stricture may include the following:

- Impaired urinary elimination secondary to urethral stricture.
- Deficient fluid volume related to lack of oral fluid intake secondary to lengthy, painful urination.

Planning and Implementation

The primary goal for the management of urethral stricture is to facilitate urinary drainage to prevent urinary stasis, which can lead to a urinary tract infection or to hydronephrosis. Treatment is usually successful, but there is a high rate of recurrence of stricture. With small strictures, urethral dilation can be accomplished by inserting gradually increasing diameter instruments into the stricture until normal diameter is achieved. A urethral stent may be placed using a cystoscopic approach (Figure 64-6). If urinary retention has developed as a result of the severity of the stricture, a suprapubic urinary catheter may be placed. **Urethrotomy** (an opening in the urethra) can decrease the stricture size, at least on a temporary basis. This procedure involves direct visualization of the urethra through an endoscope to create small longitudinal incisions through the fibrotic scar tissue.

Open **urethroplasty** may need to be performed. This procedure involves removing the diseased portion of the urethra and inserting a new urethra that is constructed using other tissue. In some cases, a urinary diversion is created so that self-catheterization can be performed through the abdominal wall. Medications are usually not helpful in treatment of urethral stricture.

Evaluation of Outcomes

Potential patient outcomes for each of the example nursing diagnoses for the patient with an urethral stricture are:

- Impaired urinary elimination secondary to urethral stricture. The patient is continent of urine or verbalizes satisfactory management.
- Deficient fluid volume related to lack of oral fluid intake secondary to lengthy, painful urination. The patient experiences adequate fluid volume and electrolyte balance as evidenced by urine output greater than 30 mL/hour, normotensive blood pressure, heart rate 100 beats/minute, consistency of weight, and normal skin turgor.

EPISPADIAS AND HYPOSPADIAS

Both epispadias and hypospadias are congenital malformations involving the location of the urethral meatus. Misplacement or malformation occurs in approximately 1 in 300 male births. When the urinary meatus is located along the superior (upper) aspect of the penis, the condition is referred to as **epispadias.** When the urinary meatus is located along the inferior (lower) aspect of the penis, the condition is referred to as **hypospadias.** Either variant can occur anywhere along the length of the penis but occur most commonly on the glans of the penis. Aside from controlling urinary flow direction, the greatest problem with epispadias and hypospadias is infertility, because sperm will be deposited in the vagina rather than near the cervix. Most cases of epispadias and hypospadias are considered a nuisance and not a threat to health.

Pathophysiology

The pathophysiology of both epispadias and hypospadias is an incomplete closure of the urethra during fetal development. The urethral opening then forms prior to the tip of the glans. The farther from the glans the urethral opening occurs, the more complex the surgical repair will be.

Assessment with Clinical Manifestations

Assessment is based on clinical findings and the patient history. The defect of both epispadias and hypospadias is apparent at birth by visualizing the location of the foreskin prepuce in relationship to the glans penis.

Diagnostic Tests

The diagnosis of epispadias and hypospadias is made on visualization and clinical assessment. Other diagnostic tests are usually not required, because diagnosis is based on clinical findings alone.

Nursing Diagnoses

Based on the information gathered, examples of nursing diagnoses in the patient with epispadias and hypospadias may include the following:

- Deficient knowledge related to the diagnosis of epispadias and hypospadias.
- Disturbed body image related to abnormal genital formation.

Planning and Implementation

The goals of care for epispadias or hypospadias are to promote acceptance of this anomaly by the parents and to facilitate normal penile function during voiding and sexual intercourse. If the defect is midshaft or lower, or if there are multiple urethral openings, surgery for urethral reconstruction is done before the child is 2 years of age. Circumcision will not be performed on infants with these defects, because the foreskin needs to be preserved so that it can be used as a tissue graft during reconstructive surgery.

Evaluation of Outcomes

Potential patient outcomes for each of the example nursing diagnoses for the patient with epispadias and hypospadias are:

- Deficient knowledge related to the diagnosis of epispadias and hypospadias. The patient should demonstrate motivation to learn, identify perceived learning needs, and verbalize an understanding of desired content.
- Disturbed body image related to abnormal genital formation. The patient demonstrates enhanced body image and self-esteem as evidenced by ability to look at, touch, talk about, and care for actual or perceived altered body part or function.

PEYRONIE'S DISEASE

Peyronie's disease is the formation of dense fibrotic scar tissue plaques in the corpora cavernosa, the tissue that engorges with blood during penile erection. These plaques lack flexibility and cause the penis to curve during erection, sometimes to the point of making intercourse impossible. This condition affects about 1 to 3 percent of men, most commonly between the ages of 40 and 65. Acute onset cases often follow trauma, but gradual onset cases often have no known history of trauma. The condition is most common in men of northern European descent, uncommon in men of African descent, and rare in men of Asian descent (Cornell University Department of Urology, 2005).

Pathophysiology

The pathophysiology of Peyronie's disease is not fully understood. It is hypothesized that trauma to the penis creates localized bleeding that, in turn, leads to inflammation. The inflammatory process becomes fibrotic plaques as the red cells are reabsorbed and the inflammation resolves. These plaques are inflexible and occur between the tunica and the corpus cavernosa. About 30 percent of men with Peyronie's disease will also develop fibrotic areas in other parts of their bodies, such as Dupuytren's contracture of the hand. There is a familial tendency toward Peyronie's (National Kidney and Urologic Diseases Information, 2003).

Assessment with Clinical Manifestations

A history of the onset of symptoms including progression must be obtained. Cases can range from a mild nuisance to those causing severe pain during erection and difficulty with penile penetration for intercourse. Symptoms can be slow in progression or develop overnight.

Diagnostic Tests

Diagnostic tests are usually not indicated, because the diagnosis is made on clinical findings. An important physical finding is inability to stretch the penis. The presence of plaques significantly decreases the ability of the penis to stretch.

Nursing Diagnoses

Based on the information gathered, examples of nursing diagnoses in the patient with Peyronie's disease may include the following:

- Deficient knowledge related to Peyronie's disease.
- Sexual dysfunction secondary to Peyronie's disease.

Planning and Implementation

The primary goal of treatment for Peyronie's disease is to maintain sexual function and activity in patients. Urologists believe that the majority of cases will resolve spontaneously within one to two years and do not require treatment (Peyronie's Disease, 2003). In severe cases, surgical removal of the plaque may be performed. Medications are generally not effective in treating Peyronie's disease.

Evaluation of Outcomes

Potential patient outcomes for each of the example nursing diagnoses for the patient with Peyronie's disease are:

- Deficient knowledge related to Peyronie's disease. The patient should demonstrate motivation to learn, identify perceived learning needs, and verbalize an understanding of desired content.

ETHICS IN PRACTICE

Aberrant Sexual Practices

The nurse must be careful and nonjudgmental in providing care for the patient with Peyronie's disease. An objective recording of the patient's description of symptoms is essential, because trauma to the penis may have been caused by aberrant sexual practices. In addition, the patient may be sensitive or embarrassed by the dysfunction and without sensitivity to communication and emotions, the patient may not feel open enough to share information with the nurse. Ethically, the nurse is bound to not have a condemning voice tone or visual responses that allow the patient to feel they are not being supported.

- Sexual dysfunction secondary to Peyronie's disease. The patient will verbalize satisfaction with the way he expresses physical intimacy.

CANCER OF THE PENIS (BOWEN'S DISEASE)

Penile cancer is usually squamous cell carcinoma. It is a rare condition, affecting about 1,000 men per year in the United States and Europe combined. Cancer of the penis accounts for 0.4 to 0.6 percent of all malignancies. However, penile cancer represents 20 to 30 percent of malignancies in Asia, Africa, and South America. About 48 percent of penile cancers occur on the glans, 21 percent occur on the prepuce, 9 percent affect the glans and the prepuce, and about 2 percent occur on the penile shaft. Up to 75 percent of patients diagnosed with this cancer also have phimosis (Brosman, 2004.) Penile cancer rarely occurs in men who were circumcised as newborns.

Pathophysiology

Genital herpes and human papillomavirus (HPV) infections are associated with increased rates of penile cancer. Penile intraepithelial neoplasia progresses to penile cancer in about 15 percent of cases. The cancer initially is a small lesion that can be flat, slightly raised, or crater-like in appearance and that enlarges over time. Lesions that are 5 cm in diameter or broader or that cover 75 percent or more of the penile shaft tend to have more metastases to lymph nodes and a lower survival rate (Brosman, 2004). The lesions tend to be painless. Because of the rich blood and lymphatic supplies to the penis, metastases occur readily. Death occurs within two years in untreated patients. Cure rates of 82 to 85 percent have been reported in patients undergoing treatment who have one to three nodes involved (Brosman, 2004).

Assessment with Clinical Manifestations

Patients reporting lesions or sores on their penis that do not heal should be examined. The patient needs to be evaluated regarding their pain level and subjective acceptance and understanding of their disorder.

Diagnostic Tests

Biopsy is used to definitively diagnose cancer. MRI or CT may be obtained in men with positive biopsies to determine lymph node involvement. The Jackson Classification system is commonly used to determine the grade of the cancer (Table 64-4).

Nursing Diagnoses

Based on the information gathered, examples of nursing diagnoses in the patient with cancer of the penis may include the following:

TABLE 64-4 Jackson Classification System That Grades Cancer of the Penis

STAGE I (A)	STAGE II (B)	STAGE III (C)	STAGE IV (D)
Confined to glans or prepuce	Extends onto shaft	Operable inguinal metastasis	Involves adjacent structures, associated with inoperable inguinal metastasis or distant metastasis

Adapted from Brosman, S. (2004). Penile cancer. *Retrieved June 23, 2006, from http://www.emedicine.com.*

- Deficient knowledge related to cancer of the penis.
- Sexual dysfunction secondary to cancer of the penis.

Planning and Implementation

The goal of penile cancer treatment is to remove the cancer while it is still in a small and localized stage retaining normal or nearly normal, residual penile function. Up to 50 percent of patients will delay seeking care when lesions develop because of embarrassment or fear. Care may not be sought until odor from necrosis and infection is evident. Treatment is determined by the size of the lesion and ranges from laser ablation to excisional biopsy to partial or total penectomy. Circumcision is recommended as a part of therapy to improve access to and visualization of lesions. Radiation therapy is often performed instead of penectomy because of the psychological aspects of such surgery. External beam radiation tends to require high doses and can result in fistula or stricture formation. Brachytherapy has fewer side effects. Cisplatin, bleomycin, methotrexate, and fluorouracil are chemotherapeutic medications that are often used either alone or in conjunction with radiation therapy.

Evaluation of Outcomes

Potential patient outcomes for each of the example nursing diagnoses for the patient with cancer of the penis are:

- Deficient knowledge related to cancer of the penis. The patient should demonstrate motivation to learn, identify perceived learning needs, and verbalize an understanding of desired content.
- Sexual dysfunction secondary to cancer of the penis. The patient will verbalize satisfaction with the way they express physical intimacy.

ERECTILE DYSFUNCTION

Erectile dysfunction (ED) is the inability to create or to maintain an erection of the penis for the purpose of intercourse. The term most commonly used for this condition is impotence, but ED is being used more often by the lay public as a result of ED medication advertising.

Etiology

Diabetes is the most common endocrine disease that leads to ED, but pituitary tumors and thyroid disease can also be culprits. Stroke, aging, and chronic renal failure also affect blood flow to the penis. Multiple sclerosis and other neuropathies damage the nerves that serve the penis and can also be associated with ED, as can Parkinson's. Medications, such as psychoactive agents and anticholinergics, and chemicals can also affect penile erection. Cigarette smoking markedly decreases penile blood flow, as do alcohol and marijuana. Beta blockers and calcium channel blockers used in the treatment of hypertension can cause ED, as can most medications used for prostate gland enlargement. About 1 percent of men with abdominal aneurysms also have ED.

Pathophysiology

The exact physiology of penile erection is only partially understood. The cause of ED can be psychogenic or physiological. Psychogenic erectile dysfunction is complex, may be related to anxiety or fatigue, and can be temporary or long term. Physiologically, parasympathetic nerve impulses and hormones, such as epinephrine, norepinephrine, acetyl choline, prostaglandins, and nitric oxide, work together to dilate small arteries in the penis sending blood to engorge the corpora cavernosa, causing the penis to become firm and stand upright. Physiological ED is often related to impaired arterial circulation. Arteries within the penis or the arteries in the pelvis leading to the penis may be partially occluded, resulting in insufficient blood flow to the corpora cavernosa to achieve or to sustain firm erection. Thus, erectile dysfunction can be an indicator of systemic atherosclerotic disease.

Assessment with Clinical Manifestations

The complex interdependent psychophysiologic nature of ED requires a detailed physical, psychological, and sexual history and examination. A history of the symptoms and the progression of symptoms is important, clarifying details as appropriate.

Diagnostic Tests

The majority of men presenting with ED do not require a detailed workup. However, a number of investigations exist to determine the cause of a patient's ED. Such investigations include: vascular testing, such as duplex ultrasound and dynamic infusion cavernosometry or cavernosography; neurological testing, such as a biothesiometry, somatosensory evoked potentials and pudendal electromyography; and nocturnal penile tumescence and rigidity analysis. Much debate has been conducted on the indications for such investigations. Adjunctive investigations are reserved for the following groups of patients: (a) patients who are potentially curable: this group includes patients with a high risk for primarily psychogenic ED, patients with endocrinopathy, young males with traumatically induced pure arteriogenic ED, and young males with isolated crural venous leak; (b) patients with penile curvature prior to undergoing penile reconstructive surgery; and (c) medicolegal cases (Cornell University Department of Urology, 2005).

Nursing Diagnoses

Based on the information gathered, examples of nursing diagnoses in the patient with ED may include the following:

- Deficient knowledge related to ED.
- Sexual dysfunction secondary to ED.

Planning and Implementation

The management for ED is complicated and requires sensitive communication and care by the nurse. In general, the overall goal of ED treatment is to achieve a functional erection. Nonpharmacological treatment options include vacuum devices that fit over the penis and when negative pressure is created, blood is drawn into the penile shaft. Once the penis is erect a constriction band is placed around the base of the shaft to maintain the firmness. Surgically placed penile implants are also available. The inflatable prosthesis has a reservoir and pump that are located in the scrotum and used to inflate or deflate the penis. The semirigid rod (Small-Carrion) prosthesis creates a permanent partial erection.

Pharmacology

Medications used to treat ED include oral selective enzyme inhibitors, such as sildenafil (Viagra), vardenafil (Levitra), and tadalafil (Cialis) taken 30 minutes to eight hours prior to sexual activity. However, 30 to 50 percent of men with low serum testosterone levels do not respond to Viagra alone and require concomitant testosterone replacement therapy. Side effects of Viagra may include headache, flushing, and blue-tinged vision. Viagra is

Skills 360°

Therapeutic Communication with Patients Who Have ED

The nurse must remember to be professional when communicating with patients who have ED. The nurse should think through his or her own feelings of either embarrassment or being uncomfortable when discussing the sexuality issues with patients who have ED. In addition, the nurse can also make referrals to sexuality counselors or social workers whose specialty is working with patients who have sexual disorders. In general, the nurse needs to appear objective, yet empathetic to the patient in open discussions regarding the ED issue.

contraindicated for patients on nitrate therapy and patients who have retinopathy. Yohimbine (Yohimbine or Yocon) must be taken for six to eight weeks to see results.

The selective enzyme inhibitors are contraindicated in patients with angina, a history of myocardial infarction or cerebrovascular accident in the last six months, unstable hypertension, and those taking nitrites or alpha blockers. Injections into the corpus cavernosa of prostaglandin (Caverject) or phentolamine (Regitine) successfully creates erection in 80 percent of patients in 5 to 15 minutes and should only be used every four to seven days. Urethral suppositories (alprostadil) containing prostaglandin (Muse) will produce erection in about 60 percent of men. Vasoactive agents, such as alprostadil or papaverine may be injected directly into the penis (Broyles, et al., 2007).

Patient and Family Teaching

Patient education regarding ED requires sensitivity from the nurse. An open and communicating relationship is essential between the patient and the health care provider. One aspect of the teaching is about potential side effects of medications used to treat ED. Information about how to contact a health care provider in case of an untoward reaction to a medication must also be provided. The patient and his partner must be supported as they learn to adapt their sexual practices to use of a prosthesis. The signs and symptoms of migration of a prosthesis must be clearly understood by the patient and his partner, and the nurse may find it useful to collaborate with a sex therapist. Referral to Impotence Anonymous (I-anon), a 10-step program, may also be indicated.

Evaluation of Outcomes

Potential patient outcomes for each of the example nursing diagnoses for the patient with ED are:

- Deficient knowledge related to ED. The patient should demonstrate motivation to learn, identify perceived learning needs, and verbalize an understanding of desired content.
- Sexual dysfunction secondary to ED The patient will verbalize satisfaction with the way they express physical intimacy.

PRIAPISM

Priapism is the presence of a prolonged, often painful, penile erection. Two types exist: arterial high-flow and veno-occlusive. Veno-occlusive priapism is seen most often in men with sickle cell disease. About 40 percent of men with sickle cell disease report having had at least one episode of priapism, with peak incidence between the ages of 19 and 21. Priapism can also occur as a side effect to the use of intracavernosal injections of medication used to treat ED.

Etiology

Conditions that are associated with the development of priapism include sickle cell, leukemia, amyloidosis, malaria, carbon monoxide poisoning, black widow spider bites, and spinal anesthesia. Many medications can also cause priapism. These include the psychotropic medications, especially chlorpromazine (Thorazine), trazodone (Desyrel), thioridazine (Mellaril), and citalopram (Celexa). Hydralazine (Apresoline), metoclopramide (Reglan), omeprazole (Prilosec), hydroxyzine (Vistaril), prazosin (Minipress), and other calcium channel blockers, have also been implicated in causing priapism. Androstenedione

(Andro), often used to enhance athletic ability, can also create priapism. Cocaine, marijuana, ecstasy, and methamphetamines are illicit drugs that can cause priapism.

Pathophysiology

In priapism, the corpora cavernosa remains engorged with blood because of malfunctioning of the valve system that controls the onset and release of erections. There are two main types of priapism: arterial high-flow priapism and veno-occlusive priapism. Arterial high-flow priapism is rare, is usually painless and occurs when a cavernosa artery has ruptured, usually secondary to penetrating or blunt trauma to the penis. Due to arterial spasm or clot formation, the priapism may not develop immediately after trauma. Veno-occlusive priapism is painful and occurs when a vein is occluded which prevents cavernosa drainage. If not treated promptly, the venous occlusion can create the formation of fibrotic tissue within a few hours, which in turn can lead to the loss of ability to achieve an erection (Carey, 2004).

Assessment with Clinical Manifestations

A thorough review of medical history, onset of symptoms, history of trauma, and current legal and illicit medication use is crucial to understanding the underlying causes of priapism. The nurse will need to use therapeutic communication carefully and support the patient while asking questions in obtaining a history of the condition.

> *Red Flag*
>
> **Priapism in the Emergency Department**
>
> The patient with priapism may seek the emergency department and when he is first admitted, the patient may be embarrassed about his condition. The nurse must solicit information from the patient, while working with the patient using good therapeutic communication skills. It is necessary to find out what medications the patient has been taking and if there are other potential causative agents that need to be identified quickly.

Diagnostic Tests

Obviously, the priapism is recognized upon observational assessment. However, laboratory studies including CBC and coagulation studies are indicated to rule out leukemia and detect coagulopathy. Doppler flow studies can help differentiate between high-flow and veno-occlusive priapism. In cases suspected to be caused by arterial high-flow, penile artery angiography may be obtained (Daniels, 2003).

Nursing Diagnoses

Based on the information gathered, examples of nursing diagnoses in the patient with priapism may include the following:

- Deficient knowledge related to priapism.
- Sexual dysfunction secondary to priapism.

Planning and Implementation

The goal of treating priapism is to resolve the condition before the fibrotic changes take place and cause permanent damage that leaves the patient unable to achieve erection in the future. Ice packs to the perineum will resolve some cases. Most cases require pharmacological intervention or other procedures. Selective embolization of problematic arteries is sometimes utilized. The treatment most commonly used is to aspirate 20 to 30 mL of blood by inserting a large-bore needle on a large syringe into the corpus cavernosa; multiple puncture sites and aspirations are usually required. This procedure is performed after penile nerve block has been achieved.

Pharmacology

There are a variety of medications used to manage priapism (Table 64-5). These medications have different results and are managed by the symptomatic response of the patient.

TABLE 64-5 Medications in Management of Priapism

MEDICATION	MECHANISM OF ACTION	DOSE
Metaraminol bitartrate	Strong arterial vasoconstrictor	100–500 mcg per dose, up to 10 doses administered in a dilute solution (1 mL of phenylephrine to 499 mL of saline 0.9%) 10–20 mL per dose via intracavernosal injection every 5–10 minutes.
Ethylene blue	Smooth muscle relaxant	1–2 mg/kg IV slowly over 5 minutes
Phenylephrine (Neo-Synephrine)	Arteriole vasoconstrictor	100–500 mcg per dose, up to 10 doses; use 10–20 mL of 20 mcg/mL solution via intracavernosal injection every 10 minutes
Metaraminol (Aramine)	Arterial vasoconstriction	0.5–1 mg intravenously; repeat after 5 minutes
Terbutaline (Brethaire, Bricanyl)	Smooth muscle relaxant	5 mg by mouth every 15 minutes for three doses 0.25–0.50 mg subcut every 15 minutes for three doses

Adapted from Broyles, B. E., Reiss, B. S., & Evans, M. E. (2007). Pharmacological aspects of nursing care *(7th ed.). New York: Thomson Delmar Learning.*

Evaluation of Outcomes

Potential patient outcomes for each of the example nursing diagnoses for the patient with priapism are:

- Deficient knowledge related to priapism. The patient should demonstrate motivation to learn, identify perceived learning needs, and verbalize an understanding of desired content.
- Sexual dysfunction secondary to priapism. The patient will verbalize satisfaction with the way he expresses physical intimacy.

KEY CONCEPTS

- Prostatitis is classified as either acute or chronic.
- BPH is a common condition affecting middle-aged and elderly men, and the greatest risk factor for BPH is age.
- Prostate cancer is the second most commonly diagnosed cancer in men.
- Painless enlargement of a testis is generally diagnostic of testicular cancer.
- Testicular torsion is a condition where the testis twists on the spermatic cord with resultant hypoxia of the testicle.
- Orchitis can be caused by viral, spirochetal, parasitic, or bacterial infections.
- Epididymitis usually develops secondary to bacterial infection in the urinary tract or prostatitis.
- Hydrocele, hematocele, and spermatocele all present with painless swelling or bulging in the scrotum.
- Varicocele is a group of varicose veins within the scrotum.
- Vasectomy is surgical sterilization of men to prevent passage of sperm to the urethra.
- Cryptorchidism is also referred to as undescended testes when it is present at birth.
- Phimosis, paraphimosis, balanitis, and posthitis are disorders of the glans penis and foreskin of the penis.
- Urethritis most commonly occurs with a genitourinary tract infection but can also be due to trauma.
- Urethral stricture causes difficulty voiding and a noticeably decreased urine stream.
- Epispadias and hypospadias are congenital malformations involving the location of the urethral meatus.
- Peyronie's disease is the formation of dense fibrotic scar tissue, which is the tissue that engorges with blood during penile erection.
- Penile cancer is a rare condition and seldom occurs in men who were circumcised as newborns.
- The cause of erectile dysfunction can be psychogenic or physiological.
- Priapism is the presence of a prolonged, often painful, penile erection.

REVIEW QUESTIONS

1. Which of the following is true concerning the diagnosis of prostatitis?
1. It is identified primarily by a 24-hour urine specimen.
2. It is diagnosed by culturing spontaneous or expressed urethral discharge or prostate fluid.
3. It is falsely diagnosed in the presence of prostatic massage.
4. It is a condition that is clearly identified with serum changes in a CBC.

2. Which of the following is true concerning the surgical treatment of benign prostatic hyperplasia?
1. TUMP is an alternative treatment that heats the prostate tissue.
2. TURP is seldom performed on the aged, due to complications.
3. TUNA involves freezing the prostate to decrease the nature of its inflammation.
4. Resection of the prostate is not normally performed if other procedures can be employed.

3. Which of the following is true concerning the staging and classification of prostate cancer?
1. The normal PSA range for under 40 years of age is less than 4 to 6 ng/mL.
2. The Gleason grading system is usually used for hematological cancers but not prostate cancer.
3. At least two separate biopsy specimens are graded based on their differentiation from normal prostate cells.
4. A score of D is less invasive than a score of B in the cancer staging system.

4. Which of the following is true concerning orchitis?
1. There is a single blood test that will test positive in the presence of orchitis.
2. Orchitis is usually asymptomatic.
3. Orchitis involves an active inflammation of the epididymis and vas deferens.
4. Antibiotics are normally given in the management of orchitis.

5. Which of the following is true concerning the condition of a varicocele?
1. It is normally present in one testicle and causes infertility.
2. It is the presence of varicose veins seen in the extremities of persons who have inguinal hernias.
3. It often causes infertility or subfertility as a clinical manifestation.
4. It can be removed with surgery and is managed this way if the patient is experiencing discomfort.

6. Which of the following is true of balanitis?
1. It is usually caused by a bacterial infection.
2. It is the entrapment of the retracted foreskin behind the glans penis of an uncircumcised male.
3. It is an inflammation of the foreskin.
4. It is the inability of the foreskin to be stretched and retracted over the glans of the penis.

7. Which of the following is true concerning a urethral stricture?
1. It is an incomplete closure of the urethra during fetal development.
2. It causes changes in the tissue that engorges with blood during penile erection.
3. It has a main symptom of difficulty voiding and a noticeably decreased urine stream.
4. It is not managed well with a urethral stent.

8. Which of the following is not true of penile cancer?
1. The Jackson classification system grades cancer of the penis.
2. Genital herpes and HPV infections are associated with increased rates of penile cancer.
3. The goal of penile cancer treatment is to leave the tumor in place, as it is slow growing and seldom causes problems.
4. Radiation therapy is often performed instead of penectomy because of the psychological aspects of such surgery.

9. Which of the following is true of ED?
1. The medications used to treat ED usually have to be administered 24 hours prior to sexual intercourse.
2. Parasympathetic nerve impulses and hormones work together to cause the penis to become firm in an erection.
3. There are no nonpharmacological measures that can be used to treat ED.
4. Prosthetic devices do not work well for most patients.

10. Which of the following is true concerning priapism?
1. It is best treated with a surgical penile implant.
2. It is often accompanied with a fever, chills, and nausea.
3. It is differentiated with the use of Doppler flow studies.
4. It is often caused as a complication of urethral surgery.

REVIEW ACTIVITIES

1. Select a patient with benign prostatic hyperplasia and discuss his knowledge of the disorder and the typical surgical interventions that are used in its management.
2. Teach a male patient to perform a TSE.
3. Write the subjective reflections that would accompany your thoughts and feelings about suddenly being diagnosed with cancer. Then, discuss with a peer how you would both approach a patient who was newly diagnosed with prostate cancer.
4. Develop a teaching plan to share with your peers for a patient with ED.
5. Describe the assessment and management for a patient with priapism.

Visit the Contemporary Medical-Surgical Nursing online companion resource at www.delmarhealthcare.com for additional content and study aids. Click on Online Companions then select the Nursing discipline.

UNIT

XVI

Special Considerations in Medical and Surgical Nursing

Chapter 65 Multisystem Failure

Chapter 66 Mass Casualty Care

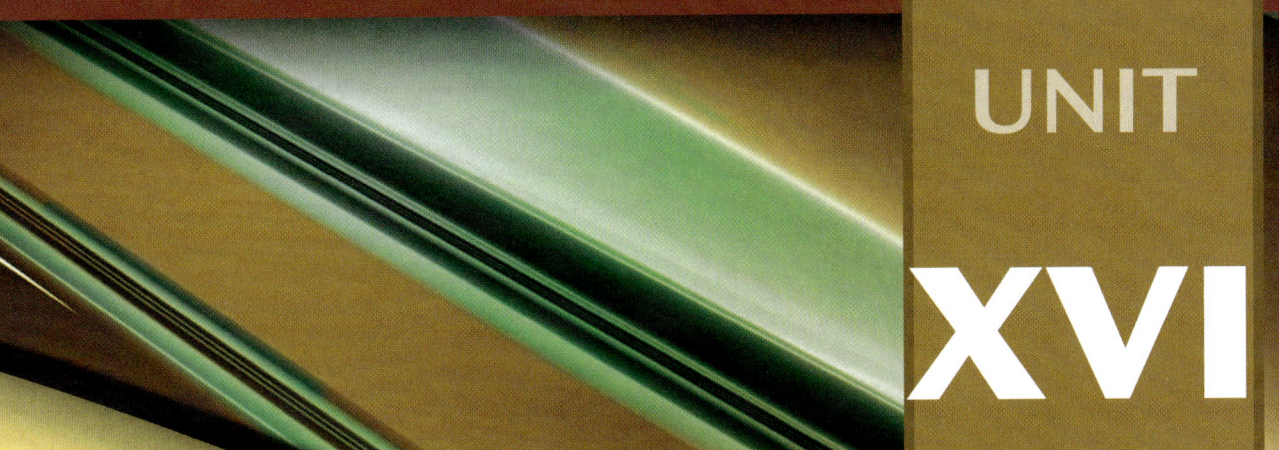

CHAPTER 65

Multisystem Failure

Ruth Grendell, MSN, RN

KEY TERMS

Absolute hypovolemia
Acute respiratory distress syndrome (ARDS)
Disseminated intravascular coagulation (DIC)
Endothelium
Hypoxemia
Inflammatory immune response (IIR)
Multiple organ dysfunction syndrome (MODS)
Phagocytosis
Primary multiple organ dysfunction
Relative hypovolemia
Secondary multiple organ dysfunction
Sepsis
Shock syndrome
Systemic inflammatory response syndrome (SIRS)
Third spacing

CHAPTER TOPICS

- Immune Inflammatory Responses
- Shock Syndrome
- Systemic Inflammatory Response Syndrome (SIRS)
- Disseminated Intravascular Coagulation (DIC)
- Acute Respiratory Distress Syndrome (ARDS)
- Multiple Organ Dysfunction Syndrome (MODS)

The human body is composed of thousands of interacting and interdependent systems that regulate body functions. Many of the cellular functions are under genetic control, including cell structure and replication. Other systems integrate the functions of different organ systems. The body fluids that surround the cells and the various organ systems provide the pathways for exchange between the internal and external environments. The physiological processes are carefully coordinated to promote homeostasis and to oppose any disruptive change. Many of these autonomic functions occur without our knowledge until something within the process is altered. On the other hand, when the body receives an insult from either the internal or external environment, certain body systems interact to counteract any detrimental effect the insult might have. If successful, the threat is minimized or eliminated and the homeostatic state returns. However, if there is widespread inflammatory response to a severe insult, several organs can be involved. An insult can be anything that triggers the body's protective inflammatory response, such as trauma, surgery, anesthesia, burns, cardiovascular disorders, renal or liver disease, pancreatitis, gastrointestinal (GI) disorders, drugs, allergic reactions, shock, infection, and various pulmonary problems. When the body systems become overwhelmed the cascade of events can be described as a domino effect, which is when one system malfunctions, the other systems are adversely affected as well.

The person is also exposed to emotional stressors, which include the possibility of hospitalization and time in the intensive care unit or surgery, receiving blood transfusions, and being without the normal intake of food and fluids. These are all events that can have consequences on recovery. Anxiety over the outcome of the illness and spiritual distress associated with the fear of suffering and possible death can also influence the patient's psychological and physiological responses. The family processes are often interrupted, causing distress and potential alterations in coping with the events surrounding the ill person's condition. Cultural influences must also be taken into consideration in the plan of care. The nurse, as an important member of a multidisciplinary team, must understand the various changes in these life-threatening situations and be able to respond promptly and appropriately to help avoid complications, secondary multiple organ dysfunction or multiple organ failure (MOF), and death. The nurse must also support the patient and family during the crisis, thus ensuring that a holistic plan of care is provided. This chapter provides an overview of the natural protective responses that are constantly defending the body from foreign substances and abnormal cells that may develop within the body, the pathophysiological responses of the body to an insult, and the current evidence-based standards for therapeutic interventions for the patient and family members.

INFLAMMATORY IMMUNE RESPONSE

The immune system is made up of several types of immune cells and the central and peripheral lymphoid bodies. The **inflammatory immune response (IIR),** is a response that is composed of several body systems, which are constantly on alert to detect nonself and harmful intruders from the normal cells and proteins in the body. The immune system also has the ability to remember a foreign agent and to develop a heightened response during a subsequent exposure. When regulation of the immune response is controlled, the response is protective; however, when the immune response is exaggerated, the consequences can be undesirable and dangerous.

The acute phase of the IIR occurs almost immediately following an insult to the body (Box 65-1). The purposes of this innate protective response are to control bleeding, remove waste products, limit infection, and promote healing. IIR responses cause local vasodilation to aid in delivering an increased blood flow and to bring neutrophils, macrophages (the major phagocytic cells of the immune system), and clotting factors to the damaged area. The body is usually economical in the use of only the required responses that will minimize tissue damage. Minor injuries or insults elicit a transient response; more serious injuries involve a sustained response that may occur for several days and can damage the vessels in the area of injury.

A prolonged response causes an increase in permeability of the capillaries. The **endothelium,** which is the cellular tissue that lines the blood and lymphatic vessels, the heart, and various other body cavities, is a prominent contributor to the activation of the IIR (Box 65-2). The endothelial cells are metabolically active and produce several compounds that affect vascular lumen and anticoagulation of platelets. Damage to the endothelium results in a loss of anticoagulation factors and can result in the development of thrombi or major hemorrhage.

Capillary permeability results in the release of several inflammatory mediators from the damaged area that attracts the elements, which will fight invading microorganisms or minimize blood loss and further injury and promote healing. Mediators are bioactive substances that stimulate physiological change in cells. The most prominent mediators are histamine, kinins, prostaglandins, and cytokines, such as interleukin-1 (IL-1). IL-1 is released by almost all nucleated cells and activates the growth and function of neutrophils, lymphocytes (including killer cells), and macrophages. Killer cells are part of the immune system

BOX 65-1

CARDINAL SIGNS OF THE INFLAMMATORY RESPONSE

The local reaction to an injury was first described by Celsus, an early Roman physician.

Cardinal signs were termed as:

Rubor (redness)

Tumor (swelling)

Calor (heat)

Dolor (pain)

The Greek physician, Galen, added a fifth cardinal sign:

Function laesa (loss of function)

BOX 65-2

CHARACTERIZATIONS OF CHRONIC INFLAMMATION

Chronic inflammation is characterized by:

- A prolonged state of inflammation that may last for weeks, months, or years usually caused by persistent irritants that are resistant to phagocytosis (digestion and destruction) and other inflammatory mechanisms.
- The release of macrophages and lymphocytes instead of neutrophils to the damaged area.
- Chronic elevation of white blood cells, low-grade fever, and pain.
- Proliferation of fibroblasts (cells involved in development of connective tissue) rather than exudates (fluids containing pus or serum).
- Great risk for scar formation and deformity (Scar tissue often replaces normal connective tissue).
- Potential formation of granuloma: a tumor or growth composed of macrophages that are unable to destroy foreign bodies and some mycobacteria, which results in the formation of a mass surrounding the foreign body that is eventually encapsulated by a dense membrane of connective tissue that isolates it.
- Causative agents include: foreign bodies, e.g., asbestos, viruses, some bacteria, fungi, and larger parasites, e.g., tubercle bacillus, mycobacterium of leprosy, treponema of syphilis, and actinomyces, and tissues surrounding healing fractures.

Adapted from Rizzo, D. (2006). Fundamentals of anatomy and physiology *(2nd ed.). New York: Thomson Delmar Learning.*

surveillance network and are automatically programmed to kill foreign cells, such as cancer and virus-infected cells. It also promotes the release of other mediators, such as the complement system (a complex cascade of more than 20 serum proteins) that influence the antigen-antibody response. The mediators increase the permeability of capillary membranes, thus leading to the classic signs of swelling, edema, redness, and heat and pain. Loss of function is because of localized swelling and the release of the chemical mediators.

When the IIR is localized as in wound healing, or systemically capable of restoring metabolic function, healing will take place without complications. However, if the IRR response is not regulated, the system goes into overdrive and is considered to be pathogenic. This heightened response can result in uncontrolled intravascular inflammation and an increase in vascular permeability. The mediators can become toxic to other cells, thus damaging tissues, vessels, and organs, and result in hypoxia. An insufficient oxygen level to meet the body's demands will result in a switch from aerobic to anaerobic metabolism by the body cells.

Anaerobic metabolism results in the formation of lactic acid as a by-product of glucose metabolism. Anaerobic metabolism is not as efficient as aerobic metabolism; waste products accumulate, and the presence of lactic acid contributes to muscle fatigue. Failure of the sodium/potassium pump due to metabolic acidosis allows sodium, which is normally in the intravascular area, to enter cells as potassium leaves cells. Fluid follows sodium into the cells causing swelling and release of intracellular enzymes, thus preventing the cells from their normal functions. Calcium also enters the cells and blocks the use of phosphorus, a component of adenosine triphosphate (ATP) that is present in all cells and needed for producing energy. The cells eventually burst and die. Hyperkalemia, or excess potassium in the blood, can cause cardiac arrhythmias

BOX 65-3

SEQUENCE OF EVENTS INVOLVING ANAEROBIC METABOLISM AND METABOLIC ACIDOSIS

Anaerobic metabolism and metabolic acidosis

Inefficient cellular metabolism, accumulation of waste products, production of lactic acid, and muscle fatigue

Failure of sodium/potassium pump

Influx of sodium and water into cell	Outflow of potassium into blood stream
Swelling and release of cellular enzymes	Hyperkalemia
Calcium enters the cells	Potential cardiac arrhythmias and muscle weakness
Phosphorus not available to form ATP to produce energy for cell functions.	

Cells eventually burst and die

Multiple organ failure process begins when a large number of cells die

Adapted from Edwards, S. (2002). Physiological insult/injury: Pathophysiology and consequences. British Journal of Nursing, 11*(4), 263–277.*

and possible muscle weakness. If the metabolic acidosis process continues and cannot be reversed, organ dysfunction and failure will occur (Box 65-3).

NEUROENDOCRINE SYSTEM RESPONSE

The neuroendocrine protective response to an insult is also closely linked to the immune response and tissue function. This response occurs as the cytokines (lymphokines and monokines) are released from the injury site. In fact IL-1 may be the linking factor between the immune response and stimulation of the neuroendocrine system. The principal elements include the sympathetic nervous system, the hypothalamus, pituitary and the adrenal glands that are involved in the typical "fight or flight" response to a threat. The sympathetic nervous system secretes the catecholamines adrenaline and noradrenaline. Adrenaline stimulates the heart and metabolic activities resulting in increased heart rate, cardiac output, metabolic rate, dilated bronchioles, and elevated blood glucose levels (Figure 65-1). Noradrenaline aids peripheral vascular constriction that helps to shunt circulating blood temporarily from nonessential organs to essential organs, such as the brain and heart, and to skeletal muscles. The major effect of the catecholamines is to increase glucose production and activation of platelets. However, if the catecholamine levels continue to rise, they could contribute to hyperglycemia, resistance to insulin, cardiac arrhythmias, and possible cardiac arrest.

The release of hormones into the blood stream is regulated by a negative feedback system. The activated sympathetic system and release of IL-1 interrupt the normal feedback process and trigger the hypothalamus to release

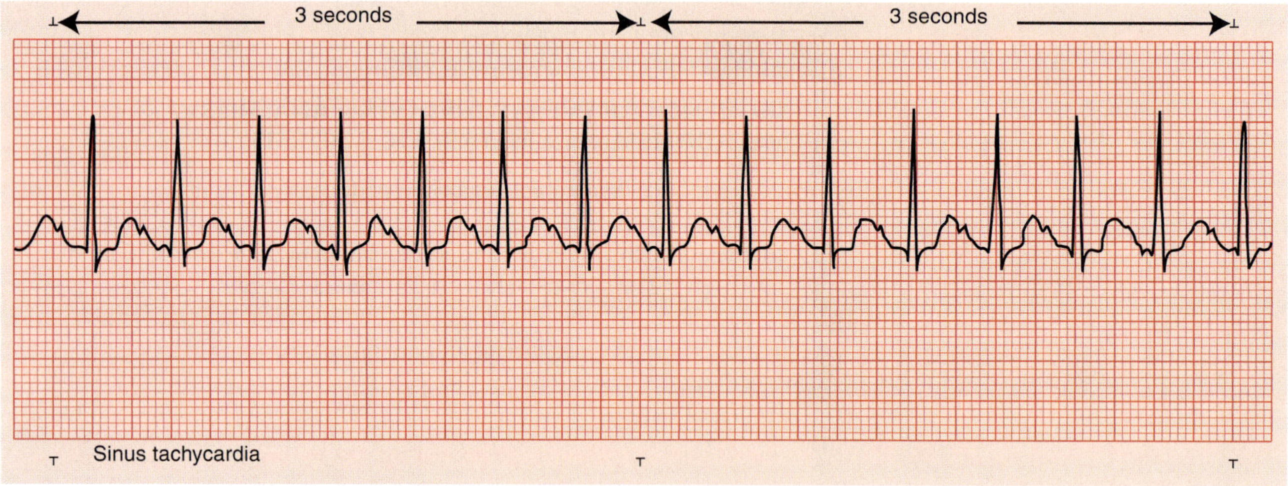

Heart rate 140 (Tachycardia)

Figure 65-1 Adrenaline causes the heart rate to develop tachycardia in the neuroendocrine response.

corticotrophin-releasing hormone (CRH). This signals the pituitary gland to secrete the adrenocorticotrophic hormone (ACTH) that stimulates the release of cortisol from the cortex of the adrenal gland. Cortisol (a) assists in the breakdown, or catabolism, of fats and proteins into simple substances; (b) assists in the synthesis of glucose from noncarbohydrate elements, such as fats and amino acids from proteins; and (c) converts glycogen that is stored in the liver into glucose. These processes take place primarily in the liver and help maintain blood glucose levels that are needed for the energy to conduct physiological processes. Cortisol also enhances adrenaline's influence on vascular constriction to aid in distribution of nutrients and energy sources where they are needed.

The purposes for the release of stress hormones following an insult to the body are to aid in restoring balance to the systems and to prevent secondary complications including loss of fluids, hypotension, and infection. The close link between the stress response and the sympathetic nervous system results in the release of a large amount of adrenaline into the blood stream in the attempt to defend the body from the stressor or insult. Stress hormones are also involved in the release of mineralocorticoids, such as aldosterone, when fluids are lost due to fluid shifts to interstitial spaces or hemorrhage. The primary function of mineralocorticoids is the regulation of the electrolyte balance, particularly potassium and sodium in the extracellular fluids.

THE RENAL RESPONSE

Loss of fluid or blood will lead to a decrease in kidney perfusion. The kidneys respond by releasing the enzyme renin. Renin splits angiotensinogen (a serum globulin formed in the liver) to angiotensin I, a vasopressor substance that is later converted in the lungs to angiotensin II. Angiotensin II stimulates the release of noradrenaline resulting in vasoconstriction, an increase in blood pressure, and thus a potential delivery of blood, nutrients, and oxygen to the deprived kidneys and other organs. Angiotensin II also stimulates the release of the mineralocorticoid aldosterone that aids the reabsorption of sodium and water by the kidneys and an increase in excretion of potassium. This process helps with an increase in intravascular volume, an increase in venous return, cardiac output, and blood pressure and clearance of potassium leaked from damaged cells. Angiotensin II also stimulates the posterior pituitary gland to release the antidiuretic hormone (ADH), which aids in water reabsorption and a decrease in urinary output (Box 65-4).

BOX 65-4

CASCADE OF PHYSIOLOGICAL EVENTS FOLLOWING AN INSULT TO THE BODY

Primary Injury

Trauma, surgery, anesthesia, burns, circulatory disorders, myocardial infarction, renal or liver disease, pancreatitis, gastrointestinal [GI] disorders, drugs, allergic reactions, shock, infection, deep vein thrombosis [DVT], and pulmonary embolism.

Systemic Inflammatory Immune Response (IIR)

Protective Measures

Release of inflammatory mediators from damaged tissue to area of need (histamine, kinins, prostaglandins, complement, and cytokines—interleukin-1).

Overdrive Response

Uncontrolled intravascular inflammation.
Increase in vascular permeability
Mediators can become toxic to other cells and contribute to hypoxic damage to organs.
Coagulation/microvascular thrombosis & altered tissue perfusion.

Secondary Response

Suppressed immune system infection—potential sepsis
Shock

Endothelial Response

The endothelium consists of flat cells that line the blood and lymphatic vessels, the heart, and various other body cavities. The cells are metabolically active and produce several compounds that affect the vascular lumen, anticoagulation and are closely linked to the IIR.

Protective Measures

Prevents excessive blood loss and isolates the injured site

Overdrive Responses

When damaged, anticoagulant properties are lost

Neuroendocrine Response

Response is to the release of cytokine (lymphokines and monokines) and other IIR mediators. Stimulation of hypothalamus, pituitary, and adrenal gland creates a highly complex series of events that affect cardiovascular system.

Protective Measures

Stimulation of sympathetic system and release of catecholamines (adrenaline and noradrenaline)

Increase in heart beat and cardiac output; metabolic rate and blood glucose dilation of bronchioles
Peripheral vasoconstriction; blood shifted temporarily from nonessential organs to brain, heart, and skeletal muscles.

Release of cortisol (as anti-inflammatory agent).
Enhances adrenaline's vasoconstrictive effects to ensure nutrients are supplied to tissues.
Release of adrenocorticotrophic hormone (ACTH) from adrenal cortex.
Release of mineralocorticoids to help regulate electrolytes.

Overdrive Responses

Excess circulating catecholamines
Increase in oxygen consumption
Rise in blood glucose
Arrhythmias, possible cardiac arrest.

Cardiovascular Response

Protective Measures

Increase in rate and strength of cardiac contractions to increase cardiac output

Overdrive Responses

Inflammatory mediators circulate and can alter endothelial integrity

Increased myocardial oxygen demand and possible arrhythmias
Cardiac depression

Systemic thrombosis or gross hemorrhage—DIC

Continued

BOX 65-4

CASCADE OF PHYSIOLOGICAL EVENTS FOLLOWING AN INSULT TO THE BODY—cont'd

Neuroendocrine Response—cont'd

Respiratory Response

Protective Measures	*Overdrive Responses*
Increase in rate and depth of breathing to enhance gas exchange and to counteract metabolic acidosis	Tachypnea $PaCO_2$ less than 32 mm Hg Alveolar damage Pulmonary edema Respiratory distress

Secondary Responses—Stress

Stress is related to increased sympathetic nervous system arousal and involves a wide physiological response. Many stressors act synergistically rather than cumulatively.

Protective Measures	*Overdrive Responses*
Presence of adrenaline in attempt to protect body from stressors (flight or fight response). Presence of cortisol	Prolonged emotional demands Can produce stress ulcers, reduced wound healing, reduced cardiac function, and reduced immune response Loss of balance between neurological, endocrine, and immune systems

Shock

The shock syndrome is a systemic condition when the peripheral blood flow is inadequate to provide sufficient blood to the heart for normal function and transport of oxygen to all organs and tissues.

Adapted from Hardaway, R. (2006). Traumatic shock. Military Medicine, 171*(4), 278–279; Ren, J., & Wu., S. (2006). A burning issue: Do sepsis and systemic inflammatory response syndrome (SIRS) directly contribute to cardiac dysfunction?* Frontiers in Bioscience, 11, *15–22.*

SHOCK SYNDROME

The **shock syndrome** is a systemic condition in which the peripheral blood flow is inadequate to provide sufficient blood to the heart for normal function and transport of oxygen to all organs and tissues. The mean arterial blood pressure (MABP) is inadequate to meet the needs of the tissues (Bench, 2004). Any factor that affects blood volume, blood pressure, or cardiac function can quickly exhaust energy resources and can initiate the complex shock syndrome. Common causes include hemorrhage, drug reaction (or allergic reaction to an antigen), trauma, pulmonary embolism, myocardial infarction, dehydration, heat stroke, and infection. There is some degree of shock with every insult or injury to the body. For example, an emotional response to an injury can induce syncope, or fainting, due to a transient inadequate blood supply to the brain.

The shock syndrome, or acute circulatory failure, has traditionally been classified according to etiology into five categories: anaphylactic, cardiogenic, hypovolemic, neurogenic, and septic (Table 65-1). A functional classification defines the types of shock as: hypovolemic, transport, obstructive, and cardiogenic. Anaphylactic, neurogenic, and sepsis shock are integrated into the transport classification. Regardless of the initiating event, there are four phases involved: initial, compensatory, progressive, and refractory. Progression from one stage to the other is dependent on the patient's health status, duration of the insult, response to therapy, and the correction of the underlying cause. The end result is always the same; tissues fail to receive oxygen and nutrients and are unable to eliminate waste products (Walsh, 2005).

TABLE 65-1 Traditional and Functional Classifications of Shock States

Impaired oxygen delivery and altered oxygen consumption is common to all shock states.

TRADITIONAL CLASSIFICATION	FUNCTIONAL CLASSIFICATION
Neurogenic—loss of sympathetic tone	*Transport*—loss of sympathetic tone, anemia, and histamine release
Low hemoglobin (a form of distributive or transport shock)	Endotoxin release
Anaphylactic—hypersensitivity reaction (a form of distributive or transport shock)	
Septic—caused by microorganisms (a form of distributive or transport shock)	
Cardiogenic—diminished forward pumping capability, ischemia, and irregularity in heart beat	*Cardiogenic*—diminished forward pumping capability, ischemia, and irregularity in heart beat
Hypovolemic—loss of intravascular volume and low cardiac output	*Hypovolemic*—loss of intravascular volume and low cardiac output
	Obstructive—barriers to blood flow
	Pulmonary embolus (artery blocked), tension pneumothorax, cardiac tamponade, or great vessels kinked

Adapted from Walsh, C. (2005). Multiple organ dysfunction syndrome after multiple trauma. Orthopaedic Nursing, *24(5), 324–335.*

The Four Stages of the Shock Syndrome

The initial stage of the shock syndrome is marked by a decrease in cardiac output and impaired tissue perfusion. In the absence of oxygen, the cells switch to the anaerobic metabolism as a source of energy. However the formation of lactic acid contributes to muscle weakness and cell damage. The body attempts to remedy the problem by initiating the homeostatic mechanisms during the compensatory stage (e.g., the person may hyperventilate to eliminate the effects of acidosis), activation of the sympathetic nervous system causes the heart to beat faster, and blood is shifted to critical organs. As the shock process progresses, cellular damage prevents cells from functioning (Figure 65-2), and every system in the body is affected and is referred to as **multiple organ dysfunction syndrome (MODS)** or MOF. Finally, during the refractory stage, the body can no longer respond to therapy. The shock condition is considered irreversible. Because of the seriousness of the shock syndrome, most hospitalized patients receive care in the specialized intensive care units. The principle collaborative treatment goals are to identify and treat the underlying cause of the shock syndrome, deliver oxygen to the tissues, promote utilization of oxygen by the tissues, maintain surveillance for complications, and provide comfort and emotional support (Box 65-5) (Bench, 2004).

Planning and Implementation

In 2003, scientists representing 11 international organizations developed research-based guidelines for treatment of severe sepsis and septic shock to improve outcomes. The guidelines are clinically tested, updated annually, and updated as often as new information becomes available (Box 65-6). In general, hospitals continue to improve their abilities to manage critical incidents with patients (see Fast Forward feature). In addition, there are general assessments and interventions for patients with the shock syndrome (Box 65-7).

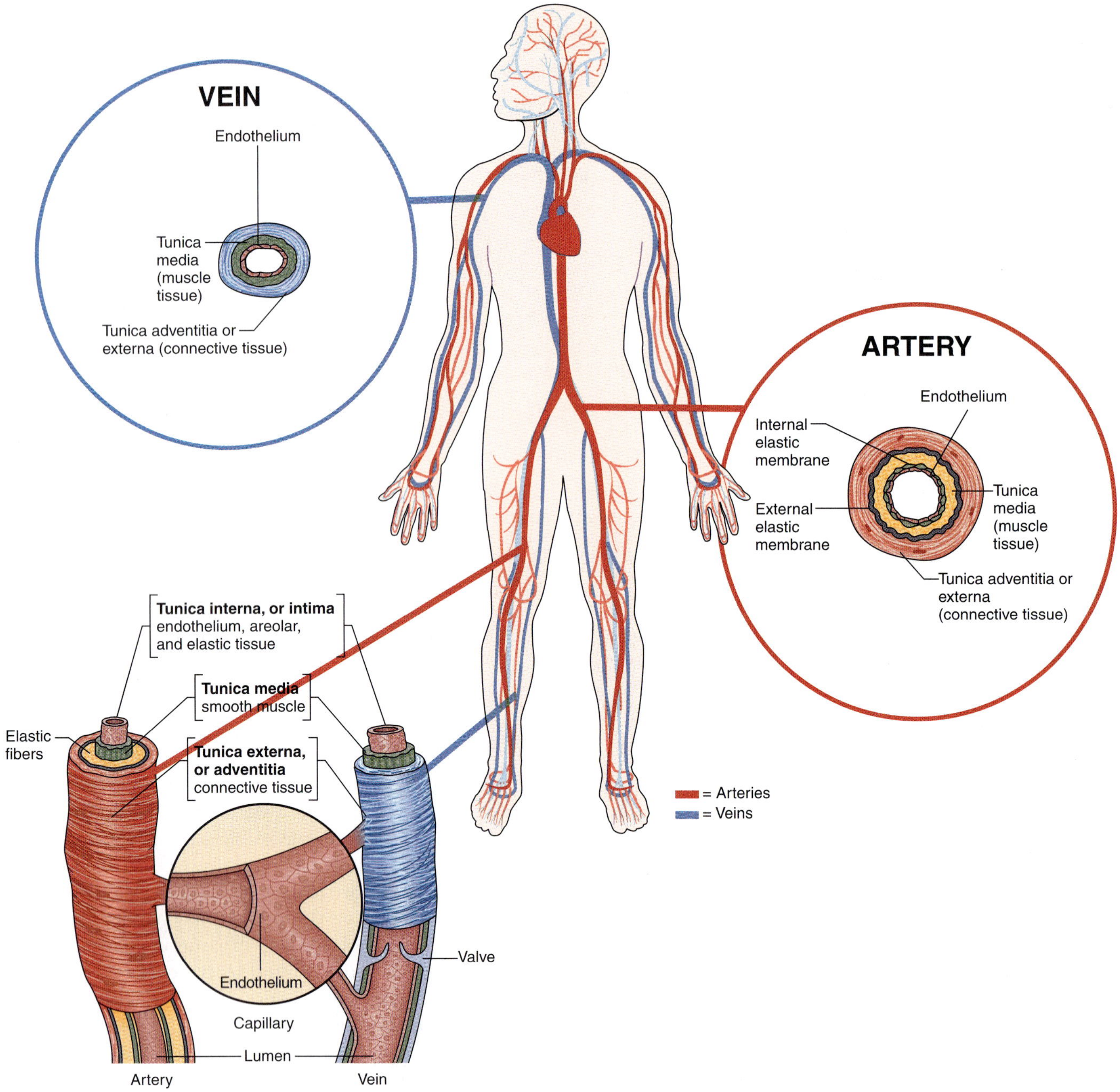

Figure 65-2 Generalized dilation of the blood vessels will cause a decrease in blood pressure as the affected fluid compartments become too enlarged.

Pediatric patients are more likely to need intubation because of low functional residual capacity and because intravenous (IV) access is difficult. Fluid resuscitation is based on weight with recommendation of 40–60 mL/kg or higher.

HYPOVOLEMIC SHOCK

The shock process is initiated by many types of injuries. These methods of initiating the shock syndrome are divided into five primary categories (hypovolemic cardiogenic, neurogenic, septic, and anaphylactic) as described in the following section. First, hypovolemic shock occurs when there is a lack of circulating fluid volume in the intravascular space. This type of shock can occur

Fast Forward ▶▶▶

100,000 Lives Campaign

The Institute for Healthcare Improvement ([IHI] 2005) reported that more than 2,600 hospitals across the United States have made a commitment to implement changes to improve patient care and to prevent avoidable deaths. The guidelines cover interventions to prevent adverse drug responses, to prevent surgical site and central venous line infections, and ventilation-associated pneumonias. Other interventions will be added and an evaluation of the outcomes of the campaign efforts is being assessed.

From IHI. (2005). 100,000 Lives Campaign. Retrieved June 14, 2006, from http://www.ihi.org.

BOX 65-5

ASSESSMENT AND DIAGNOSIS OF SHOCK

Common clinical manifestations of the shock syndrome will vary according to the underlying cause, the stage of shock, and the individual person's response to shock. The exact course of events can be variable. Each person must be assessed individually prior to any intervention.

- Regardless of the type of shock, it leads to a systolic blood pressure (SBP) less than 90 mm Hg and narrowing of pulse pressure that is inadequate to meet the tissue needs. (SBP may be elevated initially.)
- Early shock symptoms are subtle requiring close surveillance to avoid overlooking their presence.
- All persons in shock are at risk of deterioration in status. Prompt intervention is required.
- Nurses must have a clear understanding of the pathophysiology of the different etiologies of shock.
- In all instances of shock following a trauma incident, consider hypovolemia or hemorrhage unless proven otherwise.
- Shock is a frightening experience for the patient and family. Effective psychological support is essential.

Symptoms include:

- Hypothermia
- Tachycardia or bradycardia
- Rapid thready pulse, slow capillary refill, or collapse of superficial veins in extremities
- Altered mental status—dissociation from normal thought processes, detached, a feeling of numbness, and impaired sensory-emotional response. Loss of consciousness, restlessness, anxiety, irritability, and weakness may be present.
- Clinical findings correlated with organs compromised by inadequate oxygen supply and the phases of the shock syndrome.

Examples:

a. Skin: cold, clammy, cyanotic, poor capillary refill, or warm dry skin due to pooling of blood in extremities. Cyanosis (circumoral, earlobes, finger tips, or toes).
b. Kidneys: decreased urine output; anuria, or oliguria.
c. Lungs: dyspnea, crackles, or wheezes
d. GI system: thirst, dry mucous membranes; nausea and vomiting; or decreased bowel sounds

Adapted from Bench, S. (2004). Clinical skills: Assessing and treating shock: A nursing perspective. British Journal of Nursing, 13*(12), 715–721.*

with any loss of fluids in a manner that decreases the circulating plasma to effectually decrease blood pressure. A patient in hypovolemic shock can either lose fluids from the body or into different body fluid compartments and result in hypovolemic shock. Hypovolemia from whatever cause is the most common type of shock.

Etiology

Conditions that contribute to hypovolemic shock include dehydration, severe burn injuries, loss of intravascular volume, vasodilation due to neurogenic shock (loss of sympathetic tone), anaphylactic shock (release of histamine), and septic shock (release of endotoxin). Other contributing factors include

BOX 65-6

MANAGEMENT OF SEPTIC SHOCK

Research recommendations for treatment include:

The early goal-directed resuscitation procedures for the septic patient should be started during the first six hours after recognition of the problem.

- Use of diagnostic studies to identify the causative organism before administering antibiotics.
- Early administration of broad-spectrum antibiotics (usually a 7 to 10 day course).
- Ongoing physical assessment and reassessment of response to therapy.
- Administration of appropriate fluids.
- Administration of vasopressor medications.
- Administration of stress dose steroid therapy for septic shock. There is some concern about administering high-dose steroids.
- Use of recombinant activated protein C for patients with severe sepsis and at high risk for death. May be contraindicated if patient has coronary artery disease or acute hemorrhage.
- Establish hemoglobin target of 7 to 9 g/dL; appropriate use of blood products.
- Use of protective oxygen ventilation (low tidal volume) level to avoid lung damage. Follow protocols for weaning from mechanical ventilation and sedation or analgesia.
- Place patient in semirecumbent position unless contraindicated.
- Maintain blood glucose level less than 150 mg/dL after the patient is stable. Patients are at greater risk of hypoglycemia with aggressive glucose control methods.
- Monitor diagnostic studies for fluid and electrolyte balance, bicarbonate levels.
- Apply deep vein thrombosis (DVT) and stress ulcer prevention measures.

Adapted from Dellinger, R., Carlet, J., Masur, H., Gerlach, H. (2004). Surviving sepsis campaign guidelines for management of severe sepsis and septic shock. Critical Care Medicine, 32*(3), 858. Retrieved June 23, 2006, from www.survivingsepsis.com.*

vomiting, diarrhea, nasogastric suction, diuretic therapy, diabetes insipidus, trauma, surgery, and hyperglycemic osmotic diuresis.

Pathophysiology

An actual loss of fluid from the body, such as whole blood, is referred to as **absolute hypovolemia.** Normally, fluids in the intracellular and extracellular spaces remain the same and allow movement of water, electrolytes, and other substances to move back and forth. **Relative hypovolemia** refers to the shifting of fluid from the intravascular space to the extravascular, or interstitial, space that can result from a loss of intravascular integrity or increased capillary permeability or a decreased colloidal osmotic pressure.

Third spacing is the accumulation of fluid in the extracellular and intracellular spaces and in a third body, such as the intestine, that does not support circulation (Diehl-Oplinger & Kaminski, 2004). These events lead to a decrease in venous return to the heart and an eventual decrease in cardiac output and inadequate oxygen supply to body tissues.

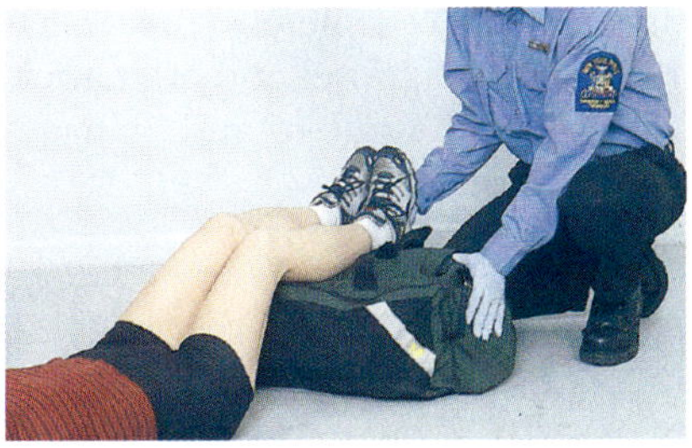

Figure 65-3 Elevation of the lower half of the body serves to allow increased blood flow to the brain and vital organs.

BOX 65-7

ASSESSMENT AND CARE OF SHOCK SYNDROME

The nurse should monitor signs and symptoms associated with alterations in body response to shock complications. Initially, the first responder should manage the patient with the immediate care interventions for patients suspected of the shock syndrome (e.g., position patient to maximize oxygen return to the brain, monitor pulse and breathing rates, keep normothermic, and administer oxygen) (Figure 65-3).

Initial Compensatory Stage

Body mechanisms are triggered to maintain adequate blood pressure and tissue perfusion. Subtle changes in baseline may be observed. Monitor heart rate and pulse, blood pressure, central venous pressure (CVP), respiratory rate core, peripheral temperature, and urinary output. Pulse oximetry may also be performed. Arterial gases are monitored for accurate assessment. Blood sampling for urea and electrolyte levels, full blood count, and glucose levels may also be performed. Elevated glucose levels are present with release of stress hormones such as cortisol.

Progressive Stage

Compensating mechanisms begin to fail. Symptoms are evident of inadequate organ perfusion. A full assessment should be done to identify any signs of blood or fluid loss, fluid shift as in ascites, infection, vomiting, or inadequate fluid intake.

Decompensated Stage

Failure of compensating mechanisms. No response to treatment. There is a great risk of cardiac arrest. A rising serum lactate is an indicator of inadequate tissue perfusion due to metabolic acidosis. Low arterial oxygen content, chest pain, cardiac dysrhythmias, altered level of consciousness (LOC), or low urinary output. MAPB cannot be maintained without assistance.

Adapted from Bench, S. (2004). Clinical skills: Assessing and treating shock: A nursing perspective. British Journal of Nursing, 13*(12), 715–721.*

Assessment with Clinical Manifestations

In hypovolemic shock, the compensatory systems attempt to maintain cardiac output. Initially, heart and respiratory rate increase and the depth of respirations increase to improve oxygenation; vasoconstriction is initiated to increase blood pressure. Later, urine output declines, and the skin becomes pale and cool with delayed capillary refill. Mental status changes due to poor oxygenation include disorientation, restlessness, anxiousness, and decreased levels of consciousness. As these compensatory mechanisms become overwhelmed (usually with the loss of 30–40 percent or 1,500–2,000 mL of fluid) tissue perfusion is impaired. Clinical manifestations include hypotension and possible orthostatic changes in blood pressure. Cardiac output will be diminished and pressures will be low in the right atrium, the pulmonary artery, and the left ventricle because of the diminished blood volume return. In shock caused by anemia or hemorrhage, hematocrit and hemoglobin levels will be low. Respiratory distress will be evident; metabolic acidosis and **hypoxemia** are present. Hypoxemia, a decreased concentration of oxygen in the blood, is measured by arterial oxygen partial pressure (PaO_2). With the loss of 40 percent or more of fluid volume, the compensatory systems fail completely (Box 65-8). Symptoms of MODS develop (Walsh, 2005). Nursing diagnoses and evaluation of outcomes are shown in Table 65-2. A listing of manifestations and management can be found in Box 65-8 and Box 65-9, respectively.

Planning and Implementation

Hypovolemic shock is treated aggressively to correct the cause and to rapidly restore perfusion to the body tissues, especially the brain and heart. Administration of fluids is usually dependent on the type of fluid that is lost.

TABLE 65-2 Examples of Nursing Diagnoses, NIC, and NOC Related to All Shock Syndromes

NANDA NURSING DIAGNOSES	NURSING INTERVENTIONS (NIC)	EXPECTED PATIENT OUTCOMES (NOC)
Airway		
Impaired gas exchange (related to specific cause) Impaired spontaneous ventilation	Shock management Airway management Airway insertion and stabilization Resuscitation Ventilation assistance	Respiratory status: Airway patency, gas exchange, ventilation stabilization
Cardiac		
Decreased cardiac output (related to specific cause)	Cardiac care, acute Cardiac precautions Vital signs monitoring	Cardiac pump effectiveness Circulation status effective
Fluids		
Deficient fluid volume Risk for deficient fluid volume Risk for fluid imbalance	Fluid and electrolyte management Acid-base management (metabolic/respiratory) Blood products administration Hypovolemia management Intravenous therapy	Electrolyte and acid-base balance Energy conservation
Tissue Perfusion		
Imbalanced nutrition, less than body requirements Ineffective tissue Perfusion (related to: renal, cerebral, cardiopulmonary, gastrointestinal, or peripheral)	Nutrition management Implement fluid management strategies	Tissue perfusion (cardiac, cerebral, peripheral, or pulmonary) Nutritional status: biochemical measures controlled
Mental		
Acute confusion Spiritual distress Anxiety Ineffective coping	Cerebral perfusion promotion Anxiety reduction Coping enhancement (patient and family)	Anxiety control Hope Coping appropriate (patient and family) Knowledge: disease process
Output		
Impaired urinary elimination	Urinary elimination management	Urinary elimination adequate

Adapted from DeLaune, S., & Ladner, P. (2006). Fundamentals of nursing *(3rd ed.). New York: Thomson Delmar Learning; Walsh, C. (2005). Multiple organ dysfunction syndrome after multiple trauma.* Orthopaedic Nursing, *24(5), 324–335.*

BOX 65-8

SELECTED MANIFESTATIONS OF HYPOVOLEMIC SHOCK

Tachycardia

Pulse pressure narrows as the diastolic increases

Tachypnea and increase in depth of respirations (may gasp for breath)

Decline in urine output

Skin pale, cool, delayed capillary refill

Jugular veins appear flat

Decreased cerebral perfusion and a change in level of consciousness (LOC)

Disoriented, confused, restless, anxious, or irritable

BOX 65-9

MANAGEMENT OF HYPOVOLEMIC SHOCK

The nurse should:

- Implement measures to minimize fluid loss.
- Monitor fluid replacement process. This includes insertion and management of large diameter intravenous (IV) catheters, IV lines and connections; administration of prescribed fluids and medications. Also, the nurse must understand the advantages, limitations, and the implications associated with the different types of fluid. Blood products can initiate a secondary shock due to infection and anaphylaxis. Observe for local or generalized rash and urticaria. Document and report findings.
- Monitor vital signs (including bradycardia or tachycardia); temperature changes, pulmonary artery pressure (PAP); pulmonary artery wedge pressure (PAWP), which measures pulmonary artery and left ventricle pressures; right atrial pressure (RAP). Positioning the patient with legs elevated, trunk flat, and head and shoulders above the chest (modified Trendelenburg position).
- Monitor for manifestations of fluid overload, such as changes in respirations or respiratory distress; assess lung sounds for crackles and rhonchi; assess changes in heart sounds and heart rate; and monitor urinary output (usually via retention catheter).
- Monitor laboratory results (Check for alterations in the coagulation process, white blood cell [WBC] level for infection and hemoglobin and hematocrit levels).
- Observe patient for signs of infection (IV insertion site and lungs).
- Monitor mental status, changes in skin condition or appearance.
- Administer analgesics.
- Provide positions for comfort; provide a calm environment.
- Limit activities to promote conservation of oxygen supply.
- Educate patient and family regarding measures to reduce anxiety.

The choices include crystalloid or colloid solutions or a combination of both. The military antishock trousers (MAST) are used in severe crisis to assist in controlling hemorrhage and to provide blood pressure support. Another garment, the pneumatic antishock garment (PASG) fits like a pair of trousers and covers the lower extremities and the trunk. This intervention is often used in the prehospital management of trauma victims.

The primary goals of are to minimize fluid loss, to enhance fluid replacement (Table 65-3), and to monitor the patient responses to interventions. Identification of patients at risk for hypovolemic shock and careful monitoring of fluid balance are important prevention strategies.

CARDIOGENIC SHOCK

Cardiogenic shock results in the failure of either the right or left ventricle or both to provide an adequate delivery of oxygen to the body tissues due to a weakened forward pumping function of the heart. Precipitating factors can be a myocardial infarction, irregular rate or rhythm, or cardiomyopathy. This type of shock commonly occurs when more than 40 percent of the myocardium is irreversibly damaged.

TABLE 65-3 Types of Parenteral Fluid Replacement

SOLUTION CLASSIFICATION	SOLUTION EXAMPLES	UTILIZATION	PRECAUTIONS
Crystalloids—solutions that mimic the body's extracellular fluid	*Isotonic* (same tonicity as plasma) 0.9% Saline Ringer's solution Ringer's lactate solution	Use for fluid losses due to vomiting, diarrhea, surgery, and prior to blood transfusion	Monitor for fluid excess or overload.
	Hypotonic 0.45% saline	To move fluid into intracellular compartment Use when sodium restriction is required	Monitor patient closely. Overload can cause intravascular fluid depletion, hypotension, cellular edema, and tissue damage.
	Hypertonic 3–5% saline Concentrated dextrose in water added to amino acid solutions.	Use to relieve cellular edema and correct hypoglycemia and provide calories	Raise risk for volume overload. Monitor closely, especially persons with heart failure.
Colloids: contain undissolved protein, sugar, and starch molecules that are too large to pass through capillary walls	Albumen (5% isotonic with no clotting components) Albumen 25%	Use to expand intravascular volume. Have same effects as hypertonic crystalloid solutions. Given in smaller volumes	Monitor closely because solutions have longer duration of action.
Blood and blood products	Whole blood	Whole blood used to replace red blood cells (RBCs), white blood cells (WBCs), platelets, and plasma	Rarely used if more than 24 hours old. Monitor for allergic reactions. *Can trigger anaphylactic shock* Administer over one to two hours or within four hours.
	Packed RBCs	Replace RBCs and delivery of oxygen to tissues	
	Plasma	Replace albumin, globulins, antibodies, proteins, and clotting factors	
Pharmaceutical plasma expanders	Dextran	Draws water into the intravascular space	Monitor closely for fluid volume deficit.
	Mannitol (sugar/alcohol substance dissolved in 0.9% saline)	Decrease intracranial pressure due to cerebral edema, reverse cerebrospinal fluid buildup; lower intraocular pressure. Produces osmotic diuresis	

Adapted from Diehl-Oplinger, L., & Kaminski, M. (2004). Choosing the right fluid to counter hypovolemic shock. Nursing, 34*(3), 52–54.*

Pathophysiology

In cardiogenic shock there is an impaired forward pumping function with a decreased stroke volume and decreased cardiac output of the left ventricle. This dysfunction results in a backup of blood into the pulmonary system causing edema and impaired gas exchange. Therefore, a reduction in oxygenated arterial blood further decreases tissue perfusion throughout the body and is followed by metabolic acidosis.

Assessment with Clinical Manifestations

Clinical manifestations of right ventricle failure are associated with systemic venous congestion (e.g., fatigue, dependent edema, jugular vein distension, liver engorgement, ascites, or cyanosis). The patient in cardiogenic shock may exhibit a heart rate greater than 100 beats per minute, a weak, thready pulse, diminished heart sounds and dysrhythmias, tachypnea and adventitious lung sounds, cool, pale, moist skin, and chest pains. Renal failure is evident by a decreased urine output, and there is a decreased level of consciousness due to hypoperfusion of brain tissue. Cardiopulmonary collapse may be the cause of death (Johnson, 2005). Review Table 65-2 for nursing diagnoses and evaluation of outcomes.

Edema and weight gain are also prominent clinical manifestations of cardiogenic shock (Box 65-10). Edema is most often developed in dependent areas of the body. Accumulation of 1 liter of fluid is evidenced by a weight gain of 1 kg or 2.2 pounds. A weight gain of 2 pounds in 24 hours or 5 pounds in a week is considered as a sign of additional heart or kidney failure. Daily monitoring of the patient's weight, intake, and output is an important assessment tool. Recall that an intake that exceeds output indicates a positive fluid balance that can result in fluid volume overload. The reverse condition occurs when output (due to fever, increased perspiration, vomiting, diarrhea, gastric suction, or diuretic therapy) exceeds fluid intake. Urine output and insensible fluid losses, such as perspiration, stool, and water vapor from lungs can vary from 750–2,400 mL/day. Elimination of 30 mL per hour or 400 mL/day is considered to be an approximate estimate of renal function. Central venous pressure (CVP) and arterial pressure measures can accurately reflect alterations in vascular volume returning to and being ejected from the heart. The nurse can also assess fluid status by assessing the skin turgor, moisture of mucous membranes, presence of edema or ascites, diaphoresis, low-grade fever, neck and hand vein engorgement, "crackles" in lungs, dyspnea, tachycardia, blood pressure changes, S_3 and S_4 sounds, headache, blurred vision, vertigo on rising, papilledema, and mental changes (Estes, 2006).

BOX 65-10

SELECTED MANIFESTATIONS OF CARDIOGENIC SHOCK

- Hypotension—Systolic blood pressure less than 90 mm Hg
- Heart rate greater than 100 beats per minute
- Weak thready pulse
- Diminished heart sounds
- Change in level of consciousness (LOC)
- Cool, pale, moist skin
- Urine output less than 30 mL/hour
- Chest pain
- Dysrhythmias
- Tachypnea
- Crackle breath sounds
- Decreased cardiac output

Planning and Implementation

Treatment includes an aggressive approach to treat the underlying cause, to enhance the pumping mechanism of the heart, and to improve tissue perfusion. Procedures are dependent on whether cardiogenic shock is caused by right-sided or left-sided heart failure. The goals of treatment for right-sided heart failure are directed toward improving right ventricular stroke volumes and to restore filling of the left ventricle. Examples include vasodilators, such as nitroglycerin, fluids, vasopressors (e.g., dopamine to support an appropriate blood pressure), and the use of IV medications, such as dobutamine, to stimulate more forceful contractions of the heart. The goals of treatment for left-sided heart failure are to increase the left ventricle contractions and to prevent the progression of right-sided heart failure. Examples of treatments include supplemental oxygen, mechanical intubation, and administration of diuretics and inotropic drugs to increase ventricle contractility and cardiac output. Cardiac monitoring and close observation are essential. Analgesics are given to relieve pain and to decrease myocardial oxygen demand. Morphine is frequently used to improve coronary perfusion by dilating the coronary vessels and to alleviate pain and anxiety. The intra-aortic balloon pump (IABP) is used to improve the oxygen supply to the myocardium. The ventricular assist device (VAD) is used as a temporary measure to replace the function of the left ventricle, allowing it to rest and heal. In some instances, coronary angioplasty and coronary artery bypass grafting is performed.

BOX 65-11

NURSING INTERVENTIONS FOR A PATIENT IN CARDIOGENIC SHOCK

The nurse should:

- Administer the prescribed fluids and medications.
- Administer supplemental oxygen and monitoring patient response.
- Monitor vital signs; observe for thready pulse, change in heart sounds, chest pain; changes in respirations or respiratory distress; assess lung sounds for crackles and rhonchi.
- Monitor patients on intra-aortic balloon pump (IABP) for complications, e.g., formation of emboli, infection, aortic rupture, improper balloon placement, function, or rupture, bleeding, and complications related to the cannulated extremity.
- Monitor laboratory results and intake and output.
- Monitor mental status, changes in skin condition or appearance.
- Administer analgesics to diminish the myocardial oxygen consumption.
- Provide positions for comfort; provide a calm environment.
- Educate patient and family regarding measures to reduce anxiety.
- Limit activities to promote conservation of oxygen supply.
- Additional interventions are similar to management of patients in hypovolemic shock.

Nursing interventions for a patient in cardiogenic shock include (a) promoting adequate supply of oxygen to the myocardium, (b) limiting myocardial consumption of oxygen, and (c) monitoring the patient's responses to interventions. For specific nursing interventions refer to Box 65-11.

ANAPHYLACTIC SHOCK

Almost any substance can cause a hypersensitivity response involving the interaction of an antibody and antigen. The antigen substances can consist of several foods including eggs and milk, shellfish, peanuts, chocolate, strawberries and tomatoes; food additives; diagnostic agents, such as iodine; blood, gamma globulin; vaccines and antitoxins; latex allergies; molds or fungus, animal dander and hair; drugs, insect stings, and venoms.

Pathophysiology

When the body is exposed to a foreign substance, or antigen, the immune system creates antibodies against it. The antibodies will recognize the specific antigen when the body is exposed to it a second time, and they attempt to destroy the antigen via **phagocytosis** (surrounding and destruction of particulate matter by phagocyte cells). This process serves as an important bodily defense mechanism against infection by microorganisms and against occlusion of mucous surfaces or tissues by foreign particles and tissue debris. Anaphylactic shock is caused by an exaggerated widespread antibody response following a previous exposure to the antigen. It can be life-threatening due to constricted bronchioles, acute respiratory distress, severe hypotension, tachycardia, hypovolemia, and inadequate blood supply to body tissues. Edema of the airways, particularly the larynx impedes airflow to the lungs.

The antibody-antigen response triggers the mast cells to release the mediators histamine, eosinophilic chemotactic factor of anaphylaxis (ECF-A), neutrophilic chemotactic factor of anaphylaxis (NCF-A), proteinases, heparin, serotonin, leukotrienes prostaglandins, and platelet-activating factor (PAF).

Assessment with Clinical Manifestations

Responses in anaphylactic shock include vasodilation, increased capillary permeability, broncho-constriction and inflammation, and stimulation of nerve endings in cutaneous tissues that produce sensations of warmth, itching, and pain. Some patients complain of abdominal cramping. Constriction of coronary vessels causes severe myocardial depression. Venous return from peripheral tissues is impaired. Decreased oxygen supply to the cellular tissues leads to impaired cellular metabolism. Death often results from airway obstruction or cardiovascular collapse or both. This is a form of transport shock in the functional classification (Walsh, 2005).

Reports of latex (natural rubber product) allergy, especially in health care, have increased in recent years. The frequent use of latex gloves to prevent the transmission of infections places individuals with hypersensitivities at risk for developing minor to serious problems. An alert was published by the National Institute for Occupational Safety and Health (NIOSH) in 1997, which provided information on the problem, and they made available a pamphlet describing prevention measures, The hypersensitivity reactions are to the proteins in the latex itself or to chemicals added to the rubber during harvesting. It is also believed that the proteins could be trapped in the powder. The most common reaction is contact dermatitis resulting in skin rashes, hives, flushing, itching, nasal, eye, or sinus problems. When the gloves are changed, the powder can become airborne and inhaled; for susceptible individuals, asthma may be the result. Some individuals with latex-induced asthma have had life-threatening anaphylactic reactions.

A comprehensive history is a valuable tool in the prevention of anaphylactic shock. A detailed description of the patient's allergies should be clearly documented and communicated to other health care personnel. Anyone can experience anaphylaxis to a foreign substance; however, it is more common in people who have a history of allergies and previous anaphylactic reactions. Patients with asthma also have a heightened immune response. The nurse must be able to anticipate the typical allergic reactions (Box 65-12) to an antigen substance and be able to intervene in this life-threatening event. Refer to Table 65-2 for nursing diagnoses and evaluation of outcomes.

BOX 65-12

CLINICAL MANIFESTATIONS OF ANAPHYLACTIC SHOCK

- Hypotension
- Tachycardia
- Decreased cardiac output
- Stridor
- Wheezing
- Rales and rhonchi
- Dysphagia
- Pruritus—Urticaria
- Erythema
- Angioedema
- Restlessness, uneasiness, apprehension, and anxiety
- Decreased level of consciousness (LOC)
- Nausea, vomiting, and diarrhea
- Incontinence or vaginal bleeding
- Complaints of feeling warm, dyspneic, itching, abdominal cramping, and pain

Planning and Implementation

The care for anaphylactic shock begins with prevention. Preventive measures include avoiding the use of latex gloves, using gloves with no powder, avoiding the use of oil-based hand creams, and washing the hands with soap and water and drying thoroughly after wearing gloves. Frequent cleaning of areas where dust containing powder should be done. Individuals with hypersensitivity to latex should wear an alert bracelet and have an Epi-Pen which is an injectable vial of epinephrine.

Nurses should be aware that other latex products are balloons, condoms, catheters, clothing elastic, carpet backing, some upholstery materials, and dishwashing gloves. Some medication vials have latex stoppers; administration of the medication can produce a severe reaction in people with hypersensitivities. Assessment of the patient's allergy history is important. Reactions are more prevalent for individuals with dermatitis, eczema, rhinitis, and asthma. Susceptible individuals may also react to avocados, bananas, chestnuts, kiwi fruit, and poinsettia plants (Hamilton, Brown, Veltri, Feroli, Primeau, Schauble, et al., 2005; Hathaway, 2005; McNulty, 2005; Smith, Wallace, & Smith-Campbell, 2004).

Nursing interventions for a patient in anaphylactic shock include a wide variety of management strategies. A priority is facilitating ventilation by ensuring a patent airway, positioning the patient, and instructing the patient to breathe slowly and deeply. Then the nurse must observe for dyspnea, hoarseness, and stridor, which are early signs of laryngeal edema. In addition, the nurse must monitor the vital signs and assess for common manifestations of decreased cardiac output (e.g., hypotension, rapid pulse, cyanosis, or dysrhythmias). The nurse also must monitor the effectiveness of prescribed oxygen therapy (Note: immediate oxygenation may be by a nonrebreather mask, and endotracheal intubation or tracheostomy may be necessary). To correct the fluid compartment issues, the nurse will likely insert a large diameter IV catheter, administering the prescribed fluids and medications, and monitor the flow of fluids. The patient must be positioned with his or her legs elevated and head and shoulders above the chest. Administration of medications may be given to relieve itching. The patient may be provided warm soaks to skin and gloves (if needed) to discourage scratching. Due to the likelihood of renal failure and renal dysfunction, the patient is monitored for a cessation of urinary output. In general the patient's and family's teaching needs are important (e.g., spiritual, psychological, and emotional needs). Last discharge planning must be implemented throughout the patient's hospitalization. The patient must be educated on how to avoid future anaphylactic reactions, instructed to wear a medical alert bracelet, and carry information that lists allergies (Smith, et al, 2004).

Goals

The primary goals of treatment include removal of the antigen if possible, reversing the effects of the biochemical mediators, and promoting adequate tissue perfusion. Support to the patient's airways is provided by administering supplemental oxygen, intubation, and mechanical ventilation if needed. In some instances, the patient may experience respiratory or cardiac arrest and cardiopulmonary resuscitation is initiated.

Pharmacology

Medications, such as IV epinephrine or via an endotracheal tube, are given to promote bronchodilation and vasoconstriction and to prevent further secretion of the mediators. Benadryl (diphenhydramine hydrochloride) is given to block the release of histamine, and corticosteroids are administered to prevent or reduce inflammation and to help stabilize the capillary membranes. Crystalloid (balanced salt solutions, such as normal saline, lactated Ringer's, and 5% glucose in water) or colloid solutions, such as hetastarch, mannitol, and dextran, which contain oncotic substances to expand intravascular volume, are given as fluid replacement. Lactated Ringer's solution contains sodium, potassium calcium chloride, and lactate. It is contraindicated for people with renal or liver disease or in lactic acidosis. Inotropic and vasoconstrictor drugs are often given to increase myocardial contraction and to reverse vasodilation. Box 65-13 includes information on pharmacological shock.

NEUROGENIC SHOCK

Neurogenic shock is usually a transient condition that occurs in the absence or suppression of sympathetic nervous system tone and is considered in the functional hypovolemic shock classification. This type of shock can be caused by anything that disrupts the transmission of an impulse to the hypothalamus, the sympathetic vasomotor center in the brain, or anything that blocks the outflow of the sympathetic response.

Pathophysiology

Loss of sympathetic tone results in massive peripheral vasodilation, loss of temperature regulation, loss of sympathetic tone to the heart, and diminished baroreceptor response to changes in blood pressure. The skin temperature becomes the same as the room temperature (poikilothermia), and because of the inability to sweat, the skin feels dry to the touch. There is an increased risk

Red Flag

Heat Stroke

Over 8,966 heat-related deaths were reported from 1979 to 2002 in the Untied States. The deadly heat wave in 2005 resulted in over 415 deaths related to dehydration and heat stroke, particularly along the Southwestern border of the United States. Many of the victims were migrants, people without shelter, and the elderly. Similar accounts were made during the heat wave across Europe in 2003. High death rates in India and southeast Asia occur annually during premonsoon high temperatures. There is a greater loss of lives worldwide because of extreme heat; yet is not classified as a natural disaster. A person's temperature is regulated by the CNS; the hypothalamus is the primary control mechanism, or thermostat. The sympathetic nervous system is responsible for vasodilation of the skin and initiates the natural sweating process to cool the body. However, profuse sweating depletes the body of essential salts and fluids. The person may experience heat exhaustion that can progress to heat stroke. The temperature can rise to 40.6°C (105° F). Hyperthermia causes increases in metabolic rate and demand for oxygen. Multiple organs are at risk of dysfunction and failure with sustained body temperature above 40°C (104° F). Manifestations of heat stroke include thirst, cessation of sweating, acute painful muscle spasms due to sodium depletion, rapid pulse and respirations, initial hypertension followed by hypotension, sudden delirium, or coma. Without prompt interventions to cool the body, replace fluids and electrolytes, the person's condition can deteriorate and death quickly follows.

BOX 65-13

PHARMACOLOGICAL SHOCK

Any drug has the potential for eliciting a shock response. Hypotension as a side effect of drugs, such as opiates, sedatives, hypnotics, beta blockers, anticholinergics, antidepressants, nitrates, and antihypertensive agents, is a major factor in initiating the shock response.

Treatment consists of (a) stopping the drug, eliminating drug from the body via gastric lavage or administration of charcoal; (b) administration of antidote naloxone for opiates; flumazenil for benzodiazepines; (c) providing airway and cardiac support; supporting fluid balance with crystalloid fluids, and vasopressors (Broyles, Reiss, & Evans, 2007). The nurse must be knowledgeable about the potential side effects of each drug being administered.

- Careful monitoring of vital signs, including alterations in cardiac, respiratory, and mental status (The frequency of monitoring will depend on the stability of the patient).

In addition, the patient may have an anaphylactic reaction to a specific drug.

- The nurse should be knowledgeable about the patient's allergy and medical history and previous response to drugs.
- Emergency equipment must be readily available (The patient may need to be moved closer to the nurse's station or intensive care unit for close monitoring).

Adapted from Bench, S. (2004). Clinical skills: Assessing and treating shock. A nursing perspective. British Journal of Nursing, 13*(12), 715–721; Hinson, G. (2005).* Shock management. *Retrieved July 6, 2006, from http://www.cdi.pub.ro.*

of developing deep vein thrombosis (DVT) in the lower extremities. Neurogenic shock often occurs with a spinal cord injury above the midthoracic region when blood vessels lose the ability to constrict, and continuing parasympathetic impulses allow vasodilation (Figure 65-4). Blood pools in the peripheral veins, venous return to the right side of the heart is inadequate, and cardiac output is decreased. Other causes include central nervous system (CNS) dysfunction, spinal anesthesia, and drugs. The end result is a decrease in delivery of oxygenated blood to body tissues.

Assessment with Clinical Manifestations

Neurogenic shock has similar clinical manifestations as those listed in the opening section of the discussion of shock syndrome. In addition, the following are typical manifestations of neurogenic shock: hypotension, bradycardia, hypothermia, warm dry skin, decreased cardiac rate and output, decreased venous return, and flaccid paralysis below spinal injury. These signifying manifestations are those that are specific to neurogenic shock and somewhat different by comparison. The paralysis and warm, dry skin are not seen commonly with the other types of shock conditions. In addition, neurogenic shock is not the same as autonomic dysreflexia, which is described in detail in chapter 36. Refer to Table 65-2 for nursing diagnoses and evaluation of outcomes.

Planning and Implementation

Fluid distribution is disrupted throughout the body; therefore the goal is to establish circulatory blood volume, administer appropriate fluids, and monitor fluid overload. Inotropic and vasoconstrictor drugs are often given to increase sympathetic tone and myocardial contraction and to reverse vasodilation if

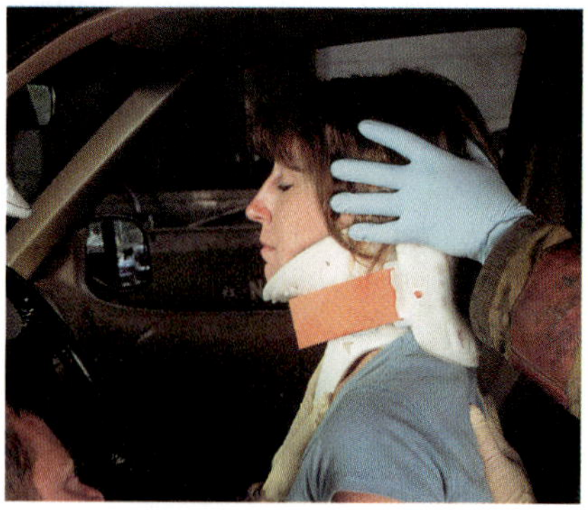

Figure 65-4 Spinal cord injuries often precede neurogenic shock.

sufficient tissue perfusion is still present. A low dose of a corticosteroid is often given to minimize inflammation (Ahrens & Vollman, 2004). Atropine is given to counteract bradycardia due to parasympathetic overstimulation of the heart. Temporary cardiac pacing may be necessary to assist in cardiac output. Assessment using the Glasgow Coma Scale is important if there is cerebral damage, and the patient must be closely monitored for further deterioration in multiple systems (Bench, 2004).

Priority nursing interventions are focused on treating the hypovolemia, promoting normal body temperature, preventing hypoxemia, and monitoring for dysrhythmias. Identification of patients at risk for neurogenic shock and careful monitoring of fluid balance are important prevention strategies. Patients are at risk of DVT because of venous pooling in the lower extremities. The nurse must administer prescribed fluids and monitor patient's response to compensate for the fluid imbalances in the neurogenic shock. The nurse must monitor for manifestations of fluid overload, such as changes in respirations or respiratory distress; assess lung sounds for crackles and rhonchi; assess changes in heart sounds and heart rate; and monitor urinary output usually via retention catheter. In addition, the nurse should monitor specific laboratory results (e.g., coagulation factors, white blood cell [WBC] levels for infection, and hemoglobin or hematocrit levels). Due to the nature of the neurogenic shock, the patient must be observed for signs of infection (e.g., IV insertion site and lungs). The nurse must monitor for evidence of DVT, including leg and foot edema and measurement of calf and thigh circumference. The application is to use prescribed antiembolic stockings or sequential pneumatic stockings, provide passive range of motion exercises, and administer prescribed anticoagulation therapy. To avoid severe complications, the nurse should also assess for signs of pulmonary embolism (e.g., shortness of breath, respiratory distress, and chest pain). Limit activities to promote conservation of oxygen supply. The patient is monitored in regard to his or her mental status, changes in skin condition and appearance. Comfort measures are employed to minimize anxiety and spiritual distress. Last, the patient and family are educated regarding measures to reduce anxiety.

SEPTIC SHOCK

Sepsis is a systemic response to infection that involves the systemic inflammatory process resulting in endothelial dysfunction and altered circulation and coagulation. Severe sepsis is associated with one or more organ dysfunctions because of hypotension or hypoperfusion of tissues. Symptoms may include lactic acidosis, oliguria, and acute changes in mental status.

Pathophysiology

Septic shock is a complex systemic response that involves action of cellular and humoral (body fluids and components of the immune system) against any type of microorganism that invades the body, including gram-negative and gram-positive bacteria, fungi, and viruses. Gram-negative bacteria are considered to be a major cause of septic shock. The microorganisms secrete endotoxins that stimulate capillary permeability and release of mediators which results in increased complement activity, leukopenia, and leukocytosis. Diagnostic studies can confirm the presence of infection; however, in some cases, the source of infection is not identified. Dilation of the vascular bed affects cardiac function and the coagulation cascade, resulting in disseminated intravascular coagulation (DIC) can be triggered by septic shock.

Assessment with Clinical Manifestations

Early symptoms may include a rising core temperature, increase in WBC count, or a rise in C-reactive protein. Manifestations often mimic the criteria established for systemic inflammatory response syndrome (SIRS). A patient

Dollars and Sense

Financial Impact of Sepsis

Severe sepsis causing multiple organ malfunctions has affected 3,234,000 people worldwide since 2001, with an estimated death rate of 927,000 people. It currently affects 750,000 Americans each year and is the cause of more than 200,000 deaths. Sepsis is the leading cause of death in intensive care units. It is estimated that annual costs in the United States are more than $15 billion. Sepsis is expected to affect one million people by the end of the decade as the population ages. It has increased for children and adults in the last 20 years. Proposed causes are overuse of antibiotics and development of drug-resistant microbes. Health care providers are also able to diagnose signs and symptoms much earlier than they were previously.

Adapted from Bridges, E., & Dukes, S. (2005). Cardiovascular aspects of septic shock: Pathophysiology, monitoring, and treatment. Critical Care Nurse, *25(2), 14–16, 18–20.*

history is important for identifying the possible etiology. Potential etiologies of septic shock include: bowel surgery, severe malnutrition, multiple antibiotic therapy or immunosuppressant therapy, prolonged hospitalization, and exposure to nosocomial infection (Kleinpell, 2005).

The patient exhibits at least two signs of SIRS and at least one organ is dysfunctional or has failed. Additional manifestations include chills, hypotension, widened pulse pressure, decreased skin perfusion, and decreased urine output. In addition, the patient with sepsis will often experience significant edema or positive fluid balance (greater than 20 mL/kg over 24 hours), a decreased capillary refill or mottling, hyperglycemia (plasma glucose greater than 120 mg/dL in the absence of diabetes, and a decreased bicarbonate (HCO_3^-), and an unexplained change in mental status (Kleinpell, 2005). Refer to Table 65-2 for the nursing diagnoses and evaluation of outcomes.

Planning and Implementation

Identification and elimination of the cause as soon as possible are paramount in the treatment of septic shock. Blood cultures are taken, and antibiotic therapy is initiated as soon as possible to prevent the progression to severe sepsis and shock. Supplemental oxygen and respiratory or ventilation support is provided, and the patient is transferred to a critical care unit if necessary. IV access is established, and fluid is administered to improve blood pressure. Inotropic medications, such as dobutamine, are often prescribed to assist with the force of cardiac contractions. Cardiac monitoring (electrocardiogram [ECG]) for possible dysrhythmias is initiated. Antipyretic therapy is administered to relieve fever after consideration is given to the stage of fever and the patient status. Strict universal precautions and prevention of secondary infection are important aspects of care. Prophylactic measures are taken to avoid DVT and stress ulcers. Steroids are administered for patients who have relative adrenal insufficiency.

Sepsis can develop quickly. The nurse must be skilled in recognizing dysfunction of any organ to prevent the progression of severe sepsis. The pulmonary and cardiovascular systems are the most common to show early signs of dysfunction. However, by the time that severe sepsis is recognized, it has already affected many areas of the body. Arterial blood pressure is the best indicator of blood flow. Appropriate tissue oxygenation is indicated by a normal blood pressure and a normal central venous pressure (about 60–75 percent). This means

Uncovering the Evidence

New Drug Reduces Mortality in Severe Sepsis

Discussion: International clinical trials were conducted to evaluate the effectiveness of drotrecogin alfa, activated (Xigris) to improve survival in severe sepsis based on the theory that the drug could minimize the affects of the inflammatory response to infection. The drug, which is a recombinant form of human activated protein C, mimics the human protein that (a) inhibits the production of thrombin and prevents clot formation, (b) inhibits the release of plasminogen activator inhibitor-1, and (c) blocks thrombin formation. Therefore, the microvascular thrombi that form can be broken down, and perfusion of tissues would be improved as well potential restoration of organ function. The study consisted of a large double-blind, placebo controlled international study. Xigris is the first drug found to improve survival in severe sepsis. There is a risk of bleeding, although only slightly higher than in patients receiving a placebo. Approximately 80 percent of the drug's effects will be cleared from the system within 30 minutes.
Implications for Practice: Although, Xigris has proven to be beneficial, the costs are prohibitive, at $6,800 for a 96-hour infusion. Strict guidelines have been established for the use of the treatment.

Adapted from Ahrens, T., & Vollman, K. (2003). Severe sepsis management: Are we doing enough? Critical Care Nurse, *24(Suppl 2), 2–16.*

that approximately 25–40 percent of oxygen is available in the blood to be extracted by the tissues to support metabolism.

The primary goals are to provide the prescribed antibiotics, fluids, and vasopressor drugs, preventing secondary infections, monitoring the fluid and electrolyte balance, and assessing the patient's response to care. The nurse must be constantly alert to subtle changes that can indicate a progression of the septic process.

Therapeutic nursing interventions for patients with septic shock include implementing standard precautions and monitoring diagnostic reports, including blood glucose levels, clotting dysfunction (e.g., activated partial thromboplastin time [APTT], and international normalized ratio [INR], or prothrombin time [PT], and platelets abnormalities). The nurse must also manage the airway, administer oxygen, supervise ventilatory support, and monitor the patient's response to airway management. The nurse must administer prescribed medications and assess the patient's response, followed by documenting the findings and providing information to appropriate team members. The administration of fluid and nutritional therapy (including blood product administration), along with monitoring and recording intake and output, is essential to the patient's positive progression. In addition, the nurse must provide comfort measures, such as warm blankets or cooling methods, and provide emotional support. Last, the patient and his or her family need education regarding the management strategies that are employed and measures to reduce anxiety.

SYSTEMIC INFLAMMATORY RESPONSE SYNDROME

Recall that infection need not be present for the IIR to be initiated. However, an uncontrolled acute inflammatory response that causes inflammation in multiple organs that are remote from the original insult is defined as the

BOX 65-14

CLINICAL MANIFESTATIONS OF SIRS

At least two or more of the following symptoms will be present in SIRS:

- Fever greater than 38° C (98.6°F) or less than 36° C (96°F) or inability to maintain a normal temperature
- Tachycardia greater than 90 beats per minute
- Tachypnea—Respiratory rate greater than 20 per minute or a $PaCO_2$ less than 32 mm Hg
- Elevated white blood cell (WBC) count (greater than 12,000 cells/μL) **or**
- Inability to create WBCs (count is less than 4,000/μL) or too many immature WBCs

systemic inflammatory response syndrome (SIRS). Conditions commonly associated with SIRS include infection, pancreatitis, ischemia, multiple trauma, hemorrhagic shock, aspiration of gastric contents, massive transfusions, and host defense deficiencies. Regardless of the cause of the insult, the body responses are similar. If the process cannot be contained, there is an increased activation of the inflammatory cells, including the neutrophils, macrophages, and lymphocytes; additional damage to the vascular endothelium, deterioration in transport of nutrients to the organs, and subsequent complication of MODS (Walsh, 2005). The symptoms defining SIRS are shown in Box 65-14.

The WBC values will vary depending on the presence of an active infection, how many of the metabolic processes occur simultaneously, and whether protein supplies are depleted. Transition from SIRS to dysfunction of multiple organs greatly increases the risk of mortality. Four factors are associated with this transition. These factors include: (a) failure to control the source of the inflammation or infection, (b) persistent hypoperfusion due to prolonged shock status, (c) the presence of necrotic tissue (e.g., an abscess), and (d) altered cellular oxygen consumption (hypermetabolism).

DISSEMINATED INTRAVASCULAR COAGULATION

Disseminated intravascular coagulation (DIC) is a pathological form of the normal localized coagulation response to injury. DIC occurs as a result of disease or injury and spreads throughout the body actually damaging organs and tissues. It alters the clotting process so that both excessive clotting and hemorrhage can occur. For example, severe crush injuries, burns, and sepsis cause cell and blood vessel injury, platelet aggregation, and release of thromboplastin into the blood stream. Circulation is impaired due to the microvascular clots. Without oxygen and nutrients, cells will die and release mediators that will activate the inflammatory process. Hypoxia and acidosis and shock occur. Systems commonly affected by DIC are the skin, lungs, kidneys, the CNS, and GI system. DIC is often associated with septic shock, some viral, bacterial, and protozoal infections, respiratory and cardiogenic shock states, hemorrhaging during pregnancy (Figure 65-5), placenta abruption, retained dead fetal tissue, heat stroke, liver disease, and some snake bites.

There may be a delay in determining internal hemorrhaging. All drainage and GI output, mucous membranes, eyes, nose, and mouth should be observed for the presence of blood. Petechiae and purpura of the skin may be early symptoms of hemorrhage. Blood pressure changes, rapid and thready pulse, decreased level of consciousness are additional indicators.

Careful handling of the patient when changing positions and performing procedures is important as these activities can produce bleeding. Avoiding sharp objects, such as razors and intramuscular injections, will be necessary. Constipation and straining should be prevented to minimize potential bleeding. Fluid replacement with crystalloid and colloid solutions and blood products are also indicated (Walsh, 2005; Edwards, 2002).

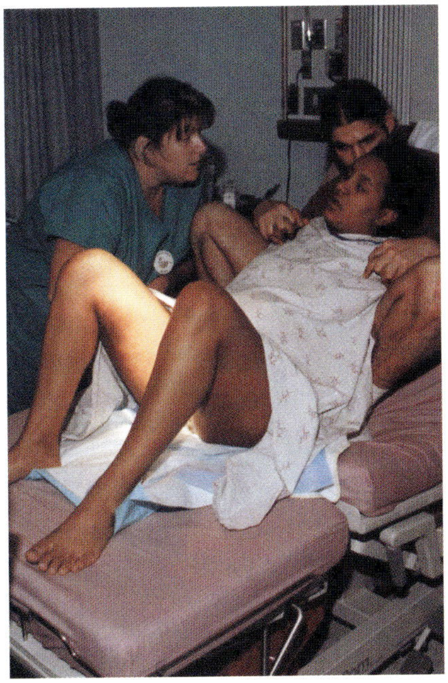

Figure 65-5 DIC can result after delivery with excess bleeding or placenta abruption.

ACUTE RESPIRATORY DISTRESS SYNDROME

Acute respiratory distress syndrome (ARDS), formerly called adult respiratory distress syndrome, is classified as noncardiac pulmonary edema with increased permeability of the alveolar-capillary membrane due to injury to the pulmonary vasculature or the airways (see chapter 32). The alveoli fill with fluid, thus minimizing or prohibiting gas exchange. It is a sudden progressive pulmonary disorder that is manifested by severe dyspnea, hypoxemia, and diffuse bilateral infiltrates.

Etiology

ARDS is caused by a variety of clinical events and often occurs in previously healthy people. (Synonyms are shock lung, wet lung, posttraumatic lung, congestive atelectasis, capillary leak syndrome, and adult hyaline membrane disease). Risk factors include direct injury from aspiration, near-drowning, inhalation of smoke and other toxic gases, pneumonia, radiation, drug toxicity, and severe chest trauma. Indirect injuries include sepsis, pneumonia, cardiopulmonary bypass (CPB), embolism, severe pancreatitis, SIRS, DIC, and shock states. ARDS is a major cause of morbidity and death in intensive care units. The risk is dependent on the condition of the host and the etiological factors. The acute phase can resolve or progress to fibrosis. Survivors are usually young, and gradual return of adequate pulmonary function may occur over a year's time. People are usually at greater risk for diminished pulmonary function, fatigue, and repeated respiratory problems (Allen & Parsons, 2005).

Diagnostic Tests

The following diagnostic criteria are recommended by the American-European Consensus Committee on ARDS based solely on pulmonary gas exchange:

- ARDS is defined by ratio of PaO_2 to fraction of inspired oxygen (FiO_2) of 200 or less regardless of positive end-expiratory pressure (PEEP) needed to support oxygenation. (a ratio less than or equal to 300 mm Hg defines acute lung injury)
- Acute (abrupt) onset.
- Development of new bilateral infiltrates on chest X-ray (CXR).
- Pulmonary artery occlusion pressure (PAOP) of 18 mm Hg or less or no clinical evidence of left atrial hypertension.

Nursing Diagnoses

Based on the information gathered, examples of nursing diagnoses in the patient with ARDS may include the following:

- Impaired gas exchange related to decreased passage of gases between the alveoli of the lungs and the vascular system.
- Decreased cardiac output related to alterations in preload.
- Imbalanced nutrition: less than body requirements related to lack of exogenous nutrients or increased metabolic demand.

Planning and Implementation

Collaborative management for ARDS consists of treating the underlying cause, promoting gas exchange, providing oxygen therapy, and preventing complications. The patient is intubated and placed on mechanical ventilation that limits and controls the amount of pressure in the lungs and helps prevent further trauma to the lungs. PEEP is used to facilitate oxygenation because the hypoxemia associated with ARDS if frequently unresponsive to oxygen therapy. Nursing management includes facilitating oxygenation and ventilation, providing comfort and emotional support, and monitoring the patient for complications.

Evaluation of Outcomes

Potential patient outcomes for each of the example nursing diagnoses for the patient with ARDS are:

- Impaired gas exchange related to decreased passage of gases between the alveoli of the lungs and the vascular system: The patient maintains optimal gas exchange as evidenced by normal arterial blood gases (ABGs) and alert responsive mentation or no further reduction in mental status.

- Decreased cardiac output related to alterations in preload: The patient maintains blood pressure within normal limits; warm dry skin; regular cardiac rhythm; clear lung sounds; and strong bilateral, equal peripheral pulses.
- Imbalanced nutrition: less than body requirements related to lack of exogenous nutrients or increased metabolic demand: The patient verbalizes and demonstrates selection of foods or meals that will achieve a cessation of weight loss and weighs within 10 percent of ideal body weight.

MULTIPLE ORGAN DYSFUNCTION SYNDROME

Multisystem failure has been called multiple system organ failure (MSOF), MOF, and MODS. Whatever the term, the meaning is the same; it is the evidence of a progressive inflammatory response in an acutely ill patient, which has caused more than one of the body's organs to fail, and homeostasis cannot be maintained without intervention (Walsh, 2005). There is usually a precipitating event, such as aspiration or septic shock, which is associated with hypotension.

Assessment with Clinical Manifestations

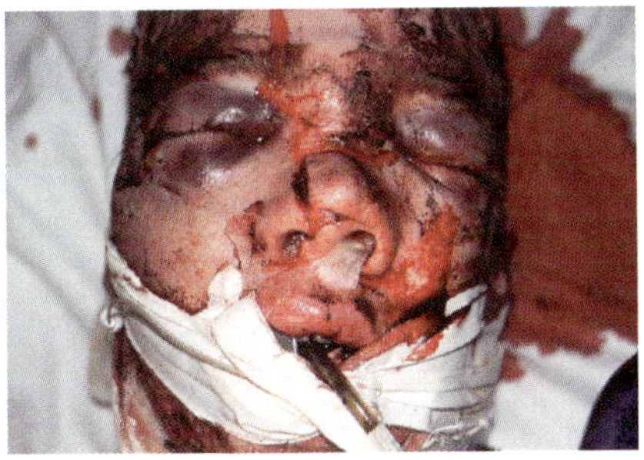

Figure 65-6 Critical head injuries often place a patient at risk for MODS. (Courtesy of Dr. Kevin Reilly, Albany Medical Center, Albany, NY.)

In MODS the patient often is in a crisis, and his or her management has included fluid administration. Following resuscitation with appropriate fluids and vasopressors, the patient appears to be doing well for a short period of time; then a sequence of systemic inflammatory events begins with manifestations of low grade fever, tachycardia, dyspnea, an increase in neutrophils and WBCs, elevated glucose levels, and then signs of infiltrates on the CXR may be seen. Renal and hepatic lab results are relatively normal in the initial stages. Dyspnea progresses and often requires mechanical intubation. Some deterioration in mental status is evident. An example of renal dysfunction includes a creatinine level more than 2 mg/dL and an output of less than 480 mL in a 24-hour period. Renal failure would require dialysis. The outcome may be irreversible, and the end is death over a period of hours to days unless the patient receives complex medical and nursing interventions, and even then, mortality is high. MODS may be responsible for approximately 80 percent of all mortality in the critical care unit and is a leading cause of late mortality after trauma (Figure 65-6).

The findings from classic studies conducted by Knaus, Draper, Wagner and Zimmerman (1986, 1993) to predict the severity of a disease and risk of death are frequently used to diagnose multiple organ dysfunctions. The acute physiology and chronic health evaluation (APACHE II) criteria includes the number of alterations in cardiac, respiratory, renal, hematological, neurological, and hepatic organ failure, age, and preexisting illnesses or diseases as predictive measures.

PRIMARY MULTIPLE ORGAN DYSFUNCTION

Primary multiple organ dysfunction is directly related to an insult, such as a major trauma to the chest or following aspiration or as the result of inhaled fumes or smoke. Primary MODS usually develops quickly. The inflammatory process can trigger the widespread SIRS that places the patient at risk for secondary organ dysfunctions.

Assessment with Clinical Manifestations

Primary MODS begins with disorders such as toxic shock. Toxic shock is a toxin-mediated multisystem disease and is a form of septic shock caused by *Staphylococcus aureus* or group A streptococcus (GAS), an aerobic gram-positive

Uncovering the Evidence

Validation of a Severity of Illness Measure

Discussion: The study purpose is to validate the effectiveness of the APACHE classification system to predict outcomes for severely ill patients admitted to the intensive care unit. The methods included collecting clinical and recorded data, which was conducted in a major U.S. hospital. The subjects were 833 severely ill patients who had been consecutively admitted on an emergency basis to a medical intensive care unit. Nonoperative patients were chosen. Data was collected 24 hours after admission by two former intensive care unit nurses. Data consisted of alterations in seven major organs. Criteria were weighted on a scale of 0 to 4. The weighted sum of 33 potential physiological measures was used as the predictive criteria. Most of the admitted patients had scores on 8–25 of the 33 potential measures, having one or more indications of individual organ failures. The study occurred over a 27-month period. Detailed information was also collected on preadmission data, including age and illnesses. Analysis of physiological data was through regression analysis, and comparison was made with the preadmission data. The findings revealed there was a significant stable association between age, severity of illness, and rate of survival. Similar findings were found with comparison of data from other hospitals. The decline in cardiopulmonary reserve capacity due to age and the incidence of chronic illnesses were closely associated with the mortality outcome predictive scores of the APACHE scale.

Implications for Practice: The APACHE scale can be a useful tool for diagnosis purposes and for suggesting appropriate interventions. The tool will also be useful in further research. Note: the APACHE scale continues to be used as a diagnostic tool and predictor of outcome for severely ill patients with organ dysfunctions.

Wagner, D., Knaus, W., & Draper, E. (1983). Statistical validation of a severity of illness measure. American Journal of Public Health, *73(8), 878–885.*

organism. The initial site of infection is the skin or soft tissue, and the infection is easily transferable. It has also occurred in children who have been exposed to the varicella virus and has occurred in young menstruating women who used vaginal tampons. Approximately half of the reported cases have occurred in men and nonmenstruating women. Initial flu-like symptoms, such as high fever, headache, vomiting and diarrhea, hyperactive bowel sounds and abdominal pain, muscle and joint pain, and general malaise, are present. The patient may have a strawberry tongue, an erythematous macular rash, which progresses to desquamation (peeling) of the skin in 7 to 10 days. The disease can cause necrotizing fasciitis (severe infection of the superficial or deep fascia that surrounds muscles of an extremity or the trunk), and spontaneous gangrene of muscle tissue that may require surgical intervention and amputation of limbs. There is a high mortality rate (Walsh, 2005).

SECONDARY MULTIPLE ORGAN DYSFUNCTION

Secondary multiple organ dysfunction is the result of failure of organs that were not affected by the initial insult. Each of the organ systems are affected by and contribute to the exaggerated inflammatory process.

Assessment with Clinical Manifestations

Typical manifestations for secondary multiple organ dysfunction are described in Box 65-15. Refer to Table 65-2 for nursing diagnoses and evaluation of outcomes.

Planning and Implementation

The goals of collaborative management of MODS are to protect the affected organs from further damage, to use aggressive management of sources of infection, to control the mediators of inflammation, and to provide nutritional support that will facilitate metabolic processes and promote homeostasis. Discussing life-sustaining therapies and end-of-life issues with family of critically ill patients is often a necessary component in the plan of care. Nurses are important in meeting these goals.

BOX 65-15

CLINICAL MANIFESTATIONS IN SECONDARY MULTIPLE ORGAN DYSFUNCTION

- Pulmonary edema due to destruction of the alveolar-capillary membrane; hypoxemia due to maldistribution of oxygenated blood; deterioration in breath sounds; and development of crackles and wheezes. Restlessness and dyspnea are evident.
- Tachycardia is initiated in attempt to increase cardiac output; hypotension is due to vasodilation; skin will be flushed, warm to touch due to vasodilation; altered level of consciousness (LOC) is result of decreased cerebral perfusion; urine output is decreased.
- Neurological dysfunction is indicated by restlessness, insomnia, or confusion that can progress to coma as result of cerebral edema. Muscles become rigid; tremors may be present.
- Gastrointestinal dysfunction results from damage to the endothelium lining; normal intestinal flora may escape into the circulation causing systemic infection, particularly of the lung; manifestations include diarrhea, bloody stools, abdominal distension, increase in stomach acidity, and development of stress ulcers.
- Manifestations of hepatic dysfunction include jaundice and impaired mental status (encephalopathy). Diagnostic tests reveal elevated bilirubin and serum glutamic-pyruvic transaminase (SGPT) or L-lactate dehydrogenase (LDH) levels, decreased albumin, and plasma proteins.
- Pancreatic dysfunction indicators include decreased insulin production and hyperglycemia; the release of proteolytic enzymes from dying cells contributes to the inflammatory process in other organs. Nausea, vomiting, and pain are present along with abdominal distension. Lipase and amylase levels are elevated.
- Renal dysfunction caused by ischemia is indicated by oliguria, elevated creatinine and BUN levels, and inability to concentrate urine, electrolyte abnormalities, hypertension, and buildup of toxins.
- Hematological dysfunction (DIC) is manifested by simultaneous bleeding and coagulation. The skin, lungs, and kidneys are the most commonly involved organs. Prothrombin time is prolonged. Signs of hypoxia are evident.

From Kidd, P. (2005). Multiple organ dysfunction syndrome. In K. Wagner & P. Kidd (Eds.), High acuity nursing *(pp. 312–324). New Jersey: Prentice Hall.*

Guidelines include ongoing careful assessment to detect manifestations of early changes in organ function, progressive inflammation and infection, and patient responses to interventions. Nursing priorities include preventing development of secondary infections, adherence to universal safety precaution standards, facilitating delivery of oxygen to the tissues, and limiting tissue oxygen demand, providing fluid and nutritional support, and providing comfort measures and emotional support (Walsh, 2005).

Severely ill patients are exposed to a variety of stressors in the critical care setting and often are unable to cope. They have a loss of autonomy and control over the environment and the loss of privacy and dignity. The feeling of powerlessness can be overwhelming. Spiritual distress is often related to the threat of death and questioning the meaning of suffering in relation to a personal belief system. The person may express anger to God or another supreme being or have self-blame feelings or express regret for being unable to practice belief rituals. Holistic care involves meeting the spiritual needs and alleviating the person's responses to stress.

Patients in intensive care are exposed to light, noise, and the general activity of the unit, which can be disturbing or even threatening. Sleep deprivation occurs due to pain, discomfort, and the environment. The patient is separated from his or her family and friends. Intubated patients cannot verbally express their needs. The sequence and accumulation of stressors, impact of medications and diminished cerebral perfusion, and fluid and electrolyte imbalances can result in acute confusion and delirium, often referred to as intensive care unit psychosis, often referred to as ICU-itis. Confused individuals may be aware of these changes in mental status and believe that they are losing their minds. Manifestations of confusion can resemble symptoms of dementia; therefore differentiation between the two conditions is more difficult (Grendell, 2004). Refer to the nursing interventions described for management of patients with septic shock.

POPULATIONS AT RISK

Several factors place individuals at risk for systemic infections, potential sepsis, and organ failure, including environmental situations, acute and chronic illnesses, hypersensitivities to antigens, genetic predisposition for altered immune function, autoimmune diseases, and acquired immune deficiency. A minor infection, such as the flu or a urinary tract infection, can be the initial source of sepsis for anyone.

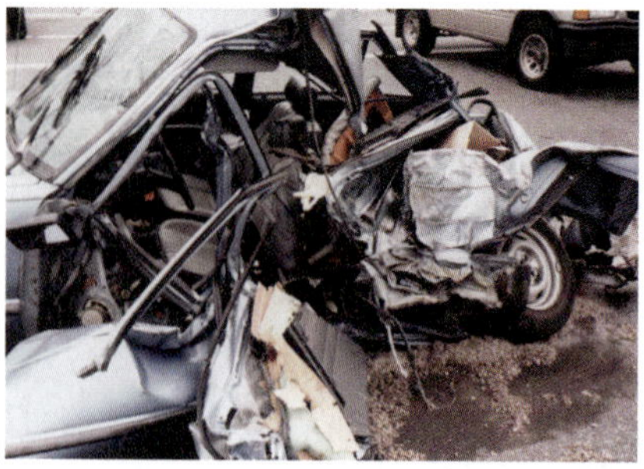

Figure 65-7 Severe motor vehicle crashes often result in multiple injuries, which creates at risk populations for shock syndromes and MODS. (Courtesy of Craig Smith)

Wounds, burns, vehicle accident injuries, and bullet wounds are also potential sources (Figure 65-7). Many trauma events involve injuries to the chest head, spinal cord, and bone fractures as well as breaks in skin integrity and hemorrhage. Burns and near-drowning incidents can cause damage to multiple organs. A trauma incident that requires surgery, blood transfusions, and other invasive measures also place the patient at risk for infection, sepsis, and secondary MODS. The hospital environment adds additional risk factors. Nosocomial (hospital acquired) infections, which are more difficult to treat than community acquired infections, are due to the presence of drug-resistant microorganisms and the compromised condition of the ill hospitalized patient (International Sepsis Forum, 2003).

Secondary, or opportunistic, infections can rapidly progress to sepsis in the extremely young (especially premature infants) and in elderly individuals who have limited immune resources to counteract infections. The immune system is also impaired by an underlying infection, addictive use of alcohol and drugs, smoking or exposure to smoke, hypersensitivities to environmental allergens, malnutrition, and chronic illnesses, such as anemia, hepatic disease, chronic fatigue, and one or more organ dysfunction. Other examples include individuals with a colostomy or ileostomy who become dehydrated due to diarrhea caused by a GI infection, individuals with a tracheostomy, and individuals with cancer who receive chemotherapy or radiation therapy.

Autoimmune diseases, such as diabetes mellitus, rheumatoid arthritis, multiple sclerosis, hemolytic anemia, glomerulonephritis, myasthenia gravis, and systemic lupus erythematosus, are conditions where the body does not recognize the tissue as a part of the self. These problems initiate their own inflammatory process in the attempt to invade and destroy the nonself tissues. Some autoimmune diseases, such as Hashimoto's thyroiditis, attack only the thyroid tissue, and non-Hodgkin's lymphoma arises directly from the thymus gland thus adversely influencing the immune system. These conditions place the individual at high risk for succumbing to infections. Other examples include acquired immune deficiency infections, such as human immunodeficiency virus [HIV] and acquired immune deficiency syndrome [AIDS], which greatly increase the individual's susceptibility to opportunistic infections. Kaposi's sarcoma, a vascular malignancy that is usually seen initially on the skin or mucous membranes, has become closely associated with AIDS. In later stages, the lungs can be affected.

Graft rejection involves the activation of the immune response against a transplanted organ that the body recognizes as nonself. Side effects of immunosuppressant therapy can be life-threatening. Infection can be a major problem following a transplant, and repeated courses in antibiotic therapy can place the patient at risk for a super infection such as *Clostridium difficile* or *Candida*, or drug-resistant bacteria. The patient is also at risk for cytomegalovirus (CMV) infection within a few months of the transplant.

KEY CONCEPTS

- An insult can be anything that triggers the body's IIR.
- The purposes of the IIR are to control bleeding, remove waste products, to limit infection, and to promote healing.
- The shock syndrome is a systemic condition when the peripheral blood flow is inadequate to provide sufficient blood to the heart for normal function and transport of oxygen to all organs and tissues.
- Manifestations of shock will vary according to the underlying cause, the stage of shock, and the individual person's response to shock. Each person must be assessed individually prior to any intervention.
- The four phases of the shock syndrome are the initial phase, the compensatory phase, multiple organ dysfunction phase, and the refractory phase.
- The principle collaborative treatment goals are to identify and treat the underlying cause of the shock syndrome, deliver oxygen to the tissues, promote utilization of oxygen by the tissues, maintain surveillance for complications, and provide comfort and emotional support.
- Hypovolemic shock occurs when there is a lack of circulating fluid volume in the intravascular space.
- Cardiogenic shock results in the failure of either the right or left ventricle or both to provide an adequate delivery of oxygen to the body tissues due to a weakened forward pumping function of the heart.
- Anaphylactic shock is caused by an exaggerated widespread antibody response following a previous exposure to an antigen.
- Neurogenic shock is usually a transient condition that occurs in the absence or suppression of sympathetic nervous system tone.
- Septic shock is a complex systemic response that involves action of cellular and humoral against any type of microorganism that invades the body including gram-negative and gram-positive bacteria, fungi, and viruses.
- An uncontrolled acute inflammatory response that causes inflammation in multiple organs, which are remote from the original insult, is defined as SIRS.
- DIC is a pathological form of the normal localized coagulation response to injury. DIC occurs as a result of disease or injury and spreads throughout the body actually damaging organs and tissues.
- ARDS is a noncardiac pulmonary edema with increased permeability of the alveolar-capillary membrane due to injury to the pulmonary vasculature or the airways. ARDS is a major cause of morbidity and death in intensive care units.
- MODS is the evidence of a progressive inflammatory response in an acutely ill patient that has caused more than one of the body's organs to fail and homeostasis cannot be maintained without intervention.

REVIEW QUESTIONS

1. Biological mediators produce:
   1. Increased capillary permeability
   2. Aspiration
   3. Hyperthermia
   4. Hypoglycemia
2. Hypovolemic shock state is produced by:
   1. Pulmonary emboli
   2. Anemia
   3. Carbon monoxide poisoning
   4. Third spacing of body fluids
3. Manifestations of anaphylactic shock include:
   1. Systolic blood pressure greater than100 mm Hg
   2. Warm, moist skin
   3. Bradycardia and hypotension
   4. Stridor and wheezing
4. Which of the following organ systems is among the most common to fail in severe sepsis?
   1. Gastrointestinal system
   2. Cardiovascular system
   3. Renal system
   4. Neurological system
5. The primary purpose for providing crystalloid solutions is to:
   1. Supplement hemoglobin concentrations
   2. Prevent right ventricular failure
   3. Restore fluid volumes and increase preload
   4. Minimize organ oxygen demand
6. DIC plays a role in the inflammatory process by:
   1. Promoting movement of bacteria into the general system
   2. Decreasing oxygen supplies to cells
   3. Limiting biological mediator release
   4. Increasing vascular resistance
7. What manifestations would indicate a reversal of the shock process?
   1. A heart rate of 90 beats per minute
   2. A blood pressure of 130/70
   3. A respiratory rate of 24 per minute
   4. A urine output of 225 cc per hour
8. All of the individuals below are at risk for developing MODS as the result of a severe insult to the body. Which one would have the greatest risk?
   1. A person who smokes
   2. A 75-year-old individual
   3. A person with congestive heart failure
   4. A person with renal dysfunction
9. Which of the following is the most important factor for increasing oxygen supply?
   1. Decreasing cardiac preload
   2. Administration of appropriate fluids
   3. Administration of vasoconstrictor medications
   4. Maximizing optimal cardiac output
10. Noncardiogenic-pulmonary edema may result from:
    1. Decrease in surfactant
    2. Shunting of blood to nonventilated areas
    3. Alterations in the alveolar-capillary membrane
    4. Increased cardiac output

REVIEW ACTIVITIES

1. What are the gastrointestinal (including hepatic, gallbladder, and pancreas) responses during the sustained IIR response and shock conditions? Use http://www.medicalfacts.org as a resource.
2. Discuss why there has been an increase in the number of sepsis cases within the last two decades.

Continued

REVIEW ACTIVITIES—cont'd

3. Get a copy of Ahrens, T., & Vollman, K. (2003). Severe sepsis management: Are we doing enough? *Critical Care Nurse* Oct. (Suppl),24(2–16).
   a. What are the ethical issues related to the use of Xigris?
   b. Read the case studies at the end of the article. Use the nursing process to develop a plan of care for these patients.
4. Access the Web site for the United States. Center for Disease Control (CDC) at: http://www.cdc. Review the links to the FEMA fact sheet and the American Red Cross Health and safety tips related to the consequences of exposure to extreme heat. Develop a plan to share this information with someone.
5. Access the Web site for the Institute for Healthcare Improvement at: http://www.ihi.org. View the PowerPoint presentation on the six-month update of the 100,000 lives campaign. Note the six changes that have been proposed to save lives. Read the press release. Listen to the informational call recording that gives an overview of the campaign.
6. Access the International Sepsis Forum Web site at: www.sepsisforum.org. You can download the free educational booklet for families. It is available in Dutch, English, French, German, Italian, Portuguese, and Spanish.
7. Access the non-Hodgkin's lymphoma Web site at: http://www.lymphomafocus.org. View videos and transcripts for information about this disease. A case study is also presented.
8. To learn more about Vytex TM, the safe latex material, access http://www.vytex.com. Read the information there that is in a pdf format.

Visit the Contemporary Medical-Surgical Nursing online companion resource at www.delmarhealthcare.com for additional content and study aids. Click on Online Companions then select the Nursing discipline.

CHAPTER 66

Mass Casualty Care

Heather Freiheit, RN, BSN, EMT-P

CHAPTER TOPICS

- Emergency Nursing
- Triage
- Mass Casualty Incidents
- Incident Command
- Hospital Operation Plans
- Personal Protective Equipment
- Hazardous Materials
- Biological Warfare
- Blast Injuries
- Stress Reactions

KEY TERMS

Acute respiratory distress syndrome (ARDS)
Anaphylaxis
Antiphagocytic
Centrifugal
Coagulopathies
Compartment syndrome
Coronavirus
Crash cart
Critical incident
Epidemiological investigation
Exanthema
High efficiency particulate air (HEPA) filter
Intradermal route
Macrophages
Macular rash
Malaise
Mass casualty incident (MCI)
Mitigation
Myalgia
Nuchal
Preparedness
Prodrome phase
Rhabdomyolysis
Rigors
Rye ergot
Stridor
Triage system
Vesicular rash

Emergency nursing is a unique aspect of the nursing profession. No matter the emergency department (ED) size, trauma level, or geographical location, the ED nurse must be ready to care for anything that comes through the doors at a moment's notice. ED nurses must be capable of providing care across the developmental continuum. This group of specialized nurses must be prepared to care for a women giving birth, care for a 70-year-old patient suffering a myocardial infarction (MI), resuscitate a 30-day-old infant, assist with a lumbar puncture, provide emotional support to the families, and everything in between. Frequently EDs are referred to as an environment of controlled chaos because of their ever-changing environment. No one can predict when the next patient will arrive, or the severity of their injury or illness; this is why EDs utilize a **triage system,** which is a method to rank or classify patient's illnesses or severity of injury.

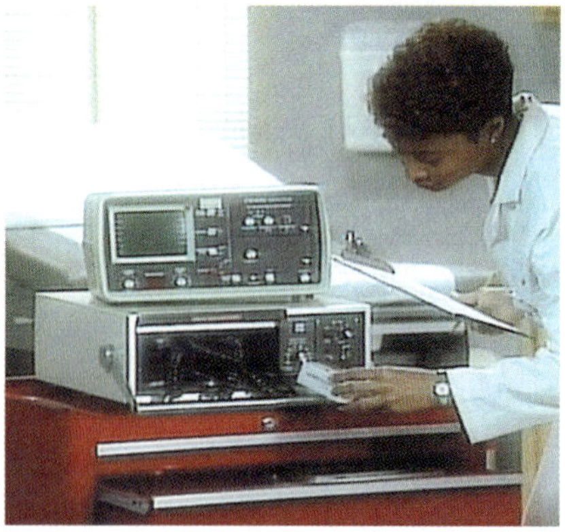

Figure 66-1 Crash cart.

EMERGENCY NURSING

EDs in the early 20th century always had dedicated nurses and were not joined by dedicated ED physicians until the 1970s. Prior to that time, many EDs were staffed by unsupervised residents, who in turn, were oriented and guided through their ED rotations by experienced ED nurses (Schriver, Talmadge, Chuong, & Hedges, 2003).

Over the last 40 years, ED nurses have been instrumental in establishing ED-specific policies and procedures. For example, registered nurse (RN) Anita Dorr developed the **crash cart** (mobile cart with defibrillator, resuscitation equipment, and medications used when patients go into cardiac arrest) (Figure 66-1), originally called the crisis cart in 1967. In 1970 the Emergency Nurses Association (ENA) was created. The ENA established the nationally recognized Certificate of Emergency Nursing and the *Journal of Emergency Nursing*, helping to establish emergency nurses as a recognized profession.

With health care in crisis, more uninsured patients than ever, a decreasing availability of medical doctors (MDs), and poor insurance reimbursement, patients are not able to establish care with a primary care physician, leaving the EDs as the safety net. Additionally, the population is growing while hospitals are closing, placing an even greater burden on emergency departments. Because of the federal regulation, Emergency Medical Treatment and Labor Act (EMTALA), hospitals cannot turn anyone away until it has been established the patient does not have a serious medical condition. These increasing patient volumes overwhelm EDs, forcing patients to be cared for on gurneys in the hallways. As hospitals build larger EDs to help care for this increasing patient population, they must be designed to allow for influxes of large numbers of patients, patients who may be contaminated with hazardous chemicals, requiring decontamination, as well as multiple trauma victims. These patients may arrive via ambulance, helicopter, taxi, or even their own private vehicles, and departments must have acceptable routes and entrances for all (Figure 66-2).

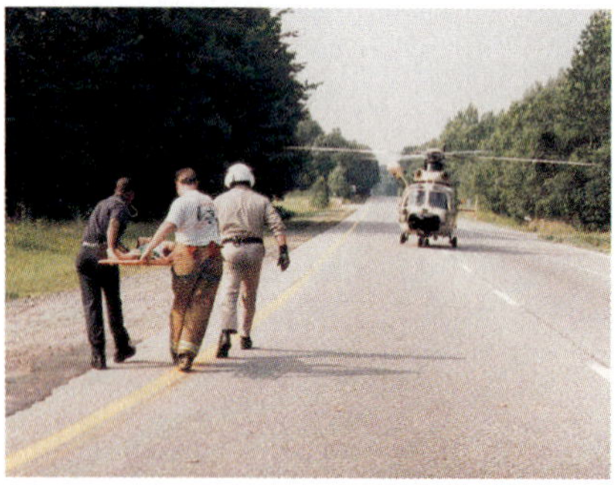

Figure 66-2 Transportation of a patient via a helicopter. Courtesy of Craig Smith.

EDs have become the major diagnostic and resuscitation site for Americans. Emergency nursing has had to keep up with the expanded role and diverse patient populations. The knowledge base, complexity, and technical skill set have grown tremendously, and emergency nurses are required to have many additional specialty certifications. These courses usually are advanced cardiac life support (ACLS), pediatric advanced life support (PALS), trauma nursing core curriculum (TNCC), or their equivalents.

The philosophy of emergency medicine is to stabilize patients, alleviate pain or symptoms, and frequently to refer the patient to a specialist for follow-up, or to admit the patient for further care. There are some minor illnesses or injuries that may not require any further follow-up, such as rashes, ear infections, strains, and sprains. Although EDs refer patients for follow-up care with a primary care physician, frequently the patient returns to the ED, because he or she has no insurance and cannot afford to pay up front to be evaluated by the referral doctor.

The nurse, patient, and the family or caregiver, must take a collaborative approach to provide the best patient management during the ED visit. The average length of stay for an ED patient is less than three hours, which creates a challenge when developing a nursing plan of care. A nurse in triage will perform a brief assessment, but the primary nurse is responsible for completing a full assessment when the patient is taken back to a room. Based on the patient's chief complaint, vital signs, and the findings from the assessment the nurse can formulate nursing diagnoses. The RN works collaboratively with the physician to decide the patient's plan of care, but the RN is responsible for implementing the plan. Throughout the implementation of the plan the RN evaluates the effectiveness of the interventions. Based on evaluations of her findings, the RN will advise the physician, and the plan will be revised. ED nurses work closely with ED physicians side by side day after day. This close work environment has helped foster comradeship between these two profes-

Uncovering the Evidence

Discussion: This one-year study looked at ambulatory visits to EDs in the United States during 2002. The data was collected from the 2002 National Hospital Ambulatory Medical Care Survey (NHAMCS), a national probability sample survey conducted by the Centers for Disease Control and Prevention (CDC) and the Health Care Statistics Division. In this study, 396 hospitals were asked to participate, and 376 completed the survey (an overall response rate of 94.9 percent). The following highlights were discovered.

ED visits increased 23 percent between 1993 through 2002, but the number of available EDs decreased by almost 15 percent.

Overall ED utilization rate per population increased by 9 percent; from 35.7 visits per 100 in 1992 to 38.9 visits per 100 in 2002.

The mean age of ED patients rose from 33 in 1992 to 35.6 in 2002; but patients over 75 years of age had the highest rate of ED visits at 61.1 visits per 100.

In 2002, abdominal pain, chest pain, fever, and headache were leading patient complaints. Two thirds of ED patients spend between 1 and 6 hours in an ED with an average of 3.2 hours.

Implications for Practice: This data shows that EDs throughout the United States are being used more frequently and are becoming busier and busier. Because 15 percent of the nation's EDs have closed over the last nine years, this has left fewer remaining open EDs to care for all of these patients, leading to longer patient wait times and stays in the ED. As a result of all of these changes, EDs are becoming more overwhelmed, including the need to divert ambulances to other EDs. More elderly patients are being seen in the EDs, and they tend to require more extensive workups and are more acutely ill than younger patients. It is becoming increasingly difficult to transfer patients out of the ED and get them admitted to an inpatient bed because of full inpatient units and limited available nurses. This leads to ED holding these patients for 24 hours or even longer. Due to EMTALA, EDs cannot turn away or refuse evaluation to any walk-in patients, which leads to overcrowded departments, long waits, patients in the hallways, ambulance diversions, and a stressful work environment for ED nurses. ED managers and educators are discovering their nurses must also have training in inpatient documentation, procedures, and care standards because they are holding these patients and care must be continued.

As these trends continue, administrators must be proactive, changing hospital-wide systems to assist EDs in obtaining beds for admissions and create system efficiencies to help reduce patient through-put times for EDs to be able to care for this continued increase in patient volume.

Source: McCaig, L., & Burt, C. (2004). National hospital ambulatory medical care survey: 2002 emergency department summary. *USDHHS Publication No. (PHS) 2004-125004-0226-0302. Hyattsville, MD: U. S. Department of Health & Human Services.*

sions and has strengthened patient care through open two-way communication channels (Figure 66-3)

TRIAGE

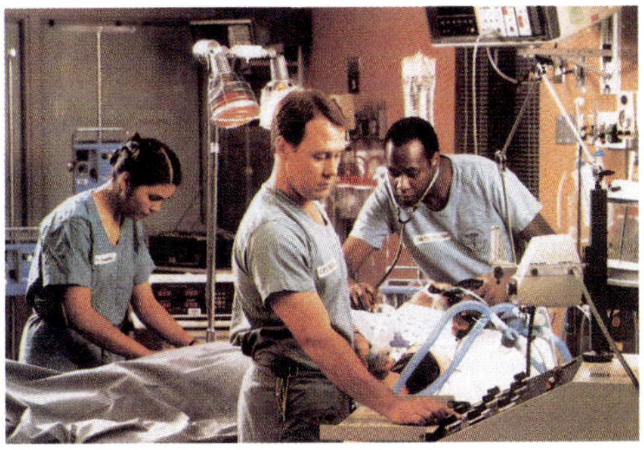
Figure 66-3 ED nurses working with a physician. Courtesy of U. S. Government, as represented by the Secretary of the Army.

Triage stems from a French word meaning "to sort." Triage is the process of rapidly assessing patients and assigning them a classification or priority for care. Triage was first used to prioritize care for injured soldiers in France in the 1800s. It was not until the 1900s, when inner city hospital EDs started to become crowded, that hospital triage was adopted in the United States (Ihlenfeld, 2003). Triage was then perfected by the American military during the Korean and Vietnam wars with Mobile Army Surgical Hospitals (MASH) units.

The objectives of a triage system are to (a) identify patients who require immediate care, (b) use space and resources efficiently, (c) facilitate patient flow into the ED, (d) provide assessment and reassessment of patients, (e) alleviate fear and anxiety of patients or visitors, (f) improve guest relations, and (g) initiate legal accountability. Triage is usually performed by a RN who completes a rapid assessment of the patient's chief complaint, vital signs, overall appearance and mentation, pain level, and psychosocial needs to

ETHICS IN PRACTICE

Family members and EDs will have different philosophies as to whether family members should be allowed to wait in the examination room during resuscitation of a cardiac arrest. Some hospitals still do not allow family to be present at all in the room during a cardiac arrest, although this practice is being challenged.

EDs are being encouraged to allow family to be present during resuscitations or at least brought in after the initial first few minutes. This practice is encouraged for a variety of reasons:

- This allows family members to see that everything is being done for their loved ones.
- This also may help loved ones choose to have the resuscitation stopped after they are educated on what has been done, the lack of patient response, and see the futility of the efforts.
- When families are present during resuscitation, they also are less apt to pursue legal actions, because they have seen what was done and had a chance to have their questions answered.

DOLLARS AND SENSE

The Financial Implications of On-Call Specialists in the ED

In November of 2003, the Centers for Medicare and Medicaid Services (CMS) revised the EMTALA regulations. In these revised regulations CMS acknowledged that the demands on health care providers are becoming overwhelming, and there is a need to balance available health care providers with ED call coverage. EDs must maintain a list of on-call health care specialists, but MDs are being allowed to take calls at more than one ED at a time. Additionally, on-call specialists are being allowed to limit the amount of call time they are available. This leniency for on-call specialist coverage combined with reduced health care provider payment from insurance companies, higher malpractice insurance, and a growing number of uninsured patients, is affecting ED patient access to specialized care in a timely fashion. Frequently, this results in patients being transferred to another ED to receive care from the needed specialist. Delays in care may lead to greater injury or disability for patients, which may have been prevented or minimized if treatment had been administered in a timely fashion. For example, a previously healthy 55-year-old male patient arrives with chest pain and ST elevation indicative of a MI. If the ED does not have a cardiologist on call, the patient cannot be immediately taken for a heart catheterization and possible intervention. If it takes two hours for the patient to be transferred to an ED with a cardiologist, the patient has two hours of cardiac muscle damage that could have been prevented. If this was extensive muscular damage and the man is disabled and can no longer be work, he begins drawing from Social Security for an injury that may have been prevented. Health care professionals, health care providers, policy makers, and the government must work together to find ways and ensure specialized physicians are on-call and available to all. This may be accomplished through capping malpractice insurance, lobbying for affordable health care, and establishing fair compensation for health care providers.

adequately determine the patient's acuity and assign him or her a priority level of care. Triage scales are based on the severity of the patient's injury or illness. There are a variety of triage scales used in EDs, but they all rate the patient's severity and classify the order in which the patient is to be seen as: Level I, II, or III; critically ill, intermediate, or low risk; and urgent, emergent, or stable (Ihenfeld, 2003).

Currently, most EDs use a three-tiered system, although this is changing to a five-tiered system because of a more reliable and consistent triage level. The five-tiered system looks not only at the patient's acuity, but it also helps to predict the number of resources the patient will require. The highest priority or the most emergent conditions involve the potential for loss of life or limb without immediate intervention. These conditions may include unresponsive patients, **anaphylaxis** (a widespread severe allergic reaction that may be life-threatening), or stroke-like symptoms. Urgent patients are defined as those having an acute condition that requires prompt evaluation and may include fractures without neurovascular compromise, abdominal pain, or nosebleeds. Nonurgent patient conditions are those in which there is not a risk of deterioration and care can be delayed. Examples include dermatitis (inflammation of the skin either from allergic reaction or direct contact with an irritant; redness, itching, and blisters may occur), medication refills, toothaches, or sprains, and strains. Triage RNs are challenged with assessing the order in which patients need to be evaluated by an ED doctor. It is the RN's responsibility to assess each patient and assign his or her triage level. These RNs are frequently challenged with an overwhelming number of patients requesting emergency care. It is recommended that the most experienced ED RNs perform triage. For some patients with life-threatening illnesses, it is an expert RN who will be able to recognize the subtle symptoms underlying the patient's complaint.

In assessing their patients, the triage nurse needs to be aware of the some risks. First, a nurse runs the risk of failing to recognize and care for patients in extreme pain, and the RN must also not judge whether the patient is or is not exaggerating his or her pain. Second, a nurse runs the risk of failing to recognize and appropriately triage high-risk chief complaints, such as chest pain, neurological changes, or headaches. Third, a nurse runs the risk of not getting complete vital signs. Fourth, a nurse runs the risk of not reevaluating patients placed in the waiting room. Last, a nurse runs the risk of incomplete or lack of documentation regarding triage assessment and reassessment.

Triage is not to be mistaken for a medical screening exam (MSE). EMTALA requires a MSE for all patients presenting to an ED requesting treatment or evaluation. EMTALA mandates that a MSE be completed to protect patients with life-threatening illnesses or injury from being refused medical treatment by ED as a result of the patient's lack of insurance coverage or inability to pay. A MSE determines whether the patient has an emergency medical condition or not. If an emergency condition exists, the patient must be treated and cannot be transferred or referred to another hospital until they are stabilized. A physician, nurse practitioner, or physician's assistant completes these exams. A MSE includes the patient's initial triage information and includes a focused examination of the appropriate system related to the chief complaint. For example, a patient with a fever and sore throat would have their throat examined to assess if there is an emergent condition, such as epiglottitis (a bacterial infection causing rapid inflammation of the epiglottis; this inflammation may completely occlude the airway and lead to death) or a peritonsillar abscess (pus collects behind the tonsils from an infection causing compression of the uvula, and this may lead to airway obstruction), before the decision can be made to refer them to a primary health care provider or clinic.

Fast Forward ▶▶▶

Nurses Future Role in the ED of Small Hospitals

Because of a decreasing availability of ED physicians in rural hospitals and an increasing patient volume, the CMS adapted their regulations and now a RN may perform a MSE, which is a new philosophy for hospitals. Currently, EDs around the nation are exploring if and how they will implement this. If ED nurses are to begin performing the MSEs, they must have a system in place that dictates which health care provider they consult if the nurse feels the patient has a life-threatening issue or if the nurse has a question.

START Method of Triage

In the early 1980s, the simple triage and rapid treatment (START) was developed as a method to quickly triage multiple patients. The START method is a nationally recognized triage system that can be initiated in the prehospital setting and carried into the hospital environment. Three patient criteria are evaluated: ventilation, pulses and perfusion, and neurological status. In the event of multiple casualties, using the START method, each patient assessment is completed in less than 60 seconds. This enables the nurse to determine the number of causalities, the severity of their injuries, and to rapidly mobilize the necessary resources.

The traditional way of triaging patients is based on caring for the most critical patients first. In dealing with a mass casualty incident (MCI), the triage philosophy is to first provide care to those patients most likely to survive (Ihlenfeld, 2003). In other words, do the greatest good for the most; patients most severely injured will be cared for last. Similarly, this MCI philosophy is similar to what is used in military triage situations. This change in philosophy may be uncomfortable to nursing personnel who want to care for all patients or to first care for those most severely injured. It is to be remembered that resources and systems will be overwhelmed during a MCI or disaster. Following the MCI philosophy, the ED will provide care to the greatest number of injured. Four colors are used to identify four categories of patients that require triaging: (a) green is used to identify patients who need minimal health care, (b) yellow is used to identify patients who need health care, but not immediately and not at a high acuity of injury, (c) red is used to identify patients who need health care immediately and are life threatened, and (d) black is used to identify patients who are going to die. As a further explanation, it is vital to identify patients who will do well with minimal care (green and some yellows), those who most likely will die even with care (black), and focus immediate resources and rapid intervention for those who will benefit the most (reds and some yellows). In disaster settings, health care providers have an obligation to treat as many people as possible that have the best chance of survive. During a MCI, in these resource-constrained situations clinicians must prioritize victims (Burkle, 2002). On the average day, ED nurses are familiar with triaging patients but during a MCI or disaster, even the most experienced triage RN will become overwhelmed.

Patients who are initially triaged at the scene of a MCI must receive the same rapid triage by a RN or MD on arrival at the ED. This assessment determines if the patient's triage criteria have changed, for example, from yellow to red.

Military Triage

Depending on the event, the military uses two different types of triage methods: tactical and nontactical. These methods are similar to other triage systems as they are intended to balance the human lives at stake, the level of resources available, and the realistic capabilities of medical personnel on the scene (Table 66-1).

MASS CASUALTY INCIDENT

Most experts agree it is not a matter of if, but rather of when the next MCI will occur. A **mass casualty incident (MCI)** is defined as an influx of victims that overwhelms the hospital and affects the institutions capability to care for this influx of victims. Unfortunately, in recent years, hospitals have had resources challenged with a rapid influx of patients: the World Trade Center bombing of 1993, the events of September 11, 2001, the anthrax events in fall of 2001, the Florida hurricanes of 2004, and the disaster associated with hurricane Katrina in 2005 (Box 66-1). Hospitals must be prepared for a MCI 24 hours a day, seven days a week. No one knows when, where, or what will be the cause of the next event. What is known is it has happened before, it will happen again, and there will be injured survivors.

The American College of Emergency Physicians defines a disaster as "when the destructive effects of natural or man-made forces overwhelm the ability of a given area or community to meet the demand of health care" (Mothershead, 2003). A MCI has large numbers of injured and dead, but the community infrastructure remains intact (Mothershead, 2003). A MCI will tax the hospital and

BOX 66-1

KATRINA DISASTER

The Katrina hurricane disaster in August 2005 was the deadliest and costliest hurricane in the history of the United States. There were 1,836 fatalities and an estimated expense of $75 billion. President George W. Bush declared a state of emergency in three states two days prior to landfall of the Class V hurricane. The mayor of New Orleans, Ray Nagin, ordered a mandatory evacuation on August 28, and the Superdome was used as a shelter for 26,000 people. Overall, Katrina revealed the difficulty in implementing a large-scale disaster plan. The Federal Emergency Management Agency (FEMA) drew tremendous criticism over the ensuing months, and people demanded a better federal plan for disasters. The Katrina disaster signaled the importance of continued progression and development of better planning for the future of mass casualty incidents.

Source: Knabb, R., Rhome, J., & Brown, D. (2005, August 23–30). Tropical cyclone report: Hurricane Katrina. National Hurricane Center. *Retrieved on May 30, 2006, from www.nhc.noaa.gov.*

TABLE 66-1 Tactical vs. Non-Tactical Triage

Tactical Triage Utilized in Combat-type Settings

Class I:	Patients with minor injuries that can be treated in an ambulatory outpatient basis.
Class II:	Patients whose injuries require immediate intervention to sustain life but require minimum amount of time, personnel, and supplies initially.
Class III:	Definitive treatment can be delayed without threat to life or limb.
Class IV:	Patients with extensive injuries that would require extensive treatment beyond the immediate medical capabilities. Caring for these victims would jeopardize other victims.

Nontactical Triage (Similar to Tactical Triage, but the Four Priority Classes Are Different)

Priority I:	Patients with correctable life-threatening illnesses or injury.
Priority II:	Patients with serious but not life-threatening injuries or illnesses.
Priority III:	Patients with minor injuries.
Priority IV:	Patients who are dead or fatally injured.

Triage during a disaster is an ongoing process that is based on trying to save the most patients possible. There will be instances when a patient may have the potential to survive but dedicating the personnel and resources to that individual most likely will compromise others.

Source: Integrated Publishing. (2004). Triage. *Retrieved June 21, 2006, from http://infodotinc.com.*

prehospital systems, whereas a mass casualty event or disaster usually destroys the community support systems and leads to the influx of an overwhelming number of patients. During a MCI or a disaster, the goal is to quickly identify those patients who have stable, minor injuries and can wait for care (green patients), those patients who will most likely die even with immediate interventions (black patients), and to focus care and resources on those patients who will benefit from rapid care and interventions (red and yellow patients).

What constitutes an MCI for one institution is not necessarily true for another. During a MCI, a hospital is challenged with a large volume of sick or injured patients, creating a discrepancy between available hospital resources and the number of patients arriving. The characteristics of the facility, such as the hospital's size, advanced preparation and training, combined with available resources, number of ED beds, radiology resources, operating room (OR) suites, and number of critical care beds, will help determine if a hospital will be overwhelmed. The facility characteristics combined with the specific event will help individual hospitals decide if they need to activate their disaster plan to manage the incident. Fortunately, the United States has never experienced an event where thousands of patients are sick or injured in one community and needing care. Unfortunately, with the current terrorist cells, it is possible this type of MCI to occur at any time and health care facilities and their communities must be prepared for this to occur (Ihlendfeld, 2003).

INCIDENT COMMAND

When a disaster or MCI occurs, it results in the hospital's normal day-to-day operations being interrupted for long periods of time and involves extensive man hours. To operate effectively and efficiently, a hospital must have preestablished response plans in place and be familiar with how to initiate and use them. The Incident Command System (ICS) is a system utilized to help manage large-scale events where areas of responsibility are assigned to personnel for coordination. Originally, the ICS was created to help manage the large numbers of firefighters utilized on wilderness fire scenes. This system was so successful it has since been restructured for hospital use, known as the hospital emergency incident command system (HEICS). The HEICS is extremely practical and creates a valid instrument for assisting hospitals during times of disasters and complex problem situations. The HEICS includes five functional branches of command, finance and planning, operations, logistics, and subunits may be established off of each branch depending on the disaster. The ICS can be implemented in varying levels, depending on the type of incident, the number of potential victims, and the estimated length of an event.

Hospital Emergency Incident Command System

The HEICS was initially tested in the early 1990s by six hospitals in Orange County, California. In 1992, HEICS was refined and distributed to hospitals around the world (Greater New York Hospital Association, 2002). Following the 1993 Northridge earthquake in California, HEICS was utilized successfully by hospitals damaged in the earthquake. Implementation of the HEICS provides the following advantages: a consistent algorithm for organizing information, controlling and coordinating the influx and movement of patients, and the distribution of required staff, supplies, and resources. HEICS also allows for a manageable span of control for the assigned group leaders and a consistent way of communication using common terminology. HEICS is a flexible program, which can be expanded on or scaled down, depending on the magnitude of the event. During large-scale events, preset roles fulfilled staffed by a variety of personnel to allow for periods of rest. HEICS also provides an organized means of successfully transferring the command process to relieve the incident command staff.

Following HEICS guidelines, the role of incident commander (IC) is preassigned, and this position is implemented immediately after notification of an event. Without an IC, staff takes independent actions that are not in coordination with one another. These uncoordinated actions lead to rapid chaos and potential patient compromise or staff injury. Depending on the type and time of the event, the IC may initially be a department manager or the house supervisor, although the IC role is transferred on to an administrator as early as possible.

Like the prehospital incident command system (ICS), the HEICS system has four components: finance, logistic, operations, and planning (FLOP). The IC appoints chiefs to these components, and the chiefs then designate directors and unit leader for each subunit. This structure and distribution of assignments limits individuals' span of control and helps obtain adequate documentation and tracking of the event. HEICS provides both a framework for standardized roles internally and allows a universal network between hospitals, police, fire, emergency medical services (EMS) agencies, and the city or county emergency operations center. This system supports effective communication between these agencies using common terminology and standardized roles (Figure 66-4). For example, during a county-wide MCI, the material and supply unit officer from one hospital can call the material and supply unit officer from another hospital to check on mask availability of N-95 masks, thus coordinating resources.

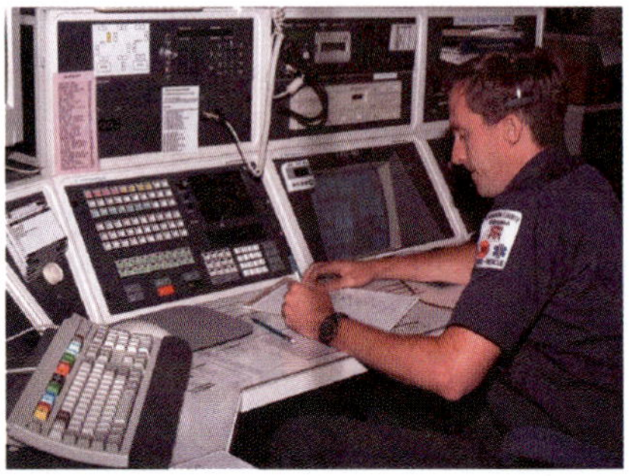

Figure 66-4 Communication among agencies is facilitated by complex technological centers.

HEICS Activator

Both internal and external events can lead to the initiation of the ICS. Internal events occur within the hospital and can prevent the hospital from functioning normally, compromising patient care. Examples of internal events include a main water pipe rupturing or fire. External events take place outside of the hospital and lead to a large influx of patients arriving at the ED. Disasters may be both internal and external, such as an earthquake or tornado. As soon as the hospital's ED receives notification of a MCI or disaster, the hospital's disaster plan is activated; this pulls additional staff from other areas of the hospital to assist ED staff in caring for the influx of sick or injured patients. In the case of possible infectious disease outbreak, as soon as the hospital's ED starts to see patients experiencing similar signs and symptoms, the disaster plan is initiated. When the hospital disaster plan is activated, outside agencies may need to be contacted so to as alert them to the hospital's limited capabilities.

Incident Command Education

It is imperative that hospitals have a preestablished incident command structure that is integrated with the hospital disaster plan. Personnel must be familiar with the hospital's ICS and understand their role during a disaster or MCI. Unless hospitals provide training and drills for staff, having a disaster plan will not be beneficial as staff will be unfamiliar with the plan. In these drills, a variety of potential scenarios must be practiced including: nuclear, biological, natural disasters, and loss of power or water. The Joint Commission on Accreditation of Healthcare Organizations ([JCAHO] 2006a) Environment of Care Standard EC.1.4 requires hospitals have an emergency management plan that addresses four phases of emergency management: **preparedness** (activities which build the hospital's capacity to manage the effects of an emergency or disaster), **mitigation** (activities a hospital undertakes to help lessen the severity and impact of potential emergencies that may affect operations or services provided by a hospital), response, and recovery. Standard EC.2.9.1 states the hospital response plan must be practiced twice a year, and at least once a year there must be an influx of victims through the ED. Following the terrorist attacks of September, 2001, JCAHO added the requirement that hospitals practice communication and coordination with other agencies and hospitals in the community in preparation for a large-scale event.

For all personnel to be included and familiar with the procedures, drills take place on day/evening/night shifts and weekends. Additionally, specific staff is trained and able to perform decontamination of patients exposed to hazardous chemicals or biological toxins and this drill is practiced at least once a year. In these drills, leadership personnel are usually placed into the IC roles, whereas patient care providers will most likely be continuing to care for patients. For the HEICS to work effectively, staff needs to understand the IC structure and needs to accept a reporting structure and different lines of authority with which they are accustomed to (Greater New York Hospital Association, 2002). Additional staff is generally sent to the ED to assist with the initial influx of patients. If hospitals have had frequent disaster drills to practice their different roles in a disaster, employees will be comfortable working in the ED to care for patients.

HOSPITAL OPERATIONS PLAN

Hospital operation plans (ps plans) are made up of many components that allow hospitals to be prepared for a variety of unusual incidents. These plans include sections on HEICS, disasters, bioterrorism, chemical, and radiation emergencies and are used by staff and IC as guides during events.

Hospital emergency operation plans need to include elements of preparedness, response, mitigation, and recovery. The plan must incorporate strategies to care for a large influx of patients for up to 72 hours, as it may be this long before assistance from the government can arrive. Additional supplies will be made available to hospitals from national stockpiles as early as 24 hours but may take as long as 72 hours. The time it takes for these resources to be mobilized and arrival depends on the extent of the event and national priority of the community requesting resources. Operation plans must also include the hospitals available supply of on site antibiotics, antidotes, ventilators, respirators, and other supplies needed to care for victims of a MCI. The plans must also have contingencies to acquire additional supplies to survive 24 to 72 hours until the arrival of federal assistance, also known as disaster medical assistance teams (DMATs). DMAT teams are made up of physicians, nurses, and EMTs who are transported to large-scale events to help in triaging, stabilization, transport, and patient treatment (Mothershead, 2003). Hospital operation plans must have established working relationships between other area hospitals, police and EMS and fire agencies, and the city or county emergency operations center. Communication plans need to have interoperability or the ability of different hospitals and public safety agencies to communicate with one another in real time. This helps to coordinate patient transport and communication with community members about the location of their loved ones. One way to help interoperability is for all entities involved to use the ICS.

A terrorist event or even a food-borne illness outbreak may be covert or overt. Hospital ops plans need to have established systems to expedite disease reporting of suspected outbreaks to both internal infection control practitioners and the county health department. Having established communication plans with the community and media prior to an event allows for quicker dissemination of important information to the general public.

In addition to hospital employees' phone numbers, these ops plans should include important external resource phone numbers, such as local health department, Federal Bureau of Investigation (FBI) field office, CDC infection control and bioterrorism branch, local hazardous materials (HazMats) team, and contracted supply and pharmaceutical suppliers. The hospital ops plan must also include the process for hospital evacuation and meeting places along with alternate care sites for the patients, supplies, and medical records (Box 66-2).

BOX 66-2

HOSPITAL OPERATION PLAN CRITERIA

Hospital disaster plans should include information on the following topics:

- Recognition and notification
- Assessment of hospital capabilities
- Personnel recall back to work
- Establishment of incident command
- Maintenance of accurate records
- Public relations
- Equipment supply and resupply

Adapted from Mothershead, J. (2003). Disaster planning. *Retrieved June 27, 2006, from http://emedicine.com; Ihlenfeld, J. (2003). A primer on triage and mass casualty events.* Dimensions of Critical Care, Nursing, 22*(5), 204–209.*

PERSONAL PROTECTIVE EQUIPMENT

Personal protective equipment (PPE) refers to the clothing and respiratory equipment required to protect staff from chemical, biological, or infectious threats. EDs must have PPE available to personnel who will be caring for these individuals. Patient care providers need access to the correct and adequate amounts of PPE. If a large-scale biological event were to occur, PPE would be needed by all ED staff with the means to rapidly replenish stock. Prior to any event, ED personnel must know how and when to correctly use the PPE and the location of where it is stored. The type of PPE required depends on the event or suspected disease. Some diseases require standard precautions, whereas others require expanded precautions. In addition to PPE, the nurse will need to follow the guidelines for standard precautions and expanded precautions (i.e., contact precautions, droplet precautions, airborne infection, and isolation precautions). Refer to chapter 11 for a review of these guidelines.

HAZARDOUS MATERIALS

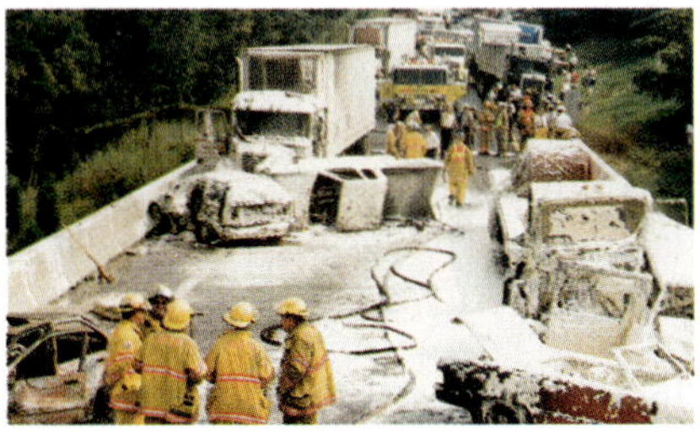

Figure 66-5 HazMats cause a type of crisis that has specific implications for health care providers and persons dispatched to the accident scene.

Hazardous materials (HazMats) are materials that have the potential to harm a person or the environment (Figure 66-5). Caring for patients who have been contaminated with HazMats is extremely challenging for staff. ED staff are required to care for contaminated patients knowing they may potentially be exposing themselves to the chemical. Even without the threat of a terrorist attack, the potential for a HazMat patient arriving at an ED is great. More than four billion tons of chemicals are transported across the United States, stemming from over 100,000 different locations, and involving over one million

BOX 66-3

COMPONENTS OF HOSPITAL HAZMAT EMERGENCY RESPONSE PLAN

- Identify local facilities producing, using or storing hazardous materials
- Have designated hospital, community, and industrial coordinators
- Have established mechanism of early notification
- Establish training programs including EMS and fire departments
- Have established decontamination area and equipment

Adapted from Cox, Robert. (2003). Hazmat. *Retrieved June 14, 2006, from http://www.emedicine.com.*

workers yearly (Cox, 2003). Review of past HazMat events show that most exposures occurred at facilities where the chemicals were stored or produced. In 13 percent of these HazMat incidences, the patients also had traumatic injuries and were taken to the trauma center. Not only do hospitals need to have decontamination plans in place and practice them, they also need to be familiar with the chemicals produced and stored in their area (Box 66-3).

ED personnel must be aware they may not have any previous warning of a contaminated patient's arrival, and these patients may come to the ED in a private vehicle. It is the triage nurse's responsibility to know how to recognize a contaminated patient and immediately direct him or her to the decontamination area. Many of these HazMat chemicals have the potential to close EDs down because of contamination from the chemical. ED nurses learn early that the top priority in dealing with a HazMat situation is to protect themselves, other patients, and the department. An ED nurse cannot help a contaminated patient if the nurse is suffering injuries from being exposed himself or herself to the contaminated substance. To assist with patient decontamination, ED staff needs to wear specific PPE to prevent their own exposure. Hospitals select which level of protection will be best for their staff based on their HazMat risk assessments, regulatory requirements, and recommendations from local experts. Level B protection will usually suffice for most hospital staff that may be involved in initial decontamination and care of contaminated patients. There are three different levels of PPE for HazMat per Occupational Safety and Health Administration (OSHA) as shown in Box 66-4.

Decontamination

Hospitals are required to have dedicated areas in which to decontaminate patients who have been exposed to chemicals. Three different decontamination tiers are required: a small designated area for a few patients, an area that can be quickly set up for medium-sized events, and an area or plan for large-scale events. Internal decontamination rooms are usually used for one to four patients and need a dedicated external entrance, negative pressure air with dedicated **High efficiency particulate air (HEPA) filters** (a filter used to remove submicron particulate matter from the air), HazMat compatible wastewater containment, tables or gurneys for washing patients, and accessible storage for staff PPE. Commonly, outdoor areas are utilized for medium to large-scale events, because these areas do not require dedicated air handling and ventilation systems. These areas will require heated water and special water containment tanks to protect the environment and the community. If the event is small, the ED will receive help from the local fire department HazMat team. During large-scale events, the local HazMat teams will be unavailable, and the EDs will need to perform patient decontamination independently.

BOX 66-4

OSHA PPE LEVELS

Level A—Provides the highest level of respiratory and skin protection. It is resistant to chemicals and impermeable to gases and vapors. This suit is used with a self-contained breathing apparatus (SCBA) or an air supplied respirator. This is the level recommended to be worn with unknown agents but is the most cumbersome for staff and is usually only worn by HazMat teams.

Level B—This suit provides respiratory protection but does not provide a fully enclosed environment. It may allow chemical vapors to permeate the suit. Although this suit is not as cumbersome as a Level A suit, it is still challenging for care providers to wear.

Level C—This suit provides splash protection and is chemical resistant, but a respirator must still be worn. With this level PPE, the chemical or agent must be known, because an agent-specific cartridge needs to be placed in the respirator to filter out that particular agent.

Adapted from Occupational Safety and Health Administration. (2005). Safety and health topics: Personal and protective equipment. *Retrieved June 24, 2006, from www.osha.gov.*

ETHICS IN PRACTICE

Preparation for an Outbreak of an Infectious Agent

Health care providers may be faced with being asked to work during an infectious agent outbreak. This may pose an ethical dilemma where they nurse is torn between staying at home, caring and protecting for her family versus going to work and potentially exposing himself or herself to a contagious disease. ED nurses must ask themselves this question in advance so they will not be in a dilemma if this situation arises. Hospitals should consider providing prophylactic medication to health care workers' families if there was an outbreak.

BIOLOGICAL WARFARE AND BIOLOGICAL AGENTS

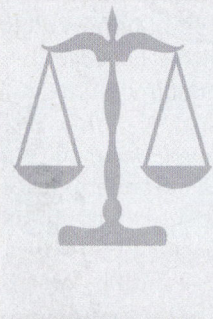

The global biological warfare threat must be taken seriously. There are at least 10 countries worldwide known to have offensive biological weapons programs. Biological warfare was used as early as the 6th century B.C. with the Assyrians poisoning enemy wells with **rye ergot** (a fungus from the rye plant causing hallucinations, gastrointestinal [GI] upset, and a form of gangrene if ingested). Since the breakup of the former Soviet Union, it is known that vials of the smallpox virus are unaccounted for and are presumed to be in the hands of possible terrorists. To protect the welfare of the health care workers, other patients, and the community, management of patients with a known or possible infectious disease must be well organized and rehearsed. The hospital operations plan needs to specify designated, preestablished areas in the hospital or an off-site location to cohort contagious patients whose illness creates a hazard to the community.

Biological weapons include bacteria, viruses, and toxins and are placed into groupings based on how dangerous they are, the ease of dissemination or transmission, and the degree of, public panic and social disruption they could cause. The A-list consists of the agents considered to be of the highest risk. The A-list bacterial agents include: anthrax, brucellosis, bubonic plague, and tularemia. Viral agents of concern are: smallpox, Venezuelan equine encephalitis, and the viral agents known to cause hemorrhagic fevers. Botulism and ricin are two biological toxins of concern.

Health care workers, especially ED personnel, may be the first people to see an increase in patients with similar signs or symptoms and become suspicious of an epidemiological outbreak. ED nurses need to be alert for these patterns and diagnostic clues that may be indicative of an outbreak, whether accidental or intentional (Box 66-5).

It is imperative that any suspicion is reported immediately to both the hospital infection control staff and the local health department so rapid diagnosing may occur. As soon as a pattern is suspected, an **epidemiological investigation** (study looking at a specific disease, its distribution, and initial source) is initiated. This investigation helps in identifying the agent, and it will also help to institute the correct medical treatment modalities as rapidly as possible and alert others of the outbreak. Treatment must begin as early as possible to provide the best chance of survival and prevent continued spread or contamination. Nurses need to be familiar with the early signs or symptoms of these infectious diseases and must know the mode of transmission to protect themselves and other patients (Table 66-2) (Stilp, 2004).

Identification of the causative agent will take longer and be more difficult if the specimen must be sent to remote laboratories for identification. Not all laboratories are able to handle suspected contagious disease specimens, especially the A-list diseases, and these specimens may need to be sent to specialized labs for diagnosis (Refer to Table 66-3). Specimen packaging and transport must be coordinated with the sending lab, CDC, and FBI to ensure safe transport. Therefore, as a result of delayed laboratory diagnosis, initial identification and treatment may rely on the presenting signs or symptoms and public health information through syndrome surveillance (Burkle, 2002).

BOX 66-5

POTENTIAL BIOLOGICAL WARFARE CLINICAL PRESENTATIONS

- Gastroenteritis of apparent infections etiology
- Pneumonia with the sudden death of a healthy adult
- Widened mediastinum in a febrile patient with no other explanation
- Rash of synchronous vesicular or pustular lesions
- Acute neurological illness with fever
- Advancing cranial nerve impairment with progressive generalized weakness
- Higher than usual number of patients with fever, urinary, and GI complaints
- Multiple patients with similar complaints from a common location
- An endemic disease appearing during an unusual time of year

Adapted from Burkle, F. (2002). Mass casualty management of a large scale bioterrorism event: An epidemiological approach that shapes triage decisions. Emergency Medicine Clinics of North America, 20*(2), 409–436.*

TABLE 66-2 Isolation Guidelines

	Bacterial Agents	Anthrax	Brucellosis	Cholera	Glanders	Bubonic plague	Pneumonic plague	Tularemia	Q fever	***Viruses***	Smallpox	Venez, equine encephalitis	Viral hemorrhagic fever	***Biological Toxins***	Botulism	Ricin
Isolation Precautions																
Standard precautions for all aspects of patient care		X	X	X	X	X	X	X	X		X	X	X		X	X
Contact precautions (gown and gloves; wash hands after each patient encounter)			X[c]	X[a]	X[a]						X		X			
Airborne precautions (negative pressure room and N-95 masks for all individuals entering the room)											X		X[b]			
Droplet precautions (surgical mask)							X									
Patient Placement																
No restrictions		X	X	X	X			X	X			X			X	X
Cohort like patients when private room unavailable				X[c]	X[a]	X	X				X		X			
Private room				X[c]	X[a]	X[a]	X				X		X			
Negative pressure											X		X[b]			
Door closed at all times											X		X[b]			
Patient Transport																
No restrictions		X	X	X	X	X		X	X			X			X	X
Limit movement to essential medical purposes only				X[c]	X[a]	X[a]	X[a]				X[a]		X			
Place mask on patient to minimize dispersal of droplets							X[a]				X[a]		X[b]			
Discontinuation of Isolation																
48 hours of appropriate antibiotic and clinical improvement							X									
Until all scabs separate											X					
Until skin decontamination completed (1 hour contact time)																
Duration of illness				X[c]	X[a]	X[a]							X			

[a]*Contact precautions needed only if the patient has skin involvement (bubonic plague: draining bubo) or until decontamination of skin is complete.*

[b]*A surgical mask and eye protection should be worn if you come within three feet of patient. Airborne precautions are needed if patient has cough, vomiting, diarrhea, or hemorrhage.*

[c]*Contact precautions needed only if the patient is diapered or incontinent.*

Adapted from Stilp, R. (2004). Biological weapons and emergency preparedness, Part I. *Retrieved June 27, 2006, from nsweb.nursingspectrum.com.*

TABLE 66-3 Laboratory Biosafety Levels

Biosafety Level I	These labs work with microorganisms not known to cause disease in healthy humans.
Biosafety Level II	These labs work with microorganisms that are of moderate risk to humans and the environment. Frequently the agents cause childhood diseases, to which the laboratory personnel have built up immunity or can be vaccinated against. Most hospital labs are biosafety level II.
Biosafety Level III	These labs work with infectious agents, which can cause serious or lethal disease, via the inhalation route. Personnel frequently wear respirators when performing these tests.
Biosafety Level IV	These labs work with infectious agents with a high potential of aerosol-transmitted diseases. Personnel wear a one-piece positive pressure suit that is ventilated by a life support system protected by HEPA filtration.

Adapted from Richmond, J. (2006). The 1, 2, 3s of biosafety levels. *Retrieved June 24, 2006, from www.cdc.gov.*

Triage stemming from a bioterrorism event (BT) will be less like standard triage and more like disaster triage. Patient care will be directed to rapidly treat those patients who have the greatest likelihood of survival as it will be difficult to successfully treat multiple patients with advanced signs or symptoms. ED staff will need to think beyond the current case, look into the future and consider the available resources and potential number of victims. Care will first be given to those with the greatest chance of survival, not necessarily the sickest. If the disease is contagious, the triage nurse's first goal will be to prevent the spread of secondary infection. To prevent secondary infection, the basic reproduction rate of the disease needs to be reduced.

Decreasing the contact rate between people will help prevent secondary infection although staff behaviors and hospital policies may need to be changed. First, adequate PPE must be worn at all times and hand washing must occur between every patient contact. Prophylactic antibiotics and vaccinations may have some benefit depending on the causative agent, and staff may be advised to receive these medications for their protection. Patients, staff, and even hospitals may need to be quarantined to help limit the epidemic (Burkle, 2002). Unlike victims of trauma, it may not always be obvious which patients were truly exposed to biological agents versus those who are worried well. Hospital ops plans must have preestablished disease-specific criteria to help assess which patients need treatment versus those who need monitoring or just emotional support. Victims who need surveillance will need to be grouped together and monitored for developing symptomatology and to initiate treatment if they become ill.

Smallpox

Smallpox is caused by the virus ortho pox and has two forms, variola major and variola minor, with major being the most common and deadly. In 1980, the World Health Organization (WHO) declared smallpox eradicated worldwide, and routine vaccination was stopped, and the supply of smallpox vaccine was destroyed. Much of the current population has not been vaccinated, or if vaccinated, they have not received routine booster shots.

Epidemiology

As a result most of the world is without smallpox immunity. Unfortunately, smallpox is thought to have the potential to become a biological weapon, and the extent of worldwide clandestine smallpox virus is unknown.

Etiology

Smallpox is usually spread through prolonged face-to-face contact and may also be spread via direct contact with contaminated items. The average incubation period for smallpox is 12 days but ranges anywhere between 7 and 19 days. Patients are contagious from rash onset until all the scabs have sepa-

Red Flag

Recognizing Smallpox

You must be prepared to recognize a **vesicular rash** (a raised blistering rash), **exanthema** (breaking out in a rash), and immediately take the appropriate isolation and droplet precautions. The hospital's infection control practitioners must be involved as early as possible, because one confirmed smallpox case could be a worldwide emergency.

rated. In some cases patients may be contagious after exposure but prior to the onset of the rash during the **prodrome phase** (the beginning clinical manifestations that a person has for an upcoming illness). It is for this reason that patients who exhibit the rash or who have been exposed are quarantined and respiratory precautions taken.

Assessment with Clinical Manifestations

Patients will initially present with an acute onset of **malaise** (a vague feeling of not being quite right or ill at ease), **rigors** (a muscular tremor caused by a chill), vomiting, headache, backache, and a high fever. This is the prodrome phase and lasts two to four days. The prodrome phase is followed by the **macular rash** (a rash with flat red spots) rash stage, which begins as small red spots on the tongue and in the mouth. These spots then break open in the patient's mouth and throat, and it is during this time that the patients are most contagious. Within 24 hours, the rash spreads to the patient's face, arms, legs, and then hands and feet. Although chickenpox and smallpox have many similarities, the distinguishing characteristic between the two is that the smallpox rash is **centrifugal** (extends outward away from the center) with a greater abundance on the extremities and face. Patients with smallpox will also have the rash on the palms of their hands and soles of their feet. Around day four the rash is raised, the lesions fill with a thick opaque fluid, develop a depression that resembles a belly button, and become round and firm to the touch. Around 10 days from the rash onset, scabs will begin to form. Approximately two-and-a-half weeks after onset, the scabs will start to fall off. After all of the scabs have fallen off, the patient is no longer contagious (CDC, 2006e).

Diagnostic Tests

Smallpox may be diagnosed by culturing the pustules, although there are only a few labs in the United States that are equipped to diagnose the ortho pox virus. The CDC will advise how the samples need to be sent (CDC, 2006e).

Nursing Diagnoses

Based on the information gathered, examples of nursing diagnoses in the patient with smallpox may include the following:

- Disturbed body image related to the smallpox rash.
- Impaired tissue integrity related to damage from the smallpox rash.
- Risk for infection related to tissue destruction from the smallpox virus.

Planning and Implementation

Smallpox is a disease that is spread from person-to-person contact. In addition, it is a highly contagious disorder with grave consequences in the event of its spread. Therefore, the plan of care is highly focused on prevention of the disease and careful assessment of potential persons who could contract the smallpox virus. Smallpox is spread via direct contact with infected body fluids or other contaminated objects, such as linen. It is also spread via the respiratory route with face-to-face contact. Individuals caring for suspected or known smallpox patients must use standard, droplet, and airborne precautions, and PPE (Box 66-6).

Pharmacology

Although at this time a smallpox vaccination does exist, there is not a large enough supply to immunize the world's population. Currently pharmaceutical companies are working to create a supply large enough for worldwide immunization. The vaccination is administered via the **intradermal route** (an injection into the skin).with a bifurcated needle, which leaves a circular scar (scarification). Refer to Figure 66-6 that shows a vaccination, which may be administered prophylactically or within seven days of a known exposure. There is no specific pharmacological treatment for smallpox, and management is supportive. In large outbreak smallpox, patients may be cared for at home with family providing the supportive care.

BOX 66-6

IMPORTANT FACTS REGARDING SMALLPOX VACCINATION

Administered by bifurcated needle.

A vesicle appears at the vaccination site five to seven days after inoculation with surrounding erythema and induration.

This lesion will scab over and heal one to two weeks later.

Common side effects include a low-grade fever and axillary lymphadenopathy.

Rare side effects include secondary inoculation of the virus to other areas, such as the face, eyelid, other people, or systemic spread of the virus (generalized vaccinia).

Adapted from Centers for Disease Control and Prevention. (2006e). Small pox disease overview. *Retrieved June 24, 2006, from www.cdc.gov.*

Patient Family Teaching

Education will need to be provided to family who will be caring for smallpox patients at home. Hospitals should have home care instructions available prior to any event in multiple languages.

Evaluation of Outcomes

Potential patient outcomes for each of the example nursing diagnoses for the patient with the smallpox virus are:

- Disturbed body image. The patient will demonstrate enhanced body image and self-esteem as evidenced by the ability to look at, touch, talk about, and care for the area of the smallpox sites.
- Impaired tissue integrity. The condition of the impaired tissue caused by the smallpox virus improves as evidenced by a decreased redness, swelling, and pain.
- Risk for infection. The patient remains free of infection, as evidenced by normal vital signs and the absence of purulent drainage from the smallpox areas. In addition, the potential area of infection is recognized early to allow for prompt treatment.

Plague

Yersinia pestis bacterium causes three forms of the plague: bubonic, septicemic, and pneumonic. The bubonic form is passed from infected fleas and then migrates into the patient's lymph nodes, known as a bubo, a swollen, painful node. Left untreated, the patient develops septicemic plague, which is often fatal. Less than 20 cases of bubonic plague are seen each year and are usually found in the southwestern United States (CDC, 2004e). During the 1950s and 1960s, the Soviet and U.S. governments worked with *Y. pestis* to create a biological weapon and were able to create an aerosolized organism. This, combined with the contagious nature of the pneumonic form, makes it particularly dangerous if it is released.

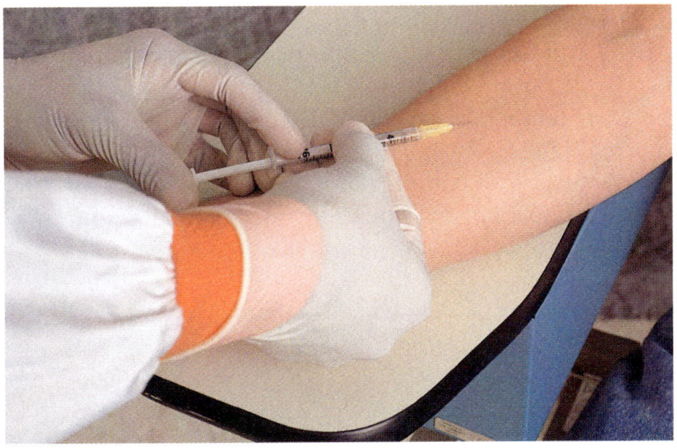

Figure 66-6 Administering vaccination.

Assessment with Clinical Manifestations

Pneumonic plague is a pulmonary infection, which arises from either inhalation of the organism, primary plague, or spreads to the lungs from septicemic plague. Symptoms develop acutely between one to six days after exposure to pneumonic plague. Symptoms include fever, chills, malaise, myalgias, headache, nausea, vomiting, diarrhea, and abdominal pain. Within 24 hours of the initial symptoms, the patient develops a cough with bloody sputum. Without treatment, the disease progresses rapidly to respiratory and circulatory collapse. The mortality of pneumonic plague is almost 100 percent, unless treatment is initiated within 24 hours of infection (Stilp, 2004).

Diagnostic Tests

Plague must be suspected with a large influx of previously healthy patients who have fulminant gram-negative pneumonia. Definitive diagnosis is made via culture of the organism from sputum and blood samples (CDC, 2004e).

Nursing Diagnoses

Based on the information gathered, examples of nursing diagnoses in the patient with the plague may include the following:

- Impaired gas exchange related to altered oxygen supply and CO_2 exchange from the plague.
- Risk for imbalanced body temperature related to the febrile condition evidenced during plague.
- Ineffective breathing pattern related to the pulmonary complications caused by plague.

Planning and Implementation

The plague is a relatively rare disorder, but when it does manifest itself, it generally presents with respiratory complications. Therefore, the care needs to initially focus on the assessment and detection of the presence of the disease. If the disease does exist in the patient, the respiratory assessment and potential oxygenation status of the patient needs managing. Because pneumonic plague is spread via droplets, these patients will need to be isolated or grouped together, and ED nurses must utilize standard and droplet precautions when caring for these patients.

Pharmacology

Antibiotic therapy must be started as soon as culture samples are taken. Streptomycin is the drug of choice, but gentamicin, tetracycline, and chloramphenicol are also effective when streptomycin is not available. Individuals who have been exposed to pneumonic plague need to be started on doxycycline as a prophylaxis (Broyles, Reiss, & Evans, 2007). Currently there is no vaccine available for plague.

Evaluation of Outcomes

Potential patient outcomes for each of the example nursing diagnoses for the patient with the plague are:

- Impaired gas exchange due to altered oxygen supply and CO_2 exchange. The patient maintains optimal gas exchange as evidenced by normal arterial blood gases (ABGs) and has alert mentation or no further reduction in mental status.
- Risk for imbalanced body temperature. The patient maintains body temperature within a normal range.
- Ineffective breathing pattern. The patient's breathing pattern is maintained as evidenced by eupnea, normal skin color, and regular respiratory rate and patterns.

Ebola

The Ebola virus is a Filovirus that has had at least 20 known outbreaks since the 1960s. This virus has been prepared as a biological weapon and is of great concern because of its extreme destructive nature and the high mortality rates associated with its occurrence.

Epidemiology

It is hypothesized that this virus is initially passed to humans via infected animals native to Africa. Initially, diagnosing Ebola may be difficult because of the non-specific symptoms, and therefore, the nurse must be astute to the patient's travel history, especially to Africa. If a large number of patients with Ebola-like symptoms are seen outside of Africa, biological warfare must be considered.

Etiology

Viral hemorrhagic fevers (VHFs) make up a group of illnesses caused by viruses from several similar families: arena viruses, Filoviruses, bunyaviruses, and flaviviruses. These four viruses are similar in that they are all RNA viruses and depend on an animal or insect host, as the natural reservoir for their survival. Humans are infected when they come into contact with one of these infected hosts (CDC, 2004b).

Assessment with Clinical Manifestation

Filoviridae virus causes Ebola hemorrhagic fever. The incubation period of Ebola ranges from 2 to 21 days. The initial symptoms begin abruptly with fever, headache, myalgias, sore throat, and weakness. Patients then develop abdominal pain, diarrhea, and vomiting (CDC, 2004b). Patients may also develop **coagulopathies** (disorders that lead to abnormal clotting of the blood), generalized internal and external hemorrhage, hypotension, and shock, because this virus targets the vascular beds.

Diagnostic Tests

A diagnosis of Ebola may be confirmed through antigen-capture enzyme linked immunosorbent assay (ELISA), IgM ELISA, and virus isolation blood tests. Because of the contagiousness of this virus, specimens must be sent to a Biolevel-4 (BL-4) lab for analysis. The CDC will advise how to package and transport the specimen.

Nursing Diagnoses

Based on the information gathered, examples of nursing diagnoses in the patient with Ebola may include the following:

- Risk for deficient fluid volume related to diarrhea and bleeding associated with Ebola.
- Diarrhea related to the Ebola virus.
- Acute pain related to the Ebola virus.

Planning and Implementation

Supportive management for a disease with no treatment or cure is the obvious recommendation from the CDC. The patient, his family, the community of focus, and health care workers need substantial teaching to illicit appropriate and timely responses to this rare but deadly disease. Ebola is spread from affected humans through direct contact with body fluids. Nurses must be cautious, because contaminated objects, such as needles, can also spread this virus. In Africa the virus has been spread from patient to caregivers who were not wearing PPE and passed via the aerosol route. Patients who are suspected of having VHF must be placed in a private isolation room with a separate anteroom for changing into PPE and patient equipment and supply storage. Standard precautions along with airborne precautions must be used for all of these patients. Additionally, if the patient has a prominent cough or loss of body fluids, the nurse must wear a respirator.

Pharmacology

There is no known specific treatment for Ebola, treatment is aimed at supportive care and treating specific symptomatology. Volume replacement may be needed for blood loss; pressor agents are frequently used to help maintain blood pressure; and ventilators may be required to help maintain oxygenation.

Evaluation of Outcomes

Potential patient outcomes for each of the example nursing diagnoses for the patient with Ebola are:

- Risk for deficient fluid volume related to diarrhea and bleeding associated with Ebola. The patient should experience fluid volume and electrolyte balance as evidenced by a urine output of greater than 30 mL/hour, normal blood pressure and heart rate, a consistency of general body weight, and normal skin turgor.
- Diarrhea related to the Ebola virus. The patient should defecate a soft, formed stool with no more than a frequency of three times a day.
- Acute pain related to the Ebola virus. The patient should verbalize an adequate relief of pain along with the ability to realistically cope with the pain if it is not completely relieved.

Anthrax

Anthrax is considered the greatest bioterrorism threat. In recent attacks, anthrax has been used as a scare tactic as well as a true threat. The organism of concern is *Bacillus anthracis,* anthrax, which is a genetic gram-positive bacterium (CDC, 2006a). The ease of obtaining the organism and relative ease of dispensing anthrax are the primary reasons for fearing this pathological threat of terrorist activity.

Epidemiology

There are three forms of anthrax: cutaneous, inhaled, and GI. Cutaneous anthrax develops from direct contact with spores usually from infected animals or animal products, such as wool. Inhalation of aerosolized anthrax spores leads to respiratory anthrax. Consumption of undercooked meat contaminated with the spores lead to the GI form. WHO estimates that if 50 kg of anthrax spores were dispersed over a 2-kilometer line upwind from a city with a population of 500,000, within three days 125,000 people would be infected and 95,000 people could die (CDC, 2006a).

Etiology

The pulmonary **macrophages** (a type of white blood cell that ingests and helps destroy foreign material) carry the spores to the tracheobronchial or mediastinal lymph nodes. This organism then produces an **antiphagocytic** (something that destroys the neutrophils and macrophages function) capsule, which produces lethal toxins leading to the release of *B. anthracis* into the blood stream, causing overwhelming septicemia. Anthrax spores resist environmental destruction, tolerate aerosolization well, and are 2 to 6 microns in diameter, the perfect setup for attachment to the respiratory mucosa.

Assessment with Clinical Manifestations

The average incubation period of inhalation of anthrax is 1 to 6 days, but it has been dormant for up to 43 days. After the incubation period, the patient complains of nonspecific flu-like symptoms, such as headache and a nonproductive cough. After 1 to 3 days, many patients have a brief period when they feel better but then rapidly deteriorate with high fever, dyspnea, **stridor** (a high-pitched harsh sound heard on inhalation due to narrowing of the airway), cyanosis, and shock. Chest x-rays (CXRs) may show a widened mediastinum. One hundred percent of inhalation anthrax patients will die if there is no treatment, and there is 95 percent mortality rate if treatment is not begun within 48 hours.

Diagnostic Tests

Anthrax should be suspected when patients present with the signs and symptoms outlined, and gram-positive bacilli are seen on peripheral blood smear. Aerobic blood culture growth of large number of gram-positive bacilli is a preliminary diagnosis of *Bacillus* species.

Nursing Diagnoses

Based on the information gathered, examples of nursing diagnoses in the patient with anthrax may include the following:

- Ineffective breathing pattern related to the respiratory problems caused by the anthrax.
- Ineffective tissue perfusion related to decreased systemic vascular resistance in anthrax condition.
- Risk for imbalanced body temperature related to the febrile condition evidenced during anthrax disorder.

Planning and Implementation

It is critical to diagnose the presence of the anthrax virus in people suspected of having the virus. The more immediate the identification of the disease, the higher the correlation of successful antibiotic therapy. In addition, the patient, family, the community of focus, and health care workers need substantial teaching to calm their fears related to a widespread contaminant and potential terrorist threat. Because anthrax has a low potential for person-to-person transmission, standard precautions are adequate.

Pharmacology

If anthrax is suspect after obtaining blood cultures, it is recommended to immediately start ciprofloxacin (Cipro) IV. Oral Cipro is recommended for postexposure treatment. This should be started as early as possible to all people exposed, including health care workers. In confirmed anthrax cases, exposed personnel should also be immunized (CDC, 2006a).

Evaluation of Outcomes

Potential patient outcomes for each of the example nursing diagnoses for the patient with the anthrax organism are:

- Ineffective breathing pattern related to the respiratory problems caused by the anthrax. The patient's breathing rhythm is maintained as shown by normal unlabored breathing, normal skin color, and verbalizing comfort in the breathing.
- Ineffective tissue perfusion related to decreased systemic vascular resistance in anthrax condition. The patient should maintain good tissue perfusion to the essential organs, as demonstrated by strong peripheral pulses, normal arterial blood gases, and an alert level of consciousness (LOC).
- Risk for imbalanced body temperature. The patient maintains body temperature within a normal range.

Severe Acute Respiratory Syndrome

Severe acute respiratory syndrome (SARS) is a newly recognized infectious disease. SARS was first recognized in the Guangdong Province in southeastern China in 2002 and is the first new infectious disease of the 21st century. WHO issued a global warning about the appearance of SARS in March of 2003 (File, 2004).

Epidemiology

This disease spread worldwide in early 2003. SARS gained global notoriety, because it is a highly contagious infectious disease with a high mortality rate and is easily transmitted to health care workers. SARS led to the disruption of health care delivery systems worldwide and has even caused hospital closures because of outbreaks (CDC, 2004f). This disease is particularly challenging because so little is known about it.

Etiology

SARS is caused by a new **coronavirus,** a virus that normally only leads to upper respiratory infection. No one understands why this virus now has turned deadly. This virus has been found in humans, in civet cats, and a raccoon dog (considered human delicacies in Guangdong Province). This suggests the virus can be passed from animal to human (File, 2004). Researchers are trying to learn why some individuals exposed to the SARS virus live, and others will die. Deaths from SARS are more prevalent in the elderly population but young, healthy individuals have also died from SARS.

Assessment with Clinical Manifestations

SARS patients initially complain of a prodrome phase with onset of fever (38° C [100.4° F] or greater), chills, rigors, **myalgia** (pain in the muscles), and headache, symptoms similar to influenza, although patients deny having sneezing or runny nose. Three to seven days later patients develop lower respiratory tract symptomatology and pneumonia with a nonproductive cough. Twenty percent of SARS patients will then develop **acute respiratory distress syndrome (ARDS)** (an acute syndrome that leads to pulmonary insufficiency from accumulation of fluid in the alveolar sacs and requires ventilatory support). After exposure, the average incubation period for developing SARS is 6 to 10 days. Because SARS is a new illness, many facts are still unknown about the disease. With each outbreak, more epidemiological, prevention, and treatments will be found.

Diagnostic Tests

The coronavirus causing SARS can be identified through a reverse transcription polymerase chain test. Blood or nasal samples are taken to look at the virus' DNA strand. Patients with SARS will also have identifiable coronavirus antibodies in their blood. The virus can also be identified via fluid or tissue culture.

Nursing Diagnoses

Based on the information gathered, examples of nursing diagnoses in the patient with SARS may include the following:

- Impaired gas exchange due to damage to alveolar-capillary membrane, change in lung compliance.
- Acute pain related to the headache condition associated with SARS.
- Fear in response to the diagnosis of SARS.

Planning and Implementation

The SARS disorder requires a worldwide preventive goal as the disease presents itself in a given region. Emphasis on patient education related to traveling and immigration should be emphasized. Once the disease is suspected, then the focus for identifying the disease and subsequent support of the patient, family, and community is necessary. ED personnel may be the first care providers to be suspicious of SARS when triaging or caring for a patient. To protect themselves, transmission of the infection must be prevented at the first point of contact. The following recommendations can be practiced for all patients visiting an ED: post signs, in appropriate language for the EDs clientele, at all entrances, asking patients to inform personnel if they have signs of a respiratory infection, to cover their mouth when coughing, to dispose of tissues, and to wash their hands frequently (Box 66-7) (CDC, 2004f). During periods of increased respiratory illnesses, triage nurses should provide masks to patients with a cough and provide a separate waiting room for these patients. Additionally, health care workers should practice droplet precautions using N-95 masks, along with standard precautions when in close contact with patients with respiratory illness. It is also theorized that the virus may be spread via contaminated objects, making it imperative that nurses practice stringent hand hygiene.

Pharmacology

There is no specific treatment for SARS, but current recommendations include supportive care (such as ventilatory support) and broad-spectrum antimicrobials.

> **Red Flag**
>
> **SARS**
>
> During periods of known SARS outbreak, triage nurses must also screen all patients with respiratory illness for the following risk factors:
>
> Within the last 10 days has the patient traveled to mainland China, Hong Kong, Taiwan, or areas where outbreak is occurring or close contact with an ill person who has traveled to these areas?
>
> Is the patient a health care worker who has been caring for patients with respiratory illness? Is the patient a laboratory staff person where live SARS virus exists? If any of these are true, the patient needs to be immediately placed in isolation with droplet precautions.

BOX 66-7

INFECTION CONTROL PRECAUTIONS FOR POTENTIAL SARS PATIENTS

Place patient in a negative-pressure isolation room.

Maintain a log of all persons who enter room.

Restrict visitors.

Restrict number of personnel caring for the patient.

All health care workers must practice hand hygiene, standard, and airborne precautions.

Limit cough inducing treatments, such as sputum induction or suction.

Avoid using noninvasive positive-pressure ventilation.

Educate all individuals caring for these patients to immediately seek treatment if they develop SARS symptoms.

Quarantine personnel who were exposed to patient without respiratory protection.

Adapted from Koller, D., Nicholas, D., Goldie, R., Gearing, R., & Selkirk, E. (2006). When family-centered care is challenged by infectious disease: Pediatric health care delivery during the SARS outbreaks. Qualitative Health Research, 16*(1), 47–60.*

Fast Forward ▶▶▶

Pharmacological Management of SARS

As with any other infectious disease it is important to educate health care workers on required infection control measures to protect themselves and others. Staff must not only understand the importance of basic infection control measures, they must practice it. During the 2003 SARS outbreak, health care workers were not following hand hygiene and isolation recommendations, and they were not using PPE correctly (CDC, 2004f). Despite worldwide research efforts, an effective treatment regimen has not been found. Recently preliminary studies found that the antiviral drug combination of lopinavir and ritonavir and ribavirin have prevented serious complications and even death. Research continues with the hope of Food and Drug Administration (FDA) approval for this use.

Evaluation of Outcomes

Potential patient outcomes for each of the example nursing diagnoses for the patient with SARS are:

- Impaired gas exchange due to damage to alveolar-capillary membrane, change in lung compliance. The patient maintains optimal gas exchange as evidenced by normal arterial blood gases (ABGs) and has alert mentation or no further reduction in mental status.
- Acute pain related to the headache condition associated with SARS. The patient should verbalize an adequate relief of pain along with the ability to realistically cope with the pain if it is not completely relieved.
- Fear in response to the diagnosis of SARS. The patient should manifest positive coping behaviors and verbalize a reduction in the amount of fear of the having this disease.

West Nile Virus

The West Nile virus (WNV) was first identified in Africa in the 1930s and was first documented in the United States in 1999. There was an epidemic in New York City in 1999, and patients were seen with what was first diagnosed as meningitis. Since that time, there have been increasing numbers of WNV reported on a worldwide basis.

Epidemiology

By 2004 all 50 states had confirmed human WNV cases totaling over 9,800 and over 250 deaths (Mayo Foundation for Medical Education and Research, 2004). Frequently individuals have been infected with the virus and have no signs or symptoms or may have complained of mild, virus-like illness. But WNV may lead to serious complications, including encephalitis, meningitis, or meningoencephalitis, and even death in the elderly and patients with other chronic medical diseases.

Etiology

WNV is a single-stranded RNA virus, a member of the Flaviviridae family. This virus survives in nature via biological transmission between blood feeding hosts (CDC, 2006f). Birds are the main reservoir for WNV. When a mosquito bites an infected bird, the mosquito then becomes the vector and passes the virus to humans via mosquito bites. Less than 1 percent of individuals bitten by an infected mosquito will become seriously ill. West Nile virus has been documented being passed from contaminated blood and organs, but it is not passed via the airborne route (Mayo Foundation for Medical Education and Research, 2004).

Assessment with Clinical Manifestations

Most people who have been bitten by an infected mosquito will have no signs or symptoms. Approximately 20 percent of bite victims will manifest a mild infection and complain of fever, headache, myalgias, backache, anorexia, GI disturbance, swollen lymph nodes, and a mild rash. One percent of patients bitten will develop a life-threatening illness manifested by high fever, stiff neck, severe headache, change in mentation, seizures, Parkinsonism, decreased coordination, partial paralysis, and coma (Mayo Foundation for Medical Education and Research, 2004).

Diagnostic Tests

The most common test for WNV is to measure for antibodies that are produced in blood. If the patient is presenting with encephalitis or meningitis symptomatology, a lumbar puncture will be performed to look for the virus presence in the patient's cerebrospinal fluid (CSF).

Nursing Diagnoses

Based on the information gathered, examples of nursing diagnoses in the patient with WNV may include the following:

- Acute pain as related to **nuchal** (a stiff painful neck due to irritated meninges) rigidity, inflammation of meninges, and headache.
- Fear in response to the diagnosis of WNV.
- Risk for imbalanced body temperature.
- Risk for infection related to the WNV.

Planning and Implementation

The WNV requires a worldwide preventive goal as the disease presents itself in a given region. Emphasis on patient education related to traveling and immigration should be emphasized. Once the disease is suspected, then the focus for identifying the disease and subsequent support of the patient, family, and community is necessary. WNV cannot be spread by direct person-to-person contact, and therefore standard precautions are all that are required when caring for a patient with WNV.

> *Red Flag*
>
> **The Use of Mosquito Repellant to Prevent WNV**
>
> Parents must be educated not to use mosquito repellent containing DEET on children less than 2 months of age. Instead, the infant's stroller should be covered with mosquito netting (CDC, 2006f).

Patient and Family Teaching

ED nurses can help provide education to patients about decreasing their risk of exposure to infected mosquitoes. Patients must be taught to use mosquito repellant with diethyltoluamide (DEET), wear long pants and long sleeve shirts during evening hours, and spend evening hours indoors in late summer and early fall. Removal of stagnate water around the house will also help decrease the number of mosquitoes.

Evaluation of Outcomes

Potential patient outcomes for each of the example nursing diagnoses for the patient with the WNV are:

- Acute pain as related to nuchal rigidity, inflammation of meninges, and headache. The patient should verbalize an adequate relief of pain along with the ability to realistically cope with the pain if it is not completely relieved.

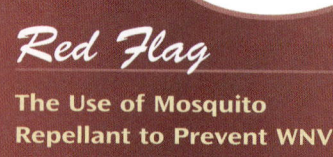

- Fear in response to the diagnosis of WNV. The patient should manifest positive coping behaviors and verbalize a reduction in the amount of fear of the having this disease.
- Risk for imbalanced body temperature. The patient maintains body temperature within a normal range.
- Risk for infection related to the WNV. The patient remains free of infection as evidenced by normal vital signs and an absence of inflammatory manifestations. In addition, an infection is recognized early for prompt management.

BLAST INJURIES

The majority of terrorist attacks in the United States, Atlanta Olympics and Oklahoma City, involve conventional weapons including bombs and missiles (CDC, 2003b). Victims of blast injuries have semipredictable injury patterns and injury severity predictors. Bombs are known to have a one third to two thirds injury split. One third of the victims will be critically injured and two thirds will be mildly injured, treated, and released.

The ED nurse must understand that injuries from explosions create a unique pattern of injury. There are four mechanisms of injury: primary, secondary, tertiary, and quaternary (Table 66-4). When a device explodes, it creates a blast wave (primary); the intense overpressurization force, which is created from the explosion of a device. This primary explosion affects the body's hollow organs.

Blast lung is the most common primary fatal injury among initial blast survivors. ED nurses will usually see this injury with the initial evaluation, but cases have been reported up to 48 hours after the event. Blast lung is characterized by a triad of apnea, bradycardia, and hypotension and produces a characteristic butterfly pattern on CXR. Abdominal injuries may be initially overlooked or hidden until the patient develops an acute abdomen or sepsis. If there is a traumatic amputation, the patient may have associated multisystem injuries. The ED nurse should not become focused on the gory injury but must perform a thorough systems assessment to rule out other injuries. Because the primary blast affects air-filled organs, air embolism is seen frequently and may present as MI, stroke, blindness, deafness, spinal cord injury (SCI), or vascular clotting. If the patient was trapped under debris, acute renal failure or **rhabdomyolysis**

TABLE 66-4 Blast Injury Patterns

CATEGORY	CHARACTERISTICS	BODY PART AFFECTED	INJURY TYPE
Primary	From blast wave	Gas-filled structures most likely the lung, GI tract, and middle ear	Blast lung (pulmonary barotraumas) tympanic rupture Abdominal hemorrhage and rupture Globe (eye) rupture Concussion
Secondary	Results from flying debris and bomb fragments	Any body part may be affected	Penetrating or blunt injuries
Tertiary	Results from patient being thrown from blast wave	Any body part may be affected	Fracture and traumatic amputation Closed and open brain injury
Quaternary	All injuries, illness not related to first, second, or third mechanism; includes exacerbation or complication of existing conditions	Any body part may be affected.	Burns Crush injury Respiratory problems due to smoke or dust Angina Hypertension

Adapted from Centers for Disease Control and Prevention (2003b). Explosion and blast injuries: A primer for clinicians. *Retrieved June 13, 2006, from www.cdc.gov/.*

(destruction of skeletal muscle cells which causes the release of myoglobin), or **compartment syndrome** (develops when muscle is damage from a traumatic event and swells cutting off circulation; if this pressure is not released, permanent muscle and nerve damage may occur) may be present. The patient may also have burn injuries from the explosive device (CDC, 2003b).

STRESS REACTIONS

Caring for victims of a MCI, whether it stems from a traumatic event, terrorism, natural disaster, or civil unrest will not only affect the victims, their families, the patient care providers, witnesses, and many others from the community. In addition to the physical injuries and depending on the event, victims may also suffer the loss of their loved ones, friends, pets, home, place of employment, and personal possessions. ED nurses will have to manage both injured disaster victim along with the worried well suffering from emotional distress, even if they were not directly affected by the event.

Traumatic events are marked by a sense of horror, helplessness, serious injury or threat of injury, or death. Following any traumatic event, it is a normal response for individuals to experience stress reactions, and the body's response to stress may affect a person's emotional, psychological, physical, or spiritual states. Individuals will have varying degrees of emotional or physical responses when exposed to a traumatic episode; these may include feelings of fear, grief, depression, nausea, vertigo, loss of appetite, change in sleep patterns, or social withdrawal (Table 66-5). These responses will be most prevalent the first days after the event and normally subside and resolve within 10 to 30 days (CDC, 2003a).

It is imperative for hospital ops plans to include established preincident crisis intervention plans that can be activated at the onset of an event to help care for their staff members. In events where there is the potential for transmission of the disease or chemical to the caregiver, staff will have the added fear of transmission or contraction of the disease. Hospital plans need to incorporate available resources and mobilization of counselors or pastors. In addition, hospitals should have coordinated preevent training with these individuals including defusing and debriefing techniques. During the event, staff who are triaging and caring for victims need to be evaluated throughout their shift to assess their emotional and physical stability. Individuals in the hospital's incident command should also be assessed for emotional stability due to the extreme pressure they can experience. Hospital plans should also include follow up for staff and victims. Postevent crisis intervention cannot be a one-time event but must be over a continuum.

The nurse plays an important role when interacting with the victims of a traumatic event and should encourage the patient to talk about their reactions

TABLE 66-5 Common Responses to a Traumatic Event

COGNITIVE	EMOTIONAL	PHYSICAL	BEHAVIORAL
Poor concentration	Shock	Nausea	Suspicion
Confusion	Numbness	Lightheaded	Irritability
Disoriented	Overwhelmed	Dizzy	Withdrawn
Memory loss	Insecure	Headaches	Silent
Indecisive	Volatile emotions	Sleeplessness	Substance abuse

Adapted from Centers for Disease Control and Prevention (2003a). Coping with a traumatic event. *Retrieved June 16, 2006, from www.cdc.gov/.*

when they are ready. Survivors respond best when the ED nurse offers eye contact, calm presence, and utilizes therapeutic listening skills. The patient needs validation that his or her reactions are normal and to be encouraged to follow normal routines, find ways to relax, eat healthy, sleep or rest quietly, and identify and utilize support systems. Frequently victims will need to have ongoing counseling to help the recovery process.

Each age-group is vulnerable to stress and may respond in different ways. Children think and process information differently than adults and will have different responses than adult patients. The age of the child will determine their understanding of the event. The nurse must understand the child's developmental stage to effectively deal with the child's psychological response. Reassurance will help children cope with traumatic events, and younger children will need a lot of cuddling. When a child asks questions, they need to be answered honestly, but do not dwell on the frightening details. Children must be encouraged to express their feelings not only through conversation, but also through drawing, painting, and play. Parents need to be encouraged to maintain normal household routines but limit children's viewing of television news coverage. Like adults, children need to be given the opportunity to discuss their feelings. The nurse should use age appropriate terms letting the child know it is okay to feel scared, sad or worried. Children respond to the emotional state of their caretaker, and the nurse needs to maintain a calm demeanor while caring for these children. It is important for the nurse to educate the child's parents that the psychological trauma does not go away immediately after the event and may continue to resurface for two years post event.

Respecting Our Differences

Cultural Backgrounds and Disasters

ED nurses must understand that patients with different cultural backgrounds may act and respond differently to disasters or traumatic events. It is imperative for the ED nurse to be familiar with the cultural groups in their communities and understand their norms, traditions, spiritual practices, and grieving process to provide the best care for these patients. Being familiar with these cultural practices will allow you to provide the best support, education, and counseling to your patients.

Posttraumatic Stress Disorder

Although it is normal for many people to experience stress reactions following a traumatic event, these responses should begin to subside within 10 days and resolve within 30 days. When these symptoms do not subside and begin interfering with a person's daily life, this is defined as posttraumatic stress disorder (PTSD). PTSD is an intense physical and psychological response to a traumatic event that lasts for weeks, months, or even years after the event. This disorder can occur in any age, socioeconomic class, gender, or any cultural group.

Pathophysiology

Both biological and physiological changes are seen with the patients suffering from PTSD. Changes are found with both the central and autonomic nervous systems; the hippocampus does not function as it should and the amygdala has abnormal activation possibly leading to flashbacks. The sympathetic nervous system becomes hyperaroused leading to sleep abnormalities and an overactive startle reflex (National Center for PTSD, 2003). Patients suffering from PTSD also have been found to have abnormal cortisol, epinephrine, and norepinephrine levels. In addition to PTSD, these patients frequently experience depression, anxiety disorder, or substance abuse which compounds their symptomatology.

Assessment with Clinical Manifestations

There are a wide variety of clinical manifestations associated with PTSD, which are illustrated in Box 66-8.

BOX 66-8

SIGNS AND SYMPTOMS OF PTSD

- Nightmares or flashbacks of the event
- Feelings of guilt
- Numbing of emotions
- Detachment or estrangement from friends and family
- Decreased interest in previous activities or hobbies
- Feelings of hopelessness or helplessness
- Difficulty concentrating
- Difficulty sleeping
- Substance abuse
- Severe depression
- Hyperarousal: panic, rage, extreme irritability

Adapted from National Center for PTSD. (2003). What is post-traumatic stress disorder? *Retrieved June 23, 2006, from www.ncptsd.org/facts.*

Planning and Implementation

PTSD is treated by a variety of psychotherapy support groups and medications. The patient should be referred to someone who is knowledgeable about trauma and disasters. The ED nurse must be aware of the signs and symptoms of PTSD and plan patient treatment with these in mind. Frequently, patients with PTSD are evaluated for depression and will need to be assessed and monitored for suicidal behaviors while in the ED. Some individuals will respond to cognitive therapy, group therapy, and exposure therapy. Selective serotonin reuptake inhibitors (SSRIs), like Prozac or Zoloft, are commonly found to be beneficial for treatment modalities for these individuals.

ED nurses have selected a highly rewarding field in which to work, but they have also selected a specialty that takes place in a demanding and stressful environment. These nurses place themselves in stressful situations daily, ranging from potential exposure to contagious disease, interacting with violent and verbally abusive patients, gruesome injuries, and traumatic deaths. ED nurses cannot choose which types of patients arrive in their department. Many of these patients die unexpectedly, and frequently these deaths involve a traumatic event. ED nurses quickly realize many of these deaths could have been prevented and were unnecessary.

Crises are a normal part of the ED nurse's day. This ongoing state of crisis places ED nurses at risk for developing PTSD. This may develop from one particular horrific event, such as caring for victims of the September 11th terrorist attack or the Columbine school shooting. Frequently though, PTSD arises from the accumulation of stress, which evolves from caring for single isolated events over time.

All people react to and respond differently to stress. These responses may be altered by a variety of things, such as the individual's psychological and emotional fatigue, coping style, and previous experiences combined with their closeness to the event. If the nurse caring for a 4-year-old critically injured child also has a child that age, it is likely that the nurse will experience increased stress compared with a nurse with no children.

Advance warning of the incoming patients and their injury or acuity level will help the ED nurse to prepare for what is arriving and begin to utilize coping strategies. When the brain receives input, it tries to file it in the appropri-

Skills 360°

Prevention of Pediatric Trauma Deaths

Up to 50 percent of the pediatric traumatic deaths are considered preventable. ED nurses commonly choose to become involved in community education to help stop these needless deaths. This may include education regarding bicycle, skateboard, and motorcycle helmet use, car seat safety, water safety, and bike rodeos. Frequently EDs give out free helmets and car seats to low-income families who visit their department. As an ED nurse it is essential you are educated on the required safety guidelines to provide injury prevention education to your patients or direct them to appropriate resources during every visit. ED nurses must take advantage of this captive audience to help promote safe and healthy children.

Respecting Our Differences

The Effects of Trauma on Children

Children are more vulnerable to the effects of an infectious disease or traumatic injury because of their physiological status. Children have a faster respiratory rate than adults, and therefore will receive more inhaled agent than adults. A child's skin is thinner, which offers less protection from absorption, and they have a larger surface to mass ratio than adults. They also have a smaller circulating blood volume with less tolerance to volume loss from bleeding, vomiting, or diarrhea (American Academy of Pediatrics, 2002). Children cannot be considered little adults, and medication and antidote doses will be different from the standard adult doses. Hospitals must have the correct pediatric and neonatal medication concentrations available. If a child requires decontamination he or she presents an even greater challenge because of his or her rapid heat loss and increased risk for hypothermia. EDs should create special treatment areas for pediatric victims. Disaster drills must include pediatric victims so staff will be familiar caring for them. Hospital operation plans need to include provisions for psychological support to these young victims.

Children depend on daily routines and when these routines are interrupted, especially because of a disaster, the child may become anxious. Following a disaster, children are fearful that the event will occur again, that they will be separated from their family, that someone will be killed, or that they will be left alone. Additionally, children may have lost a special comfort measure, such as a blanket or stuffed animal, which adults may consider insignificant, but for the child it has an emotional attachment. This loss combined with a traumatic event may lead to the child having nightmares, becoming easily upset, or even reverting to younger behaviors, such as bedwetting. The child may be afraid to leave his or her family, and some children may even believe he or she was the cause of the event.

Uncovering the Evidence

Traumatic Brain Injury

Discussion: The purpose of this study was to explore the relationship of child abuse following a natural disaster, specifically looking at traumatic brain injury (TBI). The study concluded that TBI increased in those counties most affected by Hurricane Floyd six months post disaster compared to those counties predisaster. Cases of inflicted TBI, intra-cranial injury, in children ≤ 2 years, with admission to an ICU or death from September 1998 to December 2001 in North Carolina were reviewed. A Poisson regression modeling calculated the rate ratios of injury for each geographical area by time period. It was found there was a five-fold increase for injury inflicted to children ≤ 2 years in counties more severely affected versus those less affected.

Implications for Practice: Disasters lead to increased stress related to the event. They also lead to stress from disruption of the community's social structure, loss of home, jobs, and financial hardship. Nurses need to realize the opportunities for providing parents with resources for support and need to be given immediately after the event and in the ensuing months. Parents must be educated on coping techniques and when and who to call when they are feeling overwhelmed. The ED nurse must remember to maintain a high index of suspicion when caring for children with closed head injuries or with decreased LOCs, especially in areas recently experiencing a disaster.

Citation: Keenan, H., Marshall, S., Nocera, M., & Runyan, D. (2004). Increased incidence of inflicted traumatic brain injury in children after a natural disaster. American Journal of Preventive Medicine, *26(3), 189–193.*

ate place. When the nurse knows in advance the type of patient that is coming in, the brain is better able to help the nurse prepare for the horrific case. Thus, a grotesquely disfiguring injury does not seem as bad as when the nurse has time to prepare for it emotionally.

ED nurses tend to utilize two separate sides of their brain when caring for a **critical incident** (a patient or event that causes a stress reaction in the health care worker) patient. If ED nurses were to react emotionally every time they were exposed to critical incidents, it would be extremely difficult for them to perform their job. The ED nurse utilizes their professional side to help remain calm and care for the patient at hand. All the while the nurse's emotional side is absorbing the sights, sounds, and smells of the event and is creating an imprint or memory. The professional side helps the nurse to function on autopilot at times, even relying on rote memory to achieve the desired outcomes. The professional side, all the while, is helping to keep the emotional side pushed aside or "stuffed" until it can surface after the event.

During resuscitation much of the nurse's brain is busy multitasking. The brain is taking in all that is occurring, evaluating actions, and anticipating what tasks need to be performed next. If an unanticipated sight, smell, or sound occurs, such as a parent screaming as he or she is brought into the resuscitation room, the brain cannot buffer or file this normally. This unanticipated impulse is randomly placed in the memory core of the brain, the hippocampus.

ED nurses must be proactive in trying to protect themselves from the development of PTSD. Nurses must learn how to deal with routine stress to care for themselves and coworkers. They must eat well-balanced meals, drink plenty of water, and limit caffeine and sugar intake. Regular exercise (at least 30 minutes four times a week) will help rid the body of toxic chemicals that are released dur-

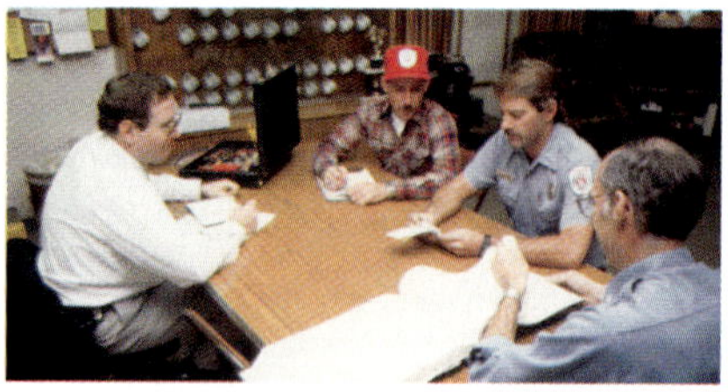

Figure 66-7 A critical incident stress management debriefing is an invaluable setting to assist health care workers, such as the phlebotomist, deal with the impact of a stressful event.

ing stressful situations. Staying rested and having consistent sleep patterns will help prevent psychological and emotional fatigue and better prepare the nurse to respond to stressful events. After being involved with the care of a patient from a critical incident, it is imperative the nurse be allowed a few minutes to decompress before moving on to care for the next patient. This will allow the nurse to cry, pray, meditate, or just have a few minutes of self-reflection and processing of the recent events. At the completion of the shift the nurse needs to take time to talk with coworkers, friends, or family to also help process the events.

Critical Incident Stress Management

Many health care professionals utilize critical incident stress management (CISM) to help decrease the stress reactions and prevent PTSD. CISM teams are made up of emergency professionals and mental health workers who have been trained in leading defusing and debriefings.

Defusing allow the staff to talk about their feelings and process their emotions and also provides an opportunity for the nurse to be educated on normal stress responses versus prolonged responses. Defusing occur as a one-on-one between a team member and the health care provider immediately or shortly after the event. This technique is employed when only one or two individuals are having difficulties with the case. Debriefings are more formalized and all health care providers are invited to attend from the EMS dispatchers to the phlebotomists (Figure 66-7). Debriefings usually occur within 24 to 96 hours after the event and take place over a two- to three-hour period. Debriefings are not critiques of the case but a chance for every team member to tell his or her story and discuss how he or she are feeling (Box 66-9). It is important for ED managers to provide support and shift coverage for any staff members to attend if they are working the day of the debriefing.

ED staff may not want to attend the debriefings, because they believe they will be considered as weak if they cannot cope. In addition, these nurses may feel that they should be able to stuff all of their emotions, because death is part of their job. If nurses do not care for themselves and take advantage of theses debriefings, they will eventually suffer from burnout and may even develop PTSD.

BOX 66-9

THE EIGHT PHASES OF A DEBRIEFING

- Introduction phase: ground rules are established, the process is explained, introductions are made, and the individuals role in the event is explained.
- Fact phase: individuals provide facts of the case. Introduction of these facts frequently fills in missing answer for other care providers.
- Thought phase: touching on the individual's emotional aspects begins in the phase.
- Reaction phase: usually felt to be the most intense phase, participants are asked to answer, "how did you react to the incident?" Individuals may just choose to listen instead of answer.
- Symptom phase: various symptoms that people are experiencing are discussed and validated.
- Teaching phase: members are educated on stress reactions and techniques to decrease these reactions are explored.
- Reentry phase: this is the closure phase.
- Follow-up phase: the CISM team may follow-up with individuals postdebriefing to ensure they are feeling better.

Adapted from Pulley, S. (2004). Critical incident stress management. *Retrieved July 6, 2006, from http://www.emedicine.com.*

BOX 66-10

MANAGING YOUR STRESS DURING A DISASTER

- Develop a buddy system with another coworker.
- Eat small, frequent, healthy snacks.
- Drink lots of water.
- Take breaks.
- Stay in touch with family or friends.
- Support your coworkers.
- Take a few minutes to defuse each shift.

Adapted from National Center for PTSD. (2003). What is post-traumatic stress disorder? *Retrieved June 23, 2006, from http://www.ncptsd.org.*

Skills 360°

Nurses Attending a Debriefing

ED nurses may not want to attend the debriefing, because they feel they are not affected by the critical event or case. All caregivers involved in the case should attend the debriefing, because they have a piece of the puzzle that may help another health care worker. For instance, the ED nurse has cared for a child involved in a house fire, the child and her sister were asleep in bunk beds. The child on the top bunk died, but the child on the bottom bunk survived. The ED nurse cannot understand why one child died and the other child lived. During the debriefing the firefighters on the scene told their part of the story and described the burned bedroom; thereby answering the nurse's questions. Ultimately this helped the nurse to cope, process, and recover form the horrific event (Box 66-10).

KEY CONCEPTS

- EDs are becoming America's safety net for patient care.
- Because of a short length of stay it is challenging for ED nurses to develop a collaborative plan of care.
- A triage system is one in which priorities for care are developed.
- The START method allows for rapid triage, less than 60 seconds, of multiple patients.
- During an MCI, the triage philosophy changes to providing care first to those most likely to survive versus providing care first to the most critical.
- A disaster is defined as the destructive effects of natural or manmade forces overwhelm the ability of a given area or community to meet the demands of health care.
- The ICS is a system utilized to help manage large-scale events.
- HEICS helps provide a consistent algorithm for organizing information, controlling and coordinating the influx of patients, distribution of required staff, supplies, resources, and communication.
- JCAHO requires hospitals to have an emergency management plan that addresses four phases: preparedness, mitigation, response, and recovery.
- Hospital ops plans need to address internal and external disasters, bioterrorism, and chemical and radiation emergencies.
- DMAT teams will be deployed to large-scale disasters and comprise MDs, nurses, EMTs, and social workers.
- HazMats have the potential to harm a person or the environment.
- There are three OSHA-approved levels of protection. Level A offers the highest level of protection.
- Biological agents include bacteria, viruses, and toxins. The A-list is those agents considered the largest threat.
- Smallpox patient are contagious until all of the scabs have fallen off.
- The mortality of *Yersinia* plague is almost 100 percent if treatment is not started within 24 hours of infection.
- If a large number of patients with Ebola-like symptoms are seen in the United States, biological warfare should be suspected.
- All of the patients suffering from inhalation anthrax will die without treatment.
- WNV is passed to humans via contaminated mosquitoes. Individuals will experience a variety of emotional and physical responses when exposed to a traumatic event.
- PTSD is an intense physical and psychological response to a traumatic event that lasts weeks, months, or years after exposure to a traumatic event.
- Defusing occurs one-on-one briefly after an event, whereas debriefings occur with larger groups after the event.

REVIEW QUESTIONS

1. Biological weapons are considered the ultimate weapon, because they:
   1. Can cause mass casualties
   2. Are inexpensive and relatively easy to produce
   3. Can be quite difficult to detect
   4. Can be disseminated at great distances
   5. All of the above
2. Which statement about smallpox is *false*?
   1. Vaccines exist for smallpox and chicken pox.
   2. Skin lesions are synchronous in development for both smallpox and chicken pox.
   3. Both diseases are contagious via the aerosol route spread between people.
   4. With smallpox, patients can develop a rash on their palms and soles of feet.
3. Patients with illnesses caused by biological warfare agents can be cared for by using standard precautions.
   1. True
   2. False
4. A patient with severe life-threatening injuries who most likely will not survive would be triaged as:
   1. Blue
   2. Yellow
   3. Black
   4. Red
5. Symptoms of PTSD usually begin to develop by:
   1. 1 week
   2. 1 year
   3. 3 months
   4. 13 months
6. All individuals who experience a traumatic event will suffer from PTSD.
   1. True
   2. False
7. Airborne precautions should be used:
   1. When the patient is coughing.
   2. At all times
   3. Never, not an infection control definition
   4. When the patient is vomiting.
8. The HEICS provides the following, except:
   1. Way organize information
   2. Controlling and coordinating patient influx and movement
   3. A new way to treat smallpox
   4. Manageable span of control
9. Pneumonic plague occurs because of:
   1. Chemical
   2. Virus
   3. Bacteria
   4. Fungi
10. Triage is the act of:
    1. Discharging a patient for follow-up
    2. Prioritizing the patient's priority for care
    3. Providing a medical screening exam
    4. Admitting a patient to the intensive care unit
11. If a patient arrives to the ED with insecticide on him or her, the ER nurse does not need to be worried.
    1. True
    2. False
12. All of the following are true about SARS except:
    1. It is caused by a virus.
    2. It is not contagious.
    3. It originated in China.
    4. Patient's complain of a prodrome phase.

REVIEW ACTIVITIES

1. Visit the ED at your next clinical rotation and ask to review their triage guidelines. See if they use a three-tiered or five-tiered system.
2. Ask your instructor to find out when the hospital is performing their next disaster drill. Ask if you can observe the ED staff during a drill.
3. Review the hospital's disaster policy or packet and review your role as a student or a new RN. Familiarize yourself with their ICS.
4. Locate the PPE on every unit you are practicing on—make sure you know what size N-95 mask you are and that you have been fit tested.
5. Research your communities CISM team members and go and talk with one of them regarding critical incident stress debriefings.
6. Ask your clinical instructor to let you have time in the ED during your rotation.

Appendix A
Concept Mapping

Concept mapping is the process of analyzing the meaning of interrelationships among several concepts. Concept mapping has many synonyms including cognitive mapping, mind mapping, concept trees, and semantic networking (Beitz, 1998). A **concept map** is a graphic design that provides a visual picture of the analytical thinking process and interpretation of the information (Kathol, Geiger, & Hartig, 1998). The major concept is usually placed in the center of the map. Concepts or words related to the major concept are situated around it in categories or clusters. The concept clusters are linked to the major concept by lines, arrows, or significant words similar to the connecting roads and topographical areas between cities on a geographical map. Concept maps have three characteristics: hierarchical structure, chains or links, and clustering (Bietz, 1998).

The mapping process is associated with problem-solving learning. Educators have found concept mapping to be an innovative teaching method that promotes critical thinking, communication, categorization of information, and self-directed learning. The tool is relatively new to nursing; however, it has been used for several years in a variety of disciplines, including education and education psychology, business, medicine, the social sciences, and research (Beitz, 1998; Kathol, et al., 1998).

In nursing education, the concept map is primarily used as an alternative to the traditional linear care plan. Visual learners particularly value the map design, because it provides a visuo-spatial illustration of patient information. Creating the map assists students in gaining a holistic perspective of the patient, the health problem, and all the contributing factors, as well as realizing the implications for each phase of the nursing process (Alexander, McDaniel, Baldwin, & Money, 2002; Beitz, 1998; Kathol, et al., 1998; Mueller, Johnston, & Bligh, 2001; Schuster, 2000).

CREATING A CONCEPT MAP

Concept maps can be simple or elaborate and creatively designed, and either handwritten or computer generated. An entire page is used, usually in landscape form. The patient's name and the reason for entering the

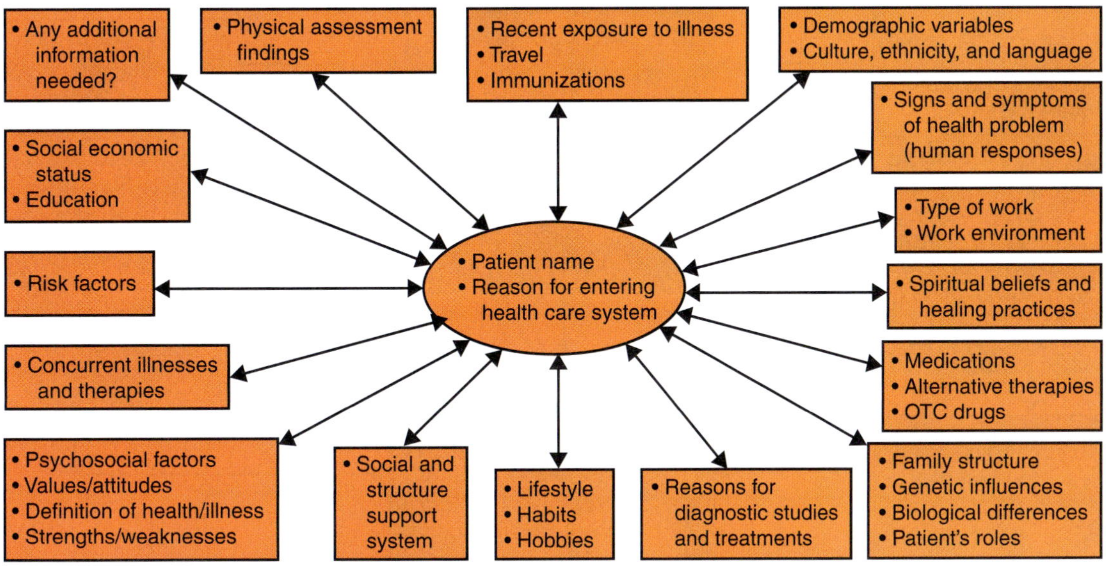

Figure A-1 Concept mapping patient information.

health care system are placed in the center of the diagram. Patient information is gathered through assessment, interviews with the patient or others, and review of the patient's record. The information can be clarified by reviewing texts, professional journal articles, and other literature. All concepts are analyzed for a possible connection to each other. Clusters of similar or related patient information are linked to the patient according to the best fit envisioned by the mapmaker. As concepts are added, the relationships and links may change (Figure A-1). Color coding is often used to sort and categorize the information and to signify priority needs and nursing actions. Arrows identify the direction of the connecting links among the various concepts and the relationship of the patient's responses to the health problem (Heinrich, Karner, Gagline, & Lambert, 2002; Kathol, et al., 1998; King & Shell, 2002).

Concept mapping also includes the organization of patient information within the phases of the nursing process to demonstrate the connections to the plan of care (Figure A-2 is an example). The end product is a unique representation "of an individual's health status as well as those concepts that affect the individual, such as social, cultural, ethnicity, and psychosocial state" (King & Shell, 2002, p. 36). Each map is considered a unique representation of the learner's ability to link theory to clinical practice.

PREPARATION FOR CONCEPT MAPPING

Students must have an understanding of the concepts and principles of the life sciences and a working knowledge of the nursing process prior to creating concept maps. Concept mapping can be introduced by mapping one's plan to visit a specific area or by creating a map of one's personal experiences and their effects on learning. These activities facilitate the transition to using nursing concepts in planning care. Case studies aid students in designing a map that illustrates the connections between clusters of information and selecting appropriate nursing diagnoses, patient outcomes, and nursing activities. Other helpful activities are mapping the effects of nursing concepts, such as immobility, oxygenation, pain, or anxiety on a patient's systems, and correlating the effects of a medication or therapy to a nursing diagnosis (King & Shell, 2002; Mueller, et al., 2001).

CLINICAL APPLICATION

Students learn the practice of clinical nursing by relating concepts, drawing on past learning and experience, and organizing conceptual meanings that make sense to them (Kathol, et al., 1998). A simple, or micromap is often used as a worksheet for a clinical day. Throughout the day, the instructor and student can evaluate where new information should be added and where changes need to be made. An updated version of the map is completed following the clinical experience.

ADVANTAGES OF CONCEPT MAPPING

Concept mapping enhances motivation and facilitates the learning process (Beitz, 1998). Critical thinking skills can be used for developing creative pictorial designs, such as placing concepts related to a respiratory problem in a lung-shaped map, inserting patient information related to a urinary problem within a kidney shape, or

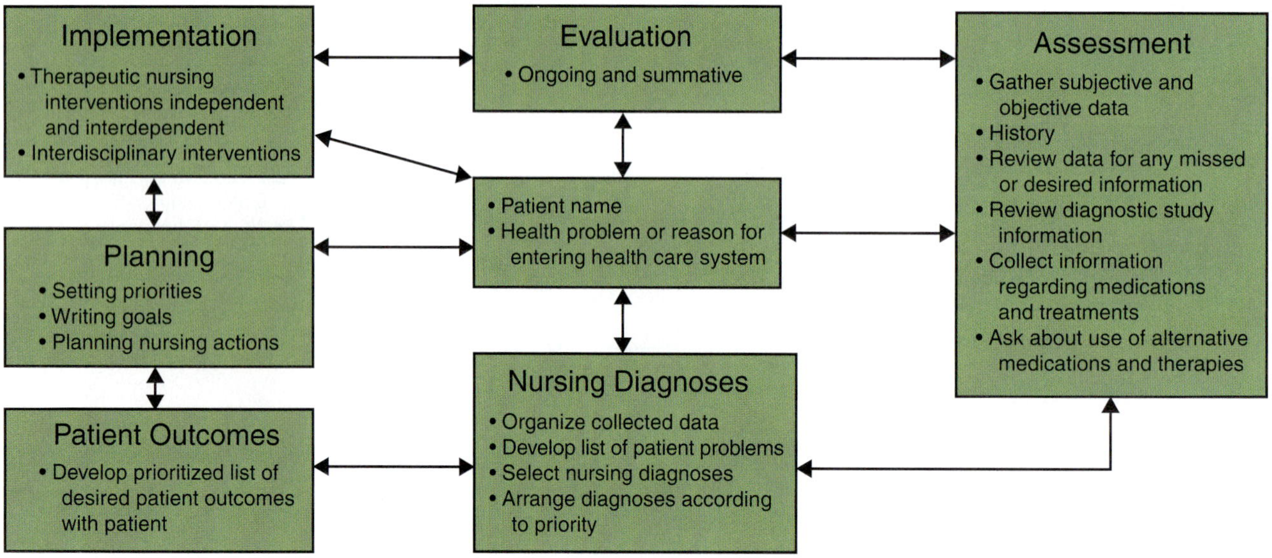

Figure A-2 Concept mapping.

drawing a map of the country of origin for content related to a patient from a different culture. Concept mapping can be an individual or group activity in the classroom or clinical settings for short-term or long-term assignments. Simple maps can be expanded throughout the curriculum to include more complex ideas, such as ethical/legal and leadership/management issues. They can also be used as study guides and for evaluation purposes. Concept mapping can be used as a curriculum matrix to track major concepts and themes, thus illustrating to faculty and students how the concepts and subject matter of the various courses are related to each other (Beitz, 1998; Heinrich et al., 2002). It also correlates well with the current emphasis on research and evidence-based practice (Burns & Grove, 2001; King & Shell, 2002).

DISADVANTAGES OF CONCEPT MAPPING

Because there are many ways to demonstrate connections between concepts, concept mapping may be difficult for individuals who believe there is only one way. The mapping process may also be challenging for people who think in a linear manner. Mapping may not be appropriate for all areas of learning. Concept mapping is a time-consuming activity; however, computer graphics facilitate the development process. Educators must value its importance and take time to prepare students to use the mapping process.

APPLICATION

Concept map case studies are included in this text to assist in learning the process of concept mapping. Statements and questions are listed as prompts for developing a concept map. However, the mapmaker is encouraged to be creative.

Appendix B English/Spanish Words and Phrases

Being able to say a few words or phrases in the patient's language is one way to show that you care. It lets the patient know that you as a nurse are interested in the individual. There are three rules to keep in mind regarding the pronunciation of Spanish words.

- If a word ends in a vowel, or in *n* or *s,* the accent is on the next to the last syllable.
- If the word ends in a consonant other than *n* or *s,* the accent is on the last syllable.
- If the word does not follow these rules, it has a written accent over the vowel of the accented syllable.

Courtesy phrases, names of body parts, and expressions of time and numbers are included in this section for quick reference. The English version will appear first, followed by the Spanish translation and Spanish pronunciation.

COURTESY PHRASES

Please	Por favor	Por-fah-**vor**
Thank you	Gracias	**Grah**-the-as
Good morning	Buenos días	Boo-**ay**-nos **dee**-as
Good afternoon	Buenas tardes	Boo-**ay**-nas **tar**-days
Good evening	Buenas noches	Boo-**ay**-nas **no**-chays
Yes/No	Sí/No	See/No
Good	Bien	Be-en
Bad	Mal	Mahl
How many?	Cuántos?	Coo-ahn-tos?
Where?	Dónde?	**Don**-day?
When?	Cuándo?	Coo-**ahn**-do?

BODY PARTS

abdomen	el abdomen	el ab-doh-men
ankle	el tobillo	el to-**beel**-lyo
anus	el ano	el **ah**-no
anvil (incus)	el yunque	el **yoon**-kay
appendix	el apéndice	el ah-**pen**-de-thay
aqueous humor	el humor acuoso	el oo-**mor** ah-coo-o-so
bladder	la vejiga	lah vah-**nee**-gah
brain	el cerebro	el thay-**ray**-bro
breast	el pecho	el **pay**-cho

buttock	la nalga	lah **nahl**-gah
calf	la pantorrilla	lah pan-tor-**reel**-lyah
cervix	la cerviz	lah ther-**veth**
cheek	la mejilla	lah mah-**heel**-lyah
chin	la barbilla	lah bar-**beel**-lyah
choroid	la coroidea	lah co-ro-e-**day**-ah
ciliary body	el cuerpo ciliar	el coo-**err**-po the-le-**ar**
clitoris	el clitoris	el **clee**-to-ris
coccyx	el coxis	el **coc**-sees
conjunctiva	la conjuntiva	lah con-hoon-**tee**-vah
cornea	la córnea	lah **cor**-nay-ah
penis	el pene	el **pay**-nay
prostate gland	la próstata	lah **pros**-ta-tah
pupil	la pupila	lah poo-**pee**-lah
rectum	el recto	el **rec**-to
retina	la retina	lah ray-**tee**-nah
sclera	la esclerótica	lah es-clay-**ro**-te-cah
scrotum	el escroto	el es-**cro**-to
seminal vesicle	la vesícula seminal	lah vay-**see**-coo-lah say-me-**nahl**
shoulder	el hombro	el **om**-bro
small intestine	el intestino delgado	el in-tes-**tee**-no del-**gah**-do
spinal cord	la médula espinal	lah **may**-doo-lah es-pe-**nahl**
spleen	el bazo	el **bah**-tho
stirrup (stapes)	el estribo	el es-**tree**-bo
stomach	el estómago	el es-**toh**-mah-go
temple	la sien	lah se-**ayn**
testis	el testículo	el tes-**tee**-coo-lo
thigh	el muslo	el **moos**-lo
thorax	el tórax	el **to**-rax
tongue	la lengua	lah **len**-goo-ah
trachea	la tráquea	lah **trah**-kay-ah
upper extremities	las extremidades superiores	las ex-tray-me-**dahd**-es soo-pay-re-**or**-es
ureter	el uréter	el oo-**ray**-ter
uterus	el útero	el **oo**-tay-ro
vagina	el vagina	lah vah-**hee**-nah
vitreous humor	el humor vítreo	el oo-**mor** **vee**-tray-o
wrist	la muñeca	lah moo-**nyay**-cah

EXPRESSIONS OF TIME, CALENDAR, AND NUMBERS

after meals	después de comer	des-poo-**es** day co-**merr**
at bedtime	al acostarse	al ah-cos-**tar**-say
before meals	antes de comer	**ahn**-tes day co-**merr**
daily	el diario	el de-**ah**-re-o

date	la fecha	lah **fay**-chah
day	el día	el **dee**-ah
every hour	a cada hora	ah **cah**-dah **o**-rah
hour (time)	la hora	lah **o**-rah
how often	cada cuánto tiempo	**cah**-dah coo-**ahn**-to te-**em**-po
noon	el mediodía	el may-de-o-**dee**-ah
now	ahora	ah-**o**-rah
once	una vez	**oo**-nah veth
today	hoy	**oh**-e
tomorrow	mañana	mah-**nyah**-nah
tonight	esta noche	**es**-tah **no**-chay
week	la semana	lah say-**mah**-nah
year	año	**a**-nyo
Sunday	el domingo	el do-**meen**-go
Monday	el lunes	el **loo**-nes
Tuesday	el martes	el **mar**-tes
Wednesday	el miércoles	el me-**err**-co-les
Thursday	el jueves	el hoo-**ay**-ves
Friday	el viernes	el ve-**err**-nes
Saturday	el sábado	el **sah**-bah-do
zero	cero	**thay**-ro
one	uno	**oo**-no
two	dos	dose
three	tres	trays
four	cuatro	coo-**ah**-tro
five	cinco	**theen**-co
six	seis	**say**-ees
seven	siete	se-**ay**-tay
eight	ocho	**o**-cho
nine	nueve	noo-**ay**-vay
ten	diez	de-**eth**

NURSING CARE SENTENCES AND QUESTIONS

What is your name?
¿Cómo se llama usted?
¿**Co**-mo say **lyah**-mah oos-**ted?**

I am a student nurse.
Soy estudiante enfermero(a).
Soy es-too-de-**ahn**-tay en-fer-**may**-ro(a).

My name is . . .
Mi nombre es . . .
Mee **nom**-bray es . . .

Do you need a wheelchair?
¿Necesita usted una silla de rueda?
¿Nay-thay-**se**-ta oos-**ted oo**-nah **seel**-lyah day roo-**ay**-dah?

How do you feel?
¿Cómo se siente?
¿**Co**-mo say se-**ayn**-tah?

When is your family coming?
¿Cuándo viene su familia?
¿Coo-**ahn**-do vee-**en**-nah soo fah-**mee**-le-ah?

This is the call light.
Esta es la luz para llamar a la enfermera.
Es-tah es lah looth **pah**-ra lyah-**mar** a lah en-fer-**may**-ra.

If you need anything, press the button.
Si usted necesita algo, oprima el botón.
See oos-**ted** nay-thay-**se**-ta **ahl**go o-pre-**ma** el bo-**tone.**

Do not turn without calling the nurse.
No se voltee sin llamar a la enfermera.
No say **vol**-tay seen lyah-**mar** a lah en-fer-**may**-ra.

The side rails on your bed are for your protection.
Los rieles del costado están para su protección.
Los re-**el**-es del cos-**tah**-do es-**tahn** **pah**-ra soo pro-tec-the-**on.**

Please do not try to lower or climb over the side rail.
Por favor no pretenda bajarlos (barjarlas) o treparse sobre ellos.
Por fah-**vor** no pray-**ten**-dah ba-**har**-los o tray-**par**-say **so**-bray **ayl**-lyos.

The head nurse is . . .
La jefa de enfermeras es . . .
La **hay**-fay day en-fer-**may**-ras es . . .

Do you need more blankets or another pillow?
¿Necesita usted más frazadas u otra almohada?
¿Nay-thay-**si**-ta oos-**ted** mahs frah-**thad**-dahs oo **o**-trah al-mo-**ah**-dah?

You may not smoke in the room.
No se puede fumar en el cuarto.
No say poo-**ay**-day foo-**mar** en el coo-**ar**-to.

Do you want me to turn on (turn off) the lights?
¿Quiere usted que encienda (apague) la luz?
¿Ke-**ay**-ray oos-**ted** day en-the-**en**-dah (a-**pah**-gay) lah looth?

Are you thirsty?
¿Tiene usted sed?
¿Tee-**en**-nah oos-**ted** sayd?

Are you allergic to any medication?
¿Es usted alérgico(a) a alguna medicina?
¿Es oos-**ted** ah-**lehr**-hee-co(a) ah ah-**goo**-nah nay-de-**thee**-nah?

You may take a bath.
Usted puede bañarse.
Oos-**ted** poo-**ay**-day bah-**nyar**-say.

Do not lock the door, please.
No cierre usted la puerta con llave, por favor.
No the-**err**-ray oos-**ted** lah poo-**err**-tah con **lyah**-vay por-fah-**vor.**

Call if you feel faint or in need of help.
Llame si usted se siente débil o si necesita ayuda.
Lyah-mah see oos-**ted** say se-**ayn**-tah **day**-bil o see nay-thay-**se**-ta ah-**yoo**-dah.

Call when you have to go to the toilet.
Llame cuando tenga que ir al inodoro.
Lyah-mah coo-**ahn**-do **ten**-gah kay eer al in-o-**do**-ro.

I will give you an enema.
Le pondré una enema.
Lay pon-**dray** **oo**-nah ay-**nay**-mah.

Turn on your left (right) side.
Voltese a su lado izquierdo (derecho).
Vol-**tay**-say ah soo **lah**-do ith-ke-**er**-do(dah) (day-**ray**-cho[cha]).

Here is an appointment card.
Aqui tiene usted una tarjeta con la información escrito.
Ah-**kee** tee-**en**-nah oos-**ted** **oo**-nah tar-**hay**-tah con lah in-for-mah-the-**on** es-**cree**-to.

You are going to be discharged (released) today.
A usted le van a dar de alta hoy.
Ah oos-**ted** lay vahn ah dar day **ahl**-tah **oh**-e.

How did this illness begin?
¿Cómo empezó esta enfermedad?
¿**Co**-mo em-pa-**tho** **es**-tah en-fer-may-**dahd?**

Is the pain better after the medicine?
Siente usted alivio depués de tomar la medicina?
¿Se-**ayn**-tah oos-**ted** al-**lee**-ve-o des-poo-**es** day to-**mar** lah may-de-**thee**-nah?

Where is the pain?
¿Qué la duele? (or) ¿Dónde le duele?
¿Kay lah doo-**ay**-le? (or) **¿Don**-day lay doo-**ay**-le?

Do you have pains in your chest?
¿Tiene usted dolores in el pecho?
¿Tee-**en**-nah oos-**ted** do-**lor**-es en el **pay**-cho?

Are you in pain now?
¿Tiene usted dolores ahora?
¿Tee-**en**-nah oos-**ted** do-**lor**-es ah-**o**-rah?

Is it constant pain or does it come and go?
¿Es un dolor constante or va y vuelve?
¿Es oon do-**lor** cons-**tahn**-tay o vah ee voo-**el**-vah?

Is there anything that makes the pain better?
¿Hay algo que lo alivie?
¿Ah-ee **ahl**-go kay lo al-**le**-ve?

Is there anything that makes the pain worse?
¿Hay algo que lo aumente?
¿Ah-ee **ahl**-go kay lo ah-oo-**men**-tay?

Where do you feel the pain?
¿Dónde siente usted el dolor?
¿Don-day se-**ayn**-tah oos-**ted** el do-**lor?**

Point to where it hurts.
Apunte usted por favor, adonde le duele.
Ah-**poon**-tay oos-**ted** por fah-**vor** ah-**don**-day lay doo-**ay**-le.

Show me where it hurts.
Enséñeme usted donde le duele.
En-**say**-nah-may oos-**ted** **don**-day lay doo-**ay**-le.

Is the pain sharp or dull?
¿Es agudo o sordo el dolor?
¿Es ah-**goo**-do o **sor**-do el do-**lor?**

Do you know where you are?
¿Sabe usted donde esta?
¿Sah-**bay** oos-**ted don**-day es-**tah?**

You are in a hospital.
Usted está en el hospital.
Oos-**ted** es-**tah** en el os-pee-**tahl.**

You will be okay.
Usted va a estar bien.
Oos-**ted** vah a es-**tar be**-en.

Do you have any drug reactions?
¿Tiene usted alguna sensibilidad a productos químicos?
¿Te-**en** nah oos-**ted** al-**goo**-nah sen-se-be-le-**dahd** a pro-**dooc**-tos **kee**-me-cos?

Have you seen another doctor or native healer for this problem?
¿Ha visto usted a otro médico o curandero tocante a este problema?
¿Ah **vees**-to oos-**ted** a **o**-tro **may**-de-co o coo-ran-**day**-ro to-**cahn**-tay a **es**-ah pro-**blay**-mah?

Have you vomited?
¿Ha vomitado usted?
¿Ah vo-me-**tah**-do oos-**ted?**

Do you have any difficulty in breathing?
¿Tiene usted alguna dificultad para respirar?
Te-**en**-nah oos-**ted** ah-**goo**-nah de-fe-cool-**tahd pah**-ra res-pe-**rar?**

Do you smoke?
¿Fuma usted?
¿Foo-**mar** oos-**ted?**

How many per day?
¿Cuántos al día?
¿Coo-**ahn**-tos al **dee**-ah?

For how many years?
¿Por cuántos años?
¿Por coo-**ahn**-tos **a**-nos?

Do you awaken in the night because of shortness of breath?
¿Se despierta usted por la noche por falta de respiración?
¿Say des-pee-**err**-tah oos-**ted** por lah **no**-chay por **fahl**-tah day res-pe-rah-the-**on**?

Is any part of your body swollen?
¿Tiene usted alguna parte del cuerpo hinchada?
¿Te-**en**-nah oos-**ted** ah-**goo**-nah **par**-tay del coo-**err**-po in-**chah**-da?

How much water do you drink daily?
Cuántos vasos de agua bebe usted diariamente?
¿Coo-**ahn**-tos **vah**-sos day **ah**-goo-ah **bay**-be oos-**ted** de-ah-re-ah-**men**-tay?

Are you nauseated?
¿Tiene náusea?
¿Te-**en**-nah **nah**-oo-say-ah?

Are you going to vomit?
¿Va a vomitar?
¿Vah a vo-me-**tar**?

When was your last bowel movement?
¿Cuánto tiempo hace que evacúa usted?
¿Coo-**ahn**-to te-**em**-po **ah**-the kay ay-vah-**coo**-ah oos-**ted**?

Do you have diarrhea?
¿Tiene usted diarrea?
¿Te-**en**-nah oos-**ted** der-ar-**ray**-ah?

How much do you urinate?
¿Cuánto orina usted?
¿Coo-**ahn**-to o-**re**-nah oos-**ted**?

Did you urinate?
¿Orino usted?
¿O-re-**no** oos-**ted**?

What color is your urine?
¿De qué color es la orina?
¿Day kay co-**lor** es lah o-**re**-nah?

Call when you have to go to the toilet.
Llame usted cuando tenga que ir al inodoro.
Lyah-mah oos-**ted** coo-**ahn**-do **ten**-gah kay eer al in-o-**do**-ro.

I need a urine specimen from you.
Necesito una muestra de orina de usted.
Nay-thay-**se**-to **oo**-nah moo-**ays**-trah day o-**re**-nah day oos-**ted**.

We will put a tube in your bladder so that you can urinate.
Le pondremos un tubo en la vejiga para que puede orinar.
Lay pon-**dray**-mos un **too**-be en lah vay-**hee**-gah **pah**-rah kay poo-**ay**-day o-re **nar**.

When was your last menstrual period?
¿Cuándo fue se última menstruación?
¿Coo-**ahn**-do foo-**ay** soo **ool**-te-mah mens-troo-ah-the-**on**?

Are you bleeding heavily?
¿Está sangrando mucho?
¿Es-tah san-**grahn**-do **moo**-cho?

Take off your clothes, please.
Desvístase usted, por favor.
Des-**ves**-tah-say oos-**ted** por-fah-**vor**.

Just relax.
Relaje usted el cuerpo.
Ray-**lah**-he oos-**ted** el coo-**err**-po.

I am going to listen to your chest.
Voy a escucharle el pecho.
Voye a es-coo-**char**-lay el **pay**-cho.

Let me feel your pulse.
Déjeme tomarle el pulso.
Day-ha-me to-**mar**-lay el **pool**-so.

I am going to take your temperature.
Voy a tomarle la temperatura.
Voye a to-**mar**-lay lah tem-pay-rah-**too**-rah.

Lie down, please.
Acuéstese, por favor.
Ah-coo-**es**-tah-say por fah-**vor**.

Do you understand?
¿Me comprende usted?
¿May com-**pren**-day oos-**ted**?

That's right.
Así. Bien.
Ah-**see. Be**-en.

You are doing very well.
Usted va muy bien.
Oos-**ted** vah **moo**-e **be**-en.

Do not take any medicine from home.
No tome usted ninguna medicina traída de su casa.
No **to**-may oos-**ted** nin-**goon**-ay may-de-**thee**-nah trah-**ee** dah day soo **cah**-sah.

I am going to give you an injection.
Voy a ponerle una inyección.
Voye a po-**nerr**-lay **oo**-nah in-yec-the-**on.**

Take a sip of water.
Tome usted un traguito de agua.
To-may oos-**ted** un trah-**gee**-to day **ah**-goo-ah.

Very good. That was fine.
Muy bien. Excelente.
Moo-e **be**-en. Ex-thay-**len**-tay.

Don't be nervous.
No se ponga nervioso(a).
No say **pon**-gah ner-ve-**o**-so(ah).

Do you feel dizzy?
¿Se siente vertigo?
¿Say see-**ayn**-tah **verr**-to-go?

Please lie still.
Quédese inmóvil, por favor.
Kay-day-say in-**mo**-veel por fah-**vor.**

You must drink lots of liquids.
Usted debe tomar muchos liquidos.
Oos-**ted day**-bay to-**mar moo**-chos **lee**-ke-dos.

Appendix C Symbols and Abbreviations

Symbols

~	similar	>	greater than
≅	approximately	<	less than
@	at	%	percent
√	check	+	positive
Δ	change	–	negative
↑	increased	♀	female
↓	decreased	♂	male
=	equals	△1 △2 △3	trimester of pregnancy (one triangle for each trimester)
#	pounds		

Abbreviations

2,3-DPG	2,3-diphosphoglycerate
AACN	American Association of Colleges of Nursing
AAOHN	American Association of Occupational Health Nurses
AARP	American Association of Retired Persons
ABG	arterial blood gas
A/C	alternative/complementary
Acetyl-CoA	acetyl coenzyme A
ADA	Americans with Disabilities Act
ADAMHA	Alcohol, Drug Abuse, and Mental Health Administration
ADH	antidiuretic hormone
ADL	activities of daily living
ADP	adenosine diphosphate
ADR	adverse drug reactions
AEB	as evidenced by
AGF	angiogenesis factor
AHA	American Hospital Association
AHNA	American Holistic Nurses Association
AHRQ	Agency for Health Care Research and Policy
AIDS	acquired immunodeficiency syndrome
AJN	*American Journal of Nursing*
AMB	as manifested by
ANA	American Nurses Association
ANS	autonomic nervous system
AONE	Association of Nurse Executives
AORN	Association for Operating Room Nurses
APN	advanced practice nurse
APRN	advanced practice registered nurse
APTT	activated partial thromboplastin time
AST	aspartate aminotransferase
AT	axillary temperature
ATP	adenosine triphosphate
ATSDR	Agency for Toxic Substances and Disease Registry
BCR	bulbocavernosus reflex
BMI	body mass index
BMR	basal metabolic rate
BN	bachelor's degree in nursing
BP	blood pressure
BScN	bachelor of science in nursing (in Canada)
BSE	breast self-examination
BSN	bachelor of science in nursing
BUN	blood urea nitrogen
C	Celsius; also called centigrade
CAT	computerized adaptive testing
CAUSN	Canadian Association of University Schools of Nursing
CBC	complete blood count
CBE	charting by exception
CDC	Centers for Disease Control and Prevention

CEUs	continuing education units
CHD	coronary heart disease
CLIA	Clinical Laboratory Improvement Act
cm	centimeter
CMS	Centers for Medicare & Medicaid Services
CNA	Canadian Nurses Association
CNATS	Canadian Nurses Association Testing Service
CNM	certified nurse midwife
CNO	community nursing organization
CNS	central nervous system
CNS	clinical nurse specialist
CO_2	carbon dioxide
COBRA	Consolidated Omnibus Budget Reconciliation Act
COPD	chronic obstructive pulmonary disease
CPK	creatine phosphokinase
CPM	continuous passive motion
CPN	central parenteral nutrition
CPR	cardiopulmonary resuscitation
CPT	chest physiotherapy
CQI	continuous quality improvement
CRNA	certified registered nurse anesthetist
CSF	cerebrospinal fluid
CST	computerized clinical simulation testing
CT	computed tomography
CVA	cerebrovascular accident
DDS	doctor of dental science
DHHS	Department of Health and Human Services
dL	deciliter; also abbreviated dl
DNR	do not resuscitate
DNSc	doctorate of nursing in science
DRGs	diagnosis-related groups
DSN	doctorate of science in nursing
DUS	Doppler ultrasound stethoscope
DVT	deep vein thrombosis
ECG	electrocardiogram (also known as an EKG)
EEG	electroencephalogram
EN	enteral nutrition
EPA	Environmental Protection Agency
EPO	exclusive provider organization
ESR	erythrocyte sedimentation rate
ET	ear canal temperature
F	Fahrenheit
FAF	fibroblast-activating factor
FAS	fetal alcohol syndrome
FDA	Food and Drug Administration
FiO_2	fraction of inspired oxygen
ft	feet
g	gram
GAS	general adaptation syndrome
GCS	Glasgow Coma Scale
gH	drop
GI	gastrointestinal
GNP	gross national product
HBD	alpha-hydroxybutyrate dehydrogenase
HBV	hepatitis B virus

HCFA	Health Care Financing Administration
Hct	hematocrit
HDL	high-density lipoprotein
HEPA	high efficiency particulate air
Hgb	hemoglobin
HIS	hospital information system
HIV	human immunodeficiency virus
HMO	health maintenance organization
HPN	home parenteral nutrition
HQIA	Healthcare Quality Improvement Act
HRSA	Health Resources and Services Administration
HSV-2	herpes simplex virus 2
HT	healing touch
IHS	Indian Health Service
IM	intramuscular
in	inch
I&O	intake and output
IOM	Institute on Medicine
IPPB	intermittent positive-pressure breathing
IRA	individual retirement account
IV	intravenous
IVP	intravenous pyelogram
JCAHO	Joint Commission on Accreditation of Healthcare Organizations
kcal	kilocalorie
kg	kilogram
LAS	localized adaptation syndrome
lb	pound
LDH	lactic dehydrogenase
LDL	low-density lipoprotein
LLQ	left lower quadrant
LOC	level of consciousness
LPN	licensed practical nurse
LUQ	left upper quadrant
LVN	licensed vocational nurse
m	meter
MA	master of arts degree
MAC	mid-upper-arm circumference
MAR	medication administration record
MD	doctor of medicine
MDR	multidrug-resistant
mEq	milliequivalent
mEq/L	milliequivalent per liter
mg	milligram
MH	malignant hyperthermia
MI	myocardial infarction
mL	milliliter; also abbreviated ml
mm	millimeter
mm Hg	millimeters of mercury
MN	master's degree in nursing
mOsm	milliosmole; also spelled milliosmol
mOsm/L	milliosmole per liter
MRI	magnetic resonance imaging
MRSA	methicillin-resistant *Staphylococcus aureus*
MSN	master of science in nursing
NACGN	National Association of Colored Graduate Nurses

NANDA	North American Nursing Diagnosis Association
NCEP	National Cholesterol Education Program
NCLEX	National Council Licensing Examination
NCLEX-PN	National Council Licensure Examination for Practical Nurses
NCLEX-RN	National Council Licensure Examination for Registered Nurses
NCNR	National Center for Nursing Research
NCSBN	National Council of State Boards of Nursing
NIC	Nursing Interventions Classification
NIH	National Institutes of Health
NINR	National Institute of Nursing Research
NLN	National League for Nursing
NMDS	Nursing Minimum Data Set
NP	nurse practitioner
NPO	*non per os* (nothing by mouth—to eat or drink)
NS	nutrition support
NST	nutritional support team
OAM	Office of Alternative Medicine
OBRA	Omnibus Budget Reconciliation Act
OR	operating room
OSHA	Occupational Safety and Health Administration
OT	occupational therapist
OT	oral temperature
OTC	over-the-counter
oz	ounce
P	pulse
PO_2	partial pressure of oxygen in a mixture of gasses, or in solution
PO_2	partial pressures of oxygen
PA	physician's assistant
PaO_2 (PAO_2)	partial pressure of oxygen dissolved in arterial blood plasma
PAP	Papanicolaou test
PAT	pulmonary artery temperature
PC	potential complication
PCA	patient-controlled analgesia
PCO_2	partial pressure of carbon dioxide dissolved in arterial blood plasma
PCP	primary care provider
PEG	percutaneous endoscopic gastrostomy
PERRLA	pupils equal, round, reactive to light, and accommodation
pH	hydrogen ion concentration of a solution
PID	pelvic inflammatory disease
PIE	problem, intervention, evaluation
PIEE	pulsed irrigation enhanced evacuation
PKU	phenylketonuria
PMR	progressive muscle relaxation
PMS	premenstrual syndrome
PN	parenteral nutrition
PNI	psychoneuroimmunology
PNS	peripheral nervous system
PO	*per os* (by mouth)
POMR	problem-oriented medical record
POR	problem-oriented record
PPN	peripheral parenteral nutrition
PPO	preferred provider organization
PPS	prospective payment system
prn	*pro re nata* (as needed)
PRO	peer review organization
PSRO	professional standards review organization
PT	physical therapist
PT	prothrombin
PT	prothrombin time
PTSD	posttraumatic stress disorder
PTT	partial thromboplastin
PURT	prompted urge response toileting
q	every
QA	quality assurance
R	respiration
RAS	reticular activating system
RBC	red blood cell
RD	registered dietitian
RDA	recommended dietary allowance
RDDA	recommended daily dietary allowances
RHC	Rural Health Clinic
RLQ	right lower quadrant
RN	registered nurse
RNA	registered nurse's assistant
ROM	range-of-motion
RPCH	rural primary care hospital
RPh	registered pharmacist
RT	rectal temperature
RT	related to
RT	respiratory therapist
RUQ	right upper quadrant
S-CDTN	Self-Care Deficit Theory of Nursing
SA	sinoatrial node
SAECG	signal-averaged electrocardiography
SaO_2	percent saturation of arterial blood (hemoglobin) with oxygen
SBC	school-based clinic
SI	*le Système International d'Unités* (the international system of units)
SL	sublingual
SLT	social learning theory
SMDA	Safe Medical Devices Act
SMI	sustained maximum inspiration
SO	source-oriented charting
SOAP	Subjective data, Objective data, Assessment, Plan
SOAPIE	Subjective data, Objective data, Assessment, Plan, Implementation, Evaluation
STD	sexually transmitted disease
SUI	stress urinary incontinence
SW	social worker
T	temperature
TEFRA	Tax Equity Fiscal Responsibility Act

TENS	transcutaneous electrical nerve stimulation
TMJ	temporomandibular joint
TNA	total nutrient admixture
TPN	total parenteral nutrition
TQM	total quality management
TSE	testicular self-examination
TT	therapeutic touch
UAP	unlicensed assistive personnel
UHDDS	uniform hospital discharge data set
USPHS	United States Public Health Service
VA	Veterans Affairs
VLDL	very low-density lipoprotein
V/Q	ventilation/perfusion mismatch
VRE	vancomycin-resistant enterococci
WBC	white blood cell
WIC	Women, Infants, and Children

Appendix D NANDA Nursing Diagnoses 2005–2006

Activity Intolerance
Risk for **A**ctivity Intolerance
Impaired **A**djustment
Ineffective **A**irway Clearance
Latex **A**llergy Response
Risk for Latex **A**llergy Response
Anxiety
Death **A**nxiety
Risk for **A**spiration
Risk for Impaired Parent/Infant/Child **A**ttachment
Autonomic Dysreflexia
Risk for **A**utonomic Dysreflexia
Disturbed **B**ody Image
Risk for Imbalanced **B**ody Temperature
Bowel Incontinence
Effective **B**reastfeeding
Ineffective **B**reastfeeding
Interrupted **B**reastfeeding
Ineffective **B**reathing Pattern
Decreased **C**ardiac Output
Caregiver Role Strain
Risk for **C**aregiver Role Strain
Impaired Verbal **C**ommunication
Readiness for Enhanced **C**ommunication
Decisional **C**onflict (Specify)
Parental Role **C**onflict
Acute **C**onfusion
Chronic **C**onfusion
Constipation
Perceived **C**onstipation
Risk for **C**onstipation
Defensive **C**oping
Ineffective **C**oping
Readiness for Enhanced **C**oping
Ineffective Community **C**oping
Readiness for Enhanced Community **C**oping
Compromised Family **C**oping
Disabled Family **C**oping
Readiness for Enhanced Family **C**oping
Risk for Sudden Infant **D**eath Syndrome
Ineffective **D**enial
Impaired **D**entition
Risk for Delayed **D**evelopment
Diarrhea
Risk for **D**isuse Syndrome
Deficient **D**iversional Activity
Energy Field Disturbance
Impaired **E**nvironmental Interpretation Syndrome
Adult **F**ailure to Thrive
Risk for **F**alls
Dysfunctional **F**amily Processes: Alcoholism
Interrupted **F**amily Processes
Readiness for Enhanced **F**amily Processes
Fatigue
Fear
Readiness for Enhanced **F**luid Balance
Deficient **F**luid Volume
Excess **F**luid Volume
Risk for Deficient **F**luid Volume
Risk for Imbalanced **F**luid Volume
Impaired **G**as Exchange
Anticipatory **G**rieving
Dysfunctional **G**rieving
Risk for Dysfunctional **G**rieving
Delayed **G**rowth and Development
Risk for Disproportionate **G**rowth
Ineffective **H**ealth Maintenance
Health-Seeking Behaviors (Specify)
Impaired **H**ome Maintenance
Hopelessness
Hyperthermia
Hypothermia
Disturbed Personal **I**dentity
Functional Urinary **I**ncontinence
Reflex Urinary **I**ncontinence
Stress Urinary **I**ncontinence
Total Urinary **I**ncontinence
Urge Urinary **I**ncontinence
Risk for Urge Urinary **I**ncontinence
Disorganized **I**nfant Behavior
Risk for Disorganized **I**nfant Behavior
Readiness for Enhanced Organized **I**nfant Behavior
Ineffective **I**nfant Feeding Pattern
Risk for **I**nfection

Risk for **I**njury
Risk for Perioperative-Positioning **I**njury
Decreased **I**ntracranial Adaptive Capacity
Deficient **K**nowledge
Readiness for Enhanced **K**nowledge (Specify)
Risk for **L**oneliness
Impaired **M**emory
Impaired Bed **M**obility
Impaired Physical **M**obility
Impaired Wheelchair **M**obility
Nausea
Unilateral **N**eglect
Noncompliance
Imbalanced **N**utrition: Less than Body Requirements
Imbalanced **N**utrition: More than Body Requirements
Readiness for Enhanced **N**utrition
Risk for Imbalanced **N**utrition: More than Body Requirements
Impaired **O**ral Mucous Membrane
Acute **P**ain
Chronic **P**ain
Readiness for Enhanced **P**arenting
Impaired **P**arenting
Risk for Impaired **P**arenting
Risk for **P**eripheral Neurovascular Dysfunction
Risk for **P**oisoning
Post-Trauma Syndrome
Risk for **P**ost-Trauma Syndrome
Powerlessness
Risk for **P**owerlessness
Ineffective **P**rotection
Rape-Trauma Syndrome
Rape-Trauma Syndrome: Compound Reaction
Rape-Trauma Syndrome: Silent Reaction
Impaired **R**eligiosity
Readiness for Enhanced **R**eligiosity
Risk for Impaired **R**eligiosity
Relocation Stress Syndrome
Risk for **R**elocation Stress Syndrome
Ineffective **R**ole Performance
Sedentary Life Style
Bathing/Hygiene **S**elf-Care Deficit
Dressing/Grooming **S**elf-Care Deficit
Feeding **S**elf-Care Deficit
Toileting **S**elf-Care Deficit
Readiness for Enhanced **S**elf-Concept
Chronic Low **S**elf-Esteem
Situational Low **S**elf-Esteem
Risk for Situational Low **S**elf-Esteem
Self-Mutilation
Risk for **S**elf-Mutilation
Disturbed **S**ensory Perception (Specify: Visual, Auditory, Kinesthetic, Gustatory, Tactile, Olfactory)
Sexual Dysfunction
Ineffective **S**exuality Patterns
Impaired **S**kin Integrity
Risk for Impaired **S**kin Integrity
Sleep Deprivation
Disturbed **S**leep Pattern
Readiness for Enhanced **S**leep
Impaired **S**ocial Interaction
Social Isolation
Chronic **S**orrow
Spiritual Distress
Risk for **S**piritual Distress
Readiness for Enhanced **S**piritual Well-Being
Risk for **S**uffocation
Risk for **S**uicide
Delayed **S**urgical Recovery
Impaired **S**wallowing
Effective **T**herapeutic Regimen Management
Ineffective **T**herapeutic Regimen Management
Readiness for Enhanced Management of **T**herapeutic Regimen
Ineffective Community **T**herapeutic Regimen Management
Ineffective Family **T**herapeutic Regimen Management
Ineffective **T**hermoregulation
Disturbed **T**hought Processes
Impaired **T**issue Integrity
Ineffective **T**issue Perfusion (Specify Type: Renal, Cerebral, Cardiopulmonary, Gastrointestinal, Peripheral)
Impaired **T**ransfer Ability
Risk for **T**rauma
Impaired **U**rinary Elimination
Readiness for Enhanced **U**rinary Elimination
Urinary Retention
Impaired Spontaneous **V**entilation
Dysfunctional **V**entilatory Weaning Response
Risk for Other-Directed **V**iolence
Risk for Self-Directed **V**iolence
Impaired **W**alking
Wandering

Appendix E
Standard Precautions

STANDARD PRECAUTIONS

FOR INFECTION CONTROL

Wash Hands (Plain Soap)
Wash after touching **blood**, **body fluids**, **secretions**, **excretions**, and **contaminated items**.
Wash immediately **after gloves are removed** and **between patient contacts**.
Avoid transfer of microorganisms to other patients or environments.

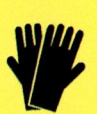

Wear Gloves
Wear when touching **blood**, **body fluids**, **secretions**, **excretions**, and **contaminated items**.
Put on **clean** gloves just **before touching mucous membranes** and **nonintact skin**.
Change gloves between tasks and procedures on the same patient after contact with material that may contain high concentrations of microorganisms. Remove gloves promptly after use, before touching noncontaminated items and environmental surfaces, and before going to another patient, and wash hands immediately to avoid transfer of microorganisms to other patients or environments.

Wear Mask and Eye Protection or Face Shield
Protect mucous membranes of the eyes, nose, and mouth during procedures and patient–care activities which are likely to generate **splashes** or **sprays** of **blood**, **body fluids**, **secretions**, or **excretions**.

Wear Gown
Protect skin and prevent soiling of clothing during procedures that are likely to generate **splashes** or **sprays** of **blood**, **body fluids**, **secretions**, or **excretions**. Remove a soiled gown as promptly as possible and wash hands to avoid transfer of microorganisms to other patients or environments.

Patient-Care Equipment
Handle used patient–care equipment soiled with **blood**, **body fluids**, **secretions**, or **excretions** in a manner that prevents skin and mucous membrane exposures, contamination of clothing, and transfer of microorganisms to other patients and environments. Ensure that reusable equipment is not used for the care of another patient until it has been appropriately cleaned and reprocessed and single use items are properly discarded.

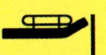

Environmental Control
Follow hospital procedures for routine care, cleaning, and disinfection of environmental surfaces, beds, bedrails, bedside equipment, and other frequently touched surfaces.

Linen
Handle, transport, and process used linen soiled with **blood**, **body fluids**, **secretions**, or **excretions** in a manner that prevents exposures and contamination of clothing and avoids transfer of microorganisms to other patients and environments.

Occupational Health and Blood-Borne Pathogens
Prevent injuries when using needles, scalpels, and other sharp instruments or devices; when handling sharp instruments after procedures; when cleaning used instruments; and when disposing of used needles.

Never recap used needles using both hands or any other technique that involves directing the point of a needle toward any part of the body; rather, use either a one-handed "scoop" technique or a mechanical device designed for holding the needle sheath.

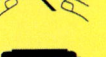

Do not remove used needles from disposable syringes by hand, and do not bend, break, or otherwise manipulate used needles by hand. Place used disposable syringes and needles, scalpel blades, and other sharp items in puncture–resistant sharps containers located as close as practical to the area in which the items were used, and place reusable syringes and needles in a puncture–resistant container for transport to the reprocessing area.

Use **resuscitation devices** as an alternative to mouth–to–mouth resuscitation.

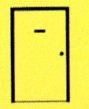

Patient Placement
Use a **private room** for a patient who contaminates the environment or who does not (or cannot be expected to) assist in maintaining appropriate hygiene or environmental control. Consult Infection Control if a private room is not available.

The information on this sign is abbreviated from the HICPAC Recommendations for Isolation Precautions in Hospitals.

Form No. **SPR** BREVIS CORP., 3310 S 2700 E, SLC, UT 84109

Courtesy of the Brevis Corporation

Glossary

12-lead electrocardiogram (ECG) A standardized recording of the electrical activity of the heart and may be used to detect heart irregularities, lack of oxygen to parts of the heart, and enlargement of the chambers.

A

A waves Plateau waves seen and related to severe intracranial hypertension. A waves have a range of 50 to 100 mm Hg.

abscess Collection or cavity of fluid, such as pus or cellular debris, which developed as result of an inflammatory response.

absolute hypovolemia Shock condition that occurs with the actual loss of fluid from the body including whole blood.

absorption A pharmacokinetic process that accounts for the movement of the drug from the site of administration into the bloodstream.

access Ability to obtain affordable health care when needed.

acculturation Process of learning the norms, beliefs, and behavioral expectations of a group.

acetylcholine A neurotransmitter in both the central and peripheral nervous system.

achalasia A motility disorder from failure of smooth muscle to relax or the absence of muscular contraction of the lower esophagus.

acidemia A decreased arterial pH, less than 7.35.

acne Results from thickening of the follicular opening, increased sebum production, the presence of bacteria, and the host's inflammatory response.

acquired immunity Refers to immunity that is not present at birth and develops as a result of exposure to pathogens; also called adaptive or specific immunity.

actin filaments The contractile part of a myofilament.

actinic keratoses Changes because of exposure to ultraviolet light (sun) Considered as premalignant lesion.

active euthanasia Someone other than the patient performs an action that ends the patient's life.

acute abdomen Refers to a constellation of clinical signs and symptoms usually best treated by surgery. Abrupt onset of abdominal pain; a potential medical emergency involving one of the abdominal organs, i.e., appendicitis.

acute respiratory distress syndrome (ARDS) Classified as noncardiac pulmonary edema with disruption of the alveolar-capillary membrane due to injury to the pulmonary vasculature or the airways (formerly called adult respiratory distress syndrome).

Adams Bending Forward Test A test used to assess for scoliosis.

adaptation (adjustment) The ongoing process of modifying one's behavior in changed circumstances or in an altered environment to fulfill psychological, physiological, and social needs.

addiction A compulsive disorder in which an individual becomes preoccupied with obtaining and using a substance, the continued use of which results in a decreased quality of life.

adducts Free radicals that can bind closely with the patient's healthy tissues and create hybrid molecules.

adenoma A benign (not malignant) tumor made of epithelial cells, usually arranged like a gland.

adjuvant A remedy that enhances the effect of another therapy.

adjuvant therapy Treatment given after the primary treatment to increase the chances of a cure. Adjuvant therapy may include chemotherapy, radiation therapy, hormone therapy, or biological therapy.

adrenergic stress response The physical and psychological responses to threatening environmental stimuli and the rapid release of epinephrine (adrenalin) from the sympathetic nervous system.

adrenocorticotropic hormone (ACTH) Hormone released from the anterior pituitary that stimulates the secretion of corticosteroids by the adrenal cortex.

adult daycare Provides health, social, and recreational services to adults who require supervision during family absence.

advance directives Written documents that allow a person to state, in advance, specific decisions about how he or she wants his or her own health care managed if he or she becomes incapacitated and is unable to communicate.

adverse effects Negative response to a drug, can range from mild to life-threatening.

aerophagia Excessive amounts of air are swallowed.

affective domain Area of learning that involves attitudes, beliefs, and emotions.

afterload The load that the ventricular muscle exerts when it is pushing its contents into the aorta.

agency Capacity for intentional action.

Agency for Healthcare Research and Quality (AHRQ) A federally funded U.S. government agency established by Congress in 1989 to support research designed to improve the quality of health care, reduce its cost, improve patient safety, decrease medical errors, and broaden access to essential health care service.

ageusia Loss or impairment of taste.

agglutination Occurs when an antibody links to the same epitope on two different antigens; appears in the blood as clumping.

agranulocytosis Severe neutropenia, with less than 200 cells/μm.

airborne transmission Infectious material trapped in dust and carried on air currents.

airway pressure release ventilation (APRV) Two levels of pressures to ventilate the patient.

akinesia The loss of movement.

alaryngeal voice Alternative methods of speaking that do not include the larynx; method used by patients who have their larynx removed.

aldosterone A mineral corticoid synthesized in the adrenal cortex; functions to maintain extracellular fluid volume.

alkalemia An increased arterial pH, more than 7.45.

allele One of two or more different genes containing specific inheritable characteristics that occupy corresponding positions on paired chromosomes.

allergen A substance that induces an allergic reaction.

allogeneic A remedy that replaces a patient's blood or bone marrow with blood or bone marrow from a donor.

allogeneic transplantation Stem cells from a sibling or unrelated donor with matching human leukocyte antigens (HLA).

allograft Skin graft.

allograft or homograft transplant *See* allogenic transplantation.

allopathic Mainstream, orthodox, conventional medical practice in the United States.

alopecia The loss of hair.

alpha-fetoprotein (AFP) A fetal protein produced in the yolk sac of the embryo for the first six weeks of gestation and then by the fetal liver.

altruism Unselfish concern for the welfare of others.

amblyopia A reduction in visual acuity caused by cerebral blockage of visual stimuli, which can develop in the eye affected by strabismus.

amenorrhea Absence of menstruation most commonly caused by an underlying hypothalamic-pituitary-endocrine dysfunction or a congenital abnormality or acquired abnormalities of the reproductive tract.

amplification The end result of the process in the formation of the erythrocyte whereby one rubriblast can form 14 to 16 erythrocytes.

amyloid Extracellular protein-like substance.

anabolism The constructive part of metabolism concerned especially with macromolecular synthesis.

analgesia Insensitivity to pain.

anaphylaxis Immediate, life-threatening hypersensitive allergic reaction.

anasarca Generalized edema is associated with malnutrition, terminal illness, and metabolic fluid overload problems.

anastomosis Surgical union of parts and especially hollow tubular parts.

androgens The male sex hormones.

anesthesia Absence of touch sensation.

anesthesia care provider Anesthesiologist or nurse anesthetist who delivers anesthesia to patients in surgical settings.

aneuploid A chromosome number that is not an exact multiple of the haploid number resulting in an extra or a missing chromosome.

aneurysm A permanent bulging and stretching of an artery, in which the dilation is two times or greater the size of the artery.

angina pectoris Pain in the chest.

angiogenesis The establishment of blood supply through formation of new blood vessels.

angioneurotic edema A condition associated with allergies and histamine release in which large welts develop below the surface of the skin, especially around the eyes and lips. The welts may also affect the hands, feet, and throat.

anion gap The portion of negatively charged ions not measured with routine laboratory studies.

anions Negatively charged particles.

ankle sprain When the ankle is displaced or a sudden force is applied, the ligaments are stretched beyond their normal stretching capacity and a sprain of the ligament occurs.

annular Ring-shaped (superficial fungal infections, such as ringworm, pityriasis rosea, seborrheic dermatitis, psoriasis, and others).

anosmia Loss or impairment of smell.

anovulation Failure to ovulate.

anthropophilic Human source.

antibodies Proteins produced by plasma cells that recognize and bind to a specific antigen.

anticipatory grieving Intellectual and emotional responses and behaviors by which individuals work through the process of modifying self-concept based on the perception of potential loss.

anticipatory stress A concern or worry about a potential problem or the uncertain outcome of a future event and the inability to control one's future.

anticoagulants Pharmaceuticals that prevent further clot formation in the body.

antidiuretic hormone (ADH) Hormone produced in the posterior pituitary and regulates the reabsorption of water in the kidneys, thereby regulating fluid volume.

antigen A substance that stimulates an immune response.

antigen presenting cells (APCs) Cells that ingest antigens, digest them, and display the epitope to stimulate immune response.

antineoplastic A drug that prevents, kills, or blocks the growth and spread of cancer cells.

antiphagocytic Something that destroys the function of the neutrophils and macrophages.

anuria Less than 50 mL per 24 hours of urine.

aphakic vision Absence of the crystalline lens of the eye.

aphasia Impairment in the ability to speak or comprehend.

apheresis Procedure that consists of withdrawal of blood from a donor, removal of one or more components (as plasma, blood platelets, or white blood cells) from the blood, and transfusion into patients with low platelet or white blood cell counts; the remaining blood is transfused back into the donor.

aphonia Loss of voice.

aphthous stomatitis Ulcerative conditions of the gums and mucous membranes; are labeled mouth ulcers.

apneustic breathing A pattern of respirations characterized by a prolonged inspiratory phase, followed by expiration apnea (the rate of apneustic breathing is usually 1:5 cycles per minute).

apoptosis An intact regulation of physiological cell death, which protects the organism from the development of a cancerous tumor.

approximated Wound edges also called borders, or margins, that are well connected without gaps.

arcus senilis Lipid deposition on the periphery of the cornea.

aromatherapy The therapeutic use of concentrated essences or essential oils that have been extracted from plants and flowers to stimulate, uplift, relax, or soothe by promoting balance between the sympathetic and parasympathetic nervous systems.

arrhythmias Deviations from normal cardiac rhythm.

arteriosclerosis Hardening of the arteries and defined as a thickening and solidifying of the endothelial lining of the walls in small arteries and arterioles.

arthroscopy A diagnostic test performed in the knee joint; an arthroscopy is an endoscopic procedure used to diagnose and repair meniscal, patellar, extrasynovial, and synovial diseases.

articulation Where a bone meets another bone to form a joint.

ASA scale Evaluation method used by anesthesiologists to determine risk of patients undergoing surgical procedures.

ascending cholangitis An infection in the gallbladder that moves in the direction of the liver.

ascites The accumulation of fluid in the peritoneal cavity.

asepsis Practice of ensuring that bacteria are excluded from open sites during surgery, wound dressing, blood sampling, and other medical procedures.

assessment The first step in the nursing process that involves the systematic collection, verification, organization, interpretation, and documentation of data for use by health care professionals.

assisted living Provides personal, social and health care, plus 24-hour supervision.

assisted suicide Similar to active euthanasia; often associated with a health care provider assisting another to end his or her own life.

astereognosis Lack of ability to identify objects by touch.

astigmatism Occurs when there is an unequal curve of the cornea and the light rays are bent unevenly.

ataxia A lack of muscle coordination.

atherogenesis Developmental process of the atherosclerotic lesion.

atherosclerosis Atherosclerosis begins as fatty streaks of the arterial wall in adolescence, progressing to hard fatty plaques that narrow and "harden" the arteries lumen in adulthood.

atopic dermatitis (AD) A hereditary and chronic skin disorder; also called eczema.

atopy A personal or familial tendency to become sensitized and produce immunoglobulin E (IgE) antibodies in response to ordinary exposure to allergens.

atresia Absence or closure of a natural passage of the body.

atypia Deviation from the standard cell form.

auditory Pertaining to the sense of hearing.

auditory learners Style of learning in which an individual learns by hearing.

aura Sensation that occurs immediately before a disorder, such as a migraine headache or a seizure.

auricle (pinna) The external ear.

auscultation Listening to sounds produced by the body, which are created by movement of air or fluid.

autoantibody An antibody that reacts against a person's own tissue.

autograft A permanent graft where a piece of skin from a remote unburned area of the body and transplants it to cover the burn wound.

autoimmunity The loss of tolerance (self-tolerance) of the body's antigenic markers on cells.

autologous The collection and storage of blood or blood components from a patient for subsequent transfusion to that same person.

autologous donation Occurs when a patient's own blood or blood products are donated 72 hours or more prior to surgery in anticipation of the need for blood or blood product replacement during surgery.

autologous transplantation Transplant of the patient's own stem cells.

autolytic debridement Uses moist wound dressings maintain a natural level of moisture, facilitating a normal inflammatory response.

automaticity When a group of cardiac cells have the ability to generate an electrical impulse spontaneously.

autonomic dysreflexia Disordered discharge of autonomic responses, which results in massive discharge of sympathetic responses.

autonomously Independent provision of primary health care.

autonomy Self-rule that is free from controlling influence by others and from limitation, such as inadequate understanding.

autosomes Any chromosome other than the sex chromosomes.

axis The imaginary line drawn between two electrodes.

ayurveda A healing system based on Hindu philosophy, which embraces the concept of an energy force in the body that seeks to maintain balance or harmony.

azoospermia Absence of spermatozoa in the semen.

azotemia A build up of nitrogenous waste products.

B

B waves Waves seen with intracranial pressures of 20 to 50 mm Hg.

balanitis Inflammation of the glans penis.

balanoposthitis A condition in which posthitis occurs concurrently with balanitis.

bariatric therapy Specialization dealing with patients who are overweight or obese.

barium An oral preparation that allows roentgenographic visualization of the internal structures of the digestive tract.

barium enema A rectal infusion of barium sulfate.

baroreceptors Pressure sensitive receptors located primarily in the arch of the aorta, which sense the pressure generated in the arteries by the pumping action of the heart.

barotrauma An injury to the lungs as a result of increased air pressure in the lungs.

basic human needs Need that must be met for survival.

basophils Granulocytes that attack fungi.

beneficence Requires that actions are of benefit to others.

bereaved People mourning a loss.

bioavailability Percentage of the drug that is available to achieve its intended effect in the body.

biofeedback A mechanism of providing feedback of physiological process to help patients learn how to manipulate those responses through mental activity.

biotechnology Use of data and techniques of engineering to solve problems related to natural organisms.

Biot's (ataxic) breathing The presence of an abnormal pattern of breathing, which is characterized by totally irregular rate and depth of respirations with periods of apnea.

blepharitis Inflammation of the hair follicles (cilia) and glands along the edges of the eyelids.

blood pressure Force exerted by the blood against the walls of the blood vessel to maintain tissue perfusion during rest and activity.

body mass index (BMI) Formula using weight and height to determine the percentage of total body fat.

bone marrow aspiration and biopsy A diagnostic test used to examine the bone marrow for abnormal tissue growth or to monitor the progress of bone marrow disease.

bone scan A diagnostic nuclear scan used to detect early bone disease, bone metastasis, and bone response to therapeutic regimens.

borborygmi sounds Loud, hyperactive bowel tones.

borborygmus Hyperactive bowel sounds.

Bouchard's nodes In rheumatoid arthritis, bony enlargements of the proximal interphalangeal joints.

brachytherapy The treatment with radioactive sources placed into or near the tumor or affected area.

bradykinesia Slowness in performing spontaneous movements.

bradypnea An abnormally slow rate of breathing.

brain dead Loss of consciousness, brainstem reflexes, and respiration with essentially flat electroencephalograms.

brash water Occurs when the mouth suddenly fills with saliva; secondary to reflex salivary secretion stimulated by acid back flow into the esophagus.

breakthrough pain Acute flares of pain when medication or therapy does not relieve all of the pain.

breast augmentation Surgical enlargement of the breasts.

bronchophony The presence of distinct, clear, and relatively loud sounds heard over areas of the lung in which the normal alveoli are filled with fluid or replaced by solid tissue.

bruit An adventitious sound of venous or arterial origin heard during auscultation.

Buerger's disease An occlusive disease mostly located in small to medium-sized arteries and occasionally in veins. Though commonly found in the upper and lower distal extremities, it is associated with clot formation and fibrosis of the vessel wall. In prolonged cases, large extremities vessels may be affected.

buffy coat An area that is light-colored and contains the mostly white blood cells seen in a test tube that is centrifuged or allowed to stand.

bullae Enlarged airspaces that do not contribute to ventilation but occupy space in the chest.

bullous myringitis The presence of an infectious vesicle and inflammation of the tympanic membrane caused by the organism *Mycoplasma pneumoniae.*

burn shock Massive fluid shifts of plasma, electrolytes, and proteins into the burn wound causing the inability of the circulatory system to meet the needs of cells, tissues, and vital organs.

burrows Linear lesions produced by tunneling of animal parasite, such as in scabies.

bursae Synovial fluid-filled sacs near a joint.

C

C waves Small waves seen with pressures less than 20 mm Hg.

cachexia A breakdown of muscle mass resulting from rapid weight loss or a general wasting due to illness or stress.

calcitonin A hormone produced by the thyroid gland when circulating calcium levels are elevated.

calculi A substance of abnormal concretion composed of mineral salts commonly produced within the renal system.

cancellous Found in the ends of the long bones and in smaller amounts in some of the flat bones.

carbuncles Aggregates of infected follicles originating deep in the dermis and subcutaneous tissue.

cardiac index The patient's cardiac output divided by the patient's body surface area.

cardiac output (CO) Total blood flow through the systemic or pulmonary circulation per minute.

cardiogenic shock Shock that occurs when inadequate oxygen and nutrients are supplied to the tissues because of severe left ventricular failure.

carditis Inflammation of the heart.

caregiver role strain Caregiver's felt difficulty in performing the family caregiver role.

carrier An individual who is heterozygous for a normal gene and an abnormal gene.

casts Accumulation of materials in a space that fills the contours of the space.

catabolism Destructive metabolism involving the release of energy and resulting in the breakdown of complex materials within the organism.

cations Positively charged particles.

cell-mediated immunity Refers to immunity that is mediated by T lymphocytes.

cellular components The parts of the blood that are derived from the stem cell. These include erythrocytes, granulocytes, platelets, B lymphocytes, and T lymphocytes.

cellulitis Generalized inflammation of the deeper connective tissue.

centering Bringing body, mind, and emotions to a quiet, focused state of consciousness; being still and nonjudgmental.

centrifugal Extends outward away from the center.

cephalalgia Headache.

cerebral perfusion pressure The pressure at which cerebral tissue is perfused. It is calculated by subtracting the intracranial pressure from the mean arterial pressure.

cerebrovascular accident ([CVA] stroke) Damage to the brain due to lack of blood flow.

cerumen A thick, wax-like substance secreted by the sweat glands within the ear canal.

chakra A concentrated area of energy of which there are seven primary centers in the physical body according to Hindu belief.

cheilosis Small fissures at the corners of the mouth.

chemoembolization An embolizing drug impregnated with chemotherapy drugs to deliver a concentrated dose directly to the area close to the tumor.

chemokines Chemicals that attract other cells, particularly leukocytes.

chemotaxis Response to a chemical stimulant to attract white blood cells to a specific site.

Cheyne-Stokes breathing The presence of an abnormal pattern of breathing, characterized by alternating periods of crescendo-decrescendo depth of breathing with periods of apnea.

cholangitis Inflammation of the bile duct.

cholecystitis Inflammation of the gallbladder.

cholelithiasis Gallstones.

cholestasis Any condition that impedes bile flowing freely through the bile ducts.

cholesteatoma A cyst that contains an accumulation of squamous epithelium, keratin, and other debris.

chondrosarcoma A cartilaginous sarcoma.

chorea Abnormal and excessive involuntary movements.

chromosomes Thread-like structures within the nucleus of a cell that carry the genes.

chyme The contents of the stomach, which are semiliquid.

climacteric The perimenopausal period.

clinical decisions Decisions that promote the optimal clinical response in a patient.

clinical ethics Ethical issues that impact patient care.

clinical practice guidelines (CPGs) Systematically developed statements to assist clinicians and patients in making decisions about appropriate health care for specific clinical circumstances.

clonus A slight involuntary pushing against the foot.

closed reduction External manipulation of a fracture, which forces it into alignment.

clubbing An abnormal enlargement of the distal phalanges.

coagulopathies Disorders that lead to abnormal clotting of the blood.

Cochrane Collaboration Global nonprofit and independent collaborative founded in 1993 in the United Kingdom that disseminates evidence summaries for use by clinicians, health policy makers, and consumers of health care.

Cochrane library Subscription service repository of full text reports and abstracts of evidence summaries.

code of ethics Principles that guide professional practice.

cognitive domain Learning by understanding the material that is presented with the mind.

colectomy Surgical operation to remove all or part of the colon.

collective bargaining Process where employer and worker representatives negotiate conditions of employment.

coma depasse Irreversible coma.

comedones Plugged secretions of horny material retain within a pilosebaceous follicle.

compartment syndrome Swelling in the soft tissues and muscles that in turn cause compromised circulation to that area.

competence Individual's demonstrated command of a body of knowledge or skills and the ability to consistently perform to a standard and achieve a desired outcome.

complement A cascade of proteins in serum that, when activated, attract more leukocytes to the site of activation, encourage phagocytosis, and lyse pathogen cell membranes.

complementary and alternative medicine (CAM) Therapy that has a focus beyond specific symptom management.

complementary therapy Otherwise known as alternative therapy; methods of medicine that are not Western based but that offer alternative ways to accomplish health care goals. Examples include massage therapy and hypnosis.

compliance The distensibility or elasticity of the lung that decreases as lung tissue becomes stiffer.

concept map A special form or diagram used for exploring knowledge and gathering and sharing information.

concussion Mild form of brain injury.

conductivity The ability of the cardiac cells to transmit an impulse.

condyloma Genital warts caused by the human papillomavirus (HPV).

conscious sedation A drug-induced depression of consciousness during which patients respond purposefully to verbal commands, either alone or accompanied by light tactile stimulation.

consensual response Pupillary constriction on the opposite pupil.

constipation Straining at stool with the production of hard stools, decreased frequency, and a feeling of not completely evacuating the colon.

contact dermatitis An acute or chronic skin inflammation triggered in the epidermis by contact with a specific antigen or irritant.

contextual features Social, economic, and cultural factors that make each person a unique individual.

continuing care Provides ongoing care for disabilities, chronic diseases, or permanent changes in functional capacity.

continuous mandatory ventilation (CMV) Breaths are delivered at preset intervals, regardless of patient effort. This mode is used most often in the paralyzed or apneic patient because it can increase the work of breathing if respiratory effort is present.

continuous positive airway pressure (CPAP) Pressure that adds to the functional residual capacity in patients who are spontaneously breathing.

continuous quality improvement (CQI) Application of scientific process analysis methods to improve quality and productivity.

contractility The capability of muscle fibers to shrink.

contracture Shortening of a muscle.

conventional medicine The common medical practice in the United States by medical doctors, doctors of osteopathy, and their adjunct practitioners: nurses, physical therapists, and social workers.

convulsion The abnormal motor response or jerking movements that occur during a seizure.

coping Conscious or unconscious methods used to deal with, and attempt to overcome, problems and difficulties such as stressful events, violence, and illness.

coping efficacy Perceived effectiveness of the coping effort to manage a stressful event.

cor pulmonale Hypertrophy or failure of the right ventricle resulting from disorders of the lungs, pulmonary vessels, or chest wall.

corneal reflex Stimulation of the trigeminal nerve (cranial nerve V) causes this protective blink.

coronary artery bypass grafting (CABG) A surgery where veins and arteries are used as conduit to bypass the coronary artery stenosis.

coronavirus A virus that normally only leads to upper respiratory infection.

cortical or compact (bone) The hard outer layer of bone surfaces.

corticosteroids Any of the hormones, except androgen, synthesized by the adrenal cortex.

cortisol A major glucocorticoid that functions in the regulation of blood glucose levels.

cough To expel air from the lungs suddenly and noisily to keep the respiratory passages free from irritating material.

counterpulsation The synchronization of the intra-aortic balloon pump to assist the heart according to the cardiac cycle.

crash cart Mobile cart with defibrillator, resuscitation equipment, and medications used when patients go into cardiac arrest.

crepitus A crinkly, crackling, or grating feeling or sound in the joints, skin, or lungs.

critical access hospital (CAH) Provides outpatient, emergency, and inpatient services in a rural area.

critical incident A patient or event that causes a stress reaction in the health care worker.

cryopexy Freezing of the retinal tear area.

cryotherapy The use of ice or cold water over an injury site to decrease inflammation.

cultural assimilation Individuals from a minority group are absorbed by the dominant culture and take on the characteristics of the dominant culture.

cultural awareness A conscious learning process in which people become appreciative of and sensitive to the cultures of others.

cultural competence The complex integration of knowledge, attitudes, and skills that enable the nurse to provide culturally appropriate health care.

cultural context Environment or situation that is relevant to the care, beliefs, values, and practices of the culture under study.

cultural diversity The difference among people that results from ethnic, racial, and cultural variables.

cultural encounter The process that encourages individuals to engage directly in cross-cultural interactions with people from culturally diverse backgrounds.

cultural knowledge The process of understanding the vital aspects of a groups' culture as it relates to health and health care practices.

cultural skill The ability to collect relevant cultural data regarding health histories and performing culturally specific assessments.

culture The knowledge, values, beliefs, art, morals, law, customs, and habits of the members of a society.

culture for caring Ideas, customs, skills, and arts of a work group that are transferred, communicated, or passed along to succeeding generations of health care workers.

Cushing response A late sign of increasing intracranial pressure with signs of slowing respirations, slowing heart rate, and increasing blood pressure.

cystectomy Removal of the bladder.

cytokines Chemicals that affect the way other cells behave.

cytotoxic (killer) T cells Lymphocytes that lyse host cells infected with a virus; also called CD8 T cells.

D

dactylitis An inflammatory affection of the fingers.

dead space That portion of ventilation that does not participate in gas exchange.

debridement A mechanical method of eliminating necrotic tissue.

deep partial-thickness burn Also called second-degree burn; a burn that involves the entire epidermis and the lower two thirds of the dermis.

deep sedation/analgesia A drug-induced depression of consciousness during which patients cannot be easily aroused but respond purposefully following repeated or painful stimulation.

deep vein thrombosis (DVT) A blood clot in a deep vein that accompanies an artery.

defibrillation Delivering an electrical shock to the heart so that it completely depolarizes the cardiac cells in an effort to terminate ventricular fibrillation.

dehiscence The separation of a wound or scar. A rupture or splitting open, as of a surgical wound or of an organ or structure to discharge its contents as splitting open.

deletion The loss of varying amounts of genetic material that is detectable at the DNA or chromosomal level.

demargination A process whereby the granulocytes can suddenly leave the peripheral tissues.

dendritic cells Large phagocytic antigen presenting cells that activate T cells.

deontology Philosophy concerned with the moral duty and obligation of an action rather than the action's outcome.

deoxyribonucleic acid (DNA) The molecular basis of heredity, consisting of purine and pyrimidine nucleotides arranged in two long strands, twisted about each other to form a double helix.

depolarization Electrical changing in the interior of an excitable cell from negative to positive, which results in an action potential.

dermatomal Localized into a dermatome supplied by one or more dorsal ganglia (herpes zoster and segmental vitiligo).

dermatome The body region supplied by a pair of a dorsal root ganglia.

detumescence The process that occurs following orgasm where the blood flow decreases and the vasocongestion is relieved.

diabetes mellitus A chronic metabolic disorder characterized by hyperglycemia (elevated blood sugar levels) related to a lack of insulin, lack of effects of insulin, or a combination.

diapedesis Cells squeeze through pores in capillary wall.

diaphoresis Profuse sweating.

diarrhea An increase in the liquid state of the stool.

diastolic blood pressure Phase in the cardiac cycle when the heart is at rest.

didelphic Duplication; usually refers to two uteri, two cervices, and two vaginas.

differentiation A process involving constant turnover of new cells of the epidermis.

diffusion The movement of solutes from an area of high concentration to an area of low concentration.

dimorphic Existing in two shapes or forms.

diploid Two complete sets of chromosomes, double the number present in gametes (ova or sperm cells). In humans, the diploid number is 46.

diplopia Double vision.

direct calorimetry A measurement of energy expended by measuring temperature changes in a closed structure.

direct contact transmission Body surface to body surface contact.

direct response Pupillary constriction on the pupil being tested.

directed or controlled coughing Cough technique to expectorate sputum and avoid fatigue associated with undirected, forceful coughing that consists of slow, maximal inspiration followed by breath holding for several seconds and then two or three coughs.

disaccharides A class of sugars, which yields two monosaccharide molecules through hydrolysis.

disease prevention or health protection Behavior motivated by a desire to actively avoid illness, detect it early, or maintain functioning within the constraints of an illness.

disequilibrium An imbalance in solute concentration across the blood brain barrier.

displaced fracture A fracture in which the bones have gone out of natural alignment.

disseminated Spread over a large area of the body, tissue, or organ.

disseminated intravascular coagulation (DIC) Clotting and bleeding disorder that results from the generation of tissue factor activity within the blood. This trigger of the coagulation cascade quickly leads to significant thrombin production, which perpetuates its own formation and results in bleeding.

distress Stressor that is perceived as negative or stress that produces a negative response; a certain level of negative stress is needed for growth and development.

distribution The movement of the drug, after absorption into the bloodstream, to the site of intended action.

diverticula Sac-like outpouches of mucosa through the muscular layer of the bowel.

diverticulosis When there are multiple infected diverticula that result in pathology.

do not resuscitate (DNR) A health care provider's order that there be no attempt to restart a failed heartbeat or apply cardiopulmonary resuscitation.

domains of nursing The four main areas of nurses' practice, which includes clinical practice, education, administrative practice, and research.

dominant culture Group whose values prevail within a society.

double effect Palliative therapy, itself, hastens death.

drawer test An assessment technique used to diagnose rupture of cruciate ligaments.

Dressler's syndrome Inflammation of the pericardium that can occur 2 to 10 weeks after a myocardial infarction.

droplet transmission Particles propelled through the air.

dual energy X-ray absorptiometry (DEXA) scans Diagnostic tests that assist with the early diagnosis of osteoporosis.

Durable Power of Attorney for Health Care (DPAHC) Advance directive that appoints an agent or proxy decision maker to make health care decisions for a person who has lost decisional capacity.

dysarthria Difficulty in oral movement to form words.

dyscrasia Nonspecific term for blood disease.

dysdiadochokinesia The inability to perform rapidly alternating movements.

dysesthesia Burning or tingling.

dysfunctional uterine bleeding (DUB) Abnormal uterine bleeding not caused by malignancy, inflammation, or pregnancy.

dysgeusia Disturbed sense of taste.

dysmenorrhea Pain associated with menstruation.

dysmetria Impaired judgment of distance, range, speed, and force of movement.

dyspareunia Painful intercourse.

dyspepsia An uncomfortable feeling in the upper abdominal region.

dysphagia Difficulty swallowing.

dyspnea Difficulty breathing.

dysrhythmia A disturbance in rhythm.

dyssynergy A lack of coordinated muscle movement.

dysthymia A low-level depression that can last at least two years, and if left untreated, can lead to more severe depression.

dysuria Painful urination.

E

echocardiogram A noninvasive test in which ultrasound is used to reflect cardiac structures. It can be performed at rest or in conjunction with a stress test.

ectopy Heartbeat arising from a location other than the sinoatrial node on a monitor screen.

ectropion When the lower eyelid is turned away from the globe of the eye.

eczematoid Lesion suggesting inflammation with tendency to thickening, oozing, vesiculation, or crusting (related to eczema).

edema An abnormal collection of fluid in the interstitial spaces between cells resulting in a lifting and separating of the layers of the skin.

effluent Waste materials.

egophony The presence of loud, nasal, and "bleating" sounds when auscultating the lungs.

ejection fraction (EF) An index that estimates contractile function of the left ventricle. The expected ejection fraction is 60 to 70 percent.

electrolytes Charged particles found in body fluids.

emboli A blood clot or other particle (plaque) that break loose and block blood vessels.

embolization Introduction of an angio catheter to visualize the internal spermatic vein, to correct dysfunction of the spermatic vein.

emmetropia In normal vision the light falls onto the retina without any distortion or abnormal bending of the light.

empowerment To assist or encourage a person to be involved in decision making and development of the plan of care; the ability to assume self-care management.

endemic Restricted to a particular region, community, or group of people.

endocarditis Inflammation of the endocardium.

endocardium The membrane that lines the cavities of the heart and forms part of the heart valves.

endocrine glands Those glands that produce hormones that are secreted into the bloodstream and travel to their target organs or tissues.

endogenous Produced or originating from within a cell or organism.

endometriosis Ectopic growth of functioning endometrial tissue.

endorphins Peptides secreted in the brain that boost mood and help fight depression and pain.

endothelium The layer that lines the blood and lymphatic vessels, the heart, and various other body cavities is a prominent contributor to the activation of the inflammatory immune response. Cells produce several compounds that affect the vascular lumen and platelets.

endotracheal intubation The passage of tube into the trachea through either the mouth or nares to maintain an open airway or facilitate mechanical ventilation.

enterokinase An enzyme that hastens effective digestion.

enterprises Organized systems of any size in any location that provide any type of health care for compensation.

enthesitis Traumatic disease occurring at the insertion of muscles where recurring concentration of muscle stress provokes inflammation with a tendency toward fibrosis and calcification.

entropia An eye that deviates inward.

entropion When the lower eyelid is turned in toward the globe of the eye.

enucleation Surgical removal of an eye.

environmental control Relationships between people and nature and a person's perceived ability to control activities of nature.

enzymatic debridement Accomplished using a chemical debriding agent.

eosinophil A granulocyte that helps to control the inflammatory process.

epidemiological investigation Study looking at a specific disease, its distribution, and initial source.

epididymitis Infection of the epididymis.

epilepsy Chronic recurrent pattern of seizures.

epiphyses The widened ends of the long bone.

epispadias The urinary meatus is located along the superior (upper) aspect of the penis.

equianalgesia The provision of equal analgesic effects in changing from one drug and/or delivery method to another or choosing a different delivery method.

ergonomics Science that seeks to adapt work or working conditions to suit the worker.

erythromelalgia A burning sensation in the digits of the extremities.

erythropoietic Relating to the formation of red blood cells.

erythropoietin (EPO) A hormone produced by the kidney in response to low oxygen states or a low hematocrit, which stimulates red blood cell production in the bone marrow.

eschar Burned skin that is dead and must be removed before healing can occur.

escharotomy Incision through full-thickness circumferential burn tissue to restore and maintain circulation or chest expansion.

esotropia Convergent strabismus.

ethics The study of philosophical ideals of right and wrong behavior.

ethics of care Belief that health care professionals have a moral obligation and duty to provide care to those in need.

ethnicity A cultural group's perception of themselves (group identity). This self-perception influences how the group's members are perceived by others.

ethnocentrism Belief that one's own culture is superior to all others.

eugenics The selection and recombination of genes already existing in the gene pool.

euglycemia A normal concentration of glucose in the blood.

euploidy A term referring to the correct number of chromosomes in a cell.

eupnea The presence of normal respirations, or normal rate and depth of breathing.

eustachian tube A tube that connects the middle ear to the nasopharynx.

eustress A certain level of positive stress that is needed for growth and survival.

euthanasia Practice in which a person other than the patient directly administers medication that causes the death of a patient.

euthenics (euphenics) The techniques for correcting defects in individuals after they have been born.

euthyroid Having a normal functioning thyroid gland.

evidence-based practice (EBP) Process through which scientific evidence is identified, appraised, and applied in health care interventions.

evidence summary Report of the state of scientifically produced knowledge that is developed using rigorous methods to synthesize knowledge across a number of research studies so that study variations and contradictory study results can be understood in a single conclusion statement.

Ewing's sarcoma A diffuse endothelioma or endothelial myeloma forming a fusiform swelling on a long bone.

exacerbation A sudden increase in the seriousness of the disease with greater intensity in signs and symptoms, which lasts from minutes to hours or days.

exanthema Breaking out in a rash.

excitability The capacity for that cell to depolarize in response to an electrical impulse.

exocrine glands Those glands that secrete substances into ducts that empty into a body cavity or onto a body surface.

exogenous Originating outside an organ.

exotropia (wall eyes) An eye that deviates outward.

expiratory reserve volume (ERV) The maximal amount of gas that can be expired at the end of a normal exhalation.

expressive aphasia (Broca's aphasia) A condition in which a patient cannot express what he or she wants to say.

extracellular fluid (ECF) The fluid located between cells and includes interstitial and intravascular fluid.

extravasation The inadvertent administration of vesicant into the surrounding tissues.

extrinsic distortion Occurs when the interpreter is improperly prepared.

exudate Accumulated fluid in a cavity.

F

fascia An inelastic connective tissue that covers and separates muscles, tendons, and ligaments.

fasciotomy Incision through a fibrous layer that separates muscles.

fast pain (rapid pain) Pain that originates in the free endings of the large myelinated nerve fibers of the skin; such pain respond to strong pressure and high temperature, thus eliciting the withdrawal reflex.

fecalith Hard mass of fecal material.

fibroadenomas Benign fibrous growths or tumors of the glandular epithelium in breast tissue.

fibromyalgia A disorder characterized by muscle pain, stiffness, and easy fatigability.

first pass effect After absorption, oral drugs are transported via hepatic portal circulation to the liver, where they are metabolized (broken down) before they can pass into the general circulation.

flatulence Gas formed within the gastrointestinal tract and expelled via the rectum.

foam cell Engorged lipid-laden macrophages that are the major component of the fatty streak.

focused assessment An assessment that is limited in scope to focus on a particular need or health care problem or potential health care risk.

folliculitis Acute inflammation of the hair follicle caused by physical irritation, infection, or chemical irritation.

fracture A break in a bone.

fremitus The feeling of vibration, which will be increased or decreased in certain conditions.

fulguration Destruction of tissue using high-frequency electric sparks.

full-thickness burn Also called third-degree burn; involves the entire epidermis and dermis that extends to subcutaneous tissue and possibly muscle and bone.

furuncles (boils) Localized bacterial infections that can manifest as painful, indurated, or fluctuant, fluid-filled masses.

G

galactorrhea Excessive secretion of milk.

gametes A mature male or female reproductive cell.

gender identity The biological sex of male, female, or intersexed.

gender role The masculine or feminine role adopted by a person, which is often culturally and socially determined.

gene A segment of a DNA molecule that is the heredity unit that occupies a fixed chromosomal locus.

gene therapy The process of treating or curing a genetic disorder by providing the affected individual with an intact, functional copy of the gene in question.

general inhibition syndrome (GIS) "Possum" response to stress because of overstimulation of the parasympathetic nervous system (PNS) as a means of survival or a paralyzing or numbing effect when facing a life-threatening event; a state of panic or freezing.

genetic counseling The interaction between health care provider and patient to manage the human problems associated with the occurrence, or risk of occurrence, of a genetic disorder in a family.

genetic engineering Changing a particular molecule in the structure of the gene, either to eliminate a certain bad trait or to improve the genotype.

genetic screening Population screening for a genetic variation or mutation, for example, PKU screening at birth.

genetic testing Testing of an individual at significant risk because of family history or because of presentation of symptoms, for example chromosome abnormalities.

genogram A family tree related to health history.

genomics The study of genome composition, structure, and function in combination with environmental factors that has led to the discovery of numerous health care products.

genotype The genetic constitution or blueprint of an individual, the gene pairs that are inherited from the parents.

global aphasia A condition in which a patient has both expressive and receptive aphasia.

globalization Organized or established worldwide.

glossitis An inflammation of the tongue.

glucagon A hormone released from the pancreas in response to low levels of blood glucose and is a counterregulatory hormone.

gluconeogenesis The process of the liver converting predominant amino acids to glucose in the fasting state.

glycogen hydrolysis Conversion of stored glycogen into usable glucose to meet the immediate energy needs of the body.

glycogen synthesis Conversion of glucose to glycogen that can be stored in preparation of times of fasting.

glycogenolysis The physiological process of the breakdown of stored glucose to raise blood sugar levels.

grading The degree of malignancy or cell differentiation of the tumor cells.

granulocytes Class of leukocytes with prominent granules.

granuloma A mass of inflamed granulation tissue.

graphesthesia Identify letters, numbers, or shapes drawn on hand.

grief resolution An adjustment to actual or impending loss.

gross domestic product (GDP) Total value of final goods and services produced in a year within the United States.

growth hormone (GH) Hormone that affects all tissues of the body, is secreted from anterior pituitary, and is one of the counterregulatory hormones.

gynecomastia Breast enlargement in men.

H

half-life The time required for the body, tissue, or organ to metabolize or make inactive half the amount of a substance taken in.

haploid One complete set of chromosomes. The haploid number in humans is 23.

haptens An antigen that does not cause an immune response unless bound to a carrier molecule.

harvesting A procedure to collect tissue such as the spongy bone marrow from inside bones containing stem cells.

healing touch (HT) An energy-based therapeutic therapy that alters the energy field through the use of touch.

health A state and a process of being and becoming an integrated and whole person.

health care Care related to all states of health from severe illness and injury to supreme good health; diagnosis and treatment of disease and strategies that maintain and improve health.

health care system Network of individuals, technologies, and processes that provide and support health care.

health insurance Insurance policy that provides payment for benefits of a covered sickness or injury. Included under this definition are various types of insurances, such as accident insurance, disability insurance, medical expense insurance, and accidental death insurance.

health maintenance Behavior directed toward maintaining a current level of health.

health maintenance activities The activities or behaviors an individual performs to maintain or improve a current level of health.

health maintenance organizations (HMOs) Type of managed care plan where access to care is controlled by a primary care provider and coverage is limited to the approved medical services, administered by a network of health care providers, hospitals, skilled nursing facilities, and other providers included in the plan. Emphasis is on prevention.

health promotion Process undertaken to increase levels of wellness in individuals, families, and communities.

heartburn (pyrosis) A substernal burning sensation often radiating to the neck that is experienced within one hour of eating or one to two hours after reclining.

Heberden's nodes Hard nodules or enlargements of the tubercles of the last phalanges of the fingers.

Heinz bodies Degraded hemoglobin.

helper T cells Lymphocytes that orchestrate the immune response; also called CD4 T cells. There are two subclasses TH1 and TH2.

hemarthrosis Untreated bleeding into the joint.

hematochezia Stools containing red blood rather than tarry stools.

hematoma Excessive bleeding that occurs around a wound site as a result of broken blood vessels from trauma or surgery.

hematomas A swelling noted in tissue, caused by extravasated blood.

hematopoiesis The ability to maintain the body's blood supply and its components.

hematopoietic Pertaining to the formation of blood or blood.

hematuria Blood in the urine.

hemiparesis Weakness on one side of the body.

hemiplegia Inability to move of one side of the body.

hemoglobinuria Hemoglobin in the urine.

hemolysis Destruction of red blood cells.

hemoptysis Indicates either the presence of frank blood or blood-streaked sputum.

hemorrhagic stroke When a blood vessel bursts leaking blood into brain tissue or surrounding spaces.

hemosiderosis A condition in which iron is toxic to the cells.

hemovac A type of surgical drain with a piece that connects to a mechanical suction device.

hepatomegaly Enlarged liver, palpated below the level of the ribs.

hereditary angioedema (HAE) An inherited abnormality of the immune system that causes swelling, particularly of the face, and abdominal cramping.

heterograft (xenograft) A graft of skin obtained from another species.

high-density lipoprotein (HDL) The substance that transports plasma cholesterol away from atherosclerotic plaques and to the liver for metabolism and excretion and is considered "good" cholesterol because increased levels decrease the tendency to CAD.

high efficiency particulate air (HEPA) filter Filter used to remove submicron particulate matter from the air.

hirsutism Condition characterized by the excessive growth of hair or the presence of hair in abnormal places.

histamine A chemical released by the immune system during allergic reactions.

histocompatibility leukocyte antigens (HLA) A complex set of proteins on the surface membrane of human nucleated cells, tissues, and blood cells (except red blood cells).

holism The concept that the whole is greater than the sum of its parts. Holism encompasses consideration of the physiological, psychological, sociocultural, intellectual, and spiritual aspects of each individual.

Homans' sign Dorsiflexing the foot, causing pain in the calf.

homeopathy Treatment of disease with minute drug doses to activate an illness that then stimulates the body's normal defense system to eliminate illness.

homeostasis Physiological and psychological equilibrium or balance.

homograft A graft of skin obtained from a cadaver 6 to 24 hours after death that is used as a temporary graft.

homonymous hemianopsia Inability to see out of one half of both eyes, and the visual field cut.

hope A feeling expressed as future-oriented, which allows the person to set goals, devise strategies for achieving the desired goals, and a sense of being in control.

hormones The chemicals produced and stored by the endocrine system that help regulate metabolism and energy, cardiac output and blood pressure, reproduction, and growth and development.

hospice Provides end-of-life care for patients and their families.

hospice care Coordinated program of palliative care services with a goal of attaining the highest possible quality of life for patients and their families at the end of life and continuing through the bereavement period.

human leukocyte antigen (HLA) MHC class I.

humectants Substances that promote moisture in skin.

humoral-mediated immunity Refers to immunity that is mediated by B lymphocytes, plasma cells, and antibodies.

hyaline Cartilage that covers the end of each bone to reduce friction and distribute weight-bearing forces.

hydronephrosis Dilation of the renal pelvis because of an obstruction of urine flow or from ureteral reflux.

hypalgesia Diminished sensitivity to pain.

hyperalgesia (allodynia) A state of neural supersensitivity where a slight painful stimulus can be interpreted as very painful.

hypercapnia An accumulation of $PaCO_2$ in the blood, indicating hypoventilation.

hypercholesterolemia High serum cholesterol.

hyperesthesia Increased sensitivity of the skin.

hypergesia Increased sensitivity to pain.

hyperglycemia An elevated blood sugar level.

hyperlipidemia Elevated blood cholesterol levels.

hyperopia (farsightedness) Occurs when the light passing through the eye is focused behind the retina when looking a close objects.

hyperplasia Increase in number.

hypersensitive response An extreme physical response to an allergen, in which large amounts of IgE are produced.

hypertension Sustained elevation of blood pressure.

hypertonic A solution with a concentration higher than that of blood.

hypertrophic Increase in size of an organ or structure secondary to inflammation or overgrowth of cells not related to tumor formation.

hypertrophy Abnormal enlargement, increase in size and mass, of a body part or organ.

hyperuricemia An abnormal amount of uric acid in the urine.

hypervolemia Excess intravascular fluid.

hypesthesia Diminished sense of touch.

hypoalbuminemia Decrease in albumin in the blood.

hypocapnia Less than normal $PaCO_2$ in the blood, indicating hyperventilation.

hypogeusia Diminished taste sensitivity.

hypokyphosis Less than normal curvature in the thoracic spine.

hypospadias The urinary meatus is located along the inferior (lower) aspect of the penis.

hypotany Low intraocular pressure.

hypotension Blood pressure lower than needed for adequate tissue perfusion and oxygenation.

hypothermia Condition where the body temperature falls to less than 36° C (96.8° F). It is classified as mild, if not less than 32° C (89.6° F).

hypotonic A solution with a concentration less than that of blood.

hypovolemia Insufficient intravascular fluid.

hypoxemia A decrease in PaO_2 below 80 mm Hg.

hypoxia A general term for decrease in tissue oxygenation.

I

icterus Yellow coloration in the sclera of the eye.

idiopathic A disease state that arises from an unknown cause.

idiopathic pain Spontaneous or unpredictable breakthrough pain.

ileus Refers to intestinal obstruction because of a partial or complete arrest of intestinal peristalsis; also known as paralytic or adynamic ileus.

illness care Care aimed at relieving the discomfort of disease.

imagery The use of one's sense to create an image in one's mind.

immune response A body response to an antigen that occurs when lymphocytes identify the antigenic molecule as foreign and induce the formation of antibodies and lymphocytes capable of reacting with it and rendering it harmless.

immunity The quality or state of being immune; a condition of being able to resist a particular disease through preventing development of a pathogenic microorganism or by counteracting the effects of its products.

immunodeficiency Inability to produce a normal complement of antibodies or immunologically sensitized T cells especially in response to specific antigens.

immunogen A particle that can cause an immune response.

immunoglobulins (IG) The class of proteins that antibodies belong to. Body manufactures five isotopes: IgM, IgD, IgG, IgA, and IgE.

immunotherapy The process of introducing allergens to the body by injection for the purpose of increasing immunity.

imperforate hymen Congenital malformation of the hymenal ring resulting in lack of a vaginal opening.

inborn error of metabolism A condition in which the metabolism of an organism is abnormal because of the presence of one, or a pair of, abnormal alleles.

incentive spirometer A machine used to allow patients a quantifiable aid in deep breathing postoperatively.

incidence The number of new cases of a condition, symptom, death, or injury that arise during a specific period of time such as a month or a year.

indirect calorimetry A method for estimating energy expenditure by measuring oxygen consumption and carbon dioxide production.

indirect contact transmission Inanimate object involved in transfer.

infertility The inability to conceive within one year when a couple is engaging in unprotected sexual intercourse at the appropriate times in the female's menstrual cycle.

infiltration Inadvertent administration of a solution into the surrounding tissues.

inflammation A nonspecific response to any foreign invader involving the immune system.

inflammatory immune response (IIR) A response that is composed of several body systems that are constantly on alert to detect nonself and harmful intruders from the normal cells and proteins in the body.

informed consent A patient's authorization for care based on full disclosure of risks, benefits, alternatives, and consequences of refusal.

innate immunity Immunity that is inherent within a species and develops regardless of exposure.

inspection Careful, systematic visual observation.

inspiratory reserve volume (IRV) The maximal amount of gas that can be inspired at the end of a normal inspiration.

insulin Hormone produced by the beta cells of the pancreas to lower blood glucose levels.

integrated care delivery system Network of organizations that provides a coordinated continuum of services to a defined population and that is willing to be held clinically and fiscally accountable for the outcomes and health status of the population served.

integrative review Alternative term for an evidence summary.

integrative therapy Therapy that combines conventional medical therapies with complementary alternative medicine (CAM) therapies for which there is some high-quality scientific evidence of safety and effectiveness.

interdisciplinary team Clearly defined group of members of specific disciplines who work collaboratively to develop a coordinated plan of care.

interferons (IFNs) Proteins formed when cells are exposed to invaders such as viruses that are able to activate other components of the immune system.

interleukins (IL) Generic name for cytokines released by leukocytes.

interstitial fluid The fluid located between cells.

interstitial space The area surrounding the nephron loops and the peritubular capillaries, which has a high osmotic pressure due to extremely high levels of sodium. The renal interstitial space facilitates the massive volume water reabsorption required to maintain fluid balance.

intra-aortic balloon pump A catheter with an oblong balloon on the end that eases the workload on the patient's heart by decreasing afterload and coronary perfusion.

intracellular fluid (ICF) The fluid located inside each cell.

intracranial pressure (ICP) The amount of pressure placed on the structures within the brain.

intractable pain Pain that is refractory or resistant to some or all forms of treatment.

intradermal route An injection into the skin.

intraductal papilloma Small benign tumor that grows within the terminal portion of a solitary milk duct of the breast.

intraoperative The operative period from entry into the operating suite through departure from the post-anesthesia care unit (PACU).

intrarenal Occurring within the kidney.

intrathecal Within the spinal canal, the space between the double-layered covering or lining of the brain and spinal cord.

intravascular fluid The fluid located inside the blood vessels, excluding the fluid inside the cells in the blood vessels.

intrinsic distortion Occurs when information is passed on from one person to another through an interpreter.

intussusception Invagination, or telescoping, of one part of the intestine into itself.

inverse ratio ventilation Ventilating the patient with a longer inspiratory time as compared to the expiratory time.

inversion stress test A physical examination test used to assess for ankle joint laxity. It is performed by bracing the heel with left hand, inverting the foot with right hand, and comparing to the opposite side.

ischemic stroke Damage to the brain due to a clogged artery.

isokinetic Exercise involving resistance through full range of movement.

isotonic Solution that has the same osmotic pressure as the referent solution (e.g., plasma).

J

jaundice Yellow pigmentation of the skin and sclera.

joint aspiration A procedure performed to examine the synovial fluid in the joint cavity and to relieve pain in the joint resulting from edema and effusion.

Joint Commission on Accreditation of Hospitals (JCAHO) An independent, not-for-profit organization that sets standards for measuring health care quality. Accredited hospitals receive an on-site review every three years.

justice Requires that like cases are treated in like fashion.

K

karyotype A photomicrograph of the chromosomes of an individual that have been arranged in the standard classifications system by group and size.

keratinization A process that is used by epidermal tissue to replenish itself.

keratitis Inflammation of the cornea.

keratometry Measurement of the cornea.

kernicterus Yellow discoloration and degenerative lesions in the central nervous system causing brain damage.

kinesthesia The ability to perceive the movement of one's body.

kinesthetic learners Learning style in which a person processes information by experiencing the information or by touching and feeling.

knowledge transformation Five sequential steps that convert primary research knowledge to evidence that a specific health care intervention achieves positive clinical outcomes.

Kupffer cells Specialized reticuloendothelial cells of the liver, which belong to the monocyte-macrophage system.

Kussmaul breathing The presence of abnormally deep and rapid respirations, with the presence of a fruity odor to the breath.

kyphoscoliosis A combination of kyphosis and scoliosis.

kyphosis An exaggeration of thoracic spine convexity.

L

labyrinth A complex, closed, fluid-filled system of interconnecting tubes in the inner ear.

lacunae Reservoirs in which the mature bone cells are embedded.

lamellar bone The thin layer of mature bone tissue.

laminar airflow Filtered air circulating in parallel-flowing planes.

lancinating Stabbing or piercing.

laparoscopic cholecystectomy A surgical procedure using a laparoscope to remove the gallbladder.

laparoscopy A diagnostic procedure where the peritoneal cavity (pelvis and abdomen) are examined.

laparotomy Surgical incision made in the wall of the abdomen.

lateral epicondylitis Pain over the lateral epicondyle of the humerus or head of the radius. Also called tennis elbow.

latex allergy An immediate type of hypersensitive reaction to latex exposure.

lavage The irrigation (wash out) of the stomach contents.

learning Process of assimilating information with a resultant change in behavior.

learning plateaus Peaks in effectiveness of teaching and depth of learning.

learning style Way in which an individual incorporates new information.

leiomyomata Benign smooth muscle tumors of the uterus commonly called fibroids.

length of stay (LOS) Length of time a patient remains hospitalized, an outcome variable that refers to the efficiency of a health care delivery system.

lentigines Flat brown spots seen on aged exposed skin.

lesions Circumscribed altered area of tissue that should be treated as abnormal finding.

leukapheresis The removal of blood to collect specific blood cells; the remaining blood is returned to the body.

leukocytes General name for all white blood cells.

leukopenia A decrease in the total circulating white blood cells.

Levine's sign Clenched fist over the chest is the universal sign for angina.

liberty Independent from coercion.

lichenification Thickening of the epidermis.

ligaments Strong bands of connective tissue that attach bone to bone or bone to cartilage.

lipodystrophy A localized complication of insulin administration characterized by changes in the subcutaneous fat at the site of the injection.

liver lobule The functional unit of the liver.

liver sweats The movement of plasma from the lymphatic system into this potential space in the abdomen.

living will (LW) Advance directive that allows a person to document specifically what medical treatment they wish, or do not wish, to have.

locus The position of a gene on a chromosome.

long-term care Extended assistance for the chronically ill, mentally ill, or disabled.

low-density lipoprotein (LDL) The main lipid component of the atherosclerotic plaque and is considered "bad" cholesterol because increased levels reflect increased tendency to CAD.

lower motor neuron Motor pathway that originates in the spinal cord and continues on as spinal nerves sending impulses to the peripheral areas of the body.

lumpectomy Wide local excision or partial mastectomy that involves excision of all cancerous tissue to microscopically clean margins.

lymphadenopathy Painless lymph node enlargements from obstruction and pressure.

lymphocytes Primary cells in the immune response.

M

macronutrients Carbohydrate, protein, and lipids.

macrophages Phagocytic cells found in tissues.

macules Flat circumscribed changes of the skin (flat nevi, café au lait spots, vitiligo, telangiectases or capillary hemangiomas).

macular rash A rash with flat red spots.

major surgery Operations that involve risk to life in some way, such as those involving multiple systems, or that require long periods of time in the operating suite.

malaise Body discomfort and fatigue.

malignant Cells that invade and destroy nearby tissues and spread to other parts of the body.

malignant hyperthermia (MH) Life-threatening, acute pharmacogenic disorder, developing during or after a general anesthesia.

malrotation Failure during embryonic development of normal rotation of all or part of an organ or system.

mammary duct ectasia Noncancerous condition of the breast in which the milk ducts beneath the nipple become dilated and sometimes inflamed.

mammoplasty Surgical procedure to increase or decrease the size or shape of the breast.

managed care organizations (MCOs) Groups implementing health care using managed care concepts including pre-authorization of treatment, utilization review, and a fixed network of care providers.

mandatory minute ventilation (MMV) A mode of ventilation that allows the ventilator to adjust its breaths based on the patient's minute ventilation.

mass casualty incident (MCI) An influx of patients that overwhelms a hospital and affects its capability to care for patients.

mastalgia Breast pain.

mastitis Inflammation or infection of the breast.

mastodynia Breast pain.

mastoidectomy An incision of the mastoid sinuses.

mastoiditis Infectious process of the mastoid sinuses.

mechanical debridement Uses gauze dressings to remove necrotic or devitalized tissue from wounds.

mechanical ventilation A means of providing ventilatory assistance by a mechanical device.

mechanism of injury The manner in which an injury occurs.

Medicaid Program that pays for medical assistance for certain individuals with low income and resources. It is jointly funded by federal and state governments.

medical futility When a particular therapy offers no medical benefit.

Medicare National health insurance program for people age 65 years and older, people under aged 65 with disabilities, and people with end-stage renal disease. Medicare provides coverage to approximately 40 million Americans.

Medicare Hospice Benefit Reimbursement benefit provided by the federal government for hospice services.

meditation A mind-body technique by which an individual can consciously quiet the mind by focusing one's attention in order to control some functions of the sympathetic nervous system.

meiosis A series of two specialized divisions of diploid germ cells to produce four gametes containing the haploid number of chromosomes.

menarche Initial menstrual period, normally occurring between 9 and 17 years of age.

menopause Permanent cessation of menstrual activity, usually occurring between 35 and 55 years of age.

menorrhagia Cyclic menstrual bleeding that is abnormally long or heavy.

menstrual cycle Periodically recurring series of changes associated with uterine endometrial growth in preparation for fertilization and shedding of endometrium when fertilization has not occurred.

meta analysis Statistical procedure used to summarize the results of research across multiple research reports.

metabolic syndrome Diagnosed when three or more factors such as high blood pressure, abdominal obesity, high triglyceride levels, low high-density lipoprotein (HDL) cholesterol and high fasting blood glucose levels are present.

metabolism or biotransformation Biotransformation process in which the drug is broken down by enzymes to a form that can be excreted from the body. The primary organ of metabolism is the liver. The chemical changes in living cells by which energy is provided for vital processes and activities, and new material is assimilated.

metastasis Spread of cancerous tumor to other distant locations.

metrorrhagia Bleeding at times other than normal menstrual cycle.

microtrauma Trauma to muscles, tendons, ligaments, and bones on a microscopic level.

minimal sedation (anxiolysis) Drug-induced state during which patients respond normally to verbal commands. Although cognitive function and coordination may be impaired, ventilatory and cardiovascular functions are unaffected.

minor surgery Operations that do not involve risk to life in some way, such as those that involve one system that can be done in a short period of time or can be performed in a health care provider's office.

minority group Ethnic, racial, or religious group that constitutes less than a numerical majority of the total population.

mitigation Activities a hospital undertakes to help lessen the severity and impact of potential emergencies that may affect operations or services provided by a hospital.

mitosis Somatic cell division resulting in the formation of two cells, each with the same chromosome complement as the parent cell.

mitral facies A florid appearance with cyanosed cheeks.

mixed venous oxygen saturation (SvO_2) A measurement of the amount of hemoglobin saturated with oxygen compared to the total amount of hemoglobin in the pulmonary artery.

modulation Alteration in the level of pain intensity (by either increasing or inhibiting it), including the processing of incoming impulses from the sensory nerve to the dorsal horn of the spinal cord; modulation also occurs via descending messages originating in the midbrain and sent to the dorsal horn.

monoclonal antibodies Genetically engineered immunosuppressive agents that are used in combination with other drugs to prevent graft rejection.

monocytes Phagocytic cells found in the blood.

monosaccharides Simple sugar molecules not decomposable by hydrolysis.

moral distress Occurs in response to awareness of the right and moral action, coupled with inability to carry out that action.

morals Customs or habits that are ethically correct.

morbidity The number of ill persons in relationship to a specific population.

mortality The ratio of the number of deaths in a given population.

mosaicism Tissue composed of cells of two different genotypes or karyotypes.

motivation The internal drive or externally arising stimulus to action or thought.

mucositis An inflammation and ulceration of the lining of the mouth, throat, or gastrointestinal (GI) tract most commonly associated with chemotherapy or radiotherapy for cancer.

Müllerian dysgenesis Malformation of the embryonic duct that becomes the fallopian tubes, uterus, and vagina.

multiple organ dysfunction syndrome (MODS) Evidence of a progressive inflammatory response has caused more than one of the body's organs to fail. The presence of altered organ function in an acutely ill patient such that homeostasis cannot be maintained without intervention.

Murphy's sign Pain on deep inspiration when an inflamed gallbladder is palpated by pressing the fingers under the rib cage.

music-thanatology A holistic and palliative method for using music to help dissipate obstacles to patients' peaceful transition to death.

mutation A permanent change in genetic material.

myalgia Pain in the muscles.

myectomy Excision of a portion of the muscle.

myelogram A diagnostic test used to determine defects in and around the spinal column.

myelosuppression A decrease in the production of red blood cells, platelets, and some white blood cells by the bone marrow. Also, inhibition of the production of blood cells, a bone marrow function.

myocardial infarction (MI) Prolonged ischemia, 20 minutes or more, that results in myocardial cellular death.

myocarditis An inflammation of the myocardium.

myoclonus Twitching or clonic spasms of a muscle or group of muscles.

myomectomy Surgical removal of fibroid tumors in the wall of the uterus.

myopia (nearsightedness) Occurs when the light passing through the eye is overbent or overrefracted.

myosin The protein that compose the thick filaments of a myofibril.

myotonia Tonic spasm of a muscle or temporary rigidity.

myringoplasty Plastic surgery of the tympanic membrane.

myringotomy Incision into the tympanic membrane.

N

nadir The period of time following chemotherapy, usually 7 to 10 days after chemotherapy, when blood counts drop, thereby increasing susceptibility to infection or bleeding.

narrative review Less rigorous form of summary process used in nursing.

nasal airway A soft, flexible tube that is inserted into the nasal passage to maintain an open airway.

National Guideline Clearinghouse Searchable database of nearly 1,500 clinical practice guidelines.

native kidney One's own kidney as opposed to a transplant graft.

negative feedback Response of a gland by increasing or decreasing the secretion of a hormone.

neoadjuvant Adjunctive or adjuvant therapy given prior to the primary (main) therapy.

neoangiogenesis Development of new blood vessels.

neoplasm An abnormal mass of cells, can be benign or malignant.

nephrectomy Surgical removal of the kidney.

nephritis Infection contained to the kidney.

nephrolithiasis Kidney stone disease.

nephropathy Disease of the kidneys.

nephrotoxic Having the ability to harm the kidney.

neuralgia Pain associated with peripheral nerves, which follows the course of nerves.

neuropathies Dysfunctions of the peripheral nervous system.

neuropeptides Amino acids produced in the brain and other sites in the body that act as chemical communicators.

neurotransmitters Chemical substances produced by the body that facilitate nerve impulse transmission.

neutropenia A decreased number of circulating neutrophils, usually less than 1,500 cells/μm.

neutrophils Chief phagocytic cell of early inflammatory response.

nociceptive pain Pain that occurs when there is normal processing of the pain impulse.

nociceptor A free nerve endings that is a receptor for painful (noxious) stimuli. Nociceptors are found in almost all types of tissue.

nocturia Urination at night.

nodules Circumscribed elevated, usually solid lesions (fibromas, neurofibromas, xanthomas, erythema nodosum, and various benign or malignant growths).

nonmaleficence Use of ability, judgment, or skill to help someone else without intent to cause injury or harm.

normovolemia State of normal blood volume.

nosocomial Infection acquired in a health care facility.

nuchal A stiff painful neck due to irritated meninges.

nutraceuticals Any natural substance found in plant or animal foods that acts as a protective or healing agent.

nystagmus An involuntary rhythmic movement of the eyes in a back and forth or cyclical movement.

O

objective data Data that are observable and measurable.

occult fracture A fracture that does not show up on plain radiographic films until the healing process begins and calcification is seen.

odynophagia Pain that is experienced when a person swallows.

oligomenorrhea Menstrual cycles occurring farther apart than usual.

oligospermic Having low sperm motility with a low semen volume.

oliguria Low urine output.

oncogenes Cancer susceptibility genes. When altered or mutated proto-oncogenes promote tumor formation or growth.

oncotic pressure Osmotic pressure because of proteins.

onycholysis The loosening of the nails starting at the border.

oocytes The early or primitive ovum before it has developed completely.

opportunistic Organism causing disease in a host whose resistance to fight infection is diminished.

oppression Rules, modes, and ideals of one group are imposed on another group.

opsonization A process that coats a foreign substance and makes it more susceptible to phagocytosis.

oral airway A stiff plastic tube that prevents the tongue from sliding back into the pharynx and blocking the airway.

orchitis Acute inflammation of the testes.

orthostatic hypotension Hypotension occurring when changing position from supine to upright.

osmolality The number of solutes per kilogram of fluid.

osmolarity The number of solutes per liter of fluid.

osmosis The movement of water from an area of low concentration of solutes (low osmolality) to an area of high concentration of solutes (high osmolality).

osmotic pressure The ability of a solution to draw fluid across a semipermeable membrane.

ossicles Three tiny bones (in the middle ear) that play a crucial role in the transmission of sound.

osteoarthritis (OA) Noninflammatory degenerative joint disease characterized by degeneration of the articular cartilage, hypertrophy of bone at the margins, and changes in the synovial membrane.

osteogenesis The process of bone formation and remodeling.

osteomalacia A condition marked by softening of the bones with pain, tenderness, muscular weakness, anorexia, and loss of weight, resulting from deficiency of vitamin D and calcium.

osteomyelitis Inflammation of the bone caused by a pyogenic organism.

osteopenia A significant amount of decrease in bone mineral density.

osteoporosis A reduction in the amount of bone mass, leading to fractures after minimal trauma.

osteosarcoma Malignant tumor of bone.

ostomy A surgically created opening made between the intestine and the abdominal wall.

otalgia Ear pain.

otitis media An inflammation of the middle ear.

otorrhea Liquid discharge or drainage from the ear.

otosclerosis A progressive hearing loss of predominately low tones.

ototoxic A substance that damages the acoustic nerve or hearing mechanism.

outcome variables Consequences of care delivery categorized as humanistic, financial, and clinical.

overuse syndrome An injury to musculoskeletal tissues affecting the upper extremity or cervical spine, resulting from repeated movement, temperature extremes, overuse, incorrect posture, or sustained force or vibration. Also called repetitive motion injuries or cumulative trauma disorders.

ovulation Periodic maturation and release of an ovum from a follicle on the ovary.

oxyhemoglobin dissociation curve A relationship between the partial pressure of oxygen in the blood and the saturation of hemoglobin with oxygen.

P

P wave Graphic representation of atrial depolarization.

Paget's mammary disease Uncommon skin cancer characterized by a chronic eczema-like rash of the nipple and adjacent areolar skin.

pain An unpleasant sensory and emotional experience arising from actual or potential tissue damage or described in terms of such damage.

pain scales scales used to quantify patient's pain so that consistent relief measures can be taken.

pain threshold The lowest intensity of a painful stimulus perceived by the individual as pain.

pain tolerance The degree of pain that an individual is willing to endure.

palliation The process of easing symptoms and maximizing quality of life when cure or control is not possible.

palliative care Active total care of patients whose disease is not responsive to curative treatment.

palpation The use of the sense of touch to assess texture, temperature, moisture, organ location and size, vibrations and pulsations, swelling, masses, and tenderness.

palpebrae Eyelids that cover and protect the eyes by covering the anterior aspect of the eyes.

panhypopituitarism Defective or absence of function of the entire pituitary gland.

papillary reflex Stimulation of cranial nerve II that causes direct and consensual reactions to light.

papilledema A swelling of the optic disc.

papules Elevated circumscribed lesions (elevated nevi, verrucae, molluscum contagiosum, and individual lesions of lichen planus).

paracentesis The aspiration of fluid from the abdominal cavity.

paraphimosis The entrapment of the retracted foreskin behind the glans penis of an uncircumcised male.

paraplegia Paralysis involving the lower extremities.

parathyroid hormone (PTH) Hormone that is secreted by the parathyroids and is not controlled by the pituitary and hypothalamus but by negative feedback.

parenchyma Functional elements of an organ.

paresthesia Numbness, tingling, or prickling sensation.

parity The number of viable births.

passive euthanasia Omission of an action, thereby allowing death to occur.

patient controlled analgesia (PCA) Devices that can be used by the patient to deliver pain medications (usually via intravenous [IV] route) as needed.

peak drug level Time it takes for the drug to reach its highest concentration in the blood.

pediculosis Infection by human lice.

pediculosis pubis Infection in pubic area by lice.

pedigrees Diagrammatic representations of a family history indicating the affected individuals and their relationship to proband or index case.

percent solution A measure of parts per hundred.

perception A person's sense and understanding of the world.

percussion Short tapping strokes on the surface of the skin to create vibrations of underlying organs.

percutaneous coronary interventions (PCI) Category of procedures performed during the cardiac angiography using catheters, balloons, and devices to treat atherosclerotic lesions (e.g., percutaneous transluminal coronary angioplasty [PTCA]).

perfusion The exchange of oxygen and carbon dioxide at the alveolar-capillary level.

pericarditis An inflammation of the pericardium.

pericardium A double-layered serous membrane that surrounds the heart.

periductal mastitis Inflammation of the breast that can occur in nonlactating older women.

perimenopause Five- to 10-year period before menopause.

perinephric Surrounding the kidney.

perioperative Inclusive term to denote preoperative, intraoperative, and postoperative periods.

periosteum The outer portion of the cortical bone that supplies nutrients and a blood supply to the bone.

peripheral vascular resistance (PVR) The pressure against the flow of blood to or from the arteries or veins outside the chest.

peristalsis Successive waves of involuntary contraction passing along the walls of a hollow muscular structure (as the esophagus or intestine) and forcing the contents onward.

petechiae Small, pinpoint hemorrhages.

phagocytosis Process by which foreign substances are ingested and destroyed.

Phalen's maneuver A physical test involving flexion of the fully extended hand at the wrist to aid in the diagnosis of carpal tunnel syndrome.

phantom limb sensation When the patient has the perception of a limb that is no longer there. If the patient feels pain it is known as phantom limb pain.

pharmaceutic Phase that an oral drug disintegrates and dissolves into a form that can be used by the body.

pharmacodynamics Phase that describes the biochemical and physiological effects the drug has on the body.

pharmacogenomics The study of how an individual's genetic inheritance affects the body's response to drugs.

pharmacokinetics Phase that describes how drugs are acted on in the body from ingestion to elimination, includes the processes of absorption, distribution, metabolism (biotransformation), and excretion.

pharmacology The scientific study of drugs and their origins, actions on, and interactions with, living things through chemical processes.

phenotype The physical, biochemical, and physiological nature of an individual as determined by the genotype and the environment. It is the outward expression of the individual's genes.

philosophy Statement of beliefs that is the foundation for one's thoughts and actions.

phimosis The inability of the foreskin to be stretched and retracted over the glans of the penis.

phlebitis Inflammation of a vein.

phlebostatic axis Location at the midpoint of the anterior and posterior chest at the fourth intercostal space. This is the point at which transducers should be leveled for hemodynamic parameters.

photoaging Degenerative changes in connective tissue caused by chronic exposure to ultraviolet A (UVA).

photoallergic Sensitivity to light that causes allergic reactions.

photochemotherapy UVA therapy combined with oral or topical 8-methoxypsoralen.

phototherapy The treatment of certain dermatological conditions with artificially produced, nonionizing UV light.

phototoxic Rapidly developing nonimmunologic skin reaction when exposed to light.

physical dependence Body is dependent on a substance and abrupt cessation or reduction in the dose may result in withdrawal symptoms.

physician-assisted suicide Medical hastening of death by a physician in consultation with a terminally ill patient.

phytonutrients Chemicals found in plants that act as protective or healing agents.

pica Craving for substances other than food, such as dirt, clay, starch, or ice cubes.

pigmentation Color of the skin (produced by melanocytes in the epidermis).

plaques Elevated disc-shaped lesions (psoriasis, lichen simplex or chronicus neurodermatitis).

plasma The liquid portion of the circulation system.

plasma half-life (t $_{1/2}$) The time required to eliminate one half of the ingested medication after administration.

plasmapheresis (plasma exchange) Plasma is removed from the patient and replaced with the fresh frozen plasma.

pleuritic chest pain Discomfort detected on expiration or inspiration caused by an inflammation of the lining of the lungs.

pneumothorax A collection of air in the pleural cavity may occur as a result of trauma, tuberculosis, or chronic respiratory diseases. This collection of air leads to a collapse of all or part of a lung.

polycystic cysts Cysts with closed sacs that develop abnormally within an organ and have a distinct enclosing membrane.

polycythemia An abnormal increase in the number of red blood cells.

polypharmacy Situation in which multiple drugs are prescribed to treat a variety of conditions.

positive end expiratory pressure (PEEP) A ventilator setting that adds pressure at the end of expiration to keep alveoli open and enable gas exchange.

posthitis Inflammation of the foreskin.

postoperative Takes the patient from the time of departing from the surgical suite through the length of their hospital stay and beyond.

postrenal Occurring after the kidney.

posttraumatic stress disorder (PTSD) A psychological reaction that occurs after experiencing a highly stressing event, such as wartime combat, physical violence, or a natural disaster.

Power of Attorney for Health Care Legal document that allows the patient to choose a person called a health care proxy or agent to make decisions about the patient's medical care when the patient is unable to do so for himself or herself.

PR interval An estimate of the amount of time it takes the impulse to travel from the SA node through the AV node, the bundle of His, and the main part of the left bundle branch.

prana The life force of the Indian culture that is believed to fill the body with a vital energy.

preferred provider organization (PPO) Type of managed care plan in which members receive more coverage if they choose health care providers approved by or affiliated with the plan.

preload The amount the myocardial fibers are stretched at the end of diastole. This stretch reflects the amount of pressure and volume in the ventricle immediately preceding systole.

preoperative Prior to the intraoperative period or events leading up to entry into the surgical suite.

preparedness Activities that build the hospital's capacity to manage the effects of an emergency or disaster.

prerenal Occurring prior to the kidney.

presbyopia A loss of near acuity (near vision) as the lens loses its elasticity and accommodation of the lens fails.

presbyphagia Dysphagia in the elderly.

prevalence The number of current cases of a disease in a specific population at a given time period.

preventive care Focuses on health promotion, including educational and preventive programs designed to promote healthy lifestyles.

priapism The presence of a prolonged, often painful, penile erection.

primary amenorrhea Failure of the menstrual cycles to begin.

primary anorgasmia Never having achieved orgasm.

primary brain tumor The growth originated in the brain or central nervous system.

primary care Basic, routine health care.

primary immune response Occurs when an antigen is initially introduced into the system. It involves both mast cell degranulation and activation of plasma proteins, i.e., complement, clotting factors, and kinin (polypeptides that increase blood flow and permeability of small blood capillaries).

primary intention Utilizes normal repair processes.

primary multiple organ dysfunction Directly related to an insult, such as a major trauma.

prions Protein-containing infectious agents.

process variables Refers to how care is provided, under what circumstances, and how patients are moved into, through, and out of the health care system.

proctocolectomy Surgical removal of the rectum together with part or all of the colon.

prodrome phase The beginning clinical manifestations that a person has for an upcoming illness.

prolactin A hormone from the anterior pituitary that stimulates the breast to cause lactation.

prophylactic Preventing or contributing to the prevention of disease.

proprioception Awareness and coordination of movement and position of the body, head, and limbs.

proptosis Forward placement of the eye.

prostatitis Inflammation of the prostate gland.

prosthesis A replacement of a missing body part, such as an extremity.

protein binding Process in which the drug, once absorbed into the bloodstream, attaches itself to a protein molecule (usually albumin) to be transported to it site of action.

proteinuria Increase in protein in the urine.

pruritus Dermatological symptom described as itching and a desire to scratch.

psoriasis T cell–mediated inflammatory disease characterized by epidermal hyperplasia (overproduction of epidermal tissue) usually localized in certain regions of the body.

psychomotor domain Area of learning that involves performance of motor skills.

psychoneuroimmunoendocrinology (PNIE) A multidisciplinary paradigm involving mind-body medicine that emerged in 1955, and is sometimes referred to as psychoneuroimmunology.

psychoneuroimmunology (PNI) An emerging field of science that studies the complex relationship between the mind and body, specifically the cognitive/affective system in the brain, the neurological system, and the immune system.

ptosis Drooping of the eyelid.

pulmonary artery (PA) catheter A long balloon-tipped catheter that is positioned in the pulmonary artery and monitors different pressures in the heart.

pulse pressure Difference between systolic and diastolic blood pressure.

pulsus alternans Alternating weak and strong heart beats.

pulsus paradoxus Pathological decrease in systolic blood pressure by 10 mm Hg or more on inspiration.

Purkinje fibers Conductive fibers that help to spread the electrical impulses of throughout the ventricular muscle. They have an inherent rate of 15 to 40 beats per minute.

purulent Containing the detritus of white blood cell activity within an infectious process usually.

purulent sputum A light green to yellowish white fluid formed in infected tissue and consists of white blood cells, cellular debris, and necrotic or dead tissue.

pustules Circumscribed elevations containing purulent exudates (pustular psoriasis, bromoderma or small pox).

pyelonephritis Infection of the ureters and kidney.

pyrosis A substernal burning sensation often radiating to the neck; commonly called heartburn.

Q

QRS complex Graphic representation of ventricular depolarization.

QT interval Graphic representation of the amount of time it takes for ventricular depolarization and repolarization.

quadriplegia (tetraplegia) Paralysis involving upper and lower extremities.

R

race A grouping of people based on biological similarities.

racism Form of oppression defined as discrimination directed toward individuals who are misperceived to be inferior because of biological differences.

radiculopathy A term used to specifically describe pain and other symptoms, like numbness, tingling, and weakness, in arms or legs that are caused by a problem with nerve roots.

radioisotope A compound that contains radioactive materials that are used in nuclear scans; the activity of these tagged materials allows the study of substances as they course through the body.

radiotherapy The use of X-rays and other forms of radiation in treatment.

Raynaud's disease Venous disease caused by unilateral vasospasm of the upper and lower extremities. Bilateral vasospasm is identified as Raynaud's disease, usually occurs in the age group over 30 and is equally distributed between genders.

rebound hypertension Rapid increase in blood pressure after abrupt stopping of medication.

receptive aphasia (Wernicke's aphasia) A condition in which a patient is unable to understand what is being said or what is written.

receptor Site on the cell membrane that can be occupied by a drug to cause an effect within the body.

recessive trait A trait that is expressed only when an individual is homozygous for that specific gene.

referred pain The transfer of visceral pain sensations and deep somatic pain via the autonomic nervous system to a body surface at a distance from the actual origin.

refractory ascites Ascites that cannot be effectively managed with normal therapies.

regeneration Replacement of damaged or lost tissue with more of the same tissue. Only the epidermis and superficial dermis are capable of regeneration.

relative hypovolemia A shifting of fluid from the intravascular space to the extravascular space that can result from a loss of intravascular integrity, increased capillary permeability, or a decreased colloidal osmotic pressure.

relaxation response A state of increased arousal of the parasympathetic nervous system, which leads to a relaxed physiological state.

remodeling A continuously occurring process in the bone that maintains the structure and integrity of the bone.

remote assessment Use of technology such as video links or teleconferencing to allow for health care personnel and patients to transmit assessment information over long distances.

renal Pertaining to the kidney.

renal parenchyma The cortex and medulla of the kidney that contain the functioning units and collecting ducts of the kidney.

repolarization Electrical change in the interior of an excitable cell following depolarization in which the inside of the cell becomes more negatively charged.

residual volume (RV) The amount remaining in the lungs and airways after a maximal expiration.

resilience Dynamic process that involves protective factors such as effective problem-solving strategies and adaptability to situations that the person cannot control or change.

resorption The removal of bone tissue by normal physiological process or as part of a pathological process, such as an infection.

resting energy expenditure A measurement of resting metabolic rate expressed as kilocalories per 24 hours.

restorative care Follow-up postoperative care, home care, and rehabilitation.

reticuloendothethial (RE) system Phagocytic system composed of monocytes and macrophages.

retroperitoneal space The space between the peritoneum (the membranous sac that surrounds the organs of the abdominal cavity) and the posterior abdominal wall that contains the kidneys and associated structures, the pancreas, part of the aorta, and inferior vena cava.

review of literature Less rigorous form of summary process used in nursing.

review of systems (ROS) A brief account from a patient of any recent signs of symptoms associated with any of the body systems.

rhabdomyolysis Destruction of skeletal muscle cells that causes the release of myoglobin.

rhinitis A seasonal or year-round immunoglobulin E (IgE)-mediated inflammation of the nasal mucosa; may be infectious, inflammatory, or allergic in nature.

rhinitis medicamentosa Rebound congestion of the nasal mucous membranes caused by overuse of decongestant nasal sprays.

rhinorrhea Thin, watery discharge from the nose.

rhonchi Bubbling or gurgling sounds heard primarily on expiration and indicate fluid in the larger airways.

RICE The acronym used for Rest, Ice, Compression, and Elevation when treating a sprain.

right to die Belief that humans have a basic right to die.

rights-based ethics Proscribes that there are specific human rights to specific human goods.

rigors A muscular tremor caused by a chill.

rotator cuff tears Refers to tears in one or more of the four muscles that form a single tendon in the shoulder. The rotator cuff is responsible for circumduction and internal and external rotation of the shoulder.

rye ergot A fungus from the rye plant causing hallucinations, gastrointestinal upset, and a form of gangrene if ingested.

S

SA node Primary pacemaker of the heart with an inherent rate of 60 to 100 beats per minute.

sacroilitis Inflammation of the sacroiliac joint.

sarcoma A form of cancer that arises in the supportive tissues such as bone, cartilage, fat, or muscle.

sarcomere The contractile unit of the muscle.

sarcopenia Age-related decreases in muscle mass.

schistocytes Fragmented red blood cells.

Schwartze's sign Rosy or reddish-blue color of the tympanic membrane related to vascular changes.

science The most reliable source of knowledge on which to base clinical decisions.

science of research synthesis Field of science that generates evidence summaries to provide state-of-the-science conclusions about knowledge thus far developed.

scoliometer An instrument for measuring curves, especially those in lateral curvature of the spine.

scoliosis An abnormal lateral curvature of the spine.

secondary amenorrhea Cessation of the menstrual cycles after they are established in the absence of pregnancy.

secondary anorgasmia Loss of the ability to achieve orgasm in a woman who was previously orgasmic.

secondary intention Heals by spread of granulation.

secondary multiple organ dysfunction The result of failure of organs that were not affected by the initial insult.

secondary or specific antibody response Includes the activation of B cells and the memory cells (IgG, IgM, IgA, and IgE); and activation of T cells, cytotoxic (killer) cells, lymphokine-producing cells, helper cells, and suppressor cells.

sedation Reduction of anxiety, stress, irritability, or excitement by the administration of a sedative agent or drug.

seizure Brief episode of abnormal electrical activity in the brain.

self-efficacy Perceived capability of mastering difficult situations and the ability to actively control one's own destiny; closely linked to a positive self-esteem and internal locus of control.

self-monitoring of blood glucose (SMBG) A method whereby a patient tests his or her own blood glucose levels.

semipermeable membranes Separation between two areas that allows movement of some fluids or solutes.

sepsis A systemic inflammatory response to an infection.

sequela Any abnormality following or resulting from a disease or injury or treatment.

serum The liquid part of blood after coagulation.

serum sickness A type III hypersensitivity reaction that results from the injection of heterologous or foreign protein or serum.

sex roles Culturally determined patterns associated with being male or female.

sexual dysfunction Unsatisfactory enjoyment of sex or inability to participate in sexual intimacy as desired because of multiple causes, including lack of sexual interest, impaired sexual arousal (erectile dysfunction in the male, lack of lubrication in the female), or inability to achieve orgasm.

sexuality Human characteristic that refers not just to gender but to all the aspects of being male or female, including feelings, attitudes, beliefs, and behavior.

shaman A folk healer priest who uses natural and supernatural forces to heal others, has an extensive knowledge of herbs, is skilled in many forms of healing, and serves as guardian of the spirits.

shamanism A form of spiritual healing that refers to the practice of entering altered states of consciousness with the intent of helping others to enhance healing and well-being. The shaman connects with spiritual guides and seeks healing on behalf of others.

shock syndrome A systemic condition when the peripheral blood flow is inadequate to provide sufficient blood to the heart for normal function and transport of oxygen to all organs and tissues.

short stay surgery Usually preplanned, nonemergency procedures with an expected hospital or surgical center stay of less than 23 hours.

shunting That portion of the cardiac output that does not exchange with alveolar air.

side effects Expected physiological effects of a drug that are not related to the desired drug effect.

sinusoids Specialized capillaries found only in the liver and are identified by specific types of cells.

slow pain Pain originating in the endings of the smaller unmyelinated nerves that has a throbbing or aching quality.

social support The person's perception of, and the degree of satisfaction with, support systems.

solutes Particles contained within the fluid that contribute to the concentration or osmolality of the fluid.

somatic (parietal) pain Pain that originates from the bone, joints, muscles, skin, or connective tissue. Sharp or knife-like in character, usually precisely located to the affected areas.

somesthesia Awareness of body; derived from the Greek words meaning body and sensation.

somnolence Prolonged drowsiness or sleepiness.

spermatocelectomy Surgical removal of the spermatocele.

spermatogenesis Formation of mature functional spermatozoa from the testes, usually beginning during puberty and continuing throughout the life of the adult male.

spinal shock A loss of all motor and sensory function, generally occurring after spinal cord injury.

spirituality Relationship with one's self, a sense of connection with others, and a relationship with a higher power or divine source.

sports medicine The application of professional knowledge to the understanding, prevention, treatment, and rehabilitation of sports- and exercise-related problems.

staging The extent or spread of the tumor within the body from the site of origin.

standard precautions Actions to be used with all patients to reduce risk of transmission of disease.

stapedectomy Removal of the stapes and replacing the stapes with a prosthetic device.

state-of-the-science review Less rigorous form of summary process used in nursing.

status asthmaticus Severe and persistent asthma that does not respond to conventional therapy and that may lead to respiratory failure.

steatorrhea Pale-yellow, greasy, fatty stool, or chronic watery diarrhea.

stereognosis Identify objects by touch.

stereotactic radiotherapy (SRS) Noninvasive use of computers and radiation to target tumor cells within the brain.

stereotyping Expectation that all people within the same racial, ethnic, or cultural group act alike and share the same beliefs and attitudes.

stomatitis The inflammation of the soft tissues in the mouth resulting in mouth sores. It is a common side effect of chemotherapy, radiation therapy, and some biological therapy.

strabismus (tropia) When one muscle is weak resulting in one eye deviating from the other when the eyes are focused on an object.

stress The body's reaction to any stimulus.

stridor Inspiratory wheezing.

structural variables Organizational features or participant characteristics that have an impact on organizational performance.

stye (hordeolum) A localized inflammatory swelling of one or more of the glands of the eyelid.

subarachnoid hemorrhage Blood that leaks into the subarachnoid space.

subclavian steal syndrome Occurs when the subclavian artery is occluded, and blood flow is diminished or obstructed to the upper extremities.

subculture Group of people within the dominant group who are functionally unified by factors, such as status, ethnic background, residence, religion, or education and whose experiences differ from those of the dominant group.

subjective data Data from the patient's point of view that may include feelings, perceptions, and concerns.

superficial burn Also called a first-degree burn; it only involves the epidural layer of the skin.

superficial partial-thickness burn Also called a second-degree burn; it involves the entire epidermis and the upper third of the dermis.

supernumerary nipples Small dark spots on the chest that may indicate undeveloped nipples and areola.

suppurative cholangitis A condition when pus is produced in the biliary tract.

surrogate decision maker Agent or proxy who is legally able to make health care decisions for another who has lost the capacity to do so for himself or herself.

sycosis Inflammation of the entire hair follicle.

sycosis barbae Inflammation of the entire hair follicle that is traumatized by shaving.

synchronized cardioversion Delivering an electrical shock to the heart that is synchronized to the patient's R wave.

synchronized intermittent mandatory ventilation (SIMV) The ventilator delivers preset breaths in coordination with the respiratory effort of the patient. Spontaneous breathing is allowed between breaths.

syndrome X Classic angina symptoms without angiographic evidence of CAD.

syndrome X (insulin resistance syndrome) A group of abnormalities of metabolism that act together to increase the risk of cardiovascular disease.

synergy model Combination of factors that each multiplies the effects of the other(s), rather than merely adding to them.

syngeneic transplant Blood or tissue donated by an identical twin.

synovium A fibrous envelope that produces a fluid to help to reduce friction and wear in a joint.

system Set of parts linked in orderly and logical interdependence that function together as a synergistic unit.

systematic review Newer term for an evidence summary.

systemic inflammatory response syndrome (SIRS) Widespread uncontrolled acute inflammatory response to a severe insult.

systolic blood pressure Blood pressure measured at the moment of contraction.

T

T wave Graphic representation of ventricular repolarization.

tachypnea An abnormally rapid rate of breathing.

Tao Traditional spiritual belief system of the Chinese. The belief that everything is the Tao, and the Tao is everything leads to the understanding of oneness in all things in nature.

target tissues Tissues or organs in the body that are affected by specific hormones.

teaching Active process in which one individual shares information with another as a means to facilitate behavioral changes.

teaching-learning process Planned interaction that promotes a behavioral change that is not a result of maturation or coincidence.

teaching strategies Techniques employed by the teacher to promote learning.

telangiectasia Dilatation of small blood vessels on the cheeks, nose, and ears, as well as pigmental changes, such as freckles from exposure to sun light.

teleology Evaluation of final causes.

tendons Connect muscle to bone and allow bone to move once the muscle has contracted.

tendosynovial Pertaining to the tendon insertion in the joint near the synovial membrane.

tenesmus Distressing but ineffectual urge to evacuate the rectum.

teratogens Agents that produces or increases the incidence of congenital malformations.

terminal illness One in which there is no possibility for a cure, resulting in the decline of the patient's physical condition and then death.

tertiary care Includes acute and complex interventions.

tertiary intention Wound requires suturing of granulation layers.

testicular self-examination (TSE) A method of a male assessing his testicles for any changes as a preventive measure against testicular cancer.

thenar Refers to the palm of the hand or the sole of the foot.

therapeutic range Serum drug level that lies between the minimum effective concentration and the toxic concentration. Level to be maintained to achieve desired affects and avoid symptoms of toxicity.

therapeutic touch (TT) Assessing alterations in a person's energy field and using a hand to direct energy to achieve a balanced energy state.

thermoregulation A patient's status in relation to internal temperature control.

third spacing The accumulation of fluid in the extracellular and intracellular spaces and in a third body, such as the intestine, that does not support circulation.

thrombophlebitis The inflammation of a vein accompanied by the formation of thrombus (blood clot), which can be dislodged and lead to pulmonary emboli. Deep vein thrombosis (DVT) is a term often used for this venous complication, which most commonly occurs in the deep veins of the lower extremities.

thrombus Blood clot that blocks a blood vessel.

thyroid-releasing hormone (TRH) The hormone that stimulates the anterior pituitary to release TSH.

thyroid-stimulating hormone (TSH) A hormone produced from the anterior pituitary that regulates the function of the thyroid.

thyroxine (T_4) The most abundant thyroid hormone; makes up approximately 90 percent of the thyroid hormone secretion.

tic douloureux Trigeminal neuralgia; dysfunction causing pain along the pathway of the fifth cranial nerve.

tidal volume (Vt) The amount of air in and out of the lungs with a normal breath.

tineas Fungal infections.

Tinel's sign A tingling sensation produced by pressing on or tapping the nerve that has been damaged or is regenerating following trauma.

tinnitus A ringing, buzzing, or jingling sound in the ear.

tolerance Occurs when a higher dose of a drug (e.g., an opioid) is required to achieve the desired effect.

tophus A chalky deposit of sodium urate occurring in gout, tophi forms most often around joints in cartilage, bone, bursae, and subcutaneous tissue and in the external ear, producing a chronic foreign body inflammatory response.

total parenteral nutrition (TPN) The intravenous (IV) administration of nutrients to patients through a central venous catheter.

total quality management (TQM) Structured systematic process for organizational planning and implementation of CQI.

toxoid A toxin that has had the active portion removed but can still be recognized by the immune system.

trabecular The porous cavity found inside the compact bone.

tracheostomy Operation of cutting into the trachea usually for insertion of a tube to overcome tracheal obstruction.

tracheostomy tube A tube placed by surgical incision into the trachea and secured by sutures to maintain an open airway or facilitate long-term mechanical ventilation.

transcellular fluid Fluid that is in neither the intracellular nor extracellular space, and includes cerebrospinal fluid, joint fluid, and the fluid within the gastrointestinal tract.

transduction The initiation of the pain stimulus.

transient ischemic attack (TIA) Temporary loss of blood flow to the brain that results in temporary loss of function.

translocation The transfer of a segment of one chromosome to a nonhomologous chromosome. When no material is lost or gained, the translocation is said to be balanced.

transmission The process of carrying the pain information along the axon of a sensory nerve to the CNS.

transmission routes Ways by which microorganisms reach the body.

tremor Rhythmic, purposeless, quivering muscle movement.

trends The general direction or prevailing tendency in following a general course.

triage system A method to rank or classify patient's illnesses or severity of injury.

triggers Cause the release of inflammatory mediators from the bronchial mast cells, macrophages, and epithelial cells and lead to recurrent episodes of wheezing, breathlessness, chest tightness, and coughing.

triiodothyronine (T_3) The most powerful thyroid hormone; 10 percent secreted by thyroid and the remainder converted from T_4 by peripheral tissues.

trisomies Three of a given chromosome instead of the usual pair.

trocar A large-bore abdominal paracentesis needle.

trough drug level Minimum blood serum level of a drug reached immediately before the next scheduled dose.

tubercles Nodules or swelling of lymphocytes and epithelioid cells that forms the lesions seen in tuberculosis.

tumor markers Substances that are expressed by the tumor or by normal tissue in response to a tumor.

tumor necrosis factor Inflammatory biochemical that is produced in response to various stressors.

tumor suppressor gene A gene that can block or suppress the development of cancer.

tumors Larger and deeper circumscribed solid lesions; they can be benign or malignant.

turgor The skin's elasticity, resilience, and hydration.

tympanometry A test performed to detect abnormalities in the middle ear, such as fluid, eustachian tube dysfunction, or problems with the ossicles.

tympanosclerosis Formation of fibrous tissue around the ossicles preventing vibratory movement.

U

upper motor neuron The descending motor pathway, which originates in the brain and synapse with lower motor neurons in the spinal cord.

uremia Accumulation of end-products of protein metabolism in the bloodstream due to renal failure.

ureteral strictures A narrowing of the lumen of the ureter.

urethral strictures A narrowing of the lumen of the urethra.

urethritis Inflammation of the urethra.

urethroplasty A procedure that removes the diseased portion of the urethra and inserts a new urethra constructed from other tissue.

urethrotomy An opening in the urethra.

urinary tract infection (UTI) An infection involving the kidneys, ureters, bladder, or urethra.

urolithiasis (calculi) Refers to stones in the urinary tract.

urticaria A hypersensitive dermatological manifestation in response to the release of histamine in an antigen-antibody reaction.

utilitarian Belief that an action should be of benefit to the greatest number of people affected by the action.

V

vaginitis Inflammation of the vagina.

valgus Bending or twisting outward from the midline of the body.

valvular regurgitation Backward flow of blood through a heart valve.

valvular stenosis A narrowing or constriction of the diameter of a bodily passage or orifice.

valvuloplasty Plastic surgery performed to repair a valve in the body.

varicocele A group of varicose veins within the scrotum.

varicocelectomy Surgical removal of the varicocele.

varicose veins Tortuous varicosities, in which the veins are dilated and lack surrounding muscle support.

varus Bending or twisting inward toward the midline of the body.

vasectomy Surgical sterilization of men through removal, ligation, or destruction of a small portion of the vas deferens to prevent passage of sperm to the urethra.

vector-borne transmission Infectious material carried by living organism tissue from base of wound.

venous stasis ulcers Erosions of the skin because of lack of blood flow to the extremity, which leads to skin necrosis, open wounds, and black, hardened skin known as eschar.

ventilation The movement of air in and out of the lungs.

ventilator weaning The gradual withdrawal of ventilatory support.

ventricular assist device (VAD) A mechanical device designed to eliminate the workload on the left ventricle, right ventricle, or both and is designed for long-term therapy unlike the intra-aortic balloon pump.

vertigo A sensation or feeling of a loss of equilibrium, sometimes referred to as spinning or whirling.

vesicant An intravenous (IV) medication that causes blisters and tissue injury when it escapes into surrounding tissue. Vesicatory refers to causing blisters.

vesicles Sharply circumscribed, elevated fluid-containing vesicle lesions (herpes, dyshidrosis, pompholyx, varicella, or contact dermatitis).

vesicoureteral reflux Backward propulsion of urine through the valve that normally closes the bladder and ureteral junction to backward flow of urine.

vesicular rash A raised, blistering rash.

visceral pain Pain that originates from any of the large interior organs that occupy a body cavity (cranial, thoracic, abdominal, or pelvic).

visual learners Style of learning in which people learn by processing information by seeing.

vital capacity (VC) The volume of air in and out of the lungs with maximal inspiratory effort and maximal expiratory effort.

volume control ventilation Delivers breaths at a preset target volume.

volvulus A twisting of the intestine on itself that causes obstruction.

W

wellness care Care focused on prevention of illness and promotion of health.

wheals Solid superficial elevations usually in response to pruritus conditions (insect bites, urticaria, or allergic reactions).

wheezes Musical sounds heard primarily on expiration and indicate narrowing of the larger airways, with either spasm or secretions.

wheezing A whistling sound when breathing out related to airway constriction.

workforce diversity Differences in attributes or belief system among members of the workforce.

X

xanthelasma A yellow, lipid-rich plaque present on the eyelids.

xenogeneic A genetic relationship between individuals of differing species.

xerosis Abnormal dryness of skin, mucous membranes, or conjunctiva.

xerostomia Dry mouth.

Z

zone of coagulation Area of the burn that has the most contact with the causative agent, causing coagulated cellular necrosis.

zone of hyperemia Area peripheral to the zone of stasis characterized by viable cells with minimal injury.

zone of stasis Area peripheral to the zone of coagulation characterized by injured viable cells with compromised blood flow.

zoophilic Animal source.

Review Questions Answers

Chapter 1

1. 3. Rationale: Historically, nurses provided comfort care. As knowledge expanded nurses took on aspects of illness care directed by physicians. Nurses then focused on wellness care as their own practice. Care directed at either illness or wellness is known as health care. Nurses now seek to provide evidence-based care.
2. 4. Rationale: As the body of scientific knowledge grew, no single physician could know all there was to know about all illnesses. Specialty practices emerged, fractionating care and the traditional close physician-patient relationship.
3. 1. Rationale: An increasing amount of legislation is regulating health care.
4. 3. Rationale: The Medicare and Medicaid amendments to the Social Security Act initiated the era of health care reform.
5. 2. Rationale: Scholarly publication is an expectation, but is not an *essential* feature of professional nursing as defined by American Nurses Associations.
6. 1. Rationale: Poultices are no longer commonly used, and the other options are bogus.
7. 4. Rationale: Food preparation, biomedical engineering, faith healing, and meditation are not required areas of knowledge or skill for nurses.
8. 2. Rationale: 1, 3, and 4 are bogus answers.
9. 3. Rationale: Although there is some evidence that fresh flowers may harbor undesirable organisms, there is currently no ban on them.
10. 3. Rationale: Blackouts related to chemical dependence are varying lengths of time when an intoxicated individual interacts with others without later memory of the interactions.

Chapter 2

1. 4. Rationale: The most reliable source of knowledge on which to base clinical decisions is state-of-the-science knowledge from integrated rigorous research.
2. 2. Rationale: The Knowledge Hurdles and Solutions matrix articulated by Stevens rates the volume and complexity of science and technology as a primary hurdle to overcome to move research into practice.
3. 4. Rationale: The primary premise underlying knowledge transformation is that such transformation is necessary before research results are useable in clinical decision making.
4. 3. Rationale: A major feature of EBP is that it is heavily interdisciplinary.
5. 3. Rationale: All of the other Web sites are bogus.
6. 4. Rationale: The ACE Star Model developed by Stevens depicts knowledge transformation through five sequential steps.
7. 2. Rationale: In 2001 Glasziou, Irwig, Bain, & Colditz articulated the six essential steps in conducting a systematic review: (a) formulate the question, (b) locate relevant studies, (c) select and appraise the studies, (d) summarize and synthesize the results across studies, (e) interpret the findings, and (f) update the review regularly.
8. 1. Rationale: Using evidence in our care increases certainty and predictability in the effect of the practice on the outcome of that practice. There are a growing number of evidence summaries available to effect transformation of evidence into use for clinical decision making by practitioners across multiple disciplines and multiple levels of practice. It is predicted that the public will soon demand that care not only be more error aversive, but that it be evidence-based.
9. 3. Rationale: While all of the answers are desirable changes in health care delivery, in 2001 the Institute of Medicine identified 20 priority areas for quality improvement according to three criteria. The number two criterion was improvability by using evidence to close gaps between best practice and usual care.

10. 1. Rationale: While the other concepts reflect the essence of the applied science of nursing, those concepts lack the essential aspects needed to make the transformation of research into practice a widespread reality.

Chapter 3

1. 2. Rationale: A learning plateau is a peak in the effectiveness of the teaching process.
2. 3. Rationale: The cognitive domain describes learning by understanding the material that is presented with the mind.
3. 4. Rationale: When the nurse allows the patient with diabetes to give an injection to a synthetic material that is similar to a real arm it is labeled a demonstration.
4. 3. Rationale: Kinesthetic learning takes place a person can physically do something.
5. 1. Rationale: Self-efficacy is when a person believes that his or her actions ("puts her mind to it") will have the desired effect.
6. 3. Rationale: Repetition is the best strategy in teaching new information for the memory impaired.
7. 2. Rationale: A lack of perception is experienced when a person does not accept the factual information regarding his or her health practices (in this instance).
8. 3. Rationale: Two basic components of health maintenance are health promotion and disease prevention.
9. 3. Rationale: Imposing a health policy that an individual must follow is not a health promotion strategy.
10. 3. Rationale: Basic human needs are the psychological dimension made up of those characteristics of self-esteem, feelings of security, and those feelings that create a sense of belonging.

Chapter 4

1. 4. Rationale: All of the elements of cultural competency result in incorporating cultural preferences into nursing practice.
2. 4. Rationale: Ethnocentrism is the belief that one's own culture is superior to all others.
3. 2. Rationale: Cultural assessment tools include assessing the family structure, traditional preferences, and medical context, all parts of the cultural assessment tool.
4. 3. Rationale: Poverty status is highly correlated with health risk factors.
5. 2. Rationale: Culture refers to the knowledge, beliefs, behaviors, ideas, attitudes, values, habits, customs, languages, symbols, rituals, ceremonies, and practices that are unique to a particular group of people.
6. 1. Rationale: All ethnic groups have shown an increase in numbers for several decades and will continue to do so.
7. 2. Rationale: Biological differences, (differences in enzymes and genetics) increase the potential for certain diseases, interactions with medications, foods (e.g., lactose intolerance).
8. 4. Rationale: Extrinsic distortion occurs when the interpreter is improperly prepared.
9. 4. Rationale: Racism is defined as a form of oppression or discrimination of people perceived as inferior.
10. 1. Rationale: A magicoreligious belief system is based on the concept that health and illness are determined by supernatural forces.

Chapter 5

1. 4. Rationale: The principle of beneficence requires that a clinical intervention benefits a patient, (e.g., in some way adds value to that patient's health).
2. 2. Rationale: Utilitarian is identified as the ethical theory that supports the "greatest good for the greatest number." This is the philosophy of giving levodopa to this patient with Parkinson's disease.
3. 2. Rationale: Professional codes of ethics focus on behavior between care providers and patients, as well as between care providers themselves. The codes seek behavior that is respectful and protects others from both external and internal harm secondary to one's behavior.
4. 1. Rationale: Moral distress in nursing occurs when the nurse is aware of the right and moral action to take in a given patient situation but is unable to carry out that action because of external restrictions.
5. 4. Rationale: This law protects patients' basic rights to privacy and their control over the disclosure of their personal health information.
6. 4. Rationale: The mother is focused on the quality of life of her child and has weighed that against medical treatments or interventions for her child.
7. 3. Rationale: The principle of double effect occurs when the intended use of palliative pain therapy has the unintended effect of hastening a person's death.
8. 5. Rationale: Advance directives for health care may be either written documents, such as a living will and durable power of attorney, or a verbal statement of preference for what a person wants done and when it is to be done.

9. 1. Rationale: The Nuremberg Code grew out of the revelations of research atrocities carried out by Nazi physicians on prisoners of war during World War II. The war ended in 1945, and the trials of war criminals followed soon after.

10. 2. Rationale: If a person has the mental capacity to make specific decisions about his or her health care, he or she is autonomous to do so, and health care providers must honor such decisions even though they may not personally or professionally agree with those decisions.

Chapter 6

1. 3. Rationale: Older adults usually underreport their symptoms. Everyone over 65 does not necessarily have two chronic health problems; not all older adults have diabetes.

2. 2 and 3. Rationale: Obesity is not primarily due to overeating; current trends indicate that obesity rates are climbing for all age-groups.

3. 1. Rationale: Smoking has been linked to persons of lower levels of education and social economic status. Smoking has actually decreased for pregnant women.

4. 1. Rationale: Most persons who attempt or commit suicide have been seen by a nonmental health care professional; symptoms are not easy to recognize, because the symptoms vary a great deal; the primary reason for suicide ideation is loss of something meaningful in the person's life, such as loss of relationship, a job, death of a loved one, and posttraumatic stress disorders.

5. 2. Rationale: The population of older women will continue to surpass the number of older men, although longevity has increased for both genders; a majority of the frail elderly will be cared for at home by family caregivers; older Hispanic (Americans) will be the largest racial/ethnic group by 2030.

6. 4. Rationale: The syndrome is related to abdominal obesity, hypertension, high triglyceride and low high-density lipoprotein (HDL) cholesterol levels, and high fasting blood glucose levels; the risk can be present at all age levels; The syndrome can contribute to coronary artery disease (CAD).

7. 2. Rationale: The other racial/ethnic groups may be at risk for hypertension, but the incidences are higher for African Americans, especially males.

8. 3. Rationale: None of the other statements ensure that safe measures will be taken. Selecting someone to perform cosmetic procedures on the basis of cost can be disastrous. Cosmetic procedures should be performed by qualified professionals (health care providers) certified by a national organization.

9. 2 and 3. Rationale: The goal is for a 50 to 75 percent of excess weight over a period of time; bariatric surgery is performed for a select group of people who meet the criteria that includes a comprehensive medical, psychological, nutritional, and surgical evaluation by a multidisciplinary team.

10. 1. Rationale: Life expectancy has increased for both genders and will continue to do so as the baby boomer generation ages. These individuals are more active and have the benefit of health promotion programs through their young and middle adult years. Women still live longer than men; the median income of older adults falls between $11,400 for females and $19,400 for males. Over 3.6 million older adults live below the poverty level, and Medicare benefits may decrease in the future.

Chapter 7

1. 4. Rationale: A tenet of hospice and palliative care is that the values and morals of the patients and families determine the best courses of action.

2. 2. Rationale: A component of therapeutic communication is an acknowledgement of difficulties faced by patients and caregivers. It is inappropriate to assume full knowledge of another person's feelings. Many individuals do not have a belief in heaven. There is no specific timeline for grief to be resolved.

3. 3. Rationale: Dyspnea is a subjective symptom best evaluated by the patient's description of the difficulty breathing.

4. 2. Rationale: A change in the breathing pattern is the universal sign of imminent death.

5. 4. Rationale: Fixed, dilated pupils are the most reliable sign of death.

6. 3. Rationale: Hospice care is indicated when the patient has a disease that is not responsive to curative treatments.

7. 1, 2, and 3. Rationale: The patient can receive hospice and palliative care services if he or she is in the hospice or home setting.

8. 1, 2, and 4. Rationale: Values and behaviors may vary among members of a given group.

9. 1, 2, 3, 4, and 5. Rationale: All listed are integral members of the team.

10. Power of Attorney for Health Care. Rationale: Advanced Directives include two documents: the Living Will and the Power of Attorney for Health Care. The Living Will provides written evidence of the patient's wishes regarding life-sustaining procedures. The Power of Attorney for Health Care allows the patient to choose an agent to make decisions about medical care when the patient is unable to do so.

Chapter 8

1. 4. Rationale: Because it is the critical nature of potential suicide.
2. 1. Rationale: There is no reason to have the patient in a patient gown to evaluate mental status.
3. 3. Rationale: Relieving the headache is an alleviating factor.
4. 2. Rationale: The patient's statement evidences this symptom as the primary reason for seeking health care.
5. 2. Rationale: The question defines an ecomap.
6. 3. Rationale: This is the best response given and is a valid nursing intervention for a spiritual problem.
7. 2. Rationale: This is the label for the definition provided in the question.
8. 4. Rationale: The elevator is not legally appropriate.
9. 1. Rationale: This test is designed for evaluating comatose patients.
10. 2. Rationale: This is the correct order for assessment.
11. 4. Rationale: This variable is the only one that can be altered.

Chapter 9

1. 1, 4; Rationale: Cri-du-chat syndrome and Down syndrome are conditions that are caused by the involvement of an entire chromosome. Neural tube defects are considered to be multifactorial, because they occur as a result of genetic and environmental factors. Sickle cell disease and achondroplasia are caused by because a defect of a single gene so they are considered to be unifactorial.
2. 3. Rationale: Answer 1 is the definition for mutation; answer 2 is the definition for phenotype; and answer 4 is the definition for karyotype.
3. 2. Rationale: Haploid refers to having one complete set of unpaired chromosomes. The haploid number in humans is 23.
4. 3. Rationale: In autosomal recessive inheritance, each parent carries a gene alteration for the condition, such as CF. Each child of those parents has a 25 percent chance to inherit the altered gene from both parents and will have manifestations of the condition.
5. 2. Rationale: An isolated neural tube defect usually occurs as a result of genetic and environmental factors and so is multifactorial in origin.
6. 3. Rationale: Genetic testing of children is indicated to make a diagnosis for conditions in which early intervention and treatment can be initiated. This is the case for Down syndrome. Being a carrier of a gene for CF does not pose a health risk to a child so is not indicated. HD is an adult-onset disorder for which there is currently no available treatment. Testing for HD is not indicated in children, until they have reached the age of 18 when such testing can be offered if risk exists.
7. 4. Rationale: Amniocentesis and CVS are prenatal diagnostic procedures. The prenatal AFP multiple marker testing is a genetic screening test to identify pregnancies at increased risk for neural tube defects and chromosomal abnormalities. Ultrasound evaluation is used to screen a pregnancy for major congenital malformations.
8. 4. Rationale: Nurses have a role in all of these activities: identifying individuals for whom genetic testing is available; referring individuals for genetic testing; and assessing the impact of genetic test results on the individual and the family.
9. 1. Rationale: BRCA1 and 2 are markers for hereditary breast and ovarian cancer not an indication of hypersensitivity to allergens. Phagocytes, eosinophils, and basophils are terms associated with white blood cells but they are not indicators of the immune system.
10. 2. Rationale: Both heredity and environmental triggers play a role in the development and expression of allergies and asthma making it a complex multifactorial disorder not a single gene disorder.

Chapter 10

1. 1. Rationale: Her behavioral response to her altered body image will be influenced by the reactions of others. There is not sufficient information in the case scenario to assume that 2, 3, or 4 is true.
2. 4. Rationale: She may be accepting the outcome as a result of fate or because external circumstances. 1, 2, and 3 are incorrect; (1) there is no indication that she is repressing her anxiety, (2) she has misinterpreted information, or (3) that she is depressed.
3. 3. Rationale: 1, 2, and 4 are incorrect. (1) Fear and depression are common reactions following discovery of a breast lump. (2) Many husbands do have problems adjusting to their wife's altered body image. (4) Married women do not have less difficulty adjusting than single women.
4. 4. Rationale: This is a major principle of self-care management. 1, 2, and 3 are incorrect. (1) Physical activity prior to bedtime does not help

to induce sleep. (2) Mild antianxiety medications can be a temporary solution that do not help to alleviate the underlying response to stress. (3) Informing the patient about hospital routines may facilitate the patient's feeling of losing control.

5. 2. Rationale: Gaining additional information will help to clarify how Jane feels and what coping mechanisms she has used to adapt to the loss of her mother and to adapt to a new manner of life. The nurse can assist Jane to make healthy decisions. 1, 3, and 4 are incorrect. (1) There is nothing to indicate that Jane is angry. (3) Asking Jane how the nurse can help her does not help Jane to search for her own inner strengths and support systems that can lead to self-care management of her life. (4) Stating that you understand how the other person feels is not totally truthful. Each person's perception of reality is unique. This is a response that can limit further expression or discussion of the person's grieving process.

6. 3. Rationale: Denial is a temporary ego defense mechanism used to protect the person from the full impact of the stressful situation/diagnosis. 1, 2, and 4 are incorrect. (1) Fantasy is an internal visualization of memories and their interpretation. (2) Undoing is an action taken to un do or to neutralize an original action. (4) Rationalization is selecting a substitute reason for the real reasons for personal behavior.

7. 4. Rationale: (1) Mr. Aiken does not have a realistic perception of his problem. (2) His perception and manner of coping are not pathological. His behavior is one of free choice. (3) He is not making a conscious secondary appraisal of the situation.

8. 2. Rationale: Rivalry with siblings is a typical behavior that occurs in normal family dynamics. Bobbie may even compete with his siblings for additional attention from his mother. (1) A drop in scholastic grades, (3) disturbance in relations with peers, and (4) a feeling of loss of personal internal control over the family situation are common responses to a stressful disintegration of the family structure.

9. 4. Rationale: (1) People often use the excuse that smoking makes them feel better for not quitting, because the initial response to nicotine is bronchodilation. (2) Refusal to quit is another frequent excuse because of the fear associated with the grieving process over loss of a pleasurable habit. (3) Denial of the severity of his condition is, also, an attempt to retain control over his life situation.

10. 3. Rationale: (1) There have been three health care revolutions over the past 30 years. (2) The current health care system is focused on illness, rather than wellness. (4) Web-based information continues to face scrutiny as to its accuracy and validity.

Chapter 11

1. 2. Rationale: Neutrophils are the first leukocytes attracted to an injured tissue.

2. 2. Rationale: This is the correct order for these events in an inflammatory response.

3. 1. Rationale: The classic sign of swelling seen in the inflammatory process results from leakage of plasma into the injured area.

4. 2. Rationale: This is the most likely cause of fever that is seen in a patient with an infectious disease.

5. 2. Rationale: Chronic inflammation is not caused by a response to a normal body substance such as low density lipoprotein lodged in excess in an arteriole wall.

6. 3. Rationale: This is a nursing teaching strategy to reduce the development of an antibiotic resistant organism.

7. 2. Rationale: A patient with a known infection must be managed by using standard precautions.

8. 4. Rationale: This is not a risk factor for delayed wound healing.

9. 3. Rationale: This fills the wound in healing by primary intention.

10. 1. Rationale: The steroid drug impedes macrophage migration, which delays wound healing if a person has been taking a steroid drug.

11. 3. Rationale: Rest and immobilization are important to wound healing because they prevent further injury to area.

Chapter 12

1. 3. Rationale: Swelling and weight gain are signs of fluid volume excess. Although the child may need increased diaper changes because of diarrhea, those are not a sign of fluid volume deficit. Depressed fontanelles occur in young children with fluid volume deficit.

2. 2. Rationale: Although all of these patients might experience fluid volume deficit, the most at risk are patients at the extreme of age, either young or old; in this case the 82-year-old patient.

3. 2. Rationale: Mental status is rarely affected in a fluid excess without a change in osmolality. Postural vital signs are most important in patients with fluid volume deficit. Urine output may be increased or decreased, depending on the cause of the fluid excess. Weight is an important indicator of fluid balance.

4. 1. Rationale: Patients with hyponatremia are at high risk for seizures. Vital sign assessment is important, but patient safety takes priority. Frequent oral care would be important in a patient with hypernatremia or fluid volume deficit. Cardiac monitoring is important in hyperkalemia or hypokalemia.

5. 2. Rationale: D_5W is a hypotonic intravenous (IV) solution. While administration of large volumes of any IV solution may result in fluid volume excess, a hypotonic IV solution also places the patient specifically at risk for hyponatremia. Fluid volume deficit is not a risk of IV fluid administration.

6. 4. Rationale: Weighing the patient and measuring edema are important interventions in patients with fluid volume excess. However, the priority intervention is to reduce the cause of the excess, in this case, the IV fluid. Capillary refill is an important assessment but is not specific for assessing fluid balance.

7. 4. Rationale: The major risk associated with a low potassium level is cardiac dysrhythmia. Chvostek's sign is associated with hypocalcemia. Although blood pressure may be affected by cardiac dysrhythmia, it is not specific to potassium balance. Edema is associated with fluid balance.

8. 1. Rationale: Kayexalate is indicated for the removal of excess potassium. K-Lor is a potassium supplement indicated for patients with hypokalemia. Kaopectate is an antidiarrheal medicine, and Keflex is an antibiotic.

9. 3. Rationale: While hypocalcemia may affect cardiac rhythm, Trousseau's sign is most specific to calcium balance. Urine output and weight are important assessment parameters for fluid balance.

10. 1. Rationale: Cardiac arrest is associated with tissue hypoxia and development of lactic acidosis. This causes a metabolic acidosis.

11. 1. Rationale: The ABGs reveal respiratory acidosis. A primary intervention is to increase ventilation through deep breathing and removal of secretions. Although vital sign and cardiac assessment are important, increasing ventilation will help resolve the problem. Leg exercises may be encouraged to prevent deep vein thrombosis, but are not related to the ABGs presented in this scenario.

12. 1. Rationale: Removal of gastric acids may result in metabolic alkalosis. The patient unable to access water is at risk for fluid volume deficit and hypernatremia. The infant is at risk for fluid volume excess. The patient experiencing a stroke is not at risk for a specific fluid, electrolyte, or acid-base imbalance.

13. 1. Rationale: The PCO_2 is low, indicating alkalosis. To compensate, the body has excreted excess bicarbonate, and the HCO_3 is low. This compensation has returned the pH within normal range.

Chapter 13

1. 1. Rationale: The cephalic vein can be a found along the thumb side of the wrist. Basilic vein can be found running along the little finger side of the arm. The vein that runs along the inner aspect of the forearm is the median vein. The dorsal metacarpal veins can be found on the back of the hand.

2. 3. Rationale: Tonicity is the ability to cause fluid movement across membranes. Osmosis is the movement of fluid through a semipermeable membrane. Hypertonicity refers to solutions that cause fluid to move out of the cell resulting in shrinking of the cells.

3. 2. Rationale: Hypotonic solution causes fluid to move into the cells leading to swelling and in some cases bursting. An isotonic solution causes no fluid shift between compartments as it has the same tonicity as plasma. Hypertonic solutions cause fluid to move out of the cell resulting in shrinking of the cells. Tonic refers to the ability to cause fluid movement across membranes.

4. 2. Rationale: Magnesium is important in the transmission of neuromuscular impulses. Too much magnesium may cause respiratory muscle depression leading to respiratory depression and arrest. Calcium is found mostly in teeth and bones and is involved in blood coagulation. It is also involved in muscle contraction and nerve impulse transmission. Potassium is necessary for the transmission of nerve impulses, cardiac rhythms, and muscle contraction. Chloride is found in the blood and in the stomach combined with other substances.

5. 4. Rationale: It is the correct steps of venipuncture.

6. 1. Rationale: Chemical phlebitis occurs when the medication itself causes irritation of the vein wall. Mechanical phlebitis occurs when the cannula causes the vein to become inflamed. Phlebitis can be present without infection and typically presents as a hard cord. Extravasation refers to the leakage of a vesicant into the surrounding tissue. A vesicant is a medication that can cause tissue damage if infused outside of the vein into the surrounding tissue. Infiltration refers to the infusion of a fluid or medication into the surrounding tissue. An occluded or blocked cannula will not cause phlebitis.

7. 3. Rationale: CDC as well as, the Infusion Nurses Society recognize the distal one third of the superior vena cava as the preferred location for a central venous catheter. All other locations are considered peripheral locations.

8. 1, 3, 4. Rationale: The other response is IV solution and not blood components.

9. 3. Rationale: The five rights are: right medication, right patient, right dose, right time, and right route.

10. 3. Rationale: The skin of an older adult is thinner, has less subcutaneous fat, and is more fragile. Consider the mental status of an older adult when obtaining consent or providing patient education. The location of an intravenous site may limit a patient's mobility, but this will not affect the nurse's assessment of the site.

11. 2. Rationale:

Ratio Proportion	Formula method	
10 mg:1 mL = 6 mg: X	X (G) = 6 mg (D)	1 = 6 = 6 ÷ 10 = 0.6 mL
10 mgX = 6 mL		
X = 0.6 mL		

12. 1. Rationale:

Ratio Proportion	Formula method
1,000 mL:24 mL = X:1 hr	1,000 mL X × mL/hour = 41.6 mL/hour or 42
24 mLX = 1,000 mL	
X = 41.6 mL/hr or 42 mL/hr	

Chapter 14

1. 4. Rationale: European herbalism is not as widely known or accepted, lacking the long tradition of Ayurvedic, TCM, and Native American shamanism.

2. 2, 4, and 5. Rationale: Integrative medicine involves the use of CAM therapies with conventional medicine. Naturopathic medicine is a form of CAM therapies that involves homeopathy, herbs, etc. Allopathic, Western, and Orthodox are all synonyms with conventional medicine, which is geared toward the use of medications or surgery to treat disease.

3. 3. Rationale: Neurobiology is a current field of study that focuses on physiology of the biology of the nervous system. Psychoimmunology and neuroimmunology omit an important component of CAM therapies—the mind-body connection. Psychoneuroimmunology studies how the mind, nervous system, and immune system all interact to promote wellness.

4. 3. Rationale: Traditional Chinese medicine and shiatsu come from Chinese origins. Shamanism comes from Native American and other indigenous peoples. Ayurvedic comes from Hindu and Indian tradition.

5. 3. Rationale: Research from the NCCAM has demonstrated acupuncture to be most cost-effective in management of osteoarthritis. It additionally improves range of motion of the knee.

6. 2, 3. Rationale: While friends may be useful in finding practitioners, they may recommend someone based on whether they liked them rather than their effectiveness or competence. Patients may be able to take herbs and prescription medications at the same time, but they should check with their pharmacists first. If they are told they cannot take both, some patients may only take herbs, denying themselves necessary medications. Patients should tell their primary care provider all CAM therapies in which they engage. They should also make sure their CAM provider is properly trained, educated, certified, or licensed.

7. American Holistic Nurses Association. Rationale: The American Holistic Nurses Association is an organization dedicated to helping nurses get education, training, and resources for integration of CAM therapies into their practice. They also provide certification for holistic nursing practice and publish a journal dedicated to holistic nursing practice.

8. 2. Rationale: Nightingale first wrote about nature acting on the patient and nursing's role in her *Notes on Nursing*. The other leaders have made major contributions to holistic nursing practice, but based on principles espoused by Nightingale.

9. 3, 4, and 5. Rationale: In most states, hypnosis requires certification, licensure, or licensure as a specified practitioner, e.g., psychologist or nurse practitioner (NP). Reiki requires attunements by a Reiki master and practitioners receive a certificate, although the states do not regulate Rciki practitioners. All states that allow acupuncture require licensure as acupuncturists, with the exception that allows health care providers or chiropractors to practice acupuncture by virtue of their medical license. Relaxation and imagery are common interventions that can be performed by any nurse and to not require any special certification or licensure.

10. 2. Rationale: Tomatoes and tomato sauce contain lycopene. Red chili peppers contain capsaicin. Apples, pears, and prunes are most beneficial for their fiber pectin. Citrus fruits, broccoli, and most other vegetables are the most common sources of ascorbic acid.

11. 5. Rationale: Aloe vera is a common ingredient in lotions and topical applications for treatment of sunburn or light skin abrasions. Evening primrose is effective for eczema, eucalyptus for respiratory decongestion, chamomile for anxiety, and celery seed for edema.

12. 4. Rationale: Milk thistle works well for persons with hepatitis or cirrhosis, both diseases of the liver.

13. 1, 4. Rationale: Gingko and brewer's yeast are known to increase bleeding risks. Aloe vera may enhance potassium loss. Licorice root may increase blood pressure and alter antihypertensive effects of some medications.

14. 2. Rationale: National Center for Complementary and Alternative Medicine was specifically developed to provide research resources for the study of the effectiveness of CAM therapies. American Holistic Nurses Association and American Association for Oriental Medicine are designed to provide a professional organization for its practitioners. National Institute of Arthritis and Musculoskeletal and Skin Diseases may provide research support for CAM therapies, but it would be incidental support. Most of its research support is for conventional medical treatment of arthritis, musculoskeletal, and skin disorders.

Chapter 15

1. 2. Rationale: T stands for size on a range from 0 to 4, 2.5 is T2 range. N represents the amount of regional lymph node involvement with a range from 0 to 4; N1 identifies involvement in one region. M represents presence of metastasis, either M0 or M1. The designation (x) for T, N, or M signifies undetermined.

2. 3. Rationale: Common sites for metastasis related to primary breast cancer are the lungs and the bone.

3. 3. Rationale: The focus of primary prevention is to prevent the disease. The focus of secondary prevention is early detection and screening to detect disease early. The focus of tertiary prevention is to prevent reoccurrence of disease or to limit disability associated with the disease. Thus, 3 is the correct answer, a focus on screening or self-exam for testicular cancer.

4. 3. Rationale: Nadir is defined as the period of time when blood counts reach their lowest point. The absolute neutrophil count is a value that represents the absolute amount of neutrophils (a type of white blood cell) in the blood.

5. 3. Rationale: Markings should not be removed until all therapy is completed. Application of cold may damage the irradiated area. This is external beam radiation therapy, not brachytherapy, therefore precautions as noted in 4 are not indicated. 3 is the best answer. Damage to the skin must be avoided and many over-the-counter creams have alcohol, or other drying agents contained. The best approach is to consult the oncology provider about which creams or lotions may be used.

6. 3. Rationale: Doxorubicin (Adriamycin) is a chemotherapeutic agent that is administered intravenously. To provide optimum safety, all intravenous (IV) chemotherapeutic agents should be managed as if all are vesicants. Therefore, special precautions should be taken, which would include use of the chemotherapy spill kit that should be present on the nursing unit.

7. 4. Rationale: In caring for a patient undergoing brachytherapy or a patient with an implanted radiotherapeutic device, the nurse must observe the three cardinal rules for radiation therapy: Time, distance, and shielding. Mrs. Brown will be on bedrest to prevent dislodgement of the radioactive implant, and all three rules must be addressed.

8. 4. Rationale: Neupogen is a colony-stimulating factor administered prior to the nadir to stimulate the production of neutrophils. Thus the focus for response would be on neutrophils, rather than red blood cells. A normal neutrophil count ranges from 2,200–7,000 mm^3. Effectiveness would be reflected in the higher neutrophil count.

9. 1. Rationale: Skin cells are naturally rapidly dividing cells, as such the normal skin cells are at risk of damage in the area which received external beam radiation therapy. When skin cells are damaged or weakened, dehiscence and evisceration are possible complications. The correct response to this item is specific to the external beam radiation and the abdominal surgery.

10. 1. Rationale: Is the only option in which all are correct according to the American Cancer Society guidelines.

Chapter 16

1. 4. Rationale: The correct response is 4, because the purpose of myelinated nerve fibers is to provide an electrical insulator to increase the speed of an impulse.
2. 3. Rationale: The correct response is 3, because the latest version of the gate control theory suggests that the control mechanism is influenced by internal analgesic substances.
3. 2. Rationale: The correct response is 2, because transduction of pain refers to the initiation of an electrical activity due to the impact of noxious stimuli.
4. 4. Rationale: The correct response is 4, because allodynia is a term that refers to hypersensitivity to a noxious stimulus.
5. 3. Rationale: The correct response is 3, because the autonomic nervous system is a major part of the CNS that regulates homeostasis or equilibrium of the body's internal environment.
6. 1. Rationale: The correct response is 1, because endogenous opioid peptides are chemicals that are released as needed to assist in modulating pain sensations.
7. 3. Rationale: The correct response is 3, because the best description for the cause of nociceptive pain is when there is no injury or malfunction of the nerve transmission process.
8. 4. Rationale: The correct response is 4, because an example of neuropathic pain is phantom limb pain.
9. 3. Rationale: The correct response is 3, because NSAIDs provide analgesia by blocking the production of prostaglandins.
10. 3. Rationale: The correct response is 3, because the cornerstone of effective pain management is patient and family education.

Chapter 17

1. 3. Rationale: The most important action the nurse can take is to check the patient's blood sugar. This data will determine the next action.
2. 4. Rationale: Glyburide is a sulfonylurea antidiabetic agent. There is a cross-sensitivity with sulfa drugs. The nurse must assess for any allergy to sulfa drugs prior to administration.
3. 2. Rationale: Anticoagulants are contraindicated for patients with potential for active bleeding. A recent history of gastric ulcers would make the patient at high risk for hemorrhage.
4. 3. Rationale: The major adverse effects of antilipemics drugs are related to altered liver function. The nurse monitors laboratory results that include elevated transaminase.
5. 1. Rationale: Theophylline is a methylxanthine bronchodilator used to treat obstructive lung diseases, such as asthma and chronic obstructive pulmonary disorder (COPD).
6. 3. Rationale: H_2 blockers are effective in blocking both volume and acidity of stomach acid. This group of drugs is used to treat duodenal ulcers, gastric ulcers, hypersecretory conditions, and gastric reflux disease (GERD).
7. 1. Rationale: The ability of digoxin to slow the heart rate is called a negative chronotropic effect. The release of calcium ions causes more forceful myocardial contraction that is termed a positive inotropic effect.
8. 4. Rationale: Unrelieved anginal pain may indicate an impending myocardial infarction (MI) and warrants emergency intervention.
9. 2. Rationale: A common side effect and potential adverse effect of diuretic therapy is hypokalemia. Potassium is frequently prescribed to prevent this adverse effect. The nurse should monitor potassium levels carefully.
10. 3. Rationale: Only drug taken by the oral route are subject to first pass metabolism in the liver.
11. 4. Rationale: Drug half-life is defined as the time it takes for half the absorbed dose to be eliminated from the body. It takes three to five half-lives to reach steady state.
12. 4. Rationale: Though age is a factor to consider, it is the function of the liver and kidneys that affect pharmacokinetic processing of medication. The nurse should obtain baseline laboratory studies of renal and liver function prior to initiating medications.
13. 2. Rationale: Ototoxicity that can include permanent hearing loss is a serious adverse effect of aminoglycoside therapy. The nurse should monitor for early signs of hearing loss.
14. 4. Rationale: Mouth sores, diarrhea, and vaginal itching are clinical manifestations of a fungal superinfection, a common adverse effect of anti-infective therapy. The nurse should notify the physician and obtain orders for treatment of this infection.

Chapter 18

1. 4. Rationale: Donabedian's classic model for evaluating quality identifies three vectors of quality: structure, process, and outcome.
2. 2. Rationale: Primary care is delivered through ambulatory outpatient agencies.

3. 1. Rationale: The three components of the synergy model are patient characteristics, nurse competencies, and safe passage.
4. 1. Rationale: Medicaid is the national health insurance program that pays for medical assistance for certain people with low income. Medicaid is administered by the state government.
5. 3. Rationale: The proportion of the gross national product dedicated to health care has been climbing for many years and currently consumes the highest percentage of all products tracked.
6. 1. Rationale: Congress passed a prescription drug payment system in the summer of 2006, but there is insufficient funding for a complete reimbursement program.
7. 3. Rationale: The hospital report card deals with measurement of acute care hospital quality and thus, tertiary care.
8. 2. Rationale: The board of trustees oversees administrative and operational processes. JCAHO evaluates clinical care processes for compliance with established standards of care for the purpose of accreditation. Positive clinical outcomes are, in part, the result of nurses accepting responsibility for providing the nursing care needed by a patient.
9. 2. Rationale: Nursing homes and hospice provide continuing care; childhood immunizations constitute preventive care.
10. 2. Rationale: Medicare is the national health insurance program for those age 65 years and over, so neither 1 nor 4 are correct.

Chapter 19

1. 2. Rationale: Sedation will help to slow the patient's respiratory rate and help the respiratory alkalosis.
2. 1. Rationale: PEEP causes increased intrathoracic pressure, which in turn decreases venous return, and can cause a pneumothorax.
3. 2. Rationale: The other situations cause the high-pressure alarm to sound.
4. 1, 3, 4, 5, 6; Rationale: 2 causes the low exhaled tidal volume alarm to sound.
5. 1. Rationale: The patient should not be requiring high amounts of oxygen prior to extubation.
6. 1. Rationale: Nitroprusside can cause rapid changes in blood pressure. Blood pressure should be monitored every five minutes.
7. 1. Rationale: The intra-aortic balloon pump deflates during systole.
8. 4. Rationale: The pulmonary artery catheter passes through the tricuspid valve and then the pulmonic valve.
9. 4. Rationale: SVR is an indirect measurement of afterload.
10. 4. Rationale: Patients who are hypovolemic will have low right atrial pressures.
11. 1. Rationale: Pulmonary artery wedge pressure is an indirect measurement of left ventricular performance.

Chapter 20

1. 2. Rationale: As an initial response, it always wise to seek clarification of complex questions, especially when the preoperative nurse is dealing with information that is likely not to have clear-cut answers. Patients may draw unusual conclusions during times that are stressful, such as the preoperative period.
2. 1. Rationale: Spirituality is the attempt to provide meaning within life's events. Religious faith has a slightly more specific definition.
3. 2. Rationale: In some cases, it might be unwise to have the preoperative patient closely examining and interpreting each vital sign reading as well as heart rhythm tracings. Nurses might want to ask for clarification of circumstances in which this would be done.
4. 4. Rationale: Electronic record keeping will always hold the potential for patients' private information to be captured by those without a need to know and without patient consent.
5. 4. Rationale: On a two-day stay and noncomplex surgery, it might be unwise for the patient to focus energy on work-related matters.
6. 2, 4, 5. Rationale: Lung removal and CABG are major surgeries because the chest cage is usually opened. Disruption to the underlying tissues, extended length of time for completion of surgery, and the likelihood of intensive care stays indicate that these are not minor. Total hip replacement also involves major tissue disruption and mobility interruption.
7. 2. Rationale: This is a recall test item. Refer to definitions within the chapter.
8. 4. Rationale: All are reasons to delay the patient's arrival in the surgery holding area. Some may lead to cancellation of surgery because the patient may not have been capable of informed consent, may not be stable physically, or may not want to go through with surgery at this time.
9. 1. Rationale: To be absolutely sure that the surgical team is positive about the correct site or correct side of the body, the patient's placing a mark is best. Lessons of the past indicate that reliance on documents or the surgeon's memory may lead to unfortunate patient consequences.
10. 3. Rationale: Only the registered nurse is permitted to perform and document physical assessment of patients.

11. 1, 2, 4. Rationale: Age, immunosuppression (even if mild at the time of surgery), and long-term respiratory compromise will increase the general risks for anesthesia and surgery.
12. 3. Rationale: This is a recall test item. Refer to discussion in the chapter.
13. 2. Rationale: There are exceptions to highest ER prioritization always centering on preservation of life. There will be instances in which the terminally ill patient will report in to the ER for ease of access to other hospital services.

Chapter 21

1. 1. Rationale: Items above the level of the draped patient are within the sterile field.
2. 1. Rationale: Shoe covers are needed for infection prevention purposes.
3. 5. Rationale: All are true for standard infection-control precautions.
4. 4. Rationale: All are methods of hand hygiene.
5. 5. Rationale: Hand washing indications include: when gloves are removed and before leaving the operating room, when hands are visibly soiled, and before patient care.
6. 1. Rationale: A jacket with long sleeves does not provide protection from blood splatter or body fluids.
7. 2. Rationale: Wearing gloves does not replace the need for hand washing.
8. 3. Rationale: All instruments need cleaning even if they do not have visible contamination.
9. 5. Rationale: All answers are true regarding monitoring the correct functioning of a sterilizer.
10. 3. Rationale: Light amplification by the stimulated emission of radiation (LASER).
11. 5. Rationale: All are early signs of MH.
12. 1. Rationale: Activation of the emergency medical code team is a main step in the emergency treatment of MH.
13. 1. Rationale: The differential diagnosis of MH includes: external heating, septicemia, thyrotoxicosis, pheochromocytoma, anaphylaxis, respiratory problems, pulmonary emboli, and myopathy
14. 4. Rationale: Monitoring of the patient suspected to have MH includes ECG, blood pressure, CO_2 monitoring, pulse oximeter, temperature, creatininase, electrolytes, and blood gas analysis.

Chapter 22

1. 2. Rationale: Not knowing a caller's identity means that the RN may be discussing confidential information with an unauthorized individual.
2. 1. Rationale: ABC's (airway, breathing, and circulation) are always the top priority to ensure preservation of life.
3. 4. Rationale: Indicates the patient is having mental status changes. Not only could this indicate fluid and electrolyte imbalance or low blood counts, it is a safety hazard.
4. 1. Rationale: Because somnolent patients often respond to simple stimulation, this should be the RN's first action, especially if family members are at the bedside
5. 2. Rationale: Indicates hematoma.
6. 2. Rationale: The nurse should medicate the patient, because the morphine given in PACU wears off in about one hour.
7. 2. Rationale: Should the patient's cardiorespiratory system be in distress from heavy blood loss, this will be indicated by signs of shock such as altered level of consciousness, rapid heart rate, and falling blood pressure.
8. 1, 2, 3. Rationale: Answers 4 and 5 are expected findings in the postoperative abdominal surgery patient.
9. 3. Rationale: This patient has early onset insulin dependent diabetes and is more likely to experience difficulty with wound healing.
10. 3. Rationale: Indicates the patient does not understand the purpose of the compression stockings.
11. 1. Rationale: The standard of care for the postoperative patients is that they will have at least 200 mL of output within six hours of surgery.
12. 1. Rationale: With the abdominal surgical patient, full (regular) diet is indicated when the patient is able to pass flatus. Flatus will be passed long before the patient is ready to have a bowel movement and indicates a functioning gastrointestinal tract.
13. 3. Rationale: The RN should try to avoid teaching when patients are distracted and involved with other activities.
14. 1. Rationale: Failure to assess the patient's readiness to learn is one of the most common mistakes made by the novice teacher.

Chapter 23

1. 1, 2. Rationale: Platelets and fibrinogen are used in hemostasis.
2. 1. Rationale: Pallor is best assessed in the mucous membranes and conjunctivae. The skin is normally a pinkish color in various skin colors.

3. 3. Rationale: The valve closing makes the loudest sound until normal physiological conditions; therefore the sound is transmitted to the chest wall.
4. 3. Rationale: Diastole is correlated with ventricular filling.
5. 4. Rationale: In children and young adults, the sound of the blood entering the ventricles may be transmitted to the chest wall, but after the early 20s the sound is associated with heart failure.
6. 2. Rationale: S_2 is the sound associated with closure of the aortic valve.
7. 1. Rationale: S_1 is the sound associated with closure of the mitral valve.
8. 4. Rationale: A physiological split of S_2 is from closure of the pulmonic valve, which is best auscultated in the second ICS on the left side of the sternum.
9. 3. Rationale: The mitral area and the apical pulse are the fifth ICS midclavicular line.
10. 2. Rationale: A scale of I to VI is the standard scale for assessing heart murmurs.

Chapter 24

1. 4. Rationale: These are all risk factors for coronary artery disease.
2. 3. Rationale: Chest pressure lasting greater than 20 minutes not relieved by rest is not a typical stable angina symptom.
3. 4. Rationale: Unstable angina, STEMI, and NSTEMI are included in the clinical spectrum of ACS.
4. 2. Rationale: The atherogenesis of coronary artery disease does not begin with unstable plaque.
5. 2. Rationale: Initial diagnostic studies in the setting of an acute MI include an ECG and exercise stress test.
6. 4. Rationale: Aspirin, beta blockers, and nitroglycerin are common medications used for CAD and ACS.
7. 5 nursing diagnoses for patients with angina and MI are:
   - Acute pain (angina) related to the imbalance between myocardial oxygen supply and demand.
   - Ineffective tissue perfusion related to myocardial ischemia and decreased cardiac output.
   - Anxiety related to pain, perceived threat of death, possible lifestyle changes, and diagnosis of CAD.
   - Activity intolerance related to angina, pulmonary congestion, fatigue, and inadequate tissue perfusion.
   - Ineffective therapeutic regimen management related to lack of knowledge related to disease process, prognosis, and treatment strategies.
8. Components of patient education for patients with stable angina are:
   - Understanding of cardiac condition
   - Chest pain management
   - Activity
   - Medications
   - Risk factor modification
   - Diet
   - Signs and symptoms to report to the physician
9. The goals of therapy for stable angina are to improve the quality of life by decreasing episodes of angina and ischemia and increase the quantity of life by preventing progression to myocardial infarction and death.
10. The goals of therapy for acute MI are to limit myocardial damage and prevent complications and recurrent events.

Chapter 25

1. 3. Rationale: Cardiac catheterization is a procedure used to help identify causes and degree of heart failure. The procedure is performed by placing a catheter through a vein that leads to the heart. An angiogram, also called a left heart catheterization, is a procedure in which the arterial system is accessed. An x-ray is taken during a cardiac catheterization procedure to allow visualization of the internal anatomy of the heart and blood vessels after the intravascular introduction of radiopaque contrast medium (dye) and can assist in measurement of pulmonary artery pressure (Murthy, 2004). A biopsy is the retrieval of a part of the heart muscle that is sent for laboratory testing.
2. 1. Rationale: Signs of left-sided heart failure may reveal dysrhythmic heart rate, tachycardia, heart murmurs, extra heart sounds, lung crackles, and decreased basilar lung sounds (Kang, 2004). An increase in the work of breathing, an increase in the rate of respirations, and an increase in the depth of respiration all indicate strain on the system in situations like heart failure. The pulse increases in an effort to pump oxygen into the body, but it will be weak and ineffective. Left-sided heart failure may present as the following symptoms: shortness of breath, paroxysmal nocturnal dyspnea, palpitations, tachycardia, cough with frothy blood-tinged mucus, fatigue, weakness, syncope, weight gain, fluid retention, and oliguria.

3. 2. Rationale: In left-sided heart failure, the left ventricle loses its ability to effectively pump oxygenated blood into the systemic circulation leaving the body starving for oxygen and nutrients (Kang, 2004).
In right-sided heart failure, the right ventricle loses its ability to pump efficiently and causes blood that would normally be pumped through the heart into the lungs, and errantly backs up into the systemic circulation. This back up of blood causes congestion that can affect the liver, the gastrointestinal tract, and the periphery (arms and legs) (Hart, 2004). The decrease in peripheral oxygenation, (not pulmonary venous congestion that the question asked about), will reveal ashen skin, cyanotic nail beds, and circumoral pallor. Eventually, the heart will not receive enough oxygen to function properly. The jugular neck veins will distend.
In heart failure in general, an increase in the work of breathing, an increase in the rate of respirations, and an increase in the depth of respiration all indicate strain on the system.
4. 4. Rationale: The more pumping and harder the heart works, the more oxygen that is required for the body to continue working hard. Respiratory support consists of nonrebreathing oxygen by mask to relieve hypoxemia and dyspnea.
5. 4. Rationale: ACE inhibitors work by decreasing the pressure the heart must overcome to eject blood from the heart by interfering with the renin-angiotensin-aldosterone system. This interference results blocking the conversion of angiotensin I to angiotensin II in the kidney, causing a decreased aldosterone, increased sodium excretion, and in peripheral vasodilatation that allows for decreased pressure-causing volume in the heart and a decrease in blood pressure (Jessup & Brozena, 2003).
6. 1. Rationale: Characteristic of acute heart failure is an abnormal accumulation of fluid in the lungs. This fluid disperses into all available lung spaces, even those that are used for oxygen exchange. This alteration in the ability of the lungs to perform their oxygenation function results in a rapid onset of symptoms such as panic, anxiety, shortness of breath, cough, and restlessness. Shortly, the pulse increases in an effort to pump oxygen into the body, but it will be weak and ineffective. A back up of blood will ensue and the jugular neck veins will distend.
7. 4. Rationale: Weight reduction is suggested for those obese HCM patients, moderation in alcohol intake is suggested, and flu vaccination is considered. HCM patients are encouraged to avoid overexertion, acute loss of body fluid volume, situations that may predispose one to fainting, hot showers or water immersion, and medication that quickly drops blood pressure.
8. 1. Rationale: Heart muscle disease is called cardiomyopathy and is a problem with the physical shape of the muscle. Heart muscle inflammatory dysfunction is called carditis; an inflammation of the heart muscle.
9. 1. Rationale: Heart transplantation is necessary for some who have severe alteration in the heart's ability to pump effectively. Still other possible treatments include electrical cardioversion, pacemaker insertion, and implantable defibrillator.
10. 2. Rationale: The lung sounds and breath sounds will become moist and noisy with frothy (sometimes pink) sputum. The patient may manifest signs of confusion. These symptoms are ominous and require immediate intervention.

Chapter 26

1. 3. Rationale: This is the appropriate method of calculating a heart rate from a strip when it is irregular. 1 and 4 are only appropriate methods to calculate heart rate when the rhythm is regular.
2. 1. Rationale: Sodium ions move into the cell to initiate depolarization.
3. 4. Rationale: The nurse should establish unresponsiveness prior to initiating CPR.
4. 4. Rationale: Asking the patient to cough may cause a vagal response, which would slow the heart rate down.
5. 1. Rationale: The electrical rhythm is normal sinus rhythm, but the patient has no pulse. The interpretation should be PEA, in which case CPR should be started.
6. 4. Rationale: The patient is not suffering from hemodynamic instability at this time. It is important to continue to monitor the patient in a sinus bradycardia.
7. 2, 4, 5. Rationale: Each of these are possible treatments for ventricular tachycardia with a pulse.
8. 2. Rationale: Epinephrine will be given after three unsuccessful defibrillation attempts in ventricular fibrillation.
9. 4. Rationale: Ventricular arrhythmias are primarily interpreted by analyzing the QRS complex as it represents ventricular depolarization.
10. 4. Rationale: The health care provider assesses and manages breathing by using positive-pressure ventilations.

Chapter 27

1. 1. Rationale: Patients with bleeding disorders need to be assessed for risks and contraindications associated with the disease prior to the start of anticoagulant therapy.
2. 3. Rationale: These are classic symptoms of thoracic-aortic aneurysm, related to the pressure of the aneurysm on the esophagus and laryngeal nerve.
3. 2. Rationale: Uncontrolled bleeding after 10 minutes must be reported to the physician, as excessive bleeding can indicate hypercoagulation.
4. 1. Rationale: INRs must be taken on a consistent basis to monitor the effectiveness of the Coumadin, and the blood level is in therapeutic and safe range.
5. 2. Rationale: The patient is demonstrating symptoms of prolonged bleeding time. Coumadin should be held and an INR drawn for evaluation.
6. 1. Rationale: Frank bleeding is a side effect of t-PA, and has a three times greater incidence of bleeding than heparin.
7. 1. Rationale: Heparin does not dissolve clots, but prevents further clot formation and is reversed quickly with protamine sulfate.
8. 2. Rationale: Venous ulcers have edema at the site, irregular margins, and pink ulcer beds.
9. 1. Rationale: Fever, abdominal pain, and dyspnea are the three major symptoms of pulmonary embolism.
10. 4. Rationale: Decreased blood flow leads to tissue necrosis and infection.

Chapter 28

1. 4. Rationale: Target organ damage that can occur from uncontrolled hypertension includes kidney dysfunction and left ventricular hypertrophy.
2. 3. Rationale: When teaching a patient how to control hypertension, the nurse must recognize that lifestyle modifications are indicated for all patients with hypertension.
3. 2. Rationale: Renin is secreted into the blood by the kidney structure known as the juxtaglomerular apparatus.
4. 1. Rationale: The secretion of antidiuretic hormone (ADH) is stimulated by decreased venous return.
5. 3. Rationale: A patient with a blood pressure of 200/141 mm Hg would have a hypertensive emergency
6. 1. Rationale: Patient teaching for modifiable risk factor reduction should include dietary factors.
7. 2. Rationale: ACE inhibitors such as captopril (Capoten) and enalapril (Vasotec) decrease both blood pressure and peripheral vascular resistance by blocking the conversion of angiotensin I to angiotensin II.
8. 2. Rationale: The interval between the first and second heart sounds is ventricular systole.
9. 3. Rationale: Afterload is the force that the left ventricle must generate to eject its blood volume.
10. 1. Rationale: Pulsus paradoxus is a sign of cardiac tamponade
11. 2. Rationale: Bupropion is a non–nicotine-containing therapy used to support smoking cessation.
12. 1. Rationale: 118/78 is considered a normal B/P according to the JNC VII guidelines.
13. 2. Rationale: A cause of secondary hypertension is hypothyroidism.

Chapter 29

1. 1. Rationale: The three components of the hematology system are: bone marrow, blood cells, and plasma.
2. 2. Rationale: As the three primary classes for anemias are: 1) bleeding, which results in RBC loss; 2) hemolytic anemia, which is caused by RBC destruction; and 3) hypoproliferative, which results from defective RBC production.
3. 2. Rationale: As thalassemia is prevalent in populations from specific areas of descent (China, Philippines, Thailand, Mediterranean ancestry, African Americans), and the other three responses are incorrect.
4. 3. Rationale: Because a cobalamin deficiency is labeled a vitamin B_{12} deficiency.
5. 1. Rationale: Because plasmapheresis is the primary treatment for thrombocytopenia.
6. 3. Rationale: Because DIC is the correct label and is described as the clotting disorder that consumes the clotting factors and causes patients to have clotting difficulties.
7. 4. Rationale: Because primary polycythemia is the type of polycythemia that is more common in European Jewish persons than the other forms of polycythemia.
8. 2. Rationale: Because acute myelogenous leukemia affects persons of all ages, and the other responses are false.
9. 3. Rationale: Because CML is characterized by the presence of the Philadelphia chromosome.
10. 2. Rationale: As bone pain is the distinguishing clinical manifestation for multiple myeloma.

Chapter 30

1. 2. Rationale: Crackles is the best description of adventitious breath sounds as described.
2. 3. Rationale: It is a false statement.
3. 4. Rationale: All four answers are correct.
4. 3. Rationale: This is the best response, because response b is false.
5. 3. Rationale: PaO_2 is the best method of assessing oxygenation status.
6. 2. Rationale: This is the correct definition for shunting.
7. 1. Rationale: The correct interpretation of the blood gases is respiratory acidosis.
8. 1. Rationale: Barrel chest can be seen in chronic obstructive lung disease and normal aging.
9. 1. Rationale: Low flow oxygen delivery systems include the use of entrainment of room air and the use of the mouth and nose as a reservoir.
10. 2. Rationale: Employment history and occupational exposure are vital data in determining prior existing conditions despite current employment status.
11. 3. Rationale: Vesicular breathing is most frequently seen in usual and normal breathing.
12. 3. Rationale: Pulsus paradoxus is described as a drop in blood pressure on inspiration.

Chapter 31

1. 3. Rationale: The most important information to give a patient about prevention with allergic rhinitis is to avoid the triggers that bring about the allergic episode. Triggers include things, such as dust, pollen, cigarette smoke, pet dander, or foods.
2. 4. Rationale: Signs and symptoms of rhinitis are the same regardless of the triggering event. Common clinical manifestations of rhinitis are rhinorrhea, nasal congestion, nasal itchiness, and sneezing are classical features. Headache and cough may be seen. If the patient presents with pyrexia (fever), further assessment should be performed to look for an infectious component.
3. 2. Rationale: The most common side effect in the second-generation antihistamines is urinary retention. The nurse should hold the medication until the health care provider can be notified.
4. 1. Rationale: Proper instructions for instilling nasal spray include tilting the head slightly forward, inhaling gently and evenly, spray once in each side of the nose and wait about 15 to 20 seconds before instilling another spray, and avoid blowing the nose after administration to enhance its effects on the mucous membranes.
5. 3. Rationale: Decongestant nasal sprays will help relieve nasal congestion by reducing the inflammation in the nasal passages. However, they should not be used for more than three consecutive days because of the risk of rhinitis medicamentosa, a rebound congestion that can be worse than the original congestion the patient was experiencing.
6. 4. Rationale: Research demonstrates the limited use of antibiotics in eradicating sinus infections. They have been overused and have lead to resistance of many bacterial organisms. Decongestants help reduce nasal swelling, loosen congestion, and promote drainage within the sinus cavities. Antihistamines have not been shown to be of benefit in treating sinusitis. There is insufficient evidence to support the use of wetting agents, mucolytics, or expectorants.
7. 3. Rationale: Fever and yellow secretions indicate the generalized response of inflammation.
8. 1. Rationale: Thick secretions are best cleared from the airways by drinking plenty of fluids to facilitate expectoration. Measures to help drain the sinuses include warm packs, irrigating the sinuses, and taking decongestants as needed.
9. 4. Rationale: It is often difficult to distinguish viral and bacterial pharyngitis. Fever and cervical adenopathy are generally more pronounced in streptococcal pharyngitis. Other characteristics that are most reliable predictors of streptococcal pharyngitis are tonsillar exudate and the absence of cough. The presence of three of these criteria has a specificity and reliability of 75 percent.
10. 3. Rationale: Patients must understand the importance of reporting frank bleeding from the surgical site. Secondary bleeding is more common than immediate postoperative bleeding and can occur 5 to 8 days after the surgery. The patient is instructed to start with liquids and progress to soft foods for the first few days. The patient should avoid gargling, coughing, straining, and smoking for 10 days.
11. 3. Rationale: Physical examination in a patient with a peritonsillar abscess reveals a displaced tonsil toward the center of the throat by the abscess, the soft palate is erythematous and swollen, and the uvula is edematous and displaced to the opposite side.
12. 3. Rationale: Complaints from a bed partner about snoring and daytime sleepiness often indicate the presence of obstructive sleep apnea. The nurse needs to ask about the onset of other symptoms, such as memory loss, personality changes, morning headaches, fatigue, nocturia, or gastric reflux.

13. 4. Rationale: The priority interventions for patients who have sustained a fracture of the nose are to control bleeding and swelling. Other important measures include pain relief, assessing for symmetry, and reducing anxiety and fear.
14. 2. Rationale: Cancer in the glottic area is usually found early because the patient complains of a change in the voice. The voice becomes raspy, harsh, or lower in pitch because of tumor impingement on the vocal cords.
15. 1. Rationale: Radiation therapy causes changes in the head and neck. Xerostomia, or dry mouth, occurs because radiation interferes with the ability of the parotid gland to produce mucus.

Chapter 32

1. 4. Rationale: *Pneumocystis carinii* pneumonia is a type of fungal infection that often affects immunocompromised patients.
2. 2. Rationale: Latent TB is diagnosed when a person presents with a positive PPD, has no clinical picture of active disease, and CXR is normal. 1 is incorrect because active disease is different than latent disease. 3 is incorrect as extrapulmonary TB disease can present within the bones but usually exist only with advanced disease circumstances. 4 is incorrect because TB disease is no longer latent if it becomes active.
3. 4. Rationale: Exposure of TB requires close frequent contact and exposure will not be present on a PPD until six weeks after inhalation of pathogen. To ensure employee safety a nurse should always report on the job injury or potential harm. Monitoring any signs or symptoms of active disease will minimize exposure to others and provide quick treatment interventions.
4. 1. Rationale: The two leading risk factors for aspiration include alcohol and mental status changes.
5. 3. Rationale: The primary reason for aspiration of pneumonia pathogens is aspiration of oropharyngeal secretions. Mechanical ventilation and enteral feedings place the patient at risk for pneumonia through aspiration or inhalation of pathogens. 1 is incorrect as the acquiring of TB disease is due to prolonged contact with a person with active disease. 2 is incorrect because there is no indication or clinical presentation that the patient has a pneumothorax. 4 is incorrect as Cor pulmonale occurs when the pulmonary blood pressure due to chronic effects of disease or pulmonary embolism.
6. 3. Rationale: A nurse should complete a patient assessment for any changes in condition, such as a soiled dressing, chest tube dislodgment, and symptoms of respiratory distress or pain. Drainage system is evaluated next and includes adequate tube connections, unclamped tubing, adequate water in the water seal chamber, and drainage amount. Next the nurse will check the water seal for air leaks and finally the suction control chamber if wall suction is being used. A gently constant bubbling should be present. Answers 2, 3, and 4 are missing aspects of the above components.
7. 4. Rationale: Chest tubes allow air or fluid to leak out on expiration but on inspiration the chest tube closes preventing fluid or air from moving into the pleural cavity. 1 is incorrect as chest tubes do not allow air and fluid to move in and out of the pleural space during both expiration and inspiration, doing so would make the chest tube dysfunctional. 2 is incorrect s chest tubes should never be clamped for longer than a few minutes and only during a chest drainage device change. 3 is incorrect, as the nurse should never reinsert chest tube devices, as this is a defined health care provider tack. Clamping of chest tubes is unacceptable practice.
8. 1. Rationale: Spontaneous pneumothorax occurs in men between the ages of 20 to 40, with thin men at high risk. Patients presenting with any trauma will have tachycardia and an elevated blood pressure as the body attempts to compensate for the injury. Swallowing breathing occurs due to the collapse lungs effects and pain with breathing. Lack of any impact injury rules out other causes for the pneumothorax. Answers 2 and 4 are incorrect, because pneumonia or tuberculosis could be a possibility but the fact that there is not a fever and the absence of cough present makes the nurse look at other options. Answer 3 is incorrect as fractured ribs could have occurred, but there is not report of trauma.
9. 2. Rationale: As a result of direct blunt force trauma to the chest and broken ribs the patient is at risk for a pneumothorax. 1 is incorrect as flail chest occurs with rib fractures of three or more ribs and an unstable or nonworking thoracic cage. 3 is incorrect as cor pulmonale is a result of a chronic disease process not an acute injury. 4 is incorrect because trauma is the reason for the ER visits not infection. However, pneumonia may occur as a complication to the pulmonary injury.

10. 4. Rationale: Includes all of the above interventions. Patients who use a medication pump are at risk and must be able to troubleshoot problems, have adequate supplies, complete routine medical workup, and know when and how to call for assistance.

Chapter 33

1. 1,950 mg; convert the patient's weight from pounds to kilograms by dividing 143 pounds by 2.2 kg. This equals 65 kg. Next multiply the 65 kg by 25 mcg. This equals 1,950 mg.
   143 lb/2.2 kg = 65 kg.
   65 kg × 25 mcg = 1,950 mg
2. 1, 2. Rationale: Signs and symptoms of right-sided heart failure include jugular venous distension and hepatomegaly. Dyspnea, crackles, and tachycardia are signs of left-sided heart failure.
3. 4. Rationale: In a patient with COPD, the stimulus to breathe is low oxygen levels. Frequent nursing observations are necessary to see how the patient tolerates low-flow oxygen administration. 1 is incorrect. Humidification is necessary, but this is not the most important nursing intervention. 2 is incorrect, because patients with COPD and hypoxemia need oxygen. 3 is incorrect, because the patient with COPD will probably need to be placed in high-Fowler's position, but this is not the most important nursing intervention.
4. 1. Rationale: The medication should be administered with food, such as milk and crackers to prevent gastrointestinal (GI) irritation. Options 2, 3, 4 are appropriate instructions regarding the use of this medication.
5. 4. Rationale: Pursed-lip breathing facilitates maximal expiration for patients with obstructive lung disease. This type of breathing allows better expiration by increasing airway pressure that keeps air passages open during exhalation. Options 1, 2, and 3 are not the purpose of this breathing.
6. 3. Rationale: The patient should be instructed to hold his or her breath at least 5 to 10 seconds before exhaling the mist. Options 1, 2, and 4 are accurate instructions regarding the use of the inhaler.
7. 3. Rationale: The development of an IgE is a strong predisposing factor for developing asthma. The other responses are false.
8. 2. Rationale: Decreased wheezing in a patient with asthma may be incorrectly interpreted as a positive sign when, in fact, it may signal an inability to move air. A "silent chest" is an ominous sign during an asthma episode. With treatment, increased wheezing may actually signal that the child's condition is improving. The normal pulse rate is 60 to 80 beats per minute. Warm, dry skin indicates improvement in condition, as the patient is normally diaphoretic during exacerbations.
9. 4. Rationale: In a sweat test, sweating is stimulated on the child's forearm with pilocarpine, the sample is collected on absorbent material, and the amounts of sodium and chloride are measured. A chloride level greater than 60 mEq/L is considered to be a positive test result. A chloride level of 40 mEq/L is suggestive of cystic fibrosis (CF) and requires a repeat test.
10. 1. Rationale: Tobramycin (TOBI) is an aerosolized medication and the best antibiotic used to treat lower respiratory tract infections in patients with CF. The other three responses are false.

Chapter 34

1. 2. Rationale: When grading muscle strength, a score of 1 indicates a trace of contraction.
2. 1. Rationale: When the nurse is performing the Romberg test he or she should instruct the patient to close his or her eyes and remain still.
3. 3. Rationale: The patient who has difficulty choosing the right words and responds hesitantly is displaying symptoms of expressive aphasia.
4. 2. Rationale: When an adult has a Babinski's it indicates upper motor neuron disease.
5. 3. Rationale: The ability to recognize an object's shape is known as stereognosis.
6. 4. Rationale: Paralysis of lateral gaze indicates a lesion of cranial nerve VI.
7. 4. Rationale: Stimulation of the parasympathetic nervous system results in relaxation of the urinary sphincters.
8. 4. Rationale: When preparing a patient for an EEG, the nurse should tell the patient that bright lights will be used during the procedure.
9. 2. Rationale: The consensual pupillary response is tested by directing a light toward one eye and observing the pupil on the opposite side.
10. 4. Rationale: One way to test the vestibular function of the acoustic nerve (CN VIII) is to rub your fingers together near the patient's ears.
11. 2. Rationale: The trapezius muscle squeeze is the technique recommended for eliciting a response to peripheral pain.
12. 1. Rationale: Cerebrospinal fluid (CSF) is reabsorbed into the venous system via the arachnoid villi.

13. 3. Rationale: The significance of the blood-brain barrier is that it limits the transmission of substances from the blood to the brain.

Chapter 35

1. 1. Rationale: The type of CVA (stroke) that occurs when a blood vessel in the brain becomes clogged, usually by plaque build up is an ischemic stroke.

2. 3. Rationale: The modifiable risk factor in the prevention of a stroke is obesity. A patient can take steps to lose weight by diet modification and exercise. Age, sex, and family history cannot be changed to prevent a stroke.

3. 4. Rationale: An important nursing intervention when caring for a patient receiving tPA is to watch for decreased level of consciousness and increase in blood pressure.

4. 2. Rationale: A CT scan is usually the radiological test first administered to a patient suspected of having a stroke.

5. 2. Rationale: A primary brain injury is caused by an external force. Often a primary brain injury is a result of direct trauma to the brain. ICPs, an abnormal growth of brain tissue, and internal force are all things that occur within the brain to cause brain damage. These are considered secondary brain injuries.

6. 1. Rationale: A moderate brain injury is characterized by a loss of consciousness ranging from a few minutes to hours to days.

7. 1. Rationale: One of the most important things to tell person teaching 7-year-olds on preventing brain injury is to always wear a helmet when riding your bike or skateboard or rollerblading.

8. 4. Rationale: When a patient is evaluated using the Glasgow Coma Scale and the patient responds only to pain by withdrawing his or her hand and cursing frequently, this patient would score a 9 (the patient responds to pain only (2), withdraws from pain (4), and curses frequently (3). $2 + 4 + 3 = 9$).

9. 3. Rationale: This patient may be developing a intracerebral bleed or cerebral edema, which is an emergency. The family should seek medical attention immediately.

10. 4. Rationale: Mannitol is an osmotic diuretic and is often used to decrease ICP.

11. 1. Rationale: Risk for infection is the most important nursing diagnosis for an open skull fracture because of the potential for bacteria to enter the brain directly through the opening.

12. 2. Rationale: Benign brain tumors are slow-growing and noncancerous tumors. Malignant brain tumors are cancerous and fast-growing.

13. 3. Rationale: A secondary brain tumor means that the cancer originated somewhere else in the body and spread to the brain.

14. 2. Rationale: The most common form of brain tumor is a glioma.

15. 3. Rationale: Stereotactic radiotherapy uses radiation with or without invasive surgery to deliver a precise dose of radiation to a specific location within the brain. It can only be used for small, benign tumors.

Chapter 36

1. 2. Rationale: A patient who has a C6 SCI will respond with "I will be able to feed myself" if the patient understands the teaching about the long-term effects of the injury.

2. 1, 3, 4. Rationale: Loss of pain and temperature sensation on the opposite side, loss of motor function (paralysis) on the same side as the injury, and loss of position sense and vibration on same side as the injury are what the patient experiences with an incomplete spinal cord injury resulting in Brown Séquard syndrome.

3. 2. Rationale: If the new SCI patient responds that there is often a period of spinal shock, and it is difficult to determine if the paralysis will be permanent. When it resolves there can be some regaining of abilities.

4. 4. Rationale: Carbamazepine (Tegretol) is the first choice of treatment for trigeminal neuralgia.

5. 4. Rationale: High-frequency hearing loss is not generally present in a patient with Ménière's disease.

6. 1. Rationale: The nurse seeing a patient with Ménière's disease in the clinic for the first time should first assess for a history of taking thyroid supplements.

7. 2. Rationale: Burning and tingling pain are worse during the nighttime in pain associated with carpal tunnel syndrome.

8. 4. Rationale: A positive Phalen's sign for carpal tunnel syndrome is indicated by pain and tingling experienced on flexion of the wrist at a right angle for one minute.

9. 1. Rationale: Emergency treatment with methylprednisolone for a patient with an SCI must be instituted within the first 8 hours after injury.

10. 1. Rationale: A patient with a cervical SCI that has an upper motor neuron lesion will need the administration of baclofen for spasticity.

11. 2. Rationale: The priority nursing action for a patient with an SCI experiencing a pounding headache and blood pressure of 220/120 indicating autonomic dysreflexia is to check for distended bladder or kinked catheter tubing.

Chapter 37

1. 4. Rationale: A patient who has a migraine headache would be sensitive to sound.
2. 2. Rationale: Nursing documentation of seizure activity should be highly descriptive and detailed.
3. 2. Rationale: The teaching plan for a patient with epilepsy should include wearing a medical alert bracelet.
4. 1. Rationale: Dairy products are food products potentially associated with migraine attacks.
5. 2. Rationale: Two distinguishing features of migraine are family history of headaches and headache-related disability.
6. 3. Rationale: The most common clinical manifestation reported by a patient with myasthenia gravis is weakness on exertion.
7. 4. Rationale: Dopamine is the neurotransmitter that is decreased in patients with Parkinson's disease.
8. 3. Rationale: The priority safety intervention when protecting the patient having a seizure is positioning the patient to prevent aspiration of secretions.
9. 1. Rationale: Atropine is the drug that must be kept at the bedside of patient's with myasthenia gravis.
10. 4. Rationale: An abnormal plantar reflex is commonly seen with upper motor neuron lesions.
11. 1. Rationale: The brief sensory experience that occurs prior to the onset of seizure is called the prodromal phase.

Chapter 38

1. 2. Rationale: A disorder of his palpebrae is a problem with the eyelids.
2. 3. Rationale: The extraocular muscles are innervated by cranial nerves III, IV, and VI.
3. 1. Rationale: The parasympathetic nervous system causes the pupils to constrict.
4. 4. Rationale: A congenital defect that causes color vision problems is due to a dysfunction in the cones.
5. 3. Rationale: The Snellen chart is responsible for testing visual acuity.
6. 2. Rationale: Yellow, lipid rich plaque lesion on the eyelid is labeled xanthelasma.
7. 3. Rationale: A left eye that does not constrict when light is shined in the right eye is labeled a problem associated with a consensual response.
8. 2. Rationale: When using the ophthalmoscope, the red numbers indicate posterior eye problems.
9. 4. Rationale: Purulent drainage coming from the ear is described as otorrhea.
10. 1. Rationale: A conduction problem of both ears is tested with a Weber test, which evaluates whether sounds are heard centrally or on one side.

Chapter 39

1. 3. Rationale: Color blindness is not one of the three main ocular movement dysfunctions.
2. 1. Rationale: Cataract describes the condition asked for in the question.
3. 3. Rationale: Tonometry is the diagnostic test used to reveal the presence of eye pressure.
4. 3. Rationale: The condition described in the question is age-related macular degeneration.
5. 2. Rationale: Assessment of the patient with an impaled object is the priority.
6. 1. Rationale: Melanoma is the most common cause of ocular cancer.
7. 2. Rationale: Keratoconus is caused by rubbing the eyes profusely.
8. 1. Rationale: Hyperopia is the condition corrected with convex corrective lens.
9. 3. Rationale: Hordeolum is the label for the condition described in the question.
10. 4. Rationale: Decreasing daily intake of water is not an appropriate nursing intervention for keratoconjunctivitis sicca.

Chapter 40

1. 2. Rationale: Patients with sensorineural hearing loss have difficulty hearing in noisy environments. The patient with conductive loss is able to hear in these environments. Mixed would also have difficulty hearing in noisy environments.
2. 4. Rationale: Patients with conductive hearing loss have difficulty hearing all pitches and therefore are able to hear in noisy environments, talk softer because they hear their voices as louder, and their speech is clear not distorted.
3. 4. Rationale: Commonly patients experience some vertigo after surgery and therefore need assistance with ambulation. The patient should lie on the unoperated ear; coughing can cause postoperative complications and should be discouraged. The patient cannot be ensured that his hearing will be normal after the operation.

4. 3. Rationale: High doses of aspirin can cause tinnitus, and the patient should report this finding to the health care provider. Tinnitus does not occur with normal aging process, increasing the sound to drown out the ringing will not solve the problem, because it is most likely caused by the aspirin. Performing a Rinne or Weber test will not detect cause of tinnitus.
5. 3. Rationale: Patients with Meniére's disease have sensorineural hearing loss and experience vertigo and tinnitus.
6. 1. Rationale: External ear canals that are blocked by cerumen should be gently irrigated. An individual should not place anything into the canal, such as cotton-tipped swabs. Curettes can cause damage to the canal or tympanic membrane and therefore should not be used. It is not necessary to refer a patient with cerumen to a specialist.
7. 1, 5. Rationale: When communicating with a person who has a hearing deficit speaking loudly or yelling will not help the patient and may cause anxiety. The light source should be placed behind the patient, not the nurse. When it is placed behind the nurse the light tends to glare into the patient's face, making it difficult to read lips or watch facial expressions. When having to repeat a word or phase, another phase should be used. Communicate in clear simple words.
8. 2. Rationale: Most hearing aids will increase the volume of sound but will not make it clearer. The hearing aid is an assistive device and will not return the patient's hearing to normal.
9. 1. Rationale: Normal hearing is measured at 0–15 dB; anything above that range indicates some loss.
10. 1. Rationale: Patient who experiences a loud blast for greater than 20 seconds can have permanent hearing loss.
11. 1, 2. Rationale: OSHA recommends that workers are tested on hiring and yearly and monitoring sound levels on a regular basis. Training and education is mandated yearly. It is not necessary for all employees to wear noise protection only the ones who are exposed to high levels.
12. 2. Rationale: Frequent attacks of vertigo, tinnitus, nausea, vomiting, and intermittent hearing loss are classic signs in Meniére's disease. Presbycusis is a degenerative hearing loss associated with the aging process and has constant loss. Otosclerosis is also a steady decrease in hearing related to the formation of spongy bones around the oval window. Mastoiditis is inflammation of the mastoid process located behind the ear, and the patient does not experience hearing loss.

Chapter 41

1. 2. Rationale: Bone marrow suppression will most likely be reflected in the immune system, but neither detecting nor signaling bone marrow is one of the immune system's roles.
2. 2, 3. Rationale: Both macrophages and dendritic cells process ingested antigen and present it to lymphocytes. Neutrophils and natural killer cells do not.
3. 1, 2, 3, 4. Rationale: Antigens are defined as a substance that can bind to a specific antibody. Haptens are a kind of antigen. Immunogens are any substance that cause an immune reaction, and therefore will eventually cause antibody production. Complement is part of the immune system and may be activated by binding to an antibody.
4. 1. Rationale: Neutrophils are phagocytes, ingesting bacteria to destroy them. Basophils and natural killer cells are exocytotic. Plasma cells produce lymphocytes.
5. 4. Rationale: Dendritic cells and macrophages both activate lymphocytes, but dendritic cells are more potent activators than macrophages.
6. 1, 4. Rationale: Bone marrow and the thymus gland are considered primary lymphoid organs, because they are the site of lymphocyte maturation.
7. 4. Rationale: The innate immune system initiates inflammation. The other answers are characteristics of the acquired immune system.
8. 2. Rationale: Family history of measles is not relevant to giving injections, although a personal history may be.
9. 4. Rationale: Angioedema is the only adverse reaction listed that is a hypersensitivity reaction.
10. 4. Rationale: Heart transplant usually results in destruction of the thymus gland either by mutilation or excision. The spleen and tonsils are both secondary lymphoid tissues.
11. 1, 2. Rationale: Both bacterial infection and MI are associated with elevated neutrophil count.
12. 1. Rationale: Health history provides the framework with which to interpret the physical examination and laboratory values.

Chapter 42

1. 3. Rationale: Patients tend to focus on lifestyle changes in the early stages of a chronic disease.
2. 4. Rationale: The goal of HAART is to avoid viral resistance for each drug.
3. 2. Rationale: The early clinical manifestations of GVHD are skin rash and pruritus.

4. 3. Rationale: Monoclonal antibodies are genetically engineered immunosuppressant drugs.
5. 3. Rationale: Hypersensitivity disorders are because of a heightened immune response to an antigen.
6. 2. Rationale: The reversible form of SLE is because of a reaction to drugs, such as oral contraceptives (e.g., Levora).
7. 1. Rationale: Cell-mediated immunity is initiated by specific antigen recognition by T cells.
8. 2. Rationale: Passive immunity involves inoculation with vaccine containing live or killed infectious organisms.
9. 2. Rationale: Sero-conversion antibodies to HIV are detected by diagnostic studies with in one to three months or more after exposure to HIV.
10. 4. Rationale: Criteria used to diagnose AIDS in an individual with HIV includes development of an opportunistic cancer.

Chapter 43

1. 1. Rationale: The elimination and challenge diet is the cornerstone for treatment of food allergy.
2. 2. Rationale: Intramuscular epinephrine (adrenaline) is the most effective drug in treating anaphylaxis. Epinephrine by inhalation is less effective.
3. 3. Rationale: Swelling around the eyes and or mouth (angioedema) is an initial response to latex allergy. The cascade of symptoms can progress rapidly to anaphylaxis.
4. 1. Rationale: Production of IgE levels to specific allergens tends to be an inherited trait.
5. 3. Rationale: Bee and wasp stings are the most common causes of anaphylaxis. The risk of hyposensitization is balanced against the much larger risk of being stung again.
6. 4. Rationale: The "wheal and flare" skin reaction is visible within 5 to 10 minutes in a positive response to an allergen.
7. 3. Rationale: Drug reactions are a common source of allergic response. The risk of a drug reaction is greater when the drug is given parenterally, rather than orally.
8. 3. Rationale: Dermatitis often appears in this distribution first.
9. 4. Rationale: The parental route gives a larger dose in a shorter period of time.
10. 3. Rationale: Bronchial hyperreactivity is a classic symptom of asthma.

Chapter 44

1. 3. Rationale: The epidermis replenishes itself by a process labeled as keratinization.
2. 4. Rationale: Cells that are responsible for skin pigmentation are melanocytes.
3. 2. Rationale: Neoangiogenesis, a process during the wound healing process is the responsibility of endothelial cells.
4. 2. Rationale: The major function of the subcutaneous tissue is to provide padding over body joints and other internal structures.
5. 3. Rationale: Regeneration of skin is accomplished by replacing damaged tissue with the same cell type.
6. 4. Rationale: Repeated or prolonged insults to tissues can result in development of pressure sores.
7. 1. Rationale: The substances that control the proliferation and differentiation of cells are known as: growth factors.
8. 2. Rationale: In assessment of an edematous area, the nurse should palpate for temperature changes, tenderness, and mobility.
9. 3. Rationale: A teenager with severe acne decides that he does not want to participate in the swimming exercises that are part of the physical education course at his school. This is an example of social isolation related to anticipatory fear of rejection.
10. 1. Rationale: Patient teaching for older adults should include information about avoiding the use of potent topical steroids because decreased vascularity in the skin decreases capacity to clear medications from the system.

Chapter 45

1. 4. Rationale: The appropriate cleansing agent is dependent on the underlying etiology of the problem. Necrotic or devitalized tissue left in the wound will impede healing. A moist wound environment must be provided and maintained for healing to take place.
2. 3. Rationale: Dermatological dysfunctions are complicated and require a multifocused care plan that may include topical and systemic medications, dietary and lifestyle adjustments, and specialized procedures of multidisciplinary team members.
3. 1. Rationale: A lesion's being visually evident does not necessarily make the etiology readily identifiable.
4. 4. Rationale: There are multiple etiologies for dermatological dysfunctions and all of the possible answers are among them.
5. 2. Rationale: Photoaging is the multiple damaging effects the ultraviolet B radiation of the sun has on skin.

6. 4. Rationale: Contact dermatitis is treated upon identification of the sensitizing substance and controlling the symptoms.
7. 1. Rationale: Fungal infections, also known as tineas, are the most common dermatological problems encountered by health care professionals.
8. 2. Rationale: Rosacea has an insidious onset, develops between 30 and 50 years of age, affects more women than men, and is more common in fair-skinned persons.
9. 3. Rationale: All other answers are fabrications.
10. 4. Rationale: Pruritus is a symptom, not a disease and can accompany both healing and infection.

Chapter 46

1. 4. Rationale: Increased capillary permeability may cause hypovolemic shock in large total body surface area burns.
2. 1. Rationale: The rule of nines refers to a method used to estimate the total body surface burned.
3. 2. Rationale: A superficial partial-thickness burn includes color pink, area moist, blisters large, and pain sensation intact.
4. 4. Rationale: Absence of skin leads to loss of protective barrier against fluid loss, hypermetabolic state increases insensible fluid loss, and increased respirations raise insensible fluid loss through moisture evaporation from the lungs.
5. 1. Rationale: Wounds that appear moist and pale with sluggish capillary refill and white in color can be classified as deep partial.
6. 1. Rationale: The fluid shift in burn shock is primarily water, electrolytes, and albumin.
7. 2. Rationale: Face = 4.5; anterior chest = 18; bilateral forearms = (4.5 + 4.5) = 9; total = 31.5 or 32 percent.
8. Formula = 4 mL × % TBSA × weight in kg. 4 mL × 32% TBSA × 70 kg = 8,960 mL.
9. Half of the total volume is to be infused over the first eight hours: 8,960/2 = 4,480.
   4,480/8 = 560 mL/hour
10. Half of the total volume is to be infused over the next 16 hours.
    8,960/2 = 4,480
    4,480/16 = 280 mL/hour

Chapter 47

1. 2. Rationale: Saliva is a product of exocrine glands in the oral cavity that lubricates the mouth and begins the digestive process.
2. 4. Rationale: The spleen is the organ that is located in the left upper quadrant.
3. 3. Rationale: Acute pain in the abdomen is labeled as an acute abdomen.
4. 4. Rationale: Auscultation is performed first when performing an abdominal assessment so that the sounds produced from percussion and palpation do not alter what is auscultated.
5. 3. Rationale: Normally the liver does not descend beyond 1 to 2 cm of the costal margin and is not palpable during an assessment.
6. 3. Rationale: Conscious sedation allows patients to respond to verbal commands throughout the procedure.
7. 2. Rationale: Murphy's sign is the assessment technique that is not used to asses for ascites.
8. 3. Rationale: A positive Murphy's sign indicates an inflammatory process associated with cholecystitis.
9. 2. Rationale: The assessment technique for flexing the patient's right leg at the hip and the knee is at a right angle and then internally and externally rotating the patient's leg and observing the patient's reaction is called an obturator muscle test.
10. 4. Rationale: The low-pitched sound that is auscultated in the abdomen and caused by turbulent blood flow is called a bruit.
11. 4. Rationale: Secretin testing is used to determine if a patient has incipient chronic pancreatitis.

Chapter 48

1. 2. Rationale: The Institute of Medicine recommended 45–65 percent of calories from carbohydrate, 20–35 percent of calories from fat, and 10–35 percent of calories from protein. The ranges allow for healthy eating with a flexible approach and allow for a higher intake from fat, provided that fat intake is mostly polyunsaturated.
2. 3. Rationale: Indirect calorimetry estimates energy expenditure by measuring oxygen consumed and carbon dioxide produced. (1) A calorie count estimates food intake over a period of one to three days; (2) there is no known blood test which determines the amount of calories burned; and (4) intake and output records are normally recorded in an acute care setting and are not related to indirect calorimetry.
3. 4. Rationale: BMI Categories: Underweight = less than 18.5, Normal weight = 18.5–24.9, Overweight = 25–29.9, Obesity = BMI of 30 or greater.
4. 3. Rationale: Maintaining a consistent intake of foods high in vitamin K will help to maintain a stable INR. Increasing or decreasing intake of foods high in vitamin K can affect the blood's

clotting ability and may result in an unnecessary change in warfarin dose.

5. 2. Rationale: A "ng" feeding is a nasogastric enteral feeding in which the tube is placed from the nose to the stomach.

6. 2. Rationale: The head of the bed should be elevated 30 degrees when a patient is being fed enterally. (1) Utilizing parenteral nutrition instead of enteral nutrition does not offer fewer complications and is not indicated when the patient can be fed enterally; and (3) blenderizing foods and putting them through a tube feeding in the hospital is contraindicated because of the potential for infection, difficulty getting the correct consistency, and decreased ability to deliver adequate nutrition to the patient.

7. 1, 2, 3, and 4. Rationale: These are indications that the patient's nutritional status is improving and are not indicators of nutrition risk.

8. 1. Rationale: Prealbumin is one of the laboratory measures of visceral protein stores. 2, 3, and 4 are abnormal lab values but are not indicators of visceral protein stores.

9. 1. Rationale: Elderly people have decreased total body water, often have impaired thirst mechanisms and may have difficulty accessing adequate food and fluid.

10. 2. Rationale: Nutrition plays a vital role in the prevention of chronic disease. (1) The incidence of obesity and diabetes are both increasing; (3) poor nutrition and overweight are risk factors for developing type 2 diabetes. Type 1 diabetes is thought to be an autoimmune disease and is not correlated with body weight; and (4) lifestyle is more a factor in the development of chronic diseases such as type 2 diabetes than genetics.

Chapter 49

1. 3. Rationale: Odynophagia is the correct label for symptoms related to erosion of the esophagus.

2. 2. Rationale: Somatic pain is the correct label for GI pain that is specific to a region of the body.

3. 3. Rationale: Burning mouth syndrome is a constant burning sensation of the tongue.

4. 4. Rationale: A PEG tube is sutured in place and has complications such as bleeding, infection, or peritonitis.

5. 2. Rationale: Pain in the esophagus from esophagitis can be confused as cardiac pain.

6. 1. Rationale: GERD is characterized by heartburn after meals, some regurgitation of fluids that are foul tasting when the patient is full, and the patient often is not able to lie down comfortably just after eating.

7. 3. Rationale: A hiatal hernia is the most likely condition when the patient is pregnant and experiencing pyrosis and regurgitation after eating her meals.

8. 1. Rationale: Fresh fruits and vegetables are appropriate foods to eat when there is a family history of stomach cancer.

9. 3. Rationale: Acute episodes of diarrhea that are sudden in occurrence; after a gastric surgery is most likely dumping syndrome.

Chapter 50

1. 3. Rationale: Intussusception is due to telescoping of a loop of bowel into a lower loop of bowel.

2. 2. Rationale: Assessment of Crohn's disease would include evidence of weight loss and anemia.

3. 3. Rationale: Teaching strategies for patients who have IBS would focus on dietary modifications.

4. 3. Rationale: IBS is best described as a functional bowel disorder with no signs of pathology present.

5. 1. Rationale: Modifications in the daily diet to alleviate IBS symptoms include a high soluble fiber diet.

6. 4. Rationale: An important change in lifestyle to aid in minimizing IBS symptoms is eating slowly.

7. 3. Rationale: Acidic chime from the stomach that flows into the duodenum is neutralized by the alkaline liquid secreted from the jejunum cells.

8. 3. Rationale: Serotonin is a neurochemical mediator that has been implicated in the transmission of pain in the GI tract.

9. 2. Rationale: IBS in the United States and other developed countries is more prevalent in women.

10. 4. Rationale: IBS symptoms can exacerbate following dietary intolerances.

Chapter 51

1. 3. Rationale: The definition of gluconeogenesis is the synthesis of glucose from amino acids during times of fasting.

2. 2. Rationale: The thymus is the organ that an endoscopic retrograde cholangiopancreatography (ERCP) does not inspect.

3. 3. Rationale: Hepatitis A is an RNA virus, spread often by food handlers infected with the virus, and has an incubation time of 15 to 50 days.

4. 1. Rationale: Wilson's disease is a hereditary disease of the liver, which is an autosomal recessive disorder related to copper metabolism.

5. 3. Rationale: A management strategy for ascites associated with cirrhosis is a surgical shunt, which diverts excessive peritoneal fluid into the venous system.

6. 3. Rationale: A hepatic abscess is usually caused by bacterial infection and is referred to as pyogenic hepatic abscess.
7. 1. Rationale: The two basic types of liver cancer are labeled primary and secondary.
8. 2. Rationale: The most common reason for children to have a liver transplant is biliary atresia.
9. 3. Rationale: The diagnosis for acute pancreatitis best made with computed tomography (CT) scanning in differentiating the pancreatitis from other abdominal issues.
10. 4. Rationale: Criteria for receiving a donated liver is rigorously defined by the United Network for Organ Sharing.

Chapter 52

1. 3. Rationale: Collect a small sample of each voiding and place in a rack for comparison over time. This allows the nurse to assess changes in color and determine the presence of blood in the urine.
2. 2. Rationale: Have the patient void and discard urine, noting this as the beginning of the 24-hour urine collection. A 24-hour urine specimen is a collection of all urine produced in 24-hour period. The collection should begin with an empty bladder.
3. 1. Rationale: Hydration, administration of acetylcysteine, or administration of IV sodium bicarbonate. Hydration is vital to protection of renal function. Patients with fluid restriction may require the additional agents.
4. 3. Rationale: Report metal screening findings to the MRI department and sedate for claustrophobia before sending him or her to the MRI department. Patients with significant exposure to metal may not be able to have an MRI.
5. 2. Rationale: Discard the specimen and collect another specimen with review of instructions. This is the only way to ensure that the specimen is not contaminated.
6. 2. Rationale: Supine position, which is critical to ensure accurate results.
7. 2. Rationale: Constipation can interfere with the viewing field, which can lead to inaccurate results.
8. 3. Rationale: The kidney receives 20 percent of the cardiac output through the renal arteries that comes directly from the aorta.
9. 4. Rationale: The patient should be encouraged to force fluids not restrict fluid intake.
10. 4. Rationale: Urine culture and sensitivity, which is used to diagnose bacterial infections of the urinary tract.

Chapter 53

1. 2. Rationale: Completely empty the bladder and do not put off the urge to urinate. Fully emptying the bladder promptly discourages the incubation of bacteria in the urinary tract.
2. 1. Rationale: Common presenting symptoms for both IC and recurrent UTI include urgency, frequency, nocturia, and dysuria.
3. 1. Rationale: Urinary retention and ascending infection of the urinary tract, both of which predispose the patient to develop a bacterial infection.
4. 3. Rationale: Nephrotic syndrome, which is 15 times more common in children than in adults.
5. 3. Rationale: Pyelonephritis is an inflammation or infection of the kidney or kidney pelvis.
6. 1. Rationale: A CT scan and ultrasound are the most appropriate methods to identify the source and extent of renal trauma.
7. 2. Rationale: Removal of the diseased organ is the best approach to treat renal cancer.
8. 3. Rationale: Bladder cancer most commonly presents without pain but with gross hematuria.
9. 1. Rationale: Continent urinary diversion uses a traditional ileal conduit.
10. 4. Rationale: Functional incontinence is likely in patients with multiple sclerosis who may experience impaired mobility.

Chapter 54

1. 3. Rationale: The oliguric period in acute renal failure usually lasts one to two weeks.
2. 2. Rationale: U waves on the electrocardiogram are associated with hypokalemia.
3. 2. Rationale: Leaking of arterial blood into an AV fistula causes the veins to enlarge, so they are easier to access for hemodialysis.
4. 4. Rationale: It is imperative for the patient to maintain an adequate fluid status as evidenced by normal weight and to remain infection free. The primary nursing goal is to help the patient maintain a positive self-image and continue to be a productive member of society.
5. 3. Rationale: Pyelonephritis is an inflammation or infection of the kidney or kidney pelvis.
6. 1. Rationale: The most common findings in acute renal failure include elevations in BUN and creatinine, metabolic acidosis, hyponatremia, hyperkalemia, hypocalcemia, and hypophosphatemia.
7. 3. Rationale: Appropriate skin care for patients with uremic frost is bathing with tepid water and applying oils to reduce dryness and itching.

8. 1. Rationale: Immediate assessments to be performed for a kidney recipient are fluid and electrolyte status, intake and output, and hypotension.
9. 2. Rationale: Peritonitis is usually caused by *Staphylococcus*. The first indication of peritonitis is cloudy dialysate.
10. 4. Rationale: Peritonitis is a life-threatening complication of continuous ambulatory peritoneal dialysis, which is manifested by abdominal pain and distension, diarrhea, vomiting, and fever. Antibiotics are given as treatment not prophylactically.

Chapter 55

1. 4. Rationale: TSH is not produced by the thyroid gland.
2. 3. Rationale: The exocrine glands are responsible for secreting substances into the ducts that empty into a body cavity or onto a body surface.
3. 4. Rationale: The hypothalamus gland secretes hormones that release or inhibit hormones from the anterior pituitary gland.
4. 1. Rationale: Epinephrine and norepinephrine are the two major hormones secreted by the adrenal medulla.
5. 1. Rationale: Circadian rhythm is an example of negative feedback is seen in the relationship between insulin and blood glucose levels.
6. 1. Rationale: The PTH is regulated by negative feedback.
7. 1. Rationale: The thyroid gland is the organ in the endocrine system that consists of two lobes, connected by an isthmus, and secretes thyroxine, calcitonin, and triiodothyronine.
8. 3. Rationale: Fever, tachycardia, and restlessness are clinical manifestations of a patient having a thyroid crisis.
9. 4. Rationale: The parathyroid gland controls serum calcium.
10. 2. Rationale: A negative feedback mechanism refers to the response of a gland by increasing or decreasing the secretion of a hormone.

Chapter 56

1. 1, 3, 4. Rationale: These are the symptoms seen in a patient with acromegaly.
2. 3. Rationale: Not having a menstrual period for a year would support a diagnosis of hyperprolactinemia.
3. 1. Rationale: Patient education for a transsphenoidal hypophysectomy would include information regarding the nasal passage being packed with gauze for 24 to 48 hours.
4. 2. Rationale: Fall prevention measures are important for the nurse to anticipate when caring for a patient with hypercortisolism.
5. 3. Rationale: Patient with Addison's disease needs to know that their glucocorticoid medications need to be increased during times of illness or stress.
6. 3. Rationale: Patients with hyperprolactinemia may experience breast engorgement.
7. 2. Rationale: Patient with pheochromocytoma needs to have their blood pressure within normal limits, as this condition causes hypertension.
8. 1. Rationale: Fine hand tremor is indicative of hyperthyroidism.
9. 1. Rationale: Patient taking methimazole (Tapazole) needs to report a sore throat and fever to their health care provider.
10. 1. Rationale: Breastfeeding is contraindicated with a patient involved in radioiodine therapy for hyperthyroidism.
11. 3. Rationale: Ionized calcium is the correct therapy for changes following a parathyroidectomy that cause numbness and tingling in the tips of the fingers and around the mouth.
12. 1. Rationale: Vasopressin causes thirst to be resolved.

Chapter 57

1. 1, 2, and 3. Rationale: Clinical manifestations of type 1 diabetes are hyperglycemia, fruity odor of breath, and tachycardia.
2. 2. Rationale: The nurse knows that more teaching is needed when the patient who is mixing insulin withdraws too much NPH insulin and injects the extra back into the Lente vial.
3. 1. Rationale: $HgbA_{1C}$ is the lab test that offers the best information about glycemic control.
4. 3. Rationale: When a patient is admitted to the hospital with DKA the nurse can anticipate that 0.9% NS will be administered.
5. 1. Rationale: Regular insulin can be administered intravenously.
6. 4. Rationale: The long term management of diabetes includes the use of a glucose lowering agent, diet, and activity.
7. 1. Rationale: The primary difference between DKA and HHNS is the absence of ketosis.
8. 4. Rationale: Clinical manifestations of hypoglycemia are irritability, increasing confusion, tremors, hunger, sweating, weakness, and visual disturbances.
9. 2. Rationale: The corresponding hyperglycemia seen in the dawn phenomena results from predawn release of counter-regulatory hormones.

10. 3. Rationale: The autonomic neuropathy conditions associated with diabetic complications lead to bowel and bladder incontinence and delayed gastric emptying.

Chapter 58

1. 2. Rationale: Wolff's law states that bone forms and remodels itself in direct proportion to the amount and the direction of physical forces placed on it.
2. 4. Rationale: In a maturing child, the epiphyseal plate, or growth plate, is where active longitudinal growth occurs (until the age of maturity). If a fracture occurs in or through the epiphyseal plate, growth in that extremity can be delayed or stopped. When maturity is reached the epiphyseal plate merges the epiphysis and the metaphysis and the epiphyseal plate completely disappears.
3. 1. Rationale: Osteoblastic activity slows down between the ages of 30 and 40. After age 40, women lose approximately 8 percent of their bone mass every decade. In men the loss is 3 percent per decade.
4. 2, 4. Rationale: The main functions of skeletal muscle are to produce movement, maintain posture and body position, support soft tissues, guard entrances and exits to the digestive and urinary tracts, and to assist in maintaining body temperature.
5. 2. Rationale: During muscle contraction, the sarcoplasm reticulum releases large amounts of calcium into the vicinity of the myofibrils. This sudden rise in calcium concentration within the sarcoplasm initiates muscle contraction by removing the tropomyosin-troponin block.
6. 3. Rationale: Ligaments help to give joints stability, guide the joint movement, and prevent excess motion within the joint.
7. 1. Rationale: Classified according to the amount of movement, three classes of joints can be identified: synarthrosis (immovable), amphiarthrosis (slightly movable), and diarthrosis (freely movable).
8. 2. Rationale: When an individual seeks assistance with a musculoskeletal complaint, it is generally because the complaint has caused a limitation in movement or pain.
9. 2. Rationale: There are three basic maneuvers used in assessing the musculoskeletal system: inspection, palpation, and assessment of range of motion (passive and active).
10. 2. Rationale: When performing a NVA you should always compare one extremity to another to observe for abnormalities.

Chapter 59

1. 2. Rationale: Acetaminophen (Tylenol) and ibuprofen (Advil) are both available over-the-counter and are relatively inexpensive. The nurse corrected Mrs. Jones perception that these were prescription medications and provided additional information.
2. 2. Rationale: Alcohol and turkey contain purine, which can aggravate gout.
3. 3. Rationale: Headaches are not a symptom of Reiter's syndrome.
4. 3. Rationale: DMARDs also reduce inflammation, as do NSAIDs, and may provide relief when NSAIDs are no longer effective.
5. 1. Rationale: A bullseye rash is the classic symptom of LD.
6. 3. Rationale: Baseline screening for fibromyalgia includes an electrolyte panel and ESR as markers of the inflammatory process that is occurring.
7. 1. Rationale: Spinal stenosis causes a narrowing of the spinal column where the nerves exit. Pressure on the nerves results in pain.
8. 4. Rationale: Small joint involvement is common in rheumatoid arthritis. All the other symptoms are seen in osteoarthritis but not rheumatoid arthritis.
9. 1. Rationale: A baseline assessment of neurological signs is made so that deviation from the database can be noted. Once a pain assessment is complete, a plan for pain management can be developed.
10. 3. Rationale: High dosage or long-term use of corticosteroids is associated with the development of gastric ulcers.

Chapter 60

1. 4. Rationale: Installing grab bars and hand rails on both sides of stairs along with improving the lighting in and around the house can decrease the risk of falling.
2. 3. Rationale: The signs and symptoms of a fracture include ecchymosis, edema, deformity, other soft tissue injury, muscle spasms, tenderness, pain, numbness, loss of function, abnormal movement, or crepitus.
3. 1. Rationale: The purpose of immobilizing or splinting the fractured limb is to minimize bleeding, edema, pain, and prevent further injury to the tissues and structures surrounding the fracture. Complications from improper handling or splinting can include increase bleeding, a significant increase in pain, and a

decrease in sensation and function, which may be temporary or permanent. The incidence of fat embolism and shock are also increased.

4. 4. Rationale: The patient may not bear weight on the cast until it is fully dry. For a plaster cast this is about 48 hours after application.

5. 1. Rationale: Fiberglass casts dry within 30 minutes of application.

6. 4. Rationale: Signs and symptoms of an infection under a cast include odor, purulent drainage, and areas of the cast that are warmer than other areas (hot spots).

7. 3. Rationale: FES is more prevalent in patients who have sustained long bone fractures, fractures of the ribs and pelvis, or multiple fractures.

8. 2. Rationale: The signs and symptoms of FES are hypoxemia, changes in mental status, petechiae on the upper body, seizures, use of accessory muscles, tachypnea, dyspnea, restlessness, apprehension, anxiety, agitation, or confusion.

9. 4. Rationale: These symptoms occur early in the disease process. The others listed (pulselessness, pallor, inability to move joints, and swelling) are late signs, and fever and erythema are indicative of an infection.

10. 1. Rationale: This test is less invasive than a pulmonary angiogram and is readily available.

11. 2. Rationale: This should be avoided, because it might cause a flexion contracture of the extremity.

Chapter 61

1. 2. Rationale: Sperm generation in the male is dependent on testosterone production, which is mediated by FSH and LH.

2. 3. Rationale: Menstruation is the result of decreasing production of estrogen and progesterone by the corpus luteum.

3. 1. Rationale: In both the male and female body, the fundamental physiological responses to effective sexual stimulation are vasocongestion and muscle tension (myotonia).

4. 4. Rationale: All of the answers are correct.

5. 4. Rationale: That question does not pertain to any prospective that might help a health care provider assess a medical situation.

6. 1. Rationale: The symptom commonly associated with sexually transmitted infections in the male is penile discharge with pain on urination.

7. 3. Rationale: The question "Violence is a problem for many women. Has someone been hurting you"? is a very important question to ask.

8. 4. Rationale: The description of vaginal discharge that is indicative of possible bacterial vaginosis is that it is copious, gray, malodorous, or "fishy" odor discharge.

9. 1. Rationale: The diagnostic tests recommended to evaluate the nodule are prostate ultrasonography, biopsy of nodule, and PSA.

10. 1. Rationale: The Pap smear examines the transformation zone between columnar epithelial cells of the cervical canal and the squamous cells covering the outer cervix.

11. 4. Rationale: The rationale for teaching an 18-year-old male how to perform self-examination of his genitals is that testicular cancer is the most common type of cancer in young men.

12. 3. Rationale: It is the best response for a female patient that has indicated she has sex with multiple partners and she does not use condoms, because she is on oral contraceptives.

Chapter 62

1. 4. Rationale: Nonprescription relief measures for dysmenorrhea include heat, exercise, and NSAIDs.

2. 3. Rationale: Dysmenorrhea that is suddenly worse may indicate the presence of endometriosis, fibroids, ovarian cysts, or infection.

3. 1. Rationale: The health implications for PCOS are insulin resistance leading to glucose intolerance and diabetes, infertility, and hyperlipidemia.

4. 2. Rationale: Weight reduction is the first priority in the management of PCOS.

5. 5. Rationale: Women experiencing vasomotor symptoms of menopause may be helped by the following interventions: wearing layered clothing, reducing the environmental temperature, increased exercise, weight reduction, smoking cessation if applicable, and relaxation techniques.

6. 3. Rationale: The most common serious complication of untreated chlamydia is infertility associated with tubal infection.

7. 5. Rationale: Educational messages for women with a diagnosis of an STD should include the following concepts:

- The only way to completely prevent transmission of STD is to abstain from sex.
- Condoms provide some protection against STDs but must be used consistently and correctly.
- Condoms are most effective in preventing infections such as human immunodeficiency virus (HIV), gonorrhea, chlamydia, and trichomoniasis transmitted by contact with mucous membranes. They are less effective in preventing those infections transmitted by skin contact, such as herpes simplex virus (HSV), human papillomavirus (HPV), and syphilis.
- If one STD is diagnosed, infection with another STD is likely and testing for all STDs is advised.

- It is important to take all the prescribed antibiotics, even after symptoms resolve.
- It is important not to have any sexual contact with an untreated infected partner.
- It is important to keep follow-up appointments.

8. 4. Rationale: Fibroids are the most common reason for hysterectomy.

9. 4. Rationale: Didelphic reproductive anomalies are generally associated with normal pregnancy outcomes, as long as there are two functional uteri, cervices, and vaginas that communicate to the outside.

10. 1. Rationale: The initial workup for infertility should include a semen analysis and charting of BBT to diagnose ovulation.

11. 4. Rationale: HPV is the virus associated with cervical cancer.

12. 3. Rationale: The decline in cervical cancer incidence is directly related to the increased use of Pap smear screening.

13. 2. Rationale: The BRCA1 and BRCA2 genes are associated with an increased risk of ovarian cancer.

14. 3. Rationale: Endometrial cancer is the most common reproductive cancer in women.

15. 1. Rationale: Urinary complications are the most common complications of FGM.

16. 4. Rationale: Lack of libido is the most common sexual dysfunction.

Chapter 63

1. 3. Rationale: The other acronyms are not hormones that act on the breast.

2. 2. Rationale: Women should be examined in the upright and supine positions; dimpling is best detected with the woman raising both arms over her head; and palpation of the breasts begins with the lymph nodes.

3. 2. Rationale: Bleeding from the nipples can be caused by trauma including fissures, as well as malignancy; fissures are associated with nipple trauma during suckling and increase the risk of mastitis; and discharge from the nipples is only normal during lactation and rarely, as a result of strong massage. Therefore, discharge under other circumstances needs to be evaluated by a health care professional.

4. 2. Rationale: Fibrocystic breast changes are typically fluid-filled cysts within the breasts; intraductal papillomas occur mainly in women between the ages of 25 and 55; and mastitis occurs primarily within the first three months after childbirth.

5. 3. Rationale: Personal or first-degree family history of any cancer is correlated with increased risk for breast cancer; exposure to various environmental pollutants such as pesticides that have chemical similarities to estrogen may behave like estrogen, increasing risk of breast cancer; and hormones are thought to increase breast cancer by effecting cell proliferation, causing DNA damage and promoting cell growth.

6. 1. Rationale: FNA biopsy of nonpalpable lesions is less useful because of sampling error; the vast majority of open biopsies are performed with either local anesthesia alone or local anesthesia with intravenous sedation; and stereotactic mammography-guided biopsy is performed only if the lesion is not visualized ultrasonographically.

7. 2. Rationale: Ductoscopy is employed to directly visualize the ductal lining of the breast; it is being evaluated for use with high-risk patients; and it is being evaluated for use in resection.

8. 3. Rationale: Lumpectomy is a wide local excision or partial mastectomy. All other procedures listed involve removal of the entire breast.

9. 3. Rationale: The histological status of the axillary nodes is the single most important predictor of outcome for breast cancer patients.

10. 2. Rationale: Cost comparisons were not provided in the chapter; fewer office visits and additional surgical interventions refers to breast reconstruction not breast augmentation; and saline implants have not been in use long enough to know how long they will last, but they may need to be replaced after 10 years.

Chapter 64

1. 2. Rationale: Prostatitis is diagnosed by culturing spontaneous or expressed urethral discharge or prostate fluid.

2. 1. Rationale: TUMP is an alternative treatment that heats the prostate tissue.

3. 3. Rationale: At least two separate biopsy specimens are graded based on their differentiation from normal prostate cells.

4. 4. Rationale: Antibiotics are normally given in the management of orchitis.

5. 4. Rationale: A varicocele can be removed with surgery and is managed this way if the patient is experiencing discomfort.

6. 1. Rationale: Balanitis is usually caused by a bacterial infection.

7. 3. Rationale: A urethral stricture has a main symptom of difficulty voiding and a noticeably decreased urine stream.

8. 3. Rationale: The goal of penile cancer treatment is to remove the tumor as soon as it is detected.
9. 2. Rationale: Parasympathetic nerve impulses and hormones work together to cause the penis to become firm in an erection.
10. 3. Rationale: Priapism is differentiated with the use of Doppler flow studies.

Chapter 65

1. 1. Rationale: Biological mediators produce increased capillary permeability.
2. 4. Rationale: Hypovolemic shock state is produced by the third spacing of fluids.
3. 4. Rationale: Manifestations of anaphylactic shock include stridor and wheezing.
4. 2. Rationale: The cardiovascular system is the most common organ system to fail in severe sepsis.
5. 3. Rationale: The primary purpose for providing crystalloid solutions is to restore fluid volumes and increase preload.
6. 2. Rationale: DIC plays a role in the inflammatory process by decreasing oxygen supplies to cells.
7. 4. Rationale: A urine output of 225 cc per hour is the manifestation that would indicate a reversal of the shock process.
8. 3. Rationale: Congestive heart failure places an individual at the greatest risk for developing MODS.
9. 4. Rationale: Maximizing optimal cardiac output is the most important factor for increasing oxygen supply.
10. 3. Rationale: Noncardiogenic-pulmonary edema may result from alterations in the alveolar-capillary membrane.

Chapter 66

1. 5. Rationale: Biological weapons may cause mass casualties. They are easy to produce and inexpensive. Currently, biological weapons cannot be easily detected and may disseminated over large areas.
2. 2. Rationale: Smallpox develops as a centrifugal rash.
3. 2. Rationale: Many agents are contagious and require contact or respiratory precautions.
4. 3. Rationale: A patient with severe life-threatening injuries who most likely will not survive would be triaged as black.
5. 3. Rationale: People still experiencing stress reactions after 3 months should seek medical or psychological follow-up.
6. 2. Rationale: Not all individuals who experience a traumatic event will suffer from PTSD.
7. 1. Rationale: Airborne precautions are used when the patient is coughing, and the suspected organism is small in diameter.
8. 3. Rationale: All other answers are true.
9. 3. Rationale: Pneumonic plague occurs because of bacteria.
10. 2. Rationale: Triage is the act of prioritizing the patient's priority of care.
11. 2. Rationale: Patients with insecticide on them are considered to be contaminated with a hazardous chemical and require decontamination. Patients with hazardous materials on them who enter an emergency department may expose everyone to a potential harmful chemical.
12. 2. Rationale: SARS is contagious.

Review Activities Answers

Chapter 1

1. This activity provides insight into the kinds of legislation that may directly or indirectly impact health care or nursing practice.
2. This activity assists the reader to gain understanding about how legislators inform the positions they take on health care bills.
3. Nurses observe shortcomings of the health care system 24/7 and are in an excellent position to identify "what if" situations. An innovation in health care delivery could be born out of this brainstorming activity.
4. It is not unusual for someone to "dump" feelings of anger, frustration, fear, or fatigue from an object of high risk for retribution to an object of lower risk for retribution. Those objects may be quite independent of each other. We all need to step back from negative situations and examine what might be influencing the negative behavior.
5. Some state boards of nursing and attorneys general take punitive action against nurses who are chemically dependent, and other states consider chemical dependence to be an illness and provide supportive assistance toward recovery. Such support may include a recovery program and long-term random testing.

Chapter 2

1. There is no specific solution to this activity, because the reader is free to pursue a questionable practice from the reader's clinical experience. The reader might choose to look for research evidence that raising the upper half of side rails is just as effective at preventing patient falls as raising the entire side rail. The activity is meant to provoke skepticism in the reader about the effectiveness of a nursing intervention and engender a spirit of curiosity about whether the activity is supported by evidence that can be found in a rigorous database.
2. Similarly, there is no specific solution to this activity, because the reader is directed to choose the topic. The activity is meant to demonstrate whether there is congruence between the databases on any identical topic.
3. A conclusion that the reader might draw is that one database is more useful to the nurse than the other. Such usefulness might be based on the breadth of subjects included, the clarity of the content, or the transferability of the content to practice.
4. If the reader finds the site useful a decision about whether a change in personal practice or a change in the practice guidelines of a health care enterprise is indicated. If a change is indicated based on solid scientific evidence, the reader will need to consider how best to implement the change.
5. It is anticipated that the reader will become aware of the value of evidence for improving nursing practice and of the potential impact that an individual nurse might make in the application of knowledge for nursing practice.

Chapter 3

1. Cognitive domain: patient understanding how the kidneys work

   Affective domain: patient having a caring attitude toward his or her spouse who is ill

   Psychomotor domain: patient is able to change his or her ostomy appliance without assistance
2. Anxiety, anger, pain, and fatigue are four barriers to learning. The following are the interventions for each:

   Anxiety: inform the patient that the surgery will cure his or her inflammation of the appendix

   Anger: allow the patient to vent his or her emotions regarding his or her new diagnosis of cancer

   Pain: ask the patient to rate his or her pain from 0 to 10

   Fatigue: schedule rest periods every hour so the patient can recover from his or her malaise

3. A combination of teaching methods increases the potential for learning.
4. Student will self-reflect on his or her own learning needs.
5. Student will develop a flow sheet that diagrams a simple teaching plan for a patient in the clinical setting
6. The student should choose two learning needs of a patient in his or her clinical setting and describe interventions for each learning need.
7. The nursing implications for Maslow are based on identifying the priority of the patient needs. This allows the nurse to set priorities and to seek interventions that will most benefit the patient.
8. The student will interview another student and ask if there is a relationship between any physical manifestations and his or her attitudes. In addition, the student will ask the peer if he or she feels better physically when he or she is mentally relaxed or vice versa.
9. The student will interview five people and ask them how they know when they are healthy. The student will also list the determinants of their health.
10. The student will list those things that motivate him or her regarding choosing healthy behaviors. In addition, the student will reflect on how these factors can assist him or her working with patients in health promotive interventions.

Chapter 4

1. Culture refers to knowledge, beliefs, behaviors, ideas, attitudes, values, habits, customs, languages, symbols, rituals, ceremonies, and practices that are unique to a particular group of people. Ethnicity, on the other hand, is a cultural group's perception of themselves or group identity. This self-perception influences how others perceive the group's members.
2. The factors that contribute to the multiculturalism environment in the United States revolve primarily around the fact that the U.S. population has shown an increase in ethnic and racial diversity during the last half of the 20th century, especially in the last three decades. Immigration from Latin America, Asia, and the Pacific Islands has contributed to the growing U.S. diversity. The population of races that are different from the Caucasian or African American populations has demonstrated significant growth, but Caucasians continue to be the most numerous race. In addition, Hispanic (Americans) are the fastest growing ethnic minority, having more than doubled from 1980 to 2000. Factors that contribute to the tremendous growth include high levels of immigration and high fertility levels. Also, the percentage of Asian (American) and Pacific Islander populations more than doubled to 3.8 percent in 2000. The Caucasian population has shown a noticeable proportional decrease in the total U.S. population. Last, the 2000 census was the first time that individuals were allowed to identify themselves as being of more than one race.
3. Discuss how a nurse can provide culturally and linguistically competent nursing care. Even when both patient and nurse speak the same language, communication problems may occur because of varying cultural contexts in which words have different meanings to different people. Therefore, the nurse needs to be aware of all aspects of communication among cultures. Also, utilizing a qualified interpreter is imperative to achieving communication when the nurse and patient do not speak the same language, regardless of the practice domain or site. In addition, the nurse must remember that nonverbal communication can be culturally misunderstood through the presence, or absence, of eye contact.
4. This is best applied in the practicum and laboratory settings. You can refer to an assessment text and develop questions to ask patients. In addition, you can discuss the topic with peers and work on the questions together.
5. This is best applied in the practicum and laboratory settings. You can refer to an assessment text and develop questions to ask patients. In addition, you can discuss the topic with peers and work on the questions together.
6. This is best applied by exploring the Web site provided (i.e., http://erc.msh.org) to learn more about Kleinman's explanatory health model. After visiting the Web site develop questions that could have been asked of the Hmong family described in *The spirit catches you and you fall down* by Ann Fadiman (1997).

Chapter 5

1. Implemented by contacting the chairperson of an IRB and discussing your impressions in class.
2. Implemented by contacting the chairperson of an ethics committee and discussing your impressions in class.
3. Performed in the practicum setting with the identification of an ethical dilemma and an appropriate ethical theory.
4. Evaluated by obtaining a copy of advanced directives, completing the form, and sharing your emotional thoughts related to filling out the form with your classmates.

5. Active euthanasia would support a person other than the patient to make the decision of do-not-resuscitate the patient. This is in contrast with passive euthanasia, which would withhold resuscitative measures from a patient who is in the terminal stages of physical life. The passive euthanasia would honor the patient's request to withhold lifesaving measures, but health care providers would not intentionally withhold treatment against the patient's desires.

Chapter 6

1. Best accomplished by accessing the Robert Havinghurst information at: http://personalwebs.oakland.edu and then interviewing a middle-aged or older adult who has or had siblings and summarizing the findings. The student will examine the interview related to the birth order of the siblings of the interviewee, the four stages of life, and the aspects of sibling relationships into the adult years.
2. Best accomplished by accessing the body mass index (BMI) measuring instrument at: http://www.consumer.gov/weightloss.bmi.htm. The BMI is calculated and then identify the risk factors you may have. In addition, determine the BMI of a family member and compare those risk factors with your own.
3. Best applied by accessing the Activity Pyramid at: http://www.mypyramid.gov/pyramid. Then design an exercise program for the inactive individual and include how to overcome potential barriers to an exercise program, such as lack of time, no convenient access to exercise center, etc.
4. Accomplished at the Activity Pyramid site, and reviewing all the topics inside the pyramid. Review the information for kids, for professionals, and my pyramid tracker and review the new dietary pyramid guidelines. Plan a menu for one day for you that meets the guidelines.
5. Best accomplished by locating the tool kit to prevent senior falls provided by the National Center for Injury and Prevention and Control at: http://www.cdc.gov/ncipc. In addition, an interview with a friend or family member who is living independently in the community is performed. And the tool kit to assess vision and balance capability is performed. Identify whether there is any assistance needed, if any, for accomplishing activities of daily living or impaired activities of daily living. Explore what safety features should be addressed in the home environment as addressed in the tool kit guidelines.
6. Applied by reviewing the tips for care of aging parents provided by the National Safety Council at http://www.nsc.org. A poster is prepared using these tips and presenting the information to a small community group (such as a church group or parent-teacher association [PTA]).
7. Accomplished by reviewing the techniques to improve patient safety (TIPS) provided by the Joint Commission Resources at: http://www.doody.com/TIPS and clicking on Obese Patients. Then a summary report of the strategies is written.
8. Best performed by accessing one of the resources and writing a brief report on the mission or services provided.

Chapter 7

1. If the nurse has been employed at the enterprise for several years, a variety of hospice and palliative care situations have probably been experienced, some particularly rewarding and perhaps others that have been quite challenging. There are patients or families who stand out in every nurse's memory, but those who stand out for the hospice and palliative care nurse may do so for reasons that are different from your experiences. Because students do not generally have an opportunity for clinical experience in a hospice or palliative care setting, learning about that aspect of nursing from someone who may feel passionately about the care could spark your interest in a unique area of practice.
2. If you choose to access a site providing health care policy information, you may discover that something you or your colleagues do routinely is actually regulated. Such a discovery ought to provoke a change in your practice or that of those nurse colleagues with whom you may share the information. In addition, your interest in health care policy may be sparked, and you may venture into the political advocacy arena.
3. One of the most advantageous ways to learn about ethnic and religious beliefs is through the firsthand application of those who hold them. Nuances, variations from region to region, and experiences that have shaped the actual practice of someone you know can put "life" into what otherwise might be considered irrelevant concepts. Consideration of others' beliefs and practices in comparison to your own might also suggest interesting practices that you may try out.

   Understanding the rationale for people's beliefs and behaviors directly from them may help you to better respect their diversity.

4. Patients and families who have a long track record of open or closed communication tend to continue that communication pattern during end-of-life interaction. If you observe closed communication that could be regretted after death, it would be appropriate for you to consult your care team colleagues and include interventions by an expert to try to support more open communication between the patient and the family.
5. The Jehovah's Witnesses forbade organ transplant in 1967 but reversed that decision in 1980. Organ transplant and organ donations are considered matters of individual choice. There is no biblical injunction against taking in body tissue or bone as there is against taking in blood.

Chapter 8

1. Health perception/health management pattern: 4, 10
   Nutrition metabolic pattern: 6
   Elimination pattern: 5
   Activity-exercise pattern: 2, 3, 7
   Sleep-rest pattern: 4
   Self-perception/self-concept pattern: 4
   Role-relationship pattern: 1, 8
   Sexuality/reproductive pattern: 1
   Coping/stress tolerance pattern: 4, 8
   Value/belief pattern: 9
2. O: "What brings you to the clinic today?"

   O: "I spoke with your primary care physician who made the referral for your hospital admission."

   W: "The last time we met, you told me you were on a diet. I see that your clothes fit much looser and that your face appears thinner. How much weight have you lost?"

   C: "I have completed the physical examination and our time is about up."
3. Open ended: "How many children do you have?"
   Open ended: "How what are your thoughts about having surgery?"
   Open ended: "What questions do you have about your new medication?"
4. The issue is her unwillingness to allow her family to be informed. The primary duty of the nurse is to the patient and to protecting her confidentiality. Professional code of conduct: If the potential for harm to another is serious, this confidentiality may be breached. A prudent and professional approach for the nurse is to explore the reasons for withholding this information from her siblings

Chapter 9

1. The nurse could explain to Martha the CF is an autosomal recessive inherited condition. Because Martha's sister has had a child with CF she is a carrier. This means that Martha's chance to be a carrier is increased (one in two chance). It would be appropriate to discuss with Martha that carrier testing for CF are available to help further define Martha's actual carrier status. If Martha decides to have carrier testing for CF and is found to be a carrier, then carrier testing would be offered to her husband. If both Martha and her husband are identified to be CF carriers, then prenatal diagnosis (e.g., amniocentesis) would be discussed. In this situation, the nurse's role is identifying individuals for whom genetic testing is available and referring individuals for genetic testing.
2. Because Mrs. R. is 35 years old, she has a higher risk for having a baby born with a chromosomal abnormality, such as Down syndrome. It would be appropriate to discuss prenatal diagnosis, such as amniocentesis. Before talking with Mrs. R. about her increased chance to have a baby with a chromosomal abnormality and the availability of prenatal diagnosis, the nurse would want to assess Mrs. R's health beliefs—how she views pregnancy, prenatal testing, and disability—whether prenatal testing is something she would consider. You could provide her with information about maternal age risks and prenatal testing in Spanish and refer her to Web sites with culturally appropriate descriptions of the testing.
3. Ann's personal and family history of depression suggests that this condition is inherited in an autosomal dominant manner with affected individuals in multiple generations. Ann is referring to pharmacogenomic testing—testing an individual to determine their particular genotype before prescribing a particular medication at a particular dose. You could respond to Ann by explaining that pharmacogenomic testing is increasingly available to individualize treatment and avoid adverse effects. You could refer Ann to her psychiatrist for further discussion about specific testing that would be appropriate for her.
4. You could explain to Susan that the constellation of congenital heart defects, cleft palate, and learning and speech issues in multiple generations does suggest the possibility of an inherited genetic condition or syndrome. You could offer Susan a referral to a geneticist for further genetic evaluation and counseling to determine whether there is an identifiable genetic condition in the

family and whether diagnostic and prenatal diagnostic testing is available to Susan.

5. Jane's family history of early-onset breast and ovarian cancer suggest the presence of a hereditary breast or ovarian cancer syndrome that is inherited in the family in an autosomal dominant manner. As the nurse practitioner, you could explain to Jane that genetic testing for hereditary breast ovarian cancer is now available to individuals and families at increased risk. You could offer Jane a referral for further genetic evaluation and counseling so that she can have the option to pursue genetic testing for hereditary breast or ovarian cancer.

Chapter 10

1. It is important to emphasize to the patient that there are common responses to stress, particularly as related to a crisis such as cancer. Describe that some of the potential physiological responses are increased heart rate, heart palpitations, diaphoresis, and rapid respirations. Educate the patient that some of the potential psychological responses are depression, worry, frustration, anger, and anxiety. In addition, explain that elderly patients are particularly prone to confusion.
2. Identifying the role of caregiver stress is essential for the family providing care to an elderly relative. Explain that stress causes a wide range of physiological and psychological as described in activity 1 and that the care providers should first accept these responses. Then describe to the family the need to adapt to their stress responses and identify constructive coping mechanisms to their stress.
3. From Orem's theory, explain that the recent surgery has caused stress, and encourage the patient to self-evaluate the surrounding stressors and the environment. Assist the patient in identifying the necessity for understanding what elements of the situation are under the patient's control. Encourage the patient to carefully follow the suggested nursing interventions that can effectively reduce stress. In addition, the nurse needs to consider the patient's self-care needs when providing patient education and implementing the plan of care.
4. Student evaluates stress level and develops a written plan for reducing stress.
5. Student evaluates their interview with a peer and writes an evaluation of the effectiveness of their coping strategies.

Chapter 11

1. This will be accomplished in student's clinical practice.
2. This will be accomplished in student's clinical practice.
3. This will be accomplished in student's clinical practice.
4. The following guidelines are to be followed when caring for any patient:
   - Nonsterile gloves must be worn when touching any body fluid, secretions, or contaminated items. Hands must be washed after removing the gloves.
   - Masks, eye protection, and face shields should be used when there is a possibility of splashes or sprays of body fluids reaching the face of the health care worker. The level of protection is determined by the degree of exposure expected.
   - Gowns should be worn to protect the health care person's skin and clothing when exposure to blood, body fluids, secretions, or excretions. The gown is to be removed prior to leaving the patient's room, and hands should be washed after removal of the gown.
   - Patient care equipment exposed to body fluids or excretions should be handled so that any contamination is removed prior to use with another patient.
   - Each facility must have procedures for the cleaning of all equipment and environmental surfaces.
   - Linens should be handled, transported, and then cleaned to prevent transfer of possible organisms to others. Adequate laundry facilities will be sufficient to destroy any possible pathogens.
   - All sharp instruments must be handled in a way to prevent injury to any person. Needles are not removed from syringes after use and are placed in a puncture-proof container.
   - Sharp instruments must be cleaned and disposed of with care.
5. a. The nurse should survey the skin of the wound area for: signs of inflammation, the type of drainage, the size, and depth of wound.
   b. The nurse should monitor the appropriate laboratory tests to monitor the process of wound healing (e.g., white blood cells/differential counts, hemoglobin/hematocrit levels, wound culture).
   c. Ensure appropriate nutrition that is vital to promoting wound healing. Protein is needed to supply the amino acids required to build new tissue.

d. Maintain a moist environment that encourages reepitheliazation and wound healing.
e. Mechanical debridement when the amount of nonviable tissue in the wound is minimal.
f. To maintain optimal conditions for wound healing, care must be taken to prevent further injury.

Chapter 12

1. One liter of fluid weighs one kilogram. A diuresis of 2,500 mL will be evidenced by a weight loss of approximately 2.5 kg. The weight today will be 59.5 kg.
2. Answers vary based on patient selected.
3. Patients with fluid volume deficit need isotonic fluid replacement. Appropriate intravenous (IV) solutions include normal saline and Ringer's lactate.
4. Patients with increased secretion of ADH will have retention of water and reduced urine output. The retention of water will dilute the bloodstream and will be indicated by a low serum osmolality and hyponatremia.
5. A patient with intracellular dehydration needs hypotonic IV solutions. This will make the extracellular fluid compartment hypotonic in relation to a concentrated intracellular space. As a result, fluid will shift from the extracellular space into the intracellular compartment correcting the intracellular dehydration.

Chapter 13

1. Practice demonstrating in a laboratory setting and then apply setting up intravenous (IV) infusion equipment in the practicum setting.
2. Infiltration is caused from fluid leaking into the interstitial space, and it causes swelling, pain, skin pallor, and coolness to touch. Phlebitis is caused by something that inflames the vein and has clinical manifestations of swelling, pain, skin redness, and warmth.
3. Correctly and accurately setting the IV rate is done first by practicing the skills in the laboratory setting and then applied in the practicum setting. The nurse preceptor or clinical faculty person should supervise the process.
4. Patients are indicated for TPN when they are not able to either mechanically eat enough to be well nourished or who are malnourished from a disease process. In addition, patients who are indicated for TPN are also those who have poor swallowing abilities and those who have some type of neurological deficiency.
5. This is evaluated in the clinical practicum setting and should be done under the supervision of the clinical faculty or nurse preceptor.

Chapter 14

1. The students will be able to know how the individual perceives acupuncture as a means to promote health or ease symptoms of illness.
2. The activity will provide new insight to the purpose of physical therapy, especially the use of therapeutic massage. Preparation of the report will assist the student to reflect on the experience, use communication skills during the interview, analyze the article(s), and practice writing skills in preparing the report.
3. This activity involves critical thinking and problem-solving skills as well as creative thinking skills in developing the case study and designing a holistic patient-centered care plan.
4. This activity involves the student in actively investigating the items that are available to the public. It also involves research to determine what interactions, if any, between the product ingredients and medications and food. Creating the poster and considering how it would create awareness is an appropriate teaching/learning strategy for fellow students or a public group.
5. The student will learn to develop appropriate questions to use in an informal survey and will be able to obtain information about the use of CAM. Higher level cognitive skills will be used in analyzing the findings. Preparing the report involves the use of critical thinking and communication skills.

Chapter 15

1. Many times the woman's activities focus around taking care of others and assuming roles as wife, mother, and possibly an employee. The woman now becomes a patient. Examine the impact of the cancer care waiting times, such as in clinics or doctors offices. Examine the effects of fatigue on running a household and taking kids to after school activities. For the woman, the usual patterns are gone, and role reversal occurs from caretaker to patient. It might help to tell others; even though the public's understanding of cancer is generally improving, some prejudices and wariness remain and she may be concerned about this for her spouse and children. Problems that occur within any family can be the most difficult to handle simply, because she cannot go home to escape them. Some family members may deny the reality of

cancer or refuse to discuss it. Her children may be asked also to behave exceptionally well, to play quietly, or contribute to household chores. The children may receive less attention, and some will fear the loss of their parent. It may help if a favorite relative or family friend can devote extra time and attention to the children, who need comfort and reassurance, affection, guidance, and discipline.

2. Effective communication is a critical skill for nurses. Nurses also need to assume responsibility for lifelong learning. Effective communication using multiple techniques expands options for continuing learning and for communicating with patients when they are outside of the clinical setting. Good communication facilitates groups and individuals sharing their ideas and experiences. E-mail, teleconferencing, and videoconferencing help to bridge some of the geographical barriers, but nurses need to become comfortable in using these tools. Identify a group, such as a class team or course section. Group members can lead review and response to selected topics in a threaded discussion format. Examples: prepare an environmental assessment of a local environment. The activity can include a comparative evaluation of the relative toxicity of common household products or selected chemotherapeutic agents the nurse may encounter on the unit. Discussion points: Using material safety data sheets (MSDS) available from the Internet; product inserts; poison control information service; include opportunities for interpretation and understanding of graphical and statistical information.

   How can we overcome the barriers or obstacles that stand in the way of pursuing good health habits and medical screening or intervention? Post a cancer case study, pose questions; accurate answers or creative problem solving questions earn points or awards. Issues: health beliefs and practices are intertwined intimately with cultural and familial traditions, how might this effect screening and early detection of breast and cervical cancer. Much emphasis of cancer care is related to screening for early detection. Many in our society have limited health care access, does this create discrimination of service. Access is more than availability. Access includes consideration of distance, trust, and cost. How might these situations impact a woman needing annual breast cancer screening?

3. Preparation is the key to a successful work reentry. Reintegration planning includes consideration of the patient, the family, and the employer.

   For the patient: have the patient keep a log so that he has some idea of how long he can tolerate activity and begin with brief time intervals at the job. Discuss how he will handle coworkers' reactions to any changes in appearance. Discuss plans for protection of exposure to office communicable illnesses. Allow time for patient to discuss concerns about returning.

   Employer: Offer to have someone from the care team contact the employer to respond to concerns. Possible work concerns: effect of medication on performance; any behavior changes from medication or treatment; anticipated physical tolerance; contact plan in case of complications; what to do if health issues occur at work; special considerations needed for return. The employee may benefit from flextime, job sharing, or telecommuting.

   Family: Talk with the family early on about the importance of communicating with friends, coworkers, and the employer during the course of the illness, so they are ready to transition the patient back. Family should have a clear contact plan that they can share if they need to be contacted suddenly on the patient's return. Other planning topics for discussion: observing for signs and symptoms of fatigue of side effects; fears they may have about the patient's ability to return to activities of daily living; and planning for dietary or treatment needs during the work shift.

4. Some risk factors for cancer (like family history) are out of your control, but you can control some of the important risk factors for most types of cancer, such as your exposure to sunlight and tanning beds. Research supports that ultraviolet (UV) light damages the deoxyribonucleic acid (DNA) in cells. Usually body repairs this damage but occasionally a cell mutates during the repair process, accumulation of these mutated cells can result in cancer.

   Fun in the sun: UV exposure; controllable; tanning beds versus outdoor exposure; skin and eye issues; sunscreens. Severe sunburn increases your risk of developing melanoma. In fact, five doses of sunburn while you are young can double your risk of developing this deadly disease later in life. Mild sunburn or tanning is also not acceptable. Myth: tanning bed exposure is safe, if you do not burn you do not do damage. There is no safe way to expose yourself to the sun without increasing your risk of skin cancer. It is actually worse to go to the tanning parlor and get a little bit each day than it is to get infrequent sunburn. Myth: if you use sunscreen you will not get skin cancer. Sunscreens are useful in reducing skin cancer risk, but they can not provide total protection from UV rays. Sunscreen is not a substitute for seeking shade, wearing protective clothing and avoiding the midday sun, when rays are strongest. In addition, sunscreen is not recommended for infants under six months of age. Skin cancer is not sexy.

Cigarette ads. Facts: Smoking causes lung cancer. As soon as you stop smoking, your risk of lung cancer starts to go down; smoking is a risk factor for all cancers associated with the larynx, oral cavity, and esophagus. Myth: smoking pipes and cigars is OK. Fact: other forms of tobacco, such as cigars, chewing tobacco, and snuff can also cause cancer; like cigarette smoking, the risks from cigar smoking increase with increased exposure. Myth: smoking low tar cigarettes is safe. Fact: research shows that people who cut back, or switch to low tar cigarettes, may often inhale more deeply and can be just as addicted to nicotine as people who smoke more; filtered and low tar cigarettes might reduce risk slightly, but most smokers cancel this out by taking more puffs, deeper puffs or smoking more cigarettes. If you smoke with your buddies, be prepared to die of cancer with your buddies.

5. This is best applied in the practicum setting by providing care for a patient with cancer. Journal your thoughts and discuss your reflections with peers in clinical seminar and laboratory settings.

Chapter 16

The activities have been structured around World Wide Web sites to encourage the reader to actively research the many resources that are available. Some of the Web sites have interactive programs. Some of the materials can be downloaded free of charge and can be used as patient instructional materials. The various activities also stimulate critical thinking and can easily be used as individual or group assignments as part of the course requirements or as extra-activities.

Chapter 17

1. Digoxin: Highly protein bound and has many drug-to-drug interactions. If given with warfarin (Coumadin, also highly protein bound), the amount of free drug is increased, and both drugs can produce adverse effects because of changes in their levels. Changes in nutritional status (decrease in albumin and decreases receptor sites) and electrolytes can affect drug levels.

   Tetracycline: Avoid administration with milk products, because it will form inactive compounds. Administer on an empty stomach. Use with caution in patients with renal impairment.
2. Develop a nursing care plan for a patient with emphasis on pharmacological interventions. Discuss the clinical manifestations of a specific medical disorder, such as congestive heart failure. Identify the selected medications used (digoxin and furosemide [Lasix]), baseline laboratory monitoring (electrolytes and renal function), informed consent and medication teaching, first dose monitoring (hypotension), and evaluation (improvement in lung sounds, respiratory effort, and edema).
3. Set up scenario for student that includes a patient (put an armband on the patient), a medication administration record (MAR), and a medication. Student should demonstrate getting the medication, checking the label, and then checking it against the MAR. The MAR should be taken to the patient, the MAR checked with the patient armband, and once again with the medication. Student should ask about allergies prior to administering medication. Administer medication. Document on the MAR and if needed in the nurses notes (for as needed medications).
4. Side effects are predictable effects of the prescribed medication. These effects can be either desirable or undesirable. An example of a desirable effect might be the sedation that results with antihistamines may help improve sleep if taken at bedtime. An undesirable effect of the same medication might be the sedation when the patient needed to be alert for daily activities. Adverse effects are not predictable or desirable. They pose potentially life-threatening problems and require the medication to be discontinued.
5. An example cited in the text was the death caused to the patient by administering intravenous (IV) medication too fast. Can be prevented by looking up the drug prior to administering to determine recommended time to push medication.

   Other errors that are documented include errors that result from drugs having similar names (wrong drug) and patients that have similar names (wrong patient).
6. Monitor drug levels. Observe patient for side effects and adverse effects. Carefully monitor drug efficacy.
7. Assess for allergies, drug, and food. If there is evidence of hypersensitivity response, stay with patient and notify physician immediately. Maintain airway and prepare to administer epinephrine. An antihistamine, such as Benadryl, may be ordered for a milder reaction. Monitor patients for a period of time after giving medications, such as penicillin.

Chapter 18

1. Individuals form opinions based on their own experiences. This activity encourages the reader to look outside of personal experiences to gain understanding about others' experiences with the

health care system and how those experiences may have promoted differing perceptions about the health care system from his or her own perceptions. It also encourages the reader to develop the habit of considering the perceptions of others.

2. As the American cultural demographic becomes more diverse, it becomes essential for health care providers to develop skills in culturally competent care. Exposing the reader to Web sites like this tool box not only gives them an enjoyable way to learn, it may also introduce them to a new resource.
3. Nurse theorists, such as Nightingale and Henderson, as well as other nurse leaders, acknowledge that the environment for care can make a significant impact on the quality of care outcomes. Nurses can gauge the tone of the environment for care through their senses and make a judgment about the level and quality of care being provided.
4. The synergy model is a relatively new concept. In striving for exemplary patient care and, perhaps, magnet status agencies ought to consider the impact that implementation of synergy concepts could make toward accomplishment of such goals. This activity provides an opportunity for the reader to teach.
5. A common concern is whether needed health care can be easily accessed. Nurses are often sought to answer such a question for patients and their families. Having such knowledge at hand can facilitate choices for care that ensure safe passage through the health care agency system.

Chapter 19

1. The patient is at risk for oxygen toxicity with the FiO_2 at 70 percent. The patient is also on too high of a tidal volume for his weight. This puts the patient at risk for respiratory alkalosis and barotrauma. Other complications associated with mechanical ventilation are ventilator-associated pneumonia, tracheal damage, anxiety, and problems with communication, stress ulcers, and fluid retention.
2. Respiratory alkalosis; possible ventilator changes may include reduction of the FiO_2, reduction of the tidal volume, or ventilator rate. Depending on the patient's respiratory rate, the patient may also need sedation.
3. The patient's room should be kept as dark as possible and quiet. Nursing cares should be spaced to allow for rest periods. The patient's vital signs should be monitored frequently to assess for changes associated with increasing intracranial pressure or changes in temperature. Complete neurological assessments should be completed to monitor for increases in intracranial pressure. The patient should be monitored for seizure activity and should be on antiepileptic medication to prevent seizures. The patient may be receiving diuretic therapy to prevent increases in cerebral edema. The patient's head should be kept in a neutral position to allow for venous drainage that helps to prevent increases in intracranial pressure. The patient's oxygenation should be carefully monitored to ensure adequate oxygenation of brain cells.
4. The family will be fearful and wanting information on prognosis and current status. The intensive care unit environment can also be intimidating to the family. The nurse can explain the intravenous (IV) lines and therapies. The nurse can give some information on current status (for example, blood pressure) and the need for mechanical ventilation. The nurse should also encourage the family to talk to the patient and let him know they are at the bedside. The physician can also be contacted to talk to the family. Financial concerns are common when the family has a loved one in the intensive care unit. The cost of intensive care unit care combined with not working can be a concern for the patient and family. Contacting social services may be helpful in this area. The family is also probably wondering if the patient will be able to work any more at all. Again, social services may be helpful. They will need teaching regarding initial home care needs and medications the patient will be started on. Information on the general floor will also be helpful. It would be helpful to have a nurse from the floor come to the intensive care unit to meet the patient and explain some of the floor routine. The patient may be fearful of having another cerebrovascular accident (CVA). The nurse can reassure the patient with regard to blood pressure control and monitoring of vital signs while the patient is on the floor.
5. The critical care nurse should acknowledge the difficulty of the situation and the grief the family members are experiencing. The nurse should then offer to arrange a meeting for the family members with the health care team to help them in making this decision. Other support services available to the family are the social services, clergy, and other medical staff. The ethics committee is also available for consult if there is indecision among family members. The role of the critical care nurse in this process is to administer analgesics and sedatives prior to extubation to prevent air hunger and distress. The nurse will also provide support and comfort to the family, information on what will

occur during the process of extubation, and what to expect after the discontinuation of life support. Comfort measures for the patient should continue to be a priority after mechanical ventilation has been withdrawn. The nurse should stay with the family as needed and until the time of death if appropriate.

Chapter 20

1. Decisional conflict, impaired comfort, risk for acute pain, risk for delayed surgical recovery, fear, and many others.
2. Some preoperative care trends would be inside-the-body biofeedback and monitoring systems with implanted chips and miniaturized intervention systems, distance monitoring leading up to the time of surgery through streaming video and digital diagnostics. Other trends will be greater levels of assertion by preoperative nurses in relation to protection of patient decision making, autonomy, and protection.
3. End-of-life and beginning-of-life issues will continue to be predominant bioethical issues. Modern technology will continue to advance to a point at which decisions will center on quality of life rather than strictly prolonging life through surgical means or medical adjustment through internal biofeedback mechanisms.
4. The nurse may safely advise the patient or family to use certain steps to investigate a health care provider or health care facility match with the patient's surgical and recovery needs. The nurse may want to avoid personally endorsing one health care provider over another. To choose a health care provider, advise the patient to trace degree-granting institutions, publications, board certification, hospitals granting staff privileges, and finally word of mouth. To choose a hospital or surgical center, investigate hospital size (recall the 300 to 500 bed sizes mentioned in the chapter), whether the hospital is university-affiliated, and whether the hospital or medical center has a national reputation. In addition look for Magnet Status, presence of a trauma center and critical care unit(s). Finally, rely on personal observation through previsits or the experience of acquaintances.
5. Recall that major surgery involves greater than minimal risk to life in some way, such as happens with surgeries involving multiple systems or that require long periods of time in the operating suite. Minor surgery involves minimal risk to life, one body system, and minimal incision length and depth. Minor surgery can be done in a short period of time, often in a health care provider's office or freestanding surgical center. Such surgical procedures as laparoscopic appendectomy or laparoscopic cholecystectomy have largely replaced the full-incision procedure. Knee arthroscopy for repair purposes may yield the same result as knee surgery requiring more extensive incision and healing time. Many dental, eye-ear-nose-throat, and urological procedures are now done in outpatient or short-stay centers as compared with the norm of 20 to 30 years ago.
6. Procedures that require long, deep incisions and full anesthesia (as a way to relax musculature) commonly require transfusion. Examples are gastrointestinal surgery and orthopedic procedures, such as hip replacement. Cardiac or respiratory procedures that require opening and spreading the bones of the thorax would also require transfusion. Family and patient will want to be informed of preoperative self-donation possibilities or family donation. Inform patients and family that modern blood-screening techniques have greatly decreased the chance of acquiring any blood-borne pathogens, such as hepatitis or human immunodeficiency virus (HIV).
7. The nurse who is teaching in the immediate period leading up to surgery will want to consult the printed or online surgical schedule to give patient and family probable time of surgery. In addition, tell the family that the patient will leave for surgery at least an hour prior to the scheduled time. Sometimes the patient's time will be delayed because of an emergency. Sometimes the time will be advanced because of a cancellation. The nurse will describe the need for diet modification and sleep assist the evening before surgery. In addition, hygiene and changing to a hospital gown without jewelry or other personal items is usually a mandate with major surgery. The patient should practice postoperative leg exercises, painless repositioning techniques, and incentive spirometry use or deep breathing. The nurse will describe IV lines, catheters, dressings or casts, pumps, monitors, and other paraphernalia that might be present in the immediate postoperative period. The nurse should be aware of whether the agency's PACU has a ward-like appearance or seems more patient-friendly.
8. Opioids, amnesiacs, anticholinergics, antacids or proton pump inhibitors, muscle relaxants, and antibiotics are some of the more commonly encountered preoperative drugs.
9. Those with pulmonary compromise; immune system suppression or compromise; neuroendocrine disorders, such as myasthenia gravis or multiple sclerosis; hepatic disease, such as

cirrhosis or hepatitis; or chronic renal problems are at increased perioperative risk. Those with diabetes mellitus and those with chronic pancreatitis are also at risk. Those with cardiovascular disorders and patients at extreme ends of the age spectrum may be at increased risk. The disabled and those who are obese, addicted, or alcoholic present challenges, as do those with unstable psychiatric situations

Chapter 21

1. Risk for infection	Limit and control traffic
	Use standard precautions
Risk for impaired skin integrity	Keep skin clean and dry
	Pad bony prominences
Risk of injury related to surgical environment	Shield from radiation sources
	Limit exposure to laser beam
Risk of hypothermia	Monitor room temperature and humidity
	Monitor patient vital signs, labs, intake and output

2. Appropriate nursing interventions for the care of patients with MH:
   - Hyperventilation with 100 percent O_2
   - Deepen anesthesia with opioids and sedatives, muscle relaxation with a nondepolarizing relaxant
   - Stop trigger, remove vaporizer
   - Prepare dantrolene perfusion
   - Antiarrhythmic therapy with beta blocker (esmolol 0.25 mg/kg intravenously.) or lidocaine (1 mg/kg intravenously.)
   - Cooling: for example, ice water through a nasogastric tube
   - Additional monitoring: arterial catheter, central venous catheter, swan-Ganz-catheter, urinary catheter
3. Errors: Surgery performed on the wrong patient, or the wrong surgical site, or the wrong side (if a bilateral option is present), or the wrong surgery is performed. Medication errors also exist as potential surgical problems.

   Prevention methods: Avoid performing multiple procedures on multiple parts of a patient during a single surgical encounter; failure to include the patient or family members and significant others when identifying the correct site; use of abbreviations related to the surgical procedure, site, or laterality; problems related to illegible handwriting; and incomplete or inaccurate communication among members of the surgical team.
4. Factors associated with electrical safety in the OR:
   - The ESU settings should always be confirmed verbally with the operator. Good practice is to always use the lowest possible power settings.
   - Manufacturer's instructions should be followed and approved instruments or electrodes should be used.
   - The ESU generator must be mounted securely on a cart or boom to prevent falling.
   - Items should not be placed on top of the generator—especially potentially dangerous items, such as fluids.
   - The ESU foot pedal should be kept in an impervious bag. Fluid from blood and irrigation solutions can cause a shock.
5. A sterile object remains sterile only when touched by another sterile object.

   Check for sterility by checking expiration dates, intactness and integrity of outer wraps, and sterilization indicators inside the package.

   Only sterile objects may be placed on a sterile field. If there is a question of sterility, it is considered contaminated or nonsterile.

   A sterile object or field out of the range of vision or an object held below a person's waist is contaminated.

   Reduce air currents around a sterile object by not reaching across a sterile field, keep doors and curtains closed, and move sterile objects as little as possible on a sterile field.

   When a sterile surface comes in contact with a wet, contaminated surface, the sterile object or field becomes contaminated by capillary action.

   Keep caps of open sterile bottles right side up; avoid splashing or spillage when pouring liquids.

   Keep tips of sterile instruments pointed down; keep hands up after performing a surgical hand scrub.
6. Factors that contribute to perioperative hypothermia:
   - Decreased metabolic heat production
   - Increased environmental heat loss
   - Redistribution of heat within the body
   - Induced inhibition of thermoregulation during surgical procedures
   - Patient's physical status
   - Type of anesthesia used
   - Body fat and length and type of surgical device

Chapter 22

1. The top priorities immediately after surgery center on airway, breathing pattern, tissue oxygenation (sensed through the pulse oximeter or with nursing observation), cardiac function, peripheral vascular

perfusion, renal perfusion, level of consciousness, body temperature regulation, and pain. Others might be electrolyte balance, correcting severe blood loss, and safety.

2. Pain and diminished sleep may be continuing problems. Nursing interventions derived from the Nursing Intervention Classification (NIC) system as described in other chapters are numerous. Medication, together with measures to decrease anxiety may be helpful with pain control. Arranging an environment free from disturbing stimuli might also be helpful. There is always the potential for wound or respiratory infection. Care with pulmonary measures, such as incentive spirometry and respiratory therapy, are helpful measures for the postoperative patient. Careful wound care and patient education are useful, and control of nutrition and fluid-electrolyte balance will help to avert infection. Delivery of ordered antibiotics is needed for those with active infection. Alterations in activity or gait problems may make it difficult for some patients to resume previous levels of independence. Consistent patient exercise by nursing or physical therapy will allow the patient to experience reassuring levels of progress in most cases. Knowledge deficit or home difficulties may make it more difficult for the recovering patient to make the transition to home care. Again, the nurse will deal with some matters directly, using consultation with social services or, in many cases, the entire discharge planning team.
3. Some possibilities include slowing your speech and activity patterns. Match your pace to that desired by the senior patient. Another style change involves carefully assessing readiness of the older patient to engage in physical activity or in learning activities. Biorhythms of the older patient may be different from those of younger people. Assess sensory changes and be sure to note vision or hearing difficulties. The older patient will often have difficulty clearing certain medications from the body. This is important in the case of antibiotics or perhaps with analgesics or soporifics. The nurse may want to allow the older patient to sleep in before the breakfast hour and to turn in for sleep earlier in the evening than what would work with a younger person.
4. List four possible complications for the patient recovering from surgery. Using the priorities list and the NANDA taxonomy, one can extrapolate likely life-threatening complications, such as ineffective breathing, airway disruption, air exchange problems, cardiovascular inefficiency, or excessive blood loss. Altered mental status may be a disturbing possibility for family and patient alike. There are many other possibilities in the immediate postoperative period. Beyond the first 24 hours, hemorrhage or hematoma may be complications. Infection of wound or respiratory system is another complication that may ensue beyond the day of surgery.
5. Typical dilemmas involve management of extended recuperation needs with senior citizens. These can be traumatic for patient and spouse. Sometimes there is a dilemma when one is unable to live free without the other. Other dilemmas might involve the delivery of negative findings and the need for later nursing support. These are difficult situations and call for thorough assessment of patient and family responses, a delicate touch, and, often, calling clergy or some of the psychologists who are familiar with assisting with adaptation under difficult circumstances. There is sometimes, although rarely, a reluctance of family to support the delivery of negative prognoses. There may be conflict when the health care provider wants to fully brief the patient on probable outcome.
6. Acute pain, hypothermia, risk for aspiration, ineffective breathing pattern, impaired gas exchange, imbalanced fluid volume (risk for), decreased cardiac output (risk for), impaired tissue integrity, and many more.
7. The best measures will be demonstration of methods for keeping the dressing dry during hygiene activities. In the hospital, plastics can be temporarily placed over the old dressing prior to showering, if the surgeon has given permission for a shower. The patient should be instructed in careful hand washing and told to do that at home prior to working with the dressing and wound. The nurse should talk the patient or designated family through a dressing change, or preferably two. In addition, the nurse will observe as the patient or family member empties the JP and recharges the vacuum. What to do in case of disrupting the drain should be covered as well as observations that necessitate a call to the health care provider.

Chapter 23

1. The formations of the cells of blood come from a stem cell that differentiates into erythrocytes, granulocytes, platelets, B lymphocytes, and T lymphocytes
2. The oxygen in the erythrocyte is carried on hemoglobin; iron is a component of the hemoglobin molecule.
3. The white blood cells include granulocytes, which include the neutrophil, eosinophils, basophils, and the lymphocytes.

4. Granulocytes are formed to respond to infections and inflammation. Phagocytosis is a method used to control foreign substance by ingesting the particle. Neutrophils respond to bacterial infections. Eosinophils are more likely to be associated with infections from parasites and are more likely to be involved in allergies. Basophils are produced in the bone marrow and go to the peripheral blood and can and migrate to the tissues; in the tissues they are called mast cells. The mast cells release prostaglandins, leukotrienes, heparin, and histamine.
5. Platelets come from megakaryocytes that form thousands of platelets, which do not have nuclei but have many receptors that respond to stimuli that make the platelet sticky for forming a platelet plug.
6. The flow of blood through the heart is as follows: The blood returns to the heart from the inferior and superior vena cave and enters into the right atrium; it then flows over the tricuspid valve into the right ventricle. It then flows through the pulmonic valve into the pulmonary arteries into the pulmonary veins and enters the left atrium. When it leaves the left atrium it travels through the mitral valve into the left ventricle. As it leaves the left ventricle it is ejected through the aortic valve into the aorta and out to systemic circulation.
7. Evaluate heart sounds on a patient in the clinical practicum setting.
8. Complete a cardiovascular assessment in the clinical practicum setting.

Chapter 24

1. Mr. Anthony has stable angina (the chest pain is relieved with rest), which is likely caused by atherosclerosis because of his genetic influences, his hypertension, and his smoking. The anginal pain is caused by the irritation of lactic acid on nerve fibers from anaerobic metabolism.
2. Evaluation of this activity will take place as the student presents his or her materials to a group of student peers.
3. This experience will enhance your ability to have knowledge about diagnostic tests and the ability to share education with patients.
4. Locating local support programs will prepare you for referring patients to appropriate programs. Attending a class will give you a better understanding of the content and location while developing valuable contacts for the future.
5. Working with an advanced practice nurse in the care of the cardiac patient will provide you with a wealth of information and practice approaches to the care of the cardiac patient. This experience will also give you a better understanding of these nursing roles.

Chapter 25

1. Heart valves function much like full-length, one-directional swinging western-style bar room doors work. They allow free flow of blood in one direction. Regurgitation occurs when the valves are unable to close appropriately because of continued pressure in the ventricles, improper fitting of the valve's leaflets because of inflammation, weakness of the valves from illness, improperly shaped leaflets because of infection, and degeneration of the surface of the leaflets. Regurgitation allows some of the blood to flow back through the valve, in the opposite direction of the way the blood is meant to flow. The term stenosis is used to describe the valve's inability to properly open. This dilemma causes a reduction in the amount of blood that is allowed through the valves and a resultant increase in blood volume that remains in the heart chamber.
2. While most cases of mitral valve prolapse remain asymptomatic, some patients have symptoms such as fatigue, shortness of breath, light-headedness, dizziness, syncope, palpitations, chest pain, and anxiety. In extreme cases, the stretching of the leaflet can expand too far, and the result is sudden death.

   Assessment of mitral regurgitation often results in the patient remaining asymptomatic. When symptoms do occur, they are often vague and nonspecific and can present as fatigue, generalized weakness, dyspnea with or without exertion, palpitations, and cough. Auscultation of the heart may (or may not) reveal a systolic murmur. Palpation of the pulse may (or may not) reveal an irregular rhythm.

   Assessment of a mitral stenosis patient may reveal no symptoms or may reveal dyspnea on exertion, fatigue, and cough with hemoptysis. History often reveals chest pain, rheumatic fever, and dysphasia (Horenstein, Petersen, & Walters, 2002). Inspection may reveal a prominent wave in the jugular venous pulse, and in late stages, signs of peripheral edema, enlarged liver, ascites, and mitral facies—a florid appearance with cyanosed cheeks (if pulmonary hypertension has developed). Palpation may reveal a displace apex beat because of the enlarged right ventricle with a right ventricular heave. Auscultation of the heart may reveal a diastolic murmur and a displace apex beat. Palpation of the pulse may reveal an irregular rhythm (Saver, Hodgson, Van Norman, & Bahler, 2004).

Assessment of aortic regurgitation often reveals an asymptomatic patient. A patient history may reveal increased dyspnea on exertion, fatigue, and paroxysmal nocturnal dyspnea. Some patients may state an awareness of forceful pulsations in the upper thorax and head regions because of an increased force with which the left ventricle is required to perform. Cardiac auscultation may reveal a diastolic murmur. Upon palpation, the nurse may be able to palpate increase in intensity of carotid and temporal pulses. A hallmark sign of aortic regurgitation is a palpable pulse that is intense and then quickly weakens. The pulse pressure, the difference between the systolic blood pressure and diastolic blood pressure, described above, widens (Singh, Sharma, Nanda, Reddy, & Strom, 2004).

Assessment of aortic stenosis often reveals an absence of symptoms, whereas advanced aortic stenosis, characterized by a decrease in blood flow to the brain, results in multiple assessment findings. Dyspnea on exertion is common. Dizziness, syncope, and angina are frequently found when oxygen supplies have decreased in aortic stenosis patients. Auscultation reveals a systolic murmur, and palpation reveals a thrill.

3. Commissurotomy, a common form of valvuloplasty, is the procedure used to separate fused valve leaflets by cutting or manually pulling apart the leaflets.

   Balloon valvuloplasty, a type of commissurotomy, is a cardiac catheterization laboratory procedure in which a balloon is inflated, which stretches the valve open, and separates the fused leaflets. Then the balloon is deflated and removed.

   Annuloplasty is a procedure used to strengthen the junction of the leaflets to the heart muscle.

   Leaflet repair is considered when the leaflets are elongated or ballooning. In the leaflet repair, the extra tissue of the leaflet is removed.

   Chordoplasty is the repair of the chordae tendineae of the mitral valve. This involves repairing the defect in the shape of the chordae tendineae that causes regurgitation.

   Valve replacement consists of removing the diseased valve and replacing it with a donor valve (prosthesis).

4. Nursing management of the heart valve repair or replacement surgical patient occurs in a critical care unit. Management consists of hemodynamic monitoring, anesthesia recovery, wound care, and patient teaching.

   Hemodynamic monitoring involves maintaining blood pressure through administration of IV fluids and hemodynamic medications. Also important to hemodynamic monitoring is the monitoring and treatment of cardiac dysrhythmias. Anesthesia recovery involves assessment of the neurological, respiratory, and cardiovascular systems. Wound assessment and management is also important.

   Patient teaching requires a simple explanation of the anatomy of heart, the functioning of coronary arteries, and explanation of surgery. Purpose of medications and side effects are also important for educating the patient. Clear explanations of the purpose for long-term anticoagulant therapy and antibiotic prophylaxis are necessary.

5. Treatment for mild symptoms includes controlling volume overload through monitoring sodium and fluid intake. Dietary restrictions of salt are recommended. Fluid intake may also be restricted. These restrictions, whether recommended in isolation or with other treatments, make up the most basic concept of volume control in the treatment of heart failure.

6. Monitoring of oxygenation via pulse oximetry and arterial blood gases is one of the more important of nursing management activities. Positioning the patient for maximum cardiovascular functioning is also important. If possible, patients should dangle legs to decrease the venous return to the heart. The head of the bed should remain elevated so that there is a decrease in the amount of lung surface area affected by the increased fluid volume. Also important in nursing management of patients with congestive heart failure is reassurance and anxiety reduction. At a time when the heart is working its hardest, anxiety can cause more work for the heart.

7. Nursing management includes assessment of symptoms: Assessment of heart failure is best accomplished through a holistic approach of gathering data from a health history, a thorough physical exam with attention paid to the cardiovascular and pulmonary systems, and objective measurement of various body parts and function.

   Oxygenation measures, respiratory effort, rate, and depth of respiration on exertion and at rest provide significant information about patients with heart failure.

   Nursing management includes administration and monitoring of therapeutic regimen; monitoring of oxygenation via pulse oximetry and arterial blood gases is one of the more important of nursing management activities.

   Nursing management includes measuring treatment effectiveness: Evaluation of therapeutic regimens is optimal when outcomes are measurable. Generally, the objective evaluation of heart failure interventions should include an increase in oxygenation, an increase in cardiac and peripheral perfusion, a cardiovascular and peripheral vascular volume balance, an increase in activity levels, a decrease in cardiac workload, a decrease in work of breathing, a decreased anxiety level, maintenance of optimal vital signs, and an increase in quality sleep and rest.

Nursing management includes providing physiological and psychological support: reassurance and anxiety reduction. At a time when the heart is working its hardest, anxiety can cause more work for the heart.

8. Dilated cardiomyopathy (DCM), a disease of the heart muscle, results in a dilated heart chamber, which expands much the way a balloon expands. DCM results in a decreased ability for the heart to pump strongly and forcefully.

   Hypertrophic cardiomyopathy (HCM) is an increase in the size and thickness of the heart muscle. The sheer size of the hypertrophic heart muscle decreases the volume of blood that can be accommodated in the heart's chambers. Likewise, the size and thickness of the hypertrophic heart muscle disallows timely cardiac relaxation that is necessary for quick blood filling of the heart chambers.

   Arrhythmogenic right ventricular cardiomyopathy (ARVC) is a disease of the cardiac muscle in which the heart muscle is replaced by fibrous scar and fatty tissue. The right ventricle is more likely to be affected. The progressive loss of heart muscle affects the hearts electrical functioning, which leads to alteration in the hearts ability to effectively pump.

   Restrictive cardiomyopathy (RCM) is a disease of the ventricular heart muscle in which the muscle walls become stiff but not necessarily thickened. The cause is not known, but metabolic disorders, sequela of radiation therapy, and family history of cardiomyopathy have been identified as causes in some people.

9. Maslow's Hierarchy of Needs for the following nursing diagnoses:
   a. Physiological: risk for ineffective respiratory function related to excessive secretions secondary to cardiopulmonary dysfunction.
   b. Safety: activity intolerance related to insufficient knowledge of adaptive techniques needed secondary to impaired cardiac function.
   c. Esteem: anxiety related to powerlessness and vulnerability.

10. Maslow's Hierarchy of Needs for the following nursing diagnoses:
    a. Physiological necessity: risk for ineffective respiratory function related to decreased respiratory depth.
    b. Physiological comfort: pain related to friction rub and inflammatory process.
    c. Safety: activity intolerance related to insufficient knowledge of adaptive techniques needed secondary to impaired cardiac function.

Chapter 26

1. Steps necessary in this activity include: (a) Take the defibrillator to the patient's bedside; (b) Attach the monitor or defibrillator pads to the patient's chest; (c) Turn the monitor power on and view rhythm; (d) Confirm ventricular fibrillation; (e) Charge the defibrillator to 200 joules; (f) Make sure everyone is clear of the patient and equipment and then deliver the shock; (g) Confirm continued presence of ventricular fibrillation then reshock. The intravenous (IV) supplies are typically kept in a drawer of the crash cart with IV solutions kept on the bottom of the crash cart. Frequently, emergency medications are kept in the top drawer of the crash cart.
2. Causes of sinus tachycardia in this patient could include pain, fever, hypoxia, and hypovolemia. The treatment of sinus tachycardia would be to identify why the patient is experiencing the rhythm, then to treat the underlying cause.
3. The steps of analyzing a rhythm strip are: (a) Determine the rate; (b) Determine the rhythm; (c) Determine the presence of P waves; (d) Measure the PR interval; (e) Measure the QRS interval; (f) Measure the QT interval.
4. This is answered by spending time in an acute care agency and observing in a telemetry or critical care setting.
5. The ventricular arrhythmias are generally more pathological for the patient, as these arrhythmias are more affecting to the cardiac output. The ventricle is the more significant muscle as associated with delivery of blood throughout the circulatory system.

Chapter 27

1. The concept map for a patient with abdominal aortic aneurysm is located on the following page.
2. Characteristics of decreased oxygen, related to peripheral vascular disease are:
   1. Altered sensation of the skin
   2. Brittle nail beds
   3. Thin/sparse hair
   4. Delayed healing
   5. Decreased or diminished pulses
   6. Skin discoloration, including pale
   7. Coolness of the skin

CONCEPT MAP

Patient: 54-Year-Old Male with Aortic Abdominal Aneurysm

1. Ineffective tissue perfusion: tissues distal to the aneurysm:

- R/T: interruption of blood flow to lower extremities
- AEB: pulsation and bruit noted in abdominal region
- AEB: neuro exam q4
- AEB: diminished pulses bilateral legs
- BP: 174/98
- AEB: need for antihypertensive medication
- AEB: lab results: list all labs R/T AAA
- AEB: abdominal X-ray demonstrating mass

2: Pain, back and abdominal

- R/T: statement of pain 8 of 10 scale
- AEB: need for quite environment
- AEB: need for antihypertensive medications
- AEB: need for pain medications
- AEB: no pressure or physical exam of the abdomen

4: Fear and anxiety:

- R/T: actual and potential serious complications
- AEB: lack of knowledge of the risk factors leading to AAA
- AEB: education of diagnostic test results
- AEB: need for education of surgical risks
- AEB: need for post-op instructions
- AEB: need for lifestyle changes

Reason for seeking health care:

Nausea, vomiting, back pain, abdominal pressure, legs bluish color

3. Risk for impaired skin integrity

- R/T: compromised tissue perfusion distal to the aneurysm
- AEB: bedrest
- AEB: diminished bilateral popliteal, dorsalis pedis, and pedal pulses
- AEB: parenthesis of lower extremities
- AEB: need to place on fall precautions

5. Imbalanced nutrition: more than body requirement:

- R/T: ht: 5'10" weight 215 lb
- AEB: high cholesterol diet history
- AEB: lack of exercise history
- AEB: list all labs R/T unbalanced diet
- AEB: need for replacement fluids and nutrients while experiencing N/V

Possible complications:

Hemorrhage
Aortic dissection
Hypovolemic shock
Decreased oxygen supply to tissues distal to the aneurysm

Preexisting conditions:

Hx of smoking
Hypertension
Diet high in cholesterol
Overweight

3. The following should be included in the nurse's assessment of the patient when being discharged:
   1. Knowledge of the plan of care
   2. Accurate return demonstration of skills needed to care for self
   3. Knowledge of self-care activities to prevent long-term complications
   4. Express the importance of health promotion activities and health screening
   5. Plan for physical support, either during recovery or continuous
   6. Financial assessment, patient has the finances to care for self
   7. Home safety assessment, prevention of falls and other hazards
4. The following are the primary teaching points for Coumadin administration:
   a. Coumadin is an anticoagulant, or blood thinner, which slows the normal blood clotting process. It can prevent clots form forming, but cannot dissolve blood clots which have already formed.
   b. Do not stop or increase your medication in any way or add other medications, including over the counter medications, without consulting your health care provider (physician or nurse practitioner). Many medications can alter the way Coumadin works, including increased bleeding, and interfere with the desired effects of your anticoagulant.
   c. Coumadin is taken once a day and your blood is tested routinely for the effectiveness of Coumadin. This monitoring is important as your health care provider will adjust the strength of your medication according to the results of the blood test.
   d. You should wear a Medic Alert bracelet stating you are taking this drug and are at an increased risk for bleeding.
   e. Common side effects include: stomach bloating and cramps; loss of hair and skin rashes; orange-yellow discoloration of the urine. If these side effects are persistent or irritating, notify your health care provider.
   f. Report the following side effects to your health care professional: unusual bleeding when brushing your teeth; excessive bleeding form an injury; excessive bruising; black, tarry stools; cloudy, dark urine; sore throat, fever, or chills; and headaches or dizziness
   g. Avoid: contact sports; using a straight razor; and foods high in vitamin K (dark green, leafy vegetables such as spinach).
5. Three NOC goals related to the following nursing diagnoses are: tissue perfusion, peripheral, ineffective.

Chapter 28

1. a. 1. Weight loss using DASH diet
   2. Aerobic exercise
   3. Smoking cessation
   4. Moderation of alcohol intake
   5. Salt restriction

   b. 1. The DASH diet is rich in grains, fruits, vegetables, and low-fat dairy products. The plan limits fat, saturated fat, and cholesterol while providing plentiful amounts of fiber, potassium, calcium, and magnesium. Multiple research studies have shown a reduction in blood pressure of 8 to 14 mm Hg in patients with hypertension who follow the DASH diet.

   2. The JNC VII advises all patients who are physically able to participate in regular aerobic physical activity for at least 30 minutes per day, most days of the week. Exercise strengthens muscles and at the same time opens up arteries to allow for more nutrients and oxygen to flow into the tissues. The combination of a stronger, more efficient heart and blood vessels that are more open leads to lower blood pressure.

   3. Tobacco is the single greatest cause of disease and premature death in the United States and is responsible for more than 400,000 deaths per year. Patients with high blood pressure who also use tobacco products are two to three times more likely to develop cardiovascular disease. Exposure to secondhand smoke, also called environmental tobacco smoke, is also a serious health hazard.

   4. Moderation is the best method for controlling alcohol intake. Excessive alcohol intake increases blood pressure and the calories have no nutritional value.

   5. It has been estimated that the average daily intake of sodium for individuals in the United States is between 4,000 and 6,000 mg. The majority of sodium intake is from food, and many foods naturally contain some sodium. Most sodium ingestion comes from commercially processed foods and meal preparation at home.

   c. Altered health maintenance R/T lack of knowledge of pathology, complications, and management of hypertension
   Ineffective coping R/T effects of chronic illness and major changes in lifestyle
   Ineffective sexuality patterns related to side effects of medications
   Risk for ineffective therapeutic regimen management R/T noncompliance with treatment
   Risk for ineffective coping R/T inability to cope with chronic disease

2\. Subjective Data / Objective Data

Subjective Data	Objective Data
a. age, height, weight, allergies	a. body build, general appearance
b. chronic diseases (DM, HTN, COPD)	b. blood pressure, heart rate, respirations
c. alcohol, tobacco, caffeine, drug use	c. level of consciousness

3\.

Causes of secondary hypertension	Diagnostic test(s)
Chronic kidney disease	Estimated GFR, MRA
Renal artery stenosis	Doppler flow study
Congenital narrowing of the aorta	CT angiography

4. Address the risk factors that apply to the patient, and identify realistic goals for the patient to decrease their hypertension. Refer to question 1b for further educational information.
5. Pharmacological therapy usually begins with a diuretic. Diuretics are divided into several classes: loop, potassium sparing, thiazide, and thiazide-like. The first diuretics usually used are thiazide diuretics. In addition, diuretics are the preferred treatment for isolated systolic hypertension in older adults. Aldosterone receptor blockers (such as spironolactone) prevent the effects of aldosterone on the kidneys and this allows the kidneys to remove the extra sodium and water.

Chapter 29

1. Iron deficiency anemia develops when there is a loss of iron that becomes inadequate for red blood cell production. It is the most common type of anemia and is particularly common in the elderly.

   Folic acid deficiency anemia results from a lack of folic acid. Folic acid deficiency anemia is found in the chronically undernourished, such as alcoholics, drug abusers, and the elderly. Consumption of alcohol increases folic acid requirements. In addition, pregnancy increases the need for folic acid.
2. The types of diagnostic tests to confirm DIC are CBC, platelet count, schistocytes (fragmented RBCs), prolonged coagulation studies (PT, PTT, thrombin time), and increased fibrin degradation products.
3. Hemophilia A, a factor VIII deficiency known as classic hemophilia, affects 1 in 10,000 males. It is transmitted to the offspring as a cross-linked recessive disorder from mothers to sons. The defect of hemophilia A on the X chromosome could cause the deficiency of factor VIII or its production.

   Hemophilia C, also known as factor XI deficiency, is also an autosomal recessive disorder. It primarily affects the population of Ashkenazi Jews and is somewhat rare based on the narrow population that is affected. The clinical manifestations are related to the prolonged partial thromboplastin time and are basically the same as for the previously other forms of hemophilia. Often these patients are identified in the perioperative arena with prolonged bleeding during or after surgery.
4. Acute leukemia is characterized by abrupt onset and rapid progression. The two types of acute leukemia are: (1) Acute myeloid leukemia (AML), which affects people of all ages, and (2) Acute lymphocytic leukemia (ALL), which most commonly affects children under 15.

   Chronic leukemia has a gradual onset, a prolonged clinical course, and relatively long survival. There are two types of chronic leukemia: (1) Chronic myeloid leukemia (CML), which affects people at all ages, and (2) Chronic lymphocytic leukemia (CLL), which rarely strikes before age 45 and most victims are over 65.
5. Autologous stem cell transplantation is a common management therapy in the cancer of the blood disorders. This procedure consists of patients undergoing peripheral stem cell collections after stimulation with granulocyte colony-stimulating factor (G-CSF), with or without a dose of mobilization chemotherapy. Once adequate stems cells are collected, high-dose melphalan is administered, followed by the infusion of the previously harvested stem cells. In general, high-dose therapy with autologous transplant may improve the survival rates of those patients who have the treatment.
6. This activity would be performed in the student nurse clinical practicum experience.

Chapter 30

1. Mrs. Hastings will require about two months to completely recover from her bout with pneumonia. Because she is weakened, her mobility and endurance may be decreased, and she is at increased risk for falls. Because her family members are unavailable during the day to assist her with activities of daily living, she may benefit from an adult daycare program or visits from a home health team. Because she may experience a relapse, she should be closely monitored for any signs of respiratory infection or increasing fatigue, alterations in mental status, or changes in overall health. By supporting her efforts to remain in her

home, her independence will be preserved while she is receiving the care she requires. She should be instructed to rest frequently, take her entire course of antibiotics, use effective hand hygiene, keep her follow-up appointment with her health care provider, and avoid crowds, those with illnesses, contact with infants and small children, hypothermia, and secondhand smoke. Referral to a case manager, social services provider, and home health nurse will be helpful in her recovery.

2. Mr. and Mrs. Myers are both experiencing health problems because of cigarette smoking. Mr. Myers is at substantially increased risk for additional lung problems because he is exposed daily to additional cigarette smoke that caused his respiratory disease. He is at risk of experiencing a respiratory emergency, because his ability to exchange oxygen at the alveolar capillary level is severely compromised. Because of his increasing dyspnea at rest, he will probably require maintenance oxygen in his home. Both Mr. and Mrs. Myers should be instructed about the importance of keeping all flames away from oxygen. Also, Mrs. Myers should be instructed to avoid any cigarette smoking inside her house and in the area adjacent to her windows in her yard. Smoking cessation should also be reexplored. Mr. Myers may develop mobility and self-care limitations because of chronic dyspnea. Further, he may become depressed because of his activity limitations. As cold weather develops, the windows in their house will probably be opened less frequently, so the accumulation of tobacco smoke in drapes, furniture, and carpets will cause additional problems. Also, heat from the furnace will dry the indoor air, making it more difficult for Mr. Myers to mobilize his respiratory secretions. He should be instructed to use a humidifier in the house all winter if the furnace is on. He should also be instructed to avoid long intervals of bed rest; avoid exposure to cold, dry air; and drink plenty of fluids to assist in mobilization of his secretions. In teaching this couple, use of visual materials and repeating instructions will be helpful. Instructions should be provided over several visits, and you should plan to follow-up with written instructions in large print that can be left in their house.

3. Because Mrs. Myers seems to have some cognitive and memory problems, she may be experiencing symptoms of confusion, delirium, hearing loss, or dementia. New learning will be difficult for her to grasp with any of these conditions. Those with problems related to thinking, memory, or hearing loss are not suitable to prepare medications for themselves or others. Mrs. Myers should be evaluated for the above problems. In the interval, Mr. Myers should receive medication assistance from a reliable family member or a home health nurse. Because of his endurance and visual problems, he should not set up his medications at this time. Whenever teaching is ongoing, all sources of distraction, such as the television or outside noise should be eliminated. Teaching in the morning may work better because fatigue set in less soon after arising.

4. Nearly every place Irma visits has known triggers for asthma. In the country or in many rural areas, pollen, dust, and molds are common. In the local grocery store, she may come in contact with those experiencing colds or flu or have secondary exposure to cleaning agents used in the store. Her weekly trip to the city library may produce breathing difficulties in the presence of smog. Further, the resale shop may cause breathing problems if mold, mildew, dust, or dry cleaning products are in the air. Exertion is a known trigger for many with asthma, so exercising at the health club may also produce wheezing and bronchospasms associated with asthma. The pet groomer is also a known trigger for asthma, because debris from fleas, dander from dog skin, and fur or hair from grooming will likely be floating in the air. Irma should be advised to medicate prior to contact with these sources of irritation, minimize contact, and consider eliminating sources of irritation from her weekly routines.

5. Ask Mr. Jeffers to hold his breath while you auscultate him.

Chapter 31

1. Nursing Diagnoses as set forth by the North American Nursing Diagnosis Association (NANDA), for a patient with upper airway infection may include the following, as well as others:
   - Activity intolerance
   - Ineffective airway clearance
   - Acute pain
   - Deficient knowledge

2. Suggested NIC for the nursing diagnoses are:

   Activity intolerance is related to fever, fatigue, or a compromised immune system. The patient experiences insufficient physiological energy to complete or endure required or desired daily activities.
   - Self-care assistance
   - Energy management
   - Environmental management
   - Sleep enhancement

Ineffective airway clearance is related to inflammation of the mucous membranes and rhinorrhea.

- Airway management
- Cough enhancement
- Fluid management

Acute pain is related to congestion, cough, and fever.

- Analgesic administration
- Environmental management
- Medication administration
- Heat/cold application

Deficient knowledge

- Health education
- Teaching—Disease process
- Teaching—Medication
- Behavior modification

3. Evidence-based medical research has shown the limited efficacy of antibiotic use in eradicating infection. This is due in part because of the overuse of antibiotics with subsequent bacterial organism resistance. Newer drugs are more costly, and studies have not demonstrated superiority of one antibiotic over another in eradicating infection. However, the amount of organism resistance in an area must be considered when selecting an antibiotic. The benefits of antibiotic therapy must be weighed against the potential for adverse effects. There is limited evidence that antibiotics (including amoxicillin, cephalosporins, and macrolides) for 7 to 10 days are effective in the treatment of radiologically or bacteriologically confirmed acute maxillary sinusitis.

   If infection with a bacterial agent is confirmed, antibiotics are indicated for 7 to 10 days. First-line drugs of choice are amoxicillin (Amoxil), and trimethoprim/sulfamethoxazole (Bactrim).

4. Standard throat cultures have fallen out of favor because of their inability to distinguish active infection from the carrier state, unpredictability between lab and user, and the fact that results are rarely available in time to decrease symptoms. On the other hand, rapid antigen testing takes about 5 to 7 minutes to obtain results and treatment can begin immediately.

5. Epistaxis is classified on the basis of the primary bleeding site as anterior or posterior. Hemorrhage is most commonly anterior, originating from the nasal septum. A common source of anterior epistaxis is Kiesselbach plexus, a network of vessels on the anterior portion of the septum just superior to the posterior end of the nasal vestibule. Posterior hemorrhage originates in the posterior nasal cavity or nasopharynx, usually below the posterior half of the inferior turbinate or roof of the nasal cavity.

   Management of nosebleeds depends on the location of the bleeding site. A nasal speculum is used to access the location of the bleeding. For nosebleeds originating from the anterior portion of the nose, direct pressure may be the only treatment that is needed. The patient is shown how to lean forward slightly while pinching the soft outer portion of the nose against the nasal septum for about five to ten minutes continuously. If this proves unsuccessful, additional treatment is indicted. If the source of bleeding can be visualized, an application of silver nitrate may help to stop the bleeding. Cotton pledgets soaked in 4% topical cocaine solution or a solution of 4% lidocaine and topical epinephrine (1:10,000) can be placed into the nasal cavity. They should remain in place for 10 to 15 minutes.

   If bleeding is occurring from the posterior portion of the nasal cavity, packing must be used to stop the bleeding. Commonly used treatments include traditional nasal packing, nasal tampons or balloons, or prefabricated nasal sponges.

   Nasal packing may be left in place for two to five days. Oral antibiotics and analgesics may be prescribed.

6. A clear association has been made between smoking, excess alcohol ingestion, and the development of laryngeal cancer. A direct correlation exists between the amount of smoking and the chance of developing laryngeal cancer. Alcohol has been found to be a synergistic agent, increasing the risk up to 100-fold in individuals who smoke and ingest alcohol over nonsmokers and nondrinkers. Other carcinogens associated with the risk of laryngeal cancer include exposure to wood dust, paint fumes, asbestos, mustard gas, tar products, leather, and metals. Other contributing factors in the development of laryngeal cancer include constant straining of the voice, a weak immune system (such as in acquired immune deficiency syndrome [AIDS]), human papillomavirus (HPV), nutritional deficiencies (such as vitamin B, A, retinoids), and gastroesophageal reflux disease (GERD).

7. Esophageal speech involves the patient being able to take air into the mouth and swallow or force the air into the esophagus by locking the tongue to the roof of the mouth. Forcing the air into the esophagus causes the walls of the esophagus and pharynx, as well as the returning air, to vibrate, producing a low-pitched sound. The tongue, lips, and mouth then form this sound into words. The process is similar to a burp or belch. The advantage

to this method is that the sound is more normal than speech produced by mechanical devices. It is less costly than other methods, because there is no equipment to buy. A disadvantage to this method it that it is more difficult to learn than speech produced with special devices and it may be harder to understand. It is important to remind the patient that it can take months to perfect this form of artificial speech.

Tracheoesophageal speech is similar to esophageal speech, but a valve is placed in the tracheal stoma to divert the air into the esophagus. The procedure is called a tracheoesophageal puncture (TEP) and may be performed at the same time as the laryngectomy. The procedure creates an opening between the trachea and the esophagus. A one-way valve is inserted into the stoma and allows air to pass from the trachea into the esophagus, while preventing food from entering the trachea. To produce speech, the patient covers the opening and forces the air into the esophagus and out of the mouth. This allows the patient to produce sound in the same way as esophageal speech, but the sound produced is much more like natural speech. Tracheoesophageal speech is successful in 80 to 90 percent of patients and is a widely accepted form of alaryngeal communication because it is fairly easy to learn. The valve can be removed and cleaned to prevent mucus from occluding the opening.

Mechanical speech may be used while the patient is learning esophageal speech or tracheoesophageal speech or if they have been unsuccessful at either of these methods. Speech production occurs by means of an electrical device that is powered by batteries (electrolarynx) or by air (pneumatic larynx). The electrolarynx is a handheld device, that when placed against the neck, causes sound to travel through the neck into the mouth. A pneumatic larynx is held over the stoma and uses air instead of batteries to make it vibrate. The sound travels to the mouth through a plastic tube. Both methods produce a mechanical sounding voice that may be difficult to understand. The advantage to mechanical speech is that communication is relatively

Chapter 32

1. This is best applied in the practicum setting with the selection of a patient that has a diagnosis of pneumonia.
2. When there is a 5-mm induration, it suggests that the patient could have one of the following: recent contact, an immunocompromised person, and an abnormal chest X-ray. When there is a 10-mm induration, it suggests that the person has diabetes mellitus, renal insufficiency, a recent gastrectomy, corticosteroid therapy, people who traveled within the past 5 years to a country with TB, and substance abusers in treatment programs. The latter is a greater severity within these potential problems.
3. The patient is assessed and diagnostic tests reveal that they have a lung abscess. Then, the treatment goals focus on minimizing further tissue damage, promoting effective airway breathing, removal of secretions, and treatment of infection. The patient will be then be prescribed antibiotic therapy to reduce the infection quickly. Bronchodilators could be used to expand the bronchi allowing removal of secretions through the use of an inhaled mist. There will also be a focus on improving his respiratory condition (e.g., oxygen therapy, rest periods when ambulating, and effective pain control) and assessing the results of the interventions. Chest physiotherapy and postural drainage will also be used to improve his condition.
4. This is be implemented in the clinical setting. Be honest with yourself and share your feelings with your classmates. Ask them and your clinical preceptor to assist you in creating strategies for your professional role with this disorder in a patient.
5. The fractured ribs can be singular in nature or multiple. The patient would have acute pain on inspiration and would naturally splint his or her rib cage area during his or her breathing. Unless the fractured ribs cause bleeding or internal organ damage, they are usually not a high priority in relationship to the viability of the patient. On the other hand, a flail chest involves the fracture of several ribs that are usually in a segment together. The patient typically has chest pain, dyspnea, tachypnea, and tachycardia. This patient will be more compromised than just fractured ribs and have more of a respiratory distressed condition.

Chapter 33

1. Tell the patient with COPD that the pulmonary rehabilitation program has educational, psychosocial, behavioral, and physical components. Identify what some of these components are. Let your patient know that he or she will set the pace. He or she will not be asked to do anything that he or she is unable to do. Let him or her verbalize his or her concerns and get his or her feelings out. Give him or her accurate information to reduce his or her fear. The patient can expect classes in anatomy and physiology of the lung, changes with COPD, medications, home oxygen therapy, nutrition, importance of regular exercise,

respiratory therapy, smoking cessation, symptom alleviation, infection prevention, sexuality, coping with COPD, communicating with the health care team, advance directives, living wills, and health care alternatives for the future.

2. This will best be answered by observation in a practicum setting. The pulmonary rehabilitation program also teaches the patient to pace activities through the day and use assistive devices to decrease energy expenditure. Measure this patient's outcomes with a tool, such as the Medical Outcomes Study Short Form.
3. This will best be applied in a practicum setting by developing a relationship with a patient and family that has cystic fibrosis (CF). In addition, accessing the Web site for the CF Foundation will complete this question.
4. This will be applied in a practicum setting by assessing and evaluating a patient with asthma.
5. This will be applied by observing a respiratory therapist in clinical setting as he or she cares for the three types of COPD patients.
6. This will be answered by evaluating CF on the identified Web site for the CF Foundation.

Chapter 34

1. The three neurotransmitters in the basal ganglia and their impact on motor function are:
   - acetylcholine—excitatory; stimulates the release of γ-aminobutyric acid (GABA);
   - GABA—excitatory and inhibitory; chorea develops with low levels;
   - dopamine—inhibits release of GABA; tremor and gait disturbances develop with low levels.
2.

SYSTEM	SYMPATHETIC RESPONSE	PARASYMPATHETIC RESPONSE
Neurological	Pupils dilated	Pupils normal size
	Heightened awareness	
Cardiovascular	Increased heart rate	Decreased heart rate
	Increased myocardial contractility	Decreased myocardial contractility
	Increased blood pressure	

Continued

SYSTEM	SYMPATHETIC RESPONSE	PARASYMPATHETIC RESPONSE
Respiratory	Increased respiratory rate	Bronchial constriction
	Increased respiratory depth	
	Bronchial dilation	
Gastrointestinal	Decreased gastric motility	Increased gastric motility
	Decreased gastric secretions	Increased gastric secretions
	Increased glycogenolysis	Sphincter dilation
	Decreased insulin production	
	Sphincter contraction	
Genitourinary	Decreased urine output	Normal urine output
	Decreased renal blood flow	

3. The six major portions of the physical assessment of the neurological system are mental status, cranial nerve exam, sensory exam, motor exam, cerebellar exam, and reflex exam.
4. The follow-up nursing interventions after a computed tomography (CT) scan are:
   a. Teaching by the nurse should begin with a description of the CT scanner. When contrast media is planned, identification of any allergies to the media, shellfish, or iodine, may require premedication. Instruct the patient on the importance of lying still during the procedure. Identify any need for sedation due to anxiety. The patient is not usually ordered to have nothing by mouth (NPO). A peripheral intravenous (IV) site may need to be implemented.
   b. The patient is placed flat on a movable table. His or her head is secured in a holding device. The table moves in and out of the cylindrical scanner. A noncontrast series of pictures are taken first. If contrast is ordered, it is administered intravenously, and the series is repeated. The entire procedure usually takes approximately 10–40 minutes.

c. If given, the nurse should monitor for any delayed reaction to contrast media When contrast media is used, the diuresis that results may require replacement fluids.

5. The student would observe several neurological diagnostic studies in the practicum setting.

Chapter 35

1. a. What type, size, and grade is the tumor? This helps to identify if the tumor is benign or malignant, the types (gliomas, meningioma, etc.), and if malignant, how much it will spread.
   b. What types of treatment options are available for this type of tumor? This question will help determine whether treatment will be surgical, radiation, chemotherapy, or a combination of all three.
   c. What is my prognosis? This helps the patient determine the next step and assist with planning.
   d. Should I see any special physicians? A patient may need to consult with a neurosurgeon, neuro-oncologist, and neuro-radiation specialist for treatments.
   e. Where can I receive this treatment? This is important for the patient to know if they will need to travel outside of the area or can remain close to family and friends for treatment.
2. Topics to include in the presentation are: (a) Helmets are an important part of recreational sports and (b) Motor vehicle crashes cause the most head injuries and is the leading cause of brain injury in teenagers. This is usually due to alcohol, drugs, inexperienced drivers, and speeding.
3. Some important nursing interventions to include are:
   a. Importance of seeking help from family, friends, and community resources.
   b. Importance of taking care of himself of herself—getting out of the house to do whatever helps the patient to relax (e.g., exercise, crafts, etc.).
   c. Promoting independence for the patients, as much is as possible.
   d. Joining support groups.
4. Some appropriate nursing interventions for this patient are: (a) Keep environment structured, (b) Orient frequently, (c) Maintain a safe environment, (d) Monitor self-care but should be able to perform with moderate assistance, (e) Keep active by attending structure programs, (f) Keep consistent with behavior modification techniques, and (g) adopt a reward system.
5. Interventions to assist a patient in modifying various risk factors for a stroke are outlined as follows:
   a. Hypertension: exercise, decrease salt intake, stress management, and administer antihypertensives.
   b. Hypercholesterolemia: decrease saturated fats in diet, increase vegetables and fruits, and administer lipid reducing medications.
   c. Atrial fibrillation: administer anticoagulants.
   d. Obesity: significant diet modification, exercise, and counseling.
   e. Smoking: participate in a smoking cessation program.
   f. Drugs and alcohol: eliminate illicit drugs and alcohol.
   g. Diabetes: control blood sugars and education regarding the complications of diabetes.

Chapter 36

1. Interviewing a patient and family members will provide an understanding of the physical limitations and psychosocial adjustments that both patients and their families must make. The physical adjustments of the living environment are significant and will help the nurse understand how to anticipate the care that patients will need when they go home. The nursing care worksheet focuses on self-care limitations and will help the nurse understand what type of self-care assistance will be needed by the patient and what the family can anticipate.
2. The improvement of neurological function after administration of methylprednisolone occurs because of the reduction of edema to the area of injury. It is also thought to occur because of the effect of the methylprednisolone on the reduction of leukocytes to the area along with a decrease in free fatty acid production. Steroid treatment also inhibits breakdown of phospholipids, improving blood flow to the spinal cord and stopping the inflammatory response, thereby avoiding further injury to the spinal cord. Methylprednisolone has been shown to counter many of the injury cascades that cause injury to the spinal cord. These injury cascades include the emergent phase of spinal shock, which includes spinal edema and inflammation processes.
3. A teaching plan should include assessment of risk factors, especially work history related to word processing and keyboarding activities. Teaching should include proper positioning of hands and wrists, proper height of keyboard, wrists off the surface of the desk and support through the use of gel devices. Teaching to athletes should emphasize rest and immobilization of the wrist if experiencing

symptoms. Nonsteroidal anti-inflammatory medications will be helpful in these situations.

4. Neurological assessment of motor and sensory function is a priority after the surgery, as well as careful assessment for the development of a headache, which may indicate a subdural hematoma. Administration of dexamethasone for the prevention and treatment of edema associated with the spinal cord tumor and surgery will be an aspect of postoperative care, along with administration of antacids to protect the gastrointestinal (GI) tract from the adverse effects of corticosteroids. Careful assessment of urinary and bowel elimination and progression to self-care activities will also be included in the postoperative care of this patient.
5. This Web site provides a wealth of information for health care providers and for patients and family members. It is important for nurses to know the research to be able to talk with patients who are knowledgeable about care.

Chapter 37

1. Tension-type headache is caused by irritation of the pain-sensitive structures of the brain. The intracranial structures include portions of the trigeminal (CN V), facial (CN VII), glossopharyngeal (CN IX), vagus (CN X), upper cervical nerves, the large arteries, and the venous sinuses. When the sensory receptors of the muscles, tendons, joints, and skin are stimulated, they transmit pain messages to the pain-sensitive areas of the brain. Tension-type headaches may be episodic or chronic.

   Migraine is characterized by vasodilation of the dural blood vessels, resulting in stimulation of the trigeminal nerve pain pathways. Then neuropeptides, involved in pain transmission, are released. The neuropeptides make the vasodilation worse and sensitize the brainstem, causing the associated symptoms of light, sound, movement, and odor sensitivity.

Medications to Treat Headaches

TENSION-TYPE HEADACHE	MIGRAINE HEADACHE	CLUSTER HEADACHE
Nonnarcotic analgesics	***Nonnarcotic analgesics***	***100 percent O_2/ facemask***
Caffeine		Ergot alkaloids
Narcotic combinations	Narcotic analgesics	Triptans
		Intranasal lidocaine
Antidepressants	Triptans	Capsaicin
	Ergot alkaloids	Nonnarcotic analgesics
		Narcotic analgesics
		Calcium channel blockers
Beta blockers	Beta blockers	Corticosteroids
	Calcium channel blockers	Anticonvulsants
	Antidepressants	

   Cluster headache is similar to a migraine headache; however, the triggers are different. The triggers include vasodilating agents (nitroglycerine), histamine, alcohol, and nicotine. Acetylcholine is believed to play a role in the parasympathetic symptoms.

2. Withholding treatment refers to never starting a treatment. Withdrawing treatment refers to stopping a treatment once it has been started. The deciding factor is whether the decision is consistent with the patient's or surrogate's interests and preferences. If the surrogate decides to withhold the tube feedings, the health care provider must respect the decision. Administering the tube feeding against the surrogate's wishes would violate their autonomy.
3. Parkinson's disease is a slowly progressive degenerative neurological disorder caused by the loss of nerve cell function in the basal ganglia. The basal ganglia includes the substantia nigra, striatum, globus pallidus, subthalamic nucleus, and the red nucleus. Loss of nerve cells in the substantia nigra causes a reduction of dopamine production. Dopamine is the neurotransmitter essential for control of posture, supporting the body in an upright position, and voluntary motions.
4. Meal planning to promote medication effectiveness; provide verbal cues to chew food thoroughly; teach caregivers the Heimlich maneuver; match food consistency to ability to swallow; and schedule meals when patient is well rested.
5. The student would compare any three of the neurological degenerative disorders described in the chapter, as related to pathophysiology.

Chapter 38

The solutions to the review activities are demonstrated in the assessment of patients in practicum settings.

Chapter 39

1. Student will accomplish this in an applied clinical setting.
2. Student will accomplish this in an applied clinical setting.
3. Student will accomplish this in an applied clinical setting.
4. Student will accomplish this in an applied clinical setting.
5. (a) Remember to assess the patient for priority injuries first, (b) leave the object in place and stabilize the patient's head, (c) place a cup over the impaled object and tape in place, and (d) transport the patient in a safe and efficient manner remembering to not allow the impaled object to move.
6. a. Myopia is nearsightedness, which occurs when the light passing through the eye is overbent or overrefracted. Objects that are viewed up close are clear and distant objects are unclear. Myopia is treated with corrective lens that redirects the light to the retina by changing the angle of the light. These corrective lens' are cut biconcave.
   b. Hyperopia, or farsightedness, occurs when the light passing through the eye is focused behind the retina when looking a close objects. As a result, images up close are unclear, but images over 20 feet distant are clear. Hyperopia is treated with convex corrective lens that redirects the light to the retina.
   c. Astigmatism occurs where the light is spread over a diffuse area. Astigmatism occurs when there is an unequal curve of the cornea, and the light rays are bent unevenly. The exact cause of astigmatism is unknown, although there is some familial pattern. Astigmatism is treated with corrective lens in a cylindrical shape.
7. Hordeolum is an inflamed sweat gland, which is reddened, swollen, and tender to touch and is also called a stye.

   Chalazion is a small benign tumor similar to a sebaceous cyst, hordeolum, or even a sebaceous carcinoma.

   Blepharitis is an inflammation of the hair follicles (cilia) and glands along the edges of the eyelids.

   Conjunctivitis, also called pink eye, can be the result of exposure to allergens or irritants and as such is not contagious.

   Keratitis is an inflammation and ulceration of the cornea.
8. Reading devices with increased bifocal power; monocular microscopes ("near telescopes"); handheld magnifiers; stand magnifiers; illuminated magnifiers; closed circuit televisions; large print newspapers, magazines, and other reading materials; dial markers on the gauges of appliances; self-threading needles; books on tape; talking clocks and watches.

Chapter 40

1. Preparing the patient for surgery is an important part of nursing care. Communicating clear expectations before surgery will help alleviate fears. Stressing that manipulation of the auditory system may interfere with hearing and take some time before hearing is restored. Other teaching should include avoiding anything that will interfere with the function of the eustachian tube (blowing nose, cough, sneeze), not lying on the surgical side, and ways in which the nurse and patient will communicate after surgery.
2. Learning as much as possible is important to be able to counsel the patient of potential resources in their own community. The nurse is a valuable contact person for patients with a hearing deficit to obtain information on what services are accessible and also make a useful tool when encountering a patient or family member who has auditory dysfunction.
3. The more information that the nurse has, the more he or she will be able to provide to the patient. The Internet has a wealth of information, and the nurse should be able to decipher fact from fiction. Many elderly patients are not computer savvy and need assistance in finding the best resource to meet their needs.
4. There are so many types of hearing aids that the nurse should become familiar with as many types as possible to assist the patient in the office or hospital. Visiting the audiologist will also give the nurse a valuable resource person when needed.
5. Putting yourself in another's shoes is an ideal way to get a picture of what the patient may be experiencing. Using both an ear muff and plugs will block out the most sound, and the nurse will be able to identify with a person having auditory dysfunction. This experience will also give the students a chance to experiment with different ways to communicate without hearing sounds.

Chapter 41

1. You should empathize with the patient, assessing her knowledge of SLE and its diagnosis. Educating the patient about both the disease and the testing is essential, as fear of the unknown is the worst kind of fear. She should be informed that the tests will show if she has inflammation not associated with an infection and whether she has antinuclear antibodies. She should also be informed that her symptoms are nonspecific, and the tests will help to determine what is wrong with her. She should be advised that although ANA is associated with SLE, it can be caused by other things.
2. Increased UTI in an elderly male patient is most likely associated with decreased urine output and decreased bladder sensitivity and possibly prostate hypertrophy. Other things that should be assessed include the urine for proteinuria, hematuria, and glycosuria (diabetes).
3. The allergy should be posted prominently in the patient's room. Nonlatex gloves should be placed in the patient's room, as well as nonlatex versions of any other bandages or instruments that may be needed in their care. Stethoscopes should be covered in a protective sleeve. The patient should be educated in the differences in appearance between common latex and nonlatex supplies. The patient should be instructed to be assertive if latex products are being used.
4. The exact requirements may vary, but your patient will most likely require proof of all the childhood immunizations, including MMR, HIB, hepatitis B, polio, tetanus, and varicella. In addition, she will also need a PPD. Booster shots will likely be needed for MMR and tetanus/diphtheria, if she did not have them when she started college as a freshman.
5. Sexual behaviors and risk should be addressed, as well as any past STDs or possible exposures. The nature of the tests to be performed should be explained as well as the procedures for picking up the results of the test. Any concerns or fears should be dealt with as empathetically as possible.

Chapter 42

1. A case study about HIV/AIDS would need to be available. Students will gain additional knowledge about the various drugs used in treatment of HIV/AIDS and also learn more about the disease process.
2. Allows students to study several diagnostic tests that are used for patients with immune disorders. In addition, the focus of patient education is beneficial to the student in addressing the practical needs of the patient.
3. Provides current update and exploration of internet resources and national guidelines for HIV/AIDS.
4. Allows student to consider the psychosocial or physical or spiritual aspects of a chronic immune disease and how to interact with patients.
5. Promotes critical thinking about safety measures for patients with immune disorders and procedures to follow for employees who have accidental exposure to HIV-contaminated fluids.
6. Provides the opportunity for students to research information on immune disorders, which are presented in this immune chapter.

Chapter 43

1. Examples of hypersensitivity type 1 allergic response are:
   a. Anaphylaxis
   b. Atopic asthma
   c. Atopic eczema
   d. Drug allergy
   e. Acute rhinitis
2. The patient and family communication should include a discussion of learning to anticipate triggers and practicing avoidance. Asthma triggers irritate the lungs and produce mucus, inflammation, and tightening of the bronchial tubes. Common triggers for asthma include:
   - Pollen: keep windows and doors closed, and use air conditioning to keep pollen out.
   - Dust mites: use special coverings for mattresses and pillows. Remove carpets, rugs and drapery in bedrooms. Wash bedding in hot water.
   - Toys should not include stuffed animals.
   - Keep humidity between 30–40 percent.
   - Use a vacuum cleaner with a filter. Change filter and bag often.
   - Animal hair and dander: Pet removal is best. If around pets, keep them out of bedrooms, and off furniture.
   - Mold: Try to eliminate mold in the environment. Dehumidifiers can help. Avoid freshly cut grass.
   - Environment: Avoid cigarette smoke and all other types of smoke. When outdoor air quality is poor, stay indoors. Cover the nose and mouth during cold weather.
   - Exercise: Perform slow warm-ups and cool-downs and be sure to use asthma medication

approximately 10 minutes before beginning an exercise routine.

3. Four categories for potential allergens that may cause anaphylaxis in hypersensitive patients are:
   - Drugs
   - Insect venoms
   - Foods
   - Animal serums
   - Blood products
   - Contrast media
4. Food allergy is treated by avoiding the foods that trigger the reaction. By excluding certain foods, (milk, soy, or wheat) from the diet, the patient with a food allergy can gradually reintroduce the eliminated foods back into the diet and evaluate potential for allergic response to the reintroduced food.
5. Exposure to an allergen initiates a humoral response. Immunoglobulin E (IgE) molecules specific to an antigen attach to cell surface receptors on mast cells. The mast cell's response includes the release of histamine, a hormone that causes vasodilation and an increase in permeability of blood vessel walls. The release of histamine creates the clinical manifestations of an allergic reaction.
6. Avoiding the allergen is the best treatment. Other treatments include treating the symptoms with antihistamines, decongestants, and corticosteroids applied by nasal spray. Secondary infections indicated by facial pain or a greenish-yellow discharge may require antibiotic therapy.
7. Atopy refers to an individual being prone to develop allergies because of a genetic state of hyper-responsiveness to sensitizing agents. If a person inherits this tendency from parents who are allergic, they have a hyper-responsive immune system that will produce large quantities of IgE on the second or subsequent exposure to an allergen. These individuals may develop a number of allergies. The spectrum of their allergic conditions may include asthma, food allergies, drug allergies, eczema, and so on.

Chapter 44

1. Best applied in the practicum setting by interviewing three persons of different cultural backgrounds. This activity permits the student to apply a holistic perspective of skin conditions and to use critical thinking skills in comparing information from different cultures.
2. Best applied with a small group of peers, either in a laboratory or practicum setting. This activity involves the use of several skills—critical thinking, problem solving, creativity—and if it is a group activity, it can be an exercise for working as a team. It also permits the student to use a holistic approach to understanding the physiological and psychosocial-spiritual aspects of an individual.
3. This activity can be done in a learning laboratory setting with peers or alone. The activity involves the student in considering the various environmental factors that contribute to skin disorders, the risks involved, and the development of patient teaching strategies.
4. This activity is best performed using an assessment text, along with interviewing or assessing an older person (e.g., friend of family or relative). It involves developing an organized approach for assessment, use of interview skills, review of information about etiology of older adult skin damage, and interaction with an older adult, and use of communication skills.
5. This activity is best performed while accessing the Web site at: http://www.aad.org. Click on Public Resource Center, then click on Skincarephysicians.com. The student can then review the information and develop an instruction pamphlet based on the answers to questions posed on the specific skin disorder.
6. This activity is best performed while accessing the Web site at: http://www.aad.org. Click on Public Resource Center, click on Kids Connection. This is an especially good activity for students who enjoy computer resources. There is a wealth of information at the American Academy of Dermatology Web site. The specific activities will increase knowledge about the various skin disorders and allow the students to be creative in completing the projects. Accessing the Web site will also provide additional resources for learning.

Chapter 45

1. Because dermatological dysfunctions are most often managed in private practices the observational experience is meant to expose the student to typical dermatological dysfunctions and to the typical management of those dysfunctions, both by physicians and by nurses. There are no right or wrong observations.
2. Examples of nursing diagnoses are:
   - Acute pain R/T contact dermatitis: Assess pain on regular basis. Teach principles of pain management. Administer pharmacological methods of pain relief.
   - Impaired skin integrity R/T radiation: Assess skin on regular basis. Remove adhesive tape and debris.

Keep bed linens clean, dry, and wrinkle free. Apply topical medications, as appropriate. Document skin condition.

- Imbalanced nutrition: Less than body weight R/T body weight 20 percent or more under ideal. Complete a nutritional assessment. Weigh patient at regular intervals. Monitor caloric and nutrient intake. Offer nutritional supplements, as needed.
- Disturbed body image R/T skin lesions: Determine patient's body image expectations. Assist patient to discuss changes. Facilitate contact with individuals with similar changes.
- Risk for infection R/T tissue destruction and increased environmental exposure: Monitor for signs and symptoms of infection. Maintain asepsis. Inspect skin and mucous membranes for redness, erythema, or drainage. Provide appropriate skin.

3. The two main herpetic infections are: (a) Herpes simplex virus-1 (HSV-1) and (b) herpes simplex virus-2 (HSV-2). HSV-1 is generally associated with oral cold sores and fever blisters, and HSV-2 is associated with genital infections. Both types of infections are becoming more common and may be related to oral-genital sexual contact. Treatment of HSV consists of cool, moist compresses of Burrow's solution, controlling secondary infections, and systemic or topical antivirals that may include Acyclovir, Famvir, or Valtrex. Treatment of herpes zoster centers on pain control and antiviral therapy. Antiviral medications must be started within 72 hours of the onset of the rash or pain. Pain can be severe enough to require nerve blocks. Selection and dosage of medications is determined according to the needs of the individual patient. The same antiviral drugs used to treat HSV are used to treat herpes zoster.
4. This is best evaluated in class and seminar settings. The strategies for treatment are the preventive strategies of covering up the areas easily burned, using protective lotions or creams to block the sun rays, and close observation of the skin for symptoms of sunburn.
5. This is applied in the seminar and laboratory settings by assessing one another and interviewing peers for their reactions and comments to their wart conditions. In addition, reviewing the pathophysiology and management strategies together can increase the knowledge level of all involved.

Chapter 46

1. Complaints of pain would be the ideal assessment indicator for distinguishing a partial-thickness from a full-thickness burn. Partial-thickness burns have intact pain receptors and nerve endings therefore pain is sensed. Pain receptors and nerve endings are destroyed in full-thickness burns and pain is not sensed (this is why escharotomy, a surgical incision, does not require an anesthetic).
2. *Withdrawal* nursing approaches include: avoid forcing patient to deal with situation, provide supportive environment, and provide ongoing information on status and care. *Denial* nursing approaches include: support patient, avoid forcing patient to deal with fears, answer questions honestly, and provide information in small doses over time. *Regression* nursing approaches include: avoid attacking and responding negatively to behavior exhibited, acknowledge patient's difficulty in coping, and encourage and reward positive behaviors and independence. *Anger and hostility* nursing approaches include: encourage verbalization of frustration, avoid responding directly to anger, provide choices and control, and assist patient to search for meaning to injury. *Depression* nursing approaches include: acknowledge the loss and focus the patient on realistic expectations.
3. Develop a fire escape plan. Keep exit routes free of clutter and have two escape routes. Do not include windows with bars in the escape routes. All windows with bars should have a quick release feature for easy removal. Keep whistle by bed to alert rescuers where you are or to warn others of fire. The fire department will place a sticker in your bedroom window to assist firefighters in locating you should a fire occur. Keep eyeglasses, keys, flashlight, and telephone near your bedside in case of an emergency. People using oxygen should not smoke or be near fire with oxygen in use. Smokers should use large deep ashtrays and never smoke in bed. Set hot water heater thermostat at 120° F or less with installation of valves in the bathrooms that regulate water temperature. Turn handles of pans to back of stove when cooking. Do not wear clothing with loose sleeves when cooking. Double-check that the stove is off after cooking.
4. Emergent phase: The goals of management include psychosocial adjustment of the patient, the prevention of scars and contractures, and the resumption of preburn activity, including work, family, and social roles. This phase may take years or even last a lifetime.
5. Appearance

Superficial Partial Injury
  Blisters that will increase in size
  Blanches with fingertip pressure and color returns when pressure returns
  Moist

Deep Partial Injury
 Blisters present slower to increase in size
 Blanching decreased, prolonged
 Less moisture
 Color

Superficial Partial Injury
 Pink

Deep Partial Injury
 Pale, mottled with dull, white, tan, cherry red areas

Healing Time

Superficial Partial Injury
 5 to 21 days, no grafting

Deep Partial Injury
 21 to 35 days without complications
 May convert to full-thickness and require grafting

Chapter 47

1. The major organs of the gastrointestinal (GI) tract include the hollow organs from the mouth to the anus; the pancreas that through its exocrine function produces digestive enzymes, and the liver and biliary systems, which achieve important metabolic, digestive, and absorption functions.
2. Perform a concise GI health history by examining the following areas:

   (a) family history, (b) past abdominal history and current problems, (c) eating habits, (d) nutritional assessment, (e)evaluating dysphagia or heartburn (pyrosis), (f) assessing nausea or vomiting, (g) assessing any abdominal pain, and (h) describing any medications taken in any form, particularly those that might influence the GI tract.
3. The physiological processes that are involved during the act of vomiting are: (a) stimulation of afferent input to the vagal fibers, which stimulates serotonin 5 via the splanchnic autonomic fibers, (b) stimulation of the vestibular system (CN VII), which increases histamine H_1 and muscarinic cholinergic receptors, (c) stimulation of the central nervous system (CNS) centers, which are located in the center dorsal part of the medulla oblongata, and (d) stimulation of the chemoreceptor trigger zone (CTZ) located in the floor of the fourth ventricle (outside of the blood-brain barrier).
4. Perform the three primary tests for appendicitis, which are:
   a. Rebound tenderness (Blumberg's sign): A positive response may mean peritoneal irritation. The tips of the fingers are pressed gently into the abdominal wall then suddenly withdrawn. A painful response is positive. Cutaneous hyperesthesia is elicited in the area of the skin over an appendix that is inflamed.
   b. Iliopsoas muscle test: The patient is asked to flex the right thigh (raises the right leg) against resistance (pushing down over the lower part of the thigh)—the patient will experience pain in the pelvis because of irritation of the iliopsoas muscle.
   c. Obturator muscle test: The patient flexes the right thigh (raises the right leg) to 90 degrees. Holding the ankle, the leg is rotated internally and externally. Pelvic pain is produced is the muscle is inflamed.
5. Choose any two of the diagnostic tests from this chapter and describe their use.

Chapter 48

1. A great resource for this patient is the American Diabetes Association at www.diabetes.org. Although this patient has not been diagnosed as being diabetic, the Web site lists community events and resources, has an online bookstore, and has a section on diabetes prevention. The patient should check with his or her health care provider to see if he or she can start a moderate exercise program. Keeping food records, decreasing portion sizes, and reading labels are actions the patient can take to improve his or her diet.
2. Utilize the BMI chart. The National Heart, Lung, and Blood Institute, www.nhlbi.nih.gov, has information on their Web site called "Aim for a Healthy Weight." Under this section, there is information on exercise, shopping, menu planning, and other helpful tips. Information can also be obtained by mail:

   NHLBI Information Center

   P.O. Box 30105

   Bethesda, MD 20824-0105

   Phone: 301-592-8573

   Fax: 301-592-8563
3. Patients with increased protein needs who might need a higher protein enteral feeding include patients with protein losses from wounds, fistulas, and hypercatabolic patients, such as burn patients.
4. If you are doing a clinical rotation or are employed by a hospital, ask for a copy of the policy on nutrition screening and assessment. JCAHO accredited hospitals are required to screen for nutrition risk and have a process in place to further assess at-risk patients.
5. Causes of the rise in childhood obesity include inadequate physical activity, along with a more sedentary lifestyle, including more hours spent

watching television. In addition, children often over-consume high calorie foods.

6. To help your elderly patients in the hospital maintain their nutritional status be on the alert for any problems with chewing, swallowing, or mouth pain and contact the health care provider when these problems are noted. Patients, who are underweight or who have had weight loss and are not diabetic, may benefit from between meal supplements. A dietitian consult can be helpful if these interventions are not successful.

Chapter 49

1. Have the patient look in a mirror and check for symmetry, the presence of lumps, swelling, or bumps. Then have him or her assess the skin on his or her face and look for moles, sores, or growths that have changed in size or color. Continue to teach the patient to check his or her neck and chin for any lumps, tenderness, or swelling. Tell the patient to assess the lips for sores or color changes and to inspect his or her mouth area with a flashlight and note areas of discoloration and to look for lumps, swelling, or bumps. Finally, instruct the patient to contact his or her dentist if he or she sees anything unusual in his or her self-exam.
2. The student would contact the speech pathology department and follow them in an observational capacity as they work with their patients.
3. The student would gain permission to watch an endoscopy and then describe the procedure.
4. The nurse should instruct the patient to (a) eat small meals at any given setting and avoid eating two to three hours before sleeping, (b) wash the throat with water after each meal, (c) sit in a semi-Fowler's position if lying down after eating, (d) avoid irritating food substances, and (e) quit smoking.
5. The patient often experiences upper epigastric pain, particularly if his or her stomach is empty. In addition, he or she may describe certain foods as causing him or her to have more pain, or he or she could describe the manifestations to be worse during stressful situations. In addition, the patient may be able to point to a specific area of the abdomen as the origin of his or her pain.
6. Initially, a genuine concerned attitude is portrayed by the nurse. Then, the nurse should express to the patient that it is important for the patient to ask whatever questions he or she has of his or her health care providers. The nurse can ask who the patient has for support systems and whether he or she would like the nurse to be there when telling these people about the new diagnosis. The nurse can move toward describing the types of supportive care that are typically presented for patients with cancer of the stomach (e.g., pharmacology, surgery). The nurse must remember to not answer with generalizations or statements, which ignore the severity of the new diagnosis.

Chapter 50

1. This will be accomplished in student classroom or lab setting.
2. This will be accomplished in the practicum setting.
3. This will be accomplished in the practicum setting.
4. The etiology of peritonitis can be a postoperative inflammatory infection, ruptured appendix, abdominal fistulas that have resulted in infection, and any other condition that allows contamination of the peritoneal area. The potential effects of peritonitis are septic shock, MODS, and SIRS. The typical clinical manifestations are hypotension, tachycardia, severe febrile condition, renal failure, and decreasing level of consciousness and mentation.
5. The etiology and risk factors for the development of herniations of the bowel are any conditions which increase intraabdominal pressure (e.g., ascites, portal hypertension), inflammatory bowel disorders, and cancer of the bowel. The management strategies for inguinal hernia repair are those that are typical for recovering abdominal surgeries (e.g., monitor vital signs for potential respiratory problems, monitor the healing of the wound area, deep breathing exercises, and active or passive range of motion. In addition, many of these surgeries are short-term surgeries and may allow the patient to be discharged within 24 hours of the surgery, which makes patient teaching important.
6. The etiology and risk factors for the development of hemorrhoids are employment that has a lack of mobility and sitting in one position for long periods of time (e.g., truck driving, grocery clerks, officer personnel); peripheral vascular disorders; and genetic predisposition to circulatory dysfunction. The clinical manifestations are internal or external bleeding of the rectal tissue, painful bowel movements with bleeding, uncomfortable when in a sitting position, chronic anemia, decreased hematocrit or hemoglobin, swelling and protrusion of the hemorrhoids in the anorectal region.

Chapter 51

1. Conjugated bilirubin (direct bilirubin) is bound to molecules while unconjugated bilirubin (indirect bilirubin) is not bound to another molecule. Total bilirubin lab tests reflect the amount of conjugated plus unconjugated bilirubin in the blood.
2. The nurse can physically palpate and percuss the liver as one method of assessing the size and location of the liver boundaries. In addition, serum tests are performed to screen patients with no symptoms. In addition, bile fluid examinations, endoscopy, liver biopsies, ultrasound, computed tomography (CT), magnetic resonance imaging (MRI), nuclear medicine, angiogram, and radiological tests can be performed.
3. Hepatitis A is spread via fecal-oral routes, is shorter in duration, and can be prevented with medical asepsis methods of care. Hepatitis B is transmitted with blood and body fluids, causes lifelong destruction to the patient and has relatively high mortality and morbidity rates.
4. Biliary cirrhosis results from blocked bile ducts, which cause congestion, inflammation, and damage to the tissue in the liver. Infants are affected when they are born with biliary atresia, which deprives the bile of avenues of exit from the liver and ultimately causing tissue damage. In adults, inflamed or blocked bile ducts can occur with scarring results.

   Cardiac cirrhosis occurs when blood flow out of the liver is restricted by severe right-sided heart failure. When that blood is not able to exit at a predictable rate, liver engorgement occurs and the pressure in the liver vasculature increases, causing venous congestion, anoxia or hypoxia, and hepatic cell necrosis.
5. The student would describe his or her feelings regarding caring for patients with alcoholism.
6. The student would describe his or her feelings if he or she were asked to donate his or her liver to a relative.
7. The laparoscopic cholecystectomy has a faster recovery time, fewer complications, and fewer bile duct injuries than the open cholecystectomy. In this operation, a small incision is made at the umbilicus plus three other puncture sites. A laparoscope with video camera and laser technology is introduced, and the gallbladder is dissected from the surrounding organs, drained of fluid and stones, and removed through the incision at the umbilicus.

   The open cholecystectomy can be performed when the laparoscopic technique fails, there are stones that are inaccessible to the laparoscope, or other surgeries are required at the same time (as in treating trauma). The gallbladder is dissected and removed, the cystic duct is ligated, and a T-tube is inserted into the common bile duct to keep it patent.

Chapter 52

1. The structures are the kidney, ureter, bladder, urethra, nephron, and tubule structure of the kidney.

   The kidney is responsible for ultrafiltration; the ureter is the structure that allows for flow of kidney fluids from the kidney to the bladder; the bladder is a small sac-like organ that collects urine; the nephron is the functional unit of the kidney; the tubule structure is responsible for the transport within the kidney.
2. Student-directed activity in a clinical setting.
3. Decreased muscle tone and elasticity in the ureters, bladder, urinary sphincter, and surrounding structures resulting in problems of incontinence; prostatic hyperplasia in the male resulting in urinary retention; decreased functioning nephrons and glomerular filtration rate. This may be reflected in slightly higher blood levels of urea nitrogen and creatinine; nocturia may become a result from problems of retention or from decreases in renal concentration.
4. Examples of diagnostic tests are renal biopsy, renal ultrasound, and intravenous pyelogram. The renal biopsy obtains a physical cellular example from the kidney for further examination. The renal ultrasound is a noninvasive test that provides images of the kidney and surrounding structures. The intravenous pyelogram is a radioactive dye study that allows for visualization of the function.
5. It is important to know the location of supplies and equipment so you can be efficient in your work in the clinical setting.

Chapter 53

1. The student will perform this activity in the clinical course arena.
2. Acute pyelonephritis presents with bacteriuria accompanied by flank pain at the costovertebral angle, fever, and chills. In addition, the patient may experience painful urination, frequency, nocturia, nausea, vomiting, and colicky abdominal pain.
3. The typical presentation of renal stones is sudden-onset unilateral flank pain, which usually causes the individual to seek medical attention. The pain does not completely remit but rather waxes and wanes. The pain is often accompanied by nausea and

occasionally vomiting. The pain can radiate to a variety of locations depending on the location of the stone. When the stone is in the upper ureter, pain may radiate anteriorly to the abdomen. When the stone is in the lower ureter, pain can radiate to the ipsilateral testicle in men or ipsilateral labium in women. If the stone is lodged at the ureterovesical junction, the major symptoms may be urinary frequency and urgency. A less common acute presentation is gross hematuria without pain. The patient may also experience the first stage of shock with cool, diaphoretic skin. In addition, the patient may develop a urinary tract infection and have the symptoms of fever, nausea, and vomiting.

4. Possible complications associated with renal injuries are secondary hemorrhage, usually due to infection (10 to 14 days after trauma), paralytic ileus (4 to 5 days) as a result of retroperitoneal hematoma, hypertension as a result of the constricting effect of reorganizing perirenal hematoma, arterio-venous fistula, renal failure, renal atrophy, hydronephrosis, chronic pyelonephritis, renal calculi, and renal artery stenosis.

5. The most commonly performed surgery to treat renal cell cancer is radical nephrectomy. During a radical nephrectomy, the whole kidney along with the cancer, the attached adrenal gland, and the fatty tissue immediately around the kidney are removed. The lymph nodes around the kidney are often removed and examined under the microscope to determine if they contain cancer. Partial nephrectomy is performed to preserve as much normal kidney tissue as possible; however its complication rate may be slightly higher than radical nephrectomy. Open partial nephrectomy is usually the treatment of choice when radical nephrectomy may result in either immediate dialysis or a high risk for subsequent dialysis. Laparoscopic radical nephrectomy is a surgical technique that is less extensive and invasive than a typical radical nephrectomy. Compared to open radical nephrectomy, laparoscopic radical nephrectomy involves longer operative time, less postoperative pain, shorter hospital stays and shorter recovery time.

Chapter 54

1. Acute pyelonephritis presents with bacteriuria accompanied by flank pain at the costovertebral angle, fever, and chills. In addition, the patient may experience painful urination, frequency, nocturia, nausea, vomiting, and colicky abdominal pain.

2. Autosomal dominant polycystic kidney disease (ADPKD) is caused by genetic mutations on chromosomes 4 and 16. A multisystem disorder, ADPKD occurs in 1 of every 500 to 1,000 individuals. Eighty-five percent of the gene carriers will evidence the disease by their seventh decade and 50 to 75 percent will advance to end-stage renal disease.

   ARPKD, on the other hand, occurs in only 1 in every 6,000 to 55,000 individuals, is more aggressive and usually causes patient death by age 15.

3.
   - Upper and lower respiratory symptoms including hoarseness, shortness of breath, cough, hemoptysis or nasal drainage; and inspect for nasal crusting or septal defect
   - Recent hearing deficit, tinnitus, pain; inspect ear for drainage, or perforation of the tympanic membrane
   - Sinus infection; pain or tenderness over the sinuses
   - Visual disturbances or conjunctivitis
   - Joint and muscle aches
   - Changes in urine quantity and quality

4. It has been demonstrated that many patients presenting with rhabdomyolysis do not admit to muscle pain or tenderness and do not present with swelling. This emphasizes the need for repeated patient questioning and thorough examination for early intervention and optimal recovery.

5. HD is more definitive in its abilities to filter the blood than CAPD. In addition, HD is monitored thoroughly by a trained clinician and is performed in a dialysis center.

   CAPD, on the other hand, is cheaper, can be performed by a family member or care provider at home, and allows the patient to be more flexible in where they perform the CAPD (e.g., the patient could travel and carry the equipment to perform the CAPD "on the road"). Potential disadvantages for CAPD include protein loss and potential for life-threatening peritoneal infection.

6. The donor should know that it is fundamental that they have disclosed everything that is pertinent and that they have been completely truthful to those asking questions prior to kidney donation (e.g., presence of HIV and illicit drugs). In addition, the donor needs to be told that they will have to undergo major surgery to have the kidney removed. However, donor nephrectomy can be accomplished by laparoscopic surgery, which involves an approximate 2 to 3 inch incision in the lower quadrant suffices for delivering the kidney.

Chapter 55

1. Endocrine glands are ductless glands that secrete specific hormones into the blood stream for circulation to their target cells. Examples of endocrine glands include the hypothalamus, pituitary, thyroid, parathyroid, thymus, adrenal glands, pancreas, ovaries in the females, and testes in the male.

   Exocrine glands empty their secretions into ducts that transport the secretions to specific locations. Examples of exocrine glands include the salivary and sweat glands. The pancreas is both an endocrine and an exocrine gland. The islets of Langerhans make up the endocrine portion of the pancreas, regulating the control of blood glucose.

   As an exocrine gland the pancreas secretes digestive enzymes through ducts that empty into the duodenum.

2. An example of negative feedback in the body is the secretion of insulin in response to rising blood glucose levels. When blood glucose levels in the body rise, insulin is secreted by the islet cells of the pancreas. Insulin acts on the cells, causing them to take up the excess glucose in the bloodstream. The blood glucose level then falls, and insulin secretion stops.

3. Hypothalamus is located at the base of the forebrain near the thalamus and regulates the anterior pituitary hormones.

   Thyroid is located in the neck, inferior to the larynx and cricoid cartilage and regulates the rate of metabolism.

   Parathyroids are located in the lobes of the thyroid and regulate levels of calcium and phosphate.

   Adrenal glands are located above each kidney and regulate metabolism, blood pressure, sodium, and potassium levels.

   Pancreas is located between the duodenum and the spleen and regulates blood glucose levels.

4. Do you have enough energy to perform your normal daily tasks?

   Have you experienced any changes in your appetite or weight?

   Have you noticed any changes in your ability to tolerate heat or cold?

   Have you noticed any changes in your sleep?

   Do you have any difficulty with concentration?

   Have you noticed any changes in the beating of your heart?

   Have you had any changes in your usual bowel patterns?

   Have you noted any changes in your skin or hair?

   Are your belts or rings tighter than normal?

5. Thyroid is not enlarged, symmetrical, smooth, and nontender.

Chapter 56

1. a. Solution: Na = 115 mmol/L
   b. Solution: Neurological. The sodium level indicates dilutional hyponatremia, which can cause cerebral edema resulting in alteration in cognitive and sensory/motor function. As the sodium level drops, the patient may even seizure.
   c. Solution: 1. Ongoing neurological and fluid volume status; 2. Implementing fluid restriction as indicated; 3. Careful monitoring of intake and output; and 4. Cautious administration of NaCl 3%.

2. a. Solution:

      Skin: Oily skin, hyperpigmentation of lower extremities, hair loss, and moist warm skin.

      Eyes: Proptosis (forward placement of the eyes), lid retraction, or puffiness in periorbital area. Blurred or double vision.

      Neuromuscular: Fine hand tremor, hyperactive reflex response, nervousness, muscular weakness.

      Respiratory: Shortness of breath, exertional dyspnea.

      GI: Weight loss even with high caloric intake; Diarrhea.

      Cardiovascular: Palpitations, tachycardia, dysrhythmias, or hypertension.

   b. Solution: TSH (Thyroid-stimulating hormone) and a T_4 (Thyroxin) are recommended for initial diagnosing of hyperthyroidism.
   c. Solution: Beta blocker, i.e., propranolol or atenolol

3. a. Solution: Change in menstrual cycle: amenorrhea or oligomenorrhea; galactorrhea; or infertility.
   b. Solution: Because of the estrogen deficiency that accompanies hyperprolactinemia, women often develop osteopenia and osteoporosis.

4. a. Solution: Potassium. In Cushing's disease, an excess of mineral corticoids leads to retention of sodium and potassium loss.
   b. Solution: 1. Cardiac dysrhythmias; 2. Muscle weakness; 3. Decrease in gastrointestinal motility; and 4. Polyuria.

5. Solution: A patient who is alert will be thirsty and request water or other drinks, thereby maintaining fluid balance. An unconscious patient will readily

become dehydrated with fluid and electrolyte replacement. Another problem is that elderly people sometimes lose their thirst sensation and are not sensitive to their need for fluids.

Chapter 57

1. Acute illnesses, even a viral infection or upper respiratory infection, can affect the blood sugar level. This occurs as the counter regulatory hormones respond to the stress of the illness. The patient should be taught to continue eating his or her regular meal plan and increase the amount of fluids that do not have calories, i.e., water and decaffeinated fluids. They should monitor their blood glucose every four hours and take their insulin or oral agents as prescribed. If the blood sugar level rises above 240 mg/dL, the urine should be checked for ketones every three to four hours. If moderate to large amounts of ketones are present in the urine, the health care provider should be contacted. If nausea and vomiting prevents the normal food intake, the glucose lowering agents should be continued as prescribed. If possible, fluids with carbohydrates should be ingested, such as regular soft drinks without caffeine, fruit juices, and soups. If the patient is not able to keep anything down, the health care provider should be notified. It is important that the patient understand to continue the glucose lowering agents during illness, either insulin or oral hypoglycemics, as the counter regulatory hormones will produce an elevation in blood glucose.
2. Feet should be inspected daily for signs of redness and pressure. If the patient is unable to do this, it should be done by a significant other. Cuts can be cleansed with warm water and mild soap. Do not use any over-the-counter antiseptics on cuts. Cover the cut with a clean dressing that does not apply pressure. Continue to observe the area for signs of infection. Socks should be white absorbent cotton or colorfast. It is important to check the temperature of the water to avoid burn injuries. Wash the feet daily in warm water using a mild soap. Dry thoroughly between the toes. Pat the feet dry, do not rub. Toenails should be cut straight across. No commercial preparations are to be used for removal of corns or calluses. Shoes should fit properly without any pressure areas and should not have open toes or heels. The patient should not go barefoot.
3. The blood sugar level is below 70 mg/dL indicating that the patient is hypoglycemic and requires immediate intervention. Because the patient is still responsive and able to swallow, 15 grams of a fast-acting carbohydrate such as 8 ounces of low-fat milk or 4–6 ounces of regular soft drink or fruit juice are given orally. Glucose tablets or gels may also be used in this situation as the patient is able to swallow. The blood sugar is reassessed 15 minutes after the carbohydrates are ingested. This is repeated until the blood sugar level rises above 70 mg/dL. The patient is then given a regularly scheduled meal or snack, and the blood glucose is reassessed in 45 minutes.
4. When patients with diabetes experience an acute illness, the body reacts to this stress by activating the counter-regulatory hormones. The counter-regulatory hormones increase blood sugar levels. It is common to see hospitalized patients on insulin therapy even though they do not require it at home. When the patient heals and returns home, he or she can expect to return to his or her usual management.
5. Polydipsia, polyphagia, and polyuria are symptoms that occur with hyperglycemia. Polyphagia (increased eating) is a result of the cells starving as there is not sufficient insulin present to move the food into the cells. Polyuria (frequent urination) and polydipsia (increased thirst) result from the osmotic effect of hyperglycemia. The thirst center is stimulated to reduce the concentration by increasing fluid intake, and the kidneys increase urination in an attempt to reduce the concentration on glucose.
6. The student will need to communicate with the diabetic educator to answer the specific questions for this question.

Chapter 58

1. Explain to the patient that a fracture goes through various stages of healing. The first stage takes several days to complete. The next stage, when new bone cells start to grow, can take up to a week to get started. The third stage occurs when the callus starts to form. The callus grows and becomes stronger for the next several weeks. By the end of the six weeks, the callus has strengthened enough to allow return to normal activity. The fracture area is still healing and may take three to four months to return to its previous strength. During this time the patient may feel tinges or aches at the healing fracture site, but this is completely normal.

   When teaching your patient about signs of circulatory and neurological impairment, review the neurovascular assessment. Show the patient how to check for proper movement in the hands and fingers or feet and toes. Teach the patient and his or her care providers how to check pulses and capillary refill. Inform the patient to report any numbness, tingling, or edema that is not relieved with 30 minutes of elevation of the extremity. Also teach the patient to feel the foot or hand for warmth. He or she should report these findings to a health care provider. Provide a handout to reinforce teaching and for discharge.

2. The quality of a nursing article depends on how applicable the information is to daily patient care. In the nursing article found, did the article address nursing assessment of the patient? Nursing articles should address nursing assessment and compare normal and abnormal findings for the particular topic investigated. The article should address what nursing interventions are done to minimize complications. Additionally, the article should address the collaboration necessary between the nurse and the health care provider or advanced practice nurse to determine the best plan of care. Also, patient or family involvement should be included during the discussion of plan of care.
3. Inform the neighbor with bursitis that a bursa is a fluid-filled sac under a tendon near the joint that provides cushioning and minimizes friction between the tendon and other structures in the joint. With bursitis the fluid-filled sac is swollen, and the cushioning over the joint is interrupted. This causes the tendon to rub on the bone, a ligament, or another tendon leading to pain.
4. During the assessment of a postoperative orthopedic patient, observe the nurse performing head-to-toe assessments. The nurse should be assessing for the following: level of consciousness; alertness and orientation; lung and heart sounds; bowel sounds; and a neurovascular assessment on the affected extremity or full neurological assessment that includes bilateral hand grasps, bilateral dorsiflexion, and plantar flexion for spine surgery. While performing the neurovascular assessment the nurse should assess both extremities to compare and contrast sides, looking for differences that may indicate neurovascular impairment related to the operative procedure.
5. Tell the patient that a magnetic resonance imaging (MRI) is the most sensitive technique for outlining structures in the body. The MRI can determine whether a tumor is within or adjacent to a bone. Computed tomography (CT) scans are not as sensitive and X-rays only show the surface structure of the bone, not what is happening inside the bone itself. In preparing the patient for the procedure, the nurse is responsible asking about metal implants and ensuring the consent form has been signed. A female patient should be asked about her pregnancy status. All patients need to remove jewelry. Explain the procedure and the length of the procedure. This depends on how many images the health care provider needs, but it generally takes 30 minutes. Determine if the patient gets claustrophobic. Some patients need to be lightly sedated because of anxiety. Unless the patient has had sedation, there are no special precautions needed after the procedure.

Chapter 59

1. Watching orthopedic surgery is like being in your father's workshop. You will see saws, hammers, screws, bolts, and other equipment. This is the equipment used to repair fractures and remove damaged bone tissue and make room for prostheses that will replace a joint surface. During join replacement you will notice that the team is dressed in what might be referred to as space suits, complete with helmets and air hoses for cooling the team member off. Because of the vascularity of the joint and susceptibility to infection, the surgeons wear these suits to protect the patient from infection. When working on an extremity, it is often suspended with tape and gauze to keep the extremity in the correct position to facilitate the surgery. Often the extremity is exsanguinated using ace wraps to minimize blood loss. The type of traction used in surgery is skin traction to keep the bone ends apart before or during the procedure.
2. Today, true orthopedic nursing units are vanishing. Quite often the service is coupled with another surgical service. Specialty hospitals are becoming more popular. There are several purely orthopaedic institutions across the United States. The types of patients seen on an inpatient unit are typically hospitalized after joint replacements or traumas. These patients are generally hospitalized, because they need special nursing care to assist in their recovery. This special care includes administration of antibiotics, establishing anticoagulant therapy, monitoring the patient's response, and ensuring the patient can perform mobility tasks safely (getting in and out of a bed or chair and ambulating with assistive devices). Other types of orthopedic surgery are generally done on an outpatient basis, because they do not require the special skills of a nurse to recover successfully. The typical length of stay for a joint replacement of the lower extremity is three to four days. These patients do not generally need to go to an extended care facility after discharge.
3. Tell your patient with osteoarthritis that although there is no cure for the disease, control can be obtained and they can live normal and active lives

with a few lifestyle changes. You can refer your patient to a local chapter of the Arthritis Foundation or other local arthritis support groups to assist in the physical and emotional coping that is required. When assessing acceptance of the information you provide, ask your patients what plans they may have to contact the organization. You can also make a follow-up phone call. You can offer support at that time and ask if she contacted the agency. Sometimes, patients just need encouragement to seek the assistance that will make their lives easier.

4. When obtaining information from the World Wide Web, you need to take many things into consideration, such as whether or not the information is from a reliable source and is accurate. Two sources that can assist in knowing about the reliability and accuracy of the information is the Health on the Net Foundation (http://www.hon.ch or http://www.hon.ch/HONcode/Conduct.html). This international foundation reviews Web sites for accuracy and reliability. They have a distinctive logo that they apply to a Web site homepage if they feel the information meets the standards of the foundation. Please visit one of the two sites to see the logo. Bobby Watchfire is a web accessibility desktop testing tool designed to help expose barriers to accessibility and encourage compliance with existing accessibility guidelines, including Section 508 of the U.S. Rehabilitation Act and the W3C's Web Content Accessibility Guidelines (WCAG). You can find this at http://www.watchfire.com. They rate Web sites according to the amount of compliance met to the Section 508 standards.

Chapter 60

1. Visiting an outpatient rehabilitation facility will give the student exposure to a wide variety of sports-related injuries not normally seen on an inpatient basis. They will be able to see firsthand what treatments are used for specific injuries and will be able to see the work involved with rehabilitation. It is also important to realize what limitations these patients must live with until their rehabilitation is complete.
2. Visiting an emergency department will expose the student to a wide variety of trauma. The student should focus on the initial treatments given in the field especially how any fractures are splinted and immobilized.
3. Visiting an inpatient orthopaedic unit will expose the student to patients who have sustained hip fractures. Describing the type of fracture along with the surgical treatment will help the student link the two together with the rationale on why that particular treatment was chosen. This activity will also help the student link which patients need to follow hip precautions.
4. Developing a teaching plan on fall prevention will help the student to focus on fall prevention strategies and to focus on how an elderly patient learns best. The student should include adult learning principles into the plan. It should also help the student to bring to fruition the risk factors that places a patient at risk for falls. Having the student list important questions will help to clarify and organize the main elements of the teaching plan.
5. It is important for the student to realize the value of being a patient advocate. To be an advocate the student must be able to find information that the patient may need and to be able to use available resources available to the nurse to bring the resources, such as a support group, and the patient together. The student must also be able to recognize quality Web sources and to be able to tell a patient how to find a quality Web source as well.

Chapter 61

1. Best applied in a laboratory setting with a peer. Use a nursing assessment text and develop a list of questions to ask in a sexual health history.
2. Best performed in a practicum setting by providing nursing care for a person of the opposite gender who is close to your age. Afterward, discuss with your peers the potential difficulties of patient education regarding self-examinations that are characteristic of reproductive function. Ideally, find a peer of the opposite gender and get his or her perspective on how he or she would feel having these types of questions asked of him or her. Remember, your goal is to increase your knowledge level to enhance your abilities to be comfortable with the topic.
3. Best applied in laboratory or seminar settings. Review the sexual response cycle before the discussion with a peer to increase your knowledge level in the content area.
4. Compare four of the varied diagnostic tests in the reproductive system that are performed with a male (e.g., urethral smear, urinalysis, semen analysis, digital rectal examination (DRE), endocrine evaluation of various hormones, and prostate-specific antigen [PSA] levels).
5. Compare four diagnostic tests in the reproductive system, which are performed with a female (e.g., mammography, blood cultures, Pap smear, colposcopy, culdoscopy, and endometrial biopsy).

Chapter 62

1. The patient education sheet should include most of the following elements:
   - Description of PCOS as an endocrine disorder with insulin resistance as its main pathology.
   - List of symptoms women may experience including hirsutism, high body mass index (BMI), acne, and infertility.
   - Descriptions of the lifestyle changes that may help relieve symptoms, including weight loss, exercise, calcium supplementation, and avoiding smoking.
   - List of medications that might be used to treat PCOS including oral contraceptives, metformin, clomiphene citrate, and topical eflornithine HCL.
   - Web sites and other patient resources.
2. Concerns for a hysterectomy patient may include:
   - Pain and pain relief issues
   - Returning to regular daily activities
   - Effects on sexual response
   - Response to loss of childbearing including grief, loss, or relief
   - Need for education about physical changes associated with hysterectomy
3. Sample nursing diagnoses for patient with PCOS:
   - Anxiety related to infertility
   - Disturbed body image related to physical changes associated with PCOS
   - Risk for situational low self-esteem related to changes in body image

   Expected outcomes for patient with PCOS:
   - Relief of anxiety
   - Improved body image
   - Improved self-esteem
4. Cervical cancer incidence by state can be found at the Centers for Disease Control and Prevention (CDC) Web site: http://www.cdc.gov/. Local cervical cancer incidence may be obtained from the American Cancer Society (ACS) or local health departments. Recommendations for improvement in cervical cancer screening programs may include screening women most at risk, e.g., those in sexually transmitted disease (STD) clinics; offering screening along with other services, e.g., mammograms or emergency department visits; and using a variety of providers to do screenings (nurse practitioners and physicians' assistants, along with physicians).
5. Postmenopausal women have a variety of attitudes about hormone therapy. Many women who were happily taking therapy in 2002 were distressed to learn about potential side effects and recommendations to reduce or stop therapy. Many other women have always been reluctant to take hormones and avoided any postmenopausal therapy. Other women are conflicted. They do not want to increase their risks for serious health conditions, but need effective relief of menopausal symptoms that interfere with activities of daily living and relationships. Interviewing postmenopausal women should give nursing students an idea of the range of opinions about hormone therapy and an insight into the controversy surrounding this topic.

Chapter 63

1. At birth there is rudimentary breast tissue that has ducts lined with epithelium. During puberty, or adolescence, there is a release of follicle-stimulating hormone (FSH), luteinizing hormone (LH), and prolactin that stimulates the release of estrogen from the ovaries. The estrogen stimulates the growth of the ductile system in the breasts, and the breast assumes the characteristic contour. During pregnancy, estrogen, progesterone and prolactin prepare the breast for lactation. At menopause, the breasts lose their glandular tissue because of decreased levels of estrogen and progesterone.
2. Patients need to first be advised that BSE should be performed once a month, eight days following menses or on any given fixed date. Advise the patient to avoid the time when her breasts might be tender because of menstruation or ovulation. Encourage her to put the BSE on her calendar and include her significant other in the process.

   Second, think B (bed): Show the patient how to palpate her breast while supine in bed using the palmar surfaces of her fingers. She should start by placing her right arm over her head and palpating the right breast with the left hand, moving in concentric circles from the periphery inward and including the periphery, tail of Spence, and areola. Finally, instruct the patient to squeeze the nipple to examine for discharge. Using the reverse procedure, she should examine the other breast.

   Third, think S (standing): Instruct the patient to repeat the above palpation method while standing.

   Fourth, think E (examination before a mirror): The patient should stand in front of a mirror with her arms at her sides, then with her arms raised over head, and finally with her hands pressed into her hips and in each position examine her breasts for symmetry, retractions, dimpling, inverted nipples, or nipple deviation.
3. This is performed in the clinical setting and should identify such topics as privacy issues, importance of

the gender of the health care provider, and clear communication encouraged by the health care provider.

4. The first surgeries for breast augmentation occurred in the 18th century with poor results. Throughout the 1990s the use of silicone implants for augmentation had varying results, but techniques have greatly improved since that time. Saline-filled implants have decreased some risks, but still have some complications. Breast augmentation surgeries continue to be evaluated and are being taken more seriously as improved techniques are employed.
5. A description needs to be given of one of the following: physical examination, mammography, ultrasonography, or biopsy.
6. A description is given for each of the following: cryotherapy, laser ablation, radiofrequency ablation (RFA), and focused ultrasound ablation. In most of these a probe is placed under the skin into the breast lesion under the guidance of an imaging modality, and tumor cell destruction is achieved by means of either heat or cold.

Chapter 64

1. This is performed in the clinical practicum setting with the selection of a patient with benign prostate hypertrophy. Discuss your findings with your peers in clinical seminar and laboratory settings.
2. Teach a TSE to a male patient. Introduce yourself in the clinical setting and describe the rationale for performing this procedure. Provide the patient time to ask questions and use information from an assessment text to support your techniques of examination.
3. Take notes in a reflective journal and perhaps selecting a patient with cancer would assist you in this activity. Then meet with a peer who shares your clinical course with you and ask open-ended questions regarding his or her feelings if he or she were to be diagnosed with cancer. Encourage open communication and be honest in stating how you would really feel if you were suddenly diagnosed with cancer.
4. This is best applied in a laboratory setting, and you can use a peer to simulate being the patient. Then share how you would bring up the initial topic of ED with the patient. Ask your peer to evaluate how you ask your questions and specifically to critique whether or not you appear to be comfortable and at ease in sharing your information.
5. This is best applied in a laboratory setting, and you can use a peer to simulate being the patient. Focus on techniques of therapeutic communication for discussing the priapism with the patient. Ask the peer to simulate asking you difficult questions and have the peer be hesitant to bring up the subject. Then, practice discussing the disorder using verbal techniques to make the patient be comfortable with this topic.

Chapter 65

The activities have been structured around World Wide Web sites to encourage the reader to actively research the many resources that are available. Some of the Web sites have interactive programs. Some of the materials can be downloaded free of charge and can be used as patient instructional materials. The various activities also stimulate critical thinking and can easily be used as individual or group assignments as part of the course requirements or as extra activities. Some of the articles include case studies related to the shock syndrome and multiple organ dysfunction.

Chapter 66

1. Reviewing an emergency department (ED) triage criteria will help one to become familiar with guidelines. This will also help to give some ideas as to what type of injuries or illnesses as triaged at what level.
2. Observing or even participating in a disaster drill is a wonderful way to see how hospitals implement their disaster policies and incident command. Disaster drill observation also will show how triage differs in a disaster versus every day triage.
3. This will allow the student to know what will be expected if he or she was in clinical if the hospital disaster plan was initiated and how the event would be run.
4. As a student, one must develop practices to protect oneself from contagious diseases. This includes knowing where to locate and how to use the appropriate personal protective equipment (PPE) for the disease.
5. Talking with CISM team members will give you a better understanding of the team members' roles. Familiarization with this process will make one more comfortable attending a debriefing if the situation arose.
6. There is no better way to experience ED nursing than have clinical time in the department.

References

Abbas, A., & Lichtman, A. (2004). *Basic immunology: Functions and disorders of the immune system* (2nd ed.). Philadelphia: W. B. Saunders Co.

Abu AlRub, R. (2004). Job stress, job performance, and social support among hospital nurses. *Journal of Nursing Scholarship,* 36(1), 73–78.

Ackley, B. J., & Ladwig, G. B. (2004). *Nursing diagnosis handbook: A guide to planning care* (6th ed.). St. Louis, MO: Mosby.

Adams, H. P., Adams, R. J., Brott, T., del Zoppo, G. J., Furlan, A., Goldstein, L. B., et al. (2003). Guidelines for the early management of patients with ischemic stroke: A scientific statement from The Stroke Council of the American Stroke Association. *Stroke, 34*(4), 1056–1083.

AdminaStar Federal. (2003). *Explanation of reimbursement rates under Critical Access Hospitals (CAH).* Washington, DC: Critical Access Hospital Certified Manual.

Aggarwal, S., (2003). Portal vein thrombosis complicating neonatal hepatic abscess. *Indian Pediatrics, 40*(10), 997–1001.

Agraharkar, M. (2004, September). *Nephrotic syndrome.* Retrieved January 25, 2006, from http://www.emedicine.com.

Ahrens, T., & Sona, C. (2003). Capnography application in acute and critical care. *AACN Clinical Issues, 14,* 123–132.

Ahrens, T., & Vollman, K. (2003). Severe sepsis management: Are we doing enough? *Critical Care Nurse, 24*(Suppl 2), 2–16.

Ahrens, T., & Vollman, K. (2004). Low dose steroid replacement in severe sepsis. *Critical Care Nurse, 24*(2), 16.

Aiken, L. H., Clarke, S. P., Sloane, D. M., Sochalski, J., & Silber, J. H. (2002). Hospital nurse staffing and patient mortality, nurse burnout, and job dissatisfaction. *The Journal of the American Medical Association, 288*(16), 1987–1993.

Ait-Khaled, N., & Enarson D. (2006). Management of asthma: The essentials of good clinical practice. *International Journal of Tuberculosis and Lung Disease, 10*(2), 133–137.

Alarcon-Segovia, D., Alarcon-Riquelme, M., Cardiel, M., Caeiro, F., Massardo, L., Villa, A., et al. (2005). Familial aggregation of systemic lupus erythematosus, rheumatoid arthritis, and other autoimmune diseases in 1,177 lupus patients form the GLADEL cohort. *Arthritis and Rheumatism, 52*(4), 1138–1147.

Alden, N., Rabbits, A., & Yurt, R. (2005). Burn injury in patients with dementia: An impetus for prevention. *Journal of Burn Care and Rehabilitation, 26*(3), 267–271.

Alderson, P., Green, S., & Higgins, J. P. T. (Eds.). (2003). Cochrane reviewers' handbook 4.2.2. In *The Cochrane Database of Systematic Reviews* (1), 2004. Chichester, UK: John Wiley & Sons.

Aldridge, M. (2005). Decreasing parental stress in the pediatric intensive care unit: One unit's experience. *Critical Care Nurse,* 25(6), 40–50.

Alexander, J., McDaniel, G., Baldwin, M., & Money, B. (2002). Promoting, applying, and evaluating problem-based learning in the undergraduate nursing curriculum. *NLN Perspectives, 23*(5), 248–254.

Allen, D. (2004). Reading the signs. *Nursing Older People, 16*(4), 6.

Allen, G. (2005). Evidence for practice. Conversion from laparoscopic to open cholecystectomy. *AORN Journal, 81*(3), 690, 693.

Allen, G., & Parsons, P. (2005). Acute lung injury: Significant treatment and outcome. *Current Opinion in Anesthesiology, 18*(2), 209–215.

The ALLHAT Officers and Coordinators for the ALLHAT Collaborative Research Group. (2002). Major outcomes in high-risk hypertensive patients randomized to angiotensin-converting enzymes inhibitor or calcium channel blocker vs diuretic: The antihypertensive and lipid-lowering treatment to prevent heart attack trial (ALLHAT). *Journal of the American Medical Association, 288,* 2981–2997.

Almefty, R., Webber, B., & Arnautovic, K. (2006). Intraneural perineurioma of the third cranial nerve: Occurrence and identification. Case report. *Journal of Neurosurgery, 104*(5), 824–827.

Alsakafi, N., & Kuznetsov, D. (2004). *Spermatocele.* Retrieved July 1, 2006, from http://www.emedicine.com.

Altizer, L. (2004). Casting for immobilization. *Orthopedic Nursing, 23*(2), 136–141.

Altizer, L. (2005). Hip fractures. *Orthopaedic Nursing, 24*(4), 283–292.

Altman, G. (2004). *Delmar's fundamental and advanced nursing skills* (2nd ed.). New York: Thomson Delmar Learning.

Altman, G. B., & Taylor, S. C. (2004). Assessing immediate postoperative care. In G. B. Altman (Ed.), *Delmar's fundamental and advanced nursing skills* (2nd ed., pp. 510–519). Albany, NY: Thomson Delmar Learning.

Amado, M., & Portnoy, J. (2006). Recent advances in asthma management. *Missouri Medicine, 103*(1), 60–64.

Ambuel, B., Hamlett, K., Marx, C., & Blumer, J. (1992). Assessing distress in pediatric intensive care environments: The comfort scale. *Journal of Pediatric Psychology, 17*(1), 95–109.

American Academy of Allergy, Asthma, and Immunology. (2002). *Practice parameters for the diagnosis and management of sinusitis.* Retrieved December 17, 2004, from http://www.aaaai.org.

American Academy of Allergy, Asthma, and Immunology. (2006). *Fact sheets.* Retrieved July 8, 2006, from www.aaaai.org.

American Academy of Dermatology. (2002). Actinic keratoses and skin cancer. *Dermatology Nursing, 16*(6), 397–399.

American Academy of Dermatology. (2006). *Aging skin.* Retrieved July 22, 2006. from http://www.aad.org.

American Academy of Orthopaedic Surgeons. (2003). *Orthopaedic fast facts.* Retrieved September 5, 2006, from http//orthoinfo.aaos.org.

American Academy of Otolaryngology-Head and Neck Surgery (AAO-HNS). (2002a). *Fact sheet: Antibiotics and sinusitis.* Retrieved December 17, 2004, from http://www.entnet.org/healthinfo/sinus/antibiotics_sinusitis.cfm.

American Academy of Otolaryngology-Head and Neck Surgery (AAO-HNS). (2002b). *Fact sheet: Sinusitis: Special considerations for aging patients.* Retrieved December 17, 2004, from http://www.entnet.org/healthinfo/sinus/aging_patients.cfm.

American Academy of Otolaryngology-Head and Neck Surgery (AAO-HNS). (2002c). *Fact sheet: Sinus surgery.* Retrieved December 17, 2004, from http://www.entnet.org/healthinfo/sinus/sinus_surgery.cfm.

American Academy of Otolaryngology-Head and Neck Surgery (AAO-HNS). (2002d). *Doctor, explain tonsils and adenoid.* Retrieved August 25, 2004 from, http://www.entnet.org/healthinfo/throat/tonsils.cfm.

American Academy of Pediatrics. (2002). *The youngest victims: Disaster preparedness to meet childrens' needs.* Retrieved June 23, 2006, from aap.org/terrorism.htm.

American Association of Clinical Endocrinologists Male Sexual Dysfunction Task Force. (2003). Medical guidelines for clinical practice for the evaluation and treatment of male sexual dysfunction: A couple's problem—2003 update. *Endocrine Practice, 9*(1), 77–95.

American Association of Colleges of Nursing. (1997). *Peaceful death document.* Retrieved June 15, 2006, from www.aacn.nche.edu/publications/deathfin.htm.

American Association of Colleges of Nursing. (October, 2004). *Position statement on the practice doctorate in nursing.* Retrieved October 3, 2005, from www.aacn.nche.edu/DNP/DNPpositionstatement.htm.

American Association of Critical Care Nurses. (2002) *Critical care nursing fact sheet.* Retrieved May 21, 2004, from www.aacn.org.

American Association of Critical Care Nurses. (2003). *General information regarding certification.* Retrieved May 7, 2004, from www.aacn.org.

American Association of Critical Care Nurses and AACN Certification Corporation. (2003). Safeguarding the patient and the profession: The value of critical care nurse certification. *American Journal of Critical Care, 12*(5), 154–164.

American Brain Tumor Association. (2004a). *A primer of brain tumors: A patient's reference* (8th ed.). Retrieved June 13, 2006, from www.abta.org.

American Brain Tumor Association. (2004b). *Focusing on treatment: Chemotherapy.* Retrieved June 14, 2006, from www.abta.org.

American Brain Tumor Association. (2004c). *Focusing on treatment: Surgery.* Retrieved June 13, 2006, from www.abta.org.

American Burn Association. (2005). *Advanced burn life support course: Provider's manual.* Chicago: Author.

American Cancer Society. (2003). Cancer reference information: Overview: Laryngeal and hypopharyngeal cancer. Retrieved June 10, 2004, from http://www.cancer.org/docroot/CRI/CRI_2_1x.asp?rnav=criov&dt=23.

American Cancer Society. (2004a). *Cancer facts and figures.* Atlanta, GA: Author.

American Cancer Society. (2004b). *Detailed guide to cervical cancer.* Retrieved August 30, 2004, from http://www.cancer.org/docroot/CRI/CRI_2_3x.asp?dt=8.

American Cancer Society. (2004c). *Detailed guide to endometrial cancer.* Retrieved October 14, 2004 from http://www.cancer.org/docroot/CRI/CRI_2_3x.asp?dt=11.

American Cancer Society. (2004d). *Ovarian cancer.* Retrieved August 30, 2004, from http://www.cancer.org/docroot/CRI/CRI_0.asp.

American Cancer Society. (2004e). *Overview: Lung cancer.* Retrieved August 16, 2006, from http://www.cancer.org.

American Cancer Society. (2004f). *Understanding radiation therapy: A guide for patients and families.* Retrieved March 22, 2005, from http://www.cancer.org.

American Cancer Society. (2004g). *What are the key statistics for brain and spinal cord tumors? Cancer Reference Information.* Retrieved June 13, 2006, www.cancer.org.

American Cancer Society. (2006a). *Stomach (gastric) cancer* (p. 1). Retrieved June 25, 2006, from www.cancer.gov.

American Cancer Society. (2006b). *Surveillance research.* Retrieved October 4, 2006, from http://www.cancer.org.

American Cancer Society. (2006c). Retrieved June 24, 2006, from www.cancersociety.com.

American Chronic Pain Association. (2004). *Nurses' pain awareness kit.* Retrieved from www.theacpa.org.

American College for Emergency Physicians. (2004). Code of ethics. Policy statement. *Annals of Emergency Medicine, 43*(5), 686–694.

American College of Obstetricians and Gynecologists. (2002). *Nonsurgical diagnosis and management of vaginal agenesis.* ACOG Committee Opinion: No. 274, 82–85.

American College of Obstetricians and Gynecologists. (2005). Urinary incontinence in women. *Obstetrics and Gynecology, 105*(6), 1533–1545.

American College of Physicians. (2005). *Lyme disease: A patient guide.* Retrieved September 5, 2006, from www.acponline.org.

American College of Rheumatology. (2004). *New pulmonary hypertension guideline challenges use of common medications.* Retrieved September 16, 2004, from http://www.rheumatology.org.

American Diabetes Association. (2006). Retrieved June 23, 2006, from www.diabetes.org.

American Heart Association. (2001). Heart association science advisory: Lyon diet heart study. Benefits of a Mediterranean-style, National Cholesterol Education Program/American Heart Association step I dietary pattern on cardiovascular disease. *#71-0202 Circulation, 1*(103), 1823–1825.

American Heart Association. (2003). *Heart disease and stroke statistics—2004 update.* Dallas, TX: American Heart Association.

American Heart Association. (2004a). *Heart disease and stroke statistics—2004 update.* Retrieved June 24, 2006, from www.aha.com.

American Heart Association (2004b). *Primary or unexplained pulmonary hypertension.* Retrieved September 16, 2004, from http://www.americanheart.org.

American Heart Association. (2004c). *Pulmonary hypertension.* Retrieved July 17, 2006, from http://www.americanheart.org.

American Heart Association. (2005). *Heart disease and stroke statistics.* Dallas: Author.

American Heart Association. (2006a). *American heart association 2005 guidelines for CPR and ECC.* Retrieved July 3, 2006, from www.americanheart.org.

American Heart Association. (2006b). *Heart failure: Understanding heart failure.* Retrieved June 26, 2006, from www.americanheart.org.

American Heart Association. (2006c). *Inflammation heart disease and stroke: The role of C-reactive protein.* Retrieved June 23, 2006, from www.americanheart.org.

American Holistic Nursing Association. (2006). (p. 14). Retrieved June 23, 2006, from www.ahna.org.

American Hospital Association. (1980). *A patient's bill of rights.* Chicago: Author.

American Hospital Association. (1992). Catalog no. 157759. Retrieved July1, 2005, from www.aha.org.

American Hospital Association. (2005, December 8). *AHA News Now.*

American Infertility Association. (2005). *Focus on fertility.* Retrieved June 23, 2006, from http://www.focusonfertility.org.

American Joint Committee on Cancer. (2002). *Staging systems.* Retrieved June 16, 2005, from http://training.seer.cancer.gov.

American Lung Association. (2003a). *Bronchietasis fact sheet.* Retrieved August 15, 2006, from http://www.americanheart.org.

American Lung Association. (2003b). *Facts about lung cancer.* Retrieved June 30, 2004, from http://www.lungusa.org.

American Lung Association. (n.d.a). *Freedom from smoking online.* Retrieved August 30, 2005, from http://www.lungusa.org.

American Lung Association. (n.d.b). *Open airways for schools.* Retrieved August 30, 2005, from http://www.lungusa.org.

American Lung Association. (n.d.c). *Special reports.* Retrieved August 30, 2005, from http://www.lungusa.org.

American Lung Association. (n.d.d). *Tobacco control and teens.* Retrieved August 30, 2005, from http://www.lungusa.org.

American Lung Association Epidemiology and Statistic Unit Research and Scientific Affairs. (2004). *Trends in lung cancer and morbidity and mortality.* Retrieved June 30, 2004, from http://www.lungusa.org.

American Medical Association. (1999). Medical futility in end-of-life care. *Journal of the American Medical Association, 281,* 937–941.

American Medical Association. (2003). Pain management: The online series. Retrieved from www.ama-cmeonline.com.

American Medical Association. (2004). News from the AMA: *Giving antibiotics within four hours of arrival at a hospital improved outcomes for older patients with pneumonia.* Retrieved September 16, 2004, from http://www.medem.com.

American Nurses Association. (1992a). *Position statement on active euthanasia.* Washington, DC: Author.

American Nurses Association. (1992b). *Position statement on nursing and the patient self determination act.* Washington, DC: Author.

American Nurses Association. (1992c). *Position statement on nursing care and do-not-resuscitate decisions.* Washington, DC: Author.

American Nurses Association. (1992d). *Position statement on foregoing nutrition and hydration.* Washington, DC: Author.

American Nurses Association. (1995). *Nursing: A social policy statement.* Washington, DC: Author.

American Nurses Association. (2001). *Code of ethics for nurses with interpretive statements.* Silver Spring, MD: American Nurses Publishing. Retrieved August 5, 2006, from www.nursingworld.org.

American Nurses Association. (2003a). *Nursing's social policy statement* (2nd ed.). Washington, DC: Author.

American Nurses Association. (2003b). *Position statement on pain management and control of distressing symptoms in dying patients.* Retrieved July 12, 2005, from Nursebooks.org.

American Nurses Association. (2003c). *Social policy statement on pain symptom management of the dying patient.* Retrieved from www.nursingworld.org.

American Nurses Association. (2006). *Code of ethics for nurses with interpretive statements.* Washington DC: American Nurses Publishing.

American Nurse Credentialing Center. (2005). Retrieved June 15, 2005, from http://www.nursingworld.org/ancc.

American Organization of Nurse Executives. (2004, April 9). *AONE eNews Update.*

American Pain Foundation. (2004). Retrieved from www.painfoundation.org.

American Sleep Apnea Association. (2004). *What is sleep apnea?* Retrieved June 10, 2004, from http://www.sleepapnea.org.

American Society for Aesthetic Plastic Surgery. (2006). *What's new in plastic surgery?* Retrieved July 26, 2006, from http://www.surgery.org.

American Society of Anesthesiologists. (2004). *Continuum of depth of sedation definitions of general anesthesia and levels of sedation/analgesia.* Oklahoma: ASA House of Delegates.

American Society of Plastic Surgeons. (2002). *National clearinghouse of plastic surgery statistics 2002 report.* Arlington Heights, IL: Author.

American Spinal Injury Association. (2004). Retrieved July 13, 2006, from http://www.asia-spinalinjury.org.

American Stroke Association. (2004, June 24). Long-term outlook good for carotid stenting to prevent stroke. Fifth World Stroke Congress meeting report. *Stroke News.* Retrieved June 13, 2006, from http://www.strokeassociation.org.

American Thoracic Society, Center for Disease Control, & Infectious Disease Society of America. (2003). *Treatment of tuberculosis.* MMWR. Retrieved September 16, 2004, from http://www.cdc.gov.

American Urologic Association. (2004, February). *Orchitis and epididymitis.* Retrieved June 1, 2006, from http://www.urologyhealth.org.

American Urological Association. (2006). *Urologic diseases in America.* Retrieved July 16, 2006, from www.auanet.org.

Analay, Y., Ozcan, E., Karan, A., Diracoglu, D., & Aydin, R. (2003). The effectiveness of intensive group exercise on patients with ankylosing spondylitis. *Clinical Rehabiliation, 17*(6), 631–636.

Andersen, B., Kallehave, F., & Andersen, H. (2004). *Antibiotics versus placebo for prevention of postoperative infection after appendectomy* [Electronic version: Cochrane Review]. Retrieved December 15, 2004, from http://www.cochrane.org.

Anderson, B. (2005). Nutrition and wound healing: The necessity of assessment. *British Journal of Nursing, 14*(19); *Tissue Viability Supplement:* S30, S32, S34.

Anderson, D., Woltman, M., Kovach, G., & Konety, B. (2004) Long-term treatment of metastatic renal-cell carcinoma with fluorouracil. *Lancet Oncology, 5*(11), 690–692.

Anderson, R. (2005). *Psychoneuroimmunoendocrinology review and commentary. Townsend Letter for doctors and patients.* Retrieved August 2, 2006, from www.learnnet.co.nz.

Anderson-Shaw, L. (2003). The unilateral DNR order—one hospital's experience. *Journal of Nursing Administration's Healthcare, Law, Ethics, and Regulation, 5*(2), 42–46.

Andres, E., Affenberger, S., Zimmer, J., Vinzio, S., Grosu, D., Pistol, G., et al. (2006). Current hematological findings in cobalamin deficiency. A study of 201 consecutive patients with documented cobalamin deficiency. *Clinical and Laboratory Haematology,28*(1), 50–56.

Andres, E., Loukili, N. H., Noel, E., Kaltenbach, G., Abdelgheni, M. B., Perrin A. E., et al. (2004). Vitamin B_{12} (cobalamin) deficiency in elderly patients. *Canadian Medical Association Journal, 171*(3), 251–259.

Andrews, E., & Fleischer, A. (2005). Sonography for deep venous thrombosis: Current and future applications. *Ultrasound Quarterly, 21*(4), 213–225.

Andrews, M. M., & Boyle, J. S. (2002). *Transcultural concepts in nursing care* (4th ed.). Philadelphia: Lippincott, Williams & Wilkins.

Andrews, M., & Boyle, J. (2003). *Transcultural concepts in nursing care* (5th ed.). Philadelphia: Lippincott, Wilkins, & Williams.

Angus, F., & Burakoff, R., (2003). The percutaneous endoscopic gastrostomy tube: Medical and ethical issues in placement. *The American Journal of Gastroenterology, 98*(200), 272–277.

Antai-Otong, D. (2003). *Psychiatric nursing: Biological and behavioral concepts.* Clifton Park, NY: Thomson Delmar Learning.

Antman, E. M., Anbe, D. T., Armstrong, P. W., Bates, E. R., Green, L. A., Hand, M., et al. (2004). ACC/AHA guidelines for the management of patients with ST-elevation myocardial infarction-executive summary. *Circulation, 110*(5), 588–641.

Anzueto, A., & Niederman, M. S. Diagnosis and treatment of rhinovirus respiratory Infections. (2003). *Chest, 123*(5), 1664–1672.

Appel, G., Radhakrishnan, J., & D'Agati, V. (2004). Secondary glomerular disease. In B. Brenner (Ed.), *Brenner and Rector's the kidney* (7th ed., vol. 1, p. 1381). Philadelphia: W. B. Saunders Co.

Aragon, D., Ring, C., & Covelli, M. (2003). The influence of diabetes mellitus on postoperative infections. *Critical Care Nursing Clinics of North America, 15*(1), 125–136.

Arnstein, P. (2005). Accurate assessment is key to effective pain management: taking the fifth (vital sign). *RN, 68*(1), 12.

Aron, D., Finding. J., & Tyrell, B. (2004a). Glucocorticoids and adrenal androgens. In F.S. Greenspan & D. G. Gardner (Eds.), *Basic and clinical endocrinology* (pp. 534–543). St. Louis, MO: Lange Medical Books.

Aron, D., Finding, J., & Tyrell, B. (2004b).Hypothalamus and pituitary. In F. S. Greenspan & D. G. Gardner (Eds.), *Basic and clinical endocrinology* (pp. 537–542). St. Louis, MO: Lange Medical Books.

Aronson, B. S., & Marquis, M. (2004). Care of the adult patient with cystic fibrosis. *Medsurg Nursing, 13*(3), 143–154; quiz 155.

Arthritis Food Guide. (2006). *Arthritis today on call: Safe foods for gout.* Retrieved September 5, 2006, from http://arthritis-guide.com.

Artinian, N. (2003). The psychosocial aspects of heart failure. *American Journal of Nursing, 103*(12), 32–41.

Artinian, N. (2004). Innovations in blood pressure monitoring. *American Journal of Nursing, 104*(8), 52–59.

Asbury, E., & Collins, P. (2005). Cardiac syndrome X. *International Journal of Clinical Practice, 59*(9), 1063–1069.

Ashworth, N. L., Chad, K. E., Harrison, E. L., Reeder, B. A., & Marshall, S. C. (2005). Home versus center based physical activity programs in older adults. *The Cochrane Database of Systematic Reviews 2005.* Art. CD004017. Pub 2. DOI:0.1002/14651858.CD004017.pub2.

Asp, A. (2005) Mechanisms of endocrine control. In K. Copstead & J. L Banasik, *Pathophysiology* (pp. 639–645). St. Louis, MO: Elsevier Saunders.

Association for the Advancement of Medical Instrumentation. (2005). *Standards. Sterilization in health care facilities (part 1) and sterilization equipment (part 2).* Arlington, VA: AAMI Publications.

Association of Operating Room Nurses. (2005a). Recommended practices for electrosurgery. In *Standards, recommended practices and guidelines* (pp. 248–250). Denver: AORN.

Association of Operating Room Nurses. (2005b). Recommended practices for surgical attire. In *Standards, recommended practices and guidelines.* Denver: AORN.

Association of Operating Room Nurses. (2006). *Standards, recommended practices, and guidelines with official AORN statements. 2006 Edition.* Denver: AORN.

Assouline-Dayan, Y., Chang, C., Greenspan, A., Shoenfeld, Y., & Gershwin, M. E. (2002). Pathogenesis and natural history of osteonecrosis. *Seminars in Arthritis Rheumatism, 32*(2), 94–124.

Astin, J. (2004). Mind-body therapies for the management of pain. *Clinical Journal of Pain, 20*(1), 27–32.

Astin, J. A., & Forys, K. (2004). Psychosocial determinants of health and illness: Integrating mind, body and spirit. *Advances in Mind-Body Medicine, 20*(4), 14–21.

Attarian, S., Vedel, J., Pouget, J., & Schmied, A. (2006). Cortical versus spinal dysfunction in amyotrophic lateral sclerosis. *Muscle and Nerve, 33*(5), 677–690.

Aufort, S., Charra, L., Lesnik, A., Bruel, J., & Taourel, P. Multidetector CT of bowel obstruction: Value of post-processing. *European Radiology, 15*(11), 2323–2329.

Ayers, D. (2004). Melanoma. *Nursing, 34*(4), 52–53.

Azziz, R., Woods, K., Reyna, R., Key, T., Knochenhauer, E., & Yildiz, B. (2004). The prevalence and features of the polycystic ovary syndrome in an unselected population. *Journal of Clinical Endocrinology and Metabolism, 89,* 2745–2749.

Bacon, P. (2005). The spectrum of Wegener's granulomatosis and disease relapse. *The New England Journal of Medicine, 352*(4), 330-332.

Bader, M., Littlejohns, L., & March, K. (2003). Brain tissue oxygen monitoring in severe brain injury II: Implications for critical care teams and case study. *Critical Care Nurse, 23*(4), 29–43.

Badesch D. B., Abman S. H., Ahearn G. S., Barst R. J., McCrory D. C., Simonneau G., et al. (2004). Medical therapy for pulmonary arterial hypertension: ACCP evidenced based clinical practice guidelines. *Chest*(1 Suppl), *126,* 35S–62S.

Badke, M. B., Shea, T. Z., Miedaner, J. A., & Grove C. R. (2004). Outcomes after rehabilitation for adults with balance dysfunction. *Archive Physical Medicine Rehabilitation, 85,* 227–233.

Baier, F. (2006). The Medicare prescription drug benefit: Understanding the benefits and the gaps in this new coverage. *American Journal of Nursing, 106*(6), 66–72.

Bailey, D., & Dresser, G. (2004). Natural products and adverse drug interactions. *Canadian Medical Association Journal, 170*(10), 1531–1532.

Bakas, T., Austin, J. K., Jessup, S. L., Williams, L. S., & Obsert, M. T. (2004). Time and difficulty of tasks provided by family caregivers of stroke survivors. *Journal of Neuroscience Nursing, 36*(2), 95–106.

Baker, D. (2005, October 5). Teens having casual sex earlier, study says. *San Diego Union Tribune,* p. A5.

Baker, J. J. (2002). Medicare payment system for hospital inpatients: Diagnosis-related groups. *The Journal of Health Care Finance, 28*(3), 1–13.

Bandman, E., & Bandman, B. (2002). *Nursing ethics through the life span* (4th ed.). Princeton, NJ: Prentice Hall.

Bandura, A. (1977). *Social learning theory.* Englewood Cliffs, NJ: Prentice Hall.

Baron, R., & Schwartzstein, R. (2004). *Diseases of the chest wall.* Retrieved June 25, 2006, from http://www.uptodate.com.

Barone, C., Pablo, C., & Barone, G. (2004). Postanesthetic care in the critical care unit. *Critical Care Nurse, 24*(1), 38–45.

Bartels, D., (2004). Adherence to oral therapy for type 2 diabetes: Opportunities for enhancing glycemic control. *Journal of the American Academy of Nurse Practitioners, 16*(1), 8–16.

Bartholomay, M., Finn, S., Rounds, A., Bigelow, R., Barrett E., & Coakley A., et al. (2006). Uncovering practice differences related to the care of indwelling and external tunneled catheters across practice settings in a large academic medical center. *Oncology Nursing Forum, 33*(2), 419–420.

Bassi, P., De Marco, V., De Lisa, A., Mancini, M., Pinto, F., Bertoloni, R., et al. (2005). Non-invasive diagnostic tests for bladder cancer: A review of the literature. *Urologia Internationalis, 75*(3), 193–200.

Battais, F., Mothes, T., Moneret-Vautrin, D., Pineau, F., Kanny, G., Popineau, Y., et al. (2005). Identification of IgE-binding epitopes on gliadins for patients with food allergy to wheat. *Allergy, 60*(6), 815–821.

Battleman, D. S., Callahan M., & Thaler, H. T. (2002). Rapid antibiotic delivery and appropriate antibiotic selection reduced length of hospital stay of patients with community acquired pneumonia. *Archives of Internal Medicine, 167*(6), 682–688.

Bee, H., & Boyd, D. R. (2003). *The developing child* (10th ed.). New York: Allyn & Bacon.

Beebe, R., & Funk, D. (2001). *Fundamentals of emergency care.* New York: Thomson Delmar Learning.

Beers, M. H., & Berkow, R. (2004). *The Merck manual of diagnosis and therapy* (17th ed.). West Point, PA: Merck & Co.

Beese-Bjurstrom, S. (2004). Hidden danger: Aortic aneurysm and dissections. *Nursing, 34*(2), 36–42.

Behin, A., Hoang-Xuan, K., Carpentier, A. F., & Delattre, J. (2003). Primary brain tumors in adults. *Lancet, 361*(9354), 323–331.

Beitz, J. (1998). Concept mapping: Navigating the learning process. *Nurse Educator, 23*(5), 35–41.

Bell, G., & Sander, J. (2002, April 11). The epidemiology of epilepsy: the size of the problem. *Seizure, 10*(Suppl A), 306–316.

Bench, S. (2004). Clinical skills: Assessing and treating shock. A nursing perspective. *British Journal of Nursing, 13*(12), 715–721.

Benisty J. I. (2002). *Pulmonary hypertension.* Retrieved September 16, 2004, from http://circ.ahajournals.org.

Benner, E., Mosley, R., Destache, C., Lewis, T., Jackson-Lewis, V., Gorantla, S., et al. (2004). Therapeutic immunization protects dopaminergic neurons in a mouse model of Parkinson's disease. *Proceedings of the National Academy of Sciences of the USA, 101*(25), 9435–9440.

Benson, A. B., III, Ajani, J. A., Catalano, R. B., Engelking, C., Kornblau, S. M., Martenson, J. A., Jr., et al. (2004). Recommended guidelines for the treatment of cancer treatment-induced diarrhea. *Journal of Clinical Oncology, 22*(14), 2918–2926.

Beral, V. (2003). Breast cancer and hormone-replacement therapy in the Million Women Study. *Lancet, 362*(9382), 419–427.

Berardino, M., Morrone, O., Sciacca, P.F., Rosato, R., Ciccone, G. & Massaro, F. (2004). Discharge criteria from intensive care unit in brain injured patients. *Acta Neurochir (Wein), 146*(5), 453–456.

Beresford, I. J. M., Parsons, A. A., & Hunter, A. J. (2003). Treatments for stroke. *Expert Opinions on Emerging Drugs, 8*(1), 103–122.

Berg, F. M., Tymoczko, J. L., & Stryer, L. (2002.) *Biochemistry* (5th ed.). New York: W. H. Freeman and Company.

Bergren, M. (2004). Information technology: HIPAA-FERPA revisited. *Public Health Nursing, 20*(2), 107–112.

Bergs, L. (2005). Immunology: Goodpasture syndrome. *Critical Care Nurse, 25*(5), 50–58.

Bergstrom, N., & Braden, B. (2002). Predictive validity of the Braden Scale among black and white subjects. *Nursing Research, 51*(6), 398–403.

Berman, B. M., Lao, L., Langenberg, P., Lee, W. L., Gilpin, A. M. K., & Hochberg, M. C. (2004). Effectiveness of acupuncture as adjunctive therapy in osteoarthritis of the knee: A randomized, controlled trial. *Annals of Internal Medicine, 141*(12), 901–910.

Berry, T., & Shooner, K. (2004). Family history: The first genetic screen. *The Nurse Practitioner, 29*(11), 14–23.

Beth Israel Deaconess Medical Center. (2004). *WebMD clinical trial services.* Retrieved June 10, 2005, from http://my.webmd.com.

Beyea, S. C. (Ed.). (2002). *The perioperative nursing data set* (2nd ed.). Denver: AORN, Inc.

Bialous, S., & Sarna, L. (2004). Sparing a few minutes for tobacco cessation. *American Journal of Nursing, 104*(12), 54–60.

Binder, I. B. (2003). Paget's disease. *Journal of Endodontics, 29*(11), 720–723.

Birgen, M., Harris, S., Lindbaek, M., & Oslo, N. (2004). Cochlear implants and health status: A comparison with other hearing-impaired patients. *Annals Otology Rhinology and Laryngology, 113,* 914–921.

Bishop, A. H., & Scudder, J. R., (Eds.). (1985). *Caring, curing, coping: Nurse, physician, patient relationships.* Birmingham, AL: University of Alabama Press.

Bisno, A. L., Gerber, M. A., Gwaltney, Jr, J. M., Kaplan, E. L., & Schwartz, R. H. (2002). Practice guidelines for the diagnosis and management of group A streptococcal pharyngitis. *Clinical Infectious Diseases; Infectious Diseases of America, 35*(2), 113–125.

Bisson, J., & Andrew, M. (2005). Psychological treatment of post-traumatic stress disorder (PTSD). *The Cochrane Database of Systematic Reviews* (2), CD003388.

Biton, V., & Tabak, N. (2003). The relationship between the application of the nursing ethical code and nurses' satisfaction. *International Journal of Nursing Practice, 55*(3), 140–157.

Black, J., & Hawks, J. (2004). *Medical-surgical nursing: Clinical management for positive outcomes* (7th ed.). Philadelphia: W. B. Saunders.

Blair, S., & Church, T. (2003). The importance of physical activity and cardiorespiratory fitness for patients with type 2 diabetes. *Diabetes Spectrum, 16*(4), 236–240.

Blais, K., Hayes, J., Kozier, B., & Erb, G. (2002). *Professional nursing practice: Concepts and perspectives* (4th ed.). New Jersey: Prentice Hall.

Blood type facts. (2006). Retrieved July 11, 2006, from http://www.bloodbook.com.

Bloom, B. S. (1977). *Taxonomy of educational objectives: The classification of educational goals, Handbook I: Cognitive domain.* New York: Longman.

Blumenthal, D., Prais, D., Bron-Harlev, E., & Amir, J. (2004). Possible association of Guillain-Barre syndrome and hepatitis A vaccination. *Pediatric Infectious Disease Journal, 23*(6), 586–588.

Blumenthal, M., Brinkman, J., Dinda, K., Goldberg, A. & Wolkschlaegear, B. (2004). *The ABC clinical guide to herbs.* New York: Hawthorne Press, Inc.

Bluvol, A. (2003). The Codman Award Paper: Quality of life in stroke survivors and their spouses: Predictors and clinical implications for rehabilitation teams. *AXON, 25*(2), 10–19.

Bodnar, L., Cogswell, M., & McDonald, T. (2005). Have we forgotten the significance of postpartum iron deficiency? *American Journal of Obstetrics and Gynecology, 193,* 36–44.

Boehm, M., Olive, M., True, A. L., Crook, M. F., San, H., Qu, X., et al. (2004). Bone marrow-derived immune cells regulate vascular disease through a p27Kip1-dependent mechanism. *Journal of Clinical Investigation, 114*(3), 419–426.

Bogardus, S. T., Yueh, B., & Shekelle, P. (2003). Screening and management of adult hearing loss in primary care: Clinical applications. *JAMA, 289*(15), 1986–1990.

Bonadonna, R. (2003). Meditation's impact on chronic illness. *Journal of Holistic Nursing Practice, 17*(6), 309–319.

Bonaiuti, D., Shea, B., Iovine, R., Negrini, S., Robinson, V., Kemper, H. H., et al. (2004). Exercise for preventing and treating osteoporosis in postmenopausal women (Cochrane review). In *The Cochrane Database of Systematic Reviews.* Chichester, UK: John Wiley & Sons, Ltd.

Bone and Joint Decade Organization. (2004, April). *Osteoporosis in Men.* Retrieved September 20, 2004, from http://www.boneandjointdecade.org.

Borneman, T., Stahl, C., Ferrell, B., & Smith, D. (2002). The concept of hope in family caregivers of cancer patients at home. *Journal of Hospice and Palliative Nursing, 4*(1), 21–33.

Boruchoff, S., & Weinstein, M. (2004). *Sputum cultures.* Retrieved June 25, 2006, from http://www.uptodate.com.

Bosen, D. M., & Flemming, M. A. (2003). Beyond ECGs: Understanding electrophysiology testing, part 1. *Nursing, 32*(11), 1–5.

Bosetti, C., Pira, E., & La Vecchia, C. (2005). Bladder cancer risk in painters: A review of the epidemiological evidence, 1989–2004. *Cancer Causes and Control, 16*(9), 997–1008.

Botstein D., & Risch N. (2003). Discovering genotypes underlying human phenotypes: past successes for Mendelian disease, future approaches for complex disease. *Nature Genetics, 33*(Suppl), 228–237.

Boudreaus, E., Edmond, S., & Race, S. (2003) Ethnicity and asthma among children presenting to the emergency department. *Pediatrics III,* (5), e615–e621.

Boyington, A. R., Wildemuth, B. M., Dougherty, M. C., Hall, E. P. (2005). Development of a computer-based system for continence health promotion. *Nursing Outlook, 52*(5), 241–247.

Boyle, E. (2006). Visual impairment reduces functional status of elderly patients. *Ocular Surgery News, 24*(1), 73–74.

Bracken, M. B. (2004). Steroids for acute spinal cord injury. *The Cochrane Database of Systematic Reviews* (2), CD001046. DOI: 10.1002/14651858.

Bradley, J., & Davis, K. (2003). Orthostatic hypotension. *American Family Physician, 68*(12), 2393–2398.

Brady, H., Clarkson, M., & Lieberthal, W. (2004). Acute renal failure. In B. Brenner (Ed.), *Brenner and Rector's the kidney* (7th ed., vol. 1, pp. 1215–1292). Philadelphia: W. B. Saunders Co.

Braimon, J. C., Naaznin, L., & Walczak, M. (2003). In T. M. Buttaro, J. Trybulski, P. P. Bailey, & J. Sandberg-Cook (Eds.), *Primary care: A collaborative practice* (pp. 112–116). St. Louis, MO: Mosby.

Brain Injury Association of America. (2004). *Support adequate finding of the traumatic brain injury act in FY 2005.* McLean, VA: Author.

Brain Injury Association of America. (2006). Retrieved June 13, 2006, from www.biausa.org.

Brain Tumor Society. (2004). *Patient resources.* Retrieved June 15, 2006, from www.tbts.org.

Braun, A., Roth, R., & McGinniss, M. (2003). Technology challenges in screening single gene disorders. *European Journal of Pediatrics,* 162(Suppl 1), S13–S16.

Brenner, M., Hoistad, D., & Hain, T. (2004). Prevalence of thyroid dysfunction in patients with Meniere's Disease. *Archives of Otolaryngology—Head and Neck Surgery, 130*(2), 226–228.

Bretler, S. J. (2004). Traumatic brain injury. *RN, 67*(4), 32–37.

Bridges, E., & Dukes, S. (2005). Cardiovascular aspects of septic shock: Pathophysiology, monitoring, and treatment. *Critical Care Nurse, 25*(2), 14–16, 18–20, 24, 26–28, 30–32, 34–36, 38–40.

Brill, J., (2004). Trends in pain syndrome diagostic technology. *Practical Pain Management, 4*(4), 12–19.

Brookes, M. J., & Green, J. R. B. (2004). Maintenance of remission in Crohn's disease: Current and emerging therapeutic options. *Drugs, 64*(10), 1069–1089.

Brooks, G. A., Butte, N. F., Rand, W. M., Flatt, J. P., & Caballero, B. (2004). Chronicle of the Institute of Medicine physical activity recommendation. *American Journal of Clinical Nutrition, 79*(5), 921S–930S.

Brors, D., & Bodmer D. (2004). New aspects of inner ear research. *Hospital Medicine, 65*(7), 392–395.

Brosman, S. (2004). *Penile cancer.* Retrieved June 23, 2006, from http://www.emedicine.com.

Brouwer-DudokdeWit, A., Savenue, A., Zoeteweij, M., Maat-Kievit, A., & Tibben, A. (2002). A hereditary disorder in the family and the family life cycle: Huntington Disease as a paradigm. *Family Process, 41*(4), 677–692.

Brown, A. E., Elting, L., Freifeld, A. G., Greene, J. N., Ito, J. I., King, E. K., et al. (2002, May). *Fever and neutropenia treatment guidelines for patients with cancer (Version 1).* Retrieved June 10, 2005, from http://www.nccn.org.

Brown, B. B., Grigsby, J., Walsh, A. C., & Kaye, K. (2002). *Mental capacity: Legal and medical aspects of assessment and treatment* (2nd ed.). New York: Clark.

Brown, B. J. (2004). Reconstructing healthcare in a global marketplace. *Nursing Administration Quarterly, 28*(2), 81–82.

Brown, C. (2003). Surgical treatment of trigeminal neuralgia. *Association of periOperative Registered Nurses, 78*(5), 743–762.

Brown, D., & McCormack, B. (2005). Developing postoperative pain management: Utilising the Promoting Action on Research Implementation in Health Services (PARIHS) framework. *Worldviews on Evidence-Based Nursing, 2*(3), 131–141.

Brown, D. R., Ludwig, R., Buck, G. A., Durham, D., Shumard, T., & Graham, S. S. (2004). Health literacy: Universal precautions needed. *Journal of Allied Health, 33*(2), 150–155.

Brown, K. (2003). *Emergency dysrhythmias: EKG injury patterns.* New York: Thomson Delmar Learning.

Brown University School of Medicine Center for Gerontology and Health Services Research. (2000). *Facts in dying: Policy-relevant data on care at the end of life.* Retrieved July 12, 2005, from www.chsr.brown.edu/dying/usa.

Browning, A. (2006). Exploring advanced directives. *Journal of Christian Nursing, 23*(1): 34–39.

Broyles, B. E., Reiss, B. S., & Evans, M. E. (2007). *Pharmacological aspects of nursing care* (7th ed.). New York: Thomson Delmar Learning.

Brunner, E., Thorogood, M., Rees, K., & Hewitt, G. (2006). Dietary advice for reducing cardiovascular risk. *The Cochrane Database of Systematic Reviews* (1), CD002128.

Buckley, J., & Herth, K. (2004). Fostering hope in terminally ill patients. *Nursing Standard, 19*(10), 33–41.

Bukstein, D., Elder, M. A., Larsen, J., & Mellon, M. (2003). *Clearing the air: Effective management of asthma and allergic rhinitis. A special edition of patient care for the nurse practitioner.* Montvale, NJ: Thomas Medical Economics Company.

Bullard, K. M., & Rothenberger, D. A. (2005). Colon, rectum and anus. In F. C. Brunicardi (Ed.), *Schwartz's principles of surgery* (8th ed., pp. 1055–1117). New York: McGraw Hill.

Bullock, S., & Manias, E. (2002). The educational preparation of undergraduate nursing students in pharmacology: a survey of lectures' perceptions and experiences. *Journal of Advanced Nursing, 40*(1), 7–16.

Bunge, M., & Pearse, D. (2003). Transplantation strategies to promote repair of the injured spinal cord.

Journal of Rehabilitation Research and Development, 40(4) (Suppl), 1–8.

Bunn, K., & Roberts, I. for the WHO Pre-Hospital Trauma Care Steering Committee. (2004). Spinal immobilization for trauma patients. *The Cochrane Database of Systematic Reviews* (2, 4), CD002803. DOI: 10.1002/14651858.

Bunnell, R. E., Nassozi, J., Marum, E., Mubangizi, J., Malamba, S., Dillon, B., et al (2005). Living with discordance: Knowledge, challenges, and prevention strategies of HIV discordant couples in Uganda. *AIDS Care, 17*(8), 999–1012.

Burden, M., (2003). Diabetes: Signs, symptoms and making a diagnosis. *Nursing Times, 99*(1), 30–32.

Burckhardt, C. S. (2005). Educating patients: Self-management approaches. *Disability and Rehabilitation, 27*(12), 703–709.

Burkhardt, M. A., & Nathaniel, A. K. (2002). *Ethics and issues in contemporary nursing* (2nd ed.). New York: Thomson Delmar Learning.

Burkle, F. (2002). Mass casualty management of a large scale bioterrorism event: An epidemiological approach that shapes triage decisions. *Emergency Medicine Clinics of North America, 20*(2), 409–436.

Burl, D., Schambelan, M., & Lo, J. (2004). Endocrine hypertension. In F. S. Greenspan & D. G. Gardner (Eds.), *Basic and clinical endocrinology* (pp. 414–438). St. Louis, MO: Lange Medical Books.

Burns, N., & Grove, S. (2001). *Cognitive mapping in the practice of nursing research conduct, critique & utilization* (4th ed.). Philadelphia: W. B. Saunders.

Burns, V. E., Carroll, D., Drayson, M., Whitham, M., & Ring, C. (2003). Life events, perceived stress and antibody response to influenza vaccination in young, healthy adults. *Journal of Psychosomatic Research, 55*(6), 569–572.

Buscemi, N., Vandermeer, B., Friesen, C., Bialy, L., Tubman, M., Ospina, M., et al. (2005). *Manifestations and management of chronic insomnia in adults. Summary, evidence report technology assessment: Number 125.* AHRQ Publication Number 05-E021-1. Retrieved June 15, 2005, from http://www.ahrq.gov/clinic/epcsums/insomnsum.htm.

Bush, N., & Griffin-Sobel, J. (2003). Acute postoperative pain management and malfunctioning epidural catheter. *Oncology Nursing Forum, 30*(2), 227–228.

Butcher, G. (2003). *An illustrated colour text: Gastroenterology.* London: Churchill Livingstone.

Butterworth, C. E. (1974). The skeleton in the hospital closet, *Nutrition Today, 9*(2), March/April, 4.

Byars, L. (2002). Neutropenia risk assessment and management in the ambulatory care setting. *Oncology Support Care, 1,* 27–39.

Byock, I. (1997). *Dying well: The prospect for growth at the end of life.* New York: Riverhead Books.

Calder, L., Balasubramanian, S., & Stiell, I. (2004). Lack of consensus on corneal abrasion management results of a national survey. *Canadian Journal of Emergency Medicine, 6*(6), 402–407.

Calgary Health Region. (2004). *Decision-making for enteral feeding tube placement in adult patients: The development of a guideline for decision making, final report.* Retrieved July 11, 2006, from http://www.crha-health.ab.ca.

Calianno, C., & Jakubek, P. (2006). Wound and skin care. Wound bed preparation: Laying the foundation for treating chronic wounds, part I. *Nursing, 36*(2), 70–71.

Calle, E., Rodriguez, C., Walker-Thurmond, K., & Thun, M. (2003). Overweight, obesity, and mortality form cancer in a prospectively studied cohort of U.W. adults. *New England Journal of Medicine, 348*(17), 1625–1638.

Calne, S., & Kumar, A. (2003). Nursing care of patient's with late-stage Parkinson's disease. *Journal of Neuroscience Nursing, 35*(5), 242–251.

Campbell, M., & Torrance, C. (2005). Coronary angioplasty: Impact on risk factors and patients' understanding of the severity of their condition. *Australian Journal of Advanced Nursing, 22*(4), 26–31.

Campbell, T. (2004). Nurses are vital to those living with a chronic disease. *Nursing Spectrum, 43*(12), 34.

Campos, L., Meng, Z., Hu, G., Chiu, D., Ambron, R., & Martin, J. (2004). Engineering novel spinal circuits to promote recovery after spinal injury. *The Journal of Neuroscience, 24*(9), 2090–2101.

Campoy, S., & Elwell, R. (2005). Pharmacology and CKD: How chronic kidney disease and its complications alter drug response. *American Journal of Nursing, 105*(9), 60–72.

Cancer Research UK. (2004). *General side effects of chemotherapy drugs.* Retrieved June 9, 2005, from http://www.cancerhelp.org.uk.

Cancer Source. (2003). *Grading toxicities from chemotherapeutic agents.* Retrieved June 10, 2005, from http://www.cancersourcern.com.

Candela, L., & Yucha, C. (2004). Renal regulation of extracellular fluid volume and osmolality. *Nephrology Nursing Journal, 31*(4), 397–404, 444.

Cannon, C. P., Braunwald, E., McCabe, C. H., Rader, D. J., Rouleau, J. L., Belder, R., et al. (2004). Intensive versus moderate lipid lowering with statins after acute coronary syndromes. *New England Journal of Medicine, 350*(15), 1495–1504.

Cantus, S. (2004). *Phimosis and paraphimosis.* Retrieved July 2, 2006, from http://www.emedicine.com.

Capriotti, T. (2004). The "alphabet" of rheumatoid arthritis therapy. *Nursing, 13*(6), 920–928.

Carding, P., Welch, A., Owen, S., & Stafford, F. (2001) Surgical voice restoration. *The Lancet, 357,* 1463–1465.

Cardiomyopathy Association. (2006). *Which cardiomyopathy?* Retrieved June 26, 2006, from www.cardiomyopathy.org.

Carey, M. (2004). *Priapism.* Retrieved August 4, 2005, from http://www.emedicine.com.

Carpenito, L. J. (2004). *Nursing diagnosis: Application in clinical practice* (10th ed.). Philadelphia: Lippincott, Williams & Wilkins.

Carpenito-Moyet, L. J. (2005). *Nursing diagnosis: Application to clinical practice* (10th ed.). Philadelphia: Lippincott, Wilkins and Williams.

Carson, J. S., Burke, F. M., & Hark, L. A. (2004). *Cardiovascular nutrition: Disease management and prevention.* Chicago: American Diabetic Association.

Carter, K., Dufour, L., & Ballard, C. (2004). Identifying secondary skin lesions. *Nursing, 34*(1), 68.

Carter-Templeton, H. (2005). Malignant hyperthermia. *Nursing, 35*(6), 88.

Carver, C. (2005). Enhancing adaptation during treatment and the role of individual differences. *Cancer, 104*(11 Suppl), 2602–2607.

Casaccia, M., Torelli, P., Fontana, I., Panaro, F., & Valente, U. (2003). Laparoscopic bilateral hand-assisted nephrectomy: End-stage renal disease from tuberculosis, an unusual indication for nephrectomy before transplantation. *Surgical Laparoscopy Endoscopy and Percutaneous Techniques, 13*(1), 59–62.

Casebeer, L., Strasser, S., Spettell, C., Wall, T., Weisman, N., Ray, M., et al. (2003). *Designing tailored web-based instruction to improve physician's preventative practices.* Retrieved September 8, 2006, from www.jmir.org.

Casseb, J., Da Silva, D., & Alberto, J. (2005). Structured intermittent therapy with 7 day cycles of HAART for chronic HIF infections: A pilot study. *AIDS Patient Care and STDs, 19*(7), 425–429.

Castro, M. G., Cowen, R., Williamson, I. K., David, A., Jimenez-Dalmaroni, M. J., Yuan, X., et al. (2003). Current and future strategies for the treatment of malignant brain tumors. *Pharmacology and Therapeutics, 98*(1), 71–108.

Catalano, J. (2003). *Nursing now! Today's issues, tomorrow's trends* (3rd ed.). Philadelphia: F. A. Davis.

Cavanaugh, B. (2003). *Nurse's manual of laboratory and diagnostic tests.* Philadelphia: F. A. Davis Company.

Celik, S., Aksoy, G., & Akyolcu, N. (2004). Nursing role on preventing secondary brain injury. *Accident and Emergency Nursing, 12*(2), 94–98.

Center for Disease Control, National Center for Infectious Diseases. (2006). *All about Hantaviruses.* Retrieved June 23, 2006, from www.cdc.gov.

Centers for Disease Control and Prevention. (2002a). Hysterectomy surveillance—United States, 1994–1999. *Morbidity Mortality Weekly Report, 51*(SS05), 1–8.

Centers for Disease Control and Prevention. (2002b). Trends in tuberculosis morbidity–United States 1992–2002. Retrieved July 31, 2004, from http://www.cdc.gov.

Centers for Disease Control and Prevention. (2003a). *Coping with a traumatic event.* Retrieved June 16, 2006, from www.cdc.gov.

Centers for Disease Control and Prevention. (2003b). *Explosion and blast injuries: A primer for clinicians.* Retrieved June 13, 2006, from www.cdc.gov.

Centers for Disease Control and Prevention. (2003c). *New pediatric growth charts.* Retrieved June 16, 2005, from http://www.cdc.gov.

Centers for Disease Control and Prevention. (2004a). *Chlamydia fact sheet.* Retrieved July 30, 2006, from http://www.cdc.gov.

Centers for Disease Control and Prevention. (2004b). *Ebola hemorrhagic fever and viral hemorrhagic fever.* Retrieved July 3, 2006, from www.cdc.gov.

Centers for Disease Control and Prevention. (2004c). *Genital herpes fact sheet.* Retrieved July 30, 2006, from http://www.cdc.gov.

Centers for Disease Control and Prevention. (2004d). Lyme disease—United States, 2001–2002. *MMWR, 53*(17), 365–369.

Centers for Disease Control and Prevention. (2004e). *Questions and answers about plague.* Retrieved June 27, 2006, from www.cdc.gov.

Centers for Disease Control and Prevention. (2004f). *Severe acute respiratory syndrome. Supplement I: Infection control in healthcare, home and community settings.* Retrieved June 11, 2006, from http://www.cdc.gov.

Centers for Disease Control and Prevention. (2004g). *Trichomonas fact sheet.* Retrieved July 30, 2006, from http://www.cdc.gov.

Centers for Disease Control and Prevention. (2005a). *Healthy people 2010: Focus areas at a glance.* Retrieved on June 29, 2006, from www.cdc.gov.

Centers for Disease Control and Prevention. (2005b). *HIV/AIDS.* Retrieved June 25, 2006, from www.cdc.gov.

Centers for Disease Control and Prevention. (2006a). *Anthrax.* Retrieved June 22, 2006, from www.bt.cdc.gov.

Centers for Disease Control and Prevention. (2006b). Asthma prevalence and control characteristics by race/ethnicity—United States 2006. *Morbidity and Mortality Weekly Report, 53*(7), 1.

Centers for Disease Control and Prevention (2006c). *CDC fast stats. Stroke and cerebrovascular disease.* Retrieved June 17, 2006, from http://www.cdc.gov.

Centers for Disease Control and Prevention. (2006d). *Skin cancer guidelines.* Retrieved July 5, 2006, from http://www.cdc.gov.

Centers for Disease Control and Prevention. (2006e). *Small pox disease overview.* Retrieved June 24, 2006, from www.cdc.gov.

Centers for Disease Control and Prevention. (2006f). *West Nile virus.* Retrieved July 11, 2006, from http://www.cdc.gov.

Centers for Medicare and Medicaid Services. (2004). *The specifications manual for national hospital quality measures.* Retrieved May 18, 2005, from http://cms.hhs.gov/quality/hospital.

Centers for Medicare and Medicaid Services. (2005). *Health United States 2005.* Retrieved March 30, 2006, from http://www.cms.hhs.gov.

Centers for Medicare and Medicaid Services. (2006). *HIPPA insurance reform.* Retrieved from http://www.cms.hhs.gov.

Centers for Medicare and Medicaid Services. (n.d.). *Statistics and data.* Retrieved August 30, 2005, from http://www.cms.hhs.gov.

Certification for adult, pediatric and neonatal critical care nurses. (2003). Retrieved May 7, 2004, from www.aacn.org.

Cesari, M., Penninx, B. W., Newman, A. B., Kritchevsky, S. B., Nicklas, B. J., Sutton-Tyrrel, K., et al. (2003). Inflammatory markers and cardiovascular disease (The Health, Aging and Body Composition [Health ABC] Study). *The American Journal of Cardiology, 92*(5), 522–528.

Chaiyakunapruk, N., Veenstra, D., Lipsky, B., & Saint, S. (2002). Chlorhexidine compared with povidone-iodine solution for vascular catheter-site care: A meta-analysis. *Annals of Internal Medicine, 136*(11), 792–801.

Chalela, J., & Kasner, S. (2004). *Cardiac and respiratory complications of stroke.* Retrieved June 25, 2006, from http://www.uptodate.com.

Chally, P. S., & Hough, M. C. (2005). Nursing ethics. In K. Chitty, *Professional nursing: Concepts and challenges* (4th ed., pp. 212–227). St. Louis, MO: Elsevier.

Chambers, S., & Isenberg, D. (2005). Anti-B cell therapy (rituximab) in the treatment of autoimmune disease. *Lupus, 14*(3), 210–214.

Champagne, C. (2006). Dietary interventions on blood pressure: The dietary approaches to stop hypertension (DASH) trials. Prevention of nutrition-related chronic diseases: Scientific foundations and community interventions. Fifth Nestle Nutrition Conference, Mexico City, Mexico, October 7–8, 2004. *Nutrition Reviews, 64* (2 Part 2): S53–56.

Chang, B. S., & Lowenstein, D. H. (2003). Practice parameter: Antiepileptic drug prophylaxis in severe traumatic brain injury. Report of the Quality Standards Committee of the American Academy of Neurology. *Neurology, 60,* 10–16. Retrieved June 13, 2006, from www.guideline.gov.

Chang, Y., Singer, D. E., Wu, Y. A., Keller, R. B., & Atlas, S.J. (2005). The effect of surgical and nonsurgical treatment on longitudinal outcomes of lumbar spinal stenosis over 10 years. *Journal of American Geriatrics Society, 53*(5), 785–792.

Chapman, E. (2002). The social and ethical implications of changing medical technologies: The views of people living with genetic conditions. *Journal of Health Psychology, 7*(2), 195–206.

Chaudhry B., Capicatto M., & O'Brien A., (2002). Mystery of the dark green sputum: Lung abcess. *Post Graduate Medicine, 112*(3), 75–76, 82.

Chavis, S., & Duncan, L. (2003). Home study program: Pain management: Continuum of care for surgical patients. *Association of Operating Room Nurses Journal, 78*(3), 382–383, 385–386, 389–394, 396–399.

Cherkin, D. C., Sherman, K. J., Deyo, R. A., & Shekelle, P. G. (2003). A review of the evidence for the effectiveness, safety, and cost of acupuncture, massage therapy, and spinal manipulation for back pain. *Annals of Internal Medicine, 138*(11), 898–906.

Childs, S. G. (2002). Anatomy and physiology of the musculoskeletal system. In A. B. Mahler, S. W. Salmond, & T. A. Pellino (Eds.), *Orthopaedic nursing* (3rd ed., pp. 152–174). Philadelphia, PA: W. B. Saunders Company.

Chiller T. M., Galgiani J. N. & Stevens D. A. (2003). Coccidioidomycosis. *Infectious Disease Clinics of North America, 17*(1), 41–57.

Chinnock, P., & Roberts, I. (2004). Gangliosides for acute spinal cord injury. *The Cochrane Database of Systematic Reviews* (3), CD004444. DOI: 10.1002/14651858.

Chobanian, A. V., Bakris, G. L., Black, H. R., & Cushman, W. C. (2003). The seventh report of the joint national committee on the prevention, detection, evaluation, and treatment of high blood pressure: The JNC 7 report. *Journal of the American Medical Association, 289*(19), 2560–2571.

Chojnowski, D. (2003). "GOLD" standards for acute exacerbation in COPD. *Nurse Practitioner, 28*(5), 26–35; quiz 36–37.

Chojnowski, D. (2005). Peripheral arterial disease: Danger! Slow blood flow ahead. *Nursing Made Incredibly Easy, 3*(4), 4–17.

Chopra, D., & Simon, D. (2002). *Grow younger, live longer. 10 ways to reverse aging.* New York: Three Rivers Press.

Chou, L., Lo, S. Kao, M., Jim, Y., & Cho, D. (2002). Ankylosing spondylitis manifested by spontaneous anterior atlantoaxial subluxation. *American Journal of Physical Medicine & Rehabilitation, 81*(12), 952–955.

Christopher, K. (2003). Transtracheal oxygen catheters. *Clinics in Chest Medicine, 24*(3), 485–510.

Chrvala, C. A., & Bulger, R. J. (1999). *Leading health indicators for Healthy People 2010: Final report.* Division of Health Promotion and Disease Prevention, Institute of Medicine. Washington, DC: National Academy Press.

Ciarleglio, L., Bennett, R., Williamson, J., Mandell, J., & Marks, J. (2003). Genetic counseling throughout the life cycle. *The Journal of Clinical Investigation, 112*(9), 1280–1286.

Cicatiello, J. (2004). Reconstructing healthcare in a global marketplace. *Nursing Administration Quarterly, 28*(2), 83–85.

Cioffi, J. (2005). Nurses' experiences of caring for culturally diverse patients in an acute care setting. *Contemporary Nurse, 20*(1), 78–86.

Civetta, J. (1996). Futile care or caregiver frustration? A practical approach. *Critical Care Medicine, 24*(2), 346–351.

Clark, P., Drain, M., & Malone, M. (2004). *Addressing patients' emotional and spiritual needs.* Oakbrook Terrace, IL: Joint Commission Resources.

Clark, P. C., & King, K. B. (2003) Comparison of family caregivers: Stroke survivors vs. persons with Alzheimer's disease. *Journal of Gerontological Nursing, 32*(5), 45–55.

Classe, J., Curtet, C., & Campion, L. (2003). Learning curve for the detection of axillary sentinel lymph node in breast cancer. *European Journal of Surgical Oncology, 29,* 426.

Cleator, J., & Wilding, J. (2003). Obesity and diabetes. *Nursing Times, 99*(15), 54–55.

Cleveland Clinic. (2004). *What you need to know about living with pulmonary hypertension.* Retrieved September 16, 2004, from http://www.clevelandclinic.org.

Cochrane Database of Systematic Reviews. (2004). *Postoperative radiotherapy for non-small cell lung cancer.* Retrieved September 16, 2004, from http://www.cochrane.org.

Cohen, J., & De LaMare, J. (2002). *Health care costs: Fact sheet.* Retrieved June 17, 2006, from www.ahcpr.gov.

Cohen, M. R. (2005). Labetalol crisis: Speed kills. *Nursing, 35*(2), 18.

Cohen, S. M., Labadie, R. F., Dietrich, M.S., & Haynes, D. S. (2004). Quality of life in hearing-impaired adults: The role of cochlear implants and hearing aids. *Otolaryngology-Head and Neck Surgery, 131,* 413–422.

Collemer, S. (2004). *Too hot to handle.* Retrieved March 18, 2006, from http://www.aanet.org.

Collins, F. S., Green, E. D., Guttmacher, A., & Guyer, M. S. (2003). A vision for the future of genomics research: A blueprint for the genomic era. *Nature, 422*(24), 835–847.

Cole, E. (2005). *The Last Word*. U.S. Food, and Drug Administration. Retrieved March 10, 2005, from www.fda.gov.

Cole, S., & Dunne, K. (2004). Continuing professional development. *Hodgkin's lymphoma. Nursing Standard, 18*(9), 46–52, 54–55.

Colombo, A., Solberg, B., Vanderhoeft, E., Ramsay, G., & Schouten, H. (2005). Measurement of nursing care time of specific interventions on a hematology-oncology unit related to diagnostic categories. *Cancer Nursing, 28*(6), 476–480.

Comer, S. (2005). *Delmar's critical care nursing care plans* (2nd ed.). Clifton Park, NY: Thomson Delmar Learning.

Commission on Classification and Terminology of the International League against Epilepsy. (1981). Proposal for revised clinical and electroencephalographic classification of epileptic seizures. *Epilepsia, 22,* 489–501.

Conboy, L., Patel, S., Koptchuk, T., Gottlieb, B., Eisenberg, D., & Acevedo-Garcia, D. (2005). Types of complementary and alternative medicines: An analysis based on nationally representative sample. *Alternative and Complementary Medicine, 11*(6), 977–994.

Conlon, P., & Giblin, L. (2003). Vascular access for dialysis. In R. Johnson & J. Feehally (Eds.), *Comprehensive clinical nephrology* (2nd ed., pp. 957–965). St. Louis, MO: Mosby.

Cook, L. (2003). Staying current on defibrillator therapy. *Nursing, 33*(11), 44–46.

Coppin, C., Porzsolt, F., Awa, A., Kumpf, J., Coldman, A., & Wilt, T. (2005). Immunotherapy for advanced renal cell cancer. *The Cochrane Database of Systematic Reviews* (4), ID #CD001425.

Corey, H. (2003). Stewart and beyond: New models of acid-base balance. *Kidney International, 64,* 777–787.

Corley, M. C., (2002). Nurse moral distress: A proposed theory and research agenda. *Nursing Ethics, 9*(6), 635–650.

Cornell University Department of Urology. (2005). *Peyronie's disease.* Retrieved June 3, 2006, from http://www.cornellurology.com.

Cowan, J., & Graham, M. (2003, November). Polycystic ovary syndrome: More than a reproductive disorder. *Patient Care Nurse Practitioner,* 6–15.

Coward, L. J., Featherstone, R. L., & Brown, M. M. (2004). Percutaneous transluminal angioplasty and stenting for carotid artery stenosis. *The Cochrane Database of Systematic Reviews (Oxford).* ID # CD000515.

Cox, Robert. (2003). *Hazmat.* Retrieved June 14, 2006, from http://www.emedicine.com.

Craigie, J., Allen, R., DellaCroce, F., & Sullivan, S. (2003). Autogenous breast reconstruction with the deep inferior epigastric perforator flap. *Clinical Plastic Surgery, 30,* 359.

Crimlisk, J., & Grande, M. (2004). Neurologic assessment skills for the acute medical surgical nurse. *Orthopaedic Nursing, 23*(1), 3–9.

Criste, A. (2002). Gender and pain. *American Association of Nurse Anesthetists, 70*(6), 475–481.

Cross, C. (2004). Seizures: Regaining control. *RN, 67*(12), 44–51.

Crowther, C. L. (2004). Structure and function of the musculoskeletal system. In S. E. Huether & K. L. McCance (Eds.), *Understanding pathophysiology* (3rd ed., pp. 1047–1070). St. Louis, MO: Mosby.

Crowther, C. L., & McCance, K. L. (2004). Alterations of musculoskeletal function. In S. E. Huether & K. L. McCance (Eds.), *Understanding pathophysiology* (3rd ed., pp. 1071–1116). St. Louis, MO: Mosby.

Cua, I. H. Y., & George, J. (2005). Non-alcoholic fatty liver disease. *Hospital Medicine, 66*(2), 106–111.

Cuddy, M. (2005). Treatment of hypertension: Guidelines from JNC 7 (The Seventh Report of the Joint National Committee on Prevention, Detection, Evaluation, and Treatment of High Blood Pressure). *Journal of Practical Nursing, 55*(4), 17–23.

Cullen, L., Titler, M., & Drahozal, R. (2003). Family and pet visitation in the critical care unit. *Critical Care Nurse, 23*(5), 62–65.

Cullen, R. D., Higgins, C., Buss, E., Clark, M., Pillsbury, H. C., & Buchman, C. A. (2004). Cochlear implantations in patients with substantial residual hearing. *Laryngoscope, 114,* 2218–2223.

Cumbie, S., Conley, V., & Berman, M. (2004). Advanced practice nursing model for comprehensive care with chronic illness: Model for promoting process engagement. *Advances in Nursing Science, 27*(1), 70–80.

Cummins, R. (2003). *Advanced cardiac life support provider manual.* Dallas: American Heart Association.

Curhan, G. (2005). Clinical crossroads: conferences with patients and doctors. A 44-year-old woman with kidney stones. *Journal of the American Medical Association, 293*(9), 1107–1114.

Curley, M. (1998). Patient-nurse synergy: Optimizing patient outcomes. *American Journal of Critical Care, 7*(1), 64–72.

Curtis, S., Kolytolo, C., & Broome, M. (2004). Somatosensory function and pain. In C. Porth (Ed.), *Pathophysiology: Concepts of altered health states,* 6th ed. (pp. 245–251). Philadelphia: Lippincott.

Czernin, J., Gambhir, S., Brunken, R., & Schelbert, H. (2004). *Tutorial: Clinical PET-Cardiology.* Retrieved September 25, 2004, from http://laxmi.nuc.ucla.edu:8000/lpp/clinpetcardio/evaluation.html#Evaluation.

D'Antonio, J. (2004). You can lessen leukemia's toll. *Nursing, 34*(7), *Hospital Nursing,* 1–4.

D'Antonio, J. (2005). Chronic myelogenous leukemia. *Clinical Journal of Oncology Nursing, 9*(5), 535–538, 561–563.

D'Arcy, Y. (2004). Using technology to help alleviate pain. *Nursing Management, 35*(11), 45–47.

D'Arcy, Y. (2005). Pain management standards, the law, and you. *Nursing, 35*(4), 17.

Daller, J. A. (2004). *Heart valve surgery.* Retrieved August 29, 2004, from http://www.nlm.nih.gov/medlineplus/ency/article/002954.htm.

Dang, D., Johantgen, M., Pronovost, P., Jenckes, M., & Bass, E. (2002). Postoperative complications: Does intensive care unit staff nursing make a difference? *Heart and Lung, 31*(3), 219–228.

Daniels, R. (2003). *Delmar's manual of laboratory and diagnostic tests.* New York: Thomson Delmar Learning.

Daniels, R. (2004). *Nursing fundamentals: Caring and clinical decision making.* New York: Thomson Delmar Learning.

Darovic, G. (2004). *Handbook of hemodynamic monitoring* (2nd ed.). St. Louis, MO: Saunders.

Davidoff, T. Q., & Cunningham, M. (2004, May). *Sinusitis, acute.* Retrieved August 5, 2004, from http://www.emedicine.com/med/topic2555.htm.

Davies, P., & Galer, B. (2004). Review of lidocaine patch 5% studies in the treatment of postherpetic neuralgia. *Drugs, 64*(9), 937–947.

Davies, S., & Gilmore, A. (2003). The role of hydroxyurea in the management of sickle cell disease. *Blood Reviews, 17,* 99–109.

Davies, S., & Williams, J. (2003). Peritoneal dialysis: Principles, techniques, and adequacy. In R. Johnson & J. Feehally (Eds.), *Comprehensive clinical nephrology* (2nd ed., pp. 1003–1011). St. Louis, MO: Mosby.

Davila, R. E., Rajan, E., Adler, D., Hirota, W. K., Jacobson, B. C., Leighton, J. A., et al. (2005). ASGE Guideline: The role of endoscopy in the diagnosis, staging, and management of colorectal cancer. *Gastrointestinal Endoscopy, 61*(1), 1–7.

Davy, A. R., & Drew, S. J. (2002). Management of shoulder dislocations—Are we doing enough to reduce the risk or recurrence? *Injury, 33,* 775–779.

de la Chica, R., Ribas, I., Giraldo, J., Egozcue, J., & Fuster, C. (2005). Chromosomal instability in amniocytes from fetuses of mothers who smoke. *Journal of the American Medical Association, 293,* 1212–1222.

Deaton, C., Bennett, J. A., & Riegel, B. (2004). State of the science for care of older adults with heart disease. *Nursing Clinics of North America, 39*(3), 495–528.

Deb, S., & Crownshaw, T. (2004). The role of pharmacotherapy in the management of behavioral disorders in traumatic brain injury patients. *Brain Injury, 18*(1), 1–31.

DeFrances, C. J., & Hall, M. J. (2004, May 21). 2002 national hospital discharge survey. *CDC Advance Data from Vital and Health Statistics, 342*(3), 1–27.

DeLaune, S., & Ladner, P. (2006). *Fundamentals of nursing* (3rd ed.). New York: Thomson Delmar Learning.

Delta Society. (2005). *Animal assisted therapy.* Retrieved August 2, 2006, from http://www.deltasociety.org.

Dellinger, R., Carlet, J., Masur, H., Gerlach, H. (2004). Surviving sepsis campaign guidelines for management of severe sepsis and septic shock. *Critical Care Medicine, 32*(3), 858. Retrieved June 23, 2006, from www.survivingsepsis.com.

Deliveliotis, C., Papatsoris, A., Chrisofos, M., Dellis, A., Liakouras, C., & Skolarikos, A. (2005). Urinary diversion in high-risk elderly patients: Modified cutaneous ureterostomy or ileal conduit? *Urology, 66* (2), 299–304.

DeMarini, D., & Preston, R. (2005). Smoking while pregnant: Transplacental mutagenesis of the fetus by tobacco smoke. *Journal of the American Medical Association, 293,*1264–1265.

Demling, R. (2005). The role of anabolic hormones of wound healing in catabolic states. *Journal of Burns and Wounds.* Retrieved May 31, 2006, from www.journalofburnsandwounds.com.

Dempski, K. M., & Killion, S. W. (2001). *Legal & ethical issues in nursing.* Thorofare, NJ: SLACK, Inc.

Denis, L., Namey, M., Costello, K., Frenette, J., Gagnon, N., Harris, C., et al. (2004). Long term treatment optimization in individuals with multiple sclerosis using disease-modifying therapies: A nursing approach. *Journal of Neuroscience Nursing, 36*(1), 10–22.

Denkins, B. A. (2005). My side. Are we really helping? The problem of dual diagnoses, homelessness, & hospital-hopping. *Journal of Psychosocial Nursing and Mental Health Services, 43*(11), 48–50.

Dennis, M. V. (2003). Digital photographs in the ED: Images of an accident can offer ED staff a clearer picture of the cause and extent of victims' injuries. *The American Journal of Nursing, 103*(12), 44–46.

Dennis, V. (2004). *Electrosurgical safety and your staff.* Retrieved July 31, 2005, from http://www.encision.com.

Denny, E. (2004). Women's experience of endometriosis. *Journal of Advanced Nursing, 46*(6), 641–648.

Deodato, F., Boenzi, S., Rizzo, C., Abeni, D., Caviglia, S., Bartuli, A., et al. (2004). Inborn errors of metabolism: An update on epidemiology and on neonatal-onset hyperammonemia. *Acta Paediatrica, S445*(93), 18–21.

DeVault, K., & Castell, D. (2005). Updated guidelines for the diagnosis and treatment of gastrointestinal reflux disease. *American Journal of Gastroenterology, 100*(1), 190–200.

Diehl-Oplinger, L., & Kaminski, M. (2004). Choosing the right fluid to counter hypovolemic shock. *Nursing, 34*(3), 52–54.

Diepgen, T., & Mahler, V. (2002). The epidemiology of skin cancer. *British Journal of Dermatology, 146*(Suppl 61), 1–6.

Dieterich, M. (2004). Dizziness. *Neurology, 10*(3), 154–164.

Dixon, L. (2002). Postoperative complications and the older adult. *Geriatric Nursing, 23*(11), 203.

DNAdirect. (2006). *Genetic testing.* Retrieved July 10, 2006, from www.dnadirect.org.

Dochterman, J. M., & Bulechek, G. M. (2004). *Nursing interventions classification (NIC)* (4th ed.). St. Louis, MO. Mosby.

Doe Report. (2005). *Burn injuries. The Doe report medical reference library.* Retrieved March 1, 2006, from http://www.doeroport.com.

Doganci, L., Odabasi, Z., & Turan, M. (2003). Dangerous to link a hepatatrophic etiology to a neurologic illness. *American Journal of Physical Medicine and Rehabilitation, 82*(7), 563.

Donabedian, A. (1966). Evaluating the quality of medical care. *Milbank Memorial Fund Quarterly, 44*(3 Suppl), 166–206.

Donabedian, A. (1998). The quality of care: How can it be assessed? *Journal of the American Medical Association, 260*(12), 1743–1748.

Doughty, D. (2004). Skin integrity and wound healing. In R. Daniels (Ed.), *Nursing fundamentals: Caring and clinical decision making* (pp. 165–170). New York: Thomson Delmar Learning.

Douglas, R. M., Chalker, E. B., & Treacy, B. (2004, February). *Vitamin C for preventing and treating the common cold.* Retrieved June 17, 2004, from http://www.cochrane.org/cochrane/revabstr/ab000980.htm.

Drake, A. D., & Carr, M. M. (2003, February). *Tonsillectomy.* Retrieved August 25, 2004, from http://www.emedicine.com/ent/topic315.htm.

Dreger, V., & Tremback, T. (2002). Optimize patient health by treating literacy and language barriers. *Association of Operating Room Nurses Journal, 75*(2), 280–293.

Dreicer, R. (2005). *Prostate cancer.* Retrieved July 19, 2006, from http://www.clevelandclinicmeded.com.

Drug prices. (2006). Retrieved July 3, 2006, from www.drugstore.com.

Drumm, C., Bruner, J., & Minutillo, A. (2004). Plague comes to New York. *American Journal of Nursing, 104*(8), 61–64.

Druz, D. (2005). Recognizing signs, symptoms could lead to a more accurate diagnosis in diplopia. *Ocular Surgery News, 23*(8), 124–125.

Duke, J. (2002). *The green pharmacy.* Emmaus, PA: Rodale Press.

Dunn, L. (2005). New blood. *Nursing Standard, 20*(4), 69.

Dweyer M. K., & Uhl T. L. (2003). A traumatic pneumothorax as a result of a rib fracture in a college baseball player. *Orthopedics, 26*(7), 726–729.

Ebersole, P., Hess, P., & Luggen, A. (2004). *Toward healthy aging* (6th ed.). St. Louis, MO: Mosby.

Eckert, M., & Jones, T. (2002). How does an implantable cardioverter defibrillator (ICD) affect the lives of patients and their families. *International Journal of Nursing Practice, 8,* 152–157.

Edelman, C. L., & Mandle, C. L. (2002). *Health promotion throughout the life span* (5th ed.). St. Louis, MO: Mosby.

Edgar, D. (2004). Advances in genetics: Implications for children, families, and nurses. *Pediatric Nursing, 16*(6), 26–29.

Edlow, J. A. (2002). Tick-borne diseases, lyme. *eMedicine Journal, 3*(4). Retrieved September 5, 2006, from http://www.emedicine.com.

Edwards, D., & Burnard, P. (2003). A systematic review of stress and stress management interventions for mental health nurses. *Journal of Advanced Nursing, 42*(2), 169–200.

Edwards, S. (2002). Physiological insult/injury: Pathophysiology and consequences. *British Journal of Nursing, 11*(4), 263–277.

Eggenberger, S., & Nelms, T. (2004). Artificial hydration and nutrition in advanced Alzheimer's disease: Facilitating family decision-making. *Journal of Clinical Nursing, 13,* 661–667.

Eggenberger, S., Grassley, J., Restrepo, E. (2006). Culturally competent nursing care for families: Listening to the voices of Mexican-American women. *The Online Journal of Issues in Nursing, 11*(3). Retrieved from www.nursingworld.org.

Ehlers, V. (2002). Republic of South Africa: Policies and politics guide nurses' application of genetic technology in public health settings. *Policy, Politics, & Nursing Practice, 3*(2), 149–159.

Eichner, J., Dunn, S., Perveen, G., Thomson, D., Stewart, K., & Stoehla, B. (2002). Apolipoprotein E polymorphism and cardiovascular disease: A huge review. *American Journal of Epidemiology, 155,* 487–495.

El-Alfy, M., & El-Sayed, M. (2004). Overwhelming postsplenectomy infection: Is quality of patient knowledge enough for prevention? *Hematology Journal, 5*(1), 77–80.

Eliopoulos, C. (2005). *Gerontological nursing* (6th ed.). Philadelphia: Lippincott Williams & Wilkins.

Elkhodair, S., Parmar, H., & Vanwaeyenbergh, J. (2005). The role of the IPSS (International Prostate Symptoms Score) in predicting acute retention of urine in patients undergoing major joint arthroplasty. *Surgeon, 3*(2), 63–65.

Emanuel, E., Crouch, R., Arras, J., Moreno, J., & Grady, C. (2003). Ethical and regulatory aspects of clinical research. Baltimore, MD: Johns Hopkins University Press.

Eng, J., Krishnan, J., Segal, J., Bolger, D., Tamariz, L., Streiff, M., Jenckes, M., & Bass, E. (2004). Accuracy of CT in the diagnosis of pulmonary embolism: A systematic literature review. *American Journal of Roentgenology, 183,* 1819–1827.

Englund, M., Roos, E. M., & Lohmander, L. S. (2003). Impact of type of meniscal tear on radiographic and symptomatic knee osteoarthritis: A sixteen-year followup of meniscectomy with matched controls. *Arthritis and Rheumatism, 48,* 2178–2187.

Enns, G., & Packman, W. (2002). The adolescent with an inborn error metabolism: Medical issues and transition to adulthood. *Adolescent Medicine, 13*(2), 315–329.

Enright, P. (2004). *Overview of pulmonary function testing.* Retrieved June 25, 2006, from http://www.uptodate.com.

Epel, E. S., Blackburn, E. H., Lin, J., Dhabhar, F. S., Adler, N. E., Morrow, J. D., et al. (2004). Accelerated telomere shortening in response to life stress. *Proceedings of the National Academy of Science USA, 101*(49), 17312–17315.

Eppes, S. C. (2003). Diagnosis, treatment, and prevention of Lyme disease in children. *Pediatric Drugs, 5*(6), 363–372.

Erikson, E. (1963). The eight stages of man. In *Childhood and society* (2nd ed.) (pp. 247–274). New York: WW. Norton.

Erlen, J. (2004). HIPAA—clinical and ethical considerations for nurses. *Orthopaedic Nursing, 23*(6), 410–413.

Estes, M. (2006). *Health assessment and physical examination* (3rd ed.). New York: Thomson Delmar Learning.

Estiarte R., Colome, J. J., Artes, E., & Jimenez, F. J. (2003). Drug utilization study in patients with Crohn's disease in Spain. *European Journal of Gastroenterology and Hepatology, 15*(4), 355–362.

Estores, I. (2003). The consumer's perspective and the professional literature: What do persons with spinal cord injury want? *Journal of Rehabilitation Research and Development, 40*(4), 1–6.

Etchegary, H. (2006). Genetic testing for Huntington's disease: How is the decision taken? *Genetic Testing, 10*(1), 60–67.

Evans, L. S., & Hancock, B. W. (2003). Non-Hodgkin lymphoma. *Lancet, 362*(9378), 139–146.

Evered, A. (2003). Hypothermia: Risk factors and guidelines for nursing care. *Nursing Times, 99*(49), 40–43.

Everett, B., & Salamonson, Y. (2005). Differences in postoperative opioid consumption in patients prescribed patient-controlled analgesia versus intramuscular injection. *Pain Management Nursing, 6*(4), 137–144.

Eysteinsdottir, J. H., Freysdottir, J., Haraldsson, A., Stefansdottir, J., Skaftadottir, I., Helgason, H., et al. (2004). The influence of partial or total thymectomy during open heart surgery in infants on the immune function later in life. *Clinical and Experimental Immunology, 136*(2), 349–355.

Fadiman, A. (1997). *The spirit catches you and you fall down.* New York: Noonday Press.

Falkenbach, A. (2003). Disability motivates patients with ankylosing spondylitis for more frequent physical exercise. *Archives of Physical Medicine and Rehabilitation, 84*(3), 382–383.

Falkiner, S., & Myers, S. (2002). When exactly can carpal tunnel syndrome be considered work related? *ANZ Journal of Surgery, 72*(3), 204–209.

Faris, R., Flather, M., Purcell, H., Henein, M., Poole-Wilson, P., & Coats, A. (2002). Current evidence supporting the role of diuretics in heart failure: A meta analysis of randomised controlled trials. *International Journal of Cardiology, 82*(2), 149–158.

Farooq, S., & Fear, C. (2003). Working through interpreters. *Advances in Psychiatric Treatment, 9,* 104–109.

Farrington, K., Greenwood, R., & Ahmad, S. (2003). Hemodialysis: Mechanisms, outcome, and adequacy. In R. Johnson & J. Feehally (Eds.), *Comprehensive clinical nephrology* (2nd ed., pp. 975–990). St. Louis, MO: Mosby.

Fecci, P. E., Mitchell, D. A., Archer, G. E., Morse, M. A., Lyerly, H. K., Bigner, D. D., et al. (2003). The history, evolution, and clinical use of dendritic cell-based immunization strategies in the therapy of brain tumors. *Journal of Neurooncology, 64*(1–2), 161–176.

Feder, B. J., & Zeller, T. (2004). *Identity badge worn under skin approved for use in health care.* Retrieved July 4, 2006, from http://www.nytimes.com.

Felberg, R. A., & Naidech, A. (2003). The five Ps of acute ischemic stroke treatment: Parenchyma, pipes, perfusion, penumbra, and prevention of complications. *The Ochsner Journal, 5*(1), 5–10.

Ferlito, A., Silver, C. E., Howard, D. J., Laccourreye, O., Rinaldo, A., & Owen, R. (2000). The role of partial laryngeal resection in current management of laryngeal cancer: A collective review. *Acta Oto-Laryngolica, 120,* 456–466.

Ferri, F. (2005). *Ferri's clinical advisor.* Philadelphia: Lippincott, Williams & Wilkins.

Ferri, F. F., Saver, D. F., Mugge, R. E., Leickly, F. E., Millman, B., & Fox, R. (2004, August). *Allergic rhinitis.* Retrieved December 17, 2004, from http://www.firstconsult.com.

Fields, L., Burt, V., Cutler, J., Hughes, J., Roccella, E., & Sorlie, P. (2004). The burden of adult hypertension in the United States 1999–2000: A rising tide. *Hypertension, 44,* 398–404.

File, T. (2004). The challenge of SARS: A clinical review. *The Journal of Respiratory Disease, 25*(4), 147–155.

Fine, P. (2005). The evolving and important role of anesthesiology in palliative care. *Anesthesia and Analgesia, 100*(1), 183–188.

Fine, R., & Mayo, T. (2003). Resolution of futility by due process: Early experience with the Texas Advance Directives Act. *Annals of Internal Medicine, 138*(9), 743–746.

Fischer, S. J. (2005). *Rotator cuff tears.* Retrieved on September 28, 2005, from http://orthoinfo.aaos.org.

Fitzgerald, P. A. (2004). Endocrinology. In L. M. Tierney, S. J. McPhee, & M. A. Papidakis (Eds.), *Current medical diagnosis and treatment* (43rd ed., pp. 1062–1145). New York: McGraw-Hill.

Fitzpatrick, L. (2003). Alternatives to estrogen. *Medical Clinics of North America, 87*(5), 1091–1113.

Flegal, K., Carroll, M., Ogden, C., & Johnson, C. (2002). Prevalence and trends in obesity among U.S. adults, 1999–2000. *Journal of the American Medical Association, 288,* 1723–1727.

Fleischmann, D., & Rubin, G. (2005). Quantification of intravenously administered contrast medium transit through the peripheral arteries: Implications for CT angiography. *Radiology, 236*(3), 1076–1082.

Flynn, B. (1997). Partnerships in health cities and communities: A social commitment for advanced practice nurses. *Advanced Practice Nursing Quarterly, 2*(4), 1–6.

Foley, E. (2005). HIV/AIDS and African immigrant women in Philadelphia: Structural and cultural barriers to care. *AIDS Care, 17*(8), 1030–1043.

Foley, M. (2004). Update on needlestick and sharps injuries. *American Journal of Nursing, 104*(8), 96.

Folgelman, I., Cook, G., Israel, O., Van der Wall, H. (2005). Positron emission tomography and bone metastases. *Seminar Nuclear Medicine, 35*(2), 135–142.

Folmer, R. L., Martin, W. H., & Shi, Y. (2004). Tinnitus: Questions to reveal the cause, answers to provide relief. *The Journal of Family Practice, 53,* 532–540.

Folstein, M., Folstein, S., & McHugh, P. (1975). Mini-mental state: A practical method for grading the cognitive state of patients for the clinician. *Journal of Psychiatric Research, 12*(3), 189–198.

Fong, D., Aiello, L., Ferris, F., & Klein, R. (2004). Retinopathy in diabetes. *Diabetes Care, 7*(1), 84–87.

Food and Nutrition Board, National Academy of Sciences. (2004). *Dietary reference intakes table.* Retrieved June 24, 2006, from http://www.iom.edu.

Forsyth, I., Shaikh, S., & Gunn, I (2005). The nurse cystoscopist: Extending the role. *British Journal of Perioperative Nursing, 15*(8), 342–345.

Fort, C. W. (2003). Can you solve the mystery? The patient might have DVT . . . or is it FES? *Nursing Made Incredibly Easy, 1*(2), 10–16.

Fortinash, K., & Holoday-Worret, P. (2004). *Psychiatric mental health nursing* (3rd ed.). St. Louis, MO: Mosby.

Frantz, R. (2004). *Chronic wound healing.* Retrieved August 13, 2004, from www.nursing.uiowa.edu/sites/chronicwound/.

Frasco, P., Sprung, J., & Trentman, T. (2005). The impact of the joint commission for accreditation of health-care organization's pain initiative on perioperative opiate consumption and recovery room length of stay. *Anesthesia-Analgesia, 100*(1), 162–168.

Frawley, P. M., & Habashi, N. (2001). Airway pressure release ventilation: Theory and practice. *AACN Clinical Issues, 12*(2), 234–246.

Frazel, J. (2004). Optimize migraine management in primary care. *Nurse Practitioner, 29*(4), 22–33.

Frazier, S., Moser, D., Daley, L., McKinley, S., Riegel, B., Garvin, B., et al. (2003). Critical care nurses' beliefs about and reported management of anxiety. *American Journal of Critical Care, 12*(1), 19–27.

Friedman, S. L., McQuaid, K. R., & Grendell, J. H. (2003). *Current diagnosis and treatment in gastroenterology* (2nd ed.). New York: Lange Medical Books.

Friedrich, M. (2002). Preserving privacy, preventing discrimination becomes the province of genetics experts. *Journal of the American Medical Association, 288*, 815–816.

Frith, M. (2006). Acne scarring: Current treatment options. *Dermatology Nursing, 18*(2), 130–134.

Fromer, M. (2005). Metastatic kidney cancer: Prognosis still poor, but new treatment options on horizon. *Oncology Times, 27*(3), 16, 19–20.

Fry, S., & Johnstone, M. (Eds.). (2002). *International Council of Nurses Ethics in nursing practice A guide to ethical decision-making.* Malden, MA: Blackwell Publishing.

Frye, R., Tamer, M. A., & Kunha, B. A. (2005). *Bacterial overgrowth syndrome.* Retrieved June 25, 2006, from http://www.emedicine.com.

Fryer, D., & McIntosh S. (2005). A simplified history of anesthesia. *Dissector, 32*(4), 14–16.

Funk, S. G., Tournquist, E. M., & Champagne, M. T. (1989). A model for improving the dissemination of nursing research. *Western Journal of Nursing Research, 11*(3), 361–367.

Furlanetto, D., Crighton, A., & Topping, G. (2006). Differences in methodologies of measuring the prevalence of oral mucosal lesions in children and adolescents. *Journal of Pediatric Dentistry, 16*(1), 31–39.

Furness, S. (2005). Shifting sands: Developing cultural competence. *Practice, 17*(4), 247–256.

Fuster, V., Alexander, R. W., O'Rourke, R. A. (2004). *Hurst's the heart* (11th ed.). New York: McGraw-Hill Medical Publishing Division.

Gaberson, K. B., Schroeter, K., Killen, A. R., & Valentine, W. A. (2003).The perceived value of certification by certified perioperative nurses. *Nursing Outlook, 51*(6), 273–277.

Gahart, B., & Nazareno, A. (2002). *Intravenous medications* (18th ed.). St. Louis, MO: Mosby.

Gaitatzis, A., & Patsalos, P. (2002). Preconception counseling of women with epilepsy. *Pulse, 62*(30), 29–32.

Gajic, O., Dzik, W., & Toy, P. (2006). Fresh frozen plasma and platelet transfusion for nonbleeding patients in the intensive care unit: benefit or harm? *Critical Care Medicine, 34*(5 Suppl), S170–S173.

Galli, B., Munver, R., Sawczuk, I., & Kochis, E. (2005). Laparoscopic radical nephrectomy in renal cell carcinoma. *Urologic Nursing, 25*(2), 83–87, 133.

Gallup Organization. (2006). Nurses top list in honesty and ethics again in Gallup poll. Retrieved June 26, 2006, from www.gallup.com.

Gambrell, M., & Flynn, N. (2004). Seizures 101. *Nursing, 34*(8), 36–41.

Gammon, R. (2004) *Measurement of arterial blood gases.* Retrieved June 25, 2006, from http://www.uptodate.com.

Ganong, W. F. (2003). *Review of medical physiology* (21st ed.). San Francisco: Lange Medical Books/McGraw Hill.

Ganong, W. (2005). *Review of medical physiology* (22nd ed.). New York: McGraw-Hill.

Ganz, P. A., Greendale, G. A., Petersen, L, Kahn, B., & Bower, J. E. (2003). Breast cancer in your women: Reproductive and late health effects of treatment. *Journal of Clinical Oncology, 21*, 4184–4193.

Garber, S. L., & Rintala, D. H. (2003). Pressure ulcers in veterans with spinal cord injury: A retrospective study. *Journal of Rehabilitation Research and Development, 40*(5), 433–442.

Gardner, D., & Greenspan, F. (2004). Endocrine emergencies. In F.S. Greenspan & D. G. Gardner (Eds.), *Basic and clinical endocrinology* (pp. 829–842). St. Louis, MO: Lange Medical Books.

Gates, G. A., Feeney, M. P., & Higdon, R. J. (2003). Word recognition and the articulation index in older listeners with probable age-related auditory neuropathy. *Journal of American Academy of Audiology, 14*(4), 574–581.

Gawande, A. A., Studdert, D. M., Orav, E. J., Brennan, T. A., & Zinner, M. J. (2003). Risk factors for retained instruments and sponges after surgery. *New England Journal of Medicine, 348*, 229–235.

Geerts, W. H., Pineo, G. F., Heit, J. A., Bergqvist, D., Lassen, M. R., Colwell, C. W., et al. (2004). Prevention of venous thromboembolism: The seventh ACCP conference on antithrombotic and thrombolytic therapy. *Chest, 126*(3 Suppl), 338S–400S.

Geetha, D. (2004, November). *Poststreptococcal glomerulonephritis.* Retrieved January 27, 2006, from http://www.emedicine.com/med/topic889.htm.

Gehrig, L. (2005). *Sprained ankle.* Retrieved on September 26, 2005 from http://orthoinfo.aaos.org.

Geisbert, T. W., Hensley, L. E., Larsen, T., Young, H. A., Reed, D. S., Geisbert, J. B., et al. (2003). Pathogenesis of Ebola hemorrhagic fever in cynomolgus macaques: Evidence that dendritic cells are early and sustained targets of infection. *American Journal of Pathology, 163*(6), 2347–2370.

Gentlesk, P. J., & McCabe, J. (2004). *Acute pericarditis.* Retrieved June 24, 2006, from www.emedicine.com.

Gentry, C. (2005). *New program lifts safety at hospital.* Retrieved October 21, 2005, from http://www.tampatrib.com/Business/MGBAJFSCOFE.html.

Germond, C., Figueredo, A., Taylor, B. M., Micucci, S., & Zwaal, C. (2004). *Postoperative adjuvant radiotherapy and/or chemotherapy for resected stage II or II rectal cancer.* Practice guideline Report #2-3. (Program in evidence-based care). Toronto, Ontario: Cancer Care.

Geslak, J. (2005). When resources are scarce, consider growing your own. *AORN Journal, 82*(2), 244, 246–249.

Ghoraych, B. (2005). *Trans-sphenoid approach to the sella turcica.* Retrieved June 23, 2006, from www.ghorayeb.com.

Giammattei, J., Blix, G., Marshak, H. H., Willitzer, A. O., & Pettitt, D. J. (2003). Television watching and soft drink consumption: Associations with obesity in 11 to 13 year old schoolchildren. *Archives of Pediatric and Adolescent Medicine, 157*(9), 882–886.

Gibson, R. L., Burns, J. L., & Ramsey, B. W. (2003). Pathophysiology and management of pulmonary infections in cystic fibrosis. *American Journal of Respiratory and Critical Care Medicine, 168*(8), 918–951.

Giger, J. N., & Davidhizar, R. E. (2004). *Transcultural nursing: Assessment and intervention* (4th ed.). St. Louis, MO: Mosby.

Gilbert, S. (2003). *Hydrocele.* Retrieved July 10, 2006, from http://www.nlm.nih.gov.

Gilbert, S. (2004). *Orchitis.* Retrieved July 19, 2006, from http://www.nlm.nih.gov.

Gilchrist, D., & Hall, J. (2002). Medical genetics: An approach to the adult with a genetic disorder. *Canadian Medical Association Journal, 167*(9), 1021–1029.

Giles, W., Thompson, M., Champion, S., Grégoire, S., Meban, D., Patel, L., et al. (2005). *MacIntosh common symptoms and signs in gastroenterology.* Retrieved July 11, 2006, from http://gastroresource.com.

Gill, D., Davies, L., Pringle, I., & Hyde, S. (2004). The development of gene therapy for diseases of the lung. *Cellular and Molecular Life Sciences, 61*(3), 355–368.

Gill, J. M., Quisel, A. M., Rocca, P. V., & Walters, D. T. (2003). Diagnosis of systemic lupus erythematosus. *American Family Physician, 68*(11), 2179–2186.

Gillespie, L. D., Gillespie, W. J., Robertson, M. C., Lamb, S. E., Cumming, R. G., & Rowe, B. H. (2005). *Interventions for preventing falls in elderly people.* Oxford, UK: The Cochrane Database of Systematic Reviews.

Gillespie, W. J., Avenell, A., Henry, D. A., O'Connell, D. L., & Robertson, J. (2004). Vitamin D and vitamin D analogues for preventing fractures associated with involutional and post-menopausal osteoporosis (Cochrane review). In *The Cochrane Database of Systematic Reviews.* Chichester, UK: John Wiley & Sons, Ltd.

Gines, P., Guevara, M., Arroyo, V., & Rodes, J. (2003). Hepatorenal syndrome. *Lancet, 362*(9398), 1819–1827.

Girman, A., Lee, R., & Kligler, B. (2003). An integrative medicine approach to premenstrual syndrome. *American Journal of Obstetrics and Gynecology, 188*(5 Suppl), S56–65.

Glass, J. M., Lyden, A. K., Petzke, F., Stein, P., Whalen, G., Ambrose, K., et al. (2004). The effect of brief exercise cessation on pain, fatigue, and mood symptom development in healthy, fit individuals. *Journal of Psychosomatic Research, 57*(4), 391–398.

Glassroth, C. (2004). Successful migraine management: Patient-customized care. *Clinician Reviews, 14*(5), 56–61.

Glasziou, P., Irwig, L., Bain, C., & Colditz, G (2001). *Systematic reviews in health care: A practical guide.* Cambridge, UK: Cambridge University Press.

Goer, T., & Lacey, S. (2005). Bone up on fat embolism syndrome. *Nursing, 23*(4), 1–4.

Golash, V., & Willson P. (2005). Early laparoscopy as a routine procedure in the management of acute abdominal pain: A review of 1,320 patients. *Surgical Endoscopy, 19*(7):882–885.

Goldberg, B. (2002). *Alternative medicine: The definitive guide.* Tiburon, CA: Future Medicine Publishing.

Goldberg, B., & Goldberg, M. (2002). *Alternative medicine: The definitive guide.* Berkeley, CA: Celestial Arts.

Goldberg, D. (2004). *Photodamaged skin.* New York: Marcel Dekker.

Goldberg, J. P., Belury, M. A., Elam, P., Finn, S. C., Hayes, D., Lyle, R., et al. (2004). The obesity crisis: Don't blame it on the pyramid. *Journal of the American Dietetic Association, 104*(7), 1141–1147.

Goldberg, S. (2004). Tuberculosis. *Clinics in Family Practice, 6*(1), 175.

Goldhaber, S. Z., Dunn, K., Gerhard-Herman, M., Park, J. K., & Black, P. (2002). Low rate of venous thromboembolism after craniotomy for brain tumor using multimodality prophylaxis. *Chest, 122*(6), 1933–1937.

Goldie, S., Kohli, M., Grima, D., Weinstein, M., Wright, T., Bosch, F., et al. (2004). Projected clinical benefits and cost-effectiveness of a human papillomavirus 16/18 vaccine. *Journal of the National Cancer Institute, 96*(8), 604–614.

Goldrick, B. (2004). Emerging infections: MRSA, VRE, and VRSA. *American Journal of Nursing, 104*(8), 50.

Gonzales, E., & Martin, K. (2003). Bone and mineral metabolism in chronic renal failure. In R. Johnson & J. Feehally (Eds.), *Comprehensive clinical nephrology* (2nd ed., pp. 873–885). St. Louis, MO: Mosby.

Goodal, D., & Etters, L. (2005). The therapeutic use of music on agitated behavior in those with dementia. *Journal of Holistic Nursing Practice, 19*(6), 97–104.

Gordon, M. (1994). *Nursing diagnosis: Process and application* (3rd ed.). St. Louis, MO: Mosby.

Gordon, M. (1997). *Manual of nursing diagnoses.* St. Louis, MO: Mosby.

Gordon, M. (2002). *Manual of nursing diagnosis* (10th ed.). St. Louis, MO: Mosby.

Gordon, P. A. (2004). Effects of diabetes on the vascular system: Current research evidence and best practice recommendations. *Journal of Vascular Nursing, 22*(1), 2–13.

Gosselin, B. J. (2004, July). *Peritonsillar abscess.* Retrieved August 25, 2004, from http://www.emedicine.com/med/topic2803.htm.

Gottlieb, M., & Furman, J. (2004). *Successful management and surgical closure of chronic and pathological wounds using Integra®.* Retrieved May 1, 2006, from http://www.journalofburnsandwounds.com.

Gowen, G. (2003). Long tube decompression is successful in 90% of patients with adhesive small bowel obstruction. *The American Journal of Surgery, 185*, 512–515.

Greco, K., & Mahon, S. (2003). Genetics nursing practice enters a new era with credentialing. *The Internet Journal of Advanced Nursing Practice, 5*(2), 1523–6064.

Grady, D. (2006). *Studies suggest two major diseases have close links: Alzheimer's, diabetes tolls seen rising.* Retrieved July 17, 2006, from http://www.alz.org.

Graham, T. A. D. (2002). Diagnosis and treatment of pharyngitis in adults. *CJEM Journal Club, 4*(6), 429–430.

Grantham, J., & Winklhofer, F. (2004). Cystic diseases of the kidney. In B. Brenner (Ed.), *Brenner and Rector's the kidney* (7th ed., vol. 2, pp. 1743–1775). Philadelphia: W. B. Saunders Co.

Grauer, K., & Ruskin, J. (2004, February). Palpitations and arrhythmias: Benign or threatening? *Patient Care,* 30–36.

Graxiottin, A., & Brotto, L. (2004). Vulvar vestibulitis syndrome: A clinical approach. *Journal of Sex and Marital Therapy, 30,* 125–139.

Gray, E. (2005). Understanding the role of the glaucoma specialist nurse. *Nursing Times, 101*(38), 32–34.

Grayson, M. (2004). The open organization. *Hospitals and Health Networks, 78*(10), 36–44.

Greater New York Hospital Association. (2002). *Do you know your incident command system*? Retrieved July 5, 2006, from http://www.gnyha.org.

Green, D., Hartwig, D., Chen, D., Soltysik, R., Yarnold, P. (2003). Spinal cord injury risk assessment for thromboembolism. *American Journal of Physical Medicine and Rehabilitation, 82*(12), 950–956.

Green, H. J., Pakenham, K. I., & Gardiner, R. A. (2005). Objective and cognitive deficits associated with cancer: Implications for health professionals. *Psychology, Health, and Medicine, 10*(2), 145–160.

Green, R. (2005). Toward a full theory of moral status. *American Journal of Bioethics, 5*(6), 44–46.

Greenland, P., Knoll, M. D., & Stamler, J., Neaton, J., Dyer, A., Garside, D., et al. (2003). Major risk factors for cardiovascular disease as antecedents of fatal and nonfatal coronary heart disease events. *Journal of the American Medical Association, 290*(7), 891–897.

Greenspan, F. S. (2004). The thyroid gland. In F. S. Greenspan & D. G. Gardner (Eds.), *Basic and clinical endocrinology* (pp. 215–294). St. Louis, MO: Lange Medical Books.

Greenspan, F. S., & Gardner, D. G. (2004). *Basic and clinical endocrinology* (7th ed.). New York: Lange Medical Books.

Greenspan, F. S., & Resnick, N. M. (2004). Geriatric endocrinology. In F. S. Greenspan & D. G. Gardner (Eds.), *Basic and clinical endocrinology* (pp. 543–548). St. Louis, MO: Lange Medical Books.

Grendell, R. (2004). Psychosocial alterations. In L. Urden, K. Stacy, & M. Lough (Eds.), *Priorities in critical care nursing* (pp. 172–181). St. Louis, MO: Mosby.

Griffin, J. E., & Ojeda, S. R. (2004). *Textbook of endocrine physiology* (5th ed.). New York: Oxford Press.

Griffiths, R., Fernandez, R., & Murie, P (2004). Removal of short-term indwelling urethral catheters: The evidence. *Journal of Wound Ostomy Continence Nurses Society, 31*(5), 299–308.

Grigsby, P. W. (2004). Thyroid. In C. Perez, E. Halperm, L. Brady, R. Schmidt-Ullrich (Eds.), *Principles and practices of radiation oncology* (pp. 211–215). New York: Lippincott, Williams & Williams.

Gronau, E., & Pannek, J. (2005). Acute urinary retention in ileum conduit urinary diversion. *Urology, 65*(3), 593.

Gruenwald, J. (2004). *PDR for herbal medicines* (3rd ed.). Montvale, NJ: Medical Economics Co., Inc.

Gruffydd, E., & Randle, J. (2006). Alzheimer's disease and the psychosocial burden for caregivers. *Community Practitioner, 79*(1), 15–18.

Grundy, S. M., Cleeman, J. I., Merz, C. B., Brewer, B., Clark, J. T., Hunninghake, D. B., et al. (2004). Implications of recent trials for national cholesterol education program adult treatment panel III guidelines. *Circulation, 110*(2), 227–239.

Gugenheim, J. J. (2004). External fixation in orthopedics. *Journal of the American Medical Association, 291,* 2122–2124.

Guillet, G., Guillet, M., & Dagregorio, G. (2005). Allergic contact dermatitis from natural rubber latex in atopic dermatitis and the risk of later Type I allergy. *Contact Dermatitis, 53*(1), 46–51.

Gundel, J.C. (2004). *Medial collateral knee ligament injury.* Retrieved on September 28, 2005, from http://www.emedicine.com/sports/topic73.htm.

Guttmacher, A. E., & Collins, F. S. (2002). Genomic medicine: A primer. *New England Journal of Medicine,* 347(19), 1512–1520.

Guyton, A., & Hall, J. (2001). *Pocket companion to textbook of medical physiology* (10th ed). Philadelphia: W. B. Saunders Company.

Guyton, A., & Hall, J. (2006). *Textbook of medical physiology* (11th ed.). Philadelphia: W. B. Saunders.

Haas, F. (2005). Clinical. Understanding the legal implications of living wills. *Nursing Times, 101*(3), 18–24, 34–37.

Haas, K. (2004). Who will make room for the intersexed? *American Journal of Law and Medicine, 30*(1), 41–68.

Habel, M. (2004, January 6). The hospitalized older adult: Entering a danger zone. *Nurseweek,* pp. 22–23.

Hadaway, L. C. (2002, August). IV infiltration, not just a peripheral problem. *Nursing, 32*(1), 36–42.

Hader, C., & Guy, J. (2004). Your hand in pain management. *Nursing Management, 35*(11), 21–27.

Hagerty, B., & Patusky, K. (2004). Mood disorders: Depression and mania. In K. Fortinash & P. Holoday-Worret (Eds.), *Psychiatric mental health nursing* (3rd ed., pp. 324–341). St. Louis, MO: Mosby.

Hall, D. (2004). Work-related stress of registered nurses in a hospital setting. *Journal for Nurses in Staff Development, 20*(1), 6–14.

Hamilton, R. G., Brown, R. H., Veltri, M. A., Feroli, E. R., Primeau, M. N., Schauble, J. F., et al. (2005). Administering pharmaceuticals to latex allergic patients from vials containing natural rubber latex closures. *American Journal of Health System Pharmacy, 62*(17), 1822–1828.

Hamilton, R. J., Bowers, B. J., & Williams, J. K. (2005). Disclosing genetic test results to family members. *Journal of Nursing Scholarship, 37*(1), 18–24.

Hanks-Bell, M., Halvey, K., & Paice, J. (2004). Pain assessment and management in aging. *Online Journals in Nursing, 9*(3), 1–18.

Hardaway, R. M. (2006) Traumatic shock. *Military Medicine, 171*(4), 278–279.

Hark, L., & Morrison, G. (2003). *Medical nutrition and disease: A case-based approach.* Malden, MA: Blackwell Publishing.

Harkness, K., Smith, K., Taraba, L., MacKenzie, C., Gunn, E., & Arthur, H. (2005). Effect of a postoperative telephone intervention on attendance at intake for cardiac rehabilitation after coronary artery bypass graft surgery. *Heart and Lung, 34*(3), 179–186.

Harman, L. (2003). Attitudes toward genetic testing: Gender, role, and discipline. *Topics in Health Information Management, 24*(1), 50–58.

Harper, D. G., Arsura, E. L., Bobba, R. K., Reddy, C. M., Sawh, A. K. (2005). Acquired color blindness in an elderly male patient from recurrent metastatic prostate cancer. *Journal of the American Geriatrics Society, 53*(7), 1265–1267.

Hart, J. A. (2004). Right-sided heart failure. Retrieved June 24, 2006, from http://www.nlm.nih.gov.

Hathaway, L. (2005). Anaphylaxis. *Nursing, 35*(1), 46–47.

Havener, G., Roth, M., Arakere, R., & Barenfanger, K. (2005). *Effective investigation and control of an aspergillosis outbreak in a regional burn unit.* Retrieved May 1, 2006, from http://www.journalofburnsandwounds.com.

Hawkley, L. C., & Cacioppo, J. T. (2003) Loneliness and pathways to disease. *Brain, Behavior, and Immunity, 17*(Suppl 1), S98–S105.

Hayes, D. (2004). Phosphorus: Here, there, everywhere. *Nursing Made Incredibly Easy! 2*(6), 36–41.

He, L., Zhou, D., Wu, B., Li, N., & Zhou, M. (2004). Acupuncture for Bell's palsy. *The Cochrane Database of Systematic Reviews* (1), CD002914.

Headley, A. A., Ogden, C. L., Johnson, C. L., Carroll, M. D., Curtain, L. R., & Flegal, K. M. (2004). Prevalence of overweight and obesity among U.S. children, adolescents, and adults, 1999–2002. *Journal of the American Medical Association, 291*(23), 2847–2850.

Health Gate Data Corp. (2003). *Dysmenorrhea.* Retrieved September 6, 2004, from http://iHerb.com.

HealthGrades. (2005). *Medical errors gap widens between best and worst hospitals: Healthgrades study.* Retrieved June 26, 2005, from www.healthgrades.com.

Healthy People 2010. (2004). *About healthy people 2010.* Retrieved May 14, 2005, from http://www.healthypeople.gov.

Heck, R. K., & Carnesale, P. G. (2003). General principles of amputations. In S. T. Canale (Ed.), *Campbell's operative orthopaedics* (vol. 1, 10th ed., pp. 537–554). Philadelphia: Mosby.

Heffner, J. E. (2003). Chronic obstructive pulmonary disease: Translating new understanding into improved patient care. *Respiratory Care, 48*(12), 1184.

Heidary, N., & Cohen, D. (2005). Hypersensitivity reactions to vaccine components. *Dermatitis, 16*(3), 115–120.

Heinrich, C., Karner, K., Gaglione, B., & Lambert, L. (2002). Order out of chaos: The use of a matrix to validate curriculum integrity. *Nurse Educator, 27*(3), 136–140.

Heinz, D. (2004). Hospital nurse staffing and patient outcomes. *Dimensions of Critical Care Nursing, 23*(1), 44–50.

Heise, L., & Garcia-Moreno, C. (2002). *Violence by intimate partners. World report on violence and health.* Geneva: World Health Organization.

Hellman, D. B., & Stone, J. H. (2004). Arthritis & musculoskeletal disorders. In L.M. Tierney, S. J. McPhee, & M. A. Papidakis (Eds.), *Current medical diagnosis and treatment* (43rd ed., pp. 1062–1145). New York: McGraw-Hill.

Henderson, V. (1939). *Principles and practices of nursing.* New York: Macmillan.

Henderson, V. (1966). *The nature of nursing.* New York: Macmillan.

Henderson, V. (1991). *The nature of nursing: Reflections after 25 years.* New York: National League for Nursing.

Henderson, V., & Nite, G. (1978). *Principles and practice of nursing* (6th ed.). New York: Macmillan.

Henneman, E., Dracup, K., Ganz, T., Molayeme, O., & Cooper, C. (2002). Using a collaborative weaning plan to decrease duration of mechanical ventilation and length of stay in the ICU for patients receiving long-term ventilation. *American Journal of Critical Care, 11*(2), 132–140.

Hennessy, B. T., Hanrahan, E. O., & Daly, P. A. (2004). Non-Hodgkin lymphoma: An update. *Lancet Oncology, 5*(6): 341–353.

Henriksson, K. G. (2003). Fibromyalgia—From syndrome to disease. Overview of pathogenic mechanisms. *Journal of Rehabilitative Medicine, 43,* 89–94.

Hess, D., & Kacmarek, R. (2002). *Essentials of mechanical ventilation* (2nd ed.). New York: McGraw-Hill.

Hicken, B., & Tucker, D. (2002). Impact of genetic risk feedback: Perceived risk and motivation for health protective behaviors. *Psychology, Health, and Medicine, 7*(1), 25–36.

Hietanen, A., Era, P. Sorri, M., & Heikkiness, N. (2004). Changes in hearing in 80 year old people: A 10 year followup study. *International Journal of Audiology, 43,* 126–135.

Highfield, M. (2000). Providing spiritual care to patients with cancer. *Clinical Journal of Oncology Nursing, 4*(30), 115–120.

Higo, R., Tayama, N., Nitou, T., Watanabe, T., & Ugawa, Y. (2003). Videofluoroscopic and manometric evaluation of swallowing function in patients with multiple system atrophy. *Annals of Otology, Rhinology & Laryngology, 112*(7), 630–636.

Hildebrandt, L., Fracchia, J., Driscoll, J., & Giroux, P. (2002). Comparison of post-pyloric versus gastric enteral formula administration. *Topics in Clinical Nutrition, 17*(3), 44–51.

Hill, M., Hughes T., & Milford C. (2005). Treatment for swallowing difficulties (dysphagia) in chronic muscle disease. *The Cochrane Database of Systematic Reviews (Oxford)* (2), CD004303.

Hillman, T., Arriaga, M., & Chen, D. (2003). Intratympanic steroids: Do they acutely improve hearing in cases of cochlear hydrops? *Laryngoscope, 113*(11), 1903–1907.

Hillman, T., Chen, D., & Arriaga, M. (2004). Vestibular nerve section versus intratympanic gentamicin for Meniere's disease. *Laryngoscope, 114*(2), 216–222.

Hinkle, J. (2004). Potential new drug for spinal cord injury. *Journal of Neuroscience Nursing, 36*(1), 49.

Hinson, G. (2005). *Shock management.* Retrieved July 12, 2006, from http://www.cdi.pub.ro.

Hitchcock, J., Schubert, P., & Thomas, S. (2003). *Community health nursing: Caring in action* (2nd ed.). New York: Thomson Delmar Learning.

Hohler, S. E. (2004). Tips for better patient teaching. *Nursing, 34*(7), 7–8.

Hobbs, F., & Stoops, N. (2002). Demographic trends in the 20th century, *U.S. Census Bureau, Census 2000*

Special Reports, Series CENSR-4. Washington, DC: U.S. Government Printing Office.

Hobbs, F., Irwin, P., & Rubner, J. (2005). Evidence-based treatment of hypertension: What's the role of angiotensin II receptor blockers? *British Journal of Cardiology, 12*(1), 65–70.

Hockenberry, M. J., & Brown, J.(2003). Conditions caused by defects in physical development. In D. Wilson, M. L. Winkelstein, & N. E. Kline. *Wong's nursing care of infants and children* (7th ed., pp. 1757–1831). St. Louis, MO: Mosby.

Hoffman, M., & Monroe, D. (2005). Rethinking the coagulation cascade. *Current Hematology Reports, 4*(5), 391–396.

Hollinworth, H. (2005). The management of patients' pain in wound care. *Nursing Standard, 20*(7), 65–66, 68, 70.

Holmes, S. B., & Brown, S. J. (2005). Skeletal pin site care: National Association of Orthopaedic Nurses guideline for orthopaedic nursing. *Orthopaedic Nursing, 24*(2), 99–107.

Holmes, T. H., & Rahe, R. H. (1967). The social readjustment rating scale. *Journal of Psychosomatic Medicine, 11*(14), 213–218.

Holoday-Worret, P. (2004). Foundations of psychiatric mental health nursing. In K. Fortinash & P. Holoday-Worret (Eds.), *Psychiatric mental health nursing* (3rd ed., pp. 225–234). St. Louis, MO: Mosby.

Homik, J., Suarez-Almazor, M. E., Shea, B., Cranney, A., Wells, G., & Tugwell, P. (2004). Calcium and vitamin D for corticosteroid-induced osteoporosis (Cochrane Review). In *The Cochrane Database of Systematic Reviews.* Chichester, UK: John Wiley & Sons, Ltd.

Homs, M., Steyerberg, E., Eijkenboom, W., & Siersema, P. (2006). Predictors of outcome of single-dose brachytherapy for the palliation of dysphagia from esophageal cancer. *Brachytherapy, 5*(1), 41–48.

Hong, Q. N, Durand, M. J., & Loisel, P. (2003). Treatment of lateral epicondylitis: Where is the evidence? *Joint Bone Spine, 71,* 369–373.

Honkus, V. (2003). Sleep deprivation in critical care units. *Critical Care Nurse Quarterly, 26*(3), 179–189.

Horenstein, M. S., Pettersen, M., & Walters, H. L. (2002). *Mitral stenosis.* Retrieved June 24, 2006, from www.emedicine.com.

Horowitz, A., Brennan, M., Reinhardt, J. P. (2005). Prevalence and risk factors for self-reported visual impairment among middle-aged and older adults. *Research on Aging, 27*(3), 307–326.

Horstman, J. (2006). *Tai Chi. Arthritis foundation news.* Retrieved August 14, 2006, from http://www.arthritis.org.

Hosalkar, H., & Dormans, J.P. (2004). Limb sparing surgery for pediatric musculoskeletal tumors. *Pediatric Blood Cancer, 42*(4), 295–310.

Hospice Foundation of America. (2003). Retrieved June 24, 2006, from http://www.hospicefoundation.org.

Hospice and Palliative Nurses Association Board of Directors. (2004). *Artificial nutrition and hydration in end-of-life care.*

Hospital Compare. (2005). *Hospital compare.* Retrieved May 18, 2005, from http://www.hospitalcompare.hhs.gov.

Hostima, A., & Hilbrands, L. (2003). Evaluation of renal transplant donor and recipient. In R. Johnson & J. Feehally (Eds.), *Comprehensive clinical nephrology* (2nd ed., pp. 1071–1091). St. Louis, MO: Mosby.

Hoyt, K. S., & Haley, R. J. (2005). Innovations in advanced practice: Assessment and management of eye emergencies. *Topics in Emergency Medicine, 27*(2), 101–117.

Huckleberry, Y. (2004). Nutritional support and the surgical patient. *American Journal of Health-System Pharmacy, 61*(7), 671–684.

Hudak, C. M., Morton, P., Galle, B., & Fontaine, D. (2005). *Critical care nursing: A holistic approach.* Philadelphia: Lippincott, Williams & Wilkins.

Hudson, M. M., Mertens, A. C., Yasui, Y., Hobbie W., Chen, H., Gurney, J. G., et al. (2003). Health status of adult long-term survivors of childhood cancer: A report from the childhood cancer survivor study. *Journal of American Medical Association, 290*(12), 1583–1592.

Huether, S. E. (2004). Alterations of hormonal regulation. In S. E. Huether & K. L. McCance (Eds.), *Understanding pathophysiology* (pp. 356–362). St. Louis, MO: Mosby.

Hultman, C., & Daiza, S. (2003). Skin-sparing mastectomy flap complications after breast reconstruction: Review of incidence, management, and outcome. *Annals of Plastic Surgery, 50*(3), 249.

Hughes, F., Bryan, K., & Robbins, I. (2005). Relatives' experiences of critical care. *Nursing in Critical Care, 10*(1), 23–30.

Hughes, S. C., & Martin, D. E. (2005). Traditional IV catheters: To be or not to be, that is the question! *American Society of Anesthesiologists, 69*(3), 14–15.

Hurlock-Chorostecki, C. (2004). Managing diabetic ketoacidosis: The role of the ICU nurse in an endocrine emergency. *Canadian Association of Critical Care Nurses, 15*(1), 18–22.

Hurskainen, R., Teperi, J., Rissanen, P., Aalto, A., Grenman, S., Kivela, A., et al. (2004). Clinical outcomes and costs with the levonorgestrel-releasing intrauterine system or hysterectomy for treatment of menorrhagia: Randomized trial 5-year follow-up. *Journal of the American Medical Association, 291,* 1456–1463.

Hurwitz, S. R. (2004). *Plantar fasciitis.* Retrieved on December 7, 2005, from http://www.emedicine.com/orthoped/topic542.htm.

Huston, J., & Brox, G. (2004). Professional ethics at the bottom line. *The Health Care Manager, 23*(3), 267–272.

Hyman, G., Malanga, G. A., & Alladin, I. (2005). *Jumper's knee.* Retrieved on September 6, 2005, from http://www.emedicine.com/sports/topic56.htm.

Ibrahim, M., Wurpel, J., & Gladson, B. (2003). Intrathecal baclofen: A new treatment approach for severe spasticity in patients with stroke. *Journal of Neurologic Physical Therapy, 27*(3), 142–148.

Ignatavicius, D., & Workman, M. (2006). *Medical-surgical nursing: Critical thinking for collaborative care* (5th ed.). St. Louis, MO: Elsevier Saunders.

Ihlenfeld, J. (2003). A primer on triage and mass casualty events. *Dimensions of Critical Care, Nursing, 22*(5), 204–209.

Imke, S. (2003). Parkinson's disease: More than meets the eye. *Advance for Nurse Practitioners, 11*(9), 42–54.

Inadomi, J., Sampliner, R., Lagergren, J., Lieberman, D. Fendrick, & Vakil, N. (2003). Screening and surveillance for Barrett esophagus in high-risk groups: A cost-utility analysis. *Annals of Internal Medicine, 138*(3), 176–186.

Inanici, F., & Yunus, B. M. (2002, August). Fibromyalgia syndrome: Diagnosis and management. *Hospital Physician,* 53–66.

Indian Health Service. (n.d.a). *About IHS.* Retrieved August 30, 2005, from p://www.ihs.gov.

Indian Health Service. (n.d.b). *Appropriations.* Retrieved August 3, 2005, from http://www.ihs.gov.

Institute for Clinical Systems Improvement. (2003). *Diagnosis and initial treatment of ischemic stroke.* Retrieved June 17, 2006, from www.guideline.gov.

Institute for Healthcare Improvement. (2005). 100,000 lives campaign. Retrieved June 25, 2006, from http://www.ihi.org.

Institute of Medicine. (2000). *To err is human: Building a safer health system.* Washington, DC: National Academy Press.

Institute of Medicine. (2001). *Crossing the quality chasm: A new health system for the 21st century.* Washington, DC: National Academy Press.

Institute of Medicine. (2002). Dietary reference intakes for energy, carbohydrate, fiber, fat, fatty acids, cholesterol, protein, and amino acids. Washington, DC: National Academy Press.

Institute of Medicine. (2003). *Priority areas for national action: Transforming health care quality.* Washington, DC: National Academy Press.

Integrated Publishing. (2004). *Triage.* Retrieved June 21, 2006, from http://infodotinc.com.

International Headache Society. (2004). The international classification of headache disorders (2nd ed.). *Cephalalgia, 24* (Suppl 1), 1–160.

International Sepsis Forum. (2003). *The critical care forum.* Retrieved June 28, 2006, from www.sepsisforum.org.

Isowa, T., Ohira, H., & Murashima, S. (2004). Reactivity of immune, endocrine and cardiovascular parameters to active and passive acute stress. *Biological Psychology, 65*(2), 101–120.

Ives, J. R. (2005). New chronic EEG electrode for critical/intensive care unit monitoring. *Journal of Clinical Neurophysiology, 22*(2), 119–123.

Izzo, J., & Black, H. (2003). *Hypertension primer* (3rd ed.). Dallas: American Heart Association.

Jablonski, A., & Wyatt, G. (2005). A model for identifying barriers to effective symptom management at the end of life. *Journal of Hospice and Palliative Nursing, 7*(1), 23–26.

Jacobs, B., Neil, N., & Aboulafia, D. (2005). Retrospective analysis of suspending HAART in selected patients with controlled HIV replication. *AIDS Patient Care and STDs, 19*(7), 429–438.

Jacox, A., Carr, D., & Payne, R. (1994). *Management of pain. Clinical practice guidelines.* No. 9, AHCPR Publication No. 94-0592. Rockville, MD: Agency for Health Care Policy and Research, U.S. Department of Health and Human Services, Public Health Service.

Jakobsson, L., Loven, L., & Hallberg, I. R. (2004). Micturition problems in relation to quality of life in men with prostate cancer or benign prostatic hyperplasia: Comparison with men from the general population. *Cancer Nursing, 27*(3), 218–229.

Janeway, C. A., Jr., Travers, P., Walport, M., & Shlomchik, M. J. (2004). *Immunobiology, the immune system in health and disease* (6th ed.). New York: Garland Science Publishing.

Janssen, I., Katzmarzyk, P., & Ross, R. (2004). Waist circumference and not body mass index explains obesity-related health risk. *American Journal of Clinical Nutrition, 79,* 379–384.

Jarzabek, J., Zbucka, M., Pepinski, W., Szamatowicz, J., Domitrz, J., Janica, J., et al. (2004). Cystic fibrosis as a cause of infertility. *Reproductive Biology, 4*(2), 119–129.

Jarzyna, D. (2005). Opioid tolerance: A perioperative nursing challenge. *MEDSURG Nursing, 14*(6), 371–377.

Jeavons, H. (2003). Prevention and treatment of vulvovaginal candidiasis using exogenous *Lactobacillus. Journal of Obstetric, Gynecologic, and Neonatal Nursing, 32,* 287–296.

Jemal, A. (2003). Cancer statistics. *CA: A Cancer Journal for Clinicians, 53*(1), 5–26.

Jenkins, J. F., & Lea, D. H. (2004). *Nursing care in the genomic era: A case-based approach.* Sudburry, MA: Jones & Bartlett Publishers.

Jenner, P., & Olanow, C. W. (2006). The pathogenesis of cell death in Parkinson's disease. *Neurology, 66*(10 Suppl 4), S24–S36.

Jeremitsky, E., Omert, L., Dunham, M., Protetch, J., & Rodriguez, A. (2003). Harbingers of poor outcome the day after severe brain injury: Hypothermia, hypoxia, and hypoperfusion. *The Journal of Trauma, Injury, Infection, and Critical Care, 54*(2), 312–319.

Jessup, M., & Brozena, S. (2003). Medical progress: Heart failure. *New England Journal of Medicine, 348*(20), 2007–2018.

Jirillo, E., Mastronardi, M. L., Altamura, M., Munno, I., Miniello, S., Urgesi, G., et al. (2003). The immunocompromised host: Immune alterations in splenectomized patients and clinical implications. *Current Pharmaceutical Design, 9*(24), 1918–1923.

Johns Hopkins Institutes. (2003). *Economic impact of the Johns Hopkins Institutes in Maryland.* Silver Springs, MD: Johns Hopkins University and Johns Hopkins Medicine.

Johnsen, J., & Davis, J. (2005). *All about vasectomy.* Retrieved July 16, 2006, from http://www.plannedparenthood.org.

Johnson, K. (2005). Shock states. In K. Wagner, P. Kidd, & K. Johnson (Eds.), *High acuity nursing.* New Jersey: Prentice Hall.

Johnson, K., Nicol, T., & Kraus, N. (2005). Brain stem response to speech: A biological marker of auditory processing. *Ear and Hearing, 26*(5), 424–434.

Johnstone, C., Farley, A. & Hendry, C. (2005). The physiological basis of wound healing. *Nursing Standard, 19*(43), 59–65.

Joint Commission on Accreditation of Healthcare Organizations (JCAHO) and National Pharmaceutical Council (NPC). (2003). Monograph: Improving the Quality of Pain Management through Measurement and Action.

Joint Commission on Accreditation of Healthcare Organizations. (2004). *2004 national patient safety goals.* Retrieved February 7, 2005, from http://jcaho.org.

Joint Commission for Accreditation of Healthcare Organizations. (2005). *Accreditation manual.* Chicago: Author.

Joint Commission on Accreditation of Healthcare Organizations (2006a). *Emergency management standards EC.1.4 and EC.2.9.1.* Retrieved June 18, 2006, from http://www.jcrinc.com.

Joint Commission on Accreditation of Healthcare Organizations. (2006b). *Focus areas.* Retrieved May 22, 2006, from http://www.soros.org/initiatives/pdia/focusareas/grants/grantees/royal1994.

Joint Commission on Accreditation of Healthcare Organizations. (n.d.). *Critical access hospitals.* Retrieved August 4, 2005, from http://www.jcaho.org.

Joint Commission on Accreditation of Hospitals and Healthcare Organizations. (2004). *Provision of care, treatment, and services. Comprehensive accreditation manual for hospitals.* Oakbrook Terrace, IL: Author.

Jones, A. (2005). The role of hope in serious illness and dying. *European Journal of Palliative Care, 12*(1), 28–31.

Jones, D. (2005). Savings sharing. *Journal of Nursing Administration, 35*(4), 199–204.

Jones, J. (1993). *Bad blood: The Tuskegee syphilis experiment.* New York: The Free Press.

Jones, L., & Bagnall, A. (2004). Spinal injuries centres (SICs) for acute traumatic spinal cord injury. *The Cochrane Database of Systematic Reviews* (4), CD: 004442.

Jones, R. (2004). Relationships of sexual imposition, dyadic trust, and sensation seeking with sexual risk behavior in young urban women. *Research and Nursing Health, 27*(3), 185–197.

Jones, R. C., Hodgson, J. M., Bahler, R. C., & Orford, J. (2004). *Mitral valve prolapse.* Retrieved June 24, 2006, from www.firstconsult.com.

Jong, P., Demers, C., McKelvie, R. S., & Liu, P. P. (2002). Angiotensin receptor blockers in heart failure: Meta-analysis of randomized controlled trials. *Journal of the American College of Cardiology, 39*(3), 463–470.

Joo, Y., Park, C., Lee, W., Kim, H., Choi, S., Cho, C., et al. (2004). Primary non-Hodgkin's lymphoma of the common bile duct presenting as obstructive jaundice. *Journal of Gastroenterology, 39*(7), 692–696.

Jubran, A. (2004). Pulse oximetry. *Intensive Care Medicine, 30*(11), 2017–2020.

Julian, D. (2001). The evolution of the coronary care unit. *Cardiovascular Research, 51*(4), 621–624.

Jungles, S. L. (2004). Video wireless capsule endoscopy: A diagnostic tool for early Crohn's disease. *Gastroenterology Nursing, 27*(4), 170–175.

Jurgens, G., & Graudal, N. (2006). Effects of low sodium diet versus high sodium diet on blood pressure, renin, aldosterone, catecholamines, cholesterols, and triglyceride. *The Cochrane Database of Systematic Reviews* (1), CD004022.

Kaiser Permanente (n.d.). *Press room.* Retrieved September 5, 2005, from https://newsmedia.kaiserpermanente.org/kpweb/homepage.do.

Kanellos, M. (2004). *Human chips more than skin deep.* Retrieved August 23, 2006, from http://zdnet.com.com.

Kang, S. (2004). *Left-sided heart failure.* Retrieved June 24, 2006, from http://www.nlm.nih.gov.

Kang, S., Bergfeld, W. Gottlieb, A., Hickman, J., Humeniuk, J., Kempers, S., et al.(2005). Long-term efficacy and safety of Tretinoin emollient cream 0.05% in treatment of photo damaged skin. *American Journal of Clinical Dermatology, 6*(4), 245–253.

Kaplan, H. S. (1985). *Comprehensive evaluation of disorders of sexual desire.* Washington, DC: American Psychiatric Press.

Kaptanoglu, E., Beskonakli, E., Okutan, O., Surucu, H., & Taskin, Y. (2003). Effect of magnesium sulphate in experimental spinal cord injury: Evaluation with ultrastructural findings and early clinical results. *Journal of Clinical Neuroscience, 10*(3), 329–334.

Karcioglu, O., Oskara, E., Civancr, M., & Ozucclik, N. (2003). Resuscitation of a Jehovah's Witness with multiple injuries without blood: Right to die? *The Internet Journal of Emergency and Intensive Care Medicine, 7*(1).

Karnath, B. (2002). Smoking cessation. *American Journal of Medicine, 112*(5), 399–405.

Karnib, H., & Badr, K. (2004). Microvascular diseases of the kidney. In B. Brenner (Ed.), *Brenner and Rector's the kidney* (7th ed., vol. 2, pp. 1601–1623). Philadelphia: W. B. Saunders Co.

Kashtan, C. (2003). Alport and other familial glomerular syndromes. In R. Johnson & J. Feehally (Eds.), *Comprehensive clinical nephrology* (2nd ed., pp. 627–637). St. Louis, MO: Mosby.

Kasper, D. L., Braunwald, E., Fauci, A. S., Hauser, S. L., Longo, D. L., & Jameson, J. L. (2005). *Harrison's principles of internal medicine* (16th ed.). New York: McGraw-Hill.

Kataria, R. K., & Brent, L. H. (2004). Spondyloarthropathies. *American Family Physician, 69*(12), 2853–2860.

Kathol, D., Geiger, M., & Hartig, J. (1998). Clinical correlation map: A tool for linking theory and practice. *Nurse Educator, 23*(4), 31–34.

Katkin, J. P. (2002). Clinical manifestations and diagnosis of cystic fibrosis. *Up to Date, 10*(1).

Katsenis, D., Bhave, A., Paley, D., & Herzenberg, J. (2005). Treatment of malunion and nonunion at the site of an ankle fusion with the Ilizarov apparatus. *The Journal of Bone and Joint Surgery, 87*-A, 302–309.

Katz, A., Davis, P., & Findlay, S. S. (2002). Ask and ye shall plan: A health needs assessment of a university population. *Canadian Journal of Public Health [Revue Canadienne de Sante Publicque], 93*(1), 63–66.

Katz, J. N., & Simmons, B. P. (2002). Carpal tunnel syndrome. *New England Journal of Medicine, 346*(23), 1807–1812.

Katz, M. J. (2004). Medical problems: Brief reviews. Glaucoma. *Journal of Pharmacy Technology, 20*(5), 318–320.

Kazzi, A. A., & Sheeks, P. (2004, August). *Peritonsillar abscess.* Retrieved August 25, 2004, from http://www.emedicine.com/emerg/topic417.htm.

Kazzi, A. A., & Tehranazdeh, A. D. (2005, October). *Acute glomerulonephritis.* Retrieved January 27, 2006, from http://www.emedicine.com/EMERG/topic219.htm.

Keany, J. E., (2005). *Femur fractures.* Retrieved on September 28, 2005, from http://www.emedicine.com/orthoped/topic193.htm.

Kee, J. L. (2002). *Laboratory and diagnostic tests with nursing implications* (6th ed.). Upper Saddle River, NJ: Prentice Hall.

Kee, J. L, Paulanka, B., & Purnel, L. (2004). *Fluid and electrolytes with clinical applications: A programmed approach* (7th ed.). New York: Thomson Delmar Learning.

Keenan, H., Marshall, S., Nocera, M., & Runyan, D. (2004). Increased incidence of inflicted traumatic brain injury in children after a natural disaster. *American Journal of Preventive Medicine, 26*(3), 189–193.

Keithley, J. K., & Swanson, B. (2004). Enteral nutrition: An update on practice recommendations. *Medsurg Nursing, 13*(2), 131–134.

Kelly, C., & Nielson, E. (2004). Tubulointerstitial diseases. In B. Brenner (Ed.), *Brenner and Rector's the kidney* (7th ed., vol. 2, pp. 1483–1511). Philadelphia: W. B. Saunders Co.

Kelly, J. P., Kaufman, D. W., Kelley, K., Rosenberg, L., Anderson, T. E., & Mitchell, A. A. (2005). Recent trends in use of herbal and other natural products. *Archives of Internal Medicine, 165,* 281–286.

Kennedy, J. M., & Zochodne, D. W. (2005). Impaired peripheral nerve regeneration in diabetes mellitus. *Journal of the Peripheral Nervous System, 10*(2), 144–158.

Kennedy, W. (2004). Beneficence and autonomy in nursing: a moral dilemma. *British Journal of Perioperative Nursing, 14*(11), 500–506.

Kerfoot, K. M. (2004). Synergy from the vantage point of the development and transformation. *Excellence in nursing knowledge.* Indianapolis, IN: Sigma Theta Tau Press.

Kerkenbush, N. (2003). The emerging role of electronic diaries in the management of diabetes mellitus. *AACN Clinical Issues, 14*(3), 371–378.

Kern, L. (2004). Postoperative atrial fibrillation: New directions in prevention and treatment. *Journal of Cardiovascular Nursing, 19*(2), 103–115.

Keshav, S. (2004). *The gastrointestinal system at a glance.* Malden, MA: Blackwell Science.

Khan, M. A. (2002). Update on Spondyloarthropathies. *Annals of Internal Medicine, 136*(12), 896–907.

Khoury, M., McCabe, L., & McCabe, E. (2003). Population screening in the age of genomic medicine. *New England Journal of Medicine, 348*(1), 50–58.

Kidd, P. (2005). Multiple organ dysfunction syndrome. In K. Wagner & P. Kidd (Eds.), *High acuity nursing* (pp. 312-324[0]). New Jersey: Prentice Hall.

Kielb, S. (2005). Stress incontinence: Alternatives to surgery. *International Journal of Fertility of Women's Medicine, 50*(1), 24–29.

Kieran, N., & Brady, H. (2003). Clinical evaluation, management, and outcome of acute renal failure. In R. Johnson & J. Feehally (Eds.), *Comprehensive clinical nephrology* (2nd ed., pp. 183–206). St. Louis, MO: Mosby.

Kim, B. W., Wang, H. J., Jeong, I. H., Ahn, S. I., & Kim, M. W. (2005). Metastatic liver cancer: A rare case. *World Journal of Gastroenterology, 11*(27), 4281–4284.

Kim, H., Schwartz-Barcott, D., Tracy, S., Fortin, J., & Sjostrom, B. (2005). Strategies of pain assessment used by nurses on surgical units. *Pain Management Nursing, 6*(1), 3–9.

King, A. B., & LeMaire, G. J. (2002). Managing anticoagulation in patients with atrial fibrillation. *Nurse Practitioner, 27*(9), 17–23.

King, I. (1971). *Toward a theory for nursing: General concepts of human behavior.* New York: John Wiley and Sons.

King, M., & Shell, R. (2002). Teaching and evaluating critical thinking with concept maps. *Nurse Educator, 27*(5), 214–216.

King, R. (2004). Nurses perceptions of their pharmacology educational needs. *Journal of Advanced Nursing, 45*(4), 392–400.

King, T. (2004). *Basic principles and techniques of bronchoalveolar lavage.* Retrieved June 25, 2006, from http://www.uptodate.com.

Kinsel, B. (2005). Resilience as adaptation in older women. *Journal of Women and Aging, 17*(3), 23–39.

Kinton, L., Johnson, M., Smith, S., Farrell, F., Stevens, J., Rance, J., et al. (2002). Partial epilepsy with pericentral spikes: A new familial epilepsy syndrome with evidence for linkage to chromosome 4p15. *Annals of Neurology, 51*(6), 740–749.

Kirkland, L. (2005). *Fat embolism.* Retrieved on October 5, 2005, from http://www.emedicine.com/med/topic652.htm.

Kleinbeck, S. V. M. (2002) Revising the perioperative nursing data set. *AORN Journal, 75*(3), 602–610.

Kleinpell, R. (2005). Working out the complexities of severe sepsis. *The Nurse Practitioner, 30*(4), 43–48.

Klijn, C. J. M., & Hankey, G. J. (2003). Management of acute ischemic stroke: New guidelines from the American Stroke Association and European Stroke Initiative. *Lancet, 2,* 698–701.

Knabb, R., Rhome, J., & Brown, D. (*2005, August 23–30*). *Tropical cyclone report: Hurricane Katrina.* National Hurricane Center. Retrieved May 30, 2006, from www.nhc.noaa.gov.

Knaus, W., Draper, E., Wagner, D., & Zimmerman, J. (1986). An evaluation of outcome from intensive care in major medical centers. *Annals of Internal Medicine, 104*(3), 410–419.

Knaus, W., Draper, E., Wagner, D. & Zimmerman, J. (1993). Variation in mortality in length of stay in ICUs. *Annals of Internal Medicine, 118*(10), 753–762.

Knisley, J., & Johnson, M. (2004). Lyme disease: Knowledge is the best prevention. *The Nurse Practitioner, 29*(8), 34–37, 39–40, 43–45.

Knoops, K. T. B., de Groot, L. C. P. G. M., Kromhout, D., Perrin, A., Moreiras-Varela, O., Menotti, A., et al. (2004). Mediterranean diet, lifestyle factors and 10 year mortality in elderly European men and women: The HALE project. *Journal of the American Medical Association, 292*(12), 1433–1439.

Knowles, J. (1977). *Doing better and feeling worse: Health in the United States.* New York: McGraw-Hill.

Knowles, M. S. (1984). *The adult learner: A neglected species* (3rd ed.). Houston: Gulf Publishing.

Koch, T., & Hudson, S. (2000). Older people and laxative use: Literature review and pilot study report. *Journal of Clinical Nursing, 9*(4), 516–525.

Koike, Y., Uhthoff, H. K., Ramachandran, N., Doherty, G.P., Lecompte, M., Backman, D.S., et al. (2004). Achilles tendinopathy. *Critical Reviews in Physical and Rehabilitation Medicine, 16*(2), 109–132.

Koller, D., Nicholas, D., Goldie, R., Gearing, R., & Selkirk, E. (2006). When family-centered care is challenged by infectious disease: Pediatric health care delivery during the SARS outbreaks. *Qualitative Health Research, 16*(1), 47–60.

Kolon, T. (2005). *Crytporchidism.* Retrieved June 2, 2006, from http://www.emedicine.com.

Koppel, R., Metlay, J., Cohen, A., Abaluck, B., Localio, A., Kimmel, S., et al. (2005). Physician order entry systems in facilitating medication errors. *Journal of the American Medical Association, 293*(10), 1197–1203.

Korsten, M., Fajardo, N., Rosman, A., Creasey, G., Spungen, A., & Bauman, W. (2004). Difficulty with evacuation after spinal cord injury: Colonic motility during sleep and effects of abdominal wall stimulation. *Journal of Rehabilitation Research & Development, 41*(1), 95–100.

Kostis, J., Wilson, A., Freudenberger, R., Cosgrove, N., Pressel, S., & Davis, B. (2005). Long-term effect of diuretic-based therapy on fatal outcomes in subjects with isolated systolic hypertension with and without diabetes. *American Journal of Cardiology, 95,* 29–35.

Kraft, M., Btaiche, I., Sacks, G., & Kudsk, K. (2005). Treatment of electrolyte disorders in adult patients in the intensive care unit. *American Journal of Health-System Pharmacy (AJHP), 62*(16), 1663–1682.

Kreiger, D. (1993). *Accepting your power to heal: The personal practice of therapeutic touch.* Santa Fe, NM: Bear & Company Publishing.

Kreiger, D. (2002). *Therapeutic touch as transpersonal healing.* New York: Lanterns Books.

Kübler-Ross, E. (1969). *On death and dying.* New York: Macmillan.

Kuehn, B. M. (2005). Inflammation suspected in eye disorders. *JAMA: Journal of the American Medical Association, 294*(1), 31–32.

Kullmann, D. (2003). Epilepsy genetics. *Drugs Today, 39*(9), 725–732.

Kumle, M., Weiderpass, E., Braatan, T., Persson, I., Adami, H., & Lund, E. (2003). Use of oral contraceptives and breast cancer risk: The Norwegian-Swedish Women's Lifestyle and Health Cohort Study. *Cancer Epidemiologic Biomarkers Preview, 11*(11), 1375–1381.

Kuppermann, M., Varner, R., Summitt, R., Learman, L., Ireland C, Vittinghoff, E., et al. (2004). Effect of hysterectomy vs medical treatment on health-related quality of life and sexual functioning: The medicine or surgery (Ms) randomized trial. *Journal of the American Medical Association, 291,* 1447–1455.

Kuwabara, S. (2004). Guillain-Barre syndrome: Epidemiology, pathophysiology and management. *Drugs, 64*(6), 597–610.

Kuziemsky, C., Laul, F., & Leung, R. (2005). A review on diffusion of personal digital assistants in healthcare. *Journal of Medical Systems, 29*(4), 335–342.

Kvist, J. (2004). Rehabilitation following anterior cruciate ligament injury: Current recommendations for sport participation. *Injury Clinic, 34*(4), 269–280.

Lafleur, K. J. (2004). Tackling med errors with technology. *RN, 67*(5), 29–35.

Laheij, R. J., Sturkenboom, M. C., Hassing, R., Dieleman, J. Stricker, H. C., Jansen, J. (2004). Risk of community-acquired pneumonia and use of gastric acid-suppressive drugs. *Journal of the American Medical Association, 292,* 1955–1960.

Lake, A., & Hafez, K. (2005). Renal cell carcinoma: Controversies in prognosticators. *Contemporary Urology, 17*(8), 13, 15–16, 19–22.

Lal, G., & Clark, O. H.(2004). Endocrine surgery. In F. S. Greenspan & D. G. Gardner (Eds.), *Basic and clinical endocrinology* (pp. 364–367). St. Louis, MO: Lange Medical Books.

Lam, G. M., & Mobarhan, S. (2004). Central obesity and elevated liver enzymes. *Nutrition Reviews, 62*(10), 394–399.

Lampert, R., McPherson, C., Clancy, J., Caulin-Glaser, T., Rosenfeld, L., & Batsford, W. (2004). Gender differences in ventricular arrhythmia recurrence in patients with coronary artery disease and implantable cardioverter-defibrillators. *Journal of the American College of Cardiology, 43*(12), 2293–2299.

Landro, L. (2006, July 26). The new force in walk-in clinics. *The Wall Street Journal,* D1, D2.

Lane, D., Lip, G., & Beevers, D. (2005). Ethnic differences in cardiovascular and all-cause mortality in Birmingham, England: The Birmingham factory screening project. *Journal of Hypertension, 23*(7): 1347–1353.

Lang, L. (2004) Environmental impact on hearing: is anyone listening? *Environmental Health Perspectives, 102,* 102–111.

Lapin, C., & Lapin, A. (2003, March). *Airway clearance techniques for the CF team.* Paper presented at the Seventeenth North American Cystic Fibrosis Conference, Anaheim, CA.

LaPointe, M., & Haines, S. (2004). Fibrinolytic therapy for intraventricular hemorrhage in adults. *The Cochrane Database of Systematic Reviews (Oxford)* (2), CD003692.

LaPointe, M., & Haines, S. (2006). Fibrinolytic therapy for intraventricular hemorrhage in adults. *The Cochrane Database of Systematic Reviews* (1), CD003692.

Larson, E., Shadlen, M., Wang, L., McCormick, W., Bowen, J., Teri, L., et al. (2004). Survival after initial diagnosis of Alzheimer's disease. *Annals of Internal Medicine, 140*(7), 501–509.

Lashley, F. (2005). *Genetics in clinical nursing practice* (3rd ed.). New York: Springer Publishing Company.

Lau, H., & Lam, B. (2004). Management of postoperative urinary retention: a randomized trial of in-out versus overnight catheterization. *ANZ Journal of Surgery, 74*(8), 658–661.

Lavelle, D. G. (2003). Delayed union and nonunion of fractures. In S. T. Canale (Ed.), *Campbell's operative orthopaedics* (vol. 3, 10th ed., pp. 3125–3165). Philadelphia: Mosby.

Lawn, C., Weir, F., & McGuire, W. (2006). Base administration or fluid bolus for preventing morbidity and mortality in preterm infants with metabolic acidosis. *The Cochrane Database of Systematic Reviews* (1), CD003215.

Lazarus, R. (1990). Theory-based stress management. *Psychological Inquiry, 1*(1), 3–13.

Lazarus, R., & Folkman, S. (1987). *Stress, appraisal and coping.* New York: Springer.

Lea, D. H., & Smith, R. S. (2003). *The genetics resource guide.* Scarborough, ME: Foundation for Blood Research.

Leber, S. (2005). *Balanitis.* Retrieved June 2, 2006, from http://www.emedicine.com.

Lebovidge, J., Stone, K., Twarog, F., Raiselis, S., Kalish, L., Bailey, E., et al. (2006). Development of a preliminary questionnaire to assess parental response to children's food allergies. *Annals of Allergy, Asthma, & Immunology, 96*(3), 472–477.

Lee, L. (2004). Improving the quality of patient discharge from emergency settings. *The British Journal of Nursing, 13*(7), 412–421.

Lee, C., Straus, W., Balshaw, R., Barla, S., Vogel, S., & Schnitzer, T. J. (2004). A comparison of the efficacy and safety of nonsteroidal antiinflammatory agents versus acetaminophen in the treatment of osteoarthritis: A meta-analysis. *Arthritis and Rheumatism, 51*(5), 746–754.

Lee, S. B. (2005). *When will we cure cancer? Sooner rather than later, for a surprising number of malignancies. Others, we may just have to live with.* Retrieved April 20, 2005, from http://www.time.com.

Lefebvre, G., Vilos, G., Allaire, C., Jeffrey, J., Arneja, J., Birch, C., et al. (2003). The management of uterine leiomyomas. *Journal of Obstetrics and Gynaecology Canada, 25,* 396–418.

Lehne, R. (2004). *Pharmacology for nursing care.* St. Louis, MO: W.B. Saunders.

Leininger, M. (1978). *Transcultural nursing: Concepts, theories, and practice.* New York: John Wiley and Sons.

Leininger, M., & McFarland, M. (2006). *Culture care diversity and universality: A worldwide nursing theory.* Sudbury, MA: Jones and Bartlett.

Lemke, D. M. (2004). Riding out the storm: Sympathetic storming after traumatic brain injury. *Journal of Neuroscience Nursing, 36*(1), 4–9.

Leon, T. G., & Pase, M. (2004, June). Essential oncology facts for the float nurse. *Medsurg Nursing, 13*(3), 165–171, 189.

Leonard, G. D., Brenner, B., & Kemeny, N. E. (2005). Neoadjuvant chemotherapy before liver resection for patients with unresectable liver metastases from colorectal carcinoma. *Journal of Clinical Oncology, 23*(9), 2038–2048.

Leonard, T. (2005, October 18). New tuberculosis drug therapy could cut treatment time. Associated Press news release *San Diego Union Tribune,* p. A8.

Leske, J. (2002). Interventions to decrease family anxiety. *Critical Care Nurse, 22*(6), 61–65.

Letizia, M., Creech, S., Norton, E., Shanahan, M., & Hedges, L. (2004). Barriers to caregiver administration of pain medication in hospice care. *Journal of Pain and Symptom Management, 27*(2), 114–124.

Levinson, D. J., Darrow, C. N., Klein, E. B., Levinson, M. H., & McKee, B. (1978). *The seasons of a man's life.* New York: Knopf.

Lewis, J. (2002). Genetics in perinatal nursing: Clinical applications and policy considerations. *Journal of Obstetric, Gynecologic, and Neonatal Nursing, 31*(2), 188–192.

LexiComp, Inc. (2005). New drugs: Ziconotide. Retrieved from www.lexi.com/web/content/newdrugs.

Leydig, E. J. (2005) Are you endangering your patients? *RN, 68*(2), 29–31.

Li, C., Malone, K., & Porter, P. (2003). Relationship between long durations and different regimens of hormone therapy and risk of breast cancer. *Journal of the American Medical Association, 289*(24), 3254–3263.

Li, W., Keegan, T., Sternfeld, B., Sidney, S., Quesenberry, Jr., & Kelsey, J. (2006). Outdoor falls among middle aged and older adults: A neglected public health problem. *American Journal of Public Health, 96*(7), 1192–1200.

Liao, D. (2003). Management of acne. *The Journal of Family Practice, 52*(1), 43–51.

Liberati, A., D'Amico, R., Pifferi, S., Torri, V., & Brazzi, L. (2004). Antibiotic prophylaxis to reduce respiratory tract infections and mortality in adults receiving intensive care (Cochrane Review). *The Cochrane Database of Systematic Reviews* (3), 2004; (1), CD000022.

Licata, A. A. (2005). Discovery, clinical development, and therapeutic uses of bisphosphonates. *The Annals of Pharmacotherapy, 39*(4), 668–677.

Lieberman, B. (2006, August 1). Vaccine may offer immunity to obesity. *San Diego Union Tribune,* p. B3, 8.

Liebert, M. (2003a). Free thyroxine (FT4) and free triiodothyronine (FT3) estimate tests. *Thyroid, 13*(1), 21–32.

Liebert, M.(2003b). Thyroid autoantibodies (TPOAb, TgAB and TRAb). *Thyroid, 13*(1), 45–56.

Liebert, M. (2003c). Thyroid fine needle aspiration (FNA) and cytology. *Thyroid, 13*(1), 80–86.

Lim, K., & Morgenthaler, T. (2005). Defining obstruction or restriction remains the goal: Pulmonary function tests. Part 1: Applying the basics. *Journal of Respiratory Diseases, 26*(1), 26–28, 29–30, 32.

Lind, D., Smith, B., & Souba, W. (2005). Breast procedures. *ACS Surgery; Principles and Practice.* Retrieved July 5, 2005, from www.WebMD.com.

Lingappa, V. R. (2003). Disorders of the hypothalamus and pituitary gland. In S. J. McPhee, V. R. Lingappa, &

W. F. Ganong (Eds.), *Pathophysiology of disease* (pp. 367–374). New York: McGraw–Hill.

Linton, M. F., Major, A. S., & Fazio, S. (2004). Proatherogenic role for NK cells revealed. *Arteriosclerosis, Thrombosis, and Vascular Biology, 24*(6), 992–994.

Lipman, M. (2005). Earlier detection of kidney problems. *Consumer Reports on Health, 17*(4), 11.

Litman, R. S., & Rosenberg, H. (2005). Malignant hyperthermia: Update on susceptibility testing. *Journal of the American Medical Association, 293*(23), 2918–2924.

Littleton, L., & Engebretson, J. (2002). *Maternal, neonatal, and women's health nursing.* Clifton Park, NY: Thomson Delmar Learning.

Livingston, E. (2004). Procedure incidence and in-hospital complication rates of bariatric surgery in the United States. *The American Journal of Surgery, 188*(2), 105–110.

Livneh, H., & Martz, E. (2003). Psychosocial adaptation to spinal cord injury as a function of time since injury. *International Journal of Rehabilitation Research, 26*(3), 191–200.

Lledo, J. B., Roig. M. P., Bertomeu, C. A., Santafe, A. S., Lafargue, M. G., & Espinosa, R. G. (2005). Preoperative predictive factors of ambulatory laparoscopic cholecystectomy. *Ambulatory Surgery, 12*(1), 45–49.

Lloyd-Jones, D. M., Nam, B. H., D'Agostino, R. M., Levy, D., Murabito, J. M., Wang, T. J., et al. (2004). Parental cardiovascular disease is a risk factor for cardiovascular disease in middle-aged adults: A prospective study of parents and offspring. *Journal of the American Medical Association, 291*(18), 2204–2220.

Loftus, B. (2005). Neuropathic pain. Retrieved from www.lofutsmd.com/articles/pain.

Logan, R., & Delaney, B. (2001). ABC of the upper gastrointestinal tract: Implications of dyspepsia for the NHS. *British Medical Journal, 323*, 675–677.

Logue, J., & McBain, C. (2005). Radiation therapy for muscle-invasive bladder cancer: Treatment planning and delivery. *Clinical Oncology (Royal College of Radiologists), 17*(7), 508–513.

Lord, S. R., Castell, S., Corcoran, J., Dayhew, J., Matters, B., Shan, A., et al. (2003). The effect of group exercise on physical functioning and falls in frail older people living in retirement villages: A randomized, controlled trial. *Journal of the American Geriatrics Society, 51*(12), 1685–1692.

Louw, G., & Pinkerton, C. R. (2005). Interventions for early stage Hodgkin's disease in children. *The Cochrane Database of Systematic Reviews (Oxford)*, (3), 34–41.

Lozano, A. (2003). Surgery for Parkinson's disease the five W's: Why, who, what, where, and when. *Advances in Neurology, 91*, 303–307.

Lubovsky, O., Liebergall, M., Mattan, Y., Weil, Y., & Mosheiff, R. (2005). Early diagnosis of occult hip fractures MRI versus CT scan. *International Journal of the Care of the Injured, 36*(6), 788–792.

Ludwig, A., Inampudi, L., O'Donnell, M., Kreder, K., Williams, R., & Konety, B. (2005). Two-surgeon versus single-surgeon radical cystectomy and urinary diversion: Impact on patient outcomes and costs. *Urology, 65*(3), 488–492.

Lumley, J., Oliver, S. S., Chamberlain, C., & Oakley, L. (2005). Interventions for promoting smoking cessation during pregnancy. *Cochrane Pregnancy and Childbirth Group, The Cochrane Database of Systematic Reviews.* Cochrane Library (3). Chichester, UK: Wiley & Sons, Ltd.

Lundin, S. C., Paul, H., & Christensen, J. (2000). *Fish! A remarkable way to boost morale and improve results.* New York: Hyperion.

Luo, C. C. (2005). Spinal cord compression secondary to metastatic non-Hodgkin's lymphoma: A case report. *Archives of Physical Medicine and Rehabilitation, 86*(2), 332–334.

Ly-Pen, D., Andreu, J. L., de Blas, G., Sanchez-Olaso, A., & Millan, I. (2005). Surgical decompression versus local steroid injection on carpal tunnel syndrome: A one year, prospective, randomized, open, controlled clinical trial. *Arthritis and Rheumatism, 52*, 612–619.

Lyndaker, C., & Hulton, L. (2004). The influence of age on symptoms of perimenopause. *Journal of Obstetric, Gynecologic, and Neonatal Nursing, 33*(3), 340–347.

Madersbacher, H., & Madersbacher, S. (2005). Men's bladder health: Urinary incontinence in the elderly (Part I). *Journal of Men's Health and Gender, 2*(1), 31–37.

Magnusson, M., Sundelin, C., & Westerlund, M. (2006). Identification of health problems at 18 months of age—a task for physicians or child health nurses? *Child: Care, Health and Development, 32*(1): 47–54.

Maher, A. B. (2002). Assessment of the musculoskeletal system. In A. B. Maher, S. W. Salmond, & T. A. Pellino (Eds.), *Orthopaedic nursing* (3rd ed., pp. 189–210). Philadelphia, PA: W. B. Saunders Company.

Maher, A. B., Salmond, S. W. & Pellino, T. A. (2002). *Orthopedic nursing.* Philadelphia: W.B. Saunders Company.

Majewski, W. (2005). Long-term outcome, adhesions, and quality of life after laparoscopic and open surgical therapies for acute abdomen: Follow-up of a prospective trial. *Surgical Endoscopy, 19*(1), 81–90.

Makoul, G., & Clayman, M. L. (2006). An integrative model of shared decision making in medical encounters. *Patient Education and Counseling, 60*(3), 301–312.

Malanga, G. A., Andrus, S. G., & Bowen, J. (2004). *Rotator cuff injury.* Retrieved on September 28, 2005, from http://www.emedicine.com/sports/topic115.htm.

Mangan, P. (2005). Recognizing multiple myeloma. *Nurse Practitioner: American Journal of Primary Health Care, 30*(3), 14–18, 23–24, 26–29.

Mangram, A. J., et al. (2005). *Guideline for prevention of surgical site infection.* Retrieved on June 21, 2006, from www.cdc.gov.

Manias, E., Bucknall, T., Botti, M. (2005). Nurses' strategies for managing pain in the postoperative setting. *Pain Management Nursing, 6*(1), 18–29.

Manoharan, M., Reyes, M., Kava, B., Singal, R., Kim, S., & Soloway, M. (2005). Is adjuvant chemotherapy for bladder cancer safer in patients with an ileal conduit than a neobladder? *BJU International, 96*(9), 1286–1289.

Mantone, J. (2005). Critical time at rural hospitals. *Modern Healthcare, 35*(10), 22.

Mapes, T., & Zembaty, J. (1986). *Biomedical ethics* (2nd ed.). St. Louis, MO: McGraw-Hill.

Maravilla, K., Cao, Y., Heiman, J., Yang, C., Garland, P., Peterson, B., et al. (2005). *Journal of Urology, 173*(1), 162–166.

Marcus, P. (2004). Anxiety and related disorders. In K. Fortinash & P. Holoday-Worret (Eds.), *Psychiatric mental health nursing* (3rd ed., pp. 112–123) St. Louis, MO: Mosby.

Marik, P., & Zaloga, G. (2003). Gastric versus post-pyloric feeding: A systematic review. *Critical Care, 7*(3), 46–51.

Marshall, M., & Golper, T. (2003). Other dialysis modalities. In R. Johnson & J. Feehally (Eds.), *Comprehensive clinical nephrology* (2nd ed., pp. 1025–1034). St. Louis, MO: Mosby.

Martin, A. (2001). Should continuous lateral rotation therapy replace manual turning? *Dimensions of Critical Care Nursing, 20*(1), 42–49.

Martinez, J. M., & Tsai, A. M. (2004). *Stress fractures.* Retrieved on September 26, 2005, from http://www.emedicine.com/orthoped/topic446.htm.

Martins, P., Pratschke, J., Pascher, A., Fritsche, L., Frei, U., Neuhaus, P., et al. (2005). Age and immune response in organ transplantation. *Transplantation, 79*(2), 127–132.

Martis, G., D'Elia, G., Diana, M., Ombres, M., & Mastrangeli, B. (2005). Prostatic capsule- and nerve-sparing cystectomy in organ-confined bladder cancer: Preliminary results. *World Journal of Surgery, 29*(10), 1277–1281.

Martynowicz M. A., & Prakash U. B. S. (2002). Pulmonary blastomycosis: An appraisal of diagnostic techniques. *Chest, 121*(3), 768–773.

Maslow, A. (1970). *Motivation and personality* (2nd ed.). New York: Harper & Row.

Mason, J. (2003). Being around for a long time: How one woman with heart failure learned to live again. *American Journal of Nursing, 103*(12), 35.

Masoudi, F. A., & Krumholz, H. M. (2003). Polypharmacy and comorbidity in heart failure. *British Journal of Medicine, 327*(7414), 513–514.

Masters, W., & Johnson, V. (1966). *Human sexual response.* Boston: Little, Brown.

Mastin, T. (2003, September). Recognizing and treating non-infectious rhinitis. *Journal of the American Academy of Nurse Practitioners, 15,* 398–409.

Mathur, P. (2004). *An overview of medial thorascopy.* Retrieved June 25, 2006, from http://www.uptodate.com.

Matsumura, N., Yamamoto, K., Hirohashi, R., & Kitano, S. (2005). Renal tuberculosis mimicking hydronephrosis. *Journal of Internal Medicine, 44*(7), 768.

Mayer, S., & Chong, J. (2002). Critical care management of increased intracranial pressure. *Journal of Intensive Care Medicine, 17*(2), 55–67.

Mayer, V. (2004). The challenges of managing dysphagia in brain-injured patients. *British Journal of Community Nursing, 9*(2), 67–73.

Mayhall, G. C. (2004). Ventilator-associated pneumonia or not? Contemporary Diagnosis. *Emerging Infectious Disease Journal, 7*(2), 11.

Mayhew, P. M., Thomas, C. D., Clement, J. G., Loveridge, N., Beck, T. J., Bonfield, W., et al. (2005). Relation between age, femoral neck cortical stability, and hip fracture risk. *Lancet, 366*(9480), 129–135.

Mayo Clinic. (2003). *Tips for coping with a cancer diagnosis.* Retrieved June 10, 2006, from http://www.cnn.com.

Mayo Clinic. (2004, October). *Chronic sinusitis.* Retrieved December 17, 2004, from http://www.mayoclinic.com.

Mayo Clinic. (2005). *Tips for coping with a cancer diagnosis.* Retrieved June 10, 2006, http://www.mayoclinic.com/health/cancer-diagnosis/HQ01306.

Mayo Foundation for Medical Education and Research. (2004). *Severe acute respiratory syndrome.* Retrieved June 17, 2006, from http://www.cnn.com.

Max, A., Gattuso, J., Hinds, P., Norman, G., Price, R., Whitmore-Sisco, L., et al. (2003). Developing nursing care guidelines for children with Hodgkin's disease. *European Journal of Oncology Nursing, 7*(4), 253–258.

McCafferty, M., Sorbellini, D., & Cianci, P. (2002). Telemetry to home: Successful discharge of patients with ventricular assist devices. *Critical Care Nurse, 22*(3), 43–51.

McCaffery, M., and Pasero, C. (2004). *Pain: Clinical Manual,* 2nd ed. St. Louis, MO: Mosby.

McCaffrey, R., Frock, T. & Garguilo, H. (2003). Understanding chronic pain and the mind-body connection. *Holistic Nursing Practice, 17*(6), 281–287.

McCaig, L., & Burt, C. (2004). *National hospital ambulatory medical care survey: 2002 emergency department summary.* USDHHS Publication No. (PHS) 2004-125004-0226-0302. Hyattsville, MD: U. S. Department of Health & Human Services.

McCain, N., Gray, D., Walter, J., & Robins, J. (2005). Implementing a comprehensive approach to the study of health dynamics using the psychoneuroimmunology paradigm. *Advances in Nursing Science, 28*(4), 320–332.

McCance, K., & Huether, S. (2005). *Pathophysiology: The biological basis for disease in adults and children* (5th ed.). St. Louis, MO: Mosby.

McCloskey, J., & Bulechek, G. (2000). *Nursing interventions classification (NIC)* (3rd ed.). St. Louis, MO: Mosby.

McCullough, F. (2005). Book review: Nutrition and the eye. *Journal of Human Nutrition and Dietetics, 18*(4), 321.

McDaniel, J. (2005). Alternative approach. CO_2 may not be the enemy. *Virginia Nurses Today, 13*(3), 9.

McDermott, F. T., Rosenfeld, J. V., Laidlaw, J. D., Cordner, S. M., & Tremayne, A. B. (2004). Evaluation of management of road trauma survivors with brain injury and neurologic disability in Victoria. *Journal of Trauma: Injury, Infection, and Critical Care, 56*(1), 137–149.

McDevitt, E. R., Taylor, D. C., Miller, M. D., Gerber, J. P. Ziemke, G., Hinkin, D. et al. (2004). Functional bracing after anterior cruciate ligament reconstruction: A prospective, randomized, multicenter study. *The American Journal of Sports Medicine, 32*(8), 1887–1892.

McDonald, J. (2005, June 7). Supreme Court decision trumps California law. *San Diego Union Tribune,* pp. A-1, 8.

McDonald, S., Hetrick, S., & Green, S. (2004). Pre-operative education for hip or knee replacement (Cochrane Review). In: *The Cochrane Database of Systematic Reviews* (4). Chichester, UK: John Wiley & Sons, Ltd.

McElligott, J. M., Greenwald, B. D., & Watanabe, T. K. (2003). Congenital and acquired brain injury. New frontiers: Neuroimaging, neuroprotective agents, and complimentary medicine. *Archives of Physical Medicine and Rehabilitation, 84*(Suppl 1), S18–S22.

McGhee, B., & Bridges, M. (2002). Monitoring arterial blood pressure: What you may not know. *Critical Care Nurse, 22*(2), 60–79.

McGlinchey, D. (2004). *Lockheed developing military health tracking system.* Retrieved June 28, 2006, from http://www.govexec.com.

McGuigan, F. X., & Aierstok, M. D. (2005). Disorders of the Achilles tendon and its insertion. *Current Opinion in Orthopaedics, 16*(2), 65–71.

McGwin, G., Hall, T. A., Searcey, K., Modjarrad, K., Owsley, C. (2005). Cataract and cognitive function in older adults. *Journal of the American Geriatrics Society, 53*(7), 1260–1261.

McHugh, J. (2004). Diabetes and peripheral sensory neurons: What we don't know can hurt us. *AACN Clinical Issues, 15*(1), 136–149.

McKelvie, R. (2003). Heart failure. In F. Godlee (Ed.), *Clinical evidence concise,* (vol. 10, pp. 19–22). London: BMJ Publishing Group.

McKenzie, S. B. (2005). Advances in understanding the biology and genetics of acute myelocytic leukemia. *Clinical Laboratory Science,18*(1), 28–37, 57–59.

McKittrick, M. (2002). Diet and polycystic ovary syndrome. *Nutrition Today, 37*(2), 63–69.

McLauchlan, G. J., & Handoll, H. G. (2005). Interventions for treating acute and chronic Achilles tendinitis. *The Cochrane Database of Systematic Reviews* (4).

McNulty, M. (2005). Vyster unveils new natural rubber latex. *Rubber and Plastic News, 35*(1), 5.

McTiernan, A., Kooperberg, C., & White, E. (2003). Recreational physical activity and the risk of breast cancer in postmenopausal women: The Women's Health Initiative Cohort Study. *Journal of the American Medical Association, 290*(10), 1331–1336.

Mechem, C. (2004). *Pulse oximetry.* Retrieved June 25, 2006, from http://www.uptodate.com.

Medline Plus. (2005a). *Energy preservation.* Retrieved July 20, 2005, from www.nlm.nih.gov/medlineplus.gov.

Medline Plus. (2005b). *National Library of Medicine: National Institutes of Health.* Retrieved from www.medlineplus.gov.

Medline Plus. (2006). *Definitions of prevalence and incidence.* Retrieved July 20, 2006, from http://www.nih.gov/medlineplus.

Mellon, J. K. (2003). Urological issues for the nephrologist. In R. Johnson & J. Feehally (Eds.), *Comprehensive clinical nephrology* (2nd ed., pp. 759–767). St. Louis, MO: Mosby.

Menzin, J., Lang, K., Earle, C., & Glendenning, A. (2004). Treatment patterns, outcomes and costs among elderly patients with chronic myeloid leukemia: A population-based analysis. *Drugs and Aging, 21*(11), 737–746.

Meric-Berstam, F., & Pollock, R. E. (2005). Oncology. In F. C. Brunicardi (Ed.), *Schwartz's principles of surgery* (8th ed., pp. 249–294). New York: McGraw Hill.

Merikangans, K., & Risch, N. (2003). Will the genomics revolution revolutionize psychiatry? *American Journal of Psychiatry, 160,* 625–635.

Merten, G., Burgess, P., Gray, L., Holleman, J., Roush, T., Kowalchuk, G., et al. (2004). Prevention of contrast-induced nephropathy with sodium bicarbonate. *Journal of the American Medical Association, 291*(19), 2328–2334.

Metules, T., & Bauer, J. (2005). Unstable angina: Is your care up to snuff? *RN, 68*(2), 22–28.

Michelson, P. E. (2005). Common visual problems: Symptoms and treatment, part I two-part article. *Annals of Long-Term Care, 13*(8), 17–22.

Middleton, L., Dimond, E., Calzone, K., Davis, J., & Jenkins, J. (2002). The role of the nurse in cancer genetics. *Cancer Nursing, 25*(3), 196–208.

Miglioretti, D., Rutter, C., Geller, C., Cutter, G., Barlow, W., Rosenberg, R., et al. (2004). Effect of breast augmentation on the accuracy of mammography and cancer characteristics. *Journal of the American Medical Association, 291*(4), 442–450.

Miller, F. G., & Moreno, J. D. (2005). The state of research ethics: A tribute to John C. Fletcher. *Journal of Clinical Ethics, 16*(4), 355–364.

Miller, K. (2004). Management of hyperprolactinemia in patients receiving antipsychotics. *CNS Spectrums, 8*(Suppl 7), 28–32.

Miller, N. R., & Newman, N. J. (2004). The eye in neurological disease. *Lancet, 364*(9450), 2045–2054.

Miller, R. H. (2003). Knee injuries. In S. T. Canale (Ed.), *Campbell's operative orthopaedics* (vol. 3, 10th ed., pp 2165–2337). Philadelphia: Mosby.

Milligan, L. (2006). Epidemiology and cancer. *Advance for Nurses, 3*(15), 15–17.

Millman, R., & Kramer, N. (2004) *Polysomnography in the diagnostic evaluation of sleep apnea.* Retrieved June 25, 2006, from http://www.uptodate.com.

Milstead, J. A., & Furlong, E. (2006). *Handbook of nursing leadership: Creative skills for a culture of safety.* Sudbury, MA: Jones and Bartlett.

Minden, P. (2002). Humor as focal point of therapy for psychiatric patients. *Holistic Nursing Practice, 16*(4), 775–786.

Mion, L. (2003). Care provided for older adults: Who will provide? *Online Journal of Issues in Nursing 1*(2), 99–109.

Mitchell, A., & Parish, T. (2005). Using combination therapy for smoking cessation. *Clinician Reviews, 15*(5), 40–45.

Mitchell, R. A., Hasbrouch, L., Ingram, M. E., Dunaway, C. & Annest, J. L. (2003). Public health and aging: Nonfatal physical assault-related injuries among persons aged > 60 years treated in hospital emergency departments United States, 2001. *Morbidity and Mortality Weekly Report, 52*(5), 812–816.

Mittal, B., Rennke, H., & Singh, A. (2005). The role of kidney biopsy in the management of lupus nephritis. *Current Opinion in Nephrology and Hypertension, 14*(1), 1–8.

Miyamoto, R., Houston, D., & Bergeson, T. (2005). Cochlear implantation in deaf infants. *Laryngoscope, 115*(8), 1376–1380.

MMWR. (2004, September 10). *Recommendations and reports: Indicators for chronic disease surveillance.* Centers for Disease Control, 53 (RR11), 1-6, Atlanta: Author.

Mohapatra, S., Lockey, R., & Shirley S. (2005). Immunobiology of grass pollen allergens. *Current Allergy and Asthma Reports, 5*(5), 381–387.

Mohr, D., & Pelletier, D. (2006). A temporal framework for understanding the effects of stressful life events on inflammation in patients with multiple sclerosis. *Brain, Behavior, & Immunity, 20*(1), 27–36.

Mokdad, A., Ford, E., Bowman, B., Dietz, W., Vinevor, F., Bales, V., et al. (2003). Prevalence of obesity, diabetes and obesity: Related health risk factors. *Journal of American Medical Association, 289,* 76–79.

Moldwin R. M., & Sant G. R. (2002). Interstitial cystitis: A pathophysiology and treatment update. *Clinical Obstetrics and Gynecology, 45*(1), 259–272.

Mollaret, P., & Goulon, M. (1959). Le coma depasse (memoire preliminaire). *Revue Neurologique (Paris), 101,* 3–5.

Monarch, K. (2002, November/December). Legal aspects of infusion practice. *Journal of Infusion Nursing, 25*(6), S21–S30.

Montague, A. (1986). *Touching: The human significance of the skin* (3rd ed.). New York: Perennial Library.

Montbriand, M. J. (2005). Herbs or natural products that may cause cancer and harm part four of a four-part series [Online exclusive]. *Oncology Nursing Forum, 32*(1). Retrieved June 10, 2005, from http://www.ons.org.

Moore, Z. & Cowman, S. (2006). Wound cleansing for pressure ulcers. *The Cochrane Database of Systematic Reviews,* CD004983.

Moran, T. A., & Viele, C. S. (2005). Normal clotting. *Seminars in Oncology Nursing, 21*(4 Suppl 1), 1–11.

Mothershead, J. (2003). *Disaster planning.* Retrieved June 27, 2006, from http://emedicine.com.

Mount, D., & Zandi-Nejad, K. (2004). Disorders of potassium balance. In B. Brenner (Ed.), *Brenner and Rector's the kidney* (7th ed., vol. 1, pp. 997–1040). Philadelphia: W. B. Saunders Co.

Mueller, A., Johnston, M., & Bligh, D. (2001). Mind-mapped care plans: A remarkable alternative to traditional nursing care plans. *Nurse Educator, 26*(2), 75–80.

Mueller, H., & Hawkins, D. (2006). Trouble-shooting hearing aid fitting issues: the case of the missing "ping." *Hearing Journal, 59*(1), 10, 12, 14–15.

Mueller, P., Hook, C., & Hayes, D. (2003). Ethical analysis of withdrawal of pacemaker or implantable cardioverter-defibrillator support at the end of life. *Mayo Clinic Procedures, 78,* 959–963.

Mukand, J. A., Guilmette, T. J., & Tran, M. (2003). Rehabilitation for patients with brain tumors. *Critical Reviews in Physical and Rehabilitation Medicine, 15*(2), 99–111.

Muller, U., & Golden D., (2004). Immunotherapy for hymenoptera venom and biting insect hypersensitivity. *Clinical Allergy Immunology, 18,* 441–559.

Mulrow, C. (1994). Rationale for systematic reviews. *British Medical Journal, 309,* 597–599.

Mulrow, C. D., & Oxman, A. D. (Eds.). (1994; updated 2004). Cochrane Collaboration Handbook. In *The Cochrane Database of Systematic Reviews. The Cochrane Collaboration.* Oxford, UK: Update Software.

Mundy, A. (2004). Clinical updates. New updates in diabetes. *The Journal of Continuing Education in Nursing, 35*(2), 54–55.

Munro, C. L., & Grap, M. J. (2004). Oral health and care in the intensive care unit: State of the science. *American Journal of Critical Care, 13*(1), 25-33.

Murphy, F. (2005). Myths and realities in acute woundcare. *Practice Nurse, 30*(4), 52–53.

Murphy, J. (2003). Pharmacological treatment of acute ischemic stroke. *Critical Care Nurse, 26*(4), 276–282.

Murphy, K., Hopp, R., Kittelson, E., Hansen, G., Windle, M., & Walburn, J. (2006). Life-threatening asthma and anaphylaxis in schools: A treatment model for school-based programs. *Annals of Allergy, Asthma, & Immunology, 96*(3), 398–405.

Murthy, T. H. (2004). *Cardiac catheterization.* Retrieved June 24, 2006, from http://www.nlm.nih.gov.

Mustalish, S. H. (2002). Avoiding allergic reactions in children from botanical medicines. *Integrative Medicine Consult, 1,* 6.

Mutsch, M., Zhou, W., Rhodes, P., Bopp, M., Chen, R., Linder, T., et al. (2004). Use of the inactivated intranasal influenza vaccine and the risk of Bell's palsy in Switzerland. *New England Journal of Medicine, 350*(4), 896–903.

Mycyk, M., & Moyer, P. (2004). *Orchitis.* Retrieved August 1, 2005, from http://www.emedicine.com.

Myer, G., Brunner, H., Melson, P., Paterno, M., & Ford, T. (2005). Specialized neuromuscular training to improve neuromuscular function and biomechanics in a patient with quiescent juvenile rheumatoid arthritis. *Physical Therapy, 85*(8), 791–802.

Mythen, M. (2004). Postoperative gastrointestinal tract dysfunction. *Anesthesia-Analgesia, 100*(1), 196–204.

Nahas, M. (2003). Progression of chronic renal failure. In R. Johnson & J. Feehally (Eds.), *Comprehensive clinical nephrology* (2nd ed., pp. 843–856). St. Louis, MO: Mosby.

NANDA International. (2005a). *Nursing diagnoses: Definitions and classification 2005–2006.* Philadelphia: NANDA International.

NANDA International. (2005b). Nursing diagnosis: Disturbed energy field. In *Nursing diagnoses: Definitions and classification 2005–2006.* Philadelphia: Author.

National acute care nurse practitioner certification exam. (2003). Retrieved May 7, 2004, from www.aacn.org.

National Association of Orthopaedic Nurses. (2006). *Osteoporosis: Bone anabolic agents revolutionize bone loss and bone disease therapies.* Retrieved September 6, 2006, from www.orthonurse.com.

National Asthma Education and Prevention Program. (2002). *Executive summary expert panel report: Guidelines for the diagnosis and treatment of asthma–update on select topics* (No. 02-5075). Bethesda, MD: National Institutes of Health.

National Cancer Institute. (2003a). *Hormone replacement.* Retrieved July 20, 2006, from http://www.cancer.gov.

National Cancer Institute. (2003b). *Laryngeal cancer.* Retrieved December 17, 2004, from http://www.nci.nih.gov/cancertopics/pdq/treatment/laryngeal/healthprofessional.

National Cancer Institute. (2003c). *What you need to know about cancer of the larynx.* Retrieved December 17, 2004 from, http://www.nci.nih.gov/cancertopics/wyntk/larynx.

National Cancer Institute. (2004a). *Antioxidants and cancer prevention: Questions and answers.* Retrieved June 10, 2005, from http://www.cancer.gov.

National Cancer Institute. (2004b). *Biological therapy.* Retrieved June 10, 2005, from http://www.nci.nih.gov.

National Cancer Institute. (2004c). *Bone marrow transplantation and peripheral blood stem cell transplantation: Questions and answers.* Retrieved June 10, 2005, from http://cis.nci.nih.gov.

National Cancer Institute. (2004d). *National Cancer Institute cancer facts radiation therapy for cancer: Questions and answers.* Retrieved March 25, 2005, from http://cis.nci.nih.gov.

National Cancer Institute. (2004e). *Radiation enteritis.* Retrieved June 10, 2005, from http://www.cancer.gov.

National Cancer Institute. (2005a). *Gastrointestinal complications (PDQ).* Retrieved June 10, 2005, from http://www.nci.nih.gov.

National Cancer Institute. (2005b). *Gastrointestinal complications: National Cancer Institute's common toxicity criteria for grading severity of diarrhea.* Retrieved June 10, 2005, from http://www.nci.nih.gov.

National Cancer Institute. (2005c). *NCI/PDQ patients: Nutrition in cancer care.* Retrieved June 10, 2005, from http://www.oncolink.com.

National Cancer Institute. (2005d). *Prostate cancer.* Retrieved July 31, 2006, from http://www.nci.nih.gov.

National Cancer Institute. (2006). *Stomach cancer: NCI Drug Dictionary.* Retrieved June 25, 2006, from www.nic.gov.

National Cancer Institute's Cancer Information Service. (2005). *HIV/AIDS prevention home: Basic statistics overview.* Retrieved June 11, 2006, from http://cis.nci.nih.gov.

National Center for Complementary and Alternative Medicine (NCCAM). (2002). *What is complementary and alternative medicine?* Publication No. D156. Bethesda, MD: Author.

National Center for Complementary and Alternative Medicine. (2005). *Get the Facts. What is complementary and alternative medicine (CAM)?* Retrieved August 26, 2006, from http://www.nccam.nih.gov.

National Center for Complementary and Alternative Medicine. (2006). (p. 11). Retrieved June 23, 2006, from http://nccam.nih.gov.

National Center for Health Statistics. (2002, October 25). *Data tables for vaccine.* Retrieved June 30, 2004, from http://www.cdc.gov.

National Center for Health Statistics. (2004). *Health, United States, 2004 with chartbook on trends in the health of Americans.* Retrieved on July 5, 2005, from http://www.cdc.gov/nchs/data/hus/hus04.pdf.

National Center for Health Statistics. (2005). *Fact sheet on mortality: Adolescent and young adults.* Retrieved July 17, 2006, from http://www.cdc.gov.

National Center for Health Statistics. (2006a). *About healthy people 2010.* Retrieved August 25, 2006, from www.cdc.gov.

National Center for Health Statistics. (2006b). *Health, United States, 2005: 29th report on the health status of the nation.* Retrieved July 12, 2006, from http://www.cdc.gov/nchs.

National Center for PTSD. (2003). *What is post-traumatic stress disorder.* Retrieved June 23, 2006, from http://www.ncptsd.org.

National Cholesterol Education Program. (2004). Implications of recent clinical trials for the national cholesterol education program adult treatment panel III guidelines. Retrieved June 24. 2006, from http://www.nhibi.nih.bov/guidelines/cholesterol.

National Collaborating Centre for Nursing and Supportive Care. (2004). *Clinical practice guideline for the assessment and prevention of falls in older people.* Retrieved June 15, 2005, from http://www.guideline.gov.

National Committee for Quality Healthcare (n.d.). *The environment right now.* Retrieved June 15, 2005, from www.ncqhc.org/execinstitute/rightnow.cfm.

National Comprehensive Cancer Network. (2005). *Clinical practice guidelines in oncology.* Retrieved June 10, 2005, from http://www.nccn.org.

National Guideline Clearinghouse. (2002, October 21). *Evidence-based guidelines for weaning and discontinuation of ventilatory support.* Retrieved September 18, 2004, from www.guideline.gov.

National Guideline Clearinghouse. (2003). *Screening for lung cancer.* Retrieved June 30, 2004, from http://www.guideline.gov.

National Health System. (2005a). *Center for evidence-based medicine. Glossary.* Retrieved July 11, 2005, from http://www.minervation.com/cebm2.

National Health System. (2005b). *Levels of evidence.* Retrieved July 11, 2005, from http://cebm.jr2.ox.ac.uk.

National Heart, Lung, and Blood Institute. (2004a). *Health information center.* Retrieved June 24, 2006, from www.nhlbi.nih.gov.

National Heart, Lung, and Blood Institute. (2004b). *What is pulmonary arterial hypertension.* Retrieved September 16, 2004, from http://www.nhlbi.nih.gov.

National Heart, Lung, and Blood Institute. (2006a). *High blood cholesterol: What you need to know.* Retrieved July 31, 2006, from http://www.nhbi.nih.gov.

National Heart, Lung, and Blood Institute. (2006b). *What is heart failure?* (pp. 1–11). Retrieved June 25, 2006, www.nhlbi.nih.gov.

National Institute of Allergy and Infectious Diseases. (2002, April). *Sinusitis.* Retrieved December 17, 2004, from http://www.niaid.nih.gov.

National Institute of Arthritis and Musculoskeletal and Skin Diseases (NIAMS). Handout on health: Systemic lupus erythematosus (pp. 1–40). Retrieved June 26, 2006, from http://www.niams.nih.gov.

National Institute of Neurological Disorders and Stroke. (2002). *Carpal tunnel syndrome fact sheet.* Retrieved on September 28, 2005, from http://www.ninds.nih.gov/disorders/carpal_tunnel/detail_carpal_tunnel.htm.

National Institute of Neurological Disorders and Stroke. (2006). Retrieved June 16, 2006, from www.ninds.nih.gov.

National Institute of Nursing Research. (n.d.). *About NINR.* Retrieved June 1, 2005, from www.ninr.nih.gov.

National Institutes of Health. (2004a). *Frequently asked questions about acupuncture.* Bethesda, MD: National Institutes of Health.

National Institutes of Health. (2004). *My Pyramid.* U.S.D.A. NIH Publication No. 04-4006, Bethesda, MD: Author.

National Institutes of Health, National Heart, Lung, and Blood Institute. (1998). *Clinical guidelines on the identification, evaluation, and treatment of overweight and obesity in adults. The evidence report.* NIH Publication No. 98-4083, Bethesda, MD: Author.

National Kidney and Urologic Diseases Information Clearinghouse. (2003). *Peyronie's disease.* Retrieved July 13, 2006, from http://kidney.niddk.nih.gov.

National Limb Loss Information Center. (2002). *Limb amputations.* Retrieved on October 15, 2005. from http://www.amputee-coalition.org.

National Marrow Donor Program. *How the NMDP helps patients* (pp. 1–4). Retrieved June 26, 2006, from http://www.marrow.org.

National Sleep Foundation. (2004). *Sleep apnea.* December 17, 2004, from http://www.sleepfoundation.org/publications/sleepap.cfm.

National Stroke Association. (2006). *People with atrial fibrillation increase stroke risk by 500%.* Retrieved June 21, 2006, from http://www.stroke.org.

Needleman, J., Buerhaus, P., Mattke, S., Stewart, M., & Zelevinsky, K. (2002). Nurse-staffing levels and the quality of care in hospitals. *New England Journal of Medicine, 346*(22), 1715–1722.

Nelson, J. (2005). Families and bioethics: Old problems, new themes. *Journal of Clinical Ethics, 16*(4), 299–302.

Nelson, R., Edwards, S., & Tse, B. (2004). Prophylactic nasogastric decompression after abdominal surgery. *The Cochrane Database of Systematic Reviews* (3), CD004929.

Nelson, S. (2004). The search for the good in nursing? The burden of ethical expertise. *Nursing Philosophy, 5*(1), 12–22.

Net income increased by 2.5% on international sales growth. (2006, July 18). *The Wall Street Journal,* A9.

Neuhauser, D. (2003). The coming third healthcare revolution: Personal empowerment. *Quality Management in Healthcare, 12*(3), 171–184.

Neuman, B. (1982). *The Neuman systems model. Application to nursing education and practice.* Norwalk, CT: Appleton-Century-Crofts.

Neurnberger, P. (1981). *Freedom from stress: A holistic approach.* Honesdale, PA: The Himalayan International Institute of Yoga Science and Philosophy.

Neville, K. (2003). Uncertainty in illness: An integrative review. *Orthopaedic Nursing, 22*(3), 206–214.

New Haven Hospice. (2006). Retrieved August 31, 2006, from www.hospice.com.

New Zealand Guidelines Group. (2003). *Prevention of hip fracture amongst people aged 65 years and over.* Retrieved June 15, 2005 from http://www.nzgg.org.nz/.

Newman, D. (2005). Assessment of the patient with an overactive bladder. *Journal of WOCN, 32*(3 Suppl 1), S5–10, S24–26.

Nguyen, L., Mohr, W., Ahrenholz, D., & Solem, L. (2004). Treatment of hydrofluoric acid burn to the face by carotid artery infusion of calcium gluconate. *Journal of Burn Care and Rehabilitation, 25*(5), 421–424.

Nicholas, J., & Geers, A. (2006). The process and early outcomes of cochlear implantation by three years of age. In P. E. Spencer & M. Marschark (Eds.), *Advances in the Development of Spoken Language by Deaf Children* (pp. 124–129). New York: Oxford University Press.

Nicholson, B. (2003). Diagnosis and management of neuropathic pain: A balanced approach to treatment. *Journal of the American Academy of Nurse Practitioners* (Suppl 150), 3–9.

Nienhuis, A., Hanawa, H., Sawai, N., Sorrentino, B., & Persons, D. (2003). Development of gene therapy for hemoglobin disorders. *Annals of the New York Academy of Science, 996*(1), 101–111.

Nietsch, H. H., & Kowdley, K. V. (2004). Review: Magnetic resonance cholangiopancreatography is accurate for diagnosing biliary disease. *ACP Journal Club, 141*(1), 25.

Nightingale, F. (1859). *Notes on nursing: What it is and what it is not.* London: Harrison Pall Mall.

Nightingale, F. (1860). *Notes on nursing: What it is and what it is not.* London: Harrison and Sons.

Nightingale, F. (1969 [1859]). *Notes on nursing what it is and what it is not.* New York: Dover Publications.

Noble, K. (2003). Name that tube. *Nursing, 33*(3), 56–62.

Noble, V., & Brown, D. (2004). Renal ultrasound. *Emergency Medicine Clinics of North America, 22*(3), 641–659.

Noga, S. J. (2004). 93-year-old man with non-Hodgkin's lymphoma. *Advanced Studies in Medicine, 4*(3B), S202–204, S207–209.

Nogueira, S., & Appling, S. (2000). Breast cancer: Genetics, risks, and strategies. *Nursing Clinics of North America, 35*(3), 663–670.

Nolan, P. (2006). What to do until the music therapist arrives: Developing therapeutic activities using music. *Journal of Holistic Nursing Practice, 20*(1), 37–40.

Norris, J., & Spelic, S. S. (2002). Supporting adaptation to body image disruption. *Rehabilitation Nursing, 27*(1), 8–11.

North American Nursing Diagnosis Association. (2005). *Nursing diagnoses: Definitions and classifications 2005–2006.* Philadelphia: Author.

North American Menopause Society (NAMS). (2004). Treatment of menopause-associated vasomotor symptoms: Position statement of the North American Menopause Society. *Menopause: The Journal of the North American Menopause Society, 11*(1), 11–33.

Norton, L. B., Peipert, J. F., Zierler, S., Lima, B., & Hume, L. (1995). Battering in pregnancy: An assessment of two screening methods. *Obstetrics and Gynecology, 85*(3), 321–325.

Nosek, L. J. (1986). Explanation of hospital stay by nursing diagnoses, medical diagnoses, and social position. *Dissertation Abstracts International,* 47(07B), 00215. (University Microfilms No. AAG8622844).

Nosek, L. J. (2004). Globalization's costs to healthcare: How can we pay the bill? *Nursing Administration Quarterly, 28*(2), 116–121.

Nosek, L. J., & Androwich, I. M. (2003). Basic clinical health care economics. In P. Kelly-Heidenthal (Ed.), *Nursing leadership and management* (pp. 32–58). Albany, NY: Thomson Delmar Learning.

Nosek, M., Hughes, R., Howland, C., Young, M. Mullen, P, & Shelton, M. (2004). The meaning of health for women with physical disabilities. A qualitative analysis [Electronic version]. *Family and Community Health, 27*(1), 6–21.

Nour, N. (2004). Female genital cutting: Clinical and cultural guidelines. *Obstetrical and Gynecological Survey, 59*(4), 272–279.

Nowlin, A. (2005). The promise of stem cells. *RN, 68*(4), 48–53.

Nurse Healers-Professional Associates, Inc. (2005). *Therapeutic touch process.* Retrieved August 2, 2006, from http://therapeutictouch.org.

Nurseweek. (2004). *A nurse's guide to pain management.* Retrieved June 14, 2006, from www.nurseweek.com.

Nursing law case on point. Nurse terminated for botching sponge count denied U.I. benefits. (2005). *Nursing Law's Regan Report, 45*(11), 4.

Nusbaum, M., Hamilton, C., & Lenahan, P. (2003). Chronic illness and sexual functioning. *American Family Physician, 67*(2), 347–354.

O'Brien, J. G., Chennubhotla, S. A., & Chennubhotla, R. V. (2005). Treatment of edema. *American Family Physician, 71*(11), 2111–2118.

O'Connell, B., Baker, L., & Prosser, A. (2003). The educational needs of caregivers of stroke survivors in acute and community settings. *Journal of Neuroscience Nursing, 35*(1), 21–28.

O'Conner, A., & Besner, G. (2004). *Burns a surgical perspective.* Retrieved April 8, 2006, from www.emedicine.com.

O'Connor, D., Marshall, S., & Massey-Westropp, N. (2005). *Non-surgical treatment (other than steroid injection) for carpal tunnel syndrome.* Retrieved on September 28, 2005, from http://www.cochrane.org/reviews/en/ab003219.html.

O'Hara, M. (2005). A case-based review of overactive bladder. *Clinical Advisor, 8*(7), 38, 40–41, 45.

O'Sullivan, D., & Torres, V. (2003). Autosomal dominant polycystic kidney disease. In R. Johnson & J. Feehally (Eds.), *Comprehensive clinical nephrology* (2nd ed., pp. 598–609). St. Louis, MO: Mosby.

Occupational Safety and Health Administration. (2005). *Safety and health topics: Personal and protective equipment.* Retrieved June 24, 2006, from www.osha.gov.

Office of the Robert Wood Johnson Foundation. (2001). *Advanced practice nurses' role in palliative care; a position statement from American nursing leaders. Promoting excellence in end-of-life care: A national program.* Bozeman, MT: University of Montana.

Olson, T. (2004). The geriatric client. In R. Daniels (Ed.), *Nursing fundamentals: Caring and clinical decision making* (pp. 83–88). New York: Thomson Delmar Learning.

Oregon Death with Dignity Act. (1997). *Oregon Revised Statute 127800-127,* 897.

Orem, D. E. (1995). *Nursing: Concepts of practice* (5th ed.). St. Louis, MO: Mosby-Yearbook.

Orens, J. B. (2004) Listing the patient: Deciding when transplantation is the only viable life-sustaining option. *Advances in Pulmonary Hypertension.* Retrieved June 30, 2004, from http://www.phassociation.org/.

Otchy, D., Hyman, N. H., Simmang, C., Anthony, T., Buie, W.D., Cataldo, P., et al. (2004). Practice parameters for colon cancer. *Diseases of the Colon and Rectum, 47*(8), 1269–1284.

Otlowski, M., & Williamson, R. (2003). Ethical and legal issues and the "new genetics." *Medical Journal of Australia, 178*(11), 582–585.

Ottem, D. P., & Teichman, J. M. (2005). What is the value of cystoscopy with hydrodistention for interstitial cystitis? *Urology, 66*(3), 494–499.

Ouellet, L., Hodgins, M., Pond, S., Knorr, S., & Geldart, G. (2003). Post-discharge telephone follow-up for orthopaedic surgical patients: a pilot study. *Journal of Orthopaedic Nursing, 7*(2), 87–93.

Owens, B. D., Murphy, K. P., & Kuklo, T. R. (2004). *Lateral epicondylitis.* Retrieved on September 7, 2005, from http://www.emedicine.com/orthoped/topic510.htm.

Oxman, M., Levin, M., Johnson, G., Schmader, K. Straus, S., Gelb, L., et al. (2005). A vaccine to prevent herpes zoster and post-herpetic neuralgia in older adults. *New England Journal of Medicine, 352,* 2271–2284.

Ozer, H., & Diasio, R. B. (2004). Perspectives in the treatment of colorectal cancer. *Seminars in Oncology, 31*(6 Suppl 15), 14–18.

Pacini, C. M. (2004). Synergy: A framework for professional development and transformation. *Excellence in nursing knowledge.* Indianapolis, IN: Sigma Theta Tau Press.

Palmer, D., Mulhall, K., Thompson, C., Severson, E., Santos, E., & Saleh, K. (2005). Total knee arthroplasty in juvenile rheumatoid arthritis. *Journal of Bone and Joint Surgery (Am), 87*(7), 1510–1514.

Papakakais, M. A. (2006). *Current medical diagnosis and treatment* (45th ed.). New York: Lange Medical Books/McGraw-Hill.

Papanek, P. (2003). The female athlete triad: An emerging role for physical therapy. *The Journal of Orthopaedic and Sports Physical Therapy, 33*(10), 594–614.

Parker, E., Donato, L., & Dalgleish, D. (2005). Effects of added sodium caseinate on the formation of particles in heated milk. *Journal of Agricultural and Food Chemistry, 53*(21), 8265–8272.

Pavlovsky, S., & Lastiri, F. (2004). Progress in the prognosis of adult Hodgkin's lymphoma in the past 35 years through clinical trials in Argentina: A GATLA experience. *Clinical Lymphoma, 5*(2), 102–109.

Payton, C. (2005). Referral diagnosis and management of dysphagia. *Pulse, 65*(8), 64–65.

Pearson, R. L., Kabongo, M. L., Ejnes, Y. D., & Bahler, R. C. (2004). *Aortic valvular stenosis.* Retrieved June 24, 2006, from www.firstconsult.com.

Peck, S. (2005). Is it really Hodgkin's disease? *CURE: Cancer Updates, Research and Education, 4*(1), 45.

Pediatric Alert. (2004). Thalidomide for severe juvenile rheumatoid arthritis. *Pediatric Alert, 29*(24), 143–144.

Peers, K. H. E., & Lysens, R. J. J. (2005). Patellar tendinopathy in athletes: Current diagnosis and therapeutic recommendations. *Sports Medicine, 35*(1), 71–87.

Pelletier, K. (2004). *The best alternative medicine.* New York: Simon & Shuster.

Pelletier, K. (2004). Mind-body medicine in ambulatory care: An evidence-based assessment. *Journal of Ambulatory Care Management, 27*(1), 25–42.

Pender, N., Murdaugh, C., & Parsons, M. (2002). *Health promotion in nursing practice* (4th ed.). Upper Saddle River, NJ: Prentice Hall.

Perez, R., Chen, J. M., & Nedzelski, J. M. (2004). The status of the contralateral ear in established unilateral Meniere's disease. *Laryngoscope, 114*(8), 1373–1376.

Perkins, C., & Kisiel, M. (2005). Renal nursing. Utilizing physiological knowledge to care for acute renal failure. *British Journal of Nursing, 14*(14), 768–773.

Perron, A. D. (2003). Chest pain in athletes. *Clinics in Sports Medicine, 22*(1), 37–50.

Persiani, R., Biondi, A., Buccelletti, F., Rausei, S., Silveri, N. (2006). Unusual acute abdomen: To operate or not to operate? *Lancet, 367*(9521), 1548.

Philipp, C. S., Faiz, A., Dowling, N., Dilley, A., Michaels, L. A., Ayers, C., et al. (2005). Age and the prevalence of bleeding disorders in women with menorrhagia. *Obstetrics and Gynecology, 105*(1), 61–66.

Phillips, M. (2003). Genetics of hearing loss. *MEDSURG Nursing, 12,* 386–390, 411.

Phillips, N. (2004). *Berry and Kohn's operating room technique* (12th ed.). New York: Mosby.

Pierce, J., Morris, D., & Clancy, R. (2002). Understanding renal dose dopamine. *Journal of Infusion Nursing, 25*(6), 365–371.

Pierie, J. P., Muzikansky, A., Tanabe, K. K., & Ott, M. J. (2005). The outcome of surgical resection versus assignment to the liver transplant waiting list for hepatocellular carcinoma. *Annals of Surgical Oncology, 12*(7), 552–560.

Pilnick, A., & Coleman, T. (2003). "I'll give up smoking when you make me better": Patient's resistance to attempts to problematise smoking in general practice (GP) consultants. *Social Science Medicine, 57,* 135–145.

Pitchford, P. (2002). *Healing with whole foods: Asian traditions and modern nutrition.* Berkeley, CA: North Atlantic Books.

Plantinga, L., Natowicz, M., Kass, N., Hull, S., Gostin, L., & Faden, R. (2003). Disclosure, confidentiality, and families: Experiences and attitudes of those with genetic versus nongenetic medical conditions. *American Journal of Medical Genetics, 199C*(1), 51–59.

Platt, T., Parrish, K., & Hostler, D. (2004). A prospective and qualitative prehospital comparison of head immobilization devices, Prehospital Care Research Forum EMS Today, JEMS supplement. Retrieved September 8, 2006, from www.jems.com.

Plewa, M., & Worthington, R. (2004). *Mitral valve prolapse.* Retrieved June 24, 2006, from www.emedicine.com.

Plomin, R., & Spinath, F. (2004). Intelligence: Genetics, genes, and genomics. *Journal of Personality and Social Psychology, 86*(1), 112–129.

Plonk, W. M. (2005). To PEG or not to PEG. *Practical Gastroenterology, 29*(7), 16–31.

Poirier, P. (2006). The relationship of sick leave benefits, employment patterns and individual characteristics to radiation therapy related fatigue. *Oncology Nursing Forum, 33*(3), 593–601.

Pollak, M., & Yu, A. (2004). Clinical disturbances of calcium, magnesium, and phosphate metabolism. In B. Brenner (Ed.), *Brenner and Rector's the kidney* (7th ed., vol. 1, pp. 1040–1076). Philadelphia: W. B. Saunders Co.

Polovich, M. (2004). Safe handling of hazardous drugs. *Online Journal of Issues in Nursing 19*(3), Manuscript 5. Retrieved June 10, 2005, from http://www.nursingworld.org.

Pontali, E. (2005). Facilitating adherence in highly active antiretroviral therapy in children with HIV infections: What are the issues and what can be done. *Pediatric Drugs, 7*(3), 137–149.

Porth, C. (2003). *Pathophysiology: Concepts of altered health states* (5th ed.). Philadelphia: Lippincott, Williams & Wilkins.

Porth, C. (2004). *Pathophysiology: Concepts of altered health states* (6th ed.). Philadelphia: Lippincott.

Porth, C. (2005). *Pathophysiology: Concepts of altered health states* (7th ed.). Philadelphia: Lippincott, Williams & Wilkins.

Potts, H. W. (2005). Online support groups: An overlooked resource for patients. *Health Information on the Internet,* (44), 6–8.

Potts, N., & Mandleco, B. (2002). *Pediatric nursing: Caring for children and their families.* New York: Thomson Delmar Learning.

Powell, H., & Gibson, P. G. (2004). Options for self-management education for adults with asthma (Cochrane Review). In *The Cochrane Database of Systematic Reviews* (1). Chichester, UK: John Wiley & Sons, Ltd.

Powers, P. (2003). Empowerment as treatment and the role of health professionals. *Advances in Nursing Science, 26*(3), 227–237.

Practice Committee of the American Society for Reproductive Medicine. (2004). Current evaluation of amenorrhea. *Fertility and Sterility, 82*(1), 266–272.

Prather, S. H., Forsyth, L. W., Russell, K. D., & Wagner, V. L. (2003). Caring for the patient undergoing transsphenoidal surgery in the acute care setting: an alternative to critical care. *Journal of Neuroscience Nursing, 35*(5), 270–275.

Prevost, S. (2004). Improve pain management. In S. Hegyvary (Ed.), *Working Paper on Grand Challenges in*

Improving Global Health. Journal of Nursing Scholarship, 36(2), 96–101.

Price compare: Antibiotics. (2006). Retrieved August 13, 2006, from destinationrx.com.

Price, D. D., & Wilson, S. R. (2005) *Dislocations, shoulders.* Retrieved on September 27, 2005, from http://www.emedicine.com/emerg/topic148.htm.

Price, P. (2004). *Surgical technology for the surgical technologist* (2nd ed.). New York: Thomson Delmar Learning.

Price, S. A., & Wilson, L. M. (2003). *Pathophysiology: Clinical concepts of disease process.* (6th ed.). St. Louis, MO: Mosby.

Prince, M., Christensen, E., & Gluud, C. (2005). Glucocorticosteroids for primary biliary cirrhosis. *The Cochrane Database of Systematic Reviews* (3), ID #CD003778.

Prochazka, A., Kick, S., Steinbrunn, C., Miyoshi, T., & Fryer, G. (2004). A randomized trial of nortriptyline combined with transdermal nicotine for smoking cessation. *Archives of Internal Medicine, 164,* 2229–2233.

The Prostate Cancer Foundation. (2004). *Report to the nation on prostate cancer.* Retrieved July 17, 2006, from http://www.prostatecancerfoundation.org.

Proust, M. (2002 [1920]). The guermantes way. Translated by M. Treharne. New York: The Penguin Group.

Pruitt, B., & Jacobs, M. (2005). Caring for a patient with asthma. *Nursing, 33*(2), 48–51.

Pruitt, W., & Jacobs, M. (2004). Take a deep breath and conquer your fear of mechanical ventilation. *Nursing Made Incredibly Easy, June/July,* 10–21.

Public broadcasting system (PBS) interview, 89.7 FM, January 4, 2006.

Puddu, P., Cravero, E., & Puddu, G., Muscari A. (2005). Genes and atherosclerosis: At the origin of the predisposition. *International Journal of Clinical Practice, 59*(4), 462–472.

Pui, C.H., Cheng, C., Leung, W., Rai, S. N., Rivera, G. K., Sandlund, J. T., et al. (2003). Extended follow-up of long-term survivors of childhood acute lymphoblastic leukemia. *New England Journal of Medicine, 349*(7), 640–649.

Pulley, S. (2004). *Critical incident stress management.* Retrieved July 6, 2006, from http://www.emedicine.com.

Pumphrey, R. S. (2003). Fatal posture in anaphylactic shock. *Journal of Allergy Clinical Immunology, 112,* 451–452.

Punch, J., Joseph, A., & Rakerd, B. (2004). Most comfortable and uncomfortable loudness level: Six decades of research. *American Journal of Audiology, 13,* 144–157.

Puntillo, K., Wild, L., Morris, A., Stanik-Hutt, J., Thompson, C., & White, C. (2002). Practices and predictors of analgesic interventions for adults undergoing painful procedures. *American Journal of Critical Care, 11*(5), 415–429.

Purnell, L. D., & Paulanka, B. J. (2005). *Guide to culturally competent health care.* Philadelphia: F. A. Davis.

Quillen, D. M., Wuchner, M., & Hatch, R. (2004). Acute shoulder injuries. *American Family Physician, 70*(10), 1947–1954.

Raak, R., & Raak, A. (2003). Work attendance despite headache and its economic impact: A comparison between two workplaces. *Headache, 43,* 1097–1101.

Radimer, K., Bindewald, B., Hughes, J., Ervin, B., Swanson, C., & Picciano, M. F. (2004). Dietary supplement use by US adults: Data from the national health and nutrition examination survey, 1999–2000. *American Journal of Epidemiology, 160*(4), 339–349.

Rakel, R. E. & Bope, E. T. (2003). *Conn's current therapy 2003.* Philadelphia: Elsevier Science.

Ramachandran, V., & Shorvon, S. (2003). Clues to the genetic influences of drug responsiveness in epilepsy. *Epilepsia, 44*(Suppl 1), 33–37.

Ramadan, H. H. (2004). Surgical management of chronic sinusitis in children. *Laryngoscope, 114*(12), 2103–2109.

Raman, S., Somasekar, K., Winter, R. K., & Lewis, M. H. (2004). Are we overusing ultrasound in non-traumatic abdominal pain? *Postgraduate Medical Journal, 80* 177–179.

Rambaldi, A., & Gluud, C. (2005). Propylthiouracil for alcoholic liver disease. *The Cochrane Database of Systematic Reviews* (3), ID #CD002800.

Ramee, S. R., Subramanian, R., Felberg, R. A., McKinley, K. L., Jenkins, J. S., Collins, T. J., et al. (2004). Catheter-based treatment for patients with acute ischemic stroke ineligible for intravenous thrombolysis. *Stroke, 35*(5), 1–3.

Randolph, T. R. (2004). Advances in acute lymphoblastic leukemia. *Clinical Laboratory Science, 17*(4), 235–245, 247–249.

Ray, R. (2004, February 9). A distressing link between chronic stress, Alzheimer's. *Nurseweek,* p. 6.

Ray, W. A., Murray, K. T., Meredith, S., Narasimhulu, S. S., Hall, K., & Stein, C. M. (2004). Oral erythromycin and the risk of sudden death from cardiac causes. *New England Journal of Medicine, 351*(11), 1089.

Razek, O. A., & Poe, D. (2004, June). *Sinusitis, chronic, medical treatment.* Retrieved December 17, 2004, from http://www.emedicine.com/ent/topic338.htm.

Redaelli A., Laskin, B. L., Stephens, J. M., Botteman, M. F., & Pashos, C. L. (2004). The clinical and epidemiological burden of chronic lymphocytic leukaemia. *European Journal of Cancer Care, 13*(3), 279–287.

Redaelli A., Laskin B. L., Stephens, J. M., Botteman, M. F., & Pashos C. L. (2005). A systematic literature review of the clinical and epidemiological burden of acute lymphoblastic leukaemia (ALL). *European Journal of Cancer Care, 14*(1), 53–62.

Reddy, L. S. (2004). Heads up on cerebral bleeds. *Nursing Made Incredibly Easy! 2*(3), 8–17.

Reeves, S., Havidich, J., & Tobin, P. (2004). Conscious sedation of children with propofol is anything but conscious. *Pediatrics, 114*(1 Suppl), e74–e76.

Registered Nurses Association of Ontario. (2005, March). *Prevention of falls and fall injuries in the older adult.* Toronto, ON: Author.

Rehabilitation Institute of Chicago. (n.d.). *Research.* Retrieved August 30, 2005, from http://www.ric.org.

Reich, C. D. (2003) Advances in the treatment of bone metastases. *Clinical Journal of Oncology Nursing, 7*(6), 641–646.

Reiche, E. M., Nunes, S. O., & Morimoto, H. K. (2004). Stress, depression, the immune system, and cancer. *Lancet Oncology, 5*(10), 617–625.

Reid, G., & Bruce, A. (2003). Urogenital infections in women: Can probiotics help? *Postgraduate Medical Journal, 79*(934), 428–432.

Reinhold-Keller, E., Herlyn, K., Wagner-Bastmeyer, R., Gutfleisch, J., Peter, H., Raspe, H., et al. (2005). Effect of Wegener's granulomatosis on work disability, need for medical care, and quality of life in patients younger than 40 years at diagnosis. *Arthritis and Rheumatism, 47*(3), 320–325.

Reis, J., Breslin, M., Lezzoni, L., & Kirschner, K. (2004). *It takes more than ramps to solve the crisis of health care for people with disabilities.* Chicago: Rehabilitation Institute of Chicago.

Ren, J., & Wu, S. (2006). A burning issue: Do sepsis and systemic inflammatory response syndrome (SIRS) directly contribute to cardiac dysfunction? *Frontiers in Bioscience,* 11, 15–22.

Rhiner, M., Palos, G., & Termini, M. (2004). Managing breakthrough pain: A clinical review with three case studies using oral transmucosal fentanyl citrate. *Clinical Journal of Oncology Nursing, 8*(5), 507–512.

Rice, J. (2002). *Medications and mathematics for the nurse* (9th ed.). New York: Thomson Delmar Learning.

Rice, K. (2005). How to measure ankle/brachial index. *Nursing, 35*(1), 56–57.

Richmond, J. (2006). *The 1, 2, 3s of biosafety levels.* Retrieved June 24, 2006, from www.cdc.gov.

Richmond, T., & Thompson, H. (2002).Quality care in challenging circumstances: A patient with a spinal cord injury. *Journal of Neuroscience Nursing, 34*(11), 44-48.

Riddington, C., & Wang, W. (2002). Blood transfusion for preventing stroke in people with sickle cell disease. *The Cochrane Database for Systematic Reviews* (1), CD003146.

Ridker, P., Cook, N., Lee, I., Gordon, D., Gaziano, J., Manson, J., et al. (2005). A randomized trial of low-dose aspirin in the primary prevention of cardiovascular disease in women. *New England Journal of Medicine, 352*(13), 1293–1304.

Riggs, J. M. (2004). New therapies for heart failure. *RN, 67*(3), 28–33.

Rintala, D., Robinson-Whelen, S., & Matamoros, R. (2005). Subjective stress in male veterans with spinal cord injury. *Journal of Rehabilitation Research and Development, 42*(3), 291–304.

Ripamonti, C., & Mercadante, S. (2004). How to use octreotide for malignant bowel obstruction. *Journal of Supportive Oncology, 2*(4), 357–364.

Ristig, M., Drechsler, H., & Powderly, W.G. (2005). Hepatic steatosis and HIV infection. *AIDS Patient Care and STDs, 19*(6), 356–365.

Ritchey, C. (2005). Advice of counsel. Documentation puts nurse on solid legal ground. *RN, 68*(2), 21, 46, 58–59.

Rizzo, D. (2006). *Fundamentals of anatomy and physiology* (2nd ed.). New York: Thomson Delmar Learning.

Robbins, J., Gangnon, R., Theis, S., Kays, S., Hewitt, A., & Hind, J. (2005). The effects of lingual exercise on swallowing in older adults. *Journal of American Geriatric Society, 53*(9), 1483–1489.

Robert Woods Johnson Hospital. (2006). *RWJUH is one of only four hospitals in the nation to be awarded Magnet Status in nursing excellence three times.* Retrieved July 9, 2006, from www.rwjuh.edu.

Roberts, J., LaRusse, S., Katzen, H., Whitehouse, P., Barber, M., Post, S., et al. (2003). Reasons for seeking genetic susceptibility testing among first-degree relatives of people with Alzheimer disease. *Alzheimer Disease and Associated Disorders, 17*(2), 86–93.

Roberts, K. (2003). Treating asthma in the zone. *American Journal of Nursing, 103*(11), 118–119.

Robinson, P. (2004). Nurse-led diabetes care. *Community Practitioner, 77*(3), 82–84.

Robinson, P. (2005). Is surgery safe for a patient with hemophilia? *Nursing, 35*(5), *Hospital Nursing,* 1–3.

Robinson-Smith, G. (2002). Self-efficacy and quality of life after stroke. *Journal of Neuroscience Nursing, 34*(2), 91–98.

Rodgers, R. W. (2004). Hearing loss and wax occlusion in older people. *Practice Nursing, 15,* 290–294.

Rodrigue, N., Cote, R., Kirsh, C., Germain, C., Couturier, C., & Fraser, R. (2002). Meeting the nutritional needs of patients with severe dysphagia following a stroke: An interdisciplinary approach. *AXON, 23*(3), 31–37.

Rodriguez, D. A. (2002). *Conceptualizations of health and illness in Mexican American children, ages 8–12: An ecological perspective.* Phd. Diss., University of California, San Francisco.

Rogers, B. (2005). Looking at lymphoma and leukemia. *Nursing, 35*(7), 56–64.

Rome, K., Handoll, H. G., & Ashford, R. (2005). *Interventions for preventing and treating stress fractures and stress reactions of bone of the lower limbs in young adults.* Retrieved on August 5, 2005, from www.tees.ac.uk.

Rosenberg, M. T., & Hazzard, M. (2005). Prevalence of interstitial cystitis symptoms in women: A population based study in the primary care office. *Journal of Urology, 174*(6), 2231–2234.

Rosenberg, S., Prusiner, S., DiMauro, R., Barchi, E., & Nestler, J. (2003). *The molecular and genetic basis of neurologic and psychiatric disease* (3rd ed.). Philadelphia: Butterworth-Heinemann.

Roth, R. (2007). *Nutrition and diet therapy* (9th ed.). New York: Thomson Delmar Learning.

Rothenhaus, T. (2003, May). *Epistaxis.* Retrieved September 7, 2004, from http://www.emedicine.com/emerg/topic806.htm.

Rothrock, J., McEwen, D., & Smith, D. (Eds.). (2003) *Alexander's care of the patient in surgery* (12th ed.). St. Louis, MO: Elsevier.

Rovig, G. W. (2004). Hearing health risk in a population of aircraft carrier flight deck personnel. *Military Medicine, 169*(6), 429–432.

Rowley, J., & Lorenzo, N. (2004, February). *Obstructive sleep apnea.* Retrieved June 10, 2004, from http://www.emedicine.com/neuro/topics419.htm.

Roxas, M. (2005). Plantar fasciitis: Diagnostic and therapeutic considerations. *Alternative Medicine Review, 10*(2), 83–93.

Roy, C., & Andrews, H. (1991). *The Roy adaptation model: The definitive statement.* Norwalk, CT: Appleton & Lange.

Roy, C., & Andrews, H. (1999). *The Roy adaptation model* (2nd ed.). Stamford, CT: Appleton & Lange.

Royal Victoria Hospital/Montreal. (2006). Retrieved August 31, 2006, from www.royalvictoriahospital/ Montreal.

Rubber ducks at sea. (2003, August 1). *USA Today,* 14A.

Rudnicke, Cheryl. (2003, January/February). Transfusion alternatives. *Journal of Infusion Nursing, 26*(1), 29–33.

Rudy, S., & Parham-Vetter, P. (2003). Percutaneous absorption of topically applied medication. *Dermatology Nursing, 15*(2), 145–152.

Russell, T. (2005). Acute renal failure related to rhabdomyolysis: Pathophysiology, diagnosis, and collaborative management. *Nephrology Nursing Journal, 32*(4), 409–417.

Rybarczyk, B., Edwards, R., & Behel, J. (2004). Diversity in adjustment to a leg amputation: Case illustrations of common themes. *Disability and Rehabilitation, 26*(14), 944–953.

Sackett, D. L., Straus, S. E., Richardson, W. S., Rosenberg, W., & Haynes, R. B. (2000). *Evidence-based medicine: How to practice and teach EBM* (2nd ed.). Edinburgh, UK: Churchill Livingstone.

Sadovich, J. (2005). Work excitement in nursing: An examination of the relationship between work excitement and burnout. *Nursing Economics, 23*(2), 55, 91–96.

Sahn, S. (2004). *Diagnostic thoracentesis.* Retrieved June 25, 2006, from http://www.uptodate.com.

Saiman, L., & Siegel, J. (2003). Infection control recommendations for patients with cystic fibrosis: Microbiology, important pathogens, and infection control practices to prevent patient-to-patient transmission. *American Journal of Infection Control, 31*(3 Suppl), S1–S62.

Saldanha, J., Heath, A., Lelie, N., Pisani, G., & Yu, M.Y. (2005). Collaborative Study Group. A World Health Organization International Standard for hepatitis A virus RNA nucleic acid amplification technology assays. *Vox Sanguinis, 89*(1), 52–58.

Sample, S. (2003). A modern-day Florence Nightingale: Hollie's story. In C. Smeltzer & F. Vlasses (Eds.), *Ordinary people, extraordinary lives: The stories of nurses* (pp. 8–9). Indianapolis, IN: Sigma Theta Tau International.

Sanderlin, B. W., & Raspa, R. F. (2003). Common stress fractures. *American Family Physician, 68*(8), 1527–1532.

Satake, K., Lou, J., & Lenke, L. (2004). Migration of mesenchymal stem cells through cerebrospinal fluid into injured spinal cord tissue. *Spine, 29*(18), 1971–1979.

Satou, G. M., & Herzbert, G. (2004). *Heart failure, congestive.* Retrieved June 24, 2006, from www.emedicine.com.

Saunders, S., & Edwards, B. (2004). How dermatology units can improve psychological wellbeing. *Nursing Standard, 18*(21), 33–37.

Saver, D. F., Demetroulakos, J. L., Groves, M. J., Millman, B., & Mugge, R. E. (2004, September). *Cancer of the larynx.* Retrieved December 20, 2004, from http://www.firstconsult.com.

Saver, D. F., Ferri, F. F., Murray, J. L., & Demetroulakos, J. L. (2004, December). *Sinusitis.* Retrieved December 17, 2004, from http://www.firstconsult.com.

Saver, D. F., Hodgson, J. M., Van Norman, G. A., & Bahler, R. C. (2004). *Mitral stenosis.* Retrieved June 24, 2006, from www.firstconsult.com.

Savoy, N. (2005). Triage decisions. Differentiating stridor in children at triage: It's not always croup. *Journal of Emergency Nursing, 31*(5), 503–510.

Sawaya, G. F., McConnell, K. J., Kulasingam, S. L., Lawson, H. W., Kerlikowske, K., Melnikow, J., et al. (2003). Risk of cervical cancer associated with extending the interval between cervical cancer screenings. *New England Journal of Medicine, 349*(16), 1501–1509.

SBAR technique for communication: A situational briefing model. (2005). Retrieved September 2, 2006[0] from www.ihi.org.

Scarlet, C. (2006). Anaphylaxis. *Journal of Infusion Nursing, 29*(1), 39–44.

Schafer, J. (2003). *Essential medical physiology.* San Diego, CA: Elsevier Academic Press.

Schaffer, S., & Yucha, C. (2004). The relaxation response can play a role in managing chronic and acute pain. *American Journal of Nursing, 104*(8), 75–82.

Scheinman, M., Calkins, H., Gillette, P., Klein, R., Lerman, B., Morady, F., et al. (2003). NASPE policy statement on catheter ablation: Personnel, policy, procedures, and therapeutic recommendations. *Pacing and Clinical Electrophysiology, 26*(3), 789–799.

Scherger, J. E., O'Hanlon, K. M., Jones, R. C., Hodgson, J. M., Bahler, R. C., & Frances, R. J. (2004). *Aortic regurgitation.* Retrieved June 24, 2006, from www.firstconsult.com.

Schieken, L. S. (2002). Asthma pathophysiology and the scientific rationale for combination therapy. *Allergy and Asthma Proceedings, 23*(4), 247–251.

Schleder, B.J. (2003). Taking charge of ventilator-assisted pneumonia. *Nursing Management, 34*(8), 27–32

Schneider, R. A., Miclau, T., & Helms, J. A. (2002). Embryology of bone. In R. H. Fitzgerald, H. Kaufer, & A. L. Malkani (Eds.), *Orthopaedics* (pp. 143–146). St. Louis, MO: Mosby.

Schrag, D., Mitra, N., Xu, F., Rabbani, F., Bach, P. Herr, H., et al. (2005). Cystectomy for muscle-invasive bladder cancer: Patterns and outcomes of care in the Medicare population. *Urology, 65*(6), 1118–1125.

Schrier, R., McFann, K., Johnson, A., Chapman, A., Edelstein, C., Brosnahan, G., et al. (2002). Cardiac and renal effects of standard versus rigorous blood pressure control in autosomal-dominant polycystic kidney disease: Results of a seven-year prospective randomized study. *Journal of the American Society of Nephrology, 13*(7), 1733–1739.

Schriver, J., Talmadge, R., Chuong, R., & Hedges, J. (2003). Emergency nursing historical, current and futures roles, *Journal of Emergency Nursing,* 29, (5).

Schroeder, K., Fahey, T., & Ebrahim, S. (2004). *Interventions for improving adherence to treatment in patients with high blood pressure in ambulatory settings.* The Cochrane Database of Systematic Reviews (2), CD004804.

Schroeter, K. (2003). Ethics in perioperative practice: Patient advocacy. *AORN Journal, 75*(6), 941–949.

Schulder, M., Sernas, T., & Karimi, R. (2003). Thalamic stimulation in patients with multiple sclerosis: Long-term follow-up. *Stereotactic and Functional Neurosurgery, 80*(1–4), 48–55.

Schulz, A., Caldwell, C., & Foster, S. (2003). "What are they going to do with the information?" Latino/Latina and African American perspectives on the Human Genome Project. *Health Education and Behavior, 30*(2), 151–169.

Schuster, P. (2000). Concept mapping: Reducing clinical care plan paperwork and increasing learning. *Nurse Educator, 25*(2), 78–91.

Schutte, D. (2002). Evidence-based protocol: Identification, referral, and support of older adults with genetic conditions. *Journal of Gerontological Nursing, 28*(2), 6–14.

Scileppi, P. A. (2005). *Values for interpersonal communication: How then shall we live?* Belmont, CA: Star Publishing Company, Inc.

Scott, A. N. & Fong, E. (2004). *Body structures and functions* (10th ed.). Clifton Park, NY: Thomson Delmar Learning.

Scully, J. A. (2000). Life event checklists: Revisiting the social readjustment rating scale after 30 years. *Educational and Psychological Measurement, 60*(6), 864–876.

Sedlak, C. A., & Doheny, M. O. (2002). Metabolic conditions. In A. B. Maher, S. W. Salmond, & T. A. Pellino (Eds.), *Orthopaedic nursing* (3rd ed., pp. 423–467). Pitman, NJ: W.B. Saunders Company.

Sellman, S. (2005). Disease of disguise: Learning about lyme. *Canadian Journal of Health and Nutrition, 275*(15), 76–78.

Selye, H. (1956). *The stress of life.* New York: McGraw-Hill.

Selye, H. (1991). History and present status of the stress concept. In A. Monat & R. Lazarus (Ed.), *Stress and coping: An anthology* (pp. 154–168). New York: Columbia University Press.

Seventh Report of Joint National Commission on Prevention, Detection and Treatment of Hypertension (JNC7). (2006). *Hypertension.* Retrieved July 29, 2006, from http://www.cdc/dhhs.

Sever, P. S., Dahlof, B., Poulter, N. R., Wedel, H., Beevers, G., Caulfield, M., et al. (2003). Prevention of coronary and stroke events with atorvastatin in hypertensive patients who have average or lower-than-average cholesterol concentrations, in the Anglo-Scandinavian cardiac outcomes trial-lipid lowering arm (ASCOT-LLA). *Lancet, 361*(9363), 1149–1158.

Shabbir, J., Ridgway, P. F., Lynch, K., Law, C. E., Evoy, D., O'Mahoney, J. B., et al. (2004). Administration of analgesia for acute abdominal pain sufferers in the accident and emergency setting. *European Journal of Emergency Medicine, 11*(6), 309–312.

Shah, R. K., & Shapshay, S. (2003, July). *Acute laryngitis.* Retrieved August 25, 2004, http://www.emedicine.com/ent/topic353.htm.

Shapiro, J., & Bowles, K. (2002). Nurses' and consumers' understanding of and comfort with the patient self-determination act. *Journal of Nursing Administration, 3210,* 503–508.

Sharp Health Care. (2004). (p. 7). Retrieved June 23, 2006, from http://www.sharp.com.

Shatnawi, N., & Bani-Hani, K. (2005). Unusual causes of mechanical small bowel obstruction. *Saudi Medical Journal, 26*(10), 1546–1550.

Shaw, S. (2006). Nursing and supporting patients with chronic pain. *Nursing Standard, 20*(19), 60–66, 68.

Sheehan, C. (2004). *Ambulances may get virtual doctors.* Retrieved July 5, 2006, from http://www.eweek.com.

Sheffield, P., Smith, A., & Fife, C. (2004). *Wound care practices.* Flagstaff, AZ: Best Publishing Company.

Sheikh, A., & Panesar, S.S. (2003). Effective prescribing for rhinitis. *Practice Nurse, 25*(9), 46–50

Sheldon, L. K. (2004). *Communication for nurses: Talking with patients.* Thorofare, NJ: Slack.

Sherman, R. T., & Thompson, R. A (2004). The female athlete triad. *The Journal of School Nursing, 20*(4), 197–202.

Shigehiko, U., Kellum, J., Bellomo, R., Doig, G., Morimatsu, H., Morgera, S., et al. (2005). Acute renal failure in critically ill patients. *Journal of the American Medical Association, 294*(7), 813–818.

Ship, A. N. (2005). Clinical crossroads: Update. A 50-year-old man with hepatitis C and cirrhosis needing liver transplantation, 18 months later. *Journal of the American Medical Association, 293*(16), 128–134.

Shortell, S., & Kaluzny, A. (2000). *Health care management: Organization design and behavior.* New York: Thomson Delmar Learning.

Shriners' Hospitals for Children. (n.d.). *Shrine facts and statistics.* Retrieved August 30, 2005, from http://www.shrinershq.org.

Shuey, K., & Brant, J. (2004). Test your knowledge. Hypercalcemia of malignancy: part II. *Clinical Journal of Oncology Nursing, 8*(3), 321–323.

Sibell, D., Colantonio, A., & Stacey B. (2005). Successful use of spinal cord stimulation in the treatment of severe Raynaud's disease of the hands. *Anesthesiology, 102*(1), 225–227.

Sidani, M., & Campbell, J. (2002). Gynecology: Select topics. *Primary Care, 29,* 297–321.

Sieger, C., Arnold, J., & Ahronheim, J. (2002). Refusing artificial nutrition and hydration: Does statutory law send the wrong message? *Journal of the American Geriatrics Society, 50*(3), 544–550.

Sigma Theta Tau International. *Arista 3 Executive Summary Report.* Retrieved June 23, 2006, from http://www.nursingsociety.org.

Simmons, P. (2003, June). A primer for nurses who administer blood products. *MedSurg Nursing, 12*(6), 184–190.

Simmons, R. (2003). Ablative techniques in the treatment of benign and malignant breast disease. *Journal of the American College of Surgery, 197*(2), 334.

Simms, L. M., Price, S. A., & Ervin, N. E. (2000). *Professional practice of nursing administration* (3rd ed.). Albany, NY: Thomson Delmar Learning.

Sims, J. M. (2003). Guidelines for treating asthma. *Dimensions of Critical Care Nursing, 22*(6), 247–250.

Sims, N., & Baron, R. (2002). Bone: Structure, function, growth and remodeling. In R. H. Fitzgerald, H. Kaufer,

& A. L. Malkani (Eds.), *Orthopaedics* (pp. 147–159). St. Louis, MO: Mosby.

Singh, G. K. & Miller, B. A. (2004). Health, life expectancy, and mortality patterns among immigrant populations in the United States. *Canadian Journal of Public Health, 95*(3), 114–121.

Singh, V. N., Sharma, R. K., Nanda, N. C., Reddy, H., & Strom, J. (2004). *Aortic regurgitation.* Retrieved June 24, 2006, from www.emedicine.com/radio/topic45.htm.

Sisk J. E., Whang, W., Butler, J. C., Sneller V. P., & Whitney, C. G. (2003). Cost effectiveness of vaccination against invasive pneumococcal disease among people 50 through 64 years of age: Role of comorbid conditions and race. *Annals of Internal Medicine, 138*(12), 960–968.

Sismanis, A. (2005). Diagnostic and management dilemma of sudden hearing loss. *Archives of Otolaryngology-Head & Neck Surgery, 131*(8), 733–734.

Skirton, H., & Patch, C. (2002). *Genetics for healthcare professionals: A lifestage approach.* Oxford, UK: BIOS Scientific Publishers Limited.

Sloman, R., Rosen, G., Rom, M., & Shir, Y. (2005). Nurses' assessment of pain in surgical patients. *Journal of Advanced Nursing, 52*(2), 125–132.

Slota, M., Shearn, D., Potersnak, K., & Haas, L. (2003). Perspectives on family-centered, flexible visitation in the ICU setting. *Critical Care Medicine, 31*(5), S362–S366.

Slote, R. J. (2002). Psychological aspects of caring for the adolescent undergoing spinal fusion for scoliosis. *Orthopaedic Nursing, 21*(6), 19–31.

Smith, B., Ivnik, M., Owens, B., McDougall, J., & Dierkhising R. (2005). Use of an interactive health communication application in a patient education center. *Journal of Hospital Librarianship, 5*(1), 41–49.

Smith, D. H., Meaney, D. F., & Shull, W. H. (2003). Diffuse axonal injury in head trauma. *Journal of Head Trauma Rehabilitation, 18,* 307–316.

Smith, H., & Connolly, M. (2003). Evaluation and treatment of dysphagia following stroke. *Topics in Geriatric Rehabilitation, 19*(1), 43–59.

Smith, J. (2006). Debridement of diabetic foot ulcers. *The Cochrane Database of Systematic Reviews* (1), CD003556.

Smith, J. E., & Perez, C. L. (2004, July). *Nasal fractures.* Retrieved August 20, 2004, from http://www.emedicine.com/radio/topic468.htm.

Smith, K., Wallace, A., & Smith-Campbell, B. (2004). What you should know about latex allergy. *Nurse Practitioner, 29*(12), 24.

Snider, G. L. (2003). Nosology for our day: Its application to chronic obstructive pulmonary disease. *American Journal of Respiratory and Critical Care Medicine, 167*(5), 678–683.

Snyder, D. L., Doggett, D., & Turkelson, C. (2004). Treatment of degenerative lumbar spinal stenosis. *American Family Physician, 70*(3), 517–520.

Snyder, M. C., & Lydiatt, W. M. (2003, October). *Glottic cancer.* Retrieved December 20, 2004, from http://www.emedicine.com/ent/topic688.htm.

Sobajima, S., Kim, J., Gilbertson, L., & Kang, J. (2004) Gene therapy for degenerative disc disease. *Gene Therapy, 11*(4), 390–401.

Söderlin, M. K., Börjesson, O., Kautiainen, H., Skogh,T., & Leirisalo-Repo, M. (2002). *Annals of the Rheumatic Diseases, 61*(1010), 911–915.

Soderman, M., Andersson, T., Karlsson, B., Wallace, M. C., & Edner, G. (2003). Management of patients with brain arteriovenous malformations. *European Journal of Radiology, 46*(3), 105–205.

Sole, M., Lamborn, M., & Hartshorn, J. (2001). *Introduction to Critical Care Nursing.* Philadelphia: W. B. Saunders Company.

Soriano-Sarabia, N., Leal, M., Delgado, C., Molina-Pinelo, S., De Felipe, B. Ruiz-Mateos, E., et al. (2005). Effect of hepatitis C virus coinfection on humoral immune alterations in naive HIV-infected adults on HAART: A three year follow-up study. *Journal of Clinical Immunology, 25*(3), 296–302.

Souryal, T., & Adams, K. (2005). *Anterior cruciate ligament injury.* Retrieved on September 29, 2005, from http://www.emedicine.com/pmr/topic3.htm.

Spandorfer, P., Alesandrini, E., Joffe, M., Localio, R., & Shaw, K. (2005). Oral versus intravenous rehydration of moderately dehydrated children: A randomized, controlled trial. *Pediatrics, 115*(2), 295–301.

Spector, R. E. (2004). *Cultural diversity in health and illness* (6th ed.). Upper Saddle River, NJ: Prentice Hall.

Spee, R., & Floyd, N. (2005). The person behind the pain. *Perspectives, 29*(3), 17–20.

Speroff, L., & Clarkson, T. (2003). Is tibolone a viable alternative to HT? *Contemporary OB/GYN, 48,* 54–68.

Spratto, G., & Woods, A. (2003). *PDR nurses' drug handbook.* Clifton Park, NY: Thomson Delmar Learning.

Spratto, G. R., & Woods, A. L. (2007). *2007 PDR Nurse's Drug Handbook.* New York: Thomson Delmar Learning.

Stabile, G., Bertaglia, E., Senatore, G., De Simone, A., Zerbo, F., Carreras, G., et al. (2003). Feasibility of pulmonary vein ostia radiofrequency ablation in patients with atrial fibrillation: A multicenter study. *Pacing and Clinical Electrophysiology, 26,* 284–287.

Stain, S. (2005). Gastrointestinal conditions. *Journal of the American College of Surgeons, 201*(6), 940–947.

Stanford Stroke Awareness. (2002). Stroke Awareness Part II: Diagnosis and treatment options. Retrieved June 24, 2006, from www.stanford.edu.

Stanik-Hutt, J. (2003). Pain management in the critically ill. *Critical Care Nurse, 23*(2), 99–103.

Stanley, M., Blair, K., & Beare, P. (1999). *Gerontological nursing. Promoting successful aging with older adults.* Philadelphia: F. A. Davis.

Stark, P. (2004). *Computed tomographic and positron emission tomographic scanning of pulmonary nodules.* Retrieved June 25, 2006, from http://www.uptodate.com.

Staylor, A. (2005). *Heart failure therapy: Past, present, and future.* Retrieved June 24, 2006, from www.medscape.com.

Steefel, L. (2004). Race against time. *Nursing Spectrum Midwest Edition, 5*(1), 8–9.

Steinberg, G. D., & Kim, H. L. (2005). *Bladder cancer.* Retrieved June 27, 2006, from http://www.emedicine.com/med/topic2344.htm.

Steiner, M., DeWalt, D., & Byerley, J. (2004). Is this child dehydrated? *Journal of the American Medical Association, 291,* 2746–2754.

Stenson, A., Charalambous, T., Divadwa, L., Pemba, L., Du Toit J. D., Baggaley, R., et al. (2005). Evaluation of antiretroviral therapy (ART) related counseling in a workplace base on ART implementation program, South Africa. *AIDS Care, 17*(8), 949–957.

Stetler, C. B., & Marram, G. (1976). Evaluating research findings for applicability in practice. *Nursing Outlook, 24*(9), 559–563.

Stone, P. (2005). ST-segment analysis in ambulatory ECG (AECG or Holter) monitoring in patients with coronary artery disease: Clinical significance and analytic techniques. *Annals of Noninvasive Electrocardiology, 10*(2), 263–278.

Stroud, M., Duncan, H., & Nightingale, J. (2003). Guidelines for enteral feeding in adult hospital patients. *Gut, 52*(Suppl VII), vii1–vii12.

Stuart, G. (2004). *Principles and practice of psychiatric nursing* (7th ed.). St. Louis, MO: Mosby.

Stuart, M., & Nagel, R. (2004). Sickle-cell disease. *Lancet, 364,* 1343–1360.

Stevens, K. R. (2004). *ACE star model of knowledge transformation.* Retrieved May 1, 2005, from www.acestar.uthscsa.edu.

Stewart, E. G., & Spencer, P. (2002). *The V book: A doctor's guide to complete vulvovaginal health.* New York: Bantam.

Stilp, R. (2004). *Biological weapons and emergency preparedness, Part I.* Retrieved June 27, 2006, from http://nsweb.nursingspectrum.com.

Stocking, J. (2005). *Initial assessment and resuscitation.* Retrieved March 5, 2006, from http://www.astna.org.

Struijs, P., & Kerkhoffs, G. (2005, November 1). *Ankle sprain. BMJ Clinical Evidence.* Retrieved November 1, 2006, from http://www.clinicalevidence.com/ceweb/conditions/msd/1115/1115_background.jsp#REF7.

Sunderamoorthy, D., & Chaudhury, M. (2003). An uncommon peripheral nerve injury after penetrating injury of the forearm: The importance of clinical examination. *Emergency Medicine Journal, 20,* 565–566.

Supportive Care Guidelines Group. (2004) Neuro-oncology Disease Site Group. Taos, N.M., Laetsch, N. S., Wong, R. K. S., & Laperriere N. Management of brain metastases: Role of radiotherapy alone or in combination with other treatment modalities [full report]. *Cancer Care Ontario (CCO)* Mar. (35), Practice guideline report; no.13–4.

Svehla, C. J., & Anderson-Shaw, L. (2006). Hospital ethics committees: Is it time to expand our access to managed care organizations? *JONA's Healthcare Law, Ethics, and Regulation, 8*(1), 15–19.

Swartz, C. (2004). *Prevention plan and model for posttraumatic stress disorder (PTSD) from burns.* Retrieved May 1, 2006, from www.journalofburnsandwounds.com.

Swearingen, P., & Keen, J. (2001). *Manual of critical care nursing.* St. Louis, MO: Mosby.

Tablan, O. C., Anderson, L. J., Besser, R., Bridges, C., & Hajjeh, R. (2004). Guidelines for preventing health care-associated pneumonia 2003: Recommendations of CDC and the Healthcare Infection Control Practices Advisory Committee. Retrieved September 16, 2004, from http://www.cdc.gov/.

Talhari, C., Angerstein, W., Becker, J., Ruzicka, T., & Megahed M. (2005). Long-standing oral ulcers. *Lancet, 365*(9463), 1002.

Talley, N. (2005). *Dyspepsia and functional dyspepsia: Unraveling an enigma. Digestive disease week; Functional gastrointestinal disorders.* Retrieved June 25, 2006, from http://www.medscape.com.

Tallia, A. F., & Cardone, D. A. (2003). Diagnostic and therapeutic injection of the ankle and foot. *American Family Physician, 68,* 1356–1362.

Talu, G. K., & Erdine, S. (2005). Intrathecal morphine and bupivacaine for phantom limb pain: A case report. *Pain Practice, 5*(4), 55–57.

Tam, A., & Geier, K. A. Psoriatic arthritis. *Orthopaedic Nursing, 23*(5), 311–314.

Tambor, E., Bernhardt, B., Rodgers, J., Holtzman, N., & Geller, G. (2002). Mapping the human genome: An assessment of media coverage and public reaction. *Genetics in Medicine, 4*(1), 31–36.

Tantravahi, U., & Wheeler, P. (2003). Molecular genetic testing for prenatal diagnosis. *Clinics in Laboratory Medicine, 23*(2), 481–502.

Taricco, M., Adone, R., Pagliacci, C., & Telaro, E. (2004). Pharmacological interventions for spasticity following spinal cord injury. *The Cochrane Database of Systematic Reviews* (2), CD:001131.

Tate, D. M. (2003). Cultural awareness: Bridging the gap between caregivers and Hispanic patients. *Journal of Continuing Education in Nursing, 34*(5), 213–217.

Taylor, S. C., & Altman, G. B. (2004). Administering preoperative care. In G. B. Altman (Ed.), *Delmar's fundamental and advanced nursing skills* (2nd ed., pp. 491–499). Albany, NY: Thomson Delmar Learning.

Terzioglu, F., & Dinc, L. (2004). Nurses' views on their role in genetics. *Journal of Obstetric, Gynecologic, and Neonatal Nursing, 33*(6), 756–764.

Theodorescu, D., & Krupski, T. (2005). *Prostate cancer: Biology, diagnosis, pathology, staging, and natural history.* Retrieved July 31, 2006, from http://www.emedicine.com.

Thomas, B. J., & Powers, R. D. (2002, July). *Pharyngitis, bacterial.* Retrieved September 25, 2004, from http://www.emedicine.com/med/topic1811.htm.

Thomas-Hawkins, C., & Zazworsky, D. (2005). Self-management of chronic kidney disease. Patients shoulder the responsibility for day-to-day management of chronic illness. How can nurses support their autonomy? *American Journal of Nursing, 105*(10), 40–48.

Thompson, B., & Hales, C. (2004). *Clinical manifestations of and diagnostic strategies for acute pulmonary embolism.* Retrieved June 25, 2006, from http://www.uptodate.com.

Thomson Micromedex Healthcare Series. Retrieved July 24, 2005, from www.thomson.com/hcs.

Thurkettle, M. (2003). Shifting the healthcare paradigm: The case manager's opportunity and responsibility. *Case Management, 8*(4), 160–165.

Tierney, L. M., McPhee, S. J., & Papadakis, M. A. (2003). *Current medical diagnosis and treatment* (42nd ed.). Stamford, CT: Lange Medical Books/McGraw-Hill.

Tierney, L. M., McPhee, S. J., & Papakakais, M. A. (2004). *Current medical diagnosis and treatment* (43rd ed.). New York: Lange Medical Books.

Tilton, D. (2006). Central venous access device infections in the critical care unit. *Critical Care Nursing Quarterly, 29*(2), 117–122.

Tolhurst, S., Rapp, D., O'Connor, R., Lyon, M., Orvieto, M., & Steinberg, G. (2005). Complications after cystectomy and urinary diversion in patients previously treated for localized prostate cancer. *Urology, 66*(4), 824–829.

Tolkoff-Rubin, N., Cotran, R., & Rubin, R. (2004). Urinary tract infection, pyelonephritis, and reflux nephropathy. In B. Brenner (Ed.), *Brenner and Rector's the kidney* (7th ed., vol. 2, pp. 423–454). Philadelphia: Saunders.

Tolkoff-Rubin, N., Cotran, R., & Rubin, R. (2004). Urinary tract infection, pyelonephritis, and reflux nephropathy. In B. Brenner (Ed.), *Brenner and Rector's the kidney* (7th ed., vol. 2, pp. 626–631). Philadelphia: W. B. Saunders Co.

Tomey, A. M., & Alligood, M. R. (1998). *Nursing theorists and their work* (4th ed.). St. Louis, MO: C. V. Mosby.

Topf, M., & Thompson, S. (2001). Interactive relationships between hospital patients' noise-induced stress and other stress with sleep. *Heart and Lung, 30*(4), 237–243.

Topol, E. J. (2005). *Acute coronary syndrome.* New York: Marcel Dekker.

Torpy, J. M. (2005). JAMA patient page: Malignant hyperthermia. *Journal of the American Medical Association, 293*(23), 2958.

Toto, R. (2004). Approach to the patient with kidney disease. In B. Brenner (Ed.), *Brenner and Rector's the kidney* (7th ed., vol. 1, pp. 1079–1106). Philadelphia: W. B. Saunders Co.

Townes, D. A. (2004). Biliary tract disease. *Emergency Medicine, 36*(2), 17–19.

Toyoda, H., Kumada, T., Kiriyama, S., Sone, Y., Tanikawa, M., Hisanaga, Y., et al. (2005). Comparison of the usefulness of three staging systems for hepatocellular carcinoma. *American Journal of Gastroenterology, 100*(8), 1764–1771.

Transitions. (2006). *Bernice Neugarten's life times theory.* Retrieved July 25, 2006. from http://www.transitionalonestop.org.

Travis, L. (2005). *Nephrotic syndrome.* Retrieved January 25, 2006, from http://www.emedicine.com.

Trethewey, P. (2004). Systemic lupus erythematosus. *Dimensions of Critical Care Nursing, 23*(3), 111–115.

Tsai, S., Lin, Y., & Wu, S. (2005). The effect of cardiac rehabilitation on recovery of heart rate over one minute after exercise in patients with coronary artery bypass graft surgery. *Clinical Rehabilitation, 19*(8), 843–849.

Tuckett, A. G. (2004). Truth-telling in clinical practice and the arguments for and against: A review of the literature. *Nursing Ethics, 11*(5), 500–513.

Tullman, D. F., & Dracup, K. (2005). Knowledge of heart attack symptoms in older men and women at risk for acute myocardial infarction. *Nursing Research, 25*(1), 33–39.

Tusaie, K., & Dyer, J. (2004). Resilience: A historical review of the construct. *Holistic Nursing Practice, 18*(1), 3–10.

Udeh, E. (2005). Alvimopan: A peripherally selective opioid mu receptor antagonist. *Formulary, 40,* 176–183.

Ullman E. A., Donley L. P., & Brady W. J. (2003). Pulmonary trauma: Emergency department evaluation and management. *Emergency Medicine Clinics of North America, 21*(2), 291–313.

United States Public Health Service. (1990). *Healthy people 2000: National health promotion and disease prevention objective.* [Conference edition summary]. Washington, DC: U.S. Government Printing Office.

The University of Alabama National SCI Statistical Center. (2006). Retrieved July 16, 2006, from http://www.spinalcord.uab.edu.

University of California Los Angeles Library (UCLA). (2004). *Gate Control Theory.* Retrieved from http://www.library.ucla.

University of California San Diego Healthcare (UCSD). (2003). Chronic pain. Retrieved from http://community.healthgate.com.

Uphold C. R., & Graham, M. V. (2003). *Clinical guidelines in adult health* (3rd ed.). Gainesville, FL: Barmarrae Books.

Uren, N., Odbert, R., & Davey, P. (2002). *Heart failure.* Retrieved June 24, 2006, from www.netdoctor.co.uk.

U.S. Bureau of the Census. (2003). *United States—Selected social characteristics.* Retrieved June 17, 2005, from http://servlet/MYPTable.

U.S. Department of Agriculture. (2005). *Dietary guidelines for Americans.* Washington, DC: Author.

U.S. Department of Health and Human Services. (2000). *Healthy People 2010: Understanding and improving health.* Retrieved May 5, 2006, from http://www.healthpeople.gov.

U.S. Department of Health and Human Services. (2000, November). Objectives for improving heart disease and stroke. In *Healthy People 2010 Part A* (2nd ed.). Retrieved June 13, 2006, from http://www.healthypeople.gov.

U.S. Department of Health and Human Services. (2003).*Cancer and the environment* (National Institute of Health Publication No. 03-2039). Retrieved June 10, 2005, from http://www.cancer.gov.

U.S. Department of Health and Human Services. (2004). *HHS Fact Sheet.* Retrieved June 17, 2005, from http://raceandhealth.hhs.gov.

U.S. Department of Health and Human Services. (2005). *Dietary guidelines for Americans.* Washington, DC: Author.

U.S. Department of Health and Human Services, Agency for Health Care Research and Quality. (2002).

Screening for breast cancer, AHRQ Pub. No. 03-507A. Retrieved June 12, 2006, from http://www.ahrq.gov.

U.S. Department of Health & Human Services, Centers for Disease Control and Prevention. (2003). *Recommendations for public health surveillance of syphilis in the United States division of STD prevention March 2003.* Retrieved July 22, 2006, from http://www.cdc.gov.

U.S. Department of Health and Human Services Office of Minority Health. (2000). *National standards for culturally and linguistically appropriate services in health care.* Retrieved June 17, 2005, from http://www.omhrc.gov.

U.S. Food and Drug Administration. (1997). Summaries of "Dear health professional" letters and other safety notifications. Retrieved March 31, 2005, from http://www.fda.gov.

U.S. Food and Drug Administration. (2006). Retrieved from www.fda.gov.

U.S. National Library of Medicine, & National Institute of Health. (2004). *Lung cancer-non small cell.* Retrieved June 30, 2004, from http://www.nlm.nih.gov.

VA Health Care. (n.d.). *Research and development.* Retrieved August 30, 2005, from http://www.1.va.gov/health.

VA Health System. (n.d.). *A history of supporting veterans.* Retrieved August 30, 2005, from http://www.va.gov/history.

VA National Center for Patient Safety. (n.d.). *NCPS.* Retrieved August 3, 2005, from http://www.patientsafety.gov.

Vakil, N., Talley, N., Moayyedi, P., & Fennerty, M. (2005). The diagnostic value of alarm features in predicting upper gastrointestinal malignancy in dyspeptic patients: Systematic review and meta-analysis. *Gastroenterology, 128*(Suppl 2), A80.

Vallerand, A., Reily-Doucet, C. Hasenau, S., & Templin, T. (2004). Improving cancer pain management by homecare nurses. *Oncology Nursing Forum, 31*(4), 809–816.

Vadhan-Raj, S., Schreiber, F., Thomas, L. C., Gandhi, J., Hong, J. J., Gregory, S. A., et al. (2003). Every-2-week darbepoetin alfa improves fatigue and energy rating scores in cancer patients undergoing chemotherapy. *Journal of Supportive Oncology, 1*(Suppl 1), 1–8.

Valk, P., Verhaak, R., Beijen, M., Erpelinck, C., van Doorn-Khosrovani, S., Boer, J., et al. (2004). Prognostically useful gene-expression profiles in acute myeloid leukemia. *New England Journal of Medicine, 350,* 1617–1628.

Values, Ethics and Rationing in Critical Care (VERICC) Task Force. (2005). *ICU cost burdens.* Retrieved from http://www.vericc.org.

Van Campen, L., Morata, T., Kardous, C., Gwin, K., Wallingford, K., Dallaire, J., et al. (2005). Ototoxic occupational exposures for a stock car racing team: I. Noise surveys. *Journal of Occupational & Environmental Hygiene, 2*(8), 383–390.

Van Dijk, M., Peters, W., & van Deventer, P. (2005). The COMFORT behavior scale. *American Journal of Nursing, 105*(1), 33–35.

Van Ophoven, A., Pokupic, S., Heinecke, A., & Hertle, L. (2004). A prospective, randomized, placebo controlled, double-blind study of amitriptyline for the treatment of interstitial cystitis. *Journal of Urology, 172*(2), 533–536.

Varcoe, C. (2002). 'The thief of womanhood': Women's experience of polycystic ovarian syndrome. *Social Science and Medicine, 54,* 349–361.

Varricchio, C. (2004). *ACS: A cancer source book for nurses* (8th ed.). Sudbury, MA: Jones and Bartlett Publishers.

Vavilala, M. S., Bowen, A., Lam, A. M., Uffman, J. C., Powell, J., Winn, H. R., et al. (2003). Blood pressure and outcome after severe pediatric traumatic brain injury. *Journal of Trauma: Injury, Infection and Critical Care, 55*(6), 1030–1044.

Verive, M. (2004). Hypokalemia. What are the causes of hypomagnesemia? [Electronic version]. *Journal of Family Practice, 54,* 174–176.

Vermeulen, H., Ubbink, D., Goossens, A., de Vos, R., & Legemate, D. (2006). Dressings and topical agents for surgical wounds healing by secondary intention. *The Cochrane Database of Systematic Reviews* (1), CD003554.

Verschuur, E., Homs, M., Steyerberg, E., Haringsma, J., Wahab, P., Kuipers, E., et al. (2006). A new esophageal stent design (Niti-S stent) for the prevention of migration: A prospective study in 42 patients. *Gastrointestinal Endoscopy, 63*(1), 134–140.

Veterans Affairs. (n.d.). *Veteran data and information.* Retrieved August 30, 2005, from http://www.va.gov/data.

Vetere, P., Putterman, S., & Kesselman, E. (2003). Major reconstructive surgery for pelvic organ prolapse in elderly women, including the medically compromised. *Journal of Reproductive Medicine, 48*(6), 417–421.

Vrabec, J. (2003). Herpes simplex virus and Meniere's disease. *Laryngoscope, 113*(9), 1431–1438.

Vuckovic, S., Gardiner, D., Field, K., Chapman, G. V., Khalil, D., Gill, D., et al. (2004). Monitoring dendritic cells in clinical practice using a new whole blood single-platform TruCOUNT assay. *Journal of Immunological Methods, 284*(1–2), 73–87.

Vorenberg, S. (2005, April 11). Chemicals released by brain signal pain. *San Diego Union-Tribune,* pp. 1–6 (from Scripps Howard News Service.).

Wagner, L. I., & Cella, D. (2004). Fatigue and cancer: Causes, prevalence, and treatment approaches. *British Journal of Cancer, 91*(5), 822–828.

Wahlgren, N. G., & Ahmed, N. (2004). Neuroprotection in cerebral ischemia: Facts and fancies-the need for new approaches. *Cerebrovascular Disease, 17*(Suppl 1), 153–166.

Waites, K. B., Canupp, K. C., Armstrong, S., & DeVivo, M. J. (2004). Effect of cranberry juice on bacteriuria and pyuria in persons with neurogenic bladder secondary to spinal cord injury. *Journal of Spinal Cord Medicine, 27*(1), 35-40.

Wakata, N., Nemoto, H., Sugimoto, H., Nomoto, N., Konno, S., Hayashi, N., et al. (2004). Bone density in myasthenia gravis patients receiving long-term prednisolone therapy. *Clinical Neurology and Neurosurgery, 106,* 139–141.

Wallach, E., & Vlahos, N. (2004). Uterine myomas: An overview of development, clinical features, and management. *Obstetrics and Gynecology, 104,* 393–406.

Walsh, C. (2005). Multiple organ dysfunction syndrome after multiple trauma. *Orthopaedic Nursing, 24*(5), 324–335.

Walsh, D., Nelson, K. A., & Mahmoud, F. A. (2003). Established and potential therapeutic applications of cannabinoids in oncology. *Support Care Cancer, 11,* 137–143.

Walters, R. (2005). What's a nurse to do? How the Health Insurance Portability and Accountability Act of 1996 impacts a nurse's (or any other healthcare provider's) ex parte discussion of protected health information in medical malpractice cases. *JONA's Healthcare Law, Ethics, and Regulation, 7*(1): 21–34.

Walton, B., & Thorton, T. (2003). Female sexual dysfunction. *Current Women's Health Reports, 3,* 319–326.

Wang, K., Wongkeesong, M., & Buttar, N. (2005). American gastroenterological association medical position statement: Role of the gastroenterologist in the management of esophageal carcinoma. *Gastroenterology, 128*(2), 1468–1470.

Wang, Y., Prentice, L. F., Vitetta, L., Wluka, A. E., & Cicuttini, F. M. (2004). The effect of nutritional supplements on osteoarthritis. *Alternative Medicine Review, 9*(3), 275–296.

Waninger, K. (2004). Management of the helmeted athlete with suspected cervical spine injury. *The American Journal of Sports Medicine, 32*(20), 1331–1350.

Ward, M. M. (2002). Predictors of the progression of functional disability in patients with ankylosing spondylitis. *Journal of Rheumatology, 29*(7), 1420–1425.

Warm, E., & Weissman, D. (2002, March). *The legal liability of undertreatment of pain. Fast facts and concepts #63. End-of-life physician resource center.* Retrieved May 17, 2005, from www.eperc.mcw.edu.

Watkins, L. O. (2004). Epidemiology and burden of cardiovascular disease. *Clinical Cardiology, 27*(6 Suppl 3), 2–6.

Watkinson, S. (2005). Visual impairment in older people: The nurse's role. *Nursing Standard, 19*(17), 45–52, 54.

Watret, L. (2005). Teaching wound management: A collaborative model for future education. *World Wide Wounds, 8*(15), 13–16.

Watson, D., & Rivkin, A. (2004, July). *Rhinoplasty, septoplasty.* Retrieved September 7, 2004, from http://www.emedicine.com/ent/topic128.htm.

WBC (nuclear) scan. (2003, October 17). *Medical Tests and Procedures.* Retrieved September 2, 2004, from http://www.mercksource.com.

Weiger, W., & Eisenberg, D. (2002). *Easing the treatment.* Retrieved May 25, 2006, from www.keepmedia.com.

Weijer, C., & Miller, P. (2004). Protecting communities in pharmacogenetic and pharmacogenomic research. *Journal of Pharmacogenomics, 4*(1), 9–16.

Weil, A. (2005). *Healthy aging: A lifelong guide to your physical and spiritual well-being.* New York: Alfred Knopf.

Weiss, G., Skurnick, J. H., Goldsmith, L. T., Santoro, N. F., & Park, S. J. (2004). Menopause and hypothalamic-pituitary sensitivity to estrogen. *Journal of the American Medical Association, 292,* 2991–2996.

Weiss, J. (2005). A journey in holistic growth. *Journal of Holistic Nursing, 23*(4), 434–440.

Wells, C. (2003). Optimizing nutrition in patients with chronic kidney disease. *Nephrology Nursing Journal, 30*(6), 637–648.

Welsh, S., & Veenstra, M. (2004). *Shoulder dislocations.* Retrieved on September 26, 2005, from http://www.emedicine.com/orthoped/topic440.htm.

Wener, K. (2004). *Endocarditis.* Retrieved June 24, 2006, from www.nlm.nih.gov.

Westerbrook, G.J. (2005, May 23). Methadone for pain management. *Nurseweek,* pp. 8–9.

Wheaton, J., & Pinkstaff, S. (2006). Atherosclerotic vascular disease and diabetes in the older adult part I: Understanding pathogenic mechanisms and identifying risk factors. *Clinical Geriatrics, 14*(1), 17–24, 25.

Wheeler, P., & Batt, M. E. (2005). Do non-inflammatory drugs adversely affect stress fracture healing? A short review. *British Journal of Sports Medicine, 39*(2), 65–69.

White, G. (2005). *Equipment theory for respiratory care* (4th ed.). Clifton Park, NY: Thomson Delmar Learning.

White, L., & Duncan, G. (2002). *Medical-surgical nursing: An integrated approach* (2nd ed.). New York: Thomson Delmar Learning.

White, R. D. (2004). Hyperthyroidism: Current standards of care. *Consultant, 44*(8), 24–27.

Whiteman, M. K., Staropoli, C. A., Benedict, J. C., Borgeest, C., & Flaws, J. A. (2003). Risk factors for hot flashes in midlife women. *Journal of Women's Studies, 12*(5), 459–472.

Whitman, S. C., Rateri, D. L., Szilvassy, S. J., Yokoyama, W., & Daugherty, A. (2004). Depletion of natural killer cell function decreases atherosclerosis in low-density lipoprotein receptor null mice. *Arteriosclerosis, Thrombosis, and Vascular Biology, 24*(6), 1049–1054.

Whitney, J., & Parkman, S. (2004). The effect of postoperative physical activity on tissue oxygen and wound healing. *Biological Research in Nursing, 6*(2), 79–89.

Whittle, A. P. (2003). Malunion of fractures. In S. T. Canale (Ed.), *Campbell's operative orthopaedics* (vol. 3, 10th ed., pp. 3071–3124). Philadelphia: Mosby.

Whyte, J., Hart. T., Vaccaro, M., Grieb-Neff, P., Risser, A., Polansky, M., et al. (2004). Effects of methylphenidate on attention deficits after traumatic brain injury. *American Journal of Physical Medicine and Rehabilitation, 83*(6), 401–420.

Wilbanks, B., Wakim, J., Daicoff, B., & Monterde, S. (2005). Hyperkalemia-induced residual neuromuscular blockade: A case report. *AANA Journal, 73*(6): 437–441.

Wilkes, G. (2004). Anemia in cancer care. *CancerSourceRN.* Retrieved June 10, 2005, from http://www.cancersourcern.com.

Wilkinson, C. (2005). Interventions for asymptomatic retinal breaks and lattice degeneration for preventing retinal detachment. *The Cochrane Database of Systematic Reviews (Oxford)* (4), ID #CD003170.

Wilkinson, J. M. (2005). *Nursing diagnosis handbook.* Upper Saddle River, NJ: Prentice Hall.

Williams, R. (2006). Have your say. *Nursing Management, 13*(4), 38.

Wills Eye. (n.d.a). *Pioneering technology.* Retrieved August 2, 2005, from http://www.willseye.org.

Wills Eye. (n.d.b). *Charitable giving.* Retrieved August 2, 2005, from http://www.willseye.org.

Wilson, B.A., Shannon, M.T., & Stang, C.L. (2005). *Nurses drug guide.* Upper Saddle River, NJ: Pearson–Prentice Hall.

Wilson, C., Anderson, D., Toms, S., Fleetwood, J. & Phelps, J. (2006). Family-witnessed resuscitation in a family-centered critical care unit. *American Journal of Critical Care, 15*(3), 343–344.

Wilson, J. (1973). *Environment and birth defects.* New York: Academic Press.

Wilson, L. M. (1999). Healthy people—a new millennium: Progress and comparison on the Healthy People 2000 and Healthy People 2010 objectives. *JONAs Healthcare Law, Ethics, and Regulation, 1*(2), 29–32.

Winearls, C. (2003). Clinical evaluation and manifestations of chronic renal failure. In R. Johnson & J. Feehally (Eds.), *Comprehensive clinical nephrology* (2nd ed., pp. 857–871). St. Louis, MO: Mosby.

Winegarden, C. (2005). From "prehypertension" to hypertension? Additional evidence. *Annals of Epidemiology, 15*(9), 720–725.

Winer, N., & Sowers, J. R. (2004). Epidemiology of diabetes. *Journal of Clinical Pharmacology: Incidence of Diabetes, 44,* 397–405.

Winslow, C., & Rozovsky, J. (2003). Effect of spinal cord injury on the respiratory system. *American Journal of Physical Medicine and Rehabilitation, 82,* 803–814.

Winters, B. D., & Dorman, T. (2006). Rapid response teams. *Contemporary Critical Care, 4*(3):1–10.

Wisniewski, A. (2003). Chronic bronchitis and emphysema: Clearing the air. *Nursing, 33*(5), 46–49.

Withrow, S. (2004). *Healthcare IT: Adopt guidelines for electronic consultations.* Retrieved June 25, 2006, from CNET_Networks_Member_Services@newsletter.online.com.

Witt, M. E., Haas, M., Marrinan, M. A., & Brown, C. N. (2003). Understanding stereotactic radiosurgery for intracranial tumors, seed implants for prostate cancer, and intravascular brachytherapy for cardiac restenosis. *Cancer Nursing, 26*(6), 494–502.

Wittig, J. C., Bickels, J., Priebat, D., Jelinek, J., Kellar-Garney, K., Shmookler, B., et al. (2002). Osteosarcoma: A multidisciplinary approach to diagnosis and treatment. *American Family Physician, 65*(6), 1123–1132.

Wlnlk, L.W. (2006, January 8). Who works hardest. Intelligence Report, *Parade,* 20.

Wojnicki-Johansson, G. (2001). Communication between nurse and patient during ventilator treatment: Patient reports and RN evaluations. *Intensive and Critical Care Nursing, 17*(1), 29–39.

Wong, P. F., Gilliam, A. D., Kuman, S., Shenfine, J., O'Dair, G. N. & Leaper, D. J. (2005). Antibiotic regimens for secondary peritonitis of gastrointestinal origin in adults. *The Cochrane Database of Systematic Reviews* (2), CD004539.

Woodruff, D. (2006). Deciphering diagnostics. Take these 6 easy steps to ABG analysis. *Nursing Made Incredibly Easy! 4*(1), 4–7.

Woods, A. (2004). Loosening the grip of hypertension. *RN, 34*(12), 36–43.

Workowski, K., & Levine, W. (2002). *Sexually transmitted disease guidelines 2002.* Retrieved August 30, 2004, from http://www.cdc.gov.

World Health Organization. (2002). *World health report 2002: Reducing risks, promoting health lifestyles.* Geneva Switzerland. Retrieved September 18, 2006, from www.who.org.

World Health Organization. (2004a). Breakthrough (episodic) vs. baseline (persistent) pain in cancer. (Interview with Dr. S. Mercadante). *Cancer Pain Release, 17*(4).

World Health Organization. (2004b). *Stroke now and in the future.* Retrieved June 12, 2006, from http://www.who.int.2.

World Health Organization. (2005a). *Palliative care.* Retrieved May 18, 2005, from www.who.int/about/en/.

World Health Organization. (2005b). *The world health report 2000—Health systems: Improving performance.* Retrieved March 21, 2005, from www.who.int/whr/2000.

World Health Organization. (2006). (p. 13). Retrieved June 23, 2006, from http://www.who.int.

Worley, C. (2004). Assessment and terminology: Critical issues in wound care. *Dermatology Nursing, 16*(5), 451–452, 457.

Worley, C. (2005). "So, what do I put on this wound?" Making sense of the wound dressing puzzle: Part I. *Dermatology Nursing, 17*(2), 143–144.

Wormald, R., Evans, J., Smeeth, L., & Henshaw K. (2005). Photodynamic therapy for neovascular age-related macular degeneration. *The Cochrane Database Systematic Reviews (Oxford)* (4), ID #CD002030.

Wozniak, R. H. (1992). *Mind and body: René Descartes to William James.* Bethesda, MD and Washington DC: National Library of Medicine and American Psychological Association.

Wright, C., Kerzin-Storrar, L., Williamson, P., Fryer, A., Njindou, A., Quarrell, O., et al. (2002). Comparison of genetic services with and without genetic registers: Knowledge, adjustment, and attitudes about genetic counseling among probands referred t three genetic clinics. *Journal of Medical Genetics, 39*(12), 84.

Wright, L. (2005). *Spirituality, suffering, and illness: Ideas for healing.* Philadelphia: F. A. Davis.

Wright, P. E. (2003). Carpal tunnel, ulnar tunnel, and stenosing tenosynovitis. In S. T. Canale (Ed.), *Campbell's operative orthopaedics* (vol. 3, 10th ed., pp. 3761–3778). Philadelphia: Mosby.

Writing Group for the Women's Health Initiative Investigators. (2002). Risks and benefits of estrogen plus progestin in healthy postmenopausal women: Principal results from the Women's Health Initiative randomized controlled trial. *Journal of the American Medical Association, 288,* 321–333.

Yamada, Y. (2005). *Handbook of gastroenterology* (2nd ed.). Philadelphia: Lippincott, Williams & Wilkins.

Yang, C., Wang, H., Wang, Z., Du, H., Tao, D., Mu, X., et al. (2005). Risk factors for esophageal cancer: A case-control study in South-western China. *Asian Pacific Journal of Cancer Prevention, 6*(1), 48–53.

Yeates, E., Singer, M., & Morton, A. (2004). Salt and water: A simple approach to hyponatremia. *Journal of the Canadian Medical Association, 170*(3), 365–369.

Yellen, E. A., & Ricard, R. (2005). The effect of a preadmission videotape on patient satisfaction. *AORN Journal, 81*(4), 831–840, 842, 845.

Yezierksi, R., Radson, E., & Vanderah, T. (2004). Understanding chronic pain. *Nursing, 34*(4), 22–23.

Yoshitatsu, S., Sambuughin, N., & Muldoon, S. (2004). Malignant hyperthermia genetic testing in North America working group meeting. *Anesthesiology, 100*(2), 464–465.

Young, M. (2003). Preparing dermatology nurses: Biologic therapies for psoriasis. *Dermatology Nursing, 15*(2), 413–423.

Yueh, B., Shapiro, N, MacLean, C. H., & Shekelle, P. (2003). Screening and management of adult hearing loss in primary care: Scientific review. *JAMA, 289*(15), 1976–1985.

Zavarella, M., Leblebicioglu, B., Claman, L., & Tatakis, D. (2006). Unilateral severe chronic periodontitis associated with ipsilateral surgical resection of cranial nerves V, VI, and VII. *Journal of Periodontology, 77*(1), 142–148.

Zepf, B. (2003). Exercise prescription for patients with claudication. *American Family Physician, 67*(5), 1072.

Zevitz, M. E. (2004). *Heart failure.* Retrieved June 24, 2006, from www.emedicine.com.

Zorn, K. E. (2001). Infections. In D. C. Schoen (Ed.), *NAON: Core curriculum for orthopaedic nursing* (4th ed., pp. 189–204). Pitman, NJ: Anthony J. Jannetti, Inc.

Index

Page numbers followed by "f" denote figures and "t" denote tables. Page numbers followed by "b" indicate boxed text.

A

- A waves, 581
- Abatacept, 1440t, 1441
- Abbreviations
  - drug administration, 490
  - mechanical ventilation, 590t
- Abdomen
  - acute. *See* Acute abdomen
  - assessments of
    - general, 1578–79
    - physical examination, 1755
    - postoperative, 697–98
  - auscultation of, 1579, 1580t, 1581
  - hematological disorders and, 745t
  - inspection of, 1580t, 1658
  - palpation of, 1579f, 1582
  - percussion of, 1580t, 1581–82
  - postoperative assessments of, 697–98
  - quadrants of, 1580t–1581t
- Abdominal pain, 1572, 1577, 1579t, 1656–58
- Abdominal paradox, 981
- Abdominal thrusts, for airway obstruction, 1043
- Abdomino-perineal resection, 1684
- Abducens nerve, 1146f, 1147t, 1152–53
- Abduction, 1944f
- Abetalipoproteinemia, 1711
- Ability to learn, 51
- Ablation
  - arrhythmias treated with, 867
  - endometrial, 2093–94
  - laser, 2153–54
  - radiofrequency, 1724
  - tumor, 1798
- ABO system, 362–63, 737
- Abrasions, corneal, 1336
- Abscess
  - breast, 2142
  - definition of, 1075, 1512
  - hepatic, 1719–21
  - lung, 1075–78
  - peritonsillar, 1036–37
  - skin, 1512
- Absence seizures, 222, 521, 1271
- Absent breath sound, 1000t
- Absolute hypovolemia, 2212
- Absolute neutrophil count, 431
- Absolute reticulocyte count, 747t
- Absorption
  - of carbohydrates, 1650
  - of drugs, 484
  - of fats, 1649–50
  - of nutrients, 1596–98, 1648–51
  - of proteins, 1650–51
- Abuse
  - burns caused by, 1540
  - domestic, 1183
  - elder, 132, 1183, 1202
- Acarbose, 1916t
- Accessory nerve, 1146f, 1147t, 1154
- Accessory respiratory muscles, 975–76
- Acculturation, 71–72
- ACE Star Model of Knowledge Transformation
  - clinical practice guidelines, 32
  - definitions, 30
  - description of, 28–29
  - evidence summary, 31
  - premises of, 30, 30b
  - schematic diagram of, 25f
  - stages of, 31–32
- Acetaminophen, 474t
- Acetohexamide, 527–28, 1916t
- Acetylcholine, 1138, 1939
- Achalasia, 1574, 1628
- Achilles tendon injuries, 2026–27
- Acid-base balance
  - compensatory mechanisms, 987
  - description of, 328–29, 986–87
- Acid-base imbalances
  - causes of, 988t
  - compensatory mechanisms, 987
  - metabolic acidosis, 330t–331t, 332–33, 989, 2205b
  - metabolic alkalosis, 331t, 333, 988f, 988t
  - respiratory acidosis, 329–31, 988f
  - respiratory alkalosis, 330t, 332
- Acidemia, 985, 988
- Acidosis
  - metabolic, 330t–331t, 332–33, 989, 2205b
  - respiratory, 329–31, 988f
- Acini cells, 1699
- Acne, 1506–7
- Acoustic nerve, 1146f, 1147t, 1154
- Acoustic neuroma, 1196, 1366
- Acquired hemolytic anemia, 932
- Acquired immunity, 1381
- Acromegaly, 1866–69
- Actin filaments, 1938
- Actinic keratosis, 1481, 1520–21
- Action potential, 837
- Activated partial thromboplastin time, 512–13, 2043
- Active euthanasia, 114
- Activities of daily intake
  - nutrition effects on, 62
  - sleep effects on, 62
- Activities of daily living, 181
- Acupressure, 387, 1264
- Acupuncture
  - Bell's palsy treated with, 1251
  - description of, 386–87
  - tension-type headaches treated with, 1264
- Acute abdomen
  - assessment of, 1656–59
  - definition of, 1654
  - diagnostic tests, 1659–61
  - epidemiology of, 1654–55
  - etiology of, 1655
  - imaging modalities for, 1660t
  - laparoscopy for, 1662
  - laparotomy for, 1662
  - medical conditions that cause, 1661–62
  - mortality from, 1654
  - nursing diagnoses, 1661
  - outcomes, 1663–64
  - pain associated with, 1656–57
  - pathophysiology of, 1655–56
  - during pregnancy, 1663
  - surgical treatment of, 1662–63
  - treatment of, 1661–63
- Acute adrenal crisis, 1877
- Acute appendicitis. *See* Appendicitis
- Acute circulatory failure. *See* Shock syndrome
- Acute colonic pseudo obstruction
  - colonoscopic decompression of, 1674
  - description of, 1669
  - etiology of, 1670
- Acute coronary syndromes
  - alternative therapies for, 796
  - assessment of, 792
  - cardiac rehabilitation, 796–97
  - case study of, 799–800
  - complications of, 791–92
  - definition of, 775, 790
  - diagnostic tests for, 792–93
  - discharge instructions, 796, 798t
  - family teaching about, 796–97
  - incidence of, 790
  - intra-aortic balloon pump for, 796, 796f–797f
  - nursing diagnoses for, 793–94
  - outcomes, 797–98
  - pain associated with
    - description of, 755t
    - management of, 794
  - pathophysiology of, 791–92
  - patient teaching about, 796–97
  - planning and implementation for, 794–97
  - population-based care, 795–96
  - surgery for, 796
- Acute lymphocytic leukemia, 950, 954–56
- Acute myeloid leukemia, 950, 954, 956–57
- Acute myocardial infarction
  - complications of, 791
  - creatine kinase levels, 793
  - discharge instructions, 796, 798t
  - idioventricular rhythm caused by, 859
  - pharmacologic agents for, 794–95
  - treatment of, 794
- Acute otitis externa, 1318–19, 1319f
- Acute pain
  - description of, 457, 464
  - inflammation, 274–75
  - management of, 468–69
- Acute pancreatitis, 1736–38
- Acute pharyngitis, 1031–34
- Acute phase response, 1395
- Acute pulmonary edema, 809
- Acute renal failure
  - alterations in, 1828t
  - assessment of, 1826–27
  - definition of, 1824
  - diagnostic tests, 1826
  - epidemiology of, 1824
  - etiology of, 1824, 1825t
  - family education about, 1831–32
  - hypervolemia in, 1829
  - intrarenal causes of, 1826
  - nursing diagnoses, 1826
  - nutritional considerations, 1830
  - outcomes, 1832
  - pathophysiology of, 1826
  - patient education about, 1831–32
  - postrenal causes of, 1826
  - prerenal causes of, 1826
  - treatment of
    - collaborative, 1827, 1829
    - continuous renal replacement therapy, 1827, 1827b
    - evidence-based, 1829–30
    - goals, 1827
    - nutrition, 1830
    - surgery, 1831
- Acute respiratory distress syndrome (ARDS), 2225–27, 2256
- Acute sinusitis
  - antibiotics for, 1027–28
  - assessment of, 1026
  - complications of, 1026
  - decongestants for, 1028
  - description of, 1025
  - diagnostic tests, 1026–27
  - epidemiology of, 1025
  - etiology of, 1025
  - nursing diagnoses, 1027
  - outcomes, 1029
  - pathophysiology of, 1025–26
  - population-based care, 1028

symptoms of, 1026t
treatment of, 1027–28
Acute stress disorder, 250
Acute tubular necrosis, 1825t
Adalimumab, 1439, 1440t
Adams Bending Forward Test, 2000
Adaptation, 249, 251
Adaptation model, 255–56, 262f
Addiction, 159–60
Adduction, 1944f
Adducts, 1709b
A-delta fibers, 1577
Adenoiditis, 1034–36
Adenomas, 1196, 1864
Adenosine
arrhythmias treated with, 862
exercise testing using, 765
Adhesion, 285
Adhesion molecules, 1392, 1840
Adjuvant therapy
colorectal cancer treated with, 1685
description of, 419
in older adults, 476
pain management, 472, 474t
Adolescents
brain injuries in, 1182t
gender differences, 191
health assessment of, 187
risk behaviors by, 252
skin in, 1481
Adrenal cortex, 1855–56
Adrenal glands
description of, 1855–56
hypersecretion of, 1879–83
hyposecretion of, 1876–79
Adrenal insufficiency, 1876–79
Adrenal medulla, 1855
Adrenal tissue transplantation, 1284t
Adrenergic stress response, 241
Adrenocorticotropic hormone, 1851t, 1852, 2206
Adult(s)
development of
Levinson's theory of, 122, 122t
stages of, 122–23
theories of, 122–23
health assessment of, 187
nursing responsibilities in care of, 138
older. *See* Older adults
Adult daycare, 544–45
Advance directives
definition of, 151
description of, 193
discussion about, 149–50
legislation regarding, 104–5
living will, 105, 149, 151
purpose of, 105
surrogate decision maker, 106–7
verbal, 106
Advanced cardiac life support, 870–71
Advanced practice nurses
in hospice care, 152
in palliative care, 152
Adventitious breath sounds, 1000–1002
Adverse effects, 485
Advocate, 101–2, 192
Aerophagia, 1576
Affective domain, of learning, 46, 47t
Affective learning, 721
Affinity maturation, 1399
African Americans
biological variations in, 84t
death beliefs, 147t
demographics of, 72b, 73
folk medicine used by, 83t
food preferences, 85t
hypertension in, 190, 909
multiple myeloma in, 961
Afterdepolarizations, 846
Afterload, 569, 752
Agency (ethics), 97
Agency for Healthcare Research and Quality
description of, 9, 33, 536
evidence summaries from, 35, 36b
systematic reviews from, 35
Age-related macular degeneration, 1310, 1332–33
Ageusia, 1153
Agglutination, by antibodies, 1390
Aging
cardiovascular system changes, 491, 753
coronary artery disease and, 771, 795
endocrine system affected by, 1856
hearing loss associated with, 1357
hematological system changes associated with, 743
immune system changes associated with, 1402t
muscular system affected by, 1939–40
musculoskeletal changes associated with, 1003
pharmacokinetic changes caused by, 491
photoaging vs., 1504, 1505t
respiratory system changes, 993, 1002–4
skeleton affected by, 1938
systemic changes associated with, 133–34, 1402t
Aging population
description of, 125–26
of nurses, 126
nutritional considerations, 188, 1615
Agonists, 471
Agranulocytosis, 498, 948
AIDS
health disparities, 79b
in homeless persons, 81t
AIDS-dementia complex, 1428
Air embolus, 360
Air flow, in operating room, 670
Air pollution, 1118t
Air trapping, 1101
Airborne transmission
description of, 276–77
precautions for, 280t, 281
Airway(s)
artificial, 697
endotracheal intubation for, 584–85
head positioning for, 583
jaw thrust method for establishing, 583
nasal, 584
oral, 583–84
postoperative care of, 697
tracheostomy for, 585
Airway obstruction
abdominal thrusts for, 1043
description of, 869
Airway pressure release ventilation, 589
Akinesia, 1281
Alanine transaminase, 1700
Albumin
cirrhosis effects on, 1713
definition of, 1698
functions of, 365
transfusion of, 365
for wound healing, 288–89
Albuterol
asthma treated with, 1120
chronic obstructive pulmonary disease treated with, 1112
description of, 1077
Alcohol consumption
blood pressure affected by, 918
breast cancer and, 2148
corticosteroids and, 1405
by diabetes mellitus patients, 1911
hypertension and, 910
quantity of, 1713b
Alcoholic cirrhosis, 1711–12
Alcoholic hepatitis, 1709
Aldolase, 1975
Aldosterone, 1855
Aldosterone receptor blockers, 923t
Alendronate, 1991t
Alkalemia, 985
Alkaline phosphatase, 1988
Alkalosis
metabolic, 331t, 333
respiratory, 330t, 332
Allele, 199
Allen's test, 571
Allergen responses, 1458
Allergens, 1450, 1455t
Allergic contact dermatitis, 1465, 1508–9
Allergic rhinitis
assessment of, 1018–19
in children, 1019
complications of, 1023–24
definition of, 1018
diagnostic tests, 1020
environmental considerations, 1020, 1021b
nursing diagnoses, 1020, 1464
occupational, 1019t
outcomes, 1023, 1465
pathophysiology of, 1018
perennial, 1019t
seasonal, 1019t
treatment of
antihistamines, 1021–22, 1022t
evidence-based, 1020
pharmacological, 1021–23
Allergies. *See also* Asthma
assessment of, 1404, 1409
atopy vs., 1453
clinical findings of, 1409
definition of, 1404, 1450, 1464
description of, 223
diagnostic tests, 1452
drug-related, 1404
food, 181, 637, 1404, 1468–69
genetic factors, 223–25, 1450
immunoglobulin E and, 223–24, 1118–19, 1451
to insulin, 1917
latex. *See* Latex allergy
nursing diagnoses, 1452
pathophysiology of, 1450–52
preoperative discussion about, 637
sensitizing agents, 1453–54, 1455b
sinusitis vs., 1026t
Allodynia, 451
Allogeneic transplantation
bone marrow, 426, 952
definition of, 951
Allograft, 1552
Allograft transplantation, 1431
Aloe vera, 393t, 395t
Alopecia, 438
Alpha-adrenergic blockers, 509
Alpha1-antitrypsin enzyme deficiency
description of, 1102, 1711
treatment of, 1112
Alpha-fetoprotein, 213–14
Alpha-glucosidase inhibitors, 1915, 1916t
Alport syndrome, 1820–21
Alternative medicine. *See* Complementary and alternative medicine
Altruism, 9
Aluminum acetate solutions, 1501
Alveolar dead space, 983
Alveolar ventilation, 982–83
Alvimopan, 1670
Alzheimer's disease
assessment of, 1286
brain findings, 1286, 1286t
caregiver stress, 254
definition of, 1285
description of, 134
diagnosis of, 222
diagnostic tests, 1286
early-onset, 221
epidemiology of, 1285
etiology of, 1285–86
familial, 221
genetic factors, 221–22
late-onset, 221
nursing diagnoses, 1287
nutritional concerns, 1288
outcomes, 1288–89
pathophysiology of, 1286, 1286t
progression of, 1286
risk factors for, 1285
stages of, 1286, 1287t
treatment of, 1288
Amantadine, 1278t, 1283t
Amblyopia, 1324
Ambulation
by burn patients, 1558
postoperative, 715, 716b
terminology associated with, 716b
Ambulatory infusion pumps, 345
Amenorrhea, 1865, 2089, 2097
American Association of Colleges of Nursing
description of, 11
Peaceful Death document, 143
professional practice, 551
synergy model adapted by, 552
American Association of Critical Care Nurses, 560
American Holistic Nurses Association, 385
American Joint Committee on Cancer, 407
American Lung Association, 538–39
American Medical Association, 116
American Nurses Association
assisted suicide views of, 150
Code of Ethics, 99, 99b, 684
American Nurses Credentialing Center, 560
American Society of Anesthesiologists, 677
American Spinal Injury Association, 1220–21
Americans with Disabilities Act, 230, 543–44
Amiloride, 923t
Aminoglycosides, 495–98
4-Aminopyridine, 1226
Amitriptyline, 474t, 1278t, 2129
Amlodipine, 924t
Amniocentesis, 212–13
Amoxicillin, 1074
Amphiarthrosis, 1940
Amphotericin B, 1072
Amputation
ankle-brachial index, 2045
assessment of, 2044

definition of, 1943, 2043
diagnostic tests, 2045
epidemiology of, 2043
etiology of, 2044
exercise after, 2048–49
family education about, 2045–46
hematoma concerns, 2044
management of, 2045–49
mangled extremity severity score, 2045, 2046t
nursing diagnoses, 2045
outcomes, 2049
pathophysiology of, 2044
patient education about, 2045–46
phantom limb sensations after, 2048
prosthesis, 2046
psychological considerations, 2045
rehabilitation after, 2048–49
stump care, 2046–48
Amsler Grid, 1332
Amygdaloid body, 1142
Amylase, 1597, 1739
Amyloid deposits, 1825t
Amyotrophic lateral sclerosis, 1292–94
Anabolism, 1599
Anaerobic metabolism, 775, 2204, 2205b
Analgesia
deep, 677
description of, 1157
nurse-controlled, 346
patient-controlled. *See* Patient-controlled analgesia
Analgesics
myths and misconceptions regarding, 158–59
nonopioid, 470, 474t
opioid. *See* Opioid analgesics
pain management uses of, 157–59
physical dependence to, 159
tolerance to, 158–59
toxicity of, 475–76
Anaphylactic shock, 494, 1462b, 2218–20
Anaphylaxis
allergens that cause, 1463
assessment of, 1462
in cancer patients, 442
clinical manifestations of, 1463t
to contrast agents, 1802
definition of, 494, 1453, 2239
description of, 1460
epidemiology of, 1460–61
etiology of, 1453–62
pathophysiology of, 1462
risk factors for, 1453b
treatment of, 1462–63, 1463t–1464t
Anasarca, 1485, 1785
Anastomosis, 1674
Androgen deprivation therapy, 423
Androgens, 2058
Anemia
assessment of, 931
cancer-related, 430–31
classification of, 431
definition of, 430, 930
diagnostic tests for, 931
epidemiology of, 930
etiology of, 930
folic acid deficiency, 937–38
hemolytic
acquired, 932
definition of, 932
glucose-6-phosphate dehydrogenase, 933–34
hereditary spherocytosis, 934
pathophysiology of, 930
sickle cell anemia, 225–26, 934–36, 1173t
thalassemia, 933
hypoproliferative, 931
hypovolemic shock and, 932
iron deficiency, 936–37, 1607
nursing diagnoses, 931
nutritional, 936–40
outcomes, 932
pathophysiology of, 930–31
planning and implementation for, 931–32
sickle cell, 225–26, 934–36
signs and symptoms of, 430–31
symptoms of, 931
vitamin B12 deficiency, 938–40
Anergy tests, 1417
Anesthesia
definition of, 677, 1157
epidural, 678t
general
description of, 677, 678t
malignant hyperthermia risks, 683
hypothermia associated with, 681
local, 678t
neurological function recovery after, 725
recovery from, 693–95
regional, 678t
risks of, 678–80
spinal, 678t
Anesthesia care provider, 677
Anesthesiologist, 656
Aneuploidy, 200
Aneurysms
assessment of, 890
classification of, 889, 889f
definition of, 888
diagnostic tests for, 890
dissecting, 889, 889f
epidemiology of, 888
etiology of, 888–89
false, 889
fusiform, 889, 889f
inflammatory, 889
mechanical, 889
mycotic, 889
nursing diagnoses for, 890
pathophysiology of, 889–90
rupture risks, 757
saccular, 889, 889f
stroke caused by, 1172
syndromes associated with, 888–89
treatment of, 890–93
ventricular, 791
Angina pectoris. *See also* Chest pain
assessment of, 776–77, 991
differential diagnoses, 777
electrocardiography evaluations, 777–78
grading of, 777t
Levine's sign, 776
patient education about, 781
precipitating factors, 776
Prinzmetal's variant, 775
silent, 775, 795
stable, 774
types of, 502, 774–75
unstable, 502, 775
Angiogenesis
definition of, 406
in metastasis, 407
tumor, 407
Angiography
cerebral, 1162–63
computed tomography, 1006
coronary
cardiovascular system assessments, 764
coronary artery disease evaluations, 780
nursing management during, 765–66
digital subtraction, 1163
magnetic resonance
description of, 1162
stroke evaluations, 1175t
musculoskeletal system evaluations, 1948–49
pulmonary, 1005–6
Angioneurotic edema, 1467–68
Angiopathy, 1922–23
Angiotensin I, 301, 2206
Angiotensin II, 301, 509, 2206
Angiotensin II receptor antagonists, 510
Angiotensin receptor blockers
description of, 784
heart failure treated with, 809
hypertension treated with, 924t
Angiotensin-converting enzyme, 912, 1753
Angiotensin-converting enzyme inhibitors
administration of, 511b
coronary artery disease treated with, 782t, 784
heart failure treated with, 809
hypertension treated with, 924t
mechanism of action, 509–10, 784
nonsteroidal anti-inflammatory drugs effect on, 511
Angiotensinogen, 301, 2206
Angle of Louis, 975
Anion gap, 333
Anions, 298
Ankle sprain, 2024–25
Ankle-brachial index, 885, 2045
Ankylosing spondylitis, 1221, 1972
Annular lesions, 1490b
Annuloplasty, 830, 831f
Anorexia
cancer-related, 435
signs and symptoms of, 435
Anorgasmia, 2127
Anosmia, 1152
Anovulation, 1865, 2089
Antacids, 1630
Antecubital fossa, 341
Anterior axillary fold, 977
Anterior chamber, 1302
Anterior cord syndrome, 1220, 1220t
Anterior cruciate ligament
anatomy of, 2020
tear of, 2020–21
Anterior drawer test, 2025, 2025f
Anterior pituitary gland, 1852, 1853f
Anthrax, for biological warfare, 2254–55
Antianginal agents, 502–4
Antiarrhythmic agents
arrhythmogenic right ventricular cardiomyopathy treated with, 817
hypertrophic cardiomyopathy treated with, 814
Antibiotic resistant organisms, 271
Antibiotics
acute sinusitis treated with, 1027–28
bronchiolectasis treated with, 1074–75
chronic obstructive pulmonary disease treated with, 1113
chronic sinusitis treated with, 1030
lung abscess treated with, 1077
pneumonia treated with, 1061
polycystic kidney disease treated with, 1819
Antibodies
agglutination by, 1390
B cell release of, 1389
definition of, 1389
effector functions of, 1398
immunoglobulin A, 1400
mechanism of action, 1390
monoclonal, 1432
neutralization by, 1390
opsonization by, 1390
production of, 1382
screening tests for, 1413
Antibody-dependent cell-mediated cytotoxicity, 1388
Anticholinergics
chronic obstructive pulmonary disease treated with, 1111
description of, 640
Anticholinesterase agents, 1291
Anticipatory grieving, 156
Anticipatory nausea and vomiting, 434
Anticipatory stress, 250
Anticoagulants
acute coronary syndromes treated with, 795
in blood collection tube, 745–46
definition of, 511
heart failure treated with, 810
heparin, 511–12
indications for, 511–12
laboratory monitoring of, 512
pharmacokinetics of, 512
pulmonary arterial hypertension treated with, 1091
Antidepressants, 472
Antidiabetic agents
insulin, 526–27
oral hypoglycemic agents, 527–28
Antidiuretic hormone
description of, 301–2
functions of, 1851t, 1852
hyponatremia and, 307, 314
osmolarity effects on, 912
renal effects of, 599
renal production of, 1852
urinary incontinence and, 1808
Antidysrhythmics, 504–6
Antiemetics, 421, 434, 473, 1198
Antiepileptic drugs, 1272, 1273t
Antifolates, 1772b
Antifungals, 1499t
Antigen, 1382, 1433, 1450
Antigen tests, 1415
Antigen-presenting cells, 223, 1385, 1392, 1396, 1478
Antihistamines
allergic rhinitis treated with, 1021–22, 1022t
interstitial cystitis treated with, 1776b
Ménière's disease treated with, 1253
Antihyperlipidemics, 810
Antihypertensive agents
indications for, 510
laboratory monitoring of, 510
nursing management of, 510–11
overview of, 508–10
types of, 922–23, 923t–924t
Anti-infective agents
aminoglycosides, 495–98
bactericidal, 492
bacteriostatic, 492
cephalosporins
administration of, 495b
adverse effects of, 494
generations of, 493
indications for, 493

laboratory monitoring of, 494
mechanism of action, 493
nursing management for, 494–95
pharmacodynamics of, 493–94
pharmacokinetics of, 493
side effects of, 494
urinary tract infections treated with, 1772b
clinical uses of, 492
fluoroquinolones, 495–98
macrolides, 495–98
penicillins
administration of, 495b
adverse effects of, 494
extended-spectrum, 493
glomerulonephritis treated with, 1783
indications for, 493
laboratory monitoring of, 494
mechanism of action, 492–93
nursing management for, 494–95
pharmacodynamics of, 493–94
pharmacokinetics of, 493
side effects of, 494
urinary tract infections treated with, 1772b
sulfonamides, 498–99
tetracyclines, 495–98
Antilipidemics
adverse effects of, 515
bile acids, 514–16
fibric acid derivatives, 514–15
HMG-CoA reductase inhibitors, 514
indications for, 514
laboratory monitoring of, 515
mechanism of action, 513–14
pharmacokinetics of, 515
side effects of, 515
Antineoplastics, 419, 1499t
Antinuclear antibodies, 1413, 1416b, 1417, 1442
Antioxidants
cancer prevention and, 408
dietary sources of, 392
Antiparasitics, 1499t
Antiplatelet agents
coagulation affected by, 744
heart failure treated with, 810
stroke treated with, 1176
Antipruritics, 1499t
Antiseizure drugs
adverse effects of, 522
barbiturates, 521–22
benzodiazepines, 521–22
carbamazepine, 521–22
hydantoins, 521–22
indications for, 521–22
laboratory monitoring of, 522
mechanism of action, 520
nursing management for, 523
pharmacokinetics of, 522
side effects of, 522
succinimides, 521–22
valproic acid, 521–22
Antiseptics, 1499t
Antithrombin III, 512
Antiulcer agents
histamine2 antagonists, 524–25
overview of, 523–25
proton pump inhibitors, 524–25
Antivirals, 1499t
Anuria, 1826
Anus, 1571
Anxiety
assessment of, 182
in critically ill patients, 565–66
in endotracheal intubation patients, 596–98
in hospice patients, 155, 164
management of, 164
in palliative care patients, 155, 164
Anxiolysis, 677
Anxiolytics, 162
AORN. *See* Association of Perioperative Registered Nurses
Aortic dissection, 888–93
pain associated with, 755t
Aortic valve
description of, 750
regurgitation of, 827–28
stenosis of, 828–30
Apgar assessment, 186
Aphakic vision, 1328
Aphasia, 1187b, 1199–1200
Apheresis, 426, 1432
Apical area, 757
Aplastic anemia, 498
Apnea, obstructive sleep, 1038–40
Apneustic breathing, 996
Apocrine glands, 1477t, 1478
Apo-ferritin, 738
Apolipoprotein E
Alzheimer disease and, 221
cardiovascular disease and, 217–18
Apoprotein, 514
Apoptosis, 1389, 1642
Appendectomy, 1666
Appendicitis
assessment of, 1665
classification of, 1665t
definition of, 1664
diagnostic tests, 1665–66
nursing diagnoses, 1666
outcomes, 1666
pain associated with, 1665
pathophysiology of, 1664–65
during pregnancy, 1663
Rovsing's sign, 1665b
signs of, 1581, 1655
treatment of, 1666
Appendix, 1571
Appetite stimulants, 436–37
Appraisal-transaction theory, 244
Aqueous pitressin, 1875
Arachnoid, 1139–40
Arcus senilis, 1305
ARDS. *See* Acute respiratory distress syndrome
Areola, 2138–39
Aromatherapy, 394–95
Arrhythmias
after acute myocardial infarction, 791
atrial, 849–52
atrial fibrillation, 500, 851–52, 1173t
atrial flutter, 850–51, 851f, 863
atrial tachycardia, 850
causes of, 845–46
definition of, 835
electrocardiography detection of, 845, 845b
heart block. *See* Heart block
junctional escape rhythm, 853
junctional rhythms, 852–53
nursing management of, 861t
premature atrial complexes, 849–50
premature junctional complexes, 852–53
premature ventricular complexes, 856f, 856–57
sinus, 848–49
sinus bradycardia, 847f, 847–48
sinus rhythms, 846–49
sinus tachycardia, 848, 848f
supraventricular tachycardia, 852, 863
torsades de pointes, 858
treatment of
ablation therapy, 867
adenosine, 862
beta blockers, 862
calcium channel blockers, 862
defibrillation, 862–64
overview of, 860–61
pacemakers. *See* Pacemakers
pharmacological, 861–62
ventricular, 856–58
ventricular fibrillation, 858–60
ventricular tachycardia, 857–58, 871
Arrhythmogenic right ventricular cardiomyopathy, 816–17
Arterial blood gases
analysis of, 987–89
description of, 333, 334b
monitoring of, 590, 1835
sampling of, 1004
Arterial occlusive disease, 885–88
Arterial system, 880f
Arteries, 340
Arteriosclerosis, 878
Arteriovenous fistula, 1836
Arteriovenous malformation, 1181
Arteriovenous nicking, 1309
Arthritis
description of, 272
osteoarthritis. *See* Osteoarthritis
psoriatic, 1973–74
rheumatoid. *See* Rheumatoid arthritis
Arthrography, 1949
Arthrometry, 1951
Arthroscopy
description of, 1951
rotator cuff tears treated with, 2013
Artificial nutrition and hydration, 113
ASA scale, 705, 705t
Asbestos, 1078
Ascending cholangitis, 1730
Ascending sensory tracts, 1144
Ascites, 1713
Ascorbic acid, 391t
Asepsis
scrub technique for, 673
of surgical environment, 664
Asian Americans
biological variations in, 84t
demographics of, 72b, 73
folk medicine used by, 83t
food preferences, 85t
Aspartate, 1138
Aspartate transaminase, 1699–1700
Aspergillosis, 1070
Aspiration
bone marrow, 1951–52
definition of, 998
joint, 1952
Aspirin
coronary artery disease treated with, 784
pain management using, 470
stroke treated with, 1178
Assessments. *See also specific condition or disorder, assessment of*
cultural, 86–88
definition of, 174
nurse's role in, 554–55
postoperative, 695
preoperative, 632–33
Assisted living facilities, 545
Assisted suicide, 115, 150
Association for the Advancement of Medical Instrumentation, 668
Association of Perioperative Registered Nurses (AORN)
description of, 659
sterilization recommendations, 668
Astereognosis, 1158
Asthma
albuterol for, 1120
assessment of, 1120, 1121b, 1456–57
atopic, 1456–60
bronchial, 225
chest x-rays of, 1122
classification of, 1119t
complications of, 1119–20
corticosteroids for, 1120
death caused by, 1120, 1126, 1456
definition of, 1116, 1455
description of, 126–27, 1100
diagnostic tests, 1120, 1122, 1457
emergency management of, 1127
epidemiology of, 1116–17, 1456
etiology of, 1117, 1117t–1118t, 1456
exacerbation of, 1116
family education about, 1124, 1126
hospitalization for, 1126
hypoxemia associated with, 1122
inflammatory nature of, 271–72
management of, 272, 1125t, 1127, 1457–60
nursing diagnoses, 1122, 1457
outcomes, 1126, 1460
pathophysiology of, 1117–20, 1456
patient education about, 1124, 1126
peak flow meter assessments, 1123, 1123f, 1456
pharmacological treatment of, 1123–24, 1459, 1459t
population-based care, 1124
prevention of, 1455
pulmonary function testing for, 1120, 1122
severe, 1119t, 1122
signs and symptoms of, 1120, 1460
symptoms of, 1455–56
triggers for, 1117t–1118t, 1457
Astigmatism, 1337
Astrocytes, 1138
Astrocytoma, 1196
Asystole, 860, 860f
Ataxia, 1156
Atelectasis, 565
Atenolol, 782t, 924t
Atherogenesis, 773–74
Atherosclerosis
assessment of, 879
definition of, 770, 878
diagnostic tests for, 879, 881
epidemiology of, 878
etiology of, 878
family education about, 883–84
genetic factors, 879
nursing diagnoses for, 881b
outcomes, 884
pathophysiology of, 774, 878–79
patient education about, 883–84
plaque formation and progression, 774
progression of, 878f
risk factors for, 878

stroke risks, 1173b
treatment of
alternative therapies, 883
evidence-based care, 881
exercise programs, 884
goals, 881
health care resources, 882–83
nutrition, 881–82
pharmacological, 882, 882t
Atopic dermatitis, 1466, 1507–8
Atopy
anaphylaxis and, 1461b
definition of, 1101–2, 1451, 1453
Atracurium, 597t
Atrial arrhythmias, 849–52
Atrial fibrillation, 500, 851–52, 1173t
Atrial flutter, 500, 850–51, 851f, 863
Atrial natriuretic peptide, 301
Atrial tachycardia, 850
Atrioventricular node, 836
Atrioventricular valves, 822
Atrium
left, 749
rhythm of, 843
right, 749
Atrophic gastritis, 1641
Atrophy, 1489f
Atropine sulfate, 848
Atypical glandular cells of undetermined significance, 2104–6
Audiometer, 1361
Auditory brainstem evoked potentials, 1166t
Auditory dysfunction. *See also* Ear(s)
cholesteatoma, 1360
complications of, 1358–76
diagnostic tests, 1360–61
hearing loss. *See* Hearing loss
mastoiditis, 1360
nursing care for, 1374–75
nursing diagnoses, 1362
otitis media. *See* Otitis media
otosclerosis, 1360
outcomes, 1375–76
surgical treatment of, 1364–65
treatment of, 1362–76
Auditory evoked potentials, 1166t
Auditory learners, 50
Augmentation mammoplasty, 2144–46, 2157, 2157f
Aura, 1267
Auricle, 1311
Auricular pain, 1316
Aurothioglucose, 1439, 1440t
Auscultation
of abdomen, 1579, 1581
breath sounds
adventitious, 1000–1002
normal, 999–1000
cervical, 1624
definition of, 184
of heart, 758
of lungs, 1756
respiratory system, 999–1002
Autism, 216
Autoantibodies
definition of, 1453
tests for, 1413, 1416b
Autograft, 1552
Autoimmune disorders
definition of, 2231
description of, 1405, 1433
hormonal supplementation, 1433–34
pathophysiology of, 1433
progressive systemic sclerosis, 1444–45
rheumatoid arthritis. *See* Rheumatoid arthritis
Sjögren's disease, 1409, 1441
systemic lupus erythematosus, 1409, 1441–44, 1781
tissues and organs affected by, 1433
Autoimmune hepatitis, 1710
Autoimmunity, 1434
Autologous transplantation
bone marrow, 425–26, 952
description of, 951, 1432
Autolytic debridement of wounds, 287, 1498
Automatic external defibrillators, 869–70
Automaticity
arrhythmias caused by enhancement of, 846
definition of, 837
Automobile driving, 137
Autonomic dysreflexia, 1229–31
Autonomic nervous system
description of, 452–53, 1145
functions of, 464
in stress response, 242
Autonomic neuropathies, 1926–27
Autonomy
definition of, 371
genetics application of, 230–32
informed consent and, 103
medical futility and, 115
principle of, 97, 192t, 229t
Autosomal dominant inheritance, 204
Autosomal recessive inheritance, 204, 205f
Autosomes, 198
Avascular necrosis, 2037
Axillary line, 753
Axis, 838
Axon, 1137
Ayurveda, 377–78
Azathioprine, 1689, 1840, 1843t
Azelastine, 1023t
Azithromycin, 1113
Azoospermia, 2078
Azotemia, 1833

B

B cell(s)
activated, 1398
assays, 1427b
description of, 741, 1389–90
B cell receptor, 1381, 1389, 1398
B waves, 582
Babinski reflex, 1229, 1229t
Babinski's sign, 1159
Baby boomers, 125–26
Bacillus anthracis, 2254
Bacillus Calmette-Guérin vaccine, 424, 1069, 1404
Back pain, 458b, 460
Back rubs, 389
Baclofen, 1235, 1278t
Bacteria
classification of, 492
description of, 271t, 492
gram-negative, 492
gram-positive, 492
Bacterial endocarditis, 818–20
Bacterial vaginosis, 2077, 2101
Bactericidal agents, 492, 667t
Bacteriostatic agents, 492, 667t
Bag-mask ventilation, 867
Balanitis, 2186–87
Balanoposthitis, 2186–87
Balloon dilatation, for achalasia, 1628
Balloon valvuloplasty, 830
Bandura, Albert, 45t, 52
Barbiturates, 521–22
Bariatric surgery, 130, 1614
Bariatric therapy, 642–43
Barium enema, 1592, 1680t
Barium studies, 1591
Baroreceptors, 300–301, 751, 912
Barotrauma, 594–95, 1120
Barrel chest, 755, 756t, 994, 1003
Barrett's esophagus, 1629–30
Bartholin's glands, 2063, 2076, 2102
Basal body temperature, 2082–83
Basal cell carcinoma, 1521
Basal cells, 1477t
Basal ganglia, 1141–42
Basal metabolic rate, 1600
Baseline data, 183
Basic life support
airway obstruction, 869
automatic external defibrillators, 869–70
cardiopulmonary resuscitation
chest compressions, 868
definition of, 867
external compressions with, 868
rescue breathing, 867–68
steps in, 868–69
certification in, 870
training in, 867
Basophils
description of, 266t, 267, 736f, 1388
diagnostic tests, 1411
functions of, 741
Battle's sign, 1316
Beclomethasone dipropionate, 1023t
Belief systems, 182
Belladonna, 395t
Bell's palsy, 1250–52
Benazepril, 924t
Beneficence, 97, 192t, 229t, 371
Benign, 405
Benign migratory glossitis, 1621–22
Benign prostatic hypertrophy, 1751, 2056–57, 2166–69
Benign tumors, 1195
Bentham, Jeremy, 98
Benzodiazepines
antiseizure uses of, 521–22
anxiety treated with, 596
pain management uses of, 472
Benztropine, 1283t
Bereaved
definition of, 147
support for, 168
Beta2 agonists
asthma treated with, 1123–24
description of, 517
Beta blockers
adverse effects of, 503–5
angina pectoris treated with, 502–3
antidysrhythmic uses of, 504–5
arrhythmias treated with, 862
coronary artery disease treated with, 781–83, 782t
heart failure treated with, 810
hypertension treated with, 509, 924t
Beta cells, 405
Beta thalassemias, 226
Beta-adrenergic agents, 517
Beta-carotene, 392
Bethanechol, 1278t
BHR, 225
Bicarbonate buffer system, 328
Biceps reflex, 1158
Biguanides, 527–28, 1915, 1916t
Bile, 1698–99
Bile acids, 514–16
Bile duct cancer, 1735–36
Bile salts, 1700
Biliary cirrhosis, 1711–12, 1733–35
Biliary tract, 1698–99, 1729
Biliary tract diseases
cholecystitis, 1732–33
cholelithiasis, 1729–32
description of, 1655, 1729
primary sclerosing cholangitis, 1733
signs of, 1729
Bilirubin, 740, 747t, 1697, 1698b
Bill of rights
of dying patients, 148, 149b
of patients, 48, 100
Bioavailability, 484
Biofeedback, 382–83, 921
Biological response modifiers, 432
Biological therapies
cancer treated with, 424–25
mechanism of action, 424
parenteral administration of, 424
side effects of, 425
Biological warfare
agents used in
anthrax, 2254–55
Ebola virus, 2252–54
identification of, 2247
overview of, 2247
plague, 2251–52
severe acute respiratory syndrome, 2255–57
smallpox, 2249–51
West Nile Virus, 2257–59
clinical presentations in, 2247b
epidemiological investigation, 2247
history of, 2246
isolation guidelines, 2248t
triage from, 2249
Biomechanical debridement of wounds, 287
Biomedical engineer, 1207t
Biopsy
bone marrow, 1951–52
brain tumor, 1197–98
breast cancer evaluations, 2149–51
cancer, 413
complete, 1415
core needle, 2150–51
definition of, 1415
fine needle aspiration, 2150
image guided core needle, 2150
lung, 1011
open, 2150–51
partial, 1415
prostate, 2079
purpose of, 413
renal, 1760–61, 1762b
sentinel lymph node, 2154–55
skin, 1415–16
stereotactic, 2151
testicular, 2079
thyroid, 1860
Biotechnology, 3
Biotransformation, 485
Biot's breathing, 996
Biperiden, 1283t
Biphenotypic leukemia, 950

Bisphosphonates
description of, 323
osteoporosis treated with, 1984
Paget's disease treated with, 1990, 1991t
Bitter taste, 1153
Bladder
abnormalities of, 1756b
anatomy of, 1749–50, 1750f
assessment of, 1583, 1756
asymmetrical, 1756b
capacity of, 1750
catheterization of, 1757
detrusor muscles of, 1750
trigone of, 1750
urinary retention, 1757, 1804–5
Bladder cancer
assessment of, 1799
diagnostic tests, 1799–1800
epidemiology of, 1798–99
etiology of, 1799
incidence of, 403t
nursing diagnoses, 1800
outcomes, 1801
pathophysiology of, 1799
surgical treatment of, 1800–1801
treatment of, 1800–1801
types of, 1798
Bladder catheter, 629–30
Bladder elimination, in spinal cord injury patients, 1232
Bladder neck, 1750–51
Bladder outlet obstruction, 1760t
Bladder training, 1807
Blast injuries, 2259–60
Blastomycosis, 1069
Bleeding time, 747t
Blended family, 77t
Blepharitis, 1340
Blindness, 1344–45
Blood. *See also* Plasma
cellular components of, 735
description of, 734
granulocyte concentration in, 740
packed red blood cells, 363–64
renal filtering of, 911
whole, 363
Blood donation, 625–26
Blood flow, 751
Blood pressure. *See also* Hypertension
age-related changes, 909
alcohol consumption effects, 918
arterial, 752
caffeine effects, 910, 918–19
classification of, 773t, 912–13, 913t
definition of, 907
diastolic, 911
diuretics effect on, 509
exercise effects on, 921
hormonal effects on, 509
measurement of
description of, 753
factors that affect, 915t
in minority populations, 509
monitoring of, 1818
postoperative maintenance of, 697
in stroke patients, 1178
systolic, 911
vasomotor center regulation of, 508–9
weight loss effects on, 916
Blood specimens, 746, 746t
Blood transfusion
albumin, 365
burns treated with, 1530
colloids, 365
cryoprecipitate, 364
crystalloids, 365–66
description of, 362
granulocytes, 364–65
informed consent for, 365
platelets, 364
process of, 366b
refusal of, 1543
risks associated with, 365–66
Blood types, 362–63, 363t
Blood urea nitrogen, 303, 914, 1754, 1759t
Blood-brain barrier
chemotherapy passage, 1204
description of, 1143
Blue bloaters, 1103
Blumberg's sign, 1581
Body image, 437
Body mass index, 124, 916–17, 1612b, 1678
Body substance isolation, 279
Body surface area
in cardiac index calculations, 568
chemotherapy administration based on, 419
intravenous therapy calculations based on, 353
Body temperature. *See also* Thermoregulation
inflammation effects on, 274
intraoperative management of, 682
measurement of, 274
normal, 698
Body water, 296
Body weight. *See also* Obesity
intravenous therapy calculations based on, 353
regulation of, 1613
Body work therapies
description of, 387–88
reflexology, 389–90
rolfing, 389
shiatsu, 389
Bone
cells of, 1936
functions of, 1938
physiological processes of, 1937
remodeling of, 1937
repair of, 1937–38, 1983f
resorption of, 1935
structure of, 1935–36
types of, 1935t
Bone marrow
biopsy of, 413
harvesting of, 426
hematopoietic cells from, 425
white blood cell production in, 266
Bone marrow aspiration and biopsy, 1951–52
Bone marrow transplantation
allogeneic, 426, 952
autologous, 425–26, 952, 1432
bone marrow sources, 226
cancer treated with, 425–27
description of, 1432
graft-versus-host disease, 426–27, 1432
Hodgkin's disease treated with, 966
leukemia treated with, 951–52
side effects of, 426
Bone scan, 1949
Bony labyrinth, 1312
Borborygmi sounds, 1644, 1658
Borborygmus, 1576
Boric acid solutions, 1502
Borrelia burgdorferi, 1967
Bosentan, 1091
Botox injections, 130, 1628
Bouchard's nodes, 1957, 1957f
Bowel elimination, in spinal cord injury patients, 1232
Bowman's capsule, 1751
Brachial plexus, 1254
Brachytherapy, 416, 418, 1081, 2171
Braden Pressure Scale, 287, 287t
Bradycardia
management of, 871–72
sinus, 847f, 847–48, 871–72
Bradykinesia, 1281
Bradykinin, 510
Bradypnea, 995
Brain
anatomy of, 452f
basal ganglia, 1141–42
blood flow to, 1174
cerebrum, 1140, 1141f
diencephalon, 1142–43
gyrus, 1140, 1141f
herniation of, 580
hypophysis, 1143
lobes of, 1142, 1142f
ventricles, 1141
Brain cancer, 403t
Brain death, 113–14, 1185t
Brain injuries
in adolescents, 1182t
assessment of, 1186–89
behavioral symptoms of, 1187b
in children, 1182t
clinical manifestations of, 1186, 1187b, 1188f
closed, 1183–84
cognitive symptoms of, 1187b
complications of, 1185–86
computed tomography of, 1189–90
concussion, 1185, 1188f
contusions, 1184, 1188f
coup/contracoup, 1188f
diagnostic tests, 1189–90
in elderly, 1182t
epidemiology of, 1182
etiology of, 1182t, 1182–83
from falls, 1183
family education about, 1193
glucose utilization affected by, 1184
headaches after, 1186
health care costs of, 1182
hydrocephalus secondary to, 1185
level of consciousness assessments, 1192
magnetic resonance imaging of, 1190
management of
body temperature monitoring, 1193
cerebral perfusion pressure monitoring, 1193
collaborative, 1192
goals, 1192
intracranial pressure monitoring, 1193
oxygen levels, 1193
pharmacological, 1194
procedures for, 1192–93
surgery, 1193
moderate, 1185
motor vehicle accidents as cause of, 1190–91
nursing diagnoses, 1190
open, 1183
outcomes, 1193–94
pathophysiology of, 1184–86
physical signs and symptoms of, 1187b
planning and implementation for, 1190–94
prevention of, 1190–91
primary, 1183
secondary, 1183
severity of, 1185, 1185t
signs and symptoms of, 1187b
sports-related, 1182–83, 1191
stroke caused by, 1186
traumatic
definition of, 1183
etiology of, 1183
types of, 1183–84
Brain mapping, 1205
Brain tumors
adenomas, 1196
assessment of, 1196–97
astrocytoma, 1196
benign, 1195
biopsy of, 1197–98
central nervous system lymphoma, 1196
chemotherapy for, 1204
computed tomography of, 1197
decision-making abilities affected by, 1199
description of, 1195
diagnostic tests, 1197–98
epidemiology of, 1195
etiology of, 1195
glioma, 1196
headache caused by, 1196–97
home discharge after, 1203
impulsiveness caused by, 1199
magnetic resonance imaging of, 1197
malignant, 1195
memory impairments associated with, 1199
meningiomas, 1196
metastasis, 1196
mobility limitations, 1200
nursing diagnoses, 1198
outcomes, 1207
pathophysiology of, 1195–97
planning and implementation for, 1198–1207
primary, 1195
problem-solving abilities affected by, 1199
schwannomas, 1196
secondary to, 1195–96
self-care deficits secondary to, 1201
sensory-perceptual deficits secondary to, 1201
treatment of
chemotherapy, 1198–99
craniotomy, 1205
gene therapy, 1204
health care provider for, 1198
pharmacological, 1204–5
photodynamic therapy, 1204–5
radiation therapy, 1206
rehabilitation after, 1206–7, 1207t
surgery, 1205–6
Brainstem, 452f
Brainstem auditory evoked response test, 1361
Brash water, 1630
BRCA-1, 219, 403, 2121
Breakthrough pain, 462–63
Breast(s)
adolescence changes, 2137
anatomy of, 2063–64, 2136–37
augmentation of, 2144–46
examination of, 2075–76, 2138–39
hormonal effects on, 2137
lymph node palpation, 2139
maturational changes in, 2137–38
menopausal changes, 2138

nipple of, 2063
palpation of, 2139
physiology of, 2136–37
pregnancy-related changes, 2137–38
pubertal changes, 2137
reduction of, 2146
shape of, 2136
Breast cancer
alcohol consumption and, 2148
diagnostic tests
biopsy, 2149–51
mammography, 2149
ultrasound, 2149
ductal carcinoma in situ, 2155
epidemiology of, 2147
estrogen and, 423
etiology of, 2147–48
incidence of, 403t
nursing diagnoses, 2151
obesity and, 2148
pathophysiology of, 2148
racial predilection, 2147
risk factors for, 410t, 2147–48
smoking and, 2148
staging of, 2148
treatment of
axillary dissection, 2155
cryotherapy, 2153
herceptin, 2152
laser ablation, 2153–54
lumpectomy, 2153
lymphatic mapping, 2154
mastectomy. *See* Mastectomy
minimally invasive ablative techniques, 2153–54
nonsurgical, 2151–52
radiation therapy, 2152
radiofrequency ablation, 2154
reconstruction after, 2156–59
sentinel lymph node biopsy, 2154–55
surgery, 2152–59
Breast disorders
abscess, 2142
cysts, 2142
fibroadenoma, 2142
fibrocystic changes, 2141–42
galactorrhea, 2142
intraductal papilloma, 2142
mammary duct ectasia, 2143
mastalgia, 2140
mastitis, 2143
mastodynia, 2140
overview of, 2135, 2139
Paget's mammary disease, 2143–44
periductal mastitis, 2143
tumors, 2143
Breast self-examination, 2075, 2139, 2140f
Breath sounds
adventitious, 1000–1002
auscultation of, 999–1002
normal, 999–1000
Breathing
apneustic, 996
biot's, 996
Cheyne-Stokes, 996
in chronic obstructive pulmonary disease patients, 1109–10
Kussmaul, 996
rate of, 995
rhythms of, 996
strategies for improving, 1109–10
Brewer's Yeast, 395t
Broca's aphasia, 1199
Broca's area, 452f
Bromocriptine, 1283t, 1866
Bronchi, 980
Bronchial asthma, 225
Bronchial breath sound, 1000t
Bronchial-associated lymphoid tissues, 1392
Bronchiectasis, 1128
Bronchiolectasis
assessment of, 1073
definition of, 1072
diagnostic tests, 1073
epidemiology of, 1073
etiology of, 1073
nursing diagnoses, 1073–74
outcomes, 1075
pathophysiology of, 1073
patient education about, 1075
planning and implementation for, 1074–75
treatment of, 1074–75
types of, 1072–73
Bronchioles, 980
Bronchiolitis, chronic, 1100
Bronchoalveolar lavage, 1010–11
Bronchodilators
asthma managed using, 1459t
chronic obstructive pulmonary disease treated with, 1111
description of, 517–19, 1075
lung abscess treated with, 1077
Bronchophony, 1002
Bronchoscopy, 1005, 1010
Bronchovesicular breath sound, 1000t
Brown-Séquard syndrome, 1220, 1220t, 1240
Bruits, 879
Bruner, Jerome, 45t
Brush biopsy, 1010
Budesonide, 1023t
Buerger's disease, 896–98
Buffers, 328, 987
Bulbar conjunctiva, 1305
Bulbospongiosus reflex, 1229, 1229t
Bulbourethral glands, 2057, 2063, 2076
Bulk-forming laxatives, 163
Bullae, 1114, 1486b, 1488f
Bullectomy, 1114–15
Bullous myringitis, 1359–60
Bumetanide, 923t
Bundle of His, 836
Burn(s)
abuse-related, 1540
acute treatment phase
assessment, 1546–47
burn unit transfer, 1548–49
collaborative care management, 1549
description of, 1533, 1546
diagnostic tests, 1546
enteral feeding, 1550
nursing diagnoses, 1547
nursing interventions, 1547–55
nutrition, 1549–51
oral feeding, 1550–51
outcomes, 1556
patient education during, 1554–55
pharmacological management, 1551–52
topical medications used in, 1551
in adolescents, 1559
assessments
during acute phase, 1546–47
during emergent phase, 1537–39
primary, 1535
during rehabilitation phase, 1556–57
secondary, 1535
blood transfusions for, 1530
burn unit referral criteria, 1536b
chemical
causative agents, 1535
hydrochloric acid, 1535
prehospital care for, 1534–35
in children, 1544
circumferential, 1542
colloid fluids for, 1543
contact, 1534
contractures, 1557
coping with, 1555
crystalloid fluids for, 1543
definition of, 1530
dementia and, 1545
depth of, 1537, 1539t
edema formation, 1542
electrical, 1535
emergency department management of, 1536–37
emergent phase
assessment, 1537–39
fluid resuscitation, 1541–43
nursing diagnoses, 1540
outcomes, 1545–46
pharmacological treatment during, 1542–43
surgical treatment during, 1543–44
thermoregulation concerns, 1541
treatment during, 1533–37, 1540–44
wound care during, 1542
epidemiology of, 1530
etiology of, 1530–31
extinguishing of fire, 1534
family education about, 1544–45, 1554–55, 1560–61
first aid for, 1534–36
flame injuries, 1534
flash injuries, 1534
fluid loss, 1532
fluid resuscitation for, 1541–43
full-thickness, 1531, 1539t
fungal infection risks, 1548
gastrointestinal system effects, 1533
governmental programs to prevent, 1545
grafts for
allograft, 1552
autograft, 1552
donor sites for, 1553–54
full-thickness, 1553
heterograft, 1552
homograft, 1552
meshing of, 1553
procedures for, 1552–53
sheet, 1553
split-thickness, 1553
hypermetabolism secondary to, 1533
hypertrophic scarring, 1559
immune system effects, 1533
immunosuppression after, 1549
infection risks, 1547–48
inflammatory response to, 1532
intravenous therapy for, 1536b
nursing diagnoses, 1540, 1547, 1557
nutrition for, 1549–51, 1560
occupational retraining, 1560
outcomes
during acute phase, 1556
during emergent phase, 1545–46
during rehabilitation phase, 1561
pain management, 1542–43, 1551–52, 1559
partial-thickness, 1531, 1539t
pathophysiology of, 1531–33
patient education about, 1544–45, 1554–55, 1560–61
physiological response to, 1532
posttraumatic stress disorder risks, 1555
prehospital care for, 1534–36
prevention of, 1544–45
psychological issues, 1554, 1557, 1559
rehabilitation phase
ambulation, 1558
assessments, 1556–57
collaborative management during, 1560–61
contractures, 1557
diagnostic tests, 1556
exercise, 1558
goals, 1558
initiation, 1533–34, 1556
nursing diagnoses, 1557
nursing interventions, 1557–60
outcomes, 1561
pain management during, 1559
patient positioning, 1557–58
splinting, 1558
rule of nines for, 1537, 1538f
scald, 1544
self-image concerns, 1555, 1558–59
severity determinations, 1537–39, 1538f
site-specific recovery, 1537–39
superficial, 1531, 1539t
superficial partial-thickness, 1531
surgical treatment for
during acute phase, 1552–54
during emergent phase, 1543–44
escharotomy, 1543–44
grafts. *See* Burn(s), grafts
systemic response to, 1532–33
tetanus prophylaxis, 1542
tissue responses to, 1531–33
total body surface area determinations, 1537
types of, 1531f
wounds
during acute phase, 1547
debridement, 1547
dressings, 1535–36, 1551, 1553
during emergent phase, 1542
grafts for. *See* Burn(s), grafts
hydrotherapy, 1547
infection risks, 1547–48
Burn shock, 1532
Burn unit, 1536b, 1548
Burning mouth syndrome, 1622
Burnout, 256
Burrows, 1486b
Bursae, 1939
Butterfly rash, 1442f
Butyrophenones, 163

C

C3, 1412
C4, 1412
C fibers, 449
C waves, 582
CA125, 2121
Cachexia, 434–35
Caffeine, 918t
Calcineurin inhibitors, 1843t
Calcitonin, 1851t, 1855, 1984
Calcium
characteristics of, 299t

deficiency of, 311t, 320–22
excess of, 311t–312t, 322–23
functions of, 299t
kidney effects on, 300
normal levels of, 1759t
osteoporosis prevention and, 1984
recommended dietary intake of, 314t
Calcium channel blockers
angina pectoris treated with, 502
arrhythmias treated with, 862
coronary artery disease treated with, 782t, 783–84
hypertension treated with, 510, 924t
hypertrophic cardiomyopathy treated with, 814
side effects of, 503–5
Calculi
gallstones. *See* Cholelithiasis
urinary tract
assessment of, 1789–90
clinical manifestations of, 1789–90
description of, 1788–89
diagnostic tests, 1790
epidemiology of, 1789
etiology of, 1789
helical computed tomography of, 1790
nursing diagnoses, 1790
nutritional considerations, 1791
outcomes, 1792
pathophysiology of, 1789
pharmacological treatment of, 1791
surgical treatment of, 1791
Calendula, 393t
Caloric intake, 289
cAMP, 517
Campylobacter jejuni, 1244–45
Cancellous bone, 1935
Cancer. *See also* Tumor(s)
anaphylaxis associated with, 442
bile duct, 1735–36
biopsy evaluations, 413
bladder. *See* Bladder cancer
body image changes, 437
breast. *See* Breast cancer
caregivers, 440–41
chemotherapy for. *See* Chemotherapy
colorectal. *See* Colorectal cancer
coping with, 440–41
definition of, 366, 401
depression secondary to, 422–23
description of, 129
diagnostic tests for, 412–13
diet and, 404
disseminated intravascular coagulation in, 442
drugs that cause, 404–5
environmental factors, 404
esophageal. *See* Esophageal cancer
etiology of, 402–5
gallbladder, 1735–36
genetic factors, 219–20
health disparities, 79b
heredity and, 403
historical descriptions of, 402
hypercalcemia caused by, 441
incidence of, 402
kidney. *See* Renal cancer
laboratory tests for, 412
laryngeal. *See* Laryngeal cancer
lifestyle factors, 404–5
liver, 1723–25
lung. *See* Lung cancer
malignant cells in, 408
mortality of, 402, 403t
ocular, 1334–36
oncological emergencies, 441–42
oncology therapy for, 366–67
ovarian, 2120–22
overview of, 402
pathophysiology of, 405–8
penile, 2192–93
planning and implementation, 413–27
prevention of, 408–12
primary prevention of, 408–9
prostate. *See* Prostate cancer
radiation therapy for. *See* Radiation therapy
radiographic tests for, 412
rectal. *See* Colorectal cancer
renal. *See* Renal cancer
risk factors for, 410t–411t, 1405
screening recommendations, 410
secondary prevention of, 409–10
septic shock caused by, 442
signs of, 409b, 1405
skin. *See* Skin cancer
smoking and, 404
stomach. *See* Stomach cancer
symptoms-related management
anemia, 430–31
anorexia, 435
cachexia, 434–35
cognitive disorders, 433
description of, 429–30
gastrointestinal, 434–35
mucositis, 434, 436–37
myelosuppression, 430–32
neuropathy, 433
neutropenia, 431–32
sleep disorders, 439
thrombocytopenia, 432
tertiary prevention of, 412
testicular, 2173–75
treatment of
biological therapies, 424–25
body image changes, 437
bone marrow transplantation, 425–27
chemotherapy. *See* Chemotherapy
clinical trials regarding, 427–28
complementary therapies, 427
complications of, 415–16
hormonal therapy, 423–24
overview of, 414
patient education about, 422
principles, 414–16
radiation therapy. *See* Radiation therapy
sexual dysfunction caused by, 437–38
surgery, 414–16
vaccines for, 408
vocal cords, 1043–44
vulvar, 2119, 2122
Cancer pain
breakthrough, 462–63
causes of, 461
intractable, 463–64, 475
management of, 440, 459
persistent, 461
Candesartan, 924t
Candida infections, 2101
Candidiasis, 1510–11, 2077
Capillary refill, 879
Capnometry, 1009
Capsaicin, 391t
Captopril, 924t
Carbamazepine
description of, 521–22
multiple sclerosis treated with, 1278t
trigeminal neuralgia treated with, 1249
Carbidopa/levodopa, 1283t
Carbohydrates
absorption of, 1650
blood glucose regulation and, 1910
for burn patients, 1550
digestion of, 1597
Carbon dioxide
cerebral blood vessels affected by, 583
description of, 1759t
regulation of, 301
Carbon dioxide narcosis, 697, 1060
Carbonic acid, 986
Carbonic anhydrase inhibitors, 506–8
Carboxyhemoglobin, 772–73
Carbuncles, 1512
Carcinoembryonic antigen screening, 1680t, 1683
Carcinogenesis, 406–7
Cardiac arrest, 677
Cardiac assist devices
intra-aortic balloon pump, 577–78, 579t
ventricular assist devices, 578–79, 2217
Cardiac catheterization
cardiovascular system assessments, 764
coronary artery disease evaluations, 780
heart failure evaluations, 808
nursing management during, 765–66
Cardiac cells, 837–38
Cardiac cirrhosis, 1711–12
Cardiac conduction system
action potential, 837
anatomy of, 843f
atrioventricular node, 836
automaticity, 837
conductivity, 838
contractility, 838
definition of, 836
depolarization, 837
electrophysiology, 837–38
excitability, 837–38
Purkinje fibers, 836–37
repolarization, 837
sinoatrial node, 836
Cardiac cycle, 570f, 751–53
Cardiac glycosides, 500–502
Cardiac index, 568, 574t
Cardiac output
burn effects on, 1532
calculation of, 752
continuous monitoring of, 575
definition of, 911
measurement of, 568, 575
normal range for, 574t
pulmonary artery catheter, 574–75
Cardiac rehabilitation, 796–97
Cardinal fields of gaze, 1305, 1306f
Cardiogenic shock, 791, 2215–18
Cardiomyopathy
arrhythmogenic right ventricular, 816–17
definition of, 812
dilated, 812–13
hypertrophic
assessment of, 814
description of, 805, 813–14
nursing diagnoses for, 814
pharmacological treatment of, 814–15
surgical treatment of, 815
restrictive, 817–18
Cardioplegia, 787
Cardiopulmonary resuscitation
chest compressions, 868
definition of, 867
description of, 560
external compressions with, 868
rescue breathing, 867–68
steps in, 868–69
Cardiovascular agents
antianginal agents, 502–4
antidysrhythmics, 504–6
antihypertensive agents. *See* Antihypertensive agents
cardiac glycosides, 500–502
diuretics, 506–8
overview of, 498–99
Cardiovascular disease
apolipoprotein epsilon and, 217–18
costs of, 883
genetic factors, 217–18
health disparities, 79b
in homeless persons, 81t
Cardiovascular system
aging-related changes, 491, 753
assessment of
auscultation, 758
chest pain, 754, 755t
description of, 806, 1410
dyspnea, 753–54
jugular veins, 757
landmarks for, 753
lower extremities, 757
percussion, 758
precordium, 757
skin color, 756–57
subjective data, 753
blood flow, 751
circulation. *See* Circulation
diagnostic tests
cardiac catheterization, 764
chest x-ray, 762–63
coronary angiography, 764
echocardiography, 763
electrocardiogram, 762
electrophysiological studies, 764
exercise testing, 762, 763t
myocardial nuclear perfusion imaging, 763–65
nursing management for, 764–66
fluid and electrolyte balance by, 300–301
heart. *See* Heart
history-taking, 756t
immune function and, 1381
Carditis
bacterial endocarditis, 818–20
definition of, 812, 818
myocarditis, 820–21
pericarditis. *See* Pericarditis
Caregivers
coping by, 440–41
dying patients, 166
role strain for, 155
stress of, 254
Carotid duplex studies, 1166–67
Carotid endarterectomy, 1180–81
Carotid sinuses, 751
Carotid stenting, 1181, 1181f
Carpal tunnel syndrome
assessment of, 2017
definition of, 2015
description of, 19, 1256–57
diabetes mellitus and, 2016
diagnostic tests, 2017

epidemiology of, 2016
etiology of, 2016, 2016f
pathophysiology of, 2016
patient education about, 2018
treatment of, 2017–18
Carrier, 198
Cartilage callus, 1937
Carvedilol, 924t
Case manager, 259b
Casts, 700, 1825t, 2036
Catabolism, 1599
Cataracts, 1308, 1310, 1327–29
Catastrophes, 250
Catechins, 391t
Catecholamines, 1138
Catechol-O-methyltransferase inhibitors, 1282, 1283t
Catheters
central venous. *See* Central venous catheters
closed-ended, 359
fractured lines, 361
implanted ports, 359
indwelling, 1237
percutaneous, 359
pulmonary artery, 568
selection of, 358
Swan-Ganz, 367, 572
troubleshooting of, 360
tunneled, 358–59
Cations, 298
Causalgia, 458b
Cavernosography, 2079
Cavernosometry, 2079
CD40, 1398
Cecum, 1571, 1670
Celecoxib, 474t
Celery seed, 393t
Cell(s). *See also specific cell*
benign growth of, 405–6
growth of, 405
malignant, 406
Cell cycle, 419f
Cell-mediated immunity, 741, 1381, 1396–98
Cellulitis, 1508
Centering, 385
Centers for Disease Control infection control guidelines, 279, 279t–280t
Centers for Medicare and Medicaid Services
health care strategy, 536
nursing home reform, 546
Central cord syndrome, 1220, 1220t
Central cyanosis, 756
Central herniation, 580
Central nervous system
autonomic nervous system, 452–53
brain. *See* Brain
brainstem, 1143
cerebellum, 1143
description of, 451–52, 1139
meninges, 1139–40, 1141f
spine, 1143–44
Central nervous system lymphoma, 1196
Central sleep apnea, 1039
Central venous catheters
closed-ended catheters, 359
implanted ports, 359
percutaneous catheters, 359
selection of, 358
tunneled catheters, 358–59
Central venous pressure, 367
Centrally acting sympatholytics, 509
Cephalalgia. *See* Headaches
Cephalosporins
administration of, 495b
adverse effects of, 494
generations of, 493
indications for, 493
laboratory monitoring of, 494
mechanism of action, 493
nursing management for, 494–95
pharmacodynamics of, 493–94
pharmacokinetics of, 493
side effects of, 494
urinary tract infections treated with, 1772b
Cerebellar tonsils, 580
Cerebellum
anatomy of, 452f, 1143
function assessments, 1156–57
Romberg's test, 1156–57
Cerebral angiography, 1162–63
Cerebral perfusion pressure, 580, 1193
Cerebrospinal fluid
analysis of, 1160t
description of, 1141
drainage of, from ear, 1316
leaking of, 1187b
Cerebrovascular accident. *See* Stroke
Cerebrum, 1140, 1141f
Certified registered nurse anesthetist, 656
Cerumen
description of, 1311–12, 1317
hearing loss and, 1357
Cervical auscultation, 1624
Cervical cancer, 411t, 2119–20
Cervical fusion, 1228
Cervical lymphadenopathy, 1512
Cervical polyps, 2110, 2115
Cervical tongs, 1224
Cervical vertebrae
description of, 1217
range of motion, 1946t
spinal cord injury at level of, 1218–19
Cervix, 2060–61, 2076
Cetirizine, 1022t
CH50, 1412
Chakra, 378
Chalazion, 1340
Chamomile, 393t
Chancroids, 2075
Cheilosis, 937
Chemical burns
causative agents, 1535
hydrochloric acid, 1535
prehospital care for, 1534–35
Chemical dependence, 20
Chemical phlebitis, 348
Chemoembolization, 1724
Chemokines, 1385, 1393
Chemoreceptor trigger zone, 1575
Chemoreceptors, 982–83
Chemotaxis, 267
Chemotherapy
acute lymphocytic leukemia treated with, 955–56
acute myeloid leukemia treated with, 957
administration routes, 420
adverse effects of, 967, 968t
bladder cancer treated with, 1800
blood-brain barrier considerations, 1204
brain tumors treated with, 1198–99, 1204
cancer treated with, 419–23
chronic lymphocytic leukemia treated with, 959
colorectal cancer treated with, 1682
cycles of, 420
description of, 419
diarrhea caused by, 434–35
fatigue caused by, 421, 439–40, 1198
gastrointestinal symptoms, 434–35
Hodgkin's disease treated with, 967
hypersensitivity reactions, 968t
liver cancer treated with, 1724
lung cancer treated with, 1080–81
multiple myeloma treated with, 963
myelosuppression secondary to, 421, 430, 958b, 968t
nausea and vomiting caused by, 420–21, 434, 968t
non-Hodgkin's lymphoma treated with, 970
osteosarcoma treated with, 1996, 1997t
outcomes, 422–23
principles of, 419–20
renal cancer treated with, 1797
safety considerations, 420
side effects, 420–22
stomach cancer treated with, 1644
thrombocytopenia caused by, 432
vesicants, 420
Chest
assessment of, 755
barrel, 755, 756t, 994, 1003
flail, 1087–88
funnel, 756t, 994
palpation of, 997–98
pigeon, 756t, 995
reference lines, 977
Chest compressions, during cardiopulmonary resuscitation, 868
Chest pain. *See also* Angina pectoris
assessment of, 754, 755t, 991–92
causes of, 755t
noncardiac, 1634–35
pleuritic, 1056
Chest tubes, 1084–85
Chest X-rays
acute abdomen evaluations, 1660t
asthma findings, 1122
cardiovascular system assessments, 762–63
chronic obstructive pulmonary disease findings, 1105
coronary artery disease evaluations, 778
Hodgkin's disease evaluations, 966
respiratory system evaluations, 1006
tuberculosis diagnosis, 1066
Cheyne-Stokes breathing, 996
Chief operating officers, 6
Child abuse, 1540
Children. *See also* Infant(s)
allergic rhinitis in, 1019
asthma in, 127
brain injuries in, 1182t
burns in, 1544
cochlear implants in, 1366–67
epiphyseal plate in, 1935
homeless, 81
immunizations for, 1403
nephrotic syndrome in, 1784–87
pain management in, 661
perioperative considerations for, 660–61
poverty effects on, 80
trauma effects on, 2262
urinary incontinence in, 1806
Chinese Americans, 148t
Chiropractic therapy, 384
Chlamydia, 271t
Chlorhexidine, 346, 1622
Chloride, 314t
Chlorofluorocarbons, 1113
Chlorpheniramine maleate, 1022t
Chlorpropamide, 1916t
Chlorthalidone, 923t
Cholangiogram, 1701
Cholangitis
definition of, 1730
primary sclerosing, 1733
Cholecystectomy
description of, 701t
laparoscopic, 1730–31, 1731f–1732f
Cholecystitis, 1663, 1732–33
Cholecystography, 1701
Cholecystokinin, 1700
Cholelithiasis, 1729–32
Cholesteatoma, 1360
Cholesterol
cellular uses of, 1597
coronary artery disease risks, 771–72
definition of, 514
description of, 1698
in erythrocyte cell membrane, 737
food sources of, 881
hepatic production of, 1698
screening of, 881t
Cholestyramine, 1734–35
Chondroitin, 1226
Chondrosarcoma, 1994–98
Chordae tendineae, 749
Chordoplasty, 830
Chorea
definition of, 1294
Huntington's, 1294–96
Chorionic villus sampling, 209, 212t
Choroid plexus, 1141
Choroidal melanoma, 1334–35
Choroids, 1302
Christmas disease, 944
Chromium, 392
Chromosomal abnormalities
chromosomal number, 199–200
description of, 199
monosomies, 200
mosaicism, 200
sex chromosomes, 202–3
structure-related, 200–201
trisomies, 200
Chromosome(s)
breakage of, 201–2
definition of, 198
deletion of, 200–201
inversion of, 201
microdeletions, 201
number of, 198
translocation of, 201
X, 198–99, 202–3
Y, 198–99, 202–3
Chromosome 6p, 224
Chronic bronchiolitis, 1100
Chronic bronchitis, 1103
Chronic diseases, 414
Chronic fatigue syndrome, 1977
Chronic illness
across life span, 252–53
assessment of, 1405–6
coping with, 251
depression associated with, 252
immune system affected by, 1405–6
stress of, 250–52
Chronic inflammation, 270
Chronic lymphocytic leukemia, 950, 957–59

Chronic myeloid leukemia, 950, 959–61
Chronic obstructive pulmonary disease
air trapping, 1101
airflow limitations in, 1101
alpha1-antitrypsin enzyme deficiency, 1102
assessment of, 1103–4, 1104t
asthma, 1100
atopy in, 1101–2
chest x-ray findings, 1105
cigarette smoking and, 1100–1101, 1107
complications of, 1102–3
computed tomography of, 1106
course of, 1103
definition of, 1100
description of, 329
diagnostic tests, 1105–6
disorders that cause, 516
dyspnea in, 1103–4
emphysema in, 1102
epidemiology of, 1100
etiology of, 1100–1101
exacerbations of, 1103, 1106, 1112–13
family education about, 1115–16
inflammatory cells associated with, 1101
influenza vaccinations, 1112
mechanical ventilation for, 1103
nursing diagnoses, 1107
outcomes, 1116
pathophysiology of, 1101–3
patient education about, 1115–16
planning and implementation for, 1107–16
prognostic factors, 1104
risk factors for, 1100
smoking and, 1100–1101, 1107
spirometry findings, 1106t
stages of
description of, 1104, 1105t
treatment based on, 1111t
symptoms of, 1100, 1103
treatment of
airflow enhancements, 1109–10
albuterol, 1112
bronchodilators, 1111
bullectomy, 1114–15
collaborative approach, 1107–10
corticosteroids, 1112
coughing, 1110
future types of, 1116
lung volume reduction surgery, 1114
mucus-clearing agents, 1112
nutrition, 1110–11
oxygen therapy, 1113–14
pharmacological, 1111–14
postural drainage, 1109
pulmonary rehabilitation program, 1107–9
recommendations, 1111t
stage-based, 1111t
surgery, 1114–15
sympathomimetics, 1111
ventilator support, 1110
viral infection risks, 1103
weight loss in, 1103
Chronic pain
coping with, 469
description of, 460–61
in elderly, 455
Chronic pancreatitis, 1738–41
Chronic renal disease
coronary artery disease and, 771
immune system affected by, 1405
Chronic renal failure
assessment of, 1834t
clinical manifestations of, 1834t
collaborative management of, 1835, 1836b
definition of, 1832
diagnostic tests, 1833
epidemiology of, 1832
etiology of, 1833
hemodialysis for, 1836–37
nursing diagnoses, 1833
nutrition for, 1839
pathophysiology of, 1833
peritoneal dialysis for, 1837–39
pharmacological treatment of, 1835, 1836b
refusal of treatment, 1835
renal transplantation for. *See* Renal transplantation
stages of, 1832t
treatment of, 1834–43
Chronic sinusitis, 1029–31
Chronic venous insufficiency, 902
Chvostek's sign, 321, 321f, 332
Chyme, 1570, 1596, 1648
Cigarette smoking. *See* Smoking
Cilia, 981–82
Ciliary body, 1302
Cimetidine, 524
Cingulate herniation, 580
Ciprofloxacin, 496
Circle of Willis, 1143f
Circulating nurse, 657
Circulation
cerebral, 1143, 1143f
coronary artery, 750–51
pulmonary, 576f
signs of, 868
spinal cord, 1144
systemic, 750
Circulatory disorders
anticoagulants for, 511–13
antilipidemics. *See* Antilipidemics
Circumcision, female, 2116–18
Circumduction, 1944f
Circumferential burns, 1542
Cirrhosis
alcoholic, 1711–12
assessment of, 1714b
biliary, 1711–12, 1733–35
cardiac, 1711–12
definition of, 1711
pathophysiology of, 1713
postnecrotic, 1711–12
surgical treatment of, 1715
treatment of, 1714–15
Cisplatin, 1997t
Clemastine, 1022t
Clindamycin, 1077
Clinical breast examination, 2080
Clinical decision making, 24
Clinical dietician, 1911
Clinical ethics, 96–97
Clinical pathways, 612
Clinical practice guidelines
description of, 32
examples of, 37b
sources for, 36–37
Clinical trials
cancer treatments, 427–28
costs of, 428
definition of, 427
legal considerations, 429
minorities in, 456
National Cancer Institute, 428
Clitoral therapy, 2130
Clitoris, 2062
Clofibrate, 514
Clomiphene citrate, 2126, 2126t
Clonic seizures, 1271
Clonidine, 923t
Cloning, 234
Clopidogrel, 784
Clorazepate, 521
Closed reduction, for shoulder dislocation, 2012
Closed-ended catheters, 359
Clotting cascade, 742–43
Clubbing, 996–97, 1103
Cluster headaches, 1265t, 1267–68
Coagulation
hypothermia effects on, 681
medications that affect, 744t
schematic diagram of, 941f
stages of, 940b
Coagulation disorders
disseminated intravascular coagulation
in cancer patients, 442
causes of, 679–80
characteristics of, 942–44
definition of, 679
description of, 2225
hemophilia. *See* Hemophilia
Coagulation factors, 742t
Coagulopathies, 2253
Cobalamin, 1648–49
Cobalamin deficiency. *See* Vitamin B12 deficiency anemia
Coccidioidomycosis, 1069–70
Coccyx, 1140f
Cochlear implant, 1366–67
Cochrane Collaboration, 31, 35
Cochrane Library
description of, 35
evidence summaries from, 35, 36b
Code of ethics, 99–100, 191, 684
Codeine, 474t
Cognitive domain, of learning, 46, 47t
Cognitive impairment
in cancer patients, 433
definition of, 433
Cognitive learning, 720–21
Cogwheel rigidity, 1281
Cold chemical sterilization, 666b
Cold knife cold biopsy, 2081
Colectomy, 1684
Collagen, 1479
Collective bargaining, 18–19
Colloids, 365, 1543, 2216t
Coloboma, 1309
Colon
anatomy of, 1571
obstruction of, 1656
perforation of
gastrointestinal obstruction and, 1672–73
in ulcerative colitis, 1691
resection of, 1683–84
Colonoscopy, 1585–86, 1680t, 1682
Colony-stimulating factors, 432
Color perception, 1339
Color vision tests, 1304
Colorblindness, 1339
Colorectal cancer
adjuvant therapy for, 1685
assessment of, 1679
chemoradiotherapy for, 1682
colonoscopy for, 1680t, 1682
description of, 1676
diagnostic tests, 1679, 1680t–1681t
diet and, 1678
digital rectal examination screenings, 1680t
endorectal ultrasonography evaluations, 1683
environmental factors, 1677
epidemiology of, 1676
etiology of, 1676–78
familial adenomatous polyposis, 1677
fecal occult blood testing, 1679, 1680t
genetic factors, 1677t
hereditary nonpolyposis, 1676
incidence of, 403t
lesions associated with, 1679f
lymph node metastasis of, 1679
nursing diagnoses, 1681
obesity and, 1678
outcomes, 1685
pathophysiology of, 1678–79, 1679f
pharmacological treatment of, 1681
prognosis for, 1685–86
radiation therapy for, 1681–82
risk factors for, 410t–411t, 1678
screening for, 1679, 1680t–1681t
sedentary lifestyle and, 1678
smoking and, 1678
staging of, 1685–86
surgical treatments for
abdomino-perineal resection, 1684
colectomy, 1684
colon resection, 1683–84
endoscopic mucosal resection, 1682
goals, 1684
ostomy after, 1684–85
overview of, 1682–83
proctocolectomy, 1683–84
snare polypectomy, 1682
treatment of, 1681–85
Colposcopy, 2080
Coma, 1185t
Coma depasse, 113
Combat trauma, 644
Comedones, 1486b, 1488f, 1507
COMFORT Behavior Scale, 465
Commissurotomy, 830
Common vehicle transmission, 277
Communication
by critically ill patients, 567
cultural considerations, 74–75
effectiveness of, 348
in endotracheal intubation patients, 595–96
extrinsic distortion, 74
facilitation of, 632
with hearing-impaired patients, 1370–71
intrinsic distortion, 74
by myasthenia gravis patients, 1291
nonverbal, 74–75
SBAR technique for, 552
stroke-related impairments, 1199–1200
verbal, 74
Community care, 89
Community Volunteers in Medicine, 81
Community-acquired pneumonia, 525, 1057
Compartment syndrome
description of, 713–14, 2039–40, 2260
in rhabdomyolysis, 1826
Competence, 13

Complement system, 268, 1393–94
Complementary and alternative medicine
acupressure, 387, 1264
acupuncture
Bell's palsy treated with, 1251
description of, 386–87
tension-type headaches treated with, 1264
annual expenditures on, 378
aromatherapy, 394–95
Ayurveda, 377–78
barriers to use of, 246
benign prostatic hyperplasia managed using, 2168
biofeedback, 382–83, 921
body work therapies, 387–90
body-movement strategies, 383–84
cancer treated with, 427, 1997
categories of, 381t
chiropractic therapy, 384
contemporary trends in, 378–79
conventional medicine vs., 376t
definition of, 156
description of, 129–30, 246
diet therapies, 391–94
digoxin interactions, 502
drug interactions, 1602
energy therapies, 384–87
exercise, 383
focus of, 246
headaches treated with, 1264–65
healing touch, 385
herbal therapy, 392–94, 393t–394t
history of, 377–78, 477
holism, 380
homeopathy, 396
in hospice care, 156
humor, 395
hypnosis, 383
imagery, 382, 382t
massage, 386, 388–89
meditation, 381–82, 920, 1265
mind-body therapies
description of, 380–83
research into, 379
music, 396
nursing and, 396–97
nutritional therapies, 391–94
pain management using, 477–78
in palliative care, 156
pet therapy, 395–96
phytonutrients, 391, 391t
popularity of, 378–79
preoperative questions about, 613–14
reflexology, 389–90
regulation of, 379
Reiki, 385–86
relaxation, 380–81
research studies of, 477
rolfing, 389
sexual dysfunction treated with, 2130
shamanic influence, 378
shiatsu, 389
spiritual therapies, 390–91
tai chi, 384, 920, 1265
tension-type headaches treated with, 1264–65
therapeutic touch, 385, 478, 596
types of, 246
vitamins, 392
yoga, 384, 920, 1265
Complete blood count with differential, 1410–12
Complete heart block, 855f, 855–56
Compliance, 981
Comprehensive assessment, 175
Computed tomography
acute abdomen evaluations, 1660t, 1659, 1661
brain injury evaluations, 1189–90
brain tumor evaluations, 1197
chronic obstructive pulmonary disease findings, 1106
female reproductive system evaluations, 2083
gastrointestinal obstruction evaluations, 1673
musculoskeletal system evaluations, 1949
nervous system assessments, 1161
nursing management for, 1007–8, 1161
pyelonephritis evaluations, 1778, 1814
renal evaluations, 1761t
renal trauma evaluations, 1794
respiratory system evaluations, 1006–8
spinal cord injury evaluations, 1221–22
stroke evaluations, 1175t
urinary tract calculi evaluations, 1790
Computed tomography colonography, 1680t
Computer-assisted instruction, 48
Concussion, 1185, 1188f
Conductive hearing loss, 1354
Conductivity, 838
Condyloma, 2075, 2104
Cones, 1302
Confidentiality
definition of, 192
description of, 102–3
of genetic screening, 207, 230
of health assessment data, 192–93
Health Insurance Portability and Accountability Act provisions, 102–3, 192–93, 694
Confrontation test, 1152, 1152f
Confusion
in hospice patients, 154–55, 163–64
in palliative care patients, 154–55, 163–64
Congestive heart failure. *See* Heart failure
Conjunctiva
anatomy of, 1302
bulbar, 1305
palpebral, 1305
Conjunctivitis, 1340
Conscious sedation, 677
Consensual response, to pupil examination, 1305
Constipation
definition of, 1577
in hospice patients, 154, 162–63
management of, 163
opioid analgesic-induced, 473
in palliative care patients, 154, 162–63
postoperative, 724–25
signs and symptoms of, 1577
Contact dermatitis
allergic, 1465, 1508–9
definition of, 1471
irritant, 1508–9
Contact lenses, 1338
Contact transmission
description of, 276
precautions for, 280, 280t
Contemporary nursing
criteria for, 10b
definition of, 10–11
domains of, 11
in United States, 9–11
Continent urinary diversions, 1802–3
Continuing care agencies, 544–46
Continuous mandatory ventilation, 586
Continuous positive airway pressure
description of, 588
obstructive sleep apnea treated with, 1039
Continuous quality improvement, 7
Continuous renal replacement therapy, 1827, 1827b
Contractility
in critically ill patients, 569
definition of, 569, 838
myocardial, 805
problems with, 568
Contractures, 1200–1201, 1557, 2048
Contrast-induced nephropathy, 1825t
Controlled coughing, 1110
Controlled Substances Act, 355
Contusion
brain, 1184, 1188f
ocular, 1333–34
renal, 1792
spinal cord, 1218
Conventional medicine, 375–77
Convulsion, 1269
Cooper's ligaments, 2136, 2136f
Coordination testing, 1156
Coping
adaptive mechanisms, 247
assessment of, 440–41
with burns, 1555
with cancer, 440–41
by caregivers, 440–41
with chronic illness, 251
with chronic pain, 469
definition of, 247
emotion-focused, 244
maladaptive mechanisms, 247
problem-focused, 244
self-efficacy and, 245
with spinal cord injury, 1237–38
unconscious mechanisms that affect, 247
Coping efficacy, 247
Cor pulmonale, 1039, 1089, 1092–94
Core needle biopsy, 413, 2150–51
Cornea
abrasions of, 1336
examination of, 1305
keratoconus of, 1336
ulceration of, 1336
Corneal reflex, 1302
Coronary angiography
cardiovascular system assessments, 764
coronary artery disease evaluations, 780
nursing management during, 765–66
Coronary arteries, 750f, 751
Coronary artery bypass grafting
coronary artery disease treated with, 786–87
description of, 701t
heart failure treated with, 811
peripheral arterial occlusive disease treated with, 887–88
Coronary artery circulation, 750–51
Coronary artery disease
assessment of, 775–77
atheroma formation, 770
case study of, 799–800
description of, 129, 769–70
diagnostic tests
cardiac catheterization, 780
chest x-ray, 778
coronary angiography, 780
electrocardiogram, 777–78
electrocardiogram stress test, 779
electron beam computed tomography, 780
Holter monitor, 778
magnetic resonance imaging, 780
nuclear scans, 779–80
positron emission tomography, 780
stress echocardiogram, 779
epidemiology of, 770
etiology of, 770–73
family education about, 787, 789t–790t
health care costs for, 771
laboratory tests, 778
nursing diagnoses, 780
outcomes, 790
pathophysiology of, 774–77
patient education about, 787, 789t–790t
planning and implementation for, 780–90
risk factors for
age, 771, 795
chronic renal disease, 771
cigarette smoking, 772–73
description of, 770–71
diabetes mellitus, 773
family education about, 787, 789t–790t
gender, 771
hyperlipidemia, 771–72
hypertension, 772
modifiable, 771–73
nonmodifiable, 771
obesity, 773
patient education about, 787, 789t–790t
physical inactivity, 773
therapeutic lifestyle changes to reduce, 788
treatment of
alternative therapies, 796
angiotensin-converting enzyme inhibitors, 782t
aspirin, 784
beta blockers, 781–83, 782t
bile acid sequestrants, 783t
calcium channel blockers, 782t, 783–84
collaborative approach, 781
coronary artery bypass grafting, 786–87
dihydropyridines, 782t, 783
fibric acid derivatives, 783t
goals, 781
HMG-CoA reductase inhibitors, 782t, 785
niacin, 783t
nitrates, 781, 782t
percutaneous coronary interventions, 785–86
pharmacological agents, 781–85
surgery, 785–87
Coronavirus, 2255
Corpus callosotomy, 1274t
Corpus callosum, 1140
Corpus cavernosa, 2062
Corpus luteum cysts, 2112
Cortical bone, 1935
Corticosteroids
adverse effects of, 1228
alcohol consumption and, 1405
asthma treated with, 1120
chronic obstructive pulmonary disease treated with, 1112
chronic sinusitis treated with, 1030
definition of, 1855
gout managed using, 1966
immunosuppressive uses of, 1843
inhaled, 519–20
intranasal, 1022, 1030
multiple sclerosis treated with, 1278t
nursing management for, 520
pain management uses of, 472
side effects of, 1501
in spinal cord-injured patients, 1227–28

topical, 1499t, 1501
urticaria treated with, 1467t
Corticotrophin-releasing hormone, 1869, 2206
Corticotropin, 1278t
Cortisol, 1855
Cortisone acetate, 1776b
Coryza, 1318
Cosmetic treatments, 130
Costochondral junctions, 975
Costochondritis, 755t
Costodiaphragmatic recess, 978
Costovertebral angle, 1747–48
Cotton wool spots, 1309
Cough, 990, 1055
Cough reflex, 982
Counterpulsation, 578
COX-2 inhibitors
description of, 471b
osteoarthritis treated with, 1959
rheumatoid arthritis treated with, 1439, 1440t
Crackles, 806
Cranial nerves, 1145, 1146f, 1147t, 1151–55
Craniectomy, 1205
Craniotomy
brain injuries treated with, 1193
brain tumors treated with, 1205
description of, 701t, 1001, 1001t
venous thromboembolism risks, 1205
Crash cart, 794, 794f, 2236
C-reactive protein
coronary artery disease evaluations, 778
definition of, 807, 1412
description of, 273
immune system evaluations using, 1412
Creatine kinase, 793, 1975
Creatinine phosphokinase, 515
Credentialing, 656
Cremasteric reflex, 1229t
Crepitus, 1957
Crescendo, 762f
Crescendo decrescendo, 760, 762f
Creutzfeldt-Jakob disease, 672
Cricoid cartilage, 979
Cricopharyngeal myotomy, 1626
Cri-du-chat syndrome, 200
Crigler-Najjar disease, 1698b, 1710, 1725
Critical access hospitals, 536, 540
Critical care nurse
description of, 560–61
extubation by, 601
Critical care patients, 561, 563–64
Critical care unit. *See also* Intensive care unit
admission criteria, 562b–563b
definition of, 559
history of, 560
interdisciplinary team in, 563–64
nursing care in, 561
transfer to
description of, 692
from postanesthesia care unit, 704–5
Critical incident, 2263
Critical incident stress management, 2264
Critically ill patients
family of, 567–68
hemodynamic monitoring of
afterload, 569
cardiac output, 568
contractility, 569
description of, 568
equipment for, 569–70
intra-arterial, 571–72
left atrial pressure, 576–77
measurements, 570–77
mixed venous oxygen saturation, 577
preload, 568–69
pulmonary artery pressure monitoring, 572–76, 574t
waveform patterns, 571
intracranial pressure monitoring
cerebral perfusion pressure, 580
description of, 579–80
types of, 580–81
waveforms, 581–82
problems experienced by
anxiety, 565–66
communication, 567
immobility, 564–65
infection, 564
nutrition, 564
pain, 565
sleep, 566–67
stress experienced by, 254
Crohn's disease, 1433, 1690–91
Cromolyn, 516
Cross-matching, 1841
Crust, 1489f
Cryopexy, 1331
Cryoprecipitate, 364
Cryopreservation, 426
Cryotherapy, 2027, 2153
Cryptorchidism, 2183–84
Crystalloid fluids
for burn patients, 1543
description of, 365–66
for shock patients, 2216t
Culdoscopy, 2080
Cullen's sign, 1658
Cultural assimilation, 72
Cultural awareness, 86t, 189
Cultural beliefs, 88
Cultural competence
definition of, 188
description of, 85–86
elements of, 86t
evaluation, 89
nursing process and, 86–89
planning and implementation, 88–89
in teaching, 89
Cultural context, 70
Cultural desire, 86t
Cultural diversity, 72
Cultural encounters, 86t, 189
Cultural knowledge, 86t, 189
Cultural skill, 86t, 189
Culture
assessment of, 86–88, 189
biological variables, 82, 84t
case study of, 90–91
characteristics of, 70, 190
death beliefs based on, 146–47, 147t–148t
definition of, 70, 188
dominant, 71
environmental control, 82
folk medicine, 82, 83t
food preferences based on, 85t
gender roles based on, 78
health assessment considerations, 188–89
health disparities, 78–84
labeling, 71
literacy rates, 75
maturation differences, 187
organizing phenomena of
communication, 74–75
overview of, 73–74
social organization, 76–78
space, 76
time orientation, 76
postoperative care and, 717
preoperative considerations, 633–34
spinal cord injury and, 1237
stereotyping based on, 71
Culture for caring, 17–19
Cushing response, 1192
Cushing's disease
assessment of, 1870
diagnostic tests, 1870
epidemiology of, 1869
etiology of, 1869
fall prevention in, 1871
nursing diagnoses, 1870
outcomes, 1873
pathophysiology of, 1869–70
treatment of
overview of, 1870–71
pharmacological, 1871
surgical, 1871–73
Cutaneous herpes simplex, 1513
Cutaneous hyperesthesia, 1581
Cutaneous T cell lymphoma, 1505–6
Cyanosis, 756
Cyclosporin, 1843t
Cyclosporine, 1841
Cylindrical bronchiolectasis, 1072
Cyst
breast, 2142
description of, 1486b
ovarian, 2112, 2114
Cystectomy, 1803
Cystic bronchiolectasis, 1072
Cystic duct, 1699
Cystic fibrosis
amenorrhea and, 2097
assessment of, 1128
bronchiolectasis and, 1073
definition of, 216, 1127
diagnostic tests, 1128
epidemiology of, 1127
family education about, 1131
genotyping for, 1129
hypoxemia associated with, 1129
infection control in, 1129
nursing diagnoses, 1129
nutritional considerations, 1129–30
outcomes, 1131
pancreatitis and, 1738
pathophysiology of, 1128
pharmacological treatment of, 1130
prenatal testing for, 212–13
prevalence of, 216
respiratory infection in, 1130
signs and symptoms of, 1128
surgical treatment of, 1130–31
treatment of, 1129–31
Cystic fibrosis transmembrane conductance regulator, 1128
Cystocele, 2110–11
Cystography, 1758t
Cystoprostatectomy, 1801
Cystoscopy, 1761–62, 1791
Cytochrome P450, 485, 1601–2
Cytokines
definition of, 1385, 1393
description of, 1393
in inflammatory response, 268–69
Cytotoxic T cells, 1391, 1397

D

Dacarbazine, 1997t
Dactinomycin, 1997t
Dactylitis, 1970
Dalton's law, 983
Dandelion, 393t
Darbepoetin, 431
Davol drain, 700t
Dawn phenomenon, 1922
DCC gene, 1677t
Dead space, 979, 983
Dead space volume, 1011
Deaf culture, 72
Death
cultural influences, 146–47, 147t–148t
grief reactions to, 168
inevitability of, 143
leading causes of, 127t, 144, 1595
overview of, 144
pronouncement of, 167
signs and symptoms of, 167
Debridement of wounds, 287–88, 903, 1496–98, 1547
Debriefing, 2264, 2264b
Decibels, 1353, 1369b
Decision making
ethical models of. *See* Ethical decision-making models
patient's ability to make decisions, 106
surrogate decision maker, 106–7
Declaration of Helsinki, 117
Decompression laminectomy, 2002
Decongestants
acute sinusitis treated with, 1028
chronic sinusitis treated with, 1030
Decontamination, 2245
Decrescendo, 760, 762f
Decubitus ulcers, 1232–34
Deep brain stimulation
multiple sclerosis treated with, 1277
Parkinson's disease treated with, 1284t
Deep breathing exercises, 921, 1074, 1081
Deep inferior epigastric perforator flaps, for breast reconstruction, 2159
Deep sedation, 677
Deep tendon reflexes
assessment of, 1226f, 1226–27
description of, 1145
rating scale for, 1158t
in spinal cord injury patients, 1226f, 1226–27
Deep vein thrombosis
description of, 662, 893–96
prevention of, 1246, 2043
Deep veins, 340
DEET, 2258
Deferoxamine, 226
Defibrillation
arrhythmias treated with, 862–64
automatic external defibrillators, 869–70
definition of, 862
electrode pads for, 863
implantable cardioverter-defibrillator, 863–64
indications for, 863
synchronized cardioversion, 863
Dehiscence, of wounds, 284, 415, 714
Delirium tremens, 644
Demargination, 740
Demerol. *See* Meperidine

Demonstration, 47
Dendrites, 1137
Dendritic cells
assays for, 1410–11
description of, 1385–87, 1396
inflammation effects on, 1399
Denver peritoneovenous shunt, 1715
Deontology, 98
Deoxyribonucleic acid
bases of, 737
definition of, 198
replication of, 220
structure of, 737
Dependence, physical, 159
Depolarization, 837
Depression
in cancer patients, 422–23
chronic illness-related, 252
in hospice patients, 155, 164
in palliative care patients, 155, 164
Dermatitis
allergic contact, 1465
atopic, 1466, 1507–8
stasis, 1518–19
Dermatological dysfunctions. *See* Skin disorders
Dermatomal lesions, 1490b
Dermatomes, 450, 450f, 1240, 1240f
Dermatomyositis, 1974–76
Dermatophytes, 1510
Dermis, 1477t, 1478f, 1479, 1482
Dermographism, 1409
Dermoid cysts, 2112
Descartes, Rene, 240, 448
Descending motor tracts, 1144
Detumescence, 2068
Developmental history, 211
Developmentally delayed patients, 53–54
Dewey, John, 45t
Dexamethasone, 1241
Diabetes insipidus, 1874–75
Diabetes mellitus
alcohol consumption, 1911
assessment of, 1906–7
carpal tunnel syndrome in, 2016
complications of
angiopathy, 1922–23
autonomic neuropathies, 1926–27
diabetic ketoacidosis. *See* Diabetic ketoacidosis
diabetic nephropathy. *See* Diabetic nephropathy
diabetic retinopathy. *See* Diabetic retinopathy
foot ulcers, 285, 1927–28
hyperosmolar hyperglycemic nonketotic syndrome, 1919–20
hypoglycemia, 1920–22
peripheral neuropathy, 1925–26
peripheral vascular dysfunction, 1927–28
coronary artery disease risks, 773
dawn phenomenon, 1922
definition of, 526, 1904
description of, 128–29
diagnostic tests, 1908
dietary guidelines for, 1910
epidemiology of, 1904
exercise for, 1915–17
familial clustering of, 218
genetic factors, 218–19
gestational, 219
glycemic control in, 1909
health disparities, 79b
home care considerations, 1909
in homeless persons, 81t
inflammatory response in, 285
insulin-dependent, 218
multifactorial nature of, 218–19
nursing diagnoses, 1908
nutritional therapy for, 1910–12
obesity and, 128, 1612
outcomes, 1917
pathophysiology of, 1904–6
perioperative myocardial ischemia and, 662
prevalence of, 128–29
Somogyi effect, 1922
stroke risks, 1173b
treatment of
alpha-glucosidase inhibitors, 1915, 1916t
biguanides, 1915, 1916t
blood glucose monitoring, 1909–10
exercise, 1915–17
insulin, 1912–15
meglitinide, 1915
overview of, 1908–9
pharmacological, 1912–15
sulfonylureas, 1915, 1916t
thiazolidinediones, 1915
type 1
characteristics of, 218, 1904–5, 1906t, 1907
nutritional therapy for, 1910
type 2, 218, 1905–6, 1906t
Diabetic ketoacidosis, 527, 1918–19
Diabetic nephropathy, 1781, 1840, 1924–25
Diabetic retinopathy, 1342–43, 1923–24
Diagnosis related groups, 612, 726–27
Dialysis
hemodialysis, 1836–37
peritoneal, 1837–39
Diapedesis, 267
Diaphoresis, 1485
Diaphragm
description of, 981
in spinal cord injury patient education about, 1233
transcutaneous electric nerve stimulation of, 1233
Diaphragmatic breathing, 921
Diaphysis, 1935
Diarrhea, 434–35, 1576–77
Diarthrosis, 1940
Diastolic blood pressure, 911
Diastolic heart failure, 804
Diastolic phase, 751
Diazepam, 1278t
Diencephalon, 452f, 1142–43
Diet. *See also* Nutrition
cancer risks and, 404
colorectal cancer and, 1678
fiber in, 1678
history-taking, 744–45, 1610, 1611f
hypertension and, 910–11
nutritionally adequate, 1598–1601
therapeutic uses of, 391–94
Dietary Approaches to Stop Hypertension, 917t, 917–18
Dietary habits, 124
Diethylstilbestrol, 2119
Dietician, 1911
Differentiation, 1476
Diffuse axonal injury, 1184
Diffuse preretinal hemorrhages, 1309
Diffuse-weighted imaging, 1190
Diffusion, 297, 297f
Digestion, 1596–98
Digital rectal examination, 1680t, 2078, 2169
Digital subtraction angiography, 1163
Digitalis toxicity
idioventricular rhythm caused by, 859
junctional tachycardia caused by, 853
Digitoxin, 500
Digoxin
description of, 500–501, 501t
heart failure treated with, 810
Dihydropyridines
coronary artery disease treated with, 782t, 783
hypertension treated with, 924t
Dihydrotestosterone, 2166
Dilated cardiomyopathy, 812–13
Dilation and curettage, 2082, 2096
Diltiazem, 924t
Dilutional hyponatremia, 307
Dimethyl sulfoxide, 1776
Dimorphic, 1070
Diphenhydramine, 1022t, 2220
2,3-Diphosphoglycerate, 739, 985
Diploid, 199
Diplopia, 1153, 1289, 1324
Diprivan, 596
Dipyridamole, 779
Direct bilirubin, 1698
Direct calorimetry, 1600
Direct contact transmission, 276
Direct Coombs' test, 1415
Direct intermittent infusion, 357
Direct observation therapy, 1067
Direct response, to pupil examination, 1305
Directed coughing, 1110
Director of surgical services, 658
Disaccharides, 1597
Disaster, 2240
Disaster medical assistance teams, 2244
Disasters, 647–48
Discussion, 47
Disease(s)
appraisal-transaction theory of, 244
biological theory of, 241
chronic, 414
early civilization theories and practices regarding, 240
germ theory of, 240–41
inflammation-induced, 272–73
Disequilibrium, 1836
Disinfection, 667t
Displaced fracture, 1947
Dissecting aneurysm, 889, 889f
Disseminated fungal infection, 1071
Disseminated intravascular coagulation
in cancer patients, 442
causes of, 679–80
characteristics of, 942–44
definition of, 679
description of, 2225
Disseminated tuberculosis, 1066
Distal splenorenal shunt, 1716
Distress, 241
Distribution, of drugs, 484
Disturbed Energy Field, 385
Disuse syndrome, 1247
Diuretics
carbonic anhydrase inhibitors, 506–8
cardiovascular uses of, 506–8
cirrhosis treated with, 1714
definition of, 506
hypertension treated with, 922–23, 923t
loop, 506–8, 923t, 1783
nephrotic syndrome treated with, 1786
osmotic, 506–8
potassium loss from, 317
potassium-sparing, 507–8, 923t
thiazide, 506–8, 923t, 1791
Diverticulitis, 1666–68
Diverticulosis, 1667
Dobutamine stress testing
coronary artery disease evaluations, 779
description of, 765
Doctor of Nursing Practice, 11
Documentation
health assessment, 194
importance of, 49–50
Domains of nursing, 11
Domestic abuse, 1183, 1191
Dominant culture, 71
Do-not-resuscitate orders, 112, 151
Dopamine
description of, 1138
replacement therapy, 1282
Doppler ultrasonography, 885–86
Dornase alfa, 1130
Dorsalis pedis, 1943
Dorsiflexion, 1944f
Dot hemorrhages, 1309
Double effect, 111
Down syndrome, 199–200, 211, 212f
Doxazosin, 924t
Doxorubicin, 1724, 1997t
Drains, for wounds, 699, 700t, 711, 723
Drawer test, 2021f
Dreiling tube, 1587
Dressings
changing of, 723
description of, 286, 699, 711
moisture retentive, 1503
Dressler's syndrome, 791–92
Driving, 137
Dronabinol, 436–37, 463
Droplet transmission
description of, 276
precautions for, 280, 280t
Drug(s). *See also specific drug*
cancer-inducing, 404–5
discharge teaching about, 724
excretion of, 485–86
first pass effect of, 485
half-life of, 486
herbal interactions with, 395t
hypersensitivity to, 475
incompatibility of, 356–57
information resources, 491
loading dose of, 486
pharmaceutic phase of, 484
pharmacodynamics of, 487
pharmacokinetics of, 484–86
preparation of, 356
side effects of, 488
therapeutic range of, 486
Drug administration
abbreviations used in, 490
description of, 473
documentation of, 488
in elderly, 490–91
ethical considerations, 491
geriatric considerations, 490–91
inhalation, 489t
intradermal, 489t
intramuscular, 489t
intranasal, 1272
mucous membranes, 489t

in older adults, 490–91
oral, 489t
parenteral, 489t
rights of, 487b, 487–89
subcutaneous, 489t
topical, 489t
transdermal, 489t
Drug allergies
description of, 475
history-taking, 180, 181
Drug concentration, 486
Drug errors
computerized physician order entry system to prevent, 536
description of, 355–56
reduction of, 487
Drug interactions, 1601–2
Drug order, 491b
Drug-eluting stents, 786
Drug-induced hepatitis, 1710
Drusen, 1309
Dry heat sterilization, 666b
Dry powder inhalers
description of, 516, 1113
directions for, 1113
Dual energy X-ray absorptiometry scan, 1949–50
Ductal carcinoma in situ, 2155
Dumping syndrome, 1640–41
Duodenal ulcers, 523
Duodenitis, 1641
Duodenum, 1570
Duplex ultrasonography, 2079
Dura mater, 1139
Durable power of attorney for health care, 105–6, 149, 151
Dust mites, 1021b
Dying. *See also* End-of-life care
active phase of, 166–68
bill of rights, 148, 149b
definition of, 144
home care during, 165–68
physiology of, 167t
spiritual considerations, 165b
Dynorphin, 454
Dysarthria, 1187b
Dyscrasia, 1040
Dysdiadochokinesia, 1156
Dysesthesia, 1157, 1243
Dysfunctional uterine bleeding, 2093–94, 2097
Dysgeusia, 1153
Dysmenorrhea, 2088, 2099–2100
Dysmetria, 1156
Dyspareunia, 2094, 2127
Dyspepsia
nonpeptic, 1574–75, 1635–38
peptic-ulcer, 1638–41
Dysphagia
assessment of, 1623–24, 1624b
cervical auscultation evaluations, 1624
definition of, 1154, 1187b, 1572–74, 1623
diagnostic tests, 1624–25
endoscopic management of, 1626, 1627f
enteral feedings for, 1626
nursing diagnoses, 1625
nutritional considerations, 1626
surgical treatment of, 1626, 1627f
treatment of, 1625–26
Dyspnea
assessment of, 753–54, 991
in chronic obstructive pulmonary disease, 1103–4
definition of, 753, 990, 1055, 1103
in hospice patients, 153–54, 162
management of, 162
in palliative care patients, 153–54, 162
in stroke patients, 1201
Dysrhythmia, 835
Dyssynergy, 1156
Dysthymia, 252
Dysuria, 1762, 1767

E

Ear(s). *See also* Auditory dysfunction; Hearing loss
anatomy of, 1351f–1352f
assessment of
history-taking, 1312–14
otoscopic, 1317–19
Rinne test, 1315, 1315f
tuning fork tests, 1314–15, 1315f
voice-whisper test, 1314
Weber test, 1314–15, 1315f
cerebrospinal fluid drainage from, 1316
embryologic development of, 1352
external
anatomy of, 1311–12, 1351f–1352f
assessment of, 1315–16
inspection of, 1315–16
otitis of. *See* Otitis externa
palpation of, 1316
external auditory canal, 1317
foreign bodies in, 1358, 1363–64
inner, 1312, 1351f–1352f
middle
anatomy of, 1312, 1351, 1352f
surgery of, 1365–66
ossicles, 1312, 1351
Ear infections
hearing loss caused by, 1358
otitis media. *See* Otitis media
Ebola virus, for biological warfare, 2252–54
Ecchymosis, 745t
Eccrine glands, 1477t, 1478
Echocardiography
acute myocardial infarction evaluations, 793
cardiovascular system assessments using, 763
definition of, 763
nursing management during, 764–65
stress, 779
transesophageal, 763–64
Ectopy, 713
Ectropion, 1305
Eczematoid lesions, 1490b
Edema
angioneurotic, 1467–68
burn-related, 1542
definition of, 1485
description of, 306
in glomerulonephritis, 1782
heart failure and, 805
spinal cord injury-related, 1227
spinal cord tumors, 1241
Edward syndrome, 200
Effleurage, 388
Effluent, 1838
Eflornithine hydrochloride, 2092
Egophony, 1002
Ejaculation
description of, 2058–59, 2067–68
retrograde, 2078
Ejection fraction, 752
Elastin, 1101
Elbow range of motion, 1946t
Elderly. *See also* Older adults
abuse of, 132, 1183, 1202
atrial fibrillation in, 852
brain injuries in, 1182t
capillary refill in, 879
chronic pain in, 455
drug administration in, 490–91
frailty of, 641
hypoglycemia in, 1921
hypothyroidism in, 1895
life span for, 71
negative life events experienced by, 252
neglect of, 132
nutrition for, 1615
patient care for, 663
perioperative considerations for, 661–63
postoperative care for, 717–18
pulmonary disease in, 662–63
pyelonephritis in, 1779
respiratory assessments in, 992–93
urine output in, 1829
visual impairments in, 1310
Elective regional lymph node dissection, 1524
Electrical burns, 1535
Electrocardiography
acute abdomen evaluations, 1659
acute coronary syndrome evaluations, 792–93
angina pectoris evaluations, 777–78
arrhythmia detection using, 845, 845b
artifacts, 841, 842t
asystole findings, 860, 860f
atrial fibrillation findings, 851f, 851–52
atrial flutter findings, 850, 851f
atrial tachycardia findings, 850
cardiac monitoring, 839–40
cardiovascular assessments, 754, 762
chronic obstructive pulmonary disease evaluations, 1106
complete heart block findings, 855f, 855–56
components of, 841
exercise, 762
first-degree heart block findings, 854, 854f
heart failure evaluations, 807
heart rate calculations, 841–43
junctional escape rhythm findings, 853
junctional tachycardia findings, 853
leads
bipolar, 840
description of, 838–39
monitoring, 839–40
placement of, 840
precordial, 839
P wave, 841, 843–44
PR interval, 841, 844
premature atrial complex findings, 850
premature junctional complex findings, 853
premature ventricular complex findings, 856, 856f
preoperative, 638
principles of, 838–39
pulseless electrical activity findings, 860
QRS complex, 841–42, 844
QRS interval, 841, 844–45
QT interval, 845
R wave, 842–43
rhythm determinations, 843–44
second-degree heart block findings, 854
sinus bradycardia findings, 847, 847f
sinus rhythm findings, 847, 847f
sinus tachycardia findings, 848, 848f
T wave, 841, 845
telemetry systems, 840, 840b
tracings, 841
troubleshooting, 841, 842t
12-lead, 762, 835, 838
ventricular fibrillation findings, 858f, 858–60
ventricular tachycardia findings, 857, 857f
Electroencephalography
description of, 1164–65
stroke evaluations, 1175t
Electrolarynx, 1047
Electrolyte balance
cardiovascular system's role in, 300–301
description of, 300–302
posterior pituitary gland's role in, 301–2
renin-angiotensin-aldosterone system's role in, 301
Electrolytes. *See also specific electrolyte*
characteristics of, 299t
definition of, 298
infusion therapy, 361–62
types of, 299t
Electromyography
description of, 1165–66
myasthenia gravis evaluations, 1290
Electron beam computed tomography, 780
Electronic health records, 616
Electrophoresis, 1413
Electrophysiological studies
cardiovascular system assessments, 764
nursing management during, 766
Electrosurgery, 675–76, 676b
Electrosurgical units, 675
E-mail, 615
Emancipated minor, 103
Embolism
definition of, 1172
pulmonary
description of, 2042–43
pain associated with, 755t, 1004
postoperative, 662
prevention of, 1246
signs of, 894
Embolization, 2181
Emergency assessment, 176
Emergency departments, 2236–37
Emergency nursing, 2236–37
Emergency surgery, 644–48
Emigrants, 72, 82, 84
Emmetropia, 1337
Emotion-focused coping, 244
Emphysema. *See also* Chronic obstructive pulmonary disease
assessment of, 1103
in chronic obstructive pulmonary disease, 1102
lung elasticity reductions caused by, 1102
lung volume reduction surgery for, 1114
panlobar, 1102
Employer value system, 17–18
Employment discrimination, 230–31
Empowerment, 63, 259, 261
Enalapril, 924t
Encephalopathy
definition of, 1698b
hepatic, 1717
Endarterectomy, 887, 1180–81
Endocarditis
bacterial, 818–20
definition of, 815
Endocardium, 748, 818
Endocrine system
adrenal glands. *See* Adrenal glands
aging effects on, 1856

anatomy and physiology of, 1849–56, 1850f
assessment of, 1856–58, 1858t
diagnostic tests, 1858–60, 1859t
hypothalamus, 1848, 1852
nervous system effects on, 1850–51
objective data, 1858
overview of, 1848–49
pancreas. *See* Pancreas
pituitary gland, 1852, 1853f
thyroid gland, 1853–55
End-of-life care. *See also* Dying
in amyotrophic lateral sclerosis patients, 1293
artificial nutrition and hydration, 113
do-not-resuscitate orders, 112, 151
double effect, 111
hospice care, 110–11
legal considerations, 1603
limitation of treatment, 112
palliative care, 110–11
right to die, 113–14
Endogenous pyrogens, 1395, 1396t
Endometrial ablation, 2093–94
Endometrial cancer, 411t, 2093, 2120, 2122
Endometriomas, 2112
Endometriosis, 2088, 2094–95, 2098
Endorectal ultrasonography, 1683
Endorphins, 383, 454, 1138
Endoscopic retrograde cholangiopancreatography, 1700, 1739
Endoscopy
dysphagia treated with, 1626, 1627f
gastrointestinal obstruction treated with, 1674–75
Endosteum, 1935
Endothelium, 2203
Endotoxins, 1709b
Endotracheal intubation
complications of
anxiety, 596–98
barotrauma, 594–95
communication, 595–96
nutrition impairments, 598–99
paralysis, 597
stress ulcers, 595
tracheal damage, 593
unplanned extubation, 593–94
description of, 584–85
indications for, 998f
suctioning of, 592, 592t
End-stage kidney disease, 1781
Enema, 1584, 1591–92
Energy, 1600
Energy expenditures, 1600
Energy field disturbance, 478
Energy therapies
acupressure, 387
acupuncture, 386–87
description of, 384–85
healing touch, 385
Reiki, 385–86
therapeutic touch, 385
Enkephalins, 454, 1138
Entacapone, 1283t
Enteral nutrition
administration of, 1605
benefits of, 1603
for burn patients, 1550
definition of, 1602
for dysphagia patients, 1626
formulas, 1603–4, 1604t
routes for, 1605, 1605f
tubes used in, 1605
Enteritis, radiation therapy, 417–18
Enterocele, 2111
Enterocytes, 1570
Enterokinase, 1570
Enterprises, 5–6
Enthesitis, 1970
Entropia, 1324
Entropion, 1305
Enucleation, 1335
Environment
asthma triggers in, 1117t
cancer etiology and, 404
Environmental control, 82
Environmental noise, 1368–69
Environmental stress, 253–54
Enzymatic debridement of wounds, 1498
Eosinophils, 267, 741, 1388
Ependymal cells, 1138–39
Ependymoma, 1238
Epicardial pacing, 865
Epicardium, 748
Epicondylitis, lateral, 2014–15
Epidemiological investigation, 2247
Epidermal growth factor, 283
Epidermis
aging effects on, 1482
anatomy of, 1476, 1477t, 1478f
appendages of, 1477t, 1478–79
cells of, 1476–78
Epididymis, 2056
Epididymitis, 2178
Epidural anesthesia, 678t
Epidural hematoma, 1188f, 1189t
Epidural probe, 581
Epiglottis, 979
Epilepsy
antiepileptic drugs for, 1272, 1273t
definition of, 1269
diagnostic criteria for, 520
epidemiology of, 1269
genetic factors, 222–23
Epimysium, 1938
Epinephrine, 912, 1463, 1851t
Epiphyses, 1935
Epispadias, 2189–90
Epistaxis, 1040–41
Epitope, 1382
Eplerenone, 923t
Epoetin alfa, 431
Epoprostenol, 1091
Eprosartan, 924t
Epstein-Barr virus, 949
Equianalgesia, 473, 475t, 710
Erb's point, 757
Erectile dysfunction, 2058, 2193–95
Erection, 2058, 2067
Ergocalciferol, 1987
Ergonomics, 19, 694
Erikson, Erik, 122
Erlotinib, 1081
Erosion, 1489f
Erythema migrans, 1621–22
Erythrocyte(s). *See also* Anemia
aging of, 739–40
bone marrow production of, 736
cell membrane of, 737
cytoskeleton of, 737
diagnostic tests of, 746, 747t
function of, 735, 737
illustration of, 736
laboratory tests, 747t
metabolic activity of, 739
Erythrocyte count, 747t
Erythrocyte sedimentation rate, 1412
Erythromelalgia, 947
Erythropoietic medications, 431
Erythropoietin, 366, 736
Eschar, 1531, 1535, 1542
Escharotomy, 1543–44
Esophageal cancer
assessment of, 1633
epidemiology of, 1632–33
incidence of, 403t
mortality rates, 1632
nursing diagnoses, 1633
obesity and, 1632
pathophysiology of, 1633
risk factors for, 1632t
screening for, 1633
treatment of, 1633–34
Esophageal dilation, 1589–90
Esophageal disorders
achalasia, 1574, 1628
description of, 1626
gastroesophageal reflux disease, 1056, 1573, 1629–31
hiatal hernia, 1631–32
Esophageal manometry, 1587
Esophageal pain, 1627–28
Esophageal speech, 1047
Esophageal varices, 1715
Esophagraphy, 1591
Esophagus
anatomy of, 1570
Barrett's, 1629–30
rupture of, 755t
Esotropia, 1306
Essential fatty acid deficiency, 361
Essential oils, 394
Estrogen
breast cancer and, 423
replacement of, 2090
Estrogen vaginal cream, 2115
Ethacrynic acid, 923t
Ethambutol, 1068t
Ethical decision-making models
contextual features, 108
integrated, 109
medical indications, 107–8
patient preferences, 108
quality of life, 108
Ethical dilemmas
brain death, 113–14
description of, 96–97
end-of-life care. *See* End-of-life care
euthanasia, 114–15
medical futility, 112, 115–16
organ donation, 113–14
pain management, 109–10
Ethical issues, 96–97
Ethical theories, 98–99
Ethics
advance directives. *See* Advance directives
clinical, 96–97
code of, 99–100, 191
confidentiality, 102–3
in data collection, 191–94
definition of, 96, 191, 371
genetic screening and testing, 193–94
informed consent, 103–4, 192
infusion therapy, 371
intraoperative, 684–86
mechanical ventilation, 589
nurse's role, 100–102
organizational, 100
perioperative, 684–86
principles of, 97, 192t
professional, 99–100
research, 116–17
rights-based, 98
Ethics of care, 98–99
Ethnic populations. *See also specific ethnicity*
older adults, 136
trends in, 126
Ethnicity
definition of, 70, 189
health assessment considerations, 189
Ethnocentrism, 71
Ethosuximide, 521
Etidronate, 1991t
Eucalyptus, 393t
Eugenics, 194
Euglycemia, 1912
Euploidy, 199
Eupnea, 995
European Americans
biological variations in, 84t
folk medicine used by, 83t
Eustachian tube
anatomy of, 1312
dysfunction of, 1358
Eustress, 241–42
Euthanasia
assisted suicide vs., 150
description of, 114–15
Euthenics, 194
Evening primrose, 393t
Eversion, 1944f
Evidence summary
analytic approach to, 34
description of, 31–34
preparation of, 34–35
sources of, 35, 36b
Evidence-based practice
ACE Star Model of. *See* ACE Star Model of Knowledge Transformation
components of, 26
definition of, 24, 138
evidence summary. *See* Evidence summary
features of, 25, 33–39
history of, 25–26
impediments to, 27, 27t
knowledge bases for, 24
in nursing, 27–28
nursing practice use of, 40
primary concept of, 26–27
priorities, 39–40
process of, 25–26
research utilization vs., 25
steps of, 138b
systematic reviews, 33–35
Evisceration, 415
Evoked potentials
multiple sclerosis evaluations, 1276
somatosensory, 1952
types of, 1166t
Excitability, 837–38
Excoriation, 1489f
Exercise
for Alzheimer's disease patients, 1288
after amputation, 2048–49
atherosclerosis prevention and, 884

blood pressure management by, 921
diabetes mellitus management by, 1915–17
energy expenditures, 1600
fibromyalgia managed using, 1979–80
osteoporosis prevention and, 1985
Paget's disease managed using, 1990
recommendations for, 921–922, 1598
respiratory adjustments during, 989
therapeutic benefits of, 383
Exercise electrocardiogram, 762
Exocrine glands, 1849
Exophthalmos, 1858f
Exostoses, 1318
Exotoxin, 289
Exotropia, 1306, 1324
Expiration, 981
Expiratory reserve volume, 1012, 1106t
Expressive aphasia, 1199
Extended family, 77t
Extended-spectrum penicillins, 493
Extension sets, 345b
External auditory canal, 1311, 1317
External ear, 1311–12
Extracellular buffers, 987
Extracellular fluid, 296, 298
Extracorporeal shock wave lithotripsy, 1791, 1792f
Extraocular muscles
anatomy of, 1301, 1301f
movement assessments, 1305–6, 1306f, 1325f
paralysis of, 1324
Extrapulmonary restrictive lung disorder, 1063–64
Extravasation, 349–50, 968t, 1394
Extremities
assessment of, 757
pulse rating in, 757b
Extrinsic distortion, 74
Extubation
by critical care nurse, 601
unplanned, 593–94
Exudate
definition of, 269
in wound, 286
Eye(s). *See also* Visual acuity
assessment of
cardinal fields of gaze, 1305, 1306f
color vision testing, 1304
extraocular examination, 1304–5
funduscopic, 1306
history-taking, 1303
ophthalmoscopic examination, 1306
posterior segment structures, 1306–11
visual acuity testing, 1303–4
visual field confrontation test, 1304
description of, 1301
diabetic retinopathy, 1342–43
external, 1301–2
extraocular muscles
anatomy of, 1301, 1301f
movement assessments, 1305–6, 1306f
health promotion, 1345
inflammatory and infectious conditions of
blepharitis, 1340
chalazion, 1340
conjunctivitis, 1340
hordeolum, 1339
iritis, 1341–42
keratitis, 1341
keratoconjunctivitis sicca, 1341
uveitis, 1341–42
internal anatomy of, 1302, 1324f
papilledema, 1342
protective barriers, 1383
refractive errors of, 1337–38
retinitis pigmentosa, 1343–44
safety concerns, 1345
Eyebrows, 1304
Eyeglasses, 1337–38
Eyelashes, 1301
Eyelids
description of, 1305
ptosis of, 1310

F

Face shields, 672
Facemask, 697, 868
Facial nerve, 1146f, 1147t, 1153–54
Factor I, 742t
Factor II, 742t
Factor III, 742t
Factor IX, 742t
Factor V, 742t
Factor V Leiden, 211
Factor VII, 742t
Factor VIII, 742t
Factor X, 742t
Factor XI
deficiency of, 944
description of, 742t
Factor XII, 742t
Factor XIII, 742t
Faith healing, 390
Fallopian tubes
agenesis of, 2113
anatomy of, 2059–60
Falls
brain injuries caused by, 1183
prevention of, 1191
False aneurysm, 889
Familial adenomatous polyposis, 1677
Familial Alzheimer's disease, 221
Family
communication uses of, 74–75
of critically ill patients, 567–68
genetic screening of, 209
postoperative instructions, 715–17, 722–25
preoperative involvement, 626–27, 633–34
Family education
acute coronary syndromes, 796–97
amputation, 2045–46
aneurysms, 892
asthma, 1124, 1126
atherosclerosis, 883–84
brain injuries, 1193
chronic obstructive pulmonary disease, 1115–16
cystic fibrosis, 1131
fibromyalgia, 1980
hypertension, 925
osteoporosis, 1984
Paget's disease, 1990–91
peripheral arterial occlusive disease, 888
Family history, 211
Family patterns, 77t
Family structure
blended, 77t
changes in, 14
extended, 77t
types of, 76, 77t
Fascia, 2039
Fasciotomy, 2040
Fast pain, 453
Fasting plasma glucose level, 1908
Fat(s)
absorption of, 1649–50
for diabetes mellitus patients, 1910
digestion of, 1597
in total parenteral nutrition, 361
Fat embolism syndrome, 2040–41
Fat soluble vitamins, 1649, 1713
Fatigue
chemotherapy-induced, 421, 439–40, 1198
hematological system abnormalities and, 744
radiation therapy-induced, 418, 439–40, 1198
Fatty liver, 1718–19
Fatty streaks, 774, 879
Febrile neutropenia, 432
Febrile seizures, 223
Fecal elimination, 181
Fecal occult blood testing, 1679, 1680t
Fecalith, 1664
Fecundity, 2069
Feeding tubes, 1590–91. *See also* Enteral nutrition; Nutrition support
Felodipine, 924t
Female genital mutilation, 2116–18
Female reproductive disorders
assessment of, 2113–14
cystocele, 2110–11
enterocele, 2111
infections. *See* Gynecological infections
leiomyomata, 2111–12
Müllerian dysgenesis, 2112
ovarian cysts, 2112, 2114
pelvic relaxation, 2110–11
polyps, 2110, 2115
rectocele, 2111, 2114
sexually transmitted diseases. *See* Sexually transmitted diseases
urethrocele, 2110–11
uterine prolapse, 2111
Female reproductive system
Bartholin's glands, 2063, 2076, 2102
breasts, 2063–64
bulbourethral glands, 2063, 2076
cervix, 2060–61, 2076
clitoris, 2062
diagnostic tests, 2080–84
external genitalia, 2061–63
fallopian tubes, 2059–60, 2113
functions of, 2059
hymen, 2062–63
labia majora, 2061–62, 2076
labia minora, 2061–62, 2076
menarche, 2064
menopause, 2064–65, 2090–91, 2096
mons pubis, 2061
ovaries, 2059, 2076
paraurethral glands, 2063
perineum, 2063
Skene's glands, 2063, 2101–2
uterus. *See* Uterus
vagina. *See* Vagina
Female sexual response, 2068–69
Fenamates, 471b
Fentanyl, 474t, 596t
Ferric ion, 738
Ferritin, 738, 747t
Ferrous ion, 738
Fertility, 2069
Fetal alcohol effect, 215
Fetal alcohol syndrome, 215, 216f
Fetoscopy, 212t, 213
Fever
diagnostic criteria for, 724
nonsteroidal anti-inflammatory drugs for, 274
postoperative, 724
Feverfew, 393t
Fexofenadine, 1022t
Fiber, 1678, 1910–11
Fiber ligands, 391t
Fiber pectin, 391t
Fibric acid derivatives, 514–15
Fibrin clot, 743
Fibrin degradation products, 743
Fibrinolytic therapy, 794–95
Fibroadenoma, 2142
Fibroblasts, 1479
Fibrocystic breast disorders, 2141–42
Fibroids, uterine, 2111–12, 2114
Fibromyalgia
assessment of, 1977–78
chronic fatigue syndrome and, 1977
definition of, 1976
diagnostic criteria for, 1978t
diagnostic tests, 1978
epidemiology of, 1976
etiology of, 1976
exercise for, 1979–80
family education about, 1980
health care resources for, 1980
hypothalamic-pituitary-adrenal axis abnormalities associated with, 1977
nursing diagnoses, 1979
nutrition in, 1979
outcomes, 1980–81
pathophysiology of, 1977
patient education about, 1980
pharmacological treatment of, 1979
physical deconditioning secondary to, 1979
syndromes associated with, 1977–78
treatment of, 1979–80
Fidelity, 192t
Fight-or-flight response, 242, 243t, 1145, 1215
Fine needle aspiration biopsy, 2150
Finger clubbing, 996–97
Fire
laser-induced, 675
in surgical environment, 675–76
First pass effect, 485
Fissure, 1489f
Flaccidity, 1155
Flail chest, 1087–88
Flash sterilization, 667, 669
Flatulence, 1576
Fleet's phospho-soda, 1585
Flexible cystoscope, 1762f
Flexible sigmoidoscopy, 1680t
Flexion, 1944f
Floating ribs, 975
Fluconazole, 1071–72
Fluid(s)
concentration regulation, 296–98
extracellular, 296, 298
gains and losses of, 296, 296t
interstitial, 296
intracellular, 296, 298
intraoperative management of, 682–83
intravascular, 296
transcellular, 296
types of, 341
Fluid balance
cardiovascular system's role in, 300–301
control of, 300–302
kidneys in, 300

overview of, 296
posterior pituitary gland's role in, 301–2
renin-angiotensin-aldosterone system's role in, 301
Fluid compartments, 296–97
Fluid imbalances. *See* Fluid volume deficit; Fluid volume excess
Fluid resuscitation
in burn patients, 1541, 1543
colloid fluids, 1543, 2215t
crystalloid fluids, 1543, 2216t
in shock patients, 2216t
volume calculations, 1543
Fluid volume deficit
assessment of, 302–3
complications of, 303
diagnostic tests for, 303
etiology of, 302
nursing diagnoses, 303–4
pathophysiology of, 302
Fluid volume excess
complications of, 306
description of, 304, 1755
diagnostic tests for, 306–7
etiology of, 304, 306
nursing diagnoses for, 307
pathophysiology of, 306
Fluid-attenuated-inversion-recovery, 1276
Fluorescein angiogram, 1923
Fluorescent in-situ hybridization
description of, 201
genetic testing uses of, 214
Fluoride, 1984
Fluoroquinolones
acute sinusitis treated with, 1028
description of, 495–98
urinary tract infections treated with, 1772b
Fluoxetine, 474t, 1278t
Fluticasone propionate, 1023t
Foam cells, 774
Focal lesionectomy, 1274t
Focused assessment, 175
Folic acid, 392, 1648
Folic acid deficiency, 1648
Folic acid deficiency anemia, 937–38
Folk medicine, 82, 83t
Follicle-stimulating hormone, 1849, 1851t, 2056, 2064, 2078
Follicular cysts, 2112, 2115
Follicular dendritic cell, 1392
Folliculitis, 1509–10
Fontaine Staging System, for peripheral arterial occlusive disease, 886, 886t
Food allergies, 181, 637, 1404, 1468–69
Food preferences, 85t
Forced expiratory volume in one second, 1101, 1106t
Forced vital capacity, 1011, 1101, 1106t
Foreign bodies
in ear, 1358, 1363–64
hearing loss caused by, 1358
ocular, 1333
Formula method, of intravenous therapy calculations, 351–52
Forward genetics, 224
Fosinopril, 924t
Fourth heart sound, 759t, 759–60
Fox sign, 1658
Fraction of inspired oxygen, 587
Fracture(s)
assessment of, 1947–48, 2033
casts for, 2036
closed, 2032, 2032f
closed reduction of, 2034
comminuted, 2032
complete, 2032
complications of, 2032
definition of, 2031
delayed union of, 2033
diagnostic tests, 2033
displaced, 1947
epidemiology of, 2031
family education about, 2034–35
fixation of, 2034, 2035b
healing of, 1937–38
hip, 2036–39
incomplete, 2032
malunion of, 2032
nasal, 1041
nonunion of, 2033
nursing diagnoses, 2033
occult, 2038
open, 2032, 2032t
open reduction of, 2034
osteoporosis-related, 1982
osteoporotic, 460
pathological, 2031, 2031b
pathophysiology of, 2031–33
patient education about, 2034–35
physical therapy for, 2035
skull, 1183
spinal cord injuries caused by, 1219
sports-related, 1947–48
stable, 1947
stress, 1947, 2029–31
treatment of, 2034
unstable, 1947
vertebral, 460
Fractured rib, 1085–87
Fragile X syndrome, 202, 205, 205f
Frailty, 135, 641
Frank-Starling's curve, 752
Frank-Starling's Law, 568
Free flaps, for breast reconstruction, 2158
Fremitus, 998
Fresh frozen plasma, 364
Frontal lobe, 452f
Fulguration, 1683
Full-thickness grafts, 1553
Full-thickness wounds, 282
Functional gastrointestinal disorders, 1635
Functional health patterns
definition of, 174
description of, 178–179
Functional incontinence, 1807b
Fungal infections
in burn wounds, 1548
opportunistic, 1069
pulmonary
aspergillosis, 1070
assessment of, 1070–71
blastomycosis, 1069
coccidioidomycosis, 1069–70
definition of, 1069
diagnostic tests, 1071
histoplasmosis, 1070
nursing diagnoses, 1071
outcomes, 1072
pathophysiology of, 1070
planning and implementation for, 1071–72
treatment of, 1071–72
skin, 1510–12
Fungi, 271t
Funnel chest, 756t, 994
Furosemide, 582, 923t, 1093–94
Furuncles, 1512
Fusiform aneurysm, 889, 889f
Fusion inhibitors, 1430b
Futility, medical, 112, 115–16

G

Gabapentin, 474t, 1278t
Gag reflex, 1624
Gagne, Robert, 45t
Gait
assessment of, 1944–45
definition of, 1156
Galactorrhea, 1865, 2142
Gallbladder
assessment of, 1583
disorders of, 1729–33
drainage of, 1699
ultrasound of, 1701
Gallbladder cancer, 1735–36
Gallstones. *See* Cholelithiasis
Gamete intrafallopian transfer, 2127
Gametes, 2056
Gamma-aminobutyric acid, 1138
Gangliosides, 1226
Garlic, 393t
Gastrectomy, 1644
Gastric cancer. *See* Stomach cancer
Gastric decompression, 1674
Gastric decompression tubes, 1588
Gastric emptying, 1636
Gastric intubation
complications of, 1588
contraindications, 1588
equipment used in, 1587–88
technique, 1589
tubes, 1587
Gastric lavage, 1587–88
Gastric lipase, 1597
Gastric lymphoma, 1643
Gastric motility agents, 1637
Gastric ulcers, 1638–41
Gastrin, 1570
Gastritis, 1641
Gastroesophageal reflux disease, 1056, 1573, 1629–31
Gastroferrin, 1570
Gastrointestinal disorders
constipation. *See* Constipation
diagnostic tests, 1584–92
diarrhea, 1576–77
obstruction. *See* Gastrointestinal obstruction
Gastrointestinal obstruction
acute colonic pseudo obstruction
colonoscopic decompression of, 1674
description of, 1669
etiology of, 1670
assessment of, 1671–72
clinical manifestations of, 1671–72
computed tomography of, 1673
description of, 1668–69
diagnostic tests, 1672–73
duodenum, 1671t
endoscopic therapy for, 1674–75
epidemiology of, 1669–70
gastric decompression for, 1674
ileus
definition of, 1669
epidemiology of, 1669–70
etiology of, 1670
postoperative, 1670
laparoscopic treatment of, 1675
large bowel, 1671t, 1672, 1675
nursing diagnoses, 1673
outcomes, 1675–76
pathophysiology of, 1671
perforation risks, 1672–73
pharmacological treatment of, 1673–76
self-expandable metal stents for, 1675
simple, 1669
small bowel
epidemiology of, 1669
etiology of, 1670, 1671t
gastric decompression for, 1674
laparoscopic treatment of, 1675
strangulated, 1669, 1671
surgical treatment of, 1675
treatment of, 1673–76
ultrasound of, 1673
Gastrointestinal system
age-related changes, 1402t
burn effects on, 1533
diagnostic tests, 1584–92
functions of, 1568
Gastrointestinal tract
anatomy of, 1569–71, 1596f
anus, 1571
appendix, 1571
assessment of
auscultation, 1579, 1581
general, 1571–73, 1578–84
observation, 1578–79
palpation, 1579, 1581
symptoms-based, 1573–76
biliary systems, 1571
cecum, 1571
colon, 1571
duodenum, 1570
esophagus, 1570
functions of, 1596
gas in, 1576
ileum, 1571
jejunum, 1571
liver. *See* Liver
motility in, 1668
nutritional processes in, 1596–98
obstruction of. *See* Gastrointestinal obstruction
pain conditions in, 1634–35
pancreas, 1570–71
rectum, 1571
stomach, 1570
Gastrokinetics, 163
Gastroplasty, 1614
Gastrostomy
feedings through, 1605
procedure for, 1590–91
Gate control theory, 449–50
Gels, 1498
Gemfibrozil, 514
Gender. *See also* Women
coronary artery disease and, 771, 795
health assessment considerations, 190–91
pain responses affected by, 455–56
physical variations related to, 190–91
Gender identity, 190
Gender research, 190
Gender role, 190
Gene(s)
definition of, 198
delivery systems for gene therapy, 233

epilepsy, 223
mutation of, 198
structure of, 198–99
Gene splicing, 234
Gene testing
advantages and disadvantages of, 208
costs of, 208
limitations of, 208
types of, 207t
Gene therapy
brain tumors treated with, 1204
definition of, 226, 233
description of, 610
gene-delivery systems, 233
hemoglobinopathies treated with, 226
principles of, 233
Gene-environment interaction, 223
General adaptation syndrome, 242
General anesthesia
description of, 677, 678t
malignant hyperthermia risks, 683
General inhibition syndrome, 242
General practitioner, 3–4
Generalized seizures, 222, 1270t, 1271
Genetic counseling, 204, 206
Genetic disorders
chromosomal. *See* Chromosomal abnormalities
cystic fibrosis, 216
mental retardation, 216
Genetic engineering, 194, 233–34
Genetic Information Nondiscrimination Act, 230
Genetic screening
confidentiality of, 207, 230
definition of, 193
ethical considerations, 193–94
family, 209
follow-up evaluation after, 207
gene testing, 207–9
insurability concerns after, 231–32
medical history used for, 211
in newborns, 207
physical examination, 211
population, 209–10
principles of, 206–7
workplace, 210–11
Genetic testing
confidentiality of, 231
definition of, 193
insurability concerns after, 231–32
insurance company access to, 231
laboratory studies used for
alpha-fetoprotein, 213
amniocentesis, 212t, 212–13
fetoscopy, 212t, 213
overview of, 211–12
percutaneous umbilical blood sampling, 212t, 213
placental biopsy, 212t
ultrasound, 214–15
research of, 217
Genetics
definition of, 198
description of, 191
ethical issues, 228–29
forward, 224
fundamentals of, 198–203
Human Genome Project, 197, 228, 232
inheritance patterns. *See* Inheritance patterns
legal issues, 229–32
neonatal conditions affected by, 215–16
nurse's role in, 235
pediatric conditions affected by, 215–16
pharmacogenomics, 234–35
positional, 224
scope of, 227–28
teratology, 206
Genogram, 179, 180f, 209f
Genome scanning, 210
Genomics
definition of, 197
nursing practice integration of, 235
Genotype, 199
Genotyping, 1129
Germ theory, 240–41
Gestational diabetes, 219
Ghon complex, 1065
Giant cells, 1398
Gigantism. *See* Acromegaly
Ginger, 393t
Ginkgo, 393t, 395t
Glabellar reflex, 1159t
Glands. *See also specific gland*
definition of, 1849
eccrine, 1477t, 1478
endocrine, 1849
exocrine, 1849
Glans, 2062
Glasgow Coma Scale, 1148, 1149t, 1186
Glatiramer acetate, 1278t
Glaucoma, 1310, 1329–30
Glaucomatous cupping, 1308
Glimepiride, 1916t
Glioma, 1196
Glipizide, 1916t
Global aphasia, 1200
Globalization, 12–13
Globulins, 738
Glomerular basement membrane disease, 1822
Glomerular filtration rate
description of, 300, 912
loop diuretics' effect on, 506
Glomerulonephritis
assessment of, 1782
chronic, 1781
definition of, 1780
diagnostic tests, 1782
edema associated with, 1782
epidemiology of, 1780
etiology of, 1780–81
nursing diagnoses, 1782
outcomes, 1784
pathophysiology of, 1781
poststreptococcal, 1780–82
symptoms of, 1782
treatment of, 1782–84
Glossitis, 430, 1621–22
Glossopharyngeal nerve, 1146f, 1147t, 1154
Glottic cancer. *See* Laryngeal cancer
Gloves, 671
Glucagon, 1851t, 1856, 1905
Glucocorticoids
endogenous, 1851t
immunosuppressive uses of, 1840
inhaled, 519–20
nephrotic syndrome treated with, 1786
Gluconeogenesis, 1697, 1905
Glucose
blood monitoring of, in diabetes mellitus, 1909–10
exercise effects on, 1917
liver metabolism of, 1697
plasma transport of, 735
self-monitoring of, 1909–10
Somogyi effect, 1922
Glucose suppression test, 1868
Glucose-6-phosphate dehydrogenase, 933–34
Glutamic acid, 1138
Glyburide, 1916t
Glycine, 1138
Glycogen, 1597, 1697
Glycogenolysis, 1905
Glycoprotein IIb/IIIb, 743
Glycoprotein IIb/IIIb receptor inhibitors, 795
Glycoproteins, 737
Glycosides, cardiac, 500–502
Glycosylated hemoglobin, 1343
Goal setting, 53
Goblet cells, 981
Goiter, 1858f, 1890
Goniometer, 1945f
Goodpasture's syndrome, 1781, 1822–23
Gout, 272, 508, 1964–66
Gowns, 672
Grafts, for burn patients
allograft, 1552
autograft, 1552
donor sites for, 1553–54
full-thickness, 1553
heterograft, 1552
homograft, 1552
meshing of, 1553
procedures for, 1552–53
rejection of, 2231
sheet, 1553
split-thickness, 1553
Graft-versus-host disease, 426, 952, 1431–32, 1496
Graft-versus-tumor effect, 426–27
Gram stain, 2077
Gram-negative bacteria, 492
Gram-positive bacteria, 492
Granulation, 711
Granulocyte(s)
basophils. *See* Basophils
blood concentration of, 740
characteristics of, 1388
definition of, 1388
eosinophils, 267, 741, 1388
inflammatory response functions of, 740
neutrophils. *See* Neutrophils
transfusion of, 364–65
Granulocyte colony-stimulating factor, 268t, 269
Granuloma, 1065, 1398
Graphesthesia, 1158
Grasp reflex, 1159t
Graves' disease
assessment of, 1884, 1885t
clinical manifestations of, 1884
diagnostic tests, 1884, 1886t
epidemiology of, 1884
etiology of, 1884
nursing diagnoses, 1885
outcomes, 1890
pathophysiology of, 1884
pharmacological treatment of, 1888–89
radioiodine therapy for, 1889
surgical treatment of, 1889–90
treatment of, 1885–90
Gray matter, 1140
Grey Turner sign, 1658
Grief
by bereaved, 168
description of, 168
resolution of, 156
Grief support groups, 168
Grieving, anticipatory, 156
Gross domestic product, 533
Group A beta-hemolytic streptococci, 1032
Growth factors, 1482–83
Growth hormone, 1851t, 1852
Growth spurt, 191
Guanadrel, 923t
Guanethidine, 923t
Guardianship, 641–42
Guillain-Barré syndrome
ascending, 1244–45
assessment of, 1244–45
autonomic dysfunction associated with, 1246
definition of, 1244
descending, 1245
diagnostic tests, 1245
disuse syndrome secondary to, 1247
epidemiology of, 1244
etiology of, 1244
neurological alterations associated with, 1247
nursing diagnoses, 1245
outcomes, 1247
pain management in, 1247
pathophysiology of, 1244
plasmapheresis for, 1246
treatment of, 1246–47
Gut-associated lymphoid tissues, 1392
Guttate psoriasis, 1516
Gynecological examination
description of, 2075–76
speculum examination, 2076–77
Gynecological infections
alternative therapies for, 2109
bacterial vaginosis, 2101
Bartholin's gland infection, 2102
menstrual. *See* Menstrual disorders
outcomes, 2110
patient education about, 2109
pelvic inflammatory disease, 2105
sexually transmitted diseases. *See* Sexually transmitted diseases
Skene's gland infection, 2102
surgical treatment of, 2108–9
toxic shock syndrome, 2105
treatment of, 2107–9
trichomoniasis, 2101–2
vaginitis, 2101–2, 2106
Gynecological malignancies
assessment of, 2121
cervical cancer, 2119–20
description of, 2118
diagnostic tests, 2121
endometrial cancer, 2120, 2122
family education about, 2123
nursing diagnoses, 2121
outcomes, 2123
ovarian cancer, 2120–22
patient education about, 2123
treatment of, 2122–23
vaginal cancer, 2119
vulvar cancer, 2119, 2122
Gynecomastia, 1698, 1865, 2138
Gyrus, 1140, 1141f

H

Hair follicles, 1477t, 1479
Half-life, 356, 486
Halo traction, 1224
Haloperidol, 597t
Hand washing

infectious disease transmission prevented through, 277, 671
presurgical, 671
recommendations for, 277
Hantavirus, 277–79
Haploid, 199
Haptens, 1382
Hard exudates, 1309
Hashimoto's thyroiditis, 1433, 1892, 2231
Hassles, 244, 246
Haversian canals, 1936, 1936f
Havinghurst, Robert, 123
Hay fever. *See* Allergic rhinitis
Hazardous materials, 2244–45
Head lice, 1514
Headaches
brain injuries as cause of, 1186
brain tumors and, 1196–97
classification of, 1262
cluster, 1265t, 1267–68
costs of, 1262
diagnostic tests, 1263
migraine, 1265t, 1266–67
nitroglycerin-related, 503
nursing diagnoses, 1264b
prevalence of, 1262
tension-type
alternative therapies for, 1264–65
assessment of, 1263, 1263b
definition of, 1262
diagnostic tests, 1263
epidemiology of, 1263
etiology of, 1263
outcomes, 1266
pathophysiology of, 1263
pharmacological treatment of, 1264, 1265t
Head-to-toe assessment, 185
Healing
factors that affect, 1482–83
nurse's role in, 397
of skin, 1481
word origin of, 380
wound. *See* Wound healing
Healing touch, 385
Health
definition of, 249
nurse's role in promoting, 60
Health assessment
of adolescents, 187
of adults, 187
age-related approaches, 186–88
care of patient after, 194
comprehensive, 175
data from
ethical considerations, 191–94
objective, 176
sources of, 176–77
subjective, 176
types of, 176
diagnostic data, 185–86
documentation, 194
emergency, 176
focused, 175
goal of, 175
head-to-toe, 185
health history, 179–82
of infant, 186
interview, 177–78
laboratory data, 185–86
of neonate, 186
of older adults, 187–88
ongoing, 175–76
physical examination. *See* Physical examination
of preschool child, 187
purpose of, 175
review of systems, 185
of school-age child, 187
of toddler, 187
types of, 175–76
Health care
access to, 533, 535
control of, 4–6
costs of, 4, 7
definition of, 3
delivery models for, 15–16
evidence-based changes in, 39–40
globalization effects on, 12–13
illness care to, transition from, 3–9
legislation effects on, 5
pharmacogenomics effect on, 235
quality measures in, 7–9
quality of, 535–36
revenues from, 16
revolutions in, 260–61
turnover rates in, 8–9
Health care agencies
continuing, 544–46
continuum of, 538f
future of, 549–50
Indian Health Services, 546–47
nurse's role in, 553–55
overview of, 536–37
practice model, 550–53
preventive, 537–39
primary care, 539–40
public, 539
restorative, 543–44
secondary, 540–41
tertiary, 541–43
Veterans Affairs Health System, 548–49
Health care enterprises, 5–6
Health care facilities
electronic advances in, 615–16
Joint Commission for the Accreditation of Healthcare Organizations inspection of, 615
selection of, 618–20
touring of, 620
Health care providers
changes in, 3–4
general practitioner, 3–4
impaired, 20
Health care systems
components of, 532
financing of, 533
goal of, 533
interrelation among, 533f
leadership of, 6
older adult use of, 136–37
Health history
description of, 179–82
heart failure evaluations, 806
hypertension assessments, 913
kidney assessments, 1754–55
Health insurance
definition of, 533
laws that prohibit discrimination, 230–31
sources of, 534f
Health Insurance Portability and Accountability Act
confidentiality provisions, 102–3, 192–93, 694
description of, 5, 178, 230
patient's rights, 177
Health maintenance
assessments, 58–59
characteristics of, 56
definition of, 55
diagnostic tests, 59
evaluation of outcomes, 64
ineffective, 60b–61b
nursing care plan, 64–65
nursing diagnoses for, 59
nutrition management behaviors, 62
planning and implementation of, 60–64
risk factor identification in, 59
self-examination techniques, 62
sleep alterations and, 62–63
Health maintenance activities, 55
Health maintenance organizations, 533
Health perception–health management, 58–59
Health professions, 25, 26b
Health promotion
care models for, 258
definition of, 56–57
global, 57
for older adults, 137–38
priorities for, 57b
strategies for, 61t
in United States, 58, 58t
Health records, 616
Health trends
aging population, 125–26
contemporary, 123–25
definition of, 123
dietary habits, 124
ethnic population, 126
in middle-aged adults, 131
minority population, 126
morbidity, 125
mortality, 125
obesity rates, 124
in older adults, 132–34
in population composition, 125–26
smoking, 125
in young adults, 131
Healthy People 2010
burn injury goals, 1545b
definition of, 138
health care access goals, 535
health disparities, 78
healthy activities addressed in, 138
objectives of, 58t
Hearing
frequency range of, 1312
physiology of, 1351–52
Hearing aids, 1372–74
Hearing loss
acquired, 1350
aging and, 1357
assessment of, 1353
cerumen production and, 1357
classification of, 1354–58
communication tools, 1370–71
conductive, 1354
congenital
cochlear implant for, 1366–67
description of, 1352–53
costs of, 1350
cultural considerations, 1371
degrees of, 1353
epidemiology of, 1350
etiology of, 1350–51
family education about, 1368–69
foreign bodies as cause of, 1358
genetic factors, 1352–53
head trauma as cause of, 1351
Ménière's disease, 1355–56
mixed, 1356–57
noise-induced, 1368–69
ototoxic medications and, 1350–51
pathophysiology of, 1351–52
patient education about, 1368–69
prevention of, 1368–69
rehabilitation for, 1372
risk factors for, 1319
sensorineural, 1355–56
surgical treatment of, 1364–65
Heart
anatomy of, 747–48, 748f, 815f
auscultation of, 758
chambers of, 747–48, 748f, 749
conduction system of. *See* Cardiac conduction system
contractile properties of, 752
electrical stimulation of, 837
fibrous skeleton of, 749
palpation of, 758f
pericardial layers of, 748–49
thoracic position of, 748f
Heart block
complete, 855f, 855–56
description of, 854
first-degree, 854, 854f
second-degree atrioventricular, 854–55
third-degree, 855f, 855–56
Heart failure
acute, 805
after acute myocardial infarction, 791
assessment of, 806–7
clinical manifestations of, 805–7
contraindicated medications for, 811t
definition of, 500, 804
diagnostic tests for
cardiac catheterization, 808
electrocardiogram, 807
magnetic resonance imaging, 808
myocardial biopsy, 808
diastolic, 804
edema associated with, 805
epidemiology of, 804
etiology of, 804
laboratory tests, 807
left-sided
clinical manifestations of, 808b
definition of, 805
nursing diagnoses for, 808
outcomes, 811–12
pathophysiology of, 804–6
planning and implementation, 808–11
in postoperative period, 662
right-sided
clinical manifestations of, 808b
definition of, 805
symptoms of, 807t
statistics regarding, 258
stress associated with, 252, 258
systolic, 804
treatment of
angiotensin receptor blockers, 809
angiotensin-converting enzyme inhibitors, 809
anticoagulants, 810
antihyperlipidemics, 810
beta blockers, 810
collaborative management, 809

digoxin, 810
diuretics, 810
nitrates, 810
overview of, 808–9
oxygenation monitoring, 809
pharmacological, 809–10
respiratory support, 808–9
surgery, 811
vasodilators, 810
tumor necrosis factor-alpha and, 807
Heart murmurs, 760–61, 761t
Heart muscle dysfunction, 813
Heart rate, 841–43
Heart sounds, 758–59, 759t
Heart transplantation
for hypertrophic cardiomyopathy, 815
immune system effects, 1406
Heart valves
anatomy of, 749–50, 815f
aortic. *See* Aortic valve
atrioventricular, 822
dysfunction and disease of. *See* Valvular dysfunction and disease
mitral. *See* Mitral valve
replacement of, 830
semilunar, 822
tricuspid, 822
Heartburn, 1572–73
Heat stroke, 2221
Heberden's nodes, 1957
Heinz bodies, 934
Helical computed tomography, 1007, 1790
Helicobacter pylori
gastritis caused by, 1575
peptic ulcer disease and, 1638–41
Helminths, 271t
Helper T cells, 1391, 1397–98
Hemarthrosis, 944
Hematocele, 2179
Hematochezia, 1679
Hematocrit, 747t, 1607, 1759t
Hematological system
age-related changes, 743
assessment of, 744–45, 744t–745t
description of, 735
diagnostic tests, 745–47
erythrocytes, 736–37
hemoglobin, 737–39
plasma, 735–36
white blood cells. *See also specific cell*
description of, 266t, 266–67
graft-versus-host disease caused by, 426–27
in packed red blood cell transfusion, 363–64
Hematology, 929
Hematoma
definition of, 745t, 1041
description of, 699
Hematopoiesis, 933
Hematopoietic cells, 425
Hematopoietic growth factor, 952
Hematuria, 1771, 1817
Heme iron, 1649
Hemilaryngectomy, 1048
Hemiparesis, 1187b, 1200
Hemiplegia, 1187b, 1200
Hemispherectomy, 1274t
Hemochromatosis, 227, 1710–11
Hemodialysis, 1836–37
Hemodynamic monitoring
of critically ill patients
afterload, 569
cardiac output, 568
contractility, 569
description of, 568
equipment for, 569–70
intra-arterial, 571–72
left atrial pressure, 576–77
measurements, 570–77
mixed venous oxygen saturation, 577
preload, 568–69
pulmonary artery pressure monitoring, 572–76, 574t
waveform patterns, 571
description of, 368
equipment for, 569–70
Hemodynamics, 568
Hemoglobin
assessment of, 1607
description of, 737–38
globulins, 738
iron in, 738
laboratory tests, 747t
oxygen binding, 738–39, 984
porphyrin, 738
structure of, 225
for wound healing, 289
Hemoglobin A, 738
Hemoglobin H disease, 225
Hemoglobin S, 934–35
Hemoglobinopathies
gene therapy for, 226
genetic factors, 225–27
Hemoglobinuria, 934
Hemolysis, 930
Hemolytic anemias
acquired, 932
definition of, 932
glucose-6-phosphate dehydrogenase, 933–34
hereditary spherocytosis, 934
pathophysiology of, 930
sickle cell anemia, 225–26, 934–36, 1173t
thalassemia, 933
Hemolytic uremic syndrome, 1825t
Hemophilia
assessment of, 944–45
categories of, 944
definition of, 944
diagnostic tests, 945
nursing diagnoses, 945
nursing measures for, 945b
outcomes, 946–47
pharmacological treatment of, 946, 946t
Hemoptysis, 991, 1044
Hemorrhagic exudate, 269
Hemorrhagic stroke, 1172
Hemosiderosis, 738
Hemostasis
components of, 741
definition of, 511
fibrin clot, 743
laboratory tests, 747t
process of, 741–43
Hemotympanum, 1318
Henderson-Hasselbalch equation, 986
Heparin
deep venous thrombosis treated with, 894, 2043
disseminated intravascular coagulation treated with, 943
laboratory monitoring of, 512
low-molecular-weight, 512
mechanism of action, 511–12
nursing management for, 513
pharmacokinetics of, 512
side effects of, 513
thrombophlebitis treated with, 894
Hepatic abscess, 1719–21
Hepatic artery thrombosis, 1728
Hepatic encephalopathy, 1717
Hepatic steatosis, 1718–19
Hepatitis
A, 1702t
acute, 1701
alcoholic, 1709
assessment of, 1701, 1708
autoimmune, 1710
B, 1703t–1704t
C, 1705t, 1712
chronic, 1701
D, 1705t–1706t
definition of, 1701
drug-induced, 1710
E, 1706t–1707t
F, 1707t
fulminant, 1701
G, 1707t
health practice to prevent against, 1708
nursing diagnoses, 1708
outcomes, 1708–9
pathophysiology of, 1701, 1702t–1707t
phases of, 1701
prevention of, 1708
toxic, 1710
types of, 1702t–1707t
Hepatitis B core antigen, 1415
Hepatitis B surface antigen, 1415
Hepatobiliary scan, 1700
Hepatocellular carcinoma, 1723
Hepatomegaly, 1719
Hepatorenal syndrome, 1717–18
Herbal therapy, 392–94, 393t–394t
Herceptin, 2152
Hereditary angioedema, 1471–72
Hereditary nonpolyposis colon cancer, 219, 1676
Hereditary spherocytosis, 934
Hermaphrodites, 190
Hernia, hiatal, 1631–32
Herniation, 580
Herpes infections
characteristics of, 1512–14
corneal ulcerations caused by, 1336
epidemiology of, 2103
sexual transmission of, 2103
signs and symptoms of, 2103
Herpes zoster, 461b, 1513–14
Hetastarch, 343t
Heterograft, 1552
Hiatal hernia, 1631–32
Hiccough, 982, 1575–76
High altitude, respiratory adjustments to, 990
High efficiency particulate air filters, 670, 2245
High pressure sterilization, 666b
High-density lipoprotein, 514, 771
High-efficiency particulate air, 281
High-flow oxygen delivery systems, 1013
Highly active antiretroviral therapy, 1429
High-molecular-weight kininogen, 742t
Hip fractures, 2036–39
Hirsutism, 1865
Hispanic (Americans)
death beliefs, 148t
demographics of, 72b, 73
family structure, 77
food preferences, 85t
His-Purkinje system, 837
Histamine, 1450
Histamine2 antagonists, 524–25
Histocompatibility leukocyte antigens, 1431
Histoplasmosis, 1070
Historic time, 123t
HMG-CoA reductase inhibitors
coronary artery disease treated with, 782t, 785
hyperlipidemia treated with, 882
indications for, 514
Hodgkin's disease
assessment of, 965–66
chemotherapy for, 967
diagnostic tests for, 966
epidemiology of, 964–65
nursing diagnoses, 966
outcomes, 967
pathophysiology of, 965
radiation therapy for, 966–67
staging of, 965b
Holism, 380
Holistic nursing care
description of, 380, 633
empowerment goals of, 259
principles of, 258–59
Holter monitor, 778
Homans' sign, 893, 1946
Home care
cultural considerations in, 89
diabetes mellitus management in, 1909
for dying patient, 165–68
emergencies in, 166
stress in, 255
Home health aides, 150
Homeless population
description of, 80–82
older adults, 135
Homeopathy, 396
Homeostasis
autonomic nervous system's role in, 452
definition of, 242, 1746
Homocystine, 879
Homograft, 1552
Homonymous hemianopsia, 1201
Hope, 248–49
Hordeolum, 1305, 1339
Hormone(s). *See also specific hormone*
adrenal, 1851t
blood pressure affected by, 509
cancer treated with, 423–24
definition of, 1849
functions of, 1848–49
pancreatic, 1851t
pituitary, 1851t
regulation of, 1850–51
small intestine affected by, 1649
thyroid, 1851t
Hormone replacement therapy, 405, 1808, 1984
Hospice care
advanced practice nurses in, 152
bereavement services, 168
definition of, 145, 545
description of, 110–11
history of, 145–46
interdisciplinary team who deliver, 144–45, 150, 152
Medicare reimbursement for, 146
mouth care, 162–63, 166
nurses involved in, 146, 150
nursing diagnoses, 155–56

overview of, 145–46
palliative care vs., 144
physical symptoms experienced in
anxiety, 155, 164
confusion, 154–55, 163–64
constipation, 154, 162–63
depression, 155, 164
dyspnea, 153–54, 162
insomnia, 154, 163–64
loss of appetite, 154, 162
nausea, 154, 163
pain, 152–53, 156–62
urinary urgency and incontinence, 154, 163
vomiting, 154
spiritual support in, 164–65
Hospital(s)
admitting areas, 619
bariatric, 642–643
electronic advances in, 615–16
hazardous materials emergency response plan of, 2245b
intermediate care unit, 704
items to bring to, 621
medical-surgical hospital unit, 620
postanesthesia care unit in. *See* Postanesthesia care unit
postsurgical unit, 704
selection of, 618, 619b
size of, 618
telemetry unit, 704
university affiliation, 618
word origin of, 3
Hospital Emergency Incident Command System, 2242–43
Hospital operations plan, 2243–44
Hospital-acquired pneumonia, 1057, 1103
Hospitalization
for asthma, 1126
stress associated with, 253
Human chorionic gonadotropin, 2064
Human Genome Project, 197, 228, 232
Human immunodeficiency virus
antibody tests, 1427b
assessment of, 1426
CD4+ T cells in, 1425
collaborative management of, 1428–29
diagnostic criteria for, 1426
diagnostic tests, 1426–28
epidemiology of, 1422
etiology of, 1423–25
health disparities, 79b
highly active antiretroviral therapy for, 1429, 1430b
Kaposi's sarcoma, 1426f
nursing care for, 1428
nursing diagnoses, 1428
occupational exposure to, 1424–25
opportunistic infections associated with, 1426
outcomes, 1430
pathophysiology of, 1425–26
pharmacological therapy for, 1429
sexual activity and, 1424
statistics regarding, 1422
systemic manifestations of, 1426
terminal care, 1428
transmission of, 1423, 1425
treatment of, 1428–29
tuberculosis caused by, 1429
types of, 1422
Human leukocyte antigens, 223, 1382, 1841
Human needs
basic, 61, 61t
Maslow's hierarchy of, 62f
overview of, 60–61
physiological, 62–63
psychological, 63
sexuality, 64
Human papillomavirus
cervical cancer and, 2119–20
characteristics of, 404, 409, 2104–5
penile cancer and, 2192
vaccination, 2120
Humectants, 1503
Humira, 1440t
Humor, 395
Humoral-mediated immunity, 1381, 1398–99
Hunner's ulcer, 1774
Hunter's glossitis, 939
Huntington disease, 216–17
Huntington's disease, 1294–96
Hyaline cartilage, 1940
Hyaluronic acid, 1959
Hydantoins, 521–22
Hydralazine, 924t
Hydration, artificial, 113
Hydrocele, 2075, 2178–80
Hydrocephalus, 1185
Hydrochloric acid
burns from, 1535
stomach production of, 1570
Hydrochlorothiazide, 509, 923t
Hydrogel, synthetic, 526
Hydronephrosis, 1748, 1765
Hydrotherapy, 1547
Hydroxychloroquine sulfate, 1443
5-Hydroxytryptophan, 743
Hydroxyurea, 226
Hygiene
postoperative, 723–24
preoperative, 627–28
Hygroton. *See* Chlorthalidone
Hymen, 2062–63
Hypalgesia, 1157
Hyperaldosteronism, 1879–83
Hyperalgesia, 451, 1157
Hypercalcemia
cancer-related, 441
description of, 311t–312t, 322–23
in Paget's disease, 1990
Hypercapnia, 984, 1039
Hypercholesterolemia
description of, 128, 1784
stroke risks, 1173b
Hypercortisolism. *See* Cushing's disease
Hyperesthesia, 1581, 1925
Hyperextension
illustration of, 1944f
injuries caused by, 1219
Hyperflexion injuries, 1219
Hyperglycemia
definition of, 1905
description of, 527
exercise-induced, 1917
Hyperinsulinemia, 1906
Hyperkalemia
characteristics of, 310t–311t, 319–21
management of, 1830b
potassium-sparing diuretics and, 508
Hyperlipidemia
causes of, 771
coronary artery disease risks, 771–72
definition of, 881
HMG-CoA reductase inhibitors for, 882
recommendations for, 789t
treatment of, 882
Hypermagnesemia, 312t–313t, 327–28
Hypernatremia, 310t–311t, 316–17
Hyperopia, 1337
Hyperosmolar hyperglycemic nonketotic syndrome, 1919–20
Hyperparathyroidism, 1895–97
Hyperphosphatemia, 314t, 324–26
Hyperprolactinemia, 1864–66
Hyperresonance, 185t
Hypersensitivity
assessment of, 1454, 1455b
definition of, 475
description of, 1433
type 2, 1453
type 3, 1453
type 4, 1453–54
type I, 1452–53
Hypertension. *See also* Blood pressure
in African Americans, 190, 909
alcohol consumption and, 910
assessment of, 912–14
caffeine and, 910, 918–19
classification of, 912–13
coronary artery disease risks, 772
definition of, 508, 907–8
description of, 128
diagnostic tests, 914–915, 915t
diet and, 910–11
Dietary Approaches to Stop Hypertension, 917t, 917–18
epidemiology of, 908
etiology of, 908, 908b
exercise for, 921
family education about, 925
genetic factors, 908–9
health history about, 913
isolated systolic, 909
nicotine and, 920
nursing diagnoses for, 915–16
obesity and, 909
pathophysiology of, 911–12
patient education about, 925
planning and implementation for, 916–25
portal, 1715–17
prevalence of, 508
rebound, 925
recommendations for, 789t
risk factors for, 508, 908–11
screening for, 915t
smoking and, 909–10, 919–20
sodium intake and, 919, 919t
stress and, 920–21
stroke risks, 1173b
treatment of
antihypertensive medications, 922–23, 923t–924t
collaborative management, 922
diuretics, 922–23, 923t
evidence-based approaches, 916–17
pharmacological, 922–24
sympatholytics, 923t–924t
Hypertensive crisis, 510
Hyperthermia
in brain-injured patients, 1187
in stroke patients, 1179–80
Hyperthyroidism
assessment of, 1884, 1885t
clinical manifestations of, 1884
definition of, 1883–84
diagnostic tests, 1884, 1886t
epidemiology of, 1884
etiology of, 1884
nursing diagnoses, 1885
outcomes, 1890
pathophysiology of, 1884
pharmacological treatment of, 1888–89
radioiodine therapy for, 1889
treatment of, 1885–90
Hypertonic solution
characteristics of, 297, 305t, 341, 342t
infiltration and, 349
Hypertrophic cardiomyopathy
assessment of, 814
description of, 805, 813–14
nursing diagnoses for, 814
pharmacological treatment of, 814–15
surgical treatment of, 815
Hypertrophic scar
in burn patients, 1559
description of, 284
Hyperuricemia, 1964
Hypervolemia
complications of, 306
definition of, 1828t
description of, 304
diagnostic tests for, 306–7
etiology of, 304, 306
nursing diagnoses for, 307
pathophysiology of, 306
in renal failure, 1829
Hypesthesia, 1157
Hyphae, 2106
Hypnosis, 383
Hypoalbuminemia, 1784
Hypocalcemia
description of, 311t, 320–22
in hypoparathyroidism, 1898
Hypocapnia, 984
Hypogeusia, 1153
Hypoglossal nerve, 1146f, 1147t, 1155
Hypoglycemia
assessment of, 1920, 1921t
beta blockers and, 505
in diabetes mellitus patients, 1920–22
in elderly patients, 1921
exercise-induced, 1917
insulin therapy and, 526
nursing diagnoses, 1921
signs of, 526
treatment of, 1921–22
Hypokalemia, 309t–310t, 317–19
Hypomagnesemia, 312t, 326–27
Hyponatremia, 307, 308t, 314–16
Hypoparathyroidism, 1897–99
Hypophosphatemia, 313t, 323–24
Hypophysis, 1143
Hypopituitarism, 1873–74
Hyposensitization, 1459
Hypospadias, 2189–90
Hypotension
definition of, 925
orthostatic, 925
Hypothalamic-pituitary-adrenal axis, 452, 1977
Hypothalamus, 1848, 1852
Hypothermia
anesthesia-related, 681
body temperature management to prevent, 682
in brain-injured patients, 1187

coagulation affected by, 681
consequences of, 681–82
definition of, 681, 698
Hypothyroidism, 1891–94
Hypotonic solutions
description of, 298, 305t, 341
in hyponatremic patients, 315
infiltration and, 349
Hypotony, 1330
Hypoventilation, 713
Hypovolemia
assessment of, 302–3
complications of, 303
definition of, 2212
delayed wound healing caused by, 284
diagnostic tests for, 303
etiology of, 302
nursing diagnoses, 303–4
pathophysiology of, 302
Hypovolemic shock
anemia and, 932
assessment of, 2213–14
clinical manifestations of, 2215b
description of, 2210–11
etiology of, 2211–12
pathophysiology of, 2212
treatment of, 2214–15, 2215b
Hypoxemia
in asthma, 1122
in cystic fibrosis, 1129
definition of, 1102, 2213
description of, 984
in hypovolemic shock, 2213
signs of, 997
Hypoxia
definition of, 984, 1039
respiratory adjustments during, 989
skin findings, 757
Hysterectomy, 2094, 2096, 2098–99
Hysterosalpingography, 2083, 2114
Hysteroscopy, 2082

I

Ibuprofen, 474t
Icterus, 1698b
Idioventricular rhythm, 859
Ifosfamide, 1997t
Ileal conduit, 1803f
Ileostomy, 1684–85
Ileum, 1571
Ileus
definition of, 1669
epidemiology of, 1669–70
etiology of, 1670
postoperative, 1670
Iliopsoas muscle test, 1582f
Illiteracy, 75–76
Illness
appraisal-transaction theory of, 244
early civilization theories and practices regarding, 240
life changes theory of, 244–45
stress effects on susceptibility to, 245
Image guided core needle biopsy, 2150
Imagery, 382, 382t
Imatinib, 960
Immobility, 564–65
Immune response
cell-mediated, 1396–98
definition of, 1431
humoral-mediated, 1398–99
inflammatory, 2203–5
innate, 1394–95
primary, 1422, 1451
secondary, 1422, 1451
triggering of, 1450
Immune system
in adults, 1401–2
age-related changes, 1401–3, 1402t
anatomy of, 1383–94
assessment of, 1401–10
burn effects on, 1533
cardiovascular health and, 1381
chemical components of, 1392–94
chemokines, 1393
chronic illness effects on, 1405–6
complement, 1393–94
diagnostic tests, 1410–17
environmental influences, 1407–8
functions of, 1380, 1421
impaired, 1408b
leukocytes. *See* Leukocytes
lifestyle influences, 1407–8
lymphocytes. *See* Lymphocytes
medications that affect, 1407
memory of, 1399–1400
in neonates, 1401
nonspecific, 1381
nursing management of, 1417
physical examination of, 1408–10
self vs. nonself distinction by, 1382
skin tests, 1416
social isolation effects, 1407
stress effects, 1406–7
surgery effects on, 1406
Immune thrombocytopenia purpura, 940
Immunity
acquired, 1381
adaptive, 1395–1401
antigen, 1382
cell-mediated, 1381, 1396–98
definition of, 1422
humoral-mediated, 1381, 1398–99
innate, 1381
Immunizations
childhood, 1403
definition of, 1400
health disparities, 79b
infection prevention using, 1403–4
mechanisms of, 1400–1401
passive, 1400
Immunodeficiency, defined, 1417
Immunodeficiency disorders
causes of, 1431
graft-versus-host disease, 1431–32
hypersensitivity disorders, 1433
immunosuppressive therapy, 1432
Immunogen, 1382
Immunoglobulin(s)
A, 1383, 1414t
assays, 1427b
definition of, 1389
E, 223–24, 1118–19, 1414t, 1451
G, 1390, 1415t, 1451
M, 1390, 1415t, 1451
Immunoglobulin A nephropathy, 1781
Immunoglobulin electrophoresis, 1413, 1414t
Immunological disorders, 1423b. *See also specific disorder*
Immunomodulators, 1500t
Immunosuppressive therapy
agents used in, 1840–41, 1843t
dermatomyositis treated with, 1975
description of, 1432
after liver transplantation, 1728–29
polymyositis treated with, 1975
Immunotherapy
bladder cancer treated with, 1800
cancer treated with, 424–25
definition of, 1020
renal cancer treated with, 1797
Impaired colleagues, 20
Imperforate hymen, 2089, 2113
Impetigo, 1514
Implantable cardioverter-defibrillator, 863–64
Implanted ports, 359
In vitro fertilization, 2126
Inborn errors of metabolism, 204, 215
Incentive spirometer, 713, 713f
Incidence
definition of, 123, 402
of suicide, 125
Incontinence
functional, 1807b
overflow, 1807b
stress, 1807b
in stroke patients, 1201–2
urge, 1807b
urinary
assessment of, 1806–7
definition of, 1805–6
diagnostic tests, 1807
epidemiology of, 1806
etiology of, 1806
health care costs, 1806
in hospice patients, 154, 163
nursing diagnoses, 1807
outcomes, 1808
in palliative care patients, 154, 163
pathophysiology of, 1806
treatment of, 1807–8
types of, 1807b
Incus, 1312
Indian Health Services, 546–47
Indigestion. *See* Dyspepsia
Indirect bilirubin, 740
Indirect calorimetry, 1600
Indirect contact transmission, 276
Indium scan, 1950
Indocin, 1966
Indoles, 471b
Indwelling catheter, 1237
Ineffective health maintenance, 60b–61b
Infant(s). *See also* Children
body water in, 296
gender differences, 191
health assessment of, 186
Infant mortality, 79b
Infection
asthma exacerbations caused by, 1118t
in burn wounds, 1548
in critically ill patients, 564
in cystic fibrosis, 1130
immunizations against, 1403–4
intravenous therapy-related, 348
wound, 286–87
Infection control
in cystic fibrosis, 1129
guidelines for, 279t, 279–81
standard precautions, 279
universal precautions, 279
Infectious diseases
hantavirus, 277–79
organisms that cause, 270–71, 271t
plague, 277–78
transmission of
airborne, 276–77, 280t, 281
common vehicle, 277
contact, 276, 280
droplet, 276, 280, 280t
hand washing to prevent, 277
nurse's role in preventing, 281
overview of, 275–76
precautions for, 280–81
vector borne, 277–79
Infectious mononucleosis. *See* Mononucleosis
Inferior petrosal sinus sampling, 1870
Infertility
assessment of, 2124
definition of, 2180
diagnostic tests, 2124
female, 2124
male, 2124
nursing diagnoses, 2124
pharmacological treatment of, 2126, 2126t
prevalence of, 2123
surgical treatments for, 2126–27
treatments for, 2125–27
Infiltration, 348–49
Inflammation
body temperature affected by, 274
chronic, 270, 2204b
dendritic cells affected by, 1399
diseases caused by, 272–73
fungal, 1510
myocardial infarction and, 273
nursing diagnoses, 273–75
nursing response, 273–75
pain caused by, 458
signs of, 269
of veins, 349
Inflammatory aneurysms, 889
Inflammatory bowel disorders
Crohn's disease, 1690–91
diagnostic tests, 1688
epidemiology of, 1688
nursing diagnoses, 1688
outcomes, 1689–90
pharmacological treatment of, 1689
smoking cessation in, 1689
ulcerative colitis, 1691
Inflammatory diarrhea, 1577
Inflammatory immune response, 2203–5
Inflammatory response
in asthma, 271–72
to burns, 1532
chemicals involved in, 268t, 268–69
concept map of, 290–91
description of, 266
diabetes mellitus effects on, 285
diseases that cause, 270–72
granulocyte functions in, 740
leukocytes, 266t, 266–67
monocytes' role in, 267
phagocytosis, 269
to tissue injury, 267–69
tissue resolution and repair, 269–70
Informal teaching, 53
Informed consent
for blood transfusions, 365
description of, 103–4, 192
for surgery, 621–23, 622f, 677

Infusion pumps, 344–46
Infusion therapy. *See also* Intravenous therapy
  add-on devices for, 345b
  administration sets for, 341
  blood. *See* Blood transfusion
  complications of
    extravasation, 349–50
    infections, 348
    infiltration, 348–49
    nerve damage, 350
    overview of, 347–48
    phlebitis, 348
    sepsis, 348
  continuous, 357
  equipment and production selection, 341, 344–46
  ethical considerations, 371
  future of, 371–72
  hemodynamic monitoring during, 367
  intermittent, 357
  legal considerations, 370–71
  nosocomial infections caused by, 340
  in older adults, 369
  pain management during, 367
  piggyback, 357
  plasma expanders, 343t–344t
  procedure for, 346–47
  rate control devices for, 341, 344
  solutions, 342t–344t
  units as related to, 352–53
  volume expanders, 342t–343t
Inguinal herniorrhaphy, 701t
Inhalers
  cost of, 1113
  dry powder
    description of, 516, 1113
    directions for, 1113
  metered dose
    description of, 516, 516f
    directions for, 1112
Inheritance patterns
  autosomal dominant, 204
  autosomal recessive, 204, 205f
  discovery of, 203
  Mendelian, 203–6
  non-Mendelian, 206
  X-linked dominant, 205
  X-linked recessive, 205–6
Injury
  inflammatory immune response, 2203–5
  neuroendocrine system response, 2205–6
  physiological events after, 2207b–2208b
  renal response to, 2206, 2207b–2208b
Innate immune response, 1394–95
Innate immunity, 1381
Inner ear, 1312
Insomnia
  in hospice patients, 154, 163–64
  in palliative care patients, 154, 163–64
Inspection
  definition of, 183
  musculoskeletal system, 1943
  respiratory system, 993–97
Inspiration, 981–82
Inspiratory reserve volume, 1012, 1106t
Institutional review board, 117
Instruments
  counts of, during surgery, 680–81
  sterilization of, 668, 669
Insulin
  administration of, 1912–14
  allergic reactions to, 1917
  characteristics of, 526–27
  for dawn phenomenon, 1922
  definition of, 1849, 1905
  diabetes mellitus treated with, 1912–15
  endogenous, 1905
  functions of, 1851t, 1856
  Lente, 1912, 1913t
  Lispro, 1912, 1913t
  management of, 527
  NPH, 1913t
  regular, 1912, 1913t
  storage of, 1913–14
  Ultra Lente, 1913t
Insulin glargine, 1913, 1913t
Insulin growth factor, 1866
Insulin pumps, 1914
Insulin resistance syndrome, 773, 1905
Integrated care delivery system, 549
Integrative medicine, 375
Integrative therapy, 379
Intellectual functioning, 63
Intensity modulated radiation therapy, 2171
Intensive care unit. *See also* Critical care unit
  admission criteria, 562b–563b
  discharge criteria, 563b
  discharge from, 702–5
  stress in, 254
  surgical, 694, 704
  transfer from postanesthesia care unit to, 704–5
Intention tremor, 1280
Intercostal space, 748
Interdisciplinary team, in hospice and palliative care, 144–45, 150, 152
Interferons
  -_, 1397
  beta-1a, 1278t
  description of, 269, 1393
Interleukins
  -1β, 1385t
  -2, 424
  -6, 807, 1385t
  -7, 1399
  -12, 1385t
  -15, 1399–1400
  description of, 268–69, 1393
Intermediate care unit, 704
Intermittent infusion loops, 345b
Intermittent infusion therapy, 357
Internal mammary artery, 786–87
Internet
  consumer access to, 261
  support groups on, 48
Interpersonal skills, 55
Interpersonal threats, 19
Interpleural space, 978
Interpreter, 74, 76
Interstitial cystitis
  assessment of, 1774
  definition of, 1771
  diagnostic tests, 1774–75, 1775b
  epidemiology of, 1771, 1773t
  etiology of, 1772
  genetic factors, 1774
  health care resources for, 1777
  nursing diagnoses, 1775
  outcomes, 1777
  pathophysiology of, 1772, 1774
  surgical treatment of, 1777
  treatment of, 1776b, 1776–77
Interstitial Cystitis Association, 1777
Interstitial fluid, 296
Interstitial space, 1752
Intervertebral discs, 1144
Intervertebral foramen, 1140f
Interview, 177–78
Intestinal decompression tubes, 1588
Intimate partner violence, 2071–73
Intra-aortic balloon pump, 577–78, 579t, 796, 796f–797f, 2216
Intraarterial drug administration, 473
Intra-arterial monitoring, 571–72
Intracavitary radiation, 418
Intracellular buffers, 987
Intracellular fluid, 296, 298
Intracerebral hemorrhage, 1172
Intracranial headache, 458b
Intracranial pressure
  cerebral tumor effects on, 442
  increased
    Cushing response, 1192
    management of, 582–83
    osmotic diuretics for, 582
    patient positioning to prevent, 582
    sedation of patients with, 583
    shunts for, 1205
    signs and symptoms of, 582
  monitoring of
    in brain-injured patients, 1193
    in critically ill patients
      cerebral perfusion pressure, 580, 1193
      description of, 579–80
      types of, 580–81
      waveforms, 581–82
    in stroke patients, 1182
Intractable pain, 463–64, 475
Intradermal test, 1416
Intradiscal electrothermal annuloplasty, 460
Intraductal papilloma, 2142
Intramuscular drug administration
  characteristics of, 489t
  description of, 473, 488, 489t
Intranasal corticosteroids, 1022
Intraocular pressure, 1329
Intraoperative, definition of, 608
Intraoperative period. *See also* Perioperative period
  body temperature management in, 682
  complications during
    hypothermia, 681–82
    malignant hyperthermia, 683–84
    retained objects, 680–81
  ethics in, 684–86
  fluid management in, 682–83
  nursing care, 659–63
  patient positioning in, 683
  patient safety in, 686–87
  transportation of patient in, 686–87
Intraparenchymal probe, 581
Intrapulmonary restrictive lung disorder, 1063–64
Intratympanic steroids, 1254
Intravascular fluid, 296
Intravenous pyelogram, 1761t, 1770t
Intravenous therapy. *See also* Infusion therapy
  administration of
    description of, 353
    flow rate calculations, 353
    guidelines, 355
    three-step method, 354–55
  air embolus during, 360
  antibiotics delivered through, 1061
  bolus, 357
  in burn patients, 1536b
  calculations
    body surface area in, 353
    body weight, 353
    description of, 350
    formula method, 351–52
    percent solutions, 352
    ratio-proportion method, 350–51
    units of measure used in, 350
  central venous catheters
    closed-ended catheters, 359
    fractured lines, 361
    implanted ports, 359
    percutaneous catheters, 359
    selection of, 358
    troubleshooting of, 360
    tunneled catheters, 358–59
  complications of
    extravasation, 349–50
    infections, 348
    infiltration, 348–49
    nerve damage, 350
    overview of, 347–48
    phlebitis, 348
    sepsis, 348
  continuous, 357
  controlled substances, 355
  drug administration through, 473
  drugs for
    incompatibility of, 356–57
    preparation of, 356
  electrolytes, 361–62
  hemodynamic monitoring during, 367
  intermittent, 357
  legal considerations, 370–71
  line insertion, 629
  medication errors, 355–56
  nurse's role in, 356–57
  nursing process applied to, 356
  in older adults, 369
  pain management during, 367
  peripheral nerve injury caused by, 1255
  pharmacology, 355–58
  prescribing of, 355
  procedure for, 346–47
  push, 357
Intraventricular catheter, 581
Intrinsic distortion, 74
Intrinsic factor, 1571, 1648
Intubation. *See* Endotracheal intubation; Nasogastric intubation
Inverse ratio ventilation, 588
Inversion, 201, 1944f
Inversion stress test, 2025, 2025f
Ionizing radiation, 416
Ipratropium bromide, 1111
Irbesartan, 924t
Iris
  anatomy of, 1302
  examination of, 1305
Iris lesions, 1490b
Iritis, 1341–42
Iron, 1649
Iron deficiency anemia, 936–37, 1607
Irritable bowel syndrome, 1686–88
Ischemic stroke, 1172
Islets of Langerhans, 1699, 1856
Isokinetic exercise, 1948
Isolated systolic hypertension, 909
Isolation, 2248t
Isoniazid, 1068t

Isosorbide dinitrate, 782t
Isotonic solution, 297, 305t, 341, 342t–343t
Isotype switching, 1398
Isradipine, 924t
Itraconazole, 1071

J

Jackson-Pratt drain, 700t
Japanese Americans, 148t
Jaundice, 1698b
Jaw-thrust maneuver, 583, 867
Jejunostomy, 1590–91
Jejunum, 1571
Job-related stress, 255–56
Johns Hopkins Hospital, 542
Joint Commission for the Accreditation of Healthcare Organizations
  end-of-life standards, 1603
  founding of, 7
  health care facility inspections by, 615
  hospice program standards, 145
  medication error prevention, 487–88
  nutrition screening standards, 1609
  pain management standards, 109, 159, 367, 467–68
  patient safety goals, 686
  quality performance dimensions, 8b
Joints
  anatomy of, 1940
  aspiration of, 1952
Jugular veins
  assessment of, 757
  distention of, 306, 806–7
  emergency use of, 341
Jumper's knee. *See* Patellar tendinopathy
Junctional escape rhythm, 853
Junctional rhythms, 852–53
Junctional tachycardia, 853
Justice, 97, 192t, 229t
Juvenile rheumatoid arthritis, 1436–37
Juxtaglomerular apparatus, 1753

K

Kaposi's sarcoma, 1409, 1426f
Karyotype, 211
Kayser-Fleisher rings, 1710
Kegel exercises, 1808, 2115, 2117
Keloid, 284, 1489f
Keratin, 1479
Keratinization, 1476
Keratinocytes, 1393, 1477t
Keratitis, 1341, 1967
Keratoconjunctivitis sicca, 1341
Keratoconus, 1336
Keratometry, 1336
Keratosis, 1490b
Kernicterus, 1698b
Ketoacidosis, diabetic, 527
Kidneys
  acid-base balance by, 328
  age-related changes, 1754
  anatomy of, 1747f, 1747–49
  assessment of
    description of, 1583, 1814
    health history, 1754–55
    medication history, 1755, 1755b
    physical examination, 1755–56
  blood filtering in, 911
  blood studies, 1757, 1759t
  blood supply to, 1748, 1753
  burn effects on, 1532
  diagnostic tests, 1757–62
  drug excretion affected by, 486
  efficiency of, 1748–49
  electrolyte balance by, 300
  fibrous capsule of, 1748
  fluid balance by, 300
  functions of, 300, 1749b, 1813
  immunological diseases of, 1820–22
  injury response of, 2206, 2207b–2208b
  juxtaglomerular apparatus of, 1753
  nephrons of, 1748, 1751, 1751f–1752f
  palpation of, 1755–56, 1756f
  percussion of, 1756f
  pH response by, 987
  radiographic studies of, 1757, 1761t
  traumatic injuries to, 1792–95
  tubules of, 1751–53
  ultrasound of, 1757, 1760
  urination patterns, 1754b
  urine studies, 1757, 1758t
  vascular diseases of, 1795, 1795t, 1820–22
Kilocalories, 1600
Kineret, 1440t
Kinesthesia, 451
Kinesthetic learners, 50
Kinin system, 267–68, 268t
Klinefelter syndrome, 202
Knee arthroscopy, 701t
Knowledge transformation
  ACE Star Model of, 25f, 28
  definition of, 30
  description of, 28
  premises of, 30, 30b
Kübler-Ross, Elizabeth, 145
Kupffer cells, 267, 1384, 1696
Kussmaul breathing, 996, 1918
Kwashiorkor, 1607
Kyphoplasty, 460
Kyphoscoliosis, 994
Kyphosis, 994, 1982, 2002

L

Labeling, 71
Labetalol, 924t
Labia majora, 2061–62, 2076
Labia minora, 2061–62, 2076
Laboratory biosafety, 2249
Labyrinth, 1312
Labyrinthitis, 1356
Laceration, ocular, 1334
Lachman's test, 2021f
Lacrimal gland, 1301
Lactase deficiency, 187, 1576, 1650b
Lactobacillus, 2107
Lactobacillus acidophilus, 2061
Lactulose, 1717
Lacunae, 1936
Lamellar bone, 1935
Laminar air flow, in operating room, 670
Laminectomies, 1242
Lancinating, 1248
Langerhans' cells, 1477t, 1478
Laparoscopically assisted vaginal hysterectomy, 2099
Laparoscopy
  acute abdomen treated with, 1662
  cholecystectomy, 1730–31, 1731f–1732f
  definition of, 701t, 1586
  gastrointestinal obstruction treated with, 1675
  radical nephrectomy, 1798
Laparotomy, 1662
Laplace's law, 1671
Laryngeal cancer
  assessment of, 1044
  description of, 1043
  diagnostic tests, 1044–45
  epidemiology of, 1043–44
  etiology of, 1044
  nursing diagnoses, 1045
  nutrition considerations, 1049
  outcomes, 1049–50
  prognosis for, 1045, 1050
  recurrence of, 1050
  speech therapy, 1047–49
  staging of, 1046b
  treatment of
    considerations for, 1045
    endoscopic transoral laser surgery, 1045
    goals, 1047
    laryngectomy. *See* Laryngectomy
    radiation therapy, 1045, 1047
Laryngeal obstruction, 1042
Laryngectomy
  laryngeal cancer treated with, 1047–48
  nutritional support after, 1049
  patient education about, 1049, 1050b
  speech therapy after, 1048–49
Laryngitis, 1037–38
Laryngopharynx, 979
Laryngoscopy, 1044–45
Laser
  fire caused by, 675
  hazards associated with, 674
  surgical uses of, 674
Laser ablation, 2153–54
Laser in situ keratomileusis, 1338
Lateral collateral ligament, 2020
Lateral epicondylitis, 2014–15
Latex allergy
  anaphylactic shock caused by, 2219
  characteristics of, 637–38, 1469–70
  definition of, 625, 633, 671, 676–77, 1404
  sources of, 2219
Latinos, 83t
Latissimus dorsi myocutaneous flaps, for breast reconstruction, 2158
Lavage, 1587
Lavender, 393t
Laxatives, 163
Leading causes of death, 127t, 144, 1595
Learning
  ability to learn, 51
  affective, 721
  assumptions about, 45
  barriers to, 45–46, 46b
  beliefs about, 45b
  cognitive, 720–21
  definition of, 44
  domains of, 46–47, 47t
  evaluation of, 55
  facilitators of, 45
  philosophy of, 44
  principles of, 46t
  psychomotor, 721
  readiness for, 51–52
  styles of, 50
Learning needs, 50–51
Learning plateaus, 45
Learning theories, 45t
Lecithin-cholesterol acyltransferase deficiencies, 1718
Left anterior descending artery, 751
Left atrial pressure, 576–77
Left heart catheterization, 808
Left ventricle, 749
Left ventricular hypertrophy, 758
Leiomyomata, 2088, 2111–12
Length of stay, 535
Lentigines, 1482
Leukapheresis, 426
Leukemia
  acute lymphocytic, 950, 954–56
  acute myeloid, 950, 954, 956–57
  assessment of, 950
  biphenotypic, 950
  bone marrow transplantation for, 951–52
  chronic lymphocytic, 950, 957–59
  chronic myeloid, 950, 959–61
  definition of, 949
  diagnostic tests for, 950
  epidemiology of, 950
  etiology of, 950
  incidence of, 403t
  nursing care for, 953b
  nursing diagnoses for, 951
  outcomes for, 953–54
  pathophysiology of, 950
  radiation therapy for, 951
  signs and symptoms of, 954–55
  stem cell transplantation for, 951–52
  surgical treatments for, 951–52
  treatment of, 951–52
Leukocytes
  definition of, 1383–84
  dendritic cells, 1385–87
  description of, 266t, 266–67, 736f
  granulocytes, 1388
  macrophages, 267, 1384
  mast cells, 1387, 1387t
  monocytes, 266–67, 736f, 1384–85
  natural killer cells, 1388
  production of, 1384
Leukocytosis, 1395
Leukopenia, 948
Leukotriene modifiers, 1124, 1459
Leukotrienes, 267
Leuprolide, 2116
LeVeen peritoneovenous shunt, 1715
Level of consciousness
  assessment of, in brain-injured patients, 1192
  postanesthesia care unit assessment of, 698
Levine's sign, 776
Levinson, Daniel, 122
Levodopa, 1282, 1283t
Levofloxacin, 496
Levothyroxine, 1894
Liberty, 97
Lichenification, 1489f, 1508
Licorice root, 395t
Life events, 244–45
Life expectancy, 136
Life review, 165
Life Structure Theory, 122
Life support
  advanced cardiac, 870–71
  basic. *See* Basic life support
  description of, 601
Life time, 123t
Life-preserving surgery, 645–46
Ligaments
  anatomy of, 1939
  injuries to, 2019–21

Limbic system, 1406
Linear lesions, 1490b
Linoleic acid, 361
Lip reading, 1371
Lipid lowering agents, 782t, 784–85
Lipids
  classification of, 772t
  digestion of, 1597
Lipodystrophy, 1914, 1917
Lipopolysaccharide, 1385
Liposome, 233
Lisinopril, 924t
Lispro insulin, 1912
Lister, Joseph, 240
Liver
  anatomy of, 1696–98
  assessment of, 1582
  blood supply to, 1696
  burn effects on, 1533
  diagnostic tests, 1699–1701
  estrogen metabolism in, 1698
  fat transport to, 1597–98
  fatty, 1718–19
  functions of, 1696
  glucose conversion by, 1697
  hereditary diseases of, 1710–11
  lobules of, 1696
  metabolism by, 1697–98
  traumatic injuries to, 1721–22
  venous drainage of, 1696, 1697f
Liver biopsy, 1700b
Liver cancer, 1723–25
Liver enzymes, 1700
Liver function tests, 1699–1701
Liver sweats, 1713
Liver transplantation
  auxiliary, 1725–26
  diagnostic tests, 1727
  donors, 1726, 1726b
  hepatic artery thrombosis after, 1728
  history of, 1725
  immunosuppressive therapy after, 1728–29
  indications for, 1725
  nursing diagnoses, 1727
  orthotopic, 1725
  outcomes, 1729
  postoperative care, 1728
  preparations for, 1727–28
  procedure for, 1725
  recipients, 1726–27, 1727b
  United Network for Organ Sharing, 1726
Living will, 105, 149, 151
Loading dose, 486
Lobar pneumonia, 1057
Lobectomy, 1274t
Local anesthesia, 678t
Locked-in syndrome, 1185t, 1293
Locus, 203
Long bones, 1935
Long-term care, 544
Loop diuretics, 506–8, 923t, 1783
Loop electrosurgical excision, 2081, 2108–9
Loop of Henle, 1752
Loratadine, 1022t
Lorazepam, 596t
Losartan, 924t
Loss of appetite
  in hospice patients, 154, 162
  in palliative care patients, 154, 162
Lotions, 1498, 1501
Lou Gehrig's disease. *See* Amyotrophic lateral sclerosis
Low vision, 1344–45
Low-density lipoproteins, 273, 510, 514, 771
Lower airway disease, 1055–56
Lower motor neurons, 1217
Lower respiratory tract, 980–81
Low-flow oxygen delivery systems, 1013
Low-molecular-weight heparin
  atherosclerosis indications, 882t
  deep venous thrombosis treated with, 894
  description of, 512
  peripheral arterial occlusive disease treated with, 887
  thrombophlebitis treated with, 894
L-selectin, 1392
Lubricants, 1503–4
Lumbar puncture
  description of, 1160
  multiple sclerosis evaluations, 1276
Lumbar spine, 1946t
Lumpectomy, 2153
Lung(s)
  acid-base balance by, 328–29
  alveoli, 979
  anatomy of, 976–79
  auscultation of, 1756
  carbonic acid regulation by, 986
  compliance of, 981
  fissures of, 977f
  left, 976
  lobes of, 977
  perfusion rates of, 983
  right, 976
  ventilation rates of, 983
Lung abscess, 1075–78
Lung biopsy, 1011
Lung cancer
  asbestos exposure and, 1078
  assessment of, 1079
  classification of, 1079
  description of, 1078
  diagnostic tests, 1079, 1080t
  epidemiology of, 1078
  etiology of, 1078–79
  incidence of, 403t
  nonsmall cell, 1079
  nursing diagnoses, 1079–80
  outcomes, 1082
  pathophysiology of, 1079
  planning and implementation for, 1080–82
  risk factors for, 410t
  small cell, 1079
  smoking and, 1078
  staging of, 1079
  treatment of
    chemotherapy, 1080–81
    evidence-based, 1081
    pharmacologic, 1081
    radiation therapy, 1081
    surgery, 1081–82
Lung transplantation
  chronic obstructive pulmonary disease treated with, 1115
  criteria for, 1116
  cystic fibrosis treated with, 1130–31
  double, 1131
Lung volume reduction surgery, 1114
Luteinizing hormone, 1851t, 2078
Lycopene, 391t
Lyme disease, 277, 1966–69
Lymph nodes
  assessment of, 1409–10
  axillary dissection of, 2155
  description of, 1392
  elective regional lymph node dissection, 1524
  mapping of, 2154
Lymphadenopathy, 965
Lymphangiography, 1427b
Lymphatic system, 965f
Lymphocytes
  characteristics of, 1389
  description of, 266t, 267, 741
  T, 1388, 1390–91
  tests for, 1411–12
  types of, 741
Lymphoid organs
  primary, 1391
  secondary, 1391–92
Lymphoid tissues, 1392
Lymphoma
  central nervous system, 1196
  gastric, 1643
  Hodgkin's disease. *See* Hodgkin's disease
  non-Hodgkin's, 403t, 965b, 969–70, 2231

M

Macrobore tubing, 341
Macrolides, 495–98
Macronutrients, 1596, 1599t
Macrophages, 267, 1384
Macropinocytosis, 1386
Macula
  age-related degeneration of, 1310, 1332–33
  assessment of, 1310–11
  description of, 1302
Macular edema, 1311
Macular rash, 2250
Macules, 1486b, 1488f
Mafenide acetate, 1551
Magnesium
  characteristics of, 299t
  deficiency of, 312t, 326–27
  excess of, 312t–313t, 327–28
  functions of, 299t
  recommended dietary intake of, 314t
Magnetic resonance angiography
  description of, 1162
  stroke evaluations, 1175t
Magnetic resonance cholangiopancreatography, 1739
Magnetic resonance imaging
  brain injury evaluations, 1190
  brain tumor evaluations, 1197
  costs of, 1163
  female reproductive system evaluations, 2083
  functional, 1162, 1190
  heart failure evaluations, 808
  multiple sclerosis evaluations, 1276
  musculoskeletal system evaluations, 1950
  myocardial infarction assessments, 780
  nervous system assessments, 1161–62
  nursing management for, 1161–62
  perfusion, 1190
  renal evaluations, 1761t
  spinal cord injury evaluations, 1221–22
  stroke evaluations, 1175t
Magnetic resonance spectroscopy, 1162
Magnetoencephalography, 1165
Major histocompatibility complex
  definition of, 1382, 1840
  dendritic cell transport of, 1386
Major surgery, 620, 693
Mal-absorption disorders, 1652
Malaise, 2250
Mal-assimilation syndromes, 1651–54
Mal-digestion disorders, 1651–52
Male reproductive disorders
  balanitis, 2186–87
  benign prostatic hypertrophy, 1751, 2056–57, 2166–69
  cryptorchidism, 2183–84
  description of, 2163
  epididymitis, 2178
  epispadias, 2189–90
  erectile dysfunction, 2058, 2193–95
  hematocele, 2179
  hydrocele, 2178–80
  hypospadias, 2189–90
  orchitis, 2177–78
  paraphimosis, 2184–85
  Peyronie's disease, 2190–92
  phimosis, 2184–85
  posthitis, 2186–87
  priapism, 2195–97
  prostate cancer. *See* Prostate cancer
  prostatitis, 2164–65
  testicular cancer, 2173–75
  testicular torsion, 2175–77
  urethral stricture, 2188–89
  urethritis, 2187–88
  varicocele, 2180–81
Male reproductive system
  androgens, 2058
  assessment of, 2074–75
  bulbourethral glands, 2057
  diagnostic tests, 2077–80
  epididymis, 2056
  functions of, 2055
  penis, 2057
  physical examination of, 2074–75
  prostate gland, 2056–57
  semen production, 2058
  seminal vesicles, 2056
  spermatogenesis by, 2055, 2057–58
  testes, 2055–56
  vas deferens, 2056
Male sexual response, 2066–68
Malignant, 405
Malignant hyperthermia, 683–84
Malignant melanoma, 1522–24
Malignant tumors
  of brain, 1195
  description of, 407–8
Malleus, 1312
Malnutrition
  assessment of, 1607
  definition of, 1606
  diagnostic tests, 1607
  epidemiology of, 1606
  etiology of, 1606
  gastric surgery and, 1644
  nursing diagnoses, 1608
  outcomes, 1608–10
  treatment of, 1608
Mammary duct ectasia, 2143
Mammograms, 410
Mammography, 2149
Mammoplasty
  augmentation, 2144–46, 2157, 2157f
  definition of, 2144
  reduction, 2146
Managed care
  cost containment model of, 260
  description of, 7

Managed care organizations, 533
Mandatory minute ventilation, 589
Mangled extremity severity score, 2045, 2046t
Mannitol, 343t, 507
Mannose-binding lectin, 1394
Manubriosternal angle, 975
Manubrium, 975
Marasmus, 1607
Marijuana, 463
Masks
  oxygen delivery using, 697
  personal protective uses of, 672
Maslow's hierarchy of needs, 62f
Mass casualty care
  biological warfare. *See* Biological warfare
  blast injuries, 2259–60
  emergency nursing, 2236–37
  overview of, 2235
  triage. *See* Triage
Mass casualty incident
  definition of, 2240
  Hospital Emergency Incident Command System, 2242–43
  hospital preparations for, 2240–41
  incident command, 2241–43
  personal protective equipment for, 2244
  posttraumatic stress disorder secondary to, 2261–64
  signs and symptoms of, 2261
  stress reactions to, 2260–65
Massage therapy, 386, 388–89
Mast cell stabilizers, 1123–24
Mast cells, 267, 268t, 741, 1387, 1387t
Mastalgia, 2140
Mastectomy
  breast reconstruction after, 2156–59
  description of, 701t, 2155–56
  modified radical, 2156
  simple, 2156
Mastitis, 2143
Mastodynia, 2140
Mastoid surgery, 1365–66
Mastoid tenderness, 1316
Mastoidectomy, 1366
Mastoiditis, 1360
Material safety data sheets, 420
Matrix metalloproteinases, 1483
McGill pain questionnaire, 450, 469
Meal planning, 1110
Mean arterial pressure, 572, 752
Mean corpuscular hemoglobin, 747t
Mean corpuscular volume, 747t
Mechanical debridement of wounds, 288, 1497
Mechanical ventilation
  abbreviations, 590t
  airway pressure release ventilation, 589
  in chronic obstructive pulmonary disease, 1110
  chronic obstructive pulmonary disease treated with, 1103
  complications of
    anxiety, 596–98
    barotrauma, 594–95
    communication, 595–96
    nutrition impairments, 598–99
    oxygen toxicity, 599
    paralysis, 597
    stress ulcers, 595
    tracheal damage, 593
    unplanned extubation, 593–94
  continuous mandatory ventilation, 586
  continuous positive airway pressure, 588
  definition of, 586
  endotracheal intubation. *See* Endotracheal intubation
  ethical considerations, 589
  goal of, 1103
  indications for, 586b
  inverse ratio ventilation, 588
  life support withdrawal, 601
  mandatory minute ventilation, 589
  negative pressure ventilation, 586
  nitrogen supplementation, 598
  nursing management during, 590–92, 591t
  positive end expiratory pressure, 588
  positive pressure ventilation, 586
  pressure control ventilation, 587–88
  pressure support ventilation, 588
  proportional assist ventilation, 589
  synchronized intermittent mandatory ventilation, 586, 600
  total parenteral nutrition in, 598
  ventilator alarms, 590
  volume control ventilation, 587–88
  weaning, 599–601
Medial collateral ligament, 2019–20
Mediastinum, 747, 978–79
Medicaid, 136–37, 545
Medical futility, 112, 115–16
Medical marijuana, 463
Medical screening examination, 2239
Medical team, 4
Medicare
  definition of, 545
  description of, 136
  Hospice Benefit, 146
Medication administration. *See* Drug administration
Medication administration record, 487–88, 712
Medication errors
  computerized physician order entry system to prevent, 536
  description of, 355–56
  reduction of, 487
Meditation, 381–82, 920, 1265
Medulla oblongata, 452f, 1146f
Medullary cavity, 1935
Megacolon, 1691
Megakaryocyte, 741
Meglitinides, 527, 1915
Meiosis, 199
Melanocytes, 1476, 1477t, 1482
Melanoma
  choroidal, 1334–35
  malignant, 1522–24
  vulvar cancer, 2119
Memory cells, 1399–1400
Memory impairments, 1199
Menarche, 2064
Mendel, Gregor, 203
Mendelian inheritance patterns, 203–6
Ménière's disease, 1252–54, 1355–56, 1363
Meninges, 1139–40, 1141f
Meningiomas, 1196
Meniscal injuries, 2022–24
Menopause
  breast changes during, 2138
  description of, 2064–65
  management of, 2090–91, 2096–97
Menorrhagia, 2093
Menstrual cycle, 2059, 2064
Menstrual disorders
  alternative therapies for, 2099–2100
  amenorrhea, 2089, 2097
  assessment of, 2095
  botanical therapies for, 2100
  diagnostic tests, 2095–96
  dysfunctional uterine bleeding, 2093–94, 2097
  dysmenorrhea, 2088, 2099–2100
  endometriosis, 2094–95, 2098
  menopause, 2064–65, 2090–91, 2096–97
  nursing diagnoses, 2096
  nutritional considerations, 2098
  outcomes, 2100–2101
  patient education about, 2100
  pharmacological treatment of, 2098
  polycystic ovary syndrome, 2092–93, 2097, 2125
  premenstrual dysphoric disorder, 2091–92, 2096–97
  premenstrual syndrome, 2091–92, 2096–97
  surgical treatment of, 2098–99
  treatment of, 2096–2100
Menstrual pain, 2088
Mental illness, 220–21
Mental retardation, 216
Mental status assessments, 1149, 1151
Meperidine, 472
Mesenchymal stem cells, 1225
Mesothelioma, 1078
Meta analysis, 33
Metabolic acidosis, 330t–331t, 332–33, 989, 2205b
Metabolic alkalosis, 331t, 333, 988f, 988t
Metabolic patterns, 181
Metabolic rate, 1599–1601
Metabolic syndrome, 127–28, 773
Metabolism, 1596–98
Metabolism, of drugs, 485–86
Metaphysis, 1935
Metaraminol bitartrate, 2197t
Metastasis
  bone tumors, 1998–99
  brain, 1196
  colorectal cancer, 1679
  definition of, 407
  sites of, 407
  spinal cord tumors, 1239, 1242
  squamous cell carcinoma, 1522
Metered dose inhalers
  description of, 516, 516f
  directions for, 1112
Metformin, 527, 765, 1916t
Methadone, 464, 474t
Methemoglobinemia, 739
Methicillin-resistant *Staphylococcus aureus*, 271, 277
Methotrexate, 1436, 1440t, 1997t
Methyldopa, 923t
Methylphenyltetrahydropyridine, 1280
Methylprednisolone
  multiple sclerosis treated with, 1278t
  in renal transplantation, 1843t
  spinal cord injury managed using, 1226–27
Methylxanthines, 517
Metolazone, 923t
Metoprolol, 503, 782t, 924t
Metronidazole, 1077
Metrorrhagia, 2093
Microaneurysms, 1309
Microarray, 210
Microbore tubing, 341
Microdeletions, 201
Microglia, 1139
Microorganisms
  antibiotic-resistant, 271
  infectious diseases caused by, 270–71, 271t
Midazolam, 597t
Midbrain, 452f
Midclavicular line, 977
Middle cerebral arteries, 1143
Middle ear, 1312
Midsternal line, 977, 978f
Miglitol, 1916t
Migraine headaches, 460, 1265t, 1266–67
Military antishock trousers, 2215
Military triage, 2240, 2241t
Milk thistle, 393t
Millimeters of mercury, 751
Mills, John Stuart, 98
Mind-body therapies
  description of, 380–83
  pain management using, 477
  research into, 379
Mineralocorticoids, 1851t
Minimal sedation, 677
Minimally responsive state, 1185t
Mini-Mental State Examination, 1151
Minor surgery, 620, 693
Minority group, 71
Minority populations
  blood pressure control in, 509
  trends in, 126
Minoxidil, 924t
Minute volume, 1106t
Mitosis, 199
Mitoxantrone, 1278t
Mitral facies, 826
Mitral regurgitation, 824–25
Mitral valve
  anatomy of, 750, 822
  replacement of, 832f
  stenosis of, 825–27
Mitral valve annuloplasty, 830, 831f
Mitral valve prolapse, 819, 823–24
Mixed hearing loss, 1356–57
Mixed sleep apnea, 1039
Mixed venous oxygen saturation, 577
Modafinil, 1278t
Modified radical mastectomy, 2156
Moexipril, 924t
Mohs micrographic surgery, 1490
Moisture retentive dressings, 1503
Moisturizers, 1503–4
Molds, 1021b
Monilial vulvovaginitis, 1511
Monoclonal antibodies, 1432, 1681
Monocyte colony-stimulating factor, 268t, 269
Monocytes, 266–67, 736f, 1384–85
Mononucleosis, 949
Monosaccharides, 1597
Monosodium glutamate, 1153
Monosomies, 200
Mons pubis, 2061, 2076
Montelukast, 1020, 1022t
Moral distress, 101
Morals, 96
Morbid obesity, 642
Morbidity, 125
Morphine sulfate
  administration of, 160–61
  characteristics of, 474t
  dosing of, 161–62
  mechanical ventilation uses of, 596t
  pain management using, 157, 159–60, 794, 1542
Mortality
  for cancer, 403t
  definition of, 125, 402
  leading causes of, 127t, 144, 1595

spinal cord injury and, 1214
in spinal cord injury patients, 1234
treatment of, 1984–85
Osteosarcoma, 1994–98
Ostomy
creation of, 1684–85
definition of, 1684
ileostomy, 1684–85
sexual intimacy affected by, 438–39
Otalgia, 1313, 1356
Otitis externa
acute, 1318–19, 1319f
description of, 1374
serous, 1319
Otitis media
acute, 1362
bacterial causes of, 1359
definition of, 1359
diagnosis of, 1359
with effusion, 1363
hearing loss caused by, 1354
prevention of, 1363
recurrent, 1354
serous, 1409
treatment of, 1362, 1374
tympanic membrane perforations caused by, 1359
Otomycosis, 1318
Otorrhea, 1313
Otosclerosis, 1354, 1360, 1363
Otoscopic assessment, 1317–19, 1360, 1360f
Ototoxic medications, 1350–51
Outcome variables, 535
Ovarian agenesis, 2112–13
Ovarian cancer, 403t, 2120–22
Ovarian cysts, 2112, 2114
Ovaries, 2059, 2076
Overflow incontinence, 1807b
Overuse syndrome, 2010, 2010b
Overweight, 1612
Ovulation, 2059
Oxicams, 471b
Oxidation-reduction reaction, 738
Oximetry. *See* Pulse oximetry
Oxybutynin, 1278t
Oxycodone, 474t
Oxygen
delivery systems for, 1013
hemoglobin binding, 738–39, 984
myocardial supply and demand, 775
supplementation of, during postoperative period, 696–97
transport of, 983–84
Oxygen free radicals, 1184
Oxygen therapy
chronic obstructive pulmonary disease treated with, 1113–14
response to, 1115
sickle cell anemia treated with, 935
Oxygen toxicity, 599
Oxygenation assessments, 806
Oxygen-hemoglobin dissociation curve, 984–86
Oxyhemoglobin, 984
Oxyhemoglobin dissociation curve, 739
Oxytocin, 1851t, 2137

P

p53, 1677t
P wave, 841, 843–44
Pacemakers
definition of, 864
dual-chamber, 865
external, 865
interventions for, 865b
malfunction of, 866–67
mechanism of action, 864–65
permanent, 866
single-chamber, 865
transvenous, 865
types of, 865
Packed red blood cells, 363–64
PACU. *See* Postanesthesia care unit
Paget's disease
alkaline phosphatase tests, 1988
assessment of, 1988
bisphosphonates for, 1990, 1991t
definition of, 1987
diagnostic tests, 1988–89
epidemiology of, 1988
etiology of, 1988
exercise for, 1990
family education about, 1990–91
hypercalcemia caused by, 1990
nursing diagnoses, 1989
outcomes, 1991–92
pathophysiology of, 1988
patient education about, 1990–91
treatment of, 1989–90, 1991t
X-ray evaluations, 1988–89
Paget's mammary disease, 2143–44
Pain
abdominal, 1572, 1577, 1579t, 1656–58
acute
description of, 457, 464
management of, 468–69
acute abdomen, 1656–57
age-related influences, 455
appendicitis-related, 1665
assessment of. *See* Pain assessment
auricular, 1316
back, 458b, 460
cancer. *See* Cancer pain
chronic
coping with, 469
description of, 460–61
in elderly, 455
in critically ill patients, 565
definition of, 448
esophageal, 1627–28
fast, 453
gastrointestinal tract, 1634–35
gate control theory of, 449–50
gender influences, 455–56
idiopathic, 462
importance of, 448
intractable, 463–64, 475
mechanisms of, 453–54
menstrual, 2088
modulation of, 450, 454
mouth, 1621–22
neuropathic, 456–57, 458b–459b
nociceptive, 456
nursing diagnoses, 467
parietal, 1656
pathophysiology of, 450–53
pattern theory of, 449
perception of, 454
phantom, 458b
physical care for, 469–70
prolonged exposure to, 466
psychogenic, 458b
reassessment of, 464, 476
referred, 456, 457f, 458b, 1578, 1578f, 1584, 1656
reporting of, 466–67
responses to, 455–56
sexual intercourse-related, 2127
slow, 453
sociocultural influences, 455
somatic, 456, 1656
specificity theory of, 448
spinal cord tumor, 1240
theories of, 448–50
tonsillitis, 1035
transduction of, 450, 453
transmission of, 450, 453–54
undertreatment of, 159, 440, 466
visceral, 456, 459t, 1656
Pain assessment
barriers to, 465–67
description of, 153b, 753, 754b
elements of, 464–65
inadequate, 466
tools for, 464–65
Pain history, 464
Pain management
acupuncture for, 386
in acute coronary syndromes, 794
acute pain, 468–69
barriers to, 160b, 465–67
in burn patients, 1542–43, 1551–52
cancer-related pain, 440, 459b
in children, 661
complementary and alternative therapies, 477–78
conventional measures for, 467–68
description of, 367
discharge teaching about, 723
ethical issues of, 109–10
in Guillain-Barré syndrome, 1247
in hospice patients, 152–53, 156–59
Joint Commission for the Accreditation of Healthcare Organizations standards, 109, 159, 367, 467–68
mind-body therapies using, 477
myths and misconceptions regarding, 158–59
nonpharmacological methods, 162, 711
nursing education about, 466
opioids for. *See* Opioid(s)
in palliative care patients, 152–53
in pediatric patients, 661
in peripheral nerve injuries, 1255
pharmacologic methods
adjuvant medications, 472, 474t
aspirin, 470
nonopioid analgesics, 470, 474t
nonsteroidal anti-inflammatory drugs, 470
opioid analgesics. *See* Opioid(s)
postoperative
in children, 661
description of, 611, 701–2, 710
principles of, 156–57, 467
World Health Organization approach, 157–58
Pain scales, 701
Pain threshold, 454–55
Pain tolerance, 454
PAINAID Scale, 465
Palliation, 414
Palliative care
advanced practice nurses in, 152
definition of, 110, 144
ethical considerations, 110–11
goal of, 144
hospice care vs., 144
interdisciplinary team who deliver, 144–45, 150, 152
mouth care, 162–63, 166
nurses involved in, 146, 150
nursing diagnoses, 155–56
spiritual support in, 164–65
World Health Organization definition of, 144
Pallidotomy, 1284t
Pallor, 1308
Palmomental reflex, 1159t
Palpation
of abdomen, 1579f, 1582
definition of, 183
of external ear, 1316
of heart, 758f
musculoskeletal system assessments, 1943
of precordium, 757
respiratory system, 997–98
technique of, 183–84, 184f
Palpebral conjunctiva, 1305
pamidronate, 1991t
Pancreas
anatomy of, 1570–71, 1699, 1856
assessment of, 1583
cells of, 1699
hormones produced by, 1851t
insulin production by, 1905
Pancreatectomy, 1740f
Pancreatic cancer, 403t
Pancreatitis
acute, 1736–38
chronic, 1738–41
Pancuronium, 597t
Panhypopituitarism, 1873
Panic disorder, 1635
Panlobar emphysema, 1102
Pap tests, 2076–77, 2080, 2104
Papillary muscle dysfunction, 791
Papillary reflex, 1302
Papilledema, 1342, 1967
Papules, 1486b, 1488f
Paracentesis, 1586–87, 1714
Para-chlorobenzoic acid derivatives, 471b
Paralysis
assessment of, 1942
neuromuscular blockers for, 597–98
Paramyxovirus, 1988
Paraphimosis, 2184–85
Paraplegia
definition of, 1218
wheelchair use after, 1233–34
Parasitic infestations
conjunctivitis caused by, 1340
in homeless persons, 81t
Parasympathetic nervous system, 1216
Parathyroid adenomas, 1896
Parathyroidectomy, 1897
Paraurethral glands, 2063
Parenteral nutrition
definition of, 1606
formulas, 1606
peripheral, 362, 362t
total
advantages and disadvantages of, 361t
definition of, 360
metabolic complications of, 362
nursing considerations for, 360b
patient selection for, 361–62
protein in, 361
Paresthesia, 1157, 1240
Parietal lobe, 452f, 1142
Mosaicism, 200
Motivation, 56
Motor evoked potentials, 1242
Motor vehicle accidents, 1190–91
Mouth
allergy-related findings, 1409
anatomy of, 1569, 1620f
inspection of, 995
physical examination of, 1755
Mouth care
for hospice patients, 162–63, 166
for mechanical ventilation patients, 594t
Mouth pain, 1621–22
Moxifloxacin, 1429
Mucociliary elevator, 981
Mucosa-associated lymphoid tissues, 1392
Mucositis, radiation therapy-related, 1047
Mucus
agents used to clear, 1112
description of, 981
Müllerian dysgenesis, 2112
Multiculturalism, 72–73
Multilumen central line, 359
Multiple marker screening, 213
Multiple myeloma
acute renal failure caused by, 1825t
in African Americans, 961
assessment of, 962
calcium imbalances in, 964
clinical features of, 961
definition of, 961
diagnostic tests for, 962–63
epidemiology of, 961
etiology of, 961
incidence of, 403t
outcomes, 964
pathophysiology of, 962
renal insufficiency associated with, 962
stem cell transplantation for, 963–64
treatment of, 963–64
Multiple organ dysfunction
primary, 2227–28
secondary, 2228–30
Multiple organ dysfunction syndrome, 2209, 2227
Multiple sclerosis
assessment of, 1275
clinical manifestations of, 1275, 1275t
deep brain stimulation for, 1277
definition of, 1274
description of, 1433
diagnostic tests, 1276–77
epidemiology of, 1274
etiology of, 1274
nursing diagnoses, 1277
outcomes, 1279
pathophysiology of, 1274–75
primary progressive, 1275
progressive-relapsing, 1275
relapsing-remitting, 1275
secondary progressive, 1275
treatment of, 1277–79, 1278t
trigeminal neuralgia and, 1248
Munchausen's syndrome, 1661
Murphy's sign, 1582, 1659
Muscle
aging effects on, 1939–40
skeletal, 1938–40
Muscle relaxants, 472
Muscle strength, 1155, 1155t, 1944, 1945f, 1946t
Muscle tone, 1944
Musculoskeletal disorders
dermatomyositis, 1974–76
description of, 1955
fibromyalgia. *See* Fibromyalgia
gout, 1964–66
Lyme disease, 1966–69
osteoarthritis. *See* Osteoarthritis
osteomalacia, 1985–87
osteomyelitis, 1992–94
osteoporosis. *See* Osteoporosis
Paget's disease. *See* Paget's disease
polymyositis, 1974–76
spondyloarthropathies. *See* Spondyloarthropathies
Musculoskeletal system
assessment of
gait, 1944–45
guidelines, 1941b
health history, 1941–42
inspection, 1943
muscle strength grading, 1944, 1946t
muscle tone, 1944
neurovascular, 1943
overview of, 1940
physical examination, 1942–45
range of motion, 1944–45, 1946t
diagnostic tests
angiogram, 1948–49
arthrography, 1949
arthrometry, 1951
arthroscopy, 1951
bone marrow aspiration and biopsy, 1951–52
bone scan, 1949
computed tomography, 1949
dual energy X-ray absorptiometry scan, 1949–50
indium scan, 1950
laboratory studies, 1948
magnetic resonance imaging, 1950
myelogram, 1950–51
nerve conduction studies, 1952
somatosensory evoked potentials, 1952
x-rays, 1951
joints, 1940
ligaments, 1939
skeletal muscles, 1938–40
skeleton, 1935–38
tendons, 1939
trauma to, 1942
Musculoskeletal trauma
Achilles tendon injuries, 2026–27
amputation. *See* Amputation
ankle sprain, 2024–25
carpal tunnel syndrome. *See* Carpal tunnel syndrome
compartment syndrome, 2039–40
fat embolism syndrome, 2040–41
fractures. *See* Fracture(s)
hip fractures, 2036–39
lateral epicondylitis, 2014–15
ligament injuries, 2019–21
meniscal injuries, 2022–24
overuse syndrome, 2010, 2010b
overview of, 2009
patellar tendinopathy, 2018–19
plantar fasciitis, 2027–29
repetitive motion injuries, 2010, 2010b
rotator cuff tears, 2012–14
shoulder dislocation, 2010–12
sports injuries, 2010
venous thromboembolism, 2042–43
Musculoskeletal tumors
chondrosarcoma, 1994–98
description of, 1994
Ewing's sarcoma, 1994–98
metastatic, 1998–99
osteosarcoma, 1994–98
primary bony, 1994–98
soft tissue, 1994–98
Music, 396
Music-thanatology, 396
My Pyramid, 1598, 1599f
Myasthenia gravis, 1289–92
Mycophenolate mofetil, 1841, 1843t
Mycoplasma, 271t
Mycoplasma pneumoniae, 1056
Mycotic aneurysms, 889
Myectomy, 815
Myelography, 1164, 1950–51
Myelosuppression, chemotherapy-related, 421, 430, 958b, 968b
Myocardial contractility, 805
Myocardial infarction
complications of, 791
creatine kinase levels, 793
definition of, 770
idioventricular rhythm caused by, 859
inflammation and, 273
non-ST segment elevation, 791, 793–94
pharmacologic agents for, 794–95
ST segment elevation, 791–94
treatment of, 794
Myocardial nuclear perfusion imaging, 763–65
Myocardial oxygen supply and demand, 775
Myocarditis, 820–21
Myocardium, 748
Myoclonic seizures, 1271
Myomectomy, 2111
Myometrium, 2060
Myopia, 1337
Myosin, 1938
Myotonia, 2066
Myringoplasty, 1366
Myringosclerosis, 1318
Myringotomy, 1365–66
Myxedema coma, 1895

N

N-Acetylcysteine, 1130
Nadir, 431
Nadolol, 924t
Nails
anatomy of, 1477t, 1479
clubbing of, 996–97
Naloxone hydrochloride, 472, 475
Nasal airways, 584
Nasal cannula, 1113
Nasal polyp, 1042, 1042f
Nasal sprays, 1024
Nasogastric intubation
complications of, 1588
contraindications, 1588
dysphagia nutrition using, 1626
equipment used in, 1587–88
technique, 1589
tubes, 1587
Nasopharynx, 979
National Center for Complementary and Alternative Medicine, 156, 246, 379, 477
National Center for Patient Safety, 549
National Comprehensive Cancer Network, 414
National Guideline Clearinghouse, 36
National Hospice Reimbursement Act, 146
National Institute of Nursing Research, 550
National Kidney Disease Education Program, 1842
National Labor Relations Act, 18
National Labor Relations Board, 18
National Quality Forum, 536
Native Americans
biological variations in, 84t
death beliefs, 147t
folk medicine used by, 83t
food preferences, 85t
Natural killer cells, 741, 1388
Nausea
anticipatory, 434
antiemetics for, 421, 434
assessment of, 1572
chemotherapy-induced, 420–21, 434, 968t
definition of, 1575
in hospice patients, 154, 163
in palliative care patients, 154, 163
Neck, 995
Necrotizing fasciitis, 289
Nedocromil, 516
Needle biopsy
of brain tumor, 1197
description of, 413
Needleless access devices, 345b
Needlestick injuries, 277, 347
Negative feedback, 1850
Negative pressure ventilation, 586
Neglect, 132
Negligence
definition of, 370
proving of, 370–71
Neoadjuvant therapy, 419
Neoangiogenesis, 1479
Neoplasm, 405
Neostigmine, 1278t
Neovascularization, 1309
Nephrectomy
definition of, 1794
radical, 1797–98
simple, 1819f
Nephrolithiasis, 1789
Nephrons, 1748, 1751, 1751f–1752f
Nephrosclerosis, 1795, 1795t
Nephrotic syndrome, 1784–87
Nephrotoxic agents, 1753, 1755b
Nervous system
age-related changes, 1146
anatomy and physiology of, 1137–46
assessment of
cerebellar function, 1156–57
description of, 1410
history-taking, 1147–48
interview, 1148, 1150b–1151b
mental status, 1149, 1151
motor function, 1155
physical examination, 1148–49, 1151–59
reflex testing, 1158–59
sensory system, 1157–58
autonomic, 1145
cells of, 1137–39
central. *See* Central nervous system
description of, 1136
diagnostic tests
carotid duplex studies, 1166–67
cerebral angiography, 1162–63
cerebrospinal fluid analysis, 1160t
computed tomography, 1161
description of, 1159
digital subtraction angiography, 1163

electroencephalography, 1164–65
electromyography, 1165–66
evoked potentials, 1166t
functional magnetic resonance imaging, 1162, 1190
lumbar puncture, 1160
magnetic resonance angiography, 1162
magnetic resonance imaging, 1161–62
magnetic resonance spectroscopy, 1162
magnetoencephalography, 1165
myelography, 1164
positron emission tomography, 1163–64
radiographic studies, 1160–64
single-photon emission computed tomography, 1164
transcranial Doppler sonography, 1167
ultrasound, 1166–67
x-rays, 1161
endocrine system functioning affected by, 1850–51
parasympathetic, 1216
parasympathetic response, 1148t
peripheral, 1144–45
sympathetic response, 1148t
Neugarten, Bernice, 123
Neural tube defects, 213
Neuralgia, 1243
Neuroendocrine system response, 2205–6
Neurofibrillary tangles, 1286
Neurogenic shock, 1228–29, 2220–22
Neuroglia, 1138–39
Neuromuscular blockers, 597–98
Neurons, 1137–39
Neuropathic pain, 456–57, 458b–459b
Neuropathies
Bell's palsy, 1250–52
carpal tunnel syndrome, 1256–57
definition of, 1243
etiology of, 1243
Guillain-Barré syndrome. *See* Guillain-Barré syndrome
Ménière's disease, 1252–54
pathophysiology of, 1243–44
peripheral, 433, 1243
trigeminal neuralgia, 1243, 1247–50
Neuropeptides, 379
Neuroreceptor, 454
Neurotransmitters
characteristics of, 1138, 1138t
definition of, 379
small intestine affected by, 1649
Neurovascular assessment, 1943
Neutralization, by antibodies, 1390
Neutropenia
biological response modifiers for, 432
in cancer patients, 431–32
definition of, 431
description of, 948–49, 1388
drug-induced, 1411–12
febrile, 432
infectious causes of, 1412b
Neutrophils
description of, 266, 736f, 1388
stem cell origin of, 740
Nicotinamide adenine dinucleotide, 739
Nicotinamide adenine dinucleotide phosphate, 739
Nicotine. *See also* Smoking
circulatory effects of, 643
physiologic effects of, 909–10
withdrawal symptoms from, 920
Nicotinic acid, 514
Nifedipine, 924t
Night driving, 1310
Nightingale, Florence
description of, 3, 6, 610
disease studies by, 240–41
disease transmission writings, 281b
healing environment provided by nurses, 551
imagery therapy, 382
nursing as viewed by, 610
palliative care principles, 158
theory of nursing by, 10
Nipple
anatomy of, 2063
dimpling of, 2139
discharge from, 2141
disorders of, 2140–41
examination of, 2139
fissures of, 2141
supernumerary, 2137
Nisoldipine, 924t
Nitrates
coronary artery disease treated with, 781, 782t
heart failure treated with, 810
indications for, 502
mechanism of action, 781
pharmacokinetics of, 502–3
side effects of, 503, 781
Nitroglycerin, 502–3, 782t
Nits, 1514
Nociceptive pain, 456
Nociceptor, 451
Nocturia, 1771
Nodules, 1486b, 1488f
Noise, 1368–70
Noncardiac chest pain, 1634–35
Noncontinent urinary diversions, 1802
Non-Hodgkin's lymphoma, 403t, 965b, 969–70, 2231
Noninflammatory diarrhea, 1576–77
Nonmaleficence, 97, 192t, 229t, 371
Nonnucleoside reverse transcriptase inhibitors, 1429, 1430b
Non-seminomas, 2173
Nonsmall cell lung cancer, 1079
Non-ST segment elevation myocardial infarction, 791, 793–94
Nonsteroidal anti-inflammatory drugs
angiotensin-converting enzyme inhibitors affected by, 511
chemopreventive uses of, 412
classification of, 471b
fever reduction using, 274
in older adults, 476
osteoarthritis treated with, 1958–59
pain management using, 157, 470
patellar tendinopathy managed using, 2019
rheumatoid arthritis treated with, 1439, 1440t
Nontoxic goiter, 1890
Nonulcer dyspepsia, 1635–38
Nonverbal communication, 74–75
Norepinephrine, 912, 1138, 1851t
Nose
allergy-related findings, 1409
anatomy of, 1018f
fractures of, 1041
hypertrophic turbinates, 1042
inspection of, 995
obstruction of, 1041–42
Nosebleeds. *See* Epistaxis
Nosocomial infections
definition of, 1779, 1815
infusion therapy-related, 340
urinary tract infections, 1767
Nuchal, 2258
Nuclear perfusion imaging
coronary artery disease evaluations, 779–80
description of, 763–65
Nucleoside reverse transcriptase inhibitors, 1429, 1430b
Nuremberg Code, 116–17
Nurse
adult care by, 138
aging workforce of, 126
altruism by, 9
critical care, 560–61
education of, 6
ethics-based role of, 100–102
hospice care, 146, 150
impaired, 20
in medical team, 4
palliative care, 146, 150
patient advocate role of, 101–2, 192
school, 259
self-awareness by, 88
Nurse case manager, 259b
Nurse-controlled analgesia, 346
Nursing
business approach to, 15
care delivery models for, 15–16
complementary and alternative therapies and, 396–97
criteria for, 10b
definition of, 10–11, 255
domains of, 11
emergency, 2236–37
future of, 261–62
transcultural, 84–85
in United States, 9–11
Nursing competencies, 551
Nursing diagnoses
for acromegaly, 1868
for acute coronary syndromes, 793–94
for acute renal failure, 1826
for allergies, 1452
for Alzheimer's disease, 1287
for amputation, 2045
for appendicitis, 1666
for asthma, 1122, 1457
for atherosclerosis, 881b
for bladder cancer, 1800
for breast cancer, 2151
for bronchiolectasis, 1073–74
for chronic obstructive pulmonary disease, 1107
for chronic renal failure, 1833
for coronary artery disease, 780
cultural competence and, 88
for Cushing's disease, 1870
for cystic fibrosis, 1129
for diabetes mellitus, 1908
for fibromyalgia, 1979
for fractures, 2033
for gastrointestinal obstruction, 1673
for glomerulonephritis, 1782
for Guillain-Barré syndrome, 1245
for gynecological malignancies, 2121
for headaches, 1264b
for health maintenance, 59
for heart failure, 808
for hepatitis, 1708
for hospice care, 155–56
for human immunodeficiency virus, 1428
for hypercalcemia, 323
for hyperkalemia, 320
for hypermagnesemia, 328
for hypernatremia, 317
for hyperphosphatemia, 325
for hypertension, 915–16
for hypertrophic cardiomyopathy, 814
for hypocalcemia, 321
for hypoglycemia, 1921
for hypokalemia, 318–19
for hypomagnesemia, 326
for hyponatremia, 315
for hypophosphatemia, 324
for inflammation, 273–75
for inflammatory bowel disorders, 1688
for interstitial cystitis, 1775
for liver transplantation, 1727
for lung cancer, 1079–80
for malnutrition, 1608
for multiple sclerosis, 1277
for obesity, 1613
for osteoarthritis, 1957–58
for Osteomyelitis, 1993
for osteoporosis, 1983–84
for Paget's disease, 1989
for pain, 467
for palliative care, 155–56
for Parkinson's disease, 1281
for perioperative period, 660
for pneumonia, 1059
for pneumothorax, 1084
for polycystic kidney disease, 1818
for portal hypertension, 1716
for prostate cancer, 2171
for pulmonary arterial hypertension, 1090
for pulmonary fungal infections, 1071
for renal cancer, 1797
for rheumatoid arthritis, 1437, 1438t
for shock, 2214t
for spinal cord tumors, 1241
for stomach cancer, 1643
for stroke, 1175
for teaching-learning process, 52
for thrombophlebitis, 894
for tuberculosis, 1066
for urinary incontinence, 1807
for urinary tract calculi, 1790
for urinary tract infections, 1771, 1773
Nursing education
description of, 11–12
genetics concepts included in, 235
Nursing Home Quality Initiative, 545
Nursing homes, 546b
Nursing models
adaptation model, 255–56
self-care theory, 257–58
systems model, 256–57
Nursing practice
education, 11–12
environment for, 17–20
family structure changes, 14
genetic, 235
globalization of, 12–13
health care agencies and, 550–53
informality of, 14
leadership, 11
risk-taking behaviors, 14
Nursing process
assessment, 50–51
cultural competence and, 86–89
intravenous therapy uses of, 356
Nutrition. *See also* Diet
in acute renal failure, 1830
for aging population, 188, 1615
for Alzheimer's disease patients, 1288
for amyotrophic lateral sclerosis patients, 1294
artificial, 113
assessments of, 181, 1607t
atherosclerosis and, 881–82
in Bell's palsy patients, 1251
for burn patients, 1549–51, 1560
in chronic obstructive pulmonary disease patients, 1110–11
for chronic renal failure, 1839
in critically ill patients, 564
in cystic fibrosis patients, 1129–30
in diabetes mellitus patients, 1910–12
drug interactions, 1601–2
dysphagia effects on, 1626
for fibromyalgia, 1979
in Graves' disease, 1886–87
health maintenance uses of, 62
for myasthenia gravis patients, 1291
for osteoarthritis, 1958
osteoporosis prevention and, 1984
in Parkinson's disease patients, 1282
postoperative, 724
in rheumatoid arthritis patients, 1439
screening of, 1607t, 1609t
therapeutic uses of, 391–94
tissue repair effects on, 275
wound healing affected by, 284, 288–89
Nutrition support
description of, 1602
enteral feedings
administration of, 1605
benefits of, 1603
for burn patients, 1550
definition of, 1602
formulas, 1603–4, 1604t
routes for, 1605, 1605f
tubes used in, 1605
gastrostomy feedings, 1605
parenteral nutrition. *See* Parenteral nutrition
Nutritionally adequate diet, 1598–1601
Nystagmus, 1152, 1306, 1324

O

Obesity
assessment of, 1612–13
body mass index calculations, 1612b
breast cancer and, 2148
cancer risks, 404
colorectal cancer and, 1678
coronary artery disease risks, 773
definition of, 773, 1612
diabetes mellitus and, 128, 1612
epidemiology of, 1612
esophageal cancer and, 1632
etiology of, 1612
fat cells, 909
hypertension and, 909
inflammatory response and, 273
morbid, 642
nursing diagnoses, 1613
outcomes, 1614
preoperative considerations, 641
prevalence of, 124
rates of, 124
recommendations for, 790t
stroke risks, 1173b
surgical treatment of, 1614
treatment of, 1613–14
upper body, 909
vaccine studies, 128
wound healing affected by, 284–85
Objective data, 176
Obstructions
gastrointestinal. *See* Gastrointestinal obstruction
laryngeal, 1042
nasal, 1041–42
Obstructive sleep apnea, 1038–40
Obturator muscle test, 1582f
Occipital lobe, 452f
Occlusive disease, 885–88
Occult fractures, 2038
Occult pneumothorax, 1083
Occupational allergic rhinitis, 1019t
Occupational stress, 254–55
Occupational therapist, 1207t
Octreotide, 1868
Ocular cancer, 1334–36
Ocular movement disorders
assessment of, 1326
description of, 1324
nystagmus, 1324
ocular muscle paralysis, 1324
strabismus, 1324
Oculomotor nerve, 1146f, 1147t, 1152–53, 1302
Odynophagia, 1044, 1573–74
Office of Alternative Medicine, 379
Off-pump coronary artery bypass grafting, 787
Ogilvie's syndrome, 1669
Ointments, 1498
OKT3, 1843t
Older adults. *See also* Elderly
age-related changes in, 476
atrial fibrillation in, 852
automobile driving by, 137
chronic illness in, 135–36
chronic pain in, 455
classification of, 369, 476
drug administration in, 490–91
ethnic, 136
frailty of, 135
health and illness trends in, 132–34
health assessment of, 187–88
health care services used by, 136–37
health conditions that affect, 134
health promotion for, 137–38
homeless, 135
hospitalization of, 253
hypothyroidism in, 1895
immune system changes in, 1402–3
infusion therapy in, 369
interactions with, 132
intravenous therapy in, 369
medication use by, 134b
needs of, 136
negative life events experienced by, 252
neglect of, 132
nonsteroidal anti-inflammatory drugs in, 476
nutrition for, 1615
patient care for, 663
perioperative considerations for, 661–63
postoperative care for, 717–18
profile of, 133b
pulmonary disease in, 662–63
pyelonephritis in, 1779
in rural areas, 135
skin care in, 369–70
stressors for, 132–33
subpopulations of, 134–36
venipuncture in, 369–70
visual impairments in, 1310
women, 135
Olfactory bulb, 1146f
Olfactory nerve, 1146f, 1147t, 1151–52
Oligodendrocytes, 1138
Oligomenorrhea, 2089
Oligospermia, 2078
Oliguria, 1782, 1826
Olmesartan, 924t
Omega-3 fatty acids, 392
Omnibus Budget Reconciliation Act, 104–5
Oncogenes, 219–20, 406
Oncogenesis, 406
Oncology therapy
chemotherapy. *See* Chemotherapy
description of, 366–67
radiation. *See* Radiation therapy
Oncotic pressure, 298, 1543
Ongoing assessment, 175–76
Onycholysis, 1973
Oocytes, 2064
Open biopsy, 2150–51
Operating room, 670
Operating room nurses, 656–58
Ophthalmopathy, 1887
Ophthalmoscope, 1306t
Ophthalmoscopic examination, 1306
Opioid analgesics
addiction concerns, 159–60
administration of, 159–60, 477, 710–11
agonist-antagonist, 474t
constipation caused by, 473
contraindications, 477
diverticulitis pain managed using, 1668
intramuscular administration of, 710–11
moderate, 474t
morphine, 157, 159–60, 474t
overdose of, 475
pain management using, 157–59, 471–72
physical dependence on, 471–72
preoperative use of, 640
respiratory depression caused by, 473
side effects of, 473, 475–76
tolerance to, 472
toxicity of, 475–76
withdrawal symptoms, 475
Opportunistic infections
fungal, 1069
HIV-related, 1426
pneumonia, 1056–57
Oppression, 71
Opsonization, 268, 1390
Optic atrophy, 1308
Optic disc, 1307f
Optic nerve, 1146f, 1147t, 1152, 1302
Oral airways, 583–84
Oral cancer, 1622
Oral cavity disorders
burning mouth syndrome, 1622
description of, 1620
dysphagia. *See* Dysphagia
etiology of, 1620
mouth pain, 1621–22
planning and implementation for, 1620–21
Oral cholecystography, 1701
Oral contraceptives, 2120
Oral glucose tolerance test, 1908
Oral hypoglycemic agents, 527–28
Oral ulcers, 1621t
Orchiectomy, 2175f
Orchiopexy, 2183
Orchitis, 2177–78
Organ donation
end-of-life care and, 113–14
ethical considerations, 685–86
Organ of Corti, 1352
Organ Procurement and Transplantation Network, 685
Organizational ethics, 100
Orgasm, 2068–69
Orgasmic disorders, 2128
Oropharyngeal dysphagia, 1574
Oropharynx, 979
Orphenadrine, 1283t
Orthostatic hypotension, 925
Osmolality, 296
Osmolarity, 296
Osmosis, 297, 297f
Osmotic diuretics
description of, 506–8
intracranial pressure lowering using, 582
Osmotic pressure, 297–98, 298f
Ossicles, 1312, 1351
Osteoarthritis
assessment of, 1957
bone spurs associated with, 1957
definition of, 1956
description of, 272
diagnostic tests, 1957
epidemiology of, 1956
etiology of, 1956
health care resources, 1959–60
nursing diagnoses, 1957–58
outcomes, 1960, 1962
pathophysiology of, 1956–57
primary, 1956
secondary, 1956
treatment of
nutrition, 1958
pharmacological, 1958–59
surgery, 1960
Osteoblasts, 1936
Osteoclasts, 1936
Osteocytes, 1936
Osteogenesis, 1935
Osteomalacia, 1985–87
Osteomyelitis, 1992–94
Osteon, 1936
Osteopenia, 1865, 1938
Osteoporosis
assessment of, 1982
bisphosphonates for, 1984
definition of, 1981
diagnostic tests, 1983
epidemiology of, 1981
etiology of, 1981
exercise for, 1985
family education about, 1984
fractures caused by, 460, 1982
health care resources, 1984
nursing diagnoses, 1983–84
nutritional considerations, 1984
outcomes, 1984
pathophysiology of, 1981–82
patient education, 1984
pharmacological treatment of, 1984
predisposing factors, 1982t
risk assessments, 1982
selective estrogen receptor modulators for, 1
skeletal anabolics for, 1984

Parietal pain, 1656
Parity, 2060
Parkinson's disease
assessment of, 1280–81
definition of, 1279
diagnostic tests, 1281
epidemiology of, 1280
etiology of, 1280
nursing diagnoses, 1281
nutritional considerations, 1282
outcomes, 1284
pathophysiology of, 1280
perioperative considerations, 663
treatment of
overview of, 1281–82
pharmacological, 1282, 1283t
surgical, 1284t
tremor associated with, 1280
Paroxysmal nocturnal dyspnea, 517
Partial laryngectomy, 1048
Partial seizures, 222, 1270t, 1272
Partial thromboplastin time, 747t
Partial-thickness wounds, 282
Passive euthanasia, 115
Passive immunization, 1400
Past medical history, 632
Pasteur, Louis, 240
Patau syndrome, 200
Patellar tendinopathy, 2018–19
Pathological reflexes, 1159, 1159t
Patient(s)
decisional capacity of, 106
empowerment of, 63, 259, 261
knowledge base of, 52
motivation of, 56
nurse's role as advocate of, 101–2, 192
perceptions of, 56
previous experience of, 52
rights of, 192
strengths of, 52
teaching of, 488–89
Patient education
acute coronary syndromes, 796–97
acute renal failure, 1831–32
amputation, 2045–46
aneurysms, 892
angina pectoris, 781
asthma, 1124, 1126
atherosclerosis, 883–84
bronchiolectasis, 1075
burns, 1544–45, 1554–55, 1560–61
carpal tunnel syndrome, 2018
chronic obstructive pulmonary disease, 1115–16
fibromyalgia, 1980
fractures, 2034–35
glomerulonephritis, 1783–84
gynecological infections, 2109
gynecological malignancies, 2123
hypertension, 925
menstrual disorders, 2100
mitral valve prolapse, 823–24
nosebleeds, 1041
osteoporosis, 1984
osteosarcoma, 1997–98
outcomes, 1069
Paget's disease, 1990–91
peripheral arterial occlusive disease, 888
pneumothorax, 1084–85
polycystic kidney disease, 1819
postoperative care, 719–25
purposes of, 44
surgery, 626
thrombophlebitis, 895–96
topics for, 44t
tuberculosis, 1069
urinary diversion, 1803
varicose veins, 902
wound care, 722–23
Patient positioning
increased intracranial pressure prevented by, 582
intraoperative, 683
in postanesthesia care unit, 698–99
postoperative, 698–99
safety in, 683
Patient Self Determination Act, 104, 134, 151, 193
Patient-controlled analgesia
description of, 345–46, 357–58, 473, 475
postoperative uses, 710
surgical uses of, 611
Patient's Bill of Rights, 48, 100, 488, 627
Patriarchal family structure, 78
Pattern reversal evoked potentials, 1166t
Pattern theory, 449
Pavlov, Ivan, 45t
Peak drug level, 497
Peak expiratory flow, 1122
Peak flow meter, 1123f
Pectoral myositis, 1003
Pectus carinatum, 756t, 994f
Pectus excavatum, 756t, 994f, 994–95
Pediatric patients. *See* Children
Pediculosis, 1514–15
Pedigrees, 235
Pelvic examination, 2114, 2114f
Pelvic inflammatory disease, 2101, 2105
Pelvic relaxation, 2110–11
Pemphigus, 1515
Penetrating trauma
ocular, 1334
renal, 1792
Penicillin G, 1033
Penicillins
administration of, 495b
adverse effects of, 494
extended-spectrum, 493
glomerulonephritis treated with, 1783
indications for, 493
laboratory monitoring of, 494
mechanism of action, 492–93
nursing management for, 494–95
pharmacodynamics of, 493–94
pharmacokinetics of, 493
side effects of, 494
urinary tract infections treated with, 1772b
Penile brachial index, 2080
Penile cancer, 2192–93
Penis
anatomy of, 2057
discharge from, 2075
ejaculation from, 2058–59, 2067–68
erection of, 2058, 2067
physical examination of, 2074
Penrose drain, 700t, 723
Pentosan polysulfate sodium, 1776, 1776b
Peppermint, 394t
Pepsin, 1570
Peptic duodenitis, 1641
Peptic ulcer disease, 523–24
Peptic-ulcer dyspepsia, 1638–41
Percent solutions, 352
Perception, 56
Percussion
of abdomen, 1580t, 1581–82
definition of, 184, 998
of kidneys, 1756f
notes obtained during, 999, 999t
of precordium, 758
respiratory system assessments, 998–99
sounds on, 184, 185t
technique for, 184, 184f, 998–99
Percutaneous catheters, 359
Percutaneous coronary interventions, 785–86
Percutaneous endoscopic gastrostomy, 1591, 1626
Percutaneous endoscopic jejunostomy, 1591
Percutaneous transluminal coronary angioplasty
coronary artery disease treated with, 785
peripheral arterial occlusive disease treated with, 887
Percutaneous umbilical blood sampling, 212t, 213
Perennial allergic rhinitis, 1019t
Perfusion, 983
Perfusion magnetic resonance imaging, 1190
Pergolide, 1283t
Perianal region, 1584
Pericardial cavity, 749
Pericardial friction rub, 760
Pericarditis
acute coronary syndromes and, 791
characteristics of, 821–22
chest pain caused by, 791
pain associated with, 755t
Pericardium, 748, 821
Perichondritis, 1316
Periductal mastitis, 2143
Perimenopause, 2090
Perindopril, 924t
Perinephric, 1842
Perineum, 2063
Perioperative, definition of, 608
Perioperative nurse
description of, 630, 653
knowledge and skills of, 654b
pediatric interactions, 660–61
role of, 654–55
Perioperative Nursing Data Set, 659–60
Perioperative period. *See also* Intraoperative period
ethics in, 684–86
geriatric considerations, 661–63
Health Insurance Portability and Accountability Act provisions, 695
nursing care, 659–63
nursing diagnoses, 660
for Parkinson disease, 663
pediatric considerations, 660–61
transportation of patient in, 686–87
Periorbital contusion, 1333
Periosteum, 1935
Peripheral arterial occlusive disease, 885–88
Peripheral blood stem cells, 425
Peripheral nerve injuries, 1254–66
Peripheral nervous system
description of, 450–51, 1144–45
dysfunction of. *See* Neuropathies
Peripheral neuropathy, 433, 1243, 1925–26
Peripheral parental nutrition, 362, 362t
Peripheral vascular dysfunction, 1927–28
Peripheral vascular resistance, 910
Peripherally acting sympatholytics, 509
Peristalsis, 1596, 1748
Peritoneal dialysis, 1837–39
Peritoneovenous shunt, 1715
Peritonitis, 1655–56, 1665
Peritonsillar abscess, 1036–37
Permanent pacing, 866
Permethrin cream, 1518
Persistent vegetative state, 1185t
Personal digital assistants, 882, 1911
Personal protective equipment, 276f, 671–72, 2244
Personal space, 76
Perspiration, 1383
Pesticides, 404
Pet therapy, 395–96
Petechiae, 745t, 819, 941
Peyronie's disease, 2190–92
pH, 987
Phacoemulsification, 1328
Phagocytic cells
description of, 1384
function tests for, 1413
Phagocytosis, 266, 269, 740, 1385, 2218
Phalen's maneuver, 2017, 2017f
Phantom pain/limb sensations, 458b, 2048
Pharmaceutic phase, 484
Pharmacodynamics, 487
Pharmacogenomics, 234–35
Pharmacokinetics
absorption, 484
aging effects, 491
bioavailability, 484
biotransformation, 485
definition of, 484
distribution, 484
metabolism, 485–86
Pharmacology, 483
Pharyngitis, acute, 1031–34
Pharynx
functions of, 1569–70
inspection of, 995
Phenobarbital, 521
Phenotype, 203
Phentermine and fenfluramine, 1088
Phenylacetic acids, 471b
Phenylephrine, 2197t
Phenytoin, 521
Pheochromocytoma, 1881–83
Philadelphia chromosome, 959
Philosophy, 44
Phimosis, 2184–85
Phlebitis
description of, 347
intravenous therapy as cause of, 348
Phlebostatic axis, 570, 572
Phlebostatic measurements, 570
Phlebotomy, 947
Phospholipids, 514
Phosphorus
deficiency of, 313t, 323–24
excess of, 314t, 324–26
normal levels of, 1759t
recommended dietary intake of, 314t
Photoaging, 1504
Photoallergic, 1504
Photochemotherapy, 1505–6
Photodynamic therapy
bladder cancer treated with, 1800
brain tumors treated with, 1204–5
Photorefractive keratotomy, 1338
Photosensitivity, tetracycline-related, 497
Phototherapy, 1504–6
Physiatrist, 1207t
Physical dependence
definition of, 159
on opioids, 471–72

Physical examination
auscultation, 184–85
baseline data collection, 183
care of patient after, 194
documentation, 194
genetic screening, 211
inspection. *See* Inspection
palpation. *See* Palpation
percussion. *See* Percussion
preparation for, 183
purpose of, 182–83
Physical inactivity
coronary artery disease risks, 773
recommendations for, 789t
Physical self-examinations, 62
Physical therapist, 1207t
Physician-assisted suicide, 150
Physicians, 4, 617–18
Physiological integrity, 255
Phytoestrogens, 391t
Phytonutrients, 391, 391t
Phytosterols, 391t
Pia mater, 1140
Pica, 937
Pigeon chest, 756t, 995
Piggyback infusions, 357
Pigmentation, 1476
Pink eye. *See* Conjunctivitis
Pink puffers, 1103
Pinna, 1311
Pituitary adenoma, 1869
Pituitary gland
anatomy of, 1146f
anterior
description of, 1852, 1853f–1854f
hypersecretion of, 1864–73
hyposecretion of, 1873–74
hormones produced by, 1851t
posterior
description of, 1852, 1854f
disorders of, 1874–76
Plague, 277–78
Plague, for biological warfare, 2251–52
Plantar fasciitis, 2027–29
Plantar flexion, 1944f
Plantar reflex, 1159t
Plaque brachytherapy, 1335
Plaque psoriasis, 1516
Plaques, 1486b, 1488f
Plasma, 735–36
Plasma exchange, 1432
Plasma expanders, 343t–344t, 2216t
Plasmapheresis
definition of, 1432
description of, 942
Guillain-Barré syndrome treated with, 1246
myasthenia gravis treated with, 1291
Plasmin, 743
Platelet(s)
activation of, 741
adenosine diphosphate release by, 743
clot formation functions of, 743
description of, 735, 740, 741
function of, 741–42
transfusion of, 364
Platelet disorders
overview of, 940
thrombocytopenia, 940–42
Platelet-activating factor, 267
Pleura, 981
Pleural cavity, 978
Pleural effusion, 442
Pleural friction rubs, 1001t, 1001–2
Pleurisy, 1003–4
Pleuritic chest pain, 1056
Pleuritic pain, 777
Plexus
brachial, 1254
definition of, 1254
Pneumatic antishock garments, 2215
Pneumatic retinopexy, 1331
Pneumococcus vaccination, 1061
Pneumocystis carinii pneumonia, 1057, 1426
Pneumocystosis pneumonia, 1069
Pneumocytes, 980–81
Pneumonia
assessment of, 1058
atypical, 1056
classification of, 1057
community acquired, 1057
community-acquired, 525
definition of, 1056
diagnostic tests, 1059
epidemiology of, 1056–57
high-risk indicators for, 1058b
in HIV-infected patients, 1062
hospital-acquired, 1057, 1103
lobar, 1057
mortality rates, 1058
nursing diagnoses, 1059
opportunistic, 1056–57
outcomes, 1063
pain associated with, 755t, 1004
pathophysiology of, 1057–58
patient education about, 1062–63
physical examination findings, 1058
planning and implementation for, 1059–63
Pneumocystis carinii, 1057, 1426
postoperative, 713
prevention of, 1059–60
in spinal cord injury patients, 1233
symptoms of, 1058
treatment of
antibiotics, 1061
evidence-based, 1060, 1061t
oxygen supplementation, 1060
pharmacological, 1060–62
postural drainage, 1060
vaccination, 1061
ventilator assisted, 1057
ventilator-associated, 593–94
viral, 1056
Pneumonia severity index, 1058
Pneumothorax
assessment of, 1083
chest tubes for, 1084–85
definition of, 1004, 1082
diagnostic tests, 1083–84
etiology of, 1082–83
fractured ribs as cause of, 1085
nursing diagnoses, 1084
occult, 1083
pain associated with, 755t, 1004
pathophysiology of, 1083
patient education about, 1084–85
risk factors for, 1082
spontaneous, 1082–83
tension, 1083
traumatic, 1083
treatment of, 1084
Pollens, 1021b
Polyarteritis, 1781
Polycystic cysts, 1755
Polycystic kidney disease
antibiotics for, 1819
assessment of, 1817
autosomal dominant, 1816
autosomal recessive, 1816–17
definition of, 1816
diagnostic tests, 1817
epidemiology of, 1816
genetic factors, 1816
nursing diagnoses, 1818
outcomes, 1819–20
pathophysiology of, 1817
patient education about, 1819
treatment of, 1818–19
Polycystic ovary syndrome, 2092–93, 2097, 2125
Polycythemia vera, 947–48, 1102
Polyethylene glycol, 1585
Polymyositis, 1974–76
Polyp
cervical, 2110, 2115
colonic, 1678
definition of, 1678
Polypectomy, 1682
Polypharmacy, 490
Polysomnography, 1009–10
Pons, 452f
Population genetics, 209–10
Populations
at-risk, 2230–31
trends in, 125–26
vulnerable. *See* Vulnerable populations
Porphyrin, 738
Portal hypertension, 1715–17
Ports, imported, 359
Positional genetics, 224
Positive end expiratory pressure, 588, 599, 2226
Positive pressure ventilation, 586, 1060
Positron emission tomography
bone tumor evaluations, 1998
coronary artery disease evaluations, 780
nervous system assessments, 1163–64
nursing management for, 1163–64
stroke evaluations, 1175t
Postanesthesia care unit (PACU)
abdominal assessments, 697–98
Aldrete system, 702, 703t
anesthesia recovery, 693–95
care units after, 704
critical care unit transfer, 704–5
description of, 692, 693
discharge from, 702–5
equipment in, 693
ergonomics in, 694
level of consciousness assessments, 698
orthopedic assessments, 702–3
oxygen supplementation, 697
pain management in, 701–2
patient positioning, 698–99
recovery in, 692–702
reports, 699
respiratory deficits in, 702
sterility of, 694
stretchers in, 694
thermoregulation in, 698
transfer from, 703–5
wound stabilization, 699–700
Postanesthesia care unit nurse, 661, 693
Posterior cord syndrome, 1220
Posterior cruciate ligament, 2020
Posterior inferior cerebral arteries, 1143
Posterior pituitary gland, 1852
Posterior tibialis, 1943
Posthitis, 2186–87
Postnecrotic cirrhosis, 1711–12
Postoperative, definition of, 608
Postoperative care
abdominal assessments, 697–98
ambulation, 715, 716b
artificial airways, 697
assessments, 695
blood pressure, 697
complications
anticipating of, 713–14
cardiovascular, 662, 713
compartment syndrome, 713–14
ectopy, 713
family education about, 715–16
neurosensory, 714
patient education about, 715–16
respiratory, 713
signs of, 724
treatment of, 714
types of, 696t
wound dehiscence, 714
cultural considerations, 717
discharge planning and teaching
description of, 719
electronic resources, 725–26
family teaching, 722–25
hygiene, 723–24
medications, 724
nutrition, 724
pain management, 723
patient teaching, 719–25
tips for, 720b
electronic resources, 725–26
family considerations, 715–17, 722–25
home planning, 718–29
hospitalization times, 701t
in-patients, 707–8
liver transplantation, 1728
monitoring during, 611
nursing care
bedding, 709
drains, 711
future of, 729–30
health care provider's orders, 712
inpatients, 707–8
pain management, 710–11
short-stay patients, 705–7
after transfer, 709–13
urinary elimination, 711
wound dressings, 711
older adults, 717–18
onset of, 691
oxygen supplementation, 696–97
pain management
in children, 661
description of, 611, 701–2
patient positioning, 698–99
physiological stabilization, 695–99
recovery
delayed, 726–27
long-term, 727–29
milestones in, 714–17
rehabilitative care, 727–28
remote monitoring, 725–26
respiratory stability, 695–96
rest, 723

short-stay patients, 705–7
transfers
description of, 708b
postanesthesia care unit, 703–5
trends in, 692
urinary elimination, 711
wounds
healing of, 705
stabilization of, 699–700
Poststreptococcal glomerulonephritis, 1780–82
Postsurgical unit, 704
Posttraumatic stress disorder
in burn patients, 1555
description of, 241, 247, 249–50, 251b, 2261–63
Postural drainage
for chronic obstructive pulmonary disease, 1109
for pneumonia, 1060
Potassium
characteristics of, 299t
deficiency of, 309t–310t, 317–19
excess of, 310t–311t, 319–21
functions of, 299t
intravenous, 318
normal levels of, 1759t
recommended dietary intake of, 314t
Potassium channel blockers, 505
Potassium iodide, 1889
Potassium permanganate, 1502
Potassium-sparing diuretics, 507–8, 923t
Potential learning needs, 51
Poverty
description of, 80
in older adults, 133b
Povidone-iodine solution, 346
Power of attorney for health care. *See* Durable power of attorney for health care
PR interval, 841, 844
Pramipexole, 1283t
Prana, 384
Prayer, 78, 390
Prazosin, 924t
Prealbumin, 598, 1607, 1607t
Precordial leads, 839
Precordium
definition of, 757
inspection of, 758
palpation of, 757
percussion of, 758
Prednisolone, 1843t
Prednisone, 1278t, 1776b, 1975
Preferred provider organizations, 533
Pregnancy
acute abdomen during, 1663
appendicitis during, 1663
breast changes during, 2063–64, 2137–38
cholecystitis during, 1663
folic acid supplementation during, 392
gestational diabetes, 219
smoking during, 125
surgical emergencies during, 1663
Pregnancy tests, 2082
Prehypertension, 913
Preimplantation genetic diagnosis, 208–9
Prekallikrein, 742t
Preload, 568–69, 752
Premature atrial complexes, 849–50
Premature junctional complexes, 852–53
Premature ventricular complexes, 856f, 856–57
Premature ventricular contractions, 504, 778f
Premenstrual dysphoric disorder, 2091–92, 2096–97
Premenstrual syndrome, 2091–92, 2096–97
Preoperative, definition of, 608
Preoperative period. *See also* Surgery
age-related considerations, 634–35
checklist for, 624f, 636–37
communication in, 632
complementary therapy evaluations, 613–14
cultural considerations, 633–34
electronic advances, 615–16
environmental safety, 635–36
family during
involvement, 626–27, 633–34
support for, 639–40
history-taking, 638
intake interview, 632–33
laboratory tests, 638
medications used in, 639
note-taking during, 631–32
NPO status during, 629
nurse-sensitive indicators, 635
patient safety, 636–39
patients
assessment of, 632–33
education of, 626–27
safety of, 636–39
personal hygiene, 627–28
pharmacology, 640
population-specific care
description of, 641
frail elderly, 641
guardianships, 641–42
obese patients, 641–42
smoking, 643
substance users, 643–44
procedures during, 626–35
remote assessment, 613
spirituality, 614
transfer strategies, 640–41
venipuncture during, 631
Preoperative preparation teams, 611
Presbyopia, 1310, 1338
Presbyphagia, 1623
Preschool child, 187
Pressure bags, 344
Pressure control ventilation, 587–88
Pressure support ventilation, 588
Pressure ulcers
description of, 285
prevention of, 287
Prevalence, 123
Preventive care
access to, 538
definition of, 537
financing of, 538
quality of, 539
Prialt. *See* Ziconotide
Priapism, 2195–97
Primary aldosteronism, 1880–83
Primary biliary cirrhosis, 1711–12, 1733–35
Primary care, 539
Primary ciliary dyskinesia, 1073
Primary intention, 282
Primary lymphoid follicles, 1392
Primary multiple organ dysfunction, 2227–28
Primary progressive multiple sclerosis, 1275
Primary research, 31
Primary sclerosing cholangitis, 1733
Primitive neuroectodermal tumors, 1196
Prinzmetal's variant angina, 775
Prion diseases, 672
Prions, 672
Probanthine, 1278t
Problem-focused coping, 244
Process variables, 535
Proctocolectomy, 1683–84
Proctosigmoidoscopy, 1586
Procyclidine, 1283t
Professional ethics, 99–100
Progesterone, 2089
Programmed instruction, 48
Progressive muscle relaxation, 381, 920–921
Progressive systemic sclerosis, 1444–45
Progressive-relapsing multiple sclerosis, 1275
Prolactin, 1851t, 2078, 2137
Prolactinomas, 1864
Prolastin, 1112, 1711
Proliferative retinopathy, 1923
Propionic acid derivatives, 471b
Propofol, 597t
Proportional assist ventilation, 589
Propranolol, 503, 924t
Proprioception, 451
Prostaglandin synthetase inhibitor, 470
Prostaglandins, 267
Prostate biopsy, 2079
Prostate cancer
androgen deprivation therapy for, 423
assessment of, 2169
biopsy evaluations, 2169–70
definition of, 2169
diagnostic tests, 2169–70
digital rectal examination assessments, 2169
epidemiology of, 2169
etiology of, 2169
grading system for, 2170, 2170t
hormonal therapies for, 423–24
incidence of, 403t
nursing diagnoses, 2171
pathophysiology of, 2169
prostate-specific antigen screening, 2169, 2170t
radiation therapy for, 2171
risk factors for, 410t
treatment of, 2171–72, 2172f
Prostate gland
anatomy of, 2056–57
fluid analysis, 2078
physical examination of, 2075
Prostate-specific antigen, 412, 2056, 2078–79, 2169, 2170t
Prostatitis, 2164–65
Prosthetic heart valves, 760
Protamine sulfate, 512
Protease inhibitors, 391t, 1430b
Protein
absorption of, 1650–51
for burn patients, 1550
for diabetes mellitus patients, 1910
digestion of, 1597
for peritoneal dialysis patients, 1839
in total parenteral nutrition, 361
Protein binding, 485
Protein C, 743
Protein electrophoresis, 1413
Protein S, 743
Proteinuria, 1784, 1821
Prothrombin time, 512, 747t, 945
Proton pump inhibitors, 470, 524–25, 1630, 1639
Proto-oncogenes, 220
Protozoa, 271t
Prozac. *See* Fluoxetine
Pruritus, 1457, 1515
Pseudoephedrine, 1022t
Pseudohermaphrodites, 203
Pseudomembranous colitis, 494
Psoriasis, 1500t, 1516–17
Psoriasis activity and severity index, 1516
Psoriatic arthritis, 1973–74
Psychic integrity, 255–56
Psychogenic pain, 458b
Psychologist, 1207t
Psychomotor domain, of learning, 46, 47t
Psychomotor learning, 721
Psychoneuroimmunoendocrinology, 245–47, 379
Psychosocial history, 182, 913
Ptosis, 1152, 1289
Public health care agencies, 539
Pulmonary angiography, 1005–6
Pulmonary arterial hypertension
assessment of, 1089
classification of, 1090
definition of, 1088
diagnostic tests, 1090
epidemiology of, 1089
etiology of, 1089
nursing diagnoses, 1090
outcomes, 1091–92
patient education about, 1091
pharmacological treatment of, 1091
planning and implementation for, 1090–91
risk factors for, 1089b
surgery for, 1091
treatment of, 1090–91
Pulmonary artery catheters
complications of, 574–75
description of, 568, 572
insertion of, 573
right ventricle displacement of, 575
types of, 572–73
Pulmonary artery pressure monitoring, 572–76
Pulmonary capillary wedge pressure, 574, 574t
Pulmonary circulation, 576f
Pulmonary edema, 809
Pulmonary embolism
description of, 2042–43
pain associated with, 755t, 1004
postoperative, 662
prevention of, 1246
signs of, 894
Pulmonary function testing
asthma evaluations, 1120, 1122
respiratory system evaluations, 1011–12
Pulmonary fungal infections
aspergillosis, 1070
assessment of, 1070–71
blastomycosis, 1069
coccidioidomycosis, 1069–70
definition of, 1069
diagnostic tests, 1071
histoplasmosis, 1070
nursing diagnoses, 1071
outcomes, 1072
pathophysiology of, 1070
planning and implementation for, 1071–72
treatment of, 1071–72
Pulmonary rehabilitation, 1107–9
Pulmonary vascular resistance, 567, 575–76
Pulmonic valve, 749–50
Pulse oximetry
description of, 592, 983, 1009
oxygen measurements using, 1113–14, 1190, 1584
Pulse pressure, 911
Pulse rating, 757b
Pulseless electrical activity, 860

Pulseless ventricular tachycardia, 871
Pulsus alternans, 792
Pulsus paradoxus, 925
Punnett Square, 203, 203f
Pupil examination, 1305
Purified-protein derivative, 1403–4
Purkinje fibers, 836–37
Purpura
  definition of, 745t
  immune thrombocytopenia, 940
  thrombotic thrombocytopenic, 940
Pursed-lip breathing, 1110
Purulent sputum, 1073
Pustular psoriasis, 1516
Pustules, 1486b, 1488f
Pyelonephritis, 1751, 1777–80, 1814–16
Pyrazolone derivatives, 471b
Pyrethrin, 1515
Pyridoxine, 1068t
Pyrosis, 1573

Q

Qi, 240
QRS complex, 841–42, 844
QRS interval, 841, 844–45
QT interval, 845
Quadrants of abdomen, 1580t–1581t
Quadriceps setting, 713
Quadriplegia
  description of, 1218
  wheelchair use after, 1233–34
Quality health care, 7–9
Quality of life
  chronic illness effects on, 250
  ethical decision making based on, 108
  prostate cancer effects on, 2167
Quinapril, 924t
Quinidine, 504

R

R wave, 842–43
Race
  definition of, 70, 189
  demographic changes, 72b
  health assessment considerations, 189–90
Racism, 71
Radial keratotomy, 1338
Radiation nephritis, 1825t
Radiation therapy
  bladder cancer treated with, 1800
  bone tumors treated with, 1999
  brain tumors treated with, 1206
  breast cancer treated with, 2152
  cancer treated with, 416–19
  colorectal cancer treated with, 1681–82
  definition of, 416
  enteritis caused by, 417–18
  external, 416–17
  fatigue caused by, 418, 439–40, 1198
  Hodgkin's disease treated with, 966–67
  internal, 416, 418
  intracavitary, 418
  laryngeal cancer treated with, 1045, 1047
  leukemia treated with, 951
  lung cancer treated with, 1081
  non-Hodgkin's lymphoma treated with, 970
  outcomes, 419
  principles of, 416–17
  prostate cancer treated with, 2171
  side effects of, 417
  skin reactions to, 418
  spinal cord tumors treated with, 1242–43
  stereotactic, 1206
Radical cystectomy, 1800
Radical neck dissection, 701t
Radical nephrectomy, 1797–98
Radiculopathy, 2013
Radioallergosorbent test, 1413
Radiofrequency ablation, 1724, 2154
Radioiodine therapy, 1889
Radiopharmaceuticals, 1007
Radon, 409
Rales. *See* Crackles
Raloxifene, 1984
Range of motion testing, 1944–45, 1946t
Rapamycin, 1841
Rapid antigen testing, 1033
Ratio-proportion method, of intravenous therapy calculations, 350–51
Raynaud's disease, 899–900
Raynaud's phenomenon, 899–900
Reactive arthritis, 1970, 1973
Readiness to learn, 51–52
Rebound hypertension, 925
Rebound tenderness, 1581, 1581f, 1655
Receptive aphasia, 1200
Recessive trait, 199
Recombinant DNA, 1432
Recombinant plasminogen activators, 794
Recommended dietary allowances, 1598
Rectal cancer. *See* Colorectal cancer
Rectocele, 2111, 2114
Rectum, 1571
Red blood cells. *See* Erythrocyte(s)
Red reflex, 1307–8
Reduced penetrance, 222
Reduction mammoplasty, 2146
Reed-Sternberg cells, 965
Reentry, 846
Referred pain, 456, 457f, 458b, 1578, 1578f, 1584, 1656
Reflex arcs, 451f
Reflex erection, 1237
Reflex testing, 1158–59
Reflexology, 389–90
Refractive errors, 1337–38
Refractory ascites, 1713
Refractory period, 837
Regional anesthesia, 678t
Registered nurse first assistant, 658
Registered nurses
  education of, 4
  staffing ratio laws, 5
Registered Nurses Association of Ontario, 37
Regurgitation, 1575
Regurgitation, valvular
  aortic, 827–28
  mitral, 824–25
  pathophysiology of, 822
Rehabilitation
  after brain tumor treatment, 1206–7, 1207t
  burn wound. *See* Burn(s), rehabilitation phase
  cardiac, 796–97
  postoperative, 727–28
  pulmonary, 1107–9
  spinal cord injury, 1231–35
  team members involved in, 1206–7, 1207t
Rehabilitation engineer, 1207t
Rehabilitation nurse, 1207t
Reiki, 385–86
Reiter's syndrome, 1970
Relapsing-remitting multiple sclerosis, 1275
Relative hypovolemia, 2212
Relaxation, 380–81
Relaxation response, 381, 477
Religious faith, 615
Remicade, 1440t
Remodeling of bone, 1937
Remote monitoring, 725–26
Renal angiography, 1761t
Renal artery
  description of, 1753
  stenosis of, 1795, 1795t, 1825t
Renal biopsy
  description of, 1760–61, 1762b
  glomerulonephritis evaluations, 1783
Renal cancer
  assessment of, 1796
  diagnostic tests, 1796–97
  epidemiology of, 1795–96
  etiology of, 1796b
  genetic factors, 1796
  incidence of, 403t
  nursing diagnoses, 1797
  outcomes, 1798
  pathophysiology of, 1796
  surgical treatment of, 1797–98
  treatment of, 1797–98
Renal cell carcinoma, 1795–96
Renal colic, 1790–91
Renal failure
  acute
    alterations in, 1828t
    assessment of, 1826–27
    collaborative treatment of, 1827, 1829
    continuous renal replacement therapy, 1827, 1827b
    definition of, 1824
    diagnostic tests, 1826
    epidemiology of, 1824
    etiology of, 1824, 1825t
    evidence-based care, 1829–30
    family education about, 1831–32
    hypervolemia in, 1829
    intrarenal causes of, 1826
    nursing diagnoses, 1826
    nutritional considerations, 1830
    outcomes, 1832
    pathophysiology of, 1826
    patient education about, 1831–32
    postrenal causes of, 1826
    prerenal causes of, 1826
    surgical treatment of, 1831
  chronic
    assessment of, 1834t
    clinical manifestations of, 1834t
    collaborative management of, 1835, 1836b
    definition of, 1832
    diagnostic tests, 1833
    epidemiology of, 1832
    etiology of, 1833
    hemodialysis for, 1836–37
    nursing diagnoses, 1833
    nutrition for, 1839
    pathophysiology of, 1833
    peritoneal dialysis for, 1837–39
    pharmacological treatment of, 1835, 1836b
    refusal of treatment, 1835
    renal transplantation for. *See* Renal transplantation
    stages of, 1832t
    treatment of, 1834–43
Renal insufficiency, 962
Renal parenchyma, 1748
Renal transplantation
  allogeneic, 1840
  allograft, 1840
  complications of, 1841–42
  description of, 1839–40
  donors, 1841
  drug therapy after, 1843t
  health care resources for, 1842
  nursing management for, 1842b
  outcomes, 1842–44
  technique for, 1841, 1842f
  xenogeneic, 1840
Renal trauma, 1792–95
Renal tuberculosis, 1787–88
Renal tubules, 1751–53
Renal vascular disorders, 1795, 1795t
Renal vein thrombosis, 1795, 1795t
Renin
  angiotensin II production stimulated by, 509
  definition of, 2206
  description of, 301
  functions of, 912
Renin-angiotensin system, 509, 1753–54
Renin-angiotensin-aldosterone system, 301, 911, 1717
Repetitive motion injuries, 2010, 2010b
Repolarization, 837
Reproductive history, 211
Rescue breathing, 867–68
Research
  ethics in, 116–17
  institutional review board for, 117
Research utilization, 25
Reserpine, 923t
Residual volume, 1003
Resilience, 247–48
Resonance, 185t
Respiration
  physiology of, 982–90
  regulation of, 982
Respiratory acidosis, 329–31, 988f
Respiratory agents
  administration of, 516
  bronchodilators, 517–19
  dry powder inhalers, 516
  inhaled corticosteroids, 519–20
  metered dose inhalers for, 516, 516f
Respiratory alkalosis, 330t, 332
Respiratory distress
  acute. *See* Acute respiratory distress syndrome
  signs of, 997
Respiratory excursion, 997
Respiratory muscles
  accessory, 975–76
  age-related changes, 1003
Respiratory system
  age-related changes in, 993, 1002–4, 1402t
  allergy-related findings, 1410
  anatomy of, 975–82
  assessment of
    in allergy patients, 1410
    auscultation, 999–1002
    chest pain, 991–92
    cough, 990
    in elderly, 992–93
    history-taking, 990–93
    inspection. *See* Respiratory system, inspection of
    palpation, 997–98

Mosaicism, 200
Motivation, 56
Motor evoked potentials, 1242
Motor vehicle accidents, 1190–91
Mouth
  allergy-related findings, 1409
  anatomy of, 1569, 1620f
  inspection of, 995
  physical examination of, 1755
Mouth care
  for hospice patients, 162–63, 166
  for mechanical ventilation patients, 594t
Mouth pain, 1621–22
Moxifloxacin, 1429
Mucociliary elevator, 981
Mucosa-associated lymphoid tissues, 1392
Mucositis, radiation therapy-related, 1047
Mucus
  agents used to clear, 1112
  description of, 981
Müllerian dysgenesis, 2112
Multiculturalism, 72–73
Multilumen central line, 359
Multiple marker screening, 213
Multiple myeloma
  acute renal failure caused by, 1825t
  in African Americans, 961
  assessment of, 962
  calcium imbalances in, 964
  clinical features of, 961
  definition of, 961
  diagnostic tests for, 962–63
  epidemiology of, 961
  etiology of, 961
  incidence of, 403t
  outcomes, 964
  pathophysiology of, 962
  renal insufficiency associated with, 962
  stem cell transplantation for, 963–64
  treatment of, 963–64
Multiple organ dysfunction
  primary, 2227–28
  secondary, 2228–30
Multiple organ dysfunction syndrome, 2209, 2227
Multiple sclerosis
  assessment of, 1275
  clinical manifestations of, 1275, 1275t
  deep brain stimulation for, 1277
  definition of, 1274
  description of, 1433
  diagnostic tests, 1276–77
  epidemiology of, 1274
  etiology of, 1274
  nursing diagnoses, 1277
  outcomes, 1279
  pathophysiology of, 1274–75
  primary progressive, 1275
  progressive-relapsing, 1275
  relapsing-remitting, 1275
  secondary progressive, 1275
  treatment of, 1277–79, 1278t
  trigeminal neuralgia and, 1248
Munchausen's syndrome, 1661
Murphy's sign, 1582, 1659
Muscle
  aging effects on, 1939–40
  skeletal, 1938–40
Muscle relaxants, 472
Muscle strength, 1155, 1155t, 1944, 1945f, 1946t
Muscle tone, 1944
Musculoskeletal disorders
  dermatomyositis, 1974–76
  description of, 1955
  fibromyalgia. *See* Fibromyalgia
  gout, 1964–66
  Lyme disease, 1966–69
  osteoarthritis. *See* Osteoarthritis
  osteomalacia, 1985–87
  osteomyelitis, 1992–94
  osteoporosis. *See* Osteoporosis
  Paget's disease. *See* Paget's disease
  polymyositis, 1974–76
  spondyloarthropathies. *See* Spondyloarthropathies
Musculoskeletal system
  assessment of
    gait, 1944–45
    guidelines, 1941b
    health history, 1941–42
    inspection, 1943
    muscle strength grading, 1944, 1946t
    muscle tone, 1944
    neurovascular, 1943
    overview of, 1940
    physical examination, 1942–45
    range of motion, 1944–45, 1946t
  diagnostic tests
    angiogram, 1948–49
    arthrography, 1949
    arthrometry, 1951
    arthroscopy, 1951
    bone marrow aspiration and biopsy, 1951–52
    bone scan, 1949
    computed tomography, 1949
    dual energy X-ray absorptiometry scan, 1949–50
    indium scan, 1950
    laboratory studies, 1948
    magnetic resonance imaging, 1950
    myelogram, 1950–51
    nerve conduction studies, 1952
    somatosensory evoked potentials, 1952
    x-rays, 1951
  joints, 1940
  ligaments, 1939
  skeletal muscles, 1938–40
  skeleton, 1935–38
  tendons, 1939
  trauma to, 1942
Musculoskeletal trauma
  Achilles tendon injuries, 2026–27
  amputation. *See* Amputation
  ankle sprain, 2024–25
  carpal tunnel syndrome. *See* Carpal tunnel syndrome
  compartment syndrome, 2039–40
  fat embolism syndrome, 2040–41
  fractures. *See* Fracture(s)
  hip fractures, 2036–39
  lateral epicondylitis, 2014–15
  ligament injuries, 2019–21
  meniscal injuries, 2022–24
  overuse syndrome, 2010, 2010b
  overview of, 2009
  patellar tendinopathy, 2018–19
  plantar fasciitis, 2027–29
  repetitive motion injuries, 2010, 2010b
  rotator cuff tears, 2012–14
  shoulder dislocation, 2010–12
  sports injuries, 2010
  venous thromboembolism, 2042–43
Musculoskeletal tumors
  chondrosarcoma, 1994–98
  description of, 1994
  Ewing's sarcoma, 1994–98
  metastatic, 1998–99
  osteosarcoma, 1994–98
  primary bony, 1994–98
  soft tissue, 1994–98
Music, 396
Music-thanatology, 396
My Pyramid, 1598, 1599f
Myasthenia gravis, 1289–92
Mycophenolate mofetil, 1841, 1843t
Mycoplasma, 271t
Mycoplasma pneumoniae, 1056
Mycotic aneurysms, 889
Myectomy, 815
Myelography, 1164, 1950–51
Myelosuppression, chemotherapy-related, 421, 430, 958b, 968b
Myocardial contractility, 805
Myocardial infarction
  complications of, 791
  creatine kinase levels, 793
  definition of, 770
  idioventricular rhythm caused by, 859
  inflammation and, 273
  non-ST segment elevation, 791, 793–94
  pharmacologic agents for, 794–95
  ST segment elevation, 791–94
  treatment of, 794
Myocardial nuclear perfusion imaging, 763–65
Myocardial oxygen supply and demand, 775
Myocarditis, 820–21
Myocardium, 748
Myoclonic seizures, 1271
Myomectomy, 2111
Myometrium, 2060
Myopia, 1337
Myosin, 1938
Myotonia, 2066
Myringoplasty, 1366
Myringosclerosis, 1318
Myringotomy, 1365–66
Myxedema coma, 1895

N

N-Acetylcysteine, 1130
Nadir, 431
Nadolol, 924t
Nails
  anatomy of, 1477t, 1479
  clubbing of, 996–97
Naloxone hydrochloride, 472, 475
Nasal airways, 584
Nasal cannula, 1113
Nasal polyp, 1042, 1042f
Nasal sprays, 1024
Nasogastric intubation
  complications of, 1588
  contraindications, 1588
  dysphagia nutrition using, 1626
  equipment used in, 1587–88
  technique, 1589
  tubes, 1587
Nasopharynx, 979
National Center for Complementary and Alternative Medicine, 156, 246, 379, 477
National Center for Patient Safety, 549
National Comprehensive Cancer Network, 414
National Guideline Clearinghouse, 36
National Hospice Reimbursement Act, 146
National Institute of Nursing Research, 550
National Kidney Disease Education Program, 1842
National Labor Relations Act, 18
National Labor Relations Board, 18
National Quality Forum, 536
Native Americans
  biological variations in, 84t
  death beliefs, 147t
  folk medicine used by, 83t
  food preferences, 85t
Natural killer cells, 741, 1388
Nausea
  anticipatory, 434
  antiemetics for, 421, 434
  assessment of, 1572
  chemotherapy-induced, 420–21, 434, 968t
  definition of, 1575
  in hospice patients, 154, 163
  in palliative care patients, 154, 163
Neck, 995
Necrotizing fasciitis, 289
Nedocromil, 516
Needle biopsy
  of brain tumor, 1197
  description of, 413
Needleless access devices, 345b
Needlestick injuries, 277, 347
Negative feedback, 1850
Negative pressure ventilation, 586
Neglect, 132
Negligence
  definition of, 370
  proving of, 370–71
Neoadjuvant therapy, 419
Neoangiogenesis, 1479
Neoplasm, 405
Neostigmine, 1278t
Neovascularization, 1309
Nephrectomy
  definition of, 1794
  radical, 1797–98
  simple, 1819f
Nephrolithiasis, 1789
Nephrons, 1748, 1751, 1751f–1752f
Nephrosclerosis, 1795, 1795t
Nephrotic syndrome, 1784–87
Nephrotoxic agents, 1753, 1755b
Nervous system
  age-related changes, 1146
  anatomy and physiology of, 1137–46
  assessment of
    cerebellar function, 1156–57
    description of, 1410
    history-taking, 1147–48
    interview, 1148, 1150b–1151b
    mental status, 1149, 1151
    motor function, 1155
    physical examination, 1148–49, 1151–59
    reflex testing, 1158–59
    sensory system, 1157–58
  autonomic, 1145
  cells of, 1137–39
  central. *See* Central nervous system
  description of, 1136
  diagnostic tests
    carotid duplex studies, 1166–67
    cerebral angiography, 1162–63
    cerebrospinal fluid analysis, 1160t
    computed tomography, 1161
    description of, 1159
    digital subtraction angiography, 1163

electroencephalography, 1164–65
electromyography, 1165–66
evoked potentials, 1166t
functional magnetic resonance imaging, 1162, 1190
lumbar puncture, 1160
magnetic resonance angiography, 1162
magnetic resonance imaging, 1161–62
magnetic resonance spectroscopy, 1162
magnetoencephalography, 1165
myelography, 1164
positron emission tomography, 1163–64
radiographic studies, 1160–64
single-photon emission computed tomography, 1164
transcranial Doppler sonography, 1167
ultrasound, 1166–67
x-rays, 1161
endocrine system functioning affected by, 1850–51
parasympathetic, 1216
parasympathetic response, 1148t
peripheral, 1144–45
sympathetic response, 1148t
Neugarten, Bernice, 123
Neural tube defects, 213
Neuralgia, 1243
Neuroendocrine system response, 2205–6
Neurofibrillary tangles, 1286
Neurogenic shock, 1228–29, 2220–22
Neuroglia, 1138–39
Neuromuscular blockers, 597–98
Neurons, 1137–39
Neuropathic pain, 456–57, 458b–459b
Neuropathies
Bell's palsy, 1250–52
carpal tunnel syndrome, 1256–57
definition of, 1243
etiology of, 1243
Guillain-Barré syndrome. *See* Guillain-Barré syndrome
Ménière's disease, 1252–54
pathophysiology of, 1243–44
peripheral, 433, 1243
trigeminal neuralgia, 1243, 1247–50
Neuropeptides, 379
Neuroreceptor, 454
Neurotransmitters
characteristics of, 1138, 1138t
definition of, 379
small intestine affected by, 1649
Neurovascular assessment, 1943
Neutralization, by antibodies, 1390
Neutropenia
biological response modifiers for, 432
in cancer patients, 431–32
definition of, 431
description of, 948–49, 1388
drug-induced, 1411–12
febrile, 432
infectious causes of, 1412b
Neutrophils
description of, 266, 736f, 1388
stem cell origin of, 740
Nicotinamide adenine dinucleotide, 739
Nicotinamide adenine dinucleotide phosphate, 739
Nicotine. *See also* Smoking
circulatory effects of, 643
physiologic effects of, 909–10
withdrawal symptoms from, 920
Nicotinic acid, 514
Nifedipine, 924t
Night driving, 1310
Nightingale, Florence
description of, 3, 6, 610
disease studies by, 240–41
disease transmission writings, 281b
healing environment provided by nurses, 551
imagery therapy, 382
nursing as viewed by, 610
palliative care principles, 158
theory of nursing by, 10
Nipple
anatomy of, 2063
dimpling of, 2139
discharge from, 2141
disorders of, 2140–41
examination of, 2139
fissures of, 2141
supernumerary, 2137
Nisoldipine, 924t
Nitrates
coronary artery disease treated with, 781, 782t
heart failure treated with, 810
indications for, 502
mechanism of action, 781
pharmacokinetics of, 502–3
side effects of, 503, 781
Nitroglycerin, 502–3, 782t
Nits, 1514
Nociceptive pain, 456
Nociceptor, 451
Nocturia, 1771
Nodules, 1486b, 1488f
Noise, 1368–70
Noncardiac chest pain, 1634–35
Noncontinent urinary diversions, 1802
Non-Hodgkin's lymphoma, 403t, 965b, 969–70, 2231
Noninflammatory diarrhea, 1576–77
Nonmaleficence, 97, 192t, 229t, 371
Nonnucleoside reverse transcriptase inhibitors, 1429, 1430b
Non-seminomas, 2173
Nonsmall cell lung cancer, 1079
Non-ST segment elevation myocardial infarction, 791, 793–94
Nonsteroidal anti-inflammatory drugs
angiotensin-converting enzyme inhibitors affected by, 511
chemopreventive uses of, 412
classification of, 471b
fever reduction using, 274
in older adults, 476
osteoarthritis treated with, 1958–59
pain management using, 157, 470
patellar tendinopathy managed using, 2019
rheumatoid arthritis treated with, 1439, 1440t
Nontoxic goiter, 1890
Nonulcer dyspepsia, 1635–38
Nonverbal communication, 74–75
Norepinephrine, 912, 1138, 1851t
Nose
allergy-related findings, 1409
anatomy of, 1018f
fractures of, 1041
hypertrophic turbinates, 1042
inspection of, 995
obstruction of, 1041–42
Nosebleeds. *See* Epistaxis
Nosocomial infections
definition of, 1779, 1815
infusion therapy-related, 340
urinary tract infections, 1767
Nuchal, 2258
Nuclear perfusion imaging
coronary artery disease evaluations, 779–80
description of, 763–65
Nucleoside reverse transcriptase inhibitors, 1429, 1430b
Nuremberg Code, 116–17
Nurse
adult care by, 138
aging workforce of, 126
altruism by, 9
critical care, 560–61
education of, 6
ethics-based role of, 100–102
hospice care, 146, 150
impaired, 20
in medical team, 4
palliative care, 146, 150
patient advocate role of, 101–2, 192
school, 259
self-awareness by, 88
Nurse case manager, 259b
Nurse-controlled analgesia, 346
Nursing
business approach to, 15
care delivery models for, 15–16
complementary and alternative therapies and, 396–97
criteria for, 10b
definition of, 10–11, 255
domains of, 11
emergency, 2236–37
future of, 261–62
transcultural, 84–85
in United States, 9–11
Nursing competencies, 551
Nursing diagnoses
for acromegaly, 1868
for acute coronary syndromes, 793–94
for acute renal failure, 1826
for allergies, 1452
for Alzheimer's disease, 1287
for amputation, 2045
for appendicitis, 1666
for asthma, 1122, 1457
for atherosclerosis, 881b
for bladder cancer, 1800
for breast cancer, 2151
for bronchiolectasis, 1073–74
for chronic obstructive pulmonary disease, 1107
for chronic renal failure, 1833
for coronary artery disease, 780
cultural competence and, 88
for Cushing's disease, 1870
for cystic fibrosis, 1129
for diabetes mellitus, 1908
for fibromyalgia, 1979
for fractures, 2033
for gastrointestinal obstruction, 1673
for glomerulonephritis, 1782
for Guillain-Barré syndrome, 1245
for gynecological malignancies, 2121
for headaches, 1264b
for health maintenance, 59
for heart failure, 808
for hepatitis, 1708
for hospice care, 155–56
for human immunodeficiency virus, 1428
for hypercalcemia, 323
for hyperkalemia, 320
for hypermagnesemia, 328
for hypernatremia, 317
for hyperphosphatemia, 325
for hypertension, 915–16
for hypertrophic cardiomyopathy, 814
for hypocalcemia, 321
for hypoglycemia, 1921
for hypokalemia, 318–19
for hypomagnesemia, 326
for hyponatremia, 315
for hypophosphatemia, 324
for inflammation, 273–75
for inflammatory bowel disorders, 1688
for interstitial cystitis, 1775
for liver transplantation, 1727
for lung cancer, 1079–80
for malnutrition, 1608
for multiple sclerosis, 1277
for obesity, 1613
for osteoarthritis, 1957–58
for Osteomyelitis, 1993
for osteoporosis, 1983–84
for Paget's disease, 1989
for pain, 467
for palliative care, 155–56
for Parkinson's disease, 1281
for perioperative period, 660
for pneumonia, 1059
for pneumothorax, 1084
for polycystic kidney disease, 1818
for portal hypertension, 1716
for prostate cancer, 2171
for pulmonary arterial hypertension, 1090
for pulmonary fungal infections, 1071
for renal cancer, 1797
for rheumatoid arthritis, 1437, 1438t
for shock, 2214t
for spinal cord tumors, 1241
for stomach cancer, 1643
for stroke, 1175
for teaching-learning process, 52
for thrombophlebitis, 894
for tuberculosis, 1066
for urinary incontinence, 1807
for urinary tract calculi, 1790
for urinary tract infections, 1771, 1773
Nursing education
description of, 11–12
genetics concepts included in, 235
Nursing Home Quality Initiative, 545
Nursing homes, 546b
Nursing models
adaptation model, 255–56
self-care theory, 257–58
systems model, 256–57
Nursing practice
education, 11–12
environment for, 17–20
family structure changes, 14
genetic, 235
globalization of, 12–13
health care agencies and, 550–53
informality of, 14
leadership, 11
risk-taking behaviors, 14
Nursing process
assessment, 50–51
cultural competence and, 86–89
intravenous therapy uses of, 356

Nutrition. *See also* Diet
in acute renal failure, 1830
for aging population, 188, 1615
for Alzheimer's disease patients, 1288
for amyotrophic lateral sclerosis patients, 1294
artificial, 113
assessments of, 181, 1607t
atherosclerosis and, 881–82
in Bell's palsy patients, 1251
for burn patients, 1549–51, 1560
in chronic obstructive pulmonary disease patients, 1110–11
for chronic renal failure, 1839
in critically ill patients, 564
in cystic fibrosis patients, 1129–30
in diabetes mellitus patients, 1910–12
drug interactions, 1601–2
dysphagia effects on, 1626
for fibromyalgia, 1979
in Graves' disease, 1886–87
health maintenance uses of, 62
for myasthenia gravis patients, 1291
for osteoarthritis, 1958
osteoporosis prevention and, 1984
in Parkinson's disease patients, 1282
postoperative, 724
in rheumatoid arthritis patients, 1439
screening of, 1607t, 1609t
therapeutic uses of, 391–94
tissue repair effects on, 275
wound healing affected by, 284, 288–89
Nutrition support
description of, 1602
enteral feedings
administration of, 1605
benefits of, 1603
for burn patients, 1550
definition of, 1602
formulas, 1603–4, 1604t
routes for, 1605, 1605f
tubes used in, 1605
gastrostomy feedings, 1605
parenteral nutrition. *See* Parenteral nutrition
Nutritionally adequate diet, 1598–1601
Nystagmus, 1152, 1306, 1324

O

Obesity
assessment of, 1612–13
body mass index calculations, 1612b
breast cancer and, 2148
cancer risks, 404
colorectal cancer and, 1678
coronary artery disease risks, 773
definition of, 773, 1612
diabetes mellitus and, 128, 1612
epidemiology of, 1612
esophageal cancer and, 1632
etiology of, 1612
fat cells, 909
hypertension and, 909
inflammatory response and, 273
morbid, 642
nursing diagnoses, 1613
outcomes, 1614
preoperative considerations, 641
prevalence of, 124
rates of, 124
recommendations for, 790t
stroke risks, 1173b
surgical treatment of, 1614
treatment of, 1613–14
upper body, 909
vaccine studies, 128
wound healing affected by, 284–85
Objective data, 176
Obstructions
gastrointestinal. *See* Gastrointestinal obstruction
laryngeal, 1042
nasal, 1041–42
Obstructive sleep apnea, 1038–40
Obturator muscle test, 1582f
Occipital lobe, 452f
Occlusive disease, 885–88
Occult fractures, 2038
Occult pneumothorax, 1083
Occupational allergic rhinitis, 1019t
Occupational stress, 254–55
Occupational therapist, 1207t
Octreotide, 1868
Ocular cancer, 1334–36
Ocular movement disorders
assessment of, 1326
description of, 1324
nystagmus, 1324
ocular muscle paralysis, 1324
strabismus, 1324
Oculomotor nerve, 1146f, 1147t, 1152–53, 1302
Odynophagia, 1044, 1573–74
Office of Alternative Medicine, 379
Off-pump coronary artery bypass grafting, 787
Ogilvie's syndrome, 1669
Ointments, 1498
OKT3, 1843t
Older adults. *See also* Elderly
age-related changes in, 476
atrial fibrillation in, 852
automobile driving by, 137
chronic illness in, 135–36
chronic pain in, 455
classification of, 369, 476
drug administration in, 490–91
ethnic, 136
frailty of, 135
health and illness trends in, 132–34
health assessment of, 187–88
health care services used by, 136–37
health conditions that affect, 134
health promotion for, 137–38
homeless, 135
hospitalization of, 253
hypothyroidism in, 1895
immune system changes in, 1402–3
infusion therapy in, 369
interactions with, 132
intravenous therapy in, 369
medication use by, 134b
needs of, 136
negative life events experienced by, 252
neglect of, 132
nonsteroidal anti-inflammatory drugs in, 476
nutrition for, 1615
patient care for, 663
perioperative considerations for, 661–63
postoperative care for, 717–18
profile of, 133b
pulmonary disease in, 662–63
pyelonephritis in, 1779
in rural areas, 135
skin care in, 369–70
stressors for, 132–33
subpopulations of, 134–36
venipuncture in, 369–70
visual impairments in, 1310
women, 135
Olfactory bulb, 1146f
Olfactory nerve, 1146f, 1147t, 1151–52
Oligodendrocytes, 1138
Oligomenorrhea, 2089
Oligospermia, 2078
Oliguria, 1782, 1826
Olmesartan, 924t
Omega-3 fatty acids, 392
Omnibus Budget Reconciliation Act, 104–5
Oncogenes, 219–20, 406
Oncogenesis, 406
Oncology therapy
chemotherapy. *See* Chemotherapy
description of, 366–67
radiation. *See* Radiation therapy
Oncotic pressure, 298, 1543
Ongoing assessment, 175–76
Onycholysis, 1973
Oocytes, 2064
Open biopsy, 2150–51
Operating room, 670
Operating room nurses, 656–58
Ophthalmopathy, 1887
Ophthalmoscope, 1306t
Ophthalmoscopic examination, 1306
Opioid analgesics
addiction concerns, 159–60
administration of, 159–60, 477, 710–11
agonist-antagonist, 474t
constipation caused by, 473
contraindications, 477
diverticulitis pain managed using, 1668
intramuscular administration of, 710–11
moderate, 474t
morphine, 157, 159–60, 474t
overdose of, 475
pain management using, 157–59, 471–72
physical dependence on, 471–72
preoperative use of, 640
respiratory depression caused by, 473
side effects of, 473, 475–76
tolerance to, 472
toxicity of, 475–76
withdrawal symptoms, 475
Opportunistic infections
fungal, 1069
HIV-related, 1426
pneumonia, 1056–57
Oppression, 71
Opsonization, 268, 1390
Optic atrophy, 1308
Optic disc, 1307f
Optic nerve, 1146f, 1147t, 1152, 1302
Oral airways, 583–84
Oral cancer, 1622
Oral cavity disorders
burning mouth syndrome, 1622
description of, 1620
dysphagia. *See* Dysphagia
etiology of, 1620
mouth pain, 1621–22
planning and implementation for, 1620–21
Oral cholecystography, 1701
Oral contraceptives, 2120
Oral glucose tolerance test, 1908
Oral hypoglycemic agents, 527–28
Oral ulcers, 1621t
Orchiectomy, 2175f
Orchiopexy, 2183
Orchitis, 2177–78
Organ donation
end-of-life care and, 113–14
ethical considerations, 685–86
Organ of Corti, 1352
Organ Procurement and Transplantation Network, 685
Organizational ethics, 100
Orgasm, 2068–69
Orgasmic disorders, 2128
Oropharyngeal dysphagia, 1574
Oropharynx, 979
Orphenadrine, 1283t
Orthostatic hypotension, 925
Osmolality, 296
Osmolarity, 296
Osmosis, 297, 297f
Osmotic diuretics
description of, 506–8
intracranial pressure lowering using, 582
Osmotic pressure, 297–98, 298f
Ossicles, 1312, 1351
Osteoarthritis
assessment of, 1957
bone spurs associated with, 1957
definition of, 1956
description of, 272
diagnostic tests, 1957
epidemiology of, 1956
etiology of, 1956
health care resources, 1959–60
nursing diagnoses, 1957–58
outcomes, 1960, 1962
pathophysiology of, 1956–57
primary, 1956
secondary, 1956
treatment of
nutrition, 1958
pharmacological, 1958–59
surgery, 1960
Osteoblasts, 1936
Osteoclasts, 1936
Osteocytes, 1936
Osteogenesis, 1935
Osteomalacia, 1985–87
Osteomyelitis, 1992–94
Osteon, 1936
Osteopenia, 1865, 1938
Osteoporosis
assessment of, 1982
bisphosphonates for, 1984
definition of, 1981
diagnostic tests, 1983
epidemiology of, 1981
etiology of, 1981
exercise for, 1985
family education about, 1984
fractures caused by, 460, 1982
health care resources, 1984
nursing diagnoses, 1983–84
nutritional considerations, 1984
outcomes, 1984
pathophysiology of, 1981–82
patient education about, 1984
pharmacological treatment of, 1984
predisposing factors, 1982t
risk assessments, 1982
selective estrogen receptor modulators for, 1984
skeletal anabolics for, 1984

spinal cord injury and, 1214
in spinal cord injury patients, 1234
treatment of, 1984–85
Osteosarcoma, 1994–98
Ostomy
creation of, 1684–85
definition of, 1684
ileostomy, 1684–85
sexual intimacy affected by, 438–39
Otalgia, 1313, 1356
Otitis externa
acute, 1318–19, 1319f
description of, 1374
serous, 1319
Otitis media
acute, 1362
bacterial causes of, 1359
definition of, 1359
diagnosis of, 1359
with effusion, 1363
hearing loss caused by, 1354
prevention of, 1363
recurrent, 1354
serous, 1409
treatment of, 1362, 1374
tympanic membrane perforations caused by, 1359
Otomycosis, 1318
Otorrhea, 1313
Otosclerosis, 1354, 1360, 1363
Otoscopic assessment, 1317–19, 1360, 1360f
Ototoxic medications, 1350–51
Outcome variables, 535
Ovarian agenesis, 2112–13
Ovarian cancer, 403t, 2120–22
Ovarian cysts, 2112, 2114
Ovaries, 2059, 2076
Overflow incontinence, 1807b
Overuse syndrome, 2010, 2010b
Overweight, 1612
Ovulation, 2059
Oxicams, 471b
Oxidation-reduction reaction, 738
Oximetry. *See* Pulse oximetry
Oxybutynin, 1278t
Oxycodone, 474t
Oxygen
delivery systems for, 1013
hemoglobin binding, 738–39, 984
myocardial supply and demand, 775
supplementation of, during postoperative period, 696–97
transport of, 983–84
Oxygen free radicals, 1184
Oxygen therapy
chronic obstructive pulmonary disease treated with, 1113–14
response to, 1115
sickle cell anemia treated with, 935
Oxygen toxicity, 599
Oxygenation assessments, 806
Oxygen-hemoglobin dissociation curve, 984–86
Oxyhemoglobin, 984
Oxyhemoglobin dissociation curve, 739
Oxytocin, 1851t, 2137

P

p53, 1677t
P wave, 841, 843–44
Pacemakers
definition of, 864
dual-chamber, 865
external, 865
interventions for, 865b
malfunction of, 866–67
mechanism of action, 864–65
permanent, 866
single-chamber, 865
transvenous, 865
types of, 865
Packed red blood cells, 363–64
PACU. *See* Postanesthesia care unit
Paget's disease
alkaline phosphatase tests, 1988
assessment of, 1988
bisphosphonates for, 1990, 1991t
definition of, 1987
diagnostic tests, 1988–89
epidemiology of, 1988
etiology of, 1988
exercise for, 1990
family education about, 1990–91
hypercalcemia caused by, 1990
nursing diagnoses, 1989
outcomes, 1991–92
pathophysiology of, 1988
patient education about, 1990–91
treatment of, 1989–90, 1991t
X-ray evaluations, 1988–89
Paget's mammary disease, 2143–44
Pain
abdominal, 1572, 1577, 1579t, 1656–58
acute
description of, 457, 464
management of, 468–69
acute abdomen, 1656–57
age-related influences, 455
appendicitis-related, 1665
assessment of. *See* Pain assessment
auricular, 1316
back, 458b, 460
cancer. *See* Cancer pain
chronic
coping with, 469
description of, 460–61
in elderly, 455
in critically ill patients, 565
definition of, 448
esophageal, 1627–28
fast, 453
gastrointestinal tract, 1634–35
gate control theory of, 449–50
gender influences, 455–56
idiopathic, 462
importance of, 448
intractable, 463–64, 475
mechanisms of, 453–54
menstrual, 2088
modulation of, 450, 454
mouth, 1621–22
neuropathic, 456–57, 458b–459b
nociceptive, 456
nursing diagnoses, 467
parietal, 1656
pathophysiology of, 450–53
pattern theory of, 449
perception of, 454
phantom, 458b
physical care for, 469–70
prolonged exposure to, 466
psychogenic, 458b
reassessment of, 464, 476
referred, 456, 457f, 458b, 1578, 1578f, 1584, 1656
reporting of, 466–67
responses to, 455–56
sexual intercourse-related, 2127
slow, 453
sociocultural influences, 455
somatic, 456, 1656
specificity theory of, 448
spinal cord tumor, 1240
theories of, 448–50
tonsillitis, 1035
transduction of, 450, 453
transmission of, 450, 453–54
undertreatment of, 159, 440, 466
visceral, 456, 459t, 1656
Pain assessment
barriers to, 465–67
description of, 153b, 753, 754b
elements of, 464–65
inadequate, 466
tools for, 464–65
Pain history, 464
Pain management
acupuncture for, 386
in acute coronary syndromes, 794
acute pain, 468–69
barriers to, 160b, 465–67
in burn patients, 1542–43, 1551–52
cancer-related pain, 440, 459b
in children, 661
complementary and alternative therapies, 477–78
conventional measures for, 467–68
description of, 367
discharge teaching about, 723
ethical issues of, 109–10
in Guillain-Barré syndrome, 1247
in hospice patients, 152–53, 156–59
Joint Commission for the Accreditation of Healthcare Organizations standards, 109, 159, 367, 467–68
mind-body therapies using, 477
myths and misconceptions regarding, 158–59
nonpharmacological methods, 162, 711
nursing education about, 466
opioids for. *See* Opioid(s)
in palliative care patients, 152–53
in pediatric patients, 661
in peripheral nerve injuries, 1255
pharmacologic methods
adjuvant medications, 472, 474t
aspirin, 470
nonopioid analgesics, 470, 474t
nonsteroidal anti-inflammatory drugs, 470
opioid analgesics. *See* Opioid(s)
postoperative
in children, 661
description of, 611, 701–2, 710
principles of, 156–57, 467
World Health Organization approach, 157–58
Pain scales, 701
Pain threshold, 454–55
Pain tolerance, 454
PAINAID Scale, 465
Palliation, 414
Palliative care
advanced practice nurses in, 152
definition of, 110, 144
ethical considerations, 110–11
goal of, 144
hospice care vs., 144
interdisciplinary team who deliver, 144–45, 150, 152
mouth care, 162–63, 166
nurses involved in, 146, 150
nursing diagnoses, 155–56
spiritual support in, 164–65
World Health Organization definition of, 144
Pallidotomy, 1284t
Pallor, 1308
Palmomental reflex, 1159t
Palpation
of abdomen, 1579f, 1582
definition of, 183
of external ear, 1316
of heart, 758f
musculoskeletal system assessments, 1943
of precordium, 757
respiratory system, 997–98
technique of, 183–84, 184f
Palpebral conjunctiva, 1305
pamidronate, 1991t
Pancreas
anatomy of, 1570–71, 1699, 1856
assessment of, 1583
cells of, 1699
hormones produced by, 1851t
insulin production by, 1905
Pancreatectomy, 1740f
Pancreatic cancer, 403t
Pancreatitis
acute, 1736–38
chronic, 1738–41
Pancuronium, 597t
Panhypopituitarism, 1873
Panic disorder, 1635
Panlobar emphysema, 1102
Pap tests, 2076–77, 2080, 2104
Papillary muscle dysfunction, 791
Papillary reflex, 1302
Papilledema, 1342, 1967
Papules, 1486b, 1488f
Paracentesis, 1586–87, 1714
Para-chlorobenzoic acid derivatives, 471b
Paralysis
assessment of, 1942
neuromuscular blockers for, 597–98
Paramyxovirus, 1988
Paraphimosis, 2184–85
Paraplegia
definition of, 1218
wheelchair use after, 1233–34
Parasitic infestations
conjunctivitis caused by, 1340
in homeless persons, 81t
Parasympathetic nervous system, 1216
Parathyroid adenomas, 1896
Parathyroidectomy, 1897
Paraurethral glands, 2063
Parenteral nutrition
definition of, 1606
formulas, 1606
peripheral, 362, 362t
total
advantages and disadvantages of, 361t
definition of, 360
metabolic complications of, 362
nursing considerations for, 360b
patient selection for, 361–62
protein in, 361
Paresthesia, 1157, 1240
Parietal lobe, 452f, 1142

Parietal pain, 1656
Parity, 2060
Parkinson's disease
assessment of, 1280–81
definition of, 1279
diagnostic tests, 1281
epidemiology of, 1280
etiology of, 1280
nursing diagnoses, 1281
nutritional considerations, 1282
outcomes, 1284
pathophysiology of, 1280
perioperative considerations, 663
treatment of
overview of, 1281–82
pharmacological, 1282, 1283t
surgical, 1284t
tremor associated with, 1280
Paroxysmal nocturnal dyspnea, 517
Partial laryngectomy, 1048
Partial seizures, 222, 1270t, 1272
Partial thromboplastin time, 747t
Partial-thickness wounds, 282
Passive euthanasia, 115
Passive immunization, 1400
Past medical history, 632
Pasteur, Louis, 240
Patau syndrome, 200
Patellar tendinopathy, 2018–19
Pathological reflexes, 1159, 1159t
Patient(s)
decisional capacity of, 106
empowerment of, 63, 259, 261
knowledge base of, 52
motivation of, 56
nurse's role as advocate of, 101–2, 192
perceptions of, 56
previous experience of, 52
rights of, 192
strengths of, 52
teaching of, 488–89
Patient education
acute coronary syndromes, 796–97
acute renal failure, 1831–32
amputation, 2045–46
aneurysms, 892
angina pectoris, 781
asthma, 1124, 1126
atherosclerosis, 883–84
bronchiolectasis, 1075
burns, 1544–45, 1554–55, 1560–61
carpal tunnel syndrome, 2018
chronic obstructive pulmonary disease, 1115–16
fibromyalgia, 1980
fractures, 2034–35
glomerulonephritis, 1783–84
gynecological infections, 2109
gynecological malignancies, 2123
hypertension, 925
menstrual disorders, 2100
mitral valve prolapse, 823–24
nosebleeds, 1041
osteoporosis, 1984
osteosarcoma, 1997–98
outcomes, 1069
Paget's disease, 1990–91
peripheral arterial occlusive disease, 888
pneumothorax, 1084–85
polycystic kidney disease, 1819
postoperative care, 719–25
purposes of, 44
surgery, 626
thrombophlebitis, 895–96
topics for, 44t
tuberculosis, 1069
urinary diversion, 1803
varicose veins, 902
wound care, 722–23
Patient positioning
increased intracranial pressure prevented by, 582
intraoperative, 683
in postanesthesia care unit, 698–99
postoperative, 698–99
safety in, 683
Patient Self Determination Act, 104, 134, 151, 193
Patient-controlled analgesia
description of, 345–46, 357–58, 473, 475
postoperative uses, 710
surgical uses of, 611
Patient's Bill of Rights, 48, 100, 488, 627
Patriarchal family structure, 78
Pattern reversal evoked potentials, 1166t
Pattern theory, 449
Pavlov, Ivan, 45t
Peak drug level, 497
Peak expiratory flow, 1122
Peak flow meter, 1123f
Pectoral myositis, 1003
Pectus carinatum, 756t, 994f
Pectus excavatum, 756t, 994f, 994–95
Pediatric patients. *See* Children
Pediculosis, 1514–15
Pedigrees, 235
Pelvic examination, 2114, 2114f
Pelvic inflammatory disease, 2101, 2105
Pelvic relaxation, 2110–11
Pemphigus, 1515
Penetrating trauma
ocular, 1334
renal, 1792
Penicillin G, 1033
Penicillins
administration of, 495b
adverse effects of, 494
extended-spectrum, 493
glomerulonephritis treated with, 1783
indications for, 493
laboratory monitoring of, 494
mechanism of action, 492–93
nursing management for, 494–95
pharmacodynamics of, 493–94
pharmacokinetics of, 493
side effects of, 494
urinary tract infections treated with, 1772b
Penile brachial index, 2080
Penile cancer, 2192–93
Penis
anatomy of, 2057
discharge from, 2075
ejaculation from, 2058–59, 2067–68
erection of, 2058, 2067
physical examination of, 2074
Penrose drain, 700t, 723
Pentosan polysulfate sodium, 1776, 1776b
Peppermint, 394t
Pepsin, 1570
Peptic duodenitis, 1641
Peptic ulcer disease, 523–24
Peptic-ulcer dyspepsia, 1638–41
Percent solutions, 352
Perception, 56
Percussion
of abdomen, 1580t, 1581–82
definition of, 184, 998
of kidneys, 1756f
notes obtained during, 999, 999t
of precordium, 758
respiratory system assessments, 998–99
sounds on, 184, 185t
technique for, 184, 184f, 998–99
Percutaneous catheters, 359
Percutaneous coronary interventions, 785–86
Percutaneous endoscopic gastrostomy, 1591, 1626
Percutaneous endoscopic jejunostomy, 1591
Percutaneous transluminal coronary angioplasty
coronary artery disease treated with, 785
peripheral arterial occlusive disease treated with, 887
Percutaneous umbilical blood sampling, 212t, 213
Perennial allergic rhinitis, 1019t
Perfusion, 983
Perfusion magnetic resonance imaging, 1190
Pergolide, 1283t
Perianal region, 1584
Pericardial cavity, 749
Pericardial friction rub, 760
Pericarditis
acute coronary syndromes and, 791
characteristics of, 821–22
chest pain caused by, 791
pain associated with, 755t
Pericardium, 748, 821
Perichondritis, 1316
Periductal mastitis, 2143
Perimenopause, 2090
Perindopril, 924t
Perinephric, 1842
Perineum, 2063
Perioperative, definition of, 608
Perioperative nurse
description of, 630, 653
knowledge and skills of, 654b
pediatric interactions, 660–61
role of, 654–55
Perioperative Nursing Data Set, 659–60
Perioperative period. *See also* Intraoperative period
ethics in, 684–86
geriatric considerations, 661–63
Health Insurance Portability and Accountability Act provisions, 695
nursing care, 659–63
nursing diagnoses, 660
for Parkinson disease, 663
pediatric considerations, 660–61
transportation of patient in, 686–87
Periorbital contusion, 1333
Periosteum, 1935
Peripheral arterial occlusive disease, 885–88
Peripheral blood stem cells, 425
Peripheral nerve injuries, 1254–66
Peripheral nervous system
description of, 450–51, 1144–45
dysfunction of. *See* Neuropathies
Peripheral neuropathy, 433, 1243, 1925–26
Peripheral parental nutrition, 362, 362t
Peripheral vascular dysfunction, 1927–28
Peripheral vascular resistance, 910
Peripherally acting sympatholytics, 509
Peristalsis, 1596, 1748
Peritoneal dialysis, 1837–39
Peritoneovenous shunt, 1715
Peritonitis, 1655–56, 1665
Peritonsillar abscess, 1036–37
Permanent pacing, 866
Permethrin cream, 1518
Persistent vegetative state, 1185t
Personal digital assistants, 882, 1911
Personal protective equipment, 276f, 671–72, 2244
Personal space, 76
Perspiration, 1383
Pesticides, 404
Pet therapy, 395–96
Petechiae, 745t, 819, 941
Peyronie's disease, 2190–92
pH, 987
Phacoemulsification, 1328
Phagocytic cells
description of, 1384
function tests for, 1413
Phagocytosis, 266, 269, 740, 1385, 2218
Phalen's maneuver, 2017, 2017f
Phantom pain/limb sensations, 458b, 2048
Pharmaceutic phase, 484
Pharmacodynamics, 487
Pharmacogenomics, 234–35
Pharmacokinetics
absorption, 484
aging effects, 491
bioavailability, 484
biotransformation, 485
definition of, 484
distribution, 484
metabolism, 485–86
Pharmacology, 483
Pharyngitis, acute, 1031–34
Pharynx
functions of, 1569–70
inspection of, 995
Phenobarbital, 521
Phenotype, 203
Phentermine and fenfluramine, 1088
Phenylacetic acids, 471b
Phenylephrine, 2197t
Phenytoin, 521
Pheochromocytoma, 1881–83
Philadelphia chromosome, 959
Philosophy, 44
Phimosis, 2184–85
Phlebitis
description of, 347
intravenous therapy as cause of, 348
Phlebostatic axis, 570, 572
Phlebostatic measurements, 570
Phlebotomy, 947
Phospholipids, 514
Phosphorus
deficiency of, 313t, 323–24
excess of, 314t, 324–26
normal levels of, 1759t
recommended dietary intake of, 314t
Photoaging, 1504
Photoallergic, 1504
Photochemotherapy, 1505–6
Photodynamic therapy
bladder cancer treated with, 1800
brain tumors treated with, 1204–5
Photorefractive keratotomy, 1338
Photosensitivity, tetracycline-related, 497
Phototherapy, 1504–6
Physiatrist, 1207t
Physical dependence
definition of, 159
on opioids, 471–72

Physical examination
auscultation, 184–85
baseline data collection, 183
care of patient after, 194
documentation, 194
genetic screening, 211
inspection. *See* Inspection
palpation. *See* Palpation
percussion. *See* Percussion
preparation for, 183
purpose of, 182–83
Physical inactivity
coronary artery disease risks, 773
recommendations for, 789t
Physical self-examinations, 62
Physical therapist, 1207t
Physician-assisted suicide, 150
Physicians, 4, 617–18
Physiological integrity, 255
Phytoestrogens, 391t
Phytonutrients, 391, 391t
Phytosterols, 391t
Pia mater, 1140
Pica, 937
Pigeon chest, 756t, 995
Piggyback infusions, 357
Pigmentation, 1476
Pink eye. *See* Conjunctivitis
Pink puffers, 1103
Pinna, 1311
Pituitary adenoma, 1869
Pituitary gland
anatomy of, 1146f
anterior
description of, 1852, 1853f–1854f
hypersecretion of, 1864–73
hyposecretion of, 1873–74
hormones produced by, 1851t
posterior
description of, 1852, 1854f
disorders of, 1874–76
Plague, 277–78
Plague, for biological warfare, 2251–52
Plantar fasciitis, 2027–29
Plantar flexion, 1944f
Plantar reflex, 1159t
Plaque brachytherapy, 1335
Plaque psoriasis, 1516
Plaques, 1486b, 1488f
Plasma, 735–36
Plasma exchange, 1432
Plasma expanders, 343t–344t, 2216t
Plasmapheresis
definition of, 1432
description of, 942
Guillain-Barré syndrome treated with, 1246
myasthenia gravis treated with, 1291
Plasmin, 743
Platelet(s)
activation of, 741
adenosine diphosphate release by, 743
clot formation functions of, 743
description of, 735, 740, 741
function of, 741–42
transfusion of, 364
Platelet disorders
overview of, 940
thrombocytopenia, 940–42
Platelet-activating factor, 267
Pleura, 981
Pleural cavity, 978
Pleural effusion, 442
Pleural friction rubs, 1001t, 1001–2
Pleurisy, 1003–4
Pleuritic chest pain, 1056
Pleuritic pain, 777
Plexus
brachial, 1254
definition of, 1254
Pneumatic antishock garments, 2215
Pneumatic retinopexy, 1331
Pneumococcus vaccination, 1061
Pneumocystis carinii pneumonia, 1057, 1426
Pneumocystosis pneumonia, 1069
Pneumocytes, 980–81
Pneumonia
assessment of, 1058
atypical, 1056
classification of, 1057
community acquired, 1057
community-acquired, 525
definition of, 1056
diagnostic tests, 1059
epidemiology of, 1056–57
high-risk indicators for, 1058b
in HIV-infected patients, 1062
hospital-acquired, 1057, 1103
lobar, 1057
mortality rates, 1058
nursing diagnoses, 1059
opportunistic, 1056–57
outcomes, 1063
pain associated with, 755t, 1004
pathophysiology of, 1057–58
patient education about, 1062–63
physical examination findings, 1058
planning and implementation for, 1059–63
Pneumocystis carinii, 1057, 1426
postoperative, 713
prevention of, 1059–60
in spinal cord injury patients, 1233
symptoms of, 1058
treatment of
antibiotics, 1061
evidence-based, 1060, 1061t
oxygen supplementation, 1060
pharmacological, 1060–62
postural drainage, 1060
vaccination, 1061
ventilator assisted, 1057
ventilator-associated, 593–94
viral, 1056
Pneumonia severity index, 1058
Pneumothorax
assessment of, 1083
chest tubes for, 1084–85
definition of, 1004, 1082
diagnostic tests, 1083–84
etiology of, 1082–83
fractured ribs as cause of, 1085
nursing diagnoses, 1084
occult, 1083
pain associated with, 755t, 1004
pathophysiology of, 1083
patient education about, 1084–85
risk factors for, 1082
spontaneous, 1082–83
tension, 1083
traumatic, 1083
treatment of, 1084
Pollens, 1021b
Polyarteritis, 1781
Polycystic cysts, 1755
Polycystic kidney disease
antibiotics for, 1819
assessment of, 1817
autosomal dominant, 1816
autosomal recessive, 1816–17
definition of, 1816
diagnostic tests, 1817
epidemiology of, 1816
genetic factors, 1816
nursing diagnoses, 1818
outcomes, 1819–20
pathophysiology of, 1817
patient education about, 1819
treatment of, 1818–19
Polycystic ovary syndrome, 2092–93, 2097, 2125
Polycythemia vera, 947–48, 1102
Polyethylene glycol, 1585
Polymyositis, 1974–76
Polyp
cervical, 2110, 2115
colonic, 1678
definition of, 1678
Polypectomy, 1682
Polypharmacy, 490
Polysomnography, 1009–10
Pons, 452f
Population genetics, 209–10
Populations
at-risk, 2230–31
trends in, 125–26
vulnerable. *See* Vulnerable populations
Porphyrin, 738
Portal hypertension, 1715–17
Ports, imported, 359
Positional genetics, 224
Positive end expiratory pressure, 588, 599, 2226
Positive pressure ventilation, 586, 1060
Positron emission tomography
bone tumor evaluations, 1998
coronary artery disease evaluations, 780
nervous system assessments, 1163–64
nursing management for, 1163–64
stroke evaluations, 1175t
Postanesthesia care unit (PACU)
abdominal assessments, 697–98
Aldrete system, 702, 703t
anesthesia recovery, 693–95
care units after, 704
critical care unit transfer, 704–5
description of, 692, 693
discharge from, 702–5
equipment in, 693
ergonomics in, 694
level of consciousness assessments, 698
orthopedic assessments, 702–3
oxygen supplementation, 697
pain management in, 701–2
patient positioning, 698–99
recovery in, 692–702
reports, 699
respiratory deficits in, 702
sterility of, 694
stretchers in, 694
thermoregulation in, 698
transfer from, 703–5
wound stabilization, 699–700
Postanesthesia care unit nurse, 661, 693
Posterior cord syndrome, 1220
Posterior cruciate ligament, 2020
Posterior inferior cerebral arteries, 1143
Posterior pituitary gland, 1852
Posterior tibialis, 1943
Posthitis, 2186–87
Postnecrotic cirrhosis, 1711–12
Postoperative, definition of, 608
Postoperative care
abdominal assessments, 697–98
ambulation, 715, 716b
artificial airways, 697
assessments, 695
blood pressure, 697
complications
anticipating of, 713–14
cardiovascular, 662, 713
compartment syndrome, 713–14
ectopy, 713
family education about, 715–16
neurosensory, 714
patient education about, 715–16
respiratory, 713
signs of, 724
treatment of, 714
types of, 696t
wound dehiscence, 714
cultural considerations, 717
discharge planning and teaching
description of, 719
electronic resources, 725–26
family teaching, 722–25
hygiene, 723–24
medications, 724
nutrition, 724
pain management, 723
patient teaching, 719–25
tips for, 720b
electronic resources, 725–26
family considerations, 715–17, 722–25
home planning, 718–29
hospitalization times, 701t
in-patients, 707–8
liver transplantation, 1728
monitoring during, 611
nursing care
bedding, 709
drains, 711
future of, 729–30
health care provider's orders, 712
inpatients, 707–8
pain management, 710–11
short-stay patients, 705–7
after transfer, 709–13
urinary elimination, 711
wound dressings, 711
older adults, 717–18
onset of, 691
oxygen supplementation, 696–97
pain management
in children, 661
description of, 611, 701–2
patient positioning, 698–99
physiological stabilization, 695–99
recovery
delayed, 726–27
long-term, 727–29
milestones in, 714–17
rehabilitative care, 727–28
remote monitoring, 725–26
respiratory stability, 695–96
rest, 723

short-stay patients, 705–7
transfers
description of, 708b
postanesthesia care unit, 703–5
trends in, 692
urinary elimination, 711
wounds
healing of, 705
stabilization of, 699–700
Poststreptococcal glomerulonephritis, 1780–82
Postsurgical unit, 704
Posttraumatic stress disorder
in burn patients, 1555
description of, 241, 247, 249–50, 251b, 2261–63
Postural drainage
for chronic obstructive pulmonary disease, 1109
for pneumonia, 1060
Potassium
characteristics of, 299t
deficiency of, 309t–310t, 317–19
excess of, 310t–311t, 319–21
functions of, 299t
intravenous, 318
normal levels of, 1759t
recommended dietary intake of, 314t
Potassium channel blockers, 505
Potassium iodide, 1889
Potassium permanganate, 1502
Potassium-sparing diuretics, 507–8, 923t
Potential learning needs, 51
Poverty
description of, 80
in older adults, 133b
Povidone-iodine solution, 346
Power of attorney for health care. *See* Durable power of attorney for health care
PR interval, 841, 844
Pramipexole, 1283t
Prana, 384
Prayer, 78, 390
Prazosin, 924t
Prealbumin, 598, 1607, 1607t
Precordial leads, 839
Precordium
definition of, 757
inspection of, 758
palpation of, 757
percussion of, 758
Prednisolone, 1843t
Prednisone, 1278t, 1776b, 1975
Preferred provider organizations, 533
Pregnancy
acute abdomen during, 1663
appendicitis during, 1663
breast changes during, 2063–64, 2137–38
cholecystitis during, 1663
folic acid supplementation during, 392
gestational diabetes, 219
smoking during, 125
surgical emergencies during, 1663
Pregnancy tests, 2082
Prehypertension, 913
Preimplantation genetic diagnosis, 208–9
Prekallikrein, 742t
Preload, 568–69, 752
Premature atrial complexes, 849–50
Premature junctional complexes, 852–53
Premature ventricular complexes, 856f, 856–57
Premature ventricular contractions, 504, 778f
Premenstrual dysphoric disorder, 2091–92, 2096–97
Premenstrual syndrome, 2091–92, 2096–97
Preoperative, definition of, 608
Preoperative period. *See also* Surgery
age-related considerations, 634–35
checklist for, 624f, 636–37
communication in, 632
complementary therapy evaluations, 613–14
cultural considerations, 633–34
electronic advances, 615–16
environmental safety, 635–36
family during
involvement, 626–27, 633–34
support for, 639–40
history-taking, 638
intake interview, 632–33
laboratory tests, 638
medications used in, 639
note-taking during, 631–32
NPO status during, 629
nurse-sensitive indicators, 635
patient safety, 636–39
patients
assessment of, 632–33
education of, 626–27
safety of, 636–39
personal hygiene, 627–28
pharmacology, 640
population-specific care
description of, 641
frail elderly, 641
guardianships, 641–42
obese patients, 641–42
smoking, 643
substance users, 643–44
procedures during, 626–35
remote assessment, 613
spirituality, 614
transfer strategies, 640–41
venipuncture during, 631
Preoperative preparation teams, 611
Presbyopia, 1310, 1338
Presbyphagia, 1623
Preschool child, 187
Pressure bags, 344
Pressure control ventilation, 587–88
Pressure support ventilation, 588
Pressure ulcers
description of, 285
prevention of, 287
Prevalence, 123
Preventive care
access to, 538
definition of, 537
financing of, 538
quality of, 539
Prialt. *See* Ziconotide
Priapism, 2195–97
Primary aldosteronism, 1880–83
Primary biliary cirrhosis, 1711–12, 1733–35
Primary care, 539
Primary ciliary dyskinesia, 1073
Primary intention, 282
Primary lymphoid follicles, 1392
Primary multiple organ dysfunction, 2227–28
Primary progressive multiple sclerosis, 1275
Primary research, 31
Primary sclerosing cholangitis, 1733
Primitive neuroectodermal tumors, 1196
Prinzmetal's variant angina, 775
Prion diseases, 672
Prions, 672
Probanthine, 1278t
Problem-focused coping, 244
Process variables, 535
Proctocolectomy, 1683–84
Proctosigmoidoscopy, 1586
Procyclidine, 1283t
Professional ethics, 99–100
Progesterone, 2089
Programmed instruction, 48
Progressive muscle relaxation, 381, 920–921
Progressive systemic sclerosis, 1444–45
Progressive-relapsing multiple sclerosis, 1275
Prolactin, 1851t, 2078, 2137
Prolactinomas, 1864
Prolastin, 1112, 1711
Proliferative retinopathy, 1923
Propionic acid derivatives, 471b
Propofol, 597t
Proportional assist ventilation, 589
Propranolol, 503, 924t
Proprioception, 451
Prostaglandin synthetase inhibitor, 470
Prostaglandins, 267
Prostate biopsy, 2079
Prostate cancer
androgen deprivation therapy for, 423
assessment of, 2169
biopsy evaluations, 2169–70
definition of, 2169
diagnostic tests, 2169–70
digital rectal examination assessments, 2169
epidemiology of, 2169
etiology of, 2169
grading system for, 2170, 2170t
hormonal therapies for, 423–24
incidence of, 403t
nursing diagnoses, 2171
pathophysiology of, 2169
prostate-specific antigen screening, 2169, 2170t
radiation therapy for, 2171
risk factors for, 410t
treatment of, 2171–72, 2172f
Prostate gland
anatomy of, 2056–57
fluid analysis, 2078
physical examination of, 2075
Prostate-specific antigen, 412, 2056, 2078–79, 2169, 2170t
Prostatitis, 2164–65
Prosthetic heart valves, 760
Protamine sulfate, 512
Protease inhibitors, 391t, 1430b
Protein
absorption of, 1650–51
for burn patients, 1550
for diabetes mellitus patients, 1910
digestion of, 1597
for peritoneal dialysis patients, 1839
in total parenteral nutrition, 361
Protein binding, 485
Protein C, 743
Protein electrophoresis, 1413
Protein S, 743
Proteinuria, 1784, 1821
Prothrombin time, 512, 747t, 945
Proton pump inhibitors, 470, 524–25, 1630, 1639
Proto-oncogenes, 220
Protozoa, 271t
Prozac. *See* Fluoxetine
Pruritus, 1457, 1515
Pseudoephedrine, 1022t
Pseudohermaphrodites, 203
Pseudomembranous colitis, 494
Psoriasis, 1500t, 1516–17
Psoriasis activity and severity index, 1516
Psoriatic arthritis, 1973–74
Psychic integrity, 255–56
Psychogenic pain, 458b
Psychologist, 1207t
Psychomotor domain, of learning, 46, 47t
Psychomotor learning, 721
Psychoneuroimmunoendocrinology, 245–47, 379
Psychosocial history, 182, 913
Ptosis, 1152, 1289
Public health care agencies, 539
Pulmonary angiography, 1005–6
Pulmonary arterial hypertension
assessment of, 1089
classification of, 1090
definition of, 1088
diagnostic tests, 1090
epidemiology of, 1089
etiology of, 1089
nursing diagnoses, 1090
outcomes, 1091–92
patient education about, 1091
pharmacological treatment of, 1091
planning and implementation for, 1090–91
risk factors for, 1089b
surgery for, 1091
treatment of, 1090–91
Pulmonary artery catheters
complications of, 574–75
description of, 568, 572
insertion of, 573
right ventricle displacement of, 575
types of, 572–73
Pulmonary artery pressure monitoring, 572–76
Pulmonary capillary wedge pressure, 574, 574t
Pulmonary circulation, 576f
Pulmonary edema, 809
Pulmonary embolism
description of, 2042–43
pain associated with, 755t, 1004
postoperative, 662
prevention of, 1246
signs of, 894
Pulmonary function testing
asthma evaluations, 1120, 1122
respiratory system evaluations, 1011–12
Pulmonary fungal infections
aspergillosis, 1070
assessment of, 1070–71
blastomycosis, 1069
coccidioidomycosis, 1069–70
definition of, 1069
diagnostic tests, 1071
histoplasmosis, 1070
nursing diagnoses, 1071
outcomes, 1072
pathophysiology of, 1070
planning and implementation for, 1071–72
treatment of, 1071–72
Pulmonary rehabilitation, 1107–9
Pulmonary vascular resistance, 567, 575–76
Pulmonic valve, 749–50
Pulse oximetry
description of, 592, 983, 1009
oxygen measurements using, 1113–14, 1190, 1584
Pulse pressure, 911
Pulse rating, 757b
Pulseless electrical activity, 860

Pulseless ventricular tachycardia, 871
Pulsus alternans, 792
Pulsus paradoxus, 925
Punnett Square, 203, 203f
Pupil examination, 1305
Purified-protein derivative, 1403–4
Purkinje fibers, 836–37
Purpura
  definition of, 745t
  immune thrombocytopenia, 940
  thrombotic thrombocytopenic, 940
Pursed-lip breathing, 1110
Purulent sputum, 1073
Pustular psoriasis, 1516
Pustules, 1486b, 1488f
Pyelonephritis, 1751, 1777–80, 1814–16
Pyrazolone derivatives, 471b
Pyrethrin, 1515
Pyridoxine, 1068t
Pyrosis, 1573

Q

Qi, 240
QRS complex, 841–42, 844
QRS interval, 841, 844–45
QT interval, 845
Quadrants of abdomen, 1580t–1581t
Quadriceps setting, 713
Quadriplegia
  description of, 1218
  wheelchair use after, 1233–34
Quality health care, 7–9
Quality of life
  chronic illness effects on, 250
  ethical decision making based on, 108
  prostate cancer effects on, 2167
Quinapril, 924t
Quinidine, 504

R

R wave, 842–43
Race
  definition of, 70, 189
  demographic changes, 72b
  health assessment considerations, 189–90
Racism, 71
Radial keratotomy, 1338
Radiation nephritis, 1825t
Radiation therapy
  bladder cancer treated with, 1800
  bone tumors treated with, 1999
  brain tumors treated with, 1206
  breast cancer treated with, 2152
  cancer treated with, 416–19
  colorectal cancer treated with, 1681–82
  definition of, 416
  enteritis caused by, 417–18
  external, 416–17
  fatigue caused by, 418, 439–40, 1198
  Hodgkin's disease treated with, 966–67
  internal, 416, 418
  intracavitary, 418
  laryngeal cancer treated with, 1045, 1047
  leukemia treated with, 951
  lung cancer treated with, 1081
  non-Hodgkin's lymphoma treated with, 970
  outcomes, 419
  principles of, 416–17
  prostate cancer treated with, 2171
  side effects of, 417
  skin reactions to, 418
  spinal cord tumors treated with, 1242–43
  stereotactic, 1206
Radical cystectomy, 1800
Radical neck dissection, 701t
Radical nephrectomy, 1797–98
Radiculopathy, 2013
Radioallergosorbent test, 1413
Radiofrequency ablation, 1724, 2154
Radioiodine therapy, 1889
Radiopharmaceuticals, 1007
Radon, 409
Rales. *See* Crackles
Raloxifene, 1984
Range of motion testing, 1944–45, 1946t
Rapamycin, 1841
Rapid antigen testing, 1033
Ratio-proportion method, of intravenous therapy calculations, 350–51
Raynaud's disease, 899–900
Raynaud's phenomenon, 899–900
Reactive arthritis, 1970, 1973
Readiness to learn, 51–52
Rebound hypertension, 925
Rebound tenderness, 1581, 1581f, 1655
Receptive aphasia, 1200
Recessive trait, 199
Recombinant DNA, 1432
Recombinant plasminogen activators, 794
Recommended dietary allowances, 1598
Rectal cancer. *See* Colorectal cancer
Rectocele, 2111, 2114
Rectum, 1571
Red blood cells. *See* Erythrocyte(s)
Red reflex, 1307–8
Reduced penetrance, 222
Reduction mammoplasty, 2146
Reed-Sternberg cells, 965
Reentry, 846
Referred pain, 456, 457f, 458b, 1578, 1578f, 1584, 1656
Reflex arcs, 451f
Reflex erection, 1237
Reflex testing, 1158–59
Reflexology, 389–90
Refractive errors, 1337–38
Refractory ascites, 1713
Refractory period, 837
Regional anesthesia, 678t
Registered nurse first assistant, 658
Registered nurses
  education of, 4
  staffing ratio laws, 5
Registered Nurses Association of Ontario, 37
Regurgitation, 1575
Regurgitation, valvular
  aortic, 827–28
  mitral, 824–25
  pathophysiology of, 822
Rehabilitation
  after brain tumor treatment, 1206–7, 1207t
  burn wound. *See* Burn(s), rehabilitation phase
  cardiac, 796–97
  postoperative, 727–28
  pulmonary, 1107–9
  spinal cord injury, 1231–35
  team members involved in, 1206–7, 1207t
Rehabilitation engineer, 1207t
Rehabilitation nurse, 1207t
Reiki, 385–86
Reiter's syndrome, 1970
Relapsing-remitting multiple sclerosis, 1275
Relative hypovolemia, 2212
Relaxation, 380–81
Relaxation response, 381, 477
Religious faith, 615
Remicade, 1440t
Remodeling of bone, 1937
Remote monitoring, 725–26
Renal angiography, 1761t
Renal artery
  description of, 1753
  stenosis of, 1795, 1795t, 1825t
Renal biopsy
  description of, 1760–61, 1762b
  glomerulonephritis evaluations, 1783
Renal cancer
  assessment of, 1796
  diagnostic tests, 1796–97
  epidemiology of, 1795–96
  etiology of, 1796b
  genetic factors, 1796
  incidence of, 403t
  nursing diagnoses, 1797
  outcomes, 1798
  pathophysiology of, 1796
  surgical treatment of, 1797–98
  treatment of, 1797–98
Renal cell carcinoma, 1795–96
Renal colic, 1790–91
Renal failure
  acute
    alterations in, 1828t
    assessment of, 1826–27
    collaborative treatment of, 1827, 1829
    continuous renal replacement therapy, 1827, 1827b
    definition of, 1824
    diagnostic tests, 1826
    epidemiology of, 1824
    etiology of, 1824, 1825t
    evidence-based care, 1829–30
    family education about, 1831–32
    hypervolemia in, 1829
    intrarenal causes of, 1826
    nursing diagnoses, 1826
    nutritional considerations, 1830
    outcomes, 1832
    pathophysiology of, 1826
    patient education about, 1831–32
    postrenal causes of, 1826
    prerenal causes of, 1826
    surgical treatment of, 1831
  chronic
    assessment of, 1834t
    clinical manifestations of, 1834t
    collaborative management of, 1835, 1836b
    definition of, 1832
    diagnostic tests, 1833
    epidemiology of, 1832
    etiology of, 1833
    hemodialysis for, 1836–37
    nursing diagnoses, 1833
    nutrition for, 1839
    pathophysiology of, 1833
    peritoneal dialysis for, 1837–39
    pharmacological treatment of, 1835, 1836b
    refusal of treatment, 1835
    renal transplantation for. *See* Renal transplantation
    stages of, 1832t
    treatment of, 1834–43
Renal insufficiency, 962
Renal parenchyma, 1748
Renal transplantation
  allogeneic, 1840
  allograft, 1840
  complications of, 1841–42
  description of, 1839–40
  donors, 1841
  drug therapy after, 1843t
  health care resources for, 1842
  nursing management for, 1842b
  outcomes, 1842–44
  technique for, 1841, 1842f
  xenogeneic, 1840
Renal trauma, 1792–95
Renal tuberculosis, 1787–88
Renal tubules, 1751–53
Renal vascular disorders, 1795, 1795t
Renal vein thrombosis, 1795, 1795t
Renin
  angiotensin II production stimulated by, 509
  definition of, 2206
  description of, 301
  functions of, 912
Renin-angiotensin system, 509, 1753–54
Renin-angiotensin-aldosterone system, 301, 911, 1717
Repetitive motion injuries, 2010, 2010b
Repolarization, 837
Reproductive history, 211
Rescue breathing, 867–68
Research
  ethics in, 116–17
  institutional review board for, 117
Research utilization, 25
Reserpine, 923t
Residual volume, 1003
Resilience, 247–48
Resonance, 185t
Respiration
  physiology of, 982–90
  regulation of, 982
Respiratory acidosis, 329–31, 988f
Respiratory agents
  administration of, 516
  bronchodilators, 517–19
  dry powder inhalers, 516
  inhaled corticosteroids, 519–20
  metered dose inhalers for, 516, 516f
Respiratory alkalosis, 330t, 332
Respiratory distress
  acute. *See* Acute respiratory distress syndrome
  signs of, 997
Respiratory excursion, 997
Respiratory muscles
  accessory, 975–76
  age-related changes, 1003
Respiratory system
  age-related changes in, 993, 1002–4, 1402t
  allergy-related findings, 1410
  anatomy of, 975–82
  assessment of
    in allergy patients, 1410
    auscultation, 999–1002
    chest pain, 991–92
    cough, 990
    in elderly, 992–93
    history-taking, 990–93
    inspection. *See* Respiratory system, inspection of
    palpation, 997–98

percussion, 998–99
sputum, 990–91, 991t
defense mechanisms of, 981–82
diagnostic tests
bronchoalveolar lavage, 1010–11
bronchoscopy, 1010
capnography, 1009
chest x-rays, 1006
computed tomography, 1006–8
laboratory tests, 1004–5
lung biopsy, 1011
oximetry, 1009
polysomnography, 1009–10
positron emission tomography, 1008–9
pulmonary angiography, 1005–6
pulmonary function testing, 1011–12
thoracentesis, 1012
thoracoscopy, 1012
transbronchial needle aspiration, 1011
ventilation-perfusion scan, 1008
exercise-related adjustments, 989
high altitude adjustments, 990
hypoxia-related adjustments, 989–90
inspection of
breathing. *See* Breathing
clubbing, 996–97
mouth, 995
skeletal deformities, 994–95
laboratory tests
arterial blood gas sampling, 1004
PaO_2/FiO_2 ratio, 1005
sputum studies, 1005
lower respiratory tract, 980–81
musculature of, 981
oxygen delivery systems, 1013
pulmonary mechanics, 981
upper respiratory tract, 979, 980f
Resting energy expenditure, 1600
Resting tremor, 1280
Restorative care agencies, 543–44
Restrictive cardiomyopathy, 817–18
Restrictive lung disease, 516, 587, 1063–64
Retained objects, during surgery, 680–81
Reticulocyte, 736
Reticulocyte count, 736, 747t
Reticuloendothelial system, 267, 739
Retina
anatomy of, 1302
assessment of, 1307–9, 1331f
color variations of, 1308t
detachment of, 1309, 1330–32
Retinal hemorrhages, 1309
Retinitis pigmentosa, 1343–44
Retinoids, 1116
Retinol binding protein, 1607, 1607t
Retinopexy, 1331
Retirement, 134
Retrograde ejaculation, 2078
Retroperitoneal space, 1747
Retropubic prostatectomy, 701t
Review of systems, 185, 633, 1484
Reye's syndrome, 470
Rh factor, 363
Rhabdomyolysis, 1823–24, 2259–60
Rheumatoid arthritis
assessment of, 1435–36
clinical manifestations of, 1435
cytokines associated with, 1435
description of, 272, 1405, 1405f
diagnostic criteria for, 1437b
diagnostic tests, 1437
epidemiology of, 1434
etiology of, 1434
juvenile, 1436–37
nursing diagnoses, 1437, 1438t
nutritional considerations, 1439
pathophysiology of, 1434–35
progression of, 1439
treatment of
COX-2 inhibitors, 1439, 1440t
goals, 1439
nonsteroidal anti-inflammatory drugs, 1439, 1440t
overview of, 1437–39
pharmacological, 1439–41, 1440t
surgery, 1441
Rheumatoid factor, 1413, 1434–35
Rhinitis
allergic. *See* Allergic rhinitis
definition of, 519, 1018
nonallergic, 1018
viral, 1024–25
Rhinitis medicamentosa, 1025
Rhinorrhea, 1018, 1268
Rhonchi, 1001, 1001t
Ribs
anatomy of, 975
floating, 975
fracture of, 1085–87
Rickettsia, 271t
Rifampin, 1068t
Right atrial pressure, 572–74
Right atrium, 749
Right to die, 113–14
Right ventricle, 574f, 749
Rights-based ethics, 98
Right-sided heart failure. *See also* Cor pulmonale
clinical manifestations of, 808b
definition of, 805
symptoms of, 807t
Rigidity
cogwheel, 1281
description of, 1155
in Parkinson's disease, 1280–81
Rigors, 2250
Rilutek, 1296
Ringer's Lactate solution, 343t
Rinne test, 1154, 1315, 1315f, 1361, 1361f
Risedronate, 1991t
Risk-taking behaviors, 14
Rituxan, 1440t, 1441
Rods, 1302
Role-playing, 47–48
Rolfing, 389
Romberg's test, 1156–57
Rooting reflex, 1159t
Ropinirole, 1283t
Rosacea, 1517
Rosenbaum near vision chart, 1304
Rotator cuff tears, 2012–14
Roth's spots, 819, 1309
Roux-en-Y gastric bypass, 1614
Rovsing's sign, 1659, 1665b
Rubriblast, 736
Rule of nines, 1537, 1538f
Rural hospitals, 540

S

Saccular aneurysm, 889, 889f
Sacroiliitis, 1970
Sacrum, 1140f
Safety
environmental, 635–36
intraoperative, 686–87
patient, 636–39
in patient positioning, 683
preoperative, 636–39
Safety cannulas, 347
Sage, 394t
Salicylates, 471b
Saline infusion sonohysterography, 2083
Saliva, 1569, 1596
Salmeterol, 1112
Salpingo-oophorectomy, 2099
Salty taste, 1153
Sanitization, 667t
Sarcoma
chemotherapy for, 1996, 1997t
chondrosarcoma, 1994–98
Ewing's, 1994–98
Kaposi's, 1426f
osteosarcoma, 1994–98
Sarcomere, 1938
Sarcopenia, 1623
Sarcoplasm, 1938
Sarcoplasmic reticulum, 1938
Sarcoptes scabiei, 1517
Scabies, 1517–18
Scald burns, 1544
Scales, 1489f
Scalp, 1139, 1139f
Scar, 1489f
Schatzki's ring, 1574
Schistocytes, 943
Schizophrenia, 220
Schlemm's canal, 1302
School nurse, 259
School-age child, 187
Schwann cells, 1226
Schwannomas, 1196
Schwartze's sign, 1363
Science of research synthesis, 33
Sclera, 1302
Scleral buckle, 1331
Scleroderma, 1444–45
Sclerotherapy, 1716, 2179–80
Scoliometer, 2000f
Scoliosis, 994, 2000–2002
Scratch test, 1416
Scrotal masses, 2075
Scrub clothes, 673
Scrub nurse, 657b, 657–58
Scrub technique, 673
Seasonal allergic rhinitis, 1019t
Sebaceous glands, 1477t, 1478–79
Sebum, 1479
Secondary care agencies, 540–41
Secondary intention, 282, 711
Secondary lymphoid follicles, 1392
Secondary multiple organ dysfunction, 2228–30
Secondary polycythemia, 948
Secondary progressive multiple sclerosis, 1275
Second-degree atrioventricular heart block, 854–55
Secretin testing, 1587
Sedation
conscious, 677
deep, 677
definition of, 677
description of, 368
of increased intracranial pressure patients, 583
minimal, 677
response to, 678
Seizures
absence, 222, 521, 1271
assessment of, 1269–72
atonic, 1271
clonic, 1271
definition of, 1269
description of, 520
epidemiology of, 1269
etiology of, 1269, 1269t
febrile, 223
generalized, 222, 1270t, 1271
myoclonic, 1271
outcomes, 1273
partial, 1270t, 1272
pathophysiology of, 1269, 1270b
patient safety during, 523
phases of, 1269–70
surgical treatment of, 1274t
tonic-clonic, 521, 1271
treatment of, 1272–73, 1273t
Selective estrogen receptor modulators, 423, 1984
Selective serotonin reuptake inhibitors
menstrual disorders treated with, 2098
neuropathic pain treated with, 472
Selegiline, 1283t
Self Determination Act, 104, 134, 151, 193
Self-care theory, 257–58
Self-concept, 182
Self-contract, 260
Self-efficacy
coping and, 245
definition of, 52, 245
Self-examinations
breast, 2075, 2139, 2140f
description of, 62
Self-image, 1484, 1555, 1559
Self-monitoring of blood glucose, 1909–10
Selye, Hans, 241–42
Semen
analysis of, 2078
anatomy of, 2058
Semicircular canals, 1312
Semilunar valves, 822
Seminal vesicles, 2056
Sensation testing, 1157
Sensorineural hearing loss, 1355–56
Sensory receptors, 1145
Sensory systems
function assessments of, 1157–58
history-taking, 181–82
Sensory-impaired patients, 54
Sentinel events, 552
Sentinel lymph node biopsy, 1523, 2154–55
Sepsis, 348, 2223
Septic shock, 442, 2212b, 2222–24
Sequela, 817
Semipermeable membranes, 296–97
Serotonin, 1138
Serous otitis externa, 1319
Serpiginous lesions, 1490b
Sertoli cells, 2056
Serum, 746
Serum cardiac markers, 793
Serum creatinine, 1759t
Serum electrophoresis with immunofixation, 962–63
Serum glutamic oxaloacetic transaminase, 1699–1700
Serum sickness, 1470–71
Serum transferrin, 1607, 1607t

Severe acute respiratory syndrome, for biological warfare, 2255–57
Sex roles, 64
Sexual abuse and assault, 2073–74
Sexual arousal disorder, 2127–28, 2130
Sexual desires, 2065–66
Sexual dysfunction
  alternative therapies for, 2130
  arousal disorders, 2127–28, 2130
  assessment of, 2127
  cancer treatment-related, 438–39
  causes of, 2127–28
  definition of, 2069, 2127
  diagnostic tests, 2127–29
  dyspareunia, 2127
  epidemiology of, 2127
  nursing diagnoses, 2129
  orgasmic disorders, 2127
  outcomes, 2131
  pain disorders, 2127
  pharmacological treatment of, 2129, 2130t
  psychological issues, 2070
  substance-induced, 2069–70
  treatment for, 2129–30
  vaginismus, 2127, 2130
  vulvar vestibulitis syndrome, 2127, 2129
Sexual intimacy, 2069
Sexual response
  definition of, 2065–66
  female, 2068–69
  male, 2066–68
Sexuality
  assessment of, 2070–77
  cancer treatment effects on, 438–39
  description of, 64
  health history of, 2071, 2072b
  history-taking, 182
  intimate partner violence, 2071–73
  medical history of, 2071
  in spinal cord injury patients, 1236–37
Sexually transmitted diseases
  assessment of, 2106
  chlamydia, 2103, 2106
  definition of, 2102
  description of, 2070–71, 2080
  diagnostic tests, 2106
  epidemiology of, 2102
  gonorrhea, 2103, 2106
  herpes simplex virus, 2103
  human papillomavirus, 2104–5
  prevention of, 2083
  screening of, 2083–84
  syphilis, 2103
  treatment of, 2107
Shaman, 378
Shamanism, 378, 390–91
Sharps
  counts of, during surgery, 680
  disposal of, 278f
Shiatsu, 389
Shingles. *See* Herpes zoster
Shock
  anaphylactic, 494, 1462b, 2218–20
  assessment of, 2211b
  cardiogenic, 2215–18
  diagnosis of, 2210b
  hypovolemic. *See* Hypovolemic shock
  neurogenic, 1228–29, 2220–22
  nursing diagnoses, 2214t
  septic, 442, 2212b, 2222–24
Shock syndrome, 2208–10, 2213b
Short stay surgery
  description of, 612–13
  nursing care after, 705–7
Shoulder
  dislocation of, 2010–12
  range of motion for, 1946t
  rotator cuff tears, 2012–14
Shunt
  Denver peritoneovenous, 1715
  distal splenorenal, 1716
  increased intracranial pressure treated with, 1205
  LeVeen peritoneovenous, 1715
  transjugular intrahepatic portosystemic, 1716
Shunting
  definition of, 983
  examples of, 983
Sickle cell anemia, 225–26, 934–36, 1173t
Sickle cell crises, 935
Side effects, 488
Sigmoid colectomy, 701t
Sign language, 1371
Sildenafil, 1237, 2058, 2194
Silver sulfadiazine, 1551
Simple mastectomy, 2156
Single-photon emission computed tomography, 1007, 1164
Sinoatrial node, 836
Sinus arrest, 849
Sinus arrhythmia, 848–49
Sinus bradycardia
  definition of, 504
  description of, 847f, 847–48
  management of, 871–72
Sinus exit block, 849
Sinus rhythms
  description of, 846–47
  normal, 847, 847f
Sinus tachycardia, 504, 848, 848f
Sinusitis
  acute
    antibiotics for, 1027–28
    assessment of, 1026
    complications of, 1026
    decongestants for, 1028
    description of, 1025
    diagnostic tests, 1026–27
    epidemiology of, 1025
    etiology of, 1025
    nursing diagnoses, 1027
    outcomes, 1029
    pathophysiology of, 1025–26
    population-based care, 1028
    symptoms of, 1026t
    treatment of, 1027–28
  chronic, 1029–31
Sinusoids, 1696
Sirolimus, 1843t
Sjögren's disease, 1409, 1441
Skeletal anabolics, 1984
Skeletal muscle cells, 405
Skeletal muscles, 1938–40
Skeleton
  aging effects on, 1938
  anatomy of, 1935–38
Skene's glands, 2063, 2101–2
Skin
  in adolescents, 1481
  age-related changes, 1402t, 1403, 1481–82
  anatomy of, 1476f, 1476–81
  assessment of, 1409, 1483–89
  barrier functions of, 1383
  cardiovascular system evaluations and, 756–57
  color assessments, 756–57
  cyanosis of, 756
  dermis, 1477t, 1479, 1482
  diagnostic tests, 1489–90
  edema, 1485
  epidermis. *See* Epidermis
  excretory functions of, 1479
  functions of, 340, 1475, 1477t
  healing of, 1480
  health care team for, 1490
  hematological problems and, 745t
  homeostatic functions of, 1479
  moisture of, 1485
  nursing diagnoses, 1490
  odor of, 1485–86
  peripheral arterial occlusive disease findings, 885
  protective functions of, 1479
  psychosocial functions of, 1480
  radiation therapy effects on, 418
  sensory perception functions of, 1480
  structures of, 1477t
  subcutaneous tissue of, 1479
  sun-damaged, 1504, 1505t
  synthetic substitutes for, 1552
  temperature of, 1485
  texture of, 1485
  thermoregulation functions of, 1479
  turgor of, 1485, 1755
  vitamin D synthesis by, 1479
  weight of, 1475
Skin biopsy, 1415–16, 1489–90
Skin cancer
  basal cell carcinoma, 1521
  incidence of, 403t
  prevention of, 408
  risk factors for, 411t
  squamous cell carcinoma, 1521–22
  treatment of, 1524
Skin disorders
  acne, 1506–7
  atopic dermatitis, 1507–8
  carbuncles, 1512
  cellulitis, 1508
  contact dermatitis, 1508–9
  description of, 1496
  folliculitis, 1509–10
  fungal infections, 1510–12
  furuncles, 1512
  herpes infections, 1512–14
  impetigo, 1514
  nursing management of, 1524
  pediculosis, 1514–15
  pemphigus, 1515
  pruritus, 1515
  psoriasis, 1516–17
  rosacea, 1517
  scabies, 1517–18
  stasis dermatitis, 1518–19
  tineas, 1510–11
  treatment methods
    lotions, 1498, 1501
    lubricants, 1503–4
    moisture retentive dressings, 1503
    moisturizers, 1503–4
    ointments, 1498
    photochemotherapy, 1505–6
    phototherapy, 1504–6
    powders, 1501
    topical, 1498
    topical corticosteroids, 1499t, 1501
    topical soaks and wraps, 1501–3
  warts, 1519
  xerosis, 1519
Skin grafts. *See* Grafts, for burn patients
Skin lesions
  arrangement of, 1487f
  assessment of, 1409
  characteristics of, 1486, 1487f–1489f
  malignant, 1520–21
Skin tests, 1416
Skinner, B. F., 45t
Skull
  bones of, 1139, 1139f
  fracture of, 1183
  radiological examination of, 1161
Sleep
  activities of daily intake affected by, 62
  by critically ill patients, 566–67
  history-taking, 181
  polysomnography evaluations, 1009–10
Sleep apnea, obstructive, 1038–40
Slow pain, 453
Small bowel resection, 701t
Small cell lung cancer, 1079
Small intestine
  anatomy of, 1570, 1596, 1648
  nutrient absorption in, 1648–51
  obstruction of
    epidemiology of, 1669
    etiology of, 1670, 1671t
    gastric decompression for, 1674
    laparoscopic treatment of, 1675
Small vessel vasculitis, 1821–22
Smallpox, for biological warfare, 2249–51
Smoke detectors, 1544
Smoking. *See also* Nicotine
  aneurysms risks and, 891
  atherosclerosis and, 883–84
  bladder cancer and, 1799
  breast cancer and, 2148
  cancer risks, 404
  carcinogens produced by, 406
  cessation of, 789t, 884t
  chronic obstructive pulmonary disease and, 1100–1101, 1107
  colorectal cancer and, 1678
  coronary artery disease risks, 772–73
  hypertension and, 909–10, 919–20
  lung cancer and, 1078
  preoperative considerations, 643
  psychological effects of, 643
  stroke risks, 1173b
  trends in, 125
Smoking cessation
  benefits of, 919–20
  description of, 789t, 884t, 1107
  inflammatory bowel disorders and, 1689
  medications for, 920t
  physiological changes after, 1108t
Snake toxin, 1400
Snare polypectomy, 1682
Snellen chart, 1152f, 1304, 1328f
Snout reflex, 1159t
Soaks, 1501–2
Social isolation, 1407
Social organization, 76–78
Social readjustment rating scale, 1406, 1406t
Social Security Act, 136
Social support, 247

Social time, 123t
Social worker, 1207t
Sociocultural history, 182
Sodium
  characteristics of, 299t
  deficiency of, 307, 308t, 314–16
  excess of, 308t–309t, 316–17
  functions of, 299t
  hypertension and, 919, 919t
  normal levels of, 1759t
  recommended dietary intake of, 314t
Solutes, 296
Solution(s)
  hypertonic, 297, 305t, 341, 342t
  hypotonic, 298, 305t, 341
  isotonic, 297, 305t, 341, 342t–343t
Somatic pain, 456, 1656
Somatomedin C, 1867, 1868
Somatosensory brainstem evoked potentials, 1166t
Somatosensory evoked potentials, 1166t, 1952
Somatostatin, 1851t
Somesthesia, 452
Somnolence, 1039
Somogyi effect, 1922
Sore throat, 1033
Sour taste, 1153
Space, personal, 76
Space of Disse, 1696
Spasticity
  description of, 1155, 1200
  in multiple sclerosis patients, 1279
  in spinal cord injury patients, 1234–35
  treatment of, 1235, 1279
Specificity theory of pain, 448
Speculum examination, 2076–77
Speech
  cochlear implant benefits for, 1367
  esophageal, 1047
  tracheoesophageal, 1047
Speech therapy, 1047–49
Speech-language pathologist, 1207t
Spermatocelectomy, 2179
Spermatoceles, 2075
Spermatogenesis, 2055, 2057–58
Spermatozoa, 2056
Spinal anesthesia, 678t
Spinal cord
  anatomy of, 1144, 1144f, 1216f
  gray matter of, 1215, 1215f
  transection of, 1218
  white matter of, 1215, 1215f
Spinal cord compression
  motor and sensory function affected by, 1239
  tumor-induced, 442
Spinal cord injury
  acute management of
    collars, 1224
    evidence-based care, 1225–27
    immobilization, 1223–24
    methylprednisolone, 1226–27
    overview of, 1222–23
    pharmacological therapy, 1226–28
    support braces, 1224
  American Spinal Injury Association Impairment Scale, 1220–21
  assessment of, 1217–20, 1226
  cervical
    acute management of, 1222–23
    description of, 1218–19
    high, 1224
    pulmonary complications, 1233
    respiratory difficulties, 1224–25
    traction for, 1224
  classification of, 1218
  collaborative management of, 1236–38
  complications of
    autonomic dysreflexia, 1229–31
    bladder dysfunction, 1231–32
    bowel dysfunction, 1231–32
    decubitus ulcers, 1232–34
    diaphragmatic, 1233
    hypothermia, 1232
    osteoporosis, 1234
    pneumonia, 1233
    spasticity, 1234–35
  computed tomography of, 1221–22
  coping with, 1237–38
  cultural considerations, 1237
  deep tendon reflex testing, 1226–27
  diagnostic tests, 1221–22
  edema secondary to, 1227
  epidemiology of, 1214
  etiology of, 1214
  family education about, 1237–38
  fractures that cause, 1219
  health care costs of, 1238
  hyperextension injuries as cause of, 1219
  hyperflexion injuries as cause of, 1219
  incomplete
    anterior cord syndrome, 1220, 1220t
    Brown-Séquard syndrome, 1220, 1220t
    categorizing of, 1220–21
    central cord syndrome, 1220, 1220t
    description of, 1218
    posterior cord syndrome, 1220
    types of, 1219–20, 1220t
  levels of, 1218–19
  life expectancy of, 1214
  lumbar, 223
  magnetic resonance imaging of, 1221–22
  management of
    acute. *See* Spinal cord injury, acute management of
    collaborative, 1236–38
  mechanism of, 1218
  muscle atrophy secondary to, 1234
  neurogenic shock and, 2222
  nontraumatic, 1221
  osteoporosis and, 1214
  outcomes, 1238, 1239t
  pathophysiology of, 1215–17
  patient education about, 1236–38
  prevention of, 1214
  psychosocial support after, 1234–35
  regeneration studies, 1225–26
  rehabilitation after, 1231–35
  secondary prevention of, 1222
  sensory assessments, 1226
  sexuality issues, 1236–37
  spinal shock after. *See* Spinal shock
  spirituality issues, 1236
  sports-related, 1214, 1223
  suicide risks, 1235
  surgical treatment for, 1228
  thoracic, 223, 1218
  transfer of patients with, 1234–35
  wheelchair use after, 1233–34
  in women, 1237
Spinal cord stimulator systems, 475
Spinal cord tumors
  assessment of, 1240
  classification of, 1238
  diagnostic tests, 1240–41
  edema associated with, 1241
  ependymoma, 1238
  epidemiology of, 1238
  etiology of, 1239
  extramedullary, 1238
  growth rate for, 1240
  laminectomies for, 1242
  metastatic, 1239, 1242
  motor evoked potentials for, 1242
  nursing diagnoses, 1241
  outcomes, 1243
  pain associated with, 1240
  pathophysiology of, 1239–40
  pharmacological treatment of, 1241
  radiation therapy for, 1242–43
  spinal cord injury secondary to, 1221
  surgical treatment of, 1242
Spinal disorders
  description of, 1999
  kyphosis, 994, 1982, 2002
  scoliosis, 2000–2002
Spinal nerves, 1145, 1216f
Spinal reflexes, 1145
Spinal shock
  definition of, 1226
  management of, 1228–29
  onset of, 1229
  reflex assessments in, 1229t
Spinal stenosis, 2002–3
Spine
  description of, 1143–44
  radiological examination of, 1161
Spiral computed tomography scanning, 1007
Spiritual support, 164–65
Spiritual therapies, 390–91
Spirituality, 63, 6146
Spirometry
  chronic obstructive pulmonary disease findings, 1106t
  description of, 1011
Spironolactone, 923t, 1714
Spleen
  anatomy of, 1391
  assessment of, 1583
Splinting, 713, 714f
Split-thickness grafts, 1553
Spondylitis, 1003
Spondyloarthropathies
  ankylosing spondylitis, 1221, 1972
  assessment of, 1970–71
  description of, 1969–70
  diagnostic tests, 1971
  etiology of, 1970
  nursing diagnoses, 1971
  outcomes, 1972
  pathophysiology of, 1970
  pharmacological treatment of, 1972
  psoriatic arthritis, 1973–74
  reactive arthritis, 1970, 1973
  treatment of, 1971–72
Sponges, 680
Spontaneous pneumothorax, 1082–83
Sports injuries
  brain injuries, 1182–83, 1191
  fractures, 1947–48
  management of, 2010
  spinal cord injuries, 1214, 1223
Sports medicine, 2010
Sputum
  characteristics of, 990–91, 991t
  directed coughing for, 1110
  purulent, 1073
  studies of, 1005
  suctioning of, 1005
Squamocolumnar junction, 2060
Squamous cell carcinoma
  of larynx, 1045
  of skin, 1520f, 1521–22
St. John's Wort, 394t
ST segment elevation myocardial infarction, 791–94
Stable fracture, 1947
Stable tachycardia, 872
Staff
  diversity of, 18
  ratio laws for, 5
Staffing, 534
Standard precautions, 279
Stapedectomy, 1363, 1366
Stapedius, 1312
Stapes, 1312
Staphylococcus aureus
  methicillin-resistant, 271, 277
  necrotizing fasciitis caused by, 289
  vancomycin-resistant, 271
Staphylococcus folliculitis, 1509
START method of triage, 2239–40
Stasis dermatitis, 1518–19
Statins, 514
Status asthmaticus, 1120
Status epilepticus, 521, 1272, 1273t
Steam sterilization, 666b
Steatorrhea, 1650, 1733
Stem cell, 735
Stem cell research, 954
Stem cell transplantation
  allogeneic, 964
  leukemia treated with, 951–52, 960–61
  multiple myeloma treated with, 963–64
  Parkinson's disease treated with, 1284t
Stents
  carotid, 1181, 1181f
  coronary artery disease treated with, 785
  drug-eluting, 786
  peripheral arterial occlusive disease treated with, 887
Stereognosis, 1158
Stereotactic biopsy, 2151
Stereotactic radiotherapy, 1206
Stereotyping, 71
Sterilization
  biological indicators of, 668–69
  chemical indicators of, 668
  definition of, 667t
  of equipment and supplies, 667
  flash, 667, 669
  of instruments, 668, 669
  mechanical indicators of, 668
  methods of, 666b, 666–67
  monitoring of, 668–69
Sterilization cycle, 669
Sternum, 975
Stethoscope, 758
Stoma, 1685
Stomach, 1570
Stomach cancer
  assessment of, 1643
  chemotherapy for, 1644
  description of, 1641–42
  diagnostic tests, 1643

epidemiology of, 1642
etiology of, 1642
nursing diagnoses, 1643
outcomes, 1644–45
pathophysiology of, 1642–43
surgical treatments for, 1644
survival rates for, 1642
treatment of, 1643–44
Stopcocks, 345b
Strabismus, 1306, 1324
Strangulated obstruction, 1669, 1671
Stratum corneum, 1477t
Streptococcus pneumoniae, 1056
Streptococcus pyogenes, 1032
Stress
adaptation model of, 255–56, 262f
anticipatory, 250
appraisal-transaction theory of, 244
assessment of, 182
behavioral responses to, 242
brain responses to, 242–44
caregiver, 254
in critically ill patients, 254
definition of, 239, 244
environmental, 253–54
fight-or-flight responses to, 242, 243t
financial effects of, 257
hassles and, 244, 246
health problems caused by, 131
in home care, 255
hospitalization-related, 253
hypertension and, 920–21
immune functioning affected by, 1406–7
job-related, 255–56
life events and, 244–45
nursing models applied to management of, 255–58
occupational, 254–55
peripheral vascular resistance affected by, 910
physiologic responses to, 242
resilience, 247–48
responses to, 246
self-care theory applied to, 257–58
stimulus-response theory of, 241–44
systems model of, 256–57
Stress echocardiography, 779
Stress fractures, 1947, 2029–31
Stress incontinence, 1807b
Stress management
critical incident, 2264
description of, 920–21, 1264–65, 1417
Stress response
description of, 255
to mass casualty incidents, 2260–65
Stress testing
adenosine, 765
cardiovascular system assessments, 762, 763t, 765
coronary artery disease evaluations, 779
dobutamine, 765, 779
electrocardiogram evaluations, 807
Stress ulcers, 595
Stressors
description of, 244
for older adults, 132–33
perception of, 262
Stress-related illnesses
acute stress disorder, 250
chronic illness, 250–53
cultural factors, 253
description of, 245
posttraumatic stress disorder, 241, 247, 249–50, 251b, 2261–63
risk factors for, 253–55
Stretchers, 694
Stridor, 1001, 1042, 1457, 2254
Stroke
assessment of, 1174
brain injuries as cause of, 1186
communication impairments caused by, 1199–1200
diagnostic tests, 1174–75, 1175t
dyspnea secondary to, 1201
epidemiology of, 1172
etiology of, 1173–74
health care costs of, 1172
health disparities, 79b
hemorrhagic, 1172
incontinence concerns after, 1201–2
ischemic, 1172
management of
algorithm, 1177f
antiplatelet agents, 1176
emergency, 1176–80
goals, 1175–76
pharmacological, 1176
surgery, 1180–81
tissue plasminogen activator, 1176–80
nursing diagnoses, 1175
outcomes, 1181–82
pathophysiology of, 1174
planning and implementation for, 1175–81
rehabilitation after, 1182
risk factors for, 1173b–1174b
spasticity secondary to, 1200
Structural variables, 535
Struvite stones, 1789
Stump care, in amputation patients, 2046–48
Stye, 1305, 1339
Subarachnoid hemorrhage, 1172, 1189t
Subarachnoid space, 1160
Subbasement membrane fibrosis, 1119
Subclavian steal syndrome, 898–99
Subculture, 72, 188
Subdural hematoma, 1188f, 1189t
Subjective data, 176
Substance P, 453, 1138
Substance-induced sexual dysfunction, 2069–70
Succinimides, 521–22
Sucking reflex, 1159t
Sudden cardiac death, 792, 863–64
Suicide
assisted, 115, 150
emergency assessment of, 177
incidence rates for, 125
physician-assisted, 150
Sulfasalazine, 1972
Sulfonamides, 498–99
Sulfonylureas, 527–28, 1915, 1916t
Sun protection, 1520
Sun protective factor, 1520
Sunburn, 1519–20
Supernumerary nipples, 2137
Support stockings, 716
Suppurative cholangitis, 1730
Supraglottic cancer. *See* Laryngeal cancer
Supraglottic laryngectomy, 1048
Suprapubic prostatectomy, 2172f
Suprasternal notch, 975
Supraventricular tachycardia, 852, 863
Surfactants, 981, 1395
Surgeon, 617–18, 656
Surgery. *See also* Postanesthesia care unit; Preoperative period
acute coronary syndromes treated with, 796
anatomic site
antimicrobial cleansing of, 673
confirmation of, 637, 639
aneurysms treated with, 892
auditory, 1364–65
bariatric, 130
blood donation for, 625–26
cancer treated with, 414–16
cataract, 1328
chronic obstructive pulmonary disease treated with, 1114–15
chronic sinusitis treated with, 1031
classification of procedures, 659t
coronary artery disease treated with, 785–87
cosmetic, 130
decision to undergo, 616–17
for disaster injuries, 647–48
emergency, 644–48
environmental safety, 635–36
flail chest treated with, 1087–88
gastrointestinal obstruction treated with, 1675
health care facilities for, 618–20
heart failure treated with, 811
hospitalization times for, 701t
immune system affected by, 1406
informed consent for, 621–23, 622f, 677
legal-ethical concerns, 646–47
life-preserving, 645–46
lung cancer treated with, 1081–82
lung volume reduction, 1114
major, 620, 693
medication history before, 625
minor, 620, 693
nonelective, 644–48
NPO status before, 629
nursing contributions in, 609–10
obstructive sleep apnea treated with, 1040
pain management after, 611
patient education about, 626
patient-controlled analgesia, 611
peritonsillar abscess treated with, 1037
planning and implementation for, 630–44
pulmonary arterial hypertension treated with, 1091
recovery after
delayed, 726–27
milestones in, 714–17
short stay, 612–13
spinal cord tumors treated with, 1242
stroke treated with, 1180–81
student observations during, 655b
time frames and tasks, 623, 625–30
trends in, 610–16
urgent, 644–48
varicose veins treated with, 901–2
weight loss before, 625
Surgical biopsy, 413
Surgical debridement of wounds, 288, 1498
Surgical environment
areas of, 664
asepsis of, 664
fire in, 675–76
operating room, 670
overview of, 663–64
patient safety in
fires, 675–76
laser, 674–75
latex allergies, 676–77
personnel movement in, 664–65
precautions in
description of, 671
hand washing, 671
personal protective equipment, 671–72
scrub technique, 673
sterile supplies, 674
sterile supplies in, 665
sterility of, 664
sterilization in. *See* Sterilization
traffic patterns in, 664–65
Surgical intensive care units, 694, 704
Surgical services education coordinator, 658
Surgical team
anesthesiologist, 656
attire of, 672–73
certified registered nurse anesthetist, 656
changes in, 611
circulating nurse, 657
operating room nurses, 656–58
registered nurse first assistant, 658
scrub nurse, 657b, 657–58
specialties, 658
surgeon, 656
Surgical technologist, 658
Surrogate decision maker, 106–7
Swallowing
description of, 1570
difficulty in. *See* Dysphagia
physiology of, 1623b
Swan-Ganz catheter, 367, 572
Sweet taste, 1153
Sycosis barbae, 1509
Sympathetic nervous system, 300–301
Sympathetic response, 1148t, 1194
Sympatholytics
description of, 509
hypertension treated with, 923t–924t
Sympathomimetics
chronic obstructive pulmonary disease treated with, 1111
description of, 517–19
Synapses, 1137–38
Synaptic knob, 1137
Synarthrosis, 1940
Synchronized cardioversion, 863
Synchronized intermittent mandatory ventilation, 586, 600
Syndrome of inappropriate antidiuretic hormone, 314, 442, 1875–76
Syndrome X, 775, 1906
Synergy model, 551–52
Syngeneic transplant, 1432
Synovial cavity, 1940
Synovium, 1940
Systematic reviews
description of, 33–34
evidence sources for, 35
Systemic circulation, 750
Systemic inflammatory response syndrome, 2224–25
Systemic lupus erythematosus, 1409, 1441–44, 1781
Systemic vascular resistance, 574t, 922
Systems model, 256–57
Systolic blood pressure, 911
Systolic heart failure, 804
Systolic phase, 751

T

T cell(s)
activation of, 1386, 1397

anergy tests, 1417
antigen presenting cell binding to, 1397
assays, 1427b
CD4+, 1425
characteristics of, 741, 1388, 1390–91
cytotoxic, 1391, 1397
description of, 1840
helper, 1391, 1397–98
memory, 1399–1400
selection process for, 1391
T cell receptor, 1381, 1388
T wave, 841, 845
Tachycardia
atrial, 850
junctional, 853
sinus, 848, 848f
stable, 872
supraventricular, 852, 863
unstable, 872
ventricular
description of, 857–58
pulseless, 871
treatment of, 871
Tachypnea, 995
Tacrolimus, 1841, 1843t
Tagamet. *See* Cimetidine
Tai chi, 384, 920, 1265
Tamoxifen, 423, 2120
Tamsulosin, 2168
Tao, 377
Tapotement, 388b
Target tissues, 1849
Tax Equity and Fiscal Responsibility Act, 7
TDD, 1374
Teaching
culturally competent, 89
definition of, 44
documentation of, 49–50
evaluation of, 55
informal, 53
legal considerations, 48–49
nursing care phases and, 49, 49t
professional responsibilities related to, 48–50
strategies for, 47–48
timing of, 53
of vulnerable populations, 53–54
Teaching-learning process
assessment stage, 50–51
definition of, 44
documentation of, 49–50
evaluation stage, 55
goal setting, 53
implementation stage, 54–55
nursing diagnoses, 52
planning stage, 52–54
Telangiectasias, 1481, 1481f, 1486b
Telemetry unit, 704
Teleology, 98
Telmisartan, 924t
Temporal lobe, 452f
Tendons, 1939
Tenesmus, 1679
Tennis elbow. *See* Lateral epicondylitis
Tensilon test, 1290
Tension pneumothorax, 594–95, 1083
Tension-type headaches
alternative therapies for, 1264–65
assessment of, 1263, 1263b
definition of, 1262
description of, 458b
diagnostic tests, 1263
epidemiology of, 1263
etiology of, 1263
outcomes, 1266
pathophysiology of, 1263
pharmacological treatment of, 1264, 1265t
Tensor tympani, 1312
Teratogens, 206, 215
Teratology, 206
Terazosin, 924t
Terbutaline, 2197t
Terminal illness
description of, 144
fluids for patients with, 304
human immunodeficiency virus, 1428
Terrorism, 13, 250
Tertiary care agencies, 541–43
Tertiary intention, 282
Testes, 2055–56
Testicular biopsy, 2079
Testicular cancer, 2173–75
Testicular self-examination, 2074, 2173–74
Testicular torsion, 2175–77
Testosterone, 2058
Tetanus, diphtheria, and pertussis immunization, 1403
Tetracyclines, 495–98
Tetraplegia, 1218
Th1, 223
Th2, 223
Thalamotomy, 1284t
Thalassemias
beta, 226
description of, 225, 933
Thalidomide, 215, 1436–37
Thallium chloride, 763
Theophylline, 517–18
Therapeutic range, 486
Therapeutic recreational therapist, 1207t
Therapeutic touch, 385, 478, 596
Thermistor, 572
Thermoregulation
in burn patients, 1541
definition of, 693
in postanesthesia care unit, 698
postoperative, 698
skin's role in, 1480
Thiazide diuretics, 506–8, 923t, 1791
Thiazolidinediones, 527, 1915
Thioamides, 1888
Third heart sound, 759, 759t
Third spacing, 2212
Third-degree heart block, 855f, 855–56
Thompson test, 2026
Thoracentesis, 1012
Thoracic cage, 975
Thoracic lines, 978f
Thoracoscopy, 1012
Thoracotomy, 701t
Thorax, 975–78
Thorndike, Edward L., 45t
Three-step method, for intravenous therapy, 354–55
Thrills, 757
Thrombin time, 747t
Thrombocytopenia, 432, 940–42
Thrombolytic agents
coagulation affected by, 744
deep venous thrombosis treated with, 895
peripheral arterial occlusive disease treated with, 887
stroke treated with, 1177f
thrombophlebitis treated with, 895
Thrombophlebitis, 893–96
Thrombotic thrombocytopenic purpura, 940–41
Thrombus, 1172
Thrush, 162–63
Thyme, 394t
Thymine, 737
Thymoglobulin, 1843t
Thyroid cancer, 403t, 1890–91
Thyroid cartilage, 979
Thyroid crisis, 1857, 1887–88
Thyroid gland
anatomy of, 1853–55
hypersecretion of, 1883–95
Thyroid nodules and neoplasms, 1890–91
Thyroid scan, 1859–60
Thyroid storm, 1887–88
Thyroid suppression therapy, 1891
Thyroiditis, 1890
Thyroid-stimulating hormone, 1851t, 1852, 1855
Thyroxine, 1851t, 1853–54, 1886t
Tibial osteotomy, 1960
Tibolone, 2091
Tic douloureux, 1247
Tidal volume, 587, 1011–12, 1106t
Tiludronate, 1991t
Time orientation, 76
Timolol, 924t
Tinea capitis, 1511
Tinea corporis, 1512
Tinea cruris, 1511
Tinea pedis, 1511
Tinea versicolor, 1510
Tinel's sign, 2017, 2017f
Tinnitus, 1357
Tiotropium bromide, 1111
Tissue macrophages, 1384
Tissue plasminogen activator
nursing management of, 1178
stroke treated with, 1176–80
Tissue typing, 1841
Tobacco. *See* Smoking
Tobramycin, 1130
Tobutamide, 1916t
Toddlers
gender differences, 191
health assessment of, 187
Todd's paralysis, 1270
Tolazamide, 1916t
Tolcapone, 1283t
Tolerance
definition of, 158–59
to opioids, 472
Tonic-clonic seizures, 521, 1271
Tonsillar hypertrophy, 1035
Tonsillectomy, 1035–36
Tonsillitis, 1034–36
Tophi, 1316
Topical administration, 489t
Topical corticosteroids, 1499t, 1501
Torsades de pointes, 858
Torsemide, 923t
Total abdominal hysterectomy and bilateral salpingo-oophorectomy, 2099
Total hip replacement, 701t, 1960f, 1961b–1963b
Total iron binding capacity, 747t
Total knee replacement, 1960f, 1961b–1963b
Total parenteral nutrition
advantages and disadvantages of, 361t
definition of, 360
in mechanical ventilation patients, 598
metabolic complications of, 362
nursing considerations for, 360b
patient selection for, 361–62
postoperative, 715
protein in, 361
Total quality management
definition of, 536
description of, 7
Touch vibrations, 388b
Toxic megacolon, 1691
Toxic shock syndrome, 2105
Toxic storm, 1887
Toxins, 19–20
Toxoid, 1400
Trabecular bone, 1935
Trabeculectomy, 1330
Trabeculoplasty, 1330
Trachea
anatomy of, 978–79
deviation of, 997
endotracheal intubation effects on, 593
Tracheoesophageal puncture, 1047, 1049
Tracheoesophageal speech, 1047
Tracheostomy, 585, 1040
Traction, 1224
Traditional Chinese medicine
acupuncture, 386
description of, 377
Transbronchial needle aspiration, 1011
Transcellular fluid, 296
Transcranial Doppler imaging, 1175t
Transcranial Doppler sonography, 1167
Transcultural nursing, 84–85
Transcutaneous electric nerve stimulation, 1233
Transduction, 450, 453
Transesophageal echocardiography, 763–64
Transfer of patient
critical care unit
description of, 692
from postanesthesia care unit, 704–5
nursing care after, 709–13
Transferrin, 738, 1607, 1607t
Transfusion. *See* Blood transfusion
Transient ischemic attacks, 1173b
Transitional cell carcinoma, 1798
Transjugular intrahepatic portosystemic shunt, 1716
Translocation, of chromosomes, 201
Transplantation
allogeneic, 951
autologous, 951
bone marrow. *See* Bone marrow transplantation
kidney. *See* Renal transplantation
liver. *See* Liver transplantation
renal. *See* Renal transplantation
Transportation of patients, 686–87
Transsphenoidal hypophysectomy, 1871, 1871f
Transthyretin, 1607, 1607t
Transtracheal aspiration, 1005
Transtracheal oxygenation, 1013
Transurethral microwave procedure, 2168
Transurethral resection of the prostate, 2167–68
Transvenous pacemaker, 865
Transverse rectus abdominis myocutaneous flaps, for breast reconstruction, 2156, 2158
Trauma. *See also* Mass casualty incident
barotrauma, 594–95, 1120
brain injuries caused by
definition of, 1183
etiology of, 1183
in children, 2262

combat, 645
to kidneys, 1792–95
liver, 1721–22
ocular
contusion, 1333–34
foreign bodies, 1333
laceration, 1334
penetrating trauma, 1334
penetrating, 1334
stress responses to, 2260t
Traumatic Brain Injury Act, 1191
Traumatic pneumothorax, 1083
Treatment(s)
bariatric surgery, 130
complementary alternative medicine, 129–30
cosmetic, 130
limitation of, ethical considerations, 112
Tremor
definition of, 1280
in Parkinson's disease, 1280
Trends
aging population, 125–26
contemporary, 123–25
definition of, 123
dietary habits, 124
ethnic population, 126
in middle-aged adults, 131
minority population, 126
morbidity, 125
mortality, 125
obesity rates, 124
in older adults, 132–34
in population composition, 125–26
smoking, 125
in young adults, 131
Trephining, 240
Treponema pallidum, 2103
Treprostinil, 1091
Triage
description of, 2237–39
military, 2240, 2241t
START method of, 2239–40
Triamterene, 923t
Trichomoniasis, 2101–2
Tricuspid valve, 750, 822
Trigeminal nerve, 1146f, 1147t, 1248f
Trigeminal neuralgia, 458b, 1243, 1247–50
Triggered activity, 846
Triglycerides, 513–14
Trihexyphenidyl, 1283t
Triiodothyronine, 1851t, 1853–54, 1886
Triple screen, 213
Triple X, 202
Trisomies, 200
Trocar, 1586
Trochlear nerve, 1146f, 1147t, 1152–53
Troglitazone, 1916t
Troponin, 735, 793
Trough drug level, 497
Trousseau's sign, 332
True vocal cords, 1043
Tubercles, 1064
Tuberculomas, 1067
Tuberculosis
assessment of, 1066
definition of, 1064
description of, 990
diagnostic tests, 1066, 1403–4
direct observation therapy for, 1067
disseminated, 1066
epidemiology of, 1064
extrapulmonary, 1065t, 1787
HIV-associated, 1429
latent infection, 1065
nursing diagnoses, 1066
pathophysiology of, 1065–66
patient education about, 1069
pharmacological treatment of, 1067–69
planning and implementation for, 1066–69
recurrence of, 1067
renal, 1787–88
secondary, 1065
treatment of, 1066–69
vaccine for, 1069
Tumor(s). *See also* Cancer
ablation of, 1798
angiogenesis of, 407
brain. *See* Brain tumors
breast, 2143
classification of, 407, 407t
definition of, 1486b, 1488f
grading of, 407–8
intracranial pressure affected by, 442
malignant, 407–8
oncological emergencies, 441–42
spinal cord. *See* Spinal cord tumors
spinal cord compression caused by, 442
staging of, 407–8
Tumor markers, 412
Tumor necrosis factor, 269, 1532
Tumor necrosis factor-_, 807, 1385t, 1395
Tumor suppressor genes, 220, 406
Tuning fork tests, 1314–15, 1315f, 1361, 1361f
Tunneled catheters, 358–59
Turgor, 1485
Turner syndrome, 200, 202
Turner's syndrome, 2112–13
Tympanic membrane
description of, 1312, 1317
disorders of, 1359–60
perforation of, 1359
retracted, 1318
Tympanometry, 1360–61
Tympanoplasty, 1366
Tympanosclerosis, 1359
Tympany, 185t
Type I hypersensitivity, 1452–53

U

Ulcer
characteristics of, 1489f
corneal, 1336
decubitus, 1232–34
duodenal, 523
gastric, 1638–41
oral, 1621t
peptic ulcer disease, 523–24
Ulcerative colitis, 1691
Ultrasound
acute abdomen evaluations, 1660t
breast cancer evaluations, 2149
of gallbladder, 1701
gastrointestinal obstruction evaluations, 1673
genetic testing using, 214–15
nervous system assessments, 1166–67
pyelonephritis evaluations, 1778, 1814
renal, 1757, 1760
stroke evaluations, 1175t
thyroid gland, 1860
Ultraviolet light, 1504
Umbilicus, 1584
Uncal herniation, 580
Unit, 352
United Network for Organ Sharing, 685, 1726
Universal precautions, 279
Unstable angina, 502, 775
Unstable fracture, 1947
Unstable tachycardia, 872
Upper esophageal sphincter dysfunction, 1574
Upper gastrointestinal study, 1592
Upper motor neurons, 1217
Upper respiratory infections, 1017
Upper respiratory tract
anatomy of, 979, 980f, 1043f
function of, 979
Uremia, 1755
Ureteral strictures, 1793
Ureters, 1749
Urethra
posterior, 1750–51
strictures of, 1793, 2188–89
Urethral meatus, 2075
Urethritis, 2187–88
Urethrocele, 2110–11
Urethroplasty, 2189
Urethrotomy, 2189
Urge incontinence, 1807b
Urgent surgery, 644–48
Uric acid stones, 1789
Urinalysis, 1769
Urinary bladder. *See* Bladder
Urinary disorders
interstitial cystitis. *See* Interstitial cystitis
pyelonephritis, 1777–80
urinary tract infections. *See* Urinary tract infections
Urinary diversion, 1801–3
Urinary elimination, 181
Urinary incontinence
assessment of, 1806–7
definition of, 1805–6
diagnostic tests, 1807
epidemiology of, 1806
etiology of, 1806
health care costs, 1806
in hospice patients, 154, 163
nursing diagnoses, 1807
outcomes, 1808
in palliative care patients, 154, 163
pathophysiology of, 1806
treatment of, 1807–8
types of, 1807b
Urinary retention, 1757, 1760t, 1804–5
Urinary system, 1402t
Urinary tract calculi
assessment of, 1789–90
clinical manifestations of, 1789–90
description of, 1788–89
diagnostic tests, 1790
epidemiology of, 1789
etiology of, 1789
helical computed tomography of, 1790
nursing diagnoses, 1790
nutritional considerations, 1791
outcomes, 1792
pathophysiology of, 1789
pharmacological treatment of, 1791
surgical treatment of, 1791
Urinary tract infections
assessment of, 1767–69, 1769t
catheter use and, 1202, 1232
definition of, 1766
description of, 498
diagnostic tests, 1769–70
epidemiology of, 1766, 1766t
etiology of, 1767, 1768t
incidence of, 1766t
nursing diagnoses, 1771, 1773t
outcomes, 1771, 1773t
pathophysiology of, 1767
predisposing factors, 1768t
prevalence of, 1766t
in spinal cord injury patients, 1232
symptoms of, 1767–68
treatment of, 1771, 1772b
upper, 1767–68
Urine collection, 1758t, 1769–70
Urine culture, 1758t, 1770b
Urine electrophoresis with immunofixation, 962–63
Urine output
by burn patients, 1541
in elderly, 1829
Urolithiasis. *See* Urinary tract calculi
Ursodeoxycholic acid, 1731, 1734
Urticaria, 1466–67
U.S. Preventive Services Task Force, 36, 39b
U.S. Public Health Service, 58
Uterine bleeding, 2081–82, 2093–94
Uterine cancer, 403t
Uterine fibroids, 2111–12, 2114
Uterine hemorrhage, 2094
Uterus
anatomy of, 2060
didelphic, 2113
prolapse of, 2111
Utilitarianism, 98
Uveitis, 1341–42

V

V region, 1389
Vaccinations. *See* Immunizations
Vagina
anatomy of, 2061, 2065
cancer of, 2119
Vaginal hysterectomy, 701t
Vaginal intraepithelial neoplasia, 2119
Vaginal mucus, 2083
Vaginismus, 2127, 2130
Vaginitis, 2101–2
Vagotomy, 1640
Vagus nerve, 1146f, 1147t, 1154
Vagus nerve stimulation, 1274t
Valerian, 394t
Valgus stress test, 2021f
Valproic acid, 521–22
Valsartan, 924t
Value-based purchasing, 550
Values, 182
Valve replacement, 830
Valvular dysfunction and disease
aortic regurgitation, 827–28
aortic stenosis, 828–30
mitral stenosis, 825–27
mitral valve prolapse, 819, 823–24
overview of, 822
pathophysiology of, 822–23
Valvular regurgitation, 819
Valvular stenosis, 819
Valvular surgery, 830–32
Valvuloplasty
definition of, 825
technique for, 830

Van Leeuwenhoek, Anton, 240
Vancomycin-resistant *Enterococcus*, 271, 277, 1767
Vancomycin-resistant *Staphylococcus aureus*, 271
Varicocele, 2180–81
Varicocelectomy, 2181
Varicose bronchiolectasis, 1072
Varicose veins, 900–902
Varus stress test, 2021f
Vas deferens, 2056
Vascular access devices, 1838b
Vascular dysfunction
  aneurysms. *See* Aneurysms
  arteriosclerosis, 878
  atherosclerosis. *See* Atherosclerosis
  Buerger's disease, 896–98
  deaths caused by, 877
  peripheral arterial occlusive disease, 885–88
  Raynaud's phenomenon, 899–900
  subclavian steal syndrome, 898–99
  thrombophlebitis, 893–96
  varicose veins, 900–902
  venous stasis ulcer, 902–3
Vasectomy, 2181–82
Vasoactive intestinal polypeptide, 1699, 2068
Vasoconstriction, 750
Vasodilators
  heart failure treated with, 810
  hypertension treated with, 509–10, 924t
Vasomotor center, 508
Vasopressin. *See* Antidiuretic hormone
Vasopressors, 1888
Vector, 233
Vector borne transmission, 277–79
Vecuronium, 597t
Vegetative state, 1185t
Veins
  anatomy of, 340
  deep, 340
  definition of, 750
  dilation of, 347
  inflammation of, 349
  superficial, 340
  varicose, 900–902
Venipuncture
  insertion site monitoring, 349
  in older adults, 369–70
  preoperative, 631
  skin effects of, 340
  veins for, 340–41
Venous Doppler imaging, 2042
Venous stasis ulcer, 902–3
Venous thromboembolism, 1205, 2042–43
Venous ulcers, 285
Ventilation
  alveolar, 982–83
  definition of, 982
  mechanical. *See* Mechanical ventilation
  regulation of, 982
Ventilation-perfusion mismatch, 983–84
Ventilation-perfusion ratio, 983
Ventilation-perfusion scan, 1008, 2042
Ventilator assisted pneumonia, 1057
Ventilator-associated pneumonia, 593–94
Ventricle
  left, 749
  right, 749
Ventricular aneurysm, 791
Ventricular arrhythmias, 856–58
Ventricular assist devices, 578–79, 2217
Ventricular end-diastolic pressure, 752
Ventricular fibrillation, 858–60
Ventricular hypertrophy, 804
Ventricular tachycardia
  description of, 857–58
  pulseless, 871
  treatment of, 871
Ventriculogram, 780
Venules, 750
Verapamil, 924t
Verbal advance directives, 106
Verbal communication, 74
Vertebrae
  cervical, 1217
  description of, 1143–44
  injuries. *See* Spinal injuries
  injuries to, 1219
Vertebral column
  anatomy of, 1139, 1140f, 1216, 1216f
  bones of, 1140f
  injuries to, 1219
Vertebral fractures, 460
Vertebroplasty, 460
Vertigo, 1356
Very-low-density lipoproteins, 510, 771
Vesicant, 349
Vesicants, 420
Vesicles, 1486b, 1488f
Vesicular breath sound, 1000t
Vestibular schwannomas, 1196
Vestibulocochlear nerve, 1146f, 1147t, 1154
Veterans Affairs Health System, 548–49
Video-assisted thoracoscopic lung surgery, 1011
Videofluoroscopy, 1625
Vincristine, 1997t
Viral rhinitis, 1024–25
Virtual colonoscopy, 1680t
Viruses, 271t. *See also specific virus*
Visceral pain, 456, 459t, 1656
Visceral pericardium, 748
Visceral pleura, 981
Visual acuity. *See also* Eye(s)
  disorders of
    cataracts, 1327–29
    description of, 1326
    glaucoma, 1329–30
    macular degeneration, 1332–33
    retinal detachment, 1330–32
  testing of, 1303–4
  traumatic injuries that affect
    contusion, 1333–34
    foreign bodies, 1333
    laceration, 1334
    penetrating trauma, 1334
Visual aids, 48
Visual electrical response, 1166t
Visual evoked potentials, 1166t
Visual field confrontation test, 1304
Visual learners, 50
Vital capacity, 1012, 1106t
Vitamin(s)
  for burn patients, 1550
  fat soluble, 1649
  therapeutic uses of, 392
Vitamin A, 1550
Vitamin B12, 1648–49
Vitamin B12 deficiency anemia, 938–40
Vitamin C, 1550
Vitamin D
  deficiency of, 1649, 1986–87
  description of, 300
  functions of, 1986
  osteomalacia and, 1986–87
  skin absorption of, 1479
Vitamin K
  deficiency of, 1649
  description of, 512–13, 1602b
Vitrectomy, 1331–32
Vitreous humor, 1302
Vocal cord cancer, 1043–44
Vocational rehab counselor, 1207t
Voice sounds, 1002
Voice-whisper test, 1314
Voiding cystometrogram, 1758t
Voiding cystourethogram, 1770t
Volume control infusion, 357
Volume control ventilation, 587–88
Vomiting
  anticipatory, 434
  antiemetics for, 421, 434
  assessment of, 1572
  chemotherapy-induced, 420–21, 434, 968t
  in hospice patients, 154
  in palliative care patients, 154
  physiology of, 1575, 1575t
von Hippel-Lindau syndrome, 1796
von Willebrand factor, 742t
von Willebrand's disease, 944, 946t
Vulnerable populations
  description of, 80
  homeless, 80–82
  poor, 80
  teaching of, 53–54
Vulvar cancer, 2119, 2122
Vulvar erythema, 2077
Vulvar intraepithelial neoplasia, 2119
Vulvar vestibulitis syndrome, 2127, 2129
Vulvectomy, 2123

W

Wald, Florence, 145
Warfarin
  deep venous thrombosis treated with, 895
  description of, 485
  food interactions, 1602
  laboratory monitoring of, 512
  mechanism of action, 512
  nursing management for, 513
  pharmacokinetics of, 512
  side effects of, 513
  thrombophlebitis treated with, 895
  valvular disorders and, 832
Warts, 1500t, 1519
Water's view, 1026
Watson, John, 45t
Weaning, ventilator, 599–601
Weber test, 1314–15, 1315f, 1361, 1361f
Wegener's granulomatosis, 1781, 1821–22
Weight loss
  blood pressure reductions secondary to, 916
  in chronic obstructive pulmonary disease, 1103
  strategies for, 916
  before surgery, 625
Wellness
  culture and, 78
  nurse's role in promoting, 60
Wellness care, 2
Wenckebach phenomenon, 854
Wernicke's aphasia, 1200
Wernicke's area, 452f
West Nile Virus, for biological warfare, 2257–59
Wheals, 1486b, 1488f
Wheelchairs, 1233–34
Wheezes, 1001, 1001t, 1120, 1456
Whipple procedure, 1740f
Whipple's disease, 1650
Whispered pectoriloquy, 1002
White blood cells. *See also specific cell*
  complete blood count with differential, 1410–12
  description of, 266t, 266–67
  graft-versus-host disease caused by, 426–27
  in packed red blood cell transfusion, 363–64
White willow, 394t
Whole blood, 363
WIC. *See* Women, Infants, and Children
Wilson's disease, 1710, 1711b
Women
  coronary artery disease in, 795
  older, 135
  spinal cord injury in, 1237
  temperature fluctuations in, 190
Women, Infants, and Children (WIC), 80
Wong-Baker Faces Scale, 464–65
Work ethics, 16
Workforce diversity, 18
Workplace
  caring in, 17–20
  genetic screening in, 210–11
  noise control in, 1368
  safety in, 19–20
  stressors in, 254–55
World Health Organization
  description of, 57
  health care access, 535
  pain management approach, 157–58
  palliative care as defined by, 144
Worldwide travel, 13
Wound(s)
  assessment of, 286–87, 723
  burn. *See* Burn(s), wounds
  casts for, 700
  chronic, 289
  cleansing of, 288
  debridement of, 287–88, 903, 1496–98, 1547
  definition of, 281
  dehiscence of, 284, 415, 714
  depth of, 282, 286
  diabetic foot ulcers, 285
  drains for, 699, 700t, 711, 723
  dressings for, 286, 699, 711, 1551, 1553
  exudates in, 286
  full-thickness, 282
  infection of, 286–87
  injury prevention, 288
  inspection of, 723
  irrigation of, 288
  management of, 287–89
  moist environment for, 288
  partial-thickness, 282
  patient education about, 722–23
  postoperative care, 699–700
  pressure ulcers, 285, 287
  size of, 286
  stabilization of, 699
  venous ulcers, 285
Wound healing
  collagen disorders effect, 284
  definition of, 281
  delayed
    factors associated with, 284–85, 711
    risk factors for, 282, 283t
  factors that affect, 1482–83
  impairments in, 711

inflammatory phase of, 283
nursing response to, 286–89
nutritional requirements, 288–89
obesity effects, 284–85
open to the air, 715
overview of, 281–82
phases of, 283–84
postoperative, 715
primary intention, 282
proliferative phase of, 283
remodeling phase of, 283–84
secondary intention, 282, 711
tertiary intention, 282
types of, 282
Wraps, 1502
Wrist range of motion, 1946t

X

X chromosome
abnormalities of, 202–3
description of, 198–99
Xanthelasma, 1305
Xanthine derivatives, 517
Xanthines, 882t
Xerosis, 1485, 1519
Xerostomia, 1047
Xiphoid, 975
X-linked dominant disease, 202
X-linked dominant inheritance, 205
X-linked recessive inheritance, 205–6
X-rays
chest. *See* Chest X-rays
hip fracture evaluations, 2038

Y

Y chromosome
abnormalities of, 202–3
description of, 198–99
Yersinia pestis, 278
Yoga, 384, 920, 1265

Z

Zafirlukast, 1022t
Zenker's diverticulum, 1574
Ziconotide, 471
Zinc, 1550
Zollinger-Ellison syndrome, 1639, 1649
Zone of coagulation, 1531
Zone of hyperemia, 1532
Zone of stasis, 1531
Zygote intrafallopian transfer, 2126
Zymogens, 1393–94

Contemporary Medical-Surgical Nursing

IMPORTANT! READ CAREFULLY: This End User License Agreement ("Agreement") sets forth the conditions by which Thomson Delmar Learning, a division of Thomson Learning Inc. ("Thomson") will make electronic access to the Thomson Delmar Learning-owned licensed content and associated media, software, documentation, printed materials, and electronic documentation contained in this package and/or made available to you via this product (the "Licensed Content"), available to you (the "End User"). BY CLICKING THE "I ACCEPT" BUTTON AND/OR OPENING THIS PACKAGE, YOU ACKNOWLEDGE THAT YOU HAVE READ ALL OF THE TERMS AND CONDITIONS, AND THAT YOU AGREE TO BE BOUND BY ITS TERMS, CONDITIONS, AND ALL APPLICABLE LAWS AND REGULATIONS GOVERNING THE USE OF THE LICENSED CONTENT.

1.0 SCOPE OF LICENSE

1.1 Licensed Content. The Licensed Content may contain portions of modifiable content ("Modifiable Content") and content which may not be modified or otherwise altered by the End User ("Non-Modifiable Content"). For purposes of this Agreement, Modifiable Content and Non-Modifiable Content may be collectively referred to herein as the "Licensed Content." All Licensed Content shall be considered Non-Modifiable Content, unless such Licensed Content is presented to the End User in a modifiable format and it is clearly indicated that modification of the Licensed Content is permitted.

1.2 Subject to the End User's compliance with the terms and conditions of this Agreement, Thomson Delmar Learning hereby grants the End User, a nontransferable, nonexclusive, limited right to access and view a single copy of the Licensed Content on a single personal computer system for noncommercial, internal, personal use only. The End User shall not (i) reproduce, copy, modify (except in the case of Modifiable Content), distribute, display, transfer, sublicense, prepare derivative work(s) based on, sell, exchange, barter or transfer, rent, lease, loan, resell, or in any other manner exploit the Licensed Content; (ii) remove, obscure, or alter any notice of Thomson Delmar Learning's intellectual property rights present on or in the Licensed Content, including, but not limited to, copyright, trademark, and/or patent notices; or (iii) disassemble, decompile, translate, reverse engineer, or otherwise reduce the Licensed Content.

2.0 TERMINATION

2.1 Thomson Delmar Learning may at any time (without prejudice to its other rights or remedies) immediately terminate this Agreement and/or suspend access to some or all of the Licensed Content, in the event that the End User does not comply with any of the terms and conditions of this Agreement. In the event of such termination by Thomson Delmar Learning, the End User shall immediately return any and all copies of the Licensed Content to Thomson Delmar Learning.

3.0 PROPRIETARY RIGHTS

3.1 The End User acknowledges that Thomson Delmar Learning owns all rights, title and interest, including, but not limited to all copyright rights therein, in and to the Licensed Content, and that the End User shall not take any action inconsistent with such ownership. The Licensed Content is protected by U.S., Canadian and other applicable copyright laws and by international treaties, including the Berne Convention and the Universal Copyright Convention. Nothing contained in this Agreement shall be construed as granting the End User any ownership rights in or to the Licensed Content.

3.2 Thomson Delmar Learning reserves the right at any time to withdraw from the Licensed Content any item or part of an item for which it no longer retains the right to publish, or which it has reasonable grounds to believe infringes copyright or is defamatory, unlawful, or otherwise objectionable.

4.0 PROTECTION AND SECURITY

4.1 The End User shall use its best efforts and take all reasonable steps to safeguard its copy of the Licensed Content to ensure that no unauthorized reproduction, publication, disclosure, modification, or distribution of the Licensed Content, in whole or in part, is made. To the extent that the End User becomes aware of any such unauthorized use of the Licensed Content, the End User shall immediately notify Thomson Delmar Learning. Notification of such violations may be made by sending an e-mail to delmarhelp@thomson.com.

5.0 MISUSE OF THE LICENSED PRODUCT

5.1 In the event that the End User uses the Licensed Content in violation of this Agreement, Thomson Delmar Learning shall have the option of electing liquidated damages, which shall include all profits generated by the End User's use of the Licensed Content plus interest computed at the maximum rate permitted by law and all legal fees and other expenses incurred by Thomson Delmar Learning in enforcing its rights, plus penalties.

6.0 FEDERAL GOVERNMENT CLIENTS

6.1 Except as expressly authorized by Thomson Delmar Learning, Federal Government clients obtain only the rights specified in this Agreement and no other rights. The Government acknowledges that (i) all software and related documentation incorporated in the Licensed Content is existing commercial computer software within the meaning of FAR 27.405(b)(2); and (2) all other data delivered in whatever form, is limited rights data within the meaning of FAR 27.401. The restrictions in this section are acceptable as consistent with the Government's need for software and other data under this Agreement.

7.0 DISCLAIMER OF WARRANTIES AND LIABILITIES

7.1 Although Thomson Delmar Learning believes the Licensed Content to be reliable, Thomson Delmar Learning does not guarantee or warrant (i) any information or materials contained in or produced by the Licensed Content, (ii) the accuracy, completeness or reliability of the Licensed Content, or (iii) that the Licensed Content is free from errors or other material defects. THE LICENSED PRODUCT IS PROVIDED "AS IS," WITHOUT ANY WARRANTY OF ANY KIND AND THOMSON DELMAR LEARNING DISCLAIMS ANY AND ALL WARRANTIES, EXPRESSED OR IMPLIED, INCLUDING, WITHOUT LIMITATION, WARRANTIES OF MERCHANTABILITY OR FITNESS OR A PARTICULAR PURPOSE. IN NO EVENT SHALL THOMSON DELMAR LEARNING BE LIABLE FOR: INDIRECT, SPECIAL, PUNITIVE OR CONSEQUENTIAL DAMAGES INCLUDING FOR LOST PROFITS, LOST DATA, OR OTHERWISE. IN NO EVENT SHALL THOMSON DELMAR LEARNING'S AGGREGATE LIABILITY HEREUNDER, WHETHER ARISING IN CONTRACT, TORT, STRICT LIABILITY OR OTHERWISE, EXCEED THE AMOUNT OF FEES PAID BY THE END USER HEREUNDER FOR THE LICENSE OF THE LICENSED CONTENT.

8.0 GENERAL

8.1 Entire Agreement. This Agreement shall constitute the entire Agreement between the Parties and supercedes all prior Agreements and understandings oral or written relating to the subject matter hereof.

8.2 Enhancements/Modifications of Licensed Content. From time to time, and in Thomson Delmar Learning's sole discretion, Thomson Delmar Learning may advise the End User of updates, upgrades, enhancements and/or improvements to the Licensed Content, and may permit the End User to access and use, subject to the terms and conditions of this Agreement, such modifications, upon payment of prices as may be established by Thomson Delmar Learning.

8.3 No Export. The End User shall use the Licensed Content solely in the United States and shall not transfer or export, directly or indirectly, the Licensed Content outside the United States.

8.4 Severability. If any provision of this Agreement is invalid, illegal, or unenforceable under any applicable statute or rule of law, the provision shall be deemed omitted to the extent that it is invalid, illegal, or unenforceable. In such a case, the remainder of the Agreement shall be construed in a manner as to give greatest effect to the original intention of the parties hereto.

8.5 Waiver. The waiver of any right or failure of either party to exercise in any respect any right provided in this Agreement in any instance shall not be deemed to be a waiver of such right in the future or a waiver of any other right under this Agreement.

8.6 Choice of Law/Venue. This Agreement shall be interpreted, construed, and governed by and in accordance with the laws of the State of New York, applicable to contracts executed and to be wholly preformed therein, without regard to its principles governing conflicts of law. Each party agrees that any proceeding arising out of or relating to this Agreement or the breach or threatened breach of this Agreement may be commenced and prosecuted in a court in the State and County of New York. Each party consents and submits to the nonexclusive personal jurisdiction of any court in the State and County of New York in respect of any such proceeding.

8.7 Acknowledgment. By opening this package and/or by accessing the Licensed Content on this Web site, THE END USER ACKNOWLEDGES THAT IT HAS READ THIS AGREEMENT, UNDERSTANDS IT, AND AGREES TO BE BOUND BY ITS TERMS AND CONDITIONS. IF YOU DO NOT ACCEPT THESE TERMS AND CONDITIONS, YOU MUST NOT ACCESS THE LICENSED CONTENT AND RETURN THE LICENSED PRODUCT TO DELMAR LEARNING (WITHIN 30 CALENDAR DAYS OF THE END USER'S PURCHASE) WITH PROOF OF PAYMENT ACCEPTABLE TO THOMSON DELMAR LEARNING, FOR A CREDIT OR A REFUND. Should the End User have any questions/comments regarding this Agreement, please contact Thomson Delmar Learning at delmarhelp@thomson.com.

StudyWare™ to Accompany Contemporary Medical-Surgical Nursing

Minimum System Requirements

- Operating System: Microsoft Windows 98 SE, Windows 2000, or Windows XP
- Processor: Pentium PC 500 MHz or higher (750 Mhz recommended)
- Memory: 64 MB of RAM (128 MB recommended)
- Screen Resolution: 800 × 600 pixels
- Color Depth: 16-bit color (thousands of colors)
- Disk Space: Minimum of 10 MB free
- Macromedia Flash Player 9. The Macromedia Flash Player is free, and can be downloaded from http://www.adobe.com/products/flashplayer/

Installation Instructions

1. Insert disc into CD-ROM drive. The StudyWare™ installation program should start automatically. If it does not, go to step 2.
2. From My Computer, double-click the icon for the CD drive.
3. Double click the *setup.exe* file to start the program.

Technical Support

Telephone: 1-800-477-3692, 8:30 A.M.-5:30 P.M. Eastern Time
Fax: 1-518-881-1247
E-mail: delmarhelp@thomson.com